OXFORD TEXTBOOK OF
CLINICAL
HEPATOLOGY

OXFORD MEDICAL PUBLICATIONS

EDITORS

JOHANNES BIRCHER
Visiting Professor
Department of Clinical Pharmacology
University of Bern
Bern, Switzerland

JEAN-PIERRE BENHAMOU
Professor of Hepatology and Gastroenterology
Hôpital Beaujon
Clichy, France

NEIL McINTYRE
Professor of Medicine
Royal Free Hospital School of Medicine
London, UK

MARIO RIZZETTO
Professor of Gastroenterology
University of Turin
Turin, Italy

JUAN RODÉS
Professor of Medicine
Chief of Liver Unit
University of Barcelona
Barcelona, Spain

OXFORD TEXTBOOK OF
CLINICAL HEPATOLOGY

SECOND EDITION

VOLUME II
Sections 14–32 and Index

Edited by

Johannes Bircher
Jean-Pierre Benhamou
Neil McIntyre
Mario Rizzetto
Juan Rodés

Oxford   New York   Tokyo
OXFORD UNIVERSITY PRESS
1999

Oxford University Press, Great Clarendon Street, Oxford OX2 6DP

Oxford New York

Athens Auckland Bangkok Bogota Buenos Aires Calcutta
Cape Town Chennai Dar es Salaam Delhi Florence Hong Kong Istanbul
Karachi Kuala Lumpur Madrid Melbourne Mexico City Mumbai
Nairobi Paris São Paolo Singapore Taipei Tokyo Toronto Warsaw

and associated companies in
Berlin Ibadan

Oxford is a trade mark of Oxford University Press

Published in the United States
by Oxford University Press, Inc., New York

First published 1991
Second edition published 1999

British Library Cataloguing in Publication Data
Data available

Library of Congress Cataloging in Publication Data

1 3 5 7 9 10 8 6 4 2

ISBN 0 19 262515 2 (Two Volume Set)
ISBN 0 19 263039 3 (Vol 1)
ISBN 0 19 263040 7 (Vol 2)
(Available as a two volume set only)

Typeset by Latimer Trend

Printed in Hong Kong

Preface to the second edition

The first edition of the *Oxford Textbook of Clinical Hepatology* enjoyed considerable success and achieved much critical acclaim; we were encouraged, therefore, to produce a new edition, not only to amplify our original aims but also to document the enormous progress made in hepatology and related fields over the last few years. All chapters have been updated, and many have been restructured and expanded. New chapters have been added on topics such as *in vitro* techniques, 'hepatitis G', overlap syndromes, glycogen storage diseases, and intracellular and extracellular lipidosis. To serve the practising hepatologist the focus on clinical medicine has been further strengthened, although the necessary basic science is still included. The initial chapters containing the latter have been directed towards newer techniques and concepts which have developed during the last few years. As before referencing throughout is comprehensive, covering both key sources from the past and the most recent literature.

We thank all our contributors: their patient work and dedication have made the production of the book possible. We also gratefully acknowledge the excellent management of Mrs Christina Wagner in the editorial office and of Dr Irene Butcher and our friends at Oxford University Press.

Johannes Bircher

January 1999

Jean-Pierre Benhamou

Neil McIntyre

Mario Rizzetto

Juan Rodés

Preface to the first edition

We all met several times, in different cities, to plan this book. We wanted to produce a comprehensive account of clinical hepatology, covering not only the common hepatological problems but also the rare conditions which are seen from time to time by hepatologists, gastroenterologists, and general physicians. We thought it important to consider how the liver may be affected in diseases of other systems, and to describe the effects of diseases of the liver on other parts of the body, as these interactions often create a confusing clinical picture; these topics occupy two large sections of the book which should be of particular value to general physicians and specialists in other diseases. We felt a need for a fuller than usual account of the effect of infections on the liver; patients with bacterial, fungal and parasitic infections, and those with viral infections other than the classical viral hepatitides, often have abnormal liver function tests, or symptoms or signs suggesting liver disease.

There are chapters on other topics which have received little attention in other texts, such as symptoms and signs, diagnostic strategy, general management, and prescribing and anaesthesia in liver disease. There are chapters on liver disease in children, in the elderly, and in drug addicts and homosexual men, and one on the history of liver disease.

We also thought it would be helpful to have some appendices: listing non-drug chemicals and toxins causing liver damage, the geographical distribution of infectious diseases, and the rare diseases in which the liver may be involved (particularly in children). Another appendix contains the excellent handouts produced for patients by the American Liver Foundation.

Colleagues often remark that it is irritating, when reading chapters with many references, to have to search at the end of the chapter to find the original sources. We therefore decided to use mainly short 'text references' to enable readers to decide quickly if they are already familiar with the source and, if not, to allow them to jot the reference down with the minimum of effort. We consider this experiment to have been worthwhile, but we hope that readers will tell us if they prefer the conventional approach.

More than 200 authors have contributed to this book; nearly all are acknowledged internationally as experts in their field(s) of interest. We are grateful to all of them. We believe that their expertise is reflected in their contributions, many of which we consider to be quite outstanding.

Our major purpose was to provide a book for practising clinicians. We hope this text will prove useful not only to hepatologists, gastroenterologists, and general physicians, but also to specialists in other fields. It was for this reason that we chose the title 'clinical hepatology'. We believe that this book will provide solutions to many of the hepatological problems which arise in clinical practice, but only our readers can tell whether our belief is justified. If, when using this book, you fail to find the information you are seeking, we would be grateful if you could draw these omissions to our attention (using the cards enclosed), so that they can be corrected in the next edition.

Our book is being brought out in English, French, and Spanish. We would like to thank the staff of the Oxford University Press, Flammarion, and of Salvat, not only for their willingness to publish it but for their help and enthusiasm during the long gestation period. We are particularly grateful to the executive editor for the book, Irene Butcher, who dealt initially with all the manuscripts, and later with the galleys and page proofs of this English edition.

Neil McIntyre
Jean-Pierre Benhamou
Johannes Bircher
Mario Rizetto
Juan Rodés

Contents

Contributors

ALFREDO ALBERTI
Professor of Internal Medicine, University of Padova, Italy
12.1.2.5 Hepatitis C

FRANCIS ANDRÉ
Vice President and Senior Medical Director, SmithKline
Beecham Biologicals, Rixensart, Belgium
12.1.3.1(a) Vaccines against hepatitis A

PETER W. ANGUS
Consultant Hepatologist in Charge, Transplant Unit,
Repatriation General Hospital, Melbourne, Victoria, Australia
*24.2 The effect of gastrointestinal disease on the liver and biliary
tract*
25.5 Effect of liver disease on the gastrointestinal tract

THOMAS ARMBRUST
Junior Scientist in the Department of Gastroenterology and
Endocrinology, Department of Internal Medicine, University
of Göttingen, Germany
2.7.1 Cytokines and the liver

VICENTE ARROYO
Hospital Clinic i Provincial, Barcelona, Spain
8.1 Pathogenesis, diagnosis, and treatment of ascites in cirrhosis
8.2 Renal dysfunction in cirrhosis
24.4 The liver in urogenital diseases
25.7 Effect of liver disease on the urogenital tract

DANIEL AZOULAY
Surgeon, Centre Hepatobiliaire, Villejuif, France
22.2.2 Malignant biliary obstruction
*30.1 General surgical aspects and the risks of liver surgery in
patients with hepatic disease*

CHARLES BALABAUD
Professor of Hepatology, CHU de Bordeaux, Université
Bordeaux II, Bordeaux, France
1.2 Liver and biliary-tract histology

VIJAYAN BALAN
Assistant Professor of Medicine, Divisions of Transplantation
Medicine, Gastroenterology and Hepatology, University of
Pittsburgh Medical Center, Pennsylvania, USA
30.5 Liver transplantation

MICHAEL BARAITSER
Consultant in Clinical Genetics, Hospital for Children,
Great Ormond Street, London, UK
32.3 Rare diseases with hepatic abnormalities

JAMES A. BARROWMAN*
Faculty of Medicine, Memorial University of Newfoundland,
St John's, Canada
2.2 Hepatic lymph and lymphatics

NATHAN M. BASS
Professor of Medicine, University of California, San Francisco
School of Medicine, and Attending Physician, UCSF Hospitals
and Clinics, USA
*2.19 In vitro techniques: isolated organ perfusion, slices, cells, and
subcellular elements*

JEAN-PIERRE BENHAMOU
Professor of Hepatology and Gastroenterology at University of
Paris 7, Service d'Hépatologie, Hôpital Beaujon, Clichy, France
5.4.1 Liver biopsy
6.2 Cirrhosis: clinical aspects
7.3 Intrahepatic portal hypertension
*11.2 Non-parasitic cystic diseases of the liver and intrahepatic
biliary tree*
19 Fulminant and subfulminant liver failure
21.3 Obstruction of the hepatic venous system
21.4 Vascular malformations
22.1.1 Liver haemangioma
22.1.2.2 Benign hepatocellular tumours
*25.1 The effect of liver disease on the cardiovascular system,
lungs, and pulmonary vasculature*

O. BERNARD
Hôpital de Bicêtre, Bicêtre, France
26 Paediatric liver disease

JACQUES BERNUAU
Consultant, Service d'Hépatologie, Hôpital Beaujon, Clichy,
France
19 Fulminant and subfulminant liver failure

H.L.C. BEYNON
Consultant Physician and Rheumatologist, Royal Free
Hospital, London, UK
24.7 Musculoskeletal diseases and the liver
25.9 Musculoskeletal problems in liver disease

PRITHI S. BHATHAL
Professor/Director of Anatomical Pathology, Royal Melbourne
Hospital and University of Melbourne, Victoria, Australia
2.6 Nerve supply and nervous control of liver function

* It is with regret that we report the death of Professor J. Barrowman during
the preparation of this edition.

PAULETTE BIOULAC-SAGE
Professor of Pathology, CHU de Bordeaux, Université de
Bordeaux II, France
1.2 Liver and biliary-tract histology

MICHEL BIOUR
Director, Centre de Pharmacovigilance Paris-Saint Antoine
and Associate Professor of Pharmacology, Medical School,
University of Paris VI, France
17.0 Drug-induced liver injury

JOHANNES BIRCHER
Visiting Professor, Department of Pharmacology, University
of Bern, Switzerland
25.8 The nervous system in liver disease
29.3 Drug treatment in patients with liver disease

HENRI BISMUTH
Professor of Surgery, Hôpital Paul-Brousse, Villejuif, France
1.1 Macroscopic anatomy of the liver
22.2.2 Malignant biliary tract obstruction
*30.1 General surgical aspects and the risks of liver surgery in
patients with hepatic disease*

NORBERT BLANCKAERT
Professor of Clinical Pathology, University Hospital
Gasthuisberg, Leuven, Belgium
2.9 Bilirubin metabolism
20.6 Hyperbilirubinaemia

ANDRES T. BLEI
Professor of Medicine, Northwestern University, Chicago,
Illinois, USA
9 Hepatic encephalopathy

P. BONNABRY
Division of Clinical Pharmacology, University Hospital,
Geneva, Switzerland
2.5 Hepatic metabolism of drugs

FLAVIA BORTOLOTTI
Senior Lecturer in Internal Medicine, University of Padova,
Italy
12.1.2.5 Hepatitis C

JAIME BOSCH
Professor of Medicine, University of Barcelona School of
Medicine and Chief of Hepatic Haemodynamic Laboratory
and Consultant Physician, Hospital Clinic, Barcelona, Spain
7.2 Pathophysiology of portal hypertension and its complications
*7.4 Clinical manifestations and management of bleeding episodes
in cirrhotics*
21.2 Obstruction of the portal vein

PIERRE M. BOULOUX
Department of Medicine, Royal Free Hospital, London, UK
24.6 The effect of endocrine diseases on liver function
25.2 The effect of liver disease on the endocrine system

J. BOYER
Ensign Professor of Medicine and Director, Liver Center,
Yale University School of Medicine, New Haven,
Connecticut, USA
23.3 Intrahepatic cholestasis

F. BRAET
Faculty of Medicine and Pharmacy, Free University of
Brussels, Belgium
1.4 Sinusoidal liver cells

SOLANGE BRESSON-HADNI
Professor of Hepatology, WHO Collaborating Centre for
Prevention and Treatment of Human Echinococcoses,
University Hospital, Besançon, France
13.4.2 Echinococcosis of the liver

PIERRE BRISSOT
Professor of Hepatology, University Hôpital Pontchalliou,
Rennes, France
2.16.1 Normal iron metabolism
20.2 Haemochromatosis

MIGUEL BRUGUERA
Senior Consultant, Hospital Clinic and Professor of Medicine,
Medical School, University of Barcelona, Spain
22.1.2.1 Benign biliary tumours
22.2.3 Malignant mesenchymal tumours of the liver
*24.5 The effect of haematological and lymphatic diseases on the
liver*

JORDI BRUIX
Liver Unit, Hospital Clinic, University of Barcelona, Spain
22.3.1 Metastatic liver disease

A.D.M. BRYCESON
Professor of Tropical Medicine, London School of Hygiene
and Tropical Medicine and Consultant Physican, Hospital for
Tropical Diseases, London, UK
13.3.3 Visceral leishmaniasis

A.K. BURROUGHS
Consultant Physician and Hepatologist, Royal Free Hospital,
London, UK
*7.4 Clinical manifestations and management of bleeding episodes
in cirrhotics*
28 Liver disease and pregnancy

ALASTAIR D. BURT
Professor of Hepatopathology, Medical School, University of
Newcastle upon Tyne, UK
15.2 Pathology of alcoholic liver disease

J.R. BUSCOMBE
Consultant in Nuclear Medicine, Royal Free Hospital,
London, UK
5.6 Radionuclide investigations of the liver

JOAN CABALLERIA
Consultant Physician, Liver Unit, Hospital Clinic, University
of Barcelona, Spain
15.4 Extrahepatic manifestions of alcoholism

LUIZ CAETANO DA SILVA
Chief, Division of Gastroenterology, Faculty of Medicine,
University of São Paulo, Brazil
13.1.2 Leptospirosis
*13.4.3 Ascariasis, visceral larva migrans, capillariasis,
strongyloidiasis, and pentastomiasis*

JOYCE CARLSON
Senior Physician, Department of Clinical Chemistry, Malmö
University Hospital, Sweden
20.3 α₁-Antitrypsin deficiency and related disorders

ELLEN CARMICHAEL
Associate Director of Strategic and Corporate Development,
Vion Pharmaceuticals, Inc., New Haven, Connecticut, USA
*2.14.1 Transcription, RNA processing, liver specific factors, RNA
translocation, translation, protein co-translocation, secretion*

ANTONI CASTELLS
Gastroenterology Department, Hospital Clinic, University of
Barcelona, Spain
22.3.1 Metastatic liver disease

R.W. CHAPMAN
Department of Gastroenterology, John Radcliffe Hospital,
Oxford, UK
*24.2 The effect of gastrointestinal diseases on the liver and biliary
tract*
25.5 Effect of liver disease on the gastrointestinal tract

P.P. CHIEFFI
Professor of Preventive Medicine, School of Medicine,
University of São Paulo, Brazil
*13.4.3 Ascariasis, visceral larva migrans, capillariasis,
strongyloidiasis, and pentastomiasis*

MARCO CIPOLLI
Consultant Physician, Gastroenterology Service, Cystic
Fibrosis Centre, Verona Hospital, Italy
20.4 The liver in cystic fibrosis

PETER COLLINS
Senior Lecturer and Honorary Consultant Cardiologist,
National Heart and Lung Institute, Imperial College London,
UK
24.1 The liver in cardiovascular and pulmonary disease
*25.1 The effect of liver disease on the cardiovascular system,
lungs, and pulmonary vasculature*

JULIET COMPSTON
Lecturer in Medicine and Honorary Consultant Physician,
University of Cambridge School of Clinical Medicine, UK
25.10 The effect of liver disease on bone

L. DA COSTA GAYOTTA
Professor of Pathology, University of São Paulo, Brazil
13.1.2 Leptospirosis
*13.4.3 Ascariasis, visceral larva migrans, capillariasis,
strongyloidiasis, and pentastomiasis*

ROBERT N. DAVIDSON
Consultant Physician, Northwick Park Hospital, Harrow,
Middlesex, UK
13.3.3 Visceral leishmaniasis

P. DAYER
Division of Clinical Pharmacology, University Hospital,
Geneva, Switzerland
2.5 Hepatic metabolism of drugs

R.B.D. DE ZANGER
Faculty of Medicine and Pharmacy, Free University of
Brussels, Belgium
1.4 Sinusoidal liver cells

FRANÇOISE DEGOS
Consultant, Service d'Hépatologie, Hôpital Beaujon, Clichy,
France
5.4.1 Liver biopsy

MARIE-HELENE DENNINGER
Head of Haemostasis Laboratory, Hôpital Beaujon, Clichy,
France
2.14.3 The liver and coagulation
25.4 Haemostasis in liver disease

VALEER J. DESMET
Emeritus Professor of Pathology, Catholic University of
Leuven, Belgium
1.5 Embryology of the liver and intrahepatic biliary tract
3.1 Histological features
3.2 Histological classification of chronic liver disease
11.1 Non-cystic malformations of the biliary tract

JULES DESMEULES
Division of Clinical Pharmacology, University Hospital,
Geneva, Switzerland
2.5 Hepatic metabolism of drugs

YVES DEUGNIER
Professor of Hepatology, Université Hôpital Pontchalliou,
Rennes, France
2.16.1 Normal iron metabolism
20.2 Haemochromatosis

DANIEL DHUMEAUX
Professor of Hepatology and Gastroenterology, University of
Paris XIl, France
14.7 The liver in graft-versus-host disease

JULES L. DIENSTAG
Associate Professor of Medicine, Harvard Medical School and
Physician, Massachusetts General Hospital, Boston, USA
12.1.2.2 Hepatitis A

TOM DOHERTY
Clinical Scientist, MRC Laboratories, Fajara, Banjul,
The Gambia
32.1 Geographic distribution of infections causing liver disease

PETER T. DONALDSON
Head of Immnogenetics, Institute of Liver Studies, King's College Hospital, London, UK
2.7.2 Immunogenetics of liver disease

JAMES S. DOOLEY
Senior Lecturer in Medicine and Honorary Consultant Physician, Royal Free Hospital, London, UK
23.2 Extrahepatic biliary obstruction: systemic effects, diagnosis, management
23.5 Cholangitis and biliary tract infections

R. HERMON DOWLING
Professor of Hepatology and Gastroenterology and Consultant Physician, United Medical and Dental Schools and Guy's Hospital, London, UK
23.4 Gallstones

GEOFFREY DUSHEIKO
Professor of Medicine, Royal Free Hospital and School of Medicine, London, UK
12.1.2.3 Hepatitis B

CHRISTOPHE DUVOUX
Physician, Service d'Hépatologie et de Gastroenterologie, Hôpital Henri Mondor, Paris, France
14.7 The liver in graft-versus-host disease

M. EDDOUKS
Faculty of Medicine and Pharmacy, Free University of Brussels, Belgium
1.4 Sinusoidal liver cells

C. EMPSEN
Faculty of Medicine and Pharmacy, Free University of Brussels, Belgium
1.4 Sinusoidal liver cells

MICHAEL J. EPPIHEIMER
Post-Doctoral Fellow, Department of Molecular and Cellular Physiology, lSU Medical Center, Shreveport, Louisiana, USA
2.2 Hepatic lymph and lymphatics

STEN ERIKSSON
Department of Medicine, University of Lund, Malmö, Sweden
20.3 α_I-Antitrypsin deficiency and related disorders

SERGE ERLINGER
Professor of Hepatology and Gastroenterology, at University of Paris 7, Service d'Hépatologie, Hôpital Beaujon, Clichy, France
6.2 Cirrhosis: clinical aspects

H. FALK
Falk Foundation, Freiburg, Germany
31.0   History of hepatology

NELSON FAUSTO
Professor and Chairman, Department of Pathology, University of Washington School of Medicine, Seattle, USA
2.8.1 Hepatic regeneration

ALBERTO FERRARI
Assistant Professor of Gastroenterology, Medical School, University of Modena, Italy
5.4.2 Laparoscopy

V.A. FERREIRA ALVES
University of São Paulo, Brazil
13.1.2 Leptospirosis

JOHAN FEVERY
Chairman, Department of Internal Medicine, University Hospital Gasthuisberg, Leuven, Belgium
2.9 Bilirubin metabolism
20.6 Hyperbilirubinaemia

JEAN-FRANÇOIS FLÉJOU
Professor of Pathology, University of Paris 7, Service d'Anatomie Pathologique, Hôpital Beaujon, Clichy, France
22.1.2.2 Benign hepatocellular tumours

NICK FRANCIS
Senior Lecturer in Histopathology, Imperial College School of Medicine at Charing Cross, London, UK
13.3.2 Malaria

F.H. FRANKEN
Professor, University of Düsseldorf, Germany
31.0 History of hepatology

M. FUCHS
Instructor in Medicine, Department of Internal Medicine, University of Lübeck, Germany
2.1 Metabolism of bile acids

PETER R. GALLE
Professor of Internal Medicine and Chairman, I. Department of Internal Medicine, University of Mainz, Germany
2.8.2 Apoptosis in the liver

JUAN CARLOS GARCÍA-PAGÁN
Liver Unit, Hospital Clinic, Barcelona, Spain
7.2 Pathophysiology of portal hypertension and its complications
21.2 Obstruction of the portal vein

JOSÉ M. GATELL
Consultant Physician, Hospital Clinic Barcelona and Associate Professor of Medicine, University of Barcelona, Spain
13.3.4 Toxoplasmosis

PAUL GENECIN
Director, Yale Health Plan and Clinical Associate Professor of Medicine (Digestive Diseases), Yale University School of Medicine, New Haven, Connecticut, USA
2.1 Hepatic blood flow

WOLFRAM H. GERLICH
Professor of Medical Virology ,Institute of Medical Virology, Justus-Leibig University of Giessen, Germany
12.1.2.1 Structure, replication, and laboratory diagnosis of hepatitis viruses

WOLFGANG GEROK
Emeritus Professor of Internal Medicine, University of
Freiburg, Germany
2.14.2 Protein secretion, degradation, and function

RICHARD GILSON
Senior Lecturer in Sexually Transmitted Diseases, Division
of Pathology and Infectious Diseases, Windeyer Institute of
Medical Sciences, University College London Medical
School, UK
*12.3 Hepatitis and human immunodeficiency virus infection in
homosexual men and injecting drug users*

PERE GINÈS
Staff Member, Liver Unit, University of Barcelona, Spain
8.1 Pathogenesis, diagnosis, and treatment of ascites in cirrhosis
8.2 Renal dysfunction in cirrhosis

PAOLO GIOANNINI
Clinica Malattie Infettive, Ospedale Amedeo di Savoia, Torino,
Italy
12.4 Exotic virus infections of the liver

JONATHAN D. GITLIN
Professor of Pediatrics and Chief, Pediatric Rheumatology,
Washington University School of Medicine, St Louis,
Missouri, USA
2.16.2 Normal copper metabolism
20.1 Wilson's disease

DERMOT GLEESON
Consultant Physician, Gastroenterology and Liver Unit,
Royal Hallamshire Hospital, Sheffield, UK
23.3 Intrahepatic cholestasis

CHRISTIAN GLUUD
Chief Physician, Copenhagen Trial Unit, Copenhagen
University Hospital, Denmark
32.4 The Cochrane Hepato-Biliary Group

D. NEIL GRANGER
Professor and Head, Department of Molecular and Cellular
Physiology, LSU Medical Center, Shreveport, Louisiana,
USA
2.2 Hepatic lymph and lymphatics

A.M. GRESSNER
Professor of Clinical Chemistry, Pathobiochemistry, and
Laboratory Medicine, Institute for Clinical Chemistry and
Pathobiochemistry, RWTH University Clinic, Aachen,
Germany
*2.15 Function and metabolism of collagen and other extracellular
proteins*
*6.1 Cellular and molecular pathobiology, pharmacological
intervention, and biochemical assessment of liver fibrosis*

PAUL GRIFFITHS
Professor of Virology, Royal Free Hospital School of
Medicine, London, UK
12.2 Systemic virosis producing hepatitis

GENY M.M. GROOTHUIS
Assistant Professor of Pharmacokinetics and Drug Delivery,
Groningen Institute for Drug Studies, University Centre for
Pharmacy, University of Groningen, The Netherlands
2.4 Hepatobiliary disposition and targeting of drugs and genes

VOLKER GROSS
Professor of Internal Medicine, University of Freiburg,
Germany
2.14.2 Protein secretion, degradation, and function

HOWARD GROSSMAN
Senior Lecturer in Pathology, University of Melbourne,
Victoria, Australia
2.6 Nerve supply and nervous control of liver function

ROBERTO J. GROSZMANN
Professor of Medicine, Yale University School of Medicine,
New Haven, Connecticut, USA
2.1 Hepatic blood flow

JORGE J. GUMUCIO
Professor of Medicine, Gastroenterology Division, University
of Michigan Medical Center and Veterans Affairs Medical
Center, Ann Arbor, Michigan, USA
2.18 Functional organization of the liver

M. HADCHOUEL
Hôpital de Bicêtre, Bicêtre, France
26.0 Paediatric liver disease

FADI G. HADDAD
Assistant Professor of Pediatric Gastroenterology and
Hepatology, University of Texas Health Science Center,
San Antonio, Texas, USA
2.1 Hepatic blood flow

STEPHANOS J. HADZIYANNIS
Professor of Medicine, Athens University School of Medicine
and Director of the National Reference Centre for
Communicable Liver Disease, Hippokration General
Hospital, Athens, Greece
12.1.2.7 The new 'hepatitis' virus G or GBV-C

A.J. HALL
Reader in Communicable Disease Epidemiology, London
School of Hygiene and Tropical Medicine, UK
32.1 Geographic distribution of infections causing liver disease

D.S. HARRY
Principal Clinical Scientist and Honorary Lecturer, Royal
Free Hospital, London, UK
2.12 Plasma lipids and lipoproteins

D. HÄUSSINGER
Professor of Internal Medicine and Director of Clinic for
Gastroenterology, Hepatology, and Infectiology, Heinrich
Heine University, Düsseldorf, Germany
2.13.2 Ammonia, urea production, and pH regulation

R.J. HAY
Professor of Cutaneous Medicine, United Medical and Dental Schools of St Thomas's and Guy's Hospital, London, UK
13.2 Fungal infections affecting the liver

JENNY HEATHCOTE
Professor of Medicine, University of Toronto and Staff Gastroenterologist, The Toronto Hospital, Ontario, Canada
14.1 Primary biliary cirrhosis
14.6 Overlap syndromes

J. MICHAEL HENDERSON
Department of General Surgery, The Cleveland Clinic Foundation, Ohio, USA
7.1 Anatomy of the portal venous system in portal hypertension

A.J.W. HILSON
Consultant in Nuclear Medicine, Royal Free Hospital, London, UK
5.6 Radionuclide investigations of the liver

K.E.F. HOBBS
Professor of Surgery, Royal Free Hospital School of Medicine, London, UK
23.6 The gallbladder and laparoscopic cholecystectomy

H.J.F HODGSON
Professor of Medicine, Imperial College School of Medicine at The Hammersmith, London, UK
22.3.2 Carcinoid tumours

A.V. HOFFBRAND
Emeritus Professor of Haematology, Royal Free Hospital, London, UK
20.7 The liver in intracellular and extracellular lipidosis

J. HUGHES
Specialist Registrar, Department of Dermatology, Royal Free Hospital, London, UK
24.3 The effect of skin diseases on the liver
25.6 The effect of liver disease on the skin

IRENE HUNG
Pediatric Rheumatology, Washington University School of Medicine, St Louis, Missouri, USA
2.16.2 Normal copper metabolism
20.1 Wilson's disease

D. GERAINT JAMES
Adjunct Professor of Medicine, Royal Free Hospital School of Medicine, London, UK
14.2 Hepatic granulomas

O.F.W. JAMES
Professor of Medicine and Head of School of Clinical Medical Science, University of Newcastle upon Tyne, UK
27 Liver disease in the elderly

P.L.M. JANSEN
Professor of Gastroenterology, University of Groningen, The Netherlands
2.4 Hepatobiliary disposition and targeting of drugs and genes

WLADIMIRO JIMÉNEZ
Hospital Clinic i Provincial, Barcelona, Spain
8.2 Renal dysfunction in cirrhosis

ALBERT L. JONES
Professor of Medicine and Anatomy, University of California, San Francisco, California, USA
1.3 Electron microscopy of the liver

REGINE KAHL
Professor of Toxicology, Institute of Toxicology, University of Düsseldorf, Germany
18.1 Toxic liver injury
32.2 Liver injury in man ascribed to non-drug chemicals and natural toxins

MARK A. KANE
World Health Organization, Geneva, Switzerland
12.1.3.1(b) Hepatitis B vaccines and immunization

EMMET B. KEEFFE
Professor of Medicine, Stanford University School of Medicine; Chief of Clinical Gastroenterology and Medical Director, Liver Transplant Program, Stanford University Medical Center, California, USA
16 Non-alcoholic fatty liver: causes and complications

S. KEIDING
Consultant Physician, Department of Hepatology V and PET Centre, Aarhus University Hospital, Denmark
5.2 Hepatic removal of circulating substances: importance for quantitative measurements of liver function

CHRISTOPHER KIBBLER
Consultant in Medical Microbiology, Royal Free Hospital, London, UK
13.1.1 Bacterial infection and the liver

K. KRAWCZYNSKI
Chief, Experimental Pathology Section, Hepatitis Branch, DVRD/NCID, Centers for Disease Control and Prevention, Atlanta, Georgia, USA
12.1.2.6 Hepatitis E

J.E.J. KRIGE
Associate Professor of Surgery, Department of Surgery and Surgical Gastroenterology, University of Cape Town and Groote Schuur Hospital, South Africa
30.4 Hepatobiliary trauma

YOLANTA T. KRUSZYNSKA
Associate Professor of Medicine, Department of Medicine, University of California at San Diego, La Jolla, USA
2.11 Carbohydrate metabolism
2.13.1 Amino acid metabolism
24.6 The effect of endocrine diseases on liver function
25.2 The effect of liver disease on the endocrine system

F. KUNSTLINGER
Consultant Radiologist, Centre Hépatobiliaire, Hôpital Paul-Brousse, Villejuif, France
1.1 Macroscopic anatomy of the liver

DOMINIQUE LARREY
Professor of Hepatology, Medical School, University of
Montpellier, France
17 Drug-induced liver injury

NICHOLAS F. LaRUSSO
Professor of Medicine and Biochemistry and Molecular
Biology, Mayo Medical School, Clinic, and Foundation,
Rochester, Minnesota, USA
14.4 Sclerosing cholangitis

BERNARD H. LAUTERBURG
Professor of Clinical Pharmacology and Internal Medicine,
University of Bern, Switzerland
*5.2 Hepatic removal of circulating substances: importance for
quantitative measurements of liver function*

BRIGITTE LE BAIL
Maître de Conference des Universités, Praticien Hospitalier
CHU de Bordeaux, Université de Bordeaux II, France
1.2 Liver and biliary-tract histology

DIDIER LEBREC
Director, INSERM, Hôpital Beaujon, Clichy, France
5.7 Splanchic haemodynamic investigations

RANDALL G. LEE
Associate Professor of Pathology, University of Pittsburgh
Medical Center, Pennsylvania, USA
16 Non-alcoholic fatty liver: causes and complications

JOSEP M. LLOVET
Liver Unit, Hospital Clinic, University of Barcelona, Spain
22.3.1 Metastatic liver disease

LAURENCE B. LOVAT
Immunological Medicine Unit (Division of Medicine),
Imperial College School of Medicine, Hammersmith Hospital,
London, UK
14.8 Amyloidosis

ANNA LUCCHINI
Clinica Malattie Infettive, Ospedale Amedeo di Savoia, Turin,
Italy
12.4 Exotic virus infections of the liver

JURGEN LUDWIG
Emeritus Professor of Pathology, Mayo Clinic and Mayo
Medical School, Rochester, Minnesota, USA
14.4 Sclerosing cholangitis
14.5 Vanishing bile duct syndrome

D. LUO
Faculty of Medicine and Pharmacy, Free University of
Brussels, Belgium
1.4 Sinusoidal liver cells

THOMAS T. LUTHER
Medical Student, Medical School, University of
Witten/Herdecke, Germany
*2.19 In vitro techniques: isolated organ perfusion, slices, cells,
and subcellular elements*

R.N.M. MacSWEEN
Professor of Pathology, University of Glasgow; Honorary
Consultant, Department of Pathology, Western Infirmary,
Glasgow, UK
15.2 Pathology of alcoholic liver disease

PIETRO E. MAJNO
Chef de Clinique Associé, Centre Hépatobiliaire,
Hôpital Paul Brousse, Villejuif, Paris, France
1.1 Macroscopic anatomy of the liver
22.2.2 Malignant biliary obstruction
*30.1 General surgical aspects and the risks of liver surgery in
patients with hepatic disease*

S.V. MALLETT
Consultant Anaesthetist, Royal Free Hospital, London, UK
30.2 Anaesthesia and liver disease

FEDERICO MANENTI
Professor of Gastroenterology, Medical School, University of,
Modena, Italy
5.4.2 Laparoscopy

MICHAEL P. MANNS
Medizinsche Hochschule Hannover, Zentrum fur Innere
Medizin und Dermatologie, Hannover, Germany
2.7.2 Immunogenetics of liver disease
5.3 Immunological investigations in liver diseases
14.3 Autoimmune hepatitis

J. WALLIS MARSH
Associate Professor of Surgery, University of Pittsburgh
School of Medicine, Pennsylvania, USA
30.5 Liver transplantation

ADOLFO MARTINEZ PALOMO
Professor of Experimental Pathology, Center for Research and
Advanced Studies, Mexico
13.3.1 Amoebiasis, giardiasis, and cryptosporidiosis

ANTONI MAS
Staff Member, Liver Unit, Hospital Clinic, University of
Barcelona, Spain
18.2 Hepatic injury due to physical agents

GIANNI MASTELLA
Professor of Paediatrics and Scientific Director, Cystic
Fibrosis Centre, Verona Hospital, Italy
20.4 The liver in cystic fibrosis

KEITH P.W.J. McADAM
Wellcome Professor of Tropical Medicine, London School of
Hygiene and Tropical Medicine and Director, MRC
Laboratories, Fajara, Banjul, The Gambia
14.8 Amyloidosis

P. AIDEN McCORMICK
Liver Unit, St Vincent's Hospital, Dublin, Ireland
*10 The spleen, hypersplenism, and other relationships between the
liver and spleen*

NEIL McINTYRE
Professor of Medicine, Royal Free Hospital School of
Medicine, London, UK
2.12 Plasma lipids and lipoproteins
2.13.1 Amino-acid metabolism
4.0 Symptoms and signs of liver disease
5.1 Biochemical investigations in the management of liver disease
5.8 Diagnostic approach to liver disease
23.1 Cholestasis
23.4 Gallstones
24.1 The liver in cardiovascular and pulmonary disease
*25.1 The effect of liver disease on the cardiovascular system,
lungs, and pulmonary vasculature*
25.3 Haematological abnormalities in liver disease
29.1 The general management of liver disease

ATUL B. MEHTA
Consultant Haematologist, Royal Free Hospital, London, UK
25.3 Haematological abnormalities in liver disease

DIRK K.F. MEIJER
Professor of Pharmacokinetics and Drug Delivery, Groningen
Institute for Drug Studies, University Centre for Pharmacy,
University of Groningen, The Netherlands
2.4 Hepatobiliary disposition and targeting of drugs and genes

HERMANN MENGER
Clinic for Neurology and Clinical Neurophysiology,
University of Witten/Herdecke, Wuppertal, Germany
25.8 The nervous system in liver disease

YVES MENU
Professor of Radiology at University of Paris 7, Service de
Radiologie, Hôpital Beaujon, Clichy, France
5.5 Imaging of the liver and biliary tract
*11.2 Non-parasitic cystic diseases of the liver and intrahepatic
biliary tree*
22.1.2.2 Benign hepatocellular tumours

KARL-HERMANN MEYER ZUM BUSCHENFELDE
Professor of Medicine, Johannes-Gutenberg Universität,
Mainz, Germany
5.3 Immunological investigations in liver diseases

J.P. MIGUET
Service d'Hépatologie et de Soins Intensifs Digestifs, CHU
Jean Minjoz, Besançon, France
13.4.2 Echinococcosis of the liver

JOSÉ M. MIRO
Consultant Physician, Hospital Clinic Barcelona and Associate
Professor of Medicine, University of Barcelona, Spain
13.3.4 Toxoplasmosis

P.K. MISTRY
Director of Comprehensive Gaucher Disease Program,
Department of Human Genetics, Mount Sinai School of
Medicine, New York, USA
20.7 The liver in intracellular and extracellular lipidosis
20.8 Glycogen storage diseases

MARSHA Y. MORGAN
Senior Lecturer and Honorary Consultant Physician,
Royal Free Hospital, London, UK
*15.3 Alcoholic liver disease: natural history, diagnosis, clinical
features, evaluation, management, prognosis, and prevention*
29.2 Nutritional aspects of liver and biliary disease

MARTINA MÜLLER
Department of Internal Medicine IV, Hepatology and
Gastroenterology, University Hospital, Heidelberg, Germany
2.8.2 Apoptosis in the liver

MIGUEL NAVASA
Faculty Member, Liver Unit, Hospital Clinic, University of
Barcelona, Spain
25.11 Infections in liver disease

DIETER NEUMANN-HAEFELIN
Professor of Virology, University Hospital, Freiburg,
Germany
12.2 Systemic virosis producing hepatitis

YVES NORDMANN
Professor of Biochemistry, Faculté Xavier Bichat, University
of Paris 7, France
2.17 Haem biosynthesis and excretions of porphyrins
20.5 Human hereditary porphyrias

ANDREAS OCHS
Department of Internal Medicine, University of Freiburg,
Germany
2.16.3 Trace elements

HIROAKI OKUDA
Assistant Professor, Institute of Gastroenterology,
Tokyo Women's Medical College, Tokyo, Japan
22.2.1 Primary liver cell carcinoma

KUNIO OKUDA
Emeritus Professor of Medicine, Chiba University School of
Medicine, Japan
22.2.1 Primary liver cell carcinoma

ALBERT PARES
Consultant Physician, Liver Unit, Hospital Clinic, University
of Barcelona, Spain
15.4 Extrahepatic manifestions of alcoholism

DOMINIQUE PESSAYRE
Director of Research, INSERM U481, Hôpital Beaujon,
Clichy, France
17 Drug-induced liver injury

RAMÓN PLANAS
Hospital Clinic i Provincial, Barcelona, Spain
8.1 Pathogenesis, diagnosis, and treatment of ascites in cirrhosis

JORGE RAKELA
Professor of Medicine and Chief, Division of
Gastroenterology and Hepatology, University of Pittsburgh,
Pennsylvania, USA
30.5 Liver transplantation

GIULIANO RAMADORI
Professor of Medicine and Chairman of Gastroenterology and
Endocrinology, Department of Internal Medicine,
University of Göttingen, Germany
2.7.1 Cytokines and the liver

JÜRG REICHEN
Professor of Medicine and Chairman, Department of Clinical
Pharmacology, University of Bern, Switzerland
2.3 Physiology of bile formation and of the motility of the biliary tree

ANTONI RIMOLA
Associate Professor, Department of Medicine, Hospital Clinic,
University of Barcelona, Spain
25.11 Infections in liver disease

MARIO RIZZETTO
Professor of Gastroenterology, University of Turin, Italy
12.1.1 Introduction
12.1.2.4 Hepatitis D
12.1.3.2 Therapy of chronic viral hepatitis
12.2 Systemic virosis producing hepatitis

JUAN RODÉS
Professor of Medicine and Chief of Liver Unit, University of
Barcelona, Spain
8.1 Pathogenesis, diagnosis, and treatment of ascites in cirrhosis
8.2 Renal dysfunction in cirrhosis
18.2 Hepatic injury due to physical agents
22.2.3 Malignant mesenchymal tumours of the liver
24.4 The liver in urogenital diseases
25.7 Effect of liver disease on the urogenital tract
30.3 Postoperative jaundice

S.B. ROSALKI
Honorary Consultant in Chemical Pathology, Royal Free
Hospital, London, UK
5.1 Biochemical investigations in the management of liver disease

TANIA ROSKAMS
Professor of Pathology, Catholic University of Leuven,
Belgium
1.5 Embryology of the liver and intrahepatic biliary tract
3.1 Histological features
3.2 Histological classification of chronic liver disease
11.1 Non-cystic malformations of the biliary tract

M. RUSTIN
Consultant Dermatologist, Royal Free Hospital, London, UK
24.3 The effect of skin diseases on the liver
25.6 The effect of liver disease on the skin

MARIE-FRANCE SAINT-MARC-GIRARDIN
Physician, Service d'Hépatologie et de Gastroenterologie,
Hôpital Henri Mondor, Paris, France
14.7 The liver in graft-versus-host disease

MIKKO SALASPURO
Professor of Alcohol Diseases, University of Helsinki, Finland
15.1 Epidemiological aspects of alcoholic liver disease, ethanol metabolism, and pathogenesis of alcoholic liver injury

JUAN M. SALMERON
Staff Member, Liver Unit, Hospital Clinic, Barcelona, Spain
30.3 Postoperative jaundice

JOSE MARIA SÁNCHEZ-TAPIAS
Consultant Physician, Liver Unit, Hospital Clinic and Associate
Professor of Medicine, Medical School, University of Barcelona,
Spain
13.1.1 Bacterial infection and the liver

GIORGIO SARACCO
Associate Professor of Gastroenterology, Azienda Ospedaliera
S. Giovanni Battista, Turin, Italy
12.1.3.2 Therapy of chronic viral hepatitis

PETER J. SCHEUER
Emeritus Professor of Histopathology, Royal Free Hospital
School of Medicine, London, UK
14.2 Hepatic granulomas

DOUGLAS L. SCHMUCKER
Associate Career Research Scientist, Veterans Administration
Medical Center; Professor of Anatomy and Senior
Investigator, Liver Center, University of California,
San Francisco, USA
1.3 Electron microscopy of the liver

J. SCHOLMERICH
Professor and Director, Klinik und Poliklinik für Innere
Medizin I, Universität Regensburg, Germany
2.16.3 Trace elements

DETLEF SCHUPPAN
Medizinische Klinik mit Poliklinik der Friedrich-Alexander
Universität, Erlangen, Germany
2.15 Function and metabolism of collagen and other extracellular proteins
6.1 Cellular and molecular pathobiology, pharmacological intervention, and biochemical assessment of liver fibrosis

SHEILA SHERLOCK
Professor of Medicine, Department of Surgery, Royal Free
Hospital, London, UK
14.1 Primary biliary cirrhosis

ANTONINA SMEDILE
Associate Professor of Gastroenterology, Azienda Ospedaliera
S. Giovanni Battista, Turin, Italy
12.1.2.4 Hepatitis D

WALTRAUD SOMMER
Scientific Assistant, University of Witten/Herdecke, Germany
29.3 Drug treatment in patients with liver disease

HERBERT SPAPEN
Physician, Medical Intensive Care Department, Academic Hospital, Free University of Brussels, Belgium
1.4 Sinusoidal liver cells

EDUARD F. STANGE
Professor of Medicine and Chief, Division of Gastroenterology, Department of Internal Medicine, University of Lübeck, Germany
2.10 Metabolism of bile acids

JOHN TERBLANCHE
Professor and Chairman, Department of Surgery, University of Cape Town; Surgeon-in-Chief, Groote Schuur Hospital Teaching Hospital Group, Cape Town, and Co-Director, Medical Research Council Liver Research Centre, University of Cape Town, South Africa
30.4 Hepatobiliary trauma

JOSEP TERÉS
Professor of Medicine, Hospital Clinic, Barcelona, Spain
21.1 Hepatic arteries

REINER THOMSSEN
Professor of Medical Microbiology and Head of Department of Medical Microbiology, University of Göttingen, Germany
12.1.2.1 Structure, replication, and laboratory diagnosis of hepatitis viruses

JONATHAN M. TIBBALLS
Consultant Radiologist, Royal Free Hospital, London, UK
5.5 Imaging of the liver and biliary tract

DOMINIQUE VALLA
Professor of Hepatology and Gastroenterology at University of Paris 7, Service d'Hépatologie, Hôpital Beaujon, Clichy, France
7.3 Intrahepatic portal hypertension
21.3 Obstruction of the hepatic venous system

J. VAN DEN BOGAERDE
Royal Free Hospital, London, UK
24.7 Musculoskeletal diseases and the liver
25.9 Musculoskeletal problems in liver disease

PETER VAN EYKEN
Consultant Pathologist, Catholic University of Leuven, Belgium
1.5 Embryology of the liver and intrahepatic biliary tract
11.1 Non-cystic malformations of the biliary tract

GIORGIO VERME
Emeritus Professor of Gastroenterology, Azienda Ospedaliera S. Giovanni Battista, Turin, Italy
12.1.2.4 Hepatitis D

D. VERMIJLEN
Faculty of Medicine and Pharmacy, Free University of Brussels, Belgium
1.4 Sinusoidal liver cells

JEAN-PAUL VERNANT
Professor of Haematology, Service d'Hématologie, Hôpital Pitié Salpêtrière, Paris, France
14.7 The liver in graft-versus-host disease

DOMINIQUE VUITTON
Professor of Clinical Immunology, WHO Collaborating Centre for Prevention and Treatment of Human Echinococcoses, University Hospital, Besançon, France
13.4.2 Echinococcosis of the liver

DAVID A. WARRELL
Professor of Tropical Medicine and Infectious Diseases and Director, Centre for Tropical Medicine, University of Oxford, UK
13.3.2 Malaria

K.S. WARREN
The Picower Institute for Medical Research, Manhasset, New York, USA
13.4.1 Blood flukes (schistomes) and liver flukes

ANTHONY F. WATKINSON
Consultant Radiologist, Royal Free Hospital, London, UK
5.5 Imaging of the liver and biliary tract

IAN WELLER
Professor of Sexually Transmitted Diseases, Division of Pathology and Infectious Diseases, Windeyer Institute of Medical Sciences, University College London Medical School, UK
12.3 Hepatitis and human immunodeficiency virus infection in homosexual men and injecting drug users

RUSSELL H. WIESNER
Medical Director, Liver Transplantation, Mayo Clinic and Professor of Medicine, Mayo Medical School, Rochester, Minnesota, USA
14.4 Sclerosing cholangitis

R.M. WINTER
Professor of Dysmorphology and Clinical Genetics, Institute of Child Health, London, UK
32.3 Rare diseases with hepatic abnormalities

EDDIE WISSE
Professor of Cell Biology and Histology, Faculty of Medicine and Pharmacy, Free University of Brussels, Belgium
1.4 Sinusoidal liver cells

GEORGE Y. WU
Professor of Medicine and Chief, Division of Gastroenterology-Hepatology, University of Connecticut Health Center, Farmington, USA
2.14.1 Transcription, RNA processing, liver specific factors, RNA translocation, translation, protein co-translocation, secretion

ELIE-SERGE ZAFRANI
University of Paris XII, France
14.7 The liver in graft-versus-host disease

14

Immune disorders of the liver

14.1 Primary biliary cirrhosis

Sheila Sherlock and Jenny Heathcote

Definition of primary biliary cirrhosis

Small intrahepatic bile ducts are progressively destroyed, probably by an immunological process. This results in slowly progressive cholestasis.

Introduction

The first descriptions were in 1851 by Addison and Gull, and in 1876 by Hanot. In 1949, the association with high levels of serum cholesterol and skin xanthomas led to McMahon and Thannhauser coining the term 'xanthomatous biliary cirrhosis'.

In 1950, Ahrens and the group from the Rockefeller Institute in New York gave the first clear description of the condition which they termed primary biliary cirrhosis. This was a misnomer as not all patients are cirrhotic, at least on initial presentation. In 1964, Rubin, Schaffner, and Popper from the Mount Sinai Hospital in New York described the disease as 'chronic non-suppurative destructive cholangitis'. This is a better term although too cumbersome to replace the popular 'primary biliary cirrhosis'.

The clinical course both in symptomatic and asymptomatic patients has been well described.[1–5]

Prevalence and epidemiology

The disease usually affects middle-aged women between 40 and 59 years old (range 22 to 80 plus). The reason for the 90 per cent female predominance is unknown. There are no particular distinguishing features when the disease affects men. The disease has been reported from all parts of the world: Asian, Caucasian, Hispanic, and blacks persons are affected. The reported prevalence rates vary, the lowest being 19 per million in Victoria, Australia and the highest 154 per million in Newcastle, England (Watson, Gut, 1995; 36:927). Death rates are difficult to assess, but are probably of the order of 0.6 to 2 per cent of those who die from cirrhosis. However, the disease is much harder to diagnose once cirrhosis has developed and, therefore, as more patients are diagnosed while alive, and subsequently die, the figures will undoubtedly change. When routine screening for serum alkaline phosphatase was conducted between 1991 and 1995 in one Italian hospital, 0.12 per cent of the women with an elevated serum alkaline phosphatase were diagnosed as having primary biliary cirrhosis (Magrini, Liver, 1996; 16:377). There is family clustering and primary biliary cirrhosis has been reported in sisters and twins (Chohan, Gut, 1973; 14:213), and in mothers and daughters (Bach, Gastro, 1991; 102:A776; Brind,

Gut, 1995; 36:618). The prevalence of circulating mitochondrial antibodies, which have an almost constant association with primary biliary cirrhosis when tested by immunofluorescence, was found to be increased in relatives of patients (Galbraith, NEJM, 1974; 290: 63); however, using more sensitive and specific testing, this was not found to be the case in another study (Caldwell, Hepatol, 1992; 16: 899). There is a weak association with class II HLA DR8 antigen (Manns, Gastro, 1991; 101:1367).

Environmental factors are suggested by the development of the disease in a daughter, her mother, and an unrelated close friend who nursed the daughter in her terminal illness (Douglas, BMJ, 1979; ii:419).

In a 3-year study (1977 to 1979) of primary biliary cirrhosis in Sheffield, England, 90 per cent of patients came from an area that had only 4 per cent of the population and who were supplied with water from one particular reservoir (Triger, BMJ, 1980; 281:772). No one so far has matched this experience, and an environmental factor in the water supply could not be identified.

Pathogenesis (Table 1)

The major diagnostic hallmark of primary biliary cirrhosis is the antimitochondrial antibody (**AMA**), but it is uncertain whether AMA are involved directly in the pathogenesis of this disease. As serum AMA may be persistently absent in some patients who otherwise appear to have all the characteristics of primary biliary cirrhosis (these patients are sometimes described as having 'auto-immune cholangitis'), a pathogenic role for AMA seems unlikely.

AMA are reactive to a number of inner mitochondrial proteins, namely the E2 subunit of the pyruvate dehydrogenase complex (**PDC-E2**), the E2 subunit of the branched-chain keto acid dehydrogenase complex (**BCKD-E2**), the E2 subunit of the 2-oxoglutaric dehydrogenase complex (**OGDC-E2**), the E1-α and the E1-β subunit of PDC, and protein X (Fussey, PNAS, 1988; 85:8654; Van de Water, JImmunol, 1988; 141:2321). Immunofluorescence studies of bile duct epithelial cells in livers affected by primary biliary cirrhosis indicate that PDC-E2, or a substance which shares a common epitope to PDC-E2, is expressed in the subluminal cytoplasmic regions of the bile duct cells. This staining is limited to the interlobular bile ducts and is not found in other chronic liver diseases of the bile ducts or in normal liver. This same staining may be found in the bile duct epithelial cells from the liver tissue of patients who appear to have primary biliary cirrhosis but are AMA seronegative (Tsuneyama, Hepatol, 1995; 22:1375). PDC-E2 is also

Table 1 Possible aetiological factors in primary biliary cirrhosis

1.	'Molecular mimicry'—mitochondrial antigens with possible infectious particles, present in interlobular bile duct epithelial cells
2.	Enhanced expression of HLA on bile duct cells
3.	Cytotoxic T-cell mediated injury to mitochondrial antigens (PDC-E2)
4.	Failure of immune regulation? Genetic?

aberrantly expressed on the apical cytoplasmic regions of the salivary ducts of patients with coexisting primary biliary cirrhosis and Sjögren's syndrome, but not in Sjögren's syndrome alone (Joplin, Hepatol, 1994; 19:1375). It is not clear why this mitochondrial protein is located in these sites and not in other parts of the biliary tree. It may not be mitochondrial protein but rather a cross-reacting substance—an example of 'molecular mimicry' (Burroughs, Nature, 1992; 258:377). The inciting antigens would most likely be infectious agents; certain bacterial polypeptides are recognized by AMA, such as rough mutants of *Escherichia coli* (Fussey, PNAS, 1990; 87:3987) and *Myobacterium gordonae* (Vilagut, JHepatol, 1994; 21:673).

In primary biliary cirrhosis, both IgA and IgM deposits can be found on the luminal aspects of bile duct epithelial cells (Krams, Hepatol, 1990; 12:306) and B cells may be present in lymphoid follicles, but most of the lymphoid cells infiltrating the biliary epithelial cells in liver tissue are T cells, both T_{H1} and T_{H2} (Van de Water, JExpMed, 1995; 181:723). Cytotoxic CD8 T-cells can only direct a response to peptides expressed by HLA class I. The expression of HLA class I on hepatocytes and biliary epithelial cells is found to be enhanced in primary biliary cirrhosis, but this expression appears somewhat later than the expression of PDC-E2 in the biliary epithelial cells (Tsuneyama, Hepatol, 1995; 21:1031). Aberrant expression of class II HLA, as well as class I, is found on the biliary epithelial cells of liver tissue in primary biliary cirrhosis and is probably induced by proinflammatory cytokines. A T-cell response to components of the pyruvate dehydrogenase complex has been observed in primary biliary cirrhosis (Van de Water, JImmunol, 1991; 146:89; Jones, Hepatol, 1995; 21:995).

There are many other observations in primary biliary cirrhosis which strongly support an immunopathogenic mechanism for this disease. Accessory molecules, known to facilitate immune reactions, are expressed on endothelial cells of damaged bile ducts, portal vein branches, and peribiliary vascular plexi (Yasoshima, JPath, 1995; 175:1319). Nevertheless, the exact sequence of events remains unclear; if PDC-E2 is an autoantigen, its location on the luminal aspect of the biliary epithelial cells is not optimal for attack by the cellular immune system. The association with HLA class II DR8 is only weak and there is some evidence suggesting that destruction of biliary epithelial cells may not be restricted to MHC class II (Martins, Hepatol, 1996; 23:988). Clinical observations suggest both genetic and environmental factors may play a role in the genesis of primary biliary cirrhosis.

Diagnosis (Table 2)
Diagnostic features

The patient is usually a middle-aged woman. Presentation nowadays tends to be early, and the patient is usually asymptomatic. She may

Table 2 Diagnosis of primary biliary cirrhosis

Clinical features
    Middle-aged female
    Fatigue
    Pruritus
    Hepatosplenomegaly
    Other autoimmune diseases
    Xanthomas
Biochemical features
    Elevated alkaline phosphatase
    Elevated γ-glutamyl transpeptidase
    Elevated cholesterol
    Normal or elevated conjugated bilirubin
Serological features
    Elevated IgM
    Positive for antimitochondrial antibody (>1:40)
Radiological features
    Normal endoscopic retrograde cholangiopancreatograph
Histological features
    Granulomatous bile duct destruction
    Bile ductular proliferation
    Chronic inflammatory cell infiltration
    Fibrosis with or without cirrhosis

be found to have a raised level of serum alkaline phosphatase and/ or total serum cholesterol, discovered at a routine check. The diagnosis may be made in patients under investigation for a condition known to be associated with primary biliary cirrhosis, such as a thyroid disorder, scleroderma, or rheumatoid arthritis. Osteoporosis may be the initial observation. Abnormal physical signs may be absent. The serum antimitochondrial antibody is always positive in a titre exceeding 1:40. In some instances AMA-positive subjects detected as part of a rheumatological work-up may have a normal level of serum alkaline phosphatase. Measurement of serum immunoglobulins generally reveals an elevated IgM value. Serum bilirubin may be normal or only minimally increased. Serum aminotransferases may also be normal, but not always.

Liver biopsy is nearly always abnormal and usually shows features consistent with primary biliary cirrhosis, even if the patient is asymptomatic and the level of serum alkaline phosphatase is normal.

The most frequent symptom of patients with primary biliary cirrhosis is fatigue. The cause remains unknown. It does not correlate with the severity of the disease (Cauch-Dudek, Hepatol, 1996; 22:108A). The second most common symptom, namely generalized pruritus, starts insidiously and patients may be referred initially to dermatologists. Jaundice may never develop but, without treatment, it appears in most patients within 2 years of the onset of itching (Plate 1). Jaundice preceding pruritus is extremely unusual, and jaundice without pruritus is only observed in endstage disease. The pruritus can start during pregnancy and the diagnosis may

Disease	No.	%
Sjögren's syndrome	182	20.8
Rheumatoid arthritis	49	5.6
Hashimoto's thyroiditis	49	5.6
Raynaud's phenomenon	35	4.0
Scleroderma	12	1.4
Ulcerative colitis	3	0.3

Table 3 Primary biliary cirrhosis: commonly associated autoimmune diseases*

* In 874 Japanese patients (from Inoue, Liver, 1995; 15:70).

then be confused with idiopathic cholestatic jaundice of the last trimester.

Clinical features

Examination shows a well-nourished woman whose jaundice is slight or absent. The liver is usually enlarged and firm and the spleen may be palpable. Scratch marks may be seen on the skin. In endstage disease (rarely seen nowadays as most suitable patients receive a liver transplant before this time) the patient becomes increasingly pigmented and jaundiced. Diarrhoea may occur due to steatorrhoea. Weight loss develops when jaundice deepens. In spite of the jaundice, patients feel surprisingly well and have a good appetite, though many are consistently fatigued. The course is afebrile and abdominal pain is unusual, although many complain of upper right quadrant discomfort (Laurin, AmJGastr, 1994; 89: 1840). Skin xanthomas develop frequently, but many patients remain free of them throughout their course. In a similar manner to the pruritus, xanthomas may disappear with disease progression. The skin may be thickened and tough over the fingers, ankles, and legs due to chronic scratching.

In men, the pruritus is less common at the time of diagnosis, there is less skin pigmentation, and fewer autoimmune features, especially the sicca syndrome. Survival is the same for men and women (Lucey, Gut, 1986; 27:1373).

Associated conditions (Table 3)
Rheumatological associations

Non-hepatic disorders are found in 69 per cent of patients (Golding, AmJMed, 1973; 55:772). Primary biliary cirrhosis is associated with many autoimmune diseases, such as rheumatoid arthritis, dermatomyositis, polymyositis, mixed connective tissue disease, and systemic lupus erythematosus (Hall, AnnIntMed, 1984; 100:388).

However, the most common association is with various manifestations of scleroderma. Primary biliary cirrhosis may be associated with full-blown scleroderma in up to 4 per cent of cases, and with just the CREST (calcinosis, Raynaud's phenomenon, (o)esophageal dysphagia, sclerodactyly, telangiectasia) syndrome in others (Reynolds, AmJMed, 1971; 50:302). Keratoconjunctivitis sicca is common (Powell, QJMed, 1987; 62:75). These patients usually have an antinuclear centromere antibody (Makinen, Arth-Rheum, 1983; 26:9141), and sometimes circulating immune complexes containing ribonuclear protein AgRo (Penner, Gastro, 1986; 90:724). The sicca complex of dry eyes and mouth, a form of

secondary Sjögren's syndrome, is present in about 75 per cent of patients, only revealed by direct questioning in some. Dysphagia is common in these patients (Mang, 1996; in press). Inconvenience may be caused by dry eyes and/or dry mouth without full-blown Sjögren's syndrome being present.

Metabolic associations

It is not unusual for thyroid disorders to antedate the diagnosis of primary biliary cirrhosis, and thyroid antibodies are found in close to 25 per cent or cases. Patients may present with hypothyroidism (Crowe, Gastro, 1980; 78:1437), but Graves' disease may be observed in a few (Nieri, AmJGastr, 1985; 7:434)

As a result of high cholesterol, xanthomas may be present, particularly early on in the disease; they tend to disappear with disease progression when the serum cholesterol falls, and so the presence of skin xanthomas may bear little relation to the height of the serum cholesterol. Rarely, xanthomas may affect peripheral nerves giving rise to a painful xanthomatous neuropathy (Turnberg, Gut, 1972; 13:976).

With the advent of reliable methods of detecting osteoporosis without resorting to bone biopsy, (see Chapter 25.10) the high prevalence of osteoporosis in both pre- and postmenopausal women with primary biliary cirrhosis has been recognized (Eastell, Hepatol, 1991; 14:296). Osteoporosis may be the initial presentation and may be the primary indication for liver transplantation, as bone density improves post-transplant after the first 6-month period (Hay, Hepatol, 1990; 12:838). The women at particular risk are those who have undergone hysterectomy and oophorectomy at a young age without being given any hormone replacement therapy. Although oestrogens are generally contraindicated in patients with chronic liver disease, especially in cholestasis, the new natural oestrogens given by the transdermal route are probably safe; one retrospective study indicated that postmenopausal women given hormone replacement therapy suffer less metabolic bone disease (Crippin, AmJGastr, 1994; 89:47). The cause of osteoporosis in primary biliary cirrhosis is unknown; osteoblast function is reduced (Hodgson, AnnIntMed, 1985; 103:855) (see also Chapter 25.10). After the menopause, osteoclastic activity increases, which compounds the problem. Vitamin D supplementation is of little value, unless serum metabolites are low; serum vitamin K levels, which affect osteocalcin activity, are normal (Aguilar, Gastro, 1993; 104:A868). An *in vitro* study suggests that unconjugated bilirubin reduces osteoblast activity (Janes, JCI, 1995; 95:2581) and this effect has been proposed as a possible mechanism for cholestasis-related metabolic bone disease.

Other bony problems include finger clubbing, which is common; hypertrophic osteoarthropathy is present occasionally (Epstein, Gut, 1981; 22:203). Periostitis may cause excruciating pain in the wrists and lower limbs.

Renal associations (Chapter 25.7)

Renal complications include IgM-associated membranous glomerulonephritis (Rai, BMJ, 1977; 1:817). Renal tubular acidosis is attributed to copper deposits in the distal renal tubule (Pares, Gastro, 1981; 80:681). Hypouricaemia and hyperuricosuria are further expressions of renal tubular damage (Izumi, Hepatol, 1983; 3:719). Bacteriuria develops in 35 per cent and may be asymptomatic (Burroughs, Gut, 1984; 25:133); it is unexplained, but it has been postulated that urinary tract organisms might be involved in the pathogenesis of primary biliary cirrhosis. In one report, serum AMA were found in 50 per cent of sera from women with recurrent urinary tract infections (Butler, BiochemMolBiolInt, 1995; 35:473).

Gastrointestinal associations (Chapter 25.5)

Primary biliary cirrhosis has been associated with selective immunoglobulin A deficiency in a family (James, Gastro, 1986; 90: 283). This indicates that the pathogenesis does not require IgA-dependent immune mechanisms. Some patients may also have coeliac disease (Behr, AmJGastr, 1986; 81:796). Ulcerative colitis is another rare accompaniment (Bush, Gastro, 1987; 92:2099). Pancreatic insufficiency is secondary to low bile flow (Ros, Gastro, 1984; 87:180) and, perhaps, to immunological damage to the pancreatic duct (Epstein, Gastro, 1982; 82:1177).

Gallstones, usually of pigment type, have been seen by endoscopy in 39 per cent of patients (Summerfield, Gastro, 1976; 70: 240). They are occasionally symptomatic but rarely migrate to the common bile duct.

Pulmonary associations (Chapter 25.1)

Abnormal pulmonary gas transfer studies are associated with an abnormal chest radiograph showing nodules and interstitial fibrosis. Pulmonary interstitial giant-cell granulomas have also been described (Wallace, Gastro, 1987; 9:431). Computed tomography shows 81 per cent of patients with enlarged lymph nodes in the gastrohepatic ligament and porta hepatis (Outwater, Radiol, 1989; 17:731). Pulmonary hypertension in primary biliary cirrhosis may be seen with and without portal hypertension.

Neurological associations

Primary biliary cirrhosis has been associated with transverse myelitis due to angiitis and necrotizing myelopathy (Rutan, Gastro, 1986; 90:206). Both autonomic and peripheral neuropathies (asymptomatic for the most part) were found in a high percentage of patients with primary biliary cirrhosis in one study (Hendrickse, JHepatol, 1993; 19:401). Neither vitamin E deficiency nor hyperlipidaemia was associated with these findings.

Dermatological associations (Chapter 25.6)

Vitiligo is common as with all autoimmune disease. Lichen planus has been described as well as capillaritis mediated by the immune complex (Graham-Brown, BrJDermatol, 1982;106:699). Thickened pigmented skin is seen in all chronic cholestatic states associated with sustained pruritus.

Malignancy in primary biliary cirrhosis

As in all patients with chronic liver disease there is probably an increased rate of primary hepatocellular carcinoma, but there is controversy as to whether there is an increase in other malignancies. There are reports of an increased rate of breast cancer (Wolke, AmJMed, 1984; 76:1075; Goudie, BMJ 1985; 291:1597), but this has not been confirmed by others (Witt-Sullivan, Hepatol, 1990; 12:98; Lööt, Hepatol, 1994; 20:101).

Investigations

Serum bilirubin values are rarely very high at the onset, usually less than 34 mmol per 100 ml (2 mg per 100 ml), especially in asymptomatic patients. Serum alkaline phosphatase and γ-glutamyl transpeptidase are raised, often to very high levels. The serum aminotransferase levels may or may not be elevated. The total serum cholesterol is increased, but not constantly (see Chapter 2.12). Serum albumin level is usually normal at presentation and the total serum globulin only moderately increased. Serum immunoglobulin M is usually raised.

Serum antimitochondrial antibody tests (Chapter 5.3)

A positive result is virtually constant in a titre greater than 1:40. Standard immunofluorescence techniques generally suffice and titres are usually high. The ELISA technique is more sensitive (Kaplan, Hepatol, 1984; 4:727; Van De Water, NEJM, 1989; 320:1377) and immunoblotting is yet more sensitive and specific (Penner, Hepatol, 1986; 90:724). Positive results are almost always diagnostic of primary biliary cirrhosis. They are absent in patients with mechanical obstruction to the bile ducts. In autoimmune cholangitis, hepatic histology suggests primary biliary cirrhosis, but AMA tested by all methods are absent and antinuclear antibodies (ANA) are present in high titre (Ben-Ari, Hepatol, 1993; 18:10; Michieletti, Gut, 1994; 35:260). Very occasionally, AMA may be found in the sera of patients who otherwise have classic autoimmune hepatitis (Czaja, Gastro, 1993; 105:1522).

Liver biopsy

The only hepatic lesion diagnostic of primary biliary cirrhosis is the granulomatous destruction of septal or interlobular bile ducts. Such ducts are not often seen in needle biopsy specimens.

The disease begins with damage to the epithelium of the small bile ducts. Histometric examinations show that bile ducts less than 70 to 80 mm in diameter are destroyed, particularly in the early stages (Nakanuma, Gastro, 1979; 76:1326).

As the bile ducts become destroyed, their sites are marked by aggregates of lymphoid cells and bile ducts begin to proliferate (Plate 2). This may be delineated using a cytokeratin stain which shows the abnormal proliferating bile ducts very clearly. Hepatic arterial branches can be identified in the portal zones, but without accompanying bile ducts. Portal venous radicals may be involved in the inflammatory process and nodular regenerative hyperplasia is a consequence (Colina, Gastro, 1992; 102:1319). Fibrosis extends from the portal tracts and there is a variable degree of interface hepatitis. Substantial amounts of copper and copper-associated protein can be demonstrated histochemically in periportal zones. The fibrous septa gradually come to distort the architecture of the liver and regeneration nodules form. These are often irregular in distribution, and cirrhosis may be seen in one part of a biopsy but not in another. In some areas, zonal architecture may be preserved for some time. Hepatocellular hyaline deposits, similar to those of alcoholic liver disease, are found in hepatocytes in about 25 per cent of cases.

The histological appearances have been divided into four stages: stage I, florid bile duct lesions; stage II, ductular proliferation; stage

III, scarring (septal fibrosis and bridging); and stage IV, cirrhosis (Scheuer, ProcRoySocMed, 1967; 60:1257). Such staging is of limited value as the changes in the liver are focal and evolve at different speeds in different parts of the liver. Stages overlap, and it is particularly difficult to separate stages II and III.

The disease has a very variable course and advanced stage III lesions or even stage IV may be seen in the asymptomatic patient. Serial biopsies have shown that, in most cases, primary biliary cirrhosis progresses histologically over a 2-year period (Lock, Hepatol, 1996; 23:52). However, an 'early' lesion histologically does not necessarily predict prognosis.

Progressive fibrosis developing into cirrhosis is likely to be multifactorial in origin. Increasing cholestasis due to loss of bile ducts, chronic inflammation, and portal and hepatic vein thrombi (Nakamura, AmJGastr, 1982; 77:405), all probably play a role in the gradual development of liver failure in primary biliary cirrhosis.

The biliary tree

Visualization of the bile ducts may be necessary in atypical patients. These include males and those with a negative serum AMA test, inconclusive liver biopsy findings, or abdominal pain. Because of the small size of the intrahepatic bile ducts, the endoscopic route is preferable to the percutaneous.

The anatomy of the main intrahepatic bile ducts is normal in primary biliary cirrhosis, and this excludes primary sclerosing cholangitis. However, when cirrhosis has developed, the intrahepatic bile ducts may look narrow and irregular, but not beaded. Gallstones may be an incidental finding.

Differential diagnosis (Table 4)

In the later stages, the differentiation from other causes of cirrhosis may be difficult; however, the pattern of serum biochemical tests is usually different.

As the AMA test is so specific, the value of liver biopsy in making a diagnosis of primary biliary cirrhosis has been brought into question, particularly as it is not very helpful as an indicator of prognosis. AMA-negative primary biliary cirrhosis (autoimmune cholangitis) is discussed in Chapter 14.6.

Primary sclerosing cholangitis may cause diagnostic difficulty, but the AMA test is always negative and cholangiography demonstrates the typical bile-duct irregularities, unless the disease is confined to the small intrahepatic ducts (Wee, AnnIntMed, 1985; 102:581).

The cholestatic form of sarcoidosis, particularly found in young black males, can be indistinguishable from primary biliary cirrhosis. Lymphadenopathy and chest radiographic changes tend to be obvious. Liver biopsy shows more granulomas, often present in the parenchyma, which tend to become fibrotic with time, and less bile duct damage is observed than in primary biliary cirrhosis. An increased level of serum angiotensin-converting enzyme may be found in any person with significant liver disease and, therefore, its measurement is not helpful in this situation. Bronchoalveolar lavage findings are similar to primary biliary cirrhosis (Spiteri, Gut, 1990; 31:280). Drug-related cholestasis, for example after chlorpromazine or antibiotics such as flucloxacillin or amoxycillin–clavulinic acid, can become chronic and produce a picture resembling primary

biliary cirrhosis (Monadpour, Hepatol, 1994; 20:1437). Biochemical tests may remain abnormal for many years. However, there is a history of taking the drug and the initial presentation is with jaundice, whereas in primary biliary cirrhosis this is delayed. Patients with autoimmune hepatitis may have biochemical cholestasis and some are AMA positive. Bile duct lesions are occasionally found on liver biopsy; these overlaps of primary biliary cirrhosis and autoimmune hepatitis are discussed in detail in Chapter 14.6.

Complications
Bone changes (Chapter 25.10)

These complicate all forms of chronic cholestasis even prior to the onset of jaundice, but are particularly severe in the deeply jaundiced patient with primary biliary cirrhosis when osteomalacia as well as osteoporosis may be present. (Hay, Gastro, 1995; 106:276) (Fig. 1). Osteoporosis may be detected even at presentation in some patients (Mitchison, Gastro, 1988; 94:463). Hence dual energy X-ray absorptiometry (DEXA) as a measure of bone density should be part of the screening in any new patient with primary biliary cirrhosis.

Serum 25-dihydroxyvitamin D levels are low in advanced cases and cholestyramine therapy further reduces the availability of vitamin D. However, osteoporosis is much commoner than osteomalacia (Atkinson, QJMed, 1956; 25:299; Herlong, Gastro, 1982; 83:103). Bone analysis demonstrates decreased osteoblastic activity which is enhanced in patients who are postmenopausal and further complicated by increased osteoclastic activity. Symptoms, such as backache, pain over the ribs, and pathological fractures are seen in the late stages, but severe disease is rare now that transplantation is the recognized therapy for endstage disease.

Malabsorption

Other deficiencies of fat-soluble vitamins may be present (Kaplan, Gastro, 1988; 95:787). Vitamin A malabsorption is associated with low levels of serum vitamin A (retinol), but symptoms such as night blindness are rare (Walt, BMJ, 1984; 288:1030). However, specific tests of dark adaptation are often abnormal.

Vitamin K deficiency is marked by prolongation of the prothrombin time and the presence of circulating abnormal prothrombin (des-g-carboxyl prothrombin).

Vitamin E deficiency is shown by low serum concentrations of the vitamin (Jeffery, JHepatol, 1987; 4:307). The neuromuscular syndrome attributed to vitamin E deficiency, described in children with prolonged cholestasis, is extremely rare in patients with primary biliary cirrhosis.

Portal hypertension (Chapter 7.2)

Bleeding oesophageal varices may be a presenting feature, even before nodules have developed in the liver (Kew, Gut, 1971; 12:830). The portal hypertension is probably presinusoidal and may be related to nodular regenerative hyperplasia. Haemorrhage from varices may also accompany the late, cirrhotic stage.

Liver failure

The terminal stages last about 1 to 2 years and are marked by deepening of jaundice, with disappearance of both xanthomas and

Table 4 Differential diagnosis of primary biliary cirrhosis

Disease	Features	Serum antimitochondrial antibody	Liver biopsy
Primary biliary cirrhosis	Female, pruritus, high serum alkaline phosphatase	Positive high titre	Bile duct lesions, lymphoid aggregates; intact lobules; periseptal cholestasis
Autoimmune cholangiopathy	" " "	Negative	" " "
Primary slcerosing cholangitis	Males predominate; associated ulcerative colitis; pruritus; cholangiography is diagnostic	Negative	Zone 1 ductular proliferation, fibrosis and cellularity; 'onion-skin' duct fibrosis
Cholestatic sarcoidosis	Equal sexes; usually black persons; high alkaline phosphatase; itching; chest radiographic abnormalities	Negative	Many granulomas all zones/often fibrotic; modest bile-duct changes
Cholestatic drug reaction	History of drug use, acute onset	Negative	Mononuclear zone 1 reaction, sometimes with eosinophils and granulomas; modest piecemeal necrosis may be followed by duct paucity
Autoimmune hepatitis	Female; high serum aminotransferases and gammaglobulin; positive serum anti-smooth-muscle and antinuclear antibodies or anti-liver-kidney-microsomal antibodies	Negative or low titre	Zone 1 mononucleosis and fibrosis; marked piecemeal necrosis; bridging necrosis; rosettes of liver cells; plasma cell infiltrates; rare bile-duct loss

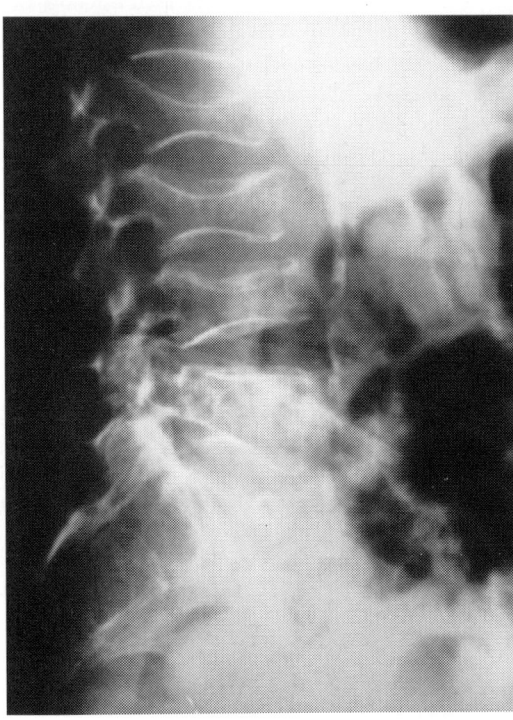

Fig. 1. Advanced primary biliary cirrhosis. Radiograph of the lumbar spine shows extreme osteoporosis with biconcave deformities and vertebral compression.

pruritus. The levels of serum albumin and total cholesterol fall. Oedema and ascites develop. Occasionally, ascites appears prior to the onset of jaundice, although this is unusual. The final events include episodes of hepatic encephalopathy and uncontrollable bleeding, usually from oesophageal varices. An intercurrent infection leading to septicaemia, generally Gram-negative, may be terminal.

The question of liver transplantation should be discussed from the outset. The asymptomatic patient should be reassured that she may never need the operation. Those whose quality of life has been reduced to the level that they are virtually housebound, with increasing jaundice or signs of hepatocellular failure, should consider the procedure early rather than late as the results will be much better (Neuberger, Gut, 1990; 31:1069). Occasionally, liver transplantation is considered an option for those with uncontrollable pruritus alone.

Natural history

Studies suggest that primary biliary cirrhosis is being diagnosed with increasing frequency (Myszar, QJMed, 1990; 75:377), most probably because of easy access to screening blood tests and an increase in physician awareness of the disease. Hence, more and more asymptomatic cases are being diagnosed (Inoue, Liver, 1995; 15:70). Early reports suggested that the survival of patients with asymptomatic primary biliary cirrhosis was no different from that of an age- and gender-matched control population (Beswick, Gastro, 1985; 89:267), but subsequent studies indicate that this is not the case (Balasubramanian, Gastro, 1990; 98:1567). A follow-up study of 279 patients with primary biliary cirrhosis indicates that the median survival for symptomatic disease is 8 years and for asymptomatic disease 16 years (Mahl, JHepatol, 1994; 20:707). Predictors of poor outcome have been sought; all the sample sizes studied have been relatively small and it would seem that no single factor is useful in predicting which asymptomatic patient will become

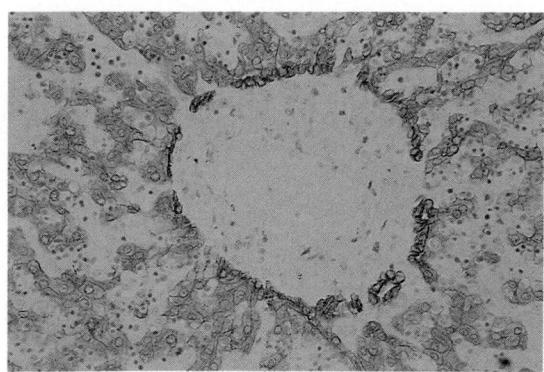

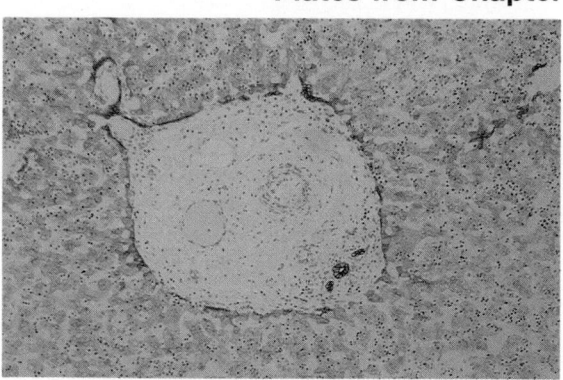

Plate 1. Embryonic ductal plate in liver tissue of a 16-week-old human fetus. The picture shows a branch of the portal vein with its accompanying mesenchyme, surrounded by the 'ductal plate'. The latter corresponds to a partly double layer of epithelial cells, which show smaller size and stronger cytokeratin expression than the surrounding epithelial cells (primitive hepatocyte precursor cells). A more dilated lumen (a tubule) develops in some segments of the ductal plate (between 3 and 4 o'clock, and at 5 o'clock).

Plate 2. Remodelling of ductal plate in liver tissue of a 25-week-old human fetus. A cross-sectioned primitive portal tract is shown, surrounded by the ductal plate which is easily recognized by its stronger cytokeratin expression (brown stain). At 5 o'clock, a tubular duct becomes detached from the ductal plate and is gradually incorporated into the portal mesenchyme, which shows a higher cellularity in that area. (Immunoperoxidase stain with anticytokeratin antibody CAM 5.2, staining cytokeratins 8, 18, and 19. Nuclear counterstain with haematoxylin, $\times 32$.)

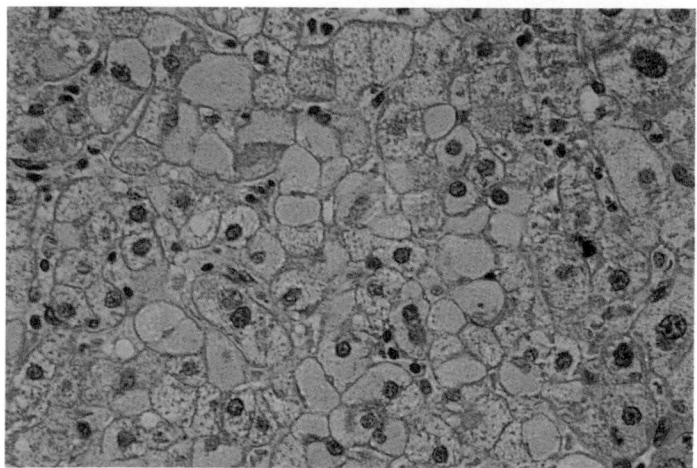

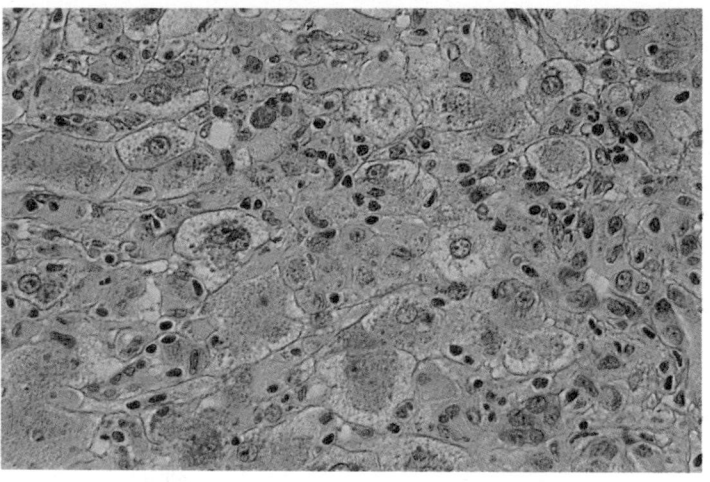

Plate 1. Liver biopsy from a patient with chronic hepatitis B. Numerous ground-glass hepatocytes with homogeneous, pale pink cytoplasm can be seen (haematoxylin and eosin $\times 65$).

Plate 2. Liver biopsy from a patient with acute hepatitis B, characterized by liver cell pleomorphism and parenchymal inflammation. Pleomorphism of hepatocytes is reflected in unequal size and staining quality. Ballooned hepatocytes appear swollen and pale, especially in the peripheral part of their cytoplasm. Two small eosinophilic apoptotic cell fragments lie close to lymphocytes (haematoxylin and eosin $\times 104$).

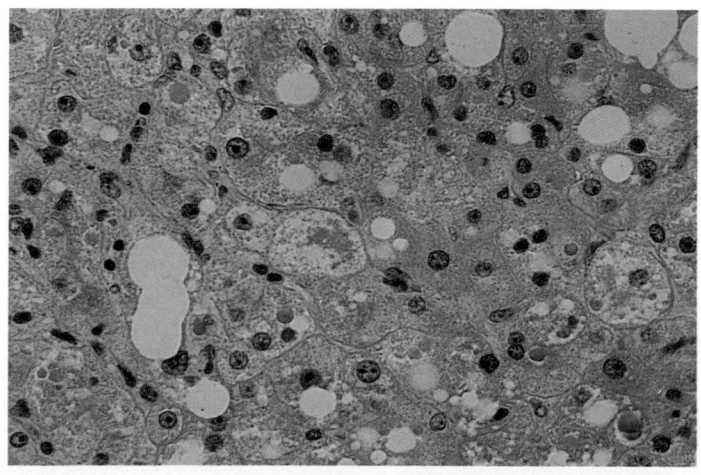

Plate 3. Liver biopsy from a patient with alcoholic liver disease. The picture shows some steatosis vacuoles, two pale, swollen hepatocytes containing an irregularly shaped Mallory body, and several parenchymal cells with one or more round, eosinophilic inclusions: megamitochondria (haematoxylin and eosin $\times 104$).

Plates from Chapter 3.1

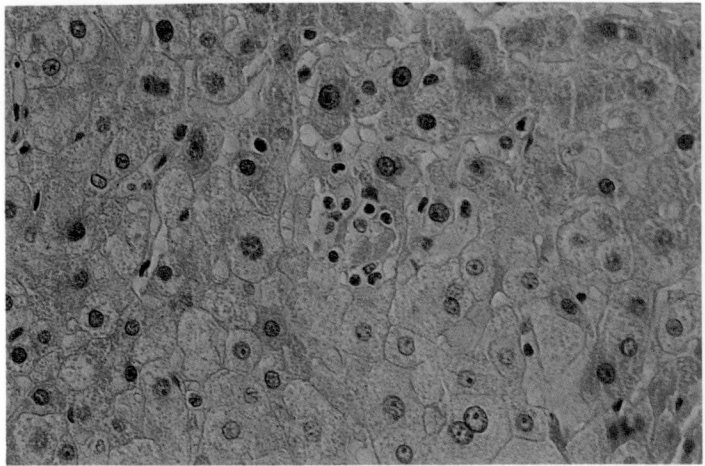

Plate 4. Liver biopsy from a patient with chronic persistent hepatitis B. Small focus of focal (or 'spotty') necrosis, with accumulation of lymphocytes and mononuclear cells around a dying liver cell, of which only two small eosinophilic fragments (apoptotic bodies) are recognizable (haematoxylin and eosin × 104).

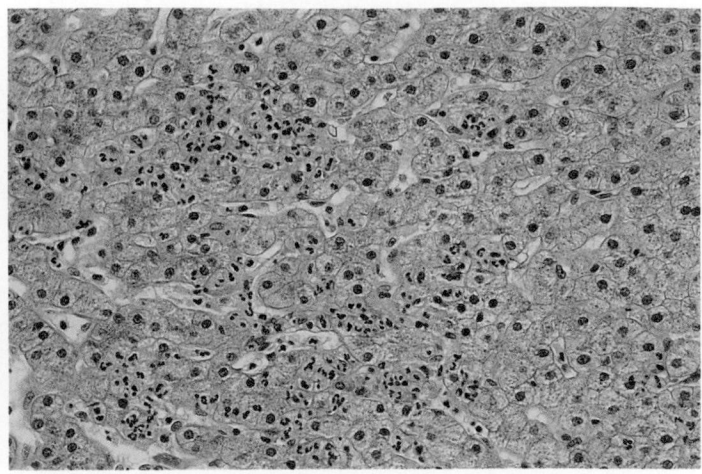

Plate 5. Surgical liver biopsy. 'Surgical necroses' are represented by clusters of accumulating polymorphonuclear neutrophils (haematoxylin and eosin × 65).

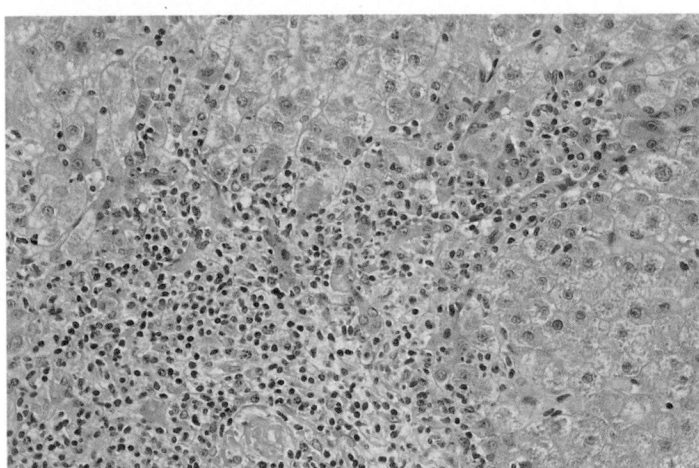

Plate 6. Liver biopsy from a patient with chronic active hepatitis B, characterized by piecemeal necrosis. The portal tract (lower left corner) shows dense mononuclear cell infiltration, which extends into the surrounding parenchyma, creating an irregular connective tissue–parenchymal interphase. A longer extension (up to right upper corner) represents an early stage of active septum formation (haematoxylin and eosin × 65).

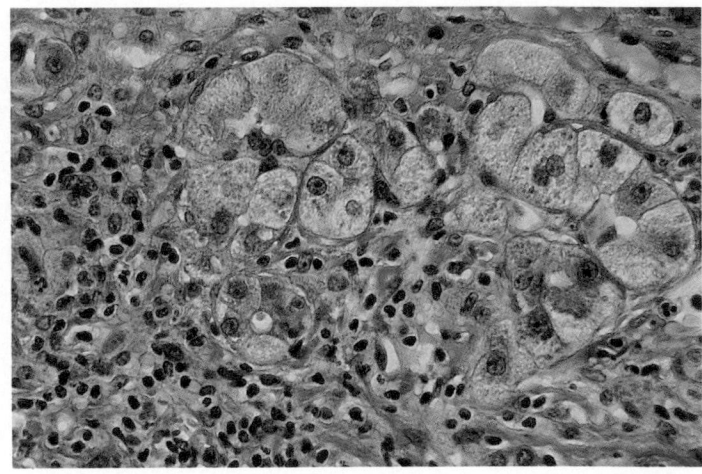

Plate 7. Liver biopsy from a patient with post-hepatitic cirrhosis. Hepatitic liver cell rosettes represent small groups of sequestrated hepatocytes, surrounded by fibrosis and inflammatory infiltration (Masson's trichrome (collagen appears blue) × 104).

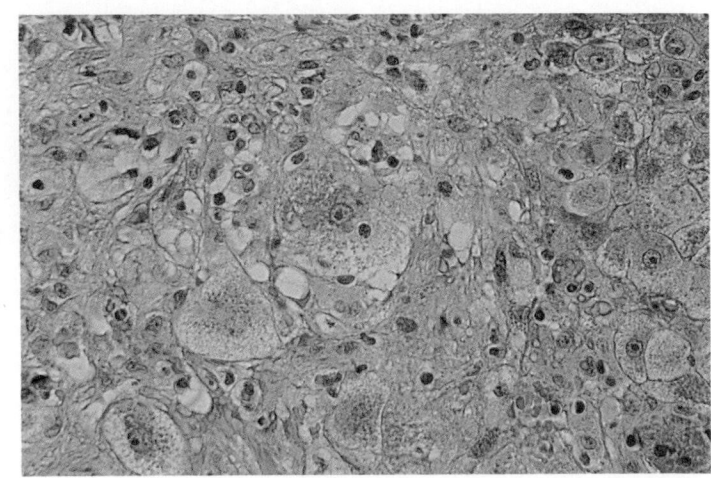

Plate 8. Liver biopsy from a patient with acute hepatitis B. The picture shows liver cell pleomorphism and ballooning, and interrupted continuity of liver cell plates. Note the presence (centre) of a lymphocyte, surrounded by a narrow clear halo, in the cytoplasm of a ballooned hepatocyte: emperipolesis (haematoxylin and eosin × 104).

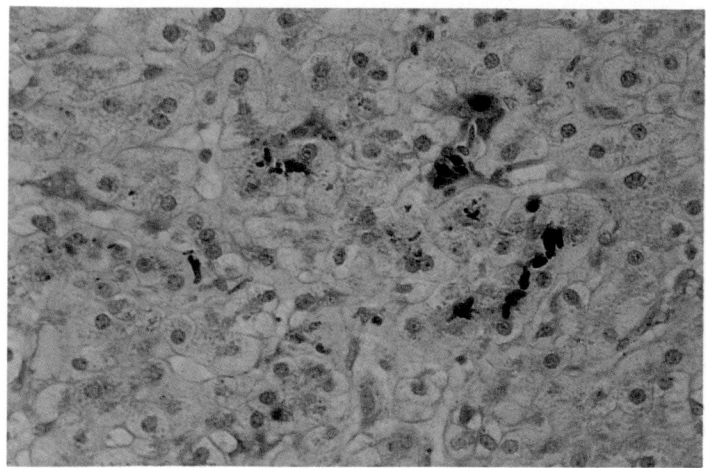

Plate 9. Liver biopsy from an infant with biliary atresia. The picture shows bilirubin granules in a couple of hepatocytes (hepatocellular bilirubinostasis), coarse bilirubin-stained casts in dilated canaliculi (canalicular bilirubinostasis), and coarse bilirubin deposits in hypertrophic, red-stained (PAS-positive) Kupffer (Kupffer cell bilirubinostasis) (PAS-Schiff after diastase digestion (PAS-D), × 104).

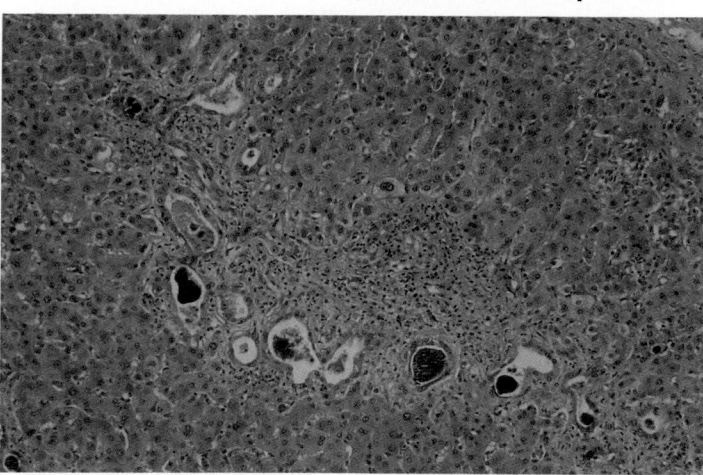

Plate 10. Liver biopsy from a severely jaundiced patient with monilia sepsis. The picture shows an obliquely cut portal tract, extending from the upper left to lower right corner. The upper and lower border is lined by a large number of extremely dilated ductules containing bile concrements in varying degree of inspissation (ductular bilirubinostasis) (haematoxylin and eosin × 26).

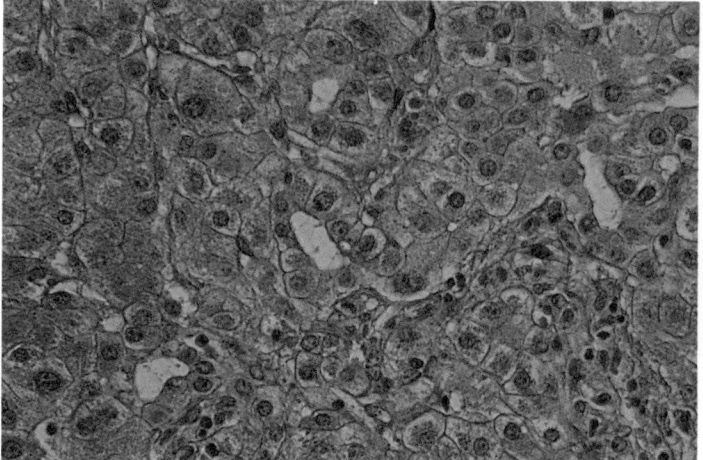

Plate 11. Liver biopsy from a 9-year-old child with incomplete obstruction of the common bile duct by annular pancreas. Chronic cholestasis is reflected in the appearance of cholestatic liver cell rosettes: groups of hepatocytes arranged around a central lumen. In this instance, there are no obvious bile concrements in the lumina (haematoxylin and eosin × 104).

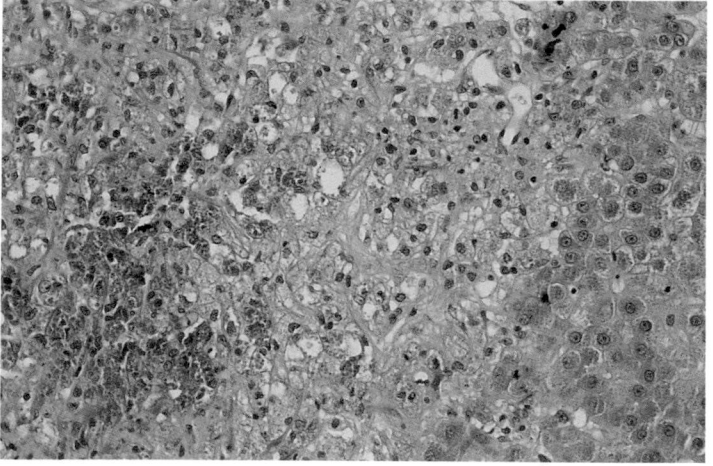

Plate 12. Liver biopsy from a patient with long-standing extrahepatic bile-duct obstruction. The picture shows part of a large paraportal bile infarct (compare with the appearance of relatively normal parenchyma on the right side). The central part of the necrotizing area (left side of picture) is most heavily impregnated with bilirubin pigment (haematoxylin and eosin × 65).

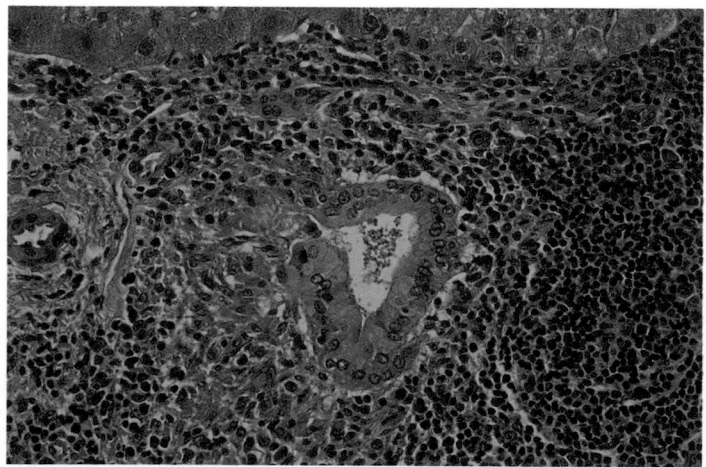

Plate 13. Liver biopsy from a patient with primary biliary cirrhosis. The pictures shows a cross-sectioned interlobular bile duct, lying amidst a densely lymphoplasmocytic infiltrate. Note the focal rupture of the bile-duct lining (near 10'clock) and the development of an epithelioid granuloma on the ruptured side of the duct (haematoxylin and eosin × 65).

Plates from Chapter 3.1

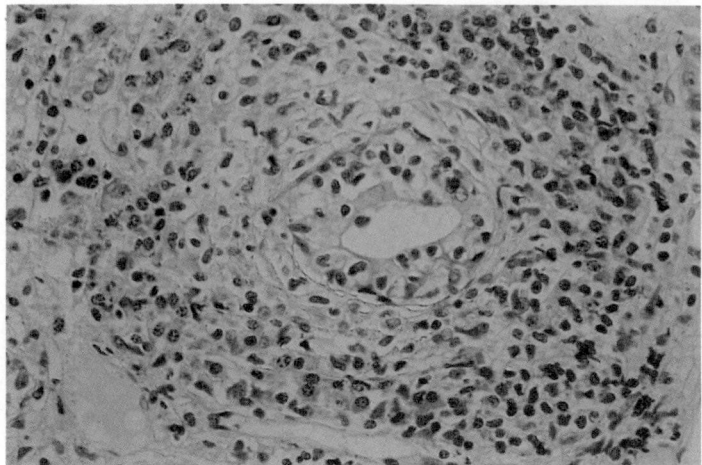

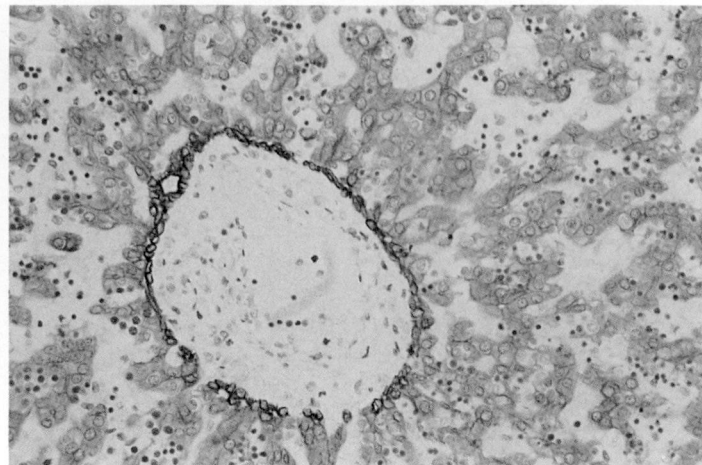

Plate 14. Liver biopsy from a patient with chronic active hepatitis. The picture shows a cross-sectioned interlobular bile duct, in a portal tract with dense infiltration by lymphocytes and plasma cells. The bile-duct lining cells appear swollen and multilayered, and are infiltrated by lymphocytes (haematoxylin and eosin × 104).

Plate 15. Liver specimen from a 16-week-old human fetus. The picture shows a portal vein branch surrounded with mesenchyme. Adjacent to the latter lies a partly double layer of smaller and darker staining cells (the ductal plate). A tubular lumen has formed in one of the double layered segments (upper left). The primitive hepatocytes are weakly stained, with stronger positivity near the cell periphery. Interspersed haematopoietic cells are keratin negative (immunoperoxidase stain for cytokeratins (antibody CAM 5.2, which stains cytokeratins nos. 8,18, and 19): counterstain with Harris haematoxylin × 65).

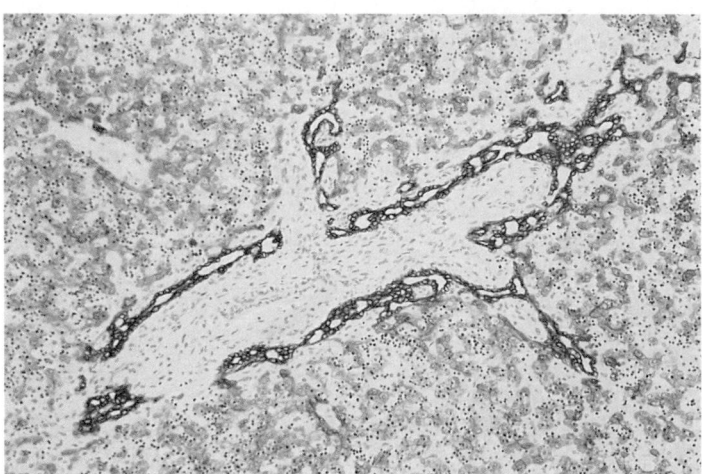

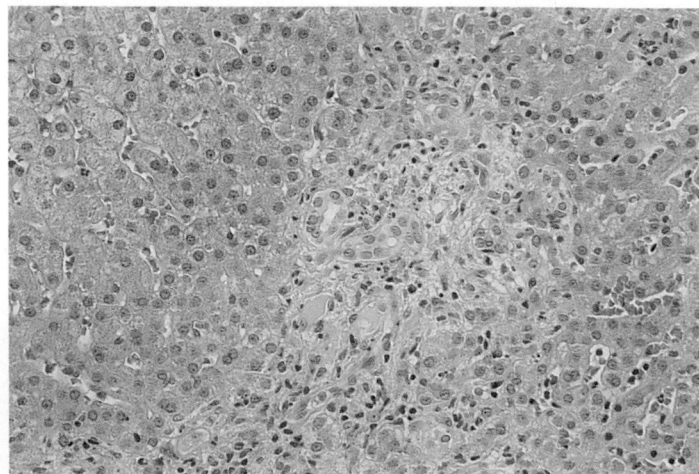

Plate 16. Liver specimen from a 20-week-old human fetus with Meckel syndrome. The picture shows a portal vein with two short side branches surrounded with mesenchyme. Adjacent to the latter lies a double layer of small, darkly-staining cells which form numerous cross-sectioned tubular structures. Persistence of these structures indicates lack of remodelling of the ductal plate, i.e. the ductal plate malformation. The primitive hepatocytes are weakly stained, with stronger positivity near the cell periphery. Interspersed haematopoietic cells are negative for keratin (immunoperoxidase stain for cytokeratins (antibody CAM 5.2, which stains cytokeratins nos. 8,18, and 19): counterstain with Harris haematoxylin, × 65).

Plate 17. Liver biopsy from a patient with primary sclerosing cholangitis. The portal tract in the centre appears oedematous; an increased number of ductular profiles can be seen extending into the surrounding parenchyma, with a sprinkling of polymorphonuclear and mononuclear inflammatory cells (cholangiolitis) (haematoxylin and eosin × 65).

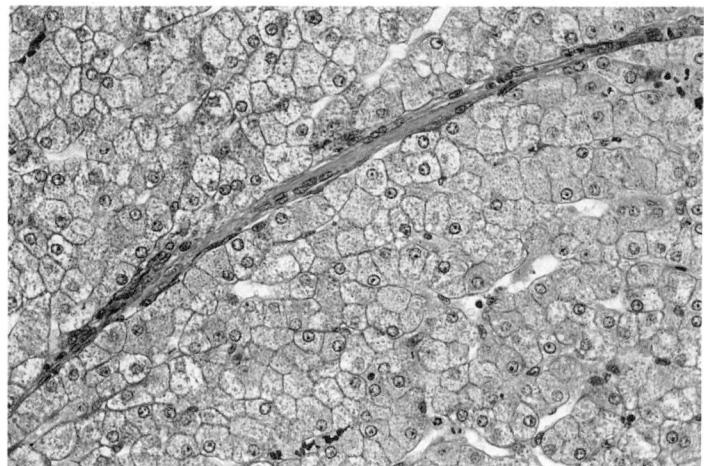

Plate 18. Liver biopsy from a patient with inactive macronodular cirrhosis. A passive septum appears as a sharply delineated blue-stained line. Note the presence of vessels and the absence of inflammatory cells in the septum. The nodular parenchyma appears hyperplastic, with plates of thickness of two or more cells (Masson's trichrome stain × 65).

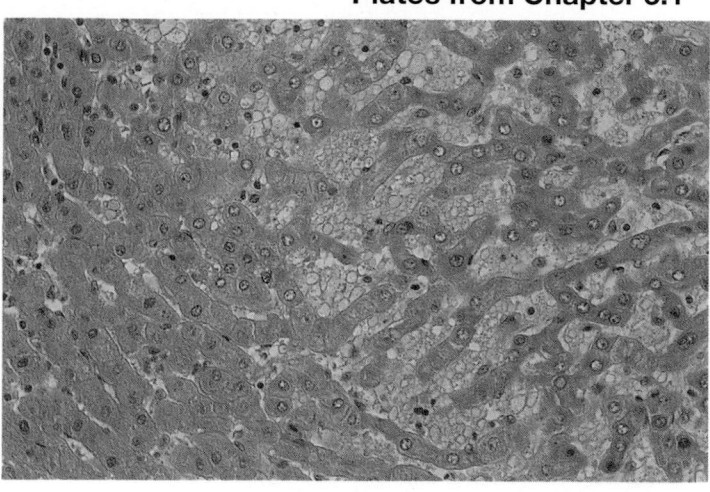

Plate 19. Liver biopsy from a patient with venous outflow block (heart decompensation). Note the dilatation of the sinusoids, engorged with erythrocytes, and the thinning of the liver cell plates in acinar zone 3 (right side of picture) (haematoxylin and eosin × 65).

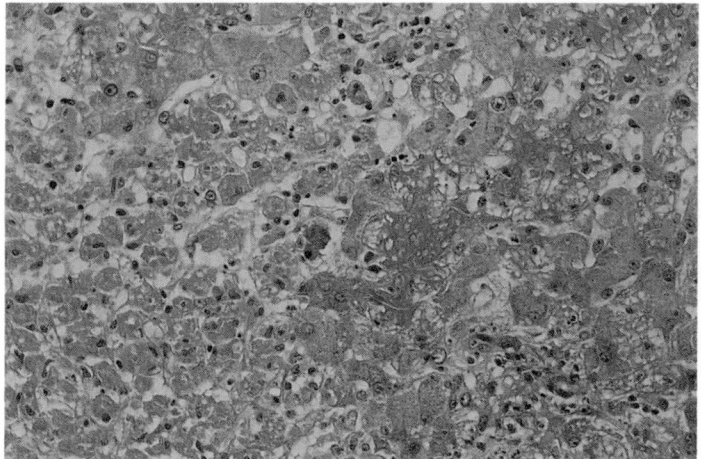

Plate 20. Liver biopsy from a pregnant patient with eclampsia. A small portal tract is located near the lower right corner. Several paraportal sinusoids are blocked with pink fibrin clots (centre and upper right). Note the early stage of ischaemic necrosis of parts of the parenchyma (left side), with increased eosinophilia of the cytoplasm and pyknosis of the nuclei (haematoxylin and eosin × 65).

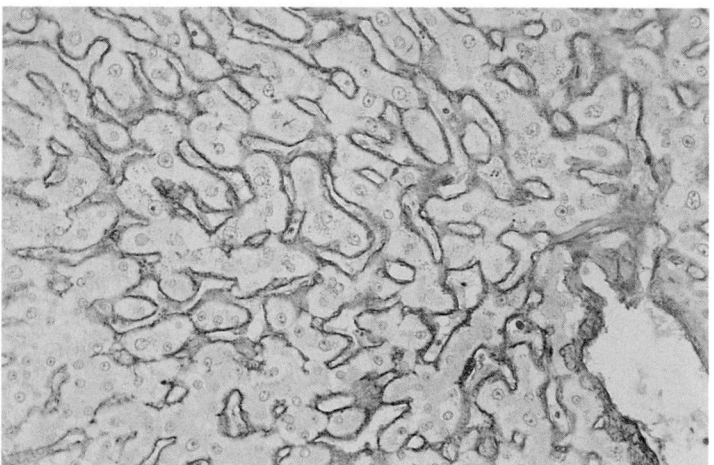

Plate 21. Liver biopsy from a patient with light chain deposit disease. A terminal hepatic venule (centre vein) is located in the lower right corner. The Disse space between sinusoidal lumina and liver cell plates contains material which is immunoreactive for kappa light chains of immunoglobulin (immunoperoxidase stain for kappa light chains: counterstain of nuclei with haematoxylin and eosin × 65).

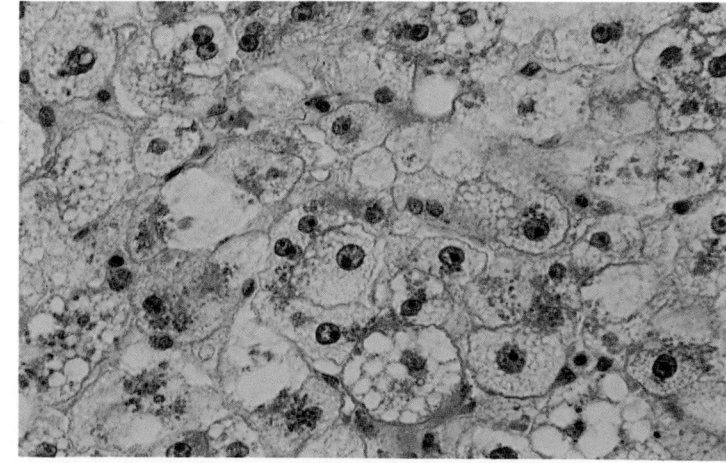

Plate 22. Liver biopsy from a patient with tetracycline intoxication. The picture shows part of the parenchyma, characterized by small droplet steatosis. The hepatocytes contain numerous small fat droplets, and retain their nucleus in central poition. Granular bilirubin pigment also accumulates between the fat vacuoles (hepatocellular bilirubinostasis) (haematoxylin and eosin × 104).

Plates from Chapter 3.1

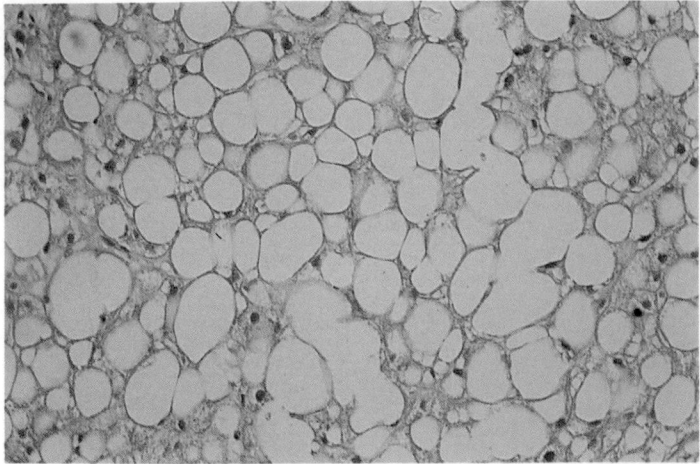

Plate 23. Liver biopsy from a patient with alcohol abuse. Most hepatocytes contain single, large fat vacuoles, pushing the nucleus to the periphery of the cell. Some adjacent vacuoles fuse to larger 'fatty cysts' (haematoxylin and eosin × 65).

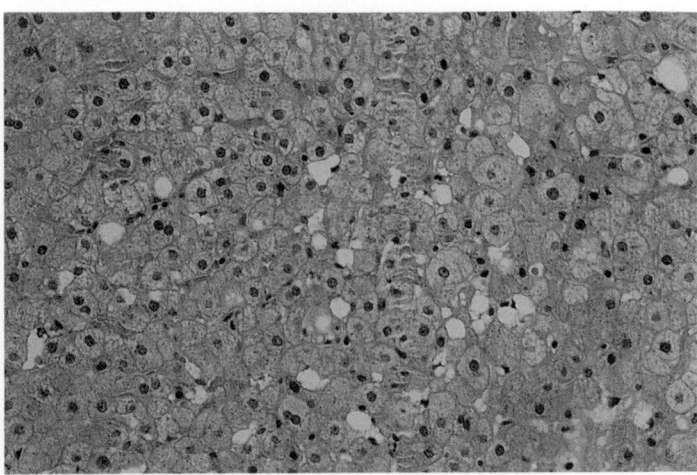

Plate 24. Liver biopsy from a patient with vitamin A intoxication. Numerous clear spaces occur between the hepatocytes: they correspond to hyperplastic Ito cells (so-called fat storing cells); they contain fat droplets in their cytoplasm which indent the contour of their nucleus (haematoxylin and eosin × 65).

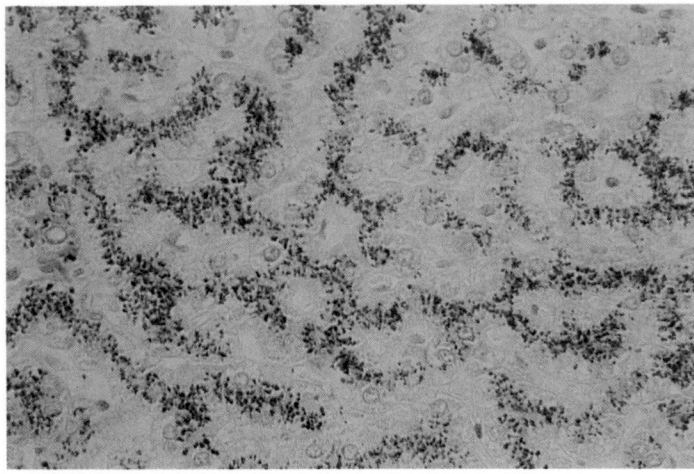

Plate 25. Liver biopsy from a patient with idiopathic (genetic) haemochromatosis. Blue-stained haemosiderin granules accumulate in the pericanalicular region of the hepatocytes (which is a typical localization of lysosomes) (Prussian blue stain for iron; neutral red counterstain, × 104).

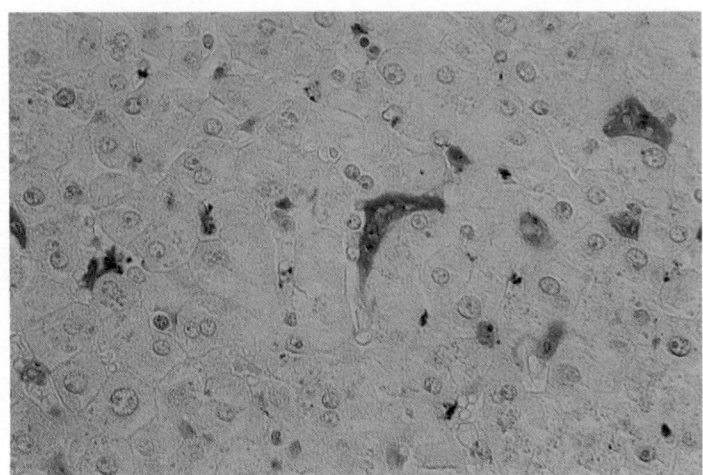

Plate 26. Liver biopsy from a patient under chemotherapy for leukaemia. Reticulendothelial siderosis: blue-stained haemosiderin granules accumulate in hyperplastic Kupffer cells; the parenchymal cells are negative (Prussian blue stain for iron; neutral red counterstain, × 104).

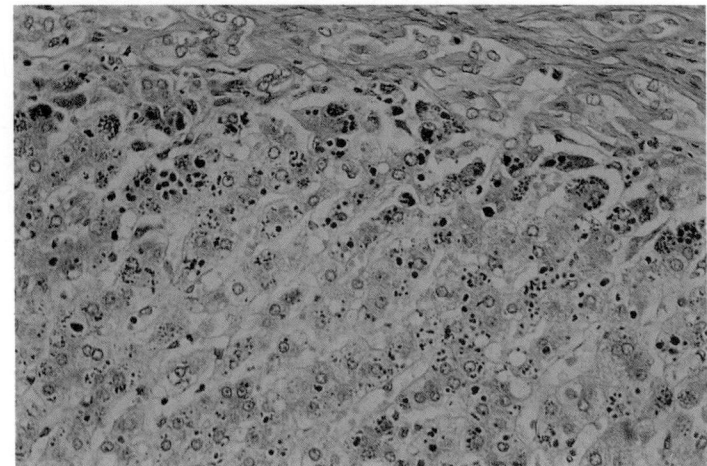

Plate 27. Liver biopsy from a patient with liver cirrhosis and α_1-antitryspin deficiency. Part of a cirrhotic nodule is shown; red-stained (PAS-positive) inclusions of variable size are present in hepatocytes, especially in the nodular periphery near a connective tissue septum (upper part) (periodic acid-Schiff after diastase digestion (PAS-D), × 65).

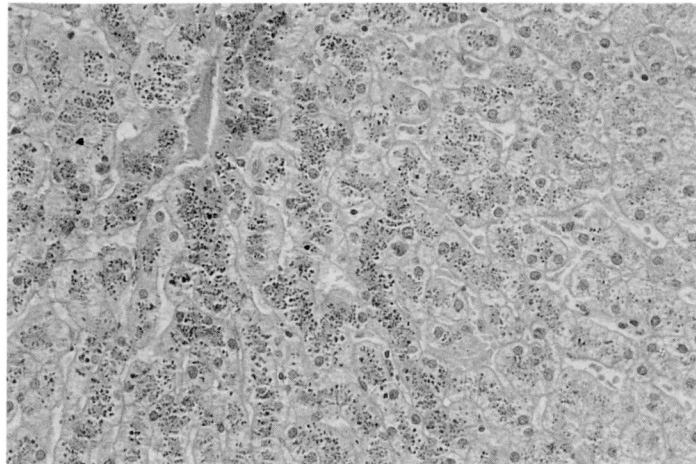

Plate 28. Liver biopsy from a patient with Dubin-Johnson syndrome. A terminal hepatic venule (central vein) is located near the upper left corner. The hepatocytes contain numerous brown pigment granules, especially in acinar zone 3 (haematoxylin and eosin × 65).

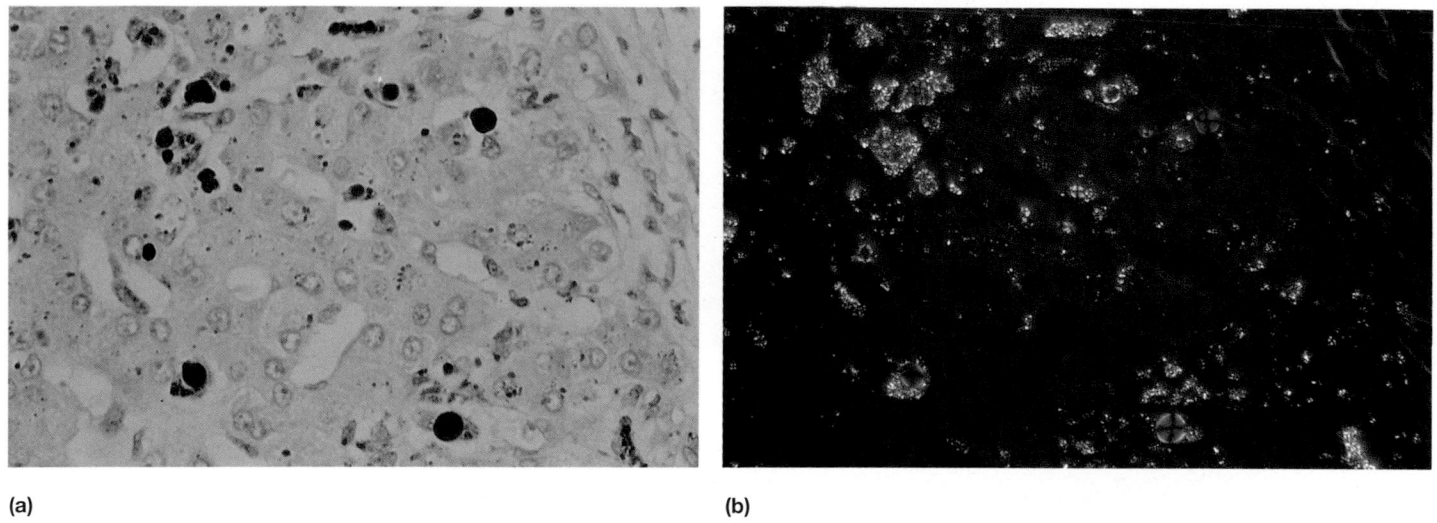

(a)

(b)

Plate 29. Liver specimen from a patient with erythropoietic protoporphyria. Brown-black deposits of variable size are seen in hepatocytes, canaliculi, and hyperplastic Kupffer cells. (a) Haematoxylin and eosin, × 104. (b) The same area under polarized light: the deposits show birefringence, in Maltese cross configuration in the larger deposits. (Specimen by courtesy of Dr B. Portmann, London.)

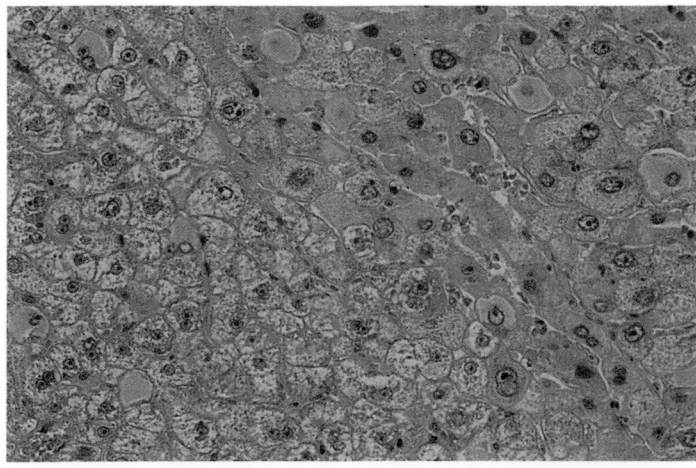

Plate 30. Liver biopsy from a patient with hepatitis B virus positive liver cirrhosis. The upper right half of the picture shows hepatocytes with enlarged cytoplasmic and nuclear size (dysplastic cells). Ground-glass change of the cytoplasm is seen in some of the dysplastic and non-dysplastic cells (haematoxylin and eosin × 104).

Plates from Section 4

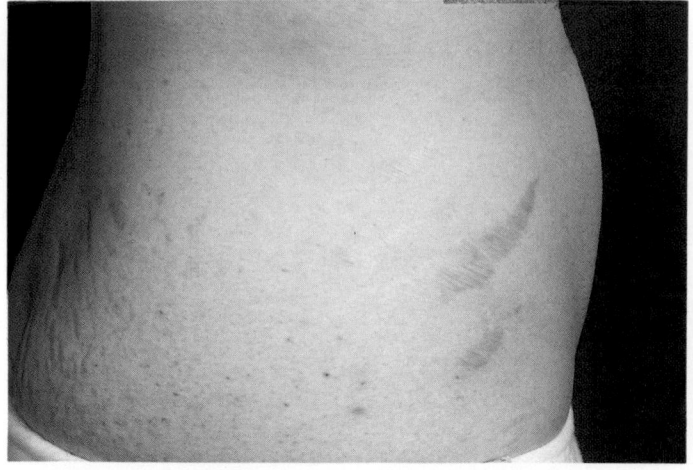

Plate 1. Abdominal striae in a young woman with autoimmune chronic active hepatitis.

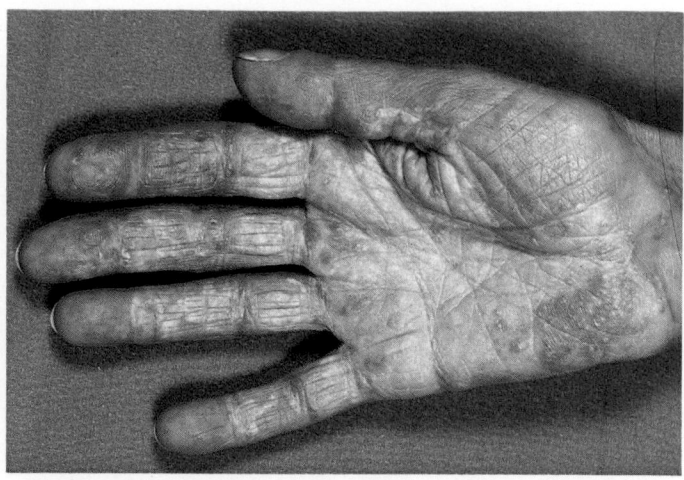

Plate 2. Palmar xanthomas in a patient with long-standing biliary obstruction due to primary biliary cirrhosis.

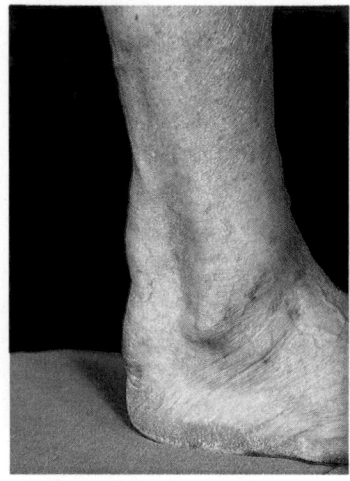

Plate 3. A tendon xanthoma in a patient with primary biliary cirrhosis.

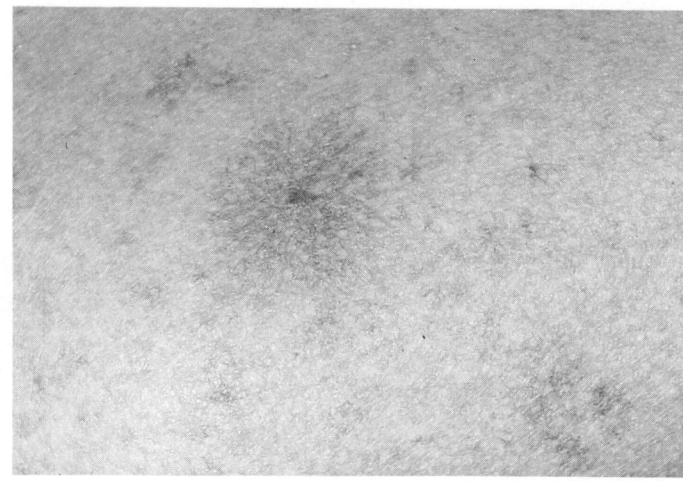

Plate 4. A classical spider naevus in a patient with alcoholic cirrhosis.

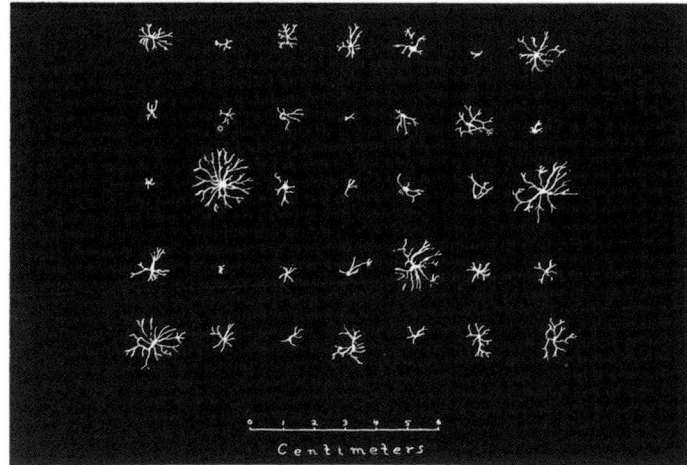

Plate 5. This figure, from Bean's classic paper (Medicine, 1945; 24: 243), illustrates the wide variation that can be seen in the appearance of 'spider naevi'.

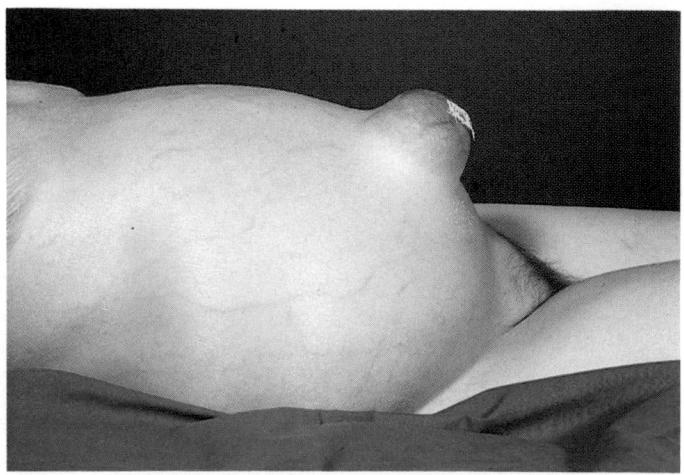

Plate 6. Gross ascites. Note the unusually large distance between the xiphisternum and the umbilicus compared with the distance between the umbilicus and the symphysis pubis.

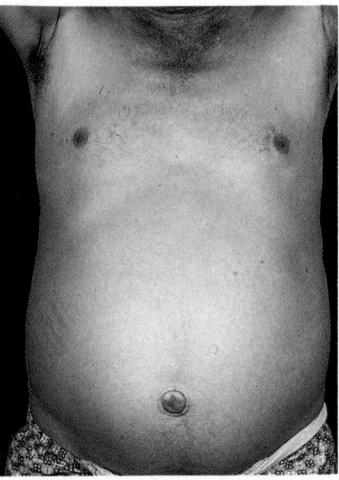

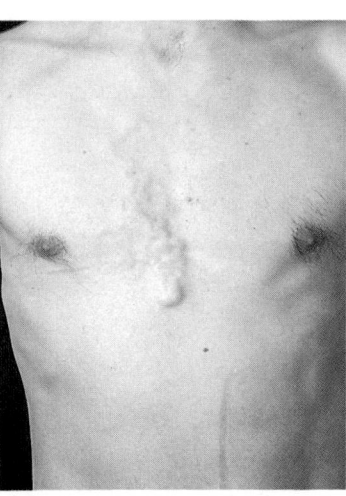

Plate 7. Abdominal collaterals, above and below the umbilicus, which have their origin in the umbilical or para-umbilical veins. They become obvious at some distance from the umbilicus.

Plate 8. Upper abdominal collaterals, close to the midline, originating in para-umbilical veins, via small veins which penetrate the rectus sheath to reach the surface.

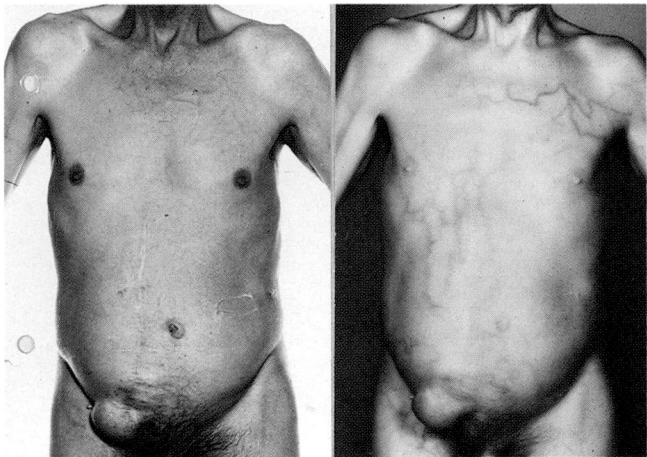

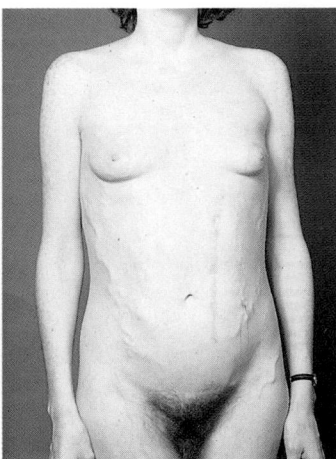

Plate 9. Abdominal collaterals appearing around a scar resulting from previous abdominal surgery, presumably due to adhesions between the viscera and the abdominal wall.

Plate 10. Prominent abdominal wall veins with inferior vena caval obstruction. The blood runs upwards even over the lower abdomen, and the veins are usually most prominent at the sides of the abdomen.

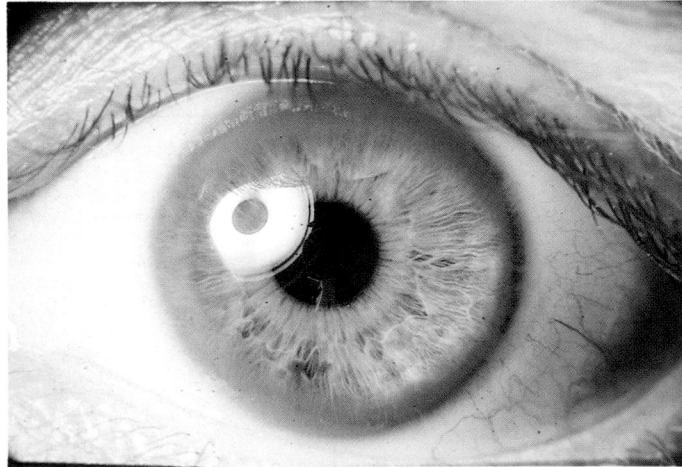

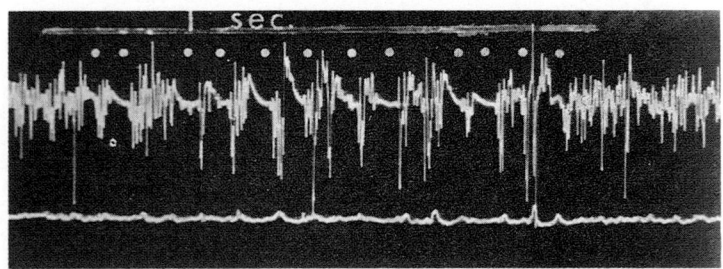

Plate 11. A Kayser–Fleischer ring. It is easy to see in this patient because of the pale iris.

Plate 12. An EMG from a patient with hepatic encephalopathy. Asterixis occurred when longer periods of electrical silence coincided in different muscles (from Leavitt, ArchNeurol, 1964; 10:360).

Plates from Chapter 5.4.2

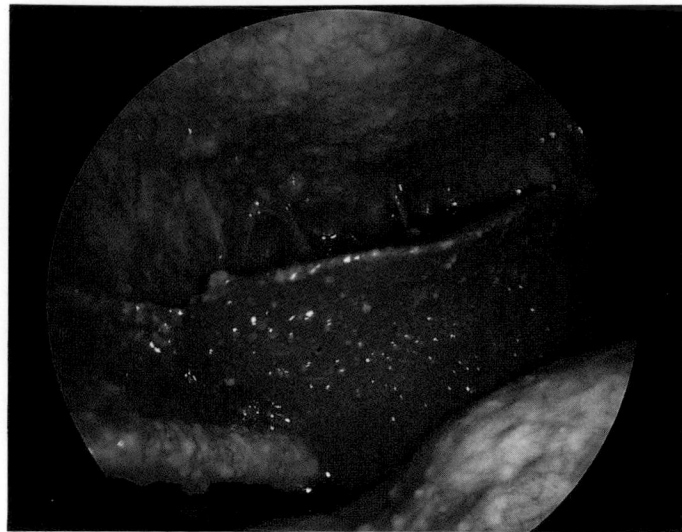

Plate 1. Peritoneal tuberculosis. The whitish nodules are present all over the peritoneal surface (parietal, hepatic, and intestinal). The ascitic fluid is clear and pale yellow.

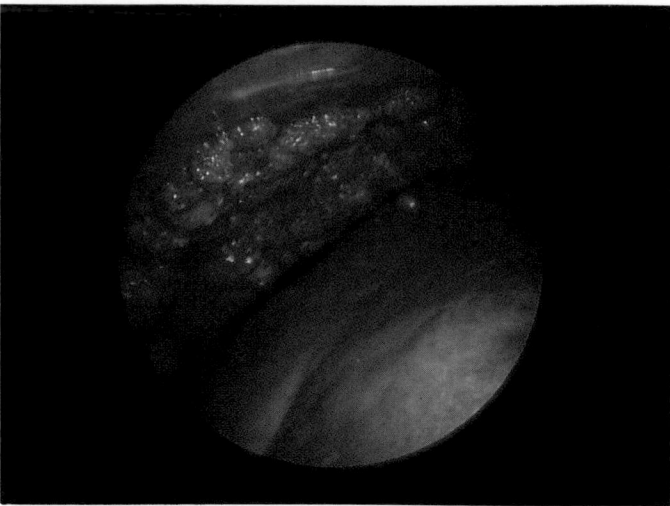

Plate 2. Peritoneal carcinosis. The nodules are irregular, red-greyish, and bigger than tubercula. The picture is strongly suggestive of the diagnosis. Often only an adequate biopsy can distinguish the real nature of the lesion.

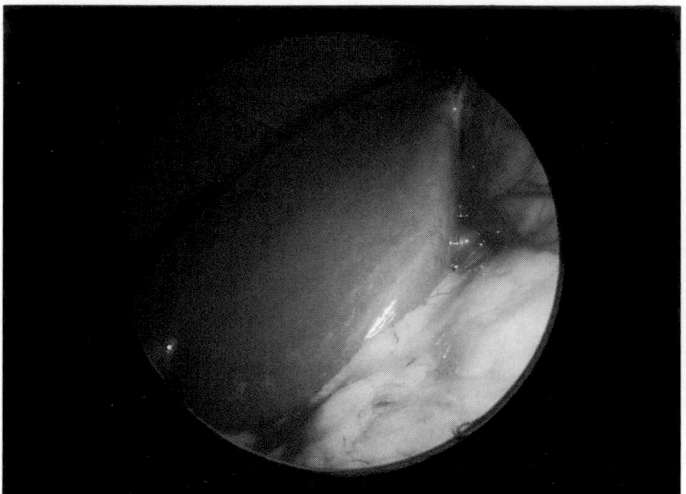

Plate 3. The normal liver (right lobe). The margin is smooth. The surface is regular and lucent with a red-purple colour.

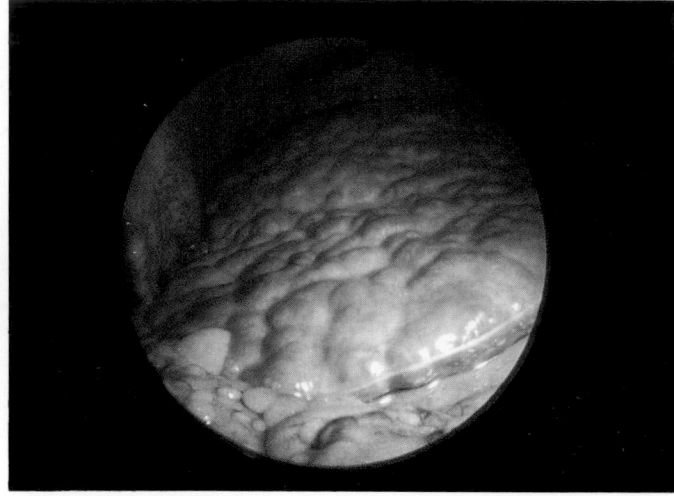

Plate 4. Macronodular cirrhosis (left lobe). The liver is large, with a thick margin, irregular surface, and evident multiple nodules.

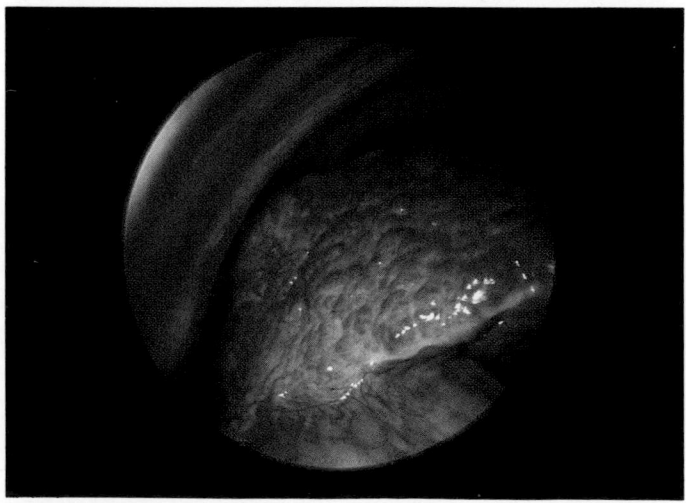

Plate 5. Secondary neoplasm. Typical volcano-like lesion with depressed central zone, surrounded by an hyperaemic halo.

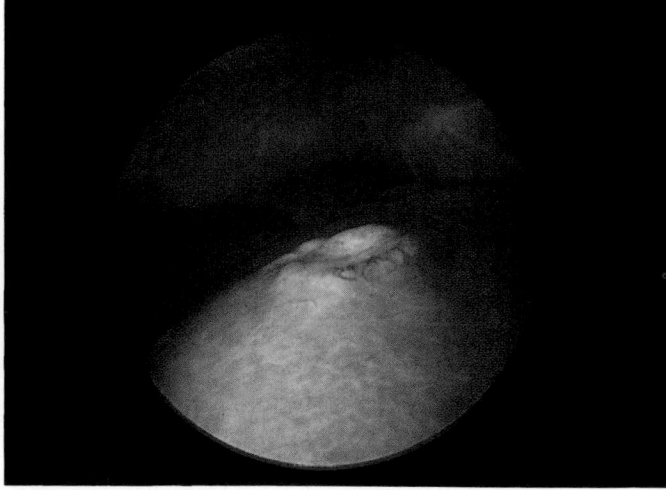

Plate 6. Carcinoma in cirrhosis. The tumour is emerging as a grey-reddish lesion on the convex surface of the right cirrhotic liver lobe.

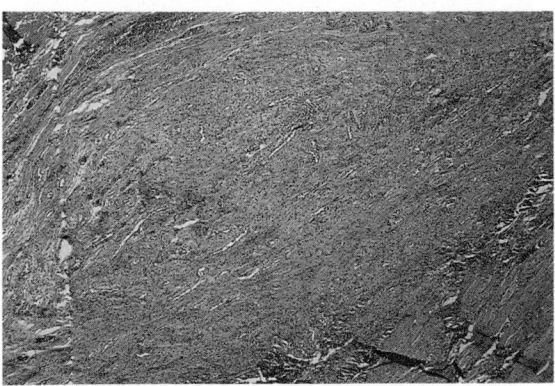

Plate 1. Atresia of extrahepatic bile ducts. Fibrous remnant 'Gautier type 1'. Cross-section through fibrous remnant of common hepatic duct which is completely obliterated and reduced to a fibrous cord (haematoxylin and eosin, × 12).

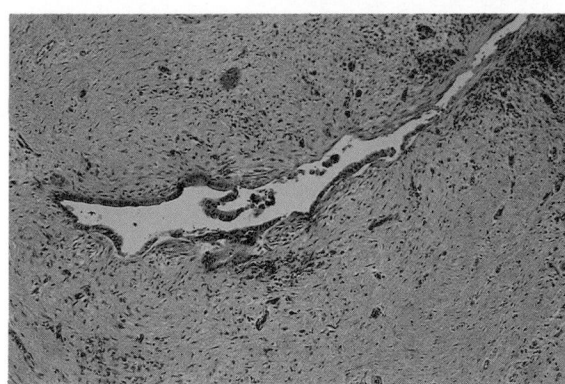

Plate 2. Atresia of extrahepatic bile ducts. Fibrous remnant 'Gautier type 3'. Cross-section through fibrous remnant of hepatic duct. The duct shows partially desquamated and damaged epithelial lining, surrounded by fibrosis and mild inflammatory infiltration (haematoxylin and eosin, × 32).

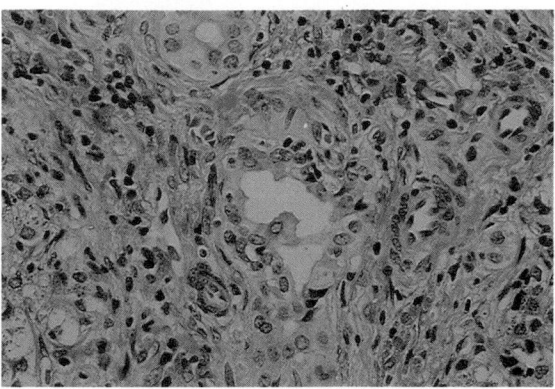

Plate 3. Atresia of extrahepatic bile ducts. Detail from liver biopsy of a baby with EHBDA, showing branches of hepatic artery and interlobular (portal) bile ducts. The duct in the centre shows irregularity and necrobiosis of its lining epithelium. There is mild inflammatory infiltration in the portal connective tissue (haematoxylin and eosin, × 128).

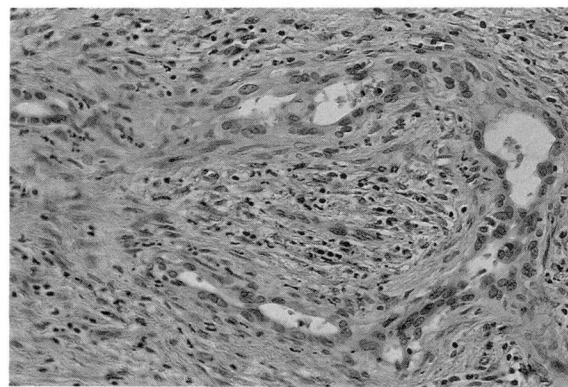

Plate 4. Atresia of extrahepatic bile ducts. Detail from liver biopsy of a 60-day-old baby with EHBDA. The picture shows a portal tract, with obliterating portal vein in the centre, and sprinkling by inflammatory cells. The bile ducts lie in an interrupted circle, corresponding to a partially remodelled ductal plate configuration. The epithelial line of thes ductal plate shows segments of flattening and involution (haematoxylin and eosin, × 80).

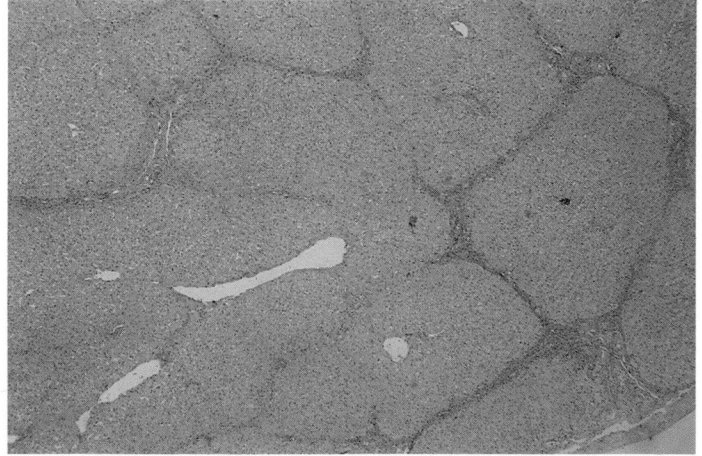

Plate 5. Atresia of extrahepatic bile ducts. Liver biopsy from a patient who is clinically well and jaundice free, 4.5 years after successful hepatic portoenterostomy. The main lesion consists of the development of some periportal fibrosis and portal–portal septa, resembling normal pig's liver (haematoxylin and eosin, × 12).

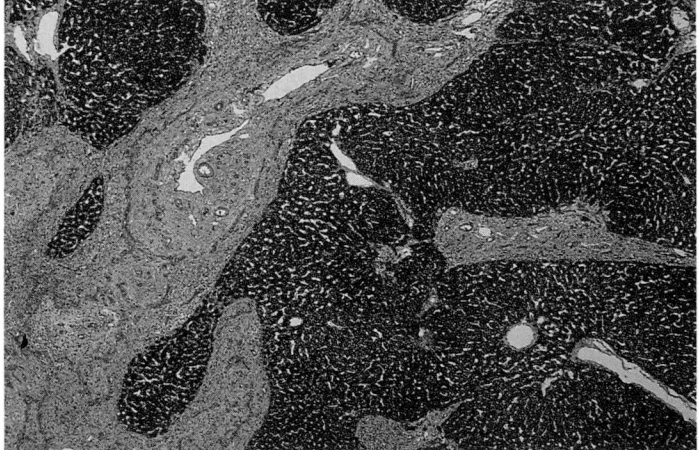

Plate 6. Atresia of extrahepatic bile ducts. Liver biopsy from a patient who is clinically well and jaundice free, 4 years after successful hepatic portoenterostomy. The lesion resembles congenital hepatic fibrosis, with broad porto–portal fibrous connections, but basically preserved lobular architecture. The broad fibrous septa carry excessive numbers of bile-duct structures, many of which appear in circular ductal plate configuration (Masson's trichrome stain (connective tissue in green), × 12).

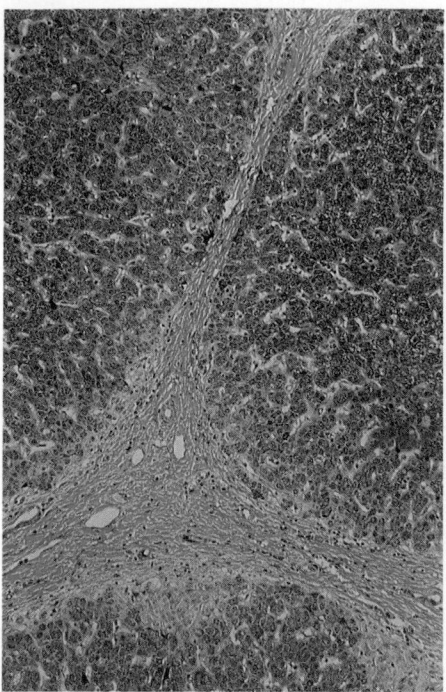

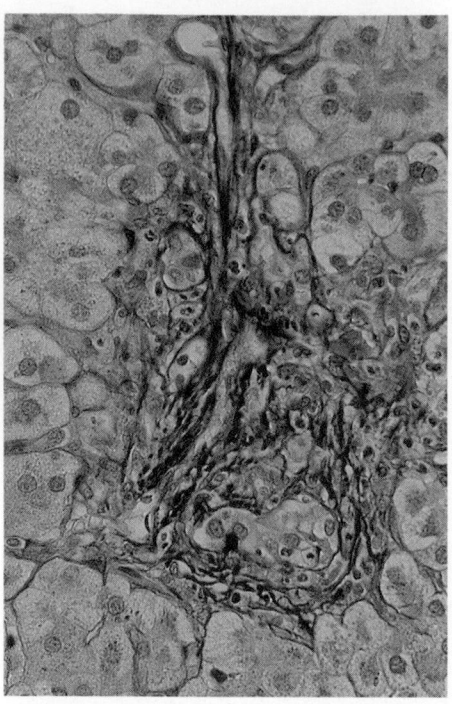

Plate 7. Atresia of extrahepatic bile ducts. Liver biopsy from a patient who is clinically well and jaundice free, 4 years after successful hepatic portoenterostomy. The liver shows advanced biliary fibrosis, with porto-portal fibrous septa. Note absence of portal bile ducts, hypoplastic size of portal veins, and occasional focus of ductular reaction (middle right) (Masson's trichrome stain (connective tissue in green), × 32).

Plate 8. Syndromatic paucity of interlobular bile ducts (Alagille syndrome). Liver biopsy from a 3-month-old baby. Several portal tracts in this biopsy do not contain an interlobular bile duct. The remaining ducts show irregularity and vacuolization of the epithelium and inflammatory infiltration (Sirius red stain (collagen appears in red), × 128).

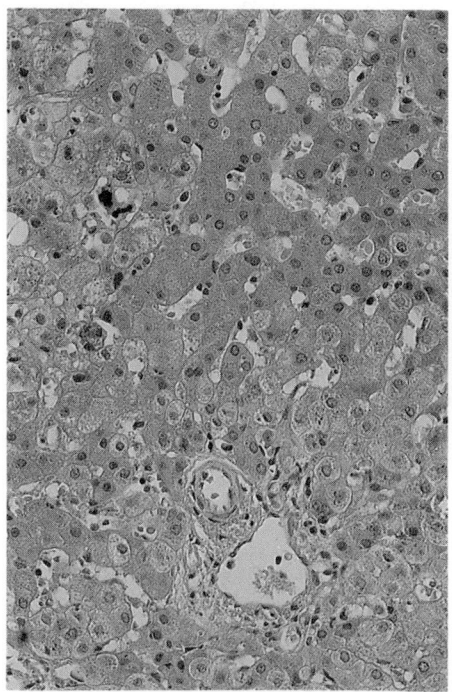

Plate 9. Paucity of interlobular bile ducts. Liver biopsy from a 73-day-old baby. Overview of portal tract (bottom) and parenchyma. The portal tract carries no interlobular bile duct, but is virtually free of inflammatory infiltration and ductular reaction. Bile plugs (bilirubinostasis) appear in the parenchyma (haematoxylin and eosin, × 80).

Plates from Chapter 12.3

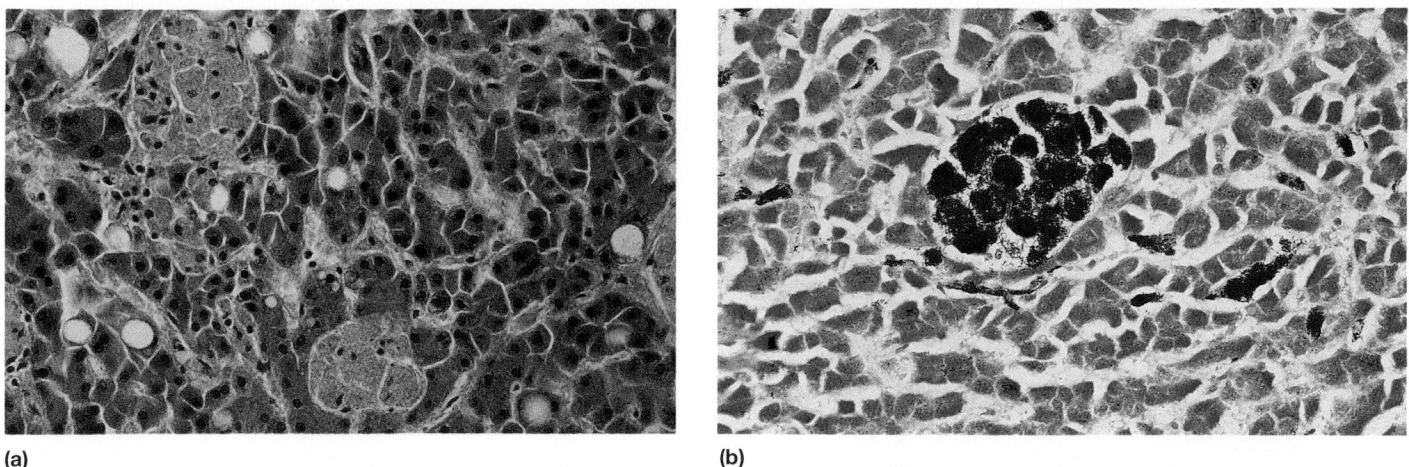

(a) (b)

Plate 1. *Mycobacterium avium-intracellulare* complex infection. (a) Discrete, non-necrotic aggregates of unactivated macrophages in the sinusoids. The haematoxyphilic cytoplasm results from the tightly packed mycobacteria (haematoxylin and eosin). (b) The same specimen stained by the Ziehl–Neilsen method showing large numbers of intracellular acid-fast bacilli. (By courtesy of Professor S. Lucas, UMDS Department of Histopathology, London, UK.)

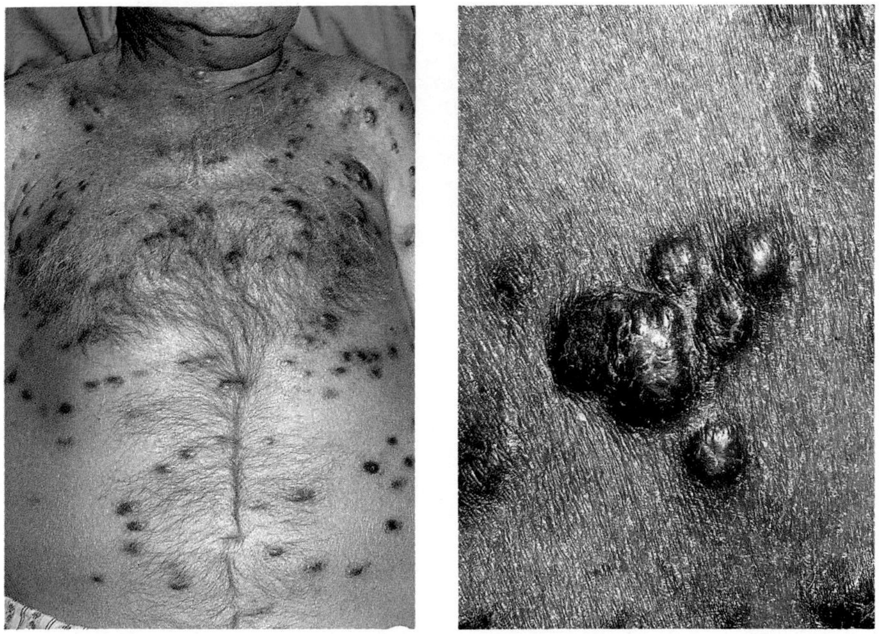

(a) (b)

Plate 2. Cutaneous Kaposi sarcoma in a patient with AIDS (by courtesy of the Photography Department, The Middlesex Hospital, London, UK).

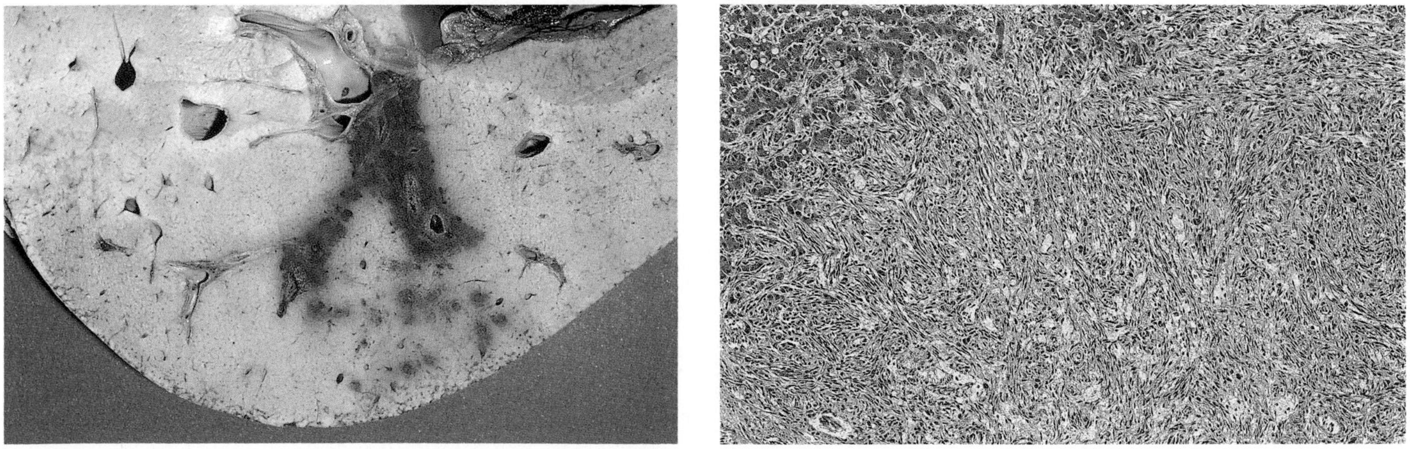

(a) (b)

Plate 3. Kaposi sarcoma in the liver. (a) Purplish lesion infiltrating the portal tracts and spreading into the parenchyma (fixed liver). (b) Interlacing bands of Kaposi spindle cells infiltrating a portal tract and extending into the parenchyma (haematoxylin and eosin) (by courtesy of Professor S. Lucas, UMDS Department of Histopathology, London, UK).

Plates from Chapter 14.1

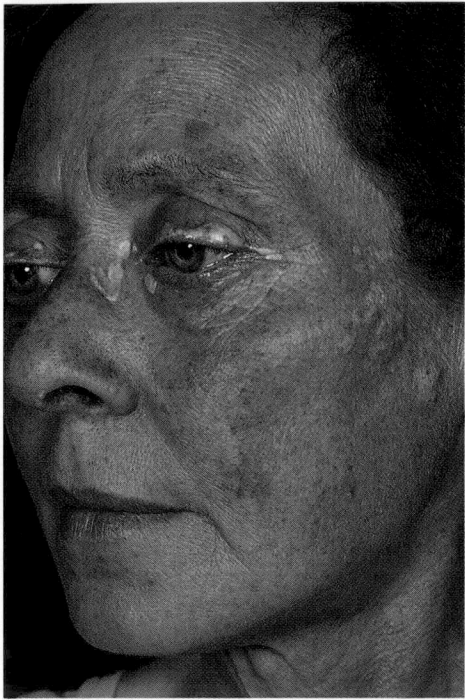

Plate 1. A patient with advanced primary biliary cirrhosis shows pigmentation, jaundice, and xanthelasma.

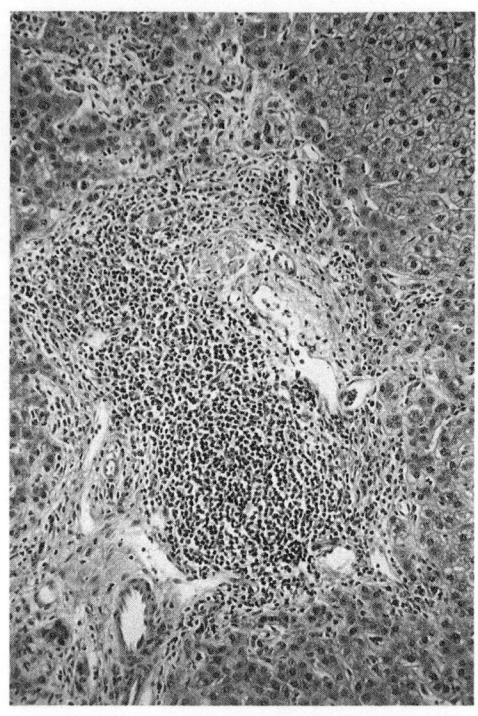

Plate 2. Primary biliary cirrhosis (later stage) shows severe portal inflammation. Portal vein tributaries and hepatic artery branches can be identified but interlobular bile ducts are absent (stained haematoxylin-eosin).

Plates from Chapter 23.6

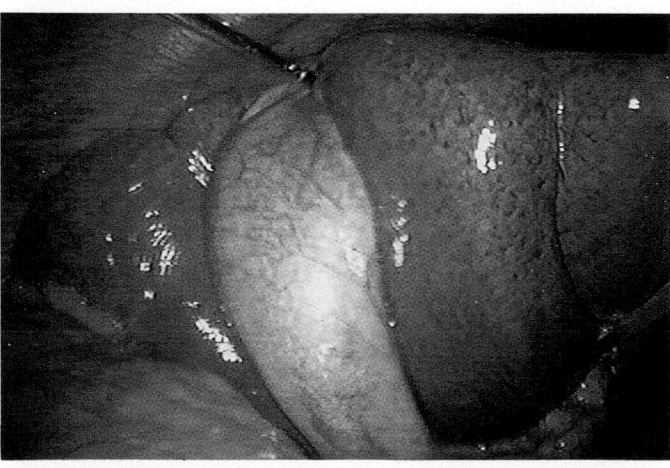

(a)

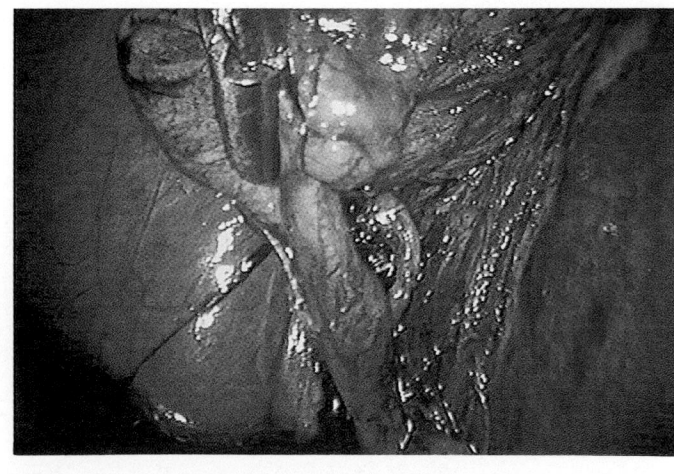

(b)

Plate 1. (a) Appearance of gallbladder and liver at the time of laparoscopy. (b) Cystic duct and artery after dissection during laparoscopic cholecystectomy.

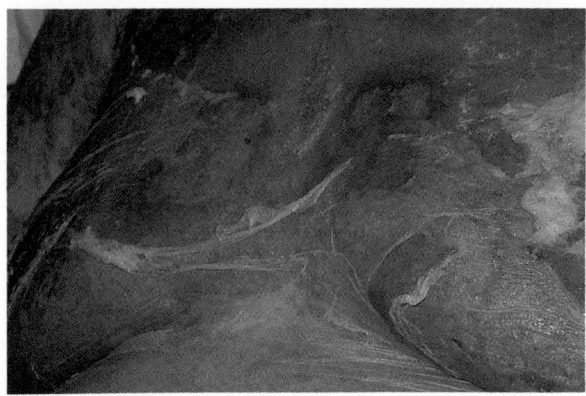

Plate 1. Toxic epidermal necrolysis. There is a background erythema with peeling of the dead epidermis leaving raw denuded dermis.

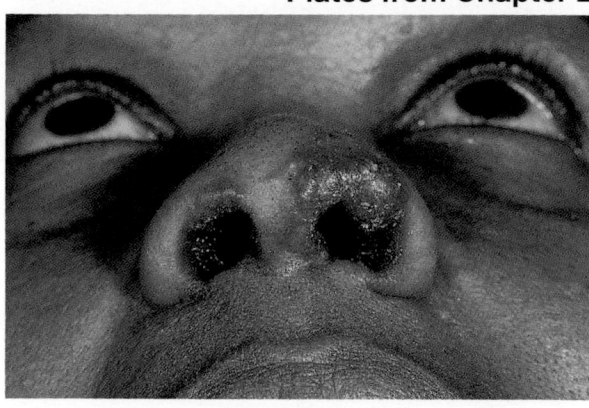

Plate 3. Cutaneous sarcoidosis. Granulomatous papules and nodules on the ala margins and on the columella.

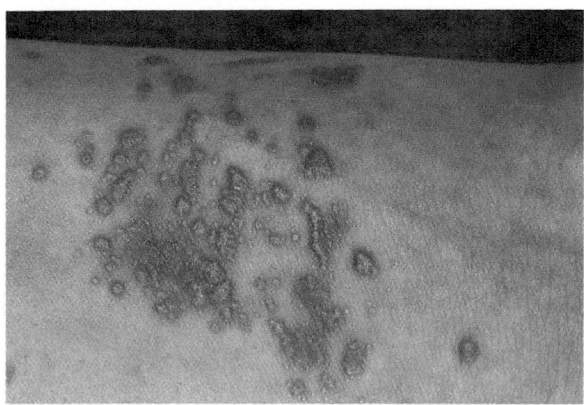

(a)

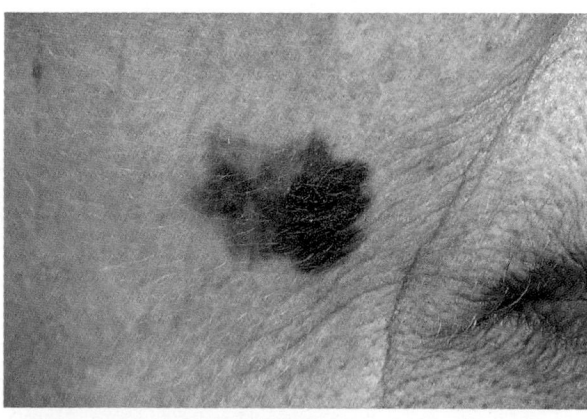

Plate 4. Malignant melanoma. The lesion on the right cheek is variably pigmented and has an irregular outline.

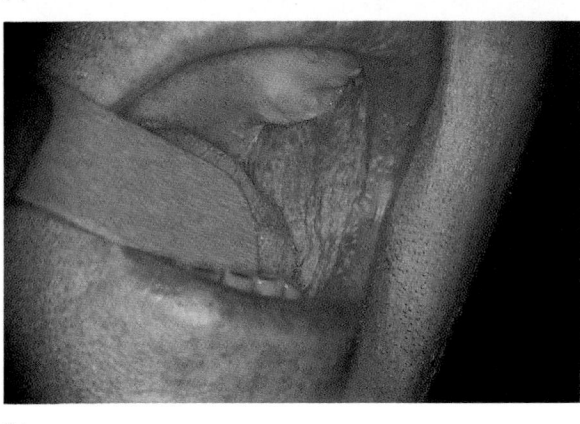

(b)

Plate 2. Lichen planus. Violaceous, polygonal, shiny, flat-topped papules on forearm, some showing evidence of koebnerization (linear lesions occurring at sites of scratching). White lace-like patterning on buccal mucosa, with some areas becoming confluent.

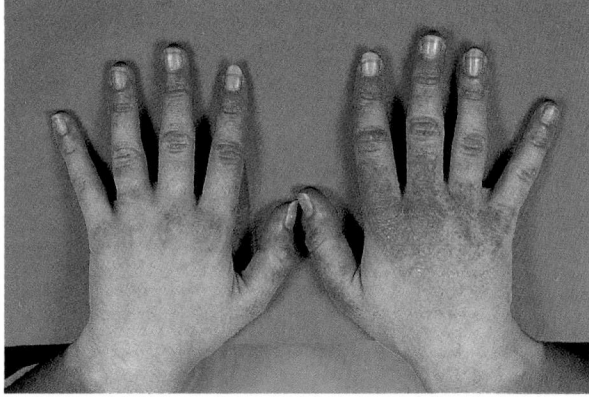

Plate 5. Dermatomyositis. Periungal erythema and papular erythema over the extensor surfaces of the fingers known as Gottron's sign.

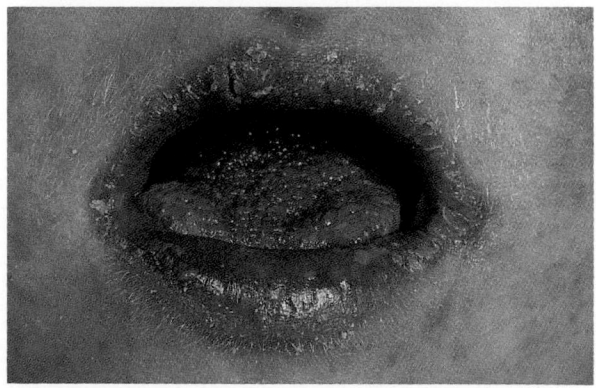

Plate 6. Kawasaki disease. Strawberry red tongue with scaling and fissuring of lips.

Plates from Chapter 25.6

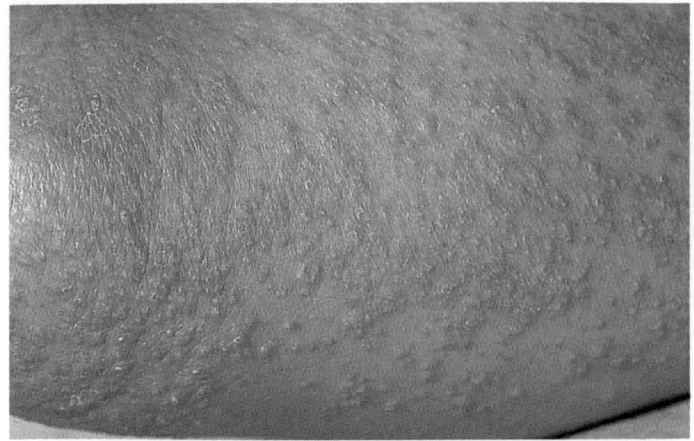

Plate 1. Giannotti–Crosti syndrome. Multiple flesh-coloured monomorphic papules on a thigh.

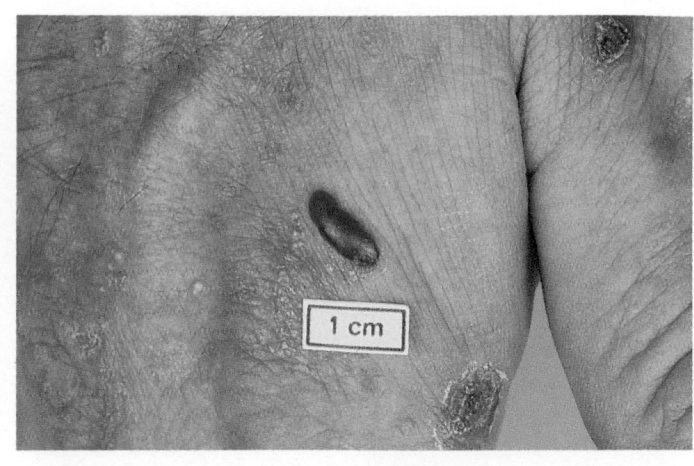

(a)

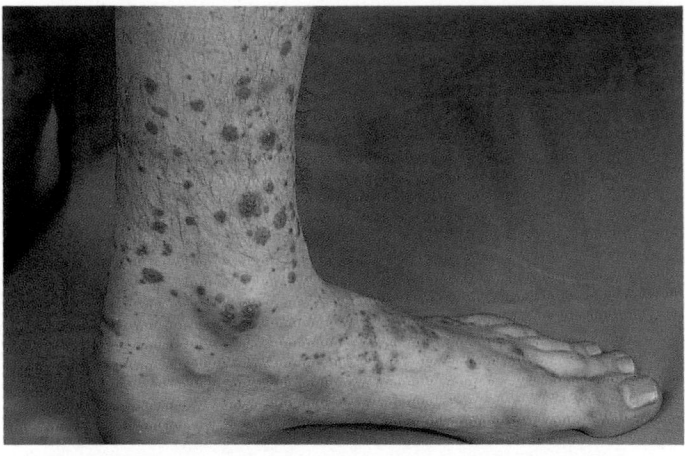

Plate 2. Cryoglobulinaemia. Purpuric areas at peripheral sites corresponding to areas of intravascular thrombosis.

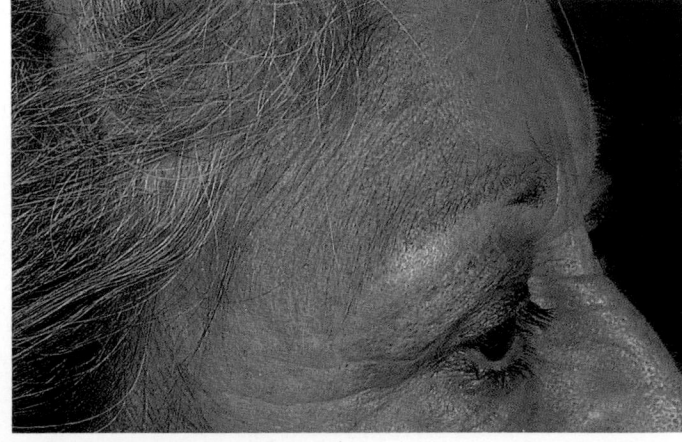

(b)

Plate 4. Porphyria cutanea tarda. Multiple milia (epidermal cysts) and a haemorrhagic blister on the dorsum of the right hand arising after minor trauma. Hypertrichosis of the temple.

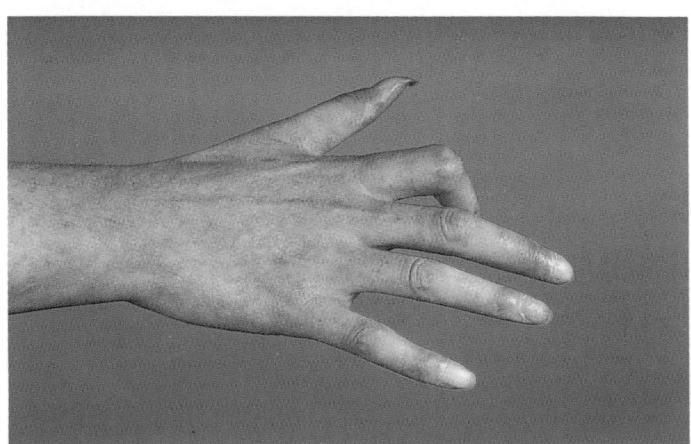

Plate 3. Systemic sclerosis. Sclerodactyly, fixed flexion deformity and loss of finger tip pulp.

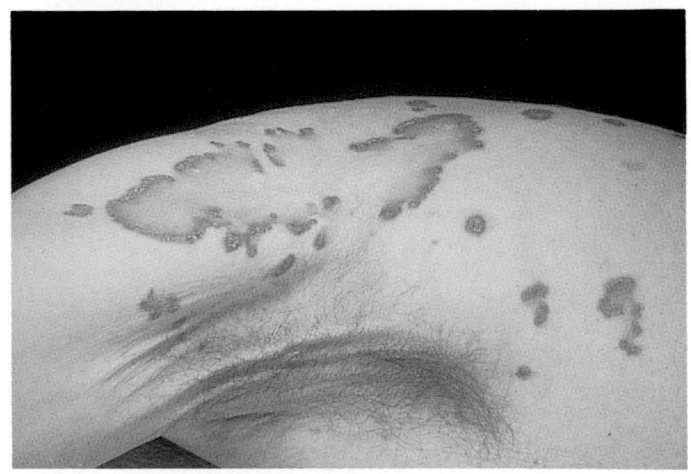

Plate 5. Pseudoxanthoma elasticum-like changes with hanging folds of skin in the axilla and lesions of elastosis perforans serpiginosa on the arm and chest wall characterized by scaly papules arranged in a serpiginous pattern.

Table 5 Independent clinical varibles predictive of survival in primary biliary cirrhosis from several prognostic models

Yale	European	Mayo	Oslo	Glasgow	Australian
Age	Age	Age	Variceal bleed	Age	Age
Bilirubin	Bilirubin	Bilirubin	Bilirubin	Bilirubin	Bilirubin
Hepatomegaly	Albumin	Albumin		Ascites	Albumin
Fibrosis/cirrhosis	Cirrhosis	Prothrombin time		Fibrosis	
	Cholestasis	Oedema		Cholestasis	
				Mallory bodies	

From Wiesner *et al*. (Hepatol, 1992; 16:1290).

symptomatic. In one study, symptoms developed in one-third of asymptomatic patients in 5 years, 10 per cent of whom died (Springer, AmJGastro, 1998; submitted).

A small study of asymptomatic patients, who were AMA positive with normal liver tests, followed for more than 10 years (Metcalf, Lancet, 1996; 348:1399) indicated that 83 per cent subsequently developed biochemical evidence of liver disease and 75 per cent became symptomatic. However, another study of healthy AMA-positive subjects suggested that few had or developed primary biliary cirrhosis (Jorde, ActaMedScand, 1986; 220:241). These authors noted that in subjects in whom the AMA titre was low, the positive result was often transient.

These studies all indicate that the rate of progression of disease is unpredictable. It is possible that some asymptomatic patients will never progress to symptomatic disease. As asymptomatic patients tend to be 2 to 10 years older than their symptomatic counterparts, asymptomatic disease does not necessarily mean presymptomatic disease.

Prognosis (Table 5)

Several prognostic models have been developed which give an indication of the outcome of a particular patient with primary biliary cirrhosis (Weisner, Hepatol, 1992; 16:1290). The only common factor in each prognostic model is serum bilirubin.

The serum bilirubin value is the easiest to use of all the indicators of prognosis (Shapiro, Gut, 1979; 20:137). Values may remain normal for many years, and once elevated may be relatively stable for the first few years of the jaundiced stage. As the liver fails, the serum bilirubin rises precipitously, especially during the last 2 years of life. If they are suitable, such patients should be referred to a transplant centre. Other features that predict decreased survival include hepatosplenomegaly, ascites and oedema, and hypo-albuminaemia (less than 3 g/dl) (Roll, NEJM, 1983; 308:1).

Of all the models that have been devised to predict survival, the Mayo Model (Weisner, Hepatol, 1992; 16:1290), which does not require a liver biopsy but rather utilizes age, serum bilirubin, albumin, prothrombin time, and the presence or absence of oedema, is the most often used. No models can yield a precise estimate of survival in the individual patient. They cannot predict a life-threatening episode such as bleeding oesophageal varices. These models are most useful for therapeutic clinical trials and for predicting the timing for liver transplantation.

Treatment

Several aspects of therapy for primary biliary cirrhosis should be considered: symptomatic, preventative, and therapeutic.

Symptomatic

The most common symptom of primary biliary cirrhosis is fatigue, and this is associated with considerable psychological dysfunction (Cauch-Dudek, Hepatol, 1995; 22:108A; Huet, Gastro, 1996; 110: 1215A). It has not been determined whether fatigue is caused by the associated depression leading to sleep dysfunction or vice versa. Fatigue, not infrequently, accompanies other chronic progressive diseases.

Pruritus is the next most common complaint of patients with primary biliary cirrhosis. The cause of the pruritus is uncertain. In the past it had always been thought that pruritus was related to elevated bile acids, as cholestyramine, which binds bile acid in the gut, often relieves this symptom. However, the bile acid theory did not explain why pruritus tends to diminish with the severe cholestasis associated with endstage disease. An imbalance of intrahepatic bile acids has been proposed (Ghent, AmJGastr, 1987; 82: 117) and this hypothesis has been used to explain the beneficial effect of rifampin therapy for the pruritus of primary biliary cirrhosis. When cholestyramine (up to 12 g daily) fails, rifampin is a second line of therapy, starting at 150 mg twice daily. For the 50 per cent of patients in whom it is effective, the benefit is felt within the first month of treatment. Increasing the dose rarely helps further. As this drug is an enzyme inducer, care must be taken with regard to potential drug interactions. Pruritus is often worse in the winter, which may explain the observed seasonal variation in presentation (Hamlyn, Gut, 1983; 24:940). Although dry skin, which is not unusual in the cold weather, may accentuate itching, it is also likely that the diminished amount of ultraviolet light leads to the worsening of this symptom. Treatment with short bursts of ultraviolet light (without sunblock) may be beneficial. Pruritus may be precipitated by pregnancy. Exogenous hormone therapy such as use of the oral contraceptive pill or hormone replacement therapy may provoke pruritus. Not surprisingly, men with primary biliary cirrhosis complain less commonly of pruritus than women (Lucey, Gut, 1986; 27:1373).

The specific cause for pruritus remains unknown. Some have suggested that circulating endogenous opioids, which are elevated in primary biliary cirrhosis (Thornton, BMJ, 1988; 297:1501), may have a central effect that leads to the sensation of pruritus (Bergasa,

AnnIntMed, 1995; 123:161). Indeed, the opioid antagonists naloxone and nalmafene have been used successfully to treat the pruritus of cholestasis, some patients develop 'withdrawal' symptoms typical of narcotic withdrawal.

Multiple xanthomas may cause a painful neuropathy which can be treated with plasmapheresis (Turnberg, Gut, 1972; 13:976). The dry eyes of the sicca syndrome may be relieved by artificial tears. The dry mouth is reduced by stimulants of salivary flow such as lemon juice or sour candy. Regular dental care should be emphasized and patients advised to take all medications in the upright position with plenty of fluid to avoid the development of drug-induced oesophageal ulcers.

Raynaud's syndrome is treated along conventional lines by avoiding immersion in cold water and the wearing of gloves. Although calcium channel blockers may help the Raynaud's syndrome, they may make scleroderma of the oesophagus symptomatic by promoting reflux. Neuropathy and bone pain (from fractures or the more rare condition of periostitis) may be treated by analgesics, but non-steroidal anti-inflammatory drugs and aspirin should be avoided, as oesophageal varices are common in primary biliary cirrhosis.

Prevention

In the jaundiced patient, the associated steatorrhoea due to intestinal bile salt deficiency leads to malabsorption of vitamins A, D, and K and these should be supplied parenterally or in the water-soluble oral form if available.

Jaundiced patients with primary biliary cirrhosis may develop osteomalacia but, more importantly, all patients with primary biliary cirrhosis are at risk for osteoporosis. Osteoporosis is difficult to treat, but calcium supplements and vitamin D derivatives are usually given and the patients should exercise. Exposure to sunlight is encouraged. Hormone replacement therapy for postmenopausal patients using transdermal therapy is unlikely to worsen cholestasis and probably prevents at least the postmenopausal component of osteoporosis (Crippin, AmJGastr, 1994; 89:47). There is insufficient data on the value of biphosphonates for the treatment of osteoporosis associated with primary biliary cirrhosis; those that are associated with the development of oesophageal ulcers are best avoided in patients with primary biliary cirrhosis with portal hypertension.

If the patient has endoscopically proven large oesophageal varices with danger signs (North Italian Endoscopic Club, NEJM, 1988; 319:983), or has bled from them, non-selective β-blockers such as propranolol or nadolol should be considered. These reduce the chances of bleeding (Poynard, NEJM, 1991; 324:1532).

Medical treatment (Table 6)

At present, no curative medical treatment can be recommended for primary biliary cirrhosis. Most reported trials have usually been too short, too small, and poorly controlled. Statistically significant long-term benefits are difficult to establish in a disease with such a long and varied natural history. However, evaluation of currently available measures should continue in the context of large controlled trials. Three groups of drugs have been used. The immunomodulators would be expected to be effective in the early stages of the disease, whereas the antifibrotics and anticholestatics

should be helpful by preventing the progression to cirrhosis and liver failure.

Azathioprine (Imuran) was of marginal benefit in improving survival (Christensen, Gastro, 1985; 89:1084) and occasionally may have serious side-effects. Corticosteroids improve well being, and may relieve pruritus. Serum alkaline phosphatase, aminotransferases, and procollagen III fall. Liver histology improves. However, the development of progressive bone thinning is always a particular concern for patients with primary biliary cirrhosis (Mitchison, JHepatol, 1992; 15:336)

Cyclosporin A reduces pruritus and fatigue, serum bilirubin and alkaline phosphatase fall, and hepatic histology improves (Lombard, Gastro, 1993; 104:519). There is no effect on survival. The beneficial effects are achieved at the expense of complications, particularly impaired renal function and systemic hypertension. The use of cyclosporin in primary biliary cirrhosis has been abandoned because of the risks of administering a toxic drug over many years.

For the same reasons, chlorambucil, shown in one small study to have a beneficial effect on liver chemistry in primary biliary cirrhosis, is not advocated—25 per cent of patients in this study needed to be withdrawn because of side-effects (Hoofnagle, Gastro, 1986; 91:1327).

Methotrexate, given by mouth in a dose of 15 mg per week, was found to result in improvement in pruritus and fatigue, and a fall in serum levels of alkaline phosphatase and bilirubin (Kaplan, Gastro, 1991; 101:1332). Liver biopsies showed a reduction in portal inflammation. The Mayo prognostic score was unchanged. No randomized, controlled studies on the use of methotrexate have been published to date. Side-effects include a downward trend in white cell count and platelets, indicating bone marrow toxicity. Interstitial pneumonitis develops in 12 to 15 per cent of patients, but responds to cessation of the drug and the giving of corticosteroids. There is no evidence that methotrexate improves survival. In a recent trial, one group of patients was given ursodeoxycholic acid plus methotrexate and compared with another who received ursodeoxycholic acid alone. There was no added benefit from the combination (Lindor, Hepatol, 1995; 22:1158).

Colchicine is an inexpensive, antifibrotic drug with few side-effects. Controlled trials showed that biochemical results and symptoms improved, but histological progression was not affected and long-term benefit was not shown (Zifroni, Hepatol, 1991; 14:990). Combination therapy (colchicine plus ursodeoxycholic acid) does not appear to enhance the effect (Poupon, Hepatol, 1996; 24:1098). D-Penicillamine, another antifibrotic, was also shown to be of no value in treating patients with primary biliary cirrhosis (Dickson, NEJM, 1985; 312:1011).

Ursodeoxycholic acid acts as a non-toxic, hydrophilic, choleretic bile acid, which may decrease the toxicity of retained bile acids in patients with cholestasis. It may stabilize hepatocyte membranes and it does increase bile acid transport across the liver cell and canaliculus (Jazrawi, Gastro, 1994; 106:134). In primary biliary cirrhosis, ursodeoxycholic acid modifies the bile acid pool so that it becomes the predominant bile acid. There have been many trials of therapy involving the use of ursodeoxycholic acid (Table 6). In a placebo-controlled trial lasting 2 years, followed by another 2 years of open-label therapy, ursodeoxycholic acid reduced the progression

Table 6 Randomized, controlled trials of therapy in primary biliary cirrhosis		
Therapy	**Reference**	**No. of patients in study**
Azathioprine	Heathcote, Gastro 1976; 70:656	45
	Christensen, Gastro 1985; 89:1084	248
Prednisone	Mitchison, J Hepatol 1992; 15:336	36
Cyclosporin	Minuk, Gastro 1988; 95:1356	12
	Wiesner, NEJM 1990; 332:1419	29
	Lombard, Gastro 1993; 104:519	349
Chlorambucil	Hoofnagle, Gastro 1986; 91:1327	24
Colchicine	Kaplan, NEJM 1986; 315:1448	60
	Warnes, Hepatol 1987; 5:1	64:
	Bodenheimer, Gastro 1988; 95:124	57
	Kershenobich, NEJM 1988; 18:1709	100
D-Penicillamine	Epstein, Lancet 1981; i:1275	87
	Matloff, NEJM 1982; 306:319	52
	Taal, Liver 1983; 3:345	24
	Dickson, NEJM 1985; 312:1011	227
	Neuberger, Gut 1985; 26:114	189
Ursodeoxycholic acid	Leuschner, Gastro 1989; 97:1268	20
	Oka, Gastro Jpn 1990; 25:774	45
	Poupon, NEJM 1991; 324:1548	146
	Battezzati, J Hepatol 1993; 17:332	88
	Lindor, Gastro 1994; 106:1284	180
	Heathcote, Hepatol 1994; 19:1149	222
	Turner, J Gastrohepatol 1974; 9:162	46
	Combes, Hepatol 1995; 22:759	151

of disease and the probability of death or the need for liver transplantation (Poupon, NEJM, 1994; 330:1342). Another trial confirmed the reduction in serum bilirubin levels, but treatment showed little effect on symptoms, liver histology, or survival (Heathcote, Hepatol, 1994; 10:1149). Results in yet another large trial showed a fall in serum bilirubin in the treated group, but there was no change in hepatic histology (Lindor, Gastro, 1994; 106:1284). The combined analysis of these three placebo-controlled trials has confirmed that ursodeoxycholic acid prolongs life and increases the time to transplantation (Heathcote, Gastro, 1995; 106:1082A). Ursodeoxycholic acid is not a panacea for the treatment of patients with primary biliary cirrhosis and one study suggested it was ineffective in patients with a serum bilirubin level of greater than 34 mmol/l (Combes, Hepatol, 1995; 22:759). It should probably be given to all patients unless they have reached the end stages and are approaching the time for transplantation. A decision to treat the early, asymptomatic patient with ursodeoxycholic acid is a difficult one and a decision must be made in each individual patient, bearing in mind the cost.

For successful treatment of primary biliary cirrhosis it is likely that therapy would be best started early, at the stage of acute bile-duct inflammation. Unfortunately, apart from screening for AMA, there is no specific marker for this disease, which may have been present for years before the diagnosis is made and currently there is no known curative medical therapy.

Liver transplantation (Chapter 30.5)

Primary biliary cirrhosis is a common indication for liver transplantation in adults. The end stages of this disease are relatively easy to recognize but, preferably, transplantation should be considered at the first indication that the hepatocytes are failing. These signs include ascites, oedema, or hepatic encephalopathy.

A serum bilirubin level between 100 and 150 mmol/l should prompt transplant referral. Although treatment with ursodeoxycholic acid causes a fall in all the serum markers of cholestasis, both the Mayo score and the serum bilirubin values remain reliable prognostic markers on treatment (Kilmurry, Hepatology, 1995; 23: 1148). Preferably, the possibility of the need for a transplant in the future should already have been discussed with the patient. Results are better in younger patients, but advanced age is not a contraindication as long as there are no serious comorbid conditions. If the transplant is delayed, so that the serum bilirubin exceeds 340 mmol/l, the prothrombin time is greater than 15 s, the creatinine exceeds 1.3 mg, and the liver is shrunken (less that 2.5 per cent body weight), survival is poor (Neuberger, Gut, 1991; 31: 1069). The 1-year survival after hepatic transplantation in patients with primary biliary cirrhosis exceeds 70 per cent, and over 80 per cent of survivors achieve full activity both vocationally and socially (Markus, NEJM, 1989; 320:709).

The transplant operation is relatively easy, particularly if there has been no previous upper abdominal surgery. The most common technical complication is fragmentation and intramural dissection of the recipient hepatic artery. This necessitates an arterial graft in 20 per cent of patients. A retransplant is required in 20 per cent or patients, usually for a non-functioning graft or hepatic artery thrombosis.

Postoperatively, the encephalopathy is cured and oesophageal varices slowly disappear. Unfortunately, despite calcium and vitamin D therapy, there is an initial worsening of the osteoporosis. This can be related to recumbency and corticosteroid and other immunosuppressive therapy. Improvement in bone density follows with prolonged survival (Eastell, Hepatol, 1991; 14:296).

It may be difficult histologically to distinguish recurrence of primary biliary cirrhosis from chronic graft rejection (Demetris, Hepatol, 1988; 88:939). Both conditions show a suppurative cholangitis with bile duct paucity. However, chronic rejection is not associated with development of pruritus.

Conclusions

There has been no significant breakthrough in the treatment of primary biliary cirrhosis and it remains a condition incurable by medicines. Ursodeoxycholic acid, as an anticholestatic agent, looks promising, but this can only be expected to delay the development of hepatocyte failure. Its early use in combination with an immunomodulating agent might give rise to more satisfactory results. Hepatic transplantation is giving excellent results in the well-chosen patient treated in a centre with a proven good record of transplant.

References

1. Sherlock S and Scheuer P. The presentation and diagnosis of 100 patients with primary biliary cirrhosis. *New England Journal of Medicine*, 1973; **289**: 674–78.

2. Kaplan MM. Primary biliary cirrhosis. *New England Journal of Medicine*, 1996; **335**: 1570–80.

3. Long RG, Scheuer PJ, and Sherlock S. Presentation and course of asymptomatic primary biliary cirrhosis. *Gastroenterology*, 1977; **72**: 1204–7.

4. Mistry P and Seymour CA. Primary biliary cirrhosis from—Thomas Addison to the 1990's. *Quarterly Journal of Medicine*, 1992; **82**: 185–96.

5. Mahl TC, Slockcar W, and Boyer JL. Primary biliary cirrhosis: survival of a large cohort of symptomatic patients followed for 24 years. *Journal of Hepatology*, 1994; **20**: 707–13.

6. Mitchison HC, *et al*. Positive antimitochondrial antibody but normal alkaline phosphatase: is this primary biliary cirrhosis? *Hepatology*, 1986; **6**: 1279–84.

Hepatic granulomas

D. Geraint James and Peter J. Scheuer

Granulomas are focal accumulations of macrophages that have undergone transformation to predominantly secretory cells in response to antigenic stimulation. They represent an example of delayed-type hypersensitivity. The transformation of macrophages and the subsequent maintenance of the granuloma are regulated by T_{H1} lymphocytes and a number of cytokines, as described below.

The term 'granuloma' is often used for lesions that do not strictly conform to the above definition, such as foreign-body reactions and accumulations of macrophages in response to ingested or injected mineral oil. 'Microgranuloma' is used to describe a focal accumulation of cells of the macrophage series, smaller than most granulomas; some of these are true granulomas whilst others are simple phagocytic reactions. Use of the term 'microgranuloma' is discouraged for this reason.[1] Terms such as 'epithelioid-cell granuloma' and 'sarcoid granuloma' are sometimes used for lesions conforming to the definition of a granuloma, in order to overcome this confusion.

Granulomas are composed of epithelioid cells, lymphocytes, and a variable mixture of other leucocytes, fibrin, fat, and extracellular matrix components. The cause of the lesion, for example mycobacteria, may also be present. The epithelioid cells, so-called because of a supposed resemblance to epithelium, may form multinucleated giant cells.

Pathologists often report the finding of granulomas in liver biopsies. Sometimes they are expected, providing confirmation of a suspected granulomatous disease such as tuberculosis or sarcoidosis. At other times the finding of a granuloma is unexpected, and may be of great diagnostic help if, as a result, a search for one of the many known causes of hepatic granulomas unearths relevant new information or leads to new interpretation of existing data. However, granulomas often remain unexplained.

Pathogenesis
Macrophage—T_{H1} granulomatous response

Delayed-type hypersensitivity and the acute granulomatous response are mediated by T_{H1} clones, which synthesize and secrete interleukins 1 and 2 (**IL-1, -2**), tumour necrosis factor, and interferon-γ. The stimulating antigens, including mycobacteria, bacteria, and viruses, seem to determine this T_{H1}-response profile, and, coupled with MHC class II macrophages and their cytokines, the progression to granuloma formation (Fig. 1). The T_{H2}-response profile is quite different; it is associated with mast cell and eosinophil growth and differentiation, as well as IgE formation by B cells,

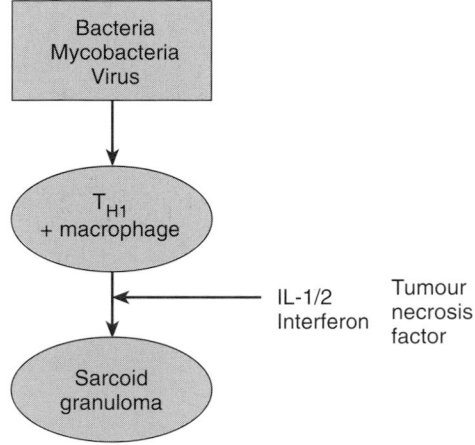

Fig. 1. The CD4-T_{H1}-type profile.

progressing to atopic allergic inflammation (Fig. 2). The T_{H2} cells secrete IL-4, -5, -10 and -13, leukotriene D_4, and platelet activating factor.

In a recent Japanese study (Kawakami, Sarcoid, 1995; 12:111), T-cell lines were established from bronchoalveolar fluid and from a sarcoid lymph node from patients with active sarcoidosis. The cells were subjected to flow cytometry, which revealed that they were T cells, and then to a proliferation assay and immunofluorescence with several monoclonal antibodies. It was shown that the cells from bronchoalveolar fluid and a sarcoid lymph node were T_{H1}-like cell lines. Moreover, cytokine assays revealed that they produced T_{H1} cytokines, namely IL-1 and -2 and interferon-γ.

Granuloma formation

This framework of a macrophage MHC class II-CD4 T_{H1}-type cell synergy with its appropriate cytokine cascade provides only a temporary springboard (Fig. 3). Adhesion molecules, matrix receptors of the integrin family, and numerous cytokines continue to remodel this framework or make it obsolete. Apart from fresh technology, it is also important to assess the following factors which influence granuloma formation.

Sarcoid diathesis

Sarcoidosis predominates in those between 20 and 50 years old and is much less frequent in children and in the elderly. It is most frequent in the black population of the United States and the West

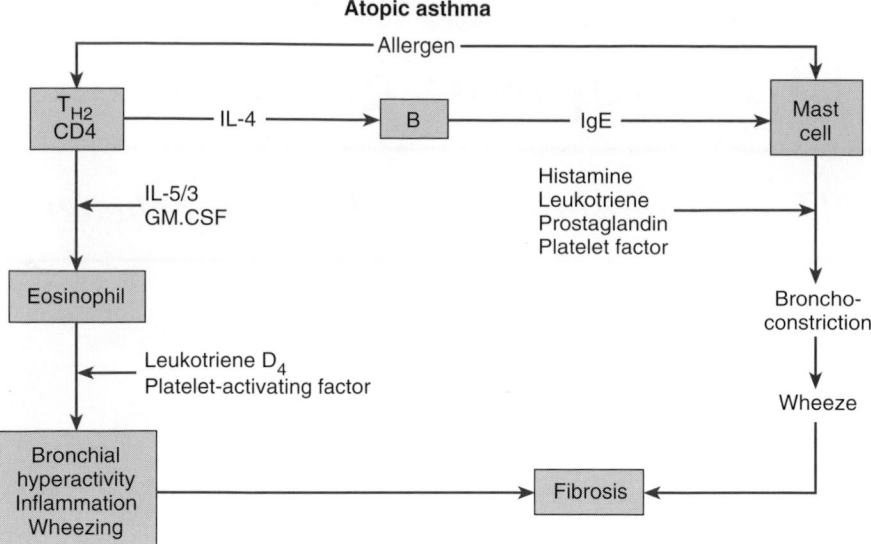

Fig. 2. The T$_{H2}$ pathway to atopic asthma.

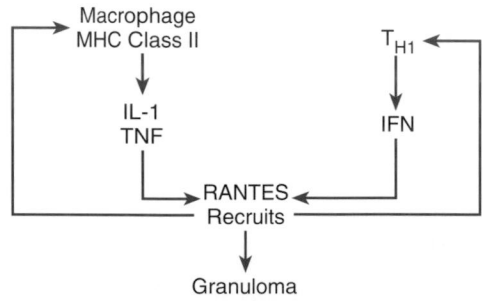

Fig. 3. Granuloma formation.

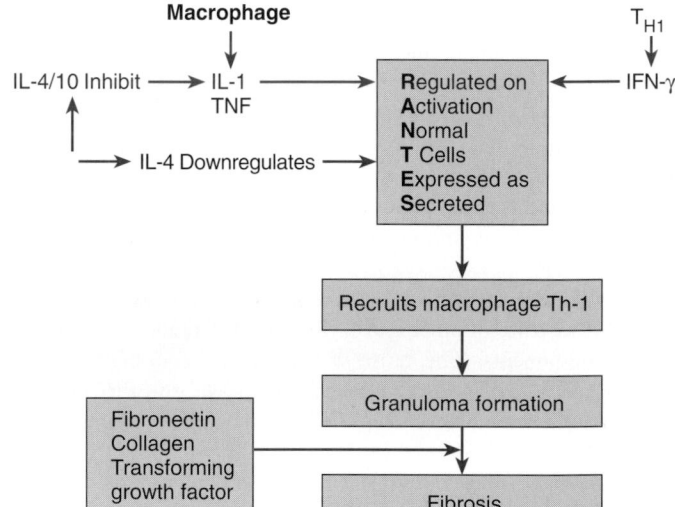

Fig. 4. The granulomatous road to fibrosis.

Indies. Erythema nodosum and hilar lymphadenopathy (Lofgren's syndrome) is commonly recognized in women aged about 25 years, and they may be pregnant or lactating. Sarcoidosis is also commonly associated with HLA B8/A1/Cw7/Dr3, with B13 in the Japanese, and with A9/B5 in Turkey. These features suggest a sarcoid diathesis or terrain, a soil which allows granulomas to proliferate until they reach clinical recognition.

Sarcoid fibrosis

Why do some patients develop severe irreversible fibrosis whereas other heal without discernible or incapacitating fibrosis? Do liver granulomas heal more inconspicuously than pulmonary granulomas? Ocular granulomas used to heal with calamitous adverse effects, including glaucoma due to involvement of the canal of Schlemm, cataracts, and blindness. Since the introduction of steroid therapy, these ocular mishaps have become rare.

The granulomatous road to fibrosis

RANTES (**R**egulated on **a**ctivation **n**ormal **T** cells **e**xpressed as secreted) is a chemokine initially recognized on the basis of its *in vitro* chemotactic properties for human CD4 memory T lymphocytes and monocytes (Schall, Nature, 1990; 347:669), but with no significant

chemoattraction for CD4+ naive T lymphocytes, CD8 T lymphocytes, B lymphocytes, or neutrophils (Fig. 3). Macrophages and T$_{H1}$-type cells contribute to the production of RANTES in the delayed-type hypersensitivity response and in sarcoid and tuberculous granulomas. In view of its chemotactic properties, RANTES may play a role in the selective accumulation of these macrophages and T$_{H1}$ lymphocytes. The T$_{H1}$ cell contributes via interferon-γ and the macrophage via IL-1 and -2 and tumour necrosis factor. Macrophages are producers as well as targets of RANTES, suggesting that their recruitment into granuloma formation is self-perpetuating and due to a cytokine cascade involving IL-1, tumour necrosis factor, and interferon-γ (Figs 3 and 4). The French group (Devergne, JExpMed, 1994; 179:1689), who promote this theory so convincingly, also provide clues to the downregulation of the process. Opposing T$_{H2}$ cells produce IL-4 and -10 which inhibit IL-1, and IL-4 also downregulates RANTES production.

Immunohistochemistry has revealed a continuing role for fibronectin, collagen, integrin receptors, and transforming growth factors in that slippery road from a healthy granulomatous response to irreversible and unchangeable fibrosis. Roman (AmJMedSci, 1995; 309:124) used the technique and provided elegant results in lungs of patients with pulmonary sarcoidosis and animals with experimental granulomatosis. Type 1 collagen was found in a circumferential pattern around sarcoid granulomas, sometimes extending between cells towards the centre. Fibronectin occurred in both the periphery and centre of granulomas. Procollagen type 1 was mainly central. Transforming growth factor is a polypeptide which is expressed in abundance and seems to promote fibrosis while diminishing inflammation. It is not known what controls the see-saw effect of inflammation and fibrosis, but recognition of its role will be salvation in this road to irreversible fibrosis.

Causes

Hepatic granulomas are most often due to infections, but causes also includes drugs and other chemicals, immunological upset, enzyme defects, and neoplasia (Table 1).

Infections

Mycobacterial and fungal infections, schistosomiasis, toxocariasis, and toxoplasmosis are singled out from the large list of infections and infestations (Table 1) because they constitute a large global problem.

Tuberculosis (Fig. 5) is a frequent worldwide cause of hepatic granulomas, and its incidence is more conspicuous as a running mate with AIDS. Acid-fast bacilli are only demonstrated in hepatic granulomas in one-tenth of immunocompetent patients. Tuberculosis should always be suspected in Asian patients, particularly if there is fever, sweating, respiratory symptoms, splenomegaly, and/or a strongly positive tuberculin skin test (Table 2). BCG vaccination, used as a prophylactic measure to prevent tuberculosis, may itself give rise to granulomas.

Schistosomiasis (due to *S. mansoni* and *S. japonicum*, and less commonly to other species) is an important cause of hepatic granulomas (see Chapter 13.4.1). It should not be overlooked in patients who have lived in endemic areas. Ova may be seen in the centre of the granuloma (Fig. 6), and may also be found by rectal biopsy. Eosinophils may be a pointer to parasitic granulomas of the T_{H2} type (Fig. 2). Histoplasmosis, blastomycosis, and coccidiomycosis may be the cause of granulomas in patients coming from areas in which these diseases are endemic.

Q fever

The hepatic granuloma in Q fever contains fibrin, producing a halo effect surrounding a central area of fat, necrosis, or inflammatory cells (Fig. 7). Similar fibrin-ring granulomas have now been described in many different conditions (Table 3) (Ponz, Gastro, 1991; 100:268; Ruel, DigDisSci, 1992; 37:1915; De Bayser, Gastro, 1993; 105:272; Yamamoto, Liver, 1995; 15:276), and cannot therefore be regarded as specific for Q fever (Marazuela, HumPath, 1991; 22: 607; Murphy, Histopath, 1991; 19:91). However, their presence in a patient with fever of unknown cause should lead to appropriate investigation for this infection.

Table 1 Causes of hepatic granulomas
Infections
Mycobacteria
Tuberculosis
Leprosy
M. Avium intracellulare
Bacteria
BCG
Brucella
Francissella tularense
Yersinia
Proprioni
Pseudomonas pseudomallei (Melioidosis)
Staphylococcus epidermidis
Whipple's disease
Spirochaetes
Treponema pallidum
Borrelia burgdorferi (Lyme disease)
Fungi
Blastomyces
Cococcidioides
Histoplasma
Cryptococcus
Protozoa
Leishmania
Toxoplasma
Metazoa
Schistosoma
Toxocara
Rickettsia
Q fever
Boutonneuse fever
Viruses
Hepatitis C
Cytomegalovirus
Epstein–Barr
Chemicals and drugs
Beryllium
Copper
Drugs (see Table 9)
Immunological upset
Sarcoidosis
Crohn's disease
Ulcerative colitis
Primary biliary cirrhosis
Hypogammaglobulinaemia
Systemic lupus erythematosus
Immune complexes
Hepatic granulomatous disease (granulomatous hepatitis)
Polymyalgia rheumatica
AIDS
Enzyme defect
Chronic granulomatous disease of children
Neoplasia
Lymphoma
Carcinoma
Miscellaneous
Talc
Cholestasis

Hepatitis C

Although not reported in several biopsy series, epithelioid-cell granulomas have been described in the livers of a minority of patients with hepatitis C (Emile, HumPath, 1993; 24:1095; Okuno, JGastroHepatol, 1995; 10:532). Their cause is uncertain, but intravenous drug abuse with consequent injection of talc should be considered in patients with hepatitis C and unexplained granulomas.

Table 2 Features distinguishing tuberculosis from sarcoidosis

Features	Tuberculosis	Sarcoidosis
Ethnic groups	Pakistani/Indian/Bangladeshi	West Indian/Irish
Age incidence (years)	Over 50	20–50
Fever	Common	Rare
Erythema nodosum	Uncommon	Common
Uveitis		
Skin involvement	Very rare	Common
Enlarged parotids		
Bone cysts		
Ulceration and sinuses	Common	No
Involvement of:		
pleura		
peritoneum		
pericardium	Common	Very rare
meninges		
small intestine		
Caseation	Maximal	Minimal
Acid-fast bacilli	Present	Absent
Tuberculin test	Positive in most	Negative in 65%
Kveim–Siltzbach test	Negative	Positive in 80%
Hypercalcaemia	No	Yes
Hypercalciuria	No	Yes
Serum angiotensin-converting enzyme	Elevated in up to 10%	Elevated in 60%
Calcification	Yes	Rare
Hilar lymphadenopathy	Unilateral	Bilateral
Pulmonary cavities	Common, early	Rare, late
Ghon focus	Yes	No
Corticosteroids	Harmful alone	Helpful
Antituberculous drugs	Treatment of choice	Unhelpful

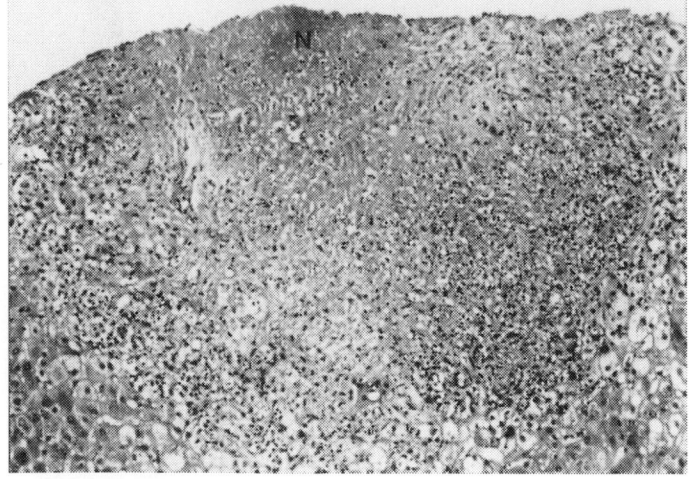

Fig. 5. Tuberculosis. A granuloma has undergone extensive necrosis of caseous type. Haematoxylin and eosin, × 112.

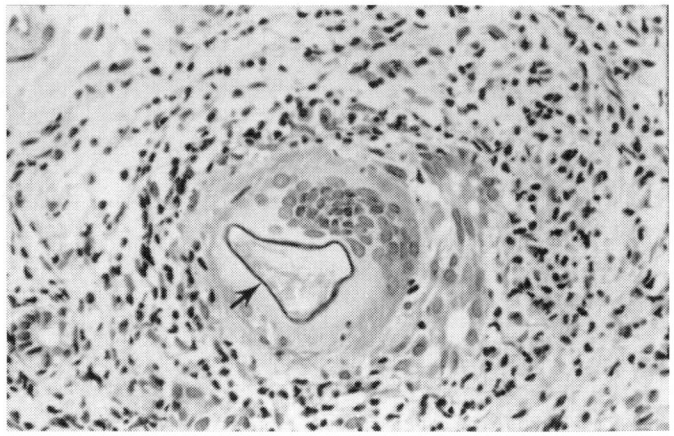

Fig. 6. Schistosomiasis. An ovum (arrow) is surrounded by a multinucleated giant cell. Ziehl–Neelsen, × 282.

AIDS

The acquired immunodeficiency syndrome (AIDS) provides an impoverished terrain which allows many different organisms—bacteria, viruses, fungi—to flourish in addition to the causative virus. Granulomas and granuloma-like accumulations of macrophages are found in various organs including the liver, often due to disseminated *Mycobacterium avium-intracellulare*, which can be visualized by diastase–periodic acid–Schiff or the Ziehl–Neelsen stain. Aspiration liver biopsy samples in suspected cases should be subjected to special stains and culture. Granulomas may be due to *M. tuberculosis* or various opportunistic mycobacteria. They may also be due to drugs, to B-cell lymphoma (Table 1), or to foreign material such as talc.

Non-infective causes of granulomas

Sarcoidosis

Hepatic granulomas are found in two-thirds of aspiration liver biopsies done on patients with sarcoidosis, although the hepatic involvement usually causes no clinical problems. The granulomas

Table 3 Recorded causes of fibrin-ring granulomas

Allopurinol hypersensitivity
Cytomegalovirus infection
Epstein–Barr virus infection
Giant-cell arteritis
Hepatitis A and C
Hodgkin's disease
Leishmaniasis
Q fever
Staphylococcal infection
Systemic lupus erythematosus
Toxoplasmosis

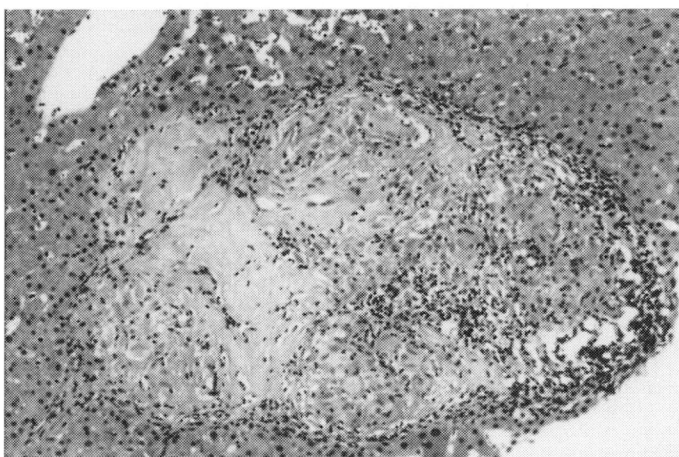

Fig. 8. Sarcoidosis. A cluster of granulomas is embedded in dense fibrous tissue. Haematoxylin and eosin, × 112.

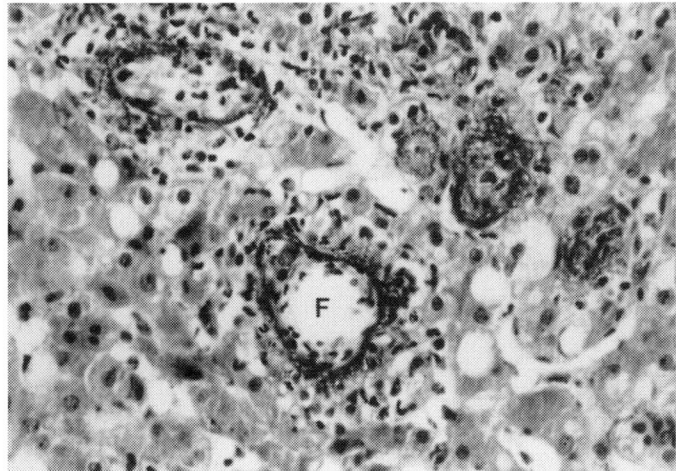

Fig. 7. Q fever. Deeply stained fibrin rings surround epithelioid cells, neutrophils, and fat (F). Trichrome, × 282.

are usually found in the portal tracts, but also in the acini, and are often in well-defined clusters with multinucleated giant cells containing inclusions (Fig. 8).[2,3] There may be associated inflammatory cells, including plasma cells and eosinophils. Central necrosis is less conspicuous than in tuberculosis and there is abundant reticulin in the granulomas. Older lesions display dense hyalinized collagen and the granuloma becomes converted into an acellular mass of hyaline material. Whereas pulmonary sarcoidosis may heal with troublesome complicating fibrosis, this is an extremely rare complication in the liver.

Patients with sarcoidosis often have splenomegaly, but hepatomegaly is uncommon although the liver is sometimes markedly enlarged and there may be a high level of alkaline phosphatase and elevated levels of aminotransferases. The two major hepatic complications of sarcoidosis are cholestasis and portal hypertension. Both are rare complications of hepatic sarcoidosis, occurring in less than 1 per cent of patients. They are most frequently seen in black males aged between 20 and 50 years, who usually have extensive fibrotic sarcoidosis in lungs and eyes.

The cholestatic form of sarcoidosis presents with jaundice, pruritus, and hepatosplenomegaly, often persists for many years, and may lead to hepatic fibrosis and cirrhosis. Its differentiation from primary biliary cirrhosis may be very difficult.

The portal hypertension is thought to be due to the involvement and narrowing of smaller portal venous radicles, and it is a pre-sinusoidal type of portal hypertension, the wedged hepatic venous pressure being normal. Haemorrhage from oesophageal varices may occur early in the course, in the absence of cirrhosis. If hepatic function is good, a portocaval shunt may be appropriate therapy. Sarcoidosis is a rare cause of the Budd-Chiari syndrome (Russi, AmJGastr, 1986; 81:71).

Long-term corticosteroid therapy is the main form of treatment for patients with hepatic sarcoidosis. It appears to have little effect on portal hypertension, but it reduces the size of an enlarged liver or spleen, and usually leads to a lowering of the levels of alkaline phosphatase and aminotransferases.

Primary biliary cirrhosis

Primary biliary cirrhosis must always be considered close second to sarcoidosis as a cause of non-infective hepatic granulomas. The granulomatous battlefield between antigen and antibody is often adjacent to bile ducts. Whereas the granulomas in sarcoidosis are abundant with rare and inconspicuous bile duct damage, the granulomas in primary biliary cirrhosis are few and may be poorly defined but bile duct damage is extensive. It is usually possible to distinguish these two conditions on the basis of the clinical picture, but the Kveim test and serum antimitochondrial antibodies are particularly helpful in differential diagnosis (Tables 4 and 5).

Primary sclerosing cholangitis

Granulomas were also seen in 7 of 100 native livers from patients who had orthotopic liver transplantation for primary sclerosing cholangitis. This is precisely the same incidence as that noted in the native livers in 100 patients with primary biliary cirrhosis with chronic ductopenic cholestatic disease. In contradistinction to the granulomas in primary biliary cirrhosis, the granulomas in primary sclerosing cholangitis did not represent granulomatous cholangitis. They may have developed as a result of leakage of bile or bile components (Ludwig, Liver, 1995; 15:307).

Lymphoma (see Chapter 24.5)

Epithelioid granulomas are sometimes found in patients with Hodgkin's disease, even in the absence of malignant deposits in the liver, and they may also be seen with other types of lymphoma. It is most

Table 4 Features distinguishing sarcoidosis from primary biliary cirrhosis

Features	Sarcoidosis	Primary biliary cirrhosis
Sex F:M	Equal	8:1
Decade of onset	3,4	5
Diagnosis over 40 years	Rare	Frequent
Erythema nodosum	Yes	No
Uveitis	Yes	No
Respiratory	Yes	No
Pruritus	No	Yes, eventually
Jaundice	No	Yes, late
Xanthomas	No	Yes, late
Clubbing	No	Yes
Hepatomegaly	Infrequent	Usually
Splenomegaly	Yes	Yes
Skin pegmentation	No	Yes
Steatorrhoea	No	Yes with jaundice
Bilateral hilar lymphadenopathy	Yes	No
Kveim–Siltzbach test	Positive in 80%	Always negative
Depression of delayed-type hypersensitivity	Yes	Yes
Circulating antimitochondrial antibodies	No	Yes (in 99%)
Calcium metabolism	Hypercalcaemia, vitamin D sensitivity	Hypocalcaemia (steatorrhoea)
Raised serum:		
alkaline phosphatase	Yes, minority	Yes, in most
angiotensin-converting enzyme	Yes, in 60%	Yes, in 16%
Liver granulomas	Yes	Yes
Corticosteroids	Helpful	Contraindicated
Vitamin D	Contraindicated	Helpful
Cholestyramine	Not necessary	Helpful
Prognosis	Very good	Variable

Table 5 Features distinguishing cholestatic sarcoidosis from primary biliary cirrhosis

Features	Sarcoidosis	Primary biliary cirrhosis
Sex	Equal	80% female
Age	Young	Middle age
Pruritus	Yes	Yes
Jaundice	Yes	Yes
Respiratory complaints	Yes	No
Hepatosplenomegaly	Yes	Yes
Serum alkaline phosphatase	Raised	Raised
Hilar lymphadenopathy	Usual	Rare
Hepatic granulomas	Clustered, portal	Mainly near bile ducts
Serum angiotensin-converting enzyme	Raised	Raised
Antimitochondrial antibody	No	Yes (98%)
Kveim–Siltzbach test	Positive	Negative
Bronchoalveolar lavage:		
lymphocytosis	Present	Present
activated macrophages	Present	Present

important that hepatic granulomas due to Hodgkin's disease are not confused with sarcoidosis, or with other types of granulomatous disease, because the consequences of mismanagement may be catastrophic. A set of criteria is presented for distinguishing granulomas associated with lymphomas from those due to sarcoidosis (Table 6).

Chronic granulomatous disease of childhood

Infective hepatic granulomas may be seen in chronic granulomatous disease of childhood; they tend to vary in size, and contain homogeneous eosinophilic material, necrotic debris, or pus. In normal subjects, the killing of many bacteria by neutrophils depends on a burst of respiratory-enzyme activity, which leads to the production of hydrogen peroxide and superoxide which are toxic to the bacteria. Neutrophils in chronic granulomatous disease of childhood are unable to kill some ingested bacteria because they are deficient in the enzymes needed for this superoxide respiratory burst.

The classic X-linked disorder occurs in boys aged about 5 years, presenting with hepatosplenomegaly, generalized lymphadenopathy, weeping granulomatous skin lesions, and diffuse miliary lung infiltration. Neutrophil leucocytes from normal patients with

Table 6 Features distinguishing sarcoidosis from Hodgkin's disease

Features	Sarcoidosis	Hodgkin's disease
Age (years)	20–40	20–40
Sex M:F	Equal	Males 3:1
Weight loss	Rare	Common
Splenomegaly	Rare	Frequent
Submental lymph nodes	Infrequent	Frequent
Erythema nodosum	Frequent	Rare
Gut symptoms	Absent	Common
Pruritus	Absent	Common
Bone lesions	'Punched out' phalangeal cysts	Sclerotis lesions of spine and pelvis
Sclerotic lesions	No	Mixed sclerotic/osteolytic in 16%
Leucocytosis, lymphopenia, and eosinophilia	Not a feature	May be present
Hilar lymphadenopathy	Bilateral	Bilateral or unilateral
Hilar gland pressure	No	Yes
Pulmonary infiltration	Common	Uncommon
Pulmonary infiltration followed by hilar adenopathy	Never	Yes
Pleural effusion	Rare	Common
Skin lesions	Distinctive histology	Specific histology with eosinophilia
Secondary infections	Rare	Common
Abdominal lymphangiogram	Normal	Abnormal
Delayed-type hypersensitivity	Depressed	Depressed
Immunoglobulins	Abnormal	Normal
Kveim–Siltzbach test	Positive	Negative
Radiotherapy	Unhelpful	Curative
Corticosteroids	Therapy of choice	Helpful
Immunosuppressive regimens	Not indicated	Indicated
Prognosis	Good	Guarded

bacterial infections reduce nitroblue tetrazolium from its colourless state to form blue-black formazan granules in the cytoplasm. This fails to occur in the leucocytes of children with chronic granulomatous disease or in the mothers of those with the X-linked variety and this reaction can be used as a diagnostic test.

Crohn's regional enteritis

Granulomas are found in the intestine, perineum, penis, and other paragenital areas, and also occasionally in the liver. The clinical picture is usually clearcut and there are several differences between the clinical pictures of sarcoidosis and Crohn's regional enteritis (Table 7).

Immune complex disease

Immune complexes are large molecular aggregates composed of antigen, antibody, and complement; they are constantly being formed in the circulation. When antigen is in excess of antibodies IgG and IgM, the complex remains soluble and may persist in the circulation. When antibody is in excess, immune complexes tend to be insoluble and are rapidly removed by the reticuloendothelial system. Immune complex tissue injury includes vasculitis, haemorrhage, thrombosis, ischaemic necrosis, and sometimes granuloma formation. Granulomas may also be found in liver and lymph nodes in patients with hypogammaglobulinaemia and with selective IgA deficiency.

Hepatic granulomatous disease ('granulomatous hepatitis')

This diagnosis should only be made when all other causes of hepatic granulomas have been excluded; in this sense it may be regarded as

an idiopathic ragbag. However, two variants of 'granulomatous hepatitis' have been described which may be distinct disorders. One is an acute febrile disease characterized by respiratory symptoms, splenomegaly, and a high count of blood lymphocytes (Eliakim, Lancet, 1968; ii: 348). The other is the chronic condition described by Simon and Wolff (Medicine, 1973; 52:1), who studied 13 patients, 9 of whom were males. All suffered high spiking fevers, rigors, and severe sweating. The illness lasted from months to years, and was often disabling, with marked weakness and loss of weight. Myalgias and arthralgias were common. In some patients, right upper quadrant pain occurred in association with hepatic tenderness. The liver was palpable in several patients, but there were few other physical signs. Jaundice and hyperbilirubinaemia occurred in only 1 patient, but several had modest elevations of aminotransferases, and the alkaline phosphatase was increased in 8 patients during the active phase; all had normal prothrombin times and 5 had mild hypoalbuminaemia. The erthrocyte sedimentation rate was markedly elevated (more than 50 mm/h) in 10 of the patients and 3 were anaemic. On liver biopsy all the patients had multiple granulomas; however, the term 'granulomatous hepatitis' is a misnomer because there is no true hepatitis but just clusters of hepatic granulomas in the portal tracts and acini resembling those found in sarcoidosis and many other conditions.

Patients with this condition, which has been described in a family (Mahido, AmJGastr, 1988, 83:42), usually undergo extensive investigations and the only striking abnormality is the presence of hepatic granulomas suggesting sarcoidosis. However, all tests for sarcoidosis are negative, including the Kveim test, as are investigations for tuberculosis. There is usually a good response to treatment with steroids, which lower the temperature to normal and cause marked improvement of liver function tests. Colchicine and

Table 7 Features distinguishing sarcoidosis from Crohn's regional enteritis

Features	Sarcoidosis	Crohn's regional enteritis
Histology	Granulomas are similar	Granulomas are similar
Involvement of:		
Intestine	Rare	Invariable
Intrathoracic region	Yes in 90%	No
Skin	Yes in 25%, but they do not ulcerate	Mucocutaneous ulceration involving genitalia
Erythema nodosum	Yes	Yes
Eyes	Yes in 25%	No
Associated		
Ankylosing spondylitis	No	Yes
Complicating:		
Malabsorption	No	Yes
Amyloidosis	No	Yes
Peritonitis	No	Yes
Hepatic granulomas	Common	Occasional
Depression of delayed-type hypersensitivity	Yes	Yes
Kveim–Siltzbach test	Positive in 80%	Negative
Abnormal calcium metabolism	Hypercalcaemia and hypercalciuria	Hypocalcaemia associated with malabsorption
Serum		
Antireticulin antibodies	Negative	Positive in 25%
Lysozyme	Raised	Raised
Angiotensin-converting enzyme	Raised	Normal
Surgical treatment	No	Yes
Corticosteroids	+	+
Azathioprine	+/−	+
Calciferol	Contraindicated	Indicated

indomethacin may also be effective in controlling the fever. We remain ignorant of the cause(s) of this condition.

Whipple's disease

This is not a common disease, but it does cause widespread alimentary tract granulomas including hepatic granulomas (Cho, Gastro, 1984; 87:941). It has been confused with both sarcoidosis and Crohn's regional enteritis. The management of these diseases is not the same and so it is important to recogize the differences between them. Whipple's disease should be considered when the patient has polyarthritis, steatorrhoea, and widespread alimentary tract granulomas. At first the patient is suspected of having tuberculosis or a lymphoma but, eventually, the benign course suggests sarcoidosis. Intestinal biopsy with the appropriate staining is definitive (Table 8). The causative organism *Tropheryma whipplei* may be detected by electron microscopy and by the polymerase chain reaction in peripheral blood leucocytes (Wilson, DigDisSci, 1989; 34:640).

Drugs

Many drugs are hepatotoxic and several produce granulomas; the possibility that a drug has caused hepatic granulomas should always be considered even if it is not included in the list given in Table 9.[4, 5] Cholestasis and hepatocellular disturbances may be additional pointers to the presence of granulomas. Drugs used to treat patients with liver disease may cause hypersensitivity liver granulomas, and this may cause considerable confusion in the practical management of the original disease.

Investigative routine

Management of granulomatous diseases depends on their cause, so investigation must be thorough. Liver histology is supplemented whenever possible by histological examination of other tissues, bacteriology of part of the submitted specimen, and radiology. The routine enquiry should include a history of drugs and geographical origins, chest radiograph, slit-lamp examination of the eyes, skin tests, and serum antibodies. It may be necessary to do CT scans and gallium uptake studies.

Angiotensin-converting enzyme (ACE) is a dipeptidyl carboxypeptidase that converts angiotensin-I to angiotensin-II. It is present in serum and the level is elevated in about 90 per cent of patients with active sarcoidosis; it is a useful method of monitoring the activity of sarcoidosis. However, the serum level of angiotensin-converting enzyme may also rise, though less commonly, in other granulomatous disorders, including primary biliary cirrhosis, and the level has been found to be increased in some patients with other acute and chronic parenchymal liver diseases.

Liver biopsy in granulomatous diseases

Liver biopsy helps to establish that a disease is granulomatous in nature and may provide information about its cause, evolution, and complications. Step sections through the biopsy specimen are usually advisable if no granulomas are found in initial sections, or if the cause of granulomas is not at first apparent. In such cases it is also necessary to do appropriate stains for mycobacteria and fungi.

In practice, granulomas are found in liver biopsies either as part of another lesion or as the main finding. The former situation is

Table 8 Features distinguishing sarcoidosis from Whipple's disease

Features	Sarcoidosis	Whipple's disease
Other names		Lipophagic intestinal granulomatosis
Sex	Equal	Males predominantly
Decade	3 and 4	4–7
Non-deforming arthritis	Yes with erythema nodosum	Characteristic, initial
Steatorrhoea	No	Severe principal feature
Diarrhoea	No	Yes
Weight loss	Infrequent	Frequent
Lymphadenopathy	27%	40%
Polyserositis	No	Yes
PAS stain of macrophages in lymph node	Negative	Positive
Duodenal biopsy	Normal	PAS-staining macrophages, PCR defines *Tropheryma*
Electron microscopy	Negative	*Tropheryma*
Tropheryma	No	In peripheral blood leucocytes
Treatment	Corticosteroids	Antibiotics

PAS, periodic-acid Schiff; PCR, polymerase chain reaction.

typified by fat granulomas around lipid vacuoles in a fatty liver, or a granulomatous reaction near damaged bile ducts in a biopsy otherwise showing typical histological features of primary biliary cirrhosis. In this situation, no further investigation is usually necessary from the point of view of the granulomas. Sometimes, however, granulomas are found unexpectedly in a biopsy showing unrelated liver disease, and it may then be appropriate to investigate the patient further in order to exclude the commoner causes of granulomas.

When granulomas are the main finding in a liver biopsy, the pathologist is faced with one of four situations:

1. The cause of the granulomas can be demonstrated histologically, and the diagnosis is established with certainty. Examples are the finding of tubercle bacilli or of ova of *Schistosoma mansoni* in

Table 9 Currently used drugs causing hepatic granulomas

Acetylsalicylic acid	Gold
Allopurinol	Halothane
Amiodarone	Hydralazine
Amoxycillin	Hydrochlorothiazide
Ampicillin	Isoniazid
Carbamazepine	Methyldopa
Cephalexin	Metolazone
Chloropromazine	Nitrofurantoin
Clorpropamide	Papaverine
Clavulanic acid	Penicillin
Clofibrate	Phenylbutazone
Contraceptive steroids	Phenytoin
Dapsone	Procainamide
Diazepam	Procarbazine
Diltiazem	Quinidine
Dimethicone	Ranitidine
Erythromycin	Sulphonamides
Fenfluramine	Sulphonylureas
Flucloxacillin	Tocainidine
Glibenclamide	Tolbutamide

the lesions (Fig. 6). Examination of the biopsy may also provide further information, for example the presence or absence of venous lesions and portal fibrosis in schistosomiasis. In fatty livers, serial or step sections may be helpful for demonstrating a fat vacuole in the centre of a fat granuloma.

2. The cause of the granulomas is not seen as such, but is obvious from other considerations. In the example of primary biliary cirrhosis already cited, a combination of typical clinical features and biochemical abnormalities, antimitochondrial antibodies, and corresponding histological changes may leave no doubt about the diagnosis, and make further investigation of the granulomas unnecessary. Similarly, granulomas with extensive central necrosis of caseous type in a febrile patient virtually establish a diagnosis of tuberculosis even if no bacilli are found (Fig. 5.)

3. The cause of the granulomas cannot be established with certainty on histological grounds, but the appearances throw strong suspicion on a particular disease. In Q fever, there are sometimes very characteristic granulomas within a fatty parenchyma; epithelioid cells, giant cells, and neutrophils surround a fat vacuole, and are themselves surrounded by a ring of fibrin (Fig. 7). Uncertainty about the diagnosis reflects the fact that other causes of these 'doughnut' or 'fibrin–ring' granulomas have been reported, including idiosyncratic reaction to allopurinol (Vanderstigel, Gastro, 1986; 90:188). In sarcoidosis, granulomas are sometimes non-specific in appearance, but in other patients give rise to a histological picture which, while not decisive, strongly supports the diagnosis; flower-like clusters of granulomas embedded in dense fibrous tissue expand the portal tracts while other, smaller granulomas are seen in the parenchyma (Fig. 8). Liver biopsy in patients with sarcoidosis also gives helpful information about the extent of hepatic fibrosis, and may reveal the rare chronic cholestatic lesion resembling primary biliary cirrhosis.

4. There are granulomas in portal tracts, parenchyma, or both, but there are no histological clues to their aetiology. This is a common situation. Further investigation of biopsy specimens and the patient is indicated. In the Western world, principal causes to be considered include sarcoidosis, tuberculosis, drug hypersensitivity,

brucellosis, Hodgkin's disease, and AIDS. In persons who abuse intravenous drugs, examination of a granuloma under polarized light may reveal birefringent spicules of injected talc.

References

1. Denk H, *et al*. Guidelines for the diagnosis and interpretation of hepatic granulomas. *Histopathology*, 1994; **25**: 209–18.

2. Devaney K, Goodman ZD, Epstein MS, Zimmerman HJ, and Ishak KG. Hepatic sarcoidosis. Clinicopathologic features in 100 patients. *American Journal of Surgical Pathology*, 1993; **17**: 1272–80.

3. James DG. *Sarcoidosis and other granulomatous disorders*. Marcel Dekker Inc, 1994.

4. Farrell GC. *Drug-induced liver disease*. Edinburgh: Churchill Livingstone, 1994: 301–17.

5. Zimmerman HJ and Ishak KG. Hepatic injury due to drugs and toxins. In MacSween RNM, Anthony PP, Scheuer PJ, Burt AD, and Portmann BC, eds. *Pathology of the liver*. 3rd edn. Edinburgh: Churchill Livingstone, 1994: 563–633.

14.3 Autoimmune hepatitis

Michael P. Manns

Introduction

Autoimmune hepatitis was first described in 1950 in young women (Waldenström, DtschZVerdauStoffwechselkr, 1950; 2:113). An association of autoimmune hepatitis with antinuclear antibodies had led to the proposed term 'lupoid hepatitis' (Mackay, Lancet, 1956; ii:1323). Because viral causes of chronic active hepatitis had not yet been identified, the concept of autoimmune hepatitis was extended in the 1960s and 1970s to encompass the spectrum of chronic active hepatitis, and the histological and biochemical features of chronic active hepatitis were arbitrarily considered as characteristic of autoimmune hepatitis. In the 1970s, autoimmune hepatitis was defined as a disease not associated with known factors for liver damage, characterized by the presence of antinuclear antibodies, periportal and bridging necrosis, hypergammaglobulinaemia, and elevated aminotransferases. However, with the subsequent discovery of the hepatitis viruses, it became clear that none of the 'classic' morphological or biochemical features of autoimmune hepatitis is specific to this disease. More confusing, it also emerged that autoantibodies, the hallmark of autoimmune hepatitis, can be present in the course of chronic viral hepatitis or may be absent in liver disorders that otherwise meet diagnostic criteria for autoimmune hepatitis, including a prompt response to steroid therapy. Thus the concept of autoimmune hepatitis has become progressively blurred and its diagnosis has become a most challenging exercise.

The issue was recently reviewed, and diagnostic guidelines proposed, by the International Autoimmune Hepatitis Group.[1] At the time of diagnosis the disease has usually been present for 6 months or more, and patients have high concentrations of aminotransferases. In full-blown disease, histological examination reveals periportal and/or periseptal hepatitis (piecemeal necrosis). The liver disease progresses further to bridging necrosis, panlobular and multilobular necrosis, and active cirrhosis. Without treatment, autoimmune hepatitis is associated with a high mortality and a low rate of spontaneous remission; 50 per cent of patients with severe autoimmune hepatitis will die in about 5 years. The diagnosis is based on particular features that are typical of autoimmune hepatitis and the exclusion of other causes of chronic hepatitis (Tables 1 and 2).[1,2] Patients with continuing infections with hepatitis viruses or excessive intake of alcohol are excluded. Features characteristic of autoimmune hepatitis are female predominance (female–male ratio 4:1), hypergammaglobulinaemia, circulating autoantibodies, benefit from immunosuppression, extrahepatic clinical autoimmune syndromes, and overrepresentation of HLA alleles –DR3 or –DR4. These features have been summarized in a provisional scoring system for the diagnosis of autoimmune hepatitis (Table 1). According to the autoantibodies found, autoimmune hepatitis has been subdivided into types 1 to 3 (Table 2).[3–5] Type 1 is characterized by antinuclear and/or antismooth-muscle autoantibodies, type 2 by antibodies specific for liver and kidney microsomes (**LKM-1** and **LKM-3**), and type 3 by autoantibodies against cytosolic liver antigens, either cytokeratins 8 or 18 (anti-SLA)[4] or antibodies to liver–pancreas antigen (LP). Further autoantibodies associated with autoimmune hepatitis are directed against the asialoglycoprotein receptor (Treichel, Hepatol, 1990; 11:606) and the liver cytosol-1 antigen (Martini, Hepatol, 1988; 8:1662).

Histopathology

Liver biopsy is important in determining the activity (grading) and degree of fibrosis (staging) of chronic hepatitis. However, histological examination is less effective for defining the aetiological background of liver diseases and in particular autoimmune hepatitis. Originally the presence of an inflammatory infiltrate was regarded as a diagnostic hallmark for autoimmune hepatitis. However, in a light-microscopic study (Dienes, ZGastr, 1989; 27:325) on liver biopsy specimens from 26 patients with well-documented autoimmune hepatitis, plasma cells were not a hallmark, at least compared with hepatitis B and non-A, non-B (nowadays identified as hepatitis C). There was no specific histological pattern of autoimmune hepatitis, and furthermore there were no specific features associated with either of its three subtypes as defined by autoantibody patterns. However, broad hypocellular areas of collapse, extending from the portal tracts into the parenchyma and encompassing groups of hepatocytes, with microacinar transformation, were found to be characteristic, as was hydropic swelling of hepatocytes. In contrast, the eosinophilic cell damage with acidophilic bodies frequently seen in non-A, non-B hepatitis (Popper, VirchArchA, 1980; 387:91; Dienes, Hepatol, 1982; 2:562) was not specific nor was it a characteristic finding in autoimmune hepatitis.

Aetiology and pathogenesis
Environmental factors and aetiology

A number of agents have been considered as triggers for the self-perpetuating autoimmune process in autoimmune hepatitis (viruses, bacteria, chemicals, drugs, genetic factors), with recent emphasis on viruses. All the major hepatotropic viruses have been implicated as a cause of autoimmune hepatitis, including measles viruses,

Table 1 Scoring system for diagnosis of autoimmune hepatitis (AIH): minimum required measures

Measure	Score
Gender	
Female	+2
Male	0
Serum biochemistry	
Ratio of elevation of serum alkaline phosphatase vs aminotransferase:	
>3.0	−2
<3.0	+2
Total serum globulin, gammaglobulin or IgG	
Times upper normal limit:	
>2.0	+3
1.5–2.0	+2
1.0–1.5	+1
<1.0	0
Autoantibodies (titres by immunofluorescence on rodent tissues)	
Adults:	
ANA, SMA or LKM-1	
>1:80	+3
1:80	+2
1:40	+1
<1:40	0
Children:	
ANA or LKM-1	
>1:20	+3
1:10 or 1:20	+2
<1:20	0
or SMA	
>1:20	+3
1:20	+2
<1:20	0
Antimitochondrial antibody	
Positive	−2
Negative	0
Viral markers	
IgM anti-HAV, HBsAg or IgM anti-HBc-positive	−3
Anti-HCV-positive by ELISA and/or RIBA	−2
Anti-HCV-positive by PCR for HCV RNA	−3
Positive test indicating active infection with any other virus	−3
Seronegative for all of the above	+3
Other aetiological factors	
History of recent hepatotoxic drug usage or parenteral exposure to blood products:	
Yes	−2
No	+1
Alcohol (average consumption):	
Male <35 g/day; female <25 g/day	+2
Male 35–50 g/day; female 25–40 g/day	0
Male 50–80 g/day; female 40–60 g/day	−2
Male >80 g/day; female >60 g/day	−1
Genetic factors, HLA-DR3, HLA-DR4 or other autoimmune diseases in patient or first-degree relatives	+1

Interpretation of aggregate scores: definite AIH, greater than 15 before treatment and greater than 17 after treatment; probable AIH, 10 to 15 before treatment and 12 to 17 after treatment.
According to Johnson and McFarlane [1].
Abbreviations: HAV, hepatitis A virus; HBsAg, hepatitis B surface antigen; HBc, hepatitis B core antigen; ELISA, enzyme-linked immunosorbent assay; PCR, polymerase chain reaction; RIBA, recombinant immunoblot assay; other abbreviations in text.

hepatitis A, hepatitis B, hepatitis C, hepatitis D, herpes simplex virus type 1, and Epstein–Barr virus.

Several observations suggest that autoimmune hepatitis can develop after acute infection with the hepatitis A virus (Vento, Lancet, 1991; 337:1183), and after hepatitis B infection (Hopf, ZGastr, 1984; 22:121; Laskus, DigDisSci, 1989; 34:1294). In the early 1990s there was lively discussion on the relation between

hepatitis C virus and the induction of autoimmune hepatitis. Hepatitis C does not appear to induce autoimmune hepatitis; however, infection with the hepatitis C virus is associated with autoimmune markers that are also seen in autoimmune hepatitis (see below).[6] Hepatitis D is also associated with a number of autoimmune reactions, in particular with several autoantibodies. However, there is no proof that hepatitis D virus can cause autoimmune hepatitis (see

Table 2 Aetiological classification of chronic hepatitis

Hepatitis type	HBsAg	HBV DNA	HDV antibody (HDV RNA)	HCV antibody (HCV RNA)	Autoantibodies
B	+	+/−	−	−	—
D	+	−	+	−	10–20% anti-LKM-3
C	−	−	−	+	2–10% anti-LKM-1
Autoimmune:					
Type 1	−	−	−	−	ANA, SMA
Type 2	−	−	−	−	LKM-1 or LKM -3, LC-1
Type 3	−	−	−	−	SLA/LP, ANA, SMA
Drug-induced	−	−	−	−	Some: ANA, LKM, LM
Cryptogenic	−	−	−	−	—

SLA, soluble liver antigen antibody; LP, liver–pancreas antigen antibody; LM, liver microsomal antibody; HB, (C) (D) V, hepatitis B (C) (D) viruses; HBsAg, hepatitis B surface antigen; ANA, antinuclear antibody; LKM, liver–kidney microsomes.
Modified according to Desmet *et al.* [2].

below). Recent interest has concentrated on hepatitis G (**GBV-C**), but this recently discovered group of viruses does not appear to be the major cause of autoimmune hepatitis (Heringlake, JHepatol, 1996; 25:980). In a recent study we found the prevalence of GBV-C RNA in autoimmune hepatitis to be between 9 and 15 per cent, depending on the serological subgroup. This is about the range seen with cryptogenic chronic hepatitis and below the prevalence of GBV-C in other liver diseases such as chronic viral hepatitis.

The major B-cell epitope of antibodies against cytochrome P450 2D6, the major LKM-1 antigen, shares sequence homology with the immediate early protein IE 175 of herpes simplex virus type 1 (Fig. 1) (Manns, JCI, 1991; 88:1370). Although some observations suggest that autoimmune hepatitis may develop after herpesvirus infection, this does not seem to be a major cause of autoimmune hepatitis. Furthermore, another peptide of cytochrome P450 2D6 shares sequence homology with the 21-hydroxylase of the adrenal gland and the carboxypeptidase H of the pancreas [Choudhury, JHepatol, 1996; 25 (Suppl. 1):70]. Therefore an exogenous agent sharing a sequence with these enzymes of different organs might trigger autoimmunity, leading to an autoimmune process attacking various tissues. The clinical presentation, however, could depend on additional factors including the genetic background of the patient.

The earlier observation that measles virus infection was associated with autoimmune hepatitis could not be confirmed (Robertson, Lancet, 1987; ii: 9). More recently, autoimmune hepatitis has been thought to be associated with Epstein–Barr virus infection (Vento, Lancet, 1995; 346:608). It is not known whether certain drugs or chemicals can cause autoimmune hepatitis. The mechanisms for immune-mediated, drug-induced hepatitis may serve as models. Drugs may be triggers of autoimmune hepatitis (see below), but no particular drug has been identified as a true aetiological agent. It is of interest that drug-metabolizing enzymes of phase I and phase II, that is, cytochromes P450 and UDP glucuronosyltransferase (**UGT**) proteins, are targets of virus- and drug-induced autoimmunity as well as of autoimmune hepatitis. It seems that different aetiological agents may trigger autoimmunity against the same molecular target. For example, P450 2D6 is a target for the autoantibodies found in autoimmune hepatitis and hepatitis C. P450 1A2 is a target in autoimmune hepatitis as part of

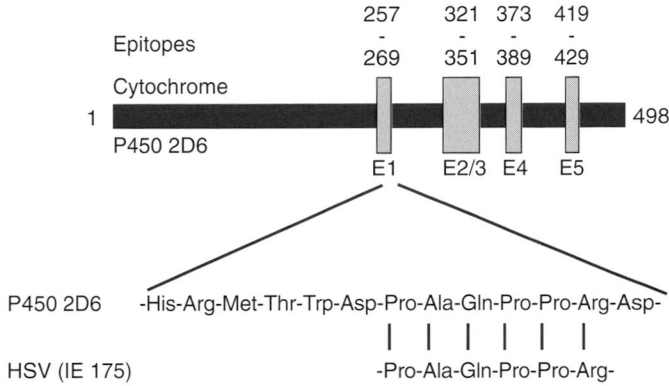

Fig. 1. Recognition of linear epitopes on cytochrome P450 2D6 in autoimmune hepatitis type 2. Data for this figure are derived from Manns (JCI, 1991; 88:1370) and Yamamoto (EurJImmun, 1993; 23: 1105). HSV, herpes simplex virus type 1; IE 175, immediate early protein, 175 kDa.

the autoimmune polyendocrine syndrome type 1, and in di-hydralazine hepatitis (see below). In any case, a specific immunogenetic background seems to be an important prerequisite for autoimmune hepatitis. Probably the manifestation of an autoimmune hepatitis is the result of multiple factors, for example a specific genetic background and a specific agent triggering the autoimmune process, which might be a virus or a chemical. Other cofactors might be necessary, for example female hormones and environmental reagents that up- or down-regulate mediators or components of the immune system, or even autoantigens. One could think of environmental reagents such as nicotine, alcohol, and nutrients that up- or down-regulate drug-metabolizing enzymes, which then become autoantigens.

Autoantibodies

Antinuclear antibodies (ANA)

Typical for autoimmune hepatitis type 1 are significant titres of antinuclear (**ANA**) and smooth-muscle (**SMA**) antibodies. The most frequent method for the detection of ANA is indirect immuno-fluorescence on Hep-2 cells. Different patterns of fluorescence are found depending on the autoantigens detected: homogeneous (58 per cent), speckled (21 per cent), homogeneous and speckled (10 per cent), centromere (9 per cent), or homogeneous perinuclear (6 per cent) (Nishioka, In *Immunology and liver*. Lancaster, UK: Kluwer, 1993; 193). Each pattern is associated with the recognition of several nuclear antigens with a wide range of molecular weights. The cut-off titre for a positive autoantibody result may vary from laboratory to laboratory, but 1:40 for ANA and 1:80 for SMA are cut-off values in many laboratories. Among ANA are autoantibodies directed against single-strand DNA, double-strand DNA, small nuclear ribonucleoproteins, tRNA, and lamin A and C. Recently, cyclin A was discovered as another species of antigens for ANA (Strassburg, JHepatol, 1996; 25:859). So far neither a liver-specific nuclear antigen nor a liver disease-specific ANA has been identified.

Smooth-muscle antibodies (SMA)

SMA autoantibodies are directed against structures of the cyto-skeleton. They are measured by indirect immunofluorescence on smooth-muscle cells, which have a well-developed cytoskeleton because of their contractile function. Antibodies to actin represent a subset of SMA antibodies found often in autoimmune hepatitis type 1. In autoimmune hepatitis, SMA are directed predominantly against F-actin (Kurki, In *Immunology and liver*. Lancaster, UK: Kluwer, 1993:206). These seem to be diagnostically more relevant in children. Recently, antiactin antibodies in autoimmune hepatitis have been further analysed (Czaja, Hepatol, 1996; 24:1068): actin antibody-positive patients were younger, and more commonly HLA-DR3-positive; death and transplantation occurred more frequently in these patients than in actin antibody-negative patients with ANA.

LKM-1 autoantibodies

Autoimmune hepatitis type 2 is characterized by the presence of LKM-1 autoantibodies.[3] These autoantibodies were first described in 1973 (Rizzetto, ClinExpImmun, 1973, 15:331) using indirect immunofluorescence on rodent liver and kidney sections. Their characteristic feature is the exclusive staining of liver tissue and of the P3 portion of the proximal renal tubules.[3] Western blots with hepatic microsomes reveal a protein band at 50 kDa. In addition to the 50-kDa protein, a 55- and a 64-kDa protein are detected less frequently (Codoner-French, ClinExpImmun, 1989; 54:232; Manns, JCI, 1989; 83:1066).

Cytochrome P450 2D6 is the major antigen for LKM-1 auto-antibodies (Zanger, PNAS, 1988; 85:8256; Gueguen, BBResComm, 1989; 159:542; Manns, JCI, 1989; 83:1066). *In vitro* the enzymatic activity of cytochrome P450 2D6 is inhibited by LKM-1 auto-antibodies. The epitopes recognized by LKM-1 autoantibodies have been characterized. In a first report (Manns, JCI, 1991; 88:1370), 11 out of 26 sera recognized a short, minimal epitope of eight amino acids spanning amino acids 257 to 269 DPAQPPRD (Fig. 1). Twelve other sera recognized the C-terminal two-thirds of P450 2D6 (Manns, JCI, 1991; 88:1370). Further work on epitope mapping resulted in the identification of three other epitopes on P450 2D6 (Yamamoto, Gastro, 1993; 104:1762). This confirmed that most patients with autoimmune hepatitis type 2 serologically recognize

the epitope of amino acids 257 to 269, including the core sequence of DPAQPPRD. However, about 50 per cent of patients with autoimmune hepatitis type 2 recognize, in addition, an epitope from amino acids 321 to 351, and some recognize an epitope of amino acids 373 to 389 or 410 to 429 (Fig. 1).

LKM-1 serum was absorbed using peptides of the four previously described linear domains (Yamamoto, Gastro, 1993; 104: 1762). The preadsorbed sera were used to inhibit P450 2D6-mediated enzyme reactions. Most of the inhibitory activity of the autoantibodies could not be abolished by saturating the binding sites for the linear peptides, and affinity-purified autoantibodies directed against these linear epitopes failed to inhibit P450 2D6-mediated enzymatic activity significantly, suggesting that the inhibitory activity was due to the presence of autoantibodies to conformational epitopes (Duclos-Vallee, DigDisSci, 1995; 40:1069), a hypothesis that was recently confirmed (Zanger, ZGastr, 1997; 35: 87). As multiple epitopes are recognized by most of the patients' sera the original immune response may be polyclonal, with a later oligoclonal response due to affinity maturation. The immunodominant sites are believed to be due to the structural and sequential characteristics of the protein and the patient's genetic background (Yamamoto, EurJImmun, 1993; 23:1105).

LKM-1 autoantibodies are widely used as diagnostic markers for autoimmune hepatitis type 2, or autoimmunity associated with hepatitis C, but their role in liver-cell injury is not known. One possible mechanism of liver-cell injury mediated by these autoantibodies could be through their direct binding to hepatocytes, resulting in cell lysis either by complement or by antibody-directed, cell-mediated cytotoxicity. A prerequisite for the activation of both of those possible mechanisms would be the expression of P450 2D6 on the surface of the hepatocyte of patients with LKM-positive autoimmune hepatitis. The topic of surface expression of cytochromes P450 has, however, been controversial for many years, though recently the surface expression of different cytochromes of family 2 has been demonstrated using a diversity of methods and controls (Loeper, Hepatol, 1990; 11:850; 1993; 104:203). One group (Robin, Gastro, 1995; 108:1110) has even succeeded in describing the route of transport to the surface membrane. Using fluorescence-activated cell-sorter analysis and electron microscopy, they have demonstrated the surface expression of cytochrome P450 2B and shown that the cytochromes follow a vesicular route from the endoplasmic reticulum to the Golgi apparatus. Interestingly, they found that cytochrome P450 2B expressed on the cytoplasmic surface of the endoplasmic reticulum was located at the outer surface of the plasma membrane; its outward surface location might suggest a pathogenetic role for autoantibodies and their antigens in autoimmune hepatitis.

LKM-2 autoantibodies

To date LKM-2 autoantibodies have only been found in drug-induced hepatitis caused by tienilic acid (see later), and not in autoimmune hepatitis (Homberg, ClinExpImmun, 1984; 55:561). LKM-2 autoantibodies are directed against cytochrome P450 2C9 (Beaune, PNAS, 1987; 84:551).

LKM-3 autoantibodies

LKM-3 antibodies were found in 10 to 20 per cent of patients with chronic hepatitis D (Crivelli, ClinExpImmun, 1983; 54:232). They are different from LKM-1 and LKM-2, and react with a 55-kDa microsomal protein. In about 10 per cent of patients with autoimmune hepatitis type 2, LKM-3 autoantibodies occur in addition to LKM-1 antibodies (Phillip, Lancet, 1994; 344:578; Durazzo, Gastro, 1995; 108:455; Obermayer-Straub, Gut, 1995; 37: A100). Owing to this low prevalence, data for only six sera with LKM-3 autoantibodies associated with autoimmune hepatitis are available in our laboratory. In five the LKM-3 was associated with LKM-1 autoantibodies; one patient was, however, positive for LKM-3 only (Strassburg, Gastro, 1996; 111:1582). Epitope mapping revealed a large, minimal epitope from amino acids 264 to 373, indicating that the autoantibody was conformation-dependent. LKM-3 autoantibodies associated with autoimmune hepatitis type 2 are usually characterized by high titres on western blot, and the sera usually recognize UGT family 1 at dilutions of 1:1000 or above.

LM autoantibodies

Antimicrosomal antibodies that react only with liver tissue are called **LM** antibodies. They were found in drug-induced hepatitis caused by dihydralazine and reacted with cytochrome P450 1A2 (Bourdi, JCI, 1990; 85:1967). Anti-P450 1A2 antibodies were also found in one patient with autoimmune hepatitis (Manns, ArchBiochemBiophys, 1990; 280:229). More recently, the finding of LM antibodies against cytochrome P450 1A2 in non-drug-induced autoimmune liver disease was identified as a diagnostic marker for liver disease as part of the autoimmune polyendocrine syndrome type 1 [Clemente, JHepatol, 1995; 23 (Suppl. 1):126]. There does not seem to be a serological overlap between LKM-1 antibodies in autoimmune hepatitis type 2 and LM antibodies in that syndrome.

Antibodies against the asialoglycoprotein receptor

Autoantibodies against the asialoglycoprotein receptor (**ASGP-R**), a liver-specific membrane receptor, are found frequently in autoimmune liver diseases and in particular in autoimmune hepatitis (McFarlane, ClinExpImmun, 1984; 55:347; Treichel, Gastro, 1994; 107:799). However, they may also be detected less frequently in primary biliary cirrhosis, viral hepatitis, and other liver diseases. Anti-ASGP-R antibodies correlate with disease activity and anti-ASGP-R antibodies against human-specific epitopes seem to be closely associated with autoimmune hepatitis (Treichel, Gastro, 1994; 107:799). T lymphocytes directed against the ASGP-R were isolated from the liver tissue of cases of autoimmune hepatitis type 1 (Löhr, Hepatol, 1990; 12:1314). The tissue expression of the ASGP-R is most evident in the periportal areas where piecemeal necrosis is found as a marker of severe inflammatory activity. ASGP-R antibodies may serve as a diagnostic marker for autoimmune hepatitis if other markers are negative and autoimmune liver disease is suspected; unfortunately, the assay requires chemically purified receptor, which is not easily available.

Other autoantibodies

Many other autoantibodies have been described in autoimmune hepatitis, but their testing is limited to research laboratories and is not generally available.[8]

Cellular immunity

Histologically the liver in autoimmune hepatitis shows dense, mononuclear infiltrates, mostly consisting of T cells. Several years ago, studies on cellular immunity had concentrated on the characterization of suppressor-cell defects, as reviewed by Vergani.[8] Aminotransferase concentrations often fluctuate in patients before immunosuppressive therapy is begun, indicating that the disease process is regulated rather than being due to a single, up-regulated, autoreactive T cell. Therefore, the concept was developed (Lohse, ClinExpImmun, 1993; 94:163) that an aberrant autoimmune response is present in autoimmune hepatitis and that attempts by the immune system to down-regulate this autoimmune process cause spontaneous immunosuppression. To prove this, patients with untreated autoimmune hepatitis type 1 were investigated and, as expected, 10/11 patients showed significant T-cell reactivity to soluble liver antigens, whereas very low, if any, reactivity could be detected in patients with hepatitis C and B virus infection. Five days after the start of immunosuppressive therapy the reactivity remained unchanged but, after remission with that treatment, T-cell reactivity to soluble liver antigens became undetectable in all 10 patients. In order to investigate whether active suppression was involved, irradiated peripheral blood lymphocytes from the remission phase were added to preremission T cells and the T-cell reactivity against soluble liver antigens determined; active suppression was detected in the T-cell response from 7/9 patients *in vitro*. Moreover, patients with autoimmune hepatitis in remission showed a lack of a T-cell proliferative response to *in vivo* immunization with tetanus toxoid while healthy individuals and patients with chronic hepatitis B or C reacted strongly. These results demonstrate that active immunosuppression is involved in the regulation of autoimmune hepatitis (Lohse, Hepatol, 1995; 22: 381).

A study of patients with autoimmune hepatitis type 2 (Löhr, ClinExpImmun, 1991; 84:297) sought to ascertain whether T cells react to the same antigens as those recognized by LKM-1 autoantibodies. One hundred and eighty-nine T-cell clones were isolated from liver biopsies of four patients, and four of these clones proliferated specifically in response to recombinant human cytochrome P450 2D6. These T lymphocytes were of the T-helper (CD4+) phenotype and were inhibited by monoclonal antibodies to major histocompatibility complex (**MHC**) class II. Furthermore, T cells with specific reactivity to ASGP-R were isolated from liver tissue (Löhr, Hepatol, 1990; 12:1314; Wen Li, Lancet, 1990; 336: 1527); ASGP-R-specific, T-helper cells were shown to facilitate ASGP-R antibody formation *in vitro*.

Immunogenetics

In Caucasian populations, autoimmune hepatitis type 1 is associated with HLA-B8 and with the *HLA-B8-DR3* haplotype (Mackay, Lancet, 1972; ii:793; Gastro, 1980; 79:95). *HLA-B8* is in linkage disequilibrium with *HLA-DR3*, resulting in a close association between autoimmune hepatitis type 1 and HLA-B8.[8] An association with HLA-DR4 was found subsequently (Donaldson, Hepatol, 1991; 13:701). Patients with the *HLA-DR3* allele are younger at the onset of hepatitis, have a more active disease than those with other HLA alleles, are less likely to enter remission, and relapse more frequently during and after withdrawal of cortico-steroid therapy (Czaja, Gastro, 1990; 98:1587; Czaja, Gastro, 1993; 105:1502; Doherty, Hepatol, 1994; 19:609). Consequently, liver transplantation is needed more often in HLA-DR3-positive patients. It seems that patients with HLA-DR4 are more likely to develop concurrent extrahepatic diseases. The situation is different in Japan where autoimmune hepatitis type 1 is rare and no as-sociation with HLA-DR3 is found, whereas there is an association with HLA-DR4 (Seki, Hepatol, 1990; 12:1300). There is also a highly significant association with HLA-B54: 45 per cent in patients with autoimmune hepatitis compared with 11 per cent in controls.

The HLA class III region has been studied in autoimmune hepatitis with particular emphasis on the genes for complement C2, C4A, C4B, and factor B. Studies on complement polymorphism revealed low concentrations of C4 in autoimmune hepatitis type 1. This was associated with deletions in the gene for C4A, responsible for an increase in the *C4A-Q0* alleles (Vergani, Lancet, 1985; 346: 608; Scully, Gastro, 1993; 104:1478). Since C4 is involved in the clearance of immune complexes, its low concentrations might indicate the involvement of a viral agent in the pathogenesis of the disease.

Only limited data are available on the genetic background of autoimmune hepatitis type 2, but an association with HLA-DR3 is reported (Lenzi, JHepatol, 1992; 16:59; Manns, Hepatol, 1992; 14: A60).[3] Further preliminary findings indicate an association with HLA-B14, HLA-DQ2, and C4A-Q0.

Recent advances in molecular biology have resulted in further progress on the immunogenetic background of autoimmune hep-atitis, in particular X-ray crystallography of the purified antigens HLA-A2 and -DR1 and the development of polymerase chain reaction-based, HLA-genotyping techniques. Patients with auto-immune hepatitis type 1 had a very high frequency of the *HLA-DRB1*0301-DRB3*0101-DQA1*0501-DQB1*0201* haplotype (52 per cent as compared to 19 per cent of controls) and there was a strong secondary association with one of the *HLA-DR4* alleles *DRB1*0401* (54 per cent of the *DRB3*0101*-negative patients compared to 23 per cent of *DRB3*0101*-negative controls) (Doherty, Hepatol, 1994; 19:609). *HLA-DRB* genes are more strongly associated with the disease than *-DQA* or *-DQB*. A strong association was found for a single amino-acid residue, lysine, at position 71 of the HLA-DRβ polypeptide (Doherty, Hepatol, 1994; 19:609). Lysine DRβ71 is encoded by *DRB1*0301* and *DRB1*0401* as well as by all of the *HLA-DRB3* alleles. The implicit involvement of DRβ71 is supported by the results of a study on patients from North America (Strettell, Gastro, 1996; 110:A1335) but not by data from Japan (Ota, Immunogenet, 1992; 36:49; Seki, Hepatol, 1993; 18:73) or Argentina (Marcos, Hepatol, 1994; 19:1371). Studies on Japanese patients indicate that basic amino acids at position 13 of the HLA-DR β-polypeptide (DRβ13) are responsible for the second HLA-DR4 association found in their late-onset, autoimmune hep-atitis type 1.

Our knowledge on the immunogenetic susceptibility to liver disease is still incomplete. However, future work will help to define better the genetic background at the amino-acid level, that is, to identify particular amino acids at the bottom of the groove of the HLA class II molecule as risk factors for the various subgroups of autoimmune hepatitis in adult and juvenile, European and Asian patients. These studies should help to identify patients at risk and

those likely to experience a severe disease course or concurrent extrahepatic syndromes. Hopefully we will better understand the pathogenetic mechanisms of tissue destruction by T lymphocytes, so that new therapeutic strategies can emerge. For further reading the reader is referred to recent review articles.[9,10]

Experimental autoimmune hepatitis

Several animal models for experimental autoimmune hepatitis have been described (Meyer zum Büschenfelde, ClinExpImmun, 1972; 10:99; Mori, Hepatol, 1985; 5:770). Most experiments have been on mice, but experiments on the rat or rabbit are also reported. In a mouse model, experimental autoimmune hepatitis was induced by intraperitoneal immunization with the $100\,000\,g$ supernatant of syngeneic liver homogenate (S100) in complete Freund adjuvant (Lohse, SemLivDis, 1991; 11:241). The most susceptible inbred mouse strain was C57Bl/6, and less susceptible were Balb/c or C3H; experimental autoimmune hepatitis could not be induced in Lewis rats (Lohse, Hepatol, 1990; 11:24). Intraperitoneal im-munization was more effective than intramuscular or subcutaneous immunization. A single injection of S100 in complete Freund adjuvant led to biochemical and histological signs of hepatitis. At week 2, alanine aminotransferase was elevated and, histologically, perivascular inflammatory infiltrates and moderate liver damage were visible. The peak of the disease was at week 4, followed by biochemical and histological recovery; aminotransferases were normal at 8 weeks, with histological recovery taking up to 6 months. In experimental autoimmune hepatitis, characteristic autoantibodies directed against only a few target proteins appeared several weeks after disease induction and titres rose continuously, even after the biochemical and histological effects had regressed. However, the targets differed from those in human autoimmune hepatitis. Based on the lateness of the development of the autoantibodies and the lack of correlation between antibody titres and severity of disease, it has been concluded that these autoantibodies are not critical to the pathogenesis of experimental autoimmune hepatitis (Lohse, JHepatol, 1992; 14:48).

In contrast, T-cell reactivity was critical for the development of experimental autoimmune hepatitis since it could be induced by the transfer of T cells from diseased to naive animals. However, the adoptively transferred disease was milder than the antigen-induced, active disease. In the course of experimental autoimmune hepatitis, T-cell reactivity to liver antigens precedes the histologically dem-onstrable disease (Araki, ClinExpImmun, 1987; 67:326). At the peak of the disease the T-cell response is already suppressed. The suppression is active and antigen-specific: 42 per cent suppression was measured *in vitro* using soluble liver antigens, while suppression was only 16 per cent when using tetanus toxoid as an irrelevant antigen. The suppressive effect was even more pronounced in *in vivo* studies with tetanus toxoid at the peak of the disease, where more than 90 per cent inhibition was found in animals with ex-perimental autoimmune hepatitis. These findings show that *in vitro* and *in vivo* immunosuppression is associated with recovery from experimental autoimmune hepatitis and they emphasize the in-volvement of immunoregulatory circuits in autoimmune hepatitis (Lohse, ClinExpImmun, 1993; 94:163). Interestingly, an analogous immunosuppression was shown in patients with autoimmune hepatitis type 1 who went into remission after immunosuppressive treatment. This indicates that in man also, active immuno-suppression facilitates recovery from autoimmune hepatitis (Lohse, Hepatol, 1995; 22:381).

Clinical features

Autoimmune hepatitis may present at any age in either sex, although it occurs most frequently in females between the ages of 10 and 30 years or in late middle age.[1] In around 30 per cent of cases the presentation is acute and may mimic that of an acute viral hepatitis. Autoantibodies may be lacking in the acute phase and appear in serum several weeks after the onset of the disease. In the remainder the onset is insidious and the disease may not be recognized until liver damage is advanced. The frequency of the various clinical manifestations has been similar in the major reported series. A significant proportion of patients will be jaundiced at presentation. Anorexia, fatigue, and amenorrhoea are common. Abdominal pain, often related to hepatic tenderness, occurs in 10 to 40 per cent; up to 20 per cent may have a fever at presentation. Most patients will have palpable hepatomegaly and 50 per cent a palpable spleen. Patients frequently have spider naevi, which may reflect changes in the activity of the disease. Between 30 and 80 per cent of patients will already have progressed to cirrhosis by the time of presentation, and 10 to 20 per cent may already have evidence of decompensated cirrhosis with ascites and, less commonly, encephalopathy. Around 20 per cent of patients will have evidence of oesophageal varices.

Extrahepatic manifestations occur frequently. In a study of 108 patients with chronic hepatitis of various causes, 63 per cent had evidence of disease in at least one organ other than the liver.[9] Arthropathy and periarticular swelling occurs in 6 to 36 per cent, affecting both large and small joints; it is usually transient and reflects disease activity but occasionally an erosive arthritis may occur. Skin rashes occur in around 20 per cent of cases and may take the form of a pleomorphic maculopapular or an acneiform rash. Allergic capillaritis, lichen planus, and leg ulcers occur commonly. Very occasionally the patient may appear cushingoid, with ab-dominal striae, before the start of any therapy. There are associations with other diseases, particularly ulcerative colitis, in which there appears to be an overlap syndrome with primary sclerosing cho-langitis. Particularly in children, primary sclerosing cholangitis may initially present as a chronic hepatitis (El-Shabrawi, Gastro, 1987; 12:1226). There is also an increased incidence of various auto-immune and other diseases including autoimmune thyroiditis, Sjög-ren's syndrome, renal tubular acidosis, fibrosing alveolitis, peripheral neuropathy, and glomerulonephritis. Hepatitis may be part of the autoimmune polyglandular syndrome type 1. In this multiorgan autoimmune endocrine disease, hypoparathyroidism, adrenal and ovarian insufficiency as well as mucocutaneous can-didiasis are the major organ manifestations. However, in 10 to 20 per cent the liver may be involved, presumably as a specific form of autoimmune hepatitis. This may present as chronic hepatitis, acute hepatitis, or even fulminant hepatic failure. This polyglandular syndrome is an autosomal-recessive genetic disorder that is endemic in Scandinavia and Sardinia. The gene locus is on chromosome 21.

Serological diagnosis

As in many other autoimmune diseases the diagnosis of autoimmune hepatitis is based on several clinical and laboratory measures. The International Autoimmune Hepatitis Group has defined the dia-gnostic criteria and has given them specific scores (Table 1): hy-pergammaglobulinaemia, female sex, genetic markers, absence of markers of viral hepatitis, and last but not least autoantibodies.

Several autoantibodies are of relevance to the diagnosis of auto-immune hepatitis. Most are listed as diagnostic criteria for auto-immune hepatitis by the International Autoimmune Hepatitis Group.[1] (Table 1). ANA, the most important and earliest-defined markers of autoimmune hepatitis type 1, are diagnostically relevant when detected by immunofluorescence at a titre of more than 1:40. As mentioned above, ANA are determined by indirect immuno-fluorescence on rodent liver and kidney tissue, but nowadays, tissue cultures with Hep 2 cells are preferred in many laboratories. They are very heterogeneous. For routine purposes their detection by immunofluorescence is sufficient and subtyping of ANA has not shown any diagnostic relevance to routine clinical practice.

Cytoskeletal antibodies are also of diagnostic relevance in auto-immune hepatitis type 1. SMA are detected by indirect immuno-fluorescence on rodent liver and kidney, with staining of vessel walls, and on stomach due to staining of the muscle layer. SMA in liver diseases, in particular autoimmune hepatitis, are directed against F-actin. A titre of more than 1:80 is regarded as dia-gnostically significant. SMA can be the only marker of autoimmune hepatitis if at high titre; this is particularly relevant in children with autoimmune hepatitis (Odievre, Hepatol, 1983; 3:407). Low SMA titres are frequently observed in chronic viral hepatitis, but usually lack F-actin specificity.

LKM antibodies are also primarily determined by indirect immunofluorescence.[11] LKM-1 antibodies are themselves hetero-geneous; they are markers of autoimmune hepatitis type 2.[3] Their main target antigen is human cytochrome P450 2D6, as explained above (Zanger, PNAS, 1988; 85:8256; Gueguen, BBResComm, 1989; 159:542; Manns, JCI, 1989; 83:1066). LM antibodies reacting with cytochrome P450 1A2 occur either in drug-induced hepatitis due to dihydralazine or in autoimmune hepatitis as part of the autoimmune polyendocrine syndrome type 1.

Antibodies to cytosolic antigens are either detectable by fluor-escence as anti-LC1 and anti-LC2 antibodies, or by Ouchterlony immunodiffusion (Martini, Hepatol, 1988; 8:1662). Antibodies to soluble liver antigen (anti-SLA), or antiliver–pancreas antigen (anti-LP) are detectable by enzyme-linked immunsorbent assay and characterize a third subgroup of autoimmune hepatitis. Anti-LC1 and -LC2 antibodies usually occur together with LKM-1 antibodies and seem to characterize autoimmune hepatitis type 2.

Other autoantibodies are directed against antigens of the liver-cell membrane, notably the ASGP-R (see above). ASGP-R is liver-specific and membrane-associated. It is of interest for pathogenetic studies. Anti-ASGP-R antibodies occur very frequently in auto-immune hepatitis type 1; in addition, they occur in primary biliary cirrhosis and in some patients with chronic viral hepatitis (McFarlane, ClinExpImmun, 1984; 55:347; Treichel, Gastro, 1994; 107:799).

Antimitochondrial antibodies, as determined by indirect immunofluorescence, are markers of primary biliary cirrhosis and should be negative in autoimmune hepatitis; they therefore received a negative score from the International Autoimmune Hepatitis Group as a diagnostic criterion for autoimmune hepatitis.

The determination of HLA phenotypes or even HLA alleles at the DNA level is usually not necessary for routine clinical practice. Certainly a few cases of autoimmune hepatitis respond to corticosteroids but are negative for all marker autoantibodies; in these cases, the finding of HLA-DR3 or HLA-DR4 would support a diagnosis of autoimmune hepatitis. Possibly more sophisticated and more specific genetic markers of the MHC locus determined at the DNA level might be even more helpful in the future.

Relevance of subtypes of autoimmune hepatitis

There is a debate as to whether autoimmune hepatitis can be further differentiated into serologically distinct subgroups. The International Autoimmune Hepatitis Group[1] thought the evidence too preliminary to justify the subtyping of autoimmune hepatitis at present, partly because of the lack of availability of sophisticated autoantibody testing in routine laboratories.

There are two possibilities for distinct subgroupings of autoimmune hepatitis.[5] The most widely used is based on autoantibody profiles. Autoimmune hepatitis type 1 is characterized by ANA with or without SMA and represents by far the most common subgroup. Although recent research in many centres has focused on autoimmune hepatitis type 2, with its anti-P450 and anti-UGT autoimmunity, one should not forget that autoimmune hepatitis type 1 is by far the commonest form. Autoimmune hepatitis type 2 characterized by LKM-1 antibodies against P450 2D6 is rarely seen in the United States, Australia, and Japan. Furthermore, most of our knowledge on the genetic background and on the treatment response, as well as on long-term outcome after liver transplantation, is based on type 1.

On the other hand several arguments support the distinction of autoimmune hepatitis type 1 from types 2 and 3. Type 2 has a more specific autoantibody profile than the heterogeneous ANA response. Furthermore, patients with type 2 seem to suffer more frequently from fulminant hepatic failure and extrahepatic syndromes; low IgA concentrations are also more common. Autoimmune hepatitis type 2 is particularly frequent in childhood/adolescent patients and the geographical difference in its prevalence argues for a different aetiological background. The case of autoimmune hepatitis type 3 is more difficult. Certainly there are cases of autoimmune hepatitis that are negative for the usual autoantibody markers (ANA, SMA, LKM-1) and anti-SLA/LP antibodies may identify such patients. However, these patients with autoimmune hepatitis type 3 share the clinical and genetic characteristics of type 1.

Another subgrouping is based on the genetic background. Patients with HLA-DR3 are younger at onset, have a more rapid disease progression, and more frequently experience relapse after treatment. HLA-DR3-positive individuals are over-represented among patients with autoimmune hepatitis who are candidates for liver transplantation. A second subgroup is associated with HLA-DR4. These patients are older at onset, have a slower disease process, and usually respond better to immunosuppression. In Japan, autoimmune hepatitis is restricted to the HLA-DR4-positive group. Further development of the DNA-based technology to identify HLA alleles and even particular amino acids as risk factors will further help to clarify the issue of subgroups of autoimmune hepatitis.

Differential diagnosis
Liver disease in the autoimmune polyendocrine syndrome type 1

The autoimmune polyendocrine syndrome type 1 is a rare, autosomal-recessive disorder characterized by a variable combination of disease components.[12] The first clinical manifestation of the syndrome usually occurs in childhood and progressively new components may appear throughout life, with most (63 per cent) of the patients suffering from three to five of them. The most frequent components are chronic mucocutaneous candidiasis, hypoparathyroidism, adrenocortical and gonadal failure in females, with autoimmune hepatitis a serious but less frequent component. In contrast to other autoimmune diseases, female predominance and linkage to HLA-DR do not exist (Ahonen, JClinEndoc, 1988; 66: 1152). The locus for the syndrome has been assigned to the long arm of chromosome 21 (Altonen, NatureGen, 1994; 8:83). Lymphocytic infiltration of the affected organs and the presence of organ-specific autoantibodies are typical features. The first hepatic autoantigen in autoimmune hepatitis related to autoimmune polyendocrine syndrome type 1 has recently been identified (Clemente, JClinEndoc, 1997; 82:1353).

Autoimmunity associated with viral hepatitis
Hepatitis C

Chronic infection with hepatitis C virus (HCV) is known to induce autoimmune reactions. Hepatitis C is associated with an array of extrahepatic manifestations, including mixed cryoglobulinaemia, membranoproliferative glomerulonephritis, polyarthritis, porphyria cutanea tarda, Sjögren's syndrome, and autoimmune thyroid disease. Not surprisingly, numerous autoantibodies are apparently associated with chronic hepatitis C. As for autoimmune hepatitis, antibodies against tissues, including ANA, SMA, LKM, and antithyroid antibodies, are found very frequently (Pawlotsky, Hepatol, 1994; 19:841). Anti-GOR is a disease-specific autoantibody that is present in at least 80 per cent of sera from patients with HCV hepatitis. The epitope recognized by anti-GOR (GRRGQKAKSNPNRPL) is located on a nuclear protein that is overexpressed in hepatocellular carcinoma (Mishiro, Lancet, 1990; 336:1400). Interestingly, anti-GOR is not associated with autoimmune hepatitis, but is specific for hepatitis induced by HCV (Michel, Lancet, 1992; 339:267). Depending on the geographical origin, a variable proportion of patients with anti-LKM-1-associated liver disease are infected with HCV. The prevalence of HCV infection among LKM-1-positive patients is about 90 per cent in Italy (Lenzi, Lancet, 1991; 338:277), about 50 per cent in France and Germany (Lunel, Hepatol, 1992; 16:630; Michel, Lancet, 1992; 339:267), and less than 10 per cent in England (Lenzi, Lancet, 1991; 338:277). Overall, 0 to 7 per cent of patients with chronic hepatitis C are positive for LKM-1 antibodies. Interferon

Table 3 Clinical features of autoimmune hepatitis type 2 and HCV-associated autoimmunity (LKM)

	Autoimmune hepatitis type 2	Chronic hepatitis C associated with LKM-1 autoantibodies
Age	Young	Older
Sex	90% female	No prevalence
ALT	↑↑↑	↑
LKM-1 titre	↑↑↑	↑
Immunosuppressive effective	+ + +	−
Interferon effective	−	(+) possibly side-effects increased
HLA-DR3	+ +	+
C4A-Q0	+	+
anti-HCV/HCV RNA	−	+

ALT, alanine aminotransferase; HCV, hepatitis C virus; LKM, liver–kidney microsomal antibodies.

seems an effective treatment, but the liver disease may worsen in some patients (Table 3).

Chronic hepatitis D

Crivelli *et al.* (JExpImmunol, 1983; 54:237) found that 11 of 81 patients with chronic hepatitis D had serum antibodies against microsomes from the liver and proximal renal tubules. Since these antibodies differed from LKM-1 and LKM-2 they were termed LKM-3. The molecular target of the LKM-3 autoantibody was identified by screening a cDNA library, which revealed UGT 1.6 as the reactant (Philipp, Lancet, 1994; 344:578). Western blotting with recombinant rabbit UGT 1.6 was used to characterize the clinical associations of LKM-3 autoantibodies. These were detected only in hepatitis D and autoimmune hepatitis, and not in hepatitis B, hepatitis C, primary biliary cirrhosis, primary sclerosing cholangitis, and lupus erythematosus.

Immune-mediated, drug-induced hepatitis

Because of its central role in xenobiotic metabolism the liver is an important target for adverse drug reactions. In the course of normal metabolism, many drugs may form unstable metabolites that bind to cellular proteins or DNA; their direct toxic effects may lead to cell death or cancer (Guengerich, AmSci, 1993; 81:440). However, if the protein adducts formed in this process are presented to the immune system as neoantigens, an immune response may eventually be induced, including the production of autoantibodies, inflammation of the liver, and necrosis. This type of immunoallergic reaction represents drug-induced hepatitis. Hepatitis induced by tienilic acid and dihydralazine has been intensively investigated and provides a hypothesis for the induction of autoantibodies and T-cell responses (Pessayre, ProgrHepatol, 1993; 23; Beaune, AdvPharm, 1994; 30:199).

Tienilic acid-induced hepatitis

Tienilic acid, a uricosuric drug used in hypertension, was withdrawn from the market because of rare cases of severe drug-induced hepatitis. The hepatitis was dose-independent and occurred with a delay ranging from 14 to 240 days after the start of drug treatment (Zimmerman, Hepatol, 1984; 4:315). Females and males were equally affected. After discontinuation of the drug liver damage resolved, but rechallenge resulted in symptoms after a shorter period. These patients produced a new specific antibody directed against unmodified liver and kidney microsomal proteins (LKM-2) (Homberg, ClinExpImmun, 1984; 55:561; Hepatol, 1985; 5:722) which were later identified as cytochrome P450 2C9, the major tienilic acid-metabolizing enzyme in the liver (Beaune, PNAS, 1987; 84:51).

Dihydralazine-induced hepatitis

Long-term treatment with the hypertensive drug dihydralazine has been associated with many reports of hepatitis.[13] This type of drug-induced hepatitis affects females more than males, the ratio being of 7:2 (Roschlau, ZKlinMed, 1986; 41:817). Most patients are of the slow-acetylator phenotype. The hepatitis is usually delayed, with a latent period of several months, and it resolves after discontinuation of the drug. Rechallenge with the drug results in recurrence (Reinhardt, DtschZVerdauStoffwechselkr, 1985; 45:283). Inflammatory infiltrates include mononuclear cells, neutrophils, and eosinophils. In several patients a positive lymphocyte transformation was reported. Dihydralazine hepatitis is associated with LM antibodies that do not stain kidney sections (Homberg, ClinExpImmun, 1984; 55:561; Bourdi, JCI, 1990; 85:1967). The target protein was identified as cytochrome P450 1A2. LM autoantibodies are very specific. Despite a high sequence homology between cytochromes P450 1A1 and P450 1A2, no cross-reaction with cloned human P450 1A1 was observed (Bourdi, JCI, 1990; 85:1967; MolPharm, 1992; 42:280).

Cryptogenic hepatitis

About 10 to 20 per cent of patients with chronic hepatitis are classified as cryptogenic since no specific cause can be identified.[2] These cases may be due either to unknown viruses or to mutants of

Table 4 Treatment of autoimmune hepatitis

	Single drug regimen	Combination regimen
Prednisolone	50 mg for 10 days; then tapering down to a maintenance dose of 20 mg or lower as required	50 mg for 10 days; taper 5 mg every 10 days; maintenance 10 mg or lower as required
Azathioprine	None	100 mg for 3 weeks; 50 mg
Upon remission (after 24 months treatment): Prednisolone	Taper 2.5 mg every week	Taper 2.5 mg every week
Azathioprine	None	Taper 25 mg every 3 weeks
Follow-up		

Test	Before therapy	During therapy (every 4 weeks)	In remission	After treatment withdrawal	
				Every 3 weeks for 3 months	Every 3 months thereafter
Physical examination	+	+	+	+	+
Liver biopsy	+		+		
Blood count	+	+	+	+	+
Aminotransferases	+	+	+	+	+
γ-Glutamyl transferase	+	+	+		
Gammaglobulin	+	+	+	+	+
Bilirubin	+	+	+	+	+
Coagulation	+	+	+	+	+
Autoantibodies	+	+/−			
Thyroid function	+	+/−			

known viruses, but may also be of autoimmune type, although negative for characteristic autoantibodies. A positive response to immunosuppression, as well as genetic markers, may help to diagnose the presence of autoimmune hepatitis.

Overlap syndromes (see also Chapter 14.6)

Primary biliary cirrhosis is usually not a diagnostic problem, owing to the detection of antimitochrondrial antibodies against acyl-transferases, in particular antibodies to the E2 subunit of pyruvate dehydrogenase. There is debate about whether antimitochondrial antibody-negative primary biliary cirrhosis exists. Several groups have observed patients with clinical and morphological characteristics of primary biliary cirrhosis who are negative for antimitochondrial antibodies but positive for ANA. Such studies do not include enough patients to draw final conclusions. These cases are called autoimmune cholangitis and seem to respond to immunosuppression (Brunner, DeutschMedWschr, 1987; 12: 1454).

The condition of another group of patients became known as the chronic active hepatitis/primary biliary cirrhosis overlap syndrome. These are patients who share the characteristics of both autoimmune hepatitis and primary biliary cirrhosis. Histologically they present with piecemeal necrosis and periductular infiltration of the portal tracts with bile-duct destruction. They are positive for antimitochondrial antibodies and ANA, and seem to profit from immunosuppressive treatment. A specific antimitochondrial antibody does not seem to be associated with this syndrome (Davis,

Hepatol, 1992; 16:1128; Palmer, JHepatol, 1993; 18:251) as had been assumed before (Berg, Lancet, 1980; ii:1329). While the overlap syndrome between primary biliary cirrhosis and autoimmune hepatitis is described in adults, overlap between primary sclerosing cholangitis and autoimmune hepatitis is described in children (Mieli-Vergani, Hepatol, 1989; 9:198). These patients show typical strictures and dilatations of the bile ducts on endoscopic retrograde cholangiography while typical histological lesions of chronic hepatitis are evident on liver biopsy. Again, high titres of ANA are the serological hallmarks.

Treatment

The treatment of choice for autoimmune hepatitis is immunosuppression. The standard treatment is either prednisolone alone or a combination of prednisolone and azathioprine (Table 4). Both prednisolone monotherapy or combination treatment are effective in inducing remission. We prefer prednisolone monotherapy in children and young females, and in adults we prefer combination therapy if there are no contraindications to the use of azathioprine, such as leucopenia or drug-induced cholestasis. Either prednisolone or prednisone can be used; prednisone is the prodrug that is converted to prednisolone in the liver. The metabolism of prednisone into prednisolone is not affected in patients with liver cirrhosis.

The standard treatment regimens have been used worldwide for many years.[14] Immunosuppression improved the survival of patients with severe autoimmune hepatitis (Kirk, Gut, 1980; 21:78). It has been suggested that cases with mild to moderate inflammatory activity need not be treated, but this view is controversial. Clinical remission is followed by biochemical and then histological remission. About 65 per cent of patients experience complete clinical, biochemical, and histological remission. Treatment should be continued for 2 years. If complete remission is not achieved within 24 months there should be no further continuation of treatment. Up to 80 per cent of responders may experience a relapse after the end of the 2-year treatment period; if so, a long-term, low-dose immunosuppressive treatment should be introduced to maintain remission. There are two alternatives, either low-dose prednisolone, between 5 and 15 mg/day, or azathioprine monotherapy, 2 mg per kg body wt.[15] While azathioprine alone does not induce remission, this drug as monotherapy can maintain remission for a long time.[15] Recent data on the long-term use of azathioprine in transplant recipients have shown that it confers less oncogenic risk and has fewer teratogenic complications than previously suspected.

There seems to be a difference in the response to standard treatment depending on the genetic background. Patients with HLA-DR3 experience full remission less frequently, and relapse rates are higher than in HLA-DR3-negative patients. Consequently, HLA-DR3 is more prevalent among transplanted patients from Europe and Northern America who had autoimmune hepatitis. If standard treatment with prednisolone alone or in combination with azathioprine fails to induce remission, other immunosuppressive drugs including cyclosporin, FK 506, Mofetil, and cyclophosphamide may be tried. However, an adequate response has been shown for only a minor proportion of such patients in single case reports.

Liver transplantation is very effective in the endstage of autoimmune hepatitis with cirrhosis (Sanchez-Urdazapal, Hepatol, 1992; 15:215), given that cirrhosis may develop despite complete biochemical remission under long-term immunosuppressive treatment. Autoimmune hepatitis is among the best indications for liver transplantation, with long-term survival rates of more than 90 per cent after 5 years. Although the recurrence of autoimmune hepatitis after liver transplantation has been reported in some cases, this does not prejudice the long-term outcome. Furthermore, immunosuppressive treatment is started immediately after liver transplantation.

Steroids which are rapidly metabolized by the liver, such as budesonide, are under clinical investigation for autoimmune hepatitis. Budesonide has a 90 per cent first-pass uptake by the liver. The idea is that the drug reaches pathogenetically relevant lymphocytes within the liver before being metabolized. Hepatic metabolism then prevents severe systemic side-effects such as bone disease. A Swedish group has shown that budesonide normalizes elevated transaminase concentrations in autoimmune hepatitis.[16] Our own studies in a limited number of patients have confirmed that budesonide is effective in reducing liver transaminases, and the concentrations of cortisol in the peripheral blood are hardly changed if the patient has not yet developed cirrhosis with portosystemic shunts.[17]

References

1. Johnson PJ and McFarlane IG. Meeting report of the International Autoimmune Hepatitis Group. *Hepatology*, 1993; **18**: 998–1005.

2. Desmet V, Gerber MA, Hoofnagle JH, Manns M, and Scheuer P. Classification of chronic hepatitis: diagnosis, grading and staging. *Hepatology*, 1994; **9**: 1513–20.

3. Homberg JC, *et al.* Chronic active hepatitis associated with anti-liver/kidney microsome antibody type I: a second type of 'autoimmune hepatitis'. *Hepatology*, 1987; **197**: 1333–9.

4. Manns M, Gerken G, Kyriatsoulis A, Staritz M, and Meyer zum Büschenfelde K-H. Characterization of a new subgroup of autoimmune chronic active hepatitis by autoantibodies against soluble liver antigen. *Lancet*, 1987; i: 292–4

5. Czaja AJ and Manns MP. The validity and importance of subtypes in autoimmune hepatitis: a point of view. *American Journal of Gastroenterology*, 1995; **90**: 1206–11.

6. Strassburg CP and Manns MP. Viral hepatitis and autoimmunity: chicken or egg? *Viral Hepatitis*, 1995; **1**: 97–102.

7. Peter JB and Schoenfeld Y. *Autoantibodies*. Elsevier, Amsterdam 1996.

8. Vergani D and Mieli-Vergani G. Autoimmune hepatitis: cellular immune reactions. In Meyer zum Büschenfelde K-H, Hoofnagle J, and Manns M, eds. *Immunology and liver*. Dordrecht: Kluwer Academic, 1993: 233–9.

9. Manns M and Krüger M. Immunogenetics in liver diseases. *Gastroenterology*, 1994; **106**: 1676–97.

10. Donaldson PT. Immunogenetics in liver disease. In Manns MP, ed. *Liver and gastrointestinal immunology*. Vol. 10. *Baillière's clinical gastroentrology*. London: Baillière Tindall, 1996: 533–49

11. Rizzetto M, Swana G, and Doniach D. Microsomal antibodies in active chronic hepatitis and other disorders. *Clinical and Experimental Immunology*, 1973; **15**: 331–44.

12. Ahonen P, Myllrniemi S, Sipil I, and Perheentupa J. Clinical variation of autoimmune polyendocrinopathy-candidiasis-ectodermal dystrophy (APECED) in a series of 68 patients. *New England Journal of Medicine*, 1990; **322**: 1829–36.

13. Stricker BHC. *Drug-induced hepatic injury*. Amsterdam: Elsevier, 1992.

14. Czaja AJ. Autoimmune hepatitis. Current therapeutic concepts. *Clinical Immunotherapy*, 1994; **6**: 413–29.

15. Johnson PJ, McFarlane IG, and Williams R. Azathioprine for long-term maintenance of remission in autoimmune hepatitis. *New England Journal of Medicine*, 1995; **333**: 958–63.

16. Danielson A and Prytz H. Oral budesonide for treatment of autoimmune chronic active hepatitis. *Alimentary Pharmacology and Therapeutics*, 1994; **8**: 585–90.

17. Schüler A and Manns MP. In Arroyo V, Bosch J, and Rodés J, eds. *Treatment in hepatology*. Barcelona: Masson, 1995: 375.

14.4 Sclerosing cholangitis

Nicholas F. Larusso, Russell H. Wiesner, and Jurgen Ludwig

Introduction

Primary sclerosing cholangitis is an incurable illness that is usually progressive and often fatal. A syndrome of unknown aetiology, it is characterized by cholestasis due to diffuse inflammation and fibrosis which may involve the entire biliary system. Delbet identified the syndrome for the first time in 1924 (Delbet, BullMemSocChirParis, 1924; 50:1144).

The pathological process leads to narrowing and obliteration of intrahepatic bile ducts and ultimately to biliary cirrhosis. The clinical course is variable, but generally there is slow progression, perhaps over decades, to portal hypertension, and eventually premature death from liver failure.

Primary sclerosing cholangitis may occur alone, but in more than 70 per cent of cases is associated with inflammatory bowel disease. Diagnosis is usually based on a combination of clinical, biochemical, and radiological abnormalities, although histological abnormalities that are highly suggestive or even pathognomonic are seen occasionally in biopsy specimens of the liver.

In years past, primary sclerosing cholangitis was generally diagnosed in its late stage, when the patient was very ill, markedly jaundiced, and usually when exploratory laparotomy was necessary to identify the diseased bile ducts and to establish the diagnosis. More recently, non-surgical diagnostic tests such as endoscopic retrograde cholangiography (**ERC**) have become available, and the syndrome can now be recognized earlier, without the need for surgery, and sometimes in the asymptomatic stage.

Definition

Sclerosing cholangitis is a clinical syndrome rather than a specific disease. It is usually characterized by progressive fatigue, pruritus, and jaundice. These symptoms are due to diffuse structural abnormalities in the bile ducts.[1] In contrast to many of the syndromes for which the commonly used terminology does not accurately depict the pathological process, the designation 'sclerosing cholangitis' is both appropriate and accurate. 'Sclerosing' indicates induration due to chronic inflammation, especially induration by hyperplasia of fibres of connective tissue. Diffuse inflammation and scar tissue are seen in bile ducts microscopically.

The literal definition of cholangitis is inflammation of the bile ducts. Thus, cholangitis is a term that accurately describes the pathological process. However, physicians also use this term in a purely clinical sense to represent episodes of fever, jaundice, and abdominal pain.

Table 1 Syndrome of sclerosing cholangitis

Primary
  With/without associated inflammatory bowel disease
Secondary
  Stones
  Stricture
  Cancer
  Drugs
  Infection
  Congenital anomalies

The syndrome of sclerosing cholangitis may be primary or it may be secondary to congenital abnormalities of the bile ducts, cholangiocarcinoma, infection, drugs, postoperative stricture, or choledocholithiasis (Table 1). This chapter will focus entirely on the primary variety. The term 'primary' is used to indicate that this form of sclerosing cholangitis is idiopathic. When sclerosing cholangitis occurs in association with inflammatory bowel disease some authors have been reluctant to use the designation 'primary' because they regard the hepatobiliary disease as secondary to the intestinal condition. However, although a complex relationship exists between sclerosing cholangitis and inflammatory bowel disease, there is no evidence that the former is caused by the latter.

The term 'pericholangitis' is often used, by both pathologists and clinicians, as a designation for chronic hepatitis in patients with chronic ulcerative colitis. In fact, pericholangitis is a descriptive morphological term most appropriately used to designate the presence of inflammation around interlobular or septal bile ducts as seen on biopsy of the liver. However, because this term is so widely misunderstood, an international panel has deleted it from its list of descriptive terms for diseases of the liver.[2]

Primary sclerosing cholangitis can be further defined in terms of involvement of the biliary system, and findings on cholangiography and liver biopsy (Table 2). Global primary sclerosing cholangitis involves the bile ducts both inside and outside the liver, is characterized by cholangiographic abnormalities of intra- and extrahepatic bile ducts, and displays typical findings on liver biopsy. Large-duct primary sclerosing cholangitis involves principally the extrahepatic ducts and those parts of the intrahepatic biliary ductal system that can be visualized cholangiographically; liver biopsy may or may not show characteristic findings. Small-duct primary sclerosing cholangitis involves the intrahepatic ducts at the microscopic level and is characterized by typical findings on liver biopsy;

Table 2 Classification of primary sclerosing cholangitis (PSC)

Diagnostic term	Cholangiography	Hepatic histology
Classic/global PSC	Typically abnormal	Typically abnormal
Small-duct PSC ('pericholangitis')	Typically not diagnostic	Typically abnormal
Large-duct PSC (extra- or intrahepatic)	Typically abnormal	Typically not diagnostic

in this condition cholangiography may show ducts of relatively normal appearance.

Epidemiology

Primary sclerosing cholangitis was once considered a rare disease; fewer than 100 cases were reported in the English language literature before 1980. Recent experience, however, suggests that it is much more common than previously thought. Many studies, particularly since the introduction of ERC in the early 1970s, have indicated an increased frequency of diagnosis of this syndrome. Whether this represents a true increase in the incidence of the syndrome, or whether it reflects, as seems more likely, increased clinical awareness and availability of diagnostic tests such as ERC, is not yet clear.

Although there are virtually no data regarding the prevalence of the disease, it is possible to make some reasonable estimates. For example, the prevalence of chronic ulcerative colitis in the United States is between 40 and 100 cases per 100 000 population. Since several studies have indicated that approximately 3 to 5 per cent of patients with chronic ulcerative colitis have primary sclerosing cholangitis (Schrumpf, ScaJGastr, 1982; 17:33), one can estimate the prevalence of the latter to be between 1 and 4 cases per 100 000 population. This estimate suggests that primary sclerosing cholangitis is considerably more common than was previously thought and that there are between 2500 and 10 000 cases in the United States at present. We suspect that this is an underestimate.

Primary sclerosing cholangitis is principally a disease of young men.[3] Seventy per cent of patients are male, and the average age at the time of diagnosis is 40 years. The age range (2 to 75 years) is the same in both sexes. The reason for this sex and age distribution is not apparent. Moreover, there appear to be no major differences between male and female patients with regard to frequency of associated inflammatory bowel disease or complications of cirrhosis and portal hypertension.

Pathophysiology

The cause of primary sclerosing cholangitis is at present unknown; genetic factors, acquired factors, or both could be involved (Table 3). Several recent observations are consistent with an important role for genetic factors. For example, the frequency of HLA B8 is significantly higher in patients with primary sclerosing cholangitis (60 per cent) than in controls (25 per cent) (Chapman, Gut, 1981; 22:871). Other studies have also established an association of primary sclerosing cholangitis with the HLA haplotype A1 B8 DR3 Drw52a (Donaldson, Hepatol, 1991; 13:129); whether or not there is an association between a particular HLA haplotype (e.g. DR4) and prognosis in primary sclerosing cholangitis is unclear (Olerup,

Table 3 Pathogenetic factors in primary sclerosing cholangitis

Genetic
HLA haplotypes
Familial occurrence
Acquired
Toxins
Infectious agents
Altered immunity

Gastro, 1995; 108:870). Also, recent reports have described the familial occurrence of both primary sclerosing cholangitis and chronic ulcerative colitis, and this is further evidence for a genetic component to the disease (Quigley, Gastro, 1983; 85:1160).

Potential acquired factors include toxins, infectious agents, or altered immunity. Although elevated hepatic copper levels, a nearly universal finding (see below), were initially thought to be potentially important in the initiation and/or perpetuation of the disease, recent negative results from a controlled trial with D-penicillamine (see below) make it unlikely that elevated hepatic copper levels are pathogenetically important.[4] Recently, extrahepatic biliary tract disease closely mimicking primary sclerosing cholangitis has been described following infusions with the chemotherapeutic agent 5-fluorodeoxyuridine (Ludwig, Hepatol, 1989; 9:215). This drug apparently causes small-vessel arteriopathy which probably leads to ischaemic bile-duct damage, fibrosis, and destruction. The syndrome, however, represents a type of secondary sclerosing cholangitis. Only a few data are available concerning the possible role of infectious agents in the aetiopathogenesis of primary sclerosing cholangitis. Results from several studies have excluded hepatitis B virus as a causative agent. It is unlikely, but possible, that the hepatitis C virus is involved. Cytomegalovirus may affect intrahepatic bile ducts, but the histological picture appears to differ from that seen in primary sclerosing cholangitis. Nevertheless, viruses could be involved. The induction of cholangitis and biliary atresia in weanling mice by reovirus type III, as well as the association of some cases of neonatal biliary atresia with reovirus type III infections, suggests a possible viral cause of hepatobiliary diseases characterized by obliterative cholangitis, including primary sclerosing cholangitis. However, reovirus infections have not so far been directly linked to its development. It is possible that portal bacteraemia may be of pathogenic importance, particularly in patients with associated inflammatory bowel disease. However, this seems an unlikely cause because portal phlebitis is mild and uncommon in liver biopsy specimens from patients with primary sclerosing cholangitis, and because no striking differences are present in liver biopsy specimens from patients with primary sclerosing cholangitis with and without inflammatory bowel disease.

The pathogenesis seems to be more closely linked with alterations in the immune system. Although serological markers, such as antimitochondrial or smooth muscle antibodies, are generally absent, other data strongly support disturbed alterations in the immune system in patients with primary sclerosing cholangitis. For example, this syndrome is associated with an increased frequency of HLA B8 and HLA DR3 haplotypes; these two haplotypes are known to be present in autoimmune diseases. Other more direct lines of evidence supporting an immunological basis include the inhibition of leucocyte migration by biliary antigens, elevated IgM levels, the presence of circulating immune complexes, decreased clearance of immune complexes, and increased complement metabolism. In addition, cells involved in the destruction of bile ducts in primary sclerosing cholangitis have recently been shown to be T lymphocytes, and abnormalities in lymphocyte subsets in peripheral blood have also been demonstrated. Finally, enhanced autoreactivity of suppressor/cytotoxic T lymphocytes from peripheral blood of patients with primary sclerosing cholangitis has been reported. All these studies support the hypothesis that alterations in the immune system are pathogenetically related to the development and/or the perpetuation of primary sclerosing cholangitis, although the exact mechanisms are still not understood.[5]

It seems plausible, therefore, that the aetiology depends on the interplay of acquired toxic or infectious agents with certain inherited factors, perhaps relating to altered immunity. Moreover, the interplay of such postulated mechanisms may also be relevant to the cause of at least some cases of inflammatory bowel disease. Indeed, the existence of a common cause and variable organ response could explain why primary sclerosing cholangitis and inflammatory bowel disease may occur alone or together, in any time sequence.

Clinical features and diagnosis
Symptoms

Like the syndrome of primary biliary cirrhosis with which it shares many features, primary sclerosing cholangitis usually begins insidiously; therefore, it is difficult to determine the time of onset of the disease with accuracy. About 75 per cent of all patients with this syndrome have symptoms for 1 to 2 years before diagnosis.

The gradual onset of progressive fatigue and pruritus followed by jaundice is the most frequent symptom complex leading to the diagnosis of primary sclerosing cholangitis; this complex is present in about two-thirds of all patients.[1,3,6] Clinical evidence of cholangitis, such as recurrent pain in the right upper quadrant, fever, and jaundice, is uncommon unless previous bile-duct reconstructive surgery has been done. In fact, recent experience suggests that symptoms of cholangitis in a patient with primary sclerosing cholangitis who has not had previous bile-duct surgery may indicate the presence of a complication of primary sclerosing cholangitis, such as choledocholithiasis or superimposed adenocarcinoma of the bile duct.

Attempts at treatment of primary sclerosing cholangitis or associated inflammatory bowel disease frequently involve surgical approaches, and approximately two-thirds of patients will undergo hepatobiliary or colonic surgery at some time during the course of their disease.

Table 4 Diseases associated with primary sclerosing cholangitis

Inflammatory bowel disease
Pancreatitis
Arthritis
Sarcoidosis
Coeliac sprue
Thyroiditis

Signs

Although some patients may have a normal physical examination, up to 75 per cent of patients have some abnormality, usually hepatomegaly, jaundice, or splenomegaly. Hyperpigmentation and xanthelasma may also be seen, but these occur much less often than in primary biliary cirrhosis.

Associated diseases

A variety of other diseases are found in association with primary sclerosing cholangitis (Table 4). The association with inflammatory bowel disease, the disease most commonly associated with this syndrome, was first noted by Thorpe and colleagues (Thorpe, Gut, 1967; 8:435). Although early studies suggested a prevalence of 25 to 30 per cent of inflammatory bowel disease in association with primary sclerosing cholangitis, more recent studies support the likelihood that as many as 75 to 85 per cent of patients with primary sclerosing cholangitis will ultimately prove to have inflammatory bowel disease.

The most common type of inflammatory bowel disease found in association with primary sclerosing cholangitis is chronic ulcerative colitis. The other major type of inflammatory bowel disease, Crohn's disease, is rarely associated with primary sclerosing cholangitis. Although most patients have symptoms of intestinal disease before developing symptoms of primary sclerosing cholangitis, the latter has been reported to occur before intestinal disease becomes clinically apparent. Indeed, in patients who have undergone total proctocolectomy for chronic ulcerative colitis, symptoms of primary sclerosing cholangitis can develop years after the operation. Recent experience suggests that patients with primary sclerosing cholangitis and inflammatory bowel disease are similar (clinically, biochemically, radiologically, and histologically) to patients with primary sclerosing cholangitis without inflammatory bowel disease.[2] Of interest are recent data suggesting that patients with primary sclerosing cholangitis and chronic ulcerative colitis have a higher risk for colonic dysplasia and colon cancer than those with chronic ulcerative colitis alone (Ahnen, Gastro, 1996; 110:628). This may be related to a very long preclinical stage of inflammatory bowel disease in patients with primary sclerosing cholangitis.

Several diseases other than chronic ulcerative colitis are found occasionally in patients with primary sclerosing cholangitis. These diseases are thought to result from altered immune mechanisms and include thyroiditis, coeliac sprue, sarcoidosis, and arthritis.

Radiographic evidence of chronic pancreatitis by pancreatography has been seen in approximately 11 per cent of patients with primary sclerosing cholangitis; clinical evidence of chronic pancreatitis, however, is much less common. Sarcoidosis occurs in

Table 5 Diagnostic criteria in primary sclerosing cholangitis

Selection
Clinical
Biochemical
Radiological
Histological
Exclusion
Causes of secondary sclerosing cholangitis

approximately 5 per cent of patients. Finally, there have been occasional case reports on the occurrence of unusual syndromes, such as retroperitoneal and mediastinal fibrosis, histiocytosis X, and pseudotumour of the orbit in association with primary sclerosing cholangitis.

Diagnostic criteria

The diagnosis is based on biochemical, radiological, and hepatic histological criteria. The major biochemical criterion is an elevated level of serum alkaline phosphatase (Table 5).

The major radiological criterion is cholangiographic demonstration of diffusely distributed multifocal strictures (Fig. 1). The strictures are characterized by irregularity of both the intrahepatic and extrahepatic bile ducts (Table 6).

Hepatic histological abnormalities are often categorized as follows: stage 1 changes, including cholangitis or portal hepatitis; stage 2 changes, including periportal fibrosis with periportal hepatitis; stage 3 changes, including septal fibrosis, necrosis, or both; and stage 4 changes, representing biliary cirrhosis.

In general, primary sclerosing cholangitis should not be diagnosed if the patient has had previous bile-duct surgery (other than simple cholecystectomy) or documented choledocholithiasis before the diagnosis of primary sclerosing cholangitis, or if there is congenital disease of the biliary tract. More generally, if a specific cause can be identified for the underlying sclerosing cholangitis, the disease cannot be confidently classified as primary. In addition, primary sclerosing cholangitis cannot be diagnosed confidently in a patient with biopsy-proven adenocarcinoma of the bile duct unless the carcinoma is a complication of primary sclerosing cholangitis. Similarly, the diagnosis should not be made in a patient in whom there have been observed radiographic changes strongly suggestive of cancer of the bile duct.

Investigations and other diagnostic considerations

Laboratory tests

Virtually all patients have a cholestatic biochemical profile. The serum alkaline phosphatase is usually abnormal, although it may

Table 6 Cholangiographic features in primary sclerosing cholangitis

Diffusely distributed, multifocal, annular strictures with intervening segments of normal or ectatic ducts
Short, band-like strictures
Diverticulum-like outpouchings

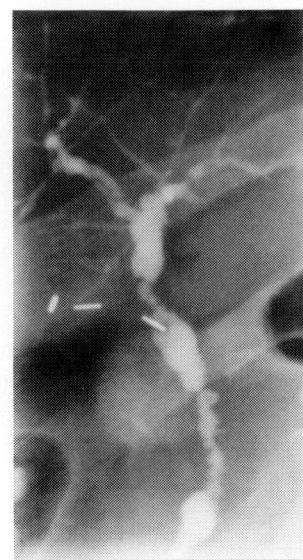

Fig. 1. Retrograde cholangiogram showing typical radiological features of primary sclerosing cholangitis, including multifocal strictures involving the intrahepatic and extrahepatic bile ducts. Diverticulum-like outpouchings in the common bile duct and focal dilated segments producing a beaded appearance are seen. Surgical clips are present. (Reproduced with permission from LaRusso NF et al., New England Journal of Medicine, 1984; **310**: 899–903.)

fluctuate occasionally to within the normal range. Most patients have an increase in the level of serum aspartate aminotransferase, but usually of a mild degree. Perhaps 50 per cent of patients with primary sclerosing cholangitis have a modest increase in total serum bilirubin at the time of initial diagnosis; in others, however, it may be normal or very high. Indeed, in an individual patient, the serum bilirubin can fluctuate markedly over time. Tests related to copper metabolism are virtually always abnormal in patients with primary sclerosing cholangitis.[3] For example, hepatic copper levels are elevated in approximately 90 per cent of patients, while urine levels are increased up to two-thirds; both are increased to levels seen in primary biliary cirrhosis and Wilson's disease. However, serum copper and caeruloplasmin levels are usually increased in patients with primary sclerosing cholangitis, but are low in Wilson's disease. It seems likely that abnormal copper metabolism is a universal feature, that hepatic copper accumulates and urinary excretion of copper increases as the disease progresses, and that these disturbances reflect the cholestatic nature of the syndrome with resulting diminished biliary copper excretion.[7]

Other laboratory abnormalities have sometimes been noted in primary sclerosing cholangitis. For example, eosinophilia of a mild degree may occasionally be observed, as in primary biliary cirrhosis (Chapter 25.3). Recently, antineutrophil cytoplasmic antibodies have been identified in the serum of approximately 70 per cent of patients with primary sclerosing cholangitis with or without associated inflammatory bowel disease (Duerr, Gastro, 1991; 100: 1385).

Cholangiographic features

Cholangiographic abnormalities may be seen in the intrahepatic and extrahepatic biliary ductal system.[8] Usually, the abnormalities

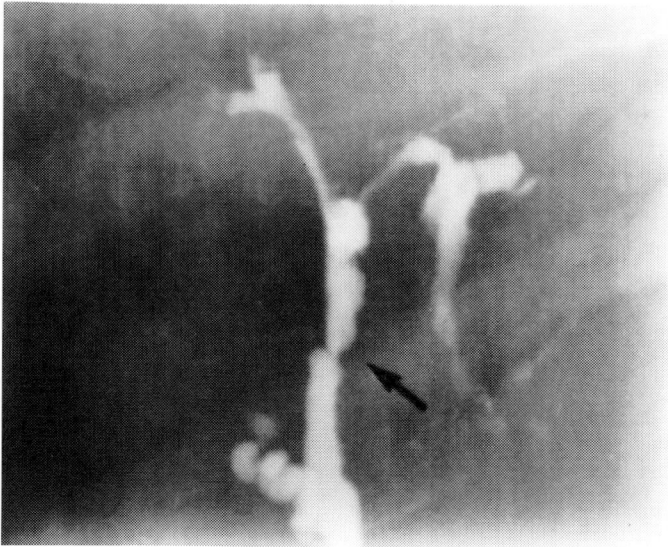

Fig. 2. Retrograde cholangiogram demonstrating a band-like stricture (arrow) in primary sclerosing cholangitis.

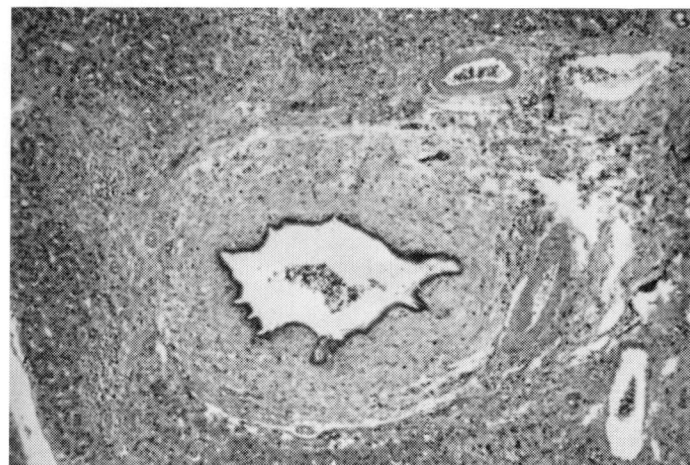

Fig. 4. Fibrous cholangitis of septal bile duct in a liver biopsy specimen in primary sclerosing cholangitis. Note periductal fibrosis and inflammation. This type of lesion tends to progress to ductal obliteration (fibrous obliterative cholangitis).

include diffusely distributed strictures which are short and annular with intervening segments of apparently normal or slightly dilated ducts producing the characteristic beaded appearance (Fig. 1). Short band-like strictures (Fig. 2) and diverticulum-like outpouchings (Fig. 3) are also found in approximately 25 per cent of patients.

Although focal dilatation of bile ducts is often seen between strictures, diffuse non-segmental dilatation is unusual. In perhaps 50 per cent of patients, coarse or fine irregularities are present which, when severe, produce a characteristic shaggy appearance. The pancreatic duct may also be abnormal, the changes resembling those seen in chronic pancreatitis; they include diffuse narrowing of the main pancreatic duct with multiple short strictures and mildly ectatic intervening segments. Occasionally, these radiological

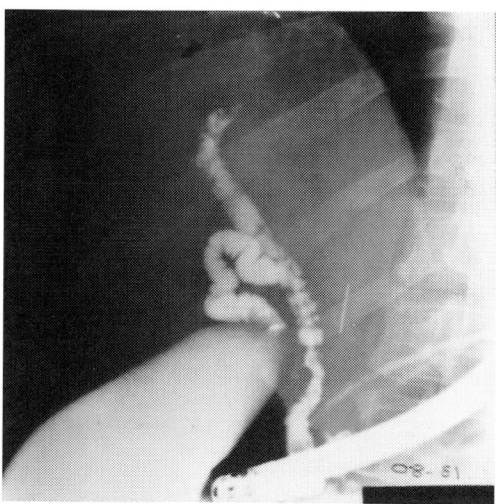

Fig. 3. Retrograde cholangiogram showing diverticulum-like outpouchings ('pseudodiverticuli'), a finding highly suggestive of primary sclerosing cholangitis. (Reproduced with permission from MacCarty RL *et al.*, *Radiology*, 1983; **149**: 39–44.)

abnormalities are accompanied by clinical evidence of chronic pancreatitis. Cholangiographic abnormalities of the cystic duct and gallbladder are also seen in a smaller number of patients.

Hepatic histology

In almost all patients, histological abnormalities can be seen in liver biopsy specimens. The characteristic features include bile-duct proliferation, periductal fibrosis and inflammation, ductal obliteration, and loss of bile ducts.[9]

The disease usually begins with enlargement of portal tracts characterized by some oedema, deposition of connective tissue, and proliferation of interlobular bile ducts. Inflammatory infiltrates are not usually prominent. Histologically this is stage 1 disease. With progression, extensions of connective tissue grow into the periportal parenchyma, again with only mild cellular inflammation (stage 2 disease). If the process results in the formation of fibrous septa, the disease is categorized histologically as stage 3. Ultimately, biliary cirrhosis develops (stage 4 disease). The pathognomonic histological changes can be found in some wedge specimens and only occasionally in needle biopsy specimens; they are characterized by fibrous obliterative cholangitis (Fig. 4), leading to replacement of ductal segments by solid cords of connective tissue. It is probable that other forms of destructive cholangitis also occur. In many instances of advanced disease, complete loss of intrahepatic bile ducts may be observed.

From a purely histological viewpoint, the differential diagnosis of the abnormalities seen in liver biopsy specimens of patients with primary sclerosing cholangitis includes small-duct primary sclerosing cholangitis without large-duct involvement ('pericholangitis'), the syndrome of primary biliary cirrhosis, prolonged extrahepatic obstruction, rare cases of chronic hepatitis, and idiopathic adulthood ductopenia (Ludwig, JHepatol, 1988; 7:193).

Examination of biopsy specimens shows that the syndrome of primary biliary cirrhosis has many histological features that overlap with those of primary sclerosing cholangitis, including periportal cholestasis, copper deposition, and granulomas. However, florid duct lesions are not seen in primary sclerosing cholangitis and are

Table 7 Distinguishing features of primary sclerosing cholangitis and primary biliary cirrhosis

Feature	Primary sclerosing cholangitis	Primary biliary cirrhosis
Average age (years)	41	53
Sex, M/F	63/37	10/90
Cholangitis (clinical) (%)	14	2
Fever (%)	32	8
Hyperpigmentation (%)	25	54
Xanthelasma (%)	3	19
Inflammatory bowel disease (%)	70	<1
Sicca syndrome	2	69
Arthritis (%)	7	19
Thyroid disease (%)	2	19
Hepatic histology	Non-suppurative obliterative cholangitis	Non-suppurative destructive cholangitis (florid duct lesion)
Cholangiography	Extrahepatic ducts usually abnormal	Extrahepatic ducts always normal

almost pathognomonic of primary biliary cirrhosis. In contrast, fibrous obliterative cholangitis, a hallmark of primary sclerosing cholangitis, has not been observed in primary biliary cirrhosis.

It seems unlikely that chronic hepatitis associated with chronic ulcerative colitis (also called pericholangitis by some workers) exists as an entity separate from primary sclerosing cholangitis and chronic active hepatitis. It is more likely that this situation reflects either small-duct primary sclerosing cholangitis or chronic active hepatitis.

Differential diagnosis

The diagnosis is usually straightforward, assuming that the clinician is aware of the syndrome and thus considers it in the differential diagnosis of conditions causing chronic cholestasis. It should be the major working diagnosis in a male with chronic cholestasis and inflammatory bowel disease. In a woman with chronic cholestasis, particularly if she is middle-aged, primary biliary cirrhosis should be excluded.[10] Although considerable overlap exists in the clinical, biochemical, and hepatic histological features of primary sclerosing cholangitis and primary biliary cirrhosis, it is usually possible to distinguish these diseases with confidence (Table 7). Indeed, the most useful diagnostic test in distinguishing the two syndromes is radiological visualization of the bile ducts. Although the intrahepatic bile ducts are radiographically abnormal in essentially all cases of large-duct primary sclerosing cholangitis,and in some patients with primary biliary cirrhosis, the extrahepatic ducts are never involved in primary biliary cirrhosis, and are thought to become abnormal eventually in most patients with primary sclerosing cholangitis. Therefore, in a patient suspected of having large-duct primary sclerosing cholangitis because of compatible clinical and biochemical findings, a suitable cholangiogram is all that is necessary for diagnosis. A liver biopsy may also be appropriate to provide confirmatory diagnostic information; however, it is primarily of value for accurate histological classification and for prognosis. If the cholangiogram is normal, liver biopsy is needed to exclude small-duct primary sclerosing cholangitis.

Other conditions which need to be considered in the differential diagnosis include secondary sclerosing cholangitis, chronic active hepatitis, and idiopathic adulthood ductopenia. Secondary sclerosing cholangitis should be the diagnosis when biochemical and radiological changes can be attributed confidently to an identifiable cause, such as a stone, stricture, or adenocarcinoma of the bile duct. An overlap syndrome between idiopathic chronic active hepatitis and primary sclerosing cholangitis has been described.[11] In these circumstances, patients who fulfil the accepted criteria for idiopathic chronic active hepatitis have ultimately been shown to have radiological changes on cholangiography which are typical for primary sclerosing cholangitis. Indeed, all patients with idiopathic chronic active hepatitis and associated inflammatory bowel disease should have a cholangiogram to exclude primary sclerosing cholangitis. Idiopathic adulthood ductopenia is a very rare, recently described syndrome characterized by unexplained absence of interlobular bile ducts and cholestasis (Ludwig, JHepatol, 1988; 7:193). Patients with this syndrome can be distinguished from patients with primary sclerosing cholangitis because they have an essentially normal cholangiogram and no associated inflammatory bowel disease.

Complications

Complications can be separated into two general categories; those common to any form of chronic liver disease and those peculiar to primary sclerosing cholangitis.

In the first category, complications include ascites, portosystemic encephalopathy, portal hypertension, diarrhoea, steatorrhoea, deficiencies of fat-soluble vitamins, liver failure, and metabolic bone disease. One or more of such problems probably occur in over 75 per cent of patients with primary sclerosing cholangitis who are followed systematically for 5 to 10 years.

In the second category are problems such as recurrent bacteraemia, gallstones, and adenocarcinoma of the bile duct. In some patients, the major incapacitating complication is recurrent episodes of bacteraemia, presumably secondary to bacterial seeding of the bloodstream from a chronically infected biliary tract. Such episodes occur in patients with primary sclerosing cholangitis, with or without associated inflammatory bowel disease, may lead to the formation of a hepatic abscess or to infection of other organs, and are unpredictable with regard to frequency and severity in an individual patient.

Nearly one-third of all patients will have undergone cholecystectomy at some time during their illness. Nevertheless, only about 20 per cent of such patients will actually have gallstones. Indeed, these gallstones are often asymptomatic, and the original indication for surgery was often obscure jaundice rather than biliary colic. Conversely, if patients with primary sclerosing cholangitis and intact gallbladders are screened by ultrasonography, approximately 25 per cent will be shown to have gallstones (Brandt, AJR, 1988; 150:571). Since most of these patients will be young men, a group in whom gallstones are relatively uncommon, this figure probably represents an increased frequency of cholelithiasis in primary sclerosing cholangitis.

Stones in the bile ducts (as opposed to the gallbladder) may also complicate primary sclerosing cholangitis. Moreover, the diagnosis of choledocholithiasis in a patient with primary sclerosing cholangitis may be very difficult, since symptoms of cholangitis can occur in the absence of biliary stone disease. Nevertheless, since choledocholithiasis may be amenable to definitive treatment, a cholangiogram to identify bile-duct stones complicating primary sclerosing cholangitis should be considered in the patient with primary sclerosing cholangitis who has symptoms that might be secondary to stones, such as recurrent episodes of cholangitis.

Although carcinoma of the bile duct has been reported in patients with known primary sclerosing cholangitis, only recently has direct evidence been generated that strongly suggests that this syndrome actually predisposes to the development of carcinoma of the bile duct.[12] For example, nearly 50 per cent of a small group of patients with primary sclerosing cholangitis who died were found at autopsy to have a carcinoma of the bile duct superimposed on primary sclerosing cholangitis. Patients whose disease is complicated by superimposed adenocarcinoma of the bile duct usually have cirrhosis, portal hypertension, and long-standing inflammatory bowel disease; they are also generally older at the time of diagnosis and progressive changes on cholangiography, such as cystic dilatation of the biliary tree, suggest the development of carcinoma superimposed on primary sclerosing cholangitis. A recent report suggests that patients with primary sclerosing cholangitis and chronic ulcerative colitis who develop colonic neoplasia are also more likely to develop cholangiocarcinoma (Broome, Hepatol, 1995; 22:1404). The value of serum tumour markers (e.g. CA19–9, CEA) in the early diagnosis of cholangiocarcinoma in patients with primary sclerosing cholangitis is a matter under active investigation (Nichols, MayoClinProc, 1993; 68:874).

Therapy
General guidelines

Management provides a real challenge to the clinician, given the array of symptoms and complications that can develop and the absence of any effective specific therapy. The first decision relates to whether any therapeutic intervention is necessary in a patient with newly diagnosed disease. In the asymptomatic patient with mild liver test abnormalities and early disease on liver biopsy, the prognosis is reasonably good; as no established specific therapy is available, simple observation is a reasonable approach. Alternatively,

therapy might be considered in the context of a randomized controlled trial with medical treatment. If a decision is made to intervene therapeutically, the goals of therapy should be clearly identified. Specifically, therapy should be directed either towards symptoms, complications, or the underlying hepatobiliary disease. The development and validation of mathematical models that address the natural history of primary sclerosing cholangitis are increasingly useful in guiding decisions regarding management (Dickson, Gastro, 1992; 103:1893).

Therapy for symptoms/complications

Pruritus and fat-soluble vitamin deficiencies are common problems in patients with primary sclerosing cholangitis; conventional approaches to management of these problems, which will not be reviewed here, are reasonable (see Chapters 14.1 and 23.2). Also, when complications such as variceal bleeding develop, appropriate intervention such as sclerotherapy should be considered.

There are, however, complications which are relatively specific for primary sclerosing cholangitis, as mentioned earlier; these include recurrent cholangitis and bacteraemia, dominant strictures, and cholangiocarcinoma.

Patients with recurrent episodes of cholangitis without dominant stricture should be treated with broad-spectrum antibiotics as needed. Prophylactic antibiotics are favoured by some for patients with frequent episodes of cholangitis, but the efficacy of this approach has not been firmly established.

Patients may develop dominant strictures in the biliary tract which can lead to rapid increases in serum bilirubin levels, account for recurrent episodes of cholangitis, and precipitate or aggravate pruritus. Consideration of dilatation of these strictures in the symptomatic patient is reasonable, particularly in patients with non-cirrhotic disease. Depending upon their location, a transhepatic or endoscopic approach with or without stent placement may be useful. Indeed, data from the transhepatic approach in symptomatic patients with primary sclerosing cholangitis and dominant strictures suggest that balloon dilatation is very effective in alleviating pruritus and in diminishing the frequency of cholangitic episodes resulting from dominant strictures (May, AJR, 1985; 145:1061).

Data reviewed earlier suggest that cholangiocarcinoma develops in perhaps 10 to 15 per cent of patients with primary sclerosing cholangitis. The management of a suspected or established cholangiocarcinoma superimposed on primary sclerosing cholangitis is complicated and is still evolving. If the cholangiocarcinoma is surgically resectable, and the patient is not a candidate for liver transplantation, an attempt at surgical resection seems reasonable. Alternatively, if the cholangiocarcinoma is not surgically resectable, or if it is but the patient has advanced liver disease, consideration should be given to orthotopic liver transplantation, although results have been poor.

Therapy for primary sclerosing cholangitis

At present there is no specific or effective treatment for the underlying hepatobiliary disease in primary sclerosing cholangitis. This reflects, in part, our lack of knowledge about the exact pathogenesis of the disease. Nevertheless, therapeutic approaches for the underlying hepatobiliary disease can be classed as mechanical, surgical, and medical (Table 8).

Table 8 Therapeutic approaches in primary sclerosing cholangitis

Mechanical
    Balloon dilatation
Surgical
    Biliary tract reconstructive procedures
    Proctocolectomy*
    Orthotopic liver transplantation
Medical
    Cupriuretic*
    Immunosuppressive
    Antifibrogenic
    Choleretic

* Study results refute these indications.

Mechanical approaches

Advocates suggest that balloon dilatation of dominant strictures may be beneficial to the natural history of the underlying hepatobiliary disease; obstruction is undoubtedly a cause of hepatic fibrosis. However, there have been no comparable studies of patients with primary sclerosing cholangitis to test the results of these procedures in terms of the development of fibrosis. Thus, it would seem reasonable, until more data are available, to restrict balloon dilatation of dominant strictures to the symptomatic relief of jaundice or pruritus and not to use it for treatment of the underlying hepatobiliary disease.

Surgical approaches

The indications for hepatobiliary surgery in primary sclerosing cholangitis remain unclear. Only occasionally is an operation required for diagnosis. However, a diagnostic laparotomy may occasionally be needed to differentiate primary sclerosing cholangitis from adenocarcinoma of the bile duct, a distinction that is often difficult even at the operating table. Because there are no specific histological abnormalities of the extrahepatic bile ducts in primary sclerosing cholangitis, bile-duct biopsy is helpful only for exclusion of carcinoma. In contrast, it seems reasonable to treat symptomatic cholelithiasis or choledocholithiasis surgically in some patients with primary sclerosing cholangitis, even though the presence of underlying parenchymal disease may result in increased operative morbidity and mortality. In some patients with primary sclerosing cholangitis and choledocholithiasis, particularly if they have had a cholecystectomy, endoscopic sphincterotomy may be preferable to surgical choledocholithotomy. Other forms of non-surgical treatment for cholelithiasis, such as direct solvent or oral dissolution agents and extracorporeal shock-wave lithotripsy, remain to be evaluated in patient with primary sclerosing cholangitis and cholelithiasis.

There are three surgical procedures that have been considered of potential benefit in the treatment of primary sclerosing cholangitis: biliary tract reconstructive procedures, proctocolectomy in a patient with primary sclerosing cholangitis and chronic ulcerative colitis, and orthotopic liver transplantation. Indeed, some surgeons have encouraged an aggressive surgical approach in the treatment of primary sclerosing cholangitis itself, using a variety of imaginative procedures for internal or external biliary drainage (Pitt, AnnSurg,

1984; 199:637). However, no controlled trials have been performed. Such procedures might provide transient and symptomatic benefit in the occasional patient with jaundice and pruritus secondary to a dominant stricture of the common bile or common hepatic ducts. However, it seems unlikely that these procedures will alter the natural history of primary sclerosing cholangitis because in most, if not all, cases the disease involves the entire biliary ductal system, including the intrahepatic ducts. Moreover, many patients already have cirrhosis at the time of operation and this will not be affected by improving biliary drainage. It seems more reasonable to consider biliary tract reconstructive procedures in the same category as balloon dilatation, that is, as palliative procedures to alleviate symptoms, but which are unlikely to affect the natural history of the disease. Unfortunately, only limited and uncontrolled published data are currently available about the role of biliary tract reconstructive procedures in the treatment of the underlying liver disease in primary sclerosing cholangitis. Finally, it is important to point out that biliary tract reconstructive procedures may make subsequent liver transplantation more difficult (see below) because of the fibrosis and scar tissue which often develops in the right upper quadrant.

Some workers have suggested that proctocolectomy in a patient with primary sclerosing cholangitis and chronic ulcerative colitis may have a favourable effect on the hepatobiliary disease. This is an important issue, not only because beneficial treatment for primary sclerosing cholangitis is needed, but because a proctocolectomy in a patient with primary sclerosing cholangitis and chronic ulcerative colitis may be associated with considerable morbidity. Moreover, proctocolectomy with a conventional or continent ileostomy results in the development of varices around the ostomy stoma in at least 25 per cent of patients with primary sclerosing cholangitis. In nearly 50 per cent of these patients, major and often life-threatening bleeding occurs from these varices. A recently published study involving patients with primary sclerosing cholangitis and chronic ulcerative colitis, which evaluated the effects of proctocolectomy on the progression of clinical, biochemical, cholangiographic, and hepatic histological features, demonstrated that the onset of new complications, serial changes in biochemical tests, histological progression on liver biopsy, and survival were not affected by proctocolectomy.[13] It was concluded from this study that proctocolectomy for chronic ulcerative colitis is not beneficial for primary sclerosing cholangitis in patients with both diseases. Clearly, however, if a patient with primary sclerosing cholangitis and chronic ulcerative colitis has accepted colitic indications for proctocolectomy, such as rectal bleeding, stricture formation, dysplasia, or intractability, then proctocolectomy should be considered.

Orthotopic liver transplantation has recently become an important therapeutic option for patients with primary sclerosing cholangitis as it has for patients with other forms of advanced liver disease. Indeed, at many major transplantation centres, primary sclerosing cholangitis is one of the three most frequent indications for liver transplantation in adults. Indications for liver transplantion in patients with primary sclerosing cholangitis are similar to indications in other chronic liver diseases and include clinical and biochemical evidence of endstage liver disease, life-threatening complications, and unacceptable quality of life from liver disease. Although data are still evolving, published (Marsh, AnnSurg, 1988; 207:21) and unpublished results suggest that the outcome of liver transplantation in patients with primary sclerosing cholangitis is no different from the survival in patients with other forms of non-infectious, non-malignant chronic liver disease, with 5-year survival rates of approximately 80 per cent. However, special problems may be encountered in patients with primary sclerosing cholangitis who undergo liver transplantation. For example, primary duct-to-duct anastomosis is always difficult, and often impossible, because of disease in the common bile duct. Therefore, the donor's bile duct is usually anastomosed to the limb of the recipient's jejunum. Such an anastomosis may create a greater number of postoperative problems than a direct duct-to-duct anastomosis. In addition, up to 60 per cent or more of patients with primary sclerosing cholangitis have undergone previous abdominal surgical procedures such as proctocolectomy or choledochoenterostomy. Such surgical procedures are likely to exacerbate the technical problems of liver transplantation. Also, patients transplanted for primary sclerosing cholangitis appear to have an increased incidence of chronic ductopenic rejection resulting in graft loss, and an increased incidence of post-transplant biliary strictures (McEntee, TransplProc, 1991; 23:1563). Not surprisingly, the risk of colon cancer in patients with chronic ulcerative colitis who undergo liver transplantion for primary sclerosing cholangitis remains; it might actually increase after liver transplantion, perhaps related to chronic immunosuppression. Recent data suggest that there may indeed be a subset of transplant patients with primary sclerosing cholangitis who rapidly develop colorectal neoplasms after transplantation (Bleday, DisColRec, 1993; 36:908).

Finally, it is important to emphasize that only limited published data are available on several other aspects of liver transplantation in patients with primary sclerosing cholangitis, including the recurrence of primary sclerosing cholangitis after successful liver transplantation, and the effect of active inflammatory bowel disease on the transplanted liver in patients with both diseases.

Medical approaches

Medical approaches for the treatment of the underlying hepatobiliary disease in primary sclerosing cholangitis have included the use of cupriuretic, immunosuppressive, antifibrogenic, and choleretic agents. Unfortunately, no medical therapy has been shown to induce complete clinical, biochemical, radiological, and histological remission in primary sclerosing cholangitis.

The finding of elevated hepatic copper levels in primary sclerosing cholangitis, and early reports showing apparent biochemical improvement induced by D-penicillamine in primary biliary cirrhosis, another chronic cholestatic liver disease with many similarities to primary sclerosing cholangitis, prompted the initiation of a therapeutic trial of D-penicillamine in 1980.[4] In a randomized, prospective, double-blind trial, 39 patients received penicillamine (250 mg, three times a day), and 31 received a placebo. The two groups were highly comparable at entry with regard to their clinical, biochemical, radiological, and hepatic histological features. Although a predictable decrease in levels of hepatic copper was achieved in patients taking penicillamine, there was no beneficial effect on disease progression or on overall survival. Progressive symptoms, deterioration in serial hepatic laboratory values, and histological progression in sequential liver biopsy specimens were similar in both groups. The development of major side-effects led

to the permanent discontinuation of penicillamine in 21 per cent of the patients taking the drug. It was concluded from this study, which is the only published randomized trial of drug therapy in primary sclerosing cholangitis, that the use of penicillamine in primary sclerosing cholangitis is not associated with a beneficial effect on disease progression or survival and has considerable toxicity.

A variety of uncontrolled studies on small numbers of patients have assessed the effect of immunosuppressive agents including prednisone, azathioprine, and most recently cyclosporin. Corticosteroids have been used both topically and systemically in several small studies in primary sclerosing cholangitis. A small controlled trial of nasobiliary lavage with corticosteroids compared with placebo gave negative results (Allen, JHepatol, 1986; 3:118). There have been uncontrolled observations that a small number of patients with a marked inflammatory component to their primary sclerosing cholangitis have shown an impressive response to orally administered corticosteroids. In one study, 7 of 10 patients with primary sclerosing cholangitis showed objective biochemical improvement and some beneficial effect on liver histology while they were receiving long-term corticosteroid therapy (Burgert, Gastro, 1984; 86:1037). Initial enthusiasm for both methotrexate and cyclosporine as a result of small, uncontrolled pilot studies has waned because the results of recent controlled trials with these drugs in primary sclerosing cholangitis (Wiesner, Hepatol, 1991; 14:63A; Knox, Gastro, 1994; 106:494) were largely negative; currently neither drug has a role in the medical treatment of this syndrome, at least when used alone. Azathioprine has been used in at least two instances without apparent benefit.

There was interest in the use of antifibrogenic agents, specifically colchicine, in primary sclerosing cholangitis, based on encouraging data on the use of colchicine in primary biliary cirrhosis (Kaplan, NEJM, 1986; 315:1448). Whether the apparent biochemical benefit will be sustained and whether this drug will prevent histological progression and improve survival in primary sclerosing cholangitis or other chronic liver diseases must await results of controlled trials.

Considerable interest has recently been directed towards the potential benefit of ursodeoxycholic acid in the treatment of chronic cholestatic liver diseases. Although the efficacy of ursodeoxycholic acid in dissolving cholesterol gallstones has been known for nearly a decade, only recently has its possible benefit in cholestatic liver diseases been appreciated. Recently, several small uncontrolled trials suggest that this agent is beneficial in primary sclerosing cholangitis. Currently, a number of controlled trials assessing the efficacy of ursodeoxycholic acid in primary sclerosing cholangitis are underway (Stiehl, AnnIntMed, 1994; 26:345).

References

1. LaRusso NF, Wiesner RH, Ludwig J, and MacCarty RL. Primary sclerosing cholangitis. *New England Journal of Medicine*, 1984; **310**: 899–903.
2. Ludwig J, Barham SS, LaRusso NF, Elveback LR, Wiesner RH, and McCall JT. Morphologic features of chronic hepatitis associated with primary sclerosing cholangitisor chronic ulcerative colitis. *Hepatology*, 1981; **1**: 632–40.
3. Wiesner RH and LaRusso NF. Clinicopathologic features of the syndrome of primary sclerosing cholangitis. *Gastroenterology*, 1980; **79**: 200–6.
4. LaRusso NF, Wiesner RH, Ludwig J, MacCarty RL, Beaver SJ, and Zinsmeister AR. Prospective trial of penicillamine in primary sclerosing cholangitis. *Gastroenterology*, 1988; **95**: 1036–42.

5. Lindor KD, Weisner RH, and LaRusso NF. Recent advances in the management of primary sclerosing cholangitis. *Seminars in Liver Disease*, 1987; **7**: 322–7.

6. Chapman RW, *et al*. Primary sclerosing cholangitis: a review of clinical features, cholangiography and hepatic histology. *Gut*, 1980; **21**: 870–7.

7. Gross JB, Ludwig J, Wiesner RH, McCall JT, and LaRusso NF. Abnormalities in tests of copper metabolism in primary sclerosing cholangitis. *Gastroenterology*, 1985; **89**: 272–8.

8. MacCarty RL, LaRusso NF, Wiesner RH, and Ludwig J. Primary sclerosing cholangitis: findings on cholangiography and pancreatography. *Radiology*, 1983; **149**: 39–44.

9. Ludwig J, LaRusso NF, and Wiesner RH. Primary sclerosing cholangitis. In Peters RL and Craig JR, eds. *Liver pathology—contemporary issues in surgical pathology*. New York: Churchill Livingstone, 1986: 193–214.

10. Wiesner RH, LaRusso NF, Ludwig J, and Dickson ER. Comparison of the clinicopathologic features of primary sclerosing cholangitis and primary biliary cirrhosis. *Gastroenterology*, 1985; **88**: 108–14.

11. Lindor KD, Wiesner RH, LaRusso NF, and Dickson ER. Chronic active hepatitis: overlap with primary biliary cirrhosis and primary sclerosing cholangitis. In Czaja AJ and Dickson ER, eds. *Chronic active hepatitis: the Mayo Clinic experience*. New York: Marcel Dekker, 1986: 171–87.

12. Wee A, Ludwig J, Coffey RJ, LaRusso NF, and Wiesner RH. Hepatobiliary carcinoma associated with primary sclerosing cholangitisand chronic ulcerative colitis. *Human Pathology*, 1985; **16**: 719–26.

13. Cangemi JR, *et al*. Effect of proctocolectomy for chronic ulcerative colitis on the natural history of primary sclerosing cholangitis. *Gastroenterology*, 1989; **96**: 790–4.

14.5 Vanishing bile duct syndrome

Jurgen Ludwig

Definition

Vanishing bile duct syndrome is the name for a group of biliary disease states with different aetiologies but one common feature—progressive loss of interlobular and proximal septal bile ducts.

Introduction

For many years, primary biliary cirrhosis in adults and paucity of intrahepatic bile ducts in paediatric patients were the only widely known liver diseases that featured loss of small bile ducts resulting in ductopenia. However, during the last 20 years, an increasing number of other ductopenic conditions have been recognized. They all may have very similar clinical, laboratory, and morphological manifestations and, therefore, use of a collective term for these diseases has proved practical. The name vanishing bile duct syndrome has diagnostic and prognostic significance; it is particularly useful in instances where the duct loss is diagnosed before the underlying disease has been recognized.

Classification

An aetiological classification of vanishing bile duct syndrome is presented in Table 1. As shown, the syndrome can be caused by several immunological or putative immunological mechanisms but

Table 1 Aetiological classification of the vanishing bile duct syndrome

Alloimmune cholangitis
  Hepatic allograft rejection
  Hepatic graft-versus-host disease
Autoimmune or putative autoimmune cholangitis
  Primary biliary cirrhosis
  Autoimmune cholangitis unrelated to primary biliary cirrhosis
  Primary sclerosing cholangitis
  Chronic cholestasis of sarcoidosis
Cholangitis with undefined immune components
  Paediatric paucity of intrahepatic bile ducts
  Drug-induced ductopenia
  Idiopathic adulthood ductopenia
Cholangitis or ductopenia caused by non-immunological mechanisms
  Ischaemic cholangitis
  Infectious cholangitis
  Neoplastic duct destruction

it can also result from conditions without a major immunological component.

Hepatic allograft rejection

This is the prototype of an alloimmune liver disease.[1] The most common form of this condition, cellular rejection (acute rejection), is by definition associated with cholangitis. Mixed inflammatory infiltrates, often with eosinophils, are found. The condition generally is reversible. In a fortunately decreasing number of cases, progressive duct destruction leads to ductopenic rejection (chronic rejection) which often is irreversible. The condition may develop in less than 2 weeks after transplantation but more often occurs after several months or even years. Foam cell arteriopathy (vascular rejection) probably can cause duct ischaemia and thus might accelerate the process. The role of persistent cytomegalovirus infection in vanishing bile duct syndrome is controversial. (See also Chapter 30.5.)

Graft-versus-host disease

In both acute and chronic graft-versus-host disease the liver may be affected. The changes closely resemble those seen in hepatic allograft rejection. Cholangitis and ductopenia after bone marrow transplantation are rather reliable diagnostic markers for graft-versus-host disease. Isolated vanishing bile duct syndrome can be a manifestation of severe acute hepatic graft-versus-host disease.[4] (See also Chapter 14.7.)

Primary biliary cirrhosis

This condition is by far the most common ductopenic disorder in adults. It is characterized by granulomatous duct destruction which occurs primarily in the early stages of the disease. Antimitochondrial antibodies are found in the majority of patients. (See also Chapter 14.1.)

Autoimmune cholangitis unrelated to primary biliary cirrhosis

Some patients with clinical and biopsy evidence of primary biliary cirrhosis had antinuclear antibodies and no antimitochondrial antibodies. Further study of some such patients suggested that their cholangitis might be unrelated to primary biliary cirrhosis. Antibodies to human carbonic anhydrase II which are uncommon or absent in other types of cholangitis[5] may be an important distinguishing feature. (See also Chapter 14.6.)

Primary sclerosing cholangitis

This is the only putative autoimmune cholangitis that often affects the entire biliary system, from interlobular bile ducts to the papilla of Vater. This observation, and the common association with inflammatory bowel disease, sets primary sclerosing cholangitis apart from the other conditions in this group. In large wedge biopsy specimens, the diagnosis of primary sclerosing cholangitis often can be confirmed by the presence of fibrous-obliterative cholangitis. Unfortunately, this feature cannot be appreciated in most needle biopsy samples. (See also Chapter 14.4.)

Chronic cholestasis of sarcoidosis

This variant of sarcoidosis is very rare. It resembles primary biliary cirrhosis clinically[6] and is the only condition that shares its main diagnostic morphological feature—destructive granulomatous cholangitis. Typically, patients with chronic cholestasis of sarcoidosis are antimitochondrial antibody negative. (See also Chapter 14.2.)

Paucity of intrahepatic bile ducts in childhood

Ductopenia (paucity of small bile ducts) in paediatric patients may be an isolated finding (non-syndromic paucity of intrahepatic bile ducts), or it may occur with a characteristic set of congenital anomalies (Alagille's syndrome; syndromic paucity of intrahepatic bile ducts). It should be noted that a host of other genetic diseases, most notably α_1-antitrypsin deficiency, also may be associated with paucity of intrahepatic bile ducts. (See also Chapters 1.5, 20.3, and Section 26.)

Drug-induced ductopenia

Cholangitis and ductopenia after administration of drugs most commonly appears to be the result of an idiosyncratic reaction. At least 20 drugs have been incriminated. Amoxicillin–clavulanate has acquired particular notoriety.[7] (See also Section 17.)

Idiopathic adulthood ductopenia

By definition, the ductopenia in idiopathic adulthood ductopenia is unexplained but circumstantial evidence suggests that those patients who are in their second or third decade of life might have delayed onset of paediatric paucity of intrahepatic bile ducts (see above). Others, mostly young adults, are thought to have isolated small-duct primary sclerosing cholangitis. Older patients, who often have non-progressive disease, might have autoimmune cholangitis without identifiable markers or viral cholangitis, as seen in some cases of chronic hepatitis C. The disease may be asymptomatic.[8]

Ischaemic cholangitis

This type of cholangitis appears to be responsible for postoperative duct necrosis and strictures, occasionally as an aftermath of cholecystectomies or intra-arterial floxuridine administration.[9] However, the majority of cases are found in hepatic allografts[10] with thrombosis or strictures of, or near, the hepatic artery anastomosis. The biliary tree, which is supplied by its own vascular network, is particularly sensitive to ischaemia and therefore ischaemic cholangitis is not always associated with parenchymal damage—that is, centrilobular necroses or infarcts.

Infectious cholangitis

Ascending bacterial cholangitis may lead to duct destruction, particularly if it is associated with duct ischaemia (see above). The main complication is septicaemia and not the, generally limited, duct loss. In patients with AIDS or genetic immunodeficiency states such as familial combined immundeficiency, infectious cholangitis is more common than in immunocompetent patients. Thus, in patients with AIDS (see Chapter 12.3), cholangitis may be caused by cryptosporidia or by *Candida albicans*. Although primary sclerosing cholangitis-type changes have been described in many AIDS patients, ductopenia does not appear to be a prominent features.

Neoplastic bile duct destruction

Primary or metastatic carcinomas rarely destroy enough hepatic tissue to elicit a ductopenic syndrome. If they do, the diagnosis is evident. However, lymphomas, in particular, Hodgkin's lymphoma, can destroy small bile ducts and in many respects imitate an inflammatory liver disease with cholangitis.[11] Similarly, the infiltrates of Langerhans' cell histiocytosis can destroy small bile ducts and cause primary sclerosing cholangitis-type changes.[12] In all these conditions, the differential diagnosis must be based on the cytological features of the infiltrate. In other cases with Hodgkin's lymphoma, vanishing bile duct syndrome developed in the absence of lymphomatous infiltrates in the affected portal tracts. In these instances, the infiltrates might have disappeared after the ducts were destroyed or humoral factors such as toxic cytokines might have caused the ductopenia.[13]

Morphological features

As expressed by the name vanishing bile duct syndrome, ductopenia is the main manifestation of this syndrome. In normal liver biopsy specimens, 70 to 80 per cent of all hepatic artery branches are accompanied by a bile duct.[14] Customarily, if more than 50 per cent of the artery branches lack an accompanying bile duct, ductopenia is diagnosed. For scientific documentation, at least 20 complete portal tracts should be evaluated before the diagnosis is considered confirmed. However, in many instances, experienced pathologists can diagnose ductopenia after review of only a few portal tracts. This is possible because the complications of duct loss are of considerable diagnostic help; they include fibrous or biliary piecemeal necrosis, periportal cholate stasis, deposition of copper, and formation of Mallory bodies in periportal hepatocytes.

The histological features of duct destruction may be of great diagnostic help. Thus, granulomatous cholangitis occurs only in primary biliary cirrhosis and in the exceedingly rare chronic cholestasis of sarcoidosis. It should be noted, however, that in the above-mentioned, equally rare, Langerhans' cell histicytosis neoplastic granulomatous aggregates may destroy small bile ducts; this process may closely resemble destructive granulomatous cholangitis.[12]

Fibrous-obliterative cholangitis is a rather specific feature of primary sclerosing cholangitis. Ischaemia, infection, and neoplastic duct destruction usually can also be diagnosed microscopically. However, in many other instances, the cholangitic changes are characterized by mixed inflammatory infiltrates with little diagnostic specificity or the ducts are absent, leaving no diagnostic clues. Depending on the clinical circumstances the diagnosis still may be straightforward, as in many paediatric patients with cholestatic syndromes or in hepatic allografts with a history of recurrent rejection.

Clinical features

As expected, the conditions that may cause vanishing bile duct syndrome have many common features because duct loss of any cause leads to severe cholestasis with itching, jaundice, and hepatic failure. They also have common biochemical findings such as high alkaline phosphatase and γ-glutamyl transferase values. The diagnostic significance of the history, for example liver transplantation or drug exposure, and of age and sex is apparent from the list of diseases that may contribute to vanishing bile duct syndrome.

Pathogenesis

In ischaemic, infectious, and neoplastic diseases, the pathogenesis of the ductopenia is evident. For most immunologically mediated biliary diseases, a specific immunoreactivity of small bile ducts must be considered since, with the exception of primary sclerosing cholangitis, only interlobular and septal bile ducts are affected. These ducts occupy only about 1 per cent of the distance to the papilla of Vater. The enormous number of small bile ducts with a correspondingly large inner surface helps to explain why even extensive duct loss can be tolerated for a long time.

Therapy

Therapeutic options are discussed with the specific conditions elsewhere. However, immunologically-mediated small duct diseases probably have common pathogenetic mechanisms which might lead to improved treatment—for instance of both rejection and primary biliary cirrhosis.

References

1. Vierling JM. Immunology of hepatic allograft rejection. In: Maddrey WC and Sorrell MF, eds. *Transplantation of the liver*, 2nd edn. Norwalk: Appleton and Lange, 1995: 335–65.
2. Paya CV, Wiesner RH, Hermans PE, *et al*. Lack of association between cytomegalovirus infection, HLA matching, and the vanishing bile duct syndrome after liver transplantation. *Hepatology*, 1992; **16**: 66–70.
3. Arnold JC, Portmann BC, O'Grady JG, Maoumov NV, Alexander GJ, and Williams R. Cytomegalovirus infection persists in the liver graft in the vanishing bile duct syndrome. *Hepatology*, 1992; **16**: 285–92.
4. Yeh KH, Hsieh HC, Tang JL, Lin MT, Yang CH, and Chen YC. Severe isolated acute hepatic graft-versus-host disease with vanishing bile duct syndrome. *Bone Marrow Transplantation*, 1994; **14**: 319–21.
5. Gordon SC, Quattrociocchi-Longe TM, Khan BA, Kodali VP, Chen J, Silverman AL, and Kiechle FL. Antibodies to carbonic anhydrase in patients with immune cholangiopathies. *Gastroenterology*, 1995; **108**: 1802–9.
6. Pereira-Lima J and Schaffner F. Chronic cholestasis in hepatic sarcoidosis with clinical features resembling primary biliary cirrhosis. *American Journal of Medicine*, 1987; **83**: 144–8.
7. Hautekeete ML, Brenard R, Horsmans Y, *et al*. Liver injury related to amoxycillin-clavulanic acid: interlobular bile duct lesions and extrahepatic manifestations. *Journal of Hepatology*, 1995; **22**: 71–7.
8. Moreno A, Carreno V, Cano A, and Gonzales C. Idiopathic biliary ductopenia in adults without symptoms of liver disease. *New England Journal of Medicine*, 1997; **335**: 835–8.
9. Ludwig J, Kim CH, Wiesner RH, and Krom RAF. Floxuridine-induced sclerosing cholangitis: An ischemic cholangiopathy? *Hepatology*, 1989; **9**: 215–18.
10. Fisher A and Miller CM. Ischemic-type biliary strictures in liver allografts: An Achilles heel revisited? *Hepatology*, 1995; **21**: 589–91.
11. Lefkowitch JH, Falkow S, and Whitlock RT. Hepatic Hodgkin's disease simulating cholestatic hepatitis with liver failure. *Archives of Pathology and Laboratory Medicine*, 1985; **109**: 424–6.
12. Ishak KG. Granulomas of the liver. *Advances in Pathology and Laboratory Medicine*, 1995; **8**: 247–361.
13. Hubscher SG, Lumley MA, and Elias E. Vanishing bile duct syndrome: A possible mechanism for intrahepatic cholestasis in Hodgkin's lymphoma. *Hepatology*, 1993; **17**: 70–7.
14. Nakanuma Y and Ohta G. Histometric and serial section observations of the intrahepatic bile ducts in primary biliary cirrhosis. *Gastroenterology*, 1979; **76**: 1326–32.

14.6 Overlap syndromes

Jenny Heathcote

The overlap syndromes refer to cases of chronic liver disease which appear to have autoimmune features but which present a mixed picture of both cholestatic and hepatitic liver disease, either simultaneously or at different times in the same patient (Table 1). In addition, infection with hepatotrophic viruses (Magrin, JHepatol, 1991; 13:56; Abnaf, JHepatol, 1993; 18:359), a hepatotoxic reaction to certain drugs, and graft-versus-host disease (Siegert, BoneM-Trans, 1992; 10:221) may be associated with the presence of non-organ specific antibodies in serum considered typical of autoimmune liver disease. Hence before concluding that autoimmune liver disease is present, these alternative possibilities need to be considered. Although graft-versus-host disease is generally specific to those who have received an allograft, it may occasionally be seen following a blood transfusion (Nishimura, BrJHaemat, 1996; 92:1011). In patients who are at risk for graft-versus-host disease there are often multiple alternative aetiologies for their liver test abnormalities (Bertheau, BoneMTrans, 1995; 16:261) which must be sought after rigorously.

Autoimmune hepatitis compared with primary biliary cirrhosis

A diagnosis of autoimmune hepatitis cannot be made without careful consideration of all the clinical, biochemical, serological, virological, and histological data. The term chronic hepatitis only refers to the persistence of abnormal levels of serum aminotransferases for a period of greater than 6 months. After excluding the most common causes, such as viral hepatitis, alcohol or other causes of drug-induced hepatotoxity, inherited metabolic diseases, and non-alcoholic hepatosteatonecrosis, it is appropriate to consider autoimmune liver disease.

Table 1 Autoimmune liver disease	
Cholestatic	**Hepatitic**
Primary biliary cirrhosis	Autoimmune hepatitis: type 1 (classic) type 2 (anti-LKM-1)
Primary sclerosing cholangitis	type 3 (anti-SLA)
'Autoimmune cholangitis'	
Overlap syndromes	

NB. May be mimicked by virus, drugs, and graft-versus-host disease.

Clinical

Patients may or may not have symptoms. Symptoms when present are generally fairly non-specific, such as fatigue, malaise, and anorexia. Secondary amenorrhoea is much more frequently seen in patients with autoimmune hepatitis. Whereas autoimmune hepatitis may present at any age, primary biliary cirrhosis has never been reported in persons under 20 years; most cases are seen in women who are postmenopausal at diagnosis. In patients with either autoimmune hepatitis or primary biliary cirrhosis, arthralgia and even arthritis may be present. Some patients with autoimmune hepatitis will present for the first time with decompensated liver disease, that is, jaundice, ascites, variceal haemorrhage, and less commonly with hepatic encephalopathy (generally in someone with burnt-out autoimmune hepatitis and cirrhosis). Whereas presentation with variceal haemorrhage is not uncommon, even in the early stages of primary biliary cirrhosis, other manifestations of hepatic decompensation are generally signs of terminal disease. It is most unusual for a patient with autoimmune hepatitis to complain of pruritus, unless pregnant or recently prescribed the oral contraceptive pill or hormone replacement therapy. Should pruritus be present then a chronic cholestatic disorder should be considered more likely. Pruritus is often the presenting symptom of primary biliary cirrhosis. Other non-hepatic autoimmune diseases may be seen in association with both autoimmune hepatitis and primary biliary cirrhosis. Thyroid disease is common with both. The connective tissue diseases, Raynaud's phenomenon, sicca syndrome, scleroderma, and CREST syndrome (calcinosis, Raynaud's phenomenon, (o)esophageal dysphagia, sclerodactyly, telangiectasia) are really only seen with primary biliary cirrhosis.

Biochemistry

The biochemical features of autoimmune hepatitis generally reflect hepatocellular injury (elevated values of serum aminotransferase); however, cholestatic features may occasionally be present, in that the alkaline phosphatase and particularly the γ-glutamyl transpeptidase are elevated. It is important first to rule out the use of any enzyme inducers which may be responsable for an elevation in γ-glutamyl transpeptidase. Usually, at first presentation, patients with primary biliary cirrhosis are anicteric and have an enzyme pattern typical of cholestasis, although a fivefold or greater elevation in serum aminotransferase levels may sometimes be observed.

There are really no specific biochemical features which suggest autoimmune liver disease, but in patients with an overlap syndrome a biochemical pattern suggestive of both hepatitis and cholestasis is usual. Cholestatic hepatitis may also be due to a number of hepatic drug reactions, and the biochemical abnormalities may persist for years although the jaundice tends to fade early (Altraif, AmJGastr, 1994; 89:1250).

Serology

Testing for several non-organ antibodies is most helpful in supporting a diagnosis of autoimmune liver disease. High-titre anti-nuclear antibodies (ANA) and/or smooth muscle antibodies (SMA) are so characteristic of classic type I autoimmune hepatitis that if they are found in combination with an elevated level of serum IgG, sometimes to extraordinary high levels (three- to fourfold elevation), the diagnosis of autoimmune hepatitis is almost secured (Johnson, Hepatol, 1993; 18:948). However, some patients who appear to have type I autoimmune hepatitis also test positive for antimitochondrial antibodies (AMA), that is, antibodies usually associated specifically with primary biliary cirrhosis (Kenny, DigDisSci, 1986; 37:705). These are generally in low titre, but are not false positives, as they can be confirmed by a more specific and sensitive method, namely immunoblotting. Therefore, some patients with otherwise typical autoimmune hepatitis appear to be AMA positive (Czaja, Gastro, 1993; 105:1522).

However, there are other patients with autoimmune hepatitis, namely the type 2 form associated with the presence of the anti-liver, -kidney, -microsomal antibody (anti-LKM), in whom a false positive AMA may be reported (Czaja, Gastro, 1993; 105:1522) as a result of misreading the immunofluorescence pattern; these patients cannot be truly referred to as having an overlap syndrome.

Histology

Confirmation of a diagnosis of autoimmune hepatitis is generally made by finding the classic features on histological analysis of liver tissue. Some patients with autoimmune hepatitis, not all of whom have cholestatic biochemical features, are nevertheless found to have duct injury on liver biopsy in addition to the more classic features of autoimmune hepatitis. However, the duct injury can generally be differentiated from that seen in primary biliary cirrhosis (Christoffersen, HumPath, 1972; 3:227). These patients are not necessarily those with autoimmune hepatitis who have a serum positive for AMA. Some patients with severe autoimmune hepatitis may have visible cholestasis on biopsy; in these instances it is particularly important to rule out any primary or superimposed drug-induced liver injury.

The typical features of primary biliary cirrhosis on liver biopsy are more likely to be seen in the patient without established cirrhosis; they are granulomatous destruction of bile ducts and bile duct proliferation. There may, in addition, be significant periportal as well as portal chronic inflammatory cell infiltration; sometimes a lobular component may be observed. The histological pattern is very different from that observed with autoimmune hepatitis.

Recently reported are patients who have the serological findings typical of type I autoimmune hepatitis but have a histological pattern indistinguishable from primary biliary cirrhosis. The first three cases to be described, in 1987, were classified as having 'immune cholangitis' (Brunner, DMedWoch, 1987; 12:1454). A subsequent paper (Ben-Ari, Hepatol, 1993; 18:10) described four similar cases and claimed, as did the initial paper, that corticosteroid therapy led to remission of disease, at least in the short term. A subsequent study (Michieletti, Gut, 1994; 35:260) described 17 subjects who had been referred to a clinical therapeutic trial for primary biliary cirrhosis, but who were excluded because their AMA test by immunofluorescence was negative. Their AMA-negative status was later confirmed by immunoblotting. When these 17 patients were compared with 17 patients with AMA-positive primary biliary cirrhosis referred to the same trial, matched for height of serum bilirubin, the only distinguishing features were significantly lower levels of serum alanine aminotransferase and IgM in the patients negative for AMA. All of the AMA-negative patients were found to have either ANA and/or SMA in their serum. Another report (Taylor, AmJSurgPath, 1994; 18:91) confirmed that some patients with otherwise typical primary biliary cirrhosis had no serological evidence of AMA, even using the most sensitive and specific tests, but all had a high titre of ANA. The term 'autoimmune cholangitis' has been used to describe these patients, but it is probably more accurate to describe them as having AMA-negative primary biliary cirrhosis. Certainly, the natural history of these AMA-negative patients and their associated autoimmune conditions, such as scleroderma, coeliac disease, Raynaud's phenomenon, sicca syndrome, rheumatoid arthritis, and thyroid disease, is much more like the picture of primary biliary cirrhosis than that of autoimmune hepatitis type 1. From the pathologist's standpoint, a retrospective study indicated that it was not unusual to observe the histological appearances of primary biliary cirrhosis when the serological findings are more typical of autoimmune hepatitis (Goodman, DigDisSci, 1995; 40:1232).

Diagnosis changing with time

The pattern of autoimmune liver disease does not always remain stable. Colombato (Gastro, 1994; 107:1839) described a patient who when first seen appeared to have obvious AMA-positive, biopsy-proven, primary biliary cirrhosis and hence was treated with ursodeoxycholic acid. Treatment resulted in a marked improvement in liver biochemistry. Subsequently, the patient developed a sudden rise in serum aminotransferase levels which coincided with the disappearance of serum AMA and appearance of ANA. Repeat liver biopsy at this time showed features of autoimmune hepatitis on a background of primary biliary cirrhosis. Ursodeoxycholic acid treatment was continued, but prednisone was added to the therapeutic regimen; this resulted in a marked improvement in liver biochemistry. Dose reduction of the steroids, but not the ursodeoxycholic acid, led to a flare-up of serum aminotransferase levels which responded to an increase in steroid dose.

Pathogenesis

It is hoped that molecular immunological techniques may clarify the pathogenesis of autoimmune liver disease in the future. Molecular genetic techniques indicate that type I autoimmune hepatitis is associated with class II HLA DR3 and DR4 (Donaldson, Hepatol, 1990; 13:701), whereas primary biliary cirrhosis has been shown by some to have a weak association with DR8 (Gregory, QJMed, 1993; 86:393). No reports on HLA associations in 'autoimmune cholangitis' have been reported. The AMA is directed against several enzyme components of the inner membrane of mitochondria. How an intracellular component induces the generation of extra-cellular antibodies is unclear. The concept of 'molecular mimicry' has been postulated (Burroughs, Nature, 1992; 358:377). Some antigenic components of rough mutants of *Escherichia coli* are common to the inner mitochondrial antigens. Curiously, these same mitochondrial antigens may be detected in the cytoplasm of the luminal side of biliary endothelial cells (but only of the interlobular bile ducts), both in typical AMA-positive primary biliary cirrhosis and in serum AMA-negative primary biliary cirrhosis (autoimmune cholangitis), (Tsuneyama, Hepatol, 1995; 34:496). This observation would suggest that AMA or its mimic may be pertinent to the liver injury which results in a histological pattern typical of primary biliary cirrhosis. To date, autoimmune hepatitis cases positive for AMA in serum have not been studied similarly. Investigations into other aspects of the immune response and targeted substrates in patients with autoimmune liver disease should be helpful in further elucidating their pathogeneses.

Therapy

The premise 'at least do no harm' is particularly relevant to the management of overlap syndromes. Treatment of symptomatic autoimmune hepatitis with corticosteroids leads to a marked improvement of survival (Cook, QJMed, 1971; 21:613; Soloway, Gastro, 1972; 63:820; Murray-Lyon, Lancet, 1973; i:735). Those patients who are cholestatic but do not have liver histology typical of primary biliary cirrhosis, despite some duct injury, should probably be treated similarly. AMA positive but otherwise classic autoimmune hepatitis should also receive steroid therapy. However, if the clinical symptoms and histology are more in keeping with primary biliary cirrhosis, it is probably wise to avoid steroid therapy and to use ursodeoxycholic acid (Kim, Hepatol, 1997; 26:22).

Autoimmune hepatitis compared with primary sclerosing cholangitis

Before the introduction of endoscopic retrograde cholangio-pancreatography (ERCP) there was no easy way to make a diagnosis of primary sclerosing cholangitis, and it is likely that many cases were misdiagnosed. A review of the liver histological findings in patients subsequently found on ERCP to have primary sclerosing cholangitis revealed a myriad of histological diagnoses ranging from autoimmune hepatitis to primary biliary cirrhosis (Chapman, Gut, 1980; 21:870).

Clinical

It is likely that many patients with primary sclerosing cholangitis remain undiagnosed, either because they have no symptoms or because they are misdiagnosed right up until the point of requiring liver transplantation. When symptoms are present they may be non-specific, as with any chronic liver disease. Pruritus may be the only feature suggesting cholestasis and which distinguishes it from autoimmune hepatitis. It is most important to keep primary sclerosing cholangitis in mind in any patient with liver disease who has inflammatory bowel disease. An ERCP may become a necessary part of the work-up in such patients who otherwise appear to have autoimmune hepatitis.

Biochemistry

Abnormal biochemistry suggestive of primary sclerosing cholangitis is most often identified during follow-up for chronic inflammatory bowel disease, usually ulcerative colitis affecting the entire colon and less commonly colonic Crohn's disease. However, chronic inflammatory bowel disease may also be associated with type 1 autoimmune hepatitis (Rabinovitz, DigDisSci, 1992; 37:1606). The biochemical pattern of both autoimmune hepatitis and primary sclerosing cholangitis may be very similar, although the findings in the latter more commonly suggest cholestasis. However, the serum alkaline phosphatase level may be entirely normal in up to 50 per cent of patients with primary sclerosing cholangitis (Wiesner, Gastro, 1980; 79:200), particularly in children (Wilschanski, Hepatol, 1995; 22:1414). In these circumstances it may be helpful to check the γ-glutamyl transpeptidase, which is virtually always elevated in primary sclerosing cholangitis, sometimes quite markedly. In both autoimmune hepatitis and primary sclerosing cholangitis, liver biochemistry can fluctuate, even the level of bilirubin, without the introduction of therapy.

Serology

It is not unusual for patients with primary sclerosing cholangitis to show the serological markers of autoimmune hepatitis, that is, to be positive for both ANA and SMA (Zauli, JHepatol, 1987; 5:14). The antineutrophil cytoplasmic antibody (ANCA), commonly found in patients with primary sclerosing cholangitis, may also be found in patients with otherwise clear-cut autoimmune hepatitis (Targan, Gastro, 1995; 108:1159); therefore, none of these non-organ specific antibodies are entirely specific for any one of the autoimmune liver diseases. A particularly high IgG level may favour autoimmune hepatitis rather than primary sclerosing cholangitis.

An ERCP may become a necessary part of the work-up in some patients who otherwise appear to have autoimmune hepatitis. The overlap of autoimmune hepatitis and primary sclerosing cholangitis occurs most commonly in children so, despite the attendant difficulties with performing an ERCP in the very young, the test needs to be done. Ultrasonography showing thickened bile ducts is not sufficiently reliable to make a firm diagnosis, but it is possible that magnetic resonance cholangiography may delineate the biliary tree sufficiently well to diagnose sclerosing cholangitis. This non-invasive diagnostic tool needs to be validated against the ERCP before its true value can be assessed.

Histology

Although duct lesions may be found on liver biopsy in subjects who appear to have autoimmune hepatitis, their presence should raise the suspicion of primary sclerosing cholangitis or small duct cholangitis (Wee, AnnIntMed, 1985; 102:581). There are no histological features which are common to all cases of primary sclerosing cholangitis; in fact, histology is not helpful in making a diagnosis of this condition. 'Onion' skin fibrosis is rarely seen (Wiesner, Gastro, 1980; 79:200) and the ERCP findings are the gold standard for diagnosis.

Pathogenesis

The only finding suggesting a common pathogenesis or risk factor for autoimmune hepatitis and primary sclerosing cholangitis seems to be their identical class II HLA association with DR3 and DR4 (Donaldson, Hepatol, 1990; 13:701; Mehal, Gastro, 1994; 106:160). Several forms of sclerosing cholangitis are secondary to ischaemic damage to the bile ducts and there has also been the finding of ischaemic changes on liver histology in autoimmune hepatitis (Kaplan, Hepatol, 1994; 20:144A); but again, ischaemia may only be a risk factor for inciting immune-mediated tissue damage.

Therapy

A trial of therapy with corticosteroids has never been used to distinguish autoimmune hepatitis from sclerosing cholangitis in the way that it has been used to distinguish autoimmune hepatitis from primary biliary cirrhosis (Geubel, Gastro, 1976; 71:444). Treatment with ursodeoxycholic acid would be expected to lead to an improvement in serum biochemistry in both conditions and hence would not be helpful (Leuschner, DigDisSci, 1985; 30:642; Stiehl, ScaJGastr, 1994; 204 Suppl.59). Therapy with corticosteroids needs to be avoided in patients with primary sclerosing cholangitis, unless essential for management of inflammatory bowel disease, as steroids may promote the development of or exacerbate bacterial cholangitis as well as enhance the risk of osteoporosis. The latter is found in patients with inflammatory bowel disease and/or sclerosing cholangitis even before the introduction of corticosteroid therapy (Compston, AlimPharmTher, 1995; 9:237; Hay, Gastro, 1995; 108:276).

There are some occasions when it would appear that autoimmune hepatitis and primary sclerosing cholangitis coexist (Minuk, CanJ-Gastr, 1988; 2:22; Rabinovitz, DigDisSci, 1992; 37:1606; Gohlke, JHepatol, 1996; 24:699). It is claimed that under these circumstances the autoimmune hepatitis features of the disease respond well to corticosteroid therapy, and hence it may be impossible to avoid the use of immunosuppressive therapy. Ursodeoxycholic acid increases the transport of retained bile acids out of the liver (Jasrawi, Gastro, 1994; 106:134), probably benefits all cholestatic patients, and may even be beneficial for inflammatory bowel disease.

Autoimmune hepatitis and/or chronic hepatitis C

Whereas in the United States the prevalence of hepatitis C in patients with autoimmune hepatitis is low (less than 3 per cent; Czaja, DigDisSci, 1995; 40:33), the association is better recognized in countries where the risk of acquiring HCV is higher.

Clinical

Both autoimmune hepatitis and viral hepatitis C (**HCV**) may be asymptomatic or associated with a variety of non-specific complaints such as fatigue, malaise, and abdominal discomfort. Petechial haemorrhages of the extremities related to cryoglobulinaemia are associated with hepatitis C, as may be membranous proliferative glomerulonephritis. Sjögren's syndrome, lichen planus, and non-Hodgkin's lymphoma (Kaupke, WestJMed, 1996; 164:442) may also

be found. Superimposed hepatoma occurs with both autoimmune hepatitis and hepatitis C, but is more common in autoimmune hepatitis complicated by infection with hepatitis C (Ryder, Hepatol, 1995; 22:718).

Biochemistry

Both autoimmune hepatitis and hepatitis C may present with an acute outset, flare-up or with low-grade chronic disease. The pattern of enzyme elevation in hepatitis C infection generally shows a higher level of alanine than of aspartate aminotransferase, before cirrhosis appears, whereas there is no specific pattern in autoimmune hepatitis. The main distinguishing feature is the marked elevation of IgG often seen in autoimmune hepatitis which is not common with hepatitis C.

Serology

The non-organ specific antibody findings may not be helpful in distinguishing autoimmune hepatitis from hepatitis C infections, as 60 per cent of patients with hepatitis C have some autoimmune markers in their serum (Clifford, Hepatol, 1995; 21:613). At least one-third are ANA and/or SMA positive and others may have anti-LKM antibodies. Anti-LKM is directed against cytochrome P450 11D6 (Yamamoto, Gastro, 1993; 104:1762). The hepatitis C genome has areas that cross-react with cytochrome P450 11D6, suggesting that the virus may induce autoimmunity. However, the target epitope for anti-LKM antibodies in hepatitis C is different from that for type 2 autoimmune hepatitis (Manns, JCI, 1991; 88:1370). Certainly, in patients with apparent autoimmune hepatitis but who give a history of a risk factor for hepatitis C or who come from a high incidence area, it is wise to check for anti-HCV, better still HCV-RNA, as sometimes a false positive ELISA for hepatitis C antibody may occur in the presence of hyperglobulinaemia (Skaug, VoxSang, 1993; 64:215).

Pathogenesis

Some workers have suggested that autoimmune hepatitis may be initiated by a viral infection (Vento, Lancet, 1991; 337:1183), and hepatitis C infection is associated with several extrahepatitic manifestations resembling autoimmune disease that would support this concept. Unfortunately, the lack of an animal model, apart from the chimpanzee, restricts further studies in this area. Study of the HLA pattern in autoimmune hepatitis and hepatitis C suggests no common associations.

Therapy

Deciding what to do for the best in a patient with chronic hepatitis with autoimmune markers and proven hepatitis C infection (RNA positive in serum) is a dilemma. Patients with a high titre of ANA (greater than 1:160) are generally advised not to receive interferon therapy for their hepatitis C, as interferon may exacerbate autoimmune disease. However, in a group of patients with proven hepatitis C who seemed to develop autoimmune hepatitis after the introduction of interferon therapy, the finding of a non-organ specific antibody before treatment did not predict who would develop interferon-associated hepatitis (Garcia-Buey, Gastro, 1995; 108:1770). Corticosteroid therapy when given to patients with hepatitis C causes an increase in viral replication (Fong, Gastro, 1994; 107:196), but a retrospective study which reviewed cases of hepatitis C inadvertently treated with steroids indicated that some patients appeared to respond well to this treatment (Thiel, AmJGastr, 1996; 91:300). When the International Autoimmune Hepatitis Scoring System (Johnson, Hepatol, 1993; 18:948) was applied to these patients, it was not helpful in predicting responders from non-responders. For the most part, it is likely that corticosteroids are not too harmful in chronic hepatitis C; patients with hepatitis C who undergo liver transplantation and develop recurrent infection have a post-transplant survival similar to uninfected transplant recipients (Gane, NEJM, 1996; 334:815), at least in the short term. However, as with chronic hepatitis B infection, sudden withdrawal of immunosuppressive therapy may lead to a flare-up and even fatal hepatitis (Vento, Lancet, 1991; 337:1183; Gruber, JIntMed, 1993; 234:223). Combination therapy of interferon and corticosteroid is without value as the latter maintains viral replication in the face of antiviral therapy.

In patients with low-titre ANA and/or SMA, absence of hyper-gammaglobulinaemia, and chronic hepatitis C, cautious interferon therapy is advised. Similarly, in patients with proven hepatitis C (RNA positive) associated with anti-LKM antibodies, interferon therapy is appropriate. However, if the patient has high-titre ANA and/or SMA with hypergammaglobulinaemia, immunosuppressive therapy may be more appropriate despite the presence of hepatitis C RNA (Bellary, AnnIntMed, 1995; 1223:32). This combination is more likely to be seen in patients who are from countries where there is a high prevalence of hepatitis C.

14.7 The liver in graft-versus-host disease

Christophe Duvoux, Marie-France Saint-Marc-Girardin, Jean-Paul Vernant, Elie-Serge Zafrani, and Daniel Dhumeaux

Introduction

Graft-versus-host disease can be defined as the clinical, bio-chemical, and histological manifestations resulting from the response of donor immunocompetent cells to the histocompatibility antigens of a recipient (Sullivan, ClinHaem, 1983; 12:775). Allogeneic bone marrow transplantation is the most common cause of graft-versus-host disease,[1] but graft-versus-host-disease has also been described after solid organ transplantation, mainly after small bowel (Schraut, Gastro, 1988; 94: 709), pancreaticosplenic (Deierhoi, Transpl, 1986; 41:544), or liver transplantations (Burdick, NEJM, 1988; 318:689) and in patients who have received non-irradiated blood products (Brubaker, VoxSang, 1983; 45:401). It is noteworthy that in graft-versus-host-disease occurring after liver transplantation, the liver is not involved in the process since the immunocompetent cells responsible for graft-versus-host disease are transmitted with the engrafted liver and share the same histocompatibility antigens. After bone marrow transplantation, graft-versus-host disease occurs in 25 to 60 per cent of recipients from HLA genoidentical, mixed lymphocyte, culture-unreactive donors (Neudorf, SemHemat, 1984; 21:91; Sullivan, Blood, 1981; 57:267).[2] In patients receiving grafts from non-related HLA phenoidentical donors or non-identical donors, the prevalence of graft-versus-host disease is even higher.[1]

At least three conditions are required for the development of graft-versus-host disease (Santos, ClinHaem, 1983; 12:611):

(1) the graft contains immunocompetent cells;

(2) the existence of a genetic disparity between host and graft so that the recipient is recognized as foreign;

(3) the inability of the host to exhibit an effective immunological reaction against the graft.

Two distinct forms of graft-versus-host disease may be observed, that is acute and chronic. They differ in chronology and in organ involvement. This chapter will focus on the hepatic manifestations of these two forms.

Acute graft-versus-host disease

Acute graft-versus-host disease is a clinicopathological syndrome that usually occurs within 6 weeks after bone marrow transplantation.[1] It consists of dermatitis with diffuse skin rash, enteritis with watery or bloody diarrhoea and abdominal pain, and liver disease.[3] Liver involvement results in cholestasis, the severity of which greatly varies from subclinical disease to overt jaundice. When clinical or biochemical signs of liver disease are observed, cutaneous lesions are evident in most cases. Rarely, liver abnormalities are the only presenting feature. There are usually no overt signs of hepatocellular failure, that is ascites and hepatic encephalopathy (Wolford, JClinGastro, 1988; 10:419).[1-3,4] An increase in serum alkaline phosphatase activity precedes hyperbilirubinaemia, is generally moderate, and is associated with mild serum alanine aminotransferase (**ALT**) and serum aspartate aminotransferase (**AST**) elevation. The increase in serum alkaline phosphatase activity is not constant as normal alkaline phosphatase activity has been reported in patients with histologically-proven graft-versus-host disease.[1] Liver biopsy is not required when hepatic abnormalities are consistent with graft-versus-host disease and associated cutaneous or intestinal involvement is established. By contrast, biopsy may be necessary when the diagnosis is doubtful. However, characteristic histological features may appear only 2 weeks after the beginning of hepatic symptoms.[3]

Hepatocytes as well as bile ducts can be altered. Marked hepatocyte necrosis was observed in six of the 15 patients reported by Snover et al.[5] and in three of the six patients of Bernuau et al.[4] Interlobular bile duct damage is a characteristic feature, although the lesions can be slight. Mild or moderate lesions consisting of lymphocytosis, cholangitis, and/or anisocytosis and anisonucleosis of biliary epithelial cells were observed in six of the 15 patients of Snover et al.[5] and in all of the five patients of Bernuau et al., in whom portal spaces were visible.[4] Lobular or portal tract inflammation is usually moderate.[4,5] Lymphocytes have been shown to be in close contact with hepatocytes and bile duct cells[4] and this probably explains necrosis of both hepatocytes and biliary cells. Endotheliitis, that is the attachment of lymphoid cells to the endothelium of central and/or portal veins, was reported in 40 per

Table 1 Grades of acute graft-versus-host disease

Grade	Definition
I	Moderate skin rash, no gut or liver involvement
II	Moderate to severe skin rash, moderate gut involvement, and/or moderate liver involvement (serum bilirubin 3.5–25.5 μmol/dl)
III	Severe skin rash and intestinal involvement, severe liver disease (serum bilirubin 5.0–25.5 μmol/dl)
IV	Severe organ involvement with serum bilirubin >25.5 μmol/dl

cent of the patients of Snover et al.[5] In summary, histological features of graft-versus-disease greatly resemble those of acute rejection after liver transplantation[6] (Alexander, Hepatol, 1990; 11:144) and even those of primary biliary cirrhosis (Shulman, Hepatol, 1988; 8:463).

Four grades of graft-versus-host disease have been defined by the Seattle group, according to the degree of organ involvement (Table 1).[1] Moderate to severe (grade II to IV) graft-versus-host disease develops in 25 to 50 per cent of the patients. Death occurs in half of the patients with graft-versus-host disease;[1] usually this is not due to liver failure but rather to the involvement of other organs, or to infectious complications directly related to immuno-suppressive therapy.

Liver involvement may require specific therapy. In addition to cyclosporin, therapy includes steroids at conventional or high dosage, with or without antithymocyte globulins or monoclonal antibodies (Neudorf, SemHemat, 1984; 21:91).[8] Additional supportive care is essential, including parenteral nutrition, gut rest, and prophylaxis against infectious diseases. However, in spite of therapy, more than 50 per cent of the patients who survive severe graft-versus-host disease will develop chronic disease.[3]

Chronic graft-versus-host disease

Chronic graft-versus-host disease is a multiorgan, autoimmune-like disease developing within 80 to 400 days after bone marrow transplantation.[9] In most cases, chronic graft-versus-host-disease is preceded by the acute disease, even if this has apparently resolved.[1,9] However, 20 to 30 per cent of chronic graft-versus host disease occurs de novo. Liver involvement is observed in most patients with chronic disease. It has been reported in 42 of 47 (89 per cent) patients with extensive disease affecting skin, eyes, mouth, and other target organs but it may also be observed in patients with more limited chronic disease.[10]

Cholestatic features are more severe in chronic than in acute graft-versus-host disease. In Shulman et al.'s series of 20 patients with chronic graft-versus-host disease, 14 (70 per cent) had marked increase in serum alkaline phosphatase (median of nine times the upper limit of normal), reaching a value of 30 times the upper limit of normal. The degree of hyperbilirubinaemia was different in patients in whom the chronic form followed progressive acute graft-versus-host disease and in patients in whom it appeared de novo or after the resolution of the acute form. Moderate hyperbilirubinaemia was observed in five of the nine patients with progressive acute disease; none of the patients in the other group developed jaundice.

The AST was also usually slightly elevated, with median values of three times the upper limit of normal (range 1–19 times normal). Among the 14 patients tested, an increase in IgG and IgM was noted in seven and four, respectively. Serum autoantibodies were studied in 17 of the patients in this series; antinuclear and anti-mitochondrial antibodies were observed in eight and three cases, respectively.[10] The presence of antiliver/kidney microsomal type I antibodies has also been reported (Homberg, GastrClinBiol, 1985; 9:622). Severe interlobular bile duct lesions, chronic destructive cholangitis and sometimes ductopenia are the most striking features in patients with chronic graft-versus-host disease.[4,5,7] In one series of eight patients,[4] marked lymphocyte and macrophage infiltration of the portal spaces was observed in six; in another series of eight patients such portal tract inflammation was noted in only three.[5] Intensity of hepatocellular necrosis varies from one case to another: it was severe in the patients reported by Bernuau et al.[4] and moderate in those of Snover et al.[5]

The prognosis of chronic graft-versus-host disease depends on the severity of the disease and the type of onset. It is better in de novo chronic graft-versus-host disease than in the chronic form following acute disease with a progressive course.[10] Among nine patients with such a progressive course, histological specimens obtained 160 days after transplantation showed degenerative changes of bile duct epithelium in four patients and ductopenia in three[10]. Six patients had periportal fibrosis[10] and cirrhosis which, although a rare complication of chronic graft-versus-host disease (Knapp, Gastro, 1987; 92:513; Yau, Transpl, 1986; 41:129), may eventually occur.[10] Indeed, it is well known that biliary cirrhosis is the ultimate stage of all diseases in which there is disappearance of interlobular bile ducts, for example primary biliary cirrhosis, primary sclerosing cholangitis, chronic sarcoidosis,[11] and idiopathic paucity of intrahepatic bile ducts (Zafrani, Gastro, 1990; 99:1823; Zafrani, AnnPath, 1995; 15:348). It is of interest that aberrant expression of HLA class II antigens on bile ducts, a factor favouring T lymphocyte-mediated bile duct injury, has been reported in patients with primary biliary cirrhosis and in those with hepatic graft-versus-host disease.[11]

The treatment of chronic graft-versus-host disease includes prednisone, cyclosporin, and eventually azathioprine or thalidomide. In patients with cholestasis who do not respond to therapy, ursodeoxycholic acid might be helpful, as it has been shown to be effective in other cholestatic syndromes with ductopenia (Chazouilleres, JHepatol, 1989; 9 Suppl. I: S138; Poupon, NEJM, 1994; 330:1342). In a preliminary study, ursodeoxycholic acid was tested for 6 weeks in 12 patients with chronic graft-versus-disease after failure of usual immunosuppressive therapy. Liver tests improved during ursodeoxycholic acid, but biochemical relapse occurred after withdrawal of therapy (Fried, AnnIntMed, 1992; 116:624). Further studies are therefore required to assess the efficacy of sustained use of ursodeoxycholic acid in graft-versus-host-disease.

Liver transplantation may also be considered in the treatment of out of the ordinary, life-threatening, graft-versus-host disease. It has been reported in at least two cases. In one patient, liver transplantation was successfully performed for end-stage secondary biliary cirrhosis, a long time after bone marrow transplantation (Rhodes, Gastro, 1990; 99:536). In the second case, liver transplantation was performed 107 days after bone marrow transplantation for acute graft-versus-host-disease leading to vanishing bile duct syndrome, but the patient died 23 days after surgery (Dowlati, Transpl, 1995; 60:106). The actual therapeutic value of liver transplantation for severe graft-versus-host-disease remains to be defined. These preliminary reports suggest a high postoperative risk when liver transplantation is performed shortly after bone marrow transplantation, due to an obvious high risk of infections; it might be safer when performed some time after bone marrow transplantation, when the immune status has improved.

Differential diagnosis

The large number of possible causes of liver dysfunction in patients with bone marrow transplant renders the diagnosis of graft-versus-host disease difficult. Furthermore, the occurrence of two or more different liver diseases in the same patient, for example viral hepatitis, drug hepatitis, and graft-versus-host disease, is not uncommon. It is not our purpose to discuss here all liver diseases that may develop after bone marrow transplantation. Since graft-versus-host disease is mainly characterized by cholestasis, we shall focus on diseases associated with a cholestatic syndrome.

Viral infections

Cytomegalovirus (CMV) infection is frequent in patients with bone marrow transplant (Preiksaitis, TransplImmunol, 1989; 9:137). Liver involvement is characterized by jaundice or isolated abnormalities of AST and alkaline phosphatases levels. Liver biopsy shows mononuclear portal and sinusoidal infiltration. Intranuclear CMV inclusions are frequent, especially in immunodeficient patients (Snover, LabInvest, 1985; 52:64A). Canalicular cholestasis and bile duct epithelium damage can also be seen. Culture of liver biopsy specimens as well as immunochemistry, may help in diagnosis. It has been shown that acute graft-versus-host disease significantly increases the risk of CMV infection, and these two diseases may thus occur together. As a result, the precise role of CMV in liver dysfunction is often difficult to ascertain.

For years, non-A non-B virus hepatitis has been a common infection in bone marrow transplant recipients because of the large transfusion requirements before and after the procedure. However, identification of C virus as the major agent of post-transfusional hepatitis and the subsequent screening of blood donors for hepatitis C virus (HCV) antibodies has resulted in a dramatic decrease in the incidence of HCV-related hepatitis after bone marrow transplantation. In one study, the incidence of HCV seroconversion after bone marrow transplantation fell from 14 per cent before screening for non-A non-B hepatitis to 1.6 per cent after blood screening for HCV antibodies (Norol, Transpl, 1994; 57:393). Acute post-transfusional hepatitis may cause moderate or marked hyper-transaminasaemia with or without jaundice, whereas the chronic form is characterized by a mild increase in serum transaminases, possibly associated with alkaline phosphatase and γ-glutamyl transferase elevation. Bile duct damage may be seen at liver biopsy (Lefkowitch, Gastro, 1993; 104:595) and histological differentiation between chronic post-transfusional hepatitis and chronic graft-versus-host disease can therefore be difficult (Shulman, Hepatol, 1988; 8:463). It has been suggested that HCV serological tests could be less sensitive in immunosuppressed patients than in patients with normal immune condition (Pawlotsky, JClinMicrobiol, 1995;

33:1357). When serological tests for HCV are negative, serum or even liver testing for HCV RNA by PCR may thus be required to rule out HCV infection, or to assess the coexistence of both graft-versus-host disease and HCV infection.

Drug-induced liver disease

Cyclosporin and azathioprine, which are used in the treatment of acute and chronic graft-versus-host disease, may be hepatotoxic. Cyclosporin hepatotoxicity is dose dependent and responsible for hyperbilirubinaemia and slight abnormalities of liver enzyme levels (Mentha, GastrClinBiol, 1986; 10:641). Azathioprine has been incriminated in cholestatic jaundice in some patients (DePinho, Gastro, 1981; 86:162; Loiseau, ClinTranspl, 1987; 1:88; Menard, Gastro, 1980; 78:142). However, withdrawal of immunosuppressive drugs should be undertaken with caution since an exacerbation of graft-versus-host disease may occur. Antimicrobial agents are commonly used in bone marrow transplant patients and can frequently be hepatotoxic. Sulphamethoxazole–trimethoprim may cause cholestasis.[12] Amoxicillin–clavulanate potassium as well as roxithromycin (Dubois, GastrClinBiol, 1989; 13:317) and erythromycin salts have been shown to be responsible for cholestatic hepatitis that is sometimes associated with interlobular bile duct lesions and simulates extrahepatic obstruction (Zafrani, DigDisSci, 1979; 24:385; Hautekeete, JHepatol, 1995; 22:71).[12]

Veno-occlusive disease of the liver

Veno-occlusive disease of the liver is the most common cause of hepatic dysfunction after bone marrow transplantation (Ganem, IntJRadiatOncolBiolPhys, 1988; 14:879). It is usually distinguished from graft-versus-host disease on clinical grounds; that is the association with:

(1) jaundice;
(2) hepatomegaly and/or right upper quadrant abdominal pains;
(3) ascites and/or unexplained weight gain.

In addition, veno-occlusive disease occurs within the first month of bone marrow transplantation, whereas hepatic manifestations of graft-versus-host disease are rarely present before 3 weeks. In doubtful cases liver biopsy, generally performed transvenously because of coagulation disorders, is helpful.

Nodular regenerative hyperplasia of the liver

This disease has been recognized as a possible cause of hepatic disorder after bone marrow transplantation (Snover, Hepatol, 1989; 9:443). It is characterized by diffuse, nodular transformation of the liver consisting of nodules of regeneration that are not encircled by fibrosis but are limited by hepatocellular plates separated by dilated sinusoids. It differs from graft-versus-host disease by its clinical (i.e. hepatomegaly, portal hypertension) and histological features.

In patients with bone marrow transplant, an increased bilirubin level may also be noted after blood transfusions and sepsis. Renal dysfunction aggravates conjugated hyperbilirubinaemia.

Problems related to liver biopsy

Biopsy is frequently required for the differential diagnosis of hepatic disease in bone marrow transplant patients. Because of the difficulties of liver biopsy in such patients, its indication should be carefully considered. In patients with a low platelet count leading to abnormal bleeding time (a frequent situation in the early period after transplantation) biopsy can be performed safely by the transjugular route. However, the sample obtained by this method is often small, with a low number of portal tracts which makes the diagnosis of graft-versus-host disease more difficult. The sensitivity and specificity of liver biopsy in the diagnosis of graft-versus-host disease must also be considered. Liver biopsy is not a sensitive procedure in the very early phase of graft-versus-host disease since the changes are simply those of mild lobular hepatitis.[3] One study has confirmed that false-negative diagnoses are more frequent when specimens are obtained within the first month following transplantation.[7] In addition, bile duct abnormalities, which are the most characteristic changes in graft-versus-host disease, are not specific (see above). It must therefore be emphasized that a definitive diagnosis, with its therapeutic implication, should always be based on rigorous clinicopathological correlations.

Prognosis

Graft-versus-host disease is a frequent and sometimes life-threatening complication following bone marrow transplantation. Although serious complications are associated with graft-versus-host disease, it is now recognized that its development after bone marrow transplantation favourably influences the prognosis of the haematological malignancy. Indeed, an inverse relationship has been found between the occurrence of graft-versus-host disease and the recurrence of leukaemia.[8] In the future, the routine use of T lymphocyte-depleted bone marrow may reduce the incidence of graft-versus-host disease.[2] This will necessitate more effective antineoplastic agents to lessen the risk of relapse. Progress may also be made by:

(1) adapting prophylaxis for graft-versus-host disease to the expected risk of this disease (Bagot, Transpl, 1986; 41:316);

(2) better donor selection; female donors with previous pregnancies, in particular, are reported to be associated with an increased risk of graft-versus-host disease.[8]

References

1. McDonald GB, Shulman H.M, Wolforo JL, and Spencer GD. Liver disease after human marrow transplantation. *Seminars in Liver Diseases*, 1987; **7**: 210–29.

2. Mitsuyasu RT *et al*. Treatment of donor bone marrow with mono-clonal anti-T-cell antibody and complement for the prevention of graft-versus-host disease. *Annals of Internal Medicine*, 1986; **105**: 20–6.

3. McDonald GB, Shulman HM, Sullivan KM, and Spencer GD. Intestinal and hepatic complications of human bone marrow transplantation. Part I. *Gastroenterology*, 1986; **90**: 460–77.

4. Bernuau D. *et al*. Histological and ultrastructural appearance of the liver during graft-versus-host disease complicating bone marrow transplantation. *Transplantation*, 1980; **29**: 236–44.

5. Snover DC, Weisdorg SA, Ramsay NK, MeGlave P, and Kersey JH. Hepatic graft versus host disease: a study of the predictive value of liver biopsy in diagnosis. *Hepatology*, 1984; **4**: 123–30.

6. Wight DGD and Portmann B. Pathology of liver transplantation. In Calne R, ed. *Liver transplantation*, 2nd edn. London: Grune and Stratton, 1987: 385–435.

7. Shulman HM, Sharma P, Amos D, Fenster LF, and McDonald GB. A coded histologic study of hepatic graft-versus-host disease after human bone marrow transplantation. *Hepatology*, 1988; **8**: 463–70.

8. Storb R. Graft rejection and graft-versus-host disease in marrow transplantation. *Transplantation Proceedings*, 1989; **21**: 2915–18.

9. McDonald GB, Shulman HM, Sullivan KM, and Spencer GD. Intestinal and hepatic complications of human bone marrow transplantation. Part II. *Gastroenterology*, 1986; **90**: 770–84.

10. Shulman HM *et al*. Chronic graft-versus-host syndrome in man. A long term clinicopathologic study of 20 Seattle patients. *American Journal of Medicine*, 1980; **69**: 204–17.

11. Sherlock S. The syndrome of disappearing intrahepatic bile ducts. *Lancet*, 1987; **ii**: 493–6.

12. Zimmerman HJ and Lewis JH. Drug-induced cholestasis. *Medical Toxicology*, 1987; **2**: 112–60.

14.8 Amyloidosis

Laurence B. Lovat and Keith P. W. J. McAdam

Introduction

Definition

Amyloidosis is the collective name given to a group of different conditions whose common feature is the extracellular deposition of insoluble amyloid fibrils. Under light microscopy the deposits have an amorphous eosinophilic appearance staining pink with Congo red dye and exhibiting a green-yellow birefringence when viewed through crossed nickel prisms under polarization microscopy. It is this characteristic histological appearance which defines amyloid. In the electron microscope, amyloid deposits are found to consist of rigid non-branching fibrils about 10 nm wide. X-ray diffraction of purified fibrils suggests that the fibril proteins are arranged in a β-pleated sheet conformation (Glenner, NEJM, 1980; 302:1283, 1333). It is known that many different proteins can assume a fibrillar structure, staining with Congo red and exhibiting green birefringence under polarized light. To date at least 16 different amyloid fibril proteins have been described in man (Table 1).

Historical perspectives

As early as 1859, Friedreich and Kekulé (who described the structure of benzene) showed that amyloid was proteinaceous in nature (ArchPathAnat, 1859; 16:60); it was given a misleading chemical name by Virchow in 1854 on account of its waxy nature and starch-like staining properties with iodine and sulphuric acid (like amylose) (Aterman, Histochem, 1976; 49:131). However, the name has stuck as the generic title for a group of different conditions which share common histochemical properties. Earlier descriptions by the famous Viennese anatomist Rokitansky in 1842 of the 'lardaceous' liver, and by Christensen in 1844 of the 'sago' spleen, in patients with chronic diseases almost certainly referred to infiltration with 'amyloid substance'. For the next century, the homogeneous eosinophilic amyloid substance remained a pathological curiosity, diagnosed by its characteristic staining properties with metachromatic cotton dyes and, in particular, with Congo red. It was not until 1959 that the ultrastructural findings of Cohen and Calkins (Nature, 1959; 183:1202) demonstrated the fibrillar structure of amyloid. Heller's suggestion (JPatholBacteriol, 1964; 88:15) that amyloid might represent a variety of diseases involving different proteins was significant as, before that time (and even since), amyloid had been assumed to be composed of a single uniform subunit.

Classification

Amyloidosis is usually an acquired condition although there are several hereditary amyloid syndromes. Deposits are sometimes localized to one site or organ, or may be systemic. Many localized forms remain asymptomatic, but some, such as β-protein amyloidosis in Alzheimer's disease, are associated with major morbidity. Without specific treatment, most forms of systemic amyloidosis are fatal.

The original clinical classifications of systemic amyloidosis were based on the presence or absence of an underlying disease process and the organ distribution of the amyloid deposits. Thus patients with amyloidosis complicating chronic diseases (secondary or reactive) were described as having a 'typical' distribution pattern of amyloid in the liver, spleen, kidneys, and adrenal glands, while those in whom no underlying cause could be identified (primary), and those with amyloidosis complicating myeloma, had an 'atypical' tissue distribution pattern involving the heart, lymph nodes, nerves, and gut. This empirical clinical classification of amyloid has been superseded by one based on the protein composition of the fibrils (Table 1).

The molecular mechanisms underlying the characteristic organ and tissue distributions of amyloid are still unknown, but might reflect the tissue content of different glycosaminoglycans, particularly heparan sulphate, which are always tightly associated with the fibrils (Nelson, BiochemJ, 1991; 275:67).

Serum amyloid P component

There is only one protein which is found in amyloid deposits of all chemical varieties, the amyloid P component (**AP**). This non-fibrillar protein is derived from and identical to serum amyloid P component (**SAP**) (Baltz, ClinExpImmun, 1986; 66:691; Pepys, PNAS, 1994; 91:5602). SAP is synthesized in the liver and circulates as a decamer (M_r 254 000) comprising two planar pentameric discs facing each other. It undergoes reversible calcium-dependent binding to all amyloid fibrils (Pepys, ClinExpImmun, 1979; 38:284) and comprises up to 15 per cent of the mass of amyloid deposits. The physiological role of SAP is not known, but it is itself highly resistant to proteolysis (Kinoshita, ProteinSci, 1992; 1:700). SAP inhibits proteolytic digestion of amyloid fibrils *in vitro* and may thereby contribute to their persistence *in vivo* (Li, ScaJImmunol, 1984; 20:219; Tennent, PNAS, 1995; 92:4299). Radiolabelled SAP has recently been developed as a nuclear medicine tracer for diagnosing amyloidosis and for quantitative

Table 1 Classification of the most common types of amyloidosis

Type	Fibril protein precursor	Clinical syndrome
AA	Serum amyloid A	Reactive systemic amyloidosis, associated with chronic inflammatory diseases. Formerly known as secondary amyloidosis
AL	Monoclonal immunoglobulin light chains	Systemic amyloidosis associated with myeloma, monoclonal gammopathy, occult dyscrasia. Formerly known as primary amyloidosis Localized deposits in bronchial tree, bladder, and other sites
AH	Monoclonal immunoglobulin heavy chains	Systemic amyloidosis Ocular amyloid
ATTR	Normal plasma transthyretin	Senile systemic amyloidosis with prominent cardiac involvement
	Genetically variant transthyretin	Familial amyloid polyneuropathy. Sometimes prominent amyloid cardiomyopathy or nephropathy
$A\beta_2M$	β_2-Microglobulin	Periarticular and, occasionally, systemic amyloidosis associated with renal failure and long-term dialysis
AApoAI	Normal plasma apolipoprotein AI	Amyloid localized to aortic intima
	Genetically variant apolipoprotein AI	Familial visceral amyloidosis, non-neuropathic. Sometimes prominent peripheral neuropathy with systemic amyloidosis
Alys	Variant lysozyme	Familial visceral amyloidosis, non-neuropathic
Afib	Variant fibrinogen α-chain	Familial visceral amyloidosis, non-neuropathic
$A\beta$	β-Protein (and rare genetic variants)	Cerebrovascular and intracerebral plaque amyloid in Alzheimer's disease. Occasional familial cases Hereditary cerebral haemorrhage with cerebral amyloidosis
AGel	Variant gelsolin	Hereditary cranial neuropathy and renal (systemic) amyloid in homozygotes
ACys	Variant cystatin C	Hereditary cerebral haemorrhage with major asymptomatic visceral amyloidosis
ACal	(Pro)calcitonin	Amyloid in medullary carcinomas of thyroid
AANF	Atrial natriuretic factor	Isolated amyloid in cardiac atria
AIAPP	Islet amyloid polypeptide	Amyloid in islets of Langerhans in type II diabetes mellitus and insulinoma
	Keratin	Amyloid localized to skin
APrP	Prion protein	Spongiform encephalopathies with or without cerebral amyloid

scintigraphic monitoring of amyloid deposits in patients (Hawkins, NEJM, 1990; 323:508).

The vitamin K-dependent clotting factors (particularly factor X, but also to a lesser extent factors IX, VIII, and II) also bind in a calcium-dependent manner to amyloid fibrils. When fibrils are in direct contact with blood, as in the splenic circulation, deficiencies of these factors can then be a clinically significant cause of bleeding, which responds dramatically to splenectomy in a number of patients (Greipp, AmJHemat, 1981; 11:443).

Many other proteins are found in association with amyloid deposits including apolipoprotein E. The apoE4 genotype is a strong risk factor for developing Alzheimer's disease (Corder, Science, 1993; 261:921) but not systemic forms of amyloidosis (Lovat, AmyloidIntJExpClinInvest, 1995; 2:163).

Clinical amyloidosis

Clinically significant amyloidosis is not rare. Localized amyloid deposits in the brain and cerebral blood vessels are key pathological hallmarks of Alzheimer's disease and amyloid is present in the islets of Langerhans in type II diabetes mellitus (O'Brien, VetPathol, 1993; 30:317). There is increasing evidence that the localized cerebral amyloid deposits contribute to the pathogenesis of Alzheimer's disease, but the role of pancreatic amyloid in diabetes mellitus is less clear. Amyloid deposition in bones, joints, and periarticular structures affects most patients receiving long-term haemodialysis (Koch, KidneyInt, 1992; 41:1416) and is a cause of serious morbidity among hundreds of thousands of such patients world-wide. Acquired systemic amyloidosis complicating myeloma and other B-cell dyscrasias (AL amyloidosis) or chronic infections and inflammatory diseases (AA amyloidosis) is important because of the difficulty often experienced in making the diagnosis, its poor prognosis, and the increasing availability of effective treatments. The commonest hereditary amyloid syndrome is familial amyloid polyneuropathy, which is very rare except in a few geographical foci; however, it is important as a model for understanding the pathogenesis of amyloid in general. Untreated, the systemic disease

Table 2 Diseases associated with reactive systemic (AA) amyloidosis

Acute recurrent and chronic infections	Chronic inflammatory diseases	Neoplastic diseases
Tuberculosis	Rheumatoid arthritis	Hodgkin's disease
Leprosy	Juvenile chronic arthritis	Renal cell carcinoma
Chronic osteomyelitis	Crohn's disease	Others:
Decubitus ulcers	Reiter's syndrome	Carcinoma of gut, lung, urogenital tract
Bronchiectasis	Ankylosing spondylitis	Malignant melanoma
Paraplegia	Psoriatic anthropathy	Basal-cell carcinoma
Cystic fibrosis	Behçet's syndrome	Hairy-cell leukaemia
Chronic skin suppuration in	Dermatomyositis	
parenteral drug abusers	Adult Still's disease	
Recurrent infection in	Systemic lupus erythematosus	
hypogammaglobulinaemia	(very rare)	
Nodular non-supportive panniculitis	Papua New Guinean amyloidosis	
Malaria	Gaucher's disease	
Leishmaniasis	Takayasu disease	
Schistosomiasis	Nieman–Pick disease	
Filariasis	Familial Mediterranean fever	
Whipple's disease	Muckle–Wells syndrome	
	Familial Hibernian Fever	

is usually fatal and the clinical findings are due to the deposition of amyloid in vital organs, which then malfunction.

It is a widely held misconception that amyloid deposits persist indefinitely. Although no treatment yet exists that specifically causes regression of deposits, therapy which reduces the supply of amyloid fibril precursor proteins is associated with marked regression of amyloid in many cases and with a significant improvement in prognosis in all forms of amyloidosis including AA, AL, $A\beta_2M$, and ATTR amyloidosis.

The liver is a frequent site for amyloid deposition. Clinical hepatic dysfunction is unusual, even in the presence of large liver deposits, but hepatomegaly or disturbance of liver enzymes can sometimes be the only presenting feature of systemic amyloidosis.

Clinical syndromes
Reactive systemic—AA amyloidosis

AA amyloidosis can develop during the course of any disease that is associated with an acute-phase response for a prolonged period. The fibrils are derived from the circulating acute-phase protein, serum amyloid A (**SAA**). SAA is predominantly synthesized in the liver under stimulation by interleukin 1 and to a lesser extent interleukin 6 and tumour necrosis factor (Woo, JBC, 1987; 262: 15790). The serum concentration of SAA rises by up to one thousandfold within 48 h of acute inflammatory stimuli (McAdam, JCI, 1978; 61:390).

Many chronic inflammatory, infective, and neoplastic disorders are associated with AA amyloidosis (Table 2) and it is likely that variations in susceptibility to developing the disorder are genetically determined. In Papua New Guinea, AA disease is very common with a prevalence at autopsy of 0.7 per cent and up to 10 per cent in one local language group. This is due to the frequency of conditions causing recurrent fever and inflammation, including leprosy reactions, tuberculosis, recurrent malaria, filariasis, or trophic ulcers (McAdam, PapuaNGuineaMedJ, 1978; 21:69).

The commonest predisposing conditions in the developed world are idiopathic inflammatory diseases. In northern Europe up to 10 per cent of patients with rheumatoid arthritis or Crohn's disease are affected, but for reasons that are not clear the incidence is much lower in the United States (Lind, ScaJGastr, 1985; 20:665; Greenstein, Medicine, 1992; 71:261). Amyloidosis is very rare in systemic lupus erythematosus and ulcerative colitis, reflecting the characteristically modest acute-phase response evoked in these inflammatory conditions (de Beer, Lancet, 1982; ii:231). AA amyloidosis is a common complication of familial Mediterranean fever (see below).

The clinical presentation is proteinuria or renal insufficiency in 95 per cent of patients, although diffuse vascular deposits are always present. The spleen is heavily infiltrated in every patient and the liver in about one-quarter, but hepatosplenomegaly is evident clinically in only 5 per cent of cases and liver function is usually well preserved. Functional hyposplenism is occasionally seen. A goitre can be found in up to 10 per cent of patients and gastrointestinal complaints can be elicited at diagnosis in one-fifth, usually with features of malabsorption or motility disturbance (Gertz, Medicine, 1991; 70:246) although gastrointestinal bleeding has also been described (Yamada, HumPath, 1985; 16:1206). Severe autonomic neuropathy is rare and suggests advanced disease.

The incidence of AA amyloidosis increases with the duration of the underlying condition, but better control of chronic inflammatory disorders has led to a decline in the developed world. Endstage renal failure is the usual cause of death and the median survival in untreated patients is approximately 5 years from diagnosis, although many patients now survive much longer with active supportive measures. Amyloid probably infiltrates the liver late in the disease and is associated with a poor prognosis (Lovat, Gut, 1998; 42:727). The aim of therapy is to suppress the underlying inflammatory process and therefore reduce the acute-phase synthesis of SAA. This is achieved particularly effectively in juvenile chronic arthritis using chlorambucil (Schnitzer, ArthRheum, 1977; 20:245).

Table 3 Clinical features of systemic AL amyloidosis
Carpal tunnel syndrome
Restrictive cardiomyopathy
Nephrotic syndrome
Peripheral neuropathy
Autonomic neuropathy
Non-thrombocytopenic purpura
Macroglossia
Large-joint arthropathy
Isolated factor IX and X deficiency
Cutaneous plaques and nodules
No predisposing inflammatory condition
Monoclonal gammapathy

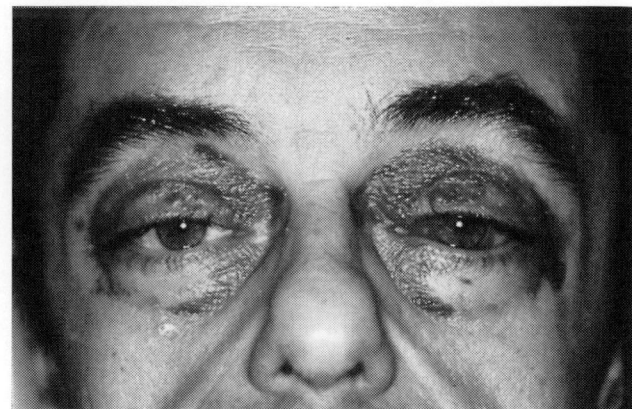

Fig. 1. A 58-year-old patient with systemic AL amyloidosis showing bilateral periorbital haemorrhages.

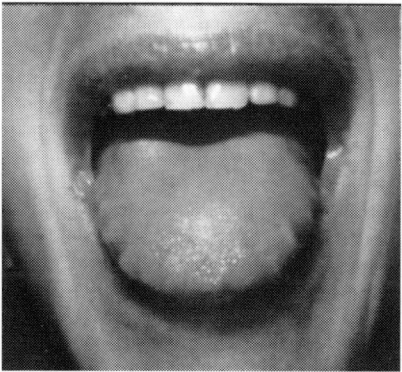

Fig. 2. A 39-year-old patient with systemic AL amyloidosis demonstrating macroglossia. The indentation marks of the teeth are easily identified.

Amyloidosis associated with immunocyte dyscrasia—AL amyloidosis

AL amyloid fibrils are derived from monoclonal immunoglobulin light chains (λ-type in 70 per cent of cases), and AL amyloidosis can occur in most clonal B-cell dyscrasias. Amyloid complicates 15 per cent of cases of myeloma but is much less common in 'benign' monoclonal gammopathy. Due to the high frequency of monoclonal gammopathies in the elderly, most patients with AL amyloidosis do not have myeloma. Indeed, in one-fifth of patients the only identifiable evidence of an immunocyte dyscrasia is the amyloid deposits themselves (Kyle, SemHemat, 1995; 32:45).

AL amyloidosis usually occurs in individuals of more than 50 years of age, but it is an occasional finding in younger adults. It is a progressive systemic disease and almost any tissue outside the brain can be involved. Clinical manifestations are therefore diverse (Table 3). There is substantial histological involvement of the heart in most cases. Restrictive cardiomyopathy is the presenting feature in one-third of patients and the cause of death in one-half. Spontaneous periorbital oedema is a characteristic sign (Fig. 1). Carpal tunnel syndrome is common and often precedes other features of the disorder by some years. Nephrotic syndrome or renal dysfunction occur in one-third of patients and peripheral and/or autonomic neuropathy in one-fifth. The gut is commonly affected. Gastrointestinal presentations include macroglossia (which is almost pathognomonic of the condition) (Fig. 2), sicca syndrome, motility disturbance, malabsorption, haemorrhage, obstruction, and perforation (Lovat, DigDis, 1997; 15:155) and a picture resembling inflammatory bowel disease is occasionally seen in the colon (Chernenkoff, CanMedAssJ, 1972; 106:567). Gastrointestinal disturbance can also be due to autonomic neuropathy. Weight loss is frequent, may be substantial, and is associated with early death.

Some patients develop a bleeding diathesis either from fragility of infiltrated vessels, hypersplenism, or sequestration of vitamin K-dependent clotting factors, usually in an enlarged spleen where blood percolates slowly over the sinusoids containing exposed amyloid fibrils to which the factors adhere. Splenectomy has been used successfully to manage this. There is some evidence that drugs also bind to amyloid fibrils, perhaps accounting for the observed sensitivity to digoxin and calcium-channel blockers, which must be administered carefully at low dose, if at all (Buja, AmJCard, 1970; 26:394). A rare but potentially fatal manifestation of AL amyloidosis is a bleeding diathesis due to acquired deficiency of factor IX or X (Kyle, MayoClinProc, 1983; 58:665).

Median survival of untreated patients with AL amyloidosis ranges from 5 months in those with heart failure to 14 months or more in those without. Patients with peripheral neuropathy as their predominant manifestation have a better prognosis, with a median survival of 54 months (Gertz, SemArthRheum, 1994; 24:124), whereas symptomatic autonomic neuropathy carries a median survival of only 7 months (Berg, Amyloid IntJExpClinInvest, 1994; 1: 39). The liver is infiltrated in one-half of patients but hepatic amyloidosis is not associated with a poorer prognosis. AL amyloidosis is a remarkably idiosyncratic disease and a small proportion of patients with extensive deposits remain in surprisingly good health for many years.

Familial amyloid polyneuropathy—ATTR amyloidosis

Familial amyloid polyneuropathy is a rare autosomal dominant syndrome that is almost always caused by point mutations in the gene for the plasma protein transthyretin (**TTR**) (Benson, JMedGenet, 1991; 28:73). More than 50 amyloidogenic variants of transthyretin have now been described. Penetrance varies and clinical disease starts at any time from the second decade. The most common transthyretin variant 'Met30' is seen predominantly in Portugal, Japan, and Sweden.

The disorder is characterized by progressive peripheral and autonomic neuropathy with varying degrees of visceral involvement affecting the gut, the vitreous of the eye, the heart, kidneys, thyroid, spleen, and adrenal glands. Circulating plasma transthyretin is synthesized almost exclusively in the liver but the amyloid deposits are rarely deposited there (Lovat, Gut, 1998; 42:727).

Familial amyloid polyneuropathy is usually fatal within 5 to 15 years of diagnosis. Gastrointestinal involvement is often severe and malnutrition contributes significantly to mortality (Suhr, JIntMed, 1994; 235:479). The outlook for patients with familial amyloid polyneuropathy related to variants of transthyretin has improved substantially following the introduction of liver transplantation (Holmgren, Lancet, 1993; 341:1113; Steen, AmyloidIntJExpClinInvest, 1994; 1:138) (see below).

Other hereditary amyloid syndromes

Other genetically variant proteins also cause hereditary systemic amyloidosis. Patients with variant apolipoprotein AI (Soutar, PNAS, 1992; 89:7389),[1] lysozyme (Pepys, Nature, 1993; 362:553), and fibrinogen (Benson, NatureGen, 1993; 3:252) usually present in middle age with visceral amyloidosis and frequently renal impairment. The liver is often infiltrated. Amyloid deposition progresses inexorably and no specific treatment yet exists. However, renal transplantation can improve the prognosis considerably. Variant gelsolin is associated with a predominant cranial neuropathy but life expectancy with this disorder is almost normal (de la Chapelle, NatureGen, 1992; 2:157).

A number of genetically linked inflammatory illnesses are associated with typical systemic AA amyloidosis. The classic 'periodic disease', familial Mediterranean fever, is an autosomal recessive disorder of unknown aetiology which predominantly affects populations originating from the southern and eastern Mediterranean coasts, particularly Sephardic Jews and Armenians. The disease may present at any age although it usually starts in childhood with recurrent self-limiting attacks of fever, peritonitis, arthritis, pleurisy, or rash together with a marked acute-phase response. Attacks may also be subclinical. Between attacks patients remain completely well. Because of its mode of inheritance, there is rarely a family history and diagnosis may be difficult and delayed. Untreated familial Mediterranean fever is complicated by systemic AA amyloidosis in a high proportion of cases (Pras, JohnsHopkMedJ, 1982; 150:22) and some patients present with AA amyloidosis before suffering any clinical attacks of inflammation. The gene frequency is 1:16 among Libyan Jews and 1:14 within the Armenian population in the western United States. The gene locus has been mapped to the short arm of chromosome 16, but the gene has not yet been identified (Gruberg, AmJReprodImmunol, 1992; 28:241).

A number of other hereditary periodic syndromes are associated with AA amyloidosis. The Muckle–Wells syndrome is inherited in an autosomal dominant fashion in families not of Mediterranean origin (Muckle, QJMed, 1962; 31:235). It is characterized by progressive sensorineural deafness, attacks of fever, arthralgia, urticaria, and amyloidosis. Sporadic cases have also been described. An acute-phase response can be present in patients with Muckle–Wells syndrome even between attacks, and systemic AA amyloidosis

occurs in up to 20 per cent of cases (Muckle, BrJDermatol, 1979; 100:87). Approximately 100 cases have been reported world-wide. Familial Hibernian fever is an autosomal dominant condition which has been described in a single Irish family. It presents with recurrent episodes of localized myalgia, painful erythema, and an acute-phase response (Williamson, QJMed, 1982; 204:469). Although AA amyloidosis was not described in the original report, members of the family have now developed it.

Dialysis-related arthropathy—$A\beta_2M$ amyloidosis

Most patients with endstage renal failure who are maintained on haemodialysis for more than 5 years develop amyloid deposits composed of β_2-microglobulin (β_2M), a plasma protein that is normally cleared and metabolized in the kidneys. The deposits are predominantly osteoarticular and cause carpal tunnel syndrome, large joint pain and stiffness, soft tissue masses, bone cysts, and pathological fractures. Clinical problems associated with β_2m amyloidosis constitute a major cause of morbidity in long-term dialysis patients and fatal systemic amyloidosis has supervened in some cases (Gal, ArchPathLabMed, 1994; 118:718). This type of amyloid also occurs in patients on continuous ambulatory peritoneal dialysis and has even been reported in a patient with renal failure who had never been dialysed. Occult bleeding is the commonest reported gastrointestinal presentation (Maher, BMJ, 1988; 297:265). Liver infiltration has not yet been described.

Senile amyloidosis

Microscopic and clinically silent amyloid deposits of various types, many of which have not yet been characterized, are common in the aged. In addition, scattered systemic deposits of amyloid derived from wild-type transthyretin are present in many elderly subjects. These may present clinically, most often as restrictive cardiomyopathy.

Cerebral amyloidosis

The brain is not affected in acquired systemic amyloidosis, perhaps because of the blood–brain barrier. However, the brain is an important site of amyloid deposition (Duchen, IntJExpPathol, 1992; 73:535). Alzheimer's disease is the commonest cause of dementia and the fourth commonest cause of death in the developed world. A precise diagnosis of Alzheimer's disease requires histological demonstration of senile plaques in the white matter and intraneuronal neurofibrillary tangles in a patient with dementia. Senile plaques have a dense amyloid core in which the fibrils are derived from β-protein, a proteolytic product of β-amyloid precursor protein (APP) (Hendriks, EurJBioch, 1996; 237:6). Most cases of Alzheimer's disease are sporadic, but familial forms exist. Some of these are associated with point mutations in the APP gene or the genes for presenilins 1 and 2 which result in overproduction of the amyloidogenic 1–42 residue form of β-protein (van Broeckhoven, EurNeurol, 1995; 35:8; Duff, Nature, 1996; 383:710).

There are a number of proposed mechanisms for brain injury in Alzheimer's disease. The amyloid cascade hypothesis argues that amyloid deposition causes the disease (Selkoe, JNeurolNeurosurgPsych, 1994; 53:438) and potential therapeutic strategies include alteration of APP metabolism, β-protein fibrillogenesis, and amyloid persistence. Markers of inflammation are expressed at increased levels in the brain of a patient with Alzheimer's disease and may potentiate β-protein neurotoxicity. A number of retrospective clinical studies suggest that prolonged use of anti-inflammatory drugs can prevent development of Alzheimer's disease (Rogers, DrugRes 1995; 45(I):439). Oxidative stress might be important, but the evidence is still limited (Frölich, DrugRes, 1995; 45(I):443).

Amyloid derived from genetically variant β-protein is an occasional cause of familial haemorrhagic stroke (Dutch type) (Haan, ClinNeurolNeurosurg, 1989; 91:285) as is cerebral amyloid derived from variant cystatin C (Ghiso, PNAS, 1986; 83:2974). Some of the prion diseases are associated with cerebral amyloid plaques including the new variant of Creutzfeldt–Jakob disease recently described in the United Kingdom (Will, Lancet, 1996; 347:921).

Diagnosis and monitoring of amyloidosis

The diagnosis of amyloidosis can be difficult because clinical features of the many amyloid syndromes are so varied and non-specific. The diagnosis is confirmed by demonstrating that amyloid deposits are present in the tissues, traditionally using histology. Amyloid-laden material stained with Congo red gives pathognomonic red–green birefringence when viewed under crossed polarized light. Immunohistochemical staining of tissue is the most straightforward method for identifying the amyloid fibril type. Congo red staining after permanganate pretreatment is not reliable for determining the fibril protein type. Radiolabelled SAP scintigraphy is a recently developed alternative technique for demonstrating tissue amyloid deposits *in vivo* that provides a macroscopic whole-body survey and permits serial prospective monitoring (Hawkins, NEJM, 1990; 323:508).

The diagnosis of amyloid is usually unexpected and prior clinical suspicion of the disease is relatively rare. However, the presence of proteinuria in any patient with chronic inflammatory conditions such as Crohn's disease or rheumatoid arthritis should alert the physician to the possibility of AA amyloidosis and clinical signs such as macroglossia and periorbital purpura are highly suggestive of AL amyloidosis.

Histology and histochemistry

Amyloid may be an incidental finding on biopsy of any affected tissue. Biopsies of subcutaneous fat (Fig. 3) (Westermark, Arch-IntMed, 1973; 132:522) or the gastrointestinal tract, usually the rectum, have long been used to make the diagnosis of systemic amyloidosis (Fentem, BMJ, 1962; i:364). In most series, subcutaneous fat or rectal biopsies have been reported to be diagnostic in about 80 per cent of cases and duodenal, gastric, and oesophageal biopsies have been found to yield similar sensitivities (Tada, Gastr-End, 1994; 40:45), but these tests may be negative in up to 50 per cent of cases in routine practice. Rectal biopsy sensitivity can be increased by obtaining adequate submucosa in the biopsy specimen, but inexperience in histochemical processing and interpretation is responsible for many false negative results and there may also be a

significant incidence of false positives (Linke, JHistochem-Cytochem, 1995; 43:863). Liver biopsy is a very sensitive method for diagnosing amyloidosis in a patient with clinical liver involvement.

Electron microscopy does not alone confirm the diagnosis of amyloid as the fibrils cannot always be conclusively identified.

Radioisotope studies—^{123}*I-SAP scintigraphy*

The development of radiolabelled SAP as a nuclear medicine tracer has been a significant advance (Hawkins, Lancet, 1988; i:1413). Quantitative scintigraphic imaging of amyloid deposits is now possible *in vivo*. SAP labelled with radioiodine localizes specifically but reversibly to amyloid deposits in proportion to the amount of amyloid present. The uptake of tracer into separate organs can be determined scintigraphically and the whole-body distribution of amyloid can be quantified and monitored serially. Parenchymal amyloid deposits in solid viscera, including the spleen, liver, kidneys, and adrenal glands can be imaged with remarkably high resolution, whereas those in blood vessels and other hollow structures such as the heart and gut cannot be visualized reliably. SAP scintigraphy is therefore diagnostic in almost 100 per cent of patients with AA amyloidosis and about 95 per cent of patients with familial forms. It is slightly less sensitive in AL type where deposits may be limited to the peripheral nerves or the heart. Studies using $^{123/125}$I-SAP have provided substantial new information on the natural history of many different forms of amyloid and their response to treatment (Hawkins, ClinSci, 1994; 87:289), although at present this remains a specialized tool of restricted availability. Encouragingly, it has recently been possible to label SAP with technetium-99m, an inexpensive and universally available isotope, to produce a tracer that gives images of quality comparable with those obtained with radioiodine.[2]

Other non-histological investigations
AA amyloidosis

As renal dysfunction is so common in systemic AA amyloidosis, dipstick testing for proteinuria is a useful screening test in patients with chronic inflammatory diseases such as juvenile chronic arthritis or Crohn's disease. The presence of Howell–Jolly bodies in the blood film suggests functional hyposplenism, and pneumococcal immunization is advisable. Adrenal amyloid deposition is common, but although hypoadrenalism is unusual it can be devastating and the possibility should always be borne in mind. AA amyloid deposits are derived from the circulating acute-phase protein SAA and reducing circulating levels is associated with amyloid regression. The acute-phase response should therefore be monitored. Commercial assays for SAA will soon be available, and meanwhile C-reactive protein is a good surrogate marker. The erythrocyte sedimentation rate is less useful.

AL amyloidosis

Renal, splenic, and adrenal function should be investigated in systemic AL amyloidosis as in the AA type. Echocardiography is a valuable but non-specific method for evaluating cardiac amyloid. Small, stiff, concentrically thickened chambers with a sparkling 'ground glass' appearance to the ventricular wall is highly suggestive

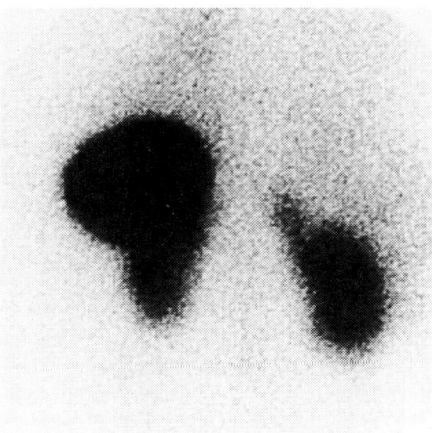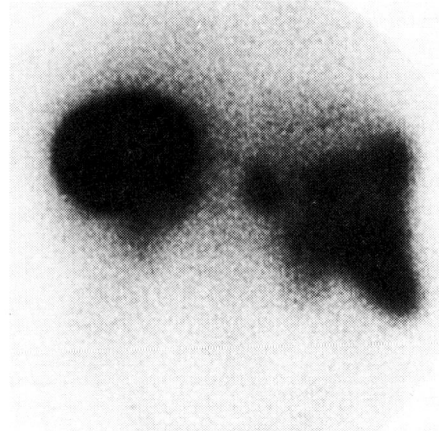

Fig. 3. Abdominal wall fat removed by aspiration biopsy, stained with Congo red, and viewed under polarization microscopy demonstrating birefringent amyloid material. Handling and interpretation of tissue stained with Congo red requires special skill as the stain must be used fresh and the amount of birefringent material is often small.

of amyloid. Suspicion of the diagnosis is supported further if these findings are associated with decreased voltages and a pseudoinfarct pattern on electrocardiography.

The presence of a circulating monoclonal immunoglobulin should be sought by serum and urine electrophoresis. The clone is often subtle and may only be detected by ultrasensitive techniques such as immunofixation of concentrated urine.

Hereditary amyloidosis

In cases of hereditary amyloidosis, the gene defect must be characterized and the variant protein demonstrated. The nature of the amyloid fibril protein can usually be identified by immuno-histochemical staining. The appropriate gene is investigated for mutations, and it is then essential to demonstrate the presence of the variant protein in the amyloid deposits by extraction of fibrillar material from deposits and amino acid sequencing.

Amyloid and the liver
Incidence of hepatic amyloidosis

Widespread vascular deposits are usual in patients with systemic amyloidosis and a diagnosis can be made on biopsies from clinically unaffected tissue, for example subcutaneous fat or rectal mucosa. Vascular amyloid is also almost universally present in the liver and is not associated with hepatic dysfunction. Parenchymal or stromal infiltration is much less common but can be associated with clinical hepatic disease (Lovat, Gut, 1998; 42:727). Using SAP scintigraphy, parenchymal or stromal amyloid deposits have been demonstrated in approximately 50 per cent of patients with systemic AL amyloidosis and 20 per cent of those with the systemic AA type. In patients on long-term dialysis, systemic amyloid deposition is a very late feature and liver infiltration has not yet been described. It is not usually seen in familial amyloid polyneuropathy caused by variant transthyretin either, even though the liver is the sole source of this protein in the plasma. Apolipoprotein AI and lysozyme amyloid deposits have been shown in the liver in all patients studied.

Pathology

Amyloid is deposited extracellularly in the liver parenchyma within the perisinusoidal space of Disse and, in advanced cases, this space is diffusely replaced by amyloid with atrophy of the hepatic cords. In a few patients the perivascular stroma of the portal triads is replaced by amyloid, but without parenchymal involvement. Deposits in the hepatic vasculature are seen in all forms of systemic amyloid but do not cause liver dysfunction (Iwata, HumPath, 1995; 26:1148). The deposits do not cause an inflammatory reaction.

When correctly processed, Congo red histology is highly specific for diagnosing hepatic amyloidosis and has a sensitivity reaching 100 per cent. Immunohistochemistry is required to identify the fibril protein.

Clinical features and investigation

Hepatic amyloidosis is usually asymptomatic but it is always part of a systemic process. When symptoms do occur they are vague and may be present for a considerable time before diagnosis. Abdominal pain and bloating are most frequent with mild and occasionally more intense fatigue. The substantial weight loss which occurs in more than one-half of patients is probably related to the general disease process rather than the liver deposits themselves. Hepatomegaly is common in systemic amyloidosis, particularly the AL type, but is often due to liver congestion in patients with restrictive cardiomyopathy and not to hepatic infiltration by amyloid (Gertz, AmJMed, 1988; 85:73). Jaundice occurs in only 5 per cent of patients with AL amyloidosis and is preterminal. No cases of jaundice complicating AA amyloidosis have been reported in the past 50 years (Rubinow, AmJMed, 1978; 64:937). Portal hypertension is exceedingly rare and spontaneous hepatic rupture has been described in only 10 cases (Harrison, Gut, 1996; 38:151).

Proteinuria, frequently within the nephrotic range (more than 5 g/day), is found in most patients at presentation. Mild derangement of liver enzymes, particularly alkaline phosphatase, is also common. Neither of these features is specific for hepatic amyloid although in a patient with undiagnosed liver disease, nephrotic syndrome, hyposplenism, or hepatomegaly disproportionate to the derangement of liver enzymes do make systemic amyloidosis more likely (Gertz, AmJMed, 1988; 85:73). Hypergammaglobulinaemia is seen in most patients with chronic liver disease and is also found in AA or hereditary amyloidosis, but in the AL type, immune paresis is more common and is usually accompanied by evidence of a monoclonal immunoglobulin in the serum or urine.

Coagulopathy is not specifically due to liver involvement in amyloidosis. A prolonged prothrombin time can be due to a factor-X deficiency but a prolonged thrombin time is much more common. It is present in approximately 60 per cent of patients with liver involvement although it is found in only 20 per cent of those without. It appears to be due to the presence of a circulating factor which inhibits conversion of fibrinogen to a fibrin clot. Dysfibrinogenaemia does not occur (Gastineau, Blood, 1991; 77: 2637).

Liver biopsy is a highly sensitive test for diagnosing all types of systemic amyloidosis with liver involvement, but significant bleeding occurs in 5 per cent of patients. This is probably due mainly to vascular wall fragility, but some patients with the AL type also have clotting disorders (such as factor-X deficiency). When a diagnosis of systemic amyloidosis is being considered, less invasive tests such as ^{123}I-SAP scintigraphy should be the initial investigation. However, this is not yet widely available; rectal biopsy is relatively safe although the poor sensitivity of the technique means negative results must be interpreted with caution.

In patients with suspected or proven amyloidosis, other manifestations of the invariable systemic involvement should be sought together with detection of the underlying cause (see below).

Prognosis

Hepatic amyloid deposition in systemic AA amyloidosis carries a poor prognosis, the predicted 5-year survival falling to 43 per cent in patients with liver involvement from 72 per cent in those without. Liver deposition probably occurs late in the evolution of systemic AA amyloidosis (Fig. 4). In contrast, hepatic involvement in the AL type does not significantly influence prognosis (Lovat, Gut, 1998; 42:727).

Role of liver transplantation in systemic amyloidosis

Supportive therapy

Clinically significant liver failure is rare and occurs in about 5 per cent of patients with systemic AL amyloidosis. It is exceedingly rare in the AA type. Liver transplantation has only been reported in a single patient with AL amyloidosis complicated by liver failure (Lovat, Gut, 1998; 42:727). He presented at 44 years with malaise, hepatomegaly, and abnormal liver function tests, and was treated with cytotoxic chemotherapy comprising vincristine, Adriamycin, and dexamethasone. Unfortunately, hepatic encephalopathy and hepatocellular failure supervened before either the clone or the amyloid had responded. He underwent orthotopic liver transplantation and remained alive at 2-year follow-up. Projected median survival with this treatment is more than 4 years and liver transplantation may, therefore, be a useful supportive treatment in

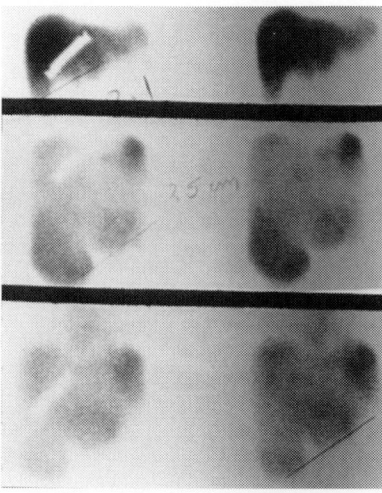

Fig. 4. Development of hepatic amyloid deposits during follow-up of a patient with systemic AA amyloidosis. Serial, posterior, abdominal, ^{123}I-labelled SAP scans of a patient with AA amyloidosis complicating rheumatoid arthritis. The scan at presentation (left) shows uptake of the tracer into amyloid deposits in the spleen, kidneys, and adrenal glands. The patient did not respond to anti-inflammatory therapy and the follow-up scan 2 years later (right) shows additional localization of tracer into the liver; reduction of the renal signal is due to endstage renal failure.

carefully selected cases providing a window of opportunity for a response to chemotherapy. The only other liver transplant for hepatic failure associated with amyloidosis was performed on a 15-year-old boy, with hereditary amyloidosis due to a variant lysozyme, who presented acutely with spontaneous hepatic rupture (Harrison, Gut, 1996; 38:151). He remained alive and well 2 years postoperatively. Spontaneous hepatic rupture is a very rare complication of amyloidosis and has only been reported in four previous cases (Ades, JClinGastrol, 1989; 11:85).

Surgical gene therapy

An exciting recent development has been the introduction of liver transplantation as a treatment for familial amyloid polyneuropathy caused by transthyretin gene mutations. Circulating transthyretin is produced exclusively by hepatocytes and liver transplantation leads to disappearance of the variant transthyretin from the plasma. The usual inexorable progression of the disease has been halted in all liver transplant recipients and most have shown some improvement, especially in symptoms related to autonomic neuropathy (Ando, NEJM, 1995; 345:195) and the gut. In those with significant visceral amyloidosis, demonstrable by SAP scintigraphy, there has also been marked regression of amyloid (Holmgren, Lancet, 1993; 341:1113) and autonomic neuropathy. This surgical form of gene therapy thus holds much promise for patients with hereditary transthyretin-related amyloidosis and has been taken up by many different centres.

Treatment
Aims of therapy

There is no treatment as yet that specifically causes amyloid deposits to resolve and the prognosis of systemic amyloidosis remains poor.

Table 4 Reducing the supply of fibril precursors in systemic amyloidosis

Disease	Aim of treatment	Example of treatment
AA amyloidosis	Suppress acute-phase response	Chlorambucil for rheumatoid arthritis and juvenile chronic arthritis Colchicine for familial Mediterranean fever Surgery for osteomyelitis and rare cytokine-producing tumours
AL amyloidosis	Suppress production of monoclonal immunoglobulin light chains	Melphalan and prednisolone Vincristine, Adriamycin and dexamethasone High-dose chemotherapy with peripheral stem-cell rescue
Hereditary amyloidosis	Eliminate source of genetically variant proteins	Orthotopic liver transplantation for transthyretin-associated familial amyloid polyneuropathy
Dialysis amyloidosis	Reduce concentration of β_2M	Renal transplantation

Presently, the rational aim of therapy is to reduce or, if possible, eliminate the supply of amyloid fibril precursor proteins (Table 4). However, because few therapeutic strategies have been evaluated, this approach to treatment remains somewhat empirical. Relatively toxic drug regimes or other radical approaches may be justified when the prognosis is otherwise poor. Previous speculation from clinical studies that amyloid deposits may sometimes regress under these circumstances has now been systematically demonstrated using SAP scintigraphy in AA (Hawkins, ArthRheum, 1993; 36: 842), AL (Hawkins, QJMed, 1993; 86:365), β_2M (Tan, KidneyInt, 1996; 50:282), and variant transthyretin amyloidosis (Holmgren, Lancet, 1993; 341:1113). Substantial clinical benefits and improvement in organ function is also seen together with improved survival.

If renal dysfunction reaches a critical level (usually when serum creatinine rises above 200 µmol/l), inexorable deterioration to end-stage renal failure is inevitable, even if amyloid deposition is halted. However, in recent years there have been substantial advances in the treatment of renal and cardiac failure which are the main causes of death in systemic amyloidosis, and supportive therapy, including dialysis and organ transplantation, remains a vital aspect of management. Several in-depth reviews of the treatment of amyloidosis have been published recently (Gertz, SemArthRheum, 1994; 24: 124; Merlini, SemHemat, 1995; 32:60; Tan, AmJKidneyDis, 1995; 26:267).

AA amyloidosis

The aim of therapy is to suppress the acute-phase response. Successful therapy has been most consistent with chlorambucil treatment in AA amyloidosis complicating juvenile chronic arthritis (Schnitzer, ArthRheum, 1977; 20:245). This cytotoxic drug effectively controls inflammation and suppresses the acute-phase production of SAA, reduces proteinuria caused by renal AA amyloid, and greatly improves survival (David, ClinExpRheumatol, 1991; 9: 73). Similar findings have been demonstrated in other conditions such as Crohn's disease (Fitchen, NEJM, 1975; 292:352; Lovat, Gastro, 1998; 42:727). SAP scans demonstrate major reduction in amyloid load in many such patients over periods as short as 12 to 30 months, although in some individuals the amyloid load just remains static instead of increasing. Indeed one of the most telling findings to emerge from use of labelled SAP is the frequent discrepancy between quantity of amyloid present and resulting organ

dysfunction. Measurement of 'target' organ function is therefore a very poor index of the amount of amyloid, and a correspondingly ineffective means of monitoring treatment aimed at promoting resolution of amyloid. In AA amyloidosis, the kidneys are usually the most seriously affected organ and haemodialysis and transplantation have long been mainstays of supportive management.

AA amyloidosis in familial Mediterranean fever

Familial Mediterranean fever is a unique example of an inflammatory disease of unknown aetiology complicated by AA amyloidosis for which a specific and effective treatment exists. Colchicine taken continuously on a prophylactic basis suppresses the inflammatory manifestations of familial Mediterranean fever in all patients sufficiently to prevent development of amyloidosis (Goldfinger, NEJM, 1972; 287:1302; Zemer, NEJM, 1986; 314: 1001). Colchicine has also been given to patients with other forms of amyloidosis, although there is little evidence to support this approach. However, the drug is safe, cheap, and well tolerated in the long term and there are grounds for further investigation of the value of colchicine in AA amyloidosis in general.

AL amyloidosis

In AL amyloidosis the aim of treatment is to suppress the abnormal B-cell clone. Drug regimens used for myeloma are usually administered but response can be difficult to achieve. Large trials at the Mayo Clinic using melphalan and prednisolone have suggested only minor benefit overall (Kyle, AmJMed, 1985; 79:708). One-fifth of individuals entered clinical remission and had prolonged survival (Gertz, Blood, 1991; 77:257). The poor response to this regime may be because suppression of the clone requires approximately 1 year of treatment and many patients will die before this. More intensive regimens characteristically using vincristine, Adriamycin, and dexamethasone cause faster suppression of the clone and appear to improve the response rate and prognosis considerably with a median survival of approximately 5 years (Persey, BrJRheum, 1996; 35(Suppl. 1):12) (Fig. 5). Preliminary reports of high-dose melphalan with rescue of blood stem cells are also encouraging (Comenzo, Blood, 1996; 88:2801). Although the disease is systemic, life-saving transplantation of heart, kidneys, or liver is a serious option in AL amyloidosis, especially in younger

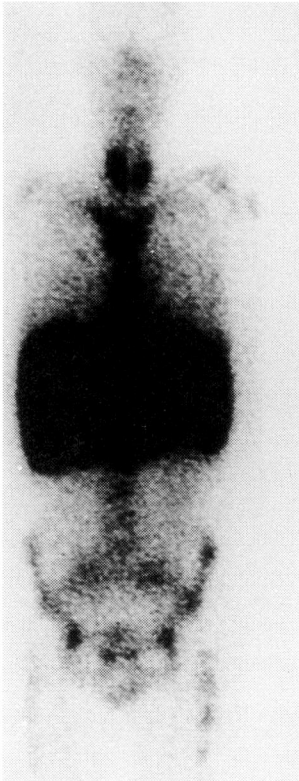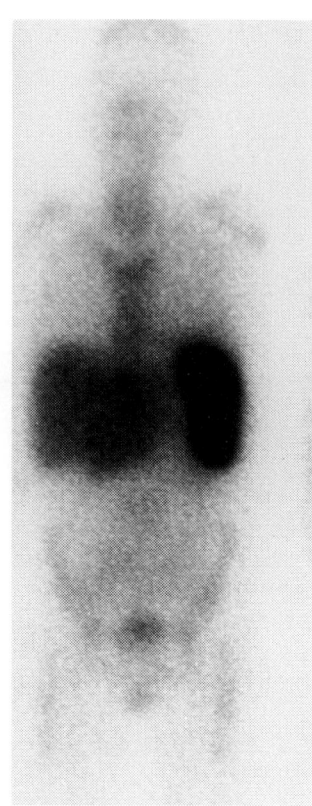

Fig. 5. Regression of hepatic amyloid deposits following chemotherapy in a patient with systemic AL amyloidosis. Serial, anterior, whole-body, ^{123}I-labelled SAP scans in a patient with AL amyloidosis who presented with hepatomegaly and liver dysfunction. The initial scan (left) shows massive uptake of tracer into amyloid deposits in the liver, spleen, and bone marrow. The follow-up scan 6 months later (right), following intensive chemotherapy, shows much less uptake of labelled SAP into the liver and bone marrow indicating substantial regression of the amyloid in these organs.

patients in whom one vital organ is particularly affected. This may also prolong survival sufficiently to enable a response to cytotoxic therapy to occur.

Hereditary amyloidosis

In familial amyloid polyneuropathy associated with transthyretin, liver transplantation is now the mainstay of treatment (see above). No specific measures exist for hereditary amyloidosis caused by other variant proteins, but general supportive measures including organ transplantation can improve prognosis considerably.

Dialysis-related amyloidosis

The only other form of amyloidosis in which the abundance of the fibril precursor protein can be sharply reduced is $\beta_2 M$ amyloidosis in dialysis patients. Successful renal transplantation lowers $\beta_2 M$ plasma concentrations immediately and is associated with rapid improvement of osteoarticular symptoms. Preliminary observations suggest that $\beta_2 M$ amyloid deposits may regress in some cases (Nelson, Lancet, 1991; 338:335). The risk of developing dialysis-related amyloidosis can be avoided altogether through early renal transplantation.(Koch, KidneyInt, 1992; 41:1416). Attempts to clear $\beta_2 M$ effectively by haemofiltration or *ex vivo* absorption have not yet led to clinical benefits.

Unfortunately these various strategies are not possible at all in many types of amyloidosis, for example Alzheimer's disease, and may fail in the systemic types of amyloidosis discussed in this review. Therefore, new approaches are still urgently required to inhibit the formation, persistence, and/or effects of amyloid deposits.

References

1. Jones LA, Harding JA, Cohen AS, and Skinner M. New USA family has apolipoprotein AI (Arg26) variant. In Natvig JB *et al.*, eds. *Amyloid and amyloidosis 1990.* Dordrecht: Kluwer Academic Publishers, 1991: 385–8.
2. Hutchinson WL *et al.* Scintigraphic imaging of amyloid deposits with ^{99m}Tc-labelled serum amyloid P component. In Kisilevsky R, Benson MD, Frangione B, Gauldie J, Muckle TJ, and Young ID, eds. *Amyloid and amyloidosis 1993.* Pearl River, New York: Parthenon Publishing, 1994: 682–4.

15

Alcoholic liver disease

15.1 Epidemiological aspects of alcoholic liver disease, ethanol metabolism, and pathogenesis of alcoholic liver injury

Mikko Salaspuro

Introduction

The association of alcohol abuse and liver damage was known by ancient Greeks and was also recognized in Indian manuscripts dealing with the Ayerveda system of medicine (Ravi Varma, QJStud-Alc, 1950; 11:484). In the 1830s the relationship between alcoholism and fatty liver was described in European medical literature. Even in the late 1940s the pathogenesis of alcoholic liver disease was regarded as being associated almost exclusively with a secondary protein and choline deficiency. Since then, however, strong evidence has emerged of a relationship between the pathogenesis of alcohol-related liver damage and the direct toxicity of ethanol, its metabolism, and its metabolites.[1] Nevertheless, many questions still remain unanswered. Although most alcoholics have at least a slight fatty liver, why do only about 20 per cent develop more severe liver injury? The reason for the individual susceptibility is, by and large, unknown. Although many toxic factors associating with ethanol metabolism have been found, the basic mechanism behind the alcohol-induced cell death has not been resolved. Although the direct hepatotoxicity of ethanol has been established in experimental animals, the role of 'supernutrients' such as S-adenosyl-L-methionine and polyenylphosphatidylcholine in the attenuation of alcohol-induced liver injury has been reported. However, the close relationship between the quantity and length of alcohol consumption and the prevalence of alcoholic liver cirrhosis is still generally accepted (Skog, ActaMedScand, 1985; 703 (Suppl.):157).

Epidemiological aspects of alcoholic liver disease

Alcohol consumption

Total alcohol consumption declined in almost all European countries from the 1870s to the Second World War. This was followed by a rather remarkable rise in consumption from the early 1950s to 1975 in most European countries as well as in the United States of America (Williams, AlcHealthResW, 1986; 10:60). In particular, the preference for beer increased strikingly in Europe. In the traditional wine-producing countries, France, Italy, Spain, and Portugal, *per capita* alcohol consumption has stayed among the highest in the world. In France, a decline in alcohol consumption began in the 1950s. A similar but less pronounced reduction in alcohol consumption started in many other European wine-drinking countries about 15 years later (Pyörälä, BrJAddic, 1990; 85:469). In the 1980s an increase in abstention and a decrease in heavier drinking was observed in the United States, especially among the employed and those with a high family income (Williams, BrJAddic, 1992; 87: 643). Long- and short-term international trends associated with alcohol consumption, beverage preference, and drinking patterns have recently been reviewed.[2] Countries with decreasing alcohol consumption from 1961 to 1990 include France, Italy, Australia, the United States, Canada, and Ireland. However, despite the marked decrease in consumption, France is still one of the leading countries in world alcohol consumption statistics. Countries with stable alcohol consumption include Austria, Norway, Sweden, and Switzerland, and countries with increasing alcohol consumption include Germany, the United Kingdom, Iceland, Poland, Japan, Denmark, and Finland.

In wine-drinking countries, wine is a component of every meal and a relatively inexpensive nutrient. In beer-drinking countries in central Europe and North America, beer is used for leisure time and to improve social contacts outside the home. In spirits-drinking countries, alcohol is used as an intoxicant. In Scandinavia, there has been a marked shift towards beer drinking during the past 2 decades. The proportion of alcohol consumption by women in European countries ranges from 18 to 38 per cent.[2] A very uneven distribution of drinking patterns can be observed in most countries. In general, the heaviest drinking 10 per cent of the population drinks about half, and the heaviest drinking 20 per cent drinks about 80 per cent of all alcohol consumed.

Mortality and prevalence of alcoholic liver cirrhosis

Most heavy drinkers and alcoholics will develop hepatomegaly and fatty infiltration of the liver. However, only 20 to 33 per cent develop a more severe liver disease—alcoholic hepatitis or liver cirrhosis.[3, 4] According to postmortem data the prevalence of cirrhosis in alcoholics is about 18 per cent; in series based on liver biopsy it ranges from 17 to 30.8 per cent.[5]

Table 1 Mortality from chronic liver diseases and cirrhosis in 1993 (*World Health Statistics Annual 1994, Causes of Death*. World Health Organization, Geneva 1995)

Country	Number of deaths/year	Number per 100 000	Alcohol intake (litres of pure alcohol/inhabitant per year)
Portugal	2742	27.8	9.9
Austria	2163	27.2	10.5
Italy	15216	26.7[b]	8.6
Germany	19447	24.0[a]	10.4
Spain	7738	19.8[b]	10.0
Luxembourg	69	17.5	12.1
France	9178	16.0[a]	11.5
Denmark	725	14.0	10.0
Belgium	1200	12.0[a]	9.1
Greece	1083	10.5[a]	8.5
Finland	521	10.3	6.8
Sweden	632	7.3[a]	5.3
Great Britain	3400	6.0	7.3
The Netherlands	778	5.1[a]	7.9
Ireland	95	2.7[a]	8.3
Total	65000	17.6	
Mortality from traffic accidents	45600	12.3	

[a] Year 1992.
[b] Year 1991.

In the early 1960s the worldwide annual mortality from cirrhosis was at least 310 000 (Steiner, TropGeogMed, 1964; 16:175). Since then mortality from cirrhosis has increased considerably. For instance, in West Germany it has increased from 6/100 000 in 1950 to 27/100 000 in 1980.[6] Similar increases in the mortality of liver cirrhosis between 1950 and 1970 to 1980 have been documented in the United Kingdom (Fig. 1), in most other European countries, in Australia, in the United States, and in Japan. Since 60 to 90 per cent of all liver cirrhosis cases can be attributed to alcohol consumption, the mortality from alcohol-related chronic liver diseases and cirrhosis is remarkable. For instance in 1993 it was higher than that from traffic accidents in European Union countries (Table 1). In many countries (for example, in England), alcoholic cirrhosis is the most common form of liver injury (Fig. 1) (Saunders, BMJ, 1981; 282:263).

In most cases, cirrhosis of the liver remains undetected during life (Schubert, ZGastr, 1982; 20:221). Accordingly, morbidity from all types of alcoholic liver diseases is much higher than mortality but no valid data about exact numbers are available. However, in Wuppertal and Tübingen the postmortem prevalence of cirrhosis of the liver was shown to be increased from about 2 per cent in 1939 to 11 per cent in 1975 (Schubert, Zgastr, 1982; 20:213).

Relation of liver cirrhosis to alcohol consumption

The volume and pattern of alcohol consumption clearly demonstrate that the prevalence of chronic liver diseases in European countries follows the trends in alcohol consumption (Fig. 2). The close relationship between alcohol consumption and liver cirrhosis mortality has been demonstrated in many studies. One of the classical examples was the effect of wine rationing in France during the Second World War.[6] From 1941 to 1946 alcohol consumption dropped drastically and this was associated with a similar decrease

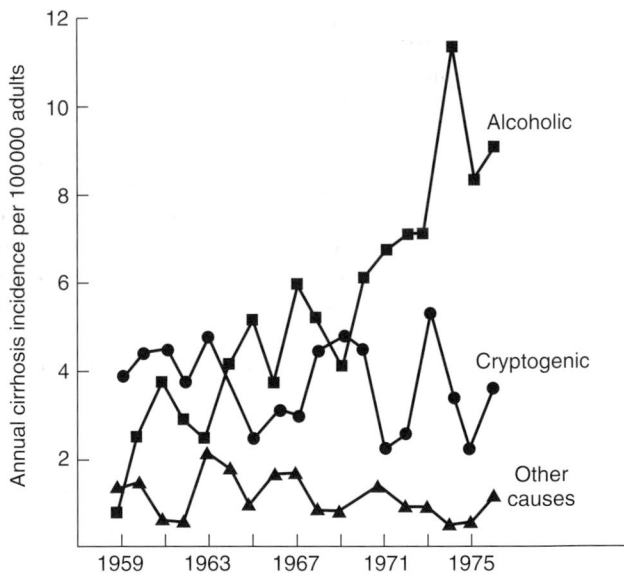

Fig. 1. Annual incidence of alcoholic, cryptogenic, and other types of cirrhosis in west Birmingham from 1959 to 1976. (Saunders, BMJ, 1981; 282:263). (From Morgan, M. Y. (1985). In Hall P, ed. *Alcoholic liver disease*. London: Edward Arnold, 193–200, with permission.)

in mortality from cirrhosis (Fig. 3). Similarly, the subsequent rise in alcohol consumption from 1946 to 1955 resulted in an even more pronounced increase in mortality caused by liver cirrhosis. From 1965, alcohol consumption has decreased equally with mortality from cirrhosis (Fig. 3).

Changes in alcohol consumption are reflected in cirrhosis mortality with a delay of 10 to 15 years. In the 1950s *per capita* wine consumption in France was 140 litres. Thereafter wine consumption started to decrease. However, annual mortality from liver cirrhosis

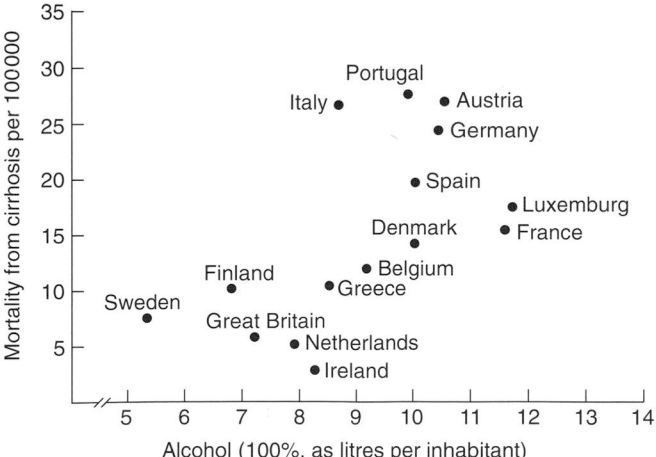

Fig. 2. Relationship between mortality from cirrhosis and alcohol consumption in European Union countries.

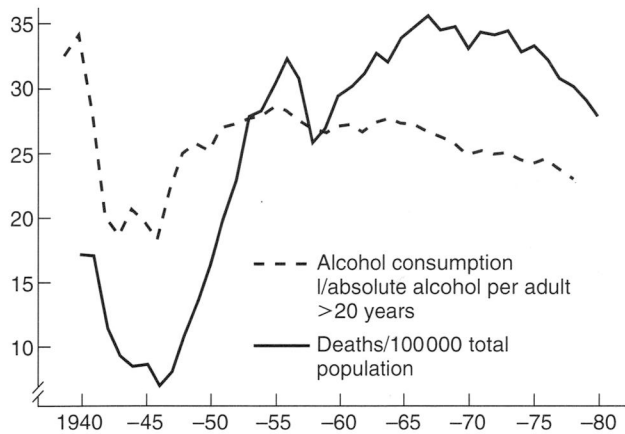

Fig. 3. Alcohol consumption (adults) and mortality from cirrhosis in France 1939 to 1980. (From Lelbach WK. In Hall P, ed. *Alcoholic liver disease*. London: Edward Arnold, 1985: 130–66, with permission.)

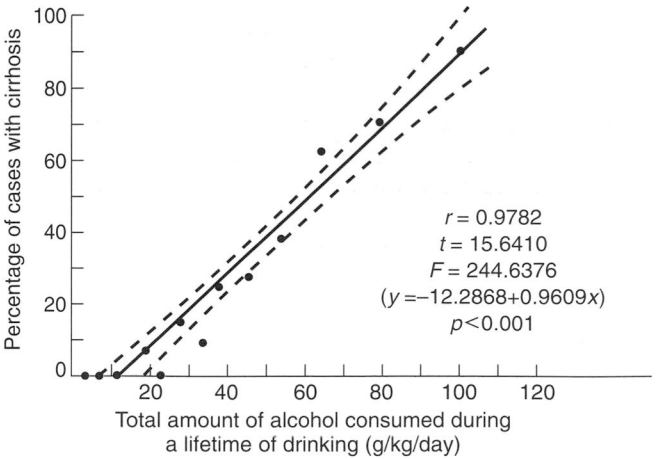

Fig. 4. Correlation between the total amount of ethanol consumed per kg body weight during a lifetime of drinking and incidence of cirrhosis of the liver (*n* = 39) in 265 alcoholics. The dotted lines represent the upper and lower confidence limits of regression. (From Lelbach WK. In Popper H and Schaffner F, eds. *Progress in liver diseases*. New York: Grune and Stratton, 1976: 494–515, with permission.)

increased until 1967 and peaked in 36 per 100 000. In the 1990s *per capita* wine consumption in France has been around 60 to 65 litres. This marked decrease in wine consumption is reflected also in the mortality from cirrhosis—16 per 100 000 in 1992, a reduction of more than 50 per cent since 1966.

The termination of alcohol rationing in Sweden in 1955 was followed by an increase in deaths attributable to cirrhosis (Norström, BrJAddic, 1987; 82:633). On the other hand, a decrease in alcohol consumption from 1976 is associated with at least an equal decrease in mortality from cirrhosis (Romelsjö, BMJ, 1985; 291:167). A highly significant positive correlation has been demonstrated between alcohol consumption and death rates from cirrhosis in 16 European countries (Schmidt, BrJAddic,1981; 76:407).

The development of alcoholic cirrhosis correlates both with the magnitude and duration of alcohol consumption (Fig. 4). For males the relative risk of cirrhosis has been estimated to be six times greater at 40 to 60 g alcohol/day than at up to 20 g/day, and 14 times greater at 60 to 80 g/day.[7] The average 'cirrhogenic' dose

has been calculated to be 180 g ethanol/day consumed regularly for approximately 25 years. According to Lelbach,[3] the probability of developing cirrhosis for an individual consuming about 210 g of ethanol daily for 22 years is 50 per cent and increases to 80 per cent after 33 years. In a case–control study in men, the relative risk for cirrhosis in men consuming 40 to 59 g absolute alcohol/day was 1.83 times the risk for men consuming less than 40 g/day.[8] The relative risk rose to 100 for men consuming over 80 g/day. Similar trends were found in women and for the risk of developing fatty liver.[8]

Most recently it has been suggested that above a rather low, but not precisely determined, level of alcohol consumption, the risk of development of cirrhosis is not further influenced by the amount of alcohol consumed (Sörensen, Lancet, 1984; ii:241; Marbet, JHepatol, 1987; 4:364). Accordingly alcohol abuse may have a permissive rather than a dose-dependent role in the development of alcoholic liver injury.[4] This concept is supported by a recent study based on an autopsy series of 210 males (Savolainen, AlcoholClinExpRes, 1993; 5:1112). Daily ingestion of ethanol below 40 g for a period of 25 years appeared not to increase the risk of alcohol-related liver disease. In contrast, a similar duration of daily intake of between 40 and 80 g increased the risk of all but fibrotic liver lesions. The incidence of both bridging necrosis and cirrhosis increased significantly only when daily alcohol intake exceeded 80 g/day. Amounts of ethanol exceeding 80 g/day did not relate to further increases in the incidence of bridging fibrosis and liver cirrhosis.

Pequignot found that the average cirrhogenic and threshold doses are lower in females than in males.[7] The increased risk of liver cirrhosis in females than in males has also been reported elsewhere[8] (Saunders, 1981; BMJ, 282:1140; Tuyns, IntJEpid, 1984; 14:53). There is no valid epidemiological or clinical evidence to suggest that drinking habits (continuous versus periodic) or the type of alcoholic beverage influence mortality from cirrhosis (Tuyns, BrJAddic, 1984; 79:389).

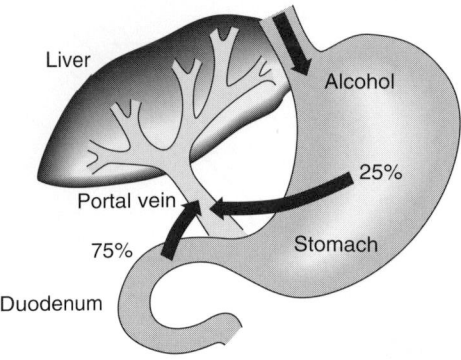

Fig. 5. Absorption of alcohol from the stomach and upper duodenum.

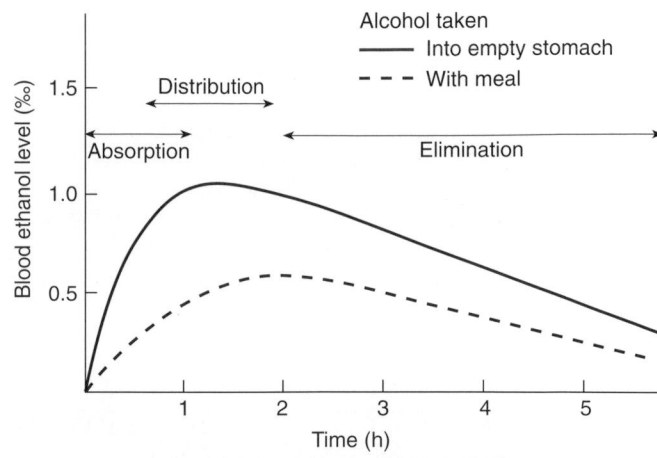

Fig. 6. The effect of a meal on the absorption of alcohol. The blood alcohol curve can be divided to three phases: absorption, distribution, and elimination.

Passage of ethanol through the body

Earlier reviews on the absorption, distribution, metabolism, and excretion of alcohol are numerous and cover different aspects of the topic (Jacobsen, PharmRev, 1952; 4:107; Hawkins, PharmRev, 1972; 24:67). In a normal man about 100 mg of ethanol/kg body weight are eliminated in an hour (7 g alcohol/hour for a 70 kg person). This may vary due to genetic, individual, and external factors. Most importantly, heavy alcohol consumption for years may increase the rate of ethanol elimination up to 100 per cent. These and other aspects of ethanol metabolism are discussed below.

Absorption

The essential features of ethanol absorption and distribution have been established for years following the studies of Mellanby,[9] Widmark,[10] and Berggren and Goldberg.[11] Ethanol is absorbed from the gastrointestinal tract by simple diffusion because of its small size, good water solubility, and low solubility in lipids. Diffusion is rather slow from the stomach and consequently most (70–80 per cent) ingested ethanol is absorbed from the duodenum and upper jejunum (Fig. 5). High ethanol concentrations, similar to those of alcoholic beverages, are reached in the mouth, oesophagus, stomach, and upper jejunum. Thereafter ethanol concentration rapidly decreases so that in the ileum ethanol levels are equal to that of the vascular space (Halsted, AmJClinNutr, 1973; 26:831).

The rate of absorption is decreased by delayed gastric emptying and by the intestinal contents. It is increased in patients with gastroenterostomies (Elmslie, SGO, 1964; 119:1256). Food delays absorption, producing a slower rise and lower peak value of the blood alcohol in fed than in fasting subjects (Fig. 6). The absorption of alcohol is slower from weak solutions such as beer and wine than from distilled beverages (Newman, Science, 1942; 96:43). High ethanol concentrations may delay gastric emptying (Rasmussen, BiochemZ, 1940; 304:358). Carbohydrates (Broitman, Gastro, 1976; 70:1101), amino acids, and dipeptides (Hajjar, Pharmacol, 1982; 23: 177) have been shown to enhance ethanol absorption in the perfused rat jejunum *in vivo*.

Distribution

The diffusion of alcohol through the cell boundaries is a rather slow process, but the distribution of alcohol is very fast by blood flow. In organs with dense vascularization and a rich blood supply, such as the brain, lungs, and liver, alcohol rapidly equilibrates with the blood. Alcohol absorbed in the blood is passed almost immediately into the brain tissue (Harger, JBC, 1937; 120:689; Hulpieu, QJStudAlc, 1946; 7:89). In contrast, the distribution of alcohol to the resting skeletal muscle is particularly slow, since only some of the capillaries are functioning under normal conditions.[12]

Alcohol is poorly lipid soluble; at body temperature tissue lipids take up only 4 per cent of the amount of alcohol that can be dissolved in a corresponding volume of water.[12] Consequently, in an obese person the same amount of alcohol per unit weight gives a higher blood alcohol concentration than in a thin person. Distribution of alcohol is mainly related to the water content of various organs and tissues. For instance, urinary alcohol concentration is slightly higher than that of blood or plasma.

Due to its easy diffusibility alcohol passes through the placental membranes and the amniotic fluid to the fetus.[13] Elimination of ethanol from the fetus is regulated primarily by maternal hepatic biotransformation of ethanol. The amniotic fluid may serve as a reservoir for ethanol *in utero*.[13]

The sex differences in ethanol pharmakokinetics are due to sex differences in body water content. The mean apparent volume of distribution of ethanol is less in women than in men, resulting in higher peak blood ethanol concentrations and greater mean areas under the ethanol concentration–time curves in women than in men (Marshall, JPharmExpTher, 1953; 109:431; Marshall, Hepatol, 1984; 3:701).

Excretion

Most of the ethanol (90–95 per cent) is oxidized and excreted as carbon dioxide and water. Other routes for elimination are urine and breath. Since alcohol is not concentrated in the urine, less than 1 per cent of ingested alcohol is removed by this route.

The distribution of ethanol between blood and expired air is 2100 : 1 (Harger, JBC, 1950; 83:197). In man under normal conditions 1 to 3 per cent (at most 5 per cent) can be eliminated through the lungs. In small animals with a higher metabolic rate (for instance, in rats), up to 10 per cent of administered alcohol can be eliminated through the lungs.

Metabolism of ethanol

Role of the liver

Early in the twentieth century Battelli and Stern (CRSocBio, 1909; 67:419) demonstrated alcohol-oxidizing capacity in both human and animal livers. The importance of the liver in the elimination of ethanol was established in several studies in the late thirties. Fiessinger et al. (CRSocBio, 1936; 122:1255) demonstrated that perfused livers effectively removed alcohol from the perfusion medium. Ethanol oxidation was shown to be reduced in the presence of liver injury (Chapheau, CRSocBio, 1934; 116:887) and almost totally abolished following evisceration (Mirsky, AmJPhysiol, 1939; 126: P587).

In cats and rats the rate of ethanol oxidation is more closely related to the size of the liver than to the size of other organs or the total body size (Eggleton, JPhysiol, 1940; 98:228; Kinard, Nature, 1959; 184:1721).

In 1938, Lundsgaard[14] and Leloir and Muñoz[15] demonstrated that ethanol could be partially oxidized in the liver. The former suggested that the depression in the respiratory quotient of the liver observed following ethanol administration indicated incomplete oxidation of ethanol. The latter reported that about two-thirds of the ethanol oxidized by liver slices could be recovered as acetic acid, and further calculated that about 75 per cent of the oxygen normally taken up by the liver is utilized for ethanol oxidation.[15]

Gastric metabolism of ethanol

Alcohol dehydrogenase is present in the mucosa of stomach, jejunum, and ileum in both the rat (Mistilis, AustAnnMed, 1969; 18: 227; Lambouef, BiochemPharm, 1981; 30:542) and man (Hempel, AlcoholClinExpRes, 1979; 3:95). These findings suggested that the stomach might contribute to the metabolism of ethanol. Subsequent studies indeed indicated that a significant fraction of ingested ethanol is metabolized in the stomach (Julkunen, LifeSci, 1985; 37:567; Caballeria,Gastro, 1989; 97:1205). Gastric metabolism of ethanol may have clinical importance, since the magnitude of gastric ethanol elimination may determine the systemic bioavailability of ethanol, and thereby play a role in the toxicity of ingested ethanol. In recent pharmacokinetic studies it has been suggested that gastric ethanol metabolism in healthy men may account for up to 20 to 30 per cent of a low dose of ingested ethanol if consumed with, or soon after, a meal (Gentry, JLabClinMed, 1994; 123:21). However, according to some contradictory opinions the liver itself may in fact account for most of the first-pass metabolism, at least in the rat (Levitt, AmJPhysiol, 1994; 267:G452).

Subnormal gastric alcohol dehydrogenase activities are found in alcoholics (Julkunen, Alcohol, 1985; 2:437; Seitz, Gut, 1993; 34: 1433) and in rats fed ethanol chronically (DiPadova, Gastro, 1987; 92:1169). This was suggested to be caused by ethanol-induced damage to gastric mucosa. In addition, alcohol dehydrogenase activity of gastric mucosa is decreased in patients with *Helicobacter pylori* associated gastritis (Salmela, AlcoholClinExpRes, 1994; 18: 1294; Thuluvath, AlcoholClinExpRes, 1994; 18:795). This may be associated with a significant decrease in the gastric first-pass metabolism of ethanol (Roine, AnnMed, 1995; 27:583). The lack of the knowledge of a possible *H. pylori*-induced gastritis and associated deficiency in gastric alcohol dehydrogenase activity may have been a confounding factor in the studies dealing with the gastric first-pass metabolism of ethanol and its inhibition by certain H2-receptor antagonists (Hernández-Muñoz, AlcoholClinExpRes, 1990; 14:946; Fraser, AlimPharmTher, 1991; 5:263; Gupta, AlcoholClinExpRes, 1995; 19:1083) or by acetylsalicylic acid (Roine, JAMA, 1990; 264:2406; Melander, PharmkinDisp, 1995; 48:151).

Bacteriocolonic pathway for ethanol oxidation

Alcohol ingested by mouth is transported to the colon by blood circulation and, after the distribution phase, intracolonic ethanol levels are equal to those in the blood (Halstedt, AmJClinNutr,1973; 26:8; Lewitt, Hepatol, 1982; 2:598). Alcohol dehydrogenase enzyme can be detected both in human (Pestalozzi, Gastro, 1983; 85: 1011) and rat colon mucosa (Tietjen, HistochemJ, 1994; 26:526). Moreover, many colonic bacteria representing the normal human colonic flora may possess high alcohol dehydrogenase activity and produce acetaldehyde from ethanol (Jokelainen, AlcoholClinExpRes, 1996; 20:967). Also, human colonic contents produce marked acetaldehyde levels when incubated *in vitro* in the presence of ethanol (Jokelainen, Gut, 1994; 35:1271). On the basis of these findings it has been suggested recently that there exists a bacteriocolonic pathway for ethanol oxidation (Jokelainen, Gut, 1996; 39:100).[16]

In this pathway intracolonic ethanol is at first oxidized by bacterial alcohol dehydrogenase to acetaldehyde.[16] Then acetaldehyde is oxidized, either by colonic mucosal or bacterial aldehyde dehydrogenase, to acetate. Some of the intracolonic acetaldehyde may also be absorbed to the portal vein and be metabolized in the liver (Matysiak-Budnik, JPath, 1996; 28:494). Due to the low aldehyde dehydrogenase activity of colonic mucosa (Koivisto, AlcoholClinExpRes, 1996; 20:551), acetaldehyde accumulates in the colon. Accordingly, during ethanol oxidation the highest acetaldehyde levels of the body are found in the colon and not in the liver (Seitz, Gastro, 1990; 98:406; Jokelainen, Gut, 1996; 39: 100).[16]

High intracolonic acetaldehyde during ethanol oxidation may contribute to the pathogenesis of alcohol-related gastrointestinal symptoms and diseases, for example diarrhoea, colon polyps, and colon cancer.[16] Furthermore, intracolonic acetaldehyde may be an important determinant of blood acetaldehyde level and a potential hepatotoxin.[16]

The total extrahepatic metabolism of ethanol has been estimated to range from 10 to 30 per cent in studies in which ethanol has been administered parenterally to experimental animals (Larsen, Nature, 1959; 184:1236; Huang, LifeSci, 1993; 53:165). In patients with cirrhosis of the liver the extrahepatic elimination has been reported to constitute about 40 per cent of total body elimination (Utne, ScaJGastr, 1980; 15:297). The contribution of the bacteriocolonic pathway to extrahepatic ethanol elimination remains to be established in future studies.

Other tissues

Small amounts of ethanol can be actively oxidized by the kidneys, [14] bone marrow cells (Wickramasinghe, ActaHaem, 1981; 66:238),

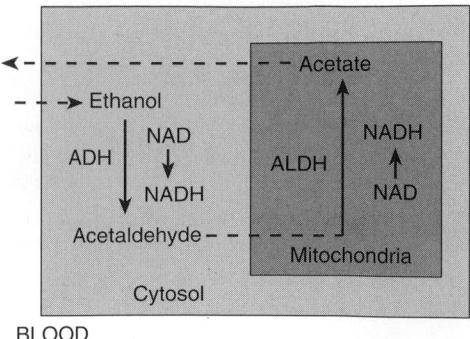

Fig. 7. Pathways of ethanol oxidation via hepatic alcohol, and aldehyde dehydrogenases.

lungs (Pikkarainen, JLabClinMed, 1981; 97:631), testis (Yamauchi, AlcoholClinExp, 1988; 12:143), and pancreas (Estival, Tox-ApplPharmacol, 1981; 61:155).

Pathways of ethanol oxidation

The hepatic metabolism of ethanol proceeds in three basic steps. First, ethanol is oxidized within the cytosol of the hepatocyte to acetaldehyde; secondly, acetaldehyde is converted to acetate, mainly in the mitochondria; and thirdly, the acetate produced in the liver is released into the blood and is oxidized by peripheral tissues to carbon dioxide, fatty acids, and water (Fig. 7). The main pathway for ethanol metabolism proceeds via the enzyme alcohol dehydrogenase. However, alternative pathways for ethanol oxidation, which are situated in other subcellular compartments, have been described.

Alcohol dehydrogenase pathway

Alcohol dehydrogenase catalyses the oxidation of alcohols, including ethanol, to their corresponding aldehydes according to the following scheme.

ADH

$$CH_3CH_2OH + NAD^+ \rightarrow CH_3CHO + NADH + H^+$$

Multiple molecular forms of alcohol dehydrogenase

The activity of hepatic alcohol dehydrogenase is low during fetal life; adult levels are reached by 5 years of age in humans (Pikkarainen, PediatRes, 1967; 1:165). Hepatic alcohol dehydrogenase is non-specific and in addition to the oxidation of alcohols it catalyses the oxidation of endogenous and exogenous sterols (Frey, PNAS, 1980; 77:924), and is responsible for the omega-oxidation of fatty acids (Björkhem, EurJBioch, 1972; 30:441; Boleda, ArchBiochemBiophys, 1993; 307:85). Endogenous steroids and/or small amounts of ethanol produced by intestinal flora (Krebs, BiochemJ, 1970; 118:635) may represent 'physiological' substrates for alcohol dehydrogenase.

The molecular weight of human liver alcohol dehydrogenase is 79 000 to 83 000 Da and each molecule contains four atoms of zinc which are vital for enzyme activity (Lange, Biochem, 1976; 15:4687). The primary structure of human alcohol dehydrogenase has

been determined (Bühler, EurJBioch, 1984; 145:447; Hempel, EurJBioch, 1984; 145:437). There is considerable polymorphism in alcohol dehydrogenase, which has been related to alcohol metabolism, alcoholism, and alcoholic liver disease.[17-20] Six different classes of mammalian alcohol dehydrogenase have been characterized.[19] Most of them are common to humans, mammals, and many vertebrates. Chromosome mapping studies have revealed that alcohol dehydrogenase genes are located on the long arm of human chromosome 4.[17] In man, the system appears to account for at least eight genes (ADH1–8), with corresponding subunits. Class I isozymes are coded by genes ADH1, ADH2, and ADH3, and are explained by the presence of three subunit types (α, β, γ) in humans. Class I enzymes have a low K_M (1–4 mmol) and high V_{max} for ethanol, and they are responsible for the bulk of ethanol oxidation (Bosron, Enzyme, 1987; 37:19).

The class II alcohol dehydrogenase isozyme is coded by ADH4 and has a markedly higher KM for ethanol (120 mmol) than class I isozymes. The class III alcohol dehydrogenase has a very high KM for ethanol (>3 M) and is not assumed to participate in the hepatic ethanol oxidation under physiological conditions.

Class IV alcohol dehydrogenase is the stomach enzyme (σ,σ-alcohol dehydrogenase) with a rather high KM, 37 mmol in man and 2.4 M in the rat (Farres, EurJBioch, 1994; 224:549). Class V alcohol dehydrogenase is found in fetal liver. Human class VI alcohol dehydrogenase has not been detected, but it has been demonstrated in rat kidneys.

Various alcohol dehydrogenase forms appear in different frequencies in different racial populations.[17-20] Furthermore, they may explain, at least in part, individual variation in the rate of ethanol elimination[20] (Martin, BehavGen, 1985; 15:93). Alcohol dehydrogenase phenotypes have been related to the production of acetaldehyde and to the extent of first-pass elimination of ethanol (vonWartburg, LabInvest, 1984; 50:5). Most recently some positive associations between alcohol dehydrogenase genotype and alcohol-related liver injury or even alcoholism have been reported (Chao, Hepatol, 1994; 19:360; Pares, Alcohol, 1994; 29:701; Sherman; BMJ, 1994; 308:341; Yamuauchi, JHepatol, 1995; 23:519; Nakamura, AlcoholClinExpRes, 1996; 20:52).

The first reaction of the bacteriocolonic pathway for ethanol oxidation is mediated by microbial alcohol dehydrogenase.[16] There are marked differences in the alcohol dehydrogenase activity and acetaldehyde producing capacity among the aerobic bacteria representing the normal human colonic flora (Jokelainen, AlcoholClin ExpRes, 1996; 20:967). The mean cytosolic alcohol dehydrogenase activity of the bacteria can be up to 30 times higher than that of the rat liver when determined under similar conditions. The highly significant positive correlation between bacterial alcohol dehydrogenase activity and their acetaldehyde producing capacity from ethanol, strongly suggests the catalytical role of microbial alcohol dehydrogenase in this reaction (Jokelainen, AlcoholClinExpRes, 1996; 20:967).

Characteristics of the alcohol dehydrogenase pathway

The pH optimum for the alcohol dehydrogenase-mediated oxidation of ethanol is about 10.8. At physiological pH the rate of reaction is only 40 per cent of the maximum. Horse and human liver alcohol dehydrogenases both have K_M values for ethanol under 1 mmol (Theorell, ActaChemSca, 1955; 9:1148; Blair, Biochem, 1966; 5:2026). This means that ethanol is effectively eliminated from the blood at a constant rate to very low concentrations, provided that acetaldehyde is also effectively removed. As the K_M for acetaldehyde is 1.4 mmol it could act as a substrate for alcohol dehydrogenase in the reverse reaction. However, the rapid transformation of acetaldehyde to acetate keeps the reaction in the forward direction.

When alcohol is oxidized to acetaldehyde via alcohol dehydrogenase, nicotinamide adenine dinucleotide (**NAD**) is required as a cofactor and is reduced to NADH during the reaction. Under normal conditions the rate of NADH production exceeds its rate of reoxidation, resulting in an increase in the liver NADH/NAD ratio (i.e. the redox state of the liver is markedly reduced) (Forsander, BiochemJ, 1965; 94:259). Most of the acute metabolic effects of ethanol, such as the inhibition of hepatic gluconeogenesis (Krebs, BiochemJ, 1969; 112:117), the decrease in the citric acid cycle activity (Forsander, BiochemJ, 1965; 94:259), and the impairment of fatty acid oxidation (Lieber, JCI, 1961; 40:394), are due to this major effect of ethanol on the intermediary metabolism of the liver.

Regulation of the alcohol dehydrogenase pathway

Several factors affect the activity of the alcohol dehydrogenase pathway for ethanol oxidation, including the activity of alcohol dehydrogenase, the intracellular acetaldehyde concentration, the activity of the shuttle mechanisms transporting reducing equivalents into the mitochondria, and the rate of the mitochondrial respiratory chain. The rate-limiting step in the alcohol dehydrogenase pathway therefore varies depending on the experimental conditions.

In fasted animals the rate-limiting step in ethanol oxidation is the availability of substrates for the hydrogen translocation shuttles (i.e. transfer of the hydrogen of the cytosolic NADH to mitochondria). Thus, addition of pyruvate (one of the possible NADH oxidizing agents) to the medium perfusing hepatocytes isolated from fasting animals increases the rate of ethanol oxidation by 153 per cent (Cederbaum, ArchBiochemBiophys, 1977; 183:638). On the other hand, in studies with hepatocytes obtained from fed animals, the rate of ethanol oxidation is regulated mainly by the capacity of the mitochondria to reoxidize reducing equivalents. However, it should be emphasized that under *in vitro* conditions—even in the presence of sufficient amounts of shuttle metabolites, uncoupling agents or pyruvate—the rate of ethanol oxidation never reaches the rate found *in vivo*.

In general, the rate of ethanol elimination *in vivo* correlates with the subject's basal metabolic rate, suggesting that the rate of mitochondrial NADH oxidation is the primary rate-limiting step in the alcohol dehydrogenase pathway. In the horse, for example, the liver contains large amounts of alcohol dehydrogenase, yet the rate of ethanol metabolism is low and relates to the animal's basal metabolic rate (Lester, LifeSci, 1967; 6:2313). In smaller animals such as the rat, although a greater proportion of total alcohol dehydrogenase activity (50–85 per cent) may be utilized for *in vivo* ethanol oxidation (Crow, Alcoholism, 1977; 1:43), the theoretical capacity of alcohol dehydrogenase to metabolize ethanol still exceeds the actual rate *in vivo* (Raskin, NatureNewBiol, 1972; 236:138).

In spontaneously hypertensive rats, derived from the Kyoto–Wistar strain, hepatic alcohol dehydrogenase activity constitutes the rate-limiting step in the alcohol dehydrogenase pathway (Rachamin, BiochemJ, 1980; 186:483). In these rats alcohol dehydrogenase activity is so low that no change is observed in the cytosolic NADH/NAD ratio after feeding with alcohol. Also protein deficiency (Horn, JPharmExpTher, 1965; 147:385; Bode, ZGesamExpMed, 1970; 152:111; Wilson, Hepatol, 1986; 6:823) and advancing age (Hahn, AlcoholClinExpRes, 1983; 7:299) result in decreased activity of hepatic alcohol dehydrogenase and a corresponding reduction in the rate of ethanol elimination.

However, these situations are the exceptions and under normal circumstances hepatic alcohol dehydrogenase is present in excess so that the most important rate-limiting step in the alcohol dehydrogenase pathway *in vivo* is the rate of NADH reoxidation. Individuals with 'atypical' alcohol dehydrogenase have enzyme activities *in vitro* that are several times higher than normal, yet eliminate ethanol at a normal rate (Edwards, ClinPharmTher, 1967; 8:824). Furthermore, in uraemic patients blood ethanol clearance is not accelerated, despite several-fold increases in liver alcohol dehydrogenase activity (Mezey, JLabClinMed, 1975; 86:931). It can therefore be concluded that while increased alcohol dehydrogenase activity may not be associated with increased rates of ethanol oxidation, reduction of alcohol dehydrogenase activity leads to a decrease in ethanol elimination.

The rate of ethanol elimination *in vivo* may be affected by several factors which indirectly affect the alcohol dehydrogenase pathway. During prolonged fasting the rate of alcohol disappearance from blood is markedly reduced, both in experimental animals and in humans (Vitale, JBC, 1953; 204:257; Dontcheff, CRSocBiol, 1973; 126:462). Originally it was suggested that this effect occurred as a result of a decrease in alcohol dehydrogenase activity (Büttner, BiochemZ, 1965; 341:300). However, since the effect of prolonged fasting on ethanol kinetics could be reversed by giving fructose, it was concluded that the rate-limiting step in the alcohol dehydrogenase pathway during fasting was the decreased capacity of the liver to reoxidize NADH (Bode, DMedWoch, 1975; 100:1849).

As the rate of ethanol oxidation depends largely on the NADH reoxidation rate, it is easy to see why attempts to increase the rate of ethanol elimination *in vivo* have, for the most part, failed. The agent known to enhance ethanol elimination both *in vivo* and *in vitro* is fructose (Tygstrup, JCI, 1965; 44:817; Thieden, BiochemJ, 1967; 102:177). This effect of fructose, which can be observed in both fasting and fed animals and in humans, occurs because the phosphorylation of fructose consumes ATP, thus increasing the capacity of the respiratory chain to oxidize NADH derived from the oxidation of ethanol and acetaldehyde (Thieden, EurJBiochem, 1972; 30:250; Scholz, EurJBiochem, 1976; 63:449).

In addition to fructose, corticosteroids have been shown to increase the rate of ethanol elimination both in experimental animals and in humans (Clark, ArchInternatPharmTher, 1966; 162:355; Fischer, BiochemPharm, 1966; 15:785; Korri, AlcAlc, 1988; 23:371). This phenomenon may be due to increased conversion of NADH to NAD as a result of enhanced gluconeogenesis.

In some situations ethanol elimination may be higher after a second dose of ethanol. This is called a swift increase in alcohol metabolism, and has been suggested to be mediated by the release of glycogenolytic hormones (Forman, AnnClinLabSci, 1988; 18:318). Ethanol elimination does not vary during the menstrual cycle

(Marshall, Hepatol, 1984; 3:701) but tends to decrease in women taking oral contraceptives (Jones, AlcoholClinExpRes, 1984; 8:24).

Alcohol dehydrogenase inhibitors

Several drugs have been shown to interfere with the metabolism of ethanol (Salaspuro, ActaMedScand, 1985; 703(Suppl.):219). Of these pyrazole and its derivatives are best characterized as alcohol dehydrogenase inhibitors. In 1963, Theorell and Yonetani (BiochemZ, 1963; 338:537) reported that pyrazole inhibits the action of horse liver alcohol dehydrogenase by forming a complex with alcohol dehydrogenase and NAD. The inhibitory effect of pyrazole and some of its substituted derivatives on human liver alcohol dehydrogenase was demonstrated subsequently (Li, Acta-ChemScand, 1969; 23:892). Pyrazole was the first compound used to inhibit alcohol dehydrogenase *in vivo*, but it proved toxic to the liver and several other organs (Lelbach, Experientia, 1969; 25:816; Lieber, LabInvest, 1970; 22:615) and was replaced by its more potent but less toxic derivative 4-methylpyrazole (Theorell, Acta-ChemScand, 1969; 23:255; Magnusson, Experientia, 1972; 28:1198). The biological effects and metabolic interactions of 4-methyl-pyrazole with ethanol have been studied extensively in rats by Blomstrand et al.[21]

In humans 4-methylpyrazole clearly decreases the rate of ethanol elimination and inhibits some of its redox-related effects on the intermediary metabolism of the liver (Salaspuro, EurJClinInvest, 1977; 7:487; Salaspuro, Metabolism, 1978; 27:631). It does not, however, prevent the development of alcohol-related liver injury in animals chronically fed ethanol. In fact 4-methylpyrazole potentiates the effects of alcohol on the liver by producing a prolonged imbalance of hepatic metabolism (Lindros, Liver, 1983; 3:79).

In addition to interfering with the metabolism of ethanol, pyrazole and its derivatives also inhibit the metabolism of other alcohols via the alcohol dehydrogenase pathway. Thus 4-methyl-pyrazole and other alcohol dehydrogenase inhibitors may have a role in the treatment of methanol and ethylene glycol poisoning.[21] 4-Methylpyrazole has also been used in the treatment of the alcohol-disulphiram reaction (Lindros, AlcoholClinExpRes, 1981; 5:528).

More recent inhibitors of alcohol dehydrogenase include a dietary supplement, acetylcarnitine (Sachan, BBResComm, 1994; 202:1496), 4-alkylpyrazoles (Echevarria, ArchPharmacol, 1994; 327:303), and bismuth compounds (Salmela, Gastro, 1993;105:325).

Microsomal ethanol oxidizing system

In 1965, a NADPH-dependent microsomal oxidase was obtained by fractionation of pig's liver, which catalysed the oxidation of methanol to formaldehyde and of ethanol to acetaldehyde (Orme-Johnson, BBResComm, 1965; 21:78). In 1968, a cytochrome P450-dependent microsomal ethanol oxidizing system (**MEOS**) was demonstrated in rats by Lieber and DeCarli.[22,23] In subsequent studies Lieber and co-workers fully characterized the MEOS pathway. The scheme of the reaction is as follows.

MEOS

$$CH_3CH_2OH + NADPH^+ + H + O_2 \rightarrow CH_3CHO + NADP^+ + 2H_2O$$

The observation that chronic consumption of ethanol leads to the proliferation of the endoplasmic reticulum (Iseri, AmJPathol,

1966; 48:535) as well as to the increased activity of several microsomal drug-metabolizing enzymes (Rubin, Science, 1968; 159:1469; Ishii, BBActa, 1973; 291:411) further supported an *in vivo* interaction between alcohol metabolism and microsomes.

The microsomal ethanol oxidizing system involves a specific form of cytochrome P450 designated as P4502E1 (**CYP2E1**) (Nebert, DNA, 1987; 6:1). In addition to ethanol, CYP2E1 oxidizes acetaldehyde and over 80 toxicologically important xenobiotics.[24,25][24,25] It is highly inducible by chronic alcohol consumption in rabbits (Koop, JBC, 1982; 257:8472), rats (Johansson, Biochem, 1988; 27:1925), and in man (Tsutsumi, Hepatol, 1989; 10:437). The induction of CYP2E1 in the human liver is due to a corresponding increase in encoding mRNA (Takahashi, Hepatol, 1993; 17:236).

The contribution of MEOS to ethanol oxidation has not yet been clarified in humans. There is recent evidence that the *c2* allele of the CYP2E1 gene may influence the rate of ethanol elimination at high ethanol levels (Ueno, AlcoholClinExpRes, 1996; 20:17). On the other hand, CYP2E1 genotypes differ neither among alcoholics or non-alcoholic controls (Iwanashi, AlcoholClinExpRes, 1995; 19:564) nor among the patients with or without alcoholic liver injury (Carr, AlcoholClinExpRes, 1995; 19:182; Chao, Hepatol, 1995; 22:1409).

In addition to liver, microsomal ethanol oxidizing capacity has been demonstrated in rats in the mucosal cells of the upper gastrointestinal tract and colon (Seitz, LifeSci, 1979; 25:1443; Seitz, NaunynSchmiedbArchPharm, 1982; 320:81) as well as in kidney and lung microsomes (Zerilli, Alcohol, 1995; 30:357).

Catalase

Catalase is a haemoprotein located in the peroxisomes of most tissues. Small amounts are also found in isolated hepatocyte microsomes, but its presence there may result from contamination (Redman, ArchBiochBiophys, 1972; 152:496). As early as 1936 Keilin and Hartree (ProcRoySocMed, 1936; 119:141) suggested that catalase may play a role in alcohol metabolism. In 1955 this was confirmed by Laser (BiochemJ, 1955; 61:122) who showed that ethanol could be effectively oxidized in the presence of hydrogen peroxide and catalase. The scheme of the reaction is as follows:

catalase

$$CH_3CH_2OH + H_2O_2 \rightarrow CH_3CHO + 2H_2O$$

xanthine

oxidase

$$Hypoxanthine + H_2O + O_2 \rightarrow xanthine + H_2O_2$$

Catalase is capable of oxidizing ethanol *in vitro* only in the presence of a hydrogen peroxide generating system (Keilin, BiochemJ, 1945; 39:293). The reaction is limited by the rate of hydrogen peroxide generation rather than by the amount of catalase itself. The physiological rate of hydrogen peroxide production is small, suggesting that catalase could account for only about 2 per cent of the *in vivo* rate of ethanol oxidation (Boveris, BiochemJ, 1972; 128:617; Sies, AngewChem, 1974; 13:706).

A strain of deermouse that lacks hepatic alcohol dehydrogenase activity has been used to study the respective roles of MEOS and catalase in ethanol oxidation. The predominant role of both MEOS

(Kato, BiochemPharm, 1988;37:2706; Alderman, ArchBiochem-Biophys, 1989; 271:33) and catalase (Handler, BiochemJ, 1987; 248:415; Handler, ArchBiochemBiophys, 1988; 265:114; Bradford, MolPharm, 1993; 43:115) has been emphasized. A possible role of mitochondrial alcohol dehydrogenase in the oxidation of ethanol in deermouse has also remained controversial (Norsten, JBC, 1989; 265:5593; Inatomi, AlcoholClinExpRes, 1990; 14:130).

Non-oxidative metabolism of ethanol

Many human organs have been found to metabolize ethanol through a non-oxidative pathway by forming fatty acid ethyl esters (Laposata, Science, 1986; 231:497). Furthermore, the authors found that the production of fatty acid ethyl esters was related to blood ethanol concentration, and consequently suggested that the non-oxidative metabolism of ethanol may explain the tissue damage seen in organs lacking oxidative alcohol metabolism. This interesting theory is awaiting confirmation and further studies.

Metabolism of acetaldehyde

Regardless of the pathway by which ethanol is oxidized, acetaldehyde is its first major 'specific' oxidation product. Acetaldehyde itself is oxidized so rapidly that under normal circumstances significant concentrations can be found only in the liver and the colon. While it has been suggested that several enzyme systems are capable of catalysing aldehyde oxidation, it is now generally accepted that the main enzyme of acetaldehyde oxidation is aldehyde dehydrogenase. Over 90 per cent of the acetaldehyde formed from ethanol is subsequently oxidized in the liver to acetate.

Aldehyde dehydrogenases

An NAD-dependent aldehyde dehydrogenase with a broad substrate specificity for aldehydes was described in 1949 by Racker (JBC, 1949; 177:883). The enzyme has a very low K_M value and a high reaction rate (Kraemer, JBC, 1968; 243:6402), which explains why, under normal circumstances, only low concentrations of acetaldehyde are found outside the liver and large bowel.

There is aldehyde dehydrogenase activity in mitochondria, cytoplasm, and microsomes (Tottmar, BiochemJ, 1973; 135:577). Several studies have shown that acetaldehyde oxidation in rat liver is entirely a mitochondrial process at the low acetaldehyde concentrations present in this organ during ethanol oxidation (Grunnet, EurJBioch, 1973; 35:236; Marjanen, BBActa, 1973; 327:238). At higher acetaldehyde concentrations (>0.4 mmol) the increase in acetaldehyde oxidation is due to the activity of extramitochondrial aldehyde dehydrogenase (Lindros, JBC, 1974; 249:7956; Parrilla, JBC, 1974; 249:4926).

Two major hepatic aldehyde dehydrogenase isozymes (ALDH1 and 2) exist in humans.[26–28] ALDH2 is predominantly of mitochondrial origin. It has a low K_M (3 μM or less) and high affinity for acetaldehyde. ALDH1, which has a relatively higher K_M, is of cytosolic origin. Aldehyde dehydrogenase enzymes of human liver are tetramers consisting of unequal subunits with molecular weights of 54 800 and 54 200 Da, respectively (Greenfield, BBActa, 1977; 483:35; Harada, LifeSci, 1980; 26:1771). The multiple molecular forms of aldehyde dehydrogenase show remarkable heterogeneity in their tissue and organ distribution.[26–28]

Interestingly, the mitochondrial isozyme (ALDH2) was found to be deficient in about 50 per cent of the liver specimens of Japanese (Goedde, HumGenet, 1979; 51:331; Agarwal, AlcoholClinExpRes, 1981; 5:12). Subsequent population genetic studies showed a wide prevalence of the isozyme deficiency among Oriental populations and South American Indian tribes but not in Caucasians and Negroes.[26–28] The homotetrameric ALDH2 enzyme is encoded by a nuclear gene located at chromosome 12q24 (Braun, HumGen, 1986; 73:365).[29] Polymorphism of this gene has been characterized for an allelic variant designated as $ALDH2^2$.[29] This allele acts dominantly by the formation of heterotetramers to reduce the enzyme activity in $ALDH2^1/ALDH2^2$ heterozygotes.[27] The deficient ALDH2 enzyme coded by the $ALDH2^2$ allele is abundant in Asian populations (Novoradovsky, AlcoholClinExpRes, 1995; 19:1105). Following alcohol consumption, $ALDH2^2$ carrier status results in alcohol flushing (i.e. symptoms of acute acetaldehyde intoxication)[26] (Harada, ProgClinBiolRes,1990; 344:289).

ALDH2-deficient liver extracts contain immunologically cross-reactive material with normal ALDH2, but with near-loss of enzyme activity. The loss of enzyme activity is due to a change of one amino acid in the enzyme molecule (Hempel, FEBSLett, 1984; 173:367; Hsu, PNAS, 1985; 82:3771).[27] Most importantly, homozygotic ALDH2 carrier status associates with a 73 to 91 per cent protection rate against alcoholism and alcohol-related liver and pulmonary diseases (Enomoto, Hepatol, 1991; 13:1071; Thomasson, AmJHumGen, 1991; 48:677; Chao, Hepatol, 1994; 19:360; Takada, AlcAlc, 1994; 29:719).

Characteristics of the acetaldehyde pathway to acetate

As stated above, the oxidation of acetaldehyde to acetate is catalysed by a low-K_M aldehyde dehydrogenase located in the mitochondrial matrix. Mitochondrial NAD functions as a coenzyme in the reaction. Consequently, oxidation of ethanol via acetaldehyde to acetate results in the reduction of both cytosolic and mitochondrial redox states, which are reflected in the increases of liver and blood lactate to pyruvate and β-hydroxbutyrate to acetoacetate ratios, respectively.[30]

As early as 1938 it was suggested that ethanol is oxidized in the liver only to intermediates.[14,15] In studies with perfused isolated rat liver, only 2 to 7 per cent of ^{14}C-labelled ethanol can be recovered as carbon dioxide.[30] In the same study it was found that the main product of hepatic metabolism of ethanol is acetic acid. This was subsequently confirmed in rats (Gordon, CanJPhysPharm, 1968; 46:609) and in humans, using liver vein catheter techniques.[31,32]

Blood acetaldehyde concentrations

Technical difficulties associated with the measurement of blood acetaldehyde levels hampered earlier studies of this topic (Stowell, BiochemMed, 1977; 8:392; Eriksson, AlcAlc, 1993; 2(Suppl.):9). In early reports blood acetaldehyde concentrations following ethanol ranged from 0 to 250 μM (Majchrowicz, Science, 1970; 168:1100; Korsten, NEJM, 1975; 292:386). Later, using improved methodology, it was shown that blood acetaldehyde concentrations during ethanol oxidation in the peripheral blood of non-alcoholic control subjects are extremely low (0–2 μM) and are often at, or below, the limit of detection (Pikkarainen, AlcoholClinExpRes, 1979; 3:259; Lindros, PharmBiochemBehav, 1980; 13:119).

These findings indicate that in normal healthy individuals almost all the acetaldehyde formed during ethanol oxidation is effectively oxidized in the liver. However, significant, although modest, concentrations of acetaldehyde (2–20 μM) can be measured in the hepatic venous blood of moderately intoxicated non-alcoholic male Caucasians at a time when peripheral venous concentrations are less than 2 μM.[33] Consequently, in addition to liver, peripheral tissues have a considerable capacity to eliminate low concentrations of acetaldehyde. However, more pronounced concentrations of acetaldehyde exist in the peripheral blood of chronic alcoholics, in Oriental individuals who suffer alcohol-related flushing, and in the presence of aldehyde dehydrogenase inhibitors.

In contrast to the situation in normal Caucasian individuals, alcohol ingestion in some Orientals results in marked elevations of blood acetaldehyde concentrations, ranging from 10 to 50 μM following alcohol ingestion (Mizoi, PharmBiochBehav, 1979; 10: 303). These individuals then develop facial flushing and tachycardia as a direct consequence of acetaldehyde-induced catecholamine release (Ijiri, JpnJStudAlc, 1974; 9:35; Inoue, PharmBiochBehav, 1980; 13:295). The acetaldehyde-mediated flushing occurs in individuals in whom the mitochondrial ALDH2 isozyme is physiologically inactive because of a genetically determined defect in protein synthesis (see above).

As mentioned above, acetaldehyde concentrations in peripheral blood are considerably lower than in hepatic venous blood.[33] Peripheral uptake of acetaldehyde accounts for 30 to 40 per cent of the concentration gradient between hepatic venous and peripheral blood.[33] In addition, red cells may bind acetaldehyde during the passage of blood through the splanchnic area and release it in the peripheral tissues (Baraona, Hepatol, 1985; 5:1048).

Both the mucosal cells of the digestive tract (Lamboeuf, BiochemPharm, 1981; 30:542) and human blood and bone marrow cells may metabolize ethanol (Bond, ActaHaem, 1983; 69:303) and produce acetaldehyde. Acetaldehyde is also produced by bronchopulmonary washings (Miyakawa, AlcoholClinExpRes, 1986; 10: 517) and by intestinal bacteria (Baraona, Gastro, 1986; 90:103). An exaggerated acetaldehyde response after ethanol administration has been demonstrated during pregnancy and lactation in rats (Gordon, AlcoholClinExpRes, 1985; 9:17). Acetaldehyde produced by the bacteriocolonic pathway for ethanol oxidation[16] may also be absorbed by the portal blood and thereby contribute to blood acetaldehyde levels (Matysiak-Budnik, JPath, 1996; 178:469).

Aldehyde dehydrogenase inhibitors

A number of chemical compounds, including several naturally occurring substances, such as those found in the fungus *Coprinus atramentarius*, are known to cause sensitizing reactions in the presence of ethanol (Barkman, ActaPharmTox, 1963; 20:43; Genest, JPharmPharmacol, 1968; 20:102). A dietary factor which inhibits aldehyde dehydrogenase has been found in the calcinated bonemeal fed to laboratory rats and has been identified as cyanamide (Lindros, LifeSci, 1975; 17:1589; Marchner, ActaPharmTox, 1976; 39:331). Phenylisothiocyanate, which is found in cabbages and other commonly ingested cruciferous vegetables, has recently been demonstrated to be a powerful inhibitor of mitochondrial aldehyde dehydrogenase (Lindros, JPharmExpTher, 1995; 275:79).

In 1937, a sensitization reaction to alcohol caused by a tetramethylthiuram mono- and disulphide was described and the suggestion was made that these compounds might be used in the treatment of alcoholism (Williams, JAMA, 1937; 109:1472). The first animal and clinical studies using the drug disulfiram appeared more than 10 years later (Asmussen, ActaPharmTox, 1948; 4:297; Hald, ActaPharmTox, 1948; 4:305; Larsen, ActaPharmTox, 1948; 4:321). Subsequently, the trade name Antabuse® was given to the compound, and the characteristics of the sensitization reaction were studied extensively (Perman, ActaPhysiolScand, 1962; 55:5). In 1956, calcium cyanamide and its citrated derivative, calcium carbimide, were proposed for clinical use in the treatment of alcoholism (Armstrong, CanMedAssJ, 1956; 74:795; Bell, CanMedAssJ, 1956; 74:797). Later, even more powerful aldehyde dehydrogenase inhibitors were developed, but they have not gained general acceptance (Suokas, AlcoholClinExpRes, 1985; 9:221).

The reaction to alcohol which occurs following use of oral antidiabetic agents of the sulphonylurea group, such as tolbutamide, carbutamide, and chlorpropamide, closely resembles the disulfiram–alcohol reaction and has also been attributed to the presence of elevated blood acetaldehyde concentrations (Czyzyk, DMedWoch, 1957; 82:1585; Groop, Diabetolog, 1984; 26:34). Other compounds known to induce alcohol-sensitizing reactions include the antioxidant, *n*-butyraldoxime (Koe, FedProc, 1969; 28:546); the antibiotic, metronidazole (Lal, QJStudAlc, 1969; 30:140); antianginal drugs (Towell, AlcoholClinExpRes, 1985; 9:438); and cefamandole (Freundt, Infection, 1986; 14:44). However, the biochemical backgrounds of the reactions caused by these agents in the presence of ethanol have not been fully established.

Metabolism of acetate

In 1960, Forsander and Räihä reported that *in vivo* administration of ethanol to rats resulted in an increase in blood acetate concentrations.[30] Lundquist observed increases in plasma acetate concentrations in humans following ethanol intake,[31] which occurred independently of blood ethanol values over a wide concentration range.[32] After intravenous or oral ethanol, blood acetate concentrations rise to a plateau, though they may vary to a degree in fasting individuals or following fructose infusion (Lundquist, ActaPharmTox, 1958; 14:265). Acetate is further oxidized to carbon dioxide and water by peripheral tissues (Karlsson, ActaPhysiolScand, 1975; 93:391). The peripheral uptake of acetate is concentration dependent (Buckley, BiochemJ, 1977; 166:539).

During ethanol oxidation blood acetate levels are higher in alcoholics than in non-alcoholic controls, and there is a highly significant positive correlation between blood acetate concentrations and the rate of ethanol elimination in chronic alcoholics (Nuutinen, Alcohol, 1985; 2:623). Consequently, increased blood levels of acetate in the presence of ethanol indicate metabolic tolerance to alcohol and can be used as a laboratory marker of alcoholism and heavy drinking (Korri, AlcoholClinExpRes, 1985; 9:468).

Alterations in metabolism of ethanol, acetaldehyde, and acetate during chronic alcohol consumption

Chronic ethanol consumption results in an increased tolerance to alcohol. This is mainly due to adaptation of the central nervous system, but in addition alcoholics develop increased rates of ethanol elimination—'metabolic tolerance'. This is caused by adaptive changes in the alcohol dehydrogenase pathway and by increased activity of the MEOS pathway, with subsequent increases in blood acetaldehyde and acetate concentrations.

Changes in ethanol metabolism

In experimental animals and in humans chronic ingestion of ethanol has been reported to decrease ethanol elimination, to increase ethanol elimination, or to have no effect on it.[34] Results of studies on the effects of chronic ethanol on the activity of liver alcohol dehydrogenase are equally controversial.[34] It can be concluded that the net effect of chronic alcohol intake on both of these variables is the result of many metabolic events whose effects are modified by a variety of genetic and environmental factors.

Most studies show that chronic alcohol consumption enhances ethanol clearance, except in the presence of significant liver damage or severe food restriction. Indeed, both experimental ethanol administration in animals (Pikkarainen, AlcoholClinExpRes, 1980; 4: 40) and chronic alcohol abuse in humans (Kater, AmJClinNutr, 1969; 22:1608; Salaspuro, AnnClinRes, 1978; 10:294) increase the rates of ethanol metabolism. The biochemical background for this phenomenon is still the subject of debate and has variably been attributed to increased alcohol dehydrogenase activity (Hawkins, CanJPhysPharm, 1966; 44:241), to increased mitochondrial re-oxidation of NADH (Videla, BiochemJ, 1970; 118:275), to a hypermetabolic state in the liver (Israel, FedProc, 1975; 34:2052), to increased microsomal ethanol oxidation,[23] and to catalase (Handler, BiochemJ, 1987; 248:415).

As indicated earlier, increased alcohol dehydrogenase activity is not associated with enhanced ethanol elimination, since under normal conditions the rate-limiting step of the alcohol dehydrogenase pathway is the rate of NADH reoxidation. In keeping with this, several reports show that alcohol dehydrogenase activity does not increase and may even decrease after chronic ethanol ingestion, although the rate of ethanol elimination simultaneously increases (Dajani, JNutr, 1963; 80:196; Kalant, CanJPhysPharm, 1975; 53:416; Panes, AlcoholClinExpRes, 1992; 17:48).[34]

An ethanol-induced increase in the activity of Na^+, K^+-ATPase, followed by enhanced ATP consumption, decreased phosphorylation potential, increased oxygen consumption, and increased mitochondrial NADH reoxidation rate provide the biochemical basis for the 'hypermetabolic state' of the liver, which has been suggested as responsible for the adaptive increase in ethanol elimination (Bernstein, BiochemJ, 1973; 134:515; Israel, FedProc, 1975; 34:2052). This theory has been implicated in the treatment of alcoholic liver injury with propylthiouracil (Orrego, NEJM, 1987; 312:1921). However, ethanol-induced increase in ATPase activity associated with increased oxygen consumption has not been confirmed by other studies (Cederbaum, Alcoholism, 1977; 1:27; Gordon, BiochemPharm, 1977; 26:1229).

The accelerated removal of cytosolic free NADH during chronic ethanol consumption may result from either increased mitochondrial reoxidation of NADH or increased coupling between NADPH/NADP and NADH/NAD systems (Veech, BiochemJ, 1969; 115:609; Cronholm, EurJBioch, 1976; 70:83). Whatever the mechanism, the accelerated removal of cytosolic NADH leads to a shift in the rate-limiting step of the pathway from the rate of NADH reoxidation to the activity of hepatic alcohol dehydrogenase. In consequence, both cytoplasmic and mitochondrial redox changes are less marked in rats (Domschke, LifeSci, 1974; 15:1327) and in baboons fed alcohol chronically (Salaspuro, Hepatol, 1981; 1:3338).

The quantitative contribution of the MEOS pathway to the adaptive increase in ethanol elimination caused by chronic alcohol consumption is not fully established and remains controversial. Nevertheless cytochrome P4502E1 is induced two- to tenfold by chronic alcohol consumption, and this associates with an increase in various constituents of the smooth endoplasmic reticulum, such as phospholipids, cytochrome P450 reductase and cytochrome P450 (Ishii, BBActa, 1973; 291:411; Joly, BiochemPharm,1973; 22:1532) as discussed earlier.

The rate of ethanol elimination may also be influenced by the presence of alcohol-related liver injury. Cirrhotic patients with jaundice who have not taken alcohol for more than 4 weeks show decreased rates of ethanol elimination (Lieberman, Gastro, 1963; 44:261). On the other hand, ethanol elimination rates are elevated even in the presence of relatively severe liver damage, if the measurement is made in the first month of abstinence (Dakruz, ActaHepatoGastroenterol, 1975; 22:369; Ugarte, DigDisSci, 1977; 22:406). Animals with chronic non-alcohol-related liver disease show decreased rates of ethanol elimination and of alcohol dehydrogenase activity (Mikata, Gastro, 1963; 44:159). In patients with alcoholic liver injury the decreased blood ethanol clearance may reflect decreased liver alcohol dehydrogenase activity (Figueroa, Gastro, 1962; 43:10), but it may also be related to hepatic function, estimated either by the aminopyrine breath test or the indocyanine green clearance test (Panes, AlcoholClinExpRes, 1992; 17:48).

Changes in acetaldehyde metabolism

Chronic alcohol consumption produces three major alterations in the hepatic metabolism of ethanol and acetaldehyde, which result in increases of both blood and tissue acetaldehyde concentrations: (1) an increase in the rate of ethanol oxidation; (2) a reduction in the capacity of mitochondria to oxidize acetaldehyde, at least in rats; and (3) a decrease in the activity of hepatic aldehyde dehydrogenase.

Early in the 1970s elevated blood acetaldehyde concentrations were reported in alcoholics, but this was interpreted to reflect the acetaldehyde contained in the administered alcohol (Majchrowics, Science, 1970; 168:1100; Magrinat, Nature, 1973; 244:234). Subsequently, markedly elevated blood acetaldehyde levels following alcohol administration were demonstrated in chronic alcoholics as compared to controls (Korsten, NEJM, 1975; 292:386). However, at that time high blood acetaldehyde levels still represented by and large the artefactual acetaldehyde formation from ethanol contained by the blood samples. However, more recent studies with a better methodology have confirmed that blood acetaldehyde concentrations may slightly increase following chronic alcohol consumption both in baboons (Pikkarainen, BiochemPharm, 1981; 30:799) and in humans (Nuutinen, AlcoholClinExpRes; 1983:7:163; DiPadova, AlcoholClinExpRes, 1987; 11:559). In these reports blood acetaldehyde values in general have correlated positively with the rates of ethanol elimination (Nuutinen, AlcoholClinExpRes; 1983; 7:163; Panes, AlcoholClinExpRes, 1992; 17:48).

Chronic alcohol consumption also results in a significant reduction in the capacity of rat mitochondria to oxidize acetaldehyde

(Hasumura, Science, 1975; 189:727). This effect has been attributed, at least in part, to a reduction in the ability of mitochondria from ethanol-fed animals to reoxidize NADH.

The effects of chronic alcohol consumption on liver aldehyde dehydrogenase activity are controversial. In experimental animals decreases, no change, and even increases in activity have been reported (Koivula, BiochemPharm, 1975; 24:1937; Horton, BiochemJ, 1976; 156:177; Lebsack, BiochemPharm, 1981; 30:2273). These discrepancies can at least in part be attributed to the variety of acetaldehyde concentrations used to determine aldehyde dehydrogenase activity. Acetaldehyde concentrations of less than 1 mmol should be used to determine the activity of the low-K_M mitochondrial aldehyde dehydrogenase. As stated before, this enzyme plays a major role in the metabolism of acetaldehyde. It can be concluded that the decrease in acetaldehyde metabolism in ethanol-fed rats more likely reflects impaired mitochondrial oxidation of acetaldehyde than decreased aldehyde dehydrogenase activity. The situation may be different in other animals and in human alcoholics.

In baboons the plasma concentration of free acetaldehyde correlates positively with the production rate of acetaldehyde and negatively with liver mitochondrial aldehyde dehydrogenase activity (Pikkarainen, BiochemPharm, 1981; 30:799). It has been suggested that the cytosolic aldehyde dehydrogenase may play a more important role in acetaldehyde metabolism in humans. Studies using subcellular fractionation techniques suggested that there could be a selective reduction of cytosolic high-K_M aldehyde dehydrogenase in patients with alcoholic liver disease (Jenkins, Lancet, 1980, i:628; Jenkins, Lancet, 1984; i:1048). However, in another study both total and mitochondrial enzyme activities were found to be decreased in chronic alcoholic patients as compared to non-alcoholic controls (Nuutinen, AlcoholClinExpRes, 1983; 7:163). Not only was hepatic activity of the enzyme decreased but a significant negative correlation existed between peak blood acetaldehyde values and the activity of mitochondrial low-K_M aldehyde dehydrogenase. In human alcoholics acetaldehyde concentrations in hepatic venous blood may be up to 160 μM after a moderate, 0.8 g/kg body weight, dose of alcohol (Nuutinen, EurJClinInv, 1984; 14:306). If these values reflect liver acetaldehyde concentrations, this supports the dominant role of low-K_M mitochondrial aldehyde dehydrogenase in acetaldehyde metabolism in humans.

In chronic alcoholics peak blood acetaldehyde levels have been shown to be directly related to the rate of ethanol elimination (Panes, AlcoholClinExpRes, 1992; 17:48). Moreover, in alcoholic patients peak blood acetaldehyde concentrations increase as blood alcohol levels increase (Arthur, ClinSci, 1984; 67:381; Watanabe, AlcoholClinExpRes, 1985; 914). In non-alcoholic controls and in some alcoholics, blood acetaldehyde concentrations increase following intravenous fructose, which accelerates the rate of ethanol elimination (Nuutinen, AlcoholClinExpRes, 1983; 7:163). All these findings support the dominant role of the rate of ethanol oxidation in the regulation of blood acetaldehyde levels in humans.

Unusually high blood acetaldehyde levels have been found in severely intoxicated patients (Watanabe, AlcoholClinExpRes, 1985; 9:14). These exceptionally high values are most probably caused by the increased rate of ethanol elimination, especially at high blood ethanol concentrations and by a decrease in liver aldehyde dehydrogenase activity, associating sometimes with both the liver injury and chronic alcohol consumption (Matthewson, Gut, 1986; 27:756; Jenkins, Lancet, 1984, i:1048).

Pathogenesis of alcoholic liver injury

In the late 1940s the pathogenesis of alcoholic liver injury was associated almost exclusively with a secondary protein and choline deficiency (Best, BMJ, 1949: 2:1001). Since then, strong evidence has been reported for the relation between the pathogenesis of alcohol-related liver damage and the direct toxicity of ethanol, its metabolism and metabolites[1] (Ishak, AlcoholClinExpRes, 1991; 15:45; French, CritRevClinLabSci, 1992; 29:83; Day, BBActa, 1994; 1215:33; Lindros, JHepatol, 1995; 23(Suppl.1):7; Rosser, Gastro, 1995; 108:252). The spectrum of alcoholic liver disease ranges from mild hepatomegaly or fatty liver to alcoholic hepatitis, fibrosis, and cirrhosis. The pathogenesis of each of these entities may involve several mechanisms.

Animal models of alcohol-related organ damage

A lot of evidence supporting the direct hepatotoxicity of ethanol has been obtained from experiments using animal models of alcohol-induced organ damage. One of the major advances has been the introduction of a technique of feeding ethanol to rats as a part of nutritionally adequate totally liquid diet (Lieber, AlcoholClinExpRes, 1986; 10:550). However, even with the 'liquid diet model' the rat will not consume more than 36 per cent of total calories as ethanol. Consequently more advanced liver lesions than fatty liver cannot be produced in rats. In some other studies the liver lesions produced by the 'Lieber–DeCarli diet' have been related to associated nutritional imbalances rather than to the direct toxicity of ethanol (Derr, MedHypothes, 1988; 27:277; Shoemaker, DrugAlcDep, 1988; 22:49).

Severe and progressive steatosis with focal necrosis and fibrosis has been produced in rats by continuous intragastric infusion of ethanol and a nutritionally defined low-fat liquid diet (Tsukamoto, Hepatol, 1985; 5:224; Tsukamoto, Hepatol, 1986; 6:814). In this animal model the severity of alcohol-induced liver injury appeared to be related to high blood alcohol levels. Furthermore in this animal model, the development of alcoholic liver injury could be potentiated by feeding to the rats a diet with high corn oil content, which is rich in polyunsaturated linoleic acid (Nanji, AlcoholClinExpRes, 1989; 13:15). On the other hand, beef fat with high content of saturated fats appeared to be protective. This finding is in line with some epidemiological observations indicating that saturated fats and cholesterol may protect against cirrhosis while polyunsaturated fats may promote it (Nanji, AlcoholClinExpRes, 1986; 10:271).

Feeding an ethanol-containing liquid diet together with a small dose of 4-methylpyrazole (an alcohol dehydrogenase inhibitor) to rats potentiates alcoholic liver injury in this animal model (Lindros, Liver, 1983; 3:79). By following blood alcohol levels, this effect could be related to uninterrupted, prolonged oxidation of ethanol. Feeding alcohol to rats subjected to jejunoileal bypass leads to marked liver injury which mimics that of alcohol-induced liver disease in man, but without zonal distribution (Bode, JHepatol, 1987; 5:75). More advanced liver lesions have been produced in minipigs which will consume voluntarily up to 40 per cent of calories as ethanol (Halsted, Hepatol, 1993; 18:954; Villanueva, Hepatol, 1994; 19:1229).

More advanced alcoholic liver disease has been produced in baboons by applying a 'liquid-diet' feeding technique (Lieber, JMedPrimatol, 1974; 3:153). The alcohol intake of these animals can be increased to 50 per cent of total calories; they are phylogenetically close to man and furthermore their life span is long enough for cirrhosis to develop. In this animal model, the biochemical and morphological alterations in the liver (even liver cirrhosis) are comparable to those seen in humans despite the fact that a complete histological spectrum of alcoholic hepatitis as seen in man has not been produced in baboons (Popper, AmJPathol, 1980; 98:695). However, some other groups have not been able to produce significant hepatic fibrosis or cirrhosis in baboons given large amounts of ethanol and an adequate diet for up to 5 years (Ainley, JHepatol, 1988; 7:85; Porto, VirchArchA, 1989; 414:299).

Hepatotoxic factors associated with ethanol and its oxidation

Toxicity of ethanol

Ethanol, like other general anaesthetics, causes physical changes in all biological membranes, including hepatic mitochondrial and endoplasmic reticulum membranes.[35-37] Ethanol directly 'fluid-izises' membrane lipid bilayers, and it has been proposed that during chronic alcohol consumption cell surface membranes may resist this effect of ethanol (i.e. 'adapt') by changing their membrane lipid composition. Chronic ethanol feeding has been shown to increase the fluidity of liver plasma membranes in rats (Yamada, Gastro, 1985; 88:1799), mice (Zysset, Hepatol, 1985; 5:531), and in cell cultures (Polokoff, Biochem, 1985; 24:3114).

With respect to the changes in membrane lipid composition, the results, obtained mainly in experimental animals, are controversial. Some have found an increase in membrane unesterified cholesterol (Mendenhall, BBActa, 1969; 189:501) and some an increase in membrane phospholipid content (Mendenhall, BBActa, 1969; 189: 501; French, QJStudAlc, 1970; 31:801), while others have reported no changes in these lipids in total liver (Takeuchi, Lipids, 1974; 9: 353), in hepatic microsomes, or in mitochondria (Wing, BiochemPharm, 1983; 31:3431). The cholesterol–phospholipid ratio has been reported to be unaltered in liver plasma membrane fractions of mice exposed to chronic ethanol (Wing, BiochemPharm, 1983; 31:3431). On the other hand, chronic alcohol results in an increase in cholesterol ester content of liver plasma membrane fractions (Kim, Hepatol, 1988; 4:735). An increased cholesterol ester content of liver plasma membrane fractions has been proposed to mediate changes in membrane fluidity.

In addition to the alterations of lipid composition in liver plasma membrane, changes in the enzyme activities of liver membranes have also been reported. These include a decrease in cytochrome *a* and *b*, succinic dehydrogenase, and cytochrome oxidase, as well as in the total respiratory capacity of the mitochondria.[36] The changes in enzyme activities may be due to the effects of both acute and chronic ethanol on either the synthesis of membrane proteins or on the transport of amino acids, or both.[36] Furthermore, chronic alcohol consumption potentiates the release of alkaline

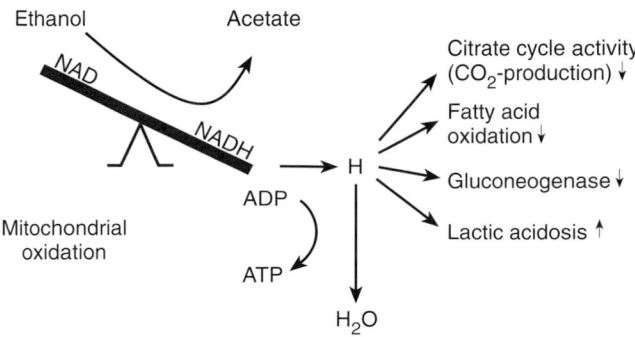

Fig. 8. The metabolic effects of the ethanol-induced increase in hepatic NADH/NAD ratio.

phosphatase from liver plasma membranes (Yamada, Gastro, 1985; 88:1799) and produces changes in the oligosaccharide chains of plasma membrane glycoproteins (Metcalf, PSEBM, 1987; 185:1).

Ethanol-induced shift in the redox state of the liver

The ethanol-induced increase in the NADH/NAD ratio is a sign of a major change in hepatic metabolism during ethanol oxidation. Many of the acute secondary changes in the intermediary metabolism of the liver can be explained by the action of ethanol on the hepatic redox state (Fig. 8). These include the inhibition of the tricarboxylic acid cycle and gluconeogenesis. The redox-related inhibition of fatty acid oxidation and the enhancement of triglyceride synthesis are the main pathogenetic mechanisms in the development of alcoholic fatty liver.

Pathogenesis of alcoholic fatty liver

Role of adipose tissue and dietary fat

An acute large dose of alcohol mobilizes fat from the adipose tissue to the liver (Brodie, AmJClinNutr, 1961; 9:432). This is mediated by chatecholamines and is associated with increased serum free fatty acids (Mallov, JStudAlc, 1961; 22:250). This mechanism plays a minor role in the development of fatty liver caused by chronic alcohol consumption.[38] Administration of ethanol together with a high fat diet, potentiates alcoholic fatty liver (Lieber, AmJClinNutr, 1970; 23:474). In this situation fatty acids accumulating in the liver resemble those of the diet (Lieber, JCI, 1966; 45:51; Mendenhall, JLipRes, 1972; 13:177). However, the decrease in fatty acid oxidation is the main cause of the deposition of dietary fat in the liver during chronic alcohol feeding to experimental animals (Lieber, JCI, 1966; 45:51).

Hepatic synthesis of lipids

Chronic alcohol does not stimulate the synthesis of fatty acids (Savolainen, BiochemJ, 1977; 164:169), but it may enhance the formation of glycerolipids (Mendenhall, BBActa, 1969; 187:501) as a consequence of the ethanol-induced increase in NADH/NAD ratio which favours the synthesis of sn-glycerol-3-phosphate (Nikkilä; PSEBM, 1963; 113:814). However, a decrease in hepatic triacylglycerol-synthesizing capacity occurs during the progression of alcoholic liver injury (Savolainen, JLipRes, 1984; 25:813). Alcohol has no effect on hepatic cholesterol and bile acid synthesis *in vivo* (Lakshman, Lipids, 1978; 13:134). The activity of phosphatidate

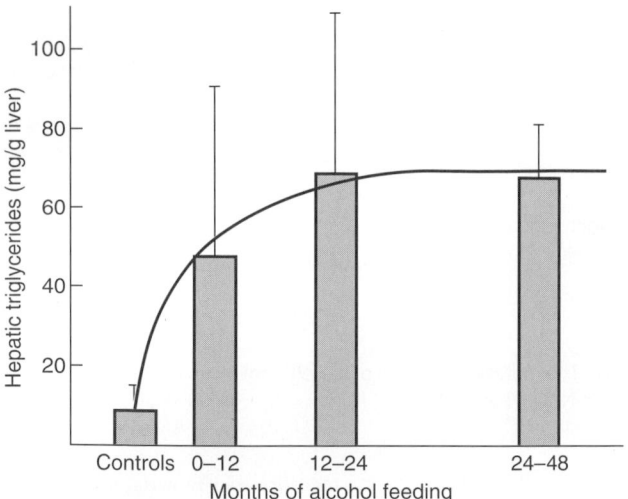

Fig. 9. Attenuation of hepatic triglyceride accumulation following chronic alcohol consumption in baboons (Salaspuro, Hepatol, 1981; 1: 3338).

phosphohydrolase, which catalyses the rate-limiting step in the synthesis of triglycerides, has recently been reported to be higher in alcoholics with severe degrees of fatty liver as compared with those with lesser degrees of fatty degeneration (Day, Hepatol, 1993; 18:823).

Oxidation of fatty acids

The inhibition of fatty acid oxidation has been demonstrated both *in vitro* and *in vivo* (Lieber, JCI, 1967; 46:1451; Blomstrand, LifeSci, 1973; 13:1131; Ontko, JLipRes, 1973; 14:78). As stated above, this is caused by the excessive generation of NADH, which suppresses the function of the citric acid cycle and β-oxidation of fatty acids (Lieber, JCI, 1967; 46:1451; Williamson, JBC, 1969; 244:5044). However, during chronic alcohol consumption, the ethanol-induced shift in the redox state of the liver is attenuated (Salaspuro, Hepatol, 1981; 1:3338) and this is also associated with the reduction of the accumulation of hepatic triglycerides (Fig. 9). This 'adaptation' during chronic alcohol consumption may explain why only a few alcoholics or heavy drinkers develop a more severe fatty liver despite continuous abuse of alcohol.

In addition to the above, alcohol has varying effects on the biliary excretion of cholesterol and bile acids. Furthermore, alcohol may interfere with the secretion of plasma lipoproteins. These factors, however, play an insignificant role in the pathogenesis of alcoholic fatty liver.[38] Alcoholic hyperlipaemia has been reviewed extensively elsewhere.[38]

Toxicity of acetaldehyde

Acetaldehyde is both pharmacologically and chemically a very potent and reactive compound, which can be a major initiating factor in the pathogenesis of alcoholic liver damage[1,39,40] (Sorrell, AlcoholClinExpRes, 1985; 9:306; Jennett, ProgLivDis, 1990; 9:325; Worrall, DigDis, 1993; 11:265). The toxicity of acetaldehyde has been related to several important metabolic and cellular factors.

Covalent binding of acetaldehyde—acetaldehyde adducts

In vitro, acetaldehyde has been shown to form adducts with phospholipids (Kenney, Alcohol, 1982; 6:412). However, most probable target macromolecules are proteins, for instance erythrocyte membrane proteins (Gaines, FEBSLett, 1977; 74:115), haemoglobin (Stevens, JCI, 1981; 67:361), plasma proteins (Lumeng, FedProc, 1982; 41:765), hepatic microsomal proteins (Nomura, BBRes-Comm, 1981; 100:131), other hepatic proteins (Medina, JLab-ClinMed, 1985; 105:5), and liver tubulin (Jennett, Hepatol, 1989; 1:57). Evidence for the formation of acetaldehyde adducts with liver proteins has also been presented *in vivo* (Barry, Gut, 1985; 26:1065; Lin, JCI, 1988; 81:615). The target molecule for acetaldehyde binding can, for instance, be the microsomal ethanol-inducible CYP2E1 (Behrens, BBResComm, 1988; 154:584) or liver collagen (Svegliati-Baroni, Hepatol, 1994; 20:111). Acetaldehyde-modified proteins can be detected in several subcellular compartments of the hepatocytes with a mean half-life of 2.3 weeks after cessation of alcohol feeding (Lin, AlcoholClinExpRes, 1992; 16:1125; Nicholls, AlcAlc, 1994; 29:149). During chronic alcohol feeding to rats protein–acetaldehyde adducts appear after 2 weeks in the perivenous zone of the hepatic acinus (Lin, Hepatol, 1993; 18:864). Later, the distribution pattern is more diffuse, but still predominant in the perivenous zone (Lin, Hepatol, 1993; 18:864). Protein–acetaldehyde adducts are detected in liver biopsy specimens of 85 per cent of patients with alcoholic and in 65 per cent of patients with non-alcoholic liver diseases (Holstege, Hepatol, 1994; 19:367). The presence of extracellular acetaldehyde adducts appeared to be correlated with the progression of liver fibrosis (Holstege, Hepatol, 1994; 19:367).

The formation of protein–acetaldehyde adducts may occur through at least three mechanisms.[40] A Schiff's base can be formed between the electrophilic carbonyl carbon of acetaldehyde and nucleophilic sites on proteins, such as the free epsilon amino group of lysine residues:

$$\text{Schiff's base: } R–NH_2 \rightarrow R–N=CHCH3$$

$$R = \text{protein}$$

$$NH_2 = \text{reactive group}$$

Schiff's base is an unstable adduct which can be stabilized by reducing agents, or even without them, to a mono- or diethylated derivative (Lin, AlcoholClinExpRes, 1995; 19:314). An alternative possibility is the formation of a cyclic imidazolidinone at the N-terminal ends of proteins or the reaction of acetaldehyde with cysteine, yielding 2-methyl-l-thiazolidine-4-carboxylic acid.[40]

The biochemical background of the possible hepatotoxicity associated with the covalent binding of acetaldehyde with tissue proteins is not yet understood. Acetaldehyde–protein adducts could:

(1) inhibit hepatic protein secretion during both acute and chronic ethanol administration (Valentine, Hepatol, 1987; 7:490);

(2) displace pyridoxal phosphate from its binding sites on proteins (Lumeng, JCI, 1978; 62:286);

(3) impair biological functions of proteins (Mauch, Hepatol, 1986; 6:263); or

(4) combine with tissue macromolecules and thereby trigger immune reactions.

Antibodies against acetaldehyde adducts

It has been shown that mice immunized by acetaldehyde adducts produce specific antibodies against binding epitopes (Israel, PNAS, 1986; 83:7293). A humoral immune response to acetaldehyde adducts is also produced in acute alcoholic liver disease (Hoerner, Hepatol, 1988; 3:569), in alcoholics without liver injury, and even in patients with non-alcoholic liver diseases (Niemelä, Hepatol, 1987; 7:1210). Serum phospholipid antibodies have been shown to reflect disease progression and correlate with disease severity (Chedid, Hepatol, 1994; 20:1465). Similar immune responses may contribute to the aggravation or perpetuation of alcoholic liver injury (Niemelä, ScaJLabClinMed, 1993; 53(Suppl.213):45).

Acetaldehyde and lipid peroxidation

As discussed later in this chapter, an enhanced lipid peroxidation caused by free radicals is one of the possible mechanisms of alcoholic liver injury. Under certain *in vitro* conditions the metabolism of acetaldehyde may mediate hepatic lipid peroxidation (Shaw, BBResComm, 1987; 143:984) by producing free radicals. In addition to mitochondrial aldehyde dehydrogenase, acetaldehyde may be oxidized to acetate via xanthine oxidase (Lewis, Lancet, 1982; ii: 188). In this reaction oxygen may be metabolized to superoxide, which is a well-known lipid peroxidative agent.

Normally, free radicals are inactivated by glutathione. However, acetaldehyde may bind with glutathione or with cysteine, which is needed in the synthesis of glutathione. This might contribute to a depression of liver glutathione with a secondary increase in lipid peroxidation (Vina, BiochemJ, 1980; 188:549; Shaw, JLabClinMed, 1981; 98:417).

Malondialdehyde is a product of lipid peroxidation which also can initiate the formation of protein–aldehyde adducts. These adducts have been demonstrated both in experimental alcoholic liver injury and in human alcoholics (Niemelä, LabInvest, 1994;70: 537). They are seen predominantly in the perivenous region and they coincide with signs of more advanced liver injury (steatonecrosis, focal inflammation, and elevated serum transaminases) (Niemelä, Hepatol, 1995; 22:1208).

Other mechanisms

In addition to above mentioned pathogenetic mechanisms, acetaldehyde has been related to the impairment of microtubular protein export, to the activation of lipocyte collagen production, and to the enhanced release of cytokines. Furthermore, there is recent evidence that acetaldehyde of extrahepatic origin (i.e. that absorbed from the gastrointestinal tract to the portal blood) may also be hepatotoxic (Matysiak-Budnik, JPath, 1996; 178:469). These aspects will be discussed below.

Hepatotoxicity associated with MEOS

Theoretically, MEOS may cause enhanced hepatotoxicity by several means.[1,24,25] MEOS contributes to the production of the potentially hepatotoxic agent, acetaldehyde. MEOS may enhance oxygen consumption, which, at least in part, may potentiate hypoxia.

Both of these factors may be more crucial in the centrilobular (perivenous) areas of the hepatic acinus, since microsomal cytochrome P450, including P4502E1, is predominantly localized in the perivenous region of the liver, both in rat and man (Väänänen, JHepatol, 1986; 2:175; Ingelman-Sundberg, BBResComm, 1988; 157:55; Tsutsumi, Hepatol, 1989; 10:437).

Other hepatotoxic agents may be metabolized into toxic intermediates by CYP2E1,[41] which itself may be induced by chronic alcohol consumption.[41] Classical examples are carbon tetrachloride (Hasumura, Gastro, 1974; 66:415) and acetaminophen (Teschke, BBResComm, 1979; 91:368). In accordance with this hypothesis, a history of ethanol consumption in humans has been shown to increase the hepatotoxicity of acetaminophen (Seef, AnnIntMed, 1986; 106:399). Included in the list are bromobenzene, isoniazide, phenylbutazone, enflurane, halothane, and nitrosamine.[41]

Both in experimental animals and in man chronic alcohol consumption has been shown to be associated with depressed hepatic vitamin A and carotenoid levels (Sato, Jnutr, 1981; 111:2015; Leo, NEJM, 1982; 37:597; Leo, Hepatol, 1993; 17:977). This is caused by microsomal degradation of the vitamin via a pathway that is inducible by ethanol and which may degrade an amount of retinol comparable to the daily intake (Leo, JBC, 1985; 260:5228). In this pathway both retinoic acid and retinol may serve as substrates, and it is mediated by NAD^+-dependent microsomal retinol dehydrogenase (Leo, ArchBiochemBiophys, 1984; 234:305; Leo, ArchBiochemBiophys, 1987; 259:241). Decreased hepatic vitamin A levels may lead to some functional and structural abnormalities in the liver (Leo, Gastro, 1983; 84:562; Ray, Hepatol, 1988; 8:1019). However, the possible therapeutic use of vitamin A in alcohol-related liver disease is complicated by its own potential hepatotoxicity (Leo, Gastro, 1982; 82:194; Leo, Hepatol, 1983; 2:1; Kim, Hepatol, 1988; 4:735).

Free radicals and lipid peroxidation

An enhanced lipid peroxidation as a mechanism of alcoholic liver injury was proposed in 1966 by Kalish and Di Luzio (Science, 1966; 152:1390). Since then several studies have been published on this topic and have been reviewed recently (Comporti, LabInvest, 1985; 53:599; Arthur, JHepatol, 1988; 6:125; Nordman, AlcAlc, 1994; 29: 513). Free radicals (superoxide and hydroxyl radicals) can damage a wide range of cellular components via lipid peroxidation, including proteins, nucleic acids, free amino acids, and lipoproteins. A great deal of evidence associates ethanol with lipid peroxidation, although the reliability of the currently available thiobutyric acid assay methods as an indicator of lipid peroxidation has been questioned (Dianzani, AlcAlc, 1985; 20:161).

The microsomal ethanol oxidizing system appears to produce active hydroxyl radicals (Cederbaum, AnnNYAcadSci, 1987; 492: 35). CYP2E1 has been shown to be able to produce superoxide anion, hydrogen peroxide, and ethanol-derived hydroxyethyl free radicals (Ekström, BiochemPharm, 1989; 38:1313; Albano, BiochemPharm, 1991; 41:1895). Reactive oxygen intermediates are also produced when acetaldehyde is oxidized to acetate via xanthine oxidase, as discussed above (Kato, Gastro,1990; 98:203). Other sources of free radical generation include NADH oxidation by aldehyde oxidase during ethanol oxidation (Mira, ArchBiochemBiophys, 1995, 318:53) and hepatic neutrophils (Williams,

Gut, 1987; 28:358). Free radicals are scavenged by superoxide dismutase and glutathione peroxidase. In rats, chronic ethanol feeding increases glutathione turnover (Morton, BiochPharm, 1985; 34:1559) and the cellular requirements for glutathione (Pierson, BiochPharm, 1986; 35:1533). Furthermore, there is an increased loss of glutathione from cells (Callans, Hepatol, 1987; 7:496), especially from mitochondria (Fernandez-Checa, JCI, 1987; 80:57). Mitochondrial glutathione originates from the cytosol by a transport system which translocates glutathione into the matrix.[42] This transport system is impaired in chronic ethanol-fed rats.[42]

In naïve rats large amounts of ethanol (5–6 g/kg) are required to produce lipid peroxidation (DiLuzio, FedProc, 1967; 26:1436; MacDonald, FEBSLett, 1974; 35:227; Teare, Gut, 1994; 35:1644), whereas a smaller dose has no effect (Shaw, JLabClinMed, 1981; 98:417; Hashimoto, ExpMolPath, 1968; 8:225). However, after chronic alcohol consumption even smaller doses of ethanol administered acutely produce lipid peroxidation, which can be partly prevented by the glutathione precursor, methionine (Shaw, JLabClinMed, 1981; 98:417). Free-radical adducts have also been demonstrated recently in the bile of rats treated chronically with intragastric alcohol (Knecht, MolPharm, 1995; 47:1028). In experimental animals, lipid peroxidation may be stimulated by iron mobilization and microsomal induction (Shaw, Alcohol, 1988; 5:135). In addition, iron appears to enhance the hepatotoxicity of ethanol in several animal models (Stal, JHepatol, 1993; 17:108; Mackinnon, Hepatol, 1995; 21:1083; Tsukamoto, JCI, 1995; 96:620).

In chronic alcoholics there is an increase both in serum and liver lipoperoxide levels (Suematsu, AlcoholClinExpRes, 1981; 5:427; Clot, Gut, 1994; 35:1637). The content of hepatic reduced glutathione is decreased, especially in patients with histological liver necrosis (Videla, ClinSci, 1984; 66:283). As an integral part of the enzyme glutathione peroxidase, selenium has a central role in the protection against the tissue damage caused by lipid peroxides. In this respect the decrease not only in blood but also in liver selenium in patients with alcoholic liver injury may also play a significant role (Välimäki, CCActa, 1987; 166:171).

Selective perivenular hepatotoxicity of ethanol

Alcoholic liver injury starts and predominates in the perivenular (also called centrilobular) region—zone 3 of the hepatic acinus, which is exposed to lowest oxygen tension. The enhanced injurious effect of ethanol at this site has been postulated to be due to hypoxia, resulting from ethanol-induced stimulation of hepatic oxygen consumption (Israel, FedProc, 1975; 34:2052). Furthermore, the livers of ethanol-fed rats have been shown to be especially vulnerable to transient hypoxia (Miyamato, Hepatol, 1988; 8:53). The low oxygen tensions existing in perivenular zones may exaggerate the ethanol-induced redox shift in this area, a change which may contribute to the exacerbation of the damage in the perivenular area of the hepatic lobule (Jauhonen, AlcoholClinExpRes, 1982; 6:350).

Results regarding the zonal distribution of the enzymes involved in the metabolism of ethanol are controversial (Bühler, AmJPathol, 1982; 108:89; Väänänen, Hepatol, 1984; 4:862; Yamauchi, Hepatol, 1988; 8:243). However, hepatocytes in zone 3 both in rat and humans contain more smooth endoplasmic reticulum and cytochrome P450 than hepatocytes of other zones, suggesting that zone 3 is the region

of maximal drug and alcohol metabolism (Väänänen, JHepatol, 1986; 2:174; Ingelman-Sundberg, BBResComm, 1988; 157:55; Tsutsumi, Hepatol, 1889; 10:437). The role of the uneven zonal distribution of the multiple microsomal functions in the pathogenesis of alcohol-related perivenular hepatotoxicity remains to be established.

Hepatocyte swelling

The enlargement of the liver is one of the earliest manifestations of hepatic damage produced by alcohol. This is caused by the accumulation of fat and protein in the liver (Baraona, Science, 1975; 190:794). The increase in hepatic protein is associated with intrahepatocytic water retention (Baraona, JCI, 1977; 60:546), which results in ballooning of the hepatocytes. In both experimental animals and humans, excessive alcohol consumption decreases liver microtubules (Matsuda, LabInvest, 1979; 41:455; Matsuda, AlcoholClinExpRes, 1985; 9:366). This leads to the accumulation of exportable proteins secondary to the impairment of microtubular polymerization (Baraona, Gastro, 1980; 79,104; Baraona, ResCommChemPathPharm, 1984; 44:265). In rats, chronic administration of ethanol decreases the rate of protein degradation (Donohue, AlcoholClinExpRes, 1989; 13:49). In addition, chronic ethanol also inhibits the secretion of hepatic glycoproteins (Sorrell, Gastro, 1983; 84:546). Some of these metabolic alterations may be due to an ethanol-induced impairment of Golgi apparatus (Guasch, AlcoholClinExpRes, 1992; 16:942).

The ethanol-induced ballooning of the hepatocytes has been related to the pathogenesis of precirrhotic portal hypertension in rats, in humans, and in alcohol-fed baboons (Orrego, Gastro, 1981; 80:546; Miyakawa, Gastro, 1985; 88:143). In accordance with this there is a dramatic reduction in the sinusoidal area in alcoholic liver damage, which is not seen in non-alcoholic liver diseases (Vindins, Hepatol, 1985; 5:408).

Alcohol and fibrogenesis

Alcohol-induced necrosis and inflammation may trigger the scarring and the development of cirrhosis. In addition, ethanol itself, its metabolism, and/or metabolites may have significant effects on collagen metabolism and fibrogenesis. This might explain why alcoholic hepatitis is not always a necessary intermediate step in the development of cirrhosis (Popper, AmJPathol, 1980; 98:695; Nakano, Gastro, 1982, 83:777; Takada, AmJGastr, 1982; 77:660). The pathophysiology of collagen metabolism in the liver and fibrogenesis has been reviewed in detail recently (Gressner, Zgastr, 1992; 30:5; McClain, SemLivDis, 1993; 13:170; Flier, NEJM, 1993; 328:1828).

The induction and proliferation of various perisinusoidal cells has been documented in alcoholic liver injury. Ito cells (perisinusoidal lipocytes, fat-storing cells) are activated to myofibroblast-like cells (hepatic mesenchymal cells or perisinusoidal stellate cells). The number of Ito cells increases and they are activated in sinusoids and scars in rats fed alcohol chronically (French, AmJPathol, 1988; 132:73). They have been suggested to produce increased amounts of type 3 collagen (Kent, PNAS, 1976; 73:3719). Ito cells contain alcohol dehydrogenase and can therefore oxidize both ethanol and retinol (Yamuchi, Gastro, 1988; 94:163).

Both perisinusoidal and perivenular cells show a morphological transition between Ito cells and myofibroblasts (Okanoue, ArchPathLabMed, 1983; 107:456). Myofibroblasts were first demonstrated in cirrhotic human livers (Bhathal, Pathology, 1972; 4:139). Later, they were isolated from baboon liver biopsies and shown to produce collagen types 1, 3, and 4 and laminin (Savolainen, Gastro, 1984; 87:777). Myofibroblasts are actively contractile cells and may contribute to scar contraction and portal hypertension in liver cirrhosis (Rudolph, Gastro, 1979; 76:704). They are predominantly present around the terminal venules and they increase in number before the development of perivenular and pericellular fibrosis (Nakano, AmJPathol, 1982; 106:145). Myofibroblast processes extend into the Disse space, although the most common cell there is the Ito cell. A proportion of Ito cells are replaced by transitional cells after chronic alcohol consumption both in baboons (Mak, Gastro, 1984; 87:188) and in man (Mak, Hepatol, 1988; 8:1027). In early alcoholic liver injury lipocytes are activated and this correlates with the degree of collagen formation in the Disse space (Horn, JHepatol, 1986; 3:333). Fibronectin formation is also activated and may form a skeleton for the new collagen formation (Junge, Gastro, 1988; 94:797).

The basic mechanisms by which chronic alcohol consumption stimulates the mesenchymal cells to produce collagen and induces their proliferation are still largely unresolved. Possible candidates are mononuclear inflammation (Nakano, Gastro, 1982; 83:777), acetaldehyde and hyperlacticacidaemia (Savolainen, Gastro, 1984; 87:777; Casini, Hepatol, 1991; 13:758; Casini, BBResComm, 1994; 199:1019), and transforming growth factor-β1 (Casini, Gastro, 1993; 105:245). Ethanol feeding has been shown to stimulate hepatic collagen synthesis in rats (Kato, ResCommChemPathPharm, 1985; 47:163). However, ethanol, acetaldehyde, and lactate do not stimulate the proteoglycan synthesis and proliferation of cultured rat liver fat-storing cells in vitro (Gressner, Gastro, 1988; 94:797).

A high fat diet has been demonstrated to sensitize hepatic lipocytes to the stimulatory effects of Kupffer cell-derived factors and thereby to enhance alcohol-induced fibrogenesis (Matsuoka, Hepatol, 1990; 11:173; Matsuoka, Hepatol, 1990; 11:599). Particularly, dietary linoleic acid has been shown to be important for the development of experimentally induced alcoholic liver injury (Nanji, LifeSci, 1989; 44:223; Takahashi, AlcoholClinExpRes, 1991; 15:1060).

Interestingly, polyunsaturated lecithin has been shown to prevent acetaldehyde-mediated hepatic collagen accumulation by stimulating collagenase activity in cultured lipocytes (Li, Hepatol, 1992; 15:373). Furthermore in long-term trials, phosphatidylcholine appeared to protect against fibrosis and cirrhosis in the baboon model of alcoholic liver injury (Lieber, Hepatol, 1990; 12:1390; Lieber, Gastro, 1994; 106:152), and also non-alcoholic hepatic fibrosis (Ma, JHepatol, 1996; 24:604).

Whatever the basic mechanism, the increased collagenization of the Disse space, associated with the reduction of fenestrations between sinusoids and the Disse space (Mak, Hepatol, 1984; 4:386; Horn, Hepatol, 1987; 7:77), may isolate the hepatocyte from its blood supply. Furthermore, these changes increase the resistance of blood flow, thereby contributing to the increased portal pressure (Miyakawa, Gastro, 1985; 88:143), often already seen in the early stage of liver injury.

Perivenular fibrosis is considered as a predictor of the progression of fibrogenesis both in baboons (VanWaes, Gastro, 1977; 73:646) and in patients who continue to drink (Nakano, Gastro, 1982; 83:777). Some authors suggested that pericellular (Disse's space) fibrosis might be more predictive for the development of cirrhosis (Nasrallah, ArchPathLabMed, 1980; 104:84). Later, both perisinusoidal and pericellular accumulation of fibronectin in the perivenous area were reported to have a definite predictive value for the development of alcoholic cirrhosis (Junge, BMJ, 1988; 296:1629). In addition to perivenular fibrosis, the presence of alcoholic hepatitis and the degree of steatosis also correlate with the later development of cirrhosis (Sörensen, Lancet, 1984; ii:241).

Role of endotoxins, Kupffer cells, and cytokines
Endotoxins

It is well known that antibiotics may protect against liver injury induced by carbon tetrachloride (Leach, ExpBiolMed, 1941; 48:361; Wilson, FedProc, 1950; 9:349) or choline deficiency (Gyorgy, AnnNYAcadSci, 1954; 57:925). However, the mechanisms of endotoxin interaction with other factors in the pathogenesis of liver injury have been, by and large, speculative.[43,44] On the other hand, plasma endotoxin concentrations have been reported to be elevated, especially in patients with alcoholic liver injury (Prytz, ScaJGastr, 1976; 11:857; Fukui, JHepatol, 1991; 12:162). This associates with high titres of antibodies to enterobacterial common antigen in patients with alcoholic cirrhosis, further supporting the role of endotoxins in the pathophysiology of alcoholic cirrhosis (Turunen, Gut, 1981; 22:949).

The pathogenesis of endotoxaemia induced by alcohol and/or liver injury is unknown.[45,46] One possibility is that chronic alcoholism increases the intestinal permeability of the gut (Bjarnason, Lancet, 1984; i:179). To that effect, one toxic candidate could be the elevated intracolonic acetaldehyde level.[16] Alternatively, heavy drinking may also alter the composition of the intestinal or faecal flora (Bode, Hepatogast, 1984; 31:30).

In rats on an alcohol diet, intravenous administration of small doses of endotoxin has been shown to produce hepatic necrosis (Bhagwandeen, JPath, 1987; 151:47). Furthermore, an acute dose of alcohol (Shibyama, ExpMolPath, 1991; 55:196) as well as its chronic administration (Arai, Hepatol, 1989; 9:846) may potentiate the hepatotoxicity of endotoxin. In experimental alcoholic liver injury plasma endotoxin levels have been shown to correlate with the severity of the liver injury (Nanji, AmJPathol, 1993; 142:367), and it was suggested that endotoxins may modulate the production of eicosanoids that contribute to the pathogenesis of alcoholic liver injury.

Most recently, antibiotics have been shown to prevent liver injury in rats following long-term exposure to ethanol (Adachi, Gastro, 1995; 108:218). This effect was related to the inhibition of endotoxin-induced activation of Kupffer cells (Adachi, Hepatol, 1994; 20:453). Supporting the endotoxin theory, feeding lactobacillus to experimental animals has been shown to reduce endotoxaemia and the severity of alcohol-induced experimental liver injury (Nanji, PSEBM, 1994; 205:243). This effect was related to an endotoxin-binding microcin provided by Lactobacillus spp. (Nanji, PSEBM, 1994; 205:243).[46]

Kupffer cells, cytokines, and endothelins

Alcoholic liver injury, especially alcoholic hepatitis, associates with increased production of cytokines.[44] This has been related to the activation of Kupffer cells by gut-derived endotoxin.[44] Kupffer cells respond by synthesizing and releasing cytokines such as tumour necrosis factor-α, interleukin-1 (**IL-1**), interleukin-6 (IL-6), and transforming growth factor-β1. Furthermore, this is associated with induced formation of platelet activating factor and reactive oxygen species. Tumour necrosis factor-α and IL-1 induce hepatocytes to secrete IL-8, which is chemotactic for neutrophils in the liver. Accordingly, serum interleukin-1 activity and tumour necrosis factor are increased in alcoholic hepatitis, which may contribute to some clinical manifestations of the disease, such as fever, anorexia, neutrophilia, and muscle catabolism (McClain, LifeSci, 1986; 39: 1479; McClain, Hepatol, 1989; 9:349). Plasma tumour necrosis factor is particularly elevated in severe cases of alcoholic hepatitis (Bird, AnnIntMed, 1990; 112:917). Highly elevated plasma interleukin-6 and -8 levels are also found in patients with alcoholic hepatitis (Devière; ClinExpImmun, 1988; 72:377; Sheron, ClinExpImmun, 1991; 84:449; Hill, Hepatol, 1993; 18:576; Huang, JHepatol, 1996; 24:337). The role of Kupffer cells in the initiation of alcoholic liver injury is further supported by the finding of reduced damage in alcohol-fed animals receiving gadolinium chloride, which inactivates Kupffer cells (Adachi, Hepatol, 1994; 20: 453).

Endothelins (**ET-1**, ET-2, and ET-3) are cytokines containing 21 amino acids. Ethanol (50–100 mmol) stimulates cultured endothelial cells to release ET-1 and ET-2 (Tsuji, AlcoholClinExpRes, 1992; 16:347). Endothelins are potent vasoconstrictors, and may therefore induce hepatic vasoconstriction and hypoxia, thereby contributing to the elevation of portal pressure (Hijioaka, BiochemPharm, 1991; 41:1551; Oshita, Hepatol, 1992; 16:1007; Oshita, JCI, 1993; 91: 1337).

All the above-mentioned factors may directly or indirectly potentiate inflammation, hepatitis, fibrosis, vasoconstriction/portal hypertension, and hypoxia associated with the progression of alcoholic liver injury.[44]

Role of immune mechanisms

It is now generally accepted that immunological reactions may contribute to the alcoholic liver disease, but the exact mechanisms are still unclear.[47]

Hypergammaglobulinaemia

In all alcohol-related liver diseases, IgA is increased and the levels correlate with the degree of injury (Iturriaga, AnnClinRes, 1977; 9: 39). The increase in serum IgA may either reflect the hepatocellular damage or be due to the interference with the transport of immunoglobulins at the bile duct level (Nagura, JImmunol, 1981; 126:587; Kuttch, Gastro, 1982; 82:184). IgA deposits along the sinusoidal walls appear to be a specific phenomenon in alcoholic liver injury (Kater, AmJClinPath, 1979; 71:51; van-de-Wiel, Hepatol, 1987; 7:95; Kaku, DigDisSci, 1988; 33:845). However, the finding is unspecific since they are also seen in diabetes-related fatty liver (Nagore, Liver, 1988; 8:281) and in some other liver injuries (Amano, AmJClinPath, 1988; 89:728). In addition to liver, IgA

deposits can be demonstrated in superficial blood capillaries of patients with alcoholic liver injury (van-de-Wiel, DigDisSci, 1988; 33:679).

Hyperglobulinaemia in alcohol-related liver disease may be contributed to by increased synthesis from both antigen-specific (monoclonal) and antigen non-specific (polyclonal) activation of B cells (van-de-Wiel, ScaJImmunol, 1987; 25:181). Recently, alcoholic liver disease has been called 'an IgA-associated disorder' (van-de-Wiel, ScaJGastr, 1987; 22:1025).

Autoantibodies and immune complexes

In alcohol-related liver disease, there is a significant increase in the prevalence of antinuclear and anti-smooth muscle antibodies (Gluud, ClinExpImmun, 1981; 44:31). Profiles of antinuclear antibodies can be used in the differentiation of autoimmune hepatitis and primary biliary cirrhosis from alcoholic liver diseases (Kurki, Hepatol, 1983; 3:297). Furthermore, patients with alcoholic cirrhosis have higher levels of ssDNA- and poly(A)-antibodies than patients with other alcoholic liver diseases (Kurki, Hepatol, 1983; 3:297).

In alcoholic liver injury, circulating antibodies to liver-specific protein and to liver membranes have been found in about one-third of the patients (Manns, Gut, 1980; 21:955; Perperas, Gut, 1981; 22: 149; Burt, Gut, 1982; 23:221). However, the latter finding was not confirmed in another laboratory (Krogsgaard, Lancet, 1982; i:1365). The presence of antibodies directed against alcoholic hyaline is equally controversial (Kanagasundaram, Gastro, 1977; 73:1368; Kehl, ClinExpImmun, 1981; 43:215). Antibodies to liver cell membrane have been demonstrated in the majority of patients with alcoholic hepatitis, but in only 60 per cent of patients with inactive cirrhosis (Kaku, DigDisSci, 1988; 33:845).

An increased prevalence of antibodies to microtubules has been demonstrated in patients with alcoholic liver disease but not in non-alcoholic liver disease (Kurki, Hepatol, 1983; 3:297; Crespi, ItalJGastr, 1986; 18:335). The production of these cytoskeleton antibodies may be due to the destruction or reorganization of the cytoskeletal structures of the liver. Furthermore, 69 per cent of patients with alcoholic liver injury have antibodies to cytokeratin filaments (Kurki, AlcoholClinExpRes, 1984; 8:212). Immune complexes are frequent in alcoholics (Thomas, ClinExpImmun, 1978; 31:150; Brown, Immunol, 1983; 49:673) and it has been suggested that alcoholic hyaline is a component of these particles (Govindarajan, ClinRes, 1982; 30:995A). Circulating IgA-containing immune complexes have also been demonstrated to be related to the severity of liver damage (van-de-Wiel, DigDisSci, 1988; 33:679).

Cellular immune mechanisms

Non-specific derangements in cellular immunity, akin to many autoimmune diseases of unknown aetiology, have been described in patients with alcoholic cirrhosis (Berenyi, AmJDigDis, 1974; 19: 199). Organ-specific changes, such as lymphocyte-mediated cytotoxicity to autologous liver cells in tissue cultures, have also been reported (Paronetto, PSEBM, 1976; 153:495; Cochrane, Gastro, 1977; 72:918). Alcohol-dependent changes in either antigenicity of liver structures or reactivity of immune reflector cells may contribute to alcoholic liver injury.

Although the neutrophilic granulocytes usually predominate in the inflammatory lesions of alcoholic liver injury, mononuclear cells are frequently seen in mild alcoholic liver damage, and the sequestration of sensitized T cells in the liver has been suggested (French, ArchPathLabMed, 1979; 103:146).

Lymphocytes with T8 (Si, AlcoholClinExpRes, 1983; 7:431) and T4 phenotype (Bergroth, ActaPMIScand, 1986; 94:337; Spinozzi, JClinLabImmunol, 1987; 23:161) are present in alcoholic hepatitis. The frequency of Ia (HLA-DR)-positive cells in mild alcoholic liver disease varies between 15 and 30 per cent of all mononuclear cells, which indicates the activation of the local T cells (Bergroth, ActaPMIScand, 1986; 94:337). This implies that T cells in alcoholic fatty liver are not only innocent bystanders but may actively participate in the local inflammatory process. Both K and T cells have been demonstrated to be involved in cytotoxicity against autologous hepatocytes (Actis, Liver, 1983; 3:8; Izumi, ClinExpImmun, 1983; 53:219; Hütteroth, Hepatol, 1983; 3:842).

An increase in the CD4 (helper, inducer)/CD8 (suppressor, cytotoxic) lymphocyte ratio has been reported in the peripheral blood of patients in the acute phase of alcoholic hepatitis (Ishimaru, AlcAlc, 1990; 25:353). However, controversial results have also been reported (Müller, ScaGastr, 1991; 26:295; Li, Hepatol, 1991; 14: 121; Roselle, JClinLabImmunol, 1988, 26:169).

Effect of alcohol on hepatocyte regeneration

In most of the studies on partially hepatectomized rats acute ethanol administration (1–6 days) has been shown to inhibit the incorporation of tritiated thymidine into hepatic DNA.[48] This indicates that both a short-term and a continuous presence of ethanol during the regeneration retards hepatic DNA synthesis and cell division. However, at the end of the experiment total liver mass and DNA content are the same as in controls (Frank, JLabClinMed, 1979; 93:402; Pösö, MedBiol, 1980; 58:329; Orrego, JLabClinMed, 1981; 97:221), indicating that liver regeneration is not inhibited. In rat hepatocyte cultures DNA synthesis is inhibited by a short-term (96 h) exposure to alcohol and this is mediated by ethanol oxidation (Carter, AlcoholClinExpRes, 1988; 12:555).

Observations on the model of chronic alcohol administration to partially hepatectomized rats generally agree with those received with the 'acute model' (Wands, Gastro, 1979; 77:528; Frank, Gastro, 1980; 78:1167; Duguay, Gut, 1982; 23:8). There is no evidence that the inhibition of hepatic regeneration may play a role in the pathogenesis of alcoholic liver damage in man.

Genetic factors

There is a large body of evidence that genetic factors are particularly important with regard to the oxidation of ethanol and acetaldehyde, as discussed earlier in this chapter. However, hereditary factors also contribute to the genesis of alcoholism and may associate with the pathogenesis of the alcoholic liver disease.[49]

The association of alcoholic cirrhosis with blood group A and colour blindness (Billington, AustAnnMed, 1956; 5:20) has not been confirmed in later studies (Cruz-Coke, Lancet, 1965; 1:1131; Fialkow, NEJM, 1966; 275:548; Reid, BMJ, 1968; 2:463; Ranek, ScaJGastr, 1970; 7:203).

In a twin study among 15 924 twin pairs, the concordance rates for cirrhosis were 14.6 (monozygotic) versus 5.4 (dizygotic)

(Hrubec, AlcoholClinExpRes, 1981; 5:207). These results suggest a genetic predisposition to alcohol-induced liver injury and accordingly has promoted the search for genetic markers and candidate genes.[49]

There is some evidence implicating a weak association between HLA antigens and the predisposition to alcoholic liver disease (Eddleston, BrMedBull, 1982; 38:13). Normally, hepatocytes do not express HLA class I antigens on their surface, which make them poor targets to immunological attacks after hepatic transplantation. However, in alcoholic hepatitis and in some other liver diseases, such HLA expression may develop (Barbatis, Gut, 1981; 22:985). There is some evidence pointing to accelerated development of alcoholic cirrhosis in patients with HLA B8, B35, and DR3 (Saunders, Lancet, 1982; 1:1381; Doffoel, Hepatol, 1986; 6:457; Marbet, Hepatogast, 1988; 35:65). Furthermore, in patients with alcoholic hepatitis increased associations of B8 in England, Cw3 in Japan and of A2 in Switzerland have been found (Morgan, JClinPath, 1980; 33:488; Shigeta, PharmBiochBehav, 1980; 13:89, Bron, Hepatogast, 1982; 29:183).

Contradictory results have been reported with respect to the polymorphism of collagen genes and the risk for alcoholic cirrhosis (Weiner, MolAspMed, 1988; 10:159; Day, Hepatol, 1990; 12:293). The results regarding the associations between the genes coding the alcohol metabolizing enzymes and the risk of alcoholic liver injury are not conclusive, as discussed above.

Nutritional factors

Although the direct hepatotoxic effect of ethanol has been indisputably proven, the role of potentiating nutritional factors has not been fully excluded. If the fat content of ethanol-containing liquid diet is decreased from 32 to 25 per cent, hepatic triglyceride accumulation significantly decreases (Lieber, AmJClinNutr, 1970; 23:474). In addition, the replacement of dietary triglycerides containing long-chain fatty acids by fat containing medium–chain fatty acids markedly reduces the capacity of alcohol to produce fatty liver in rats (Lieber, JCI, 1967; 46:1451).

Excess weight is a risk factor or a predictive sign of histological liver damage in alcoholics (Iturriaga, AmJClinNutr, 1988; 47:235). In epidemiological studies the amount of pork consumed has been shown to correlate with mortality from cirrhosis (Nanji, Lancet, 1985; 1:681). Further evaluation suggested that both saturated fat and cholesterol protect against alcoholic cirrhosis, while polyunsaturated fats promote cirrhosis (Nanji, AlcoholClinExpRes, 1986; 10:271). In accordance with this finding, a high-fat diet appeared to potentiate, and beef fat to prevent, ethanol-induced hepatic fibrosis and alcoholic liver disease in the rat (Tsukamoto, Hepatol, 1986; 6:814; French, AlcoholClinExpRes, 1986; 10:13S; Nanji, AlcoholClinExpRes, 1989; 13:15).

Deficiencies in lipotrophic factors (choline and methionine) can produce fatty liver and cirrhosis in growing rats (Best, BMJ, 1949; 2:1001; Daft, PSEBM, 1941; 48:228). In later studies hepatic injury induced by choline deficiency was suggested to be primarily an experimental disease of rats with little, if any, relevance to alcoholic liver injury, particularly in humans.[1] More recently, rats have been shown to be more resistant to choline deficiency than humans, since humans have a reduced ability to produce betaine (main donator of methyl groups) from choline (Barak, LifeSci, 1985; 37:

789). Therefore betaine (the first metabolite of choline) has been suggested for the treatment of alcoholic liver injury in humans (Barak, AlcAlc, 1988; 23:73).

It has not been possible to relate ethanol-induced experimental liver injury in rats to vitamin or mineral deficiencies. In fact, vitamin and mineral supplementation fails to affect the ethanol-induced lipid accumulation and microsomal changes produced in the rat by the standard totally liquid diet (ethanol 36 per cent of total energy) (Lieber, AlcoholClinExpRes, 1989; 13:142). However, the balance between carbohydrate and fat in liquid diets may have an effect on the development of fatty liver, as discussed earlier in this chapter.

The results in subhuman primates are controversial. The entire spectrum of alcoholic liver disease (steatosis, mild alcoholic hepatitis, and cirrhosis) has been produced in baboons by Lieber and co-workers (Lieber, JMedPrimatol, 1974; 3:153; Popper and Lieber, AmJPathol, 1980; 98:695). However, others have failed to produce fibrosis and cirrhosis in primates (Mezey, Hepatol, 1983; 3:41; Ainley, JHepatol, 1988; 7:85; Porto, VirchArchA, 1989; 414:299).[50] The discrepancy in the results has been related to the differences in the choline contents of the diets. It was suggested that chronic alcohol feeding may exaggerate choline requirements of the monkeys (Mezey, Hepatol, 1983; 3:41). However, in subsequent studies additional choline failed to prevent the development of fibrosis in baboons (Lieber, Hepatol, 1985; 5:561). The failure to produce cirrhosis in monkeys was related to the small number of animals studied, species differences, and to a relatively lower alcohol intake of the monkeys as compared with baboons (Lieber, Hepatol, 1985; 5:561).

Information about the nutritional status of alcoholics and of patients with alcoholic liver injury is equally controversial. This is largely due to the difficulties associated with reliable dietary assessment, especially in chronic alcoholics. However, without doubt, heavy alcohol consumption has profound effects on nutrient economy and may produce nutritional imbalance even in subjects eating normal diets (Morgan, BrMedBull, 1982; 38:21; Quartini, Alcologia, 1995; 7:101).

It has been claimed that alcoholic liver disease is frequently recognized among well-nourished alcoholic individuals manifesting no nutritional deficiency. On the other hand, cirrhotic alcoholics were reported to have a significantly lower total food calorie intake and a significantly lower daily protein intake than non-cirrhotic chronic alcoholics (Patek, ArchIntMed, 1975; 135:1053). Using established criteria to diagnose and classify protein–calorie malnutrition, all 248 patients with alcoholic liver disease were shown to have some evidence of malnutrition (Mendenhall, AmJMed, 1984; 76:211). The prevalence of the malnutrition correlated closely with the severity of the liver disease, with a prevalence of 72 per cent for both kwashiorkor and marasmus in those with severe disease. However, it should be noted that in neither study was the causal relationship between malnutrition and liver disease established; malnutrition, at least in part, may have been secondary to the liver injury and not its cause.

Data on the nutritional status of middle-class heavy drinkers is also controversial. Only subtle nutritional alterations have been documented in several studies (Hurt, AmJClinNutr, 1981; 34:386; Goldschmith, JAmCollNutr, 1983; 2:215; Neville, AmJClinNutr, 1986; 21:1329; Rissanen, AmJClinNutr, 1987; 45:456). Nevertheless, these drinkers also frequently develop laboratory signs of alcoholic liver injury (Rissanen, AmJClinNutr, 1987; 45:456). In some other studies a significantly decreased protein, fat, and cholesterol intake has been documented in heavy drinkers (Jones, AmJClinNutr, 1982; 35:135; Hillers, AmJClinNutr, 1985; 41:356). There is some epidemiological and clinical evidence pointing to the possible protective effect of a high protein diet on alcohol-induced cirrhosis (Raymond, SchMedWoch, 1985; 115:998; Mendenhall, AlcoholClinExpRes, 1995; 19:635).

Role of enteric bacteria

Liver injury, morphologically identical to alcohol hepatitis, often follows jejunoileal bypass surgery (Moxley, NEJM, 1974; 290:921; Peters, AmJClinPath, 1975; 63:318; Craig, Gastro, 1980; 79:131). As with alcoholic liver injury, histological evidence of pericentral fibrosis in these patients identifies those at risk of developing steatonecrosis and cirrhosis (Haines, Hepatol, 1981; 1:161). In addition to parenteral or enteral hyperalimentation (Heimburger, AmJSurg, 1975; 129:229; Ames, JAMA, 1976; 235:1249; Galambos, ArchPathol, 1976; 100:229; Lockwood, AmJClinNutr, 1977; 30:58), these patients have been treated successfully with antibiotics, chloramphenicol, and metronidazole (Baker, Gastro, 1980; 78:1593; Drenick, Gastro, 1982; 82:535). On this basis, the pathogenesis of the liver injury associated with jejunoileal bypass has been related to bacterial overgrowth in the excluded segment.

As stated previously, alcohol ingested per orally is transported to the colon by blood circulation and, after the distribution phase, intracolonic ethanol levels are equal to those in the blood. In the large bowel, ethanol is oxidized by a bacteriocolonic pathway.[16] Due to the low aldehyde dehydrogenase activity of colonic mucosa, acetaldehyde accumulates in the colon. Accordingly, during ethanol oxidation the highest acetaldehyde levels of the body are found in the colon and not in the liver. Intracolonic acetaldehyde can be absorbed to the portal vein and, accordingly, be a possible hepatotoxin (Matysiak-Budnik, JPath, 1996; 178:469). In addition to acetaldehyde, gut-derived endotoxin is another potential candidate in the pathogenesis of alcohol-related liver injury, as stated above.

Role of hepatitis B and C

The potential role of hepatitis viruses in the pathogenesis of alcoholic liver disease was suggested in early 1970s (Pettigrew, Lancet, 1972; 2:725).[51] Several studies have revealed the higher prevalence of markers of hepatitis B virus in alcoholics than in matched controls (Mills, JClinPath, 1979; 32:778; Hislop, JClinPath, 1981; 34:1017; Orholm, JClinPath, 1981; 34:1378; Periente, AmJClinPath, 1981; 76:299; Gluud, JClinPath, 1982; 35:693; Chevilotte, Gastro, 1983; 85:141; Inohue, Liver, 1985; 5:247). An increased prevalence of anti-hepatitis B virus antibodies has also been observed both in outpatient alcoholics and in patients in hospital with alcoholic liver disease (Gluud, Infec, 1982; 12:72). In some studies the highest prevalence of hepatitis B virus has been found in cirrhotics (Mills, JClinPath, 1979; 32:778; Hislop, JClinPath, 1981; 34:1017). In a prospective study in Italy, hepatitis B virus carriers were found to have a greater risk of developing hepatomegaly and raised liver enzymes than controls when drinking up to 80 g alcohol daily, suggesting that the presence of hepatitis B virus could be a contributing factor in the development of alcoholic liver injury (Villa, Lancet, 1982; ii:1243). However, this has not been confirmed in later studies (Fong, Hepatol, 1988; 8:1602; Mendenhall, Hepatol, 1991; 14:581). Nevertheless hepatitis B virus may play a role in liver cell carcinoma in alcoholic liver disease (Bréchot, NEJM, 1982; 306:1384; Nalpas, JHepatol, 1985; 1:89).

The prevalence of hepatitis C virus in patients with alcoholic liver disease ranges from zero to 73 per cent[51] (Esteban, JHepatol, 1993, 17(Suppl.3):67; Befritz, ScaJGastr, 1995; 30:1113; Bird, EurJGastroHepatol, 1995; 7:161; Coelho-Little, AlcoholClin-ExpRes, 1995; 19:1173). A high incidence of hepatitis C virus infection is found in countries with a high prevalence of hepatitis C virus in the population. Hepatitis C virus is unlikely to complicate alcoholic liver disease in a population with a low background prevalence of hepatitis C virus (Bird, EurJGastroHepatol, 1995; 7: 161). For instance, in Japan alcohol has been found to be the sole known factor in only 10 per cent of patients with liver disease (Shiomi, CJGastrHepatol, 1992; 7:274). In patients with alcoholic hepatitis the severity of liver disease and degree of liver pathology have been reported to be identical in hepatitis C virus-positive and hepatitis C virus-negative (Mendenhall, GastrJap, 1993; 28(S5):95). The combined presence of hepatitis C virus and alcohol injury appeared not to increase the mortality, but did significantly increase the number of referrals to hospital (Mendenhall, GastrJap, 1993; 28(S5):95). As in the case of hepatitis B virus, alcohol potentiates the risk of hepatocellular carcinoma in patients with hepatitis C virus (Miyakawa, AlcAlc, 1993; 1A:85). The magnitude of lifetime alcohol intake and anti-hepatitis C virus status have been shown to be additive—but not multiplicative—with regard to the risk of cirrhosis (Corrao, EurJEpid, 1992; 8:634).

It has been concluded that moderate alcohol intake during covalescence from acute viral hepatitis does not seem to be harmful (Tozun, Lancet, 1991; ii:1079), but chronic liver damage with its possible evolution is a different story.[51]

References

1. Lieber CS. Alcohol and the liver: 1994 update. *Gastroenterology*, 1994; **106**: 1085–106.
2. Simpura J. Trends in alcohol consumption and drinking patterns: lessons from world-wide development. In Holder HD and Edwards G, eds. *Alcohol and public policy. Evidence and issues*. Oxford: Oxford University Press, 1995: 9–37.
3. Lelbach WK. Epidemiology of alcoholic liver disease. *Progress in Liver Diseases*, 1976; **5**: 494–515.
4. Sörensen TIA. Alcohol and liver injury: dose-related or permissive effect? *British Journal of Addiction*, 1989; **84**: 581–9.
5. Lelbach WK. Leberschäden bei chronischem Alkoholismus. I-III. *Acta Hepato-Splenologica*, 1966; **13**: 321–49.
6. Lelbach WK. Epidemiology of alcoholic liver disease; Continental Europe. In Hall P, ed. *Alcoholic liver disease*. London: Edward Arnold, 1985: 130–66.
7. Pequignot G, Tuyns AJ, and Berta JL. Ascitic cirrhosis in relation to alcohol consumption. *International Journal of Epidemiology*, 1978; **7**: 113–20.
8. Coates RA, Halliday ML, Rankin JG, Feinman SV, and Fisher MM. Risk of fatty infiltration or cirrhosis of the liver in relation to ethanol consumption: A case-control study. *Clinical and Investigative Medicine*, 1986; **9**: 26–32.
9. Mellanby E. *Alcohol: its absorption into and disappearance from the blood under different conditions*. Medical Research Committee, Special Report Series No. 31. London: HM Stationery Office, 1919: 48.
10. Widmark EMP. Die theoretischen Grundlagen und die praktische Verwendbarkeit der gerichtlich-medizinishen Alkoholbestimmung. In Abderhalden E, ed. *Fortschritte der Naturwissenschaftlichen Forschung, Heft II*. Berlin: Urban und Schwarzenberg, 1932: 140.
11. Bergren S and Goldberg L. The absorption of ethyl alcohol from the gastrointestinal tract as a diffusion process. *Acta Physiologica Scandinavica*, 1940; **1**: 246–70.
12. Harper RN and Hulpieu HR. The pharmacology of alcohol. In Thompson GN, ed. *Alcoholism*. Springfield: Charles S. Thomas, 1956: 103–232.
13. Brien JF, Clarke DW, Richardson B, and Patrick J. Disposition of ethanol in maternal blood, and amniotic fluid of third-trimester pregnant ewes. *American Journal of Obstetrics and Gynecology*, 1985; **152**: 583–90.
14. Lundsgaard E. Alcohol oxidation in the liver. *CR Travaux Labor Carlsberg Serie Chimie*, 1938; **22**: 333–7.
15. Leloir LF and Muñoz JM. Ethyl alcohol metabolism in animal tissues. *Biochem Journal*, 1938; 32: 299–307.
16. Salaspuro M. Bacteriocolonic pathway for ethanol ethanol oxidation: Characteristics and implications. *Annals of Medicine*, 1996; **28**: 195–200.
17. Smith M. Genetics of human alcohol and aldehyde dehydrogenases. *Advances in Human Genetics*, 1986; **15**: 249–90.
18. Cotton RW and Goldman D. Review of the molecular biology of human alcohol dehydrogenase genes and gene products. *Advances in Alcohol and Substance Abuse*, 1988; 7: 171–82.
19. Jörnvall H and Höög J-A. Nomenclature of alcohol dehydrogenases. *Alcohol*, 1995; **30**: 153–61.
20. Thomasson HR, Beard JD, and Li T-K. ADH2 gene polymorphism are determinants of alcohol pharmacokinetics. *Alcoholism Clinical and Experimental Research*, 1995; 19: 1494–9.
21. Blomstrand R, Ellin Å, Löf A, and Östling-Wintzell H. Biological effects and metabolic interactions after chronic and acute administration of 4-methylpyrazole and ethanol to rats. *Archives of Biochemistry and Biophysics*, 1980; **199**: 591–605.
22. Lieber CS and DeCarli LM. Ethanol oxidation by hepatic microsomes: adaptive increase after ethanol feeding. *Science*, 1968; **162**: 917–18.
23. Lieber CS and DeCarli LM. Hepatic microsomal ethanol oxidizing system: *in vitro* characteristics and adaptive properties *in vivo*. *Journal of Biological Chemistry*, 1970; **245**: 2505–12.
24. Ingelman-Sundberg M, *et al.* Ethanol-inducible cytochrome P450E1: genetic polymorphism, regulation, and possible role in the etiology of alcohol-induced liver disease. *Alcohol*, 1993; **10**: 447–52.
25. Ingelman-Sundberg M, *et al.* Genetic polymorphism of cytochrome P450. Functional consequences and possible relationship to disease and alcohol toxicity. *EXS*, 1994; **71**: 197–207.
26. Goedde HW and Agarwal DP. Polymorphism of aldehyde dehydrogenase and alcohol sensitivity. *Enzyme*, 1987; **37**: 29–44.
27. Crabb DW, Edenberg HU, Bosron WF, and Li TK. Genotypes of aldehyde dehydrogenase deficiency and alcohol sensitivity. The inactive ALDH2(2) allele is dominant. *Journal of Clinical Investigation*, 1989; **83**: 314–16.
28. Yoshida A. Molecular genetics of human aldehyde dehydrogenase. *Pharmacogenetics*, 1992; **2**: 139–47.
29. Raghunathan L, Hsu LC, Klisak I, Sparkes RS, Yoshida A, and Mohandas T. Regional localization of the human genes for aldehyde dehydrogenase-1 and aldehyde dehydrogenase-2. *Genomics*, 1988; **2**: 267–9.
30. Forsander OA and Räihä NC. Metabolites produced in the liver during alcohol oxidation. *Journal of Biological Chemistry*, 1960; **235**: 34–6.
31. Lundquist F. Production and utilization of free acetate in man. *Nature*, 1962; **193**: 579–80.
32. Lundquist F, Tygstrup N, Winkler K, Mellemgaard K, and Munck-Petersen S. Ethanol metabolism and production of free acetate in human liver. *Journal of Clinical Investigation*, 1962; **41**: 955–61.
33. Nuutinen HU, Salaspuro MP, Valle M, and Lindros KO. Blood acetaldehyde concentration gradient between hepatic and antecubital venous blood in ethanol-intoxicated alcoholics and controls. *European Journal of Clinical Investigation*, 1984; **14**: 306–11.
34. Eriksson CJP and Deitrich RA. Metabolic mechanisms in tolerance and physical dependence on alcohol. In Kissin B, and Begleiter H, eds. *The pathogenesis of alcoholism: biological factors*. New York: Plenum Press, 1983: 253–83.
35. Goldstein DP and Chin JH. Interaction of ethanol with biological membranes. *Federation Proceedings*, 1981; **40**: 2073–6.

36. Taraschi TF and Rubin E. Biology of disease. Effects of ethanol on the chemical and structural properties of biologic membranes. *Laboratory Investigation*, 1985; **52**: 120–31.

37. Dawidowicz EA. The effect of ethanol on membranes. *Hepatology*, 1985; **4**: 697–9.

38. Baraona E. Ethanol and lipid metabolism. In Seitz HK, and Kommerell B, eds. *Alcohol Related Diseases in Gastroenterology*. Berlin: Springer Verlag, 1985: 65–95.

39. Salaspuro M and Lindroos K. Metabolism and toxicity of acetaldehyde. In Seitz HK, and Kommerell B, eds. *Alcohol related diseases in gastroenterology*. Berlin: Springer-Verlag, 1985: 106–23.

40. Lauterburg BH and Bilzer M. Mechanism of acetaldehyde hepatotoxicity. *Journal of Hepatology*, 1988; **7**: 384–90.

41. Lieber CS. Mechanisms of ethanol-drug-nutrition interactions. *Clinical Toxicology*, 1994; **32**: 631–81.

42. Fernandez-Checa JC, Hirano T, Tsukamoto H, and Kaplowitz N. Mitochondrial glutathione depletion in alcoholic liver disease. *Alcohol*, 1993; **10**: 469–75.

43. Nolan JP. Intestinal endotoxins as mediators of hepatic injury. *Hepatology*, 1989; **10**: 887–91.

44. Lands WEM. Cellular signals in alcohol-induced liver injury: A review. *Alcoholism: Clinical and Experimental Research*, 1995; **19**: 928–38.

45. Triger DR. Endotoxemia in liver disease—time for re-appraisal? *Journal of Hepatology*, 1991; **12**: 136–8.

46. Schenker S and Bay MK. Alcohol and endotoxin: another path to alcoholic liver injury? *Alcoholism: Clinical and Experimental Research*, 1995; **19**: 1364–6.

47. Paronetto F. Immunologic reactions in alcoholic liver disease. In Lieber CS, ed. *Medical and nutritional complications of alcoholism*. New York: Plenum Publishing Corporation, 1992: 283–305.

48. Joly J-G and Duguay L. Ethanol and hepatic cell regeneration. In Seitz HK, and Kommerell B, eds. *Alcohol related diseases in gastroenterology*. Berlin: Springer-Verlag, 1985: 253–68.

49. Lumeng L and Crabb DW. Genetic aspects and risk factors in alcoholism and alcoholic liver disease. *Gastroenterology*, 1994; **107**: 572–8.

50. Rogers AE, Fox JG, and Gottlieb LS. Effect of ethanol and malnutrition on nonhuman primate liver. In Berk PD, and Chalmers TCh, eds. *Frontiers in liver disease*. New York: Georg Thieme Verlag, 1981: 167–75.

51. Andreone P, Gramenzi A, Cursaro C, and Gasbarrini G. Alcoholic liver disease and hepatitis viruses. *Alcologia*, 1994; **6**: 7–10.

15.2 Pathology of alcoholic liver disease

Alastair D. Burt and R. N. M. MacSween

Introduction

Alcohol causes a spectrum of morphological changes in the liver; this includes fatty liver (steatosis), alcoholic hepatitis, and cirrhosis. This is a spectrum in which there is considerable overlap. Thus, fatty liver, the earliest recognizable histological feature of disease in the alcoholic, may persist in the later stages of alcoholic hepatitis and cirrhosis. Several additional patterns of alcohol-induced liver disease have also been described including foamy degeneration, perivenular fibrosis, hepatic vein lesions, and chronic hepatitis.

Fatty liver (alcoholic steatosis)

Fatty liver is the earliest recognizable lesion of alcoholic liver disease. This change has been observed in up to 90 per cent of chronic alcoholics (Edmondson, Medicine, 1967; 46:119). Fatty liver will develop following moderate alcohol ingestion and appears within a few days.[6] The change is reversible; following alcohol withdrawal the fat is rapidly mobilized and will disappear within 3 to 4 weeks. It is not possible, however, on a morphological basis, to be sure whether fat accumulation in the liver is due to alcohol or may be due to other aetiologies.

The pathogenesis of alcohol-induced fatty liver is explicable on a biochemical basis and is dealt with elsewhere in the text (Chapter 15.3). Histologically, affected hepatocytes are typically distended by a single large lipid droplet which displaces the nucleus, an appearance referred to as macrovesicular steatosis. This occurs principally in perivenular zones although the distribution may vary. Rarely, the change may be panacinar. This is sometimes associated with gross hepatomegaly, cholestasis, and, occasionally, fulminant hepatic failure. This clinical presentation is rare but occurs most frequently in middle-aged women (Morgan, ScaJGastr, 1978; 13: 299). Biopsies from such cases will, in addition to steatosis, show features of cholestasis-bilirubinostasis, a ductular reaction, and cholangiolitis (Fig. 1).

In uncomplicated fatty liver there are generally only minimal reactive inflammatory changes. The extrusion of lipid from hepatocytes may evoke a granulomatous response. Such lipogranulomas comprise a focal aggregate of lymphocytes, macrophages, eosinophils, and, occasionally, multinucleate giant cells surrounding an extracellular collection of lipid (Christofferson, ActaPMIScand, 1971; 79:150). Lipogranulomas are most often seen in the perivenular zones where they may rarely form confluent aggregates. A mild degree of fibrosis may occur in response to such foci. There is no evidence, however, that such fibrosis is of any pathological

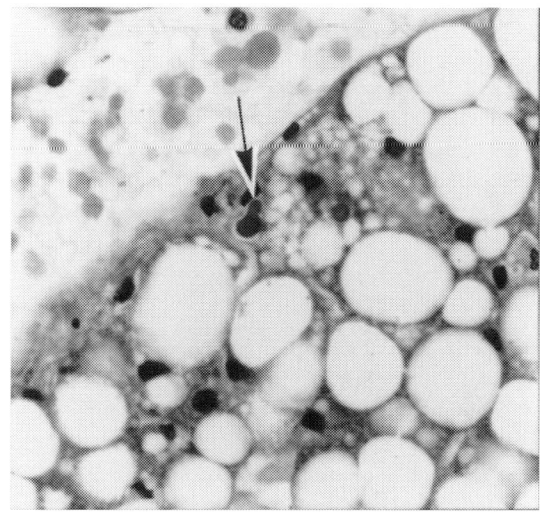

Fig. 1. Fatty liver with cholestasis. Most of the hepatocytes show macrovesicular steatosis; a canalicular bile plug can be identified (arrow).

significance or leads to progressive scarring. In some biopsies a mixed macrovesicular–microvesicular pattern of steatosis may be observed. In a recent longitudinal study, this histological pattern was identified in index biopsies as an independent predictor of the progression of liver disease (Teli, Lancet 1995; 346:987).

A variant of fatty liver, in which there is predominantly microvesicular lipid accumulation, has been described in alcoholics (Uchida, Gastro, 1983; 84:683) and has been termed alcoholic foamy degeneration. In addition to the perivenular microvesicular steatosis, there is bilirubinostasis, focal liver cell necrosis, and macrovesicular steatosis may be seen in other zones (Fig. 2). There may be mild perivenular fibrosis but there is negligible inflammation and no Mallory bodies (see below). These appearances are seen in only a minority of alcoholic patients. In Uchida's series, it was generally observed as the first episode of hepatic decompensation and occurred in the absence of encephalopathy or portal hypertension. There was marked clinical jaundice with a persistent elevation of serum alkaline phosphatase and cholesterol but, in contrast to alcoholic hepatitis, no pyrexia and no peripheral blood leucocytosis. In most cases the lesion resolves following the cessation of alcohol.

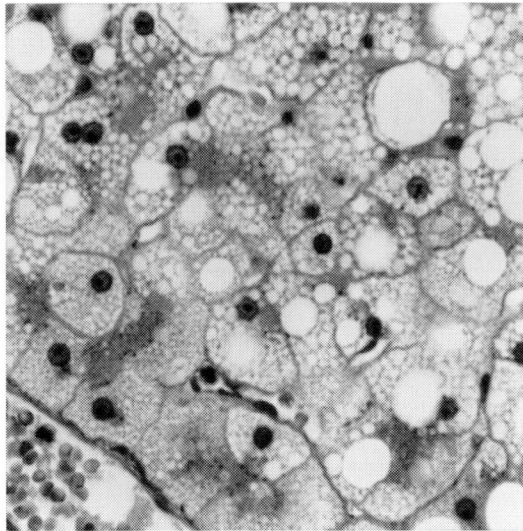

Fig. 2. Alcoholic foamy degeneration. All of the hepatocytes in this perivenular area contain numerous small lipid droplets—microvesicular steatosis.

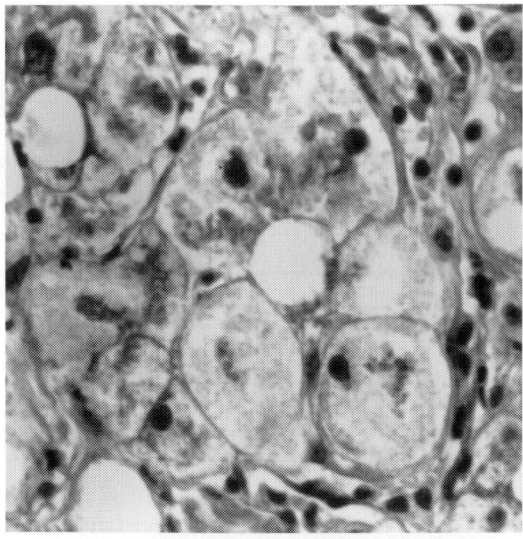

Fig. 3. Alcoholic hepatitis. Perivenular hepatocytes show ballooning degeneration. Aggregates of amorphous eosinophilic material can be seen within their cytoplasm; these are Mallory bodies.

Alcoholic hepatitis

Alcoholic hepatitis (or steatohepatitis) has been estimated to occur in approximately 40 per cent of chronic alcoholics (Hislop, QJMed, 1983; 206:232). Histologically, the lesion occurs in the perivenular areas, all of which are usually affected. It comprises a constellation of changes, of which the essential features are (i) liver cell injury with ballooning and necrosis and often with Mallory bodies, (ii) an inflammatory cell infiltrate, predominantly (but not exclusively) composed of neutrophil polymorphs, and (iii) pericellular fibrosis. In some cases there may be areas of confluent liver cell loss with central–central bridging necrosis. This may be associated with dense fibrous scarring. A range of other histological features, including giant mitochondria, hepatic vein lesions, and ductular metaplasia (Ray, Liver 1993; 13:36) may be seen, but these are not considered essential for the diagnosis. The changes may occur in various combinations and with variable degrees of severity. There is evidence of geographical variation in the incidence of the individual features (Karasawa, ActaHepatolJpn, 1979; 20:115). Thus, Mallory bodies are apparently much less frequent in biopsies from Japanese patients compared with those from Western countries.

The cytoplasm of the ballooned hepatocytes has a finely granular appearance; in some it is broken up into finely dispersed particles producing a wispy, cobweb-like appearance. This ballooning degeneration is thought to be the result of microtubule dysfunction with consequent impaired protein secretion accompanied by fluid retention. The hepatocyte swelling may contribute to clinical hepatomegaly and some authors have suggested that it may produce a sinusoidal pressure effect contributing to the development of portal hypertension (Blendis, Hepatol, 1982; 2:539). Ballooned hepatocytes may contain homogeneous, eosinophilic, perinuclear inclusions, the Mallory bodies (Figs 3 and 4). These are composed, at least in part, of aggregates of cytokeratin (**CK**) polypeptides including CK7, 18, and 19, ubiquitin together with heat shock, and tau proteins; Mallory bodies also contain high quantitites of ε (γ) glutamyl-lysine dipeptides possibly due to enhanced activity within

the hepatocytes (Jensen, Hepatol, 1994; 20:1330). Immunohistochemistry can be used to detect small, not readily apparent Mallory bodies (Ohata, LabInvest, 1988; 59:848; Yoshioka, AmJGastr, 1989; 84:535; Van Eyken, Liver, 1993; 13:113).

Ultrastructurally, three distinct types of Mallory bodies have been described (Yokoo, AmJPathol, 1972; 69:25). The most frequently recognized form in alcoholic hepatitis comprises clusters of randomly orientated fibrils of 5 to 20 nm diameter. Mallory bodies are not invariably seen in alcoholic hepatitis and are not pathognomonic of the condition (see below). The inflammatory infiltrate of alcoholic hepatitis is predominantly composed of neutrophil polymorphs which accumulate around necrotic liver cells and

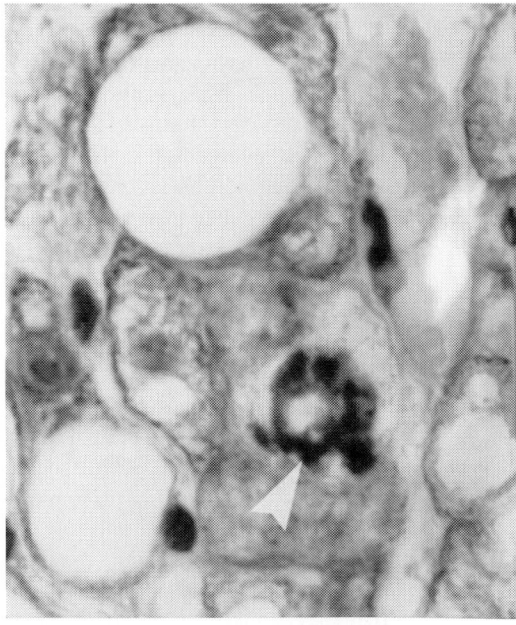

Fig. 4. Mallory bodies show immunoreactivity with antibodies to intermediate filaments of the cytokeratin type (arrowhead).

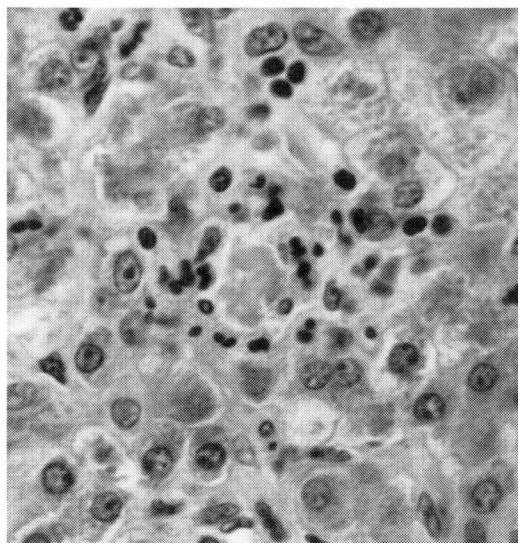

Fig. 5. Mallory body-containing hepatocytes in alcoholic hepatitis are frequently surrounded by polymorphs—so-called satellitosis.

Mallory body-containing hepatocytes. Occasionally, macrophages and lymphocytes form a significant proportion of the inflammatory cells. Characteristically, the polymorphs surround injured liver cells ('satellitosis') (Fig. 5); the intensity of the infiltrate may be related to the number of Mallory bodies. There is evidence that they are chemotactic for neutrophils (Dhinghra, Gastro, 1980; 79:1013), but other factors are thought to be involved in the recruitment of the inflammatory cells including chemokines such as interleukin-8 and the expression of adhesion molecules by sinusoidal endothelial cells in response to cytokines such as tumour necrosis factor-α (**TNF-α**) (Adams, Hepatogast, 1996; 43:32; Thompson, Hepatogast, 1996; 43:15).

Giant mitochondria may be observed within balloned hepatocytes; they may also occur in uncomplicated fatty liver (Bruguera, Gastro, 1977; 73:1383). They are identified by light microscopy as globoid, eosinophilic bodies (Fig. 6). Ultrastructurally, they have

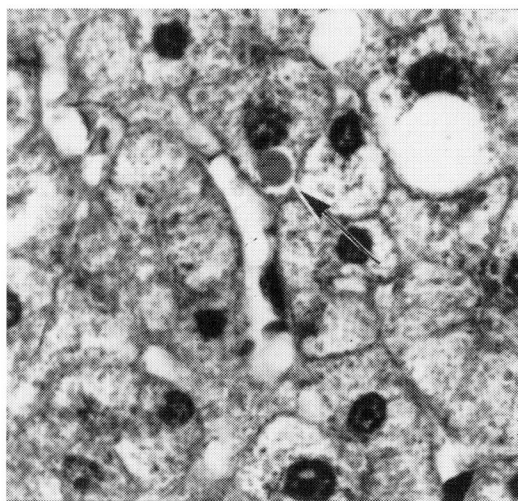

Fig. 6. Giant mitochondria are seen as globoid, eosinophilic inclusions within hepatocytes (arrow).

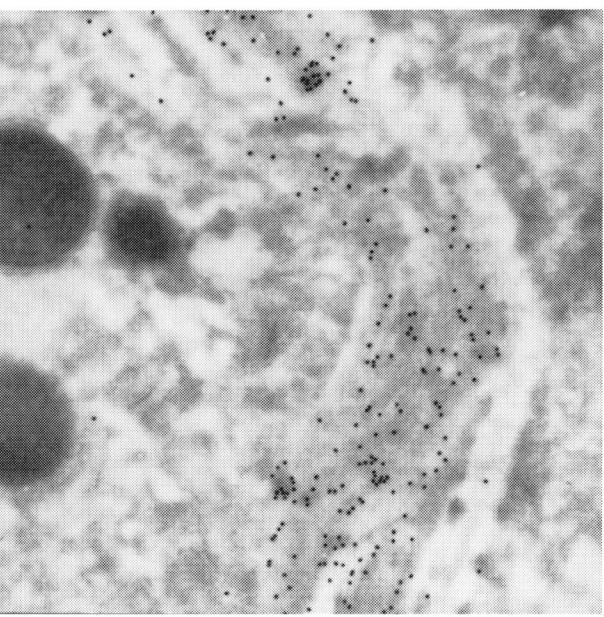

Fig. 7. Immunogold labelling for type III collagen in alcoholic hepatitis using ultrathin frozen sections (Burt, Histopathol; 1990; 16:53). Strong labelling can be seen for this protein in a pericellular distribution.

abnormal cristae and frequently contain paracrystalline inclusions. Other less common features in alcoholic hepatitis include acidophil bodies (see Chapter 15.3) and so-called induced hepatocytes which resemble classical hepatitis B virus (**HBV**)-associated, ground-glass hepatocytes but do not stain positively with Shikata's orcein; their morphological appearances result from the proliferation of the smooth endoplasmic reticulum.

Fibrosis is an early and constant feature of alcoholic hepatitis. Extracellular matrix proteins including interstitial collagens (types I and III) and fibronectin are deposited in a perisinusoidal distribution (Fig. 7). Individual hepatocytes or groups of hepatocytes become surrounded by this fibrous tissue producing a so-called chicken-wire pattern. Although not pathognomonic, it is a highly characteristic feature. There is now strong evidence that myofibroblasts and 'transitional cells' derived from the hepatic stellate cells of the space of Disse represent the major cell types involved in the process (Nakano, Gastro, 1982; 83:777; Minato, Hepatol, 1983; 3:599; Friedman, Hepatol, 1990; 12:609; Mathew, Hepatogasto, 1996; 43:72).

In addition to pericellular fibrosis there is often fibrous thickening around hepatic vein radicles, a process which has been referred to as phlebosclerosis (Fig. 8). The severity of this lesion increases with progressive liver injury. There is obliteration of vein branches making it difficult to identify the terminal hepatic vein radicles. Less common hepatic vein lesions have also been described in alcoholic liver disease (Goodman, Gastro, 1982; 87:930; Burt, JClinPath, 1986; 39:63). These comprise veno-occlusive lesions with intimal proliferation and a lymphocytic phlebitis. They are generally seen in advanced disease.

Perivenular fibrosis

The association of pericellular and perivenular fibrosis with alcoholic hepatitis has long been recognized and they have been

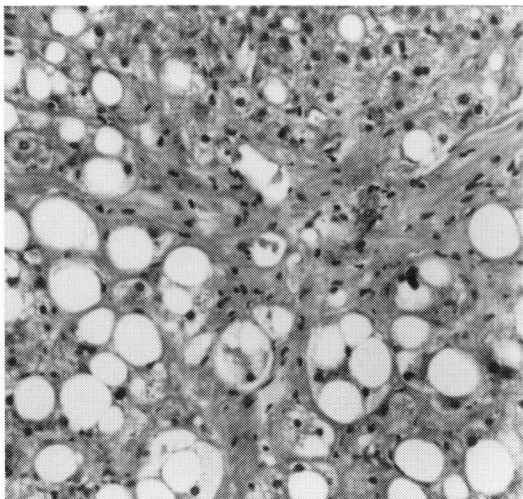

Fig. 8. Severe pericellular and perivenular fibrosis can be seen in this case of alcoholic hepatitis. The fibrotic process has resulted in the obliteration of a terminal hepatic vein radicle—phlebosclerosis.

regarded as important lesions in the progression to cirrhosis. Several groups have demonstrated that perivenular fibrosis, usually accompanied by pericellular fibrosis, may occur in the absence of hepatitis, that is in the absence of inflammation, Mallory bodies, or liver cell necrosis (Van Waes, Gastro, 1977; 73:646; Nasrallah, ArchPathLabMed, 1980; 104:84; Worner, JAMA, 1985; 254:627; Maher, SemLivDis, 1990; 10:66). Lieber's group identified patients with fatty liver and perivenular fibrosis and, in a prospective study, demonstrated that they were at greater risk of progression to irreversible liver disease than patients with fatty liver alone. Three out of 19 subjects with simple fatty liver showed progressive liver injury during a follow-up period of 1 to 4 years. In marked contrast, 13 out of 15 patients with perivenular fibrosis showed progressive fibrosis with the development of cirrhosis in four cases. More recently, evidence has been produced that perivenular fibrosis may occur in the majority of moderate and heavy drinkers, but in only a minority of these in their progression to cirrhosis (Savolainen, JHepatol, 1995; 23:524). The importance of these observations, however, is to suggest that alcohol may have a direct fibrinogenic effect and, consequently, that alcoholic hepatitis may not be the only precirrhotic lesion in the liver. This concept is supported by experiments with baboons in which it was shown that alcoholic cirrhosis could develop without preceding hepatitis, although perivenular fibrosis was identified (Popper, AmJPathol, 1980; 98:695).

Non-alcoholic steatohepatitis

The entire spectrum of features constituting alcoholic hepatitis may be seen in individuals abusing alcohol. The term non-alcoholic steatohepatitis (**NASH**) is now widely accepted for this entity (Ludwig, ProcMayoClinic, 1980; 55:434). The diseases associated with NASH are shown in Table 1 and Table 2 lists the drugs that have been reported to produce a similar pattern of liver injury. In some patients, however, no recognized associations are present and a diagnosis of NASH is made on liver biopsy findings during the investigation of mild disturbances of liver function tests and after careful exclusion of alcohol abuse (Lee, HumPath, 1989; 20:594).

The histological features may be indistinguishable from alcoholic hepatitis (Diehl, Gastro, 1988; 95:1056). However, the injury tends to be less severe, Mallory bodies may be present in small numbers, and, occasionally, in type 2 diabetes (Nagore, JPath, 1988; 156:155) and in some of the drug-related cases a periportal distribution of the lesions has been reported. Follow-up studies have shown that NASH may pursue a slow progressive course which ultimately results in cirrhosis (Powell, Hepatol, 1990; 11:34). Cirrhosis has also been reported with both nifedipine (Pessayre, Gastro, 1979; 76: 170) and amiodarone (Bach, MtSinaiMedJ, 1989; 56:293).

Alcoholic cirrhosis

With progressive injury, fibrous septa develop linking the hepatic vein branches and hepatic veins to the portal tracts. This disturbance of the liver architecture is accompanied by regenerative activity and the formation of nodules. Ultimately, a true cirrhosis develops. This is generally micronodular with nodules of 3 mm or less in diameter (Figs 9 and 10). The degree of nodular regenerative activity in advanced alcoholic liver disease may not be marked in that alcohol *per se* may inhibit hepatocyte regeneration (Duguay, Gut, 1982; 23: 8). The proliferative activity usually increases when alcohol is withdrawn, with a consequent transition towards a macronodular pattern of cirrhosis (Rubin, ArchPathol, 1973; 73:40). Steatosis and alcoholic hepatitis may be seen in the cirrhotic liver; their presence usually indicates continued alcohol abuse. Conversely, with alcohol withdrawal the features indicating an alcohol aetiology disappear. Useful features in an endstage inactive cirrhotic liver which may indicate an alcohol aetiology include the presence of fat, lipid-laden macrophages in portal tracts and severe architectural disturbance with an irregular distribution of fibrous septa. Accumulations of copper-associated protein and α_1-antitrypsin may be seen in periseptal hepatocytes and are secondary to the cirrhosis.

Other changes in alcoholic liver disease
Chronic hepatitis

Several groups have suggested that chronic hepatitis, characterized by predominantly portal and periportal lymphocytic inflammation with interface hepatitis (piecemeal necrosis), may be a consequence of alcohol abuse (Hodges, Lancet, 1982; 1:550; Crapper, Liver, 1983; 3:327). Strict criteria must be applied to establish this diagnosis; other causes of chronic hepatitis, for example HBV or HCV virus infection and drugs, must be excluded. Nevertheless, the existence of alcohol-induced chronic hepatitis is supported by the observation that the inflammatory activity may resolve following abstinence (Sakai, ActaHepatolJpn, 1988; 29:673). The prevalence of this lesion is uncertain. Our own experience and that of an international group of hepatopathologists[2] is that it is an uncommon feature of alcoholic liver disease although there may, however, be geographical differences. The role of concomitant hepatitis B or hepatitis C infection in determining the severity of alcoholic liver disease is controversial (Cooksley, JGastroHepatol, 1996; 11:187), although there is some evidence that the latter may be associated with more severe injury and, in particular, with increased intra-acinar inflammation (Paris, Hepatol, 1990; 12:1295; Rosman, ArchIntMed, 1993; 153:965).

Table 1 Diseases associated with NASH

Cause	Report
Obesity	Ludwig (ProcMayoClinic, 1980; 55:434) and Silverman (AmJGastr, 1990; 85:1349)
Diabetes mellitus	Ludwig (ProcMayoClinic, 1980; 55:434), Falchuk (Gastro, 1980; 78:535) and Silverman (AmJGastr, 1990; 85:1349)
Jejunoileal bypass, gastroplasty, and various other surgical procedures for treatment of massive obesity	Peters (JClinPath, 1975; 63:318), Hamilton (Gastro, 1983; 85:722) and Peura (Gastro, 1980; 79:128)
Pancreatoduodenectomy for pancreatic carcinoma	Nakanuma (ActaPathJpn, 1987; 37:1953)
Small intestinal diverticulosis with bacterial overgrowth	Nazim (Hepatogast, 1989; 36:349)
Limb lipodystrophy	Powell (Gastro, 1989; 97:1022)
Abetalipoproteinaemia	Partin (Gastro, 1974; 67:107)
Weber–Christian disease	Kumura (Gastro, 1980; 78:807)

Table 2 Drugs producing NASH

Cause	Report
Amiodarone	Lewis (Hepatol, 1989; 9:679) and Bach (MtSinaiMedJ, 1989; 56:293)
4′4′-Diethylaminoethoxyhexoestrol	Itoh (ActaHepato-Gastroenterol, 1973; 20:204)
Glucocorticoids	Itoh (Acta Hepato-Gastroenterol, 1997; 24:415)
Insulin	Wanless (ModPathol, 1989; 2:69)
Nifedipine	Babany (JHepatol, 1989; 9:252)
Perhexilene maleate	Pessayre (Gastro, 1979; 76:170) and Poupon (Digestion, 1980; 20:145)
Synthetic oestrogens	Seki (GastrJap, 1983; 18:197)
Tamoxifen	Pinto (JHepatol, 1995; 23:95)
Total parenteral nutrition	Craig (Gastro, 1980; 79:131)

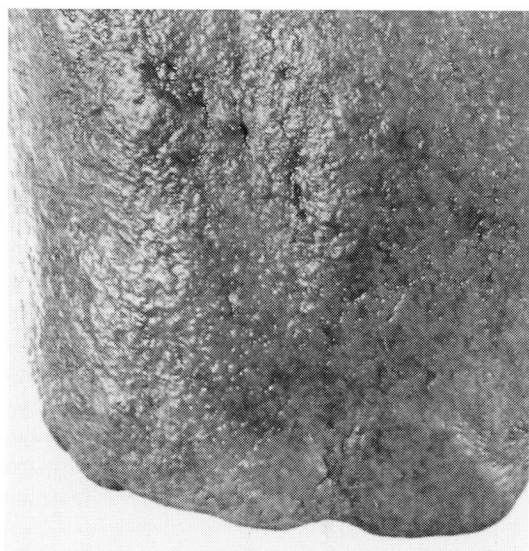

Fig. 9. Micronodular cirrhosis. Small nodules can be seen on the capsular surface of this liver.

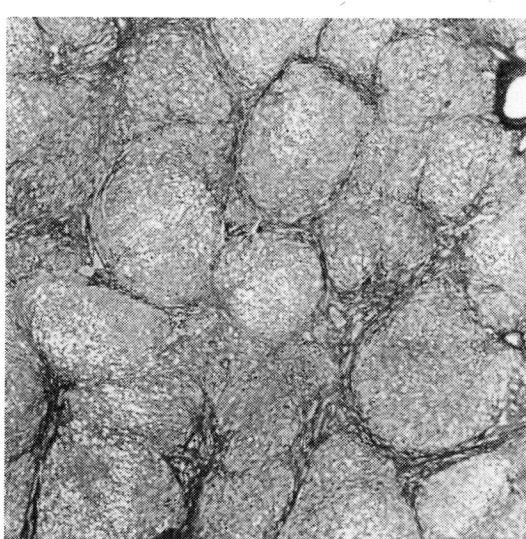

Fig. 10. Histological appearances of a micronodular cirrhosis. The presence of fibrous bands surrounding parenchymal nodules is demonstrated using a reticulin stain.

Hepatocellular carcinoma

Hepatocellular carcinoma arises in 5 to 15 per cent of patients with alcoholic cirrhosis (Lee, Gut, 1966; 7:77). It is seen more frequently accompanying a macronodular rather than a micronodular cirrhosis. The possibility that alcohol *per se* may play a role in hepato-carcinogenesis has been raised in view of reports of hepatocellular carcinoma arising in non-cirrhotic alcoholic patients.[12] There is, however, no firm evidence that alcohol is a direct carcinogen. It may act as a promoter by inducing Cyp 2E1 with the resultant production of electrophilic derivatives of chemicals (Lieber, Gastro, 1994; 106: 1085) or as a co-carcinogen with HBV or HCV (Brechot, NEJM, 1982; 306:1384; Nalpas, JHepatol, 1991; 12:70).

Hepatic siderosis

Iron deposition in hepatocytes and Kupffer cells, haemosiderosis, is often seen in alcoholic liver disease. This may be due to the high iron content of many alcoholic beverages, although alcohol itself may enhance the absorption of iron from the small intestine. Haemosiderosis is frequently observed in the later stages, where there is established cirrhosis, but is rarely severe, grade 3/4 iron deposition being seen in less than 10 per cent of cases (Jacobovitis, DigDisSci, 1979; 24:305). Where there is severe siderosis, a diagnosis of primary haemochromatosis complicated by alcoholic liver disease should be considered; a hepatic iron index (hepatic iron concentration divided by the patients age) is helpful in making this distinction (Sallie, Gut, 1991; 32:207) as is genotyping for the HLA-M gene (Chapter 20.2).

Hepatic siderosis may also be observed in patients with porphyria cutanea tarda, a condition which is exacerbated by alcohol. The liver tissue from such patients characteristically manifests red autofluorescence under ultraviolet light; birefringent acicular inclusions may be identified within the hepatocytes (Cortes, Histopathol, 1980; 4:471).

Liver biopsy in the management of alcoholic liver disease

Liver biopsy plays an important role in the clinical assessment of the alcoholic patient with abnormal liver function tests. First, it may be used to establish a diagnosis of alcoholic liver disease. This in itself is important as up to 20 per cent of such patients will have non-alcoholic disease (Levin, AmJMed, 1979; 66:429). Secondly, it is essential in determining the stage of the disease as clinical and biochemical indices are poor predictors of the extent and severity of liver injury. Finally, a liver biopsy may provide some indication of the prognosis (Chedid, AmJGastr, 1991; 86:210; Nissenbaum, DigDisSci, 1990; 35:891). The role of the histopathologist in predicting the clinical outcome, however, remains limited. In most cases it should be possible to suggest whether the changes are reversible, based on an assessment of the extent of the hepatitis, the amount of pericellular and perivenular fibrosis, and the degree of architectural distortion. Steatosis and features of hepatitis, including Mallory bodies, will disappear on alcohol withdrawal. Some resolution of the fibrosis may also occur but this takes longer and persistence of the scarring will result in microcirculatory disturbance and the evolution of a true cirrhosis.

References

1. Popper H, Thung SN, and Gerber MA. Pathology of alcoholic liver disease. *Seminars in Liver Disease*, 1981; 1: 203–16.
2. Baptista A and International Hepatopathology Group. Alcoholic liver disease: morphological manifestations. Review by an international group. *Lancet*, 1981; i: 707–11.
3. Scheuer PJ. The morphology of alcoholic liver disease. *British Medical Bulletin*, 1982; 38: 63–5.
4. MacSween RNM and Burt AD. Histologic spectrum of alcoholic liver disease. *Seminars in Liver Disease*, 1986; 6: 221–32.
5. Hall PM de la. Alcoholic liver disease. In: MacSween RNM, Anthony PP, Scheuer PJ, Burt AD, and Portmann BC, eds. *Pathology of the liver*, 3rd edn. Edinburgh: Churchill Livingstone, 1994: 317–48.
6. Rubin E and Lieber CS. Alcohol-induced hepatic injury in non-alcoholic volunteers. *New England Journal of Medicine*, 1968; 278: 869–76.
7. Sherlock S. Alcoholic liver disease. *Lancet*, 1995; 345: 227–9.
8. Day CP and Yeaman SJ. The biochemistry of alcohol-induced fatty liver. *Biochemica et Biophysica Acta*, 1994; 1215: 33–48.
9. Zimmerman HJ and Ishak KG. Non-alcoholic steatohepatitis and other forms of pseudoalcoholic liver disease. In: Hall P, ed. *Alcoholic liver disease. Pathology and pathogenesis*, 2nd edn. London: Edward Arnold, 1995: 175–98.
10. Bacon BR, Farahvash MJ, Janney CG, and Neuschwander-Tetri BA. Non-alcoholic steatohepatitis: an expanded clinical entity. *Gastroenterology*, 1994; 107: 1103–9.
11. Pinto HC, Baptista A, Camilo ME, Valente A, Saragossa A, and De Moura MC. Nonalcoholic steatohepatitis. Clinicopathological comparison with alcoholic hepatitis in ambulatory and hospitalized patients. *Digestive Diseases and Sciences*, 1996; 41: 172–9.
12. Bassendine MF. Alcohol and hepatocellular carcinoma. *Journal of Hepatology*, 1985; 2: 513–19.

15.3 Alcoholic liver disease: natural history, diagnosis, clinical features, evaluation, management, prognosis, and prevention

Marsha Y. Morgan

Alcohol is the most common cause of liver disease in the Western world today. It has also become an important cause of liver injury in a number of developing countries as economies improve, urbanization spreads, and traditional cultural and religious indictments against drinking are removed. In many countries worldwide the incidence of alcoholic liver disease is increasing at a time when the incidence of other liver disorders remains steady or is falling.

Alcoholic liver disease is classified on a morphological basis as fatty change, alcoholic hepatitis, and alcoholic cirrhosis. A number of other alcohol-related liver lesions have been described, and individuals abusing alcohol may develop liver injury of alternative aetiological backgrounds. The clinical spectrum of alcohol-related liver injury varies from asymptomatic hepatomegaly to profound hepatocellular failure with portal hypertension. Although the clinical picture tends to be more florid in individuals with more advanced liver injury, the correlation between clinical features, laboratory test results, and liver histology is poor. Liver biopsy is therefore mandatory for the diagnosis and staging of the liver disease.

Alcoholic liver disease may arise in the absence of physical dependency on alcohol and of alcohol-related emotional, social, or psychological harm; it may, in contrast, arise together with a vast panoply of other alcohol-related medical and social problems. Successful management depends on treating the alcoholic liver disease in the context of the whole patient and not in isolation. The most important therapeutic manoeuvre is the maintenance of abstinence from alcohol and this is achieved with varying degrees of difficulty. The long-term outlook for patients with alcoholic liver disease is determined to a large extent by their ability to remain free of alcohol.

Alcoholic liver disease is a preventable disorder; it is unreasonable to suppose that it will ever be eradicated but its prevalence could be reduced if governmental and personal controls were exercised over alcohol consumption.

Natural history[1–9]

In susceptible individuals the risk of developing significant alcohol-related liver injury increases above intake thresholds, variously reported, of between 20 to 80 g/day in men and of between 12 to 60 g/day in women (Lelbach, AnnNYAcadSci, 1975; 252:85; Pequignot, IntJEpid, 1978; 7:113; Tuyns, IntJEpid, 1984; 13:53; Coates, ClinInvestMed, 1986; 9:26; Norton, BMJ, 1987; 295:80; Batey, MedJAust, 1992; 156:413; Klatsky, AmJEpid, 1992; 136: 1248; Corrao, JClinEpid, 1993; 46:601; Savolainen, AlcoholClinExpRes, 1993; 17:1112; Becker, Hepatol, 1996; 23: 1025).[7] In the majority of studies the risk is shown to increase with increasing intake, but in some studies the hepatotoxic effects of alcohol have appeared permissive rather than dose-related (Savolainen, AlcoholClinExpRes, 1993; 17:1112).[7]

Alcoholic liver injury appears to progress from fatty change through alcoholic hepatitis to cirrhosis.[3] The majority of individuals who misuse or abuse alcohol will develop fatty change in their liver at some stage of their drinking career (Edmondson, Medicine, 1967; 46:119). However, only approximately 20 per cent of such individuals will develop cirrhosis.[1,2] The prevalence of cirrhosis among individuals abusing alcohol varies from 9 to 18 per cent in autopsy studies, and from 12 to 31 per cent in liver biopsy series.[1,2,5]

Fatty change is the most common lesion to develop but, although fat accumulation indicates a profound metabolic disturbance within the liver, it is not necessarily harmful. Certainly, cirrhosis may develop in an individual abusing alcohol who has never had fatty change and isolated fatty change has not been shown to proceed directly to cirrhosis.[9] Alcoholic hepatitis develops in only a proportion of drinkers, even after decades of alcohol abuse, and is assumed to be a precirrhotic lesion, although its natural history is not well understood (Lelbach, AnnNYAcadMed, 1975; 252:85).[8] Thus, in approximately 50 per cent of individuals, alcoholic hepatitis may persist for several years, and in 10 per cent of individuals the lesion may heal despite continued alcohol abuse (Galambos, Gastro, 1972; 63:1026). It has therefore been suggested that, although alcoholic hepatitis may contribute, when present, to the evolution towards cirrhosis, it is not an essential for such progression.[4] A number of alternative precursor lesions of cirrhosis have been suggested, including perisinusoidal fibrosis (Nasrallah, Arch-PathLabMed, 1980; 104:84), occlusive lesions in the terminal hepatic venules (Goodman, Gastro, 1982; 83:786), and perivenular fibrosis (Van Waes, Gastro, 1977; 73:646; Nakano, Gastro, 1982; 83:777; Worner, JAMA, 1985; 254:627).

Cirrhosis is generally considered to be an irreversible lesion. Once established it may remain asymptomatic for many years, but decompensation tends to develop at the rate of 10 per cent per annum.[10] The 10-year probability of developing decompensated disease is 58 per cent (Ginés, Hepatol, 1987; 7:122); the complication most frequently observed is ascites. The risk of developing decompensated disease increases significantly with daily intakes of alcohol in excess of 125 g (Arico, Liver, 1995; 15:202). Overall 5-year survival rates in patients with alcoholic cirrhosis vary from 0 to 70 per cent; prognosis is adversely affected by the presence of decompensated disease and continued alcohol abuse (Powell, AmJMed, 1968; 44:406). Approximately 75 per cent of patients with alcoholic cirrhosis die as a result of their liver disease; hepatocellular carcinoma develops in approximately 20 per cent of individuals with alcoholic cirrhosis and may account for up to one-third of the 'liver deaths'.[10-12]

The effects of drinking behaviour

Once the diagnosis of alcohol-related liver disease has been established its subsequent course depends on several factors including the severity of the initial lesion and subsequent drinking behaviour (Leevy, Medicine, 1962; 41:249; Alexander, AmJGastr, 1971; 56:515; Lischner, AmJDigDis, 1971; 16:481; Borowsky, Gastro, 1981; 80:1405; Davidson, SemLivDis, 1981; 1:173; Parrish, JSubsAbuse, 1991; 3:325; Arico, Liver, 1995; 15:202; Harris, AlcAlc, 1995; 30:591).[7–9]

Alcoholic fatty liver

Alcoholic fatty liver may develop after the consumption of large amounts of alcohol over short periods of time (Rubin, NEJM, 1968; 278:869). In individuals who abstain from alcohol, however, clinical and laboratory abnormalities return rapidly to normal (Devenyi, AmJGastr, 1970; 54:597; Christoffersen, ActaPMScandA, 1972; 80:557; Marshall, Alcoholism, 1983; 7:312);[7] histological evidence of fatty change normally disappears within 2 to 6 weeks, depending on its severity (Leevy, Medicine, 1962; 41:249).[7] A pronounced clearing of fat may be observed in individuals who substantially reduce their alcohol intake though do not necessarily abstain from alcohol (Colman, Gut, 1980; 21:965; Marshall, Gut, 1982; 23:1088). However, in some individuals, fatty change disappears despite continued alcohol abuse. Fatty change tends to persist in individuals who continue to abuse alcohol, and in a proportion of these, progression to alcoholic hepatitis and cirrhosis is observed (Leevy, Medicine, 1962; 41:249).[7] Fatty change may persist despite abstinence from alcohol in individuals abusing alcohol who are obese, prediabetic, or have severe pancreatitis.

Alcoholic hepatitis

The effects of subsequent drinking behaviour on the natural history of alcoholic hepatitis, once established, are not well researched, mainly because of the difficulty of monitoring cohorts of individuals who are abusing or misusing alcohol and persuading them to submit

Drinking behaviour (n)	Liver histology n (%)		
	Minimal change	Alcoholic hepatitis	Cirrhosis
Abstinent (13)	9 (69.2)	0	4 (30.8)
Reduced intake (4)	3 (75.0)	1 (25.0)	0
Continued abuse (9)	0	4 (44.4)	5 (55.6)

Table 1 Liver histology in 26 patients with alcoholic hepatitis in relation to their subsequent drinking behaviour

Data extracted from Parés, JHepatol, 1986; 2: 33.

to serial liver biopsies. There are therefore only a handful of studies on which to base conclusions and these are, in general, suboptimal in design and execution.

In one study (Galambos, Gastro, 1972; 63:1026), serial liver biopsies were obtained in 61 patients with alcoholic hepatitis over a period of 6 months to 9 years. Overall, 38 per cent developed cirrhosis, 52 per cent retained the hepatitic lesion, while in 10 per cent the liver lesion regressed completely. Normal liver histology was only observed in individuals who had been abstinent from alcohol, but abstinence did not guarantee regression of the lesion. Thus, of the patients who abstained from alcohol, 27 per cent showed normal histology, 55 per cent retained the hepatitic lesion, and 18 per cent developed cirrhosis.

In a later study,[8] serial liver biopsies were obtained in 26 patients with alcoholic hepatitis over a period of 1 to 3 years. Overall, 35 per cent developed cirrhosis, 19 per cent retained the hepatitic lesion, and 46 per cent showed minimal changes only or else normal histology. Again, only patients who abstained or significantly reduced their alcohol intake showed significant regression of the liver lesion, but cirrhosis was still observed in just under one-third of the individuals who stopped drinking (Table 1). Thus, although subsequent drinking behaviour has a major influence on the progression of alcoholic hepatitis, it is not the only variable to affect outcome.

Within this study population,[8] cirrhosis developed in 58.3 per cent of women, and did so independently of drinking behaviour, whereas it developed in only 14.3 per cent of men and then inevitably in relation to continued drinking. Similarly, cirrhosis developed in 66 per cent of individuals with severe alcoholic hepatitis on their initial biopsy, and did so independently of drinking behaviour, whereas progression was observed in only 20 to 30 per cent of individuals with mild or moderate alcoholic hepatitis, and then invariably in relation to continued abuse of alcohol. Thus, in men with mild to moderate alcoholic hepatitis, subsequent drinking behaviour is the major factor influencing outcome, whereas in women, and in individuals with severe alcoholic hepatitis, of both sexes, progression to cirrhosis is more likely to occur and is less influenced by subsequent drinking behaviour.

Data from two long-term studies in which patients with alcoholic hepatitis were followed with serial liver biopsies over 3 to 13 years confirm that the effects of abstinence from alcohol on the progression of alcoholic hepatitis are not entirely predictable.[7,9] In both studies there was evidence that, over a given threshold, the risk of developing cirrhosis was unrelated to the average daily intake of alcohol. One of these studies[9] also confirmed the earlier findings[8] that progression to cirrhosis was more likely to occur in women and in individuals with severe alcoholic hepatitis, irrespective of subsequent drinking behaviour.

Alcoholic cirrhosis

Surprisingly little information is available on the natural history of alcoholic cirrhosis and the effects of drinking behaviour on morbidity. This may be explained by the fact that approximately two-thirds of these individuals already have decompensated disease by the time of presentation.[10,11]

The natural history of compensated cirrhosis was investigated over a median of 63 months in 293 patients, of whom 122 (42 per cent) had alcohol-related liver injury; 10 years after diagnosis the probability of developing decompensated disease was 58 per cent; ascites was the first complication observed and overall the most common (Ginés, Hepatol, 1987; 7:122). The study did not, however, provide any information on the effects of drinking behaviour on morbidity in the patients with alcoholic cirrhosis.

The natural history of cirrhosis was also investigated in 1155 cirrhotic patients, 33 per cent of whom had alcohol-related disease; [10] approximately one-third of the patients had compensated cirrhosis at the time of presentation and this population developed features of decompensation at a rate of 10 per cent per annum; no attempt was made to relate the development of decompensation to drinking behaviour in the patients with alcoholic cirrhosis. Again, ascites was the first complication observed and overall the most common.

In a case-control study involving 439 patients with decompensated cirrhosis and 233 with compensated cirrhosis, the risk of decompensation was significantly related to the average lifetime daily alcohol intake; the risk of decompensation increased significantly with daily alcohol intakes in excess of 125 g (Arico, Liver, 1995; 15:202).

In a 20-year follow-up study of 100 patients with chronic liver disease and established portal hypertension, a cohort of 20, six of whom had alcoholic cirrhosis, was identified who over a 13-year period showed spontaneous regression of their oesophageal varices (Muting, JHepatol, 1990; 10:158); all the patients with alcoholic cirrhosis had been abstinent from alcohol throughout. In a study in which 58 men with alcoholic cirrhosis were followed for a median of 31 months from diagnosis, 21 per cent developed variceal haemorrhage; no comment was made on the relation, if any, to drinking behaviour (Gluud, Hepatol, 1988; 8:222).

More information is available on the effects of drinking behaviour on mortality in patients with alcoholic cirrhosis. Overall, survival is significantly adversely affected by continued alcohol abuse. Thus, in general, 5-year survival rates in patients with alcoholic cirrhosis who stop drinking are of the order of 50 to 75 per cent, whereas survival rates in patients continuing to drink rarely exceed 40 per cent (Powell, AmJMed, 1968; 44:406).[10,11,14]

Up to 20 per cent of individuals with alcoholic cirrhosis develop hepatocellular carcinoma.[11–13] It develops more frequently in men and in individuals who have abstained from alcohol (Lee, Gut, 1966; 7:77; Kato, JpnJGastr, 1990; 87:1829).

Approximately 75 per cent of patients with alcoholic cirrhosis die as a result of their liver disease, mainly from hepatocellular failure or, less often, gastrointestinal bleeding; hepatocellular carcinoma may account for up to one-third of the liver-related deaths.[10–12]

Diagnosis

Patients with alcoholic liver disease most commonly present with a variety of non-specific symptoms, such as abdominal pain, morning retching, vomiting, anorexia, diarrhoea, weight loss, lethargy, and fatigue. A surprisingly high proportion, up to 30 per cent in some series, are asymptomatic, and are referred because of the incidental finding, made at a routine medical examination or when consulting for some other complaint, of hepatomegaly and/or abnormal liver-function test results. Much less commonly, patients present with specific symptoms such as jaundice, ascites, or gastrointestinal bleeding. In all of these instances a history of chronic alcohol abuse may or may not be available. Conversely, patients may be referred with a drinking problem, may present with other alcohol-related disorders, such as pancreatitis or peripheral neuropathy, or may develop symptoms of alcohol withdrawal when admitted following an accident or with an illness such as pneumonia. In these instances the presence of liver injury is sought as part of a full assessment. There is surprisingly little variation in the mode of presentation in relation to the severity of the liver injury.

The diagnosis of alcoholic liver disease is made on the basis of a history of chronic alcohol abuse and the presence of compatible clinical, laboratory, and preferably histological evidence of liver injury. While in theory this is a two-step procedure, in practice it usually involves eliciting a history of alcohol abuse from individuals with established liver disease or detecting liver injury in individuals with a known history of alcohol abuse.

History

In obtaining a drinking history it is only necessary, for purposes of diagnosing the presence of liver disease, to establish that the individual concerned has regularly consumed an amount of alcohol likely to have caused harm. It is often stated that individuals abusing alcohol consistently under-report their alcohol intake and it is generally believed that this is deliberate. It is much more likely, however, that these individuals cannot remember exactly how much they have drunk over the past 10 to 20 years, although they should be able to give an accurate account of their current intake. Patients who drink solely at home are better able to estimate the amount they consume, as they will be directly responsible for its purchase. Individuals who drink in company and/or in public places may have greater difficulty in providing an accurate record, as they may buy only a proportion of the alcohol they consume or else may only consume a proportion of the alcohol they buy.

It is useful at the outset to obtain a brief inventory of the major life-events of the individual to use for referencing or prompting when taking the actual drinking history. Thus, information should be sought on the age at which they left school, further education or vocational training, employment, and dates of important events such as marriage, births of children, divorce, and deaths of close relatives. It is useful at this time to enquire about the drinking habits of partners and family members.

Using this information as background an attempt should be made to determine (i) the age of onset of regular drinking, defined as the establishment of a regular pattern of daily or weekly drinking, independently of the amount consumed, (ii) the age of onset of alcohol abuse, defined as the establishment of a pattern of regular drinking in excess of 60 g (7 units) daily for men and of 40 g (5 units) daily for women, and (iii) details of the current drinking behaviour. If a pattern of 'binge' drinking is reported, then details should be obtained of the length of each 'binge', the amount of alcohol consumed during the 'binge', the time periods between 'binges', the drinking behaviour between 'binges', and possible precipitating factors for drinking.

The alcohol content of the various beverages available differs widely. The alcohol content of a given beverage is, however, easily calculated from its percentage alcohol content by volume (per cent ABV), which is clearly marked on the container, taking the specific gravity of alcohol into account, viz.:

$$\text{per cent ABV} \times 0.78 = \text{g alcohol/100 ml}$$

The absolute amount of alcohol in a given drink can then be calculated by reference to its volume.

In order to simplify quantification and hence to facilitate assessment of alcohol intake, a system, based on defining quantities of beverages containing equivalent amounts of alcohol, has been devised for use in Great Britain. A 'unit' of alcohol, as originally defined, was the amount of alcohol contained in 1/2 pint of beer, a single 'pub' measure of spirits, and a single glass of table wine; it approximates to 10 ml or 8 g of absolute alcohol.

This system is now used widely by the lay public, by 'alcohol agencies', and by physicians alike. It is, however, quite seriously flawed and, as currently publicized, greatly oversimplified. First, the alcohol content of beers and lagers varies considerably, so that a pint of beer (568 ml) may contain from 2 to 5 units of alcohol depending on its strength; second, beer, particularly for off-licence consumption, is sold in cans in volumes varying from 330 to 440 or 500 ml that bear little relation to the pint measure; third, until recently the standard 'pub' measure of spirits varied by region from $\frac{1}{6}$ to $\frac{1}{4}$ gill (24 to 37 ml); European Community directives have now ensured that the measure is standardized to 25 or 35 ml; fourth, there is no standardized measure for wine; a 'glass' may therefore contain anything from 4 to 12 fluid ounces (114 to 342 ml); fifth, measures of drinks consumed at home differ from 'standard' measures; beer is consumed from bottles or cans in varying volumes, wine measures tend to be larger, while measures of spirits tend to exceed optic measures by a factor of 2.5 to 3.0. Finally, the unit system is essentially parochial and does not lend itself to international comparisons. In Australia and New Zealand, for example, a 'standard' drink contains 10 g of ethanol whereas in the United States of America a 'standard' drink contains 12 g of ethanol.

It is, however, relatively easy to improve the accuracy of the 'unit' system by taking differences in beverage strengths and volumes into account. Thus, the exact number of units of alcohol in a given beverage volume can be calculated from the per cent ABV using the information that 10 ml of absolute alcohol is equivalent to 1 unit of alcohol.

Thus, a half-litre can of 8 per cent ABV lager would contain 40 ml of absolute alcohol (5 × 8), which is equivalent to 4 units; likewise, a 750 ml bottle of 14 per cent ABV wine would contain 105 ml of absolute alcohol (7.5 × 14) or approximately $10\frac{1}{2}$ units (Table 2).

Table 2 The alcohol content of various beverages

Beverage type	Alcohol by volume (%) ABV	Measure	Alcohol content (units)
Beers/lagers/stouts/ciders:			
Alcohol-free	<0.05	440 ml	0
		Pint	0
Low alcohol	0.5–1.0	440 ml	0.4
		Pint	0.6
Standard strength	3.0–4.0	Pint	1.7–2.3
Premium strength	5.0–6.0	440 ml	2.2–2.6
		Pint	2.8–3.4
Super strength	8.0–11.0	440 ml	3.5–5.0
'Alcopops'	5.0–6.0	330 ml	1.7–2.0
Wines	8.0–13.0	750 ml	6.0–10.0
Fortified wines (sherry, vermouth, cinzano)	14.0–20.0	750 ml	10.5–15.0
Spirits:			
Light (gin, vodka, white rum)	37.5	700 ml	26.3
Dark (whisky, brandy, dark rum)	40.0	700 ml	28.0
Liquers	14.0–40.0	700 ml	10.0–28.0

In recent years, new ranges of fortified wines, such as MD 20/20 and Mad Dog, strong white ciders, such as Diamond White and Ice Dragon, fruit-flavoured lagers and ciders, such as Desperados and Maxblack, and alcoholized soft drinks, the so-called Alcopops, such as Hooch alcoholic lemon, have been marketed. The fortified wines have sweet fruit flavours such as cherry, banana, and strawberry, and a per cent ABV of between 13 and 21. The white ciders, which are filtered to remove colour and some flavours, have a per cent ABV of between 8 and 9. The lagers and ciders, which are additionally flavoured with citrus fruits or blackcurrant, and the 'Alcopops', which are essentially soft drinks that have been 'fortified' with alcohol, have a per cent ABV of between 5 and 6. These drinks are attractively packaged, often in small volumes that may nevertheless contain several units of alcohol. Their obvious appeal to young people is of mounting public concern.

Evidence of physical dependency should always be sought because of the management implications; early morning retching and tremor, ingestion of alcohol before midday, and the development of amnesia and black-outs are all suggestive; the occurrence, severity, and treatment of any previous episodes of alcohol withdrawal should be recorded. Information should always be obtained on previous advice, counselling, or other treatments received for the drinking problem.

Although an alcohol history should be obtained as soon after first contact with the patient as possible, it may be necessary to postpone taking a detailed history until they are free of withdrawal symptoms and medication, and have had a chance to 'get their story straight'. Ideally, the history should be taken on more than one occasion, preferably by more than one person; this is particularly usefully done when the results of the various investigations are to hand. Confirmation of the alcohol history should always be obtained, provided the patient agrees, from as many additional sources as possible.

Many patients, even with established alcoholic liver disease, may be asymptomatic or only complain of non-specific symptoms referable to the gastrointestinal tract. A history of specific symptoms should be sought, in particular a history of jaundice, ascites, and gastrointestinal bleeding. Details of all previous investigations and treatments of relevance should be obtained. In addition, as patients who abuse alcohol may develop non-alcoholic liver disease, information on exposure risks for viral or drug-related hepatitis, and any family history of liver disease should be documented.

Clinical features[12–16]

Individuals with alcoholic liver disease may present with evidence of recent alcohol consumption; they may smell of alcohol; they may be flushed with bloodshot eyes, excitable, and tremulous; they may be overtly intoxicated; scars and bruises, sustained as a result of accidental or intentional injuries, may be present. They may also show a constellation of skin and other abnormalities including spider naevi, cutaneous telangiectasia, acne rosacea, palmar erythema, finger clubbing, Dupuytren's contractures, facial mooning, parotid enlargement, gynaecomastia, and testicular atrophy. Some of these abnormalities, in particular spider naevi, palmar erythema, and finger clubbing, may be seen in patients with non-alcoholic liver disease and in this context they are termed 'signs of chronic liver disease'. In individuals abusing alcohol, however, these signs, although often more florid in the presence of alcoholic hepatitis and decompensated alcoholic cirrhosis, may equally be present in the absence of significant liver damage. In this context, therefore, they are best referred to as 'signs of chronic alcohol abuse'. Many of these features will regress with prolonged abstinence from alcohol.

The clinical spectrum of the liver injury may extend from asymptomatic hepatomegaly to profound hepatocellular failure with jaundice, ascites, and portal hypertension. Clinical signs cannot be relied upon to differentiate the various forms of alcoholic liver disease. Thus, patients with profound hepatocellular failure may have alcoholic hepatitis and/or alcoholic cirrhosis on liver biopsy but very occasionally may have only severe fatty change. Equally, patients with simple fatty change and patients with well-compensated alcoholic cirrhosis may be clinically indistinguishable. Alcoholic and non-alcoholic liver disease arising in individuals abusing alcohol cannot be distinguished on clinical grounds (Levin, AmJMed, 1979; 66:429).

There may also be considerable interobserver error in the interpretation of the physical signs of alcoholic liver disease. For example, in an evaluation of the agreement between six physicians in the assessment of 18 clinical signs in 50 alcohol abusers, 34 of whom had documented alcoholic liver disease, the concordance was good for ascites and splenomegaly, fair for jaundice, Dupuytren's contracture, and vascular spiders but poor for white nails and the consistency of the liver (Espinoza, DigDisSci, 1987; 32:244). As might be expected, agreement was better among senior rather than junior physicians. Thus, a diagnosis of alcoholic liver disease made on the basis of physical findings alone must be treated with caution.

Laboratory tests[17–22]

Laboratory tests can facilitate the recognition of chronic alcohol abuse, even when it is denied, and can be used to detect the presence of liver disease; they are, however, of little use in determining the degree of alcohol-related liver injury.

Markers of recent alcohol consumption

Measurement of ethanol concentrations in breath and body fluids can be used to confirm suspicions of excess drinking, which, particularly if denied, may draw attention to the possibility of chronic alcohol abuse. Blood ethanol concentrations in excess of 100 mg/100 ml (22 mmol/l) at routine medical examination, above 150 mg/100 ml (33 mmol/l) without signs of intoxication, and above 300 mg/100 ml (65 mmol/l) at any time, should be regarded as highly suspicious of alcohol abuse (Criteria Committee, National Council on Alcoholism, New York, AnnIntMed, 1972; 77:249). However, in general, random measurements of blood ethanol are of limited diagnostic value in individuals attending for assessment of liver disease. In one study, ethanol was found in the blood of 13 per cent of attenders at a morning clinic, although 36 per cent gave a history of heavy drinking (Hamlyn, Lancet, 1975; ii:345); at least three determinations were required in order to obtain a 50 per cent chance of detecting ethanol in the blood of patients with a history of alcohol abuse.

Methanol can be detected for longer in blood following ingestion of alcoholic beverages than can ethanol; it is therefore a more sensitive marker of recent alcohol consumption (Roine, AlcoholClinExpRes, 1989; 13:172; Jones, AlcAlc, 1992; 27:641).

Likewise, the urinary ratio of the serotonin metabolites 5-hydroxytryptophol and 5-hydroxyindole-3 acetic acid (5-HTOL:5-HIAA) increases after ethanol consumption (Voltaire, AlcoholClinExpRes, 1992; 16:281), and remains elevated for 5 to 15 h after blood ethanol has fallen to baseline concentrations (Helander, LifeSci, 1993; 53:847; ClinChem, 1996; 42:618).

Of these three markers of recent alcohol consumption the urinary 5-HTOL:5-HIAA ratio is the most sensitive (Helander, ClinChem, 1996; 42:618; AlcAlc, 1997; 32:133).

Markers of chronic alcohol abuse

The profound metabolic and toxic effects of alcohol are reflected in biochemical disturbances, which, although not specific for alcoholism, are nevertheless useful for its identification; abnormalities that arise in serum enzymes of hepatic origin are probably the most valuable in this regard.

γ-Glutamyl transferase

Elevation of serum γ-glutamyl transferase activity (formerly γ-glutamyl transpeptidase) is perhaps the most common biochemical abnormality observed in individuals abusing alcohol. This enzyme is of hepatic origin and its synthesis is induced by alcohol [Rosalki, Lancet, 1971; ii:376; Ishii, Gastro, 1976; 71: 913 (Abstr.)]. In some series, increased serum γ-glutamyl transferase activity was found in up to 80 to 90 per cent of chronic heavy drinkers (Rollason, CCActa, 1972; 39:75; Rosalki, CCActa, 1972; 39:41; Wu, AmJGastr, 1976; 65:318; Gjerde, ScaJCLI, 1988; 48:1; Stetter, AlcoholClinExpRes, 1991; 15:938). In general, the enzyme activity averages two to three times the upper reference range but values up to five times this limit are frequently observed (Rosalki, AdvClinChem, 1975; 17:53). Serum γ-glutamyl transferase activity decreases with abstinence from alcohol, usually in an exponential fashion (Lamy, CCActa,

1974; 56:169); in general, the activity is reduced by 50 per cent within 2 weeks and normal values are usually attained within 5 weeks (Rosalki, CCActa, 1972; 38:41).

Increased serum γ-glutamyl transferase activity is not specific for alcohol excess, since elevated values may be observed in patients taking enzyme-inducing drugs such as phenobarbitone and phenytoin (Rosalki, Lancet, 1971; ii: 376; Keeffe, DigDisSci, 1986; 31: 1056), and in patients with cholestasis or hepatocellular injury (Rosalki, AdvClinChem, 1975; 17:53; Salaspuro, ScaJGastr, 1989; 24:769). However, a rapid reduction in serum enzyme activity during the first week of a stay in hospital strongly suggests that the elevated activity was secondary to alcohol abuse (Orrego, AlcoholClinExpRes, 1985; 9:10; Pol, Alcoholism, 1990; 14:250), although a very rapid fall in serum γ-glutamyl transferase activity may be observed following relief of biliary obstruction (Krastev, ItalJGastr, 1992; 24:185). Serum activity of this enzyme may fall in patients with decompensated alcoholic cirrhosis even if they continue to drink, and also tends to fall in individuals who have been abusing alcohol for 20 years or more (Skude, ActaMedScand, 1977; 201:53); some heavy drinkers never show elevated serum γ-glutamyl transferase activity (Penn, BMJ, 1983; 286:531; Moussavian, DigDisSci, 1985; 30:211; Matsuda, AlcAlc, 1993; (Suppl. 1B): 27).

The increase in serum γ-glutamyl transferase activity in individuals abusing alcohol is independent of the degree of liver injury (Wu, AmJGastr, 1976; 65:318). However, the serum enzyme activity does correlate with the degree of hepatic inflammation and necrosis found histologically, so that the highest activities are found in patients with severe alcoholic hepatitis.

Several forms of γ-glutamyl transferase appear in serum (Moss, AdvBiochemPharmacol, 1982; 3:41). To date, the mechanisms used to effect iso-γ-glutamyl transferase separation have been laborious and poorly reproducible (Artur, AdvBiochemPharmacol, 1982; 3: 61; Nemesanszky, ClinChem, 1985; 31:797), and there has been little consensus on the nomenclature for the fractions obtained or on the interpretation of the different patterns found (Nemesanszky, ClinChem, 1985; 31:797; Sacchetti, Electrophoresis, 1989; 10:619; Okuyama, KeioJMed, 1993; 42:149).

However, one group now appears to have overcome some of the difficulties of estimating serum iso-γ-glutamyl transferase (Bellini, AlcAlc, 1997, 32:259). Multiple forms are separated by rapid gel electrophoresis and the resulting trace is then examined visually to identify fractions and the overall fraction pattern. In alcohol abusers the electrophoretic pattern differed significantly from the patterns obtained in healthy volunteers and in patients with non-alcoholic liver disease but was indistinguishable from that observed in individuals taking antiepileptic medication. Significant differences were observed in iso-γ-glutamyl transferase fractions in alcohol abusers in relation to the degree of liver injury.

This technique is still only semiquantitative and further methodological refinement is needed.

Aspartate aminotransferase

Serum aspartate aminotransferase activity is elevated in approximately 45 to 70 per cent of individuals abusing alcohol but rarely exceeds five times the upper reference limit (Bradus, AmJMedSci, 1963; 246:35; Konttinen, ActaMedScand, 1970; 188: 257; Skude, ActaMedScand, 1977; 201:53; Galizzi, ScaJGastr, 1978;

13:827). Although the elevation in serum aspartate aminotransferase activity reflects hepatocellular injury, its degree does not reflect the overall severity of the liver disease, at least in individuals who are abusing alcohol. Although the serum enzyme activity is elevated in from 60 to 80 per cent of individuals with alcoholic cirrhosis who are actively drinking, increased activity is observed in a similar proportion of individuals with less severe liver injury and to a similar degree. Thus, elevated serum aspartate aminotransferase activity has been observed in 73 per cent of individuals abusing alcohol without significant liver disease (Skude, ActaMedScand, 1977; 201:53), and in 64 per cent of a group of alcohol abusers with biopsy-proven minimal liver injury (Galizzi, ScaJGastr, 1978; 13: 827). Serum enzyme activity falls by approximately 50 per cent within 1 week of abstinence from alcohol (Rosalki, AdvClinChem, 1975; 17:53). Serum activity of this enzyme is also increased in individuals with non-alcohol-related hepatobiliary disease and in patients with disorders of skeletal and cardiac muscle. Thus its specificity as a marker for alcohol abuse is relatively low.

A disproportionate increase in the mitochondrial isoenzyme of aspartate aminotransferase is found in the serum of heavy drinkers, reflecting the specific tendency of alcohol to cause mitochondrial injury (Panteghini, CCActa, 1983; 128:133). It has now been shown, using a sensitive immunochemical technique, that the serum activity of mitochondrial aspartate aminotransferase and the ratio of mitochondrial to total enzyme activity are sensitive markers of chronic alcohol abuse, independently of the presence of liver disease (Nalpas, Hepatol, 1986; 6:608). Thus, the mean serum mitochondrial isoenzyme and the isoenzyme:total enzyme activities were significantly elevated during active drinking, with a sensitivity for the ratio of 81 per cent in individuals with normal routine liver-function tests, 85 per cent in individuals with precirrhotic liver disease, and 66 per cent in individuals with alcoholic cirrhosis. The enzyme ratio was raised in only 4.8 per cent of individuals with alcoholic cirrhosis currently abstinent from alcohol and in only 11 per cent of patients with non-alcoholic liver disease. Serum mitochondrial aspartate aminotransferase activity decreased by more than 50 per cent after 1 week's abstinence from alcohol. Others have found elevated serum activity of this isoenzyme in 92 per cent of individuals abusing alcohol but also in 48 per cent of individuals with non-alcoholic liver disease; the enzyme ratio differentiated these two groups with a sensitivity of 92 per cent but a specificity of only 70 per cent (Kwoh-Gain, ClinChem, 1990; 36:841).

Alanine aminotransferase

Serum alanine aminotransferase activity is elevated significantly less often in individuals abusing alcohol than serum aspartate aminotransferase activity (Bradus, AmJMedSci, 1963; 246:35). Indeed, serum activity of this enzyme may be normal or only minimally elevated in patients with severe alcohol-related liver injury. In contrast, its activity usually exceeds that of serum aspartate aminotransferase in patients with non-alcoholic liver disease. Thus, the ratio of serum aspartate:serum alanine aminotransferase activities has been used to distinguish alcoholic from non-alcoholic liver disease: in 80 to 90 per cent of individuals with alcoholic liver disease this ratio exceeds 1 (Clermont, Medicine, 1967; 46:197), while in 70 per cent of individuals with alcoholic hepatitis or active alcoholic cirrhosis it exceeds 2 (Cohen, DigDisSci, 1979; 24:835).

In contrast, the ratio is usually less than 1 in patients with a variety of non-alcoholic liver diseases (Kawachi, NZMedJ, 1990; 103:145). In one study the mean serum aminotransferase ratio in patients with alcoholic hepatitis (1.47) was significantly lower than the mean ratio in patients with alcoholic hepatitis and cirrhosis (2.68) (Nanji, Enzyme, 1989; 41:112). Similarly, in another study the majority of patients with chronic viral hepatitis had serum aspartate:alanine aminotransferase ratios of less than 1, but there was a statistically significant correlation between the ratio and the presence of cirrhosis, the mean ratio being 0.59 in patients without cirrhosis and 1.02 in those with cirrhosis (Williams, Gastro, 1988; 95:734). Other investigators have confirmed serum enzyme ratios of less than 1 in patients with hepatitis B infection and non-malignant, obstructive jaundice, but found a mean ratio of 1.25 in patients with hepatocellular carcinoma (Kawachi, NZMedJ, 1990; 103:145). Interestingly, in that series, the mean serum enzyme ratio in individuals abusing alcohol who had normal serum aminotransferase activities was 1.64 compared with a ratio of 1.50 in individuals with raised serum aminotransferase activities. In practice, measurements of this ratio are probably not of great diagnostic value.

Glutamate dehydrogenase

Glutamate dehydrogenase is a mitochondrial enzyme whose activity may be induced by alcohol. Serum glutamate dehydrogenase activity may be increased in 50 to 60 per cent of heavy drinkers, averaging about twice the upper reference limit and rarely exceeding five times this limit (Van Waes, BMJ, 1977; 2:1508; Mills, BMJ, 1981; 283:754; Jenkins, JClinPath, 1982; 35:207). Increased serum glutamate dehydrogenase activity falls by 50 per cent within 48 h of alcohol withdrawal (Schellenberg, AnnBiolClin, 1983; 41:255). Some investigators have claimed that serum glutamate dehydrogenase activity correlates well with the presence and histological severity of alcoholic hepatitis (Van Waes, BMJ, 1977; 2:1508) but this has not been confirmed by others (Mills, BMJ, 1981; 283:754; Jenkins, JClinPath, 1982; 35:207). The methods for assaying serum glutamate dehydrogenase activity are not entirely satisfactory, which limits its routine use.

D-Glucaric acid

Alcohol induces the microsomal enzymes responsible for the metabolism of glucuronic acid, resulting in enhanced urinary excretion of its metabolites, especially D-glucaric acid (Hunter, Lancet, 1971; i:572). Mean values for urinary D-glucaric acid are significantly increased in individuals chronically abusing alcohol but the proportion of individuals showing abnormal results varies with the technique used for measurement (Spencer-Peet, BrJAddic, 1975; 70:359; Mezey, ResCommChemPathPharm, 1976; 15:735; Tutor, ClinBioch, 1988; 21:193). Unfortunately, the greatest incidence of abnormalities is detected with methods too complex for routine laboratory use. Urinary D-glucaric acid excretion falls within a few days of abstinence from alcohol (Mezey, ResCommChemPathPharm, 1976; 15:735; Tutor, ClinBioch, 1988; 21:193). Excretion of this metabolite is also increased in individuals taking other enzyme-inducing agents and in patients with liver disease; thus its specificity for detecting alcohol abuse is low.

Aminopyrine breath test

Alcohol also induces the microsomal drug-metabolizing enzymes. Chronic alcohol abuse is associated with increased hepatic clearance of certain drugs, and this forms the basis of the aminopyrine breath test, which has been used to detect chronic alcohol abuse (Kawasaki, ClinPharmTherap, 1988; 44:217). Radiolabelled aminopyrine is injected intravenously and labelled carbon dioxide is measured in the breath over time. However, hepatocellular injury is associated with impairment of drug excretory mechanisms and, in consequence, a decrease in aminopyrine clearance (Lewis, JClinPath, 1977; 30:1040). This duplicity of effects limits the usefulness of this test in unselected populations of chronic alcohol abusers. Thus, hepatic clearance of aminopyrine is increased in approximately one-third of individuals abusing alcohol who have little or no liver injury (Lewis, JClinPath, 1977; 30:1040; Galizzi, ScaJGastr, 1978; 13:827; Rodzynek, ArchIntMed, 1986; 146:677), whereas clearance is decreased in over 75 per cent of individuals with cirrhosis, independently of its aetiological background (Lewis, JClinPath, 1977; 30:1040; Rodzynek, ArchIntMed, 1986; 146:677; Urbain, NuclMedComm, 1990; 11:289).

Plasma proteins

A number of abnormalities in plasma proteins may be observed in individuals abusing alcohol, whether or not they have liver disease. These changes are generally non-specific and include reductions of plasma albumin, orosomucoid, haptoglobin, and transferrin concentrations, and elevations in plasma concentrations of α_2-macroglobulin, caeruloplasmin, and immunoglobulins A, G, and M (Agostoni, CCActa, 1969; 26:351; Akdamar, AnnNYAcadSci, 1972; 197:101; Murray-Lyon, CCActa, 1972; 39:215). Plasma albumin is usually normal in individuals abusing alcohol who have minimal liver damage but reduced in approximately 50 per cent of individuals with alcoholic cirrhosis (Hobbs, ProcRoySocMed, 1967; 60:1250; Pollak, JAlc, 1974; 9:135; Perier, ClinChem, 1983; 29:45). Similarly, plasma IgA concentrations are increased, up to twice the upper reference limit, in less than 30 per cent of individuals with minimal alcoholic liver disease but are increased to, on average, three times the upper reference limit in 60 per cent of individuals with alcoholic cirrhosis (Bailey, BMJ, 1976; 2:727; Morgan, JClinPath, 1980; 33:488). Plasma IgA concentrations may remain elevated for many months after abstinence from alcohol (Akdamar, AnnNYAcadSci, 1972; 197:101). Plasma orosomucoid may be increased in patients with minimal alcoholic liver disease but concentrations fall as liver injury progresses (Perier, ClinChem, 1983; 29:45).

Carbohydrate-deficient transferrin

Chronic alcohol abuse is associated with changes in the microheterogeneity of serum transferrin, reflecting variable loss of its terminal trisaccharides. Carbohydrate-deficient transferrin is the collective term used to describe the variously desialyated isoforms. Serum carbohydrate-deficient transferrin is elevated in 40 to 100 per cent of individuals recently abusing alcohol, but test performance varies with the method employed. Thus the more sophisticated 'research' techniques, such as high-performance liquid chromatography, perform better than the 'commercial' test kits which are based on microcolumn technology (Allen, AlcoholClinExpRes, 1994; 18:799; Gordon, AlcRes, 1997; 2:54).[22] Abstinence from alcohol is accompanied by a reduction in serum carbohydrate-deficient transferrin into the reference range over a period of about 10 to 14 days.

The performance of serum carbohydrate-deficient transferrin as a marker of recent alcohol abuse is considerably inferior in women than men for reasons that are unclear (Anton, ClinChem, 1994; 40: 364; AlcoholClinExpRes, 1994; 18:747); it also performs poorly in adolescents and young adults of both sexes (Chan, DrugAlcDep, 1989; 23:13; Nyström, AlcoholClinExpRes, 1992; 16:93).

A significant number of false-positive results occur, most commonly amongst individuals with chronic liver disease; prevalences as high as 40 per cent have been reported (Bell, AlcoholClinExpRes, 1993; 17:246; Bean, ClinChem, 1995; 41:858). False-positive results are also found in individuals who are iron deficient, in those with the rare transferrin D phenotype, and in those with the rare, genetically determined glycoprotein syndrome and in 25 per cent of healthy carriers of this disorder (Kristiansson, ArchDisChild, 1989; 64:71; Stibler, ActaPaedScandSuppl, 1991; 375:22). False-negative results are found in up to 31 per cent of men and 83 per cent of women recently abusing alcohol (Anton, AlcoholClinExpRes, 1994; 18:747; 1996; 20:841), in individuals with genetic haemochromatosis, and in those with the rare transferrin B variant.

There can be little doubt that serum carbohydrate-deficient transferrin, when measured using 'research' techniques in clearly defined populations in whom drinking behaviour is widely divergent, is a sensitive and specific marker for recent alcohol abuse. However, the performance of the commercially available test kits is disappointing and a number of issues need to be addressed if this marker is to realize its full potential (Gordon, AlcRes, 1997; 2:54).

High-density lipoproteins

Changes occur in plasma lipid concentrations in individuals abusing alcohol. Thus, plasma high-density lipoproteins are increased in 70 to 80 per cent of such individuals when actively drinking (Johansson, ScaJCLI, 1969; 23:231; Johansson, ActaMedScand, 1974; 195:273; Castelli, Lancet, 1977; ii:153; Fraser, Atheroscl, 1983; 46:275; Lieber, AlcoholClinExpRes, 1984; 8:409; Tatosyan, CCActa, 1985; 14:211). The elevated plasma lipoproteins return to reference concentrations in 50 per cent of patients after 3 days' abstinence from alcohol and in the majority after 7 days' abstinence (Johansson, ActaMedScand, 1974; 195:273; Lamisse, AlcAlc, 1994; 29:25). Plasma high-density lipoprotein concentrations tend to be normal or low in patients with significant liver injury, even in the presence of active drinking (Sabesin, Gastro, 1977; 72:510; McIntyre, Gut, 1978; 19: 526; Nestel, Metabolism, 1980; 29:101; Devenyi, AmJMed, 1981; 71: 589), and this limits the usefulness of this potential marker for chronic alcohol abuse.

Triglycerides

Hypertriglyceridaemia is found in the majority of individuals abusing alcohol (Lieber, TrAAP, 1963; 76:289; Losowsky, AmJMed, 1963; 35:794; Schapiro, NEJM, 1965; 272:610); plasma concentrations return to reference values within 1 week of abstinence from alcohol (Chait, Lancet, 1972; ii: 62). The highest concentrations of plasma triglycerides are observed in individuals abusing alcohol who have an underlying primary disorder of lipid

metabolism (Friedman, PSEBM, 1965; 120:696; Kudzma, JLabClinMed, 1971; 77:384; Avogaro, Metabolism, 1975; 24:1231). Plasma triglycerides are also influenced by the presence and degree of liver damage; the highest concentrations are found in patients with fatty change, while they may be within the reference range in patients with alcoholic cirrhosis, despite continued alcohol abuse [Borowsky, Gastro, 1976; 70: 978 (Abstr.)].

Uric acid

Elevated serum uric acid concentrations are found in approximately 40 to 50 per cent of individuals abusing alcohol (Olin, QJStudAlc, 1973; 34:1202; Drum, ArchIntMed, 1981; 141:477), either because the synthesis of urate is increased (Faller, NEJM, 1982; 307:1598) or because renal excretion of uric acid is impaired (Lieber, JCI, 1962; 41:1863). On abstaining from alcohol the expected decline towards the reference range is not observed, for reasons that are not entirely clear (Olin, QJStudAlc, 1973; 34:1202); this limits the use of this potential marker for monitoring drinking behaviour, at least in the short term. Interpretation of the results is also complicated by the fact that serum uric acid concentrations vary with age, sex, weight, and drug ingestion (Mikkelsen, AmJMed, 1965; 39:242; Drum, ArchIntMed, 1981; 141:477).

δ-Amino-laevulinic acid dehydratase

The erythrocyte enzyme, δ-amino-laevulinic acid dehydratase, catalyses formation of porphobilinogen from δ-amino-laevulinic acid in the porphyrin biosynthetic pathway. Chronic alcohol abuse is associated with a significant decrease in its activity (Moore, Alcoholism, 1975; 54:101; Flegar-Mestric, ClinBioch, 1987; 20:81), particularly in patients with little or no liver disease; values may be within the reference range in individuals with more significant liver injury, even if they are actively drinking (Hamlyn, CCActa, 1979; 95:453). Acute alcohol intoxication will also reduce enzyme activity (Moore, ClinSci, 1971; 40:81), as will exposure to environmental toxins such as lead (Bortoli, ArchEnvironHlth, 1986; 41:251). The method for measuring this enzyme is complex; its sensitivity in the presence of alcohol-related liver disease is poor so that, although it is a relatively specific marker for alcohol abuse, the test has found little diagnostic application (Aubin, AddicBiol, 1997; 2:225).

Cupro-zinc superoxide dismutase

Increased activities of the erythrocyte enzyme, cupro-zinc superoxide dismutase, have been reported in individuals chronically abusing alcohol (Del Villano, Alcoholism, 1979; 3:291; Ledig, Alcohol, 1988; 5:387; Rooprai, AlcAlc, 1989; 24:503). Increased production of this enzyme has been attributed to the formation of the substrate superoxide from the oxidation of acetaldehyde. In one study, increased erythrocyte superoxide dismutase activity was found in 68 per cent of a group of black individuals who were abusing alcohol (Del Villano, Alcoholism, 1979; 3:291). In another, significantly increased erythrocyte enzyme activity was found in French individuals abusing alcohol, although mainly in those with decompensated cirrhosis (Ledig, Alcohol, 1988; 5:387). In a British study, individuals chronically abusing alcohol had erythrocyte superoxide dismutase activity either above or below the reference range, for reasons that are not clear (Rooprai, AlcAlc, 1989; 24:503). Further studies are obviously needed.

β-Hexosamine

The serum activity of β-hexosamine, an hepatic lysosomal glycoside, is elevated in at least 85 per cent of chronic alcohol abusers (Hultberg, CCActa, 1980; 105:317; Kärkkäinen, Alcohol-ClinExpRes, 1990; 14:187). However, serum β-hexosamine activity is also increased in individuals with liver disease, in women taking the oral contraceptive pill, and during pregnancy (Hultberg, CCActa, 1981; 113:135; Enzyme, 1981; 26:296; Kärkkäinen, AlcoholClinExpRes, 1990; 14:187).

Erythrocyte abnormalities

Macrocytosis is common in individuals abusing alcohol (Unger, AmJMedSci, 1974; 267:281; Wu, Lancet, 1974; i:829; Buffet, ArchFrMalAppDig, 1975; 64:315; Morgan, ClinLabHaemat, 1981; 3: 35; Savage, Medicine, 1986; 63:322). Its development probably reflects a toxic effect of alcohol on maturing erythrocytes (Sullivan, JCI, 1964; 43:2048; Lindenbaum, SemHemat, 1989; 17:119). The erythrocyte mean corpuscular volume returns to within reference values approximately 3 months after cessation of alcohol (Morgan, ClinLabHaemat, 1981; 3:35). The presence of macrocytosis does not relate to the severity of the liver injury. Thus it has been observed in 100 per cent of alcohol abusers with little or no liver damage, in 82 per cent of individuals with alcoholic hepatitis, and in 89 per cent of patients with alcoholic cirrhosis (Buffet, ArchFrMalAppDig, 1975; 64:315). There is a significant sex-related difference in the incidence of macrocytosis in individuals abusing alcohol; thus in one series macrocytosis was observed in 86 per cent of women but in only 63 per cent of men (Morgan, ClinLabHaemat, 1981; 3:35).

Macrocytosis may also be observed in approximately one-fifth of individuals with non-alcoholic liver disease, but invariably the erythrocyte mean corpuscular volume does not exceed 100 fl; it exceeds this value in at least 50 per cent of individuals abusing alcohol (Morgan, ClinLabHaemat, 1981; 3:35). Macrocytosis is also observed in association with folic acid deficiency, vitamin B_{12} deficiency, and hypothyroidism; these conditions can, however, be easily distinguished.

If the blood of individuals abusing alcohol is examined by scanning electron microscopy, a high proportion of morphologically abnormal erythrocytes is observed. The finding of triangulocytes is characteristic for alcohol abuse; these cells make up 1.2 to 18.0 per cent of total red cells in alcohol abusers compared with 0 to 0.5 per cent in healthy controls and 0 to 1.3 per cent in individuals with non-alcoholic liver disease (Homaidan, BloodCells, 1986; 11:375). The number of morphologically abnormal red blood cells, including triangulocytes, decreases after withdrawal of alcohol. The technique for assessing morphological change in erythrocytes, although apparently sensitive and specific, is slow and laborious, and this limits its application.

Erythrocyte haemolysates prepared from the blood of individuals abusing alcohol show increased concentrations of minor haemoglobin fractions that migrate rapidly on cation-exchange resin chromatography (Stevens, JCI, 1981; 67:361). However, the value of these minor haemoglobins as markers for chronic alcohol abuse is disputed and more studies are needed (Hoberman, Alcoholism, 1982; 6:260; Homaidan, ClinChem, 1984; 30:480).

Other markers

A number of other potential markers for chronic alcohol abuse are currently being evaluated, including serum d,l-2,3-butanediol (Casazza, AdvAlcSubstAb, 1988; 7:33), urinary dolichols (Roine, AlcoholClinExpRes, 1987; 11:525), acetaldehyde adducts with haemoglobin, cellular and extracellular proteins (Niemelä, LabInvest, 1992; 67:246; Sillanaukee, JLabClinMed, 1992; 120:42; Hoffmann, AlcoholClinExpRes, 1993; 17:69), antibodies to acetaldehyde-modified epitopes (Israel, SemLivDis, 1988; 8:81; Niemelä, JCI, 1991; 87:1367; Worrall, EurJClinInv, 1991; 21:90; AlcAlc, 1994; 29:43), and blood phosphatidylethanol (Hansson, AlcoholClinExpRes, 1997; 21:108).

Markers of alcohol-related liver injury[21]

A number of potential markers of hepatocellular injury and/or fibrosis have been described that might be used to distinguish the various histological stages of alcohol-related liver injury. The best researched are the procollagen peptides (Hahn, JHepatol, 1984; 1: 67).

Procollagen peptides and other connective-tissue markers

The serum aminoterminal propeptide of type III procollagen (**PIIINP**) has been the most extensively studied. In general, there is agreement that serum PIIINP concentrations are elevated in patients with alcohol-related liver disease but little agreement on the relation between serum PIIINP and the histological severity of the injury (Niemelä, Gastro, 1983; 85:254; Savoläinen, Alcoholism, 1984; 8: 384; Tanaka, DigDisSci, 1986; 31:712; Annoni, Hepatol, 1989; 9: 693; Bell, ScaJGastr, 1989; 24:1217; Robert, AlcoholClinExpRes, 1989; 13:176; Niemelä, AlcoholClinExpRes, 1992; 16:1064; Trinchet, AlcoholClinExpRes, 1992; 16:342). The problem is further confounded by the fact that serum PIIINP is elevated, albeit modestly, in individuals actively abusing alcohol who do not have liver disease (van Zanten, CCActa, 1988; 177:141), and that its concentrations fall significantly after withdrawal from alcohol only to increase again when drinking resumes (Niemelä, Gastro, 1990; 98:1612).

Serum concentrations of the carboxyterminal propeptide of type I procollagen (**PICP**) and of type I collagen degradation products (**CI**) are also elevated in patients with alcoholic liver disease but not to the same extent as serum PIIINP; the relation between serum PICP and C1 concentrations and the histological degree of liver injury is unclear (Savoläinen, Alcoholism, 1984; 8:384; Niemelä, AlcoholClinExpRes, 1992; 16:1064; Trinchet, AlcoholClinExpRes, 1992; 16:342).

Serum CI and PIIINP concentrations were measured in 96 patients with alcoholic liver disease and their relation to histological scores for both fibrosis and alcoholic hepatitis assessed (Trinchet, AlcoholClinExpRes, 1992; 16:342). There were significant correlations between serum CI concentrations and the scores for fibrosis ($r = 0.27$; $p < 0.01$), and between serum PIIINP concentrations and the scores for alcoholic hepatitis ($r = 0.46$; $p < 0.0001$) and, to a lesser extent, the scores for fibrosis ($r = 0.25$; $p < 0.02$). During a follow-up of between 3 and 6 months, there were significant reductions in both serum PIIINP and the score for alcoholic hepatitis but the correlation between individual variations of the two was not significant; no significant changes were observed in either serum CI or the score for fibrosis over the same period. Thus, these markers of collagen metabolism might be useful in assessing the evolution of liver injury over time.

Other collagen and non-collagen connective-tissue markers have also been investigated in patients with alcohol-related liver injury, including the carboxyterminal propeptide of type IV procollagen and type VI collagen (Niemelä, AlcoholClinExpRes, 1992; 16:1064; Shahin, Hepatol, 1992; 15:637; Fabris, AnnClinBioch, 1997; 2:151), the glycoprotein laminin (Nouchi, AlcoholClinExpRes, 1987; 11: 287; Annoni, Hepatol, 1989; 9:693; Lotterer, JHepatol, 1992; 14:71; Niemelä, AlcoholClinExpRes, 1992; 16:1064), and the proteoglycan hyaluronate (Ueno, Gastro, 1993; 105:475).

Serum PICP, PIIINP, the 7s domain of type IV collagen, and laminin fragment PI concentrations were measured in 35 alcohol abusers, and their relation to the degree of histological liver injury assessed (Niemelä, AlcoholClinExpRes, 1992; 16:1064). Serum PICP, PIIINP, type IV collagen, and laminin were elevated in 58, 90, 85 and 77 per cent of individuals, respectively; the highest concentrations were found in those with the most severe disease. The correlation with the histological degree of severity was strongest for serum PIIINP and weakest for serum PICP. During the follow-up period, serum concentrations of PIIINP, type IV collagen, and laminin fell in the patients who reduced their alcohol consumption but remained high in those who continued to drink. In contrast, serum PICP fell irrespective of drinking behaviour. The investigators suggested that as PICP and PIIINP are metabolized by different hepatic pathways, use of the serum PIIINP:PICP ratio might improve the sensitivity of these measurements for detecting significant liver injury.

Serum concentrations of PIIINP, PICP, type IV collagen, and serum prolyl hydroxylase activity were measured in 100 patients with cirrhosis and 71 patients with non-cirrhotic chronic liver disease (Fabris, AnnClinBioch, 1997; 34:151). Patients with cirrhosis had significantly higher mean values for all four markers, even after stratification for alcohol intake. Both serum PIIINP and type IV collagen were independently associated with the presence of cirrhosis and more clearly differentiated the cirrhotic patients from their non-cirrhotic counterparts than either serum PICP or prolyl hydroxylase.

Cytokines

Tumour necrosis factor is a peptide secreted by monocytes, macrophages, and lymphocytes; it is a major immune modulator. Its plasma concentrations are significantly raised in patients with severe alcoholic hepatitis (McClain, Hepatol, 1989; 9:349; Bird, AnnIntMed, 1990; 112:917; Felver, Alcoholism, 1990; 14:255). No overlap was found between the plasma concentrations of this peptide in patients with severe alcoholic hepatitis and in alcohol abusers with little or no liver disease (Bird, AnnIntMed, 1990; 112:917). However, there was a degree of overlap in plasma concentrations between patients with severe alcoholic hepatitis and those with alcoholic cirrhosis who were abstinent from alcohol.

Interleukin 8 is a cytokine that also has a role in neutrophil activation. It is generated by a variety of cells including hepatocytes; its release is stimulated by endotoxin, interleukin 1, and tumour necrosis factor. Serum interleukin-8 concentrations are markedly elevated in patients with severe alcoholic hepatitis (Sheron, Hepatol,

1993; 18:14). However, elevated concentrations, albeit not of the same degree, are also observed in alcohol abusers with little or no liver disease, and in patients with inactive alcoholic cirrhosis (Sheron, Hepatol, 1993; 18:14).

Serum F protein

It has been suggested that serum F protein may be a sensitive and specific marker for hepatocellular damage (Foster, CCActa, 1989; 184:85). F protein is a 44-kDa protein found in the liver that circulates in low concentration in serum, where it can be detected using a radioimmunoassay. F protein has been measured in patients with a variety of disorders and significantly raised concentrations found only in those with hepatocellular damage (Foster, CCActa, 1989; 184:85). In these individuals the serum F protein concentration was a more sensitive and specific marker of liver damage than conventional liver function tests, and showed a highly significant correlation with the histological grade of liver injury. More information is required.

Intracellular adhesion molecule I

Intracellular adhesion molecule I mediates the migration of lymphocytes from the circulation to sites of inflammation. Serum concentrations of the circulating, soluble form of the molecule are elevated in patients with alcohol-related liver disease and correlate significantly with the histological severity of the liver injury (Douds, JHepatol, 1997; 26:280). Further studies are needed.

Other laboratory tests

It is obviously important that potential indicators of non-alcoholic liver disease, such as serum viral markers, autoantibodies, iron, percentage transferrin saturation and ferritin, α_1-antitrypsin, and copper and caeruloplasmin are also measured.

Choice of laboratory tests[17–22]

There are a large number of laboratory variables whose values increase or decrease in individuals chronically abusing alcohol. However, there is no one marker that is sufficiently sensitive or specific to provide a 'gold standard' for detecting chronic alcohol abuse. Combining the results of several tests may yield a greater incidence of abnormalities than when each test is used individually, thereby increasing sensitivity and diagnostic specificity. Commonly used combinations of test results include serum γ-glutamyl transferase and erythrocyte mean corpuscular volume (Chick, Lancet, 1981; i:1249; Pol, Alcoholism, 1990; 14:250), serum γ-glutamyl transferase, serum aspartate aminotransferase, and erythrocyte mean corpuscular volume (Morgan, BrJAlcAlc, 1981; 16:167), the serum aspartate:alanine aminotransferase ratio and erythrocyte mean corpuscular volume (Kawachi, NZMedJ, 1990; 103:145), the serum aspartate:alanine aminotransferase ratio and serum IgA, and, more recently, combinations including serum carbohydrate-deficient transferrin (Anton, AlcoholClinExpRes, 1996; 20:841; Helander, AlcAlc, 1996; 31:101; 1997; 32:133). Use of these test combinations can detect chronic alcohol abuse with sensitivities and specificities in excess of 90 per cent.

A number of sophisticated mathematical techniques have been used, involving multiple laboratory-test results, to try to improve the detection rate of chronic alcohol abuse. For example, quadratic discriminant analysis has been applied to the results of 18 commonly requested biochemical tests, measured on a multichannel analyser, together with measurements of serum γ-glutamyl transferase activity and erythrocyte mean corpuscular volume, to try to distinguish between individuals who are abusing alcohol and non-habitual drinkers (Eckardt, JAMA, 1981; 246:2707). The combination of serum γ-glutamyl transferase activity and erythrocyte mean corpuscular volume correctly categorized patients with an accuracy of 77 per cent, whereas a combination of all routine liver function tests, urea, and electrolytes correctly categorized patients with 95 per cent accuracy. In general, multiple tests and combination analyses identify more alcohol abusers than single procedures. However, in most instances, the use of a combination of two or three simple, automated procedures should suffice.

Laboratory test results will not readily distinguish the degree of histological alcohol-related liver injury. However, a simple index has been devised, based on laboratory test results, to determine the severity of alcohol-related liver injury, thereby, it has been asserted, dispensing with the need for liver biopsy (Poynard, Gastro, 1991; 100:1397). The results of the three test variables, namely the prothrombin (P) time, the serum γ-glutamyl transferase (G) activity, and the serum apolipoprotein-A_1 (A) concentration are scored from 0 (no abnormality) to 4 (severe abnormality). The so-called **PGA** index is the sum of the three individual scores and so can range from 0 to 12. When the PGA index is less than 2, the probability of cirrhosis is zero while the probability of a normal or minimally damaged liver is 83 per cent; conversely, when the PGA index equals or exceeds 9, the probability of cirrhosis is 86 per cent while the probability of a normal or minimally damaged liver is zero. While this index might be useful for screening purposes, it is unlikely that its use will obviate the need for a tissue diagnosis.

Alcohol-related and non-alcoholic liver disease arising in individuals who abuse alcohol may also be biochemically indistinguishable. However, sophisticated mathematical techniques have been applied to various laboratory tests to aid in their distinction. For example, the results of 25 haematological and biochemical tests from patients with alcohol-related and non-alcohol-related liver disease were assessed by quadratic discriminant analysis; serum γ-glutamyl transferase activity was not measured (Ryback, JAMA, 1982; 248:2261). With this technique, 96 per cent of patients with alcohol-related and 89 per cent of patients with non-alcohol-related liver disease were correctly classified. Using only the nine 'best' tests, which were the routine liver function tests, urea, glucose, and erythrocyte and leucocyte counts, the percentage of patients correctly classified fell to 92 and 80 per cent, respectively. However, a similar degree of discrimination to that obtained with the nine 'best' tests could be obtained by simply using the ratio of the serum asparate:alanine aminotransferase activities.

Discriminant function analysis has been used to distinguish individuals with alcohol-related liver disease from those with non-alcohol-related liver disease and from non-habitual drinkers attending a gastroenterology clinic (Chalmers, Gut, 1981; 22:992). The best discriminant was a combination of serum γ-glutamyl transferase activity, serum alkaline phosphatase activity, and erythrocyte mean corpuscular volume, use of which correctly allocated more than 80 per cent of the patients. However, discrimination was better among women than men. Thus, 92 per cent of women with

Histological findings	Patients (n)	Clinical and biochemical findings	
		None	Hepatomegaly ± biochemical abnormalities
Normal liver	38	30	8
Fatty change	50	21	29
Alcoholic hepatitis	11	2	9
Chronic hepatitis	12	5	7
Cirrhosis	9	2	7
Others	34	25	9
Totals	154	85	69

Table 3 Comparison of clinical, biochemical, and histological findings in 154 individuals chronically abusing alcohol

Data extracted from Bruguera, ArchPathLabMed, 1977; 101: 644.

alcoholic liver disease, 87 per cent with non-alcoholic liver disease, and 100 per cent attending a gastroenterology clinic were correctly identified; the corresponding figures for men were 80, 71, and 100 per cent.

Thus multiple tests and combination analyses will allow better discrimination between alcohol-related and non alcohol-related liver disease but this approach may not be cost-effective.

Histology [23–26]

Histological examination of liver tissue will allow, first, confirmation of a diagnosis of alcoholic liver disease, second, accurate staging of the degree of liver injury, and third, exclusion of other or additional liver diseases.

Patients who have regularly misused or abused alcohol over a period of years may well have sustained liver injury. However, neither the presence of injury nor its severity can be assessed accurately from clinical and laboratory variables alone (Ricketts, Gastro, 1951; 17:184; Green, AustAnnMed, 1965; 14:111; Bruguera, ArchPathLabMed, 1977; 101:644; Rankin, Alcoholism, 1978; 2: 327). Thus, in a study in which liver biopsies were obtained in 154 individuals admitted to an alcoholism treatment unit, no clinical or biochemical evidence of liver disease was found in 85 patients yet the liver biopsy was abnormal in 55 (65 per cent) (Bruguera, ArchPathLabMed, 1977; 101:644). The remaining 69 patients had hepatomegaly and/or abnormal biochemical test results but the liver biopsy was normal or showed only minimal change in eight (12 per cent) (Table 3).

In another study, 50 per cent of individuals with alcoholic cirrhosis were found to have minimal or, at most, moderate clinical and laboratory abnormalities, while approximately 10 per cent of individuals abusing alcohol who had no clinical or laboratory evidence of liver disease had a histological diagnosis of cirrhosis (Rankin, Alcoholism, 1978; 2:327). Liver biopsy is therefore mandatory for accurate diagnosis.

The concordance for intra- and interobserver assessments of liver histology from individuals abusing alcohol is generally excellent. In one study, intraobserver error in the histological assessment of two needle biopsies taken simultaneously from 70 consecutive patients was evaluated (Baunsgaard, ActaPMScandA, 1979; 87:51). Unidentified samples were dispatched to the pathologist on separate days and the results of the semiquantitative assessments compared. The concordance for features such as cirrhosis, cholestasis, and steatosis was high, while the concordance for some of the more minor features, such as acidophilic bodies and bile-duct proliferation, was low. Allowance has to be made for the fact that, although the biopsies were taken simultaneously, there may still have been sampling errors.

Independent evaluations made by two pathologists of liver biopsies from 362 individuals chronically abusing alcohol have also been compared (Bedossa, Alcoholism, 1988; 12:173). There was perfect concordance for the presence of cirrhosis and hepatocellular carcinoma, and substantial concordance for fibrous septa, size of nodules, and liver-cell regeneration. In terms of overall diagnosis the concordance was substantial for cirrhosis with acute alcoholic hepatitis, cirrhosis without alcoholic hepatitis, acute alcoholic hepatitis, and normal liver histology. Concordance was moderate for steatosis and slight for fibrosis alone.

Individuals who chronically abuse alcohol may develop nonalcoholic liver injury. In one study 20 per cent of a group of individuals with a history of alcohol abuse and disturbed liver function tests had histological evidence of non-alcoholic liver disease including, cholangitis, viral hepatitis, granulomas, congestion, and tumours (Levin, AmJMed, 1979; 66:429). The patients with non-alcoholic liver disease were indistinguishable both clinically and by their laboratory test results from those with alcoholic liver injury. This study has been criticized (Atterbury, JClinGastr, 1988; 10: 605), because both the 'alcohol' histories and the prebiopsy work-up of the patients were thought to be suboptimal; as a result it has been suggested that the proportion of individuals abusing alcohol who have non-alcoholic liver disease was overestimated. Nevertheless, the fact remains that some individuals who abuse alcohol develop non-alcoholic liver disease that is not discernible other than on liver biopsy.

It has been suggested that liver biopsy may not be necessary for the diagnosis of alcoholic liver disease. In one study, 108 consecutive patients admitted for evaluation of potential liver injury were assessed (Talley, JClinGastr, 1988; 10:647). A clinical diagnosis was made, based on data obtained from interview and examination, including an alcohol history, and from laboratory data, including liver function tests, erythrocyte mean corpuscular volume, serum ferritin, and hepatitis B serology. The clinical diagnosis was then compared with the histological diagnosis made on liver biopsy material.

A clinical diagnosis of primary alcoholic liver disease was made in 27 individuals and this was confirmed histologically in 25; in the remaining two there was histological evidence of either haemochromatosis or common bile-duct obstruction. A clinical diagnosis of mixed alcoholic and non-alcoholic liver disease was made in eight patients; histological examination revealed primary alcoholic liver disease in seven and haemochromatosis in one. A clinical diagnosis of non-alcoholic liver disease was made in 73 patients; in five the histological diagnosis was of primary alcoholic liver disease while in a further four there was evidence of mixed alcoholic and non-alcoholic liver injury (Table 4).

The investigators concluded, on the basis of their data, that liver biopsy is not necessary to identify patients with alcoholic liver disease. If anything, however, their data emphasize the need to undertake this procedure. In 37 patients the primary histological diagnosis was of alcoholic liver disease; this was correctly diagnosed on clinical grounds in 25 (71 per cent) but was completely missed in 5 (13.5 per cent); in the remaining seven patients (18.9 per cent), additional clinical diagnoses were made. In six patients the histological diagnosis was of mixed alcoholic and non-alcoholic liver disease; the clinical diagnoses were of alcoholic liver disease in two and non-alcoholic liver disease in four. One individual with haemochromatosis was erroneously diagnosed on clinical grounds as having alcoholic liver disease. Although they correctly diagnosed alcohol-related liver injury in 71 per cent of patients on the basis of clinical and laboratory findings, they were not able to determine the degree of liver injury. Of greater concern was the fact that they missed the diagnosis of alcoholic liver disease in 8 per cent of individuals overall, and missed significant non-alcoholic lesions in 8 per cent of alcohol abusers. This argues strongly in favour of histological diagnosis.

The usefulness of percutaneous liver biopsy was determined in 90 patients with chronically elevated serum aminotransferase or γ-glutamyl transferase activities by comparing diagnoses made before and after the procedure (Van Ness, AnnIntMed, 1989; 111:473). Clinical diagnoses included alcoholic liver disease (26), non-alcoholic fatty liver (19), necroinflammatory conditions (25), and miscellaneous (20). Overall, 88 per cent of the patients subsequently diagnosed as having alcoholic liver disease were correctly identified, but the degree of liver injury was consistently underestimated. In five patients (19 per cent) diagnosed clinically as having alcoholic liver disease, liver biopsy revealed a variety of non-alcohol-related conditions, all requiring specific therapy. The investigators concluded that liver biopsy material should be examined in order to achieve maximum diagnostic accuracy.

Liver biopsy should be performed in all individuals who are actively abusing alcohol and who have hepatomegaly and/or disturbed liver function tests. The biopsy should not be undertaken by the percutaneous route unless the prothrombin time is within 3 s of control and the platelet count exceeds $80\,000 \times 10^9/l$. The specimen obtained with a Menghini needle is usually adequate. If there are concerns about the safety of a blind needle procedure because of coagulopathy and/or ascites, then the biopsy can be undertaken under radiological guidance, plugging the biopsy site in

Table 4 Comparison of diagnoses made in patients with chronic liver disease before and after liver biopsy

Clinical diagnosis	Patients (n)	Histology	Patients (n)
Alcohol-related	27	Alcohol-related	25
		Alcohol-related plus haemochromatosis or biliary obstruction	1 1
Mixed alcohol- and non-alcohol-related	8	Alcohol-related	7
		Haemochromatosis	1
Non-alcohol-related	73	Alcohol-related	5
		Mixed alcohol- and non-alcohol-related	4
		Non-alcohol-related	64

Data extracted from Talley, JClinGastro, 1988; 10: 647.

the liver on exit, or can be obtained by the transjugular route or at peritoneoscopy.

Other procedures

A number of other procedures have been used to diagnose the presence and severity of alcohol-related liver disease, including ultrasonography and computerized tomographic liver imaging, and magnetic resonance spectroscopy.

Ultrasound scanning was used to assess 85 patients with histologically proven liver disease, 50 of whom were abusing alcohol (Saverymuttu, BMJ, 1986; 292:13). Steatosis was identified with a sensitivity of 94 per cent and a specificity of 84 per cent, but fibrosis was less reliably detected with a sensitivity of 57 per cent and a specificity of 88 per cent. Abnormal scanning results were obtained in 94 per cent of the 50 patients known to have alcoholic liver disease. The investigators suggest that ultrasound scanning might be usefully employed to screen individuals presenting with non-specific gastrointestinal symptoms who deny alcohol misuse or abuse.

A quantitative, real-time ultrasonographic method, in which the degree of echogenicity of the patients' hepatic parenchyma is compared with that of a tissue-mimicking phantom, was used to assess patients with chronic liver disease (Medhat, Gastro, 1988; 94:157). The mean density ratio of the phantom to patients' liver was 1.04 in 30 reference individuals, 1.23 in 26 patients with early alcoholic liver disease, and 1.54 in 74 patients with cirrhosis. The differences in the mean density ratios between the groups were significant, and there was also a significant correlation between the density ratio and the functional grade of cirrhosis assessed using a modified Child's classification (Pugh, BrJSurg, 1973; 60:646).

In patients with alcoholic hepatitis, ultrasonography may show the so-called pseudoparallel channel sign. These parallel tubular structures are formed within the liver subsegments by juxtaposition of a dilated hepatic arterial branch and an adjacent portal venous branch. This sign was observed in 90 per cent of patients with biopsy-proven alcoholic hepatitis and in 23 per cent of individuals with other forms of alcohol-related liver injury, only less extensively (Sumino, Gastro, 1993; 105:1477). This feature was not observed in healthy volunteers or in patients with non-alcoholic liver disease. The sensitivity and specificity of this sign for diagnosing alcoholic hepatitis were 82 and 87 per cent, respectively. Further studies are warranted.

In patients with alcoholic liver disease, liver and spleen volumes, as assessed by computed tomography, are increased. The liver volume increases progressively with increasing severity of liver injury (Tarao, Hepatol, 1989; 9:589) and is significantly greater in patients with alcoholic rather than non-alcoholic liver disease (Sato, JHepatol, 1989; 8:150). The increase in hepatic volume is attributed to ballooning of hepatocytes and to an increase in fibrous tissue. Spleen volumes are increased in individuals with advanced liver disease, independently of its cause, presumably as a result of congestion secondary to portal hypertension. The correlation between liver and spleen volumes varies depending on the aetiological background of the liver injury, being negative in non-alcoholic and positive in alcoholic liver injury (Sato, JHepatol, 1989; 8:150). Abstinence from alcohol is associated with a decrease in the volumes of both organs. It has been suggested that computed tomographic

assessment of liver and spleen volumes could be used to identify the presence of advanced liver disease and to delineate its aetiological background (Sato, JHepatol, 1989; 8:150).

It has also been suggested that computed tomographic scanning might provide a convenient non-invasive method to screen for fatty liver in individuals misusing or abusing alcohol (Allaway, JRSocMed, 1988; 81:149). The mean attenuation value of the liver (CT number) is reduced in individuals with fatty change because of the associated reduction in liver density. A rise in CT number is observed when fatty change regresses.

At present neither ultrasonographic nor computed tomographic scanning can be used to differentiate accurately between the various stages of alcoholic liver disease or to exclude the presence of non-alcoholic liver injury; technological advances may improve their diagnostic potential (Sugano, DigDisSci, 1992; 37:220).

In vivo hepatic magnetic resonance spectroscopy can be used to assess the degree of liver injury in patients chronically abusing alcohol. Hepatic ^{31}P magnetic resonance spectroscopy was undertaken in 26 individuals chronically abusing alcohol who had liver disease of varying severity (Menon, Gastro, 1995; 108:776). The initial spectra clearly distinguished between individuals in relation to the severity of their liver injury (Fig. 1). The spectral changes in individuals with minimal liver injury reflected alterations in hepatic redox potential and induction of the hepatocyte endoplasmic reticulum; abstinence from alcohol resulted in reversal of the changes within 2 weeks. In patients with more significant liver injury the effects on redox potential and the endoplasmic reticulum were attenuated as hepatocytes were replaced with fibrous tissue, while further changes were observed that reflected alterations in cell-membrane components related to the regenerative process; abstinence from alcohol was associated with evolution of the spectral changes to a pattern of residual but stable abnormality, the degree of abnormality being determined by the degree of hepatic decompensation.

The hepatic triglyceride content can also be quantified accurately and non-invasively in individuals abusing alcohol by either localized ^{1}H magnetic resonance spectroscopy with simulated echoes (Thomsen, MagResImag, 1994; 12:487) or ^{13}C magnetic resonance spectroscopy with lipid phantoms (Petersen, Hepatol, 1996; 24:114).

Magnetic resonance spectroscopy is a technique that has great potential for assessing the degree of liver damage in patients with alcohol-related liver injury and for monitoring progress over time. However, it is expensive, labour-intensive, intrinsically insensitive, and currently relatively inaccessible. These factors limit its application.

A number of techniques may be used to obtain important diagnostic information in patients already suspected or known to have alcoholic liver disease. Upper gastrointestinal endoscopy may reveal oesophageal varices and/or hypertensive gastropathy, thereby confirming the presence of portal hypertension and, most likely, advanced liver disease. Psychometric tests and electroencephalography may be used to detect hepatic encephalopathy; its presence indicates significant liver disease and/or extensive portal–systemic shunting of blood. Ultrasonographic and computed tomographic scanning may be used to confirm the presence of a collateral circulation, to assess the biliary and pancreatic systems when cholestasis is prominent, and to search for space-occupying lesions within the liver. Endoscopic cholangiopancreatography or

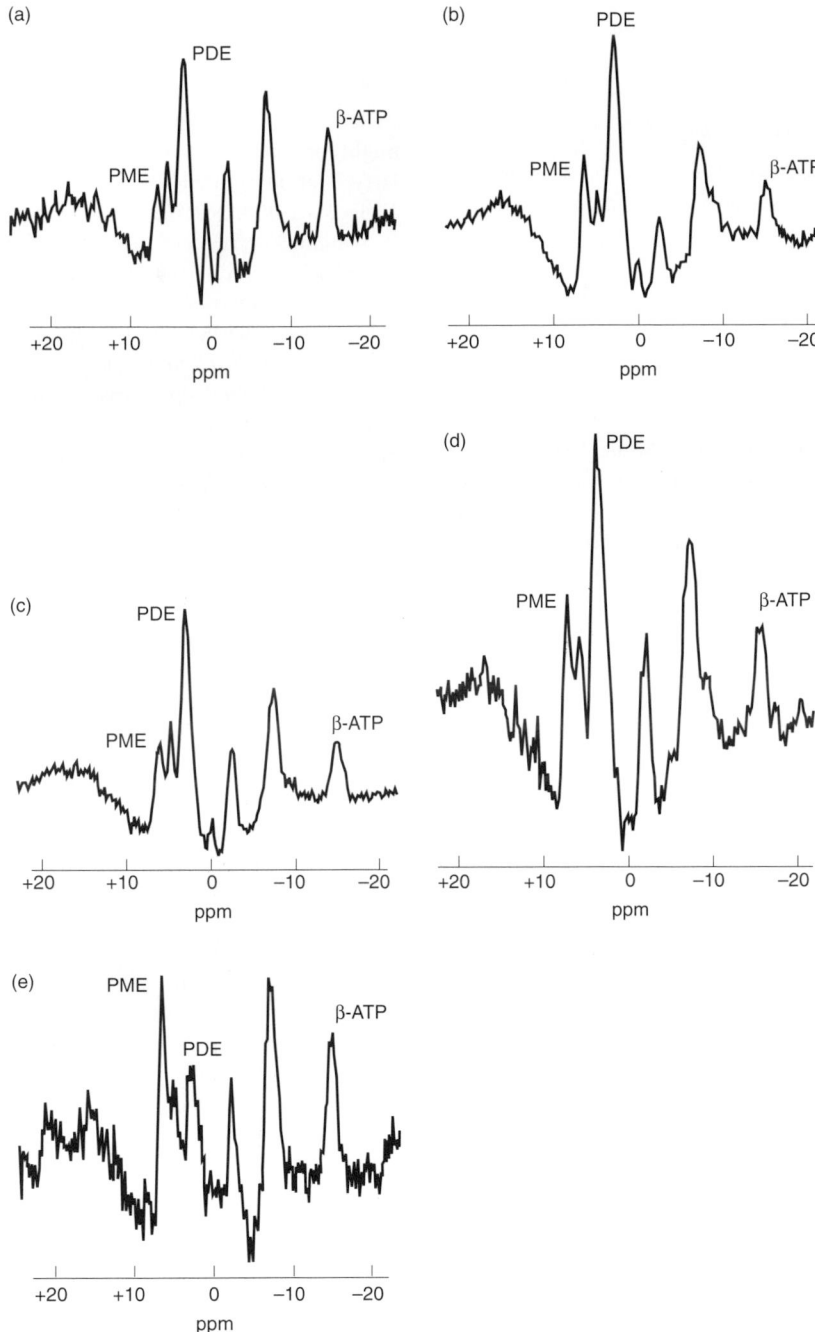

Fig. 1. Localized hepatic ^{31}P magnetic resonance spectra acquired from (a) a healthy male, (b) a woman with hepatic steatosis actively abusing alcohol, (c) a woman with alcoholic hepatitis actively abusing alcohol, (d) a man with compensated alcoholic cirrhosis actively abusing alcohol, and (e) a man with decompensated alcoholic cirrhosis actively drinking alcohol. PME, phosphomonoesters; PDE, phosphodiesters; ATP, adenosine triphosphate.

percutaneous cholangiography may be needed to investigate cholestasis further, while angiography, peritoneoscopy, and guided liver biopsy may be needed to determine the exact nature of any intrahepatic space-occupying lesions.

Clinical presentation[12–16]

Chronic alcohol abuse is associated with the development of three, distinct, histological lesions in the liver—alcoholic fatty change,

alcoholic hepatitis, and alcoholic cirrhosis—although these may overlap. The symptoms and signs associated with these histological lesions are not, however, distinct so that patients cannot easily be distinguished on the basis of clinical and laboratory data alone. Thus, although clinical presentation is usually described in relation to the underlying histological lesion, it is important to realize that the whole clinical spectrum of alcoholic liver disease, which extends from asymptomatic hepatomegaly to profound hepatocellular failure, can be observed in relation to any histological subtype. It is also important to recognize that the degree of clinical 'illness' associated with the development of alcoholic liver disease can vary enormously. Thus, patients with almost identical histological lesions may present with widely differing clinical pictures; in general, women present more floridly than men.

Most individuals with alcoholic liver disease, irrespective of its histological subtype, present in middle age. The male:female ratio is generally 3:1, despite the fact that the number of women abusing alcohol is said to have increased in recent years. The majority of these individuals have been drinking regularly for more than 10 years, with daily alcohol intakes averaging 180 to 200 g in men and 120 to 150 g in women. They present most often with non-specific digestive symptoms; hepatomegaly is the most common physical sign and increased serum γ-glutamyl transferase activity is the most frequently observed laboratory abnormality.

Alcoholic fatty liver

The majority of patients with simple fatty liver are asymptomatic, although some complain of right upper-quadrant pain or non-specific digestive symptoms such as nausea, anorexia, epigastric discomfort, or bowel disturbances. Approximately 30 to 50 per cent of such individuals are referred with an incidental finding of hepatomegaly and/or raised serum aminotransferases. Fatty change may be associated with quite marked cholestasis (Leevy, Arch-IntMed, 1953; 92:527; Ballard, AmJMed, 1961; 30:196), which is predominantly intrahepatic in origin (Popper, Gastro, 1956; 31: 683). Rarely, fatty liver may be complicated by hyperlipidaemia, haemolytic anaemia, and jaundice—the so-called Zieve syndrome (Zieve, AnnIntMed, 1958; 48:471); exceptionally fatty liver may be accompanied by profound hepatocellular failure (Morgan, ScaJ-Gastr, 1978; 13:299).

Hepatomegaly is the most common physical finding (Leevy, Medicine, 1962; 41:249);[12–16] the liver edge may extend only a few centimetres below the costal margin or may reach the iliac crest; the liver is smooth, regular, relatively firm, and only minimally tender. There is no correlation between the size of the liver and the severity of the clinical symptoms. Spider naevi, cutaneous telangiectasia, palmar erythema, parotid enlargement, Dupuytren's contractures, gynaecomastia, and testicular atrophy may be present. Jaundice, ascites, and splenomegaly are observed in a very small minority of patients.

The most common biochemical abnormalities are elevation of the serum γ-glutamyl transferase and aspartate aminotransferase activities.[12–16] The serum bilirubin may be mildly increased in 20 to 30 per cent of individuals, while elevation of serum alkaline phosphatase is observed in about 50 per cent. Blood urea and serum potassium concentrations are often low; the serum urate is often elevated and there may be hyperlipidaemia. The serum albumin is normal or low, and significant elevations of serum IgA and occasionally of serum IgM may be seen. Up to one-third of patients are mildly anaemic and there may be thrombocytopenia, which can be profound. Macrocytosis is commonly observed; the prothrombin time may be prolonged but is easily corrected with parenteral vitamin K_1. The majority of laboratory abnormalities show marked improvement, if not complete reversal, with abstinence from alcohol, in a relatively short period of time. The liver biopsy shows accumulation of triglycerides that may be mild, moderate, or severe in extent.

Alcoholic hepatitis

Alcoholic hepatitis may vary in its presentation from a mild anicteric illness with hepatomegaly to a fulminant illness with jaundice, ascites, gastrointestinal bleeding, and hepatic coma, which may be fatal (Lischner, AmJDigDis, 1971; 16:481; Gregory, AmJDigDis, 1972; 17:479). Approximately 60 per cent of individuals with mild to moderate alcoholic hepatitis on liver biopsy present with non-specific symptoms such as anorexia, fatigue, lethargy, and epigastric or right hypochondrial pain, or with an incidental finding of hepatomegaly and/or raised serum aminotransferases; some 10 to 15 per cent will present with jaundice.[8–12] Patients with severe alcoholic hepatitis on liver biopsy tend to present with more specific symptoms suggestive of hepatocellular failure, such as jaundice, ascites, and hepatic encephalopathy, or with variceal haemorrhage (Reynolds, AnnIntMed, 1969; 70:497).[12–16] Many patients with the more severe form of the illness report a reduction in food intake in the weeks or months before presentation, and possibly an increase in alcohol intake.

Overall, patients with alcoholic hepatitis are more ill than those with simple fatty liver. Women generally present with more florid illness than men, and in both sexes the severity of the clinical signs increases with the histological severity of the liver lesion (Harinasuta, Gastro, 1971; 60:1036).[12–16] The majority of individuals have hepatomegaly; the liver is mild to moderately enlarged and may be tender on palpation; an arterial bruit may be heard over the liver area in the more severely ill patients. Ascites is present in from 30 to 60 per cent of patients, and splenomegaly in present in approximately 15 per cent. At least 50 per cent of patients are jaundiced. A proportion of the more severely ill patients will show evidence of hepatic encephalopathy and/or portal hypertension. Fever is a feature in 50 per cent of patients and may be prominent. Spider naevi, cutaneous telangiectasia, and palmar erythema are usually present and may be florid; parotid enlargement, Dupuytren's contractures, gynaecomastia, and testicular atrophy are present in 10 to 20 per cent of patients. Cutaneous bruising may be marked, particularly at intravenous puncture sites; healing is generally poor. Central cyanosis is observed in the more severely ill patients and results, primarily, from intrapulmonary arteriovenous shunting of blood (Berthelot, NEJM, 1966; 274:291).

Serum γ-glutamyl transferase and aspartate aminotransferase activities are invariably increased, and are generally higher than in other forms of alcoholic liver disease; nevertheless, concentrations are still modestly elevated in relation to the degree of hepatocellular necrosis, with serum aspartate aminotransferase rarely exceeding 10 times the upper reference limit.[12–16] Two-thirds of patients will show increased serum bilirubin and alkaline phosphatase concentrations. Blood urea and serum potassium levels tend to be low unless renal failure supervenes; serum sodium concentrations are in the low reference range. Serum urate and plasma lipids are variously elevated. Approximately 50 per cent of individuals are hypo-albuminaemic, while serum IgA and IgM concentrations are raised. Over half of the patients are anaemic and macrocytosis is prominent. There is a polymorphonuclear leucocytosis in all but the most mildly ill. The platelet count is reduced and the prothrombin time is prolonged, and is, in the more severely ill patients, incompletely reversed by parenteral vitamin K_1. Approximately 15 to 20 per cent

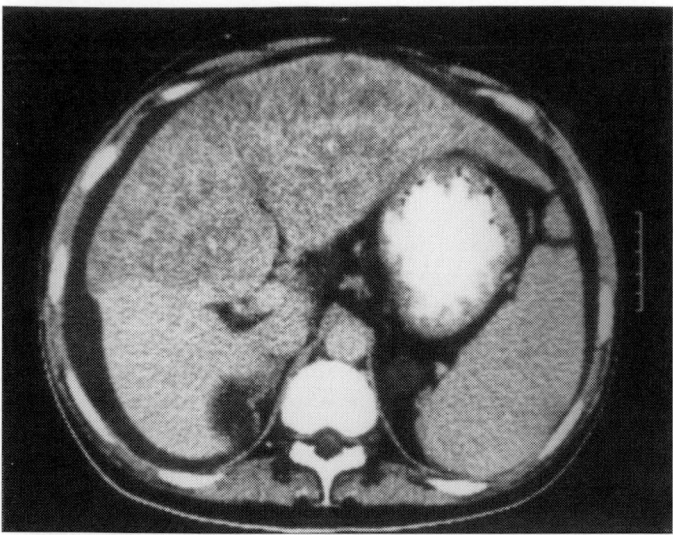

Fig. 2. Computed tomographic scan of the liver of a patient with severe alcoholic hepatitis showing a 'pseudotumour' appearance (illustration kindly provided by S. Sherlock).

of individuals will show significant serum titres of smooth-muscle and/or antinuclear antibodies.

Patients with alcoholic hepatitis may show a sudden and quite marked deterioration in their clinical condition once admitted to hospital (Hardison, NEJM, 1966; 275:61; Helman, AnnIntMed, 1971; 74:311; Lischner, AmJDigDis, 1971; 16:481; Sabesin, Gastro, 1978; 74:276; Marshall, Alcoholism, 1983; 7:312). Some form of deterioration is seen in up to 40 per cent of individuals with moderate or severe alcoholic hepatitis on liver biopsy, generally within 2 weeks of admission. In the majority this is manifest as a deterioration in laboratory-test results, but some develop gastro-intestinal bleeding, ascites, or encephalopathy. The most likely explanation for this deterioration is the sudden withdrawal of alcohol, with its associated metabolic and nutritional consequences. In the weeks or months before admission many of these patients will have relied on alcohol as their main energy source; when it is withdrawn they rapidly starve.

The combination of fever, jaundice, tender hepatomegaly, and marked leucocytosis in an acutely ill patient may lead to an erroneous diagnosis of hepatic abscess or biliary-tract disease. Errors in diagnosis such as these can have disastrous consequences for patients, particularly if, as a result, they are subjected to surgery (Mikkelsen, AmJSurg, 1968; 116:266; Orloff, AnnNYAcadSci, 1975; 252:159). The results of ultrasonographic and computed tomographic scanning, and of liver biopsy, will differentiate these conditions. The presence of an hepatic arterial bruit in a malnourished patient may suggest a diagnosis of hepatocellular carcinoma. Further investigations can be misleading, for the appearance on computed tomographic scanning and on angiography may suggest multiple tumours (Fig. 2).

This 'pseudotumour' appearance arises because of intense focal regenerative hyperplasia of liver tissue (Nagasue, Cancer, 1984; 54:2487; Kong, JClinGastr, 1990; 12:437). Serum α-fetoprotein concentrations may also be raised in patients in the regenerative phase of alcoholic hepatitis, although they rarely exceed three times the upper reference limit. Liver biopsy is mandatory to differentiate

these conditions. The centrizonal lesion of acute alcoholic hepatitis, with liver-cell swelling, focal inflammation with neutrophil infiltration, pericellular fibrosis, and varying degrees of steatosis, necrosis and cholestasis, is characteristic.

Alcoholic cirrhosis

The clinical spectrum of alcoholic cirrhosis, as with other forms of alcohol-related liver disease, varies widely from anicteric, asymptomatic hepatomegaly to profound hepatocellular failure with portal hypertension.[12–16] However, whereas patients who present with fatty change and alcoholic hepatitis have usually been abusing alcohol up to the time of presentation, patients presenting with cirrhosis may not have abused alcohol for many years. Under these circumstances they usually present with an incidental finding of hepatomegaly and/or raised serum aminotransferases, perhaps detected at a screening medical examination, or else with one of the major complications of cirrhosis such as ascites or variceal haemorrhage; they may present initially with symptoms and signs of hepatocellular carcinoma. Patients with alcoholic cirrhosis who are actively abusing alcohol are more likely to present with features of decompensation, probably because of the presence of superimposed alcoholic hepatitis.

Patients with alcoholic cirrhosis tend to present differently to specialist and non-specialist units.[12–16] Thus, in Great Britain, 10 to 20 per cent of patients with alcoholic cirrhosis presenting to District General Hospitals are diagnosed at autopsy. Of those diagnosed during life, 40 to 90 per cent present with features of hepatocellular failure such as jaundice, ascites and hepatic encephalopathy; a further 10 to 15 per cent present with gastrointestinal bleeding. In contrast, 30 to 50 per cent of patients with alcoholic cirrhosis diagnosed at specialist centres present with either non-specific digestive disorders or with hepatomegaly and/or raised serum aminotransferase activities; rather fewer present with jaundice, fluid retention, or encephalopathy; under 20 per cent present with gastrointestinal bleeding.

Patients with well-compensated cirrhosis may be asymptomatic or else complain of non-specific symptoms such as anorexia, malaise, and lethargy. Patients with decompensated cirrhosis develop major clinical symptoms in relation to the complications of cirrhosis, including jaundice, peripheral oedema, ascites, and gastrointestinal haemorrhage. The development of profound weight loss, pain in the right upper quadrant of the abdomen, an hepatic arterial bruit, rapidly accumulating ascites, and massive, uncontrollable gastrointestinal haemorrhage may signal the presence of hepatocellular carcinoma.

The most common physical sign in patients with alcoholic cirrhosis is hepatomegaly.[12–16] The liver is usually mild to moderately enlarged, firm with an irregular outline and surface; it may be tender in the presence of superadded alcoholic hepatitis, and substantially enlarged and irregular in the presence of hepatocellular carcinoma. Splenomegaly is not a prominent feature, the spleen being palpable in less than 25 per cent of patients; the presence of marked splenomegaly should prompt a search for other disorders. Other features of portal hypertension, such as collateral veins in the abdominal wall and oesophageal varices, will be present in at least 60 per cent of patients. Jaundice is observed in one-third of patients, and ascites and peripheral oedema in 30 to 40 per cent; a minority of patients will develop a right-sided pleural effusion (Johnson, AnnIntMed, 1964; 61:385). Features of hepatic encephalopathy, such as cerebral impairment and a flapping tremor, may be present in up to one-third of patients, although considerably more will show evidence of subclinical hepatic encephalopathy on psychometric testing (Gitlin, JHepatol, 1986; 3:75). A low-grade, continuous fever is common in patients with decompensated disease (Tisdale, NEJM, 1961; 265:928).

Other features, such as spider naevi, cutaneous telangiectasia, bruising, and palmar erythema, are observed in a large proportion of individuals; parotid enlargement, Dupuytren's contractures, gynaecomastia, and testicular atrophy are seen less frequently. Central cyanosis secondary to intrapulmonary arteriovenous shunting of blood may occur in the more seriously ill patients (Berthelot, NEJM, 1966; 274:291) and, rarely, features of primary pulmonary hypertension may arise (McDonnell, AmRevRespDis, 1983; 127:437).

Patients with alcoholic cirrhosis who are abstinent from alcohol may show few, if any, laboratory abnormalities.[12–16] Individuals who are actively drinking may have a constellation of abnormalities, which, while not in themselves diagnostic, may, when taken together with the clinical findings, provide strong presumptive evidence for the presence of significant alcohol-related liver injury. In these patients, serum γ-glutamyl transferase and aspartate aminotransferase activities are invariably increased. Serum bilirubin and alkaline phosphatase levels are increased, usually modestly, in 50 to 80 per cent of individuals; more marked increases occur in patients with hepatocellular carcinoma. Blood urea and serum potassium concentrations are low and serum sodium levels tend to be in the low reference range. Serum urate concentrations may be high; plasma lipids levels are variable depending on the degree of hepatic decompensation. Plasma albumin concentrations are low in approximately half of the patients, while plasma concentrations of IgA, IgM, and IgG are raised. There may be evidence of hypersplenism, with anaemia, leucopenia, and thrombocytopenia, although the white-cell count may be raised in approximately 30 per cent of patients. Macrocytosis is common; the prothrombin time may be prolonged and may not be corrected by vitamin K_1 in patients with decompensated disease. Approximately one-third of patients show significant circulating titres of smooth-muscle and/or antinuclear antibodies. Plasma α-fetoprotein concentrations are increased in the majority of patients who develop hepatocellular carcinoma.

The liver biopsy shows micronodular cirrhosis. Varying degrees of fatty change and alcoholic hepatitis may be seen within the nodules in patients who are actively drinking. Later, particularly with abstinence from alcohol, these features disappear and a macronodular cirrhosis develops that is histologically indistinguishable from other forms of 'burnt-out' cirrhosis. The presence of hepatocellular carcinoma may be confirmed on biopsy.

Evaluation[27–30]

Individuals may develop alcoholic liver disease in the absence of a history of physical dependence on alcohol and in the absence of alcohol-related social, emotional, and psychological harm. Alternatively, the presence of alcoholic liver disease may be accompanied by a wide range of other alcohol-related social and medical disorders. All patients with alcoholic liver disease should be carefully evaluated in order to determine whether they have other alcohol-related problems, as these may have a direct bearing on their immediate management and both direct and indirect effects on their subsequent rehabilitation.

Initial enquiry should be made into the patient's domestic, social, financial, and employment status. It is important to try to gauge the degree of support that the individual might receive from family and friends in their endeavours to achieve and maintain abstinence from alcohol. It is important to find out whether their job is safe or in jeopardy, or, if they are currently unemployed, what their employment prospects are. The financial burden of their alcohol habit is likely to have been substantial and many will have serious financial problems. Finally, careful enquiry must be made into their dealings with the law, for even the most respectable may have 'proceedings pending'. All of these factors must be taken into account when devising a management plan.

There are few, if any, organs or systems in the human body that escape the toxic effects of alcohol.[27–30] Pancreatitis occurs in 20 to 30 per cent of chronic alcoholic abusers (Marin, Gastro, 1969; 56:727). These patients present, characteristically, with episodes of acute pancreatitis, but functional abnormalities persist and repeated attacks occur. The late stage of the disease is associated with intermittent or persistent abdominal pain, pancreatic calcification, malabsorption, and diabetes (Sarles, ScaJGastr, 1992; 27:71). Gastrointestinal symptoms are prominent, with approximately 30 per cent of individuals reporting weight loss and a similar proportion reporting vague epigastric pain. Morning nausea and vomiting are features of alcohol dependency but may also reflect the presence of gastritis (Joske, QJMed, 1955; 24:269; Iber, Gastro, 1971; 61:120). Although alcohol undoubtedly has effects on intestinal structure and function, these have surprisingly little clinical relevance (Langman, BrMedBull, 1982; 38:71). Similarly, although it is widely believed that chronic alcohol abuse is associated with an increase in the incidence of peptic ulceration, there is no real evidence to support this contention (Friedman, NEJM, 1974; 290:469; Paffenbarger, AmJEpid, 1974; 100:307). Indeed, alcohol abusers tend to have a lower prevalence of infection with *Helicobacter pylori*, a major causal factor in the development of peptic ulcer disease [Dumont, Gut, 1994; 35 (Suppl.4): PA143]; it has even been suggested that alcohol may have an important anti-*H. pylori* effect (Weisse, BMJ, 1995; 311:1657). There is also no evidence that alcohol consumption has a deleterious effect on ulcer healing (Piper, Gut, 1978; 19:419; Thomas, Digestion, 1980; 20:79).

A wide variety of neurological abnormalities can be found in patients chronically abusing alcohol. Individuals may develop tolerance to the intoxicating effects of alcohol and may develop an acute withdrawal syndrome when their alcohol intake is suddenly reduced or stopped altogether. Structural changes suggestive of cerebral atrophy may be observed on cerebral computed tomographic scanning or magnetic resonance imaging, and these may be accompanied by evidence of impaired mental functioning (Moore, JHepatol, 1989; 9:319; Jernigan, AlcoholClinExpRes, 1991; 15:418). The term 'alcoholic dementia' has been used in relation to these findings, but this is not entirely satisfactory because the alcohol-related cerebral lesion may improve with abstinence from alcohol (Carlen, Science, 1978; 200:1076; Muuronen, AlcoholClinExpRes, 1989; 13:137), whereas the word 'dementia' implies a progressive disorder. It is unclear whether the changes observed on cerebral imaging reflect loss of neuronal cells (Harper, JNeurolSci, 1989; 92: 81; Jensen, Lancet, 1993; ii:1201).

Chronic alcohol abuse is also associated with the development of the Wernicke–Korsakoff syndrome (Joyce, BrMedBull, 1994; 50: 99), alcoholic cerebellar degeneration (Torvik, JNeurolSci, 1986; 75:43), central pontine myelinolysis (Charness, AlcoholClinExpRes, 1993; 17:2), alcoholic myelopathy (Sage, ArchNeurol, 1984; 41: 999), the Marchiafava–Bignami syndrome (Hauw, Brain, 1988; 11: 843), and movement disorders (Neiman, Neurology, 1990; 40:741). The incidence of cerebral infarction and subarachnoid haemorrhage is also increased in individuals chronically abusing alcohol (Ben-Shlomo, Stroke, 1992; 23:1093).

Alcoholic polyneuropathy is reported in varying proportions of alcohol abusers and is probably underdiagnosed (Juntunen, Acta-MedScandSuppl, 1985; 703:265); it is essentially a sensorimotor neuropathy, often with motor predominance, and mainly affects the lower limbs. Individuals chronically abusing alcohol may also develop an acute myopathy (Haller, MedClinNAm, 1984; 68:91); acute toxic rhabdomyolysis is rare but subclinical acute muscle damage is relatively common. The incidence of chronic myopathy, which results in painless progressive wasting and weakness of proximal skeletal muscles, particularly in the legs, is probably underestimated (Martin, BrMedBull, 1982; 38:53; Urbano-Márquez, AnnNeurol, 1985; 17:418).

Alcohol consumption is associated with increases in both systolic and diastolic blood pressure that appear to be dose-related (Klatsky, Circulation, 1986; 73:628; Marmot, BMJ, 1994; 308:1263; Puddey, AddicBiol, 1997; 2:159). In most individuals the blood-pressure readings fall to within normal limits on withdrawal of alcohol. Chronic alcohol abuse may cause subclinical cardiotoxicity in a high percentage of alcohol abusers (Dancey, Lancet, 1985; i:1122; McCall, CurrProbCardiol, 1987; 12:353; Bertolet, DrugAlcDep, 1991; 28:113), but clinically overt cardiomyopathy, which is characterized by congestive cardiac failure, is relatively uncommon; conversely, the prevalence of heavy drinking amongst individuals with dilated cardiomyopathy is extremely high (Gillet, AlcAlc, 1992; 27:353).

Prolonged alcohol abuse is associated with significant effects on sexual function and reproductive capacity in both men and women (Morgan, BrMedBull, 1982; 38:43; Klassen, ArchSexBehav, 1986; 15:363; Villalta, AlcoholClinExpRes, 1997; 21:128); alcohol is also associated with sometimes profound effects on the developing fetus (Jones, Lancet, 1973; ii:999; Morgan, BrMedBull, 1982; 38:43; Streissguth, JAMA, 1991; 265:1961). Various disturbances of endocrine function are also observed in chronic alcohol abusers but the majority are of only minor clinical importance (Morgan, BrMed-Bull, 1982; 38:35).

There is a strong association between alcohol abuse and the development of cancer of the mouth, pharynx, larynx, and oesophagus (*IARC monograph on the evaluation of the carcinogenic risk to humans*, Vol. 44, *Alcohol drinking*. Lyon: IARC, 1988; Tuyns, BrJC-anc, 1991; 64:415). Individuals with alcoholic cirrhosis have an increased risk of developing hepatocellular carcinoma but the exact nature of the association is unclear (Bassendine, JHepatol, 1986; 2: 513). Alcohol abuse has also been associated with the development of malignancies at other sites but the evidence for these associations is, at present, equivocal.

The presence of other alcohol-related disorders must be adequately documented. Allowance for their investigation and treatment must be made in the management plan. The likely effects of these other disorders on outcome must be considered, in particular the effects of cerebral damage on comprehension and hence compliance.

Management

A number of management issues arise in individuals who abuse alcohol and develop liver injury. The liver disease and its complications cannot be treated in isolation, and physicians involved in the care of these patients often find themselves facing problems with which they may feel ill-equipped to deal, such as acute intoxication, alcohol withdrawal, the long-term maintenance of abstinence from alcohol, and a variety of social, financial, and psychosexual issues. Although the patient may need to be referred to several individuals or agencies for advice or help, there can be no doubt that the needs of the patient are best served if the physician takes overall charge and, in this key role, orchestrates the therapeutic efforts of the others involved.

Alcohol intoxication

Individuals who chronically abuse alcohol develop cerebral tolerance to its effects. Thus, they may appear relatively sober with blood ethanol concentrations normally associated with significant cerebral impairment. In consequence, it is unusual for individuals who are chronically abusing alcohol to present with acute alcohol intoxication. However, if an habitual drinker is abstinent for a period of time and then returns to drinking at a former level, they may very quickly become intoxicated. Equally, while metabolic rates for alcohol may increase initially in heavy drinkers, they decline with the development of alcohol-related liver injury; this may be accompanied by an apparent decrease in tolerance. Finally, the development of tolerance may be race-related in that certain ethnic groups, in particular Asian Indians, continue to become intoxicated after relatively small amounts of alcohol even after years of abuse (Clarke, AlcAlc, 1990; 25:9).

The features of acute intoxication are well known and include specific neurological effects, for example ataxia, dysarthria, amnesia, and impairment of attention and memory, specific psychological effects, for example mood lability, loquacity, irritability, and disinhibition, and maladaptive behaviour, such as aggression, violence, and impaired social functioning. Concentrations of blood alcohol in excess of 400 mg/100 ml (80 mmol/l) may lead to coma and to death. Coma in a patient with a blood alcohol much below 400 mg/100 ml should lead to a search for other causes of impaired consciousness, such as cerebral injury, particularly concussion, subdural, extradural or subarachnoid haemorrhage (Galbraith, BrJSurg, 1976; 63:128; Niizuma, Stroke, 1988; 19:852), the use of other narcotic or sedative drugs, hypoglycaemia, or opportunistic infection, especially meningitis.

Seriously intoxicated individuals may suffer accidental or intentional injury, hypothermia, heat stroke, cardiac arrhythmias, venous thromboembolism, fat embolism, and hypoglycaemia. Death, when it occurs, usually results from respiratory depression or inhalation of vomitus.

Mild, uncomplicated degrees of intoxication can be managed satisfactorily in relatively simple surroundings with the minimum of medical support (Whitfield, JAMA, 1978; 239:1409). Patients whose intoxication is severe or complicated require admission to hospital and should be managed in specialist units equipped to provide close monitoring and respiratory support. Gastric lavage is not required unless other agents have been ingested. Careful observation of the level of consciousness is necessary, urine output should be recorded, blood sugar should be measured at least hourly, and blood ethanol concentrations, plasma electrolytes, and preferably blood gases should be monitored 4-hourly until recovery is assured.

Intravenous fluids should be provided to counter dehydration and to maintain urine output; plasma expanders may be required if circulatory collapse occurs. Assisted ventilation may be needed if respiration is severely depressed. Analeptics, such as nikethamide and amphetamines, have been advised but are rarely, if ever, indicated; they are of questionable value and their use is associated with the development of cardiac arrhythmias, hypertension, and convulsions. The opiate antagonist naloxone has been reported to reduce the effects of alcohol toxicity by effecting arousal from ethanol-induced coma (Jeffcoate, Lancet, 1979; ii:1157; Jefferys, Lancet, 1980; i:308; Dole, AlcoholClinExpRes, 1982; 6:275). It is given in a dose of 1 ml (0.4 mg) intravenously, repeated as necessary. The aim of treatment is to achieve a modest lightening of coma, as too rapid a reversal may induce withdrawal symptoms. A safe 'sleeping-off' state is the desired condition.

Haemodialysis has been used in severe alcohol-induced coma. It may have a place in the management of patients with very high blood ethanol concentrations, especially if other dialysable drugs have been ingested or if metabolic acidosis develops (Koch-Weser, NEJM, 1976; 294:757).

Substances that might reverse the acute effects of alcohol, so-called amethystic agents, have been widely tested, but despite many claims there are no agents that consistently accelerate ethanol breakdown (Alkana, *Biochemistry and pharmacology of ethanol*, Vol. 2. New York: Plenum, 1979:349). Hence, there is no good evidence that adrenaline, thyroxine, pyruvate, pyridoxine, dinitrophenol, glucose, or oxygen substantially change the elimination rate of ethanol, though it might increase slightly following infusions of insulin or amino acids (Victor, *Acute drug abuse emergencies: a treatment manual*. New York: Academic, 1976:197). Fructose will significantly increase the rate of ethanol metabolism whether given orally (Soterakis, AmJClinNutr, 1975; 28:254; Mascord, AlcAlc, 1991; 26:53) or intravenously (Brown, Lancet, 1972; ii: 898; Spandel, NutrMetab, 1980; 24:324). However, there is marked interindividual variation in its effects on ethanol metabolism and its use may be complicated by the development of lactic acidosis, hyperuricaemia, and an osmotic diuresis (Woods, Lancet, 1972; ii: 1354; Levy, ArchIntMed, 1977; 137:1175). In practical terms, once a patient is no longer deeply comatose, there is little to be gained by marginally increasing the rate of ethanol elimination.

Respiratory infections commonly develop in intoxicated patients because of immobility and inhalation or aspiration. The acute infection is less well tolerated if superimposed on obstructive airways disease. Antibiotics and vigorous physiotherapy are mandatory.

Acute ketoacidosis or lactic acidosis are rare complications of alcohol intoxication and tend to occur in malnourished individuals who have been vomiting. Individuals who develop these complications should be managed in an intensive-care or high-dependency unit with cardiac and central venous-pressure monitoring. Maintenance of blood sugar levels and the cautious use of intravenous bicarbonate solutions are the mainstays of therapy, although the management of this situation is difficult. Blood gases, pH, electrolytes, and sugar levels should be measured 2- to 4-hourly. Cardiac arrhythmias may develop and further complicate the situation. Hypoglycaemia may complicate ketoacidosis or present as a problem in its own right.

Secretion of antidiuretic hormone is suppressed when blood ethanol concentrations are rising but rebound secretion may occur when the blood ethanol begins to fall; thus, overhydration may occur.

Hyperpyrexia is a rare complication of alcohol intoxication; its aetiological background is unknown and it is managed empirically.

Pathological intoxication or excitation is characterized by a severely excitable and combative state requiring urgent restraint. Unfortunately, restraint stimulates further excitement and may make it impossible to administer the necessary sedation. Short-acting benzodiazepines are the treatment of choice for managing this condition; barbiturates should not be used as, paradoxically, they may increase excitement, and their metabolism may be impaired if the patient has significant alcoholic liver disease.

Acute alcohol withdrawal

Approximately 40 per cent of individuals who abuse alcohol develop a physical withdrawal syndrome when they abruptly stop or substantially reduce their alcohol intake. Most manifest a 'minor symptom complex or syndrome' that may start as early as 6 to 8 h after an abrupt change in alcohol intake (Wolfe, *Recent advances in studies of alcoholism*. Washington DC: US Government Printing Office, 1972:188; Foy, QJMed, 1997; 90:253). It may include any combination of generalized hyperactivity, anxiety, tremor, sweating, nausea, retching, tachycardia, hypertension, and mild pyrexia. These symptoms usually peak between 10 to 30 h and subside by 40 to 50 h. Fits may occur in the first 12 to 48 h and only rarely after this; they may arise singly, but typically occur in bursts of two to six; status epilepticus is not a feature. Less frequently, auditory and visual hallucinations arise that are characteristically frightening and may last for 5 to 6 days.

Delirium tremens occurs uncommonly, perhaps in less than 5 per cent of individuals withdrawing from alcohol (Victor, ResPublResNervMentDis, 1953; 32:526; Foy, QJMed, 1997; 90:253). The syndrome usually starts some 60 to 80 h after cessation of drinking, and is characterized by coarse tremor, agitation, fever, tachycardia, profound confusion, delusions, and hallucinations. Convulsions may herald the onset of the syndrome but are not part of the symptom complex. Hyperpyrexia, ketoacidosis, and profound circulatory collapse may develop, and the syndrome, if untreated, carries a mortality of up to 15 per cent (Wolfe, *Recent advances in studies of alcoholism*. Washington DC: US Government Printing Office, 1972:188); the mortality in treated patients is less than 1 per cent (Gross, *The biology of alcoholism*. New York: Plenum, 1974: 191).

Table 5 Differential diagnosis of acute alcohol-withdrawal syndrome in man

Diagnostic variable	Differential diagnoses				
	Alcohol withdrawal	Wernicke's syndrome	Subdural haematoma	Hepatic encephalopathy	Hypoglycaemia
Conscious level	Heightened	Variable	Fluctuant	Lowered	Variable
Hallucinosis	Yes	Yes	No	No	No
Anxiety	Yes	No	No	No	Yes
Speech	Rapid	Slurred	Normal	Slurred	Slurred
Pulse rate	Raised	Raised	Slow	Normal	Raised
Blood pressure	Raised	Normal	Raised	Normal or low	Low
Sweating	Yes	No	No	No	Yes

The diagnosis of acute alcohol withdrawal is not usually difficult once a history of alcohol abuse in the near past has been obtained. However, there is great variability in the severity of the symptoms and careful distinction must be made from other disturbances of behaviour and consciousness that may complicate alcohol abuse, including the Wernicke–Korsakoff syndrome, subdural haematoma, hepatic encephalopathy, and hypoglycaemia (Table 5). Not only may the distinction prove difficult but these conditions may also coexist. Occasionally, patients with hepatic encephalopathy may develop an acute psychotic state, manifest by agitation, paranoia, and delusions, that closely resembles delirium tremens but can be differentiated because of the absence of tremor, sweating, and possibly tachycardia.

Minor degrees of alcohol withdrawal are commonly encountered and sufferers can be managed without recourse to specific therapy (Rossall, BrJPsychiat, 1978; 133:479; Whitfield, JAMA, 1978; 239: 1409). However, those with moderate or severe symptoms of alcohol withdrawal should be sedated to prevent exhaustion and injury; the drugs most commonly used are the benzodiazepines (Shaw, AlcAlc, 1995; 30:765) and chlormethiazole (Morgan, AlcAlc, 1995; 30:771). These should be given in daily reducing doses to avoid undue accumulation and hence oversedation; this is particularly likely to occur in patients with liver disease in whom the metabolism of both benzodiazepines (Wilkinson, ActaPsychScandSuppl, 1978; 274:56) and chlormethiazole (Pentikäinen, BMJ, 1978; 2:861) is altered, and in whom cerebral sensitivity to sedative drugs is increased (Hoyumpa, AnnRevMed, 1982; 33:113).

Chlordiazepoxide is the benzodiazepine most commonly used in the treatment of this condition but diazepam, oxazepam, and lorazepam are also used. The benzodiazepines vary little in their efficacy, but they do differ in their speed of onset, half-lives, metabolite activity, and reliability of absorption when given intramuscularly (Bird, AnnPharmacother, 1994; 28:67).

Diazepam and chlordiazepoxide have long half-lives and, following oxidation in the liver, produce active metabolites. Their plasma half-lives increase in the presence of significant liver injury and the proportion of free drug may increase in the presence of hypoalbuminaemia. As a result, these drugs may accumulate and cause excessive drowsiness, ataxia, diplopia, and confusion, symptoms that may mirror those of the Wernicke–Korsakoff syndrome. Both drugs are absorbed erratically from intramuscular sites; diazepam has the more rapid onset of action; chlordiazepoxide is safer than diazepam if taken in overdosage in combination with alcohol (Serfaty, BrJPsychiat, 1993; 163:386).

Lorazepam and oxazepam have intermediate half-lives, are eliminated following glucuronidation, and have inactive metabolites; lorezepam is well absorbed from intramuscular injection sites. These drugs show no tendency to accumulate but their use is associated with a higher rate of fitting late in the withdrawal phase than with the longer-acting drugs (Hill, JSubsAbuseTreat, 1993; 10:449). Lorezepam is believed to induce dependency more readily than diazepam and chlordiazepoxide, but it is less likely to be fatal if taken in overdose (Serfaty, BrJPsychiat, 1993; 163:386).

The benzodiazepines can be used to procure sedation either rapidly or in a more graduated fashion. The rapid method employs the longer-acting drugs: diazepam is given orally at a rate of 10 to 20 mg hourly or, alternatively, intravenously at a rate of 5 mg every 5 min until the patient is satisfactorily sedated. If preferred, chlordiazepoxide, infused at a rate of 12.5 mg/min, can be substituted to the same end-point. Thereafter, no further medication is given, reliance being placed on the long half-life and active metabolites to ensure smooth withdrawal. These regimens are not recommended for use in patients with significant liver disease.

More usually the drugs, either short- or long-acting, are given in high dosage on days 1 to 3, and tapered off over the next 4 to 7 (or more) days in response to the patient's condition. Patients' requirements are extremely variable and the dosage difficult to predict accurately. Fixed schedules are not therefore advised. As a guide, the daily dosages commonly employed in the early phase of treatment are chlordiazepoxide 200 mg, diazepam 40 mg, or lorazepam 8 mg. After the third day a daily dose reduction of at least 25 per cent is recommended (Shaw, AlcAlc, 1995; 30:765).

Little or no modification of dosage is required in patients with minimal liver disease, but in patients with more significant liver injury the initial dosage of the longer-acting benzodiazepines should be reduced by 25 per cent.

Chlormethiazole is, for many physicians, the drug of choice for treating acute alcohol withdrawal because overdosage is less likely to occur than with the benzodiazepines. However, it is not generally available. Oral chlormethiazole undergoes extensive first-pass metabolism and has a high hepatic-extraction ratio. In patients with cirrhosis its systemic bioavailability increases substantially but its elimination rate is relatively unchanged (Pentikäinen, BMJ, 1978; 2: 861). Intravenous dosing eliminates this variation in bioavailability.

As with the benzodiazepines, little or no dosage adjustment is required in patients with fatty liver, who should be given between 9 to 12 capsules, each containing 192 mg of chlormethiazole base, on the first day, in divided doses, and then stepwise reducing doses for the next 6 days. Alternatively, the drug may be dispensed as a syrup containing 250 mg of chlormethiazole edisylate in 5 ml, in a dosage equivalent of 5 ml of syrup to one capsule. If withdrawal symptoms are severe then the drug can be administered as an intravenous solution containing 8 mg/ml of chlormethiazole, which is usually infused, using a drop counter, at a rate of 8 to 32 mg/min, reducing to 4 to 6 mg/min for maintenance. Patients should be changed to oral medication after 36 to 48 h. In individuals with alcoholic hepatitis and/or cirrhosis the initial oral dose of chlormethiazole should be reduced by 25 to 50 per cent depending on the degree of hepatic dysfunction; the dosage can then be titrated against the response, although this is probably best done using the intravenous preparation.

Treatment for acute alcohol withdrawal may need to be initiated before information is available on the state of the patient's liver. In these instances it is probably wise to start treatment with two-thirds of the normal dosage and then to titrate the dose against the response. Although chlordiazepoxide and chlormethiazole are equally effective in controlling withdrawal symptoms, chlormethiazole is the more flexible drug (Burroughs, AlcAlc, 1985; 20: 263).

If an individual is known to be physically dependent on alcohol, as evidenced by a history of previous episodes of withdrawal symptoms or of morning retching and tremor relieved by alcohol, then their withdrawal from alcohol should be covered with benzodiazepines or chlormethiazole in the doses employed to treat minor withdrawal symptoms, reducing over 4 to 6 days.

Convulsions can be successfully treated with either intravenous diazepam, 10 mg/kg body wt, infused at a rate of not more than 50 mg/min, or intravenous chlormethiazole infused at an initial rate of 12 to 20 mg/min, reducing to 4 to 6 mg/min for maintenance. Hallucinations are best treated with oral haloperidol, 2.5 mg every 3 to 4 h.

A number of non-sedative drugs have been used to treat alcohol withdrawal, including β-adrenergic blockers (Worner, AmJDrugAlcAb, 1994; 20:115), α-adrenergic agonists, such as clonidine (Baumgartner, SouthMedJ, 1991; 84:312; Adinoff, AlcoholClinExpRes, 1994; 18:873), and anticonvulsants such as carbamazepine (Malcolm, AmJPsychiat, 1989; 146:617). They can alleviate some of the more distressing autonomic symptoms that accompany alcohol withdrawal, such as sweating, tremor, and tachycardia, but have little effect on insomnia and anxiety, and no action against seizures and delirium.

There is no evidence that 'alternative' therapies such as acupuncture confer any benefit in patients withdrawing from alcohol (McLellan, JSubsAbuseTreat, 1993; 10:569).

Care must be taken to maintain the patient's general condition during the withdrawal period. Dehydration should be corrected whenever necessary by use of oral fluids; intravenous fluids should be avoided as overhydration is a serious potential hazard. Several biochemical abnormalities may be observed during the withdrawal period, such as hypokalaemia and hypomagnesaemia, but these are usually transient and do not need specific correction unless fits develop and prove difficult to control. The patient should be encouraged to eat a nutritious diet as soon as possible; supplemental feeds may be needed in the first 48 h if anorexia and nausea are severe. Many physicians prescribe high-potency parenteral vitamin supplements. There is little evidence that these confer benefit

(Brown, AlcAlc, 1983; 18:157) but equally they probably cause no harm and are generally inexpensive. Many authorities advise routine prescription of broad-spectrum antibiotics but this is not universally accepted practice.

Treatment of alcohol-related liver disease[31–35]

In general, no treatment is required for patients with alcoholic fatty liver other than abstinence from alcohol and the provision of a well-balanced diet. It might be argued, for different reasons, that no treatment other than maintenance of abstinence is required or is likely to benefit patients with established cirrhosis, although this view has been challenged (Kershenobich, NEJM, 1988; 318:1709). In the main, therefore, most therapeutic effort has been directed towards patients with alcoholic hepatitis and a variety of agents have been used to treat this condition.

It is obviously difficult to evaluate the effectiveness of drugs in a condition such as alcoholic liver disease that tends to progress slowly, that may spontaneously heal, and that is so profoundly affected by other variables such as drinking behaviour (Blake, ClinChem, 1991; 37:5). In addition, patients who are unable to control their drinking habits are unlikely to be compliant with treatment, making the evaluation of any therapeutic effect more difficult still.

Steroid therapy

Corticosteroids

Corticosteroids stimulate the appetite, increase hepatic albumin production, and inhibit the production of type I and type IV collagen. In addition, they possess both anti-inflammatory and immunosuppressive properties. As such they may benefit patients with alcoholic hepatitis.

Between 1971 and 1992 the results of 13 randomized, controlled trials of corticosteroids in patients with alcoholic hepatitis were published (Tables 6 and 7). The severity of the liver lesion varied considerably between study populations, reflected in the short-term mortality rates in the control populations, which ranged from 10 to 100 per cent. Histological confirmation of the diagnosis was obtained in 30 to 100 per cent of individuals in the various series: between 50 to 93 per cent of the individuals biopsied had established cirrhosis. Inclusion and exclusion criteria varied between studies: histological proof of diagnosis was an inclusion criterion in only three (Helman, AnnIntMed, 1971; 74:311; Bories, PressMed, 1987; 16:769; Ramond, NEJM, 1992; 326:507); patients with gastrointestinal bleeding were excluded in most studies. Treatment regimens varied both in terms of the drugs used, the dosage and reducing schedules, and the time periods employed. However, the usual treatment regimen was prednisolone, 40 mg daily, given orally for 4 to 6 weeks (Table 6). In all 13 studies the endpoint was death, usually in relation to the trial period or the hospital inpatient stay, although survival rates at 3 months or beyond were reported in some .

In the first study (Helman, AnnIntMed, 1971; 74:311), 37 patients with alcoholic hepatitis, 76 per cent of whom had underlying cirrhosis, were randomized to treatment with either prednisolone, 40 mg daily, reducing over 6 weeks, or to a placebo

Table 6 Controlled trials of corticosteroids in patients with alcoholic hepatitis of all grades of severity

First author	Year	Daily drug dosage	Treatment period (days)	Control group Patients n	Control group Deaths[a] n (%)	Steroid group Patients n	Steroid group Deaths[a] n (%)
Helman	1971	40 mg prednisolone reducing	42	17	6 (35)	20	1 (5)*
Porter	1971	40 mg methylprednisolone IV reducing oral	10 35	9	7 (78)	11	6 (55)
Campra	1973	0.5 mg/kg prednisone reducing	42	25	9 (36)	20	7 (35)
Blitzer	1977	40 mg prednisolone reducing	26	16	2 (13)	12	2 (8)
Shumaker	1978	30 mg methylprednisolone IV reducing oral	4–7 21–24	15	7 (47)	12	6 (50)
Lesesne	1978	40 mg prednisolone reducing	44	7	7 (100)	7	2 (29)*
Maddrey	1978	40 mg prednisolone reducing	28–32	31	4 (13)	24	1 (4)
Depew	1980	40 mg prednisolone reducing	42	13	7 (54)	15	8 (53)
Theodossi	1982	1 g methylprednisolone IV	3	28	16 (57)	27	17 (63)
Mendenhall	1984	60 mg prednisolone reducing	30	88	18 (20)	90	19 (21)+
Bories	1987	40 mg prednisone	30	21	2 (10)	24	1 (4)
Carithers	1989	32 mg methylprednisolone oral/IV reducing	42	31	11 (35)	35	2 (6)*
Ramond	1992	40 mg prednisolone	28	29	16 (55)	32	4 (13)*
Totals				330	112 (34)	329	76 (23)**

[a] At end of trial period except Helman (3-month mortality rates) and Theodossi (30-day mortality rates).
* Trials in which treatment conferred significant benefit.
+ Values extrapolated from trial data and other publications.
** Combined results suggest significant treatment effect.
IV, intravenous.

Table 7 Effect of treatment with corticosteroids in patients with severe alcoholic hepatitis and spontaneous hepatic encephalopathy included in randomized, controlled clinical trials

First author	Year	Control group Patients n	Control group Deaths[a] n (%)	Steroid group Patients n	Steroid group Deaths[a] n (%)
Helman	1971	6	6 (100)	9	1 (11)*
Porter	1971	8	7 (88)	7	6 (86)
Campra	1973	10	8 (80)	8	4 (50)
Blitzer	1977	2	1 (50)	3	2 (66)
Shumaker	1978	6	4 (67)	6	2 (33)
Lesesne	1978	7	7 (100)	7	2 (29)*
Maddrey	1978	10	6 (60)	5	1 (20)
Depew	1980	13	7 (54)	15	8 (53)
Theodossi	1982	14	10 (71)	20	19 (95)
Mendenhall	1984	58	13 (22)	61	13 (21)+
Carithers	1989	19	9 (47)	14	1 (7)*
Ramond	1992	10	6 (60)	9	3 (33)*
Totals		163	84 (52)	164	62 (38)**

[a] At end of the trial period except Helman (3-month mortality rates) and Theodossi (30-day mortality rates).
* Trials in which treatment conferred significant benefit.
+ Values extrapolated from trial data and other publications.
** Combined results suggest significant treatment effect.

preparation (Table 6). Details were not provided of the mortality rate at 1 month; however, the 3-month mortality rate was significantly lower in the steroid-treated patients (5 per cent) than in the controls (35 per cent) ($p<0.001$) (Table 6). Maximum benefit was observed in those most severely ill: thus the mortality rate in patients with spontaneous hepatic encephalopathy given steroids was 11 per cent compared with 100 per cent in their counterparts given the placebo preparation (Table 7).

This study has been criticized for a number of reasons, but particularly because oral energy intakes in the patients who received the placebo preparation were substantially lower than in the steroid-treated individuals. A second trial was therefore undertaken by workers from the same department, restricted to patients severely ill with alcoholic hepatitis, in which they ensured comparable daily energy intakes in both the control and steroid-treated groups (Lesesne, Gastro, 1978; 74:169) (Table 6). In this trial, the mortality rate at the end of the treatment period was also significantly lower in the patients receiving steroid (29 vs 100 per cent; $p<0.01$) (Table 7). However, although the two groups of patients appeared balanced at randomization, the steroid-treated patients were probably less severely ill, and were certainly significantly younger than those in the control group; both these factors will have affected the outcome.

Between 1971 and 1987, a further nine studies of the effects of corticosteroids in patients with alcoholic hepatitis were published, none of which showed treatment benefit (Porter, NEJM, 1971; 284: 1350; Campra, AnnIntMed, 1973; 79:625; Blitzer, AmJDigDis, 1977; 22:477; Maddrey, Gastro, 1978; 75:193; Shumaker, AmJGastr, 1978; 69:443; Depew, Gastro, 1980; 78:524; Theodossi, Gut, 1982; 23:75; Mendenhall, NEJM, 1984; 311:1464; Bories, PressMed, 1987; 16:769) (Tables 6 and 7). Four of these studies warrant separate mention.

In the first, 45 patients with alcoholic hepatitis were randomized to treatment with either prednisolone, 0.5 mg/kg daily, reducing over 6 weeks, or a placebo preparation (Campra, AnnIntMed, 1973; 79:625) (Table 6). At the end of the treatment period the mortality rates in the control (36 per cent) and steroid-treated groups (35 per cent) were similar (Table 6). However, patients with severe alcoholic hepatitis complicated by the development of spontaneous hepatic encephalopathy appeared to benefit selectively from treatment: in this subpopulation the mortality rates were 80 per cent in the controls and 50 per cent in the steroid-treated patients (Table 7). This observation prompted workers from the same department to undertake a second study including only patients with severe alcoholic hepatitis complicated by the presence of hepatic encephalopathy (Depew, Gastro, 1980; 78:524). However, treatment did not confer significant benefit: the within-trial mortality rate was approximately 50 per cent in both control and steroid-treated patients, with deaths occurring at similar rates and for similar reasons in both groups (Table 7).

In the next study, 55 patients with alcoholic hepatitis of varying severity were randomized to treatment, for approximately 1 month, with either prednisolone, 40 mg daily, or a placebo preparation (Maddrey, Gastro, 1978; 75:193) (Table 6). The 30-day mortality rates in the control (13 per cent) and steroid-treated patients (4 per cent) were similar (Table 6) as were the hospital inpatient mortality rates of 19 per cent and 13 per cent, respectively. Nevertheless, all deaths occurred in the most severely ill patients (Table 7), and discriminant function analysis showed that treatment had a significant effect on survival. Further, these investigators found that the formula:

$$\text{Discriminant function} = 4.6 \times \text{prothrombin time [s]} + \text{serum bilirubin [mg/dl]}$$

was useful in predicting survival; all deaths occurred in patients in whom the discriminant function exceeded 93 on entry into the study.

In the largest short-term study to date (Mendenhall, NEJM, 1984; 311:1464), 178 patients with alcoholic hepatitis were randomized to treatment with either prednisolone, 60 mg daily, reducing over 30 days, or a placebo preparation (Table 6). The 30-day mortality rates were similar in both control (20 per cent) and steroid-treated (21 per cent) groups (Table 6). Approximately two-thirds of the trial population had hepatic encephalopathy at the time of enrolment and of these approximately 20 per cent died; again, however, steroids had no effect on outcome in this subpopulation (Table 7).

More recently, two extremely well-designed and well-executed studies have been published, both of which report a significant effect of treatment with corticosteroids on outcome (Carithers, AnnIntMed, 1989; 110:685; Ramond, NEJM, 1992; 326:507). In the first, 66 patients with alcoholic hepatitis, recruited from four centres, were randomized to treatment with either 32 mg of methylprednisolone daily, given orally or intravenously for 4 weeks, tapering over a further 2 weeks, or a placebo preparation (Carithers, AnnIntMed, 1989; 110:685) (Table 6). All patients had severe disease, evidenced by the presence of either spontaneous hepatic encephalopathy or a discriminant function of greater than 32, calculated from the modified formula:

$$\text{Discriminant function} = 4.6 \times (\text{prothrombin time-control time}) \text{ (s)} + \text{serum bilirubin } (\mu\text{mol/l})/17.1$$

The 28-day mortality rate in the steroid-treated patients (6 per cent) was significantly lower than in the patients receiving the placebo preparation (35 per cent) ($p<0.006$) (Table 6). In the

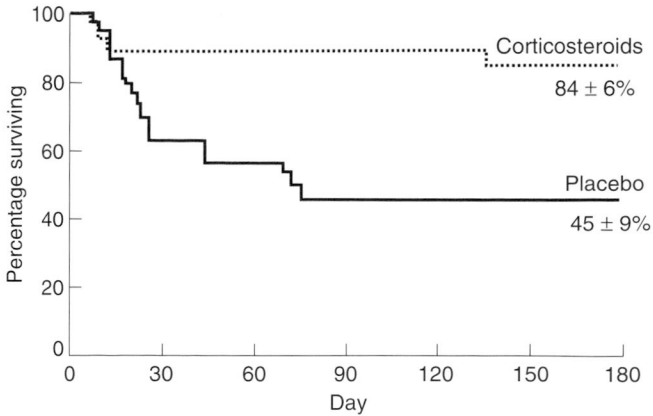

Fig. 3. Survival in 61 patients with alcoholic hepatitis randomly assigned to receive either prednisolone, 40 mg daily for 28 days, or a placebo preparation (Ramond, NEJM, 1982; 326:507).

subgroup of patients with spontaneous hepatic encephalopathy, the mortality rate in the steroid-treated patients (7 per cent) was again significantly lower than in the controls (47 per cent) ($p<0.02$) (Table 7). This was a well-conducted study but it has been criticized because the diagnosis of alcoholic hepatitis was not confirmed histologically nor were data provided on outcome beyond the study period.

The most recent study (Ramond, NEJM, 1992; 326:507), employed the same inclusion criteria and utilized a similar treatment regimen to those used in the earlier study (Carithers, AnnIntMed, 1989; 110:685). In addition, however, the diagnosis of alcoholic hepatitis was confirmed histologically in all patients and the follow-up period was prolonged beyond 6 months. Sixty-one patients were randomized to treatment with either prednisolone, 40 mg daily, or a placebo preparation, for 28 days (Table 6). During the study there were significantly fewer deaths among the steroid-treated patients (13 per cent) than among controls (55 per cent) ($p<0.001$) (Table 6). Equally, the mean cumulative survival rates at 2 and 6 months were significantly higher in the steroid-treated patients (88 and 84 per cent) than in those who had received the placebo preparation (45 and 45 per cent) (Fig. 3).

Subgroup analysis showed that the use of steroids conferred significant benefit, independently of the presence of hepatic encephalopathy (Fig. 4).

This group further examined the long-term survival of the patients who had received prednisolone in the original study and of an additional cohort treated openly using the same regimen (Mathurin, Gastro, 1996; 110:1847). At 1 year the survival in the steroid-treated patients was significantly greater than in both matched and simulated controls (70 vs 45 per cent; $p<0.05$). However, there were no differences in survival rates at 2 years. Treatment was particularly beneficial in patients with neutrophilia and marked hepatic polymorphonuclear infiltration.

Between 1989 and 1995, five separate meta-analyses of available studies were undertaken to determine whether treatment with corticosteroids affects short-term mortality in patients with alcoholic hepatitis [Reynolds, GastrInternat, 1989; 2:208; Imperiale, AnnIntMed, 1990; 113:299; Daures, GastrClinBiol, 1991; 15:223; Poynard, Hepatol, 1991; 14: 234(Abstr.); Christensen, Gut, 1995; 37:

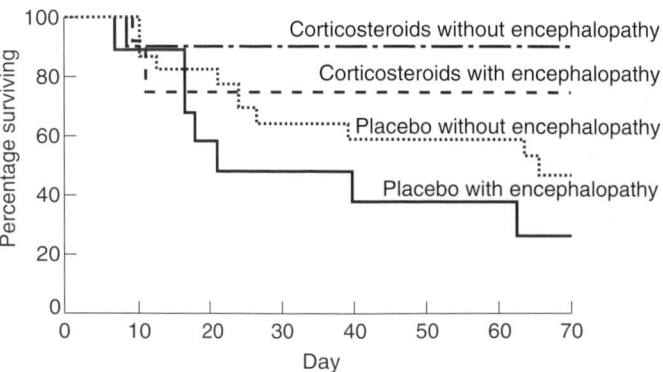

Fig. 4. Survival in 61 patients with alcoholic hepatitis randomly assigned to receive either prednisolone, 40 mg daily for 28 days, or a placebo preparation; relation to the presence or absence of hepatic encephalopathy (Ramond, NEJM, 1982; 326:507).

113]. The results of these meta-analyses are conflicting. Thus one concluded that, provided patients with gastrointestinal bleeding are excluded, steroids reduce the short-term mortality in patients with acute alcoholic hepatitis and hepatic encephalopathy (Imperiale, AnnIntMed, 1990; 113:299). Another concluded that steroids significantly reduce mortality in patients with severe alcoholic hepatitis independently of the presence of hepatic encephalopathy [Poynard, Hepatol, 1991; 14:234(Abstr.)], while a third concluded that steroids have no significant effect on mortality in patients with alcoholic hepatitis, whether or not they have hepatic encephalopathy (Christensen, Gut, 1995; 37:113), although in this study the data from the patients with severe disease were not analysed separately.

The results of these meta-analyses must be viewed with caution, bearing in mind the results of the two most recent studies, both of which show that treatment confers significant benefit in patients with severe disease (Carithers, AnnIntMed, 1989; 110:685; Ramond, NEJM, 1992; 326:507). Thus overall it would appear that, while corticosteroids do not affect outcome in patients with mild to moderate alcoholic hepatitis, they may significantly improve outcome in a small subgroup of patients with severe disease identified as having a discriminant function in excess of 32. Such individuals are, however, encountered infrequently: in one study (Carithers, AnnIntMed, 1989; 110:685) only 66 patients fulfilling these criteria were recruited from four centres in 5 years, while in another (Ramond, NEJM, 1992; 326:507), only 61 such patients were recruited from two centres in 3 years. Once identified, these individuals should be given 40 mg of prednisolone daily for 4 weeks, followed by 20 mg daily for 1 week and then 10 mg daily for a final week. The complications of treatment are surprisingly few but patients must be carefully monitored.

Steroids should be withheld in patients with gastrointestinal bleeding until they are haemodynamically stable, and in patients with severe infection until antibiotic therapy is instituted and the infection is under control. The prognosis in patients with severe alcoholic hepatitis and renal failure is extremely poor so it is unlikely that they will benefit from treatment.

The treatment regimen may need to be modified in patients with evidence of past or present infection with hepatitis B or C. Corticosteroids may reactivate or increase viral replication in these patient, and this may have clinical consequences (Wands, Gastro,

1975; 68:105; Lok, Gastro, 1991; 100:182; Magrin, Hepatol, 1994; 19:273); equally, withdrawal of corticosteroid treatment may be associated with the development of an acute hepatitis or even hepatic failure (Rakela, Gastro, 1983; 84:956; Thung, ArchIntMed, 1985; 145:1313). If these patients are to be treated at all, then the prednisolone dosage should probably be reduced and its withdrawal prolonged beyond 6 weeks.

The effect of corticosteroids on long-term survival in patients with alcoholic hepatitis is unclear. In one study its effect on survival was monitored in 99 cirrhotic patients with superimposed alcoholic hepatitis from a group of 483 cirrhotic patients observed at seven cooperating hospitals in Copenhagen (Schlichting, ScaJGastr, 1976; 11:305). Patients were assigned to treatment not randomly but on the basis of date of birth, and this is obviously a potential source of bias. Forty-four patients received prednisolone, 40 mg daily, for 4 to 8 weeks, followed by 10 to 15 mg daily for 5 to 12 years; 45 patients received a placebo preparation. The median survival time for the steroid-treated patients was 38 months, and for patients receiving the placebo 34 months.

The effects of corticosteroids on the course and outcome of alcoholic cirrhosis have been examined by the Copenhagen Study Group for Liver Disease (Schlichting, ScaJGastr, 1976; 11:305; Juhl, ActaMedScandSuppl, 1985; 703:195); they found that 10 to 15 mg of prednisolone daily had no effect on survival in men with alcoholic cirrhosis and a detrimental effect on survival in women with alcoholic cirrhosis.

Anabolic steroids

Anabolic steroids might benefit patients with alcohol-related liver disease because of their effects on nucleic acid and protein synthesis. A number of trials have been undertaken to assess the efficacy of these drugs in patients with alcohol-related liver injury of varying severity, but there is no consensus as to their value.

Anabolic steroids have been shown to accelerate the removal of fat from the liver by some investigators (Jabbari, Medicine, 1967; 46:131; Mendenhall, AmJDigDis, 1968; 13:783) but not by others (Fenster, AnnIntMed, 1966; 65:738). However, as fat will clear rapidly from the liver with abstinence from alcohol, the use of anabolic steroids is unjustified in this condition.

To date, three randomized, controlled studies have been undertaken on the effects of anabolic steroids in patients with alcoholic hepatitis (Mendenhall, NEJM, 1984; 311:1464; Bonkovsky, AmJGastr, 1991; 86:1200; 1991; 86:1209; Mendenhall, Hepatol, 1993; 17:564). In the first study, 173 men with moderate to severe alcoholic hepatitis were randomized to treatment with either oxandrolone, 80 mg daily for 30 days, or to a placebo preparation (Mendenhall, NEJM, 1984; 311:1464). The 30-day mortality rate was 13 per cent in the moderately ill and 29 per cent in the severely ill patients; treatment with oxandrolone did not affect the short-term outcome. In the individuals with moderately severe alcoholic hepatitis who survived the first 30 days, there was a significant reduction in the 6-month mortality rate in relation to treatment (3.5 vs 20 per cent; $p<0.02$). No such beneficial effect was observed in individuals with severe alcoholic hepatitis, and overall survival rates at 30 months were similar in the oxandrolone and placebo groups.

In a later study, 39 patients with moderate to severe alcoholic hepatitis were randomized to 21 days' treatment with either oxandrolone 80 mg daily, oxandrolone plus intravenous amino acid

Table 8 Mortality rates in patients with alcoholic hepatitis in relation to their degree of malnutrition, their daily energy intake, and treatment with oxandrolone

Oxandrolone	Moderate malnutrition		Severe malnutrition	
	<2500 (kcal/day)	>2500	<2500 (kcal/day)	>2500
Yes	30%	4%	59%	21%
No	33%	28%	45%	13%

Adapted from Mendenhall, Hepatol, 1993; 17: 564.

supplementation, intravenous amino acid supplementation alone, or to so-called standard therapy (Bonkovsky, AmJGastr, 1991; 86: 1200; 1991; 86:1209). No significant differences in outcome were observed between the four groups, although improvement in laboratory variables was most marked in the individuals who received both oxandrolone and nutritional supplementation.

Most recently, Mendenhall and associates (Hepatol, 1993; 17: 564), randomized 273 men with moderate to severe alcoholic hepatitis to treatment with either oxandrolone, 80 mg daily, for 30 days then 40 mg daily for 60 days, or to a placebo preparation. The oxandrolone-treated patients received, in addition, a branched-chain amino acid-enriched oral supplement that provided 60 g of protein and 1600 kcal daily for 30 days, and then 45 g of protein and 1200 kcal daily for the remaining 60 days. Overall the 6-month cumulative mortality rate was 35 per cent in patients receiving oxandrolone and nutritional supplementation and 39 per cent in controls. No selective beneficial effect was observed in relation to disease severity, as in the original study carried out by this group (Mendenhall, NEJM, 1984; 311:1464). However, a selective beneficial effect of treatment was observed in relation to the degree of malnutrition. Thus, in patients with moderate malnutrition, the 6-month mortality rate was significantly lower in those receiving the active-treatment than the control regimen. No such effect was observed in the patients with severe malnutrition.

In order to reconcile the results of their two trials and to try to separate the beneficial effects of nutritional supplementation from those of oxandrolone, Mendenhall and co-workers combined their two study populations and re-analysed their data (Alcohol-ClinExpRes, 1995; 19:635). They showed that patients with alcoholic hepatitis who were moderately malnourished benefited from treatment with oxandrolone, provided that their oral intake, whether supplemented or not, exceeded 2500 kcal/day (Table 8). In these individuals, the 6-month mortality rate was 4 per cent, compared with rates of between 28 and 33 per cent in their counterparts whose dietary intake was inadequate or who were not given the anabolic steroid (Table 8). In patients with alcoholic hepatitis and severe malnutrition, oxandrolone had no effect on outcome, but mortality was significantly lower in those consuming in excess of 2500 kcal/day (19 vs 51 per cent; $p<0.001$) (Table 8).

These workers finally concluded that patients with alcoholic hepatitis need vigorous nutritional support and, if they are moderately malnourished, they should also be given oxandrolone, although they did not suggest a treatment regimen. Oxandrolone is a relatively inexpensive drug and its use in the studies to date has

been associated with few side-effects. It probably deserves further study in patients with alcoholic hepatitis.

Three long-term, controlled studies have been undertaken to assess the effects of anabolic steroids on outcome in patients with alcoholic cirrhosis. The earliest (Wells, Lancet, 1960; ii:1416) was a trial of anabolic steroids in a group of patients with cirrhosis, 34 per cent of whom had abused alcohol. Patients were randomized to receive either 100 mg of testosterone propionate intramuscularly on alternate days for 4 weeks, followed by 300 mg once every 2 weeks for a total of 6 months, or a placebo preparation. At the end of the trial period, 31 per cent of the steroid-treated patients had died compared with 55 per cent of controls; this difference was not significant.

The next study (Islam, BrJClinPract, 1973; 27:125) used a similar trial design to examine the effects of testosterone on outcome in 70 cirrhotic patients, a minority of whom had abused alcohol. Patients were randomized to receive either testosterone propionate, 100 mg intramuscularly, on alternate days for 4 weeks, followed by 300 mg every third week for 6 to 9 months, or a placebo preparation. The 4-year survival rate in the treated group was 65.6 per cent compared with 36.8 per cent in the control group ($p<0.05$). The number of patients with alcohol-related cirrhosis in this series is, however, far too small to allow comment on the efficacy of testosterone in this subgroup.

In the most recent study (The Copenhagen Study Group for Liver Diseases, Hepatol, 1986; 6:807), 221 men with alcoholic cirrhosis were randomized to treatment with 600 mg of micronized testosterone daily, in divided doses, or to a placebo preparation. By skewed randomization, 134 patients received testosterone and 87 placebo. Patients were followed for a median of 28 months (range 8–62 months). There was no significant difference in survival between those treated with testosterone (75 per cent) and those receiving the placebo preparation (79 per cent); one patient treated with testosterone developed diffuse hepatic sinusoidal dilatation and one a Budd–Chiari syndrome (Gluud, AmJGastr, 1987; 82:660).

Colchicine

Colchicine inhibits the migration of granulocytes into areas of inflammation and interferes with the degradation of polymorphonuclear leucocytes. It also inhibits microtubular assembly and the transcellular movement of collagen, and increases collagenase activity. Thus, on theoretical grounds, it might attenuate the inflammatory response associated with alcohol-related hepatocyte injury, and might diminish collagen deposition and enhance its dissolution.

To date, two randomized, controlled studies of colchicine in the treatment of alcoholic hepatitis have been undertaken, neither of which reports benefit (Trinchet, GastrClinBiol, 1989; 13:551; Akriviadis, Gastro, 1990; 9:811). In one of these studies (Akriviadis, Gastro, 1990; 9:811), 72 patients with severe alcoholic hepatitis were randomized to treatment with either colchicine, 1 mg daily, or a placebo preparation, for 30 days. There was no significant difference in 'within hospital' mortality rates between the patients given colchicine (19 per cent) and the controls (17 per cent). There was also no significant effect of treatment with colchicine on 4-month survival rates.

In the other study (Trinchet, GastrClinBiol, 1989; 13:551), 67 patients with histologically proven alcoholic hepatitis, 50 per cent of whom had cirrhosis, were randomized to receive either 1 mg of colchicine daily or else a placebo preparation. Liver biopsies were repeated at 3 and 6 months; a scoring system was used to evaluate the initial and repeat biopsies. Nineteen patients (28 per cent) were lost to follow-up at 3 months and 39 (58 per cent) at 6 months. Thirty-nine patients (58 per cent) were abstinent from alcohol at 3 months and 33 (50 per cent) at 6 months. One patient died of liver failure. No significant overall effect was observed on clinical, laboratory, or histological variables between the two groups. However, the improvement in biopsy scores at 3 months was greater in the colchicine-treated group. The investigators suggest that a larger study, perhaps including some 260 patients, might detect differences in the course of alcoholic hepatitis in colchicine-treated patients.

In a preliminary study, colchicine appeared to confer benefit in individuals with alcoholic cirrhosis (Rojkind, Lancet, 1973; i:38). In consequence, a double-blind, controlled trial was undertaken in which 43 cirrhotic patients, 25 (58 per cent) of whom abused alcohol, were randomized to receive either colchicine, 1 mg daily, 5 days a week, or else a placebo preparation (Kershenobich, Gastro, 1979; 77:532). The results were analysed in 1979, by which time patients had been treated for periods of up to 4 years. Those who had received colchicine showed greater clinical improvement and their serial liver biopsies showed a reduction in the degree of fibrosis. However, there was no significant difference in mortality rate between the colchicine-treated patients (17 per cent) and those receiving the placebo preparation (40 per cent). Details were not provided of the drinking behaviour of the patients during the trial, although it is believed that the majority continued to abuse alcohol.

This trial has now been extended to include 100 cirrhotic patients, 45 of whom had a significant history of alcohol abuse (Kershenobich, NEJM, 1988; 318:1709). The histological diagnosis proved incorrect in eight patients, leaving a study population of 92 individuals, 50 of whom were randomized to treatment with 1 mg of colchicine daily for 5 days a week for a minimum of 3 years, while the remaining 42 received a placebo preparation. Repeat liver biopsies were undertaken every 12 to 24 months. The cumulative survival rates in the colchicine-treated group were 73 per cent at 5 years and 51 per cent at 10 years, compared with rates of 24 per cent and 9 per cent in the control group ($p<0.001$). The median survival time in the patients treated with colchicine was 11.0 years compared with 3.5 years in the patients who received the placebo preparation. Cox's proportional hazards regression analysis was employed to take account of confounding variables, such as the severity of the liver lesion and the cause of the liver injury, and confirmed significant improvement in survival in those individuals receiving active treatment. The data from patients with alcoholic cirrhosis were not analysed separately but the investigators state that outcome was not influenced by the aetiological background of the liver disease. Thirty patients receiving colchicine underwent repeat histological examination and significant histological improvement was observed in nine. In contrast there was no evidence of histological improvement in the repeat liver biopsies obtained from 14 patients who had received the placebo preparation.

While at first sight the results of this trial look impressive, some care must be exercised in their interpretation. Thus, at the time of entry into the trial, there were a number of differences between the treated and untreated groups. There were, for example, more women and more individuals with oesophageal varices in the placebo group and, overall, these patients had higher serum aminotransferase activities and lower serum albumin concentrations than their treated counterparts. However, adjustments were made for these baseline inequalities in the groups, using Cox's regression model, and the difference in survival between the two groups was still significant.

A total of 22 patients were withdrawn from the study and 19 patients were non-compliant with treatment for prolonged periods. The overall study population was therefore reduced to 51. Of the 22 patients lost from the study, three (two colchicine, one placebo) developed peptic ulceration and were withdrawn 'alive' at the time of the incident, while the remaining 19 patients were lost to follow-up (10 colchicine, nine placebo) and were considered to have withdrawn from the study 'alive' at the time of their last visit to the clinic. These data were analysed on an intention-to-treat basis. However, the method of analysis used to deal with non-compliance or premature withdrawal of treatment is not clearly detailed. It was known that patients often discontinued the study medication for months at a time, and that 14 (six colchicine, eight placebo) did not take the study medication for periods of 6 or more months. In addition, medication was permanently discontinued in five treated patients by their attending physicians. No discussion is included as to how these problems were dealt with during analysis of the study results. Information is provided that seven patients (five colchicine, two placebo) out of the 45 with alcoholic cirrhosis continued to drink heavily, but no information is given on the drinking behaviour of the other 38 patients and its effects, if any, on compliance or survival.

At present, therefore, although the results of this Mexican study look promising (Kershenobich, NEJM, 1988; 318:1709), more trials are needed before firm recommendations can be made about the use of this drug in patients with alcohol-related liver disease. The clearance of colchicine is significantly impaired in patients with cirrhosis (Leighton, Hepatol, 1991; 14:1013), thus great care must be taken in determining drug schedules especially for long-term use.

D-Penicillamine

D-Penicillamine inhibits the cross-linkage of newly formed collagen, thus rendering its fibres more susceptible to the effects of collagenase. It might therefore reduce or impede hepatic fibrogenesis.

In one study, 40 patients admitted to hospital with moderately severe, precirrhotic, alcoholic hepatitis were randomized to 8 weeks of treatment with either 1 g of D-penicillamine daily or a placebo preparation (Resnick, Digestion, 1974; 11:257). Liver biopsies were obtained, in a small number of patients, before and after treatment. Similar improvements were observed in serum bilirubin and aspartate aminotransferase in both groups during the trial, and no difference was observed in mortality rates: 16 per cent of the patients treated with D-penicillamine and 19 per cent of those receiving the placebo died. There were reductions in the degree of hepatocellular necrosis and in the active disposition of collagen in liver biopsies obtained from both groups of patients, but the changes appeared greater in those who had received the active drug. However, the number of paired pre- and post-treatment biopsies was too small for adequate statistical analysis of these histological changes in relation to treatment.

Further short- and long-term studies of D-penicillamine in patients with alcohol-related liver disease are needed.

Propylthiouracil

The liver damage produced by both alcohol and hypoxia occurs predominantly in the centrizonal region. Thus it has been suggested that chronic alcohol consumption might induce a hypermetabolic state within the liver, resulting in an increased demand for oxygen, and ultimately leading to centrizonal hypoxia. Support was gained for this suggestion from a series of studies (Israel, BiochemJ, 1973; 134:523; FedProc, 1975; 34:2052) which showed that oxygen consumption rates were increased in animals with alcohol-induced hepatic injury and that these animals developed centrilobular necrosis if their liver oxygen supply was reduced. These changes could be suppressed by thyroidectomy and abolished by use of propylthiouracil (Bernstein, JPharmExpTher, 1975; 192:583; Israel, PNAS, 1975; 72:1137).

To date, four randomized, controlled, short-term trials of propylthiouracil in the treatment of alcoholic hepatitis have been undertaken [Orrego, Gastro, 1979; 76:105; Hallé, Gastro, 1981; 82: 925; Serrano-Cancino, AmJGastr, 1981; 76: 194 (Abstr.); Peirrugues, Gastro, 1989; 96: A644(Abstr.)]. In the first study, 133 patients with alcohol-related liver disease, 38 (29 per cent) of whom had alcoholic hepatitis, were randomized to treatment with either propylthiouracil, 300 mg daily, or to a placebo preparation for 6 weeks (Orrego, Gastro, 1979; 76:105). The data in the patients with fatty change could not be interpreted and no beneficial effects of treatment were seen in patients with alcoholic cirrhosis. In patients with alcoholic hepatitis, treatment was said to be associated with more rapid improvement in a number of clinical and laboratory variables. However, very few data were provided to support this contention.

In the remaining three, short-term studies, however, treatment with propylthiouracil was reported to be of little benefit. In one study, for example (Hallé, Gastro, 1981; 82:925), 67 patients with severe alcoholic hepatitis were randomized to treatment with either 225 mg of propylthiouracil daily, for 6 weeks, or to a placebo preparation; there was no significant difference in mortality rates between treated and control participants (23 vs 19 per cent) while four patients given propylthiouracil became hypothyroid.

The results of a long-term study of propylthiouracil in 360 patients with alcohol-related liver disease of varying severity have also been reported (Orrego, NEJM, 1987; 317:1421). The diagnosis was based on a history of alcohol abuse and on clinical and laboratory evidence of liver disease, and was confirmed in 293 patients (81 per cent) by histological examination of liver biopsy material: 25.6 per cent of individuals showed fatty change or non-cirrhotic fibrosis, 17.4 per cent alcoholic hepatitis, 9.9 per cent cirrhosis, and 47.1 per cent cirrhosis with superimposed alcoholic hepatitis. The patients were allocated to treatment with propylthiouracil, 300 mg daily, or to a placebo preparation, for a maximum of 2 years. Because of the risk of hypothyroidism, patients receiving propylthiouracil were automatically switched to placebo for 1 month out of every four. Patients were instructed to send daily morning urine samples to the trial centre; these were tested for ethanol and for the riboflavin added to the trial medication to assess compliance. Patients were deemed to be non-compliant if riboflavin was detected in less than 50 per cent of urine samples. The majority of individuals continued to drink; alcohol was detected in the urine of more than 95 per cent of patients at some stage during the trial.

A total of 50 patients (25 propylthiouracil, 25 placebo) were non-compliant and so were excluded from the primary analysis. A further 194 patients (104 propylthiouracil, 90 placebo) dropped out of the study, the drop-out rate being highest in the first 3 months. Thus, overall, 244 (68 per cent) of the original cohort of 360 patients defaulted in some way.

The cumulative mortality rate in the 310 compliant patients (157 propylthiouracil, 153 placebo) was 13 per cent in the patients treated with propylthiouracil and 25 per cent in the patients receiving the placebo ($p < 0.05$). In the 213 patients with mild to moderate disease (101 propylthiouracil, 112 placebo), treatment with propylthiouracil conferred no benefit. In the 97 patients with severe disease (56 propylthiouracil, 41 placebo), the cumulative mortality rate was 25 per cent in those treated with propylthiouracil and 55 per cent in those receiving placebo ($p < 0.05$). In the subgroup of patients with alcoholic hepatitis (90 propylthiouracil, 70 placebo), the cumulative mortality among those who were compliant with treatment was 13 per cent in the propylthiouracil group and 30 per cent in the placebo group ($p = 0.05$).

Of the 122 patients followed for a minimum of a year, 68 (56 per cent) had mean morning urinary ethanol concentrations of less than 8 mmol. In this subgroup the mortality rate was 2.8 per cent in those treated with propylthiouracil and 25 per cent in those who received the placebo ($p < 0.02$). However, in those with mean morning urinary ethanol concentrations in excess of 8 mmol, the mortality rates in the propylthiouracil- and placebo-treated patients were similar (22 vs 26 per cent).

Proportional hazards stepwise regression analyses indicated that only treatment with propylthiouracil, the prothrombin time, the haemoglobin level, and the mean daily urinary ethanol concentration significantly affected mortality. The hazards ratio for the complete group indicated that the mortality in the propylthiouracil group was only 38 per cent that of the placebo group. None of the treated patients became hypothyroid.

The patients who were non-compliant and those who dropped out of the study were followed to determine survival. The 50 non-compliant patients had a higher proportion of alcohol-positive urine samples than the compliant patients. The cumulative mortality rate in the non-compliant group was 24 per cent in the patients treated with propylthiouracil and 20 per cent in those receiving the placebo. The cumulative mortality rate in the 149 patients who dropped out of the study was 19 per cent in the propylthiouracil group and 20 per cent in the placebo group.

The design of this study is unnecessarily complex, and the reporting and interpretation of the data are selective. Almost a quarter of the patients had minimal liver injury which would not be expected to progress over a 2-year period, even in the presence of continued alcohol abuse. Indeed, the analyses showed no benefit for propylthiouracil in this subgroup. Their inclusion is difficult to justify on therapeutic and ethical grounds. It is unclear when the decision to exclude non-compliant patients from the analysis was made. In a study such as this, data are usually analysed on an intention-to-treat basis and it is difficult to justify deviation from this course, although the investigators have subsequently attempted

Table 9 Effect of treatment with insulin and glucagon in patients with alcoholic hepatitis included in randomized, controlled clinical trials

First author	Year	Trial duration (weeks)	Insulin (U/24 h)	Glucagon (mg/24 h)	Control group		Treatment group	
					Patients n	Deaths n (%)	Patients n	Deaths n (%)
Baker	1981	3	24	2.4	25	6 (24)	25	3 (12)
Mirouze	1981	2	36	4.0	12	7 (58)	14	6 (43)
Radvan	1982	2	48	4.8	15	7 (47)	16	4 (25)
Fehér	1987	3	30	3.0	33	14 (42)	33	5 (15)*
Bird	1991	3	30	3.0	43	14 (33)	43	15 (35)
Trinchet	1992	3	30	3.0	35	5 (14)	37	10 (27)
Totals					163	53 (33)	168	43 (26)

* Trial in which treatment conferred significant benefit.

to justify their 'per protocol' approach to the analysis (Orrego, JHepatol, 1994; 20:343).

Overall, it would appear from the data that propylthiouracil might benefit patients with severe alcoholic liver disease who significantly reduce their daily alcohol intake. However, the likelihood of patients complying with long-term treatment is poor; in the study under discussion almost 50 per cent of the patients discontinued treatment, often within the first few months.

Further studies are obviously needed, bearing in mind that propylthiouracil can itself induce hepatic necrosis (Limaye, AmJ-Gastr, 1987; 82:152), although, in general, the incidence of hepatotoxicity with this drug is low (Werner, AmJMedSci, 1989; 297:216).

Hepatotrophic factors

A number of factors are known to control hepatic regeneration in animals, of which the best studied are insulin and glucagon (Baker, ActaMedScandSuppl, 1985; 703:201). It is reasonable to assume that the mechanisms controlling hepatic regeneration in man are similar to those in animals, and the use of hepatotrophic factors in the treatment of liver disease in man is based on this assumption. To date, six randomized, controlled trials of insulin and glucagon in the treatment of alcoholic hepatitis have been undertaken (Baker, Gastro, 1981; 80:1410; Mirouze, GastrClinBiol, 1981; 5: 1187Abstr.; Radvan, Gastro, 1982; 82: 1154 (Abstr.); Fehér, JHepatol, 1987; 5: 224; Bird, Hepatol, 1991; 14:1097; Trinchet, Hepatol, 1992; 15: 76) (Table 9).

The results of the first trial (Baker, Gastro, 1981; 80:1410) were encouraging, if inconclusive. Thus, although mean serum bilirubin concentrations and prothrombin times improved to a significantly greater degree in the patients receiving insulin and glucagon, the 21-day mortality rates in the control (24 per cent) and treated patients (12 per cent) were not significantly different (Table 9). Although patients were not stratified according to disease severity at the start of the trial, only one (7 per cent) in the treatment group, whose prothrombin time was significantly prolonged, died, compared with six such patients (32 per cent) in the control group; again, this difference is not significant.

Similarly encouraging, but more conclusive, results were reported in another study (Fehér, JHepatol, 1987; 5:224); here the mean serum bilirubin concentration, serum aspartate aminotransferase and γ-glutamyl transferase activities, and prothrombin

time improved significantly in the treatment group whilst only the mean serum bilirubin improved in the control group, and then to a lesser degree. In addition, the 21-day mortality rate in the treated patients (15 per cent) was significantly less than in the controls (42 per cent) ($p < 0.02$) (Table 9). No significant benefits of treatment were, however, reported in the remaining four studies (Table 9).

Hypoglycaemia was observed, as a complication, in all of these studies and resulted in the death of at least one treated patient (Baker, Gastro, 1981; 80:140). In addition, a number of difficulties arose in maintaining intravenous access for prolonged periods of time. Given the potential complications and complexity of this form of treatment, and the limited evidence of its efficacy, its use is not recommended.

A better understanding of the mechanisms controlling hepatic regeneration, in man, might result in the development of more specific treatment regimens.

Alcohol dehydrogenase inhibitors

The redox state of the liver is significantly reduced during ethanol metabolism and most of the acute metabolic effects of alcohol reflect changes in intermediary metabolism (Lieber, NEJM, 1973; 288: 356). In addition, ethanol metabolism results in the production of acetaldehyde, which is a significant hepatotoxin in its own right (Lauterburg, JHepatol, 1988; 7:384). It has therefore been suggested that drugs which inhibit alcohol dehydrogenase might prevent or limit alcohol-related liver damage.

Pyrazole and its 4-substituted derivatives are potent and well-characterized competitive inhibitors of alcohol dehydrogenase (Lelbach, Experientia, 1969; 25:816; Theorell, ActaChemScand, 1969; 23:255; Lieber, LabInvest, 1970; 22:615; Magnusson, Experientia, 1972; 28:1198). They suppress ethanol oxidation and several ethanol-induced, redox-related changes in the liver. However, if rats are fed pyrazole or 4-methylpyrazole, together with ethanol, over a prolonged period, the hepatotoxic effects of the ethanol are, if anything, potentiated (Lelbach, Experientia, 1969; 25:816; Kalant, BiochPharm, 1972; 21:811; Lindros, Liver, 1983; 3:79). Human studies using these compounds are not therefore warranted.

Inhibitors of alcohol dehydrogenase may have a role, however, in the treatment of methanol poisoning (Bromstrand, PNAS, 1979; 76:3499; McMartin, ArchBiochemBiophys, 1980; 199:606) and ethylene glycol poisoning (Mundy, ToxApplPharmcol, 1974; 28:

Table 10 Results of seven double-blind controlled trials of (+)-cyanidanol-3 in alcohol-related liver disease

First author	Year	Liver disease	Patients (*n*)	Drug dosage (g/day)	Treatment period (months)	Alcohol monitored	Trial outcome
Colman	1980	Precirrhotic	40	2.0	3.0	Yes	No additional benefit
Henning	1981	Alcoholic hepatitis	70	3.0	0.5	Abstinent	No additional benefit
Palmas	1981	Compensated cirrhosis	31	3.0	5.0	No	Treatment group benefit at 3 months
Sanchez-Tapias	1981	Alcoholic hepatitis	27	1.4	3.0	No	No additional benefit
Ugarte	1981	'Compensated'	25	2.0	?	No	Serum enzymes ↓ in treatment group
		'Decompensated'	37	2.0	?	No	No additional benefit
Abonyi	1984	Precirrhotic	74	1.5–2.0	12.0	Yes	Serum enzymes ↓ in treatment group
World	1984	Precirrhotic (86 per cent)	50	2.0	6.0	Yes	No additional benefit

320; van Stee, JPharmExpTher, 1975; 192:251; Beasley, VetHumTox, 1980; 22:255), and in the management of the alcohol–disulfiram reaction (Lindros, Alcoholism, 1981; 5:528).

Hepatoprotective agents

The outcome of alcohol-related liver disease is determined largely by the patients' subsequent drinking behaviour. While approximately 50 per cent of patients do manage to abstain, or at least significantly reduce their alcohol intake, the remainder continue to drink (Katz, JStudAlc, 1981; 42:136). It has therefore been suggested (Thomson, BrJAlcAlc, 1980; 15:58) that drugs capable of preventing alcohol-related liver injury, or of limiting and repairing the damage already sustained, might play an important role in the management of these individuals. A number of so-called hepatoprotective agents are available and are extensively used, particularly in continental Europe (Morgan, Alcohol and disease. *Acta Medica Scandinavica Symposium Series, No. 1.* Uppsala: Almquist and Wiksell, 1985:225). However, the evidence that their use confers any substantial benefit is poor.

(+)-Cyanidanol-3

(+)-Cyanidanol-3 (Catechin) is the best known and most extensively investigated hepatoprotective drug. It is a naturally occurring bioflavinoid that has antioxidant and membrane-stabilizing properties, and an ability to scavenge free radicals. It has been shown to normalize the NADH:NAD ratio, to increase ATP concentrations, and to stabilize lysosomal membranes in the livers of rats with alcohol-related liver injury. It also has a beneficial effect on collagen synthesis in rats given lathyrogenic drugs.

Seven randomized, double-blind trials in which (+)-cyanidanol-3 was used to treat alcohol-related liver disease have been reported to date (Table 10). In six studies, treatment with (+)-cyanidanol-3 conferred no benefit (Colman, Gut, 1980; 21:965; Henning, *International workshop on (+)-cyanidanol-3 in diseases of the liver.* London: Grune and Stratton, 1981:177; Sanchez-Tapias, *International workshop on (+)-cyanidanol-3 in diseases of the liver.* London: Grune and Stratton, 1981:173; Ugarte, *International workshop on (+)-cyanidanol-3 in diseases of the liver.* London: Grune and Stratton, 1981:181; Abonyi, ActaPhysiolHung, 1984; 64:455; World, AlcAlc, 1984; 19:23). In the remaining study (Palmas, *International workshop on (+)-cyanidanol-3 in diseases of the liver.* London: Grune

Table 11 Changes in hepatic histology over 3 months in relation to drinking behaviour and treatment with (+)-cyanidanol-3 or placebo

Treatment	Overall histological assessment *n* (%)		
	Unchanged	Improved	Deteriorated
(+)-Cyanidanol-3:			
Abstinent (9)	2 (22)	5 (55)	2 (22)
Drinking (10)	3 (30)	7 (70)	
Placebo:			
Abstinent (7)	2 (28)	5 (72)	
Drinking (13)	4 (30)	9 (70)	

Adapted from Colman, Gut, 1980; 21: 965.

and Stratton, 1981:167), patients with cirrhosis, mainly of alcoholic origin, who received (+)-cyanidanol-3 in a dose of 3 g daily for 5 months showed some improvement in laboratory variables from the third month onwards. The results of this trial are not readily interpreted, however, as no information is provided on the patients' drinking behaviour during the trial period.

The biochemical, haematological, and histological improvements seen in patients with alcohol-related liver disease who abstain or significantly reduce their alcohol intake are so pronounced that, unless drinking behaviour is monitored, any additional benefit conferred by treatment with a hepatoprotective agent might escape attention. In only two of these seven studies (Colman, Gut, 1980; 21:965; World, AlcAlc, 1984; 19:23) were trial outcomes analysed taking drinking behaviour into account. In the first trial, improvements were noted in mean values for serum enzyme activities and erythrocyte mean corpuscular volume in both treatment and control groups (Colman, Gut, 1980; 21:965;). However, when the drinking behaviour of the patients during the trial period was taken into account, it became clear that significant changes in laboratory variables only occurred in those patients who remained abstinent from alcohol. No separate or additional benefit was conferred by treatment with (+)-cyanidanol-3 (Fig. 5). The changes in liver histology over the 3-month period differentiated the drinking and abstinent patients less clearly, but again no beneficial effect from treatment with the drug was observed (Table 11). Similarly, in the

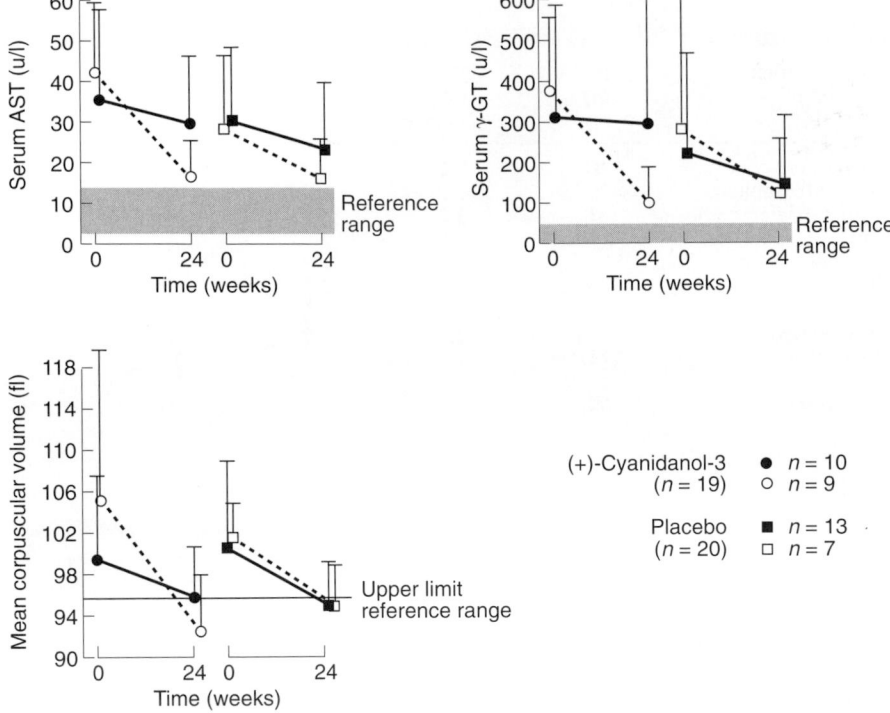

Fig. 5. Changes occurring in mean (± 1 SD) values for serum aspartate aminotransferase (AST), γ-glutamyl transferase (γ-GT), and erythrocyte mean corpuscular volume in alcohol abusers either continuing to drink (—) or abstinent from alcohol (---) during treatment with (+)-cyanidanol-3 or placebo (Colman, Gut, 1980; 21:965).

later trial (World, AlcAlc, 1984; 19:23), no benefits were observed in laboratory test results or liver histology in the treatment group other than those resulting from a reduction in alcohol intake.

Thioctic acid (α-lipoic acid)

Thioctic acid is a naturally occurring compound that is a cofactor in the pyruvate dehydrogenase and α-ketoglutarate dehydrogenase enzyme complexes forming part of the citric acid cycle; it also increases prostaglandin synthesis by an action on prostaglandin cyclo-oxygenase. Apart from some evidence to suggest that it may be of use in treating liver failure following *Amanita phalloides* poisoning (Frimmer, KlinWschr, 1968; 46:1288; Zulik, Lancet, 1972; ii:228), reports of its beneficial effects in liver disease are largely anecdotal (Thompson, AmJMed, 1956; 21:131; Moller, MedKlin, 1967; 62:380; Glaeser, Therapiewoche, 1980; 30:5585).

In a randomized, double-blind trial of thioctic acid, 300 mg daily, against placebo over a 6-month period, in 40 patients with precirrhotic, alcohol-related liver disease, improvements were noted in mean values for serum enzyme activities and erythrocyte mean corpuscular volume in both treated and control groups (Marshall, Gut, 1982; 23:1088). However, significant changes in laboratory variables were only observed in those patients who remained abstinent from alcohol. No separate or additional benefit was conferred by treatment (Fig. 6). The number of patients showing histological improvement was similar in both groups; improvement was seen predominantly in those who had abstained from alcohol. At present, therefore, there is no evidence to suggest that thioctic acid protects the liver from alcohol-related injury.

Silymarin

Silymarin is a compound, extracted from the fruit *Silybium marianum*, that consists of a complex of three isomeric compounds of the phenylchromanone group. There is experimental (Hahn, ArzForsch, 1968; 18:698; Castigli, PharmResComm, 1977; 9:59) and clinical evidence (Benda, WienMedWoch, 1973;123:512; Fassati, CasLekCesk, 1973; 112:865; Benda, WienMedWoch, 1980; 92:678; Reutter, Praxis, 1975; 64:1145) to suggest that silymarin may have a favourable effect on the course of various hepatic disorders.

A 4-week, randomized, double-blind trial of silymarin, 420 mg daily, against placebo, was undertaken in 97 patients admitted to hospital because of persistent elevation of serum aminotransferases (Salmi, ScaJGastr, 1982; 17:517). The majority were young soldiers, 78 per cent of whom reported regular daily alcohol consumption. Liver biopsy showed fatty change in 48 per cent, acute or subacute hepatitis in 30 per cent, and was normal in 22 per cent. Alcohol intake was forbidden during the first week in hospital, but some difficulty was encountered in monitoring intake during the rest of the trial. Nevertheless, patients treated with silymarin showed significantly greater decreases in serum aminotransferase activities during the trial than those receiving the placebo (Fig. 7). In addition, 73 per cent of the treated and 29 per cent of the control patients who underwent rebiopsy showed clear improvement in liver histology. In the absence of details of the patients' drinking behaviour during the trial, these findings are difficult to interpret.

In another trial [Salvagnini, JHepatol, 1985;1 (Suppl.): S142 (Abstr.)], 122 alcohol abusers with abnormal liver function tests were randomized to treatment with either silymarin, 420 mg daily,

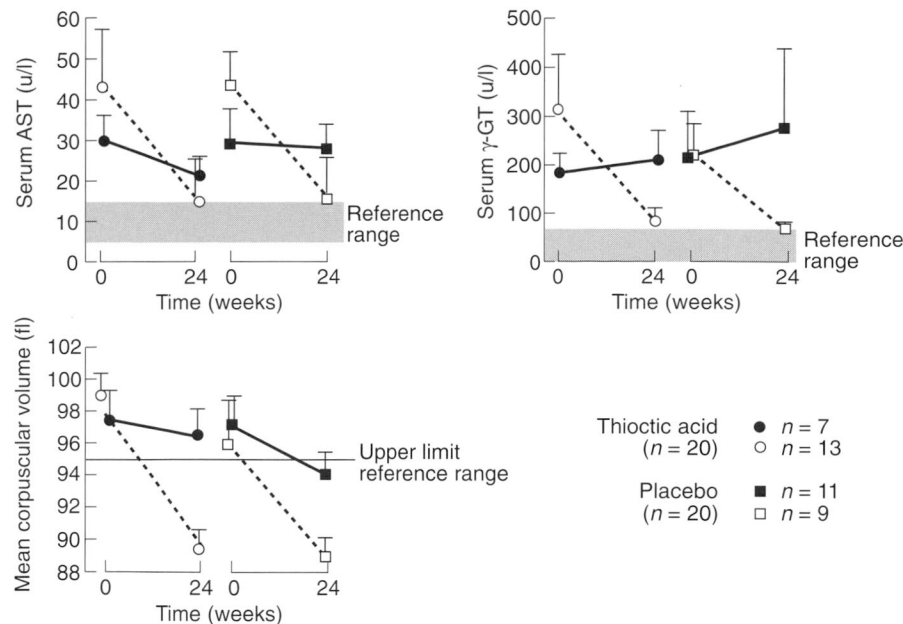

Fig. 6. Changes occurring in mean (±SEM) values for serum aspartate aminotransferase (AST), γ-glutamyl transferase (γ-GT), and erythrocyte mean corpuscular volume in alcohol abusers either continuing to drink (—) or abstinent from alcohol (---) during treatment with thioctic acid or placebo (Marshall, Gut, 1981; 23:1088).

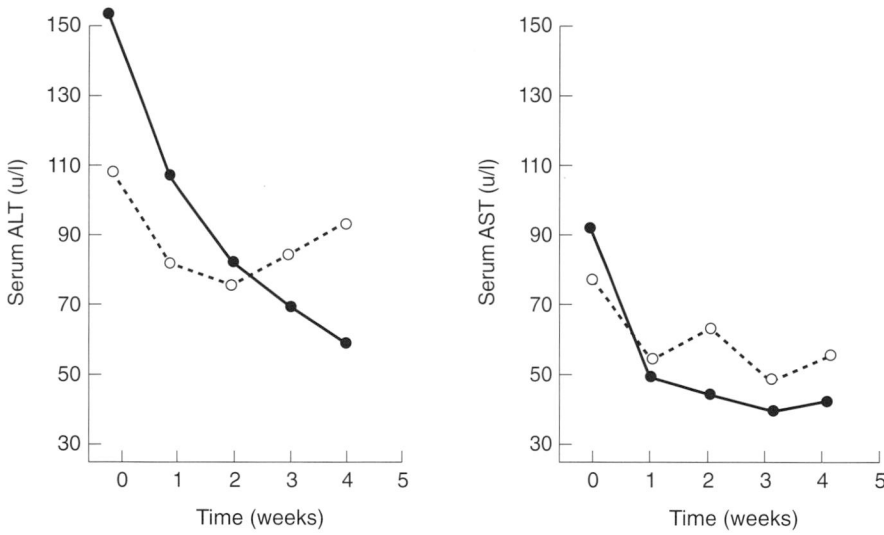

Fig. 7. Changes occurring in mean serum aspartate (AST) and alanine (ALT) aminotransferase activities in individuals receiving either silymarin (n = 50; ●—●) or a placebo preparation (n = 47; ○---○) for treatment of persistent enzyme abnormalities (Salmi, ScaJGastr, 1982; 17:517).

or a placebo preparation, for a period of 45 days. During this time, 28 per cent of the patients receiving silymarin and 35 per cent of those receiving placebo drank small amounts of alcohol daily. At the end of the trial, significantly greater improvements were observed in values for erythrocyte mean corpuscular volume and serum aspartate aminotransferase activity in the silymarin-treated patients. Further details of the separate effects of abstinence from alcohol and treatment with silymarin are not given.

In a further study (Láng, ItalJGastr, 1990; 22:283), 40 patients with well-compensated alcoholic cirrhosis were randomized to treatment, for 1 month, with either silymarin, 420 mg daily in divided doses, or a placebo preparation. Patients in both groups substantially reduced their alcohol intake during the trial period. Patients receiving the active drug showed significant reductions in their serum bilirubin concentrations, and their serum aspartate and alanine aminotransferase and γ-glutamyl transferase activities, whereas no significant changes were observed in these variables in those receiving the placebo preparation.

In a long-term, double-blind, controlled trial, 170 cirrhotic patients, 87 (61 per cent) of whom had abused alcohol, were randomized to treatment with either silymarin, 420 mg daily in divided doses, or to a placebo preparation, for periods of up to 2 years (Ferenci, JHepatol, 1989; 9:105). All patients completing the study were maintained on the trial preparations until the last one to enter had completed 2 years of treatment. Fourteen patients in the active treatment group and 10 in the placebo group were lost to follow-up. The 4-year survival rate in the patients receiving the silymarin was 58 per cent compared with 39 per cent in the patients receiving the placebo ($p = 0.04$). Analysis of the subgroups showed that treatment was only effective in patients with alcoholic cirrhosis ($p = 0.01$) and those with well-compensated liver disease at the time of entry into the trial ($p = 0.03$). Information was not provided on the drinking behaviour of the patients with alcoholic cirrhosis so that no really firm conclusion can be drawn about the efficacy of treatment with this compound.

Further studies are required.

Malotilate

Malotilate (di-isopropyl 1,3-dithiol-2-ylidenemalonate) reduces liver injury in animals exposed to a variety of toxins, including alcohol (Dumont, JHepatol, 1986; 3:260; Matsuda, Alcohol-ClinExpRes, 1988; 12:665). Results of an early placebo-controlled trial of malotilate in patients with alcoholic liver disease suggested that this drug might have beneficial effects on hepatic protein synthesis (Takase, Alcohol, 1989; 6:219). However, no beneficial effects of treatment with malotilate were observed in a large European, multicentre study in patients with alcoholic hepatitis (Mutimer, Hepatol, 1988; 8: 1411 (Abstr.)). More recently, in a multicentre, double-blind, randomized trial in patients with alcoholic liver disease of varying severity, treatment with malotilate in a dose of 750 mg daily for a minimum of 6 months was associated with a significant improvement in survival at 1 year and beyond (Keiding, JHepatol, 1994; 20:454). No such benefit was observed, however, in individuals receiving malotilate 1500 mg daily. The first-pass elimination of this drug is significantly reduced in patients with cirrhosis (Buhrer, EurJClinPharm, 1986; 30:407), and this might explain the 'dose paradox', although there was no relation between the severity of the liver injury and the response to treatment. Further studies could be justified.

Other compounds

A number of other compounds are available that might have hepatoprotective properties, for example naftidrofuryl, which has been shown to increase hepatic ATP production [Majumdar, Gut, 1979; 20: A449(Abstr.)] and S-adenosyl-l-methionine, which is known to increase hepatic glutathione production (Vendemiale, ScaJGastr, 1989; 24:407) and which attenuates alcohol-induced liver injury in baboons (Lieber, Hepatol, 1990; 11:165). Ursodeoxycholic acid has been shown to benefit patients with cholestatic, non-alcoholic liver disease; benefit may also be observed in patients with alcohol-related liver injury. Thus in one study 11 individuals with alcoholic cirrhosis who were continuing to abuse alcohol were randomized to treatment with ursodeoxycholic acid in a dose of 15 mg/kg daily for 4 weeks

or to a placebo preparation (Plevris, EurJGastroHepatol, 1991; 3: 653); treatment was associated with a significant fall in serum bilirubin and in serum alanine aminotransferase and γ-glutamyl transferase activities. Use of the Ayurvedic drug LIV.52 is associated with improvement in the results of liver function tests in patients with chronic liver disease, but has recently been shown to have a detrimental effect on survival in patients with decompensated alcoholic cirrhosis. Individuals compliant with treatment had a 2-year survival rate of 40 per cent compared with a rate of 81 per cent in individuals receiving a placebo preparation (Fleig, JHepatol, 1997; 26 (Suppl.): 127 P/CO8/04 (Abstr.)).

Nutritional therapy[36,37]

Very little information is available on the nutritional requirements of patients with alcoholic liver disease (Müller, ClinNutr, 1994; 13: 31; Nompleggi, Hepatol, 1994; 19:518). In one of the few investigations available (Weber, DigDisSci, 1982; 27:103), metabolic balance investigations were undertaken in patients with alcoholic hepatitis, and it was observed that daily protein intakes of 30 g were associated with negative nitrogen balance while daily intakes in the region of 70 to 100 g protein ensured positive nitrogen balance. It is also likely that daily energy requirements are increased in this patient population (Levine, Hepatol, 1994; 20: 318(Abstr.)).

Dietary intake may be limited by anorexia and nausea, with the result that a high percentage of total daily energy may be consumed as alcohol (Morgan, ActaChirScandSuppl, 1981; 507:81). These patients are, in consequence, frequently malnourished and this has a detrimental effect on survival (Mendenhall, AlcoholClinExpRes, 1995; 19:635; Merli, Hepatol, 1996; 23:1041). There is therefore a clear rationale for the provision of nutritional support in this population.

In a small number of studies, nutritional supplements were provided for patients with alcoholic hepatitis by the oral or enteral routes (Calvey, JHepatol, 1985; 1:141; Mendenhall, JPEN, 1985; 9: 590; Soberon, Hepatol, 1987; 7:1204; Keans, Gastro, 1992; 102: 200).

In one such study, the effects of oral nutritional support on outcome in 57 patients with moderate to severe alcoholic hepatitis were assessed (Mendenhall, JPEN, 1985; 9:590). Thirty-four patients were given a standard hospital diet and were allowed to eat *ad libitum*. The remaining 23 patients were given the same diet together with a supplement high in calories, protein, and branched-chain amino acids. Both groups were monitored over 30 days. At the end of the trial period the patients receiving the enteral supplement showed improvements in six of the nine variables used to assess nutritional status, whereas these variables were either unchanged or else had deteriorated in the patients given the hospital diet alone; mortality rates were similar in the control (21 per cent) and supplemented (17 per cent) groups. These two dietary regimens were obviously not comparable as they were neither isocaloric nor isonitrogenous. Thus it is impossible to draw any conclusions, from this study, about the benefits of nutritional supplementation over provision of a diet adequate in calories and protein consumed *ad libitum*.

In a more detailed study, 64 patients with severe alcoholic hepatitis were provided with a basic daily diet containing 1800 to 2400 kcal, 40 to 80 g of protein and 22 mmol of sodium (Calvey,

JHepatol, 1985; 1:141). Twenty-one received an additional 65 g of conventional protein and 2000 non-protein calories daily, while a further 21 received 45 g of conventional protein, 25 g of branched-chain amino acids, and 2000 non-protein calories daily. These supplements were given orally, enterally or, if necessary, intravenously, for approximately 3 weeks. At the end of the trial period no differences were observed in mortality rates between the control (32 per cent) and supplemented (38 per cent) groups. Overall, the mortality rate was significantly higher in the patients who failed to achieve positive nitrogen balance, independently of the dietary regimen used (58 vs 3 per cent; $p<0.001$). This confirms the observation that survival is significantly decreased in patients with chronic liver disease who are unable to maintain nitrogen balance (Fiaccadori, ItalJGastr, 1993; 25:336).

In a more recent study, 31 patients with alcoholic hepatitis were randomized to receive, for 28 days, either a standard hospital diet or else the same diet supplemented with a casein-based, enteral feed (Keans, Gastro, 1992; 102:200). During the trial period, patients in the supplemented group showed a more rapid clearing of their encephalopathy, a significant fall in their mean serum bilirubin concentration and a significant increase in their mean antipyrine clearance. The mortality rates in the supplemented (13 per cent) and non-supplemented (27 per cent) groups were not, however, significantly different. This study has been criticized because the energy intake in the non-supplemented group met only 80 per cent of predicted requirements, whereas the intake in the supplemented group exceeded predicted requirements by 70 per cent; likewise, the daily protein intakes in the non-supplemented and supplemented groups were widely disparate, viz 50 compared to 103 g. Thus it is difficult to draw conclusions. However, these workers were able to show that it is possible to feed these patients enterally and that enteral feeds are well tolerated. Similar conclusions were drawn by others (Soberon, Hepatol, 1987; 7:1204).

To date, a total of seven controlled trials of the effects of parenteral nutritional supplementation in patients with alcoholic hepatitis have been undertaken (Nasrallah, Lancet, 1980; ii:1276; Diehl, Hepatol, 1985; 5:57; Naveau, Hepatol, 1986; 6:270; Achord, AmJGastr, 1987; 82:871; Simon, JHepatol, 1988; 7:200; Bonkovsky, AmJGastr, 1991; 86:1020; Bonkovsky, AmJGastr, 1991; 86:1209; Mezey, Hepatol, 1991; 14:1090) (Table 12).

Overall the number of treated patients is small. The majority appear to have had mild to moderate alcoholic hepatitis as evidenced by the mortality rates in the control populations, which ranged from 0 to 22 per cent. Histological confirmation of the diagnosis was obtained in from 0 to 100 per cent of patients in the various studies; between 0 to 100 per cent of the individuals biopsied had established cirrhosis. Inclusion and exclusion criteria varied. All participants were given a well-balanced hospital diet that provided at least 30 kcal/kg and 1 g protein/kg daily, and received oral vitamin and mineral supplements. The experimental groups received, in addition, a parenteral infusion of standard amino acids with or without glucose and lipid. In two of the studies the control group received an intravenous infusion of glucose in addition to the standard diet, while in a third, individuals in the control group received an enteral supplement in addition to the standard diet. Treatment was continued for between 21 to 30 days. A wide range of variables were used to assess both liver function and nutritional

status, and these varied considerably between studies. In all seven studies, however, the end-point was death (Table 12).

Several of these studies warrant further description. The earliest study was the only one in which treatment conferred significant benefit in terms of outcome (Nasrallah, Lancet, 1980; ii:1276). The study population comprised 35 patients with biopsy-proven alcoholic hepatitis, one-third of whom had cirrhosis. All patients were given a daily diet containing 100 g of protein and 3000 kcal. The 17 patients allocated to the treatment group received, in addition, approximately 40 g/day of an intravenous, balanced amino-acid mixture for 3 days, followed by 80 g/day for a further 25 days. No placebo infusion was used (Table 12).

Dietary intakes were similar in both control and treatment groups, but were significantly less than the amounts originally provided. During the trial period, significant improvements were seen in serum bilirubin and plasma albumin concentrations in the patients receiving the nutritional supplement. The difference in survival between the control and supplemented groups was significant (0 vs 22 per cent; $p<0.01$) (Table 12). However, some caution must be exercised in interpreting these results in view of the difference in the sex ratio of patients in the two groups. Women with alcoholic liver disease generally have a worse prognosis than men and in this study there were proportionately more women in the control group. Nevertheless, the results were encouraging.

In the next study to be undertaken, 15 patients with biopsy-proven alcoholic hepatitis all ingested a hospital diet *ad libitum*; in addition, five received a parenteral amino acid–glucose solution daily for 1 month, while the remaining ten received intravenous glucose alone (Diehl, Hepatol, 1985; 5:57) (Table 12). Total calorie intakes were similar in the two groups but the mean daily protein intake in the group receiving the intravenous amino acids was 139 g compared with only 98 g in the control group. Clinical and biochemical abnormalities improved significantly in both groups. A greater improvement was seen in nitrogen balance in the patients given parenteral amino acids, but no changes were observed in the various anthropometric measures. Fatty infiltration resolved more quickly in the patients given the additional nitrogen, but otherwise there was little effect on hepatic histology. These investigators found significant correlations between certain clinical, laboratory, and histological abnormalities and the quantity of alcohol consumed before admission, and appear to suggest that the outcome of the trial was more influenced by the severity of the initial illness than by the use of parenteral amino-acid supplements.

In a further trial, 28 patients with a clinical or histological diagnosis of alcoholic hepatitis, approximately 57 per cent of whom had established cirrhosis, were randomized to treatment, for 21 days, with either conventional therapy alone or conventional therapy supplemented with a daily intravenous infusion of an amino acid–glucose solution (Achord, AmJGastr, 1987; 82:871) (Table 12). The mortality rates in the control and supplemented groups were not significantly different (21 vs 7 per cent). Significant intragroup improvement was observed in serum bilirubin and aspartate aminotransferase levels in the patients receiving conventional therapy, and in serum bilirubin, aspartate aminotransferase, and albumin levels in those receiving the supplement. Alcoholic hyaline was observed in six of eight initial liver biopsies in both groups. At the end of the study, hyaline was observed in five (83 per cent) of six biopsies from control participants but in only one (17 per cent) of six biopsies

Table 12 Effect of parenteral nutritional supplementation in patients with alcoholic hepatitis included in randomized, controlled clinical trials

First author	Year	Trial duration (days)	Control regimen (daily)	Experimental regimen (daily)	Control group Patients n	Control group Deaths n (%)	Treatment group Patients n	Treatment group Deaths n (%)
Nasrallah	1980	25	Standard diet	Standard diet + IV 80 g a.a	18	4 (22)	17	0 (0)*
Diehl	1985	30	Standard diet + IV 130 g glucose	Standard diet + IV 52 g a.a + 130 g glucose	10	0 (0)	5	0 (0)
Naveau	1986	28	Standard diet	Standard diet + IV 90 g a.a + 2800 kcal as glucose and lipid	20	1 (5)	20	1 (5)
Achord	1987	21	Standard diet	Standard diet + IV 43 g a.a + 200 g glucose	14	3 (21)	14	1 (7)
Simon	1988	28	Standard diet + 132 g protein + 3200 kcal orally	Standard diet + IV 70 g a.a + 100 g glucose/50 g lipid	18	3 (17)	16	4 (25)
Bonkovsky	1991	21	Standard diet	Standard diet + IV 70 g a.a + 100 g glucose	12	0 (0)	9	0 (0)
Mezey	1991	30	Standard diet + IV 130 g glucose	Standard diet + IV 52 g a.a + 130 g glucose	26	5 (19)	28	6 (21)

IV, intravenous; a.a, amino acids.
* Trial in which the experimental regimen conferred benefit.

from the supplemented patients; these figures are too small to allow for statistical comparison.

In another small study, 12 patients with moderate and 22 with severe alcoholic hepatitis were randomized to 28 days of treatment with either standard therapy alone or standard therapy plus parenteral nutrition (Simon, JHepatol, 1988; 7:200) (Table 12). None of the patients with moderate hepatitis died and no significant treatment effects were observed in this group. There was no significant difference in mortality between patients with severe alcoholic hepatitis treated with standard therapy (25 per cent) and those given additional nutritional support (40 per cent), but the use of parenteral nutrition was associated with a greater improvement in serum bilirubin and transferrin concentrations.

Finally, both short- and long-term outcomes were assessed in 54 patients with severe alcoholic hepatitis randomized to receive either 2 l of a parenteral dextrose–amino acid mixture daily for 1 month or intravenous dextrose alone; all patients received a standard hospital diet (Mezey, Hepatol, 1991; 14:1090) (Table 12). Nitrogen balance improved in the treated but not in the control patients, as did the serum aspartate aminotransferase activity and the prothrombin time. However, there were no differences in either the short-term mortality rates between the control and treated patients (19 vs 21 per cent), or in the 2-year mortality rates (38 vs 42 per cent).

The results of these studies are extremely difficult to interpret because it is often unclear what comparisons the investigators were trying to make. In several, the comparison made was ostensibly of the effects on outcome of a nutritionally adequate diet and a regimen providing excess protein and energy. However, in the majority of these studies, voluntary food intake was appreciably less than the amount offered and less than the amount required to sustain adequate nutritional status. In consequence, the comparisons made were effectively between regimens that were either nutritionally adequate or nutritionally inadequate.

Because of the difficulties inherent in the interpretation of these data, conclusions cannot be drawn. However, a number of observations can be made: first, voluntary food intake is likely to be poor in patients with moderate to severe alcoholic hepatitis, with the result that they may not be able to attain optimal nutrient intake unaided; second, provision of adequate energy and protein intakes will result in improvement in nutritional status and liver function, even in patients who are severely ill, but has little effect on short-term mortality; and third, no appreciable adverse events are associated with the provision of high-energy, high-protein nutritional supplements—these regimens are well-tolerated by even the most severely ill patients without exacerbation of fluid retention, azotaemia, or hepatic encephalopathy.

Thus it would seem essential to ensure that all patients with alcoholic hepatitis are adequately nourished. They should receive a minimum of 1.2 to 1.5 g of protein/kg daily and this should be given, whenever possible, by the oral or enteral route; if difficulties are encountered in meeting requirements, then a proportion of the required intake can be given parenterally, preferably via a peripheral vein.

Patients with cirrhosis have increased protein requirements; positive nitrogen balance is generally only achieved with intakes in excess of 1.2 g/kg daily (Gabuzda, AmJClinNutr, 1970; 23:479; Swart, ClinNutr, 1989; 8:329; Nielsen, BrJNutr, 1993; 69:665; BrJNutr, 1995; 74:557). Mild to moderately malnourished patients with cirrhosis retain dietary protein when their intake is increased almost as efficiently as healthy underweight individuals (Nielsen, BrJNutr, 1995; 74:557). It is therefore surprising that very little information is available on the effects of nutritional therapy on outcome in patients with alcoholic cirrhosis.

In one study, 35 severely malnourished cirrhotic patients, 66 per cent of whom were alcoholic, were randomized to either enteral tube feeding as their sole nutritional support or to a supposedly isocaloric, isonitrogenous, low-sodium diet, for a period of approximately 24 days (Cabré, Gastro, 1990; 98:715). The enteral feed provided a daily total of 2115 kcal, 71 g of whole protein enriched with branched-chain amino acids, 38 g of fat, mainly as medium-chain triglycerides, and 367 g of carbohydrate as maltodextrin; vitamins and trace elements were included at the upper limit of recommended daily allowances. The feed, which was energy-dense, providing 1.4 kcal/ml and hence only 1 litre of free water daily, was infused continuously into the stomach through a fine-bore nasogastric feeding tube using a peristaltic pump. The standard, low-sodium hospital diet supplied approximately 2200 kcal and 70 to 80 g of protein daily.

During the trial period the incidence of major complications of liver disease, such as gastrointestinal haemorrhage, fluid retention, and serious bacterial infection, was similar in both groups. However, significantly fewer patients receiving the enteral feed died as a result of these complications than patients receiving the standard diet (12 vs 47 per cent; $p = 0.02$). The investigators speculated that continuous nutrient infusion into the gastrointestinal tract might have reduced the catabolic response to injury in the enterally fed patients, thus helping them to cope better with septic complications.

Although impressive, these results must be interpreted with caution because, contrary to the design of the study, the dietary intakes in the two groups were neither isocaloric nor isonitrogenous. Thus, the mean estimated daily energy intake in the control group was only 1320 kcal compared with 2115 kcal in the experimental group ($p<0.0001$). The mean serum albumin concentration increased significantly in the group receiving the enteral feed, and it is likely that the improvement in survival observed in these patients reflected the beneficial effects of increasing nutrient intake rather than a specific effect of the feeding regimen itself.

In a controlled trial of the long-term effects of nutritional supplementation on outcome in patients with decompensated alcoholic cirrhosis, 51 outpatients were randomized either to an experimental group receiving a casein-based enteral supplement, which provided 1000 kcal and 34 g of protein daily for 1 year, or to a control group receiving a daily placebo capsule for a similar period (Hirsch, JPEN, 1993; 17:119). The within-study mortality rates in the control and experimental groups were not significantly different (24 vs 11.5 per cent). However, the rate of hospital admissions during the year was significantly lower in the experimental group, most probably reflecting a lower incidence of severe infection within this population. Dietary energy and protein intakes were, as expected, significantly higher in the supplemented patients, but improvements were observed throughout the study period in a number of biochemical and anthropometric variables in both study populations, although they tended to occur earlier in those receiving the nutritional supplement. Thus the improvements observed in disease morbidity in association with nutritional supplementation cannot be attributed solely to improvement in nutritional status.

However the findings of these two studies are interpreted, they serve to emphasize the importance of ensuring an adequate nutrient intake in patients with chronic liver disease. Enteral feeding is an excellent adjunct to oral feeding in compromised patients (Heymsfield, AnnIntMed, 1979; 90:63; Cabré, JClinNutrGastro, 1986; 1: 97).

Symptomatic treatment of the complications of liver disease

The principles of treatment of the major complications of established alcoholic liver disease, such as variceal haemorrhage, hepatic encephalopathy, fluid retention, and spontaneous bacterial peritonitis, are similar to those applied in individuals with other forms of chronic liver disease. In individuals who are actively drinking until the time of admission, management of these complications may be compromised by the presence of alcohol withdrawal.

Liver transplantation[38–41]

Liver transplantation is associated with a 5-year survival of approximately 70 per cent; it therefore provides an excellent therapeutic option for many patients with endstage chronic liver disease (Neuberger, BMJ, 1989; 299:693; Starzl, NEJM, 1989; 321:1014; Bird, BMJ, 1990; 301:15; Lucey, GastrClinNAm, 1993; 22:243; Berlakovich, Transpl, 1996; 61:554). The suitability of patients with alcoholic liver disease as candidates for liver transplantation has been debated since the advent of transplantation programmes, and clear guidelines are still lacking (Atterbury, JClinGastr, 1986; 8:1; Bird, BMJ, 1990; 301:15; Lucey, GastrClinNAm, 1993; 22:243; Sherman, AlcAlc, 1995; 30:141).[38–41]

There can be little doubt that abstinence from alcohol is associated, in the majority of patients, with improved liver function and prolonged survival.[11] It is also apparent that some patients develop progressive impairment of liver function despite abstinence from alcohol,[8] and that subsequent drinking behaviour may have little effect on outcome in patients presenting with advanced portal hypertension (Soterakis, Lancet, 1973; ii:65; Pande, Gastro, 1978; 74:64; McCormick, JHepatol, 1992; 14:99). Equally, there are, at present, no effective methods for treating decompensated alcoholic cirrhosis. Given, therefore, that alcoholic liver disease is the most common form of liver disease in the Western world today, it would seem reasonable to consider patients with endstage alcoholic cirrhosis for transplantation.

A number of objections have, however, been raised to the inclusion of such patients in transplant programmes. First, they may have other alcohol-related medical problems, such as cardiomyopathy, pancreatitis, neuropathy, and malnutrition, which might impede their management and worsen overall prognosis; second, patients who have abused alcohol for many years may have a variety of emotional, financial, and social problems, and may be relatively isolated in society, so lacking the support necessary to withstand the rigors of the transplant procedure and the months thereafter; third, they might resume alcohol misuse/abuse after transplantation and this might be associated with non-compliance with management regimens, thereby jeopardizing the allograft; and finally, inclusion of such patients in transplant programmes might adversely affect donor recruitment and might result in deferment of treatment for patients with non-alcoholic liver disease.

In the early days of liver transplantation, patients with alcoholic liver disease were excluded as candidates, probably because of those concerns (Starzl, Hepatol, 1982; 2:614; Rolles, Hepatol, 1984; 4 (Suppl.):50S). In 1983 the United States National Institute of Health convened a consensus development panel to devise guidelines for transplantation. They decided that liver transplantation could be considered for patients with alcoholic liver disease in whom there was evidence of progressive liver failure despite medical treatment and abstinence from alcohol (JAMA, 1983; 250:2961). No optimal time for surgery was stated and there was no recommended period of abstinence from alcohol before surgery.

A number of centres now offer transplant services to patients with alcoholic liver disease. Where transplantation has been undertaken, outcomes are good in terms of survival and do not differ substantially from those reported in patients with non-alcoholic chronic liver disease. Thus, survival rates of 66 to 80 per cent at 1 year, 71 to 83 per cent at 2 years, and 63 to 68 per cent at 5 years have been reported (Bird, BMJ, 1990; 301:15; Kumar, Hepatol, 1990; 11:159; Knechtle, Surgery, 1992; 112:694; Lucey, Gastro, 1992; 102:1736; McCurry, ArchSurg, 1992; 127:772; Berlakovich, Transpl, 1994; 58:560; Poynard, Lancet, 1994; 344:502; Berlakovich, Transpl, 1996; 61:554). Survival figures are higher in the later series, undoubtedly reflecting advances in surgical techniques, improvement in immunosuppressive regimens, and better selection of patients.

There appears to be no significant difference in resource utilization between patients transplanted for alcoholic and non-alcoholic cirrhosis (McCurry, ArchSurg, 1992; 127:772). Indeed, there is evidence that patients with alcoholic cirrhosis suffer significantly fewer episodes of acute cellular rejection post-transplantation than their non-alcoholic counterparts (Berlakovich, Transpl, 1996; 61:554; Farges, Transpl, 1996; 23:240).

Where data are available they show that the degree of social rehabilitation and quality of life achieved by recipient survivors is excellent and similar to that achieved by individuals transplanted for non–alcoholic cirrhosis (Kumar, Hepatol, 1990; 11:159; Knechtle, Surgery, 1992; 112:694; Gish, AmJGastr, 1993; 88:1337; Berlakovich, Transpl, 1994; 58:560).

The National Institute of Health Consensus Guidelines (JAMA, 1983; 250:2961) suggested that transplant candidates with alcoholic liver disease should be abstinent from alcohol before the procedure is undertaken but did not specify or recommend a particular abstinence period. In an early series, however, 1-year recidivism rates were low, even in individuals drinking up to the time of transplantation (Starzl, JAMA, 1988; 260:2542). Subsequently, other investigators warned that early recidivism rates should be treated with caution as in their series the early recidivism rate of 11.5 per cent rose to 32 per cent in the 3 years after the procedure (Campbell, ProcAmSocTransplSurg, 1993; A131). In many of the series reported up to that time, recidivism rates were consistently higher in individuals who were drinking immediately before transplantation than in those who were abstinent beforehand. Indeed, in one study, the single most important predictor of abstinence post-transplantation was abstinence before the transplant procedure (Osorio, Hepatol, 1994; 20:105). However, this view was challenged by others following a controlled assessment of 20 individuals who had been transplanted for alcoholic liver disease some 1 to 6 years previously (Howard, QJMed, 1994; 87:731). All remained abstinent from alcohol in the 7 to 10 months immediately after surgery, when medical supervision was at its most intense, but thereafter 80 per cent had returned to drinking. Their mean alcohol intake was 25 g daily; 40 per cent were drinking above 'low-risk' levels, defined as 112 g/week for women and 168 g/week for men, 50 per cent were 'binge' drinking, while 15 per cent were drinking heavily and

regularly. In this study there was no relation between alcohol consumption following the procedure and the duration of abstinence before surgery.

The return to drinking after transplantation is not without consequence. In one study, 18 per cent of the transplant recipients required admission to hospital for their drinking problem (Campbell, ProcAmSocTransplSurg, 1993; A131). Perhaps more disturbing is the observation that severe alcohol-related injury develops rapidly in the grafted liver in individuals who return to drinking. Thus, in a series of 23 graft recipients who continued to abuse alcohol after transplantation, histological evidence of alcoholic hepatitis was observed in all 23 within 77 to 579 days of the procedure, while cirrhosis was observed in four (Baddour, Gastro, 1992; 120: A777(Abstr.)). In a report on liver biopsies taken a mean of 36 months after transplantation in eight patients, cirrhosis was evident in the biopsies obtained from two who had returned to regular heavy drinking (Howard, QJMed, 1994; 87:731). Paradoxically, it has been reported that the rates of both acute and chronic graft rejection are significantly higher in individuals transplanted for alcoholic cirrhosis who remain abstinent from alcohol than in those who admit to continued alcohol use (Van Thiel, AlcoholClinExpRes, 1995; 19:1151).

The majority of patients with alcoholic liver disease who are transplanted have endstage cirrhosis. There are very few reports of transplantation being undertaken in patients with alcoholic hepatitis. Experience of transplanting cirrhotic individuals with and without superadded alcoholic hepatitis has, however, been documented by one group (Bonet, AlcoholClinExpRes, 1993; 17:1102). The 1-year survival rates in the patients with cirrhosis alone (81 per cent) and in those with cirrhosis and alcoholic hepatitis (89 per cent) were similar. However, the sobriety rate 1 year after transplantation was 89 per cent in the patients with cirrhosis alone but only 51 per cent in those with superadded alcoholic hepatitis. No details were given of the patients' drinking behaviour before transplantation but it is reasonable to assume that those with alcoholic hepatitis were more likely to have been abusing alcohol up to the time of the procedure.

The results of this study have resulted in the suggestion that the use of transplantation as a treatment option for patients with alcoholic hepatitis has no place outside the setting of a well-designed controlled trial (Miller, AlcoholClinExpRes, 1994; 18:224), or that it should be abandoned altogether (Sorrell, AlcoholClinExpRes, 1994; 18:2225).[41]

Alcoholic liver disease is the most common cause of liver disease in the Western world today and is a leading cause of death in the United States. In many centres, alcoholic cirrhosis has become one of the most common indications for transplantation. However, currently only a minority of the vast numbers of patients with endstage alcoholic cirrhosis are referred for consideration. The services, particularly in the United States, are already overburdened, as the requirement for donor organs currently exceeds the supply. Any further expansion of the services to patients with alcoholic liver disease might therefore overwhelm the system completely.

In Great Britain there are only seven centres designated by the Department of Health and the Scottish Office to undertake liver transplantation. The decision as to which patient receives a donor liver, when it becomes available, is made by clinicians in the individual centres selecting from their own waiting lists, basing their decision on the probability of benefit irrespective of the aetiological background of the liver disease (Neuberger, BMJ, 1997; 314:1140). There is broad agreement between centres as to the priorities for graft allocation. Financial concerns are not of prime importance as the cost of a successful procedure can be offset, at least in part, against the costs incurred in managing the complications of endstage liver disease (O'Grady, AlimPharmTher, 1997; 11:445).

In the United States there are more than 100 transplant centres and transplantation is a 'for profit' procedure. Since 1986, the United Network for Organ Sharing (UNOS), a non-profit organization, has operated the National Organ Procurement and Transplantation Network on a Federal contract. Ultimate responsibility for the Network lies with the Department of Health and Human Services. The criteria used by UNOS for allocating livers, such as the priorities allocated to patients and the geographical area for distribution, have been severely criticized and have created considerable animosity and mutual mistrust between centres (Neuberger, BMJ, 1997; 314:1140; Steinbrook, NEJM, 1997; 336:436).

In November 1996, UNOS modified their allocation policies by redefining those patients who should be given highest priority and by setting criteria for entry on to waiting lists. Priority is to be given to individuals with fulminant hepatic failure, patients with graft failure within 7 days of their first transplant, and to children. The first two categories of patients are already given priority in Great Britain by mutual agreement between the designated centres, but children are not given priority over adults.

UNOS has now defined minimal listing criteria for each disease category. Those who do not fulfil these criteria may appeal to a regional review board. It is widely believed that patients with 'self-inflicted' liver injury such as alcoholic cirrhosis will be disadvantaged by this system. Indeed, a proposal requiring a minimum of 6 months' abstinence from alcohol has already been withdrawn by the Network's Board of Directors (Steinbrook, NEJM, 1997; 336:436). Further reviews are expected by both the Federal Government and the Department of Health and Human Services to decide whether there should be additional changes in the liver allocation policies. This furore has, if nothing else, served to highlight the shortage of donor organs that is, to a large extent, responsible for the need for rationing policies. It is to be hoped that this problem will be addressed in any future policy decisions.

In view of the continuing controversy over liver allocation to patients with alcoholic liver disease, it is incumbent upon the medical community to improve the selection of patients for transplantation in order to maximize benefit. The first consideration must be whether the patient has liver disease of sufficient severity to warrant transplantation, to be certain that no alternative treatment would suffice, and that they are otherwise fit for the procedure.

The medical criteria for selecting patients have been clearly defined (Lucey, GastrClinNAm, 1993; 22:243). However, there is evidence that patients are still not being selected as carefully as they might be. In one study, for example, the efficacy of liver transplantation for alcoholic cirrhosis was assessed by comparing survival rates in 169 transplant recipients with those in two control groups treated conservatively, one matched and one simulated (Poynard, Lancet, 1994; 344:502). Overall, the 2-year survival rate in the transplanted patients (73 per cent) did not differ from that in either the matched (67 per cent) or simulated (67 per cent) control samples. However, when patients were stratified in relation to disease severity, only those retrospectively categorized as being at severe risk benefited from transplantation in terms of survival. No benefit was observed in patients categorized as of medium or low risk, suggesting that they had been transplanted 'too early'. These investigators underline the danger of using inadequate or inappropriate comparison groups to define selection criteria for transplantation. Thus, in their study, survival rates were significantly better in the low- and medium-risk patients than in the severe-risk patients. Thus, if transplant selection were based on 'best outcome', then the patient at severe risk might not have been transplanted yet paradoxically they were the ones who benefited most. Survival comparisons should not, therefore, be made within subgroups of patients selected for transplantation but with appropriate matched or simulated control groups treated conservatively.

The major controversy surrounding the selection of patients with alcoholic liver disease for transplantation is the risk of recidivism. Many centres have stipulated that patients must be abstinent from alcohol for a set period, often arbitrarily set, before being accepted for assessment; a premise no doubt based on the finding (Osorio, Hepatol, 1994; 20:105) that the best predictor of abstinence after surgery is abstinence in the pretransplant period. However, the ethics of setting an arbitrary period of abstinence as a criterion for selection has been challenged (Beresford, Psychosomatics, 1990; 31:241), and this challenge is supported by the finding in another study (Howard, QJMed, 1994; 87:731) that there is no relation between pre- and post-transplant drinking behaviour.

It should be possible, however, to identify a subgroup of patients with a low risk of recidivism using data from the body of patients already transplanted. To date, two centres have published details of such selection criteria and of their outcome data (Lucey, Gastro, 1992; 102:1736; Gish, AmJGastr, 1993; 88:1337).

One of these centres has developed a multidisciplinary approach to the selection process (Lucey, Gastro, 1992; 102:1736). Criteria for acceptance on to the transplant waiting list include severe endstage liver disease for which no alternative medical or surgical treatment is available, a clear understanding by the patient of the risks and benefits of the procedure, a favourable psychiatric report, and favourable prognostic factors for future sobriety, the latter determined using the University of Michigan Alcoholism Prognosis Scale (Table 13). This scale addresses insights into alcoholism and the presence of prognostic indices for sobriety (Vaillant, AmJMed, 1983; 75:455) and social stability (Strauss, QJStudAlc, 1951; 12: 231). It is used as a guide rather than as an absolute arbiter for selection in that no threshold score has been determined. Drinking during the assessment period or while on the waiting list results in exclusion from the programme.

The results of this approach to selection have now been published (Lucey, Gastro, 1992; 102:1736) for the period May 1985 to December 1989. Of the 99 potential candidates only 45, that is, less than half, were accepted for transplantation; the remaining 54 were refused for a number of reasons (Table 14). Survival data are available for all patient groups but data on post-selection drinking behaviour are only available for transplant recipients.

The 1- and 2-year survival rates in the transplanted patients mirrored those reported by other groups. During the follow-up period, five of the transplanted patients drank alcohol, although only two reported episodes of uncontrollable, symptomatic drinking; the

Table 13 The University of Michigan Alcoholism Prognosis Scale for major organ transplant candidates

Variable	Points awarded	
Acceptance of alcoholism:	(1–4)	
Patient and family	4	
Patient only	3	
Family only	2	
Neither	1	
Prognostic indices:	(4–12)	
Substitute activities	No 1	Yes 3
Behavioural consequences	No 1	Yes 3
Hope/self-esteem	No 1	Yes 3
Social rehabilitation	No 1	Yes 3
Social stability:	(0–4)	
Steady job	1	
Stable residence	1	
Does not live alone	1	
Stable marriage	1	
Total	5–20	

Adapted from Lucey, Gastro, 1992; 102:1736.

investigators considered this incidence of recidividism acceptable. The survival rates in those 'too well' for transplantation exceeded 90 per cent for 18 months and then fell precipitously between 18 to 24 months, indicating that these individuals should remain under constant surveillance. The high mortality rates in the group 'too ill' for transplantation were as expected. The high mortality rates in those considered unfit for transplantation because of a poor prognosis for future sobriety are unexplained, but may well reflect continued alcohol abuse.

The investigators suggest that use of a selection process which utilizes medical, surgical, and psychiatric variables allows fair assessment of transplant candidates. However, their assessment was undertaken in part retrospectively and further data collected prospectively are needed in order to assess fairly their multidisciplinary approach.

The other centre has also used a multidisciplinary approach to devise a selection scheme based on the risks of recidivism and non-compliance for patients with alcoholic cirrhosis referred for liver transplantation (Gish, AmJGastr, 1993; 88:1337). Recidivism is defined as any consumption of alcohol during the period of evaluation, while on the waiting list or following transplantation. Compliance is defined as abstinence from alcohol, correct use of prescribed medication, fulfilling the requirements of the Alcohol Rehabilitation Contract, prompt physician contact for medical problems, and clinic attendance.

Patients undergo extensive medical, psychiatric, and psychosocial evaluation. They are required to sign an Alcohol Rehabilitation Contract committing them to attend meetings of Alcoholics Anonymous and psychiatric follow-up clinics, although the programme is individualized for each patient. No absolute period of abstinence from alcohol preceding evaluation is either stipulated or required.

At the end of the evaluation period, patients are categorized, in relation to their likelihood of recidivism and non-compliance, as low, moderate, or high risk (Table 15). Patients in the low-risk category are enrolled into an alcohol rehabilitation programme and listed for transplantation; those in the moderate-risk group are enrolled into an alcohol rehabilitation programme but their listing for transplantation is deferred for between 2 to 6 months to allow for reappraisal; those categorized as being at high-risk are offered alcohol rehabilitation but refused transplantation.

A prospective analysis of the results in 47 patients clearly showed that pretransplant risk-group assignment accurately predicted both pre- and post-transplant recidivism and non-compliance (Table 16).

This scheme could readily be applied in other centres provided the necessary psychiatric expertise were available.

Potential therapeutic approaches[32]

A number of potential therapeutic approaches to the treatment of alcoholic liver disease have been identified, some of which are currently under investigation.

Table 14 Characteristics and outcome of patients referred for liver transplantation

Category	Patients (n)	Abstinence (months) Median (range)	Prognostic score (5–20) Median (range)	Survival (%)	
				1 year	2 year
Selected:					
Transplanted	45	12 (0–170)	16 (8–18)	78	73
Not selected:*					
'Too well'	17	12 (1–72)	14 (10–19)	93	59
Psychiatrically unstable	17	6 (0–72)	11 (7–15)	65	0
'Too ill'	19	8 (0–60)	12 (8–18)	0	

* One patient refused.
Data extracted from Lucey, Gastro, 1992; 102:1736.

Table 15 Criteria employed to assign patients with alcoholic cirrhosis into risk groups for recidivism and non-compliance post-transplantation

Low risk
- Documented abstinence >6 months
- No previous failures at alcohol rehabilitation
- Never told that alcohol was affecting health
- Signed 'Alcohol Rehabilitation Contract'
- Good social support system
- No psychiatric disorder

Moderate risk
- Documented abstinence 1 to 6 months
- Previous failure(s) at alcohol rehabilitation
- Signed 'Alcohol Rehabilitation Contract'
- Willing to enter alcohol rehabilitation programme (if medically stable)
- Minimal social support system
- Relative psychiatric contraindication[+]

High risk
- Period of abstinence <1 month
- Multiple failures to remain abstinent despite medical complications of liver disease
- Refusal to sign 'Alcohol Rehabilitation Contract'
- Poor or absent social support system
- Absolute psychiatric contraindication[++]

[+] Polysubstance abuse, moderate personality disorder, major mood disorder.
[++] Severe personality disorder, severe mental retardation, dementia, chronic psychosis, overt non-compliance.
Modified from Gish, AmJGastr, 1993; 88:1337.

Table 16 Recidivism and non-compliance rates from evaluation, and survival rates in liver transplant candidates, by risk category

Risk category	Patients (n)	Transplanted (n)	Recidivism and non-compliance rates (%)	Actuarial survival at 42 months (%)
Low	31	29	14	18
Medium	10	2	90	66
High	6	0	80	20

Adapted from Gish, AmJGastr, 1993; 88:1337.

The development of hepatic fibrosis is a key pathological event in the genesis of cirrhosis. It may be possible to prevent the formation of fibrous tissue by inhibiting collagen synthesis, for example by use of proline analogues. Alternatively, it might be possible to enhance collagen degradation by enhancing collagenase activity or by the insertion of exogenous DNA-encoding amino or carboxyterminal peptides of procollagen into hepatocytes (Wu, JBC, 1986; 261:10 482).

Oral supplementation with phosphatidylcholine prevents the development of alcohol-related fibrosis and cirrhosis in non-human primates (Lieber, Gastro, 1994; 106:152). The active agent has been identified as dilinoleoylphosphatidylcholine (Lieber, Gastro, 1994; 106:152); it most likely produces its beneficial effects by promoting collagen breakdown, although additional translational or post-translational effects on collagen synthesis cannot be excluded (Li, Hepatol, 1992; 15:373).

This dietary supplement is easy to administer, has high bioavailability, and is well tolerated. In a preliminary study (Panos, EurJGastrolHepatol, 1990; 2:351) involving 104 patients with alcoholic hepatitis, treatment with phosphatidylcholine for upwards of 2 years was associated with a tendency towards improved survival. More extensive trials are now under way. Treated patients will, however, need to be very carefully monitored beyond the trial period, given that rebound increases in hepatic fibrosis have been observed in baboons withdrawn from the supplement who continue to take ethanol (Lieber, Hepatol, 1990; 12:1390).

Cytokines such as tumour necrosis factor may enhance hepatic necrosis and fibrosis and have been implicated in the genesis of alcoholic hepatitis (McClain, SemLivDis, 1993; 13:710). The use of agents that inhibit cytokine production or their peripheral effects might be of therapeutic benefit. Likewise, the development of antibodies to the relevant cytokines or to their receptors might provide a useful therapeutic approach. In a preliminary randomized, placebo-controlled trial in 22 patients with severe alcoholic hepatitis [McHutchison, Hepatol, 1991; 14:96A, 195 (Abstr.)], treatment with pentoxifylline, which inhibits tumour necrosis factor and interleukins *in vivo*, was associated with a significant decrease in the incidence of renal failure.

Free radicals have been implicated in the genesis of alcohol-related liver injury (Di Luzio, Physiologist, 1963; 6:169; Nordman, FreeRadicBiolMed, 1992; 12:219), so that steps taken to either block their formation or enhance their metabolism might prove therapeutically beneficial (Nordmann, AlcAlc, 1994; 29:513). The generation of free radicals causes alteration in antioxidant balance and hence oxidative stress. This might be amenable to treatment with antioxidants such as vitamin E, vitamin A, ascorbate, selenium, N-acetylcysteine, desferrioxamine, and allopurinol given selectively or in combination (Situnayake, Gut, 1990; 31:1311).

Finally, once the factors governing hepatic regeneration have been fully identified, it might be possible to stimulate the process and so enhance recovery.

A rational approach to treatment

The most important therapeutic manoeuvre in the management of individuals with alcohol-related liver injury, irrespective of severity, is the maintenance of abstinence from alcohol; this is achieved with varying degrees of difficulty.

Individuals with minimal non-specific liver injury or hepatic steatosis need little in the way of specific therapy other than to abstain from alcohol. Their nutritional status may be suboptimal and may need attention.

The majority of individuals with mild to moderate alcoholic hepatitis will improve significantly following abstinence from alcohol and the provision of a diet sufficient to meet their nutritional needs, that is, a minimum of 30 kcal/kg and 1 g protein/kg body wt daily. Dietary intake should be monitored carefully and additional oral supplements provided as indicated.

Patients with severe alcoholic hepatitis are less easily managed as the majority will already have developed cirrhosis. Many present with severe hepatocellular failure and/or the complications of portal hypertension. Deterioration in their clinical status and laboratory variables is commonly seen following admission; the development of renal failure usually heralds a fatal outcome.

These patients should be managed in a specialist centre with the facilities to undertake their investigation and treat the complications of their liver disease. They should be provided with a minimum of 40 to 50 kcal/kg and 1.2 to 1.5 g of protein/kg body wt daily; dietary intake should be carefully monitored and additional oral supplements provided as indicated. If an adequate oral intake is not achieved in the first 48 h following admission, then nasogastric or nasojejunal feeding should be instituted. If nutritional requirements still cannot be met, then parenteral supplementation may be necessary, preferably using a long peripheral line. A small subgroup of these patients, carefully selected, may benefit from treatment with corticosteroids. No firm recommendations can be made about the value of other methods of treatment at present. The place of hepatic transplantation for these extremely sick patients is still debated.

Patients with well-compensated alcoholic cirrhosis require no specific therapy other than to maintain abstinence from alcohol. They should take a high-energy, high-protein diet providing daily intakes of 30 to 40 kcal and 1.0 to 1.5 g of protein/kg body wt, depending on their nutritional status. Patients with decompensated alcoholic liver disease should also maintain abstinence from alcohol and may require treatment for the complications of their liver disease. Particular attention should be paid to their nutritional status, using the same approach as for patients with severe alcoholic hepatitis. No specific therapy for the liver injury can be recommended at present. These patients are potential candidates for liver transplantation and should be monitored accordingly.

Management of the drinking problem[31, 42–44]

There can be little doubt that the outcome for patients who abuse alcohol, whether they have significant liver injury or not, improves significantly with abstinence from alcohol. It is incumbent upon the physician primarily responsible for the patients' care and welfare to ensure that they are offered the best possible chance of achieving this goal. How involved the physician becomes in this process is determined by a number of variables including personal preference, the 'medical' needs of the patient, and the range and availability of support and counselling services and their ease of access. It is likely that physicians will become more involved the greater the 'medical' needs of the patient and the poorer the access to, and the availability of, alternative services.

No matter how good the available support services the physician should never abdicate complete responsibility for the management of their patients' drinking problems to others. At the very least, they should present the patient with the biochemical and histological evidence of the damage done, in a factual and non-judgemental way, and should provide, as far as possible, information on the likely outcome of continued drinking and of abstinence. Clear and unambiguous advice to abstain from alcohol should be given to the patient and they should be provided with information on Alcoholics Anonymous and on appropriate local or regional treatment or specialist agencies. An offer to monitor progress by means of regular outpatient attendance should be made.

Some physicians may choose to be more closely involved in the management of their patients' drinking problems or may find they have little alternative but to be involved if there is a paucity of local help. An enthusiastic worker may, over time, build up a simple but effective support service for such individuals that produces results similar to those achieved by dedicated units.

A number of treatment alternatives are available that, for descriptive purposes, are best divided into simple advice, which can be administered by most interested primary health-care workers, and specialist treatments, which are provided by trained individuals, usually in a specialist setting. In practice these two approaches are not distinct as many specialist counsellors find that they can achieve excellent results by dispensing nothing more than simple advice.

Simple advice

Advice based on a careful appraisal of the patient's needs has been shown to be as effective as more elaborate and complex forms of treatment (Heather, AlcAlc, 1995; 30:287). Clear advice, coupled with monitoring of laboratory variables and review of the patient's drinking diary, will often be sufficient to help establish abstinence from alcohol (Kristenson, Alcoholism, 1983; 7:203). This type of support can readily be provided in a primary health-care setting (Wallace, BMJ, 1988; 297:663; Anderson, BrJAddic, 1992; 87:891), a general hospital (Katz, JStudAlc, 1981; 42:136; Chick, BMJ, 1985; 290:965), or in special outpatient clinics (Maheswaran, Hypertension, 1992; 19:79). This approach is said to work best in individuals whose alcohol abuse is discovered inadvertently; that is, in non-treatment-seeking populations (Heather, AlcAlc, 1995; 30: 287).

Simple advice may fail for a number of reasons (Heather, AlcAlc, 1995; 30:287). The patient may, for example, lack motivation, although this is an ill-defined concept that may be used erroneously, by the professional involved, to explain non-compliance or poor treatment outcome. Simple advice may not suffice for patients who have been using alcohol as a means of coping with intrapsychic or interpersonal conflicts; it is essential that such problems be recognized and treated, for they militate against effective treatment of the drinking problem.

Specialist therapy

Patients with alcohol-related problems may be offered a wide range of specialist treatment options. The diversity of such treatments shows that no single regimen is superior to any other. It also reflects the need to match patient and treatment method carefully.[45]

Behavioural approaches

Evidence suggests that many individuals who have previously abused alcohol relapse because they cannot cope with frustration or anger, or with the social pressures to drink.[46,47] By asking patients to list the personal and environmental cues to their drinking, likely triggers to relapse may be identified so that new ways of coping with them can be devised. A number of specific coping techniques may be used to modify behaviour, including contingency management (Hunt, BehavResTher, 1973; 11:91), social skills training (Foy, JStudAlc, 1976; 37:1340), assertiveness training (Ferrell, IntJAddict, 1981; 16:959), and relaxation therapy (Litman, QJStudAlc, 1974; 35:131).

Psychological approaches

Most forms of psychotherapy have been used in individuals abusing alcohol but their value has not been demonstrated conclusively

(Emrick, JStudAlc, 1975; 36:88). This does not mean that psychodynamic principles are of no relevance to treatment, as they often help elucidate the patient's intrapsychic conflicts. When excessive drinking is symptomatic of an underlying neurosis or character disorder, a psychotherapeutic or counselling approach is often helpful.[48]

Group therapy, whether based on an inpatient programme or in an outpatient setting, has been one of the mainstays of treatment of individuals abusing alcohol. The group approach gives individuals an opportunity to identify with others who have similar problems. Most groups comprise eight to 10 individuals who meet regularly, together with an experienced therapist and an observer (Yalom, AnnNYAcadSci, 1974; 233:85). Despite their popularity, particularly in inpatient specialist units, the value of group techniques in therapy remains largely unproven.

Excessive drinking may profoundly disturb marital relationships and family well-being;[49] marital and family therapy may be required if relationships and family systems have been disrupted or else have adjusted in a pathological way. A number of specialist techniques have been used but none has been effectively evaluated.[50]

Self-help groups

There are a number of self-help groups of which Alcoholics Anonymous and its sister organizations Al-Anon, which caters for the spouses of alcohol abusers, and Al-Ateen, which caters for their teenage children, are the best known. The organization, which was founded in the United States in 1935, now has groups in virtually every country in the world and, in many countries, in almost every town. Membership is open to all who admit they have an alcohol problem. Much of the strength of the organization rests in the sense of fellowship and identification it offers.

The essence of the Alcoholics Anonymous programme is the 12 steps that experienced members regard as marking their own progress through the organization.[51] Alcoholics Anonymous obviously 'works' for many people, though others cannot identify with its rituals and abstinence goal.

Follow-up studies on individuals attending Alcoholics Anonymous have shown a correlation between attendance and successful treatment outcome. Thus, in one study, the 6-month abstinence rate, following initial treatment, was 73 per cent in individuals attending meetings weekly, but only 45 per cent in individuals attending, on average, once a month, and 33 per cent in non-attenders (Hoffmann, IntJAddict, 1983; 18:311). Similarly, in another study, individuals who attended meetings regularly had a 1-year abstinence rate of 70 per cent compared with a rate of less than 50 per cent in individuals who did not attend regularly (Miller, AlcoholTreatQ, 1995; 12:41).

The relation between attendance at meetings and abstinence from alcohol is not necessarily causal. Indeed, an extensive review (Emrick, *Research on alcoholics anonymous*. New Brunswick, Canada: Alcohol Research Documentation, Inc., 1993:41) concluded that while many claim that Alcoholics Anonymous is an effective organization, there are very few systematic data to support this view. Thus it is extremely difficult to compare the efficacy of this organization with that of other treatments. It remains, however, a valuable and low-cost resource (Glaser, BrJAddic, 1982; 77:123).

A number of other national and local self-help groups have been set up, based on self-management techniques for controlling and monitoring drinking behaviour. Their efficacy remains to be assessed.

Pharmacotherapy

Treatment may be required for an underlying psychiatric illness. Great care must be taken to evaluate the patient fully before making a judgement about the coexistence of an affective disorder. If depression is evident then treatment with conventional antidepressants may be helpful, although patients should be monitored very carefully (Ciraulo, JClinPsychpharm, 1981; 1:146). Occasionally, alcohol misuse may accompany hypomania, which may be effectively treated, even in this setting, with lithium (McMillan, BrJAddic, 1981; 76:245).

Drug therapy may be directed at controlling the alcohol abuse itself (Sellers, NEJM, 1981; 305:1255; Kristenson, AlcAlc, 1995; 30:775). The drugs most commonly used are the alcohol-sensitizing agents, disulfiram (Antabuse), calcium carbamide and its citrated derivatives (Dispan, Temposil), and cyanamide (Colme). These drugs are inhibitors of hepatic aldehyde dehydrogenase; if individuals taking these drugs imbibe alcohol their blood acetaldehyde concentrations will rise significantly, producing a flushing reaction that is accompanied by nausea, vomiting, tachycardia, hypotension, dyspnoea, dizziness, and headache. This reaction is more marked with disulfiram than with the other agents but varies in intensity depending on the amount of drug and alcohol taken; the combination of these agents with alcohol can be fatal (Jacobsen, QJStudAlc, 1952; 13:16).

Although these drugs were introduced into clinical practice many years ago, surprisingly few studies of their efficacy have been undertaken (Hughes, Addiction, 1997; 92:381). A randomly allocated study showed that a combination of supervised disulfiram and behavioural therapy, focused on learning to cope with specific potential drinking situations, proved significantly more effective than traditional approaches (Azrin, JBehavTherExpPsych, 1982; 13:105). In another study, 128 alcoholic men were randomized to receive disulfiram or a placebo preparation for 1 year; while the outcomes at 3 and 6 months favoured treatment with disulfiram, the proportion maintaining abstinence at 1 year did not differ between the disulfiram-treated (23 per cent) and control (12 per cent) groups (Fuller, AnnIntMed, 1979; 90:901). In a larger study, the same workers showed no overall difference in abstinence rates between individuals taking the active drug or the placebo preparation, but the patients receiving disulfiram reported fewer drinking days (Fuller, JAMA, 1986; 256:1449). In a study of 126 patients randomly allocated to treatment, over a 6-month period, with either disulfiram, 200 mg daily, or vitamin C, 100 mg daily, in which treatment was supervised by a nominated observer, the use of disulfiram was associated with fewer drinking days, a reduction in weekly alcohol consumption, and a fall in mean serum γ-glutamyl transferase activity (Chick, BrJPsychiat, 1992; 161:84). The results of these studies indicate that, in general, alcohol-sensitizing agents should only be used as an adjunct to other therapies aimed at effecting more long-term change (Hughes, Addiction, 1997; 92: 381).

Disulfiram is usually taken orally in a dose of 250 mg daily, preferably in the evening because it causes drowsiness. Higher doses may be required in approximately 50 per cent of patients, the dose being titrated against the response to an alcohol challenge (Brewer, AlcAlc, 1993; 28:383). An effervescent formulation is available in Scandinavia that has three times the bioavailability of the standard formulation (Kristenson, AlcAlc, 1995; 30: 775 (Abstr.)); thus, in these countries, regimens employing twice-weekly or alternate-daily dosing with 400 mg of the alternative formula are commonly employed. Compliance rates with treatment may be as low as 20 per cent (Fuller, JAMA, 1986; 256:1449).

Use of these drugs is absolutely contraindicated during pregnancy and in patients with florid psychoses and established hypersensitivity. They should not to be used in patients with seriously impaired cardiac, respiratory, or hepatic function and should be avoided in patients who are impulsively suicidal or brain damaged; they are relatively contraindicated in patients with diabetes, epilepsy, and hypercholesterolaemia. In all circumstances their use should be carefully explained to the patient, who should be provided with a card detailing the nature of the therapeutic regimen. Individuals should be in control of their own treatment but there are benefits in agreeing a contract whereby a relative, close friend, or work colleague supervises the taking of the medication. These drugs should never be given to a patient without their knowledge or consent.

The most frequent side-effects of treatment with disulfiram are drowsiness, headache, gastrointestinal symptoms, an unpleasant taste in the mouth, and impotence. A number of more serious side-effects, including confusion, peripheral neuropathy and hepatitis, have also been reported (Peachey, JClinPsychpharm, 1981; 1:21; Poulsen, ActaPsychScand, 1992; 86:59). The peripheral neuropathy is sensorimotor in type and its development is probably dose-dependent (Frisoni, AlcAlc, 1989; 24:429); symptoms typically arise after about 3 months of treatment but will develop earlier in individuals exposed to higher doses of the drug. Evolution of the neuropathy ceases if the drug is discontinued; the rate and extent of the subsequent recovery reflects the initial degree of impairment; simultaneous use of chloral hydrate potentiates development of disulfiram-related neurotoxicity.

Disulfiram hepatotoxicity develops after a latency of 2 weeks to 6 months, with a peak at 60 days; its development is idiosyncratic and not dose-related (Poulsen, ActaPsychScand, 1992; 86:59). The risk of death is 1 in 25 000 treated patients per year; if the drug is stopped early then recovery is usually complete, but in approximately half the adequately documented cases drug treatment was continued, resulting in the development of massive liver-cell necrosis and death (Iber, AlcoholClinExpRes, 1987; 11:301; Wright, JClinPsych, 1988; 49:430; Berlin, AlcAlc, 1989; 24:241); hypersensitivity phenomena are occasionally observed (Mason, DICP, 1989; 23:872; Kahn, SouthMedJ, 1990; 83:833). The liver biopsy shows hepatocellular degeneration, focal or extensive necrosis, and bridging. Inclusions consisting of glycogen and degenerated organelles, that bear some resemblance to ground-glass hepatocytes, may be found, predominantly in zone I hepatocytes; portal or periportal inflammation may be present (Vázquez, Diagnos-Histopath, 1983; 6:29). The toxic effects of disulfiram probably reflect excess accumulation of toxic metabolites, most likely carbon disulphide.

Little is known about the incidence of disulfiram-related toxicity but it is likely to be underdiagnosed. Difficulty might arise in diagnosis because alcohol abuse itself is associated with the development of both peripheral neuropathy and hepatic dysfunction. Indeed, a survey of the results of liver function tests in 438 patients taking part in a placebo-controlled trial of disulfiram therapy found that when those taking the active drug developed abnormal test results it was invariably associated with a return to drinking (Iber, Alcoholism, 1987; 11:301). However, these findings should not induce complacency, for although the toxic reactions are uncommon they can be associated with a significant morbidity and, in the case of the hepatotoxicity, with a significant mortality. Disulfiram also inhibits the metabolism of several drugs including phenytoin, warfarin, chlordiazepoxide, and diazepam, leading to accumulation and typical overdose reactions.

The risk of death following deliberate overdosage is low. Lasting neurological damage can occur after attempted suicide, particularly if the drug was taken in high dosage together with alcohol (Krauss, MovementDisorders, 1991; 6:166). Severe or life-threatening alcohol-disulfiram reactions may be treated with the alcohol dehydrogenase inhibitor pyrazole and its 4-substituted derivatives (Lindros, Alcoholism, 1981; 5:528).

Disulfiram should always be prescribed in the lowest possible dose and patients should be directly questioned about possible adverse effects. Liver function tests should be obtained before treatment and then at 2-weekly intervals for the first 2 months of treatment and 4- to 6-weekly thereafter (Wright, JClinPsych, 1988; 49:430). Treatment should be discontinued after 6 months, although some physicians believe the drug should be continued indefinitely (Brewer, AlcAlc, 1993; 28:383).

Calcium carbamide has a short duration of action and so is prescribed in a dose of 50 mg twice daily. The side-effects of treatment are similar to those observed with disulfiram but are invariably less frequent and less severe (Peachey, JClinPsychpharm, 1981; 1:21). Cyanamide is prescribed in a dose of 30 to 75 mg daily. The liver lesions induced by cyanamide are more impressive than those produced by the other agents (Fig. 8); they represent a predictable lesion (Vázquez, Liver, 1983; 3:225; Bruguera, Liver, 1987; 7:216) that may progress to resemble biliary cirrhosis (Moreno, Liver, 1984; 4:15).

In recent years a number of novel pharmacotherapeutic approaches to the treatment of alcohol abuse have been suggested, based on knowledge of the effects of chronic alcohol abuse on cerebral neurotransmitter systems and neurotransmitter balance. To date, most pharmacological approaches to the treatment of alcohol dependency have focused on modifying the activity of the specific neurotransmitters thought to be involved in the regulation of alcohol consumption.

5-HT reuptake inhibitors

Chronic alcohol abuse is associated with a reduction in cerebral serotonin (5-hydroxytryptamine, **5-HT**) release; thus, drugs that enhance serotonin neurotransmission, such as the 5-HT reuptake inhibitors, might be useful in the treatment of alcohol dependency, perhaps by decreasing the desire to drink alcohol [Lejoyens, AlcAlc, 1996; 31 (Suppl.1): 69]. In general, the selective serotonin reuptake inhibitors, such as zimeldine, citalopram, and fluoxetine, confer little if any benefit (Naranjo, ClinPharmTher, 1990; 47:490; Gorelick, AlcoholClinExpRes, 1992; 16:261; Naranjo, ClinPharmTher,

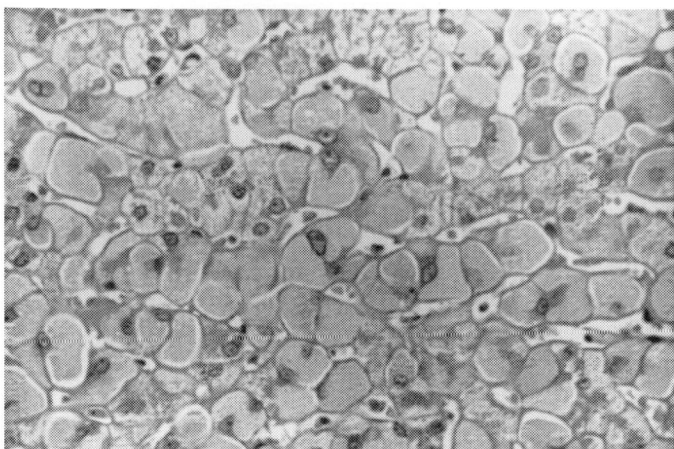

Fig. 8. Cyanamide hepatotoxicity. The hepatocytes contain pale inclusions consisting of glycogen and degenerated organelles. The resulting appearance bears some resemblance to 'ground-glass' hepatocytes. (Haematoxylin and eosin, × 530; illustration kindly provided by J.J. Vázquez.)

1992; 51:729; Balldin, AlcoholClinExpRes, 1994; 18:1133; Kranzler, AmJPsychiat, 1995; 152:391).

At least seven different types and numerous other subtypes of 5-HT receptors have been identified, each of which is involved in the regulation of specific behavioural or physiological responses (Martin, Neuropharmacol, 1994; 33:261). The selective serotonin reuptake inhibitors are non-specific in action and this may explain their relative ineffectiveness in treating alcohol dependency. Interest has therefore focused on the use of more specific serotoninergic agents in this patient population. Ritanserin, which is primarily a 5-HT$_2$ receptor antagonist, although shown in preliminary studies to be of potential use in the treatment of alcohol dependency, was found to be ineffective in a double-blind, randomized, controlled trial [Anton, AlcAlc, 1996; 31 (Suppl.1): 43]. Ondansetron, however, which is a 5-HT$_3$ antagonist, was found to be effective in reducing alcohol consumption in a group of problem drinkers with early alcohol dependency (Sellers, AlcoholClinExpRes, 1994; 18: 879).

The identification of the specific 5-HT receptor(s) involved in the regulation of alcohol intake may allow more effective therapies to be developed (Buydensbranchey, AlcoholClinExpRes, 1997; 21: 220).

Opioid antagonists

Chronic alcohol abuse is associated with an increase in brain opioid receptors and hence enhancement of opioidergic activity. Opioid antagonists, such as naltrexone and nelmefene, might therefore prove useful in the treatment of alcohol dependency by reducing the reinforcing effects of alcohol and the incentive to drink [O'Malley, AlcAlc, 1996; 31 (Suppl. 1):77]. A small number of carefully controlled, double-blind, randomized clinical trials have provided evidence that these agents are effective in preventing relapse in drinking behaviour when offered as part of a comprehensive treatment programme (O'Malley, ArchGenPsychiat, 1992; 49:881; Volpicelli, ArchGenPsychiat, 1992; 49:876; Mason, AlcoholClin ExpRes, 1994; 18:1162). Patients treated with opioid antagonists have fewer drinking days, lower rates of resumed heavy drinking,

and reduced alcohol craving compared with individuals given placebo preparations [O'Malley, AlcAlc, 1996; 31 (Suppl.1): 77].

Overall, treatment with the opioid antagonists results in a significant but modest effect on drinking behaviour in carefully selected patients admitted to intensive treatment programmes. Trials in less selected populations are obviously needed; in addition, attempts should be made to characterize those patients who might benefit most from this form of adjuvant therapy.

The central opioid system is highly complex, involving several ligands, receptors, and receptor subtypes (Khachaturian, TrendsNeurosci, 1985; 8:111). Clearer identification of the elements most closely involved in the control of drinking behaviour would allow more specific agents to be developed.

Acamprosate

The γ-aminobutyric acid (**GABA**) neurotransmitter system is thought to play a fundamental part in modifying the effects of alcohol and alcohol-drinking behaviour (Koob, TrendsPharmacolSci, 1992; 13:177). GABAergic agents might therefore have a role in the treatment of alcohol dependency (Chick, AlcAlc, 1995; 30:785). Acamprosate (calcium acetylhomotaurinate), a synthetic derivative of homotaurinate, which is a naturally occurring structural analogue of GABA, has been shown to be a useful adjuvant treatment for preventing relapse in drinking behaviour in alcohol-dependent individuals (Lhuintre, Lancet, 1985; i:1015; AlcAlc, 1990; 25:613; Paille, AlcAlc, 1995; 30:239). Patients treated with acamprosate had longer cumulative periods of abstinence, defined as the total number of days of abstinence during the trial period, than those receiving placebo preparations.

Not all patients benefit from medication with acamprosate and the characteristics of the responders have yet to be identified. The amount and type of preceding and collateral psychosocial and pharmacotherapy that best facilitates response to this drug have yet to be defined.

Choice of treatment approach

Over recent years the emphasis in the treatment of drinking problems has moved towards simpler and earlier intervention by front-line agencies, whether this is a primary health-care team, hospital ward, or social-work department. Part of this changed perspective came in response to a series of evaluation studies which demonstrated, first, that the length of inpatient treatment in a specialist unit did not significantly affect outcome (Ritson, BrJPsych, 1968; 114:1019), second, that outpatient treatment was as effective as inpatient treatment (Edwards, Lancet, 1967; i:555), and, third, that carefully chosen advice was as effective as more long-term therapies, at least in selected patient populations (Heather, AlcAlc, 1995; 30: 287).

Most reviews of evaluation studies demonstrate that rather more than half of the patients will show improved drinking behaviour without treatment and that the remission rate at 6 months quite accurately predicts subsequent outcome. Remission is much more likely in individuals who have a sound premorbid personality and are employed, married, and generally socially stable. Outcome is not influenced by the sex or age of the patient, the degree of physical dependence on alcohol, or the severity of the liver injury (Katz, JStudAlc, 1981; 42:136), and is relatively uninfluenced by treatment method; certainly there is no convincing evidence that more costly and intensive therapies are more effective (Polich, JStudAlc, 1980; 41:397).

Community studies show that two-thirds of individuals with alcohol-related problems remit over a 2-year period. Change of job, a new relationship, criticism from family or friends, a disturbing illness are all commonly given reasons for such 'spontaneous remissions' (Chick, BMJ, 1982; 285:3).

It is often necessary for physicians caring for individuals who abuse alcohol to arrange for their admission with urgent medical problems. It is just as appropriate for them to arrange admission during a social or emotional crisis relating to a period of relapse or withdrawal from alcohol. Boundaries must be drawn, however, particularly where resources are in short supply. It is therapeutically nihilistic to provide facilities for 'crisis intervention' but nothing more.

Monitoring abstinence[17–22,52]

The outcome in patients with alcohol-related liver disease is determined largely by their ability to remain abstinent from alcohol. Unfortunately, accurate data on alcohol consumption are difficult to obtain from patients with a history of alcohol abuse (Orrego, Lancet, 1979; ii:1354; Fuller, AlcoholClinExpRes, 1988; 12:201; Ness, JAMA, 1994; 272:1777); equally, family and friends cannot necessarily be relied upon to provide an accurate assessment of current intake. Monitoring for continued alcohol misuse is perhaps one of the more challenging tasks facing the physician charged with the care of these individuals.

Many experienced clinicians seem to know instinctively when a patient has returned to drinking. Their intuitive feelings are probably based on subjective, most likely subconscious, assessments of appearance, demeanour, and behaviour. This is not to say that physicians can unfailingly identify the patient who has returned to drinking without recourse to objective measurements, but instincts may prove useful, particularly when objective data are lacking or non-contributory.

The patient should, of course, be questioned about their drinking behaviour, in a non-judgemental way, and their account should be checked with a relative or friend whenever possible.

Physical signs, such as spider naevi, acne rosacea, facial mooning, gynaecomastia, jaundice, hepatomegaly, and fluid retention, tend to regress with abstinence from alcohol and will return if drinking resumes. The changes in facial appearance with abstinence from alcohol are often striking, particularly in women. These signs should be routinely monitored; clinical photographs provide an objective record.

Measurement of ethanol concentrations in breath, blood, urine, and sweat has been used to confirm recent alcohol intake and hence to monitor claimed abstinence from alcohol. When urinary ethanol concentrations were measured daily for 6 months in 37 patients with alcoholic liver disease, ethanol was detected in over 50 per cent of the samples tested (Orrego, Lancet, 1979; ii:1354). Of the patients who tested positive, 25 per cent denied drinking at all times, 17 per cent admitted to drinking at all times, while the remainder admitted to drinking on 52 per cent of occasions. In another study (Caballería, AlcAlc, 1988; 23:403), urinary ethanol concentrations were measured in morning samples obtained from 103 patients with alcoholic

Table 17 Relation between self-reported data on last alcohol consumption and markers of recent alcohol consumption

Last reported consumption (h)	Plasma ethanol	Plasma methanol (% positive)	Urinary 5-HTOL/5-HIAA*
<12	38	23	64
12–24	0	0	20
24–48	8	15	20
>48	13	10	19

* 5-hydroxytryptophol/5-hydroxy-3-indoleacetic acid.
Data extracted from Helander, AlcAlc, 1997; 32:133.

liver disease attending a follow-up clinic, and in one morning and two evening samples, obtained in the same week, from a further 78 patients. Approximately one-third of the patients who provided the morning urine samples admitted consuming alcohol and ethanol was detected in a similar proportion of samples; however, urine analysis indicated alcohol consumption in 7 per cent of individuals who had denied drinking. Approximately 36 per cent of individuals who provided serial urine samples admitted drinking whereas ethanol was detected, usually in the evening samples, in 54 per cent. Ethanol was detected in the urine of 51 per cent in women, whereas only 7.4 per cent admitted alcohol consumption. Thus, the results of serial measurements of urinary ethanol concentrations usefully complement personal interview in monitoring claimed abstinence from alcohol.

Measurements of blood methanol and the urinary 5-HTOL:5-HIAA ratio have also been used to monitor recent drinking behaviour (Helander, ClinChem, 1996; 421:618; AlcAlc, 1997; 32:133). In a large, multinational study, plasma ethanol and methanol concentrations and the urinary 5-HTOL:5-HIAA ratio were used to validate the accuracy of self-reported data on recent alcohol consumption in a total of 120 individuals (Helander, AlcAlc, 1997; 32:133). The markers were positive in varying proportions of individuals who reported alcohol consumption in the 12 h before testing; the urinary 5-HTOL:5-HIAA ratio was the most sensitive, detecting 64 per cent of recent consumers (Table 17). Conversely, elevation of one or more of the three markers was observed in several individuals who denied drinking in the 48 h before sample collection (Table 17).

These markers of recent alcohol consumption are useful in detecting relapse at an early stage; they can be used in the validation of markers of chronic alcohol abuse and in the evaluation of costly treatment programmes.

Of the various laboratory markers purported to be of use in monitoring chronic alcohol abuse, the three most valuable, especially when used in combination, are the serum γ-glutamyl transferase, the serum aspartate aminotransferase, and the erythrocyte mean corpuscular volume. Some promising data are also available on the use of serum carbohydrate-deficient transferrin for monitoring purposes.

Increased serum γ-glutamyl transferase activity is observed in approximately 80 to 90 per cent of individuals abusing alcohol (Rosalki, CCActa, 1972; 39:41; Stetter, AlcoholClinExpRes, 1991; 15:938). The incidence of enzyme elevation is largely independent of the degree of liver damage (Wu, AmJGastr, 1976; 65:318). Serum γ-glutamyl transferase activity decreases with abstinence from alcohol, usually in an exponential fashion (Lamy, CCActa, 1974; 56: 169); in general, activity reduces by 50 per cent within 2 weeks of abstinence from alcohol while normal values are attained within 5 weeks (Rosalki, CCActa, 1972; 39:41). In patients in whom initial serum enzyme values were less than five times the upper reference range the fall in serum activity with abstinence may be delayed (Wadstein, ActaMedScand, 1979; 205:317); more persistent elevation may be observed in patients with cirrhosis (Morgan, BrJAlcAlc, 1981; 16:167). Serum γ-glutamyl transferase activity increases fairly rapidly following relapse in drinking behaviour, although the level of daily alcohol consumption required to increase enzyme activity varies considerably from individual to individual.

Serum aspartate aminotransferase activity is elevated in approximately 45 to 70 per cent of individuals abusing alcohol (Bradus, AmJMedSci, 1963; 246:35; Galizzi, ScaJGastr, 1978; 13:827); the incidence of enzyme elevation is largely independent of the degree of liver injury (Skude, ActaMedScand, 1977; 201:53); values rarely exceed five times the upper reference limit. Serum enzyme activity falls by approximately 50 per cent within 1 week of abstinence from alcohol (Rosalki, AdvClinChem, 1975; 17:53); resumption of drinking is associated with further increases in enzyme activity, although the degree of daily alcohol consumption required to produce this response varies considerably from individual to individual.

Macrocytosis has been observed in from 60 to 90 per cent of individuals abusing alcohol (Wu, AmJGastr, 1976; 65:318; Morgan, ClinLabHaemat, 1981; 3:35), independently of the presence of liver disease. In one study (Wu, Lancet, 1974; i:829), macrocytosis was observed in 89 per cent of a small group of individuals abusing alcohol; over the following 3 months the erythrocyte mean corpuscular volume decreased in the three individuals who stopped drinking but remained unchanged in the four who continued to drink. In another study (Buffet, ArchFrMalAppDig, 1975; 64: 309), macrocytosis was observed in a minimum of 82 per cent of individuals abusing alcohol; the elevated values of erythrocyte mean corpuscular volume fell to within the reference range within 15 days of admission to hospital, then remained within the reference range in those who abstained from alcohol but further increased in those who resumed drinking. It has also been shown that the erythrocyte mean corpuscular volume might fall significantly following reduction, but not necessarily cessation, of alcohol intake (Morgan, ClinLabHaemat, 1981; 3:35). The rate of change of erythrocyte mean corpuscular volume with abstinence from alcohol is considered by some to be too slow to be useful for short-term monitoring of alcohol abuse (Shaw, AlcoholClinExpRes, 1979; 3:297; Morgan, ClinLabHaemat, 1981; 3:35).

Serum carbohydrate-deficient transferrin concentrations are elevated in from 40 to 100 per cent of chronic alcohol abusers; abstinence from alcohol is accompanied by a reduction in serum concentrations into the reference range over a period of approximately 10 to 14 days; serum concentrations will increase again following ingestion of alcohol in amounts exceeding 60 g/day for a minimum of 1 week (Allen, AlcoholClinExpRes, 1994; 18:799; Gordon, AlcRes, 1997; 2:54).[22]

Serum carbohydrate-deficient transferrin was sequentially measured, monthly over a 9-month period, in 86 male alcohol abusers

Table 18 Relation between self-reported data on alcohol consumption, serum carbohydrate-deficient transferrin concentrations and the urinary 5-HTOL:5-HIAA ratios in 15 male alcohol abusers			
Drinking behaviour	Self-reported drinking behaviour	Urinary 5-HTOL/ 5-HIAA* (n)	Serum CDT**
Frequent drinking	3	4	3
Sporadic drinking	5	11	3
Abstinent	7	0	9

* 5-Hydroxytryptophol/5-hydroxy-3 indolacetic acid.
** Carbohydrate-deficient transferrin.
Data extracted from Voltaire Carlsson, AlcoholClinExpRes, 1993; 17:703.

taking part in a hepatitis B vaccination programme (Rosman, AlcoholClinExpRes, 1995; 19:611). During the study, serum carbohydrate-deficient transferrin concentrations were elevated, on one or more occasions, in 28 (76 per cent) of the 38 patients who reported relapses in their drinking behaviour: in 16 (42 per cent) of these 38 individuals the increase in serum concentrations of the marker preceded self-reported drinking. Serum carbohydrate-deficient transferrin concentrations were, however, also elevated is 10 (21 per cent) of the 48 individuals with corroborated denial of drinking during the study; three of these individuals had cirrhosis. The investigators concluded that monitoring patients in this way will result in earlier detection of a relapse in drinking behaviour than with other markers, but they cautioned that test performance might be suboptimal in patients with significant liver disease.

Thrice-weekly, self-reported alcohol consumption and weekly measurements of serum carbohydrate-deficient transferrin were compared in 15 male alcohol abusers over a 6-month period (Voltaire Carlsson, AlcoholClinExpRes, 1993; 17:703); measurement of the urinary 5-HTOL:5-HIAA ratio was undertaken daily as an independent marker of alcohol consumption. Patients' drinking behaviour over the 6 months was categorized, on the basis of their self-reports, as abstinent, or as sporadic or frequent drinking. The urinary 5-HTOL:5-HIAA ratio was elevated at some time during the study in all 15 participants, indicating that none was entirely abstinent from alcohol; levels indicated frequent drinking in four individuals and sporadic drinking in the remaining eleven (Table 18). Both self-reports and the measurements of serum carbohydrate-deficient transferrin underestimated the incidence and degree of relapse (Table 18).

Measurements of serum γ-glutamyl transferase and aspartate aminotransferase activities, and of carbohydrate-deficient transferrin concentrations, are not sensitive or specific enough, when considered in isolation, to monitor drinking behaviour: sensitivities range from 33 to 40 per cent, specificities from 85 to 94 per cent (Helander, AlcAlc, 1997; 32:133). However, combining the results of these three tests will enable a more accurate assessment of drinking behaviour to be made. If test results are to be used in this way it should be remembered that there is marked interindividual variation in the sensitivities of the individual markers.

To date, few comparative studies of these monitoring variables have been undertaken. In one study, weekly measurements were made of both serum carbohydrate-deficient transferrin and serum

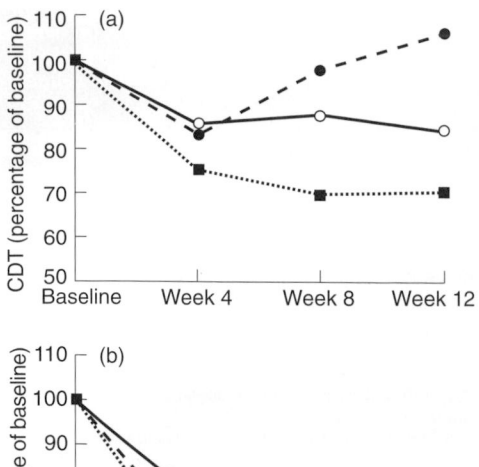

Fig. 9. Percentage changes in (a) serum carbohydrate-deficient transferrin (CDT) concentrations and (b) serum γ-glutamyl transferase (GGT) activities in 35 male alcohol abusers during a 12-week treatment trial in relation to their drinking behaviour during the trial, viz. ■ abstinent (n = 14); ○ 'slip' (n = 11); ● relapse (n = 10) (Anton, AlcoholClinExpRes, 1996; 20:841).

γ-glutamyl transferase in 10 male outpatients enrolled in a 6-month treatment programme (Helander, AlcAlc, 1996; 31:101). Relapse was assessed from self-reports and from daily determinations of the urinary 5-HTOL:5-HIAA ratio. At presentation, six individuals had elevated serum carbohydrate-deficient transferrin concentrations, one had elevated serum γ-glutamyl transferase activity, two showed elevation of both markers, and one of neither. During follow-up only one participant was abstinent from alcohol, four drank sporadically, while the remaining five drank frequently. No changes were observed in the serum levels of either marker in the abstinent patient and in those drinking sporadically; in the five frequent drinkers, significant elevations were observed in serum carbohydrate-deficient transferrin concentrations in three, and in serum γ-glutamyl transferase activities in two. The investigators concluded that use of these two markers in combination will increase the probability of detecting relapses in drinking behaviour.

Serum carbohydrate-deficient transferrin and γ-glutamyl transferase were measured monthly in 35 male alcohol abusers entering a 12-week treatment programme (Anton, AlcoholClinExpRes, 1996; 20:841). Drinking behaviour was classified on the basis of self-reported intake as abstinent, 'slip' drinking, or relapse. At entry, 17 (49 per cent) had elevated serum carbohydrate-deficient transferrin concentrations while 18 (51 per cent) had elevated serum γ-glutamyl transferase activities; a total of 27 (77 per cent) patients had elevated levels of one or both markers. During follow-up, serum carbohydrate-deficient transferrin performed better than serum γ-glutamyl transferase in detecting relapse (Fig. 9). Nevertheless, the investigators recommended that both markers should be used to facilitate the monitoring process.

There is general agreement at present that detection of relapse is improved if serum carbohydrate-deficient transferrin is used in combination with other markers (Bell, AlcoholClinExpRes, 1994; 18:1103), and that the sensitivity of this marker may be further enhanced by using higher cut-off values than for screening (Borg, AlcoholClinExpRes, 1995; 19:961; Rosman, AlcoholClinExpRes, 1995; 19:611).

The assay for serum carbohydrate-deficient transferrin is considerably more expensive than the other tests used for monitoring; it is also less accessible. However, the cost of monitoring and hence the early detection of relapse may well be offset by the costs of further admissions to hospital for patients in whom relapse detection is delayed. Cost–benefit considerations should be addressed in all future studies.

Changes also occur with abstinence from alcohol in the appearances of the liver on ultrasonographic and computed tomographic scans, and these may be useful for monitoring drinking behaviour (Allaway, JRSocMed, 1988; 81:149; Medhat, Gastro, 1988; 94:157). Hepatic ^{31}P magnetic resonance spectroscopy is an extremely sensitive method for detecting changes in drinking behaviour but it is too expensive and the technique too inaccessible for routine use (Morgan, Gastro, 1995; 108:776). Histological examination of the liver serially over time is hard to justify outside the confines of a therapeutic clinical trial. However, repeat biopsies should be undertaken in patients with previous alcoholic hepatitis, particularly if there is a suspicion of continued alcohol abuse.

Special management problems

Particular difficulties arise when individuals with alcoholic liver disease require surgery or drug treatment for associated illness. These problems are compounded if the individual has recently been abusing alcohol.

Anaesthesia

The anaesthetist called upon to deal with an habitual drinker faces several problems. Little or no information may be available on recent alcohol consumption, or on the presence or degree of liver damage, particularly when individuals are encountered as an emergency; it may not be possible, under these circumstances, to predict accurately the effects of any drugs administered. Difficulties are less likely to occur when such individuals are encountered either electively or semi-electively.

Habitual drinkers who have developed metabolic tolerance to alcohol are likely to display cross-tolerance to a number of drugs used in anaesthetic practice. Modest increases in the dosage of a variety of intravenous induction agents may therefore be necessary. The response to the inhalation agents used for induction is less predictable: some patients will display severe excitement while others lose latent hyperexcitability; in consequence, the use of these agents is best avoided. These individuals are relatively resistant to the effects of non-polarizing, curare-like relaxants; this resistance probably reflects increased binding of these drugs to circulating globulins. Their sensitivity to depolarizing relaxants such as suxamethonium is, however, increased, most likely because of a reduction in circulating concentrations of pseudocholinesterase. Thus the choice of relaxant may be difficult; non-depolarizing relaxants that are not metabolized in the liver may be the drugs of choice.

During maintenance anaesthesia, special care should be taken to avoid hypotension, hypoxia, or deep planes of anaesthesia because of the dangers of precipitating liver failure in patients with significant liver injury (Shackman, ClinSci, 1953; 12:307). Autonomic circulatory reflexes may be impaired in these patients, with the result that hypotension, syncope, and collapse may occur unexpectedly because warning signs, such as tachycardia and sweating, may be absent.

Hepatic glycogen stores tend to be low or absent in individuals with cirrhosis and in those who are malnourished. Hypoglycaemia may develop very rapidly in these individuals, particularly if they were drinking heavily before admission to hospital; hypoglycaemia may be very difficult to recognize in an anaesthetized patient and monitoring of blood sugar concentrations is advised.

Total exchangeable sodium is almost invariably raised in patients with cirrhosis even though serum sodium may be low. Saline infusions should therefore be avoided during anaesthesia and in the postoperative period because of the danger of precipitating pulmonary oedema. Many patients with alcoholic liver disease are hypokalaemic and in some instances this may reflect true potassium deficiency. Changes of hypokalaemia, such as depression of the S–T segments and inversion of T-waves, may be apparent on the electrocardiograph before surgery, and every attempt must be made to correct this electrolyte imbalance with appropriate intravenous therapy.

Hypoxia is a risk during surgery in patients with established liver disease because of the presence of intrapulmonary shunting and arterial desaturation. In addition, many heavy drinkers are also heavy smokers and so may have associated lung disease. Chronic alcohol abuse is also associated with the development of congestive cardiomyopathy that is often subclinical, although the presence of flattened T-waves on the electrocardiograph, together with a variety of atrial arrhythmias, may be suggestive. Under these circumstances, anaesthetic agents, such as halothane, that increase myocardial contractility are best avoided, as they might precipitate dangerous arrhythmias.

If the patient was drinking heavily up to the time of admission, then the development of withdrawal symptoms in the postoperative period should be anticipated and the patient monitored accordingly. It may, however, be very difficult to distinguish the symptoms of alcohol withdrawal from those of postoperative restlessness associated with pain and discomfort, and the tachycardia and fever of an associated infection. Difficulty might also arise in distinguishing the early signs of withdrawal from those of hypoglycaemia and hepatic encephalopathy. It will obviously be necessary to sedate the patient withdrawing from alcohol and this is probably best done with intravenous chlormethiazole, which can be carefully titrated against the response.

Surgery

As a rule, individuals with alcoholic liver disease tolerate surgery poorly, particularly if they have recently been drinking (Mikkelsen, AmJSurg, 1968; 116:266; Orloff, AnnNYAcadSci, 1975; 252:159). Patients with significant liver disease develop coagulation abnormalities and thrombocytopenia; chronic alcohol abuse is associated with a reduction in platelet numbers and function. Surgery in these patients may therefore be complicated by the development

of severe intra- and postoperative bleeding. This possibility can be minimized by giving vitamin K_1, 10 mg intravenously, 4 h before surgery, and by infusing two to three units of fresh frozen plasma intravenously during surgery, and one to two further units daily for the first three postoperative days; it may be necssary to use platelet concentrates, both during surgery and in the early postoperative period, and fresh blood.

Surgery may precipitate hepatic failure, particularly in patients with alcoholic hepatitis, resulting in the development of fluid retention and hepatic encephalopathy. The presence of ascites will impair lung function and may precipitate dehiscence of abdominal wounds with detrimental loss of fluid and protein. Early removal of drains, closure of drain sites, and abdominal binding are advisable. The neuropsychiatric abnormalities of hepatic encephalopathy may be mistaken for the effects of oversedation and their presence may impair management. Every effort should be made to keep the bowel empty and non-absorbable disaccharides should be prescribed routinely.

These patients are often uncooperative and non-compliant, and maintenance of drips, drains, and dressings in the postoperative period may be difficult. Wound healing tends to be poor, particularly in malnourished individuals; wound and chest infections are common; opportunistic infections are easily overlooked in the postoperative period.

Perioperative morbidity and mortality are high in this group of patients (Aranha, ArchSurg, 1986; 121:275). Thus surgical procedures should not be undertaken unless absolutely necessary and, even then, not without careful preoperative assessment within the confines of surgical urgency. Elective abdominal procedures should be avoided, if at all possible, in individuals who may be candidates for orthotopic liver transplantation (Gholson, AmJGastr, 1990; 85: 487).

Drug treatment

In general it is best to avoid medication in patients who habitually abuse alcohol and who may, in addition, have significant liver injury, for the interplay between alcohol, drugs, and impairment of hepatic function is both extensive and complex (Hoyumpa, AnnRevMed, 1982; 33:113).

The metabolism of drugs normally occupying the cytochrome P450-dependent, microsomal drug-metabolizing enzyme system, such as phenytoin, barbiturates, tolbutamide, and warfarin, will be competitively impaired in individuals who are acutely intoxicated. However, the elimination of these drugs is enhanced in individuals who chronically abuse alcohol, because of induction of the microsomal drug-metabolizing system. The effects of these drugs are therefore unpredictable in these individuals and so are best avoided.

The actions of a number of drugs may be enhanced by alcohol because of additive or potentiating effects. Thus, the hypoglycaemic effects of sulphonylureas are enhanced in the presence of alcohol, as is the propensity of the biguanides to produce lactic acidosis. Alcohol enhances the cerebral depressant effects of narcotics, sedatives, and hypnotics, and also of analgesics, especially dextropropoxyphene, antihistamines, antitussives, and anticonvulsants. Alcohol also enhances the inhibitory effects of tricyclic antidepressants on gastrointestinal motility, the hypotensive effects of certain antihypertensive agents, and the peripheral vascular effects of vasodilatory drugs.

Alcohol specifically interacts with drugs that inhibit the activity of aldehyde dehydrogenase, the best known of which are disulfiram and citrated calcium carbamide. The resultant accumulation of acetaldehyde leads to the development of flushing, tachycardia, headache, vomiting, and dyspnoea; severe hypotension, collapse, and even death might ensue. A number of other drugs may induce a mild 'Antabuse-like' effect including chloramphenicol, metronidazole, β-lactam antibiotics, moxalactam, griseofulvin, mepacrine, procarbazine, and the sulphonylureas.

Alcohol may enhance the toxicity of other drugs. Thus it appears to increase the gastric mucosal irritant effects of salicylates and other non-steroidal anti-inflammatory drugs. Alcohol appears to increase the risk of gastrointestinal haemorrhage associated with aspirin use (Needham, Gut, 1971; 12:819) and potentiates the effects of aspirin on the bleeding time (Deykin, NEJM, 1982; 306: 852).

Individuals abusing alcohol have an increased risk of developing paracetamol-related liver injury with doses of the drug that are within, or only moderately above, the recommended therapeutic range (Seeff, AnnIntMed, 1986; 104:399; Maddrey, JClinGastr, 1987; 9:180). This can occur either because activation of the drug to its toxic metabolites is increased as a result of alcohol-related induction of the cytochrome P450 system, or because conjugation of the toxic metabolites with glutathione is impaired following depletion of hepatic glutathione stores. The metabolic activation of paracetamol is not, however, substantially increased in individuals abusing alcohol (Lauterberg, Gut, 1988; 29:1153), but hepatic glutathione concentrations may be decreased both in alcohol abusers and in individuals with liver disease (Altomare, LifeSci, 1988; 43: 991). Individuals abusing alcohol should be cautioned against use of this drug.

The hepatic clearance of a drug depends on the hepatic intrinsic clearance, which is an index of hepatocellular enzyme activity, and on hepatic blood flow. If intrinsic clearance is very low it becomes rate-limiting, whereas if intrinsic clearance is very high, blood flow becomes rate-limiting. The presence of chronic liver disease may affect drug handling, for a number of reasons. First, liver blood flow is reduced in the presence of cirrhosis and this might impair elimination of drugs with a high first-pass extraction; second, portal–systemic shunting of blood will allow increased passage of drugs normally cleared on first-pass into the systemic circulation; third, reduction in functioning liver-cell mass will result in impairment of the metabolism of drugs dependent on hepatic elimination; fourth, hypoalbuminaemia may result in impaired protein binding of drugs, and may alter drug distribution and penetration; and, finally, the sensitivity of a number of tissues to the actions of drugs may be altered—for example, patients with cirrhosis may show increased sensitivity to a number of centrally-acting drugs (Laidlaw, Gastro, 1961; 40:389).

In practice, hepatic drug-metabolizing capacity is largely preserved, even in the presence of severe liver disease, so that the reduction in liver blood flow and portal–systemic shunting of blood are probably more important determinants of altered drug metabolism in these patients than is hepatocellular function.[53]

In patients with cirrhosis the degree to which the metabolism of a given drug is altered reflects the magnitude of its 'first-pass' extraction by the liver. Drugs that are at least 60 per cent extracted on 'first-pass' by the healthy liver, such as glyceryl trinitrate, propoxyphene, propranolol, labitolol, verapamil, and domperidone, will accumulate in high concentration in the circulation of patients with significant liver disease and their oral dose will need to be significantly reduced. Drugs that are less than 30 per cent extracted on first-pass, for example paracetamol, diazepam, chlordiazepoxide, theophylline, and rifampicin, may accumulate if used in standard doses over a prolonged period. Drugs that do not undergo appreciable first-pass metabolism, such as naproxen, oxazepam, frusemide, spironolactone, digoxin, prednisolone, tolbutamide, cimetidine, and ampicillin, may be prescribed in standard doses with little danger of toxicity, even in patients with severely deranged liver function.

Drug therapy may be difficult in patients abusing alcohol for a number of other reasons, including poor compliance because of low motivation and impaired comprehension, lack of available finance, social instability, gastrointestinal intolerance because of the presence of alcohol dependence and/or gastritis, and impaired absorption because of small-bowel damage.

Prognosis

A number of difficulties arise in assessing the data on prognosis and outcome in patients with alcoholic liver disease, for a variety of reasons (Harris, AlcAlc, 1995; 30:591): first, patient populations are often small and poorly characterized; second, the methods for determining the degree of liver injury are not standardized; third, the starting points for calculating survival are often arbitrarily and inconsistently set; fourth, little if any information is provided on patients' subsequent drinking behaviour, although it is one of most important outcome variables; fifth, confounding variables such as sex, nutritional status, and ethnic origin are incompletely accounted for; sixth, drop-out rates are often high so that the numbers available for subsequent analysis may be too small for meaningful results; and finally, study end-points are inconsistently set and are therefore non-comparable. The data on prognosis and outcome should therefore be viewed with these caveats in mind.

Alcoholic fatty liver

In the majority of patients, fatty liver is a benign lesion that will reverse completely following abstinence from alcohol. Exceptionally such patients die, either as a result of hypoglycaemia due to profound depletion of glycogen stores (Graham, BullJHopHosp, 1944; 74:16) or from multiple cerebral and/or pulmonary fat emboli released from the liver (Durlacher, AmJPathol, 1954; 30:633), or as a result of hepatic failure associated with cholestasis (Morgan, ScaJGastr, 1978; 13:299).

A 70 per cent 2-year survival was reported in 26 alcohol abusers with biopsy-proven hepatic steatosis;[54] no information was provided on interval drinking behaviour; none of the deaths observed was related to the presence of liver disease. A 46 per cent 10- to 13-year survival was reported in 258 alcohol abusers, 248 (96 per cent) of whom had biopsy- proven hepatic steatosis.[7] In contrast, a 72 per cent 10-year survival was reported in 212 alcohol abusers with biopsy-proven alcoholic fatty liver.[55] Details of interval drinking behaviour and on causes of death were not provided in either of these long-term studies and there is no obvious explanation for the discrepancy in survival figures between them.

Alcoholic hepatitis

The short-term outcome in patients with alcoholic hepatitis is variable and depends essentially on the severity of the liver lesion as assessed by clinical, laboratory, and histological variables. Thirty-day mortality rates of from 1.5 to 17 per cent have been reported in individuals with alcoholic hepatitis who were sufficiently ill to require admission to hospital yet well enough to permit liver biopsy (Green, ArchIntMed, 1963; 112:67; Christoffersen, ScaJGastr, 1970; 5:633; Harinasuta, Gastro, 1971; 60:1036; Lischner, AmJDig-Dis, 1971; 16:481; Mendenhall, ClinGastr, 1981; 10:417).[8] On the other hand, the 30-day mortality rate in patients in whom the prothrombin time was too prolonged to permit liver biopsy was of the order of 42 per cent (Galambos, ProgLivDis 1972; 4:567). In the Veterans Administration Cooperative Study (Mendenhall, *Alcohol related diseases in gastroenterology*. Berlin: Springer-Verlag, 1985:304), the short-term mortality rate in patients with a mild histological lesion was 1 per cent, with a moderate lesion 12 per cent, and with a severe lesion 34 per cent. Approximately two-thirds of these deaths occurred within the first 2 weeks after admission to hospital, with a mean survival time of 16 days.

Poor short-term prognosis is associated with high serum bilirubin and creatinine concentrations, prolongation of the prothrombin time to greater than 5 s over control, and the presence of hepatic encephalopathy, hypoalbuminaemia, and ascites (Maddrey, Gastro, 1978; 75:193; Orrego, Hepatol, 1983; 3:896). Poor short-term prognosis is also associated with increased circulating concentrations of tumour necrosis factor (Bird, AnnIntMed, 1990; 112:917) and interleukin 8 (Sheron, Hepatol, 1993; 18:41), and low circulating concentrations of coagulation factor V (Pereira, AlcAlc, 1992; 27:55).

Treatment with corticosteroids may significantly improve short-term survival rates in a carefully selected subpopulation of patients with severe alcoholic hepatitis characterized by a discriminant function in excess of 32 (Maddrey, Gastro, 1978; 75:193; Carithers, AnnIntMed, 1989; 110:685). In these patients, treatment is associated with a short-term survival rate in excess of 80 per cent compared with survival rates of less than 50 per cent in untreated individuals (Ramond, NEJM, 1992; 326:507).

The long-term outcome in patients with alcoholic hepatitis depends on several factors, including their sex and age, the severity of the initial lesion, its characteristics, its evolution to cirrhosis, and the patients' subsequent drinking behaviour.

A marked survival benefit has been reported in men with non-cirrhotic alcoholic liver disease compared to women, together with an increase in relative mortality of 57 per cent for both sexes with each decade increase in age.[55] In the Veterans Administration Cooperative Study (Mendenhall, *Alcohol related diseases in gastroenterology*. Berlin: Springer-Verlag, 1985:304), the 1-year survival rate in patients with mild disease was 91 per cent, in patients with moderate disease 70 per cent, and in patients with severe disease 42 per cent. An earlier study in 164 patients with biopsy-proven alcoholic hepatitis showed that, while those with mild alcoholic hepatitis had a 70 per cent 5-year survival with no increase in mortality after the first 3 years, those with severe alcoholic hepatitis has a 50 per cent 5-year survival with mortality increasing throughout the observation period (Alexander, Gastro, 1972; 63:1026).

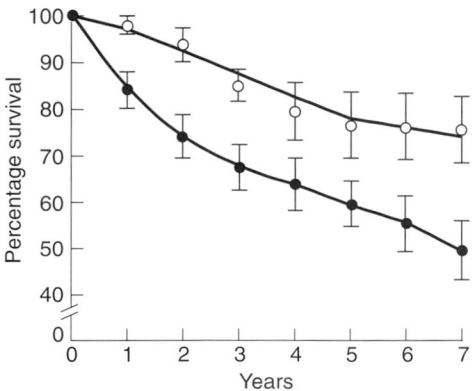

Fig. 10. Survival rates in patients with histologically proven alcoholic hepatitis who either significantly reduced their alcohol intake (*n* = 59; ○—○) or continued to drink unabated (*n* = 98; ●—●) (Alexander, AmJGastr, 1971; 56:515).

The presence of tissue cholestasis may also affect outcome. Thus in patients with alcoholic hepatitis with little or no cholestasis on their initial liver biopsy the 5-year survival was 54 per cent compared with 22 per cent in patients with moderate to severe cholestasis (Nissenbaum, DigDisSci, 1990; 35:891).

Patients with alcoholic hepatitis who subsequently develop cirrhosis have a lower survival rate than those in whom the liver lesion does not progress. Thus, in the Veterans Administration Cooperative Study (Goldberg, AmJGastr, 1986; 81:1029), patients with mild alcoholic hepatitis who developed cirrhosis had a 2-year survival rate of 70.6 per cent compared with a survival rate of 80.8 per cent in those in whom the liver lesion did not progress.

Abstinence from alcohol favourably affects outcome. Thus an 80 per cent 7-year survival rate was reported in patients with alcoholic hepatitis who reduced their alcohol intake compared with a 50 per cent 7-year survival rate in those who continued to drink (Alexander, AmJGastr, 1971; 56:515) (Fig. 10).

A 58 per cent 2-year survival was reported in 106 alcohol abusers with biopsy-proven alcoholic hepatitis, with a median survival of 55.7 months.[54] A 57 per cent 10-year survival was reported in 82 individuals with biopsy-proven alcoholic hepatitis.[55] In neither study were details provided on interval drinking or on cause of death.

Alcoholic cirrhosis

The prognosis in patients with alcoholic cirrhosis is determined by the clinical and histological severity of their liver disease at the time of presentation and by subsequent drinking behaviour (Powell, AmJMed, 1968; 44:406; Resnick, Lancet, 1974; i:138; Borowsky, Gastro, 1981; 80:1405; Schlichting, Hepatol, 1983; 3:889; Ginés, Hepatol, 1987; 7:122; Orrego, Gastro, 1987; 92:208; Gluud, Hepatol, 1988; 8:222).[10–14] Prognosis may also be influenced by the sex of the patient (Schlichting, Hepatol, 1983; 3:889; Ginés, Hepatol, 1987; 7:122),[12,13] and by their ethnic origin (Mendenhall, AlcAlc, 1989; 24:11), and is significantly affected by the development of hepatocellular carcinoma.[10–12]

Poor outcome is associated with increasing age, continued alcohol ingestion, the presence of hepatic encephalopathy, elevated serum bilirubin and creatinine concentrations, decreased plasma albumin

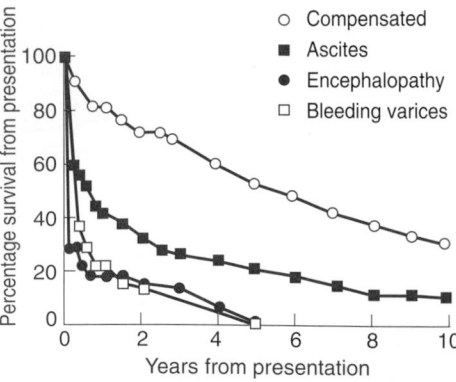

Fig. 11. Percentage survival from presentation in patients with alcoholic cirrhosis in relation to the degree of functional impairment at presentation.

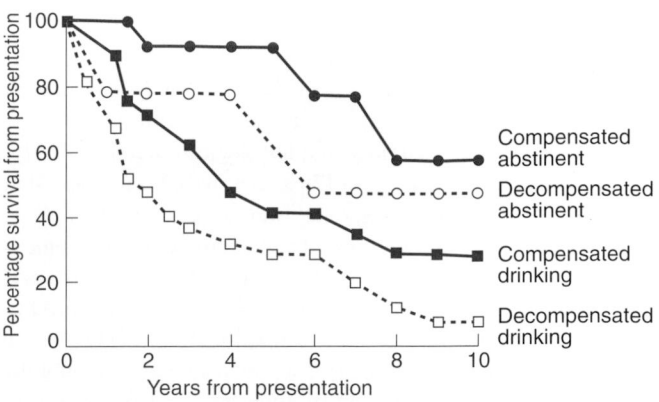

Fig. 12. Percentage survival from presentation in patients with alcoholic cirrhosis in relation to the degree of functional impairment at presentation and their subsequent drinking behaviour.

concentration, an aminopyrine breath test of less than 2 per cent, an hepatic venous pressure gradient in excess of 14 mmHg, and the presence of large oesophageal varices (Orrego, Hepatol, 1983; 3: 896; Gastro, 1987; 92:208; Gluud, Hepatol, 1988; 8:222; Adler, DigDisSci, 1990; 35:1; Poynard, Lancet, 1994; 344:502; Urbain, JHepatol, 1995; 22:179).[54]

Survival rates in patients with alcoholic cirrhosis 5 years from presentation vary from 0 to 80 per cent.[10,11,13,14] Survival is significantly reduced in patients who present with decompensated disease. In one study, for example, the 10-year cumulative survival in patients with alcoholic cirrhosis was 30 per cent in those who had presented with well-compensated disease, 10 per cent in those presenting with ascites, and 0 per cent in those presenting with variceal haemorrhage or hepatic encephalopathy (Fig. 11).[11]

In 1155 consecutive cirrhotic patients, 33 per cent of whom had alcohol-related disease, the 6-year survival rate in the patients with compensated disease was 54 per cent compared with 21 per cent in the patients with decompensated disease; there was no relation between survival and the aetiological background of the liver injury.[10] In 293 cirrhotic patients, 122 (42 per cent) of whom had alcohol-related injury, the median survival in patients with compensated disease was 8.9 years but was only 1.6 years in patients with decompensated disease (Ginés, Hepatol, 1987; 7:122). In this study the survival probability rate for patients with compensated cirrhosis was 47 per cent at 10 years whereas the rate for patients with decompensated cirrhosis was 16 per cent at 5 years; the cause of the liver disease was not an independent predictor of outcome. The overall improvement in survival figures between these studies, which were undertaken in 1981 and 1987 respectively, undoubtedly reflects better management of the complications of chronic liver disease.

Survival in patients with alcoholic cirrhosis is adversely affected by the presence of alcoholic hepatitis. In 140 patients with alcoholic cirrhosis the overall 1-year mortality rate was 20.7 per cent and the 5-year mortality rate 41.8 per cent (Orrego, Gastro, 1987; 92:208). However, at 1 year the mortality rate in the patients with 'hepatitis' (16.5 per cent) exceeded that in the patients without 'hepatitis' (7.1 per cent), while at 5 years the mortality rate in the patients with 'hepatitis' (46.9 per cent) was double that in the patients without 'hepatitis' (31.0 per cent). In another study, a 2-year survival rate of

49 per cent was reported in patients with alcoholic cirrhosis and of 35 per cent in patients with alcoholic cirrhosis with superimposed alcoholic hepatitis. It was calculated that an individual with alcoholic cirrhosis complicated by alcoholic hepatitis had a 1.9 times greater risk of dying than one with either of the lesions in isolation. It was also shown that survival in this group was independent of subsequent drinking behaviour.[54]

In the majority of studies, survival rates are significantly higher in patients who remain abstinent from alcohol, or who substantially reduce their alcohol intake, than in those who continue to drink. In general, the 5-year survival rates in patients with alcoholic cirrhosis who stop drinking are of the order of 50 to 75 per cent, whereas survival rates in those continuing to drink rarely exceed 40 per cent (Powell, AmJMed, 1968; 44:406; Borowsky, Gastro, 1981; 80: 1405).[10,11,14] The beneficial effects of abstinence from alcohol on survival are observed even in individuals who present with decompensated disease, although their survival overall is reduced (Fig. 12).[11]

The cumulative effects of the severity of the liver injury at presentation and the subsequent drinking behaviour on survival in patients with alcoholic cirrhosis are most clearly seen in a study of 283 patients (Powell, AmJMed, 1968; 44:406), in which the 5-year survival in patients with compensated cirrhosis was 89 per cent in those who stopped drinking but 68 per cent in those continuing to drink. In patients with decompensated cirrhosis, the 5-year survival was 60 per cent in the abstinent but only 34 per cent in those continuing to abuse alcohol. Abstinence from alcohol was associated with improved survival in patients who were jaundiced or who had ascites but not in those who had suffered variceal bleeding (Table 19). Others have also shown that survival in patients with alcoholic cirrhosis and established portal hypertension is independent of drinking behaviour (Soterakis, Lancet, 1973; ii:65; Pande, Gastro, 1978; 74:64; McCormick, JHepatol, 1992; 14:99) (Fig. 13).

Sex-related differences in survival in patients with alcoholic cirrhosis have been recorded in several studies but the data are inconsistent. Thus, in one study[13] it was reported that women have a lower percentage survival than men (Fig. 14), whereas in three others the opposite was observed (Schlichting, Hepatol, 1983; 3:889; Ginés, Hepatol, 1987; 7:122).[55] Ethnicity may also be a significant predictor of outcome in patients with alcoholic cirrhosis,

Table 19 The 5-year survival rates in patients with alcoholic cirrhosis relative to the severity of liver disease and subsequent drinking behaviour		
	Survival (%)	
	Abstinent	Drinking
Compensated	88.9	68.2
Decompensated:	60.1	34.1
Jaundice	57.5	33.3
Ascites	52.4	32.7
Haematemesis	35.3	20.7
Overall	63.0	40.5

After Powell, AmJMed, 1968; 44:406.

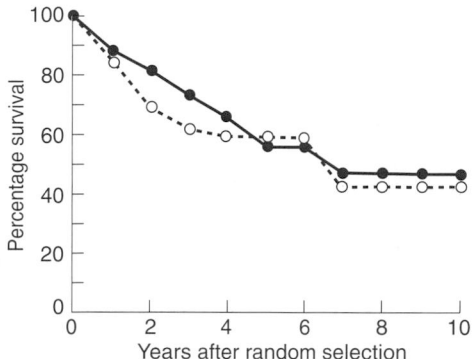

Fig. 13. Survival rates in patients with alcoholic cirrhosis and advanced portal hypertension who were abstinent from alcohol ($n = 77$; ●—●) or continued to abuse alcohol ($n = 69$; ○---○) (Soterakis, Lancet, 1973; ii:65).

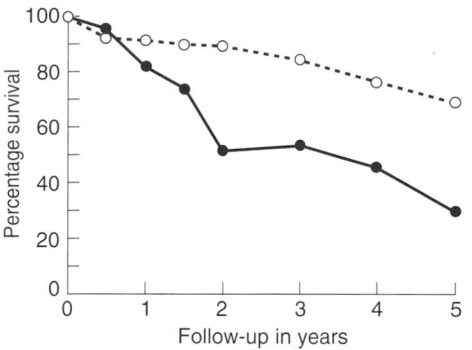

Fig. 14. Five-year survival rates in men (○---○) and women (●—●) with alcoholic cirrhosis who continue to abuse alcohol.[13]

with or without alcohol hepatitis: in a series of 437 male veterans followed over 4.5 years, survival rates at 42 months were 66 per cent in Afro-Americans, 40 per cent in Caucasians, and 28 per cent in Hispanics (Mendenhall, AlcAlc, 1989; 24:11). There is also anecdotal evidence that morbidity and mortality rates are greater in Asian Indians with alcoholic cirrhosis than in their Caucasian counterparts.

The development of hepatocellular carcinoma significantly reduces survival; the majority of patients die within weeks or, at most, months of diagnosis.[10–12] The lifetime risk of a patient with alcoholic cirrhosis developing hepatocellular carcinoma is between 3 and 25 per cent (Johnson, Gut, 1978; 19:1022; MacSween, BrMedBull, 1982; 38:31). This tumour is three times more common in men than women and is more likely to develop in individuals who have maintained abstinence from alcohol (Lee, Gut, 1966; 7: 77; Kato, JpnJGastro, 1990; 87:1829).

Individuals with alcoholic cirrhosis do not necessarily die as a result of their liver disease. Between 60 and 90 per cent will die a 'liver death', most likely as a result of hepatocellular failure and, less frequently, from gastrointestinal haemorrhage; up to one-third of the 'liver deaths' result from the development of hepatocellular carcinoma. Otherwise these individuals show an excess of deaths associated with other complications of alcohol abuse, particularly extrahepatic malignancies (*IARC monograph on the evaluation of carcinogenic risks to humans*. Lyon: IARC, 1988:4; Prior, AlcAlc, 1988; 23:163; Tuyns, *Alcohol misuse. A European perspective*. Amsterdam: Harwood Academic, 1996:163), accidents, homicide, and suicide (Adelstein, PopTrends, 1976; 6:7; Lester, AlcAlc, 1995; 30: 465).

In patients with alcoholic cirrhosis, liver transplantation is associated with 5-year survival rates of around 70 per cent (Kumar, Hepatol, 1990; 11:159; Berlakovich, Transpl, 1996; 61:554); it therefore provides an excellent therapeutic option for many patients with endstage chronic liver disease. The suitability of patients with alcoholic liver disease as candidates for transplantation has been debated since the advent of transplantation programmes and, as explained above, clear guidelines are still lacking. Nevertheless, the availability of this therapeutic option will undoubtedly influence survival figures, particularly in individuals with decompensated disease.

Prevention[56–58]

It is unreasonable to suppose that alcoholic-liver disease will ever be eradicated. It is reasonable to hope, however, that its prevalence can be reduced if governments control the amounts of alcohol available to populations, and individuals exercise control over their own consumption.

Primary prevention

There is a clear relation between the prevalence of alcohol-related liver disease and per capita alcohol consumption. Efforts at primary prevention should therefore focus on reducing both average per capita consumption of alcohol and the quantities consumed by individuals. Such efforts include controlling the availability of alcoholic beverages, public education, decreasing the incentives to drink, and the provision of alternatives to drinking. This remains an enormous and daunting task, and the prospect of achieving the World Health Organization objective in *Health For All 2000*—a reduction of overall consumption of 24 per cent between 1980 and 2000—seems unattainable.

There has been a significant increase in the worldwide commercial production of alcoholic beverages in recent years. It is not known whether small-scale local production of alcoholic beverages, for example by individual tribes or families in developing countries, has changed with the increase in large-scale commercial production, and little information is available on the production of home-brewed or distilled beverages in the Western world.

There has been no effective international action to control the availability of alcoholic beverages, although suggestions have been made concerning limitations on international trade. On a more regional level, the European Community seems rather more concerned with emphasizing free-trade practices than limiting production and availability. In many individual countries, however, the production and trade in alcoholic beverages are controlled by regulations and legislation, and in some countries steps have been taken to try to limit either production or trade.

Legislation aiming at total prohibition has been passed, at various times, in the United States, most Canadian provinces, and in many European countries. However, with time in all of these countries, enforcement became less stringent and public pressure led to repeal. Prohibition of the production, importation, sale, and consumption of alcoholic beverages is still enforced in Iran, Kuwait, Libya, Qatar, Saudi Arabia, and in the Yemen; in Bahrain, Pakistan, and Indonesia, prohibition applies to nationals but importation of alcoholic beverages by foreigners for their own use is allowed. An attempt was made at prohibition in all states of India, but this was halted and partially reversed following a change of government.

Steps have been taken in some countries to limit alcohol production and trade. Thus in India and in some parts of Africa, importation, particularly of spirits, has been banned, partly, at least, to economize on foreign exchange. France has attempted to reduce its production of alcoholic beverages by concentrating on quality rather than quantity but there is a danger that this attempt will be frustrated by free-trade agreements. Legislation in the former USSR limited the alcohol content of vodka, although increased production of wine and beer was encouraged.

Price controls are among the most effective methods for limiting alcohol consumption and in some countries, for example Scandinavia, are used successfully. In others, prices are narrowly controlled by governments, who receive a substantial income from the taxation of beverages and who are often powerfully lobbied by the 'drinks' industry. In consequence, in Britain and in many other countries, the effective price of alcohol has actually fallen in recent years. Governments are often reluctant to shape policies even to keep alcohol prices in line with inflation.

Controls on the times and places of sale of alcoholic beverages, if carefully thought out and enforced, may help to reduce drinking or, if less carefully exercised, may simply result in changes in drinking patterns.

The effectiveness of legislative, administrative, and fiscal controls aimed at changing drinking behaviour is difficult to assess, but enforcement of a number of small measures is, in general, likely to be followed by a reduction in consumption.

Perhaps even more difficult to assess are the effects of education and social controls on alcohol consumption. In general, the effects of educational campaigns have been disappointing in that, while they may increase knowledge of the potential hazards of excess alcohol consumption, they usually have little or no effect on drinking behaviour (Moskowitz, JStudAlc, 1989; 50:54; May, HealthEducJ, 1991; 50:195). In recent years, educational programmes have been devised to broaden information about all aspects of health, not just the effects of alcohol. These aim to inculcate individuals with a sense of responsibility for their own health and safety, and that of

the community. They are designed, for example, to assist individuals to decide whether to drink, under what circumstances, and in what quantities, clear in the knowledge of the consequences of their actions. It remains to be seen whether this new approach will be more effective in bringing about change.

Society imposes its own subtle controls on drinking behaviour, which are difficult to identify and even more difficult to quantify. In recent years, for example, attitudes to drinking and driving have changed dramatically and individuals who indulge in this sort of behaviour are now considered socially unacceptable. This change in attitude has occurred gradually over time and cannot be attributed to any specific event or series of events. Such changes in social attitudes have a powerful but unmeasurable effect on behaviour. Whether social attitudes to other aspects of excessive or irresponsible drinking will change over time, and influence behaviour, remains to be seen.

Every year the 'drinks' industry spends vast sums of money advertising and promoting their wares. In this they are sometimes aided by governments who are interested in maintaining revenue. However, several governments are now beginning to take action against advertising, but the task is a difficult one given the resources and power of the industry. In some countries, for example Egypt, all advertising of alcoholic beverages is prohibited by law, and in others, advertising may be banned or limited through certain media such as television or in relation to certain social functions such as sporting events. In many countries there is a voluntary or semi-enforceable code of practice that prevents targeting of certain vulnerable groups such as young people, and that prevents portrayal of alcohol or alcohol drinking as beneficial to health, vitality, or social standing. In some countries the 'drinks' industry has been involved, with governments, in establishing an ethical code of conduct in relation to advertising and sales promotion, and a number of voluntary 'watchdog' organizations are involved in monitoring performance to ensure conformity to the agreed regulations and codes. In the developing countries, however, governments are in a much weaker position to resist revenue incentives and there are few, if any, restraints on advertising and promotion, with the result that commercially produced alcoholic beverages are often the first consumer goods to reach even the most remote of rural areas.

Alternatives to drinking, such as increased cultural and sporting activities, have been proposed in an attempt to reduce consumption. Similarly, proposals have been made to change the traditional image of drinking places by increasing their appeal to families by provision of alternative beverages, food, and facilities for children. Many attempts have been made to carry out such schemes but so far there has been no assessment of their effects on drinking behaviour. It is unlikely, however, that any such effects would be obvious in the short term.

On a more positive note, there can be little doubt that the greater availability and acceptability of the low or non-alcoholic beverages has had a beneficial effect on drinking behaviour, particularly in relation to drinking and driving, although this has yet to be formally evaluated. There can also be little doubt that if these beverages were more fairly priced their advent would have had an even greater impact. However, even this positive move has now been countered by the arrival on the drinks market of a range of fortified wines, strong white ciders, fruit-flavoured lagers, and alcoholized soft drinks. These so-called Alcopops are attractively packaged, often in small volumes that may nevertheless contain high concentrations of alcohol. Their obviously appeal to young, often underaged, drinkers is a cause for concern, although the industry denies that these individuals have been specifically targeted.

Secondary prevention

Efforts at secondary prevention are usually directed at high-risk groups and are aimed at early diagnosis and intervention. In the context of alcohol-related liver injury, high-risk groups would include persons who consume amounts of alcohol known to be associated with the development of liver injury over time, and individuals who for a variety of genetic, social, or constitutional reasons appear to be either unduly susceptible or else are unduly exposed to the effects of alcohol, for example women, the young, those racially predisposed such as Asian Indians, and those in occupations that allow them free or easy access to alcohol. As the risk of developing liver injury increases significantly with daily intakes of alcohol in excess of 20 g in women and 40 g in men (Coates, ClinInvestMed, 1986; 9:26; Norton, BMJ, 1987; 295:80; Batey, MedJAust, 1992; 156:413), large proportions of the adult population in many countries fall into these high-risk categories. Therefore, the efforts of secondary prevention, in this context, largely overlap with those of primary prevention.

A number of campaigns have been undertaken, for example National Drinkwise Days in the United Kingdom, designed to increase awareness among the public at large and among individuals in the high-risk groups of the levels of alcohol consumption associated with the development of physical harm. These are repeated at intervals and certainly increase awareness and knowledge, but the effects on behaviour are less well documented. Health-care screening is becoming more popular in many countries, and as these schemes address several aspects of health they tend to be more appealing and less threatening than schemes designed to screen selectively for excess alcohol consumption. In the United Kingdom, all patients registered with a general medical practitioner undergo regular health-care screening undertaken either by the practitioner or else contracted out to health education specialists. Individuals who are found to be misusing or abusing alcohol can be alerted and can be given simple advice about reducing intake. Many industrial companies operate an alcohol policy aimed at the early detection of alcohol-related problems and early and effective intervention aimed at preserving the workforce. Other companies, while not operating an alcohol policy as such, arrange for middle and senior management to undergo comprehensive health-screening medicals, usually on an annual basis, thereby providing opportunity for early detection of alcohol-related problems.

Tertiary prevention

Tertiary prevention, in the context of alcoholic liver disease, is more or less synonymous with treatment; it is aimed at ensuring future abstinence from alcohol and preventing the development of the complications of liver disease. Many physicians have a pessimistic and negativistic attitude towards patients with alcoholic liver disease that is usually based on their experience of recidivist 'incurables' who return with recurrent variceal haemorrhages or else episodes of hepatocellular failure. These physicians are generally unaware that many patients with alcoholic liver disease achieve abstinence from alcohol after receiving simple advice to do so, and that they neither need nor require intensive follow-up. It is a pity that physicians' ignorance, antipathy, and pessimism can sometimes preclude individuals with alcoholic liver disease from receiving the help they need.

References

1. Lelbach WK. Leberschaden bei chronischem Alcoholismuss I–III. *Acta Hepatosplenologica*, 1966; **13**: 321–49.
2. Leevy CM. Cirrhosis in alcoholics. *Medical Clinics of North America*, 1968; **52**: 1445–51.
3. Lieber CS. Liver disease and alcohol: fatty liver, alcoholic hepatitis, cirrhosis and their interrelationships. *Annals of the New York Academy of Science*, 1975; **252**: 63–84.
4. Popper H. The pathogenesis of alcoholic cirrhosis. In Fisher MM, and Rankin JG, eds. *Alcohol and the liver*. New York: Plenum, 1977: 289–306.
5. Galambos JT, ed. *Major problems in internal medicine*, Vol. 17, *Cirrhosis*. Philadelphia: Saunders, 1979.
6. Schenker S. Alcoholic liver disease: evaluation of natural history and prognostic factors. *Hepatology*, 1984; **4**: 36S–43S.
7. Sørensen TIA, Orholm M, Bentsen KD, Høybye G, Eghøje K, and Christoffersen P. Prospective evaluation of alcohol abuse and alcoholic liver injury in men as predictors of development of cirrhosis. *Lancet*, 1984; **ii**: 241–4.
8. Parés A, Caballería J, Bruguera M, Torres M, and Rodés J. Histological course of alcoholic hepatitis. Influence of abstinence, sex and extent of hepatic damage. *Journal of Hepatology*, 1986; **2**: 33–42.
9. Marbet UA, Bianchi L, Meury U, and Stalder GA. Long-term histological evaluation of the natural history and prognostic factors of alcoholic liver disease. *Journal of Hepatology*, 1987; **4**: 364–72.
10. D'Amico G, Morabito A, Pagliaro L, and Marubini E. Survival and prognostic indicators in compensated and decompensated cirrhosis. *Digestive Diseases and Sciences*, 1986; **31**: 468–75.
11. Saunders, JB, Walters JRF, Davies P, and Paton A. A 20-year prospective study of cirrhosis. *British Medical Journal*, 1981; **282**: 263–6.
12. Morgan MY and Sherlock S. Sex-related differences among 100 patients with alcoholic liver disease. *British Medical Journal*, 1977; **1**: 939–41.
13. Krasner, N, Davis M, Portmann B, and Williams R. Changing pattern of alcoholic liver disease in Great Britain: relation to sex and signs of autoimmunity. *British Medical Journal*, 1977; **1**: 1497–500.
14. Brunt PW, Kew MC, Scheuer PJ, and Sherlock S. Studies in alcoholic liver disease in Britain. *Gut*, 1974; **15**: 52–8.
15. Levi AJ and Chalmers DM. Recognition of alcoholic liver disease in a district general hospital. *Gut*, 1978; **19**: 521–5.
16. Hislop WS *et al.* Alcoholic liver disease in Scotland and Northeastern England: presenting features in 510 patients. *Quarterly Journal of Medicine*, 1983; **206**: 232–43.
17. Morgan MY. Markers for detecting alcoholism and monitoring for continued abuse. *Pharmacology, Biochemistry and Behaviour*, 1980; **13** (Suppl. 1): 1–8.
18. Mihas AA and Tavassoli M. Laboratory markers of ethanol intake and abuse: a critical appraisal. *American Journal of the Medical Sciences*, 1992; **303**: 415–28.
19. Rosman AS. Utility and evaluation of biochemical markers of alcohol consumption. *Journal of Substance Abuse*, 1992; **4**: 277–97.
20. Goldberg DM and Kapur BM. Enzymes and circulating proteins as markers of alcohol abuse. *Clinica Chimica Acta*, 1994; **226**: 191–209.
21. Rosman AS and Lieber CS. Diagnostic utility of laboratory tests in alcoholic liver disease. *Clinical Chemistry*, 1994; **40**: 1641–51.
22. Conigrave KM, Saunders JB, and Whitfield JB. Diagnostic tests for alcohol consumption. *Alcohol and Alcoholism*, 1995; **30**: 13–26.

23. Desmet VJ. Alcoholic liver disease. Histological features and evolution. *Acta Medica Scandinavica Supplementum*, 1984; **703**: 111–26.

24. French SW *et al*. Pathology of alcoholic liver disease. *Seminars in Liver Disease*, 1993; **13**: 154–69.

25. Scheuer PJ and Lefkowitch JH, eds. Fatty liver and lesions in the alcoholic. In *Liver biopsy interpretation*. 5th edn. London: Saunders, 1994: 81–101.

26. Hall P de la M. Pathological spectrum of alcoholic liver disease. In Hall P, ed. *Alcoholic liver disease: pathobiology and pathogenesis*. 2nd edn. London: Edward Arnold, 1995: 41–68.

27. Sherlock S, ed. Alcohol and disease. *British Medical Bulletin*, 1982; **38**: 1–108.

28. Tygstrup N and Olsson R, eds. Alcohol and disease. *Acta Medica Scandinavica symposium series No. 1*. Uppsala: Almquist and Wiksell, 1985.

29. Edwards G and Peters TJ, eds. Alcohol and alcohol problems. *British Medical Bulletin*, 1994; **50**: 1–234.

30. Peters TJ, ed. *Alcohol misuse: a European perspective*. Amsterdam: Harwood Academic, 1996.

31. Saunders JB. Treatment of alcoholic liver disease. *Ballière's Clinical Gastroenterology*, 1989; **3**: 39–65.

32. Mezey E. Treatment of alcoholic liver disease. *Seminars in Liver Disease*, 1993; **13**: 210–16.

33. Morgan TR. Treatment of alcoholic hepatitis. *Seminars in Liver Disease*, 1993; **13**: 384–94.

34. Ramond M-J, Rueff B, and Benhamou J-P. Medical treatment of alcoholic liver disease. *Ballière's Clinical Gastroenterology*, 1993; **7**: 697–716.

35. Morgan MY. The treatment of alcoholic hepatitis. *Alcohol and Alcoholism*, 1996; **31**: 117–34.

36. Müller MJ, Böker KHW, and Selbeg O. Are patients with liver cirrhosis hypermetabolic? *Clinical Nutrition*, 1994; **13**: 131–44.

37. Nompleggi DJ and Bonkovsky HL. Nutritional supplementation in chronic liver disease: an analytical review. *Hepatology*, 1994; **19**: 518–33.

38. Lucy MR. Liver transplantation for alcoholic liver disease. *Ballière's Clinical Gastroenterology*, 1993; **7**: 717–27.

39. Krom RA. Liver transplantation and alcohol: who should get transplants? *Hepatology*, 1994; **20**: 28S–32S.

40. Webberley M and Neuberger J. Changing indications in liver transplantation. *Ballière's Clinical Gastroenterology*, 1994; **8**: 495–515.

41. Shelton W and Balint JA. Fair treatment of alcoholic patients in the context of liver transplantation. *Alcoholism Clinical and Experimental Research*, 1997; **21**: 93–100.

42. Nace EP, ed. *The treatment of alcoholism*. New York: Brunner/Mazel, 1987.

43. Saunders JB. The management of patients with alcohol problems. In Beaumont PJV and Hampshire RB, eds. *Australian textbook of psychiatry*. Melbourne: Blackwell Scientific, 1989: 156–71.

44. Edwards G. *The treatment of drinking problems*. London: Blackwell Scientific, 1987.

45. Glaser FB. Anybody got a match? Treatment research and the matching hypothesis. In Edwards G and Grant M, eds. *Alcoholism treatment in transition*. London: Croom Helm, 1980: 178–96.

46. Cummings C, Gordon JR, and Marlett GA. Relapse: prevention and prediction. In Miller WR, ed. *The addictive behaviours: treatment of alcoholism, drug abuse, smoking, and obesity*. Oxford: Pergamon, 1980: 291–321.

47. Marlett GA and Parks GA. Self-management of addictive disorders. In Kardy P and Kanfer FH, eds. *Self management and behaviour change: from theory to practice*. New York: Pergamon, 1982: 443–8.

48. Zimberg S, Wallace J, and Blume JB. *Practical approaches to alcoholism psychotherapy*. New York: Plenum, 1978.

49. Jacob T and Seilhamer RA. The impact on spouses and how they cope. In Orford J and Harwin H, eds. *Alcohol and the family*. London: Croom Helm, 1982: 114–26.

50. Harwin JH. The excessive drinker and the family: approaches to treatment. In Orford J and Harwin H, eds. *Alcohol and the family*. London: Croom Helm, 1982: 201–40.

51. Alcoholics Anonymous. *Twelve steps and twelve traditions*. New York: Harper, 1953.

52. Keso L and Salaspuro M. Laboratory tests in the follow-up of treated alcoholics: how often should testing be repeated. *Alcohol and Alcoholism*, 1990; **25**: 359–62.

53. Bircher J. Altered drug metabolism in liver disease—therapeutic implications. In Thomas HC and MacSween RNM, eds. *Recent Advances in Hepatology*, Edinburgh: Churchill Livingstone, 1983; **1**: 101–13.

54. Chedid A, Mendenhall CL, Gartside P, French WS, Chen T, Rabin L, and the VA Cooperative Study Group. Prognostic factors in alcoholic liver disease. *American Journal of Gastroenterology*, 1991; **86**: 210–16.

55. Bouchier IAD, Hislop WS, and Precott RJ. A prospective study of alcoholic liver disease and mortality. *Journal of Hepatology*, 1992; **16**: 290–7.

56. Moser J. *Prevention of alcohol-related problems: an international review of preventive measures, policies and programmes*. Toronto: Addiction Foundation, 1980.

57. Moser J. Is alcoholic liver disease preventable? In Hall P, ed. *Alcoholic liver disease: pathobiology, epidemiology and clinical aspects*. London: Edward Arnold, 1985; 304–13.

58. Brunt PW. The prevention of alcoholic liver disease. *Ballière's Clinical Gastroenterology*, 1993; **7**: 729–49.

15.4 Extrahepatic manifestations of alcoholism

Albert Pares and Joan Caballeria

Alcohol may affect most organs and systems of human beings. The mechanisms by which it produces deleterious effects are variable. These effects may be produced by alcohol *per se*, by its metabolites, or by the consequences of alcohol metabolism, including nutritional deficiencies. In this chapter the pernicious effects of alcoholism in different organs and systems are summarized.

Gastrointestinal tract

Since the gastrointestinal tract is exposed to high concentrations before ethanol enters the portal circulation, it is not surprising that alcohol may directly or indirectly damage these organs. Thus, derangements in the different parts of the alimentary tract after acute and chronic ethanol intake have been described (Table 1).

Oesophagus

Both acute and chronic alcohol administration produce oesophageal motor dysfunction characterized by a decrease in upper and lower oesophageal sphincter pressure, and a decrease in peristalsis without changes in the propagation velocity for oesophageal contractions (Hogan, JApplPhysiol, 1972; 32:755; Mayer, Gastro, 1978; 75:1133).

Table 1 Effects of alcohol on the gastrointestinal tract

Oesophagus
  Motor dysfunction with lowered sphincter pressure
  Oesophagitis reflux and its complications
  Oesophageal cancer
Stomach
  Acute gastritis
  Chronic gastritis
  Delayed gastric emptying
Small intestine
  Impairment of duodenal and jejunal mucosa
  Decrease in synthesis of brush border enzymes
  Changes in motor activity
  Depressed mechanisms of transport
  Malabsorption
Colon
  Colonic varices
  Changes in colonic motility
  Impairment of rectal mucosa

These changes are usually seen in chronic alcoholics who have also had peripheral neuropathy.

The consequences of motor dysfunction are gastro-oesophageal reflux (Kaufman, Gut, 1978; 19:336), oesophagitis, Barrett's oeso-phagus, and ulcers of the lower third of the oesophagus. Other factors involved in the pathogenesis of alcoholic oesophagitis are a direct effect of alcohol that enhances the penetration of cytotoxic agents and the effect of alcohol on the salivary glands. Alcohol intake causes a reduction of salivary secretion and also increases the viscosity of salivary secretions. Nausea and vomiting are frequent in chronic alcoholics and may induce Mallory–Weiss tears of the cardio-oesophageal area (Knauer, Gastro, 1976; 71:5). Although alcohol abuse *per se* may produce an increased risk of cancer, the interaction seen between drinking and smoking suggests that the main effect of ethanol is to act as a co-carcinogen. Nutritional factors such as iron, zinc, and vitamin A deficiencies can also be involved in the pathogenesis of oesophageal cancer (Garro, AnnRevPharmTox, 1990; 30:219).

Stomach

Acute gastritis is very common after alcohol exposure and usually resolves completely after a few days of abstinence. The endoscopic lesions of acute gastritis include mucosal erythema, erosions, petechiae, and haemorrhage. The severity of gastritis is related to the degree of alteration of the mucosal barrier and to the concentration of acid with which the mucosa comes into contact. Chronic alcohol ingestion also leads to gastritis, both the chronic superficial variety and atrophic gastritis with hypochlorhydria (Dinoso, ArchIntMed, 1972; 130:715; Parl, HumPath, 1979; 10:45). Recently, a high prevalence of *Helicobacter pylori* infection has been found among chronic alcoholics, favouring the development of chronic gastritis (Hauge, AlcoholClinExpRes, 1994; 18:886). Disruption of the mucosal barrier allows the back-diffusion of hydrogen ions, with resultant cellular damage. The mechanism of the gastric mucosal barrier damage is not well known and may occur because of diminished gastric mucus production, changes in mucosal blood flow, inhibition of active ion transport, increased cellular permeability, disruption of the cell membrane, hyperosmolarity, reduction of intracellular prostaglandins, and decreased cAMP. Probably the association of several of these factors is responsible for the disruption of the mucosal barrier. A protective effect against the gastric mucosa damage induced by alcohol has been described for prostaglandins (Tarnawski, Gastro, 1985; 88:334), somatostatin (Diel, RegulPeptides, 1986; 13:235), sucralfate (Cohen, Gastro, 1989; 96:292), and ebrotidin (Konturek, ScaJGastr, 1992; 27:438). Despite these well-established effects on gastric mucosa, there is no evidence of a higher prevalence of peptic ulcer in chronic alcoholics.

The effects of alcohol on gastric emptying are controversial and appear to be concentration dependent. After the acute administration of a low dose of ethanol, both acceleration and delay in gastric emptying have been reported, whereas acute administration of a higher concentration of ethanol diminished gastric contractions and delayed gastric emptying. Recent reports show that gastric emptying is normal in chronic alcoholics without peripheral neuropathy (Keshavarzian, Alcoholism, 1986; 10:432).

Small intestine

The small bowel is also exposed to high concentrations of ethanol and haemorrhagic lesions in duodenal villus tips have been produced in humans after ingestion of alcohol at relatively small doses. In chronic alcoholics there is a shortening of duodenal and jejunal villi with a decreased number of mucosal cells, and an increase of cell numbers in crypts because of a replacement of normal by less mature cells (Baraona, Gastro, 1974; 66:266; Rubin, Gastro, 1972; 63:801). A decrease in synthesis of brush-border enzymes, increased permeability to water and solutes, and changes in small-intestinal motor activity are the mechanisms involved in the diarrhoea commonly seen in chronic alcoholics (Robles, JohnsHopkMedJ, 1974; 135:17; Mezey, AnnNYAcadSci, 1975; 252:215).

Alcohol has direct deleterious effects on epithelial cell function and upon the active transport systems present within the small bowel. These structural alterations may account for the defective absorption of nutrients such as D-xylose, glucose, amino acids, folic acid and other vitamins, and minerals (Krasner, Gut, 1976; 17:245). By contrast, fat absorption is not affected by ethanol directly. Pancreatic, hepatic, and nutritional complications of chronic alcoholism are the causes of fat malabsorption.

Colon

Haemorrhoids and colonic varices may be a manifestation of the portal hypertension found in patients with alcoholic cirrhosis (Pickens, AmJGastr, 1980; 73:73). Although rare, varices of the colon may be an unexpected cause of rectal bleeding in these patients. Furthermore, alcohol has been shown to have direct effects on colonic motility and morphology. In the rectal mucosa of chronic alcoholics with recent alcohol intake, a dense mononuclear infiltrate was seen on light microscopy, whereas electron microscopy revealed swollen mitochondria and dilated endoplasmic reticulum (Brozynski, DisColRec, 1978; 21:329). The association between alcohol consumption and colonic cancer is not clear (Hamilton, CancerRes, 1987; 47:4305).

Pancreas[4]

Several epidemiological studies have demonstrated a close relationship between alcohol consumption and chronic pancreatitis. Diet also contributes to the incidence of chronic pancreatitis, and the risk of pancreatitis increases in proportion both to the amount of daily alcohol and protein intake (Durbec, Digestion, 1978; 18: 337). Alcohol usually causes a chronic, recurrent, calcifying pancreatitis, and a period of 6 to 12 years of alcohol consumption seems to be necessary before pancreatic symptoms occur.

The exact pathogenic mechanism for pancreatitis remains unknown. Classically a dysfunction of the sphincter of Oddi was implicated in the pathogenesis of alcoholic pancreatitis. It has been postulated that pancreatitis resulted from an excess of pancreatic flow against ductal resistance due to alcohol-induced spasm in the sphincter of Oddi. However, in animal models there are no convincing evidence supporting this theory (Pirola, AmJDigDis, 1970; 15:583). Another concomitant factor could be a reflux of bile into the pancreatic duct, and it has been shown that bile from chronically alcohol-fed rats, when injected into the pancreatic ducts of normal rats, produced pancreatic lesions, whereas the bile from non-alcohol-fed rats did not. Whether the toxic substance is alcohol, acetaldehyde, or alcohol-induced changes in biliary lipids has not been elucidated.

Chronic alcohol consumption also produces changes in pancreatic secretion. An increase in protein concentration has been suggested to explain ductular precipitates of protein and calcium carbonate (Sarles, Gastro, 1974; 66:604). These precipitates may obstruct the ducts. Whether the protein plugs precede the development of pancreatitis or are a consequence of pancreatic inflammation has not been completely elucidated. In human chronic pancreatitis it has been suggested that the precipitation of hyperconcentrated protein may be favoured by an increased concentration of the iron-binding protein lactoferrin. Alcohol has direct effects on the composition and fluidity of membranes, which can contribute to the pathogenesis of pancreatitis (Noronha, AmJGastr, 1981; 76: 114). The role of diet in the pathogenesis of pancreatitis is uncertain. The fact that malnutrition favours the development of pancreatitis is supported by the observation of poor nutrition in patients with alcoholic pancreatitis (Mezey, AmJClinNutr, 1988; 48:148) and the return to normal of impaired pancreatic secretion with a correct diet, even with continued alcohol intake (Mezey, JohnsHopkMedJ, 1976; 138:7). On the other hand, several studies have demonstrated an increased intake of fat and protein in patients with alcoholic pancreatitis (Uscanga, DigDisSci, 1985; 30:40).

In chronic alcoholics, symptoms of acute pancreatitis usually develop after functional and histological changes of chronic pancreatitis are well established (Skinazi, GastroClinBiol, 1995; 19: 266). The clinical course is characterized by recurrent attacks, precipitated by alcohol abuse. When the disease progresses, these episodes tend to be more frequent but less severe, and complications such as malabsorption, pseudocyst formation, jaundice, and diabetes become more prominent. However, in some patients the clinical course is insidious and the illness progresses to pancreatic insufficiency without acute inflammatory episodes (Ammann, Pancreas, 1986; 1:195; Capitane, SchMedWoch, 1988; 118:817). The diagnosis of chronic pancreatitis is made by pancreatic function tests and imaging. The pancreatic imaging techniques most used are ultrasonography, computer-assisted tomography (Hessel, Radiol, 1982; 143:129), and endoscopic retrograde cholangiopancreatography (Niederau, Gastro, 1985; 88:1973).

Carcinoma of the pancreas may occur with increased frequency in alcoholic patients (Burch, ArchIntMed, 1968; 122:273), although it correlates better with cigarette smoking than with alcohol consumption (Ghadirian, Cancer, 1991; 67:2664). Most patients with pancreatic cancer also had lesions of chronic pancreatitis, and the exclusion of pancreatic carcinoma in a patient with chronic alcoholic pancreatitis may be a difficult diagnostic problem. Besides the conventional imaging tests, endoscopic ultrasonography might be of help in the diagnosis of pancreatic carcinoma.

Nervous system

Acute and chronic alcohol abuse and its withdrawal may produce a variety of neurological syndromes. Their pathogenesis includes direct effects of ethanol and acetaldehyde, and nutritional deficiencies. The mechanisms of ethanol toxicity on the brain are still unclear, but changes in protein or lipid components, or both, of the neuronal membrane, thus increasing its fluidity, may play a relevant role.

Alcoholic intoxication

The symptoms of alcoholic intoxication reflect the depressant effect of alcohol on neurones of the central nervous system (Sellers, NEJM, 1976; 294:757). According to the degree of intoxication, the common symptoms are excitement, loss of restraint, loquacity, behaviour irregularities, incoordination of movements and gait, irritability, stupor, and coma. The amount of alcohol necessary to produce intoxication varies considerably from one person to another, depending on alcoholic habits, sex, and age. Alcohol affects all kind of motor performance as well as the efficiency of cognitive functions. Mild to moderate intoxication does not require special treatment, whereas alcoholic coma represents a real medical emergency, especially because of depression of respiratory function.

Alcohol withdrawal syndrome[6]

The alcohol withdrawal syndrome is the consequence of physical alcohol dependence (Behnke, HospPract, 1976; 11:79). The major clinical manifestations of alcohol withdrawal are tremulousness, hallucinations, convulsions, and delirium. Tremor is the most common withdrawal symptom and appears within a few hours of discontinuation of drinking. The tremor mainly affects the upper limbs, lips, and tongue, and is usually associated with nausea, sweating, irritability, and weakness. Transient auditory or visual hallucinations are present in about 25 per cent of patients with severe tremulousness. Hallucinations occur within 24 to 48 hours after cessation of ethanol intake and disappear within a few days. However, about 20 per cent of these patients develop chronic auditory hallucinosis and a clinical picture similar to that of schizophrenia. Alcohol may precipitate fits in epileptic patients during a heavy drinking episode and convulsions in non-epileptic individuals in the early withdrawal period. Delirium tremens is a serious manifestation of alcohol withdrawal, characterized by confusion, hallucinations, tremor, agitation, tachycardia, dilated pupils, profuse perspiration, and fever. No specific neurological signs or characteristic laboratory findings are available. Sedation by clomethiazole or benzodiazepines is required to avoid exhaustion (Feuerlein, ActaPhysiolScand(Suppl), 1986; 329:120). Recovery usually occurs after several days, although patients with associated diseases such as liver disease, pancreatitis, trauma, or aspiration pneumonia, may have a poor prognosis.

Wernicke–Korsakoff syndrome

The Wernicke–Korsakoff syndrome is a nutritional disorder caused by thiamine deficiency. Wernicke's encephalopathy represents the acute phase, whereas Korsakoff's psychosis is the chronic phase.

Wernicke's encephalopathy is characterized by oculomotor disturbances, cerebellar ataxia, and mental confusion (Reuler, NEJM, 1985; 312:1035). The ocular disturbances are nystagmus, various types of gaze palsy, or total ophthalmoplegia. The ataxia affects the trunk and lower extremities. Mental confusion is characterized by disorientation, inattention, and poor responsiveness. Stupor and coma are frequent in underdiagnosed presentations of Wernicke's encephalopathy. Treatment consists of parenteral thiamine.

Most patients who do not recover in 48 to 72 hours develop Korsakoff's psychosis. Korsakoff's psychosis is characterized by various degrees of both antegrade and retrograde amnesia with relative preservation of other intellectual functions. The disease is potentially reversible by early treatment with thiamine, but in more than 50 per cent of cases recovery is incomplete.[7]

Alcoholic cerebellar degeneration[8]

Degeneration of the cerebellar cortex, mainly the anterior and superior vermis and adjacent hemispheric folia, is often found in autopsies of chronic alcohol abusers. The disease is characterized by various degrees of gait and truncal ataxia, whereas co-ordination of upper extremities is usually not affected. The disease evolves slowly over a period of years, and may improve with nutritional replacement and cessation of alcohol intake. The pathogenesis of alcoholic cerebellar degeneration is unknown, although nutritional depletion, and direct toxic effects of alcohol and acetaldehyde have been implicated. Clinical diagnosis is not difficult and may be confirmed by high-resolution computed tomography.

Central pontine myelinolysis

Central pontine myelinolysis is a rare demyelinating disease characterized by a neuronal dysfunction centred at the pontine levels (Messert, Neurology, 1979; 29:147). Clinical manifestations are progressive quadriparesis, pseudobulbar palsy, and partial or complete paralysis of horizontal eye movements. The disease is often fatal in 2 to 3 weeks, and the diagnosis is frequently missed in the living patient. The pathogenesis is not known. It has been suggested that an acute change in serum sodium level while correcting electrolyte imbalances and water depletion may play a major role (Kleinschmidt-DeMasters, Science, 1981; 211:1068). No specific treatment is available.

Marchiafava–Bignani syndrome

The Marchiafava–Bignani syndrome is a very rare demyelinating disease of the corpus callosum encountered almost exclusively in chronic alcoholics. The disease is characterized by symptoms of bilateral involvement of the frontal lobes and acute bilateral hemispheric dysfunction (Koeppen, Neurology, 1978; 28:290). The aetiology of Marchiafava–Bignani syndrome is unknown, although the association with central pontine myelinolysis or Wernicke's disease suggests a possible common nutritional factor (Ghatak, Neurology, 1978; 28:1295).

Alcoholic dementia

Cognitive deficits caused by cortical atrophy from alcohol abuse remain a subject of controversy (Carlen, Neurology, 1981; 31:377). The brain weight of chronic alcoholics at autopsy is less than that of age-matched controls, and computed tomographic scans have shown a high incidence of cortical atrophy in alcoholics (Ron, Brain, 1982; 105:497). The syndrome of alcoholic dementia is probably a combination of the Wernicke–Korsakoff syndrome and the direct toxicity of alcohol to neurones.

Alcoholic polyneuropathy[9]

Polyneuropathy is probably the most common nutritional complication affecting the nervous system in alcoholics. Symptoms begin distally and the legs are always affected first and often exclusively. The course is insidious and progressive. Patients complain of pain, paraesthesiae, and weakness. In severe cases, symmetric, distal motor deficits are seen, and significant atrophy may be encountered. The Achilles reflex is depressed or absent even in the asymptomatic stage. Clinical diagnosis is clear, and may be supported by electrophysiological studies. Treatment consists of vitamin B complex supplementation, abstinence from alcohol, and improvement of the nutritional state. However, recovery is slow and often incomplete (Thomson, BrMedBull, 1982; 38:87).

Skeletal muscle disease

According to several studies, skeletal muscle disease occurs in between one- and two-thirds of all chronic alcohol abusers (Martin, QJMed, 1985; 55:233; Urbano-Marquez, NEJM, 1989; 320:409). However, physicians in general pay little attention to this disorder because overt clinical disease is rare and because most of the symptoms, such as cramps, muscle weakness, difficulties in gait and mobility, ataxia, incoordination and pain, are attributed to damage of the nervous system.[10]

Acute alcoholic myopathy

Acute alcoholic myopathy is a syndrome of acute muscle necrosis which occurs in heavy-drinking alcoholics (Pittman, Neurology, 1971; 21:293). The severity ranges from rhabdomyolysis with myoglobinuria to asymptomatic, transient elevations of enzymes.[11] Muscular damage is reflected in the serum by elevated activities of several enzymes released from myocytes, such as aldolase, aspartate aminotransferase, lactate dehydrogenase, and creatine kinase. The skeletal (MM) fraction of creatine kinase is the most specific indicator (Lafair, ArchIntMed, 1968; 122:417).

Acute skeletal rhabdomyolysis is characterized by a sudden onset of muscle pain, swelling, and weakness of one or more muscle groups, marked elevation of serum creatine kinase, myoglobinuria, and scattered muscle fibre necrosis. A preceding heavy bout of drinking is usual. The symptoms are maximal when the patient is first seen. Pain lasts a few days, but weakness can persist longer.

Diagnosis is based on the presence of either typical muscle symptoms, histological evidence of muscle fibre necrosis, raised serum creatine kinase, or myopathic features on electromyography (Martinez, JNeurolSci, 1973; 20:245).

The most serious complication of alcoholic rhabdomyolysis is myoglobinuria-induced acute tubular necrosis and renal failure. However, in most cases the disease is self-limited, with recovery occurring within days or weeks of abstinence. Recurrent episodes have been described in several patients. The incidence of acute skeletal muscle injury in not known since significant elevation of serum creatine kinase occurs in a high proportion of alcoholics in the absence of clinical symptoms.[12]

Chronic alcoholic myopathy[13]

This form of alcoholic myopathy consists of progressive and usually painless wasting and weakness of the proximal muscle groups, particularly in the legs. Most patients have no preceding history suggestive of acute myopathy, but a long history of ethanol intake is frequent. Coexisting peripheral neuropathy is usually evident. Histochemical techniques show a selective atrophy of type IIb fibres (Langhor, JNeurolNeurosurgPsych, 1983; 46:248). As in acute myopathy, the incidence is not known. Type II muscle fibre atrophy, the major histological feature of the disease, is also common in alcoholics without symptoms of muscle disease, sustaining the concept of a subclinical chronic alcoholic myopathy (Martin, QJMed, 1985; 218:233).

The direct role of alcohol or its metabolites in the pathogenesis of muscle disease is well established (Urbano-Marquez, NEJM, 1989; 320:409). However, the contribution of nutritional deficiencies is still controversial. Recently, evidence has been presented suggesting that coexisting malnutrition may exacerbate the disease (Conde, AlcAlcl, 1992; 27:159), whereas experimental studies in chronically alcohol-fed rats showed that a direct effect of ethanol and its metabolite acetaldehyde on protein synthesis is implicated in the pathogenesis of alcoholic myopathy (Preedy, BiochemJ, 1989; 259:261). It is well known that neurological disorders can induce skeletal muscle changes and that ethanol inhibits neuromuscular transmission (Wali, AlcAlc, 1988; 23:299). However, ethanol, and not a concomitant neuropathy, seems to be the primary precipitating factor for the development of myopathy (Mills, AlcAlc, 1986; 21:357). The management of alcoholic muscle disease consists in abstinence from alcohol and appropriate treatment of nutritional deficiency, associated mineral or electrolyte imbalances, and complicating renal disease.

Heart

The association between excessive alcohol intake and congestive cardiomyopathy was reported over a century ago. However, this association was attributed to nutritional deficiencies or toxic additives rather than to alcohol itself. Several recent studies excluding alcoholics with malnutrition, have established a direct relationship between alcohol consumption and cardiac damage (Dancy, Lancet, 1985; 1:1122).

The acute administration of ethanol can produce alterations of both mechanical function and electrophysiological properties of the heart. These effects are usually subclinical. However, in chronic alcoholics and in patients with heart disease, acute ingestion of ethanol may produce disturbances of clinical significance (Kupari, BrHeartJ, 1983; 49:174; Lang, AnnIntMed, 1985; 102:742).

Chronic alcohol consumption can lead to progressive cardiac dysfunction, resulting in congestive cardiomyopathy. Excessive daily alcohol intake of over 10 years or more is required for the development of cardiac decompensation. The clinical onset of alcoholic cardiotoxicity is insidious, with non-specific fatigue, chest discomfort, palpitations, or an isolated episode of atrial fibrillation (Steinberg, AmHeartJ, 1981; 101:461). As the cardiomyopathy progresses, manifestations of overt right and left heart failure become apparent. Orthopnoea, paroxysmal nocturnal dyspnoea, elevated right atrial pressure with distension of jugular veins, and peripheral oedema may appear. Persistent alcohol ingestion results in death from cardiac failure or its complications 2 to 4 years after onset of clinical manifestations. Sudden death may result from ventricular arrhythmia.

Laboratory findings are related to the extent of the disease and are not different from those obtained in patients with congestive cardiomyopathy due to other causes. Electrocardiography shows a variety of ST and T wave abnormalities, widened P waves, atrioventricular block, hemiblocks and bundle branch blocks, and atrial and ventricular arrhythmias.

Echocardiography may demonstrate four-chamber enlargement, left ventricular hypertrophy, and decreased left and right ventricular contractile function (Mathews, AmJCard, 1981; 47:570). Cardiac catheterization reveals depressed cardiac output, elevated left and right ventricular filling pressures, and markedly depressed indices of contractility. Left ventriculography shows a dilated hypokinetic chamber.

Treatment of alcoholic cardiomyopathy consists of alcohol abstinence combined with supportive therapy for associated heart failure and arrhythmias. Prognosis is related to the duration and severity of symptoms before the onset of abstinence (Schwartz, AmJCard, 1975; 36:963; Kupari, PostgradMedJ, 1984; 60:151).

Haematological complications

Haematological manifestations are very common in alcoholics with liver disease as well as in those without significant hepatic damage. These abnormalities are mainly observed in red blood cells, including megaloblastosis and haemolytic disturbances, as well as in leucocytes, and platelets (Table 2). Alcohol consumption also induces some derangements in haemostasis.[23]

Erythrocytes

Most alcoholics have enlarged erythrocytes in peripheral blood, as manifested by increased mean cellular volume (Wu, Lancet, 1974; ii:829). This abnormality is associated with alcohol consumption and usually disappears after some weeks of abstinence, when peripheral cells are replaced by a new, smaller cell population produced after alcohol withdrawal. Although folate deficiency is common in alcoholics, simple macrocytosis is unrelated to this deficiency or other vitamin deficiencies, and is therefore considered a consequence of the direct toxic effect of alcohol or its metabolites on developing erythroblasts, which are vacuolated similarly to those

Table 2 Effects of alcohol on blood

Red cells
  Direct effect on erythropoiesis
  Folate deficiency
  Derangement of iron metabolism (sideroblastic anaemia)
  Haemolysis
  Abnormal structure of membranes (acanthocytes, stomatocytes, etc.)
  Hypophosphataemia
Leucocytes
  Neutropenia
  Impairment of adherence and chemotaxis
  Impairment of macrophage function
  Impairment of lymphocyte function
Platelets
  Thrombocytopenia
  Abnormal function

observed in chloramphenicol toxicity. However, alcoholics may present vitamin deficiencies which result in megaloblastosis.

Thus, megaloblastic anaemia occurs in those cases with nutritional folate deficiency, although vitamin B_{12} and gastric and intestinal dysfunction may play a role in this type of anaemia. Likewise, sideroblastic anaemia is frequently found in alcoholics with severe folate deficiency, but abnormal pyridoxine function or decreased enzyme activity involved in haem synthesis may also contribute to this type of anaemia, as well as derangement of iron metabolism.

Alcoholics may present haemolytic anaemias, although they are more frequent in those cases who have already developed severe liver disease. A variety of haemolytic syndromes have been described in patients with alcoholic liver disease as a consequence of red cell derangement, or congestive splenomegaly resulting from liver disease and portal hypertension. Changes in erythrocyte membrane lipid composition and in plasma lipoproteins secondary to alcohol consumption may reduce membrane fluidity and lead to acanthocytosis. Additionally, anaemia associated with target cells, stomatocytes, knizocytes, and triangulocytes has also been described in alcoholics. The pathogenesis of these morphological abnormalities is uncertain at present. Haemolytic anaemia has been observed in alcoholics with severe hypophosphataemia, which may cause low levels of adenosine triphosphate, required to maintain the red cell metabolic activity.[19]

Some alcoholics with severe alcoholic hepatitis may present with haemolysis associated with hyperlipoproteinaemia, as first reported by Zieve in 1958 (Zieve, AnnIntMed, 1958; 118:471). Cases with similar associations were reported later, although evidence of acute haemolytic anaemia was, in most cases, equivocal since the anaemia could have been secondary to changes in hydration, or to recovery from marrow failure, or having a low grade of haemolysis associated with liver disease. Therefore this syndrome is, at present, questionable.[21]

Leucocytes

Granulocytopenia and impairment of granulocyte adherence, mobilization, and chemotaxis, as well as disturbances in macrophage and lymphocyte function, may be present in alcoholic patients, and may explain, in part, the decreased resistance to infection. The prevalence of these abnormalities is not well known, since most data are taken from patients with varying degrees of liver disease, or from experimental studies in animals.

Likewise, the respective roles of malnutrition, various acute illnesses, liver disease, and ethanol itself have not been elucidated. However, since impaired macrophage and lymphocyte function may be restored to normal after several days of withdrawal from alcohol, it could be suggested that these abnormalities were caused by alcohol consumption. In this respect lymphocyte proliferation responses are lower in alcoholic patients without liver disease (Mutchnick, AlcoholClinExpRes, 1988; 12:155).

Platelets

Thrombocytopenia is a well-known consequence of alcohol ingestion, although in most cases it is mild and without clinical consequences (Lindenbaum, AnnIntMed, 1968; 68:526). Usually platelet counts return to normal within a week of ethanol withdrawal, but occasionally there is a rebound in the platelet count. These effects on platelets seem to be due to a direct inhibitory effect of alcohol on thrombocytopoiesis, since thrombocytopenia may occur in the absence of folate deficiency or splenomegaly. Ethanol also has a role in abnormal platelet function, even in the absence of thrombocytopenia. Thus, chronic alcoholics have prolonged bleeding times, decreased platelet aggregation tests, and decreased thromboxane A_2 release from platelets, abnormalities that returned to normal after 1 to 3 weeks of alcohol withdrawal. The mechanisms of platelet dysfunction are not well known. However, alcohol may interfere with membrane function of circulating platelets and megakaryocytes, and may shorten platelet lifespan.[21]

Haemostasis

There are no significant changes in coagulation as a result of acute or chronic ingestion of alcohol without marked liver disease, since coagulation factors are usually within normal limits. In chronic alcoholics, however, antithrombin III may be diminished and may thereby explain spontaneous thrombosis in some patients. When alcoholics present abnormal bleeding times, it is mainly due to abnormal platelet function. These abnormalities are particularly prominent in patients with severe liver disease, who additionally have conspicuous reductions in the levels of all vitamin K-dependent factors, as discussed elsewhere. However, it is possible that not all the coagulation abnormalities in alcohol abusers are caused by inadequate hepatic synthesis, since deranged coagulation may be the result of interaction of acetaldehyde with coagulation proteins (Batista, DigDisSci, 1994; 39:2411) (see Chapters 24.5 and 25.3).

Endocrinological consequences

The gonadal effects of alcohol consumption are common extrahepatic abnormalities observed in alcoholics (Van Thiel, Alcoholism, 1978; 2:265) (Table 3).[26] Although gonadal effects have been considered as a consequence of hepatic dysfunction, it is now well established that alcohol per se may induce sexual dysfunction, particularly in men who experience hypoandrogenization with decreased libido, impotence, or both (Gordon, Alcoholism, 1978; 2:

Table 3 Clinical manifestations of the endocrine abnormalities observed in alcoholics
Hypogonadism
Loss of libido
Testicular atrophy
Menstrual problems
Hyperoestrogenism
Gynaecomastia
Loss of body hair
Vascular spiders
Pseudo-Cushing's syndrome

250). The pathogenesis of such abnormalities is not completely known, although it has recently been demonstrated that alcohol or its metabolites may directly affect testicular function by decreasing the production of testosterone and by interfering with gonadotrophin binding to testicular tissue (Mendelson, Alcoholism, 1978; 2:255). Additionally, alcohol may directly affect the hypothalamic–pituitary–gonadal axis; thus alcoholics have inappropriately low plasma gonadotrophin concentrations for the degree of gonadal failure. Alcoholics may also experience hyperoestrogenization manifested by palmar erythema, spider angioma, and gynaecomastia which are associated with biochemical changes including increases in sex steroid-binding globulin and oestrogen-responsive neurophysin. Plasma total oestradiol concentrations are usually normal in alcoholic men, with or without liver disease, although total and free plasma concentrations of oestrone are raised regardless of the presence of liver disease. Likewise, alcohol may induce changes in peripheral testosterone and oestrogen metabolism as well as changes in oestrogen receptors, an effect that may be of particular importance in cases with severe liver disease and portal-systemic shunting. There are studies suggesting that alcohol may be a cause of infertility. Likewise, abnormal spermatogenesis is more prevalent in heavy drinkers than in non-alcoholic subjects (Pajarinen, IntJAndrol, 1994; 17:292) which corroborates the close association between alcohol intake and male infertility. Thus, semen of alcoholics often shows abnormalities including decreased numbers and motility of spermatozoa, and increased proportions of abnormal forms. In a survey,[26] a significant relationship was found between alcohol ingestion and male infertility. Although less known, alcohol may also damage ovarian architecture as reported in rats fed ethanol, and may, in part, explain infertility of alcoholic women. The clinical studies of alcohol-dependent women suggest that they have higher prevalence of amenorrhoea, anovulation, dysfunction in the postovulative phase of the menstrual cycle, and accelerated onset of menopause, indicating that repeated or sustained episodes of alcohol intoxication suppress hormonal activity in women. Moderate alcohol use, however, has been demonstrated as an important factor for postmenopausal oestrogen status and may offer a partial explanation for the reported protective effect of moderate alcohol consumption with respect to postmenopausal cardiovascular disease risk (Gavaler, AlcoholClinExpRes 1992, 16:87).

Another endocrinological abnormality observed in chronic alcoholics is the 'pseudo-Cushing's syndrome' characterized by typical moon face, muscle wasting, abdominal striae, weakness, fatigue, excessive bruising, and hypertension (Frajria, Lancet, 1977; i:1050). This syndrome can be indistinguishable from true Cushing's syndrome with elevated plasma cortisol levels, and increased urinary steroid output and failure of dexamethasone to suppress cortisol secretion. However, the 'pseudo-Cushing's syndrome', reverts after drinking is interrupted and may recur with resumption of alcohol abuse. The pathogenesis seems to be related to the effect of alcohol intoxication on cortisol secretion, possibly mediated through the stimulation of the hypothalamic–pituitary–adrenal axis. However, this hypothesis has been questioned because ethanol *per se* can induce most of the clinical manifestations as in the so-called pseudo-Cushing's syndrome, such as central adiposity, hypertension, myopathy, osteoporosis, depression, and psychosis (Jeffloate, Lancet, 1993; 341:676).

Changes in growth hormone have also been described in alcoholics, particularly in those with liver disease, although they are without clinical relevance. However, impairment in growth hormone release, may contribute to the hypoglycaemia associated with fasting and alcohol ingestion. Elevated basal prolactin levels and exaggerated prolactin responses to the thyrotrophin-releasing hormone have been described in alcoholics, effects that are more prominent in patients with liver cirrhosis.[27]

Alcoholics without significant liver disease have no noticeable changes in the pituitary–thyroid axis, but in those with liver disease a decreased conversion of T_4 to T_3 and variable alterations of thyroxine-binding proteins have been reported (Israel, Gastro, 1979; 76:116), although usually without clinical relevance. A decreased thyroid size in alcoholic cirrhotics but not in patients with non-alcoholic cirrhosis suggests that alcohol may have a toxic effect on the thyroid gland regardless of the degree of liver damage (Hegedus, ClinExpMet, 1988; 37:229). Acute increases in parathormone levels in man after alcohol ingestion have been described; however, it is generally accepted that parathyroid function is not markedly disturbed in chronic alcoholics, although hypomagnesaemia secondary to increased urinary magnesium loss can result in parathormone resistance.[27]

Hypoglycaemia and ketoacidosis

Hypoglycaemia is an uncommon complication of alcohol abuse. It usually develops after prolonged fasting or in severely malnourished individuals who ingest a large amount of ethanol (Freinkel, JCI, 1963; 42:1112; Williams, MedClinNAm, 1984; 68:33). Stupor and coma are generally present and in some cases other neurological findings, such as conjugated deviation of the eyes, rigidity of extremities, convulsions, and the Babinski reflex, are present.

The pathogenesis of this hypoglycaemia is attributed mainly to inhibition of hepatic gluconeogenesis by alcohol in the presence of marked depletion of hepatic glycogen storage (Freinkel, JCI, 1963; 42:1112). However, derangement of endogenous glucocorticoid secretion may be a contributory factor.

Alcoholic ketoacidosis occurs in chronic ethanol abusers, commonly malnourished, who after a recent binge develop abdominal pain and vomiting which lead to acute starvation (Freinkel, JCI, 1963; 42:1112; Palmer, ClinEndMetab, 1983; 12:381). In fact, most patients with alcoholic ketoacidosis have not been able to drink alcohol for 1 to 3 days before admission to hospital, and therefore blood alcohol levels can be negative. Thus, alcoholic ketoacidosis is more common in chronic malnourished patients (Wrem, AmJMed, 1991; 91:119). Patients have tachypnoea and ketone odour of the breath, with variable abdominal findings, commonly reflecting acute gastritis (Fullop, EndMetClinMedNAm, 1993; 22:209).

Dehydration and delirium tremens may also be present. Arterial blood gas studies usually reveal moderate metabolic acidosis, although blood pH may be elevated because of coexisting respiratory alkalosis and/or metabolic alkalosis due to severe vomiting. Serum ketones are markedly elevated, and serum lactate levels may be slightly raised (Fulop, Alcoholism, 1986; 10:610). The ketosis usually disappears after a few hours of intravenous administration of glucose and saline. The pathogenesis of this syndrome is attributed to the interruption of alcohol ingestion which leads to release of an alcohol-induced block in ketogenesis.

Hyperuricaemia

Alcohol consumption has been associated with hyperuricaemia and with gout attacks in susceptible patients. The mechanism of hyperuricaemia is a decrease in the urinary excretion of uric acid, secondary to hyperlactacidaemia (Lieber, JCI, 1962; 41:1863).

Lactate competitively inhibits uric acid clearance by the proximal tubule, and consequently reduces urate excretion. In addition, in gout patients with increased production of uric acid, alcohol intake may exacerbate urate synthesis by an accelerated degradation of adenine nucleotides (Faller, NEJM, 1982; 307:1598; Nishinura, Metabolism, 1994; 43:745).

Osteoporosis

Loss of bone manifested by increased incidence of fractures in alcoholics has been reported for many years, although the influence of trauma and the association with liver disease were considered to be main factors. However, recent studies indicate that alcoholics may present osteopenia without significant liver disease (Peris, CalcifTissInt, 1995; 57:111), and it is possible that alcohol may have a direct toxic effect on osteoblasts and bone remodelling (Spencer, AmJMed, 1986; 80:393; Labib, AlcAlc, 1989; 24:141).[28] Thus, although alcoholics may present nutritional deficiencies and malabsorption of calcium and vitamin D, and abnormal parathyroid function, the low levels of osteocalcin (also known as bone γ-carboxyglutamic acid-containing protein, which is a sensitive marker of bone formation) found in alcoholics without liver disease suggest that alcohol may be directly toxic to osteoblasts (Labib, AlcAlc, 1989; 24:141). The rapid increase of serum osteocalcin levels in abstainers suggests that reduced spinal and femoral bone mass in alcoholics results from a direct toxic effect of ethanol on osteoblast function (Peris, AlcAlc, 1992; 27:619). Moreover, bone mass recovers after 2 years of abstinence.[29] The influence of endocrine factors, such as hypogonadism or hypercorticism, as well as nutritional deficiencies, in osteoporosis of chronic alcoholism has not been completely clarified.[30]

Cancer

The relationship between alcohol consumption and human cancer is based on epidemiological studies which have demonstrated a clear association of heavy alcohol drinking with cancer of mouth, larynx, and oesophagus (Keller, AmJEpid, 1977; 106:194; Schottenfeld, Cancer, 1979; 43:1962; Tuyns, CancerRes, 1979; 39:2840). Heavy drinkers were found to have a tenfold increased risk of developing cancer of the mouth and larynx.

Similar data regarding cancer of the oesophagus have been published in alcoholics, who are also often heavy smokers (Tuyns, IntJCanc, 1983; 32:443). Other sites of cancer linked with alcohol drinking include the pancreas, colon, and liver. In fact, alcohol abuse has long been recognized as an important risk factor for cancer of the liver, although hepatitis virus infections may also have a relevant role. Thus, an incidence of 30 per cent for hepatocellular carcinoma has been reported in patients with alcoholic cirrhosis, and hepatocellular carcinoma may be seen in alcoholics without cirrhosis. The combined effect of heavy smoking for the development of cancer of the mouth and larynx in heavy alcoholics is important, and recent analyses indicate that alcohol is as important as tobacco. In these cancers, other factors such as hot beverages, vitamin A and C deficiencies, and poor dental hygiene, seem to be less relevant than alcohol and tobacco.

The role of alcohol for developing cancer of the oesophagus is still more important since the relative risk for oesophageal cancer rises logarithmically with increasing alcohol consumption, even when corrected for tobacco abuse. Besides the direct effect of high alcohol concentration on the digestive mucosa, nutritional deficiencies may be implicated in the pathogenesis of oesophageal cancer, including iron and zinc as well as vitamin A deficiency. Other sites of cancer in the digestive tract such as the rectum and stomach may be related to the type of alcoholic beverage. Beer consumption has been found to be associated with cancer of rectum (Jensen, IntJCancer, 1979; 23:454), and the relative risk for gastric carcinoma seems to be increased in patients who consume red wine (Hoey, AmJEpid, 1981; 113:668).

Since there is no evidence that alcohol is carcinogenic *per se*, other mechanisms may contribute to carcinogenesis. Thus, alcohol may increase the susceptibility of various tissues to chemical carcinogens by activating these carcinogens, altering their metabolism, inducing nutritional deficiencies, and modifying the immune response. In addition, the presence of contaminant carcinogens in alcoholic beverages should be considered.

Blood pressure

Most studies of cross-sectional association of blood pressure and alcohol consumption have indicated that among persons whose reported average alcohol consumption was three to four drinks per day, systolic blood pressure was 3 to 4 mmHg greater and diastolic blood pressure was 1 to 2 mmHg greater than in non-drinkers. These elevations are more prominent in persons consuming five to six drinks per day, thus providing evidence of a dose–response relationship between blood pressure and alcohol consumption (Saunders, Lancet, 1981; ii:653; Puddley, Hypertension, 1985; 7: 707; MacMahon, AnnIntMed, 1986; 105:124). The mechanisms by which alcohol consumption may lead to blood pressure elevation remains unclear, but withdrawal phenomenon, biological effects on cardiovascular regulation, a direct effect on the central nervous system, and changes in calcium metabolism should be taken into

account (Beilin, AlcAlc, 1984; 19:191). Chronic alcoholics undergoing withdrawal may have transient marked hypertension, and it is most likely that increased blood pressure during the withdrawal phase is related to sympathetic nervous system and renin–angiotensin–aldosterone system activation (Criqui, Alcoholism, 1986; 10:564).

References

1. Chey WJ. Alcohol and gastric mucosa. *Digestion*, 1972; **7**: 239–51.
2. Gottfried EB, Korsten MA, and Lieber CS. Alcohol-induced gastric and duodenal lesions in man. *American Journal of Gastroenterology*, 1978; **70**: 587–92.
3. Burbige EJ, Lewis DR Jr, and Halsted CH. Alcohol and the gastrointestinal tract. *Medical Clinics of North America*, 1984; **68**: 77–89.
4. Geokas MC. Ethanol and the pancreas. *Medical Clinics of North America*, 1984; **68**: 57–75.
5. Charness ME, Simon RP, and Greenberg DA. Ethanol and the nervous system. *New England Journal of Medicine*, 1989; **321**: 442–54.
6. Shaw GK. Alcohol dependence and withdrawal. *British Medical Bulletin*, 1982; 38: 99–102.
7. Butters N. Alcoholic Korsakoff's syndrome: an update. *Seminars in Neurology*, 1984; **4**: 226–44.
8. Torvik A, Lindboe CF, and Rodge S. Brain lesions in alcoholics. *Journal of Neurological Sciences*, 1982; **56**: 233–48.
9. Victor M. Polyneuropathy due to nutritional deficiency and alcoholism. In Dyke PJ, Thomas PK, and Lambert EH, eds. *Peripheral neuropathy*. Philadelphia: WB Saunders, 1975: 1030–66.
10. Preedy VR, Salisbury JR and Peters TJ. Alcohol muscle disease: features and mechanisms. *Journal of Pathology*, 1994; **173**: 309–15.
11. Martin FC, Slavin G, and Levi AJ. Alcoholic muscle disease. *British Medical Bulletin*, 1982; **38**: 53–6.
12. Haller RG, and Knochel JP. Skeletal muscle disease in alcoholism. *Medical Clinics of North America*, 1984; **68**: 91–103.
13. Martin F and Peters TJ. Alcoholic muscle disease. *Alcohol and Alcoholism*, 1985; **20**: 125–36.
14. Alderman EL and Coltard DJ. Alcohol and the heart. *British Medical Bulletin*, 1982; **38**: 77–80.
15. Segel LD, Klausner SC, Gnadt JTH and Amsterdam EA. Alcohol and the heart. *Medical Clinics of North America*, 1984; **68**: 147–61.
16. Regan T. Alcoholic cardiomyopathy. *Progress in Cardiovascular Disease*, 1984; **27**: 141–52.
17. Eichner ER and Hillman RS. The evolution of anemia in alcoholic patients. *American Journal of Medicine*, 1971; **50**: 218–32.
18. Chanarin I. Haemopoiesis and alcohol. *British Medical Bulletin*, 1982; **38**: 81–6.
19. Larkin EC and Watson-Williams EJ. Alcohol and the blood. *Medical Clinics of North America*, 1984; **68**: 105–20.
20. Savage D and Lindenbaum J. Anemia in alcoholics. *Medicine*, 1986; **65**: 322–38.
21. Lindenbaum J. Hematologic complications of alcohol abuse. *Seminars in Liver Disease*, 1987; **7**: 169–81.
22. Liu YK. Effects of alcohol on granulocytes and lymphocytes. *Seminars in Hematology*, 1980; **17**: 130–6.
23. Rubin R and Rand ML. Alcohol and platelet function. *Alcoholism: Clinical and Experimental Research*, 1994; **18**: 105–10.
24. Lester R and Van Thiel DH. Gonadal function in chronic alcoholic men. *Advances in Experimental Biology and Medicine*, 1977; **85A**: 399–414.
25. Wright J. Endocrine effects of alcohol. *Clinical Endocrinology and Metabolism*, 1978; **7**: 351–67.
26. Morgan MY. Sex and alcohol. *British Medical Bulletin*, 1982; **38**: 43–52.
27. Noth RH and Walter RM. The effects of alcohol on the endocrine system. *Medical Clinics of North America*, 1984; **68**: 133–46.
28. Bikle DD, Genant HK, Cann C, Recker RR, Halloran BP and Strewler GJ. Bone disease in alcohol abuse. *Annals of Internal Medicine*, 1985; **103**: 42–8.

29. Peris P, *et al*. Bone mass improves in alcoholics after 2 years of abstinence. *Journal of Bone and Mineral Research*, 1994; **9**: 1607–12.

30. Laitinen K and Valimaki M. Alcohol and bone. *Calcified Tissue International*, 1991; **49**: 570–3.

31. Lieber CS, Garro A, Leo MA, Mak KM, and Worner T. Alcohol and cancer. *Hepatology*, 1986; **5**: 1005–19.

32. Anderson LM, Chhabra SK, Nerurkar PV, Souliotis VL, and Kyrtopoulos SA. Alcohol-related cancer risk: a toxicokinetic hypothesis. *Alcohol*, 1995; **12**: 97–104.

16

Non-alcoholic fatty liver: causes and complications

16 Non-alcoholic fatty liver: causes and complications

Randall G. Lee and Emmet B. Keeffe

Introduction

Fatty change (or steatosis) denotes the excess accumulation of lipids within hepatocytes. Although it can be defined in a biochemical sense as total lipids exceeding 5 per cent of liver weight, in practice steatosis is recognized primarily by the presence of fat droplets in histological sections. It therefore represents a morphological rather than a clinical diagnosis, and indeed, is one of the more commonly encountered findings in liver biopsy specimens.

The accumulated lipid in most instances is predominantly triglyceride, although other lipids may be deposited in certain inherited metabolic disorders or hepatotoxic drug reactions. For example, increased accumulation of cholesterol esters characterizes Wolman's disease and cholesterol ester storage disease; various sphingolipids are deposited in Gaucher's disease, Niemann–Pick disease, Tay–Sach's disease, and Farber's disease; and phospholipid collections can result from therapy with therapeutic agents such as amiodarone or perhexiline maleate. In contrast to the typical triglyceride-related steatosis, these abnormal lipids tend to collect in Kupffer cells in addition to hepatocytes.

Fatty change generally indicates some disruption of the normal physiology of triglyceride synthesis and secretion but the precise pathogenetic mechanisms are incompletely defined. Depending on the exact cause, multiple factors are likely responsible. Potential pathophysiological mechanisms include enhanced delivery of fatty acids to the liver from adipose tissue or diet, increased endogenous fatty acid synthesis, decreased mitochondrial fatty acid β-oxidation, and deficient incorporation or export of triglycerides in the form of very low density lipoproteins.

Typically, two basic histological patterns of fatty liver are recognized. In the commonplace macrovesicular variety, a single large lipid vacuole distends the liver cell and displaces the nucleus to the side; whereas in the less common microvesicular steatosis, lipid accumulates in numerous small lipid vacuoles that surround the centrally positioned nucleus. These two patterns appear to represent sequential phases in the accumulation of hepatic lipid. Initially fat collects in the form of small droplets, which are seen microscopically as microvesicular fatty change, and these subsequently coalesce into the larger globules of macrovesicular fat. The two patterns therefore reflect the tempo and duration of lipid accumulation and, depending on the cause and time course of the fatty change, both types can coexist in the same liver.

The histological patterns of steatosis, at least in their prototypic forms, also carry broadly different clinical implications. Macrovesicular steatosis occurs in a wide range of disorders and is generally considered an innocuous process with little risk of progression to advanced liver disease. Microvesicular steatosis, on the other hand, develops in a more limited set of conditions and, in its pure form, can be associated with generalized mitochondrial dysfunction and secondary metabolic disruption; accordingly it connotes a more ominous clinical picture that may entail hepatic failure, encephalopathy, coma, and death.

A distinction also needs to be drawn between the usual non-inflammatory steatosis and its necroinflammatory complication referred to as steatohepatitis. Steatohepatitis is best recognized with alcoholic liver disease (alcoholic hepatitis), but it can also develop in non-alcoholic settings (non-alcoholic steatohepatitis). In either case, steatohepatitis can lead to significant fibrosis or cirrhosis and serious hepatic dysfunction.

Macrovesicular steatosis
Causes

Macrovesicular steatosis is a non-specific finding that is the result of many nutritional, metabolic, inherited, toxic or drug-induced, and miscellaneous disorders (Table 1). Chronic alcohol consumption is the best characterized association with steatosis. In individuals who do not abuse alcohol, the most common causes of steatosis include obesity, diabetes mellitus, and nutritional abnormalities.

Fatty liver is common in obese patients, with a reported frequency ranging from 60 to 90 per cent, and women are more often affected than men.[1-4] In general, the degree of steatosis correlates with the severity of obesity. The mechanism by which obesity produces fatty liver or more progressive hepatic lesions remains unexplained.

Only a few patients with obesity and fatty liver have symptoms or signs of significant hepatic dysfunction. Mild elevations of serum aspartate aminotransferase (**AST**), alanine aminotransferase (**ALT**), alkaline phosphatase (**ALP**), or γ-glutamyltranspeptidase (**GGT**) levels are the most frequent laboratory abnormalities found in patients with steatosis, and liver biopsy typically shows non-inflammatory, predominantly macrovesicular fat accumulation. However, approximately 20 to 40 per cent of markedly obese

Table 1 Causes of macrovesicular steatosis

Alcohol consumption
Obesity
Diabetes mellitus
Nutritional alterations
   starvation
   protein–calorie malnutrition
   jejunoileal bypass
   total parenteral nutrition
Drugs and toxins
   see Table 2
Inherited metabolic disorders
   see Table 3
Miscellaneous
   hepatitis C
   acquired immune deficiency syndrome (AIDS)
   hepatic adenoma
   hepatocellular carcinoma
   hepatic ischaemia

Table 2 Drugs and toxins associated with macrovesicular steatosis[a]

Amiodarone
Asparaginase
Bleomycin
Carbon tetrachloride
Cisplatin
Clometacin
Corticosteroids
Dantrolene
Ethionine
Etretinate
Flurazepam
Halothane
Ibuprofen
Indomethacin
Isoniazid
Methimazole
Methotrexate
Methyldopa
Nitrofurantoin
Oestrogens (high dose)
Paracetamol (acetaminophen)
Phosphorus
Rifampicin
Sulindac
Tamoxifen

[a] Partial listing.

subjects have additional histological abnormalities on liver biopsy compatible with non-alcoholic steatohepatitis. There are no reliable clinical or biochemical criteria that distinguish patients with simple fatty liver versus non-alcoholic steatohepatitis; liver biopsy is required if this distinction is important for management. Limited follow-up studies of patients with simple non-inflammatory steatosis associated with obesity and unrelated to alcohol reveal no progression to cirrhosis.[5] Weight reduction may be associated with both reversal of the fatty liver by histological analysis and return of aminotransferases to normal.[6]

The prevalence of steatosis in diabetes mellitus varies, but it has been reported in approximately 50 per cent of individuals with type II (non-insulin-dependent) diabetes.[1,7] Many of these individuals will also be obese, and it is difficult to dissect the relative contributions of obesity versus diabetes to the development of steatosis. Moreover, the majority of obese patients with fatty liver also have abnormal glucose metabolism, and frank diabetes mellitus occurs in approximately 25 per cent of subjects with fatty liver. It is likely that obesity rather than diabetes mellitus is the major factor associated with fatty liver, since steatosis is found almost exclusively in adult type II diabetics and not in juvenile type I diabetics. Histological studies have demonstrated that patients with diabetes mellitus exhibit a spectrum of hepatic abnormalities, including macrovesicular steatosis (approximately 50 per cent), glycogen infiltration of the nucleus (approximately 50 per cent), non-alcoholic steatohepatitis (frequency in diabetics uncertain), and micronodular cirrhosis (approximately 15 per cent). The relatively high prevalence of cirrhosis is based on autopsy studies and may be the end result of steatohepatitis.

Other prominent causes of steatosis are nutritional abnormalities with relative degrees of malnutrition or malabsorption, as seen with protein–calorie malnutrition, particularly kwashiorkor, and also jejunoileal bypass and possibly other operations for obesity.[1] Starvation with marasmus is less frequently associated with steatosis. In kwashiorkor the hepatocellular fat accumulates first in the periportal hepatocytes and has a predominantly macrovesicular pattern. The mechanism of lipid accumulation in kwashiorkor most likely results from an imbalance in hepatic carbohydrate, protein, and lipid metabolism.[8] Kwashiorkor in developing regions of the world is associated with mild AST or ALT elevations and hepatomegaly. Kwashiorkor does not appear to progress to cirrhosis. There is also a mild to moderate increase in hepatocellular fat during starvation, although prolonged fasting is ultimately associated with a reduction in hepatic fat.

Total parenteral nutrition (**TPN**) is often associated with steatosis, which is one of the most frequent morphological changes found on liver biopsies.[8,9] Fatty liver that develops in patients on TPN may resolve or, in a small number of patients, progress to cholestasis and steatohepatitis with progressive liver disease. The infusion of large amounts of glucose is probably an important factor in the development of liver disease in these subjects.

Jejunoileal bypass is associated with a large number of postoperative complications, including several hepatic abnormalities, and thus has been abandoned as a treatment of obesity. Hepatocellular fat, which is usually present before surgery, accumulates in the initial months after bypass surgery and then returns to the baseline amount of steatosis. Some patients progress to non-alcoholic steatohepatitis, with hepatic failure developing in 2 to 5 per cent of cases.[1] The frequency of steatosis with the various gastric bypass operations remains unknown but appears to be less than with jejunoileal bypass surgery.

Many drugs and toxins are reported to cause macrovesicular steatosis (Table 2). In general, with discontinuation of the specific drug, steatosis will improve. The deposition of fat may occur as an isolated hepatic abnormality or be associated with other histological drug-induced abnormalities. Corticosteroids are the most widely used drugs that are associated with steatosis, which is invariably mild and not associated with either symptoms or biochemical abnormalities. Macrovesicular steatosis can also be a feature of numerous inherited metabolic disorders (Table 3). The histological

Table 3 Inherited metabolic disorders associated with macrovesicular steatosis[a]

Abetalipoproteinaemia
Cystic fibrosis
Familial hepatosteatosis
Familial hyperlipoproteinaemias
Galactosaemia
Glycogen storage disease type I
Homocystinuria
Hereditary fructose intolerance
Porphyria cutanea tarda
Refsum's disease
Schwachman's syndrome
Systemic carnitine deficiency
Tyrosinaemia
Wilson's disease

[a] Partial listing.

features of these entities are noted in Section 3 and extensively reviewed elsewhere.[10,11] Patients with heterozygous forms of these conditions, such as heterozygous hypobetalipoproteinaemia, may also present with elevated liver enzymes and fatty liver (Wishingrad, AmJGastr, 1994; 89:1106). In the latter condition, total cholesterol levels range from 50 to 150 mg/dl (3.9–6.5 mmol/l), and low density lipoprotein (**LDL**) levels are usually 25 to 45 mg/dl (0.65–1.2 mmol/l), one-third to one-quarter of normal.

Macrovesicular steatosis can also be seen as a minor, secondary feature in several miscellaneous disorders (Table 1) including chronic hepatitis C (Dhillon, Histopath,1995; 26:297). Fatty liver is also common in patients with acquired immune deficiency syndrome (**AIDS**), with one study showing a hyperechoic liver in 46 per cent of patients (Beale, ClinRadiol, 1995; 50:761; Freiman, AIDS, 1993; 7:379). Liver biopsy is required to distinguish the many other, predominantly infectious, disorders that occur in these patients. Steatosis can also been seen in hepatocellular neoplasms, both adenomas and carcinomas.

Clinical aspects

Fat is generally not directly toxic to hepatocytes, and fat accumulation in the liver is initially associated with normal hepatic function and liver biochemistry and no symptoms. The diagnosis of fatty liver usually follows a clinical suspicion in a patient with a known cause such as alcohol abuse, obesity, or diabetes mellitus who exhibits hepatomegaly and/or minor abnormalities of hepatic biochemical tests without an obvious alternative aetiology.[12] Most patients with uncomplicated macrovesicular steatosis are asymptomatic; however, patients with more severe steatosis may complain of right upper quadrant discomfort or fullness. In rare circumstances, steatosis has been associated with acute liver failure. On physical examination, the liver is often enlarged and smooth with a blunt edge. Standard liver tests such as AST, ALT, ALP, and GGT are either normal or show mild elevation. Elevated serum aminotransferase levels are a common but non-specific finding; the levels seldom exceed two or three times the upper limits of normal.[12] The AST–ALT ratio is typically less than or equal to 1. Elevations of GGT have been found to correlate with the amount of hepatic fat (Ikai, JHumHypert, 1994; 8:95). Serum bilirubin and serum albumin are usually normal. Overall, however, liver test abnormalities correlate poorly with the severity of the steatosis and the presence or absence of non-alcoholic steatohepatitis (Galambos, Gastro, 1978; 74:1191).

Several studies of patients with chronic and asymptomatic mild-to-moderate elevation of AST or ALT have demonstrated that fatty liver is the most common diagnosis. A Scandinavian investigation of 149 asymptomatic patients who had elevation of liver enzymes for more than 6 months and underwent liver biopsy demonstrated: (1) fatty liver in 63 per cent; (2) chronic hepatitis in 20 per cent; and (3) miscellaneous liver disease in 17 per cent (Hultcrantz, ScaJGastr, 1986; 21:109). Fatty liver was associated with high body weight, alcohol intake, hyperlipidaemia, and diabetes mellitus. It is important to note that this study was performed prior to the availability of serological testing for hepatitis C virus. In a study of the cause of an elevated serum ALT in 100 blood donors, which represents a different population from patients referred to a medical centre, presumptive fatty liver was the most common diagnosis based on exclusion of viral, autoimmune, and genetic diseases, and on the association with daily alcohol use and/or obesity (Friedman, AnnIntMed, 1987; 107:137). Liver biopsies were not performed as part of the evaluation of these patients. Anti-hepatitis C virus testing was later performed by RIBA-2 and was detected in 17 of the 100 blood donors (Katkov, AnnIntMed, 1991; 115:882). Chronic hepatitis C was more often the explanation of elevated ALT levels in individuals who were not obese and did not use alcohol, while anti-hepatitis C virus was likely to be negative in those subjects who were obese or drank alcohol regularly; these latter patients were presumed to have fatty liver. In another study, 90 patients underwent evaluation of abnormal liver tests that were more than 1.5 times normal for more than 3 months.[13] This study included a heterogeneous group of patients, many of whom were symptomatic and had advanced liver disease. Final diagnoses included steatosis or non-alcoholic steatohepatitis in 19 per cent, alcoholic liver disease in 23 per cent, probable chronic viral hepatitis in 26 per cent, and miscellaneous liver diseases in 24 per cent. Recent studies of the significance of mild aminotransferase elevations in asymptomatic patients have been performed with the addition of anti-hepatitis C virus testing to the previously available diagnostic tests and liver biopsy (Knoll, Gastro, 1992; 102:A17; Knoll, AmJGastr, 1992; 87:235). In a thorough evaluation of 62 patients with increased liver enzymes, 60 patients had an abnormal biopsy; 34 per cent of patients demonstrated steatosis or non-alcoholic steatohepatitis, and 45 per cent showed chronic hepatitis or cirrhosis (Knoll, Gastro, 1992; 102:A17). Twenty-two subjects were anti-hepatitis C virus positive, and all but two subjects with a positive hepatitis C antibody had chronic hepatitis or cirrhosis. These same authors later analysed a smaller group of 12 asymptomatic patients who had chronic elevation of liver enzymes with completely negative testing for an aetiology by standard virological and immunological tests (Knoll, AmJGastr, 1992; 87:235). In these subjects, 10 of 12 liver biopsies were abnormal; four patients had steatosis, two patients had non-alcoholic steatohepatitis, three patients had chronic active hepatitis (CAH), and one patient had primary sclerosing cholangitis. In this small group, mean serum ALT levels were higher in patients with chronic hepatitis than in those with steatosis.

In a large prospective study of French blood donors from 1987 to 1989, non-A, non-B hepatitis was assessed with third-generation tests for anti-hepatitis C virus and hepatitis C virus RNA by polymerase chain reaction (**PCR**) (Marcellin, JHepatol, 1993; 19: 167). In this study, 184 subjects (1.7 per cent) had elevated ALT (twice normal) over 6 months and 88 agreed to follow-up. Of these, 45 subjects had persistently elevated ALT over 6 months and underwent liver biopsy. Findings included:

(1) fatty liver in 29/45 (65 per cent), with 23 cases explained by alcohol, obesity or hyperlipidaemia; ALT returned to normal in 22 patients with dietary management; and

(2) chronic hepatitis in 16/45 (35 per cent); 12 of 16 patients had documented chronic hepatitis C, but four patients remained unexplained, suggesting the possibility of another virus (non-A, non-B, non-C virus).

In summary, the studies cited above document that steatosis, and possibly non-alcoholic steatohepatitis, are the most frequent causes of mild elevations of serum AST or ALT (as well as ALP and GGT). Moreover, fatty liver is often associated with obvious underlying conditions such as obesity, alcohol abuse, hyperlipidaemia, or diabetes mellitus.

Fatty liver can often be suggested by several different radiographic imaging studies. Ultrasonography demonstrates increased echogenicity, with a sensitivity that improves as the extent of steatosis increases.[14–16] A moderate amount of fat must be present in the liver for detection by ultrasonography; minimal steatosis cannot be identified in this way. Fat can usually be distinguished from fibrosis by ultrasonography. Computed tomography (**CT**) is characterized by low attenuation of the liver when compared with the spleen; these values are inversely correlated with the degree of steatosis as assessed histologically.[16,17] Magnetic resonance imaging (**MRI**) also can detect steatosis and correlates well with CT findings (Kreft, JMRI, 1992; 2:463; Longo, InvestRadiol, 1993; 28:297). Although fatty liver can be suggested by all of these imaging tests, a specific diagnosis is not possible and non-alcoholic steatohepatitis or other aetiologies of chronic liver disease cannot be defined. However, these imaging studies can detect evidence of subclinical cirrhosis with portal hypertension (e.g. collateral vessels, splenomegaly, ascites) before it becomes clinically apparent.

The definitive diagnosis of fatty liver requires liver biopsy, which is the most sensitive and specific test for documenting steatosis and distinguishing simple fatty liver from non-alcoholic steatohepatitis with or without fibrosis or cirrhosis. The role of liver biopsy in patients strongly suspected as having steatosis remains uncertain. In conditions that are transient or can be easily treated, such as by discontinuation of total parenteral nutrition or a drug that is associated with fatty liver, biopsy is not warranted. Asymptomatic patients with obesity, type II diabetes mellitus or hyperlipidaemia who have mild elevation of aminotransferase levels and no or minimal hepatomegaly might best be followed during treatment of their underlying condition. Likewise, incidental detection of steatosis by hepatic imaging studies in patients with normal liver enzymes does not require liver biopsy. On the other hand, steatosis may coexist with inflammation, fibrosis, or cirrhosis, and liver biopsy is the only way to make the distinction between simple fatty liver and non-alcoholic steatohepatitis. A liver biopsy may also be warranted in patients with symptoms or more striking hepatomegaly, particularly if biopsy will impact medical management.

Focal fatty change

Although hepatic steatosis is generally a diffuse process, it may also display an irregular or focal distribution called focal fatty change[18,19]. These lesions are often discovered incidentally on imaging or postmortem examination. Most affected individuals have an underlying condition associated with macrovesicular steatosis, such as obesity, diabetes, or malnutrition. In patients with focal fatty change, diffuse macrovesicular steatosis may or may not be present elsewhere throughout the liver. The reason for the localized accumulation of the fat in these cases is not known, but regional tissue hypoxia is often held responsible[16,18]. Hepatic imaging with ultrasonography shows an area of increased echogenicity and CT shows an area of low attenuation, characteristically with a fan-shaped or geographic profile. The lesions are usually subcapsular, often adjacent to the falciform ligament, and may be single or multiple; typically they are several centimeters in diameter, but may range up to 10 cm. Lesions with a more spherical profile, however, can be mistaken for more ominous space-occupying masses; guided liver biopsy may be required to confirm the diagnosis (Clain, Gastro, 1984; 87:948; Yoshikawa, AJR, 1987; 149:491). The primary importance of this entity is in the differential diagnosis of space-occupying lesions of the liver.

Natural history and treatment

Macrovesicular steatosis, whatever its cause, is generally a benign and self-limited process that resolves once the inciting cause is removed.[5] In one study, the impact of weight loss in treating overweight adults with abnormal serum aminotransferase levels and presumed steatosis (no primary liver disease by clinical evaluation or specific virological and immunological testing) demonstrated that weight reduction of 10 per cent or more corrected abnormal serum ALT levels and decreased hepatosplenomegaly.[6] These authors recommend that, after other causes of liver disease are eliminated by clinical and biochemical evaluation, weight reduction should be tried in obese patients with presumed fatty liver before proceeding with more expensive and invasive tests such as liver biopsy. Further evaluation might be limited to those patients who have lost 10 per cent or more of body weight without return of liver tests to normal or those who are unable to lose weight.

Controversy exists as to whether long-term steatosis can result in cirrhosis. Although cirrhosis cannot be excluded in every case, this complication is generally seen only when steatosis has been complicated by non-alcoholic steatohepatitis with fibrosis.

Non-alcoholic steatohepatitis

Non-alcoholic steatohepatitis is the term currently applied to the necroinflammatory complication of macrovesicular steatosis. Although histologically this condition resembles alcoholic hepatitis, it occurs in the absence of alcohol abuse. Several synonyms have been used, including fatty liver hepatitis, alcohol-like liver disease, pseudoalcoholic liver disease, and diabetic hepatitis. Several series detail the clinicopathological features of this disorder.[20-24]

Exact incidence figures are not available, but non-alcoholic steatohepatitis is seen in approximately 6 per cent of non-alcoholic patients at autopsy and accounts for up to 20 per cent of liver biopsy

Table 4 Conditions associated with non-alcoholic steatohepatitis

Obesity
Diabetes mellitus
Gastrointestinal surgery
   jejunoileal bypass
   small bowel resection
   gastroplasty
   biliopancreatic diversion
Drugs
   amiodarone
   4,4'-diethylaminoethoxyhexoestrol (Coralgil)
   diethylstilboestrol
   glucocorticoids (long-term)
   nifedipine
   perhexiline maleate
   tamoxifen
Total parenteral nutrition
Miscellaneous disorders
   Weber–Christian disease
   abetalipoproteinaemia
   limb lipodystrophy
Fasting/bulimia
Idiopathic

specimens in patients with chronically elevated serum amino-transferases.[13,25]

Causes

Non-alcoholic steatohepatitis has been complicated by most causes of macrovesicular steatosis (Table 4), but two disorders—obesity and diabetes mellitus—account for the preponderance of cases in most series. Obesity is noted in more than 70 per cent of reported patients, with body weights ranging from 110 per cent to over 200 per cent of ideal. Conversely, approximately 1 to 4 per cent of obese patients are discovered to have non-alcoholic steatohepatitis at liver biopsy, and the risk tends to correlate roughly with the degree of obesity. Diabetes is identified in some 25 to 75 per cent of reported patients with non-alcoholic steatohepatitis, and other individuals may manifest, or later develop, glucose intolerance. The combination of diabetes and obesity leads to a greater risk of non-alcoholic steatohepatitis (Wanless, Hepatol, 1990; 12:1106; Silverman, PatholAnn, 1989; 24(pt 1):275).

Other associations centre around gastrointestinal surgical procedures to control morbid obesity, of which the best known example is jejunoileal bypass surgery. This procedure can exacerbate pre-existing non-alcoholic steatohepatitis as well as initiate the process in unaffected livers, and can result in acute liver failure and death (Peters, AmJClinPath, 1975; 63:318; Vyberg, Liver, 1987; 7:271).

Of the handful of drugs associated with non-alcoholic steatohepatitis, most have represented unusual, isolated instances described in case reports. The major exception is amiodarone, an iodinated benzofuran derivative used for refractory ventricular arrhythmias. Asymptomatic aminotransferase elevations are seen in approximately a quarter of treated patients, with symptomatic non-alcoholic steatohepatitis developing in approximately 1 to 3 per cent (Guigui, Hepatol, 1988; 8:1063; Lewis, HumPath, 1989; 21:59; Lewis, Hepatol, 1989; 9:679).

Rarely, other disorders have been related to non-alcoholic steatohepatitis, but in some cases none of the above associations apply[24]

Clinical aspects

The typical patient with non-alcoholic steatohepatitis is a middle-aged woman. The male–female ratio among reported cases is 1 : 3, and the peak age is about 50 years, although cases are reported at all ages, including childhood (Moran, AmJGastr, 1983; 78:374). The female predominance probably reflects the greater prevalence of women among obese individuals being studied (Wanless, Hepatol, 1990; 12:1106).

Clinically the disease is often mild and inapparent. Patients are most often asymptomatic or have only non-specific systemic complaints, even with advanced disease, and the disorder is detected incidentally, when abnormal liver tests or hepatomegaly are noted during evaluation of other medical problems. Hepatomegaly is commonly present, but jaundice, ascites, oesophageal varices, or encephalopathy are noted in only a minority of patients.

Usual laboratory features include modest elevations of serum aminotransferases (typically up to four times the upper limit of normal) and normal or mildly increased alkaline phosphatase levels. Hyperlipidaemia is also occasionally noted, but hyper-bilirubinaemia, prolonged prothrombin times, and hypo-albuminaemia are infrequently seen.

By definition, affected patients should have no history of alcohol abuse. There are no absolute laboratory features that allow this determination, although elevated serum levels of γ-gluta-myltransferase, desialyated transferrin, or mitochondrial isozyme of asparate aminotransferase or an increased mean corpuscular volume have been employed to suggest the possibility of undisclosed alcohol usage (Fletcher, Hepatol, 1991; 13:455).

Pathological features

The histological hallmark of non-alcoholic steatohepatitis is its resemblance to alcoholic hepatitis, as discussed in greater detail in Section 4 and Chapter 15.2. The extent to which it parallels alcoholic hepatitis varies, although in general it tends to favour the milder, low-grade end of the spectrum.

Drug-related non-alcoholic steatohepatitis is often distinguished by minimal steatosis in the face of prominent Mallory bodies and neutrophilic infiltration. In addition, amiodarone, Coralgil, and perhexiline malate induce in the majority of recipients a distinctive type of fatty liver characterized by phospholipid accumulation (Guigui, Hepatol, 1988; 8:1063; Lewis, Hepatol, 1989; 9:679). This phospholipidosis is manifest by enlarged, granular hepatocytes and Kupffer cells, corresponding to whorled, lamellated inclusions representing phospholipid deposits within lysosomes (Shepard, JClinPath, 1987; 40:418).

Natural history and treatment

The prognosis is generally good, as the disease tends to progress slowly and cirrhosis or decompensated liver function evolves in only a fraction of patients.[22,23] In one study, the 5- and 10-year survival rates were 67 per cent and 59 per cent, lower than figures for a matched general population and contrasting sharply with the

Table 5 Causes of microvesicular steatosis

Acute fatty liver of pregnancy
Reye's syndrome
Alcoholic foamy degeneration
Drugs and toxins
  amiodarone
  didanosine
  hypoglycin A ('Jamaican vomiting sickness')
  ketoprofen
  Margosa oil
  pirprofen
  salicylates
  tetracycline
  tolmetin
  valproic acid
Congenital metabolic conditions
  urea cycle enzyme deficiencies
  defects in fatty acid oxidation
  lysosomal acid lipase deficiency
Miscellaneous
  hepatic ischaemia (especially cold ischaemia)
  fulminant hepatitis D
  fatal exertional heatstroke
  toxic shock syndrome
  sudden death

38 per cent and 15 per cent rates for alcoholic hepatitis (Propst, Gastro, 1995; 108:1607).

Because of this natural history, it has been difficult to evaluate the efficacy of treatment options. Usual recommendations include gradual and sustained weight reduction and good control of diabetes.[6] However, rapid weight loss with starvation has provoked or aggravated non-alcoholic steatohepatitis, so that a controlled, judicious means of weight loss is important (Capron, DigDisSci, 1982; 27:265).

Microvesicular steatosis

The major causes of microvesicular steatosis are summarized in Table 5. In some of these conditions, the accumulation of small-droplet fat is an expression of an underlying mitochondrial dysfunction and therefore carries serious clinical implications and a poor prognosis (Sherlock, Gut, 1983; 24:265). However, microvesicular steatosis can also be seen in patients without this prototypic clinical picture, so the histological picture must be correlated with appropriate clinical and laboratory data (Bonnell, AmJDisChild, 1986; 140:30; Fraser, ModPathol, 1995; 8:65).

Most of the disorders associated with microvesicular steatosis are discussed elsewhere in the book, but a few comments on Reye's syndrome are in order.

Reye's syndrome

Reye's syndrome is an acute and potentially life-threatening disorder of childhood characterized by microvesicular steatosis and metabolic encephalopathy. It affects infants and children of all ages, with a range from 6 months to 15 years, although rare cases have also been reported in adults.[26] The annual incidence in several population-based studies varies from 0.16 to 0.88 per 100 000 children, with striking regional variations; since the mid-1980s, the disease has become less common.[27]

The clinical findings typically follow a biphasic course. A prodromal febrile illness, usually influenza or varicella, is followed after 3 to 6 days by the abrupt onset of vomiting and varying degrees of neurological impairment. Initially the patients are alert but irritable and drowsy; these alterations may progress through increasing lethargy, obtundation, agitation, delirium, and seizures to deepening coma and death from cerebral oedema. Up to three-quarters of the patients display only milder neurological abnormalities and do not develop further deterioration. The degree of encephalopathy represents a major prognostic indicator, and a variety of clinical staging systems based on neurological findings have been proposed.

Other than hepatomegaly, there are few clinical signs or symptoms of hepatic disease, and liver dysfunction is manifest principally by laboratory test abnormalities. Serum aminotransferases are increased from three to 30 times normal; serum ammonia levels are frequently elevated, especially among comatose patients; and hypoglycaemia is noted in severe cases. The prothrombin time can be mildly prolonged, but the serum bilirubin is generally normal. Many other metabolic abnormalities can also be seen, including lactic acidosis, hypophosphataemia, azotaemia, and elevated levels of amino acids or short-chain fatty acids. Liver biopsy specimens demonstrate diffuse microvesicular steatosis in the absence of other signficant abnormalities, although mild portal inflammation or swelling or necrosis of periportal hepatocytes is noted in some instances (Bove, Gastro, 1975; 69:685).

Treatment consists of general supportive care directed at correcting the metabolic alterations and controlling cerebral oedema. The overall mortality is approximately 20 to 30 per cent, but the prognosis varies with the degree of encephalopathy, thus emphasizing the need for early recognition. Children who present with the milder stages of the disorder generally recover completely after 2 or 3 days, and long-term neurological sequelae are uncommon (Lichtenstein, NEJM, 1983; 309:133).

One of the most intriguing aspects of Reye's syndrome is its association with salicylate exposure. This association has been confirmed by several well-designed epidemiological investigations, each of which concluded that the use of aspirin during the antecedent viral illness was a signficant risk factor for developing Reye's syndrome (Hurwitz, EpidRev, 1989; 11:249). The widespread publicity generated by these studies led to lessened use of salicylates in treating febrile children; concomitantly the incidence of Reye's syndrome declined sharply.

Reye's syndrome can be confused with several inherited metabolic diseases that share many of its clinical and laboratory features. Among these differential considerations are disorders of fatty acid oxidation (for example, medium-chain acyl CoA dehydrogenase deficiency), organic acidaemias, and urea cycle disorders (for example, ornithine transcarbamylase deficiency) (Treem, SemLivDis, 1994; 14:236). These disorders should be suspected if features unusual for classic Reye's syndrome are present: lack of biphasic illness, age less than 2 years, previously history of Reye's syndrome-like symptoms, or a positive family history. Determination of urine organic acid and plasma and urine amino acid levels can aid in the distinction from Reye's syndrome, with the definite diagnosis established by appropriate gas chromatographic and mass spectrometric techniques (Green, ArchDisChild, 1992; 67:1313; Greene, JPediat, 1988; 113:156).

The aetiology and pathogenesis of Reye's syndrome are not completely understood, but the chief focus of the disorder is the mitochondrion.[27] Acute and reversible mitochondrial dysfunction appears to account for most of the clinical and biochemical abnormalities, although the processes triggering the injury remain unclear. Ultrastructurally, the mitochondria show characteristic alterations in size, shape, and internal architecture, and, correspondingly, the activities of mitochondrial enzymes located within the matrix and inner membranes are reduced. These changes have been proposed to result from depletion of mitochondrial ATP levels and subsequent interference with intramitochondrial enzyme processing[26]. The ensuing compromise of mitochondrial function would render hepatocytes and neurones incapable of maintaining their metabolic homeostasis, with overt Reye's syndrome the ultimate consequence.

References

1. Schaffner F and Thaler H. Nonalcoholic fatty liver disease. *Progress in Liver Diseases*, 1986; **8**: 283–98.
2. Clain D, and Lefkowitch J. Fatty liver disease in morbid obesity. *Gastroenterological Clinics of North America*, 1987; **16**: 239–52.
3. Klain J, *et al.* Liver histology abnormalities in the morbidly obese. *Hepatology*, 1989; **10**: 873–6.
4. Faloon W. Hepatobiliary effects of obesity and weight-reducing surgery. *Seminars in Liver Disease*, 1988; **8**: 229–36.
5. Teli M, James O, Burt A, Bennett M, and Day C. The natural history of nonalcoholic fatty liver: A follow-up study. *Hepatology*, 1995; **22**: 1714–19.
6. Palmer M and Schnaffner F. Effect of weight reduction on hepatic abnormalities in overweight patients. *Gastroenterology*, 1990; **99**: 1408–13.
7. Stone B and Van Thiel D. Diabetes mellitus and the liver. *Seminars in Liver Disease*, 1985; **5**: 8–28.
8. Quigley EMM, Marsh MN, Shaffer JL, and Markin RS. Hepatobiliary complications of total parenteral nutrition. *Gastroenterology*, 1993; **104**: 286–301.
9. Klein S, and Nealon W. Hepatobiliary abnormalities associated with total parenteral nutrition. *Seminars in Liver Disease*, 1988; **8**: 237–46.
10. Ishak K, and Sharp H. Metabolic errors and liver disease. In MacSween R, Anthony P, Scheuer P, Burt A, and Portmann B, eds. *Pathology of the liver*, 3rd edn. Edinburgh: Churchill Livingstone, 1994: 123–218.
11. Lee RG. Storage and metabolic disorders. In *Diagnostic liver pathology*. St. Louis: Mosby, 1994: 237–80.
12. Keeffe E. Abnormal liver function tests: a problem solver's delight. In Barkin J and Rogers A, eds. *Difficult decisions in digestive diseases*, 2nd edn. St. Louis: Mosby, 1994: 165–70.
13. Van Ness MM and Diehl AM. Is liver biopsy useful in the evaluation of patients with chronically elevated liver enzymes? *Annals of Internal Medicine*, 1989; **111**: 473–8.
14. Davies R, Saverymuttu S, Fallowfield M, and Joseph A. Paradoxical lack of ultrasound attenuation with gross fatty change in the liver. *Clinical Radiology*, 1991; **43**: 393–6.
15. Lin T, Ophir J, and Potter G. Correlation of ultrasonic attenuation with pathologic fat and fibrosis in liver disease. *Ultrasound in Medicine and Biology*, 1988; **14**: 729.
16. el-Hassan A, Ibrahim E, al-Mulhim F, Nabhan A, and Chammas M. Fatty infiltration of the liver: Analysis of prevalence, radiological and clinical features and influence on patient management. *British Journal of Radiology*, 1992; **65**: 774–8.
17. Jain K and McGahan J. Spectrum of CT and sonographic appearances of fatty infiltration of the liver. *Clinical Imaging*, 1993; **17**: 162–8.
18. Brawer M, Austin G, and Lewin K. Focal fatty change of the liver, a hitherto poorly recognized entity. *Gastroenterology*, 1980; **87**: 247–52.
19. Kester N and Elmore S. Focal hypoechoic regions in the liver at the porta hepatis: Prevalence in ambulatory patients. *Journal of Ultrasound Medicine*, 1995; **14**: 649–52.
20. Ludwig J, Viggiano TR, McGill DB, and Ott BJ, eds. *Nonalcoholic steatohepatitis. Mayo Clinic experience with a hitherto unnamed disease*, 1980.
21. Diehl AM, Goodman Z, and Ishak KG. Alcohol like liver disease in nonalcoholics. A clinical and histologic comparison with alcohol-induced liver injury. *Gastroenterology*, 1988; **95**: 1056–62.
22. Lee RG. Nonalcoholic steatohepatitis: A study of 49 patients. *Human Pathology*, 1989; **20**: 594–8.
23. Powell EE, Cooksley WGE, Hanson R, Searle J, Halliday JW, and Powell LW. The natural history of nonalcoholic steatohepatitis: A follow-up study of forty-two patients for up to 21 years. *Hepatology*, 1990; **11**: 74–80.
24. Bacon BR, Farahvash MJ, Janney CG, and Neuschwander-Tetri BA. Non-alcoholic steatohepatitis: An expanded clinical entity. *Gastroenterology*, 1994; **107**: 1103–9.
25. Hay JE, Czaja AJ, Rakela J, and Ludwig J. The nature of unexplained chronic aminotransferase elevations of mild to moderate degree in asymptomatic patients. *Hepatology*, 1989; **9**: 193–7.
26. Van Coster R, DeVivo D, Blake D, Lombes A, Barrett R, and DiMauro S. Adult Reye's syndrome: A review with new evidence for a generalized defect in intramitochondrial enzyme processing. *Neurology*, 1991; **41**: 1815–21.
27. Heubi J, Partin J, Partin J, and Schuber W. Reye's syndrome: current concepts. *Hepatology*, 1987; **7**: 115–64.

17

Drug-induced liver injury

17 Drug-induced liver injury

Dominique Pessayre, Dominique Larrey, and Michel Biour

Introduction

Drug-induced liver injury is a major challenge, both for the pharmaceutical industry, because hepatic injury is a frequent cause of drug recall, and for the physician, who can cure his patient by establishing the diagnosis and withdrawing the drug, whereas failure to recognize the liver disease and/or its drug aetiology may lead either to the worsening of the acute liver lesions or the progressive development of chronic liver lesions. Drug-induced liver injury is not uncommon, and may indeed be the main cause of hepatitis in elderly subjects receiving many drugs.[1] Early recognition of hepatic drug reactions is therefore a major concern for physicians.

Acquiring some knowledge of drug-induced liver lesions may seem a formidable task, however. Indeed, a thousand drugs may be hepatotoxic,[2] and this list is ever increasing as new molecules are steadily released on the market. Furthermore, drugs may damage the liver through different mechanisms, and hepatic drug reactions may mimic almost any kind of liver disease.[3] Clearly, the human mind cannot memorize all these data, nor can it be fitted into the frame of a single chapter. It is necessary, therefore, to have at least some direct knowledge of the several types of drug-induced liver lesions, the main mechanisms of hepatotoxicity, and the main drugs producing such effects. This chapter is an attempt to summarize this basic knowledge. Readers may find more exhaustive descriptions of the type of hepatitis produced by each individual drug in books that are entirely devoted to this topic.[2–4]

General considerations
Marketing of hepatotoxic drugs

Each year several drugs are marketed that subsequently turn out to be hepatotoxic, and some of them have to be recalled. Animal trials may have shown no hepatic lesion whatsoever, or they may have disclosed lesions but at very high doses that were thought meaningless for the much lower doses employed in humans. Studies in cultured human hepatocytes may have concluded that there was no toxicity at clinically relevant concentrations, although hepatitis eventually occurs in humans due to immune reactions. Clinical trials may have disclosed some patients with slightly impaired liver function tests, but this also may have occurred in a few of the patients receiving the placebo or a reference drug.

The main reason, however, for the steady release of hepatotoxic drugs is that clinical trials are extremely expensive and are therefore restricted to several hundred or a few thousand patients. If the frequency of clinical hepatitis is low (1/1000 or less) it will go undetected in these clinical trials. Additional factors may further contribute to the inefficiency of clinical trials in the detection of hepatotoxicity. Some drugs may be intended for short use (e.g. antibiotics) and clinical trials are accordingly devised. When, however, the drug is released on the market, some patients may start taking it for longer periods. This will leave more time for immunization to occur, for example, and cases of immunoallergic hepatitis may then appear. Release of the drug on the market may also expose patients that had been excluded, or included in small numbers, during the clinical trials but subsequently turn out to display particular susceptibility (e.g. very young children for valproate hepatotoxicity; elderly subjects for benoxaprofen hepatotoxicity; patients with renal insufficiency for several drugs eliminated by the kidney). It therefore seems inescapable that hepatotoxic molecules will continue to be marketed each year. Progress in pharmacovigilance should insure that their hepatotoxic potential is then quickly recognized. The responsibility of physicians in reporting all adverse events encountered with newly marketed drugs should be emphasized.

Frequency of adverse drug reactions among recipients

Once a drug is recognized as being hepatotoxic, one would like to know the frequency of this adverse effect. This can be determined accurately when the drug produces relatively frequent (e.g. 1/100) clinical manifestations. Large, post-marketing cohort studies can then gather a sufficient number of clinical cases to estimate this frequency reliably. For drugs, however, which produce clinical hepatotoxicity in 1/10 000 recipients or less, cohort studies would require a staggering number of patients and are therefore rarely conducted. The frequency of clinical hepatotoxicity often remains undetermined.

Theoretically, one should be able to estimate this frequency from the number of prescriptions and the spontaneous reports of adverse drug reactions. Although this reporting is supposed to be mandatory in several countries, there are many reasons why it tends to be neglected. In addition to the time spent in gathering the data and filling out the form, this report may lead to subsequent harassment by request(s) for more information made by the national drug agency, the drug company, or both. Furthermore, there are plenty of convenient excuses to soothe one's guilt for not doing so: 'the hepatotoxicity of the drug is already known'; 'its responsibility in the present case is far from certain'; 'this is a minor adverse reaction'; 'I shall report it later, once I have ascertained that there is sustained normalization of liver function tests'. Although none of these excuses should be considered as valid, it is clear that frequencies estimated from the spontaneous reporting of adverse events by physicians probably represent gross underestimates of the real frequencies.

Prevalence of adverse drug reactions among various causes of liver disease

One would like also to know what is the proportion of patients with drug-induced hepatic injury among all patients affected with liver disease at a given time. Surveys conducted among patients admitted to liver units have given proportions ranging from 2 to 5 per cent of cases of jaundice (Bjornhoe, ActaMedScand, 1967; 182:491; Koff, ClinRes, 1970; 18:680; Miller, ArchIntMed, 1974; 134:219) and about 10 per cent of cases of hepatitis.[1] However, liver units may give a biased view because only patients with difficult management problems may be referred to hepatologists. General practitioners are now well trained in suspecting adverse hepatic reactions and quickly withdraw potentially hepatotoxic drugs. Patients improve without ever seeing hepatologists.

An estimate is possible, however, in cases that are necessarily sent to the hospital, such as cases of fulminant hepatitis. In a large survey of causes for fulminant hepatitis, 10 to 15 per cent of cases were probably drug induced.[5] The proportion is much higher (50 per cent) in England, due to the popularity of paracetamol as a means of attempting suicide in this country (O'Grady, Gastro, 1989; 97:439).

Diversity of drug-induced liver diseases

Drugs may produce diverse liver lesions (Table 1), that correspond to different mechanisms of hepatotoxicity (Table 2).

Duration of the liver injury required to produce these lesions

The time interval between the onset of the treatment and the recognition of the liver disease corresponds to the sum of two periods: an initial period during which the drug is well tolerated and a second period of incipient, and then variably progressing, liver injury. Unless liver tests have been monitored, we do not know the actual duration of the liver injury which has led to a given liver lesion. A corollary is that terms such as 'subacute' or 'chronic' hepatitis, for example, should be understood as meaning the presence of histological lesions classified as such, rather than meaning any precise time definition. Obviously, chronic hepatitis defined by a duration of 3 or 6 months should not be seen with drugs, because the drugs should have been withdrawn as soon as the liver injury was detected.

Albeit hypothetical, Table 3 gives some tentative estimates of the probable duration of the liver injury required to produce various hepatocellular liver lesions and the possible consequences of these lesions.

Multiplicity of hepatotoxic drugs

Any list of hepatotoxic drugs represent a soon out-dated snapshot, as new drugs are constantly released on the market and many of those which cause frequent liver injury either are recalled, or fall into disrepute. Furthermore, space limitation does not allow tabulation of the thousand drugs that may cause liver injury.[2] The most frequently hepatotoxic drugs and the hepatic lesions they produce are indicated in Table 4. The reader is referred to Stricker's book for an exhaustive compilation.[2]

Diagnosis of drug-induced liver injury

Diagnosis of drug-induced liver injury can be obvious in some cases but is often difficult. A useful rule is to consider systematically the possibility of an adverse drug reaction when faced with almost any kind of liver disease.

The first step of the diagnosis relies on establishing the list of medications. This may be particularly time consuming in elderly patients who may have faltering memories, and often suffer from several ailments for which they consult various specialists. As each specialist often prescribes several drugs, the patients may end up with a dozen frequently changing drugs. Insistent questioning, and a look at the medical prescriptions, may disclose treatments that were initially forgotten. In all patients, specific inquiries should be made of treatments that may not be considered as drugs by the patient (herbal remedies, over-the-counter analgesics, oral contraceptives), and also of compounds that tend to be forgotten or concealed because of the patient's uneasiness in admitting their use or abuse (ecstasy, cocaine, hypnotics, antidepressants, neuroleptics, anabolics).

Once the list of ingested drugs has been established, the chronology of each treatment should be compared with that of the liver disease. As a general rule, the drugs which have been recently introduced in the patient's treatment should be most suspected. Nevertheless, several pitfalls must be avoided. The first would be to incriminate drugs which have been recently prescribed but for symptoms that actually heralded incipient liver injury. The second would be to neglect drugs which have been taken for many months without adverse effects. In an individual patient, even acute liver lesions may still occur under such circumstances. The third pitfall is to exclude all drugs that have been withdrawn before the onset of the liver injury. With some drugs, for example, iproniazid or the amoxicillin/clavulanic acid combination, jaundice may not occur until a fortnight after interruption of the treatment. Similarly, drugs which are retained for a long time in the liver (amiodarone, perhexiline, vitamin A) may continue to damage the liver and may lead to chronic liver lesions long after they have been stopped. A last pitfall would be to exclude recently-marketed drugs under the assumption that they are not known to be hepatotoxic. Instead, newly-marketed drugs should always be suspected of being potentially hepatotoxic, because recognition of their hepatotoxic potential (if any) often requires several years of widespread utilization.

The second step of the diagnosis relies on the gathering of information that may either strengthen the case for a iatrogenic reaction (previous adverse effects with the drug or related analogues, presence of immunoallergic manifestations) or may instead favour

Table 1 Diversity and proposed classification of drug-induced liver disease

Classification	Main lesion(s)
Acute hepatitis	
Cytolytic hepatitis	Lobular hepatocyte necrosis + lobular and portal inflammation
Cholestatic hepatitis	Cholestasis + portal inflammation
Cholestatic hepatitis with cholangiolitis and cholangitis	Cholestasis + portal inflammation + acute lesions of intraportal bile ducts
Mixed hepatitis	Necrosis + cholestasis + inflammation
Granulomatous hepatitis[a]	Hepatic granulomas + inflammation
Bland cholestasis	Cholestasis without other lesions
Lipid storage liver disease	
Macrovacuolar steatosis	Single large fat vacuole
Microvesicular steatosis	Multiple small fat vesicles
Phospholipidosis	Enlarged lysosomes with pseudomyelinic figures
Steatohepatitis	Steatosis, necrosis, mixed inflammatory infiltrate (with neutrophils), Mallory bodies, fibrosis
Subacute hepatitis, chronic hepatitis, and postnecrotic cirrhosis	
Subacute hepatitis	Acute hepatitis + bridging necrosis + fibrosis
Chronic hepatitis	Periportal necrosis + portal inflammation + portal fibrosis
Cirrhosis	Disorganized architecture + extensive fibrosis + regenerative nodules
Perisinusoidal fibrosis	Collagen deposition in the space of Disse; can lead to cirrhosis
Prolonged cholestasis	
Vanishing bile duct syndrome	Rarefaction of intraportal bile ducts
Sclerosing cholangitis	Strictures on large bile ducts
Vascular and related lesions	
Portal veins	Thrombosis
Hepatic artery	Intimal hyperplasia or angiitis
Sinusoidal dilation	Dilation of sinusoids
Peliosis	Haphazardly distributed blood-filled cavities
Veno-occlusive disease	Non-thrombotic obstruction of centrilobular veins
Budd–Chiari syndrome	Thrombosis of large hepatic veins
Periportal fibrosis	Portal fibrosis without cirrhosis
Nodular regenerative hyperplasia	Nodules without fibrosis
Tumours	
Hepatocellular adenoma	Benign tumour without central fibrous scar
Focal nodular hyperplasis	Benign hamartoma with central fibrous scar
Hepatocellular carcinoma	Malignant tumour derived from parenchymal cells
Angiosarcoma	Malignant tumour derived from endothelial cells

[a] The term should be restricted to cases where granulomas are the outstanding liver lesion.

another diagnosis (alcohol intake, blood transfusions, intravenous drug abuse, arrhythmia, cardiac failure).

The third step of the diagnosis relies on a comparison of the patient's disease with the type of liver disease produced by the potentially hepatotoxic drugs ingested by the patient. Indeed, the pattern of hepatotoxicity often differs with different drugs, with considerable differences in frequencies, times of onset, types of liver disease, associated extrahepatic features, and outcome. As one may have difficulty in memorizing all these data, it is useful always to have at hand a book such as that by Stricker (which provides this information in a concise and practical way)[2] and another book providing a more academic approach, such as that by Farrell;[3] these will indicate which drugs might be responsible for the liver injury.

Once a drug or several drugs are suspected, usually they should be withdrawn immediately. As a general rule, they were not necessary. In the surprisingly rare instance when these treatments were really needed, alternative drugs are often available.

At the same time, investigations are started to rule out other diagnoses (viral serologies and, in cholestatic cases,

ultrasonography) or strengthen the case for drug-induced liver injury. A differential white count may show eosinophilia. Nonspecific autoantibodies (antinuclear, antismooth muscle), at relatively low titres that regress after interruption of the treatment, may strengthen a diagnosis of drug-induced acute or chronic hepatitis. Specific serological markers are available with only a few drugs: antitrifluoracetylated proteins in halothane hepatitis; antimitochondrial type 6 (anti-M_6) autoantibody in iproniazid hepatitis, antiliver kidney microsomes type 2 (anti-LKM_2) autoantibody in tienilic acid hepatitis, antiliver microsomes autoantibody in dihydralazine hepatitis.[3] Lymphocyte proliferation assays performed in the presence of an inhibitor of prostaglandin synthesis (because prostaglandins inhibit immune reactions), and using either the parent compound itself or the patient's sera (to include metabolites) have recently been reported to be frequently positive in immunoallergic drug-induced hepatitis (Victorino, ClinExpMed, 1992; 87:132; Maria, JHepatol, 1994; 23:151). A liver biopsy can be dispensed with in most cases of acute liver injury. In difficult or severe cases, however, liver biopsy is perfectly justified and may, at times, be very helpful for the diagnosis (e.g. centrilobular necrosis

Table 2 Main mechanism of diverse liver lesions

Liver lesion	Main mechanism	Examples
Acute cytolytic hepatitis	Metabolite-mediated toxicity	Acetaminophen
	Metabolite-mediated immunoallergy	Halothane, sulphonamides
	Metabolite-mediated autoimmunity	Dihydralazine, tienilic acid
Acute cholestatic/mixed hepatitis	Metabolite-mediated immunoallergy (?)	Macrolides, phenothiazines
Granulomatous hepatitis	Allergy	Phenylbutazone, sulphonamides
Acute bland cholestasis	Interference with bile secretion	Anabolic steroids, oestrogens
Macrovacuolar steatosis	Decreased lipid secretion by the liver (?)	Methotrexate
Microvesicular steatosis	Inhibition of the β-oxidation of fatty acids	Tetracyclines, valproic acid
Phospholipidosis	Inhibition of lysosomal phospholipases	Amiodarone, perhexiline
Steatohepatitis	Lipid peroxidation due to steatosis and increased formation of reactive oxygen species	Amiodarone, perhexiline
Subacute and chronic hepatitis	Metabolite-mediated immune reaction (?)	Iproniazid, methyldopa
Vanishing bile duct syndrome	Autoimmune destruction of bile ducts (?)	Ajmaline, chlorpromazine
Sclerosing cholangitis	Arterial thrombosis leading to ischaemia (?)	Floxuridine
	Direct toxicity to bile ducts	Formaldehyde, hypertonic saline
Perisinusoidal fibrosis	Hypertrophy and activation of Ito cells	Methotrexate, vitamin A
Vascular lesions	Endothelial injury (?)	Chemotherapeutic agents
Adenomas	Growth-promoting effects (?)	Oral contraceptives
Carcinomas	Promoting effects; genotoxic effects (?)	Anabolic steroids, oestrogens

Table 3 Probable duration of the liver injury before the appearance of some liver diseases

Initial lesion	Days or weeks	Weeks or months	Months or years
Necrosis	Acute cytolytic hepatitis	Subacute or chronic hepatitis	Cirrhosis
Cholestasis	Acute cholestatic hepatitis		Prolonged cholestasis
Steatosis	Acute steatosis	Chronic steatosis	Steatohepatitis

in halothane-hepatitis; hepatic granulomas with allopurinol, quinidine, or sulphonamides; eosinophilic infiltration of the liver in several cases of allergic hepatitis). Suspected chronic liver lesions usually require a liver biopsy, as this is the only way of establishing the diagnosis.

The last step of the diagnosis is based on the improvement of the liver disease (usually within the weeks following the interruption of the treatment). This improvement will permit a probable diagnosis. Although readministration of the suspected drug would afford a certain diagnosis, this is usually unethical. However, when several drugs have been withdrawn but only one is reasonably suspected, readministration of these other, non-suspected drugs may be less unethical and may permit a definite diagnosis. This is important because an uncertain diagnosis may entice the patient into taking the offending drug again.

Differential diagnoses may include essentially all other causes of liver diseases, as drugs may produce the whole spectrum of the liver pathology. However, these differential diagnoses are more restricted (and shall be considered below) in the context of each particular drug-induced liver lesion.

Acute hepatitis
Liver lesions and terminology

Acute hepatitis is by far the most common drug-induced liver lesion. The gold standard for the classification of drug-induced hepatitis is the liver histology. In all cases of acute hepatitis,

there is at least some degree of inflammation, without fibrosis. Inflammation consists mostly of mononuclear cells, but may also include neutrophils or eosinophils and sometimes granulomas ('granulomatous' hepatitis). Inflammation is present at least in the portal tracts and, often, in the lobule also.

This inflammation may be associated with necrosis (or apoptosis) of the hepatocytes ('cytolytic' hepatitis), with cholestasis ('cholestatic' hepatitis), or with both necrosis and cholestasis ('mixed' hepatitis). In some forms of cholestatic hepatitis, there are lesions of bile ductules and interlobular bile ducts ('cholangiolitis' and 'cholangitis').

Because a liver biopsy is rarely necessary for the diagnosis, and therefore is rarely performed, it is useful nevertheless to be able to classify these cases from the maximal increase in serum alanine aminotransferase (**ALT**), a marker of hepatocyte damage or 'cytolysis', and that of alkaline phosphatase (**AP**), a marker of cholestasis, and from the ratio of ALT/AP, each activity being expressed in multiples of the upper limit of normal (**N**):[6]

1. The liver injury is termed 'cholestatic', if only alkaline phosphatase is increased (>2N) or, when both ALT and AP are increased, if the ALT/AP ratio is 2 or less.
2. The liver injury is designated as 'mixed' when both ALT and AP are increased and the ALT/AP ratio is between 2 and 5.
3. The liver injury will be classified as 'hepatocellular' if only ALT is increased (>2N) or, when both activities are increased, if the ALT/AP ratio is 5 or more.[6] In this case, however, one cannot

Table 4 Main drugs causing liver injury (at least 10% of biological abnormalities or 5 publication reporting liver injury)*

Aceclofenac (acute, R⁺)
Acetohexamide (cyt)
Acitretin (30%, cyt)
Acivicin (64%)
Aclarubicin (26%, R⁺)
Acyclovir (50%)
Ajmaline (chol, R⁺)
Albendazole (100%, acute, R⁺)
Allopurinol (cyt, chol, mix, severe, gran, steat, R⁺)
Alphadolone+alphaxalone (15%)
Alpidem (cyt)
Alprazolam (acute, R⁺)
Alrestatin (11%)
Alteplase (21%, R⁺)
Amidopyrine (cyt)
Amikacin (15%)
Amineptine (cyt, chol, mix, R⁺)
Aminobenzoic acid (35%)
Aminoglutethimide (67%, acute, R⁺)
Aminolaevulinic acid (57%, R⁺)
Aminosalicyclic acid (10%, cyt, severe, R⁺)
Amiodarone (55%, cyt, chol, chro, cirrh, steat, R⁺)
Amitriptyline (26%, cyt, chol, mix, severe, R⁺)
Amodiaquine (cyt, mix, severe, R⁺)
Amonafide (44%)
Amoxicillin (chol)
Amoxicillin+clavulanic acid (15%, chol, gran, steat, R⁺)
Amphotericin B (43%, chol, R⁺)
Ampicillin (20%, chol)
Amrinone (33%, acute, R⁺)
Amsacrine (41%, severe)
Aprindine (mix, chol, R⁺)
Arbekacin (25%)
Arsphenamide (acute, R⁺)
4-ASA (35%)
Asparaginase (63%, steat)
Aspirin (66%, cyt, severe, chro)
Aspoxicillin (40%)
Atovaquone (12%, R⁺)
Azacitidine (62%)
Azathioprine (28%, cyt, chol, mix, cirrh, vasc, R⁺)
Azithromycin (40%)
Azlocillin (11%)
Aztreonam (60%)
Balofloxacin (29%)
BCG therapy (gran)
Bendazac (acute, R⁺)
Benzarone (cyt, R⁺)
Bezafibrate (10%)
Biapenem (40%)
Bisantrene (49%)
Bromocriptine (22%, R⁺)
Buprenorphine (71%, R⁺)
Busulphan (100%, cyt, acute, severe, vasc)
Captopril (cyt, chol, R⁺)
Carbamazepine (22%, cyt, chol, mix, severe, gram, R⁺)
Carbarsone (acute)
Carbenicillin (56%, cyt, R⁺)
Carbetimer (18%)
Carbimazole (chol, R⁺)
Carboplatin (27%, vasc)
Carbutamide (30%, acute)
Carmustine (26%, cyt, acute, vasc)
Carprofen (56%)
Carumonam (22%)
Cefacetrile (29%)
Cefaclor (10%)
Cefalexin (cyt, chol, gran)
Cefalotin (acute)
Cefamandole (75%)

Cefazolin (43%)
Cefcapen+pivoxil (33%)
Cefclidin (40%)
Cefdinir (29%)
Cefditoren+pivoxil (37%)
Cefeprime (37%)
Cefetamet+pivoxil (23%)
Cefixime (33%)
Cefluprenam (37%)
Cefmenoxime (12%)
Cefminox (17%)
Cefodizine (44%)
Cefonicid (29%)
Cefoperazone (20%)
Cefoperazone+sulbactam (60%)
Ceforanide (43%)
Cefoselis (25%)
Cefotaxime (23%, acute)
Cefotetan (37%)
Cefotiam (33%)
Cefotiam+hexetil (29%)
Cefoxitin (26%)
Cefpimizole (19%)
Cefozopran (50%)
Cefpiramide (10%)
Cefpirome (33%)
Cefpodoxime (33%)
Cefprozil (25%)
Cefradine (24%)
Cefsulodin (18%)
Ceftazidime (36%)
Ceftibuten (14%)
Ceftizoxime (35%, acute)
Ceftriaxone (30%, acute)
Cefuroxime (29%)
Cefuroxime+axetil (20%)
Cefuzonam (14%)
Chenodeoxycholic acid (37%, acute R⁺)
Chlorambucil (acute, R⁺)
Chloramphenicol (46%, acute, R⁺)
Chlordiazepoxide (11%, acute, R⁺)
Chlormezanone (chol, R⁺)
Chloroquine (acute)
Chlorothiazide (chol)
Chlorozotocin (33%)
Chlorpromazine (42%, cyto, chol, chro, cirrh, R⁺)
Chlorpropamide (25%, cyto, chol, R⁺)
Chlortetracycline (acute)
Cholestyramine (30%)
Ciamexon (14%)
Cimetidine (38%, cyto, chol, mix, R⁺)
Ciprofloxacin (46%, cyto, chol)
Cisplatin (93%, R⁺)
Clarithromycin (50%, acute, R⁺)
Clindamycin (52%, acute)
Clofazimine (16%)
Clofibrate (20%)
Clometacin (cyto, chol, mix, severe, chro, cirrh, R⁺)
Clomipramine (11%, acute)
Clopenthixol (19%)
Clotrimazole (20%)
Cloxacillin (25%, chol, R⁺)
Clozapine (60%, cyto, R⁺)
Colchicine (29%)
Conjugated oestrogens (23%)
Cortisone (steat)
Cotrimoxazole (54%, cyt, chol, severe)
Coumarin (cyt, acute, R⁺)
Cromoglycate (17%)
Cyanamide (chro)

Table 4 continued

Cyclofenil (55%, acute, R⁺)
Cyclophosphamide (85%, cyto, severe, vasc, R⁺)
Cycloserine (13%)
Cyclosporin (94%, chol, R⁺)
Cyproheptadine (acute)
Cyproterone (17%, cyt, severe, mal.tum)
Cytarabrine (75%, acute, severe, vasc, R⁺)
Dacarbazine (50%, acute, severe, vasc)
Dactinomycin (12%, cyt, severe, vasc, R⁺)
Danazol (40%, cyt, chol, ben.tum, R⁺)
Dantrolene (cyt, chol, severe, R⁺)
Dapsone (20%, cyt, chol, mix)
Dapsone + trimethoprim (20%)
Datelliptinium (67%)
Daunorubicin (68%)
Deferiprone (44%)
Delmopressin (20%)
Desciclovir (15%)
Desflurane (11%)
Desipramine (cyt)
Dexamethasone (24%)
Dexrazoxane (13%)
Dextran (44%)
Dextrothyroxine (40%)
Diazepam (chol, R⁺)
Diaziquone (50%)
Dibekacin (14%)
Dichloromethotrexate (17%)
Diclofenac (25%, cyto, chol, mix, severe, chro, R⁺)
Dicloxacillin (acute)
Didanosine (38%, acute, R⁺)
Didemnin B (32%)
Dideoxythymidine (30%)
Difebarbamate (cyt, R⁺)
Diflunisal (acute)
Dihydralazine (cyt, chol, chro, R⁺)
Diltiazem (cyt, chol, R⁺)
Dirithromycin (29%)
Disopyramide (cyt, chol, mix, R⁺)
Disulfiram (26%, cyt, severe, R⁺)
Docetaxel (20%)
Doxorubicin (85%, acute, vasc, R⁺)
Doxycycline (10%)
Droxicam (cyt, chol)
Echinomycin (29%, acute)
Edatrexate (30%)
Elsamitrucin (13%)
Enalapril (cyt, chol, R⁺)
Enflurane (58%, cyt, mix, severe, R⁺)
Enoxaparin (36%)
Ergotamine (36%)
Erythromycin (38%, cyt, chol, mix, R⁺)
Erythropoietin (20%)
Esperamicin (11%)
Ethambutol (acute, R⁺)
Ethionamide (37%, cyt, chol, R⁺)
Etoposide (50%, severe, vasc)
Etretinate (33%, cyt, chro, steat, R⁺)
Exifone (cyt, severe)
Famotidine (acute, R⁺)
Fazarabine (46%)
Febrabamate (cyt, R⁺)
Felodipine (20%)
Fenbufen (25%, acute, R⁺)
Fengabide (54%)
Fenofibrate (27%, cyt, mix, chro, R⁺)
Fenretinide (13%)
Fentiazac (35%)
Filgrastim (75%, R⁺)

Fipexide (acute)
Flecainide (37%)
Flesinoxan (12%)
Flomoxef (33%)
Floxuridine (100%, chol, cirrh, R⁺)
Flucloxacillin (chol, R⁺)
Fluconazole (83%, cyt, chol, R⁺)
Flucytosine (18%, acute)
Fludarabine (43%)
Fluorindione (acute)
Fluorouracil (61%, severe, R⁺)
Fluoxetine (12%, acute)
Fluoxymesterone (vasc)
Fluperlapine (23%)
Fluphenasine (chol, R⁺)
Flupirtine (10%)
Fluroxene (30%, acute)
Flutamide (12%, cyt, chol, severe, R⁺)
Fluvastatin (55%)
Foscarnet (12%)
Fotemustine (31%)
Frentizole (70%)
Fropenem (20%)
Frusemide (acute)
Ftorafur (17%)
Fumarate (19%)
Fusidic acid (31%, acute)
Gallium (29%)
Ganciclovir (55%, R⁺)
Gemcitabine (39%, acute)
Gemfibrozil (10%)
Genaconazole (33%)
Gentamicin (14%)
Glafenine (cyt, severe, chro, cirrh, R⁺)
Glyburide (chol, R⁺)
Gold salts (17%, cyt, chol, severe)
Glossypol (93%)
Grepafloxacin (14%)
Griseofulvin (50%, acute)
Guanoxan (30%)
Hepatitis B vaccine (acute, R⁺)
H-interferon-alpha (58%)
H-interferon-alpha-N1 (42%)
Halofantrine (29%)
Halopemide (27%)
Haloperidol (20%, chol, R⁺)
Halothane (33%, cyt, severe, R⁺)
Heparin (90%)
Heparin LMW (25%)
Hepsulpham (25%)
Homoharringtonine (15%)
Hycanthone (severe)
Hydralazine (cyt, gran, R⁺)
Hydrocortisone (25%)
Hydroxychloroquine (11%)
Ibufenac (40%)
Ibuprofen (16%, cyt, R⁺)
Idarubicin (18%)
Ilmofosine (71%)
Imipenem + cilastatin (50%)
Imipramine (22%, cyt, chol, R⁺)
Indicine-N-oxide (62%, cyt, severe)
Indomethacin (25%, cyt, severe, R⁺)
Interleukin-1 (75%)
Interleukin-2 (100%, cyt, chol, R⁺)
Interleukin-2-FT (27%)
Interleukin-3 (21%)
Interleukin-4 (100%)
Interleukin-5 (55%)

Table 4 continued

Iodopamide (18%, cyt, R⁺)
Iprindole (chol, R⁺)
Iproniazid (30%, cyt, severe, R⁺)
Iproplatin (27%)
Irinotecan (13%, R⁺)
Isaxonine (cyt, severe, R⁺)
Isepamicin (30%)
Isocarboxazid (acute)
Isoflurane (cyt, R⁺)
Isoniazid (20%, cyt, severe, R⁺)
Isotretinoin (44%)
Itraconazole (15%, cyt, chol)
Ivermectin (23%)
Josamycin (20%, cyt, chol)
Kebuzone (27%, cyt, chol)
Ketamine (23%)
Ketoconazole (50%, cyt, chol, mix, severe, R⁺)
Ketoprofen (acute)
Labetalol (20%, cyt, R⁺)
Lansoprazole (10%)
Latamoxef (36%)
Leflunomide (18%)
Lenampicillin (22%)
Lergotrile (63%, cyt, R⁺)
Leustatin (13%)
Levamisole (61%, steat, R⁺)
Levodopa (acute)
Levofloxacin (30%)
Liblomycin (23%)
Lofepramine (46%, R⁺)
Lomefloxacin (18%)
Lomustine (39%)
Loracarbef (15%)
Lovastatin (27%, acute, R⁺)
Maprotiline (25%, mix)
Mebendazole (30%, R⁺)
Meciadanol (35%)
Megestrol (12%)
Meloxicam (11%)
Melperone (12%)
Menogaril (17%)
Mercaptopurine (53%, cyt, chol, severe, R⁺)
Meropenem (48%)
Mesalazine (21%, cyt, acute, R⁺)
Metahexamide (24%, cyt, mix, R⁺)
Methenolone (acute, R⁺)
Methicillin (19%)
Methimazole (chol, R⁺)
Methotrexate (88%, cyt, chro, cirrh, gran, steat, mal.tum, R⁺)
Methotrimeprazine (acute)
Methoxyflurane (cyt, severe, R⁺)
Methyldopa (35%, cyt, chol, mix, severe, chro, cirrh, gran, R⁺)
Methyltestosterone (32%, chol, vasc, mal.tum, R⁺)
Metoprolol (32%, R⁺)
Metronidazole (25%, cyt)
Mezlocillin (25%)
Mianserin (26%, chol, R⁺)
Mifepristone (10%)
Milacemide (70%)
Minocycline (42%, cyt, severe, chro, R⁺)
Mirtazapine (10%)
Misoprostol (17%)
Mitoguazine (18%)
Mitomycin (58%, acute, vasc)
Mitozantrone (80%)
Molgramostim (20%)
Moxisylyte (cyt, R⁺)
Mustine (100%)
N-Methylformamide (75%, acute)
Nafcillin (25%, acute)
Naltrexone (20%)
Nandrolone (acute)

Naproxen (cyt, chol, severe)
Naxagolide (11%)
Nebracetam (11%)
Nedaplatin (19%)
Nefopam (14%)
Netilmicin (29%)
Nicotinic acid (52%, cyt, chol, severe, R⁺)
Nicoumarol (acute)
Nifedipine (16%, cyt, chol, R⁺)
Niflumic acid (cyt, R⁺)
Nisoldipine (12%)
Nitrendipine (18%)
Nitrofurantoin (cyt, chol, severe, chro, cirrh, R⁺)
Nitroprusside (41%)
Nomifensine (cyt, chol, gran, R⁺)
Norethandrolone (24%, chol, R⁺)
Norethisterone (23%, chol)
Norfloxacin (acute)
Novobiocin (40%, acute)
Nystatin (33%)
Octreotide (18%, R⁺)
Ofloxacin (42%, acute)
Olanzapine (10%)
Olsalazine (15%)
Omeprazole (47%, acute)
Ondansetron (33%, R⁺)
Oral contraceptives (chol, vasc, ben.tum, mal.tum, R⁺)
Ormaplatin (53%)
Oxacillin (81%, cyt, R⁺)
Oxaprozin (20%)
Oxymetholone (50%, chol, vasc, ben.tum, mal.tum, R⁺)
Oxyphenbutazone (acute, gran)
Oxyphenisatin (acute, chro, cirrh, R⁺)
Oxytetracycline (60%, steat)
Paclitaxel (33%)
Panipenem + betamipron (38%)
Papaverine (53%, cyt, mix, chro, R⁺)
Paracetamol (<11 g/day) (50%, cyt, severe, chro, cirrh, R⁺)
Paraffin (steat)
Paroxetine (11%)
Pazufloxacin (10%)
Pefloxacin (17%)
Pemoline (cyt, severe, R⁺)
Penicillamine (chol, steat, R⁺)
Penicillin (13%, chol)
Pentamethylmelamine (31%)
Pentamidine (43%, R⁺)
Pentosan polysulphate (75%, R⁺)
Pentostatin (81%)
Perazine (43%)
Perhexiline (30%, cyt, severe, cirrh, steat)
Perphenazine (acute)
Phenacemide (cyt, severe)
Phencyclidine (50%)
Phenelzine (severe)
Phenindione (chol, R⁺)
Pheniprazine (cyt, severe)
Phenobarbitone (cyt, severe, R⁺)
Phenprocoumon (37%, chol, R⁺)
Phenylbutazone (cyt, chol, chro, gran, R⁺)
Phenytoin (90%, cyt, chol, mix, severe, chro, gran, R⁺)
Phytomenadione (acute)
Piperacetazine (93%)
Piperacillin (26%, R⁺)
Piperacillin + tazobactam (33%)
Piribedil (10%)
Piritrexim (12%)
Piroxicam (73%, cyt, chol, mix, severe, R⁺)
Pirprofen (cyt, severe, R⁺)
Pivmecillinam (17%)
Plafibride (20%)
Plicamycin (100%, cyt)

Table 4 continued

Potassium aminobenzoate (38%)
Povidone iodine (80%)
Prajmalinium (chol, R⁺)
Pravastatin (22%)
Praziquantel (18%)
Prednisone (80%)
Procainamide (chol, gran, R⁺)
Prochlorperazine (chol)
Progabide (30%, cyt, severe)
Progesterone (13%)
Promazine (chol)
Propafenone (10%, chol, R⁺)
Propoxyphene (14%, chol, mix, R⁺)
Propranolol (10%, acute)
Propylthiouracil (28%, cyt, chol, severe, R⁺)
Prothionamide (13%, cyt)
Prulifloxacin (33%)
Pyrazinamide (26%, cyt, mix, severe, R⁺)
Pyricarbate (10%, cyt, mix, R⁺)
Pyrimethamine (29%)
Pyrimethamine + sulphadoxine (cyt, chol, R⁺)
Pyritinol (chol, R⁺)
Quazolast (13%)
Quinapril (10%)
Quinidine (cyt, chol, gran, mix, R⁺)
Quinine (15%, R⁺)
Raloxifene (17%)
Raltifrexed (10%)
r-Interferon-alpha-2a (92%, acute, R⁺)
r-Interferon-alpha-2b (87%, acute, severe, R⁺)
r-Interferon-beta (40%)
r-Interferon-alpha-2c (10%)
r-Interferon-gamma (60%, R⁺)
Ranitidine (19%, cyt, chol, mix, R⁺)
Retinol (33%, chro, cirrh, vasc, steat)
Rifamixin (27%)
Rifampicin (23%, chol, mix, R⁺)
Rifamycin (10%)
Riluzole (17%)
Rioprostil (10%)
Ritipenem-acoxil (20%)
Ritonavir (30%)
Roxindole (10%)
Roxithromycin (23%, cyt, chol)
Salsalate (15%)
Saquinavir (27%)
Saramycin (40%)
Seroquel (15%)
Sevoflurane (40%)
Simvastatin (52%, cyt, R⁺)
Sparfloxacin (20%)
Spirogermanium (27%)
Stanozolol (26%, acute)
Stavudine (11%, cyt)
Stibocaptate (82%)
Stibogluconate (47%)
Stilboestrol (chol, mal.tum)
Streptokinase (75%, acute, R⁺)
Streptozotocin (67%, R⁺)
Succimer (57%)
Sulphadiazine (acute)
Sulphafurazole (acute)
Sulphamethizole (acute)
Sulphamethoxypyridazine (cyt)
Sulphanilamide (cyt, severe)
Sulphasalazine (cyt, chol, mix, severe, gran, R⁺)
Sulindac (15%, cyt, chol, mix, steat, cirrh, R⁺)
Suloctidil (15%, cyt, cirrh, R⁺)
Sulofenir (80%, acute)
Sultamicillin (43%)
Suramin (63%)

Swainsonine (53%)
Tacrine (54%, cyt, gran, R⁺)
Tacrolimus (37%)
Tamoxifen (14%, acute, steat, R⁺)
Tannic acid (cyt, severe)
Tegafur (acute, R⁺)
Teicoplanin (21%)
Teloxantrone (37%)
Temafloxacin (44%)
Tenidap (19%)
Teniposide (24%)
Tenoxicam (27%)
Terbinafine (37%, acute)
Terfenadine (19%)
Testosterone (vasc)
Tetracycline (chol, severe, steat)
Theophylline (56%, R⁺)
Thiabendazole (36%, chol, R⁺)
Thiacetazone (18%, cyt)
Thioguanine (11%, acute, vasc)
Thiopentone (87%)
Thioridazine (chol)
Thiouracil (acute, R⁺)
Thorium oxide (cirrh, mal.tum)
Tiazofurin (62%)
Ticarcillin + clavulanic acid (33%, R⁺)
Ticlopidine (10%, cyt, chol, mix)
Tienilic acid (cyt, chol, mix, severe, chro, cirrh, R⁺)
Tinzaparin (35%)
Tiopronin (chol)
Tiratricol + retinol (cyt, R⁺)
Tobramycin (23%)
Tocainide (mix)
Tolazamide (acute, R⁺)
Tolbutamide (chol, R⁺)
Tolmetin (15%)
Tolrestat (15%)
Topiramate (23%)
Trazodone (acute)
Tretinoin (85%, acute)
Triacetyloleandomycin (83%, chol, R⁺)
Tribavirin (33%)
Tribromoethyl alcohol (cyt, severe, steat)
Trichloroethylene (cyt, severe)
Trifluoperazine (chol)
Trimethoprim (chol, R⁺)
Trimetrexate (25%)
Tropisetron (41%)
Trospectinomycin (33%)
Urethane (cyt, severe, R⁺)
Valaciclovir (18%)
Valproic acid (67%, cyt, chol, mix, severe, steat, R⁺)
Vancomycin (50%)
Velnacrine (32%)
Verapamil (17%, acute, R⁺)
Vidarabine (17%)
Vigabatrin (10%)
Vinblastine (23%)
Vincristine (acute, vasc, R⁺)
Vinorelbine (24%)
Warfarin (chol, R⁺)
Zalcitabine (15%)
Zaltidine (94%)
Zidovudine (25%, cyt, severe, steat, R⁺)
Zileuton (20%)
Zimeldine (20%, acute, R⁺)
Zopolrestat (12%)
Zorubicin (52%)
Zotepine (35%)
Zoxazolamine (cyt)

%, highest reported frequency of liver test abnormalities during clinical trials; cyt, cytolytic acute hepatitis; chol, cholestatic hepatitis; mix, mixed hepatitis; acute, acute hepatitis; severe, severe acute hepatitis; chro, chronic hepatitis chro, chronic hepatitis; cirrh, cirrhosis; steat, steatosis; vasc, vascular lesions; mal.tum, malignant tumour; ben.tum, benign tumour; R⁺, positive rechallenge.

equate this 'hepatocellular' injury with 'cytolytic' hepatitis because many other lesions (e.g. microvesicular steatosis, Budd–Chiari syndrome, veno-occlusive disease, low cardiac output, etc.) may also give such a liver test profile.

Mechanisms of drug-induced acute hepatitis

Much progress has been made in recent years in the understanding of the toxic and immune mechanisms leading to drug-induced acute hepatitis. In some instances, the therapeutic effect of the drug itself may be involved in hepatotoxicity. For example, inhibitors of hydroxymethylglutaric coenzyme A reductase inhibit the synthesis of mevalonate and, because mevalonate is a precursor in the synthesis of cholesterol, these drugs are useful in the treatment of hypercholesterolemic patients. Mevalonate, however, is also a precursor of a host of important isoprenoid derivatives, including ubiquinone and heme a (two fundamental components of the mitochondrial respiratory chain), and others which serve in the isoprenylation of regulatory proteins (e.g. some low molecular weight G proteins) or structural proteins (e.g. nuclear lamins). Inhibition of isoprenoid biosynthesis appeared as the mechanism of lovastatin-induced apoptosis in an *in vitro* system (Perez-Sala, BBResComm, 1994; 199:1209).

Usually, however, drug-induced hepatitis is ascribed to the formation of reactive metabolites. Indeed, many drugs that cause hepatitis are transformed by cytochrome P-450 into reactive, potentially hepatotoxic metabolites (Table 5).

The formation and hepatotoxicity of these reactive metabolites can be viewed as the untoward consequence of two xenophobic systems: the cytochrome P-450 system which has evolved in animals to eliminate small, alien molecules ('xenobiotics') and the immune system which has evolved to eliminate foreign micro-organisms.[7] Formation of reactive metabolites by cytochrome P-450 may lead to direct toxicity, while the combination of the cytochrome P-450 and the immune system may lead to the immune destruction of hepatocytes.[7]

The cytochrome P-450 system

For a billion years, animals have been subjected to relentless biological warfare mounted by the plants that they ingested, as these plants have progressively developed new toxins.[8] Many of these plant toxins were liposoluble and could not be excreted as such in urine or bile. Clearly, animals which could develop systems able to transform these liposoluble xenobiotics into water-soluble metabolites, that could be excreted in urine or bile, benefited from an important survival advantage. This evolutionary pressure probably accounted for the development of a wide array of cytochrome P-450s able to metabolize xenobiotics in animals.[8] By duplication of an ancestral cytochrome P-450 gene, divergent evolution of these two genes, and so forth, surviving animals have been endowed with a whole panoply of cytochrome P-450s able to metabolize and eliminate essentially all liposoluble xenobiotics in the environment, as well as most drugs used at present.

These various cytochrome P-450s share the same oxidizing centre (the haem moiety) and a similar general architecture, but differ by their protein moieties (Fig. 1). Each cytochrome P-450 metabolizes partially overlapping, but largely different, sets of xenobiotics (Fig. 1).

Cytochrome P-450 is first reduced by NADPH-cytochrome P-450 reductase and may then bind molecular oxygen as a sixth ligand of the reduced haem iron. After introduction of a second electron, a reactive iron oxo complex is formed which can oxidize many substrates. Cytochrome P-450 mediates an initial functionalization (e.g. a hydroxylation) of the substrate ('phase I' of drug metabolism). This creates a 'handle' onto which a polar molecule may then be added by conjugating enzymes ('phase II' of drug metabolism), so that the resulting hydrosoluble conjugate can now be excreted in urine or bile (Fig. 1).

The cytochrome P-450s which metabolize xenobiotics are located in many organs but are particularly abundant in the liver. This disposition is probably not fortuitous. Indeed, the liver has the advantage of being both voluminous and richly vascularized, and, more importantly, of draining the blood coming from the intestine. Therefore, after the intestine (which also contains some cytochrome P-450s), the liver can metabolize ingested xenobiotics even before they reach the systemic circulation. A further refinement of the system is that the endothelial cells of the hepatic sinusoids are unique in being perforated by fenestrae. Liposoluble xenobiotics circulate in the plasma thanks to their binding to plasma proteins. The sinusoidal fenestrae allow proteins (and the xenobiotics they carry) to come into direct contact with the hepatocytes. This facilitates the removal of these xenobiotics, enabling the liver to metabolize totally some xenobiotics in a single pass through the hepatic sinusoid.

Formation of reactive metabolites

The development of the hepatic P-450 system as a means to eliminate xenobiotics had a major drawback. Although several xenobiotics are transformed by cytochrome P-450s into stable metabolites, many others are oxidized into unstable, chemically reactive, intermediates (Fig. 1).[9] These downright molecular 'bombs' can attack hepatic constituents (DNA, unsaturated lipids, proteins, glutathione) and can lead to either cancer or liver cell demise.

Reactive metabolites are mainly formed through oxidative reactions. However, cytochrome P-450 in its reduced form (ferrous iron) may also catalyze the reductive dehalogenation of several haloalkanes (such as carbon tetrachloride or halothane) to the corresponding free radicals (Mansuy, Biochim, 1978; 60:969). Furthermore, NADPH-cytochrome P-450 reductase itself may reduce some drugs into free radicals: for example the formation of semiquinone radicals from quinones (O'Brien, ChemBiolInterac, 1991; 80:1); formation of nitro anion radicals from nitroarenes (Berson, JPharmExpTher, 1991; 257:714). These drug radicals may in turn reduce molecular oxygen to the superoxide anion radical ($O_2^\bullet$), leading to other reactive oxygen species (H_2O_2, $\bullet OH$) (Berson, JPharmExpTher, 1991; 257:714).

Therefore, the cytochrome P-450 system, albeit remarkably adapted to the elimination of an infinite array of liposoluble xenobiotics, nevertheless had the serious inconvenience of forming potentially toxic metabolites. Clearly this system would not have been viable without the concomitant development of a variety of protective mechanisms.

Suicidal inactivation of cytochrome P-450

A first protective mechanism, which is automatically included in the system, is the inactivation of cytochrome P-450 by some reactive

Table 5 Main drugs transformed into reactive metabolites and causing cytolytic, mixed, or cholestatic hepatitis

Amineptine (Genève, BiochemPharm, 1987; 36:323)
Amitriptyline? (Prox, DrugMedDisp, 1987; 15:890)
Amodiaquine (Maggs, BiochemPharm, 1987; 36:2061)
Benoxaprofen (van Bremen, DrugMetDisp, 1985; 13:318)
Carbamazepine? (Lertratangkoon, DrugMedDisp, 1982; 10:1)
Carmustine (Gombard, BiochemPharm, 1980; 29:2639)
Chloramphenicol (Halpert, MolPharm, 1983; 23:445)
Chloroform (De Mol, BiochemPharm, 1980; 29:3271)
Chlorpromazine (De Mol, ChemBiolInteract, 1984; 52:79)
Cocaine (Roberts, DrugMedDisp, 1991; 19:1046)
Cyclosphamide (Martinello, CancerRes, 1984; 44:4615)
Cyproterone (Neumann, Carcinogenesis, 1992; 13:373)
Dantrolene? (Roy, ResCommChemPathPharm, 1980; 27:507)
Dapsone (Vage, ToxApplPharm, 1994; 129:309)
Dextropropoxyphene (Peterson, BiochemPharm, 1979; 28:1783)
Diclofenac (Kretz-Rommel, ToxApplPharmacot, 1993; 120:155)
Diflunisal (Dickinson, BiochemPharm, 1991; 42:2301)
Dihydralazine (Bourdi, MolPharm, 1994; 45:1287)
Disulphiram (Yourick, BiochemPharm, 1991; 42:1361)
Enflurane (Christ, DrugMetDisp, 1988; 16:135)
Erythromycin (Danan, JPharmExpTher, 1981; 218:509)
Flutamide (Berson, JPharmExpTher, 1993; 265:366)
Fluroxene (Murphy, ToxApplPharmacol, 1980; 52:69)
Germander (Loeper, Gastro, 1994; 106:464)
Halothane (Sipes, JPharmExpTher, 1980; 214:716)
Hydralazine (Sinha, BBResComm, 1982; 105:1044)
Imipramine (Kappus, BiochemPharm, 1975; 24:1079)
Indomethacin (van Bremen, DrugMetDisp, 1985; 13:318)
Iproniazid (Nelson, JPharmExpTher, 1978; 206:574)
Isaxonine (Lettéron, JPharmExpTher, 1984; 229:845)
Isoflurane (Christ, DrugMetDisp, 1988; 16:1351)
Isoniazid (Timbrell, JPharmExpTher, 1980; 213:364)
Ketoprofen (Dubois, DrugMetDisp, 1993; 21:617)
Lomustine (Gombar, BiochemPharm, 1980; 29:2639)
Methimazole (Lee, DrugMetDisp, 1978; 6:591)
Methoxsalen (Tinel, BiochemPharm, 1987; 36:951)
Metronidazole (Rosenkrantz, BBResComm, 1975; 66:520)
α-Methyldopa (Dybing, MolPharm, 1976; 12:911)
Nilutamide (Berson, JPharmExpTher, 1991; 257:714)
Nitrofurantoin (Boyd, BiochemPharm, 1979; 28:601)
Paracetamol (Mitchell, JPharmExpTher, 1973; 187:211)
Phenylbutazone (Reed, MolPharm, 1985; 27:109)
Phenytoin (Pantarotto, BiochemPharm, 1982; 31:1501)
Propylthiouracil (Hunter, BiochemPharm, 1975; 24:2199)
Sulphonamides (Cribb, DrugMetDisp, 1991; 19:900)
Tacrine (Woolf, DrugMetDisp, 1993; 21:874)
Tianeptine (Larrey, BiochemPharm, 1990; 40:545)
Tienilic acid (ticrynafen) (Lopez Garcia, EurJBioch, 1993; 213:223)
Troleandomycin (Pessayre, BiochemPharm, 1981; 30:553)
Trichloroethylene (Allemand, JPharmExpTher, 1978; 204:714)
Valproic acid (Rettenmeier, DrugMetDisp, 1985; 13:81)

intermediates. Indeed, a reactive intermediate which has just been formed inside the hydrophobic active site of cytochrome P-450 may directly attack cytochrome P-450 itself and destroy it (Fig. 1). This may occur in several ways. Some intermediates (e.g. the nitrosoalkane metabolites of macrolides) may form stable, inactive complexes with the iron(II) of cytochrome P-450 (Pessayre, BiochemPharm, 1982; 31:1699). Other metabolites may covalently bind to an aminoacyl residue of the active site of P-450 (Labbe, JPharmExpTher, 1989; 250:1034), or to a nitrogen of the haem molecule (Ortiz de Montellano, JBC, 1981; 256:4395). Free radicals may form an unstable adduct with a vinyl group of haem that then covalently binds to the cytochrome P-450 protein (Davies,

ArchBiochemBiophys, 1986; 244:387). Whatever its molecular mechanism, this 'suicidal' inactivation prevents further formation of the reactive intermediate.

Glutathione conjugation and other protective mechanisms

The tripeptide glutathione (L-γ-glutamyl-L-cysteinyl-glycine) is synthesized by the successive action of γ-glutamylcysteine synthase and glutathione synthetase (Meister, PhamTher, 1991; 51:155). The first enzyme functions at less than maximal rate due to feedback inhibition by glutathione. Thus, when the consumption of

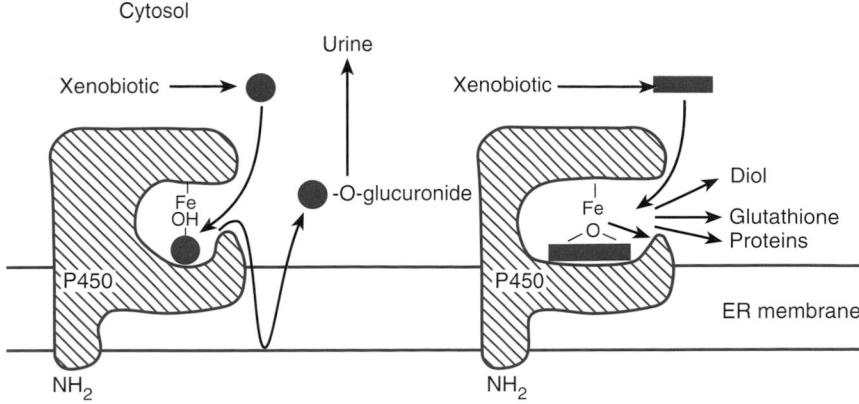

Cytosol

Lumen of the endoplasmic reticulum (ER)

Fig. 1. Structure and function of cytochrome P-450s. The different cytochrome P-450s have the same catalytic centre (the haem iron) but differ by their protein moieties and their affinities for various substrates.

glutathione increases, and its hepatic concentration tends to decrease, the liver can markedly increase the synthesis of glutathione. Although hepatic glutathione is continuously secreted in both the hepatic sinusoid (serving as a precursor of cysteine for other organs) and in bile, its active synthesis normally maintains a 10 mmol concentration of glutathione within hepatocytes (with distinct cytosolic, mitochondrial, and nuclear pools). Glutathione exerts several protective functions within hepatocytes. One of these functions is to serve as a molecular sink for electrophilic metabolites. Indeed, electrophilic metabolites spontaneously react with the SH-group of glutathione, preventing the alkylation of more critical hepatic constituents. This spontaneous reaction is greatly accelerated by several cytosolic and microsomal glutathione *S*-transferases (Mannervik, BiochemJ, 1992; 282:305). The resulting glutathione conjugates are then excreted in bile by the multispecific organic anion transporter (Pikula, JBC, 1994; 44:27566).

Several other enzymes may catalyse the rearrangement of reactive metabolites into stable metabolites. For example microsomal, cytosolic, and nuclear epoxide hydrolases speed up the hydration of reactive epoxides into diols (Oesch, Xenobiot, 1972; 3:305). Superoxide dismutase, catalase, glutathione peroxidase, and glutathione reductase act in concert to decrease the toxicity that could result from the formation of the superoxide anion by free radicals arising from the metabolism of xenobiotics. Vitamin E, vitamin C, glutathione, and glutathione peroxidases limit the initiation and propagation of lipid peroxidation (Frei, AmJMed, 1994; 97:3A). Multiple DNA repair systems allow for the reparation of damaged DNA, before a round of DNA replication can lead to somatic mutations (Sancar, Science, 1994; 266:1954).

Thanks to these protective mechanisms, recourse to the cytochrome P-450 system as a means to eliminate xenobiotics became tolerable, inasmuch as both the formation of reactive metabolites and their reaction with hepatic constituents could be partly limited. Only massive doses of these foreign substances and/or the extensive metabolism of a particular xenobiotic may then lead to direct toxicity.

In situ reaction of reactive metabolites

Some reactive metabolites (e.g. acetaldehyde or acyl-glucuronides) react slowly with tissue components and, therefore, can leave their site of formation and react elsewhere. Most reactive metabolites, however, are so highly unstable that they react *in situ* in the very organ that forms them.[10] The abundance of cytochromes P-450 in the liver, and the *in situ* reaction of reactive metabolites, explain the major role of these metabolites in drug-induced hepatitis. The centrilobular location of most cytochrome P-450s accounts for the frequently pericentral zonation of these lesions.

Molecular and cellular lesions leading to direct toxicity

A first type of molecular lesion, which is observed with drugs transformed into free radicals, is lipid peroxidation.[11] The first step in this process is the formation of lipid radicals (Link, BiochemJ, 1984; 223:577). Either the addition of a reactive drug radical ($R\bullet$) on a carbon of an unsaturated lipid, or the abstraction by this radical of an hydrogen atom, leads in both cases to a lipid radical (lipid$\bullet$). This radical quickly adds molecular oxygen to form a peroxyl radical (lipid-OO$\bullet$). This peroxyl radical may react with another lipid molecule (lipid$_2$-H) to form a hydroperoxide and a new lipid radical:

$$\text{lipid}_1\text{-OO}\bullet + \text{lipid}_2\text{-H} \rightarrow \text{lipid}_1\text{-OOH} + \text{lipid}_2\bullet$$

Lipid peroxidation may thus extend from one lipid to the other, or along the same lipid chain. Eventually, unsaturated lipids are oxidized and cut into small fragments (alkanes, malondialdehyde, alkenals). The last two compounds are themselves reactive and bind covalently to proteins.

A second type of molecular lesion is observed mainly with electrophilic metabolites. These metabolites react with, and covalently bind to, several nucleophilic groups of proteins (e.g. the SH-group of a cysteine residue or the ε-NH$_2$-group of a lysine residue), on which they remain attached by a covalent bond.

These electrophilic metabolites also react with the SH-group of glutathione, and this is an important protective mechanism which prevents reaction with more critical cellular targets. However, when large amounts of the reactive metabolite are formed, the extensive formation of glutathione conjugates then exceeds the capacity of the liver to increase the synthesis of glutathione. The resulting depletion of glutathione, together with the direct covalent binding to protein

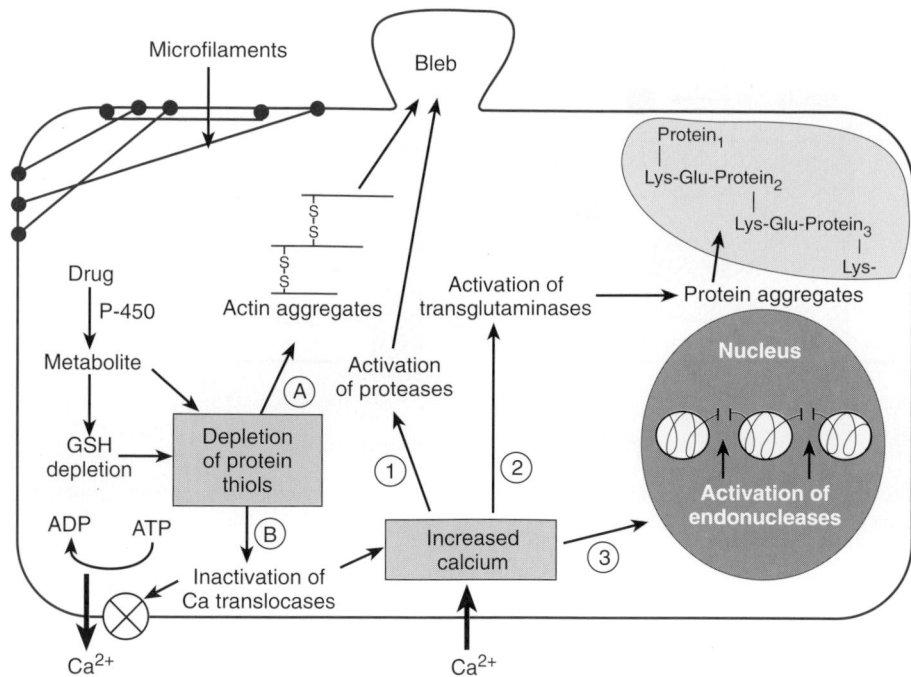

Fig. 2. Cellular mechanisms for the cytotoxicity of electrophilic metabolites.

thiols, and/or the direct oxidation of protein thiols, all tend to decrease protein thiols (Fig. 2). Depletion of protein thiols has severe toxicological consequences (Fig. 2):[7,12]

1. A first consequence is the formation of disulphur bonds between different molecules of actin, forming inactive actin aggregates.[13] This destroys the microfilamentous network that is located beneath the plasma membrane and normally maintains the shape of this membrane through its attachment to integral plasma membrane proteins. Destruction of this network allows the formation of fragile plasma membrane blebs (Fig. 2).
2. A second consequence of the oxidation of protein thiols is to decrease the activity of plasma membrane calcium translocases, whose role is constantly to extrude calcium from the hepatocytes.[14] The resulting increase in cellular Ca^{2+} activates calcium-dependent proteases (which further damage the cytoskeleton), calcium-dependent transglutaminases (which form a cross-linked protein scaffold), and calcium-dependent endonucleases (which cut DNA between nucleosomes) (Fig. 2).[7]
3. A last consequence of the oxidation of protein thiols is to permeabilize the mitochondrial inner membrane, and this decreases the mitochondrial membrane potential and the formation of ATP.[15]

The end result of these various molecular lesions may be either unscheduled apoptosis or necrosis. Apoptosis, or 'programmed cell death', is a complex physiological process responsible for the 'natural' cell death that occurs in embryogenesis, tissue atrophy, senescent cells, thymus selection, and cell-mediated cytotoxicity. Typically, apoptosis is characterized by:

(1) the activation of calcium-dependent transglutaminases leading to the formation of a cross-linked protein scaffold;

(2) the activation of calcium-dependent endonucleases leading to internucleosomal DNA fragmentation;

(3) typical ultrastructural changes including condensation of the cytoplasm, rim-like or crescent-like condensation of chromatin beneath the nuclear membrane, and the formation of large cellular blebs that initially contain ultrastructurally unaltered cellular organelles.[16] This is followed by segmentation of both the cytoplasm and the nucleus, with the formation of apoptotic bodies.

As explained above, reactive metabolites, probably by increasing Ca^{2+}, may interfere with this system, and may produce unscheduled, but otherwise typical, apoptosis.[17,18] Much progress needs to be made, however, in understanding the mechanisms of this drug-induced apoptosis, and the reasons why the formation of reactive metabolites may lead to either apoptosis or necrosis. Possibly, necrosis may develop instead of apoptosis when the various molecular lesions are both so extensive and sudden (with, for example, major and rapid ATP depletion) that the cell dies before the slower process of apoptosis can develop.[19]

Genetic and acquired factors involved in direct toxicity

The direct toxicity of reactive metabolites concerns drugs for which the formation of the reactive metabolite is low enough to ensure the absence of hepatitis in most recipients of therapeutic doses (therefore allowing the marketing of the drug), but still high enough to lead to severe toxicity in some metabolically susceptible subjects. Both genetic and acquired factors may explain the susceptibility of these few recipients.

Genes may influence both the formation and the inactivation of reactive metabolites. The cytochrome P-450 isoenzymes are under genetic control, and the hepatic level of a given isoenzyme is considerably different in different people (Shimada, JPharm-ExpTher, 1994; 270:414). While some reactive metabolites are formed by several cytochrome P-450s,[20] other reactive metabolites are mainly formed by a particular isoenzyme.[21,22] A subject with a high genetic expression of this cytochrome P-450 might be at increased risk of developing hepatitis. In contrast, a deficiency of some cytochrome P-450 isoenzymes is observed in the poor metabolizer phenotypes of several polymorphisms of drug oxidation.[23,24] Such poor metabolizers should be protected against the toxicity of reactive metabolites that are normally formed by this deficient isoenzyme.[25]

Genetic factors may also modify the inactivation of reactive metabolites. Indeed, subjects with a deficit in glutathione synthetase were more susceptible to the toxicity of paracetamol, at least when investigated in an artificial *in vitro* system.[26]

Physiological, nutritional, or therapeutic modifications of drug metabolism may also explain the susceptibility of some subjects:

1. Pregnancy, for example, may decrease the capacity of the liver to resynthesize glutathione and markedly increases the hepatotoxicity of paracetamol in mice.[27] It is not known whether similar effects also occur in women.

2. Fasting, or protein denutrition, decreases hepatic glutathione content, and dramatically increases the hepatotoxicity of paracetamol in rats.[28] In humans, hepatitis has been observed after high therapeutic doses of paracetamol in a few subjects with malnutrition (Barker, AnnIntMed, 1977; 87:229; Ware, AnnIntMed, 1978; 88:267).

3. Microsomal enzyme induction by drugs administered concurrently may increase the formation of the reactive metabolite, and the susceptibility to hepatitis. Thus, rifampin, a microsomal enzyme inducer (Pessayre, BiochemPharm, 1976; 25:943), apparently increases the hepatotoxicity of isoniazid.[29] Drugs used for premedication and general anaesthesia may induce microsomal enzymes,[30] and may potentiate isoniazid hepatotoxicity.[29] Likewise, recent introduction of microsomal enzyme inducers may have triggered fulminant hepatitis in three patients receiving prolonged treatment with iproclozide.[31] Chronic ethanol ingestion increases a particular isoenzyme of cytochrome P-450 (P-450 2E1) that activates paracetamol. This potentiates the hepatotoxicity of therapeutic doses of paracetamol in humans.[32] Ethanol also tends to decrease hepatic glutathione concentration (Shaw, DigDisSci, 1983; 28:585), an effect which may also contribute to increased paracetamol toxicity. Indeed, inducers and fasting had additive effects on the hepatotoxicity of paracetamol in rats.[33]

Clinical features of hepatitis due to direct toxicity

Hepatitis caused by direct toxicity is not associated with hypersensitivity manifestations, and an inadvertent rechallenge does not lead to a prompter recurrence. The liver injury may have a relatively high frequency, consistent with direct toxicity. As explained above, it may be favoured by either genetic or acquired metabolic factors. It is important, however, to realize that metabolic factors will also influence immunologically mediated hepatitis.

For many drugs the formation of reactive metabolites may be so low that, even in metabolically susceptible subjects, this formation

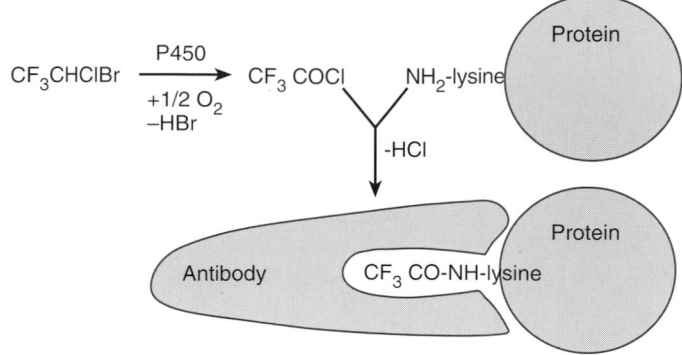

Fig. 3. Metabolism of halothane into neoantigens. Oxidation of halothane by cytochrome P-450 leads to a reactive trifluoroacetyl chloride which triflouroacetylates hepatic proteins on their lysine residues. In patients with halothane hepatitis, there are antibodies that recognize trifluoroacetylated hepatic proteins.

may at most cause mild transaminitis, but no major cell demise. Such drugs will not produce toxic liver cell necrosis. They may nevertheless produce severe hepatitis in a few subjects by interacting with the second xenophobic system of animals, namely the immune system.

The immune system

The necessity of fighting bacterial, fungal, or viral infections has led to the development of the macrophagic and immune systems in animals. The latter is based:

(1) on the acquisition, during evolution, of major histocompatibility complex molecules that can each present different sets of peptides on the cell surface;

(2) on the development, in each individual, by somatic mutation, of a whole panoply of helper T lymphocytes able to recognize among these peptides those which are foreign.[34]

The ability of viruses directly to transfect neighbouring cells has required that one of the effector strategies of the immune system should be the immunological destruction of the infected cells.

The superposition of the cytochrome P-450 and the immune system created an additional problem for animals. Indeed the covalent binding of a reactive metabolite to proteins modifies the Self of the individual. In some subjects, this modification may 'mislead' the immune system into mounting an immune attack against hepatocytes.[7] This immune attack may be directed either against the modified Self or against the unmodified Self.

Immune attack directed against the modified Self: hypothetical mechanisms

The best studied example of immunoallergic drug-induced hepatitis is the severe form of halothane hepatitis. Halothane is oxidized by cytochrome P-450 into a reactive acyl chloride (CF_3COCl) that reacts with the ε-NH_2-group of the lysine residues of proteins to form trifluoroacetylated proteins (CF_3CO-lysine-proteins) (Fig. 3).[35] In the serum of patients with severe halothane hepatitis, one finds antibodies which are directed against the parts of hepatic proteins that are modified by the covalent attachment of the trifluoroacetyl group (Fig. 3).[36,37]

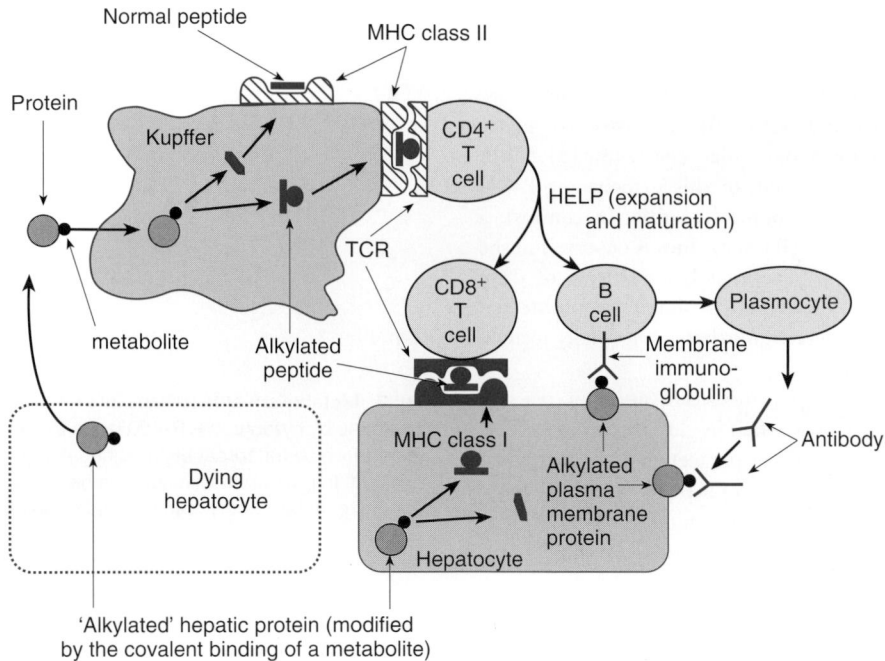

Fig. 4. Hypothetical mechanisms of immunization by, and against, the modified Self.

It remains unknown how these antibodies appear. Figure 4, nevertheless, shows a possible scenario.[7]

In order to stimulate CD4+ helper T lymphocytes, immunogenic peptides must first be presented on the cell surface by major histocompatibility complex class II molecules.[34] Major histocompatibility complex class II molecules are not normally expressed by hepatocytes,[38] but are expressed by Kupffer cells, sinusoidal endothelial cells (Rieder, JHepatol, 1992; 15:237), and B lymphocytes. It is therefore tempting to speculate on the following mechanism.[7] During the turnover of hepatocytes, and particularly if this normally slow turnover is accelerated by mild, direct toxicity of the metabolite, proteins from dying hepatocytes may be phagocytosed by antigen presenting cells, such as macrophages (Fig. 4). Inside these cells the protein is degraded into small peptides, some of which are then presented on the cell surface by major histocompatibility complex class II molecules (Fig. 4).

If a subject has taken a drug leading to the 'alkylation' of hepatic proteins (i.e. the covalent binding of a reactive metabolite to these proteins), degradation of these alkylated proteins will form not only normal peptides, but also alkylated peptides (Fig. 4).

Normal peptides are not recognized by helper T lymphocytes, because autoreactive T lymphocytes are normally deleted. In contrast, alkylated peptides are different from the Self of the individual. In the enormous pool of different helper T cells, some of them may be able to recognize these modified structures on the surface of the antigen-presenting cell (Fig. 4).

This recognition may stimulate the helper T lymphocyte, which will provide local help (through the release of cytokines) to effector immune cells that are also present because they have been able to recognize modified structures on hepatocytes.

A first type of effector cells that might be locally present are cytotoxic CD8+ T lymphocytes (Fig. 4). Indeed, hepatocytes express major histocompatibility complex class I molecules on their surface, and this expression is further increased as soon as the inflammatory reaction develops.[38] These major histocompatibility complex class I molecules may present alkylated peptides, that might serve as molecular anchors for the attachment of CD8+ cytotoxic T lymphocytes (Fig. 4). Local help provided by the neighbouring helper T cells may then lead to the clonal expansion of these cytotoxic T lymphocytes.

A second type of effector cells that might be locally present are immature B lymphocytes expressing on their surface a membrane immunoglobulin able to recognize alkylated proteins on the plasma membrane (Fig. 4). After exposure to halothane, trifluoroacetylated proteins are found on the surface of hepatocytes.[39] Similarly, after exposure to isaxonine (another drug transformed into reactive metabolites and causing immunoallergic hepatitis) there are alkylated proteins on the plasma membrane.[40] Some B lymphocytes might have an immunoglobin able to recognize these neoantigens on the hepatocyte surface. The local help which is provided by the neighbouring helper T cells may then lead to the clonal expansion of these immature B lymphocytes and their maturation into plasmocytes. These plasmocytes will secrete an antibody with the same specificity as that of the initial membrane immunoglobulin, and therefore directed against the alkylated plasma membrane proteins (Fig. 4).

These alkylated plasma membrane proteins may then serve as antigenic targets for the antibodies (antialkylated proteins) that are secreted by the plasmocytes (Fig. 4). Indeed, the incubation of hepatocytes from rabbits exposed to halothane (leading to the trifluoroacetylation of plasma membrane proteins) with sera from patients with halothane hepatitis (containing antibodies against trifluroacetylated proteins) that had been previously adsorbed to untreated rabbit hepatocytes (thereby removing any antibody against normal rabbit hepatic proteins), followed by the addition of peripheral blood mononuclear cells from normal subjects, led to the immune destruction of the halothane-treated hepatocytes.[37] A similar antibody-dependent, cell-mediated cytotoxicity was reported with the sera of patients with hepatitis due to α-methyldopa,[41] tienilic acid,[42] or clometacin.[43]

Immune attack directed against the Self: anticytochrome P-450 autoantibodies

With a few drugs, the immune attack is directed, in part, against normal, unmodified epitopes of proteins. Some of these autoantigens are cytochrome P-450s themselves. Cases of drug-induced hepatitis associated with anticytochrome P-450 auto-antibodies have been classified as 'autoimmune' hepatitis (although the relationship between these autoantibodies and the destruction of hepatocytes remains to be proven).

Tienilic acid-induced hepatitis is associated with a particular antiliver/kidney microsome autoantibody, the anti-LKM$_2$ auto-antibody.[44] This antibody is specifically directed against human cytochrome P-450 2C9, that is the isoenzyme which transforms tienilic acid into a reactive metabolite that covalently binds to the cytochrome P-450 2C9 protein.[44] Similarly, dihydralazine hepatitis is associated with antiliver microsome autoantibodies directed against cytochrome P-450 1A2,[45] that is the isoenzyme which oxidizes dihydralazine into reactive radicals that covalently bind to the cytochrome P-450 1A2 protein.[46] These antibodies exhibit a high affinity for the non-alkylated cytochromes P-450 of untreated subjects, and are therefore clearly autoantibodies.

Presence of cytochrome P-450 on the plasma membrane

Cytochrome P-450 is synthesized on polyribosomes attached to the endoplasmic reticulum membrane, and is cotranslationally inserted in this membrane, where it remains anchored by at least one transmembrane fragment (Fig. 1). There is an extensive flow of vesicles going from the endoplasmic reticulum to the Golgi apparatus, and from there to the plasma membrane, thanks to molecular motors that draw these vesicles along microtubules (Pryer, AnnRevBiochem, 1992; 61:471). Neosynthesized cytochrome P-450 partly follows this vesicular route to reach the plasma membrane in rats.[47]

When various anticytochrome P-450 autoantibodies were added to uncut, non-permeabilized, and fixed rat or human hepatocytes (thus, under conditions precluding the entry of the antibody into the cells), immunofluorescent and immunoperoxidase labelling of the plasma membrane was obtained,[48,49] showing that these autoantibodies recognized cytochrome P-450 epitopes expressed on the surface of hepatocytes. It is thus tempting to speculate that these autoantibodies might participate in the immunological destruction of hepatocytes.[49]

Hypothetical mechanism for the appearance of anticytochrome P-450 autoantibodies

Mechanisms leading to anticytochrome P-450 autoantibodies remain entirely unknown. The hypothesis presented in Fig. 5 is nevertheless attractive.[7,50]

It is known that some B lymphocytes may be autoreactive, but remain normally quiescent because they are not stimulated by helper T cells (as shall be explained later).

Let us consider such an autoreactive B cell that would express on its surface a membrane immunoglobulin recognizing a normal, unalkylated epitope of cytochrome P-450 2C9 (Fig. 5). After the death of a hepatocyte and the release of its contents, the autoreactive B cell may then cap the cytochrome P-450 2C9 protein (by binding to its normal epitope). If the subject has taken tienilic acid, the cytochrome P-450 2C9 protein will be alkylated by a reactive metabolite of tienilic acid on its active site and, therefore, in a position likely to be different from that of the epitope recognized by the autoreactive B cell (Fig. 5). After internalization and fragmentation of the cytochrome P-450 protein, the B lymphocyte will express on its surface (on major histocompatibility complex class II molecules) both normal peptides and alkylated peptides (Fig. 5).

Normally, there are no helper T cells able to recognize the normal peptides, which explains why the immature autoreactive B cell normally remains quiescent. In contrast, the alkylated peptides (modified Self) may be recognized by some helper T cells. This will lead to the clonal expansion of the B lymphocyte and its maturation into plasmocytes. These plasmocytes will secrete an antibody with the same specificity as that of the initial immunoglobulin, and therefore directed against the normal epitope of cytochrome P-450 2C9 (Fig. 5). Albeit hypothetical, this mechanism might explain the appearance of an immune reaction directed against the unmodified Self when part of the molecule has been modified by the covalent binding of a metabolite (modified Self).

Mixed immune reactions

Thus, the presence of the modified Self may trigger an immune attack directed against either the modified Self (Fig. 4) or the unmodified Self (Fig. 5). It is therefore not surprising that a single drug, such as tienilic acid or halothane, may concomitantly give rise to both types of immune reactions.[50]

Because mechanisms leading to the destruction of hepatocytes may be intertwined, the distinction between 'immunoallergic' hepatitis (reaction against the modified Self) and 'autoimmune' hepatitis (reaction against the Self) may be largely academic.

Discrete direct toxicity as a permissive factor for severe immune hepatitis

Suggested mechanisms for immunization (Figs 4 and 5) presuppose the release of alkylated hepatic proteins (modified Self) and their uptake by antigen presenting cells. If this is correct, any mild toxic effect of the metabolite (leading to the release of alkylated hepatic proteins) should greatly increase the likelihood of immunization. Indeed, many drugs (including halothane), that produce immunoallergic hepatitis in a few patients, also lead to a mild increase in serum transaminase activity in a much larger proportion of recipients, suggesting direct toxicity. The view might be held, therefore, that discrete direct toxicity may be a permissive (but not sufficient) factor for immunization to develop. This might account, in part, for the role of genetic, metabolic factors in the frequency of immune hepatitis.

Genetic factors influencing drug-induced immune hepatitis

Although all subjects probably form the reactive metabolite to some extent, only a few develop immunoallergic and/or autoimmune

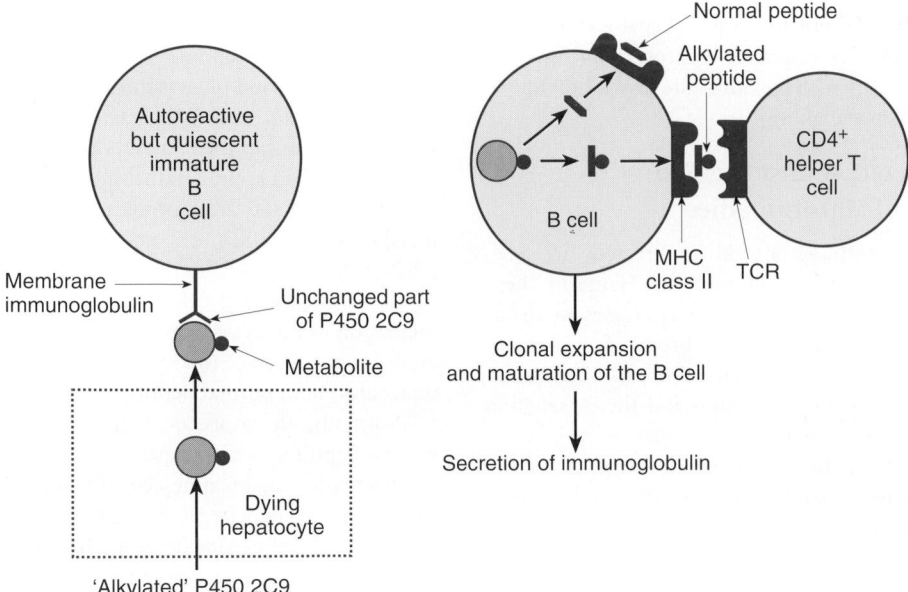

Fig. 5. Hypothetical mechanism whereby the modified Self may lead to immunization against the Self (anticytochrome P-450 autoantibodies).

hepatitis. Two types of genetic factors may explain the particular susceptibility of these few subjects.

A first type of genetic factor may affect hepatic drug metabolism. As explained above, the modification of Self due to the covalent binding of the reactive metabolites may be the initial stimulus leading to immunization. If some subjects are deficient in a metabolic pathway that normally diverts the drug away from the formation of reactive metabolites, or that normally inactivates this reactive metabolite, these deficient subjects may undergo extensive alkylation of their hepatic proteins. Perhaps more importantly, defects in protective mechanisms might allow the threshold to be crossed between a total lack of direct toxicity and a discrete form of direct toxicity that will lead to the release of alkylated hepatic proteins and their uptake by antigen presenting cells.

In rapid acetylators, dihydralazine,[46] and sulphonamides[51] are detoxified by acetylation. In slow acetylators, however, this protective pathway is deficient and a greater proportion of the dose is now transformed by cytochromes P-450 into reactive metabolites, leading to a higher incidence of immune hepatic reactions.[46,51]

Using a lymphocyte cytotoxicity assay, it has been suggested that some inherited deficit(s) in the inactivation of the reactive metabolites may favour immune drug-induced hepatitis.[51–54] Lymphocytes are very poor in cytochrome P-450 so that the reactive metabolite has to be formed by an artificial extracellular system (drug + murine microsomes + NADPH + air). Being standardized, this system produces a constant amount of reactive metabolite. Human lymphocytes are exposed to this metabolite-generating system. Although poor in cytochrome P-450, lymphocytes contain all the protective systems (such as epoxide hydrolase, glutathione, glutathione S-transferases, glutathione peroxidase, and vitamin E). If the lymphocytes of some subjects are deficient in some of these protective mechanisms, they will not detoxify the metabolite as well and will suffer increased lethality. The deficiency, being genetic, should be observed not only in subjects with drug-induced hepatitis, but also in their family members. With this technique, it has been reported that immunoallergic hepatitis due to phenytoin, sulphonamides, halothane, and amineptine may occur selectively in subjects with a genetic deficiency in a protective mechanism.[51–54] Since the deficit has never been delineated, however, one may wonder whether the test does indeed reflect deficits in inactivating mechanisms (as it is supposed to do), or instead reflects the inherited ability of lymphocytes to present alkylated peptides and undergo activation-triggered apoptosis.[7]

A second type of genetic factor that may modify the susceptibility of subjects to develop immune reactions is the polymorphism of major histocompatibility complex molecules. Major histocompatibility complex molecules, also termed human leucocyte antigen (**HLA**) molecules in humans, are extremely polymorphic. Each HLA molecule presents different, largely non-overlapping, sets of peptides.[34] Having one or another HLA molecule may favour or not favour the presentation of an alkylated immunogenic peptide. Indeed, drug-induced hepatitis may occur more frequently in subjects with a particular HLA molecule: HLA A11 in hepatitis due to halothane, tricyclic antidepressants, or diclofenac; HLA DR6 in hepatitis caused by chlorpromazine or nitrofurantoin; HLA B8 in clometacin hepatitis.[55]

Clinical characteristics of immunoallergic and autoimmune hepatitis

Hepatitis due to immune mechanisms has a low frequency (but this may be true also in idiosyncratic hepatitis due to direct toxicity). The frequency of immunologically mediated hepatitis (as that of hepatitis due to direct toxicity) may be influenced by either genetic or acquired metabolic factors (such as defects in protective mechanisms or microsomal enzyme induction).

However, immunoallergic hepatitis is frequently associated with hypersensitivity manifestations, such as fever, rash, and blood eosinophilia, and a marked inflammatory cell infiltrate in the liver, with, sometimes, eosinophils or granulomas. Immunoallergic hepatitis promptly recurs after an inadvertent drug rechallenge, sometimes after a single tablet. In some cases (halothane, tienilic acid, clometacin, α-methyldopa) the patients' sera have been shown to contain antibodies directed against hepatic neoantigens.

Cases of 'autoimmune' drug-induced hepatitis have related characteristics. However, hypersensitivity manifestations might be less frequent, and chronic liver lesions more common, in autoimmune hepatitis than in immunoallergic hepatitis.[7] Autoantibodies against hepatic proteins are present. Although corticosteroids have seemed helpful in individual cases, their efficacy remains unproven. First, no controlled trial has been reported. Second, the mere interruption of the treatment suppresses the initial stimulus for immunization (the modification of Self due to the covalent binding of the reactive metabolite), and is associated both with a progressive decrease in the autoantibody titres and with the patient's recovery.

Overview of the role of the cytochrome P-450 and immune systems

Animals are fundamentally xenophobic. They have evolved two systems to eliminate, respectively, the xenobiotics contained in the plants that they ingest (the hepatic cytochrome P-450 system) and the micro-organisms that attacked them (the immune system).

The strategy used by the first system relies on a whole array of cytochrome P-450s able to metabolize and thereby eliminate liposolube xenobiotics (and drugs). Although this system has the inconvenience of forming reactive metabolites, their adverse consequences are largely prevented by a host of protective mechanisms. Only huge amounts of the xenobiotic, the extensive metabolism of a particular xenobiotic, or genetic or acquired susceptibility factors will lead to direct toxicity and either apoptosis or necrosis.

Investigational molecules that would lead to extensive alkylation of hepatic constituents, and constant hepatitis at therapeutic doses, are not marketed. Drugs are released for human use only when the alkylation of hepatic constituents remains below the threshold for liver cell demise, at least in most recipients. In a few metabolically susceptible patients, however, this threshold may be exceeded with some drugs, producing severe hepatitis due to direct toxicity.

Most marketed drugs, however, may never reach the threshold for massive liver cell demise, although the threshold for mild toxicity may be reached in a few metabolically susceptible subjects. In most of these subjects, this will just produce a mild, asymptomatic increase in ALT activity. In a minority of these few subjects, however, the release of hepatic neoantigens may interfere with the immune system.

The immune system has evolved to recognize and destroy micro-organisms and/or cells that harbour them. The system is based on the presentation of peptides on the cell surface and the recognition of those that are foreign by lymphocytes. A reactive metabolite that has been formed by cytochrome P-450 and has covalently bound to hepatic proteins may be considered as 'foreign'. The immune system may then apply its programme for the immunological destruction of the 'infected' cells, leading to drug-induced immunoallergic or autoimmune hepatitis. These immune reactions may represent the main cause of drug-induced hepatitis. They may lead to cytolytic, cholestatic, or mixed hepatitis.

Acute cytolytic hepatitis

Elevated serum transaminase activity is the main hallmark of acute 'cytolytic' hepatitis, reflecting the release of intracellular enzymes from dying hepatocytes. Other features are more variable and depend on the severity of the disease. Indeed, with increasing degrees of liver cell necrosis, four patterns can be distinguished, each being characterized by the addition of new symptoms above those already present in milder forms:

(1) 'transaminitis' (isolated increases in ALT activity, without any clinical sign);
(2) 'anicteric hepatitis' (nausea, vomiting, abdominal pain, fever, anorexia, or asthenia, but without jaundice);
(3) 'icteric hepatitis' (with jaundice, but without encephalopathy);
(4) 'fulminant hepatitis' (with hepatic encephalopathy). When, at the same time, factor V becomes less than 20 per cent of normal, the spontaneous prognosis is usually very poor and liver transplantation must be considered. This possibility of severe liver damage is the main concern in this type of drug-induced liver disease.

Fortunately, these various forms of cytolytic hepatitis do not have the same frequency. As a general rule, asymptomatic increases in ALT activity may be 10 times more frequent than icteric cases, which may themselves be 10 times more frequent than fulminant ones. With some drugs (e.g. alpidem, iproniazid), however, the proportion of fulminant cases may be higher.

Features which distinguish cases due to direct toxicity from those involving immune reactions have been described above (in the section dealing with mechanisms of acute hepatitis).

A liver biopsy is rarely performed in obvious or mild forms, but may be useful in difficult, severe cases. The main liver lesion is hepatocellular necrosis. With some drugs, such as halothane[4] or paracetamol,[56] necrosis is characteristically centrilobular. With other agents, however, such as α-methyldopa,[57] liver cell necrosis may have a more diffuse pattern, resembling that of viral hepatitis. In some cases, macrovacuolar steatosis may also be present. As in all cases of hepatitis, there is at least some degree of inflammation; this may be moderate in hepatitis due to direct toxicity and extensive in cases due to immune reactions; in the latter case, eosinophils and, sometimes, granulomas may be present.

The differential diagnosis of acute drug-induced hepatitis is mainly concerned with viral hepatitis. This is made easier nowadays with the availability of serological markers for hepatitis A, B and C, Epstein-Barr virus (EBV), and cytomegalovirus, and the possible detection of HBV DNA and HCV RNA in serum. Some cases may be more difficult, however. Hepatitis E should be considered in patients returning from a trip to Asia or Africa. The anti-HCV antibody may be absent at the onset of the liver disease and only appear on a subsequent sample. Persons with chronic viral disease are not immune against drug-induced hepatitis. Sudden deterioration of liver tests in these patients may be due to drugs as well as reactivation, seroconversion, or surinfection.

Another important differential diagnosis is a transient low output syndrome, producing liver ischaemia and centrilobular liver cell necrosis. The episode of shock may have been transient and unrecorded. This diagnosis should be suspected in elderly patients with cardiac arrhythmias or cardiac failure, particularly when the liver failure is associated with azotaemia. Rapid improvement of the liver and kidney function once the cardiac output is restored may be striking. Careful questioning about a possible episode of arrhythmias and/or shock, and results of the ECG, cardiac ultrasonography, and haemodynamic investigations may suggest the diagnosis that can be confirmed by a transvenous liver biopsy.

Drugs causing acute hepatitis

Many drugs may cause acute hepatocellular necrosis (Table 4) but only the most commonly involved drugs (either because they are frequently hepatotoxic or because they are widely used) are discussed individually below. The reader must also consult the section concerning drugs that produce mixed hepatitis, as several of those drugs can also produce hepatocellular damage in an individual patient (for example captopril, cimetidine, lovastatin, simvastatin, oxacillin, tricyclic antidepressants, phenindione, phenylbutazone, sulphonamides, and verapamil).

Acebutol

Six cases of hepatitis possibly due to this β-adrenergic receptor antagonist had been reported to the Food and Drug Administration in 1988 (Tanner, AnnIntMed, 1989; 111:533). Hepatitis exhibited a hepatocellular or mixed pattern, and was usually associated with fever. Two patients were rechallenged, with recurrence within 2 days, suggesting an immune mechanism.

Acitretin

This aromatic retinoid is the non-esterified analogue (and a metabolite) of etretinate. Like etretinate, it is teratogenic. Pregnancy must be avoided during and long after its administration, owing to its prolonged retention in the body. As with etretinate, monitoring of liver function tests is advised. Acitretin may increase ALT activity in 17 per cent of recipients, and a few cases of clinical hepatitis have been observed.[2]

Alpidem

Because of its hepatotoxic potential, this anxiolytic agent had to be recalled. Cytolytic hepatitis was not alarmingly frequent but it frequently had a severe, subfulminant course leading to liver transplantation or death.

Allopurinol

Allopurinol can occasionally cause liver injury, particularly in persons receiving diuretics or those with compromised renal function.[58] Hepatitis occurs mostly during the first month of treatment. The liver injury is predominantly hepatocellular. Fulminant hepatitis is possible. Hepatic granulomas are observed in about 50 per cent of cases. These granulomas, and the frequent occurrence of fever, rash, and eosinophilia (both peripheral and hepatic) suggest an allergic mechanism.

Amodiaquine

This antimalarial drug may cause hepatocellular jaundice and even fulminant hepatitis.[59] It is not clear whether hepatitis is due to direct toxicity, immunoallergy, or possibly both (in different patients). Amodiaquine undergoes autoxidation into a reactive quinoneimine (Maggs, BiochemPharm, 1987; 36:2061).

Aspirin

The hepatotoxicity of aspirin has been reviewed by Zimmerman.[60] Hepatitis occurs after one to several weeks of treatment with full doses of aspirin. It is due to the toxic effects of the salicylate moiety. Salicylate levels higher than 25 mg/dl are likely to lead to hepatic injury, while levels lower than 15 mg/dl rarely do.[60] Hepatic injury is often silent, or at least anicteric; liver histology shows ballooning and focal necrosis. However, a few severe cases, with hepatic encephalopathy, have been described.[60]

Utilization of aspirin during viral infections favours the secondary development of Reye's syndrome in children (see 'Microvesicular steatosis').[61]

Clometacin

This analgesic was a frequent cause of hepatitis in France. Hepatitis occurred mainly in elderly females, possibly reflecting greater use in this group. The drug caused acute hepatocellular jaundice,[62] as well as chronic hepatitis or cirrhosis. Occurrence of fever, rash, eosinophilia, thrombocytopenia, interstitial nephritis, antismooth muscle, and antidouble-stranded DNA autoantibodies, and the frequency of the HLA B8 antigen in affected patients, all suggested an allergic mechanism. The drug is no longer used in France.

Cocaine

It is thought that 22 million Americans have used cocaine at least once and 5 million use it regularly (Kothur, ArchIntMed, 1991; 151:1126). Fifteen per cent of hospitalized, non-parenteral cocaine users presented mild elevation of liver enzyme level (Kothur, ArchIntMed, 1991; 151:1126). Acute cocaine intoxication may also lead to a severe syndrome that typically associates hyperpyrexia, hypotension, disseminated intravascular coagulation, acute renal failure, rhabdomyolysis, and severe hepatic dysfunction (Silva, JHepatol, 1991; 12:312). In these patients, a massive increases in ALT activity occurs within the first 48 h after admission, and liver lesions consist of both pericentral coagulative necrosis and periportal microvesicular steatosis (Silva, JHepatol, 1991; 12:312). Although both hypotension and hyperthermia may participate in the pathogenesis of these lesions, a direct toxicity of cocaine has been demonstrated in several in vitro studies (reviewed in Mallat, JHepatol, 1991; 12:275).

Cocaine is transformed by cytochrome P-450 into norcocaine, which is further oxidized to N-hydroxynorcocaine, norcocaine nitroxide, and norcocaine nitrosonium ion. These metabolites may cause an oxidative stress and lipid peroxidation in hepatocytes (Mallat, JHepatol, 1991; 12:275). In animals, toxicity is enhanced by inducers (phenobarbital, ethanol) of cytochrome P-450 and is prevented by cytochrome P-450 inhibitors (Mallat, JHepatol, 1991; 12:275).

Cyproterone acetate

This synthetic steroid, which is used in oral contraceptives and antiandrogen formulations, may produce minor abnormalities in liver function tests. However, in several elderly patients treated for either prostatic or breast cancers, it has instead produced fulminant hepatitis without clinical or biochemical manifestations of hypersensitivity (Hirsh; IsrJMedSci, 1994; 30:238). The drug may also lead to hepatocellular carcinoma (see hepatic tumours).

Dantrolene

Prolonged administration of dantrolene increased serum transaminase activity in 1 to 8 per cent of recipients, and produced jaundice in 0.6 per cent.[63] Hepatitis usually occurred from the second to the fifth month of treatment, but not during the first.[63] The injury was mainly cytolytic, with a pattern of either acute, subacute, or chronic hepatitis and a fatality rate of 28 per cent.[63] Hypersensitivity manifestations were uncommon.

Diclofenac

Diclofenac is among the most widely used anti-inflammatory drugs, worldwide. Due to this enormous use, several hundreds of cases of hepatitis have been observed, although the frequency appears low.[64] Hepatitis due to diclofenac is mainly hepatocellular, although some forms may be mixed or cholestatic. Hypersensitivity manifestations have been observed in a few patients, but are relatively uncommon. It remains unknown at present whether hepatitis is due to direct toxicity, immune mechanisms, or both.

Dihydralazine

Dihydralazine hepatitis occurs a few weeks to several months after the onset of treatment with this antihypertensive drug.[65] Hepatitis is hepatocellular. It may be associated, in a few cases, with fever, or blood eosinophilia, and may recur quickly after an inadvertent drug rechallenge. Antismooth muscle, antimitochondrial, and antimicrosomal autoantibodies have been observed. The antimicrosomal antibodies are directed against the cytochrome P-450 1A2 isoenzyme which transforms dihydralazine into reactive radicals.[45,46] Slow acetylators are at increased risk of developing hepatitis.[46]

Disulfiram

Use of this drug in alcoholics (as an antiabuse agent) has long delayed recognition of its hepatotoxicity. Disulfiram-induced liver injury has occurred, however, in non-alcoholic patients, and has been proven by rechallenge in many alcoholics.[3] Disulfiram is widely used in some countries and was the fourth leading cause of drug-induced liver injury in a Danish study (Friis, JIntMed, 1992; 232:133). The drug is transformed into reactive metabolites (Yourick, BiochemPharm, 1991; 42:1361), and causes abnormal liver biochemistry in 25 per cent of recipients during the first weeks of the treatment.[3] This high incidence suggests some direct toxicity.

However, clinically relevant liver cell necrosis occurs in a few subjects only. The onset is usually within the first 2 months of treatment, but may be more delayed. Disulfiram hepatitis is usually hepatocellular, and at least 10 cases of fulminant hepatitis have been reported (Forns, JHepatol, 1994; 21:853). There is a mixed cell infiltrate, usually including eosinophils. Although extrahepatic hypersensitivity manifestations are usually absent, this eosinophilic infiltrate, and the prompt and exaggerated response after rechallenge, may suggest an immune mechanism in these severe cases.

'Ecstasy' (3,4-methylenedioxymethamphetamine)

This illicit, synthetic amphetamine derivative, known as 'ecstasy', is increasingly used as a recreational drug. Its use combined with vigorous exercise at all-night dance sessions can produce a syndrome reminiscent of that caused by cocaine intoxication, with hyperthermia, hypotension, disseminated intravascular coagulation, rhabdomyolysis, acute renal failure, acute hepatic failure, and death (Brown, JAMA, 1987; 258:780). Ecstasy-induced liver injury may also present independently, a few days to 4 weeks after ingestion of the drug, as mixed hepatitis in young patients (Dyskhuizen, Gut, 1995; 36:939). Ecstasy use should be specifically sought in all young patients with 'unexplained' jaundice.

Enflurane

Hepatitis caused by this volatile anaesthetic closely resembles halothane hepatitis.[66] Like halothane, enflurane is transformed into reactive acyl halide metabolites which can lead to immunoallergic hepatitis (Christ, DrugMetDisp, 1988; 16:135).

Etretinate

Like acitretin, this aromatic retinoid is used in the treatment of psoriasis. Like acitretin, it is teratogenic, and pregnancy must be avoided during, and long after, its administration (its half-life is 120 days). It is also hepatotoxic and liver function tests must be monitored.[3] The drug produces liver function test abnormalities in 10 to 25 per cent of subjects and has been responsible for several cases of severe liver cell necrosis. Fever may be present in some cases, and the inflammatory infiltrate of portal tracts may contain eosinophils; positive rechallenges to small doses of etretinate have been observed. Due to the drug's long half-life, features of hepatitis can appear and/or the patient's condition may deteriorate after discontinuation of the treatment, with the possible development of chronic hepatitis and cirrhosis.[3] Corticosteroids have seemed helpful in some of these deteriorating cases.

Felbamate

This antiepileptic drug may cause frequent cytolytic hepatitis in addition to severe blood dyscrasias. Its use has been largely restricted to patients whose seizures are not prevented by the other, much safer, antiepileptic drugs.

Fipexide

This cognition activator is proposed in asthenia and memory disorders. The drug has produced fulminant hepatitis in three patients (Durand, JHepatol, 1992; 15:144).

Germander and other medicinal plants

Germander had been used since ancient time as a 'medicinal' drug. However, soon after its marketing and large-scale utilization as an 'adjuvant' to weight control regimens in France, an epidemic of acute hepatitis has led to the recall of all preparations containing this plant.[67] The furano neo-clerodane diterpenoids of germander are transformed by cytochromes P-450 3A into hepatotoxic metabolites.[22]

The list is rapidly growing of supposedly harmless herbal remedies which have been found to be hepatotoxic in humans. In addition to the pyrrolizidine alkaloids that cause veno-occlusive disease and shall be considered in another section, the list includes mistletoe (Harvey, BMJ, 1981; 282:186), skullcap (MacGregor, BMJ, 1989; 299:1156; Miskelly, PostgradMedJ, 1992; 68:935), chaparral leaf (Katz, JClinGastro, 1990; 12:203), senna fruit extracts (Beuers, Lancet, 1991; 337:372), and various Chinese herbal remedies used to treat eczema and psoriasis (Davies, Lancet, 1990; 336: 177; Perharic-Walton, Lancet, 1992; 340:673) or the Jin Bu Huan Anodyne tablets that are sold as a sedative and analgesic (Woolf, AnnIntMed, 1994; 121:729). Clearly, herbal remedies should be subjected to the same exhaustive premarketing tests and post-marketing surveillance as man-made chemicals. The actual composition, safety, and importation of folklore herbal remedies from developing countries should be better controlled.

Glafenine

This analgesic has produced hepatocellular jaundice in a few patients.[3] This adverse effect and other allergic manifestations have led to its recall.

Halothane

Halothane accounted for 25 per cent of the cases of drug-induced hepatitis reported to the Danish committee on adverse drug reactions between 1978 and 1987 (Friis, JIntMed, 1992; 232:133). Halothane is transformed by cytochrome P-450 via both an oxidative and a reductive pathway (Sipes, JPharmExpTher, 1980; 214:716). Both pathways lead to reactive metabolites. The reductive pathway produces a reactive radical ($CF_3\bullet CHCl$) which, under special conditions (usually microsomal enzyme induction plus hypoxia) may lead to direct hepatotoxicity in animals (Ross, Anesthesiol, 1979; 51:327). Conceivably, this toxic mechanism may also explain the silent increase in transaminase activity seen in a number of human recipients (Wright, Lancet, 1975; ii:817).

The oxidative pathway forms a reactive acyl chloride (CF_3COCl) which binds covalently to hepatic proteins, including plasma membrane proteins (see section on mechanisms of acute hepatitis). These trifluoroacetylated proteins can lead to immunization and to the severe form of hepatitis seen in exceptional subjects.

This severe form of hepatitis has all the characteristics of an allergic phenomenon:[4]

1. It is extremely uncommon (1/10 000) after a first anaesthesia and occurs within 2 weeks of this first procedure.
2. Jaundice is more frequent (7/10 000) after a repeated exposure and occurs sooner. The mean interval between exposure and onset of jaundice is 12 days after a first exposure, 7 days after a second, and 5 days after a third exposure.[4]
3. Jaundice is frequently associated with fever (75 per cent) and eosinophilia (40 per cent).
4. Sera from patients with severe halothane hepatitis contain antibodies against trifluoroacetylated plasma membrane proteins.[36, 37]

Halothane hepatitis is hepatocellular in type, and may lead to fulminant hepatitis requiring transplantation. Prevention may be obtained by preferring isoflurane (which may cause hepatitis, but less frequently) or, at least, by avoiding repeated exposure to halothane, particularly at short intervals.[68] These precautions are not always adhered to, and halothane hepatitis is still a major problem in some countries, including France.

Hydralazine

This antihypertensive drug may cause hepatocellular jaundice.[69] Fever, rash, eosinophilia, and, at times, hepatic granulomas (Jori, Gastro, 1973; 64:1163) may be seen in some patients. The acetylation of hydralazine is under genetic control; slow acetylators are at higher risk of developing anti-DNA autoantibodies and a systemic lupus erythematosus-like syndrome (Ludden, ClinPharmacokin, 1982; 7: 185). The role of the acetylator phenotype, if any, in the hepatotoxicity of hydralazine is unknown, however.

Hydralazine forms reactive free radicals (Sinha, BBResComm, 1982; 105:1044).

Isoniazid given alone or in combination with rifampicin

Isoniazid given alone increases serum transaminase activity in 10 per cent of patients, and causes clinical hepatitis in 1 per cent.[70] The peak incidence of hepatitis occurs during the second month of therapy.[70] Hepatitis is cytolytic, usually without hypersensitivity manifestations.

Isoniazid is transformed into a reactive metabolite toxic to the liver (Mitchell, Gastro, 1975; 68:392). Isoniazid is first acetylated into acetylisoniazid, which is hydrolysed into acetylhydrazine. Acetylhydrazine may be either acetylated again, into the non-toxic diacetylhydrazine, or may be transformed by cytochrome P-450 into the reactive acetyl radical which binds covalently to hepatic proteins (Timbrell, ClinPharmTher, 1977; 22:602).

The acetylation of isoniazid (and several other drugs) is under genetic control. About 40 per cent of Caucasians and Negroes, but 90 per cent of Japanese, are rapid acetylators of isoniazid (Ellard, ClinPharmTher, 1976; 19:608). The acetylator phenotype influences both the acetylation of isoniazid and that of acetylhydrazine. Thus, rapid acetylators form acetylhydrazine at a faster rate, but at the same time, detoxify it to diacetylhydrazine at a faster rate (Timbrell, ClinPharmTher, 1977; 22:602). This complex situation may explain why divergent findings have been obtained regarding the influence of the acetylator phenotype on the hepatotoxicity of isoniazid.

Rifampicin (rifampin) given alone, is not, or is seldom, hepatotoxic (Emerit, RevFrMalResp, 1974; 2:565), and mainly produces cholestatic liver injury. However, in patients receiving both rifampicin and isoniazid, the incidence of cytolytic hepatitis is higher than with isoniazid alone, reaching 5 to 8 per cent, and hepatitis occurs sooner, mainly during the first month of treatment (Emerit, RevFrMalResp, 1974; 2:565; Lees, Tubercle, 1971; 52:182). Fulminant isoniazid–rifampicin hepatitis develops even earlier, after about 1 week of treatment.[29]

It has been suggested that rifampicin, a microsomal enzyme inducer (Pessayre, BiochemPharm, 1976; 25:943), might increase the formation of the reactive isoniazid metabolite, and might thereby potentiate the hepatotoxicity of isoniazid in humans. This hypothesis has not been proved, however, and other explanations might be involved.

We believe that liver function tests should be monitored in patients receiving these antituberculous drugs, including during the first days of the treatment, then every week during the first month, and every month thereafter. Isoniazid should be withdrawn, temporarily or definitively, if ALT activities exceed three times the upper limit of normal.

Iproniazid

Although withdrawn from clinical use in the United States, iproniazid is still used in some countries, including France. The drug may lead to cytolytic jaundice, which occurs mainly during the first 3 months of treatment.[71] Interestingly, hepatitis may start 4 weeks after the discontinuance of iproniazid.[71] Although interruption of the treatment led to recovery in 80 per cent of affected patients, in the remainder, however, the disease continued to progress, eventually leading to death.[71] Iproniazid hepatitis is usually associated with a particular antimitochondrial autoantibody, the anti-M_6 autoantibody.[72,73] Iproniazid is transformed by cytochrome P-450 into the reactive isopropyl radical which binds covalently to hepatic proteins (Nelson, JPharmExpTher, 1978; 206:574). Iproniazid is also activated into reactive metabolites by the mitochondrial monoamine oxidase, and this may account for the development of the anti-M_6 autoantibodies. Whether these autoantibodies have a pathogenic role remains to be determined. However, an autoimmune component might explain the possible progression of the disease despite discontinuance of the treatment.[73]

Ketoconazole

This antifungal imidazole derivative produces silent elevations of serum transaminase activity in 6 per cent of recipients, and may lead to symptomatic hepatic injury in one of 10 000 or 15 000 recipients.[74] Monitoring of liver function tests is recommended. Hepatitis is more frequent in females (ratio 2:1). It occurs after 1.5 to 26 weeks of treatment. Hepatitis is usually hepatocellular, with some cases of fulminant hepatitis (Bercoff, Gut, 1985; 26:636). Mixed or cholestatic hepatitis can also occur.[74] Hypersensitivity manifestations are usually absent, suggesting a toxic, idiosyncratic mechanism. Ketoconazole inhibits bromosulphthalein transport in the isolated perfused rat liver (Gaeta, Naunyn-Schmiedb-ArchPharmacol, 1987; 335:697) and decreases the uptake of bile acids by isolated rat hepatocytes (Azer, JPharmExpTher, 1995; 272:1231). Ketoconazole, in high doses, is hepatotoxic in experimental animals,[74] and the drug produces toxicity in primary cultures of rat hepatocytes (Rodriguez, Toxicol, 1995; 96:83).

The average length of time required for laboratory values to return to normal after cessation of the treatment was 7 weeks (Benson, DigDisSci, 1988; 33:240). In several cases, however, liver test abnormalities have continued to deteriorate, jaundice has become more pronounced during the first 1 to 2 weeks after the drug was withdrawn, and the final recovery has been long delayed (Benson, DigDisSci, 1988; 33:240).

Labetalol

Eleven cases of hepatitis due to this adrenergic receptor antagonist have been reviewed (Clark, AnnIntMed, 1990; 113:210), nine of which occurred in women, and with two fatalities. Features of hypersensitivity were infrequent. Hepatic necrosis was present in the five cases with a histopathological assessment.

Methyldopa

Administration of methyldopa may increase ALT activity in up to 6 per cent of recipients (Elkington, Circul, 1969; 40:589). Clinical hepatitis is much less common. It predominates in females (70 per cent). Hepatitis occurs mainly during the first 4 weeks of treatment, but a later onset (several years) is possible.[57] Hepatitis is usually hepatocellular, rarely mixed or cholestatic. In one-third of patients, hepatitis is heralded by fever, but eosinophilia is uncommon. The direct Coombs' test may be positive and there may be antinuclear or antismooth muscle autoantibodies.[57] Readministration may lead to prompt recurrence, but there are exceptions.

Methyldopa is transformed into chemically reactive metabolites (Dybing, MolPharm, 1976; 12:911). It is possible that these metabolites may lead to either direct toxicity or allergic hepatitis in different patients. Indeed, 50 per cent of sera from patients with methyldopa hepatitis contained antibodies against methyldopa-altered rabbit hepatocytes; these sera became cytotoxic in the presence of normal human mononuclear cells.[41]

Nicotinic acid (niacin)

This lipid-lowering agent causes minor and transient elevations of serum ALT (Christensen, JAMA, 1961; 177:546; Knopp, Metabolism, 1985; 34:642), sometimes associated with decreased synthesis of clotting factors (Dearing, ArchIntMed, 1992; 152:861). Several cases of clinically overt acute hepatitis (Clementz, Gastro, 1987; 9:582; Mullin, AnnIntMed, 1989; 111:253; Hodis, JAMA, 1990; 264:181) and some cases of mixed or cholestatic hepatitis (Einstein, AmJDigDis, 1975; 20:282; Kohn, AmJMedSci, 1969; 258:89; Sugerman, JAMA, 1974; 228:202; Patterson, SouthMedJ, 1983; 76:239) have been reported. With the crystalline form, hepatitis usually occurs after weeks or months of treatment with daily doses of 3 g or more. With time-release preparations, hepatitis may occur both sooner and after lower daily doses (Etchason, MayoClinProc, 1991; 66:23).

Nifedipine

Compared with the widespread use of this dihydropyridine calcium channel blocker, relatively few cases of drug-induced hepatitis have been reported. Hepatitis is mainly hepatocellular, rarely mixed.[3] Fever and blood eosinophilia are frequent, and there is rapid recurrence on rechallenge, suggesting an immunoallergic mechanism.

Paracetamol (acetaminophen)

Paracetamol is extensively used worldwide because of its good analgesic and some antipyretic properties and its availability without prescription.

Paracetamol is detoxified through the conjugation of its hydroxyl group with either sulphate or glucuronic acid. Although a small fraction of the paracetamol dose is transformed by cytochrome P-450 (particularly, cytochromes P-450 1A2, 2E1, and 3A) into N-acetyl-p-benzoquinoneimine, the formation of this reactive metabolite remains limited after therapeutic doses and, furthermore, the metabolite is efficiently detoxified by conjugation with glutathione (Mitchell, JPharmExpTher, 1973; 187:211). Accordingly, paracetamol, taken at recommended doses (0.5–3 g/day), is a safe analgesic. Taken at higher doses, however, paracetamol may produce hepatitis. At these higher doses, conjugating pathways may become partly saturated and a higher fraction of the dose will undergo metabolic activation by cytochrome P-450. Extensive formation of the reactive quinoneimine then depletes hepatic glutathione stores. Once this has occurred, the quinoneimine depletes protein thiols, increases cellular calcium, and causes liver cell demise by either necrosis or apoptosis.

The hepatotoxicity of paracetamol can occur in two circumstances. After ingestion of excessive doses (4–10 g/day) for therapeutic purposes, toxicity may occur in some patients that are rendered susceptible by factors which either increase the formation of the reactive metabolite and/or decrease its inactivation by glutathione. Hepatitis (and renal failure) have been observed in chronic alcoholics (Kaysen, ArchIntMed, 1985; 145:2019) who display high levels of cytochrome P-450 2E1 and low hepatic glutathione stores.[32] Isoniazid administration also induces cytochrome P-450 2E1, and cases of severe paracetamol-induced hepatotoxicity have been observed (Murphy, AnnIntMed, 1990; 113:799; Moulding, AnnIntMed, 1991; 114:431). High therapeutic doses of paracetamol may also be hepatotoxic in those with anorexia nervosa or starvation, which may decrease hepatic glutathione stores (Barker, AnnIntMed, 1977; 87:299; Ware, AnnIntMed, 1978; 88:267).

Another circumstance leading to paracetamol hepatotoxicity is the intentional ingestion of large overdoses in a manipulative or suicidal attempt. Indeed, following extensive press coverage of the first cases of paracetamol-induced suicide in the late 1960s, paracetamol ingestion has become one of the most popular ways of attempting to take one's life. The fad started in the United Kingdom, and later extended to the United States and other English-speaking countries. Paracetamol ingestion is particularly in vogue among adolescent or young adult females, often as a means to elicit guilt, help, and care from estranged relatives or loved ones. Fortunately, even before the use of antidotal treatments, most patients did not absorb enough to cause liver damage.[56] Less than 8 per cent developed severe liver damage and less than 1 per cent died.[56] Hepatotoxicity becomes possible when a single dose of more than 7.5 g (150 mg/kg) has been ingested but (with the notable exception of alcoholics) death is unlikely unless 20 g or more have been taken.

Because the ingested dose may be wrongly estimated and because vomiting (or the gastric lavage which is often made within the first 4 h) may have decreased the amount actually absorbed, it is useful to measure paracetamol plasma levels, starting 4 h after the ingestion (earlier measurements may be misleading due to still incomplete absorption). Those patients whose plasma paracetamol concentrations are above a line joining points of 150 mg/l at 4 h and 30 mg/l at 12 h after ingestion (on a semilogarithmic plot) are at risk of developing severe liver damage and must be treated with N-acetylcysteine (Vale, Lancet, 1995; 346:547). Because alcoholic patients and those with eating disorders are more susceptible, a lower 'treatment line', joining plots of 100 mg/l at 4 h to 15 mg/l at 15 h is recommended in these patients.

Both the intravenous[56] and the oral[75] routes of administration have been shown to be similarly and remarkably effective when started during the first 12 h, but also, to some extent, up to 24 h[75] after the ingestion of paracetamol. Even at the time of overt liver failure, N-acetylcysteine administration may still afford

some benefit (Keays, BMJ, 1991; 303:1026) and is now recommended (Vale, Lancet, 1995; 346:547). When administered early, N-acetylcysteine liberates cysteine, allowing resynthesis of hepatic glutathione, and thus preventing liver injury. Later, it might accelerate the recovery of protein thiols and improve the outcome of the liver disease.

In practice, a European panel has issued recommendations that may be summarized as follows (Vale, Lancet, 1995; 346:547):

1. For patients seen less than 15 h after the overdose, take blood for plasma paracetamol measurement, and (after 8 h) for determination of prothrombin time, ALT, AST, creatinine, bilirubin, acid–base status, and blood counts. Give 50 g of activated charcoal to adult patients if less than 1 h has elapsed since a substantial overdose. If plasma paracetamol concentration is above the 'treatment line' indicated above for normal subjects, or alcoholic/malnourished subjects, respectively, start intravenous N-acetylcysteine (150 mg/kg in 200 ml of 5 per cent dextrose over 15 min; 50 mg/kg in 500 ml 5 per cent dextrose over 4 h; 100 mg/kg in 1l 5 per cent dextrose over 16 h). If the plasma paracetamol concentration is not yet available by 8 h after the overdose, begin N-acetylcysteine if more than 150 mg/kg of paracetamol has been ingested; this treatment may be discontinued when the plasma paracetamol concentration is eventually obtained and falls below the treatment line. On completion of the N-acetylcysteine treatment, repeat the above mentioned investigations (except paracetamol concentration). If the patient is asymptomatic and the investigations are normal, the patient may be discharged.

2. For patients seen after 15 h, take blood on admission for the above mentioned investigations, as well as glucose and phosphate determination. If the patient has ingested more than 150 mg/kg, is symptomatic, or has abnormal investigations, give course of N-acetylcysteine. Repeat investigations at the end of N-acetylcysteine treatment and consider continuing it (100 mg/kg in 1 litre of 5 per cent dextrose over 16 h, repeated until recovery) if the investigations are abnormal or the patient is symptomatic.

When given intravenously, N-acetylcysteine may elicit various adverse effects in up to 10 per cent of recipients. These adverse effects may be due to a dose-related release of histamine and they therefore resemble anaphylactoid reactions, with nausea, flushing, urticaria, and pruritus as the most common manifestations, and angio-oedema, respiratory distress, and hypo- or hypertension, as rare complications (Vale, Lancet, 1995; 346:547). The oral route leads to lower initial plasma levels of N-acetylcysteine and is better tolerated, but then it may favour vomiting. Whatever the route, N-acetylcysteine is a remarkable antidote, with no death observed in more than 2000 patients treated within 16 h of paracetamol ingestion.[75]

A few patients, however, really intend to die, take large overdoses of paracetamol, and conceal this ingestion until it is too late for N-acetylcysteine to be 100 per cent effective (although this antidote is nevertheless attempted). After a period of possible vomiting during the first 12 h, the patient may be essentially symptom free until the second or third day, when anorexia, nausea, vomiting, and malaise may herald the onset of the liver disease, followed by dark urine and jaundice. Serum ALT levels are extremely high. Hypoglycaemia is relatively frequent, and should be prevented by infusions of glucose. The haemogram may be normal or may show hyperleucocytosis and thrombocytopenia. Metabolic acidosis with hyperlactataemia is relatively common. Hypophosphataemia with phosphaturia, oliguria, anuria, and high creatinine levels may be due to associated acute tubular necrosis. Associated myocardial injury may lead to cardiac arrhythmia and left ventricular failure.

The following management has been recommended in patients with hepatic failure (Vale, Lancet, 1995; 346:547). Give a course of N-acetylcysteine (if not previously administered) and/or continue with 100 mg/kg in 1 litre of 5 per cent dextrose over 16 h until recovery. Administer intravenous 10 per cent dextrose to prevent hypoglycaemia and monitor blood glucose regularly. Give an H_2 receptor antagonist to prevent gastrointestinal haemorrhage. Correct severe acidosis (pH <7.2) and monitor acid–base status regularly. Give intravenous phosphate if severe hypophosphataemia is present. Dialysis or haemofiltration should be instituted if renal failure occurs. We think it is best to avoid both sedatives and fresh frozen plasma whenever possible, because these would obscure useful criteria for liver transplantation. If hepatic encephalopathy develops (in the absence of sedatives) and/or factor V drops below 20 per cent of normal, expert advice should be sought and emergency liver transplantation should be considered.

Phenprocoumon

Although other coumarin derivatives are essentially devoid of hepatotoxic effects, this particular derivative has increased ALT activity in 37 per cent of recipients (Renschler, Deutsch-ArchKlinMed, 1963; 208:524). Hepatitis has occurred from 2 to 6 months after starting the drug. The type of injury has been mainly hepatocellular, but cholestasis has also been observed. In one case, cross-sensitivity seemed to exist with acenocoumarol.

Phenytoin

Administration of phenytoin, a microsomal enzyme inducer, commonly increases serum γ-glutamyl transpeptidase activity (Keeffe, DigDisSci, 1986; 31:1056), and may lead to minor increases in serum ALT and alkaline phosphatase activity in some recipients.

Clinical hepatitis is much less common.[4] It occurs within the first 6 weeks of therapy, and is usually associated with fever, rash, lymphadenopathy, lymphocytosis (sometimes with atypical lymphocytes), and eosinophilia, suggesting an allergic mechanism. The pattern may resemble infectious mononucleosis. An autoantibody against a 53-kDa microsomal protein has been reported (Leeder, JPharmExpTher, 1992; 163:360). Hepatitis is predominantly hepatocellular, but sometimes mixed. Granulomas may be present.

Phenytoin is transformed into a reactive 3,4-epoxide (Pantorotto, BiochemPharm, 1982; 31:1501; Moustafa, DrugMetDis, 1983; 11: 574). It has been suggested (but not proven) that subjects with a deficiency in a protective mechanism (perhaps in epoxide hydrolase) might be uniquely susceptible.[52] For yet unknown reasons, black people appear to be particularly susceptible (Edeki, DrugMetDisp, 1995; 27:449).

Pirprofen

Prolonged administration of this non-steroidal anti-inflammatory compound (more than 2 months) has led to hepatocellular necrosis[76] and even fulminant hepatitis.[77] Hypersensitivity manifestations were absent, suggesting an idiosyncratic, toxic mechanism.

In some patients with pirprofen-induced hepatocellular jaundice, microvesicular steatosis accompanied liver cell necrosis (see 'microvesicular steatosis'). The drug has been recalled.

Propylthiouracil

Unlike other antithyroid drugs which produce either cholestatic or mixed hepatitis, propylthiouracil can produce cytolytic, sometimes fatal, hepatitis (Jonas, JPediatGastrNutr, 1988; 7:776). The reaction is uncommon, however.

Pyrazinamide

Pyrazinamide, even in the lower doses used nowadays, may produce hepatocellular jaundice, particularly when the drug is continued in excess of the 2 months of treatment that are normally recommended.[78]

Monitoring of serum transaminases should be performed in patients receiving this drug.[78] In tuberculous patients who receive isoniazid, rifampicin, and pyrazinamide and then develop hepatitis, the difficult question arises of whether isoniazid, pyrazinamide, or both should be withdrawn. In mild cases, the duration of the treatment may help in this difficult decision. Isoniazid–rifampicin hepatitis occurs mainly during the first month of the treatment, whereas pyrazinamide hepatitis is usually associated with longer treatments.[78] In severe cases of hepatitis, however, it may be safer to initially withdraw isoniazid, pyrazinamide, and rifampicin.

Combined treatments with rifampicin, isoniazid, and pyrazinamide can lead to fulminant and subfulminant hepatitis.[78] Two different patterns have been distinguished.[78] Patients with a time interval greater than 15 days between the onset of treatment and the onset of fulminant or subfulminant hepatitis frequently exhibited a subfulminant course with a poor spontaneous prognosis. In contrast, when fulminant hepatitis occurred earlier, patients exhibited a good spontaneous prognosis. This was reminiscent of the good prognosis of fulminant cases seen within the first 2 weeks of treatments by isoniazid and rifampicin without pyrazinamide. In patients receiving these three drugs concomitantly, it has been hypothesized that the late-onset cases (with a poor prognosis) were actually due to pyrazinamide, whereas those occurring early (and with a good prognosis) were actually due to the isoniazid–rifampicin combination.[78]

The hepatotoxicity of pyrazinamide is not associated with hypersensitivity manifestations and is probably due to direct toxicity. Its molecular mechanism remains unknown, however.

Tacrine

This reversible cholinesterase inhibitor is used in the symptomatic treatment of Alzheimer's disease. Careful monitoring of serum ALT levels and tolerance-dependent, stepwise escalation of the doses are recommended, because the drug increases ALT activity in approximately 50 per cent of recipients.[79] In most patients, the rise in ALT occurs abruptly, usually at about 6 weeks of treatment, without an upward drift in the preceding weeks.[79] Most affected subjects have mild ALT increases, without clinical manifestations. This extremely high incidence of liver dysfunction suggests direct toxicity rather than immunoallergy. The weak base tacrine is taken up by mitochondria, where it may cycle back and forth across the mitochondrial inner membrane, uncoupling respiration and wasting energy without ATP production (Berson, Gastro, 1996, 110:1878). These effects are initially compensated by adaptive mitochondrial responses leading to enhanced respiratory rates. However, the drug accumulates within hepatic lysosomes, and exhibits time-dependent accumulation and toxicity in cultured hepatocytes. This may account for the delayed liver dysfunction *in vivo*. First-pass metabolism in the liver may spare other organs, explaining why the liver is selectively injured (Berson, Gastro, 1996, 110:1878).

After interruption of the treatment in patients with ALT values above three times the upper limit of normal, and recovery, a precocious rechallenge often produces an almost immediate recurrence of the increase in ALT (possibly due to the persistence of the drug in lysosomal depots and the quicker achievement of hepatotoxic intrahepatic concentrations). The elevation in ALT is often lower on rechallenge than during the initial exposure to the drug, and most patients subsequently show normalization of their ALT levels despite continuation, and even escalation, of the doses.[79] This noticeable exception to the general rule that rechallenges should be avoided further supports the direct toxicity of tacrine rather than a metabolite-mediated immunoallergic phenomenon.

Although tacrine-induced liver injury remains mild in most patients, 2 per cent of recipients develop ALT values greater than 20 times the upper limit of normal, and a few liver biopsies have shown liver cell necrosis.[79] Fever and rash are infrequent, but eosinophilia is present in 35 per cent of those with ALT more than 20 times the upper limit of normal. Tacrine is transformed by cytochrome P-450 1A2 into reactive metabolites (Table 5). Through the immunization of some subjects, these metabolites might be involved in this severe form of hepatitis.

Tienilic acid (ticrynafen)

This drug has been withdrawn from clinical use in the United States, followed, later, by other countries. Hepatitis usually occurred after 1 to 3 months of treatment.[80] The main liver lesion was liver cell necrosis. Prompt recurrence following a challenge dose of the drug suggested an immune mechanism. Tienilic acid hepatitis was associated with an antimicrosomal autoantibody (the anti-LKM$_2$ autoantibody) directed against P-450 2C9, the isoenzyme which transforms the drug into a reactive metabolite.[44]

Acute cholestatic hepatitis

Cholestasis (etymologically, stasis or stagnation of bile) is defined as the failure of bile to reach the duodenum.[81] In cholestatic hepatitis, the dysfunction is located at the level of the bile canaliculus (canalicular cholestasis) and/or small bile ducts (see next section).

Cholestasis often predominates in the centrilobular area (zone three of the acinus). Histologically, the hepatocytes contain brownish bile granules in their cytoplasm, while canaliculi are often dilated and also contain brown bile-pigment material. In cholestatic hepatitis, there must be some degree of portal inflammation (hence, the term of hepatitis) and liver necrosis should be either absent or very mild. Should inflammation be absent, the condition should be classified, instead, as pure (bland) cholestasis. Should liver necrosis

be more prominent, the liver injury should be referred to as mixed hepatitis.

The full-blown clinical picture of cholestasis consists of jaundice and pruritus, with pale stools and dark urine. In mild forms, however, jaundice and even pruritus may be lacking, and only the biochemical abnormalities are then present. A first biochemical consequence of cholestasis is an increased plasma concentration of bile constituents such as conjugated bilirubin and bile acids. There is also increased synthesis and transfer into blood of canalicular membrane enzymes, such as alkaline phosphatase and γ-glutamyl transferase.[81] In addition, there may be some leakage of cellular enzymes, such as aminotransferases, whose activity may be slightly increased in the serum. Ultrasonography and radiology show a normal biliary tree in this intrahepatic form of cholestasis.

Hypersensitivity manifestations such as fever, rash, or blood eosinophilia are often present, consistent with an immune mechanism for this drug-induced disease. Indeed, several drugs producing cholestatic hepatitis are known to be transformed into reactive metabolites (Table 5), that might lead to immunization. Which antigens may be involved in these cholestatic cases remain totally unknown, however. Abdominal pain and a tender liver may also occur in drug-induced cholestatic hepatitis and this may confuse the diagnosis.

Indeed, the main differential diagnosis of drug-induced cholestatic hepatitis is with jaundice due to biliary obstruction. In the past, several patients who presented with abdominal pain and fever, followed by jaundice and pruritus, have been operated upon with an erroneous clinical diagnosis of choledocolithiasis. Nowadays, however, the recourse to ultrasonography in all cases of cholestatis makes this distinction much easier, and avoids these surgical misadventures. A second differential diagnosis is with the rare, but possible, cholestatic forms of viral hepatitis, particularly hepatitis A. Viral hepatitis is detected by the viral serologies. Alcoholic hepatitis may also present as cholestasis in some cases. Questioning of the patient and his family, clinical stigmata of alcoholism, an increased mean corpuscular volume, and a markedly enlarged liver will suggest the diagnosis, confirmed by a liver biopsy.

Acute cholestatic hepatitis with cholangiolitis and cholangitis

After having been secreted by the hepatocytes into the bile canaliculus (a space between two adjacent hepatocytes), and after having flowed through this canalicular network towards the periphery of the lobule, bile then enters the bile ductules (or cholangioles), which are lined by flat epithelial cells. Bile is then collected by the portal (interlobular) bile ducts lined by columnar ductal cells.[81]

Some cases of cholestatic (or mixed) hepatitis are associated with lesions of these bile ducts and ductules. It is probable that, in the past, these lesions have been neglected in many short reports of cholestatic hepatitis. These bile duct lesions should be explicitly mentioned in case reports, because they may contribute to the pathogenesis of some cholestatic episodes and may help explain the subsequent development of the vanishing bile duct syndrome.

'Cholangiolitis' refers to inflammation of the ductules and is characterized by ductular proliferation, with oedema and infiltration by polymorphonuclear leucocytes in and around the ductules.[81] 'Cholangitis' refers to oedema and acute inflammatory changes in

Table 6 Main drugs causing acute intrahepatic duct lesions

Ajmaline	Etretinate	Difetarsone
Amitiptyline	Glibenclamide	Gold salts
Amoxicillin/clavulanic acid	Chlorothiazide	Hydralazine
Ampicillin	Chlorpromazine	Interleukin-2
Allopurinol	Chlorpropamide	Methahexamide
Azathioprine	Clometacin	Methytestosterone
Barbiturates	Dantrolene	D-Penicillamine
Carbamazepine	Dextropropoxifene	Sulindac
Cefoperazone	Diazepam	Troleandomycin

and around the portal bile ducts.[81] Cholangitis is the prominent lesion, and is generally associated with cholangiolitis. In some cases the lesions are marked. The bile ducts are dilated and the epithelial cells are swollen or necrotic. The inflammatory infiltrate is usually polymorphic, and contains lymphocytes, neutrophils, and sometimes eosinophils.[81]

The mechanism for acute cholangiolitis and cholangitis is unknown. However, the presence of eosinophils in the inflammatory infiltrate and the association with granulomas in several patients, as well as the frequent association with hypersensitivity manifestations, are all suggestive of an immune mechanism.[81]

The outcome of drug-induced cholangitis is generally good, with recovery occurring rapidly after discontinuation of the causative drug. However, it may be followed by prolonged cholestasis due to the vanishing bile duct syndrome in a few patients.

Acute cholangiolitis and cholangitis have been mainly observed after administration of ajmaline, the amoxicillin–clavulanic acid combination, flucloxacillin, chlorpromazine, carbamazepine, and propoxyphene (dextropropoxyphene).[81] Occasional instances have occurred with other drugs (Table 6).

Drugs causing acute cholestatic hepatitis (with or without cholangitis)

Only the most frequently involved drugs are discussed below, while some other drugs are listed in Table 4. The reader is also referred to the section on mixed hepatitis, because drugs that usually lead to this lesion may also produce a mainly cholestatic episode in an individual patient.

Ajmaline

Jaundice has occurred after 8 to 16 days of treatment with this antiarrhythmic agent.[82] Chills, fever, and abdominal pain often preceded icterus, simulating obstructive jaundice.[82] Eosinophilia was frequent, however, and the presumed mechanism was immunoallergy. Although jaundice usually subsided within 3 months after cessation of the treatment, prolonged cholestasis due to rarefaction of bile ducts occurred in several patients, as discussed in a subsequent section. The drug has been abandoned in many countries.

Amoxicillin–clavulanic acid

Although the risk of developing significant hepatic injury may be less than 1 in 100 000 with this drug combination, this is nevertheless a frequent cause of cholestatic hepatitis, because of the large number of prescriptions. A series of 15 cases has been reported.[83] The

disease mainly affected elderly males. Cholestatic hepatitis occurred from 7 to 89 days after starting the treatment. Prolonged treatments (for 10 days or more) appeared as a predisposing factor. Interestingly, in 11 of these 15 patients, the drug had already been stopped 1 to 4 weeks before the first symptoms appeared.[83] Five patients had eosinophilia and five had low titres of antismooth muscle, antinuclear, or antimitochondrial antibodies. More recent reports show that cholangiolitis is frequently present in these patients.[84]

Because readministration of amoxicillin alone has usually been well tolerated, it is thought that the drug combination (probably the clavulanic moiety) is responsible.[3] In performing such rechallenges, however, one must beware that amoxicillin given alone also has the potential to produce cholestasis, including the vanishing bile duct syndrome (Davies, JHepatol, 1994; 20:112).

Azathioprine

Azathioprine rarely causes cholestatic jaundice. A series of seven cases has been reported.[85] These renal transplant recipients developed jaundice 33 to 88 months after starting azathioprine, together with low doses of glucocorticoids. Centrilobular cholestasis was associated with fatty liver in five of these seven patients, and with sinusoidal dilation in three. Clinical and laboratory manifestations disappeared within 1 month after stopping azathioprine. Reintroduction of azathioprine in three patients led to recurrence within 1 month.[85] The drug also produces a variety of vascular lesions that are discussed below.

Chlorpromazine

Chlorpromazine is one of the first drugs known to cause cholestatic hepatitis, and has long served as a paradigm for this conditon.[4] Jaundice usually occurs within the first 5 weeks of therapy.[4] Pruritus is frequent. Serum alkaline phosphatase values are markedly elevated (more than three- or fourfold) in 50 to 70 per cent of cases, whilst aminotransferases are moderately increased. Serum cholesterol is frequently augmented.

Prodromal signs, with fever or influenza-like symptoms, nausea or vomiting, and abdominal pain occur in 70 to 80 per cent of cases. The syndrome may thus mimic extrahepatic obstruction, and a number of patients have been subjected to laparotomy.[86] However, signs of hypersensitivity (fever, eosinophilia) occur in up to 70 per cent of patients, and a skin rash is reported in 3 to 5 per cent. Antinuclear antibodies are found in 40 per cent of cases.[4] Ultrasonography shows a normal bilary tree. The typical histological picture includes cholestasis with relatively little hepatocellular injury, and a marked portal inflammatory infiltrate.[86] Eosinophils are seen in 25 to 50 per cent of cases. Cholangiolitis occurs in approximately 25 per cent of cases, with infiltration of cholangioles with neutrophils and eosinophils.[81]

Approximately one-third of patients recover within 4 weeks after cessation of treatment, and another third in 4 to 8 weeks. The remainder may have a more prolonged course. Prolonged cholestasis and even biliary cirrhosis may ensue. Treatment is symptomatic. Corticosteroids do not influence the course.

Chlorpromazine may form reactive metabolites (De Mel, ChemBiolInteract, 1984; 52:79), and this might lead to metabolite-mediated immunoallergic hepatitis. Cross-sensitivity between chlorpromazine and several other phenothiazines has been observed.[81]

Chlordiazepoxide

This benzodiazepine has mainly caused cholestatic jaundice. Hepatitis occurs within the first 6 weeks of treatment with this anxiolytic agent (Abbruzzese, NEJM, 1965; 273:321; Lo, AmJDigDis, 1967; 12:845). A few cases of mixed or even cytolytic hepatitis have also occurred. No extrahepatic hypersensitivity manifestations were reported, although the inflammatory infiltrate contained prominent eosinophils in one case.

Erythromycins

Not only erythromycin estolate,[87] but also erythromycin ethylsuccinate, erythromycin propionate, clarithromycin, and roxithromycin, may all cause hepatitis. Hepatitis occurs mainly during the first 2 weeks of treatment. The condition is frequently associated with abdominal pains (80 per cent), fever (60 per cent), and eosinophilia (45–80 per cent).[88] Hepatitis is cholestatic or mixed, usually with a good prognosis.[89]

The liver injury often recurs within 24 to 48 h after rechallenge with the same erythromycin derivative.[88] It may or may not recur after administration of another erythromycin derivative.[88] The erythromycins are demethylated and oxidized by cytochrome P-450 into nitrosoalkane metabolites in rats and humans (Danan, JPharmExpTher, 1981; 218:509; Larrey, BiochemPharm, 1983; 32:1063). These unstable, electrophilic intermediates may react with the SH-group of glutathione or cysteine (Pessayre, JPharmExpTher, 1983; 224:685), and may bind covalently to proteins. This might lead to immunization in some patients.[90] The antigenic targets remain unknown, however.

Flucloxacillin

The hepatotoxicity of flucloxacillin is reminiscent of that of the amoxicillin/clavulanic acid combination. Flucloxacillin is a frequent cause of cholestatic hepatitis, not because of a high frequency of this adverse effect, but because of the large use of this antibiotic, at least in some countries (Derby, MedJAust, 1993; 158:596). Older patients and those receiving the drug for longer than 2 weeks are at increased risk (Fairley, BMJ, 1993; 306:233). However, females rather than males may be more frequently affected by the flucloxacillin-mediated hepatitis. In a series of 11 cases, symptoms mainly appeared within 10 to 30 days after starting the drug (Koek, Liver, 1994; 14:225). Four of these patients had cholangitis or cholangiolitis.

Although the outcome is usually favourable, prolonged cholestasis due to the vanishing bile duct syndrome may occur in a few patients (Olsson, JHepatol, 1992; 15:154; Davies, JHepatol 1994; 20:112).

Gold salts

Intrahepatic cholestasis is a rare complication of gold salt therapy.[91,92] It is observed after administration of the various gold salts used in therapy. Jaundice occurs within 5 weeks of the first administration and within 1 week of the last administration.[91] It may mimic extrahepatic obstruction, and several patients have had surgery.[91] Hepatitis, however, may be associated with proteinuria, rash and eosinophilia, and ultrasonography shows a normal biliary tree. Cholestasis is predominantly centrilobular. Recovery may take several months. Gold salts can also induce either mixed or cytolytic acute hepatitis, and even chronic hepatitis.

Penicillamine

Several cases of cholestatic jaundice have been recorded in patients taking penicillamine.[2] Jaundice appears after 3 to 5 weeks of treatment. Some cases have been associated with fever and rash, suggesting hypersensitivity. Resolution occurs in 3 to 4 weeks.

Troleandomycin

Administration of this antibiotic for 2 weeks or longer produced silent hepatic dysfunction in 50 per cent of recipients and jaundice in 4 per cent.[93] While the frequent liver dysfunction was probably due to direct toxicity, it remains unclear whether clinical hepatitis was due to direct toxicity or immunoallergy.

Troleandomycin is transformed by cytochrome P-450 into an unstable metabolite.[90] This nitroso derivative (or its nitrone precursor) may react with the SH group of glutathione and cysteine, and accordingly may bind covalently to hepatic proteins, which might lead to hepatitis.[90]

Mixed hepatitis

Mixed hepatitis is characterized by the presence of both hepatocellular necrosis and cholestasis in the same patient. When necrosis is extensive, however, such cases are best classified as cytolytic hepatitis. Accordingly, clinical and biochemical signs of mixed hepatitis are variable combinations of those of cholestatic hepatitis and mild hepatocellular damage.

Only those drugs which are most commonly involved are considered below, while some other drugs are listed in Table 4. It must be recalled that several drugs that typically produce mixed hepatitis can also lead to either acute hepatitis or cholestasis in an individual patient.

Drugs causing mixed hepatitis

Amineptine

This tricyclic antidepressant is widely used in France and several other countries. The drug was reported to cause 80 per cent of the cases of hepatitis due to tricyclic antidepressants in France (Lefébure, Therapie, 1984; 39:509). Administration of therapeutic doses of amineptine may produce two types of liver injury:

1. By far the most frequent type is mixed, or purely cholestatic, hepatitis.[2] The disease occurs during the first 3 months of treatment. It may be associated with fever and blood eosinophilia, and it promptly recurs after a rechallenge, suggesting an immunoallergic mechanism.[2] Amineptine resembles several other antidepressant drugs in having a tricyclic structure. Like imipramine (Kappus, BiochemPharm, 1975; 24:1079), amineptine is activated by cytochrome P-450 (probably on its tricyclic structure) into a chemically reactive metabolite (Genève, BiochemPharm, 1987; 36:2421). The reactive metabolite, however, is efficiently detoxified by glutathione and does not lead to direct toxicity. Presumably, it can cause immunoallergic hepatitis in some human subjects.

2. In a few patients receiving amineptine, the liver lesion has been that of microvesicular steatosis. This may be due to inhibition of mitochondrial β-oxidation by the heptanoic side chain of amineptine, as discussed in another section.

Amitriptyline

This tricyclic antidepressant causes mixed hepatitis, usually with a marked necrotic component.[94] Hypersensitivity manifestations are seen in some patients.[94]

Benoxaprofen

This non-steroidal anti-inflammatory drug had to be withdrawn because of its hepatotoxic and nephrotoxic potential, mainly in elderly females.[2] Hepatitis was mixed. Benoxaprofen may be transformed into a reactive metabolite (Mitchell, Hepatol, 1983; 3: 308).

Captopril

Compared with the widespread use of this angiotensin converting enzyme inhibitor, there have been relatively few reports of hepatic adverse reactions due to captopril. A review of 14 cases has been published, however (Rahmat, AnnIntMed, 1985; 102:56). Symptoms usually appeared between 1 and 8 weeks after starting the drug. All cases had jaundice. Fever, rash, and eosinophilia were common. Nine cases were classified as cholestatic, four as mixed, and one as hepatocellular. A more recent report cites nine cases of hepatocellular injury, including two deaths (Bellary, Lancet, 1989; ii:514).

Carbamazepine

This anticonvulsant drug may produce hepatitis within the first 6 weeks of treatment. Hepatitis is mixed. There may be acute cholangitis (Levy, AnnIntMed, 1981; 95:64; Larrey, DigDisSci, 1987; 32:554). The possible occurrence of fever, rash, eosinophilia, pancytopenia, agranulocytosis, thrombocytopenia, lymphadenopathy, and hepatic granulomas, as well as the prompt recurrence upon rechallenge, all suggest an allergic mechanism. Carbamazepine is transformed into the stable 10,11-epoxide, but also into several other (probably unstable) epoxides (Lertratanangkoon, DrugMetDisp, 1982; 10:1).

Carbimazole

This antithyroid drug is metabolized into methimazole and also produces mixed, mostly cholestatic, hepatitis, sometimes with bile duct damage. The liver injury occurs in the first 6 weeks of treatment. It may be associated with fever and blood eosinophilia, and may immediately recur upon rechallenge.

Clorpropamide

Chlorpropamide is rarely used nowadays because this long acting hypoglycaemic agent sometimes causes severe and prolonged hypoglycaemia. It has been responsible in the past for several cases of mixed (mainly cholestatic) hepatitis presumably due to immunoallergy.

Cimetidine

Asymptomatic increases in serum transaminase activity have been observed in a few patients on cimetidine, particularly those on 1.6 g/day (Blackwood, Lancet, 1976; 2:174).

Clinical hepatitis due to cimetidine appears extremely uncommon (Villeneuve, Gastro, 1979; 77:143; Van Steenbergen, JHepatol, 1985; 1:359). Hepatitis has occurred 2 to 120 days after starting the treatment (Van Steenbergen, JHepatol, 1985; 1:359). It is mixed in type. Hypersensitivity manifestations (fever, rash) and a prompt recurrence on rechallenge may suggest an allergic mechanism, at least in some patients.

Clofibrate and other fibrates

Mild and often transient increases in serum ALT levels, usually without any clinical manifestations, may occur in patients on clofibrate. In some patients, the serum transaminase elevation may be part of a myalgia syndrome (with elevated serum creatine kinase). The drug causes hepatomegaly and peroxisomal proliferation in rodents. Hepatomegaly might also occur in humans (Martini, CurrTherRes, 1982; 31:354) but without peroxisomal proliferation. Clofibrate administration also increases the saturation of bile and the incidence of gallstones (Coronary Drug Project Research Group, NEJM, 1978; 299:314).

The same types of effects may be observed with bezafibrate, fenofibrate, and gemfibrozil.

Clozapine

This neuroleptic has transformed the life of some schizophrenic patients, and is therefore maintained despite its propensity to produce agranulocytosis, which requires frequent monitoring of the haemogram. The drug may also increase ALT activity in 4 to 30 per cent of users, and two cases of cholestatic hepatitis have been reported.[2]

Dapsone

This antileprosy drug is also used in dermatis herpetiformis and in the treatment of *Pneumocystis carinii* infections in patients with the acquired immune deficiency syndrome. Like other sulphonamides, the drug may be detoxified by acetylation of its NH_2-groups. As there are two such groups in dapsone, however, both the parent compound and monoacetyldapsone can be oxidized by cytochrome P-450 to hydroxylamine derivatives that can cause methaemoglobinaemia (Vage, ToxApplPharmacol, 1994; 129:309). Hyperbilirubinaemia due to haemolysis may occur. Dapsone may also cause cholestatic or hepatocellular jaundice, which may be part of the 'sulphone syndrome' consisting of fever, malaise, hepatic necrosis, exfoliative dermatitis, lymphadenopathy, methaemoglobinaemia, and haemolytic anaemia.[95]

Enalapril

Like captopril, this angiotensin converting enzyme inhibitor infrequently produces mixed hepatitis.

Haloperidol

Although mild increases in alkaline phosphatase activity may occur in 70 per cent of users, symptomatic cases have been infrequent. Fever, jaundice, and sometimes blood eosinophilia appeared within 5 weeks of starting the treatment.[2] The disease is mainly cholestatic, although mild necrosis is often associated, and one case of mainly cytolytic hepatitis has been reported.

Imipramine

Administration of imipramine may cause jaundice, usually within the first 2 months of the treatment. Hypersensitivity manifestations (fever, rash, eosinophilia) are seen in some patients. Hepatitis is usually mixed, although either the cholestatic or the necrotic component may predominate in some patients.[4] Prolonged cholestatis and progressive hepatic fibrosis have been reported following imipramine therapy. Imipramine is transformed into a reactive metabolite, possibly leading to immunoallergic hepatitis (Kappus, BiochemPharm, 1979; 24:1079).

Iprindole

This antidepressant may cause mixed (mostly cholestatic) liver injury within the first 3 weeks of treatment (Ajdukiewics, Gut, 1971; 12:705).

Methimazole (thiamazole)

Cases of hepatitis caused by this antithyroid drug have had mainly cholestatic features, but both a predominantly hepatocellular pattern or a granulomatous form can also occur. Rash, eosinophilia, leucopenia, or agranulocytois may be associated.

Nitrofurantoin

Jaundice due to this urinary tract antiseptic affects mainly middle-aged or elderly females. This may reflect both high use in this group and higher susceptibility. Acute hepatitis occurs mainly during the first 5 weeks of treatment, and is associated with fever (60 per cent), rash (30 per cent), and blood eosinophilia (70 per cent); it is mixed in type.[4] Nitrofurantoin may also lead to chronic hepatitis. Nitrofurantoin is transformed into reactive metabolites (Boyd, BiochemPharm, 1979; 28:601) that might lead to immunoallergic hepatitis.

Phenindione

This anticoagulant may produce mixed hepatitis, usually associated with a general hypersensitivity syndrome consisting of fever, rash, eosinophilia, lymphocytosis, renal injury, and, at times, thrombocytopenia.[4] The drug has been largely abandoned in favour of the coumarin derivatives.

Phenylbutazone

Therapeutic doses may lead to hepatitis, occurring usually during the first weeks of treatment. Phenylbutazone-induced hepatitis may be classified as mixed. However, the hepatocellular component predominates in most patients, while a few have instead a mainly cholestatic pattern. Hepatitis is frequently associated with fever and/or rash, sometimes with eosinophilia and hepatic granulomas.[96] Intoxication with overdoses of phenylbutazone may produce a toxic type of hepatitis in the following days.[96] Phenylbutazone is transformed by prostaglandin H synthase into a reactive free radical (Reed, MolPharm, 1985; 27:109).

Propoxyphene (dextropropoxyphene)

This analgesic has caused increases in γ-glutamyl transferase activity in 14 per cent of recipients in one study (Persson, Lakartid, 1985; 82:491). The drug may also cause symptomatic hepatic injury. Hepatitis is mixed (mainly cholestatic), sometimes with cholangitis. The disease is probably due to hypersensitivity. Fever, rash, and blood eosinophilia were present in some cases, and rechallenges have led to relapses within 4 days. Propoxyphene is transformed into a reactive nitroso derivative (Peterson, BiochemPharm, 1979; 28:1783).

Quinidine

Initiation of treatment with this antiarrhythmic agent may produce fever and a mixed type of hepatitis (usually anicteric) 6 to 12 days later. Hepatic granulomas are frequent.[97] Readministration leads to prompt recurrence of fever and elevated transaminase levels. These features suggest an allergic mechanism.

Ranitidine

Clinical hepatitis due to ranitidine is probably uncommon (Black, AnnIntMed, 1984; 101:208; Proctor, JAMA, 1984; 251:1554; Souza Lima, AnnIntMed, 1984; 101:207). Hepatitis has occurred 2 to 45 days after the onset of the treatment. Hepatitis is mixed. In some cases, the presence of fever, chills, blood eosinophilia, and the prompt recurrence on rechallenge have suggested an allergic mechanism (Souze Lima, AnnIntMed, 1984; 101:207).

Sulindac (and other non-steroidal anti-inflammatory drugs)

Hepatitis due to sulindac occurs mainly in women, usually within 6 weeks of the initiation of treatment.[98] Fever is frequent (70 per cent), but eosinophilia is usually absent. Hepatitis is mixed, but predominantly cholestatic. Binucleated hepatocytes may be present. Leucopenia, lymphopenia, or thrombocytopenia may be associated. Rechallenge leads to recurrence within a few days. These various features suggest an allergic mechanism.

Many other anti-inflammatory drugs may produce mixed or cholestatic hepatitis (Table 4). In contrast, the hepatitis caused by either pirprofen or diclofenac is mainly hepatocellular, as mentioned above.

Sulphonamides

Sulphonamides may be detoxified by N-acetylation or may be transformed by cytochrome P-450 into reactive hydroxylamines

(Cribb, DrugMetDisp, 1995; 23:406). Administration of sulphonamides may lead to hepatitis, usually within the first month of therapy.[99] Hepatitis may be heralded by fever and rash. Hepatitis is usually mixed in type, but either the hepatocellular or the cholestatic component may predominate in other patients. Hepatic granulomas may be present. Readministration leads to prompt recurrence. The mechanism is probably allergic.

Only subjects that are slow acetylators appear to be affected.[51] As discussed above, the enhanced toxicity of reactive sulphonamide metabolites towards the patients' lymphocytes has suggested that these patients may have an additional defect in some protective mechanism.[51] However, this defect has never been characterized, and other interpretations are possible (see section on mechanisms of acute hepatitis).

Patients with the immune deficiency syndrome frequently receive the trimethoprim–sulphamethoxazole combination for the treatment of *Pneumocystis carinii* infections. These patients appear to be particularly susceptible to sulphonamide reactions, possibly because of impaired drug acetylation, due to metabolic dysfunction rather than genetic deficiency (Deloménie, BrJClinPharm, 1994; 38:581).

Terbinafine

This newly developed antifungal drug has produced several cases of mixed hepatitis (Van't Wout, JHepatol, 1994; 21:115).

Tolazamide and tolbutamide

These hypoglycaemic sulphonylureas have produced instances of mixed hepatitis. They share this adverse effect with several other analogues, including acetohexamide, carbutamide, chlorpropamide, glibenclamide, glipizide, and metahexamide.

Granulomatous hepatitis

Small rounded foci of epithelioid cells and round cells, with, at times, multinucleated giant cells are present in the liver.[100] These drug-induced hepatic granulomas are always non-caseous. They may be surrounded by eosinophils. Granulomas may be located in the portal tract, the lobule, or both.

The term of granulomatous hepatitis should be reserved for cases where hepatic granulomas are the main liver lesion, as in some cases of hepatitis due to allopurinol, carbamazepine, hydralazine, penicillin, phenylbutazone, quinidine, or sulphonamides. When hepatic granulomas are just an epiphenomenon in the context of severe liver cell necrosis, as in some cases of hepatitis due halothane or α-methyldopa, these cases must be classified as cytolytic hepatitis (with hepatic granulomas). Similarly, when granulomas accompany both liver cell necrosis and cholestasis, as in some cases of hepatitis due allopurinol, phenylbutazone, quinidine, or sulphonamides, the liver disease should be classified as mixed hepatitis (with hepatic granulomas).

Pure granulomatous hepatitis may be silent or sometimes announced by general symptoms, pruritus, mild icterus, and an enlarged liver. Serum alkaline phosphatase activity may be increased. Drugs causing hepatic granulomas are listed in Table 7.[100]

Outcome of acute drug-induced hepatitis
Outcome of hepatocellular injuries

If not already dying (or transplanted) because of fulminant hepatitis, the patient usually recovers quickly after withdrawal of the offending drug. There are a few exceptions, however. Some patients with hepatitis due to iproniazid or tienilic acid may continue to worsen despite discontinuation of the treatment (Rosenblum, GastrClinBiol, 1985; 9:255; Poupon, NouvPresseMed, 1980; 9 :1181). It is noteworthy that with these two drugs, there are specific autoantibodies directed against normal cell constituents.[44,72] Conceivably, removal of the initiating drug will not stop such autoimmunity immediately. Slow aggravation of the liver disease, with development of subfulminant hepatitis despite interruption of the treatment, was also a feature in several patients with alpidem-induced hepatitis; the mechanism of this drug-induced hepatitis remains unknown, however.

When the offending drug is not removed, liver cell necrosis may either worsen (and secondarily lead to fulminant or subfulminant hepatitis) or it may persist for a prolonged period (possibly leading to the development of chronic liver disease, as discussed below).

Outcome of granulomatous, mixed, or cholestatic hepatitis

Hepatitis usually has a good prognosis. In a few cases of cholestatic hepatitis, however, cholestasis may persist for several years after discontinuance of the offending drug (see 'Prolonged cholestasis' below).

Pure hepatocellular cholestasis

In this uncommon entity, cholestasis is due to a specific interference of the drug with bile secretion, without hepatitis. Cholestasis is the only liver lesion, without inflammation or necrosis. In the typical case, there is jaundice and pruritus, but either one or both may be absent in milder cases. Typically, alkaline phosphatase and γ-glutamyl transpeptidase activities are increased, with normal or slightly increased ALT values. The biliary tree is morphologically normal.

Oestrogens and oral contraceptives

Oestrogens interfere with bile secretion in experimental animals and man. At least three mechanisms may be involved, although their respective roles still remain to be clarified. Prolonged administration of oestrogens increases the permeability of the paracellular pathway, possibly leading to the back diffusion of materials from bile canaliculi to blood.[101] Prolonged administration of oestrogens increased the activity of lecithin cholesterol acyl transferase, leading to the accumulation of cholesterol esters in plasma membranes.[102] This may decrease membrane fluidity and inhibit $Na^+,K^+ATPase$ activity.[102] Finally, oestrogens are quickly transformed into D-ring glucuronides which exhibit an immediate and extremely potent cholestatic effect.[103]

Clinically, cholestasis has occurred in women taking the high-dosage oral contraceptives that were used in the past. Even at that time, the overt disease was extremely uncommon. Its prevalence was estimated to be approximately 1:10 000 in Europe or North

Table 7 Main drugs causing hepatic granulomas

Allopurinol	Feprazone	Phenprocoumon
Amiodarone	Flumequine	Phenylbutazone
Amoxicillin–clavulanic acid	Glibenclamide	Phenytoin
Aprindine	Gold salts	Piroxicam
Aspirin	Halothane	Prajmaline
Bacillus Calmette–Guérin	Hydralazine	Procainamide
Carbamazepine	Isoniazid	Procarbazine
Carbimazole	Methimazole	Quinidine
Carbutamide	Methotrexate	Quinine
Cephalexin	Methyldopa	Ranitidine
Chlorpromazine	Nitrofurantoin	Sulphadiazine
Chlorpropamide	Nomifensine	Sulphadimethoxine
Clofibrate	Oestroprogestatives	Sulphadoxine
Co-trimoxazole	Oxacillin	Sulphamethoxazole
Cromoglycic acid	Oxyphenbutazone	Sulphanilamide
Dapsone	Papaverine	Sulphathiazole
Diazepam	Penicillin	Sulphazalazine
Diclofenac	Penicillamine	Tacrine
Diflunisal	Perhexiline	Tocainide
Diltiazem	Phenazone	Tolbutamide
Disopyramide		

America, and 1:4000 in Chile or Scandinavia.[104] All drugs containing oestrogens have been incriminated, especially the 17-ethinyl-substituted derivatives.

It appeared that clinically overt cholestasis developed predominantly in women with an exaggerated genetic susceptibility to the normal cholestatic effects of oestrogens.[104] This was suggested by the higher prevalence of cholestasis in some ethnic groups (Chile and Scandinavia) and by the familial clustering of both cholestasis of pregnancy and cholestasis due to oral contraceptives. The reason for this enhanced susceptibility is unknown. However, women with cholestasis of pregnancy exhibited an increase in the urinary excretion of oestriol-16-glucuronide and oestriol-3-sulphate-16-glucuronide, two D-ring glucuronides (Adlercreutz, JClinEndoc, 1974; 38:51).

In addition, administration of oestrogens may aggravate other cholestatic conditions. Patients with primary biliary cirrhosis, the asymptomatic relatives of patients with benign recurrent intrahepatic cholestasis (DePagter, Gastro, 1976; 71:202) and heterozygous carriers of Byler disease (Whitington, JPediatGastrNutr, 1994; 18:134) may be more susceptible to the cholestatic effects of oral contraceptives. The two latter conditions might be related genetic diseases (different alleles of a same gene?) that cause impaired biliary transport of bile salts (Carlton, HumMolGenet, 1995; 4:1049).

Oral contraceptive-mediated cholestasis usually occurred within the first six cycles, and most commonly during the first or second.[104] Malaise, anorexia, nausea, vomiting, and weight loss were frequent, but pruritus could be the only sign. Dark urine and jaundice followed after a few days. There was no fever, rash, or abdominal pain. Jaundice was usually mild, and serum bilirubin rarely exceeded 170 μmol/l. Serum alkaline phosphatase was increased in only one-third of patients, while serum transaminase activity was moderately elevated in about two-thirds of patients.[104] When available, the liver histology showed bile-pigment material in the canaliculi and within hepatocytes, with little or no hepatocellular damage or inflammation. Bile ducts were normal. Electron microscopy showed mitochondrial alterations, and dilated bile canaliculi exhibiting bile pigment deposits and distorted microvilli (Larsson-Cohn, ActaMedScand, 1967; 181:257). Clinical and biochemical signs usually resolved 1 to 3 months after cessation of oral contraceptives, without chronic sequelae. However, worsening for up to 3 months with prolonged cholestasis and recovery after 6 months has been reported (Lieberman, JClinGastro, 1984; 6:145). Recurrence was frequent, perhaps constant, if the drug was resumed (Orellana-Alcade, Lancet, 1966; 2:1278).

Hepatologists rarely see this adverse effect nowadays, because of the lower oestrogen content of the oral contraceptives that are now used. Nevertheless, drug interactions may still trigger the syndrome. An epidemic of bland cholestasis has been observed in women taking troleandomycin while receiving oral contraceptives.[105] Jaundice with this drug combination was observed much more commonly than jaundice due to oral contraceptives alone or jaundice due to troleandomycin alone. It has been suggested that troleandomycin administration may somehow sensitize women to the cholestatic effects of oral contraceptives.[105] Indeed, troleandomycin forms an inactive complex with cytochrome P-450 3A and thereby decreases the oxidation of oestradiol to catechol oestrogens in rats.[106] It has been suggested that decreased oxidative metabolism of oestrogens by cytochrome P-450 may perhaps allow their enhanced conjugation into cholestatic D-ring glucuronides.[106]

Anabolic steroids

Anabolic–androgenic steroids with a C-17 alkyl substituent also interfere with bile secretion in experimental animals.[107] As with oestrogens, several mechanisms have been demonstrated.[107] Anabolic–androgenic steroids may inhibit $Na^+,K^+ATPase$.[107] This effect might reduce bile acid uptake, because this uptake utilizes the Na^+ gradient generated by this pump for the cotransport of bile acids. Anabolic–androgenic steroids also act at the canalicular level, producing a selective interference with the excretion of conjugated bilirubin into the canaliculi.[107] These agents finally lead to injury to the pericanalicular microfilamentous network (Philips, AmJPathol, 1978; 93:729). This injury may impair contractions of bile canaliculi and contribute to cholestasis.

Cholestasis due to anabolic–androgenic steroids has been extensively reviewed by Ishak and Zimmerman.[107] The anabolic steroids that can cause jaundice have an alkyl group in the C-17 position.[107] These include methyltestosterone, norethandrolone, oxymetholone, metenolone, metandienone, danazol, and stanozolol.[81] Testosterone and 19-nortestosterone, which are not alkylated in the C-17 position, have led to rare instances of hyperbilirubinaemia, but hardly ever to jaundice.[107]

Only a small minority of subjects receiving therapeutic doses of anabolic steroids become jaundiced, although the majority develop hepatic dysfunction.[107] Jaundice typically does not develop until the drug has been taken for at least 1 month, and often several months. Surprisingly, pruritus is uncommon, occurring in about 10 per cent of subjects only. Approximately one-third of patients have normal alkaline phosphatase values, and 50 per cent have values slightly above normal.[107] Liver biopsy shows bilirubin casts in canaliculi and bile-staining of the hepatocytes, mainly in centrilobular areas. Electron microscopy shows dilated canaliculi, with blunting and loss of microvilli.

Subsidence of jaundice may require weeks or months. With a few exceptions (see section on prolonged cholestasis) complete recovery occurs.

Cyclosporin

Cyclosporin administration decreases bile flow in rats, particularly the bile salt-dependent fraction (Stone, Gastro, 1987; 93:344). The drug inhibits both the sinusoidal uptake and the canalicular secretion of bile acids.[108] It also decreases the hepatic uptake and biliary secretion of bromosulphophthalein, and the biliary excretion of bilirubin in rats.[109]

In humans that receive cyclosporin for conditions other than liver transplantation, the drug clearly interferes, in a dose-related manner, with the hepatic clearance of bile salts, bilirubin, and bromosulphophthalein.[109] In most patients, however, these effects lead at most to mild increases in serum bilirubin and/or bile salts, with absent or mild increases in serum alkaline phosphatase and/or ALT activity.[109] These biochemical abnormalities occur 2 weeks to 3 months after the onset of the treatment.[109] They usually regress upon reduction of the dose.[109]

With the widespread use of cyclosporin after organ transplantation, some cases of cholestasis have been reported (Klintmalm, Transpl, 1981; 32:488; Schade, TransplProc, 1983; 15:2757; Leimanstoll, DMedWoch, 1984; 109:1989). The small number of reported cases and the large number of recipients suggest that the incidence of marked cholestasis is low. Another consequence, however, of the effects of cyclosporin on bile secretion is to increase the incidence of bile stones (Lorber, Transpl, 1987; 43:35).

Lipid storage liver diseases

Lipid storage liver diseases are characterized by the deposition of either phospholipids ('phospholipidosis') and/or triglycerides ('steatosis') in the liver (Table 8). Depending on the size and number of lipid droplets in a hepatocyte, steatosis can be further subdivided into 'macrovacuolar' and 'microvesicular' steatosis, although there are frequent associations and possible transitions between these two forms. Finally, chronic steatosis may be associated with a number of pseudo-alcoholic liver lesions, described under the term of 'steatohepatitis' lesions.

Macrovacuolar steatosis

Features and general mechanism

The hepatocyte contains a single, large, droplet of fat which displaces the nucleus to the periphery of the cell. In the absence of other liver lesion, macrovacuolar steatosis by itself is a relatively benign condition, at least in the short term. There may be slight increases in ALT and/or γ-glutamyl transferase activities, without clinical manifestations. The liver may or may not be slightly enlarged on clinical examination, and it is usually hyper-reflective on ultrasonogaphy.

Macrovacuolar steatosis may result from the combination of different mechanisms. These may include increased mobilization of fat from adipose tissue, a moderate decrease in their oxidation in the liver (if this effect is major, it will instead produce microvesicular steatosis), and an impaired egress of lipids out of the liver.[4] Triglycerides leave the liver in the form of lipoproteins. Their apoprotein moieties are glycoproteins which are synthesized in the rough endoplasmic reticulum and are glycosylated both there and in the Golgi apparatus.[4] Decreased output of triglycerides may result from a specific biochemical lesion, as with methotrexate which impairs protein synthesis. It may also occur as a consequence of structural lesions to the endoplasmic reticulum, Golgi, and plasma membrane. This may explain why macrovacuolar steatosis may be associated, at times, with hepatitis produced by many drugs (such as allopurinol, halothane, isoniazid, and α-methyldopa).[4]

Drugs causing macrovacuolar steatosis as the predominant lesion

Ethanol

Ethanol is probably the most widely used anxiolytic agent and is the most common cause of macrovacuolar steatosis due to exogenous agents. Macrovacuolar steatosis due to ethanol abuse may be related to increased mobilization of peripheral fat, and a mild decrease in fat oxidation.[110] When the β-oxidation of fat is severely impaired, microvesicular steatosis may instead develop.[111]

Glucocorticoids

Glucocorticoids, particularly in large doses, lead to macrovacuolar steatosis of the liver.[4] The disease is clinically silent, although hepatomegaly may be present. Glucocorticoids may enhance the mobilization of lipids from adipocytes in high doses, and may inhibit protein synthesis.[4]

Methotrexate

This potent inhibitor of dihydrofolate reductase impairs the metabolic transfer of 1-carbon units in a variety of biochemical reactions (Bleyer, Cancer, 1987; 41:36), leading to decreased DNA, RNA, and protein synthesis. The last effect may perhaps explain steatosis produced by this antineoplastic agents.[112] Methotrexate administration may also lead to fibrosis and cirrhosis (see below).

Table 8 Lipid-storage liver diseease and main causative drugs

Macrovacuolar steatosis	Steatohepatitis with phospholipidosis
Ethanol	Amiodarone
Glucocorticoids	Diethylaminoethoxyhexestrol
Methotrexate	Perhexiline
Microvesicular steatosis	Steatohepatitis without phospholipidosis
Amineptine	Diethylstilboestrol
Amiodarone	Diltiazem
Asparaginase	Glucocorticoids
Aspirin	Hexoestrol
Ethanol	Nifedipine
Didanosine	Tamoxifen
Fialuridine	
Glucocorticoids	
Ibuprofen	
Ketoprofen	
Tetracyclines	
Tianeptine	
Perhexiline	
Pirprofen	
Valproate	
Zalcitabine	
Zidovudine	

Microvesicular steatosis
Features and general mechanism

In this condition, hepatocytes are occupied by numerous, small lipid vesicles, that leave the nucleus in the centre of the cell, and give the hepatocytes a 'foamy', 'spongiocytic' appearance. When discrete, this lesion may be missed by a non-specialized pathologist. An Oil Red O stain clearly shows, however, the small reddish lipid vesicles that fill out the hepatocytes. Microvesicular steatosis affecting some hepatocytes may be associated with macrovacuolar steatosis in other hepatocytes. Patients exhibiting both lesions should be classified as cases of microvesicular steatosis (with associated macrovacuolar steatosis).

Whatever its cause, microvesicular steatosis is constantly related to severe impairment of the mitochondrial β-oxidation of fatty acids.[111] This occurs in several genetic defects affecting transporters or enzymes that are involved in the mitochondrial β-oxidation of fatty acids,[113] and in the mitochondrial cytopathies that are due to inborn defects of the respiratory chain.[114] The latter defects impair the mitochondrial reoxidation of NADH into NAD$^+$. The reduced availability of NAD$^+$ then inhibits mitochondrial β-oxidation, which requires NAD$^+$ as a necessary cofactor.[115] Genetic defects in urea cycle enzymes increase the levels of ammonium, and this impairs fatty acid oxidation.[116] The impairment of β-oxidation may also be acquired. Reye's syndrome is caused by an acquired mitochondrial insult (De Vivo, Neurology, 1978; 28:105), possibly caused by the adverse effects of cytokines (or viruses?) on mitochondrial function.[111] Pregnancy and/or female sex hormones cause ultrastructural and functional lesions of mitochondria.[117,118] Together with other genetic or acquired factors, these hormonal effects may contribute to the development of acute fatty liver of pregnancy in some women. Similarly, all drugs known to produce microvesicular steatosis impair the mitochondrial β-oxidation of fatty acids (Fromenty, JHepatol, 1997; 26 (suppl.1): 13).

Because non-esterified fatty acids are poorly oxidized by mitochondria, they undergo increased esterification into triglycerides, which represent the main form of lipids that are accumulated in these conditions (Fromenty, JHepatol, 1997; 26 (Suppl.1):13). Nevertheless, there is a residual increase in non-esterified fatty acids (Fromenty, JHepatol, 1997; 26 (Suppl.1):13). It has been suggested that these amphiphilic compounds may form an emulsifying rim around a core of neutral triglycerides (Fromenty, JHepatol, 1997; 26 (Suppl.1):13). Emulsification might explain the deposition of microvesicular fat in this condition (Fromenty, JHepatol, 1997; 26 (Suppl.1):13). The accumulated free fatty acids might also impair the assembly, cellular transport, and secretion of very low density lipoproteins by the liver. This may represent an additional factor leading to fat deposition in these conditions (Fromenty, JHepatol, 1997; 26 (Suppl.1):13).

Depending on the causative drug, liver cell necrosis may be absent (as with tetracycline) or present (as with valproic acid). Even in the absence of liver cell necrosis, extensive microvesicular steatosis is, by itself, a serious condition. Although serum transaminase and bilirubin levels are only moderately increased, the prothrombin time may be prolonged. Development of haemorrhagic episodes, attacks of syncope, hypotension, and shock may mark the seriousness of the entity, and may be followed by profound lethargy and coma.[4] Hypoglycaemia may occur. Azotaemia and pancreatitis may be associated, contributing to the poor overall prognosis.

Microvesicular steatosis is the morphological hallmark of a serious metabolic condition that may cause a severe energy crisis (Fromenty, JHepatol, 1997; 26 (Suppl.1):13):

1. Impairment of the β-oxidation of fatty acids deprives the cell of an important source of energy.
2. Not only is lipid oxidation unavailable as a source of energy, but the recourse to glucose as an alternative fuel is also compromised. Normally, the acetyl-coenzyme A formed by β-oxidation is an important allosteric activator of pyruvate carboxylase, a rate

limiting step in gluconeogenesis from lactate and pyruvate (Fromenty, JHepatol, 1997; 26 (Suppl.1):13). Furthermore, fatty acyl-CoAs inhibit glucose 6-phosphatase, which catalyzes the terminal reaction of gluconeogenesis (Filceri, BiochemJ, 1995; 307:391). When β-oxidation is impaired, the decreased levels of acetyl-coenzyme A may reduce pyruvate carboxylase, while the increased levels of acyl-CoAs may impair glucose 6-phosphatase activity. These effects limit the recourse to glucose formation and subsequent oxidation as an alternative source of energy.

3. Furthermore, the accumulation of non-esterified fatty acids and their dicarboxylic acid derivatives uncouple oxidative phosphorylation. Thus, not only are fuels less oxidized (fats) or less available (carbohydrates), but their oxidation is also wasted in vain, to produce heat instead of ATP (Fromenty, JHepatol, 1997; 26 (Suppl.1):13).

Drugs causing microvesicular steatosis

Amineptine

As explained above, this tricyclic antidepressant is a frequent cause of immunoallergic, mixed hepatitis, possibly due to the metabolic activation of its tricyclic moiety into reactive metabolites. Amineptine, however, is peculiar due to the presence of an heptanoic side chain. This 7-carbon side chain is metabolized in vivo by β-oxidation into the 5- and 3-carbons derivatives.[119] In the process, these unnatural fatty acid analogues reversibly inhibit the β-oxidation of the medium- and short-chain fatty acids.[119] This may explain why microvesicular steatosis of the liver has been observed in a few patients receiving this antidepressant (Martin, GastrClinBiol, 1981; 5:1071; Ramain, GastrClinBiol, 1981; 5:469).

Amiodarone and perhexiline

These cationic amphiphilic drugs inhibit mitochondrial function and cause microvesicular and macrovacuolar steatosis of the liver. Steatosis may be part of a more complex set of liver lesions (phospholipidosis and steatohepatitis) that are considered in another section.

L-Asparaginase

L-Asparaginase decreases the amino acid L-asparagine by hydrolysing it to L-aspartic acid and ammonia. Unlike normal cells, leukaemic cells cannot synthesize L-asparagine and are therefore selectively affected. E. coli L-asparaginase also has glutaminase activity. It therefore depletes both asparagine and glutamine (Du, CancerRes, 1983; 43:1602). As a consequence, protein synthesis decreases markedly. This explains the antineoplastic activity of this enzyme preparation, but it also causes a decrease in plasma albumin, clotting factors, and plasma lipoproteins, and the development of fatty liver. Steatosis has been found in 50 to 90 per cent patients treated with this agent.[3,4] Serum transaminase and plasma bilirubin are increased. Blood levels of ammonia are also increased, at times strikingly. Associated adverse effects may include pancreatitis, central nervous system disturbances, hypersensitivity to this bacterial product, and disseminated intravascular coagulopathy (Haskell, NEJM, 1969; 281:1028). A glutaminase-free asparaginase from Vibrio succinogenes is less toxic in animals (Durden, CancerRes, 1983; 43:1602).

Aspirin and Reye's syndrome

Reye's syndrome is a severe form of microvesicular steatosis that occurs after viral infections (in particular influenza and varicella), most often, but not exclusively, in children. Cytokines impair mitochondrial function and may be, in part, responsible for the disease.[111] Hypothetically, some viruses may also directly impair mitochondrial function. However, these mitochondrial effects are, at best, very moderate in liver cells. The vast majority of viral infections are well tolerated. Other factors are thus probably required additively to impair mitochondrial function and trigger the syndrome in the infected subjects.

A first potentiating factor has been the intake of aspirin in febrile children. In the past, 93 per cent of cases of Reye's syndrome had occurred in children receiving aspirin, and the frequency of aspirin use was higher in those that subsequently developed this syndrome than in children with similar viral diseases not followed by Reye's syndrome.[61]

Aspirin is quickly hydrolysed into salicylic acid. This carboxylic metabolite is actively transformed by mitochondria (probably on their outer membrane) into the salicylyl-coenzyme A derivative. Extensive formation of this thioester sequesters extramitochondrial coenzyme A. The latter is no longer available for the activation of long chain fatty acids, whose entry in mitochondria and subsequent β-oxidation is therefore decreased.[120] The drug-induced impairment of fatty acid oxidation (added to the effects of infection) probably helped to trigger the syndrome in children receiving aspirin for viral infections. Indeed, recommendations for the avoidance of aspirin in febrile children have led to a parallel decline in the use of aspirin and the incidence of Reye's syndrome in the United States (Fromenty, JHepatol, 1997; 26 (Suppl.1):13).

Nevertheless, a few cases of Reye's syndrome are still being observed. A second factor that may help trigger Reye's syndrome is a previously latent defect in mitochondrial β-oxidation enzymes.[111] The anorexia, vomiting, and fever associated with the infectious disease, together with the fast imposed by some ill-advised mothers, may then increase peripheral lipolysis. This may start a vicious circle, by increasing the fatty acid burden of the liver. The liver may be unable to handle this increased load of fatty acids, because the inborn defect is further aggravated by the impairment of β-oxidation resulting from the infectious process. Now that the use of aspirin has been curtailed in febrile children, residual cases of Reye's syndrome mainly occur in children with a previously latent genetic defect in β-oxidation (Rowe, JAMA, 1988; 260:1167).

Calcium hopantenate (pantoyl-γ-aminobutyrate)

This analogue of panthotenic acid may inhibit mitochondrial β-oxidation (Nakanishi, CCActa, 1990; 188:85) and has caused Reye-like syndromes in Japan (Nodan, JNeurolNeurosurgPsych, 1988; 51:582).

Cocaine

As already mentioned, cocaine-induced liver lesions may combine both centrilobular necrosis and periportal microvesicular steatosis. Cocaine analogues, such as bupivacaine decrease the mitochondrial membrane potential (Grouselle, BiochemJ, 1990; 271:269).

Ethanol

An uncommon form of alcohol-induced liver lesion is alcoholic foamy degeneration, a severe condition resembling Reye's syndrome, and characterized by massive accumulation of both microvesicular and macrovacuolar fat.[111] Such patients may present with jaundice and hepatomegaly, but no major hepatic failure. Nevertheless, lethargy, coma, and death may occur a few hours or days after admission.[111] On electron microscopy, mitochondria display diverse abnormalities such as atrophy, disorganization of the matrix, loss of cristae, or striking enlargement (megamitochondria).[111] A milder form of microvesicular steatosis is less exceptional; patients have high serum transaminase activities as compared to those with macrovacuolar steatosis, and exhibit centrilobular foamy hepatocytes, but their short-term prognosis remains good.[111]

Mitochondrial DNA (**mtDNA**) is 10 to 16 times more prone to oxidative damage than nuclear DNA, due to the attachment of mtDNA to the mitochondrial inner membrane (which is the main source of reactive oxygen species in the cell), to the lack of protective histones in mtDNA, and to less efficient repair processes in the mitochondrion than in the nucleus.[121] Oxidative damage to mtDNA produces single strand breaks and may favour slipped mispairing of repeated sequences during replication, thus leading to mtDNA deletions.[121] Oxidative damage of DNA may also cause formation of 8-hydroxy-deoxyguanosine.[121] This modified base leads to misreading during replication, producing a variety of point mutations. Because mtDNA lacks introns, any oxidative damage will involve a functionally important gene. However, as there are several hundreds of copies of the mitochondrial genome in a single cell, cells may accumulate a limited amount of various mtDNA mutations without initial detrimental effects. The mtDNA may thus serve as a molecular clock of the ageing process.[121] Accumulation of 8-hydroxy-deoxyguanosine, mtDNA deletions, and mtDNA point mutations spontaneously occur in old age, resulting in a slow, progressive deterioration of mitochondrial function.[121]

Ethanol consumption increases the generation of oxygen radicals in rat liver mitochondria.[122] Alcoholism might, therefore, accelerate the oxidative ageing of mtDNA, and this might in turn impair mitochondrial function and lead to microvesicular steatosis of the liver.[123] Indeed, a 4977-base pair mtDNA deletion was found in four of five patients (80 per cent) with lethal microvesicular steatosis, and in two of five patients (40 per cent) with regressive microvesicular steatosis. The deletion was uncommon (5 per cent) in alcoholics with other liver lesions, and absent in 62 non-alcoholic patients of similar age, with either various liver diseases or a normal liver histology.[123]

The metabolism of ethanol to acetate leads to the reduction of NAD^+ into NADH. In subjects with a normal respiratory chain, NADH is, for a large part, reoxidized back to NAD^+, thus allowing continued activity of 3-hydroxyacyl-CoA dehydrogenase (an NAD^+-dependent enzyme involved in the third step of the mitochondrial β-oxidation process).[123] Subjects with multiple mutations of the mtDNA genome might poorly reoxidize NADH in mitochondria.[123] This would lead to a considerable decrease in the NAD^+/NADH ratio, marked inhibition of mitochondrial β-oxidation, and development of alcoholic foamy degeneration. According to this view, alcoholic foamy degeneration would represent,

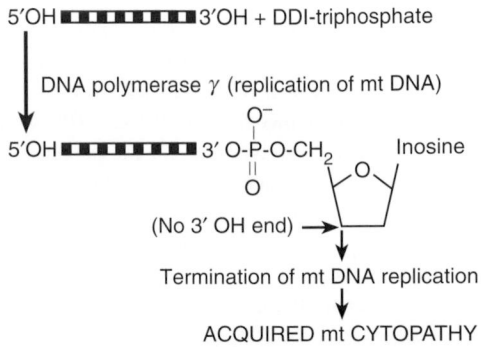

Fig. 6. Effects of dideoxynucleoside analogues on mitochondrial DNA. The analogue, didanosine (DDI)-triphosphate in this example, is incorporated by DNA polymerase γ into a growing chain of mitochondrial (mt) DNA, leading to termination of mitochondrial DNA replication, and an acquired form of mitochondrial cytopathy.

at least in some patients, an acquired form of a mitochondrial cytopathy.[123]

Dideoxynucleoside antiviral agents (zidovudine, zalcitabine, and didanosine)

3′-Azido-2′,3′-dideoxythymidine (zidovudine or AZT), 2′,3′-dideoxycytidine (zalcitabine, ddC), and 2′,3′-dideoxyinosine (didanosine, ddI) are 2′,3′-dideoxynucleosides that are used in patients with human immunodeficiency virus (**HIV**) infection.[111] The sugar analogue of these dideoxynucleosides possess the normal 5′-hydroxyl group of deoxyribose. After activation to the triphosphate derivative, the analogue can thus be incorporated (in place of a natural nucleotide) into a growing chain of DNA. In contrast, the 3′-hydroxyl group of deoxyribose is absent in these sugar analogues. Once the nucleotide analogue has been added at the end of a growing chain of DNA, the DNA chain now lacks a 3-hydroxyl end, and no other nucleotide can be incorporated, thus terminating DNA replication (Fig. 6).

Therefore, the effects of these compounds depend on the ability of various polymerases to incorporate these analogues into DNA. The HIV reverse transcriptase is able to perform this incorporation, thus impairing the reverse transcription of the viral RNA into the HIV DNA.[124] The mammalian DNA polymerases which are involved in nuclear DNA replication do not incorporate the dideoxynucleoside triphosphates into the growing chain of DNA. The replication of nuclear DNA is not impaired, allowing utilization of these compounds as therapeutic agents.[125]

The problem is that the mammalian DNA polymerase γ, which acts in mitochondria, can, like the viral reverse transcriptase, incorporate the dideoxynucleoside triphosphates into the growing chain of mtDNA, thus impairing mtDNA replication (Fig. 6).[125] Unlike the nuclear DNA, mtDNA keeps replicating, even in post-mitotic tissues. When its replication is impaired, there occurs a progressive loss of mtDNA, leading to an acquired equivalent of a mitochondrial cytopathy (Fromenty, JHepatol, 1997; 26 (Suppl.1): 13). As in the inborn mitochondrial cytopathies, the clinical manifestations may be extremely polymorphic. Although each analogue may selectively affect certain organs rather than others (for reasons that remain presently unknown), taken together the 2',3'-di-deoxynucleoside analogues may lead to bone marrow suppression with anaemia, neutropenia and thrombocytopenia, pancreatitis, peripheral neuropathy, myopathy, or microvesicular steatosis of the liver.[3,126]

Fialuridine

Recently, another type of antiviral agent, namely fluoroiodoarauracil (fialuridine, FIAU), has induced several cases of fatal microvesicular steatosis of the liver, leading to immediate interruption of these clinical trials.[127] Fialuridine has been shown to be incorporated into genomic DNA and to deplete mtDNA *in vivo*.[128] A 3'-OH group is present in the sugar moiety of this analogue. The incorporation of several adjacent fialuridine nucleotides into mtDNA inhibits DNA polymerase γ and mtDNA replication (Lewis, PNAS, 1996; 93:3592).

Glucocorticoids

Although glucocorticoids are mainly known as producing macro-vacuolar steatosis in humans, they inhibit the mitochondrial β-oxidation of fatty acids and produce microvesicular steatosis of the liver in mice (Lettéron, AmJPhysiol, 1997; 272;G1141). We have observed several patients with microvesicular steatosis due to gluco-corticoids. Prolonged treatments with high doses of glucocorticoids have led to steatohepatitis lesions in humans (Itoh, Acta-HepatoGastroent, 1977; 24:884).

Ibuprofen

Like the other 2-arylpropionate derivatives, this non-steroidal anti-inflammatory drug is transformed into slightly reactive acyl-glu-curonides that slowly covalently bind to hepatic proteins and might be responsible for the few cases of mixed hepatitis that may occur with these compounds. In a few patients, however, the liver lesion has been that of microvesicular steatosis.[3] Ibuprofen is a mixture of two enantiomers, both of which inhibit the β-oxidation of medium- and short-chain fatty acids.[129]

Ketoprofen

Also a 2-arylpropionate derivative, this non-streroidal anti-in-flammatory drug has produced a few instances of microvesicular steatosis (Dutertre, EurJGastroHepatol, 1991; 3:953).

Tetracycline derivatives

Tetracycline itself and the various tetracycline derivatives produce extensive microvesicular steatosis of the liver in experimental animals. This is due to the dual effect of these antibiotics, which inhibit both the mitochondrial β-oxidation of fatty acids and the hepatic secretion of very low density lipoproteins.[130,131] The latter effect occurs at doses which do not inhibit protein synthesis, suggesting impairment of the assembly and/or vesicular transport of these lipoproteins.[132]

At currently administered oral doses, tetracycline may produce minor degrees of hepatic steatosis of no clinical concern in humans.[4] However, severe microvesicular steatosis has occurred in the past during the intravenous administration of tetracycline, usually in high doses.[4] Predisposing factors included impaired renal function (which decreased tetracycline elimination) and pregnancy (which impaired mitochondrial function). The syndrome usually appeared after 4 to 10 days of tetracycline infusion.[4] The disease resembled Reye's syndrome. Renal failure and pancreatitis were frequently associated. Most of the reported cases have died, but milder cases may have gone unrecognized or unreported. Microvesicular steatosis has also been observed after intravenous administration of several other tetracycline derivatives.[4]

Tianeptine

This analogue of amineptine has a related tricyclic moiety and an identical heptanoic side chain. Like amineptine, it is activated by cytochrome P-450 into reactive metabolites. Like amineptine, it is metabolized mainly by β-oxidation of its heptanoic side chain, and it reversibly inhibits the mitochondrial β-oxidation of medium- and short-chain fatty acids (Fromenty, BiochemPharm, 1989; 38:3743). Unlike amineptine, however, tianeptine is used in much lower doses, and only one case of both hepatitis and microvesicular steatosis has been reported with this derivative (Le Bricquir, JHepatol, 1994: 21:771).

Pirprofen

This 2-arylpropionate non-steroidal anti-inflammatory drug had to be recalled because of its hepatotoxic potential. In some patients, microvesicular steatosis accompanied liver cell necrosis.[77] Like ibuprofen, this 2-arylpropionate anti-inflammatory drug inhibited the mitochondrial β-oxidation of fatty acids, and produced microvesicular steatosis of the liver in mice.[133]

Valproate

Administration of this anticonvulsant may produce silent increases in serum transaminase activity in 16 to 67 per cent of recipients.[134] Overt liver disease is much less common. It occurs mainly in young individuals (with highest risk in children under 3 years of age) and is favoured by the concurrent administration of phenobarbital or phenytoin, two microsomal enzyme inducers.[3] Prodromes include lethargy, lassitude, anorexia, nausea, vomiting, oedema, and facial puffiness, as well as a frequent change in the pattern of convulsions.[134] The fully developed syndrome is usually marked by jaundice, sometimes with ascites, and haemorrhagic phenomena. The disease may end up in coma, associated with azotaemia in 50 per cent of cases.[134] Serum transaminase activity is moderately increased. The prothrombin time is prolonged. Serum ammonia levels are elevated. Hypoglycaemia may occur. Microvesicular steatosis is often associated with necrosis and, at times, with cirrhosis and cholestasis.[134]

Valproic acid is a branched chain fatty acid (Fig. 7). Like natural fatty acids, it forms the acyl-coenzyme A derivative. Extensive formation of valproyl-coenzyme A inside the mitochondria depletes the intramitochondrial pool of coenzyme A, and thereby decreases the oxidation of long-, medium-, and short-chain fatty acids.[111] In addition to the sequestration of coenzyme A, another mechanism has been suggested (Fig. 7). Cytochrome P-450 (in particular phenobarbital-inducible isoenzymes) desaturate the ultimate and penultimate carbons of valproate, forming Δ_4-valproate (Rettie, Science, 1987; 235:890). This metabolite is further metabolized in mitochondria, where its β-oxidation then produces the diene

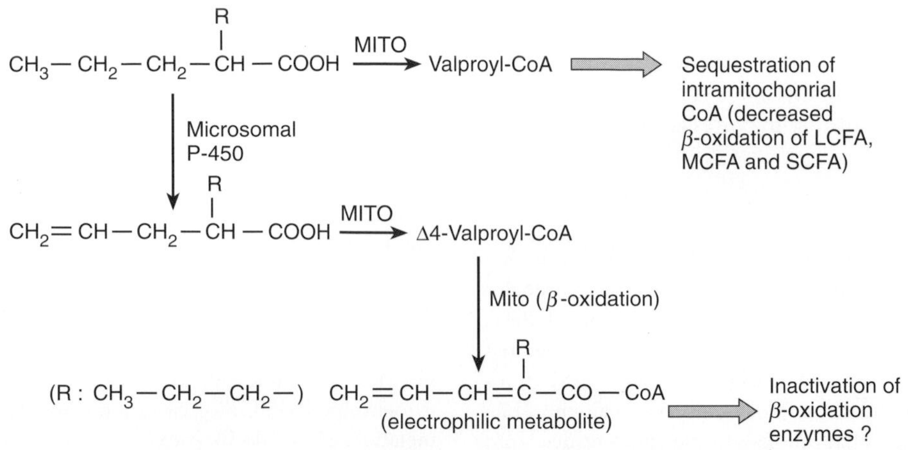

Fig. 7. Sequestration of coenzyme A by valproate and possible inactivation of mitochondrial enzymes by an electrophilic metabolite formed by the successive action of microsomal cytochrome P-450 and mitochondrial β-oxidation enzymes.

derivative: Δ_4, Δ_2-valproyl-coenzyme A. This is an electrophilic metabolite that reacts with glutathione, and might inactivate β-oxidation enzymes.[111] Although this inactivation remains to be demonstrated, this scheme would account for the increased hepatotoxicity of valproate during the concomitant administration of cytochrome P-450-inducing drugs.

Prevention of valproate hepatotoxicity relies mainly in the avoidance of this drug in children under 3 years of age or those taking other anticonvulsants.[3] These two precautions have led to a fourfold decline in the frequency of fatal liver injury.[3] Monthly monitoring of liver tests during the first 6 months of therapy is also recommended, but its efficacy remains unproven because there is a high incidence of liver enzyme elevations which are often transient, and because severe hepatotoxicity may obviously develop between the scheduled tests. Indications to stop the drug may include persisting ALT abnormalities (particularly if they exceed three times the upper limit of normal), and certainly, any abnormality in coagulation factors, bilirubin or albumin, or the appearance of lethargy, malaise, anorexia, nausea, or vomiting.[3]

Phospholipidosis and steatohepatitis

These liver lesions are considered together because they may occur concomitantly in patients receiving antianginal drugs that have a cationic amphiphilic structure. The resulting uptake of the drug by lysosomes leads to phospholipidosis, while their mitochondrial uptake leads to chronic steatosis and its possible sequel, steatohepatitis.

Features and mechanisms
Phospholipidosis

Hepatic phospholipidosis is characterized by the accumulation of phospholipids within liver cell lysosomes.[135,136] In humans, phospholipidosis has been mainly observed with the three antianginal drugs: 4,4′-diethylaminoethoxyhexestrol,[137,138] perhexiline maleate,[139–142] and amiodarone.[143–146] These drugs are cationic amphiphilic compounds with a lipophilic moiety and an amine function which can become protonated (and thus positively charged).[135,136] The uncharged, lipophilic form easily crosses the lysosomal membrane. Inside the lysosome, the pH is acidic due to the presence, on the lysosomal membrane, of H^+-ATPases that accumulate H^+ within the lysosome. Because of this acidic intralysosomal milieu, the unprotonated drug molecule is protonated within lysosomes. The protonated form is more hydrosoluble and is less able to cross back through the lysosomal membrane, leading to its accumulation within lysosomes.[136]

Lysosomes are the waste disposal system of the cell. During the process of autophagy (for example during fasting), evaginations of the hepatic endoplasmic reticulum membrane engulf and then isolate, in a double-membrane structure, whole parts of the cytoplasm (including cytosol, endoplasmic reticulum fragments, and mitochondria). These eventually end up into lysosomes for final digestion. The phospholipids of these internal membrane structures are normally degraded by intralysosomal phospholipases.

The problem is that the protonated form of amiodarone, perhexiline, or diethylaminoethoxyhexestrol forms non-covalent but tight complexes with phospholipids. Indeed, the lipophilic moiety of the protonated drug molecule may form hydrophobic bonds with the fatty acid moieties of phospholipids, while the protonated (positively charged) amine group may undergo electrostatic interaction with the negatively charged phosphate group of phospholipids.[135,136] These tight interactions hamper the action of intralysosomal phospholipases.[135,136] Phospholipids are not degraded, and they progressively accumulate, together with the bound drug molecules, within lysosomes. The accumulation of the drug–phospholipid complexes generates enormous lysosomes filled with pseudomyelinic figures.

The accumulation of phospholipids can be detected by histochemistry,[141] but confirmation of the diagnosis requires electron microscopy. On ultrastructural examination, lysosomes are both abundant and increased in size, and they contain lamellar, reticular, or pseudomyelinic figures. Phospholipidosis may affect not only the liver but also many other organs such as skin, myocardium, lungs, and blood cells.[135,136]

Phospholipidosis is extremely frequent, perhaps constant after the administration of these drugs.[147] It has probably no clinical consequence, since it occurs in many patients without clinical symptoms and either no, or little, biochemical disturbances.[147]

After withdrawal of the causative drug, phospholipidosis regresses slowly because of the very slow dissociation of the drug–phospholipid complexes. Consequently, the drug may still be detectable in plasma many months after discontinuation of treatment.[143] This protracted retention influences the outcome of the second possible liver lesion, namely steatohepatitis.

Steatohepatitis (alcohol-like lesions)

In a few patients receiving these drugs (amiodarone, perhexiline, diethylaminoethoxyhexestrol) for several months or years, a more severe form of liver disease, termed 'alcohol-like liver lesions' or 'steatohepatitis', may develop. The incidence of these lesions is related to the duration of the treatment and thus the cumulative dose. Generally, the disease develops insidiously and may be revealed by hepatomegaly or a moderate increase in serum ALT activity. In severe forms, jaundice, ascites, and encephalopathy may be observed. Histological lesions are similar to those observed in alcoholic liver disease and may include microvesicular and macrovacuolar steatosis, Mallory bodies, a mixed inflammatory cell infiltrate (containing neutrophils), fibrosis, and even cirrhosis. Despite the discontinuation of therapy, the disease may worsen and fatal cirrhosis may occur.[139] This secondary aggravation is probably related to the protracted persistence of the drug in its lysosomal deposits (see above).

The induction of steatosis and, possibly, the other lesions that characterize the steatohepatitis syndrome may be related to the ability of these drugs to interfere with mitochondrial function (Fig. 8).[111] Let us recall that the mitochondrion has two membranes, and that the transfer of electrons through complexes I, III, and IV of the respiratory chain (located on the mitochondrial inner membrane) results in the translocation of protons from the matrix into the intermembranous compartment.[111] This creates an important electrochemical gradient across the mitochondrial inner membrane. The potential energy of this gradient is utilized secondarily to generate ATP. When protons re-enter the matrix via the F_0 moiety of ATP synthase (complex V), the energy released by this re-entry is harnessed in the synthesis of ATP by the F_1 portion of complex V. An analogy of this system would be the pumping up of water by a thermal engine (the respiratory chain) up into a reservoir, followed by the harnessing of this energy by hydroelectric turbines (ATP synthase) (Fromenty, JHepatol, 7; 26 (Suppl.1):13). Amiodarone, [148,149] perhexiline,[150] and diethylaminoethoxy-hexoestrol (unpublished experiments) produce similar effects on mitochondria, so that a common concept may be proposed (Fig. 8).[111] The unprotonated form of these drugs is lipophilic, and easily crosses the mitochondrial outer membrane. In the intermembranous space, due to the abundance of protons in this space, the drug molecule is protonated. The latter molecule is positively charged, and is therefore 'pushed' inside the mitochondria by the high electrochemical potential existing across the mitochondrial inner membrane (with the outside being positively charged). In the relatively alkaline matrix, the protonated molecule dissociates into a proton and the uncharged parent compound (amiodarone, perhexiline, or diethylaminoethoxyhexestrol). The re-entry of a proton in the mitochondrial matrix (bypassing ATP synthase) decreases the membrane potential and wastes energy, while the accumulation at high concentration of the lipophilic unprotonated molecule inside

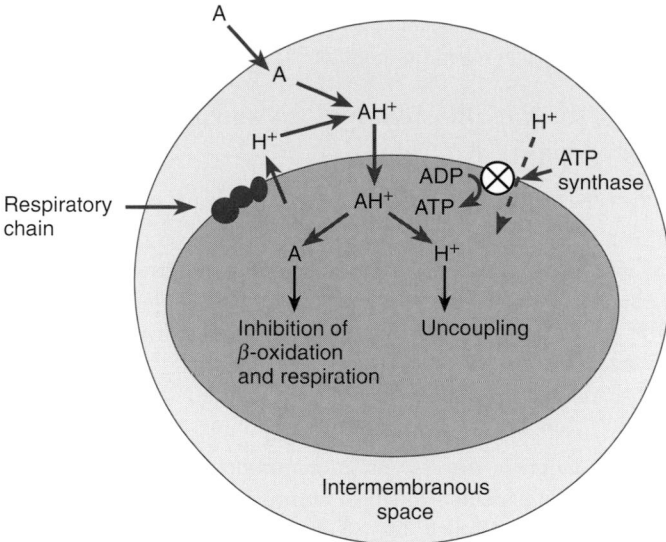

A=Unprotonated drug (amiodarone, perhexiline, or diethylaminoethoxyhexoestrol)

Fig. 8. Mitochondrial effects of amiodarone, perhexiline, and diethylaminoethoxyhexestrol. The drug is protonated in the acidic intermembranous space of the mitochondrion. The protonated drug is then translocated, along the mitochondrial potential, into the mitochondrial matrix, where it dissociates into a proton and the unprotonated molecule, whose accumulation leads to inhibition of β-oxidation and respiration.

the mitochondria probably interferes with membranous phospholipids and polypeptides and inhibits both electron transfer through the respiratory chain and the β-oxidation of long-, medium-, and short-chain fatty acids, thus explaining steatosis (Fig. 8).[148–150]

In addition to chronic steatosis, prolonged administration of these compounds may also cause necrosis, fibrosis, a neutrophil infiltrate, and Mallory bodies. Similar steatohepatitis lesions may occur in obesity, diabetes, prolonged corticosteroid administration, jejunoileal bypass, or Wilson's disease (Fromenty, JHepatol, 1996, in press). All these conditions are characterized by chronic steatosis. It seems, therefore, inescapable that chronic steatosis may be somehow involved in the possible development of these other liver lesions.

Steatosis, whether acute or chronic, leads to lipid peroxidation in mice.[151] With amiodarone, perhexiline, and 4,4′-diethyl-aminoethoxyhexestrol, lipid peroxidation is further increased due to the enhanced formation of reactive oxygen species resulting from the inhibition of the respiratory chain. Chronic lipid peroxidation might account for the diverse liver lesions regrouped under the term of steatohepatitis:[151]

1. Peroxidation may lead to cell demise (accounting for necrosis).
2. Peroxidation releases malondialdehyde and 4-hydroxynonenal.[11] Both stimulate collagen production by Ito cells (hence, fibrosis).[151]
3. 4-Hydroxynonenal is also a strong chemoattractant for neutrophils (hence the neutrophil infiltrate).[151]
4. Malondialdehyde is a bifunctional alkylating agent ($CHO-CH_2-CHO$) that cross-links proteins by reacting with the ε-amino

groups of lysine residues from two polypeptidic chains.[11] Hypothetically, it might similarly cross-link cytokeratins[151] (possibly accounting for the Mallory bodies that are formed of cross-linked cytokeratin monomers[152]).

Drugs causing phospholipidosis and alcoholic-like liver lesions

4,4′-Diethylaminoethoxyhexoestrol

This coronary vasodilatator has been recalled after being responsible for more than 100 cases of alcoholic-like liver disease associated with phospholipidosis in Japan.[4] The disease appeared usually after treatments lasting 6 months or more.[4] Fatal cirrhosis has occurred in some patients.[4]

Perhexiline maleate

An asymptomatic increase in serum aminotransferases occurs in 30 per cent of patients treated by perhexiline maleate.[142] Clinical manifestations are much less frequent and are generally observed after several months or years of treatment.[139–141] Liver lesions then associate features of alcohol-like hepatitis and phospholipidosis. Cirrhosis may occur,[141] sometimes despite discontinuation of the treatment.[139] The outcome is fatal in 50 per cent of patients with cirrhosis.[141] Liver damage is frequently associated with weight loss, peripheral neuropathy, and hypoglycaemia. Like steatohepatitis, these effects may be explained by the mitochondrial effects of this drug.[149]

The toxicity of perhexiline maleate is mainly observed in subjects with a genetic impairment in drug oxidation capacity.[153] Perhexiline is oxidized by cytochrome P-450 2D6 (i.e. the form involved in debrisoquine oxidation).[153] This isoenzyme is deficient in the liver of 3 to 10 per cent of Caucasians.[154] In deficient subjects, perhexiline oxidation is impaired and the drug accumulates anormally.[153] Oxidation phenotyping before perhexiline maleate administration should help to detect subjects that are particularly prone to develop adverse drug reactions.

Amiodarone

Mild increases in serum aminotransferase activity have been reported in 15 to 55 per cent of patients receiving this antiarrhythmic agent.[146] Phospholipidosis appears to be almost constant.[147] However, overt liver disease with alcohol-like liver lesions is uncommon.[143-146] It occurs after several months or years of treatment, and may continue to worsen after amiodarone withdrawal because of the persistence of this drug for many months in the liver.[143] Histological lesions induced by amiodarone tend to predominate in periportal areas whereas those caused by alcohol are mainly located in centrilobular areas (Poucell, Hepatol, 1985; 5: 995). Liver injury may be associated with other adverse effects of amiodarone including thyroid dysfunction, pulmonary fibrosis, neuropathy, skin discoloration, and corneal deposits (Mason, NEJM, 1987; 316:455). Amiodarone toxicity appears to be dose related, which may explain its higher incidence and earlier onset in North American countries, where daily doses have been higher than in Europe (400–600 mg versus 200 mg) (McArthur, BMJ, 1983; 287: 910). The morphological expression of phospholipidosis appears to correlate with the storage of amiodarone in liver tissue (Pirovino,

Hepatol, 1988; 8:591). Amiodarone accumulation may be assessed either by specific dosage in the liver or, non-invasively, by computed tomography scanning, thanks to the high iodine content of the drug.[146]

Steatohepatitis without phospholipidosis

A few cases of alcohol-like liver disease, without phospholipidosis, have been observed alter the administration of diltiazem (Beaugrand, GastrClinBiol, 1987; 11:76) and nifedipine (Babany, JHepatol, 1989; 9:252), two calcium-channel-blocking agents.

Steatohepatitis has been also observed after administration of several synthetic oestrogenic drugs, including hexestrol, a synthetic oestrogen resembling 4,4′-diethylaminoethylhexestrol but devoid of amphiphilic cationic properties (Seki, GastrJap, 1983; 18:197), diethylstilboestrol (Coe, Hepatol, 1983; 4:489), and tamoxifen (Cortez Pinto, JHepatol, 1995; 23:95; Prat, AnnIntMed, 1995; 123: 236).

Subacute hepatitis, chronic hepatitis, and postnecrotic cirrhosis

Prolonged damage to hepatocytes (whatever its initial mechanism) may lead to chronic hepatitis and cirrhosis. This is well demonstrated in experimental animals which develop cirrhosis after repeated administration of many compounds that produce liver cell necrosis, such as carbon tetrachloride, dimethylnitrosamine, or galactosamine.[4] In humans, prolonged drug-induced necrosis may also lead to subacute and chronic hepatitis, or even cirrhosis.

Prolonged necrosis may occur in humans in four circumstances:

1. Most frequently the liver lesion develops silently over a period of several months, but is only responsible for mild and nonspecific symptoms such as asthenia. Therefore, the liver injury remains unrecognized and the treatment is continued. When the disease is eventually detected, chronic lesions are already present.
2. In some cases, acute hepatitis is diagnosed, but the causative drug is not recognized and its administration is continued.
3. In other patients, the causative drug has been initially withdrawn but has then been readministered (or ingested again by the patient) before complete recovery from the initial episode, leading to subacute hepatitis.
4. In a few cases, finally, the process leading to the liver injury has continued despite the withdrawal of the offending drug. This has been observed with some drugs, such as tienilic acid, that trigger an autoimmune response directed against normal hepatocyte constituents.[44]

Prolonged necrosis may lead to three main types of liver diseases: subacute hepatitis, chronic hepatitis, and postnecrotic cirrhosis.

Unless there has been a medical fault (continued administration despite awareness of the liver disease), the duration of the liver disease remains unknown. This precludes using any time-based definition for these drug-induced liver diseases. Therefore terms such as drug-induced 'subacute or chronic hepatitis' are employed only to indicate the presence of particular liver lesions on liver biopsy at the time of diagnosis, without any time connotation.

Subacute hepatitis

Subacute hepatitis occurs mainly when the administration of the causative drug has been continued despite overt liver disease, or when it has been readministered before complete recovery from the initial acute episode. Clinical and biochemical manifestations persist, or even worsen, within a few weeks or a few months following the onset of jaundice. In some cases, ascites, encephalopathy, hypoalbuminaemia, and hypoprothrombinaemia develop. Histologically, subacute hepatitis is characterized by the concomitant presence of lesions at three different stages of evolution:

1. Acute lesions consist of the lobular necrosis and the lobular inflammation seen in acute hepatitis.
2. Secondary lesions consist of 'bridging necrosis', a term describing bands of parenchymal collapse (due to necrosis and subsequent cell drop-out) that link either two portal tracts together or a portal tract and a central vein.
3. Late lesions are suggestive of a chronic process, with portal fibrosis and portal inflammation, with, in some cases, the presence of nodules of regeneration.

Chronic hepatitis

Generally, clinical symptoms are absent or non-specific over a long period, sometimes up to the time of the liver biopsy. In other cases, jaundice and manifestations of hepatic failure may then arise suddenly or progressively. Serum aminotransferase activity is increased whereas alkaline phosphatase activity is usually normal. Serum gammaglobulin level is increased.

Drug-induced chronic hepatitis is histologically characterized by peripheral hepatocyte necrosis (piece-meal necrosis), and by portal inflammation and portal fibrosis which may both extend into the peripheral parenchyma.

Postnecrotic cirrhosis

The clinical manifestations are extremely variable. Cirrhosis may be recognized fortuitously or may be revealed by jaundice, ascites, hepatic encephalopathy, hepatomegaly, or complications of portal hypertension. Serum ALT activity is generally moderately increased. Hypoalbuminaemia and hypoprothrombinaemia are commonly observed.

Histologically, cirrhosis is characterized by a destruction of lobular architecture, extensive fibrosis, and nodules of regeneration. These lesions may be associated with those of subacute hepatitis or of chronic hepatitis.

Autoantibodies

Subacute hepatitis, chronic hepatitis, and postnecrotic cirrhosis are frequently associated with autoantibodies. Some of these antibodies, such as the antinuclear or antismooth muscle antibodies, have no specificity and are observed with different drugs, in particular clometacin, methyldopa, and papaverine.[155] In contrast, other autoantibodies appear to be more specifically associated with a particular drug-induced liver injury. The type 2 antiliver/kidney microsomes antibodies (anti-LKM$_2$) are observed in patients with

Table 9 Main drugs causing subacute hepatitis, chronic hepatitis, or cirrhosis as a result of prolonged hepatocyte necrosis

Acetohexamide (Goldstein, NJEM, 1966; 275:97)
Amodiaquine[59]
Aspirin (Seaman, AnnIntMed, 1974; 80:1)
Benzarone (Babany, JHepatol, 1987; 5:332)
Busulphan (Foadi, PostgradMedJ, 1977; 53:267)
Chlorambucil (Amromin, Gastro, 1962; 42:401)
Clometacin[157]
Dantrolene[63]
Diclofenac[64]
Fenofibrate (Bernard, GastrClinBiol, 1994; 18:1048)
Frentizole (Sobharwal, ArthRheum, 1980; 23:1376)
Germander (Ben Yahia, GastrClinBiol, 1993; 17:919)
Glafenine (Stricker, Liver, 1986; 6:63)
Halothane (Klastskin, NEJM, 1969; 280:515)
Iproniazid[4]
Isoniazid[70]
Metahexamide (Unger, AnnNYAcadSci, 1959; 82:510)
Methyldopa[158]
Nicotinic acid (Kohn, AmJMedSci, 1969; 258:94)
Nitrofurantoin[160]
Oxyphenisatin (Dietrichson, ScaJGastr, 1975; 10:617)
Papaverine (Poupon, GastrClinBiol, 1978; 2:305)
Phenytoin (Roy, DigDisSci, 1993; 38:740)
Paracetamol (Johnson, AnnIntMed, 1977; 87:302)
Propylthiouracil (Weiss, ArchIntMed, 1980; 140:1184)
Suloctidil (Perrin, GastrClinBiol, 1983; 7:1042)
Tienilic acid[80]
Trazodone (Beck, AnnIntMed, 1993; 118:791)
Urethane (Jonstam, ActaMedScand, 1961; 170:701)
Valproate[134]

liver injury caused by tienilic acid.[44] Antiliver microsome autoantibodies are found with dihydralazine.[45] The anti-M$_6$ antimitochondrial antibodies are found in patients with iproniazid-induced liver injury.[72]

As opposed to the autoantibodies that are observed in idiopathic autoimmune hepatitis, these drug-induced autoantibodies slowly regress with time, once the treatment is withdrawn.

Drugs causing subacute hepatitis, chronic hepatitis, and cirrhosis

Only the drugs which cause liver damage through prolonged hepatocyte necrosis are considered in this section and in Table 9. Drugs causing fibrosis or cirrhosis in the context of steatohepatitis (e.g. amiodarone and perhexiline) have been discussed above, while drugs causing cirrhosis as a consequence of either perisinusoidal fibrosis (e.g. methotrexate, vitamin A), or chronic cholestasis (e.g. chlorpromazine, flucloxacillin) are considered in subsequent sections.

Amodiaquine

Subacute hepatitis has been observed in some patients who had continued to take the drug for more than 4 weeks after the first manifestations. Recovery was very slow.[59]

Clometacin

This analgesic has been a major cause of drug-induced chronic liver disease, particularly in France,[156] but has now been recalled.

Liver injury often developed silently, so that 30 per cent of the patients with clometacin-induced liver injury already had chronic liver disease when a liver biopsy was performed; chronic hepatitis was observed in 25 per cent of these patients and cirrhosis in 5 per cent.[156] Clometacin liver injury was associated with hypersensitivity manifestations (fever, rash, blood eosinophilia) in 70 per cent of patients. Serum autoantibodies were found in 66 per cent; these were mainly antismooth muscle or antinuclear antibodies, and, less frequently, antimitochondrial or anti-DNA antibodies.[156] Giant multinucleated hepatocytes have been observed in some patients.[157] Although non-pathognomonic of this condition, this particular histological feature was helpful in the diagnosis of clometacin-induced liver disease.[157]

Dantrolene

Several cases of chronic active hepatitis and cirrhosis have been observed after the administration of this myorelaxant for more than 2 years.[63]

Diclofenac

Among 21 patients undergoing a liver biopsy for diclofenac-induced liver injury, six had chronic hepatitis.[64]

Germander

This 'medicinal' plant has produced instances of chronic hepatitis or cirrhosis (Ben Yahia, GastrClinBiol, 1993; 17:959).

Iproniazid

Fibrosis and cirrhosis may develop after the administration of this antidepressant.[4] Liver injury may worsen despite the discontinuation of the drug. Iproniazid liver injury appears to be specifically associated with the presence of anti-M_6 antimitochondrial autoantibodies.[72]

Isoniazid

Although isoniazid induces mainly acute hepatitis, chronic hepatitis and cirrhosis can also occur.[70]

Methyldopa

This antihypertensive compound was one of the most important cause of subacute hepatic necrosis,[158] particularly in patients who continued to take the drug for several weeks after the onset of the first symptoms (Toghill, BMJ, 1974; 3:545). Chronic active hepatitis or cirrhosis were also observed (Balacz, Hepatogast, 1981; 28:199). Antismooth muscle and antinuclear antibodies were frequently present.[155] Liver damage was sometimes associated with haemolytic anaemia and a positive Coombs' direct antiglobulin test.[57] About 70 per cent of patients with methyldopa-induced liver injury were female, which suggested some predisposition. With the availability of the new antihypertensive agents, the drug is now used much less.

Nitrofurantoin

This anti-infectious agent has been responsible for many cases of chronic liver injury.[159,160] At the time of the liver biopsy, 33 per cent of patients with hepatic injury exhibited lesions of chronic hepatitis or cirrhosis.[160] Most cases were in women. In addition to the more frequent use of urinary antiseptics in this gender, sex-related susceptibility was suggested. The duration of nitrofurantoin administration before the recognition of the disease exceeded 6 months in more than 85 per cent of patients with chronic liver lesions.[159,160] Serum antinuclear and antismooth muscle antibodies were present in most patients. HLA DR2 and HLA DRw6 antigens were found more frequently in patients than in a control population, although statistical significance was not reached.[160] The association with HLA B8 antigen suggested by previous reports has not been confirmed.[160]

Tienilic acid (ticrynafen)

Chronic active hepatitis and cirrhosis accounted for about 7 and 15 per cent, respectively, of cases of liver damage caused by tienilic acid.[80] Hypersensitivity manifestations were frequently observed. As already mentioned, tienilic acid-induced liver injury was associated with specific antimicrosomal autoantibodies. These anti-LKM_2 autoantibodies were directed against the isoenzyme of cytochrome P-450 (the 2C9 isoenzyme) that transforms tienilic acid into a reactive metabolite.[44] The drug has been withdrawn.

Oxyphenisatin

Prolonged administration of this laxative, usually for more than 6 months, has been a major cause of chronic hepatitis and cirrhosis in the past (Dietrichson, ScaJGastr, 1975; 10:617). This drug has been abandoned.

Papaverine

Chronic hepatitis or cirrhosis may develop in patients receiving long-term therapy. Antinuclear and antismooth muscle antibodies may be present (Poupon, GastrClinBiol, 1978; 2:305).

Other drugs

Other drugs that have caused chronic active hepatitis and/or cirrhosis are listed in Table 9. Conceivably, most drugs responsible for acute hepatocellular injury might produce chronic liver damage under conditions leading to protracted liver cell necrosis (see above).

Outcome of subacute hepatitis, chronic hepatitis, and postnecrotic cirrhosis

These drug-induced liver lesions generally improve after withdrawal of the causative drug (with a few exceptions as mentioned above). Clinical manifestations disappear quickly and serum aminotransferases decrease markedly within the first weeks, but further improvement may be slower. Similarly, autoantibodies tend to disappear progressively. Complete recovery may take several months and is not constant. Mild liver test abnormalities as well as fibrosis and inactive cirrhosis (without necrosis or inflammation) may persist as late sequelae.

Perisinusoidal fibrosis and cirrhosis
Features and mechanism

On electron microscopy, perisinusoidal fibrosis is characterized by the accumulation of collagen fibres within the space of Disse (i.e.

the space located between the endothelial sinusoidal cells and hepatocytes). Perisinusoidal fibrosis may remain asymptomatic or may lead to hepatomegaly and/or portal hypertension. It may eventually evolve into frank cirrhosis.

Perisinusoidal fibrosis is mainly observed with two drugs, namely methotrexate and vitamin A. In patients receiving these drugs, Ito cells are transformed into myofibroblastic cells that actively synthesize collagen and release it into the space of Disse. Perisinusoidal fibrosis can be viewed as a consequence of this drug-induced 'Itopathy'. However, the molecular mechanism(s) whereby methotrexate and vitamin A activate Ito cells remain poorly understood.

Causative drugs

Methotrexate

Methotrexate has been widely used for many years in patients with severe psoriasis, and is now also indicated in patients with severe rheumatoid arthritis. Its potential to induce liver lesions is mainly known in the former indication. Excessive alcohol ingestion is relatively common in patients with severe psoriasis, and is the most important predisposing factor to methotrexate hepatotoxicity. Methotrexate hepatotoxicity is also enhanced by obesity and diabetes mellitus (which both also favour fat accumulation), and renal dysfunction (which may delay methotrexate elimination).[3,161]

Prolonged administration of methotrexate to psoriatic patients can induce fibrosis or cirrhosis.[161] The risk of developing such lesions increases with the time of exposure, being low for administrations shorter than 1 year, but exceeding, in some studies, 12.5 and 25 per cent after 2 and 5 years of treatment, respectively (Nyfors, ActaPMIScand, 1976; 84:262; Zachariae, BrJDermatol, 191; 102:407). The incidence of liver injury also increases with the cumulative dose, particularly when it exceeds 2 or 4 g of methotrexate.[161] For the same cumulative dose, the incidence of liver injury was higher in the patients who had received methotrexate on a daily rather than an intermittent schedule.[161]

Fibrosis due to methotrexate (or the methotrexate–ethanol combination) may be associated with macrovacuolar steatosis, mild portal inflammation, fat-storing cell (Ito cell) hyperplasia (Horvath, Digestion, 1978; 17:488), and Kupffer cell proliferation. Electron microscopy shows deposition of collagen fibres in the space of Disse, as well as fat deposition, abnormalities of lysosomes and mitochondria, and hypertrophy of the smooth endoplasmic reticulum in hepatocytes.[3]

The disease develops insidiously. Although liver tests are usually slightly impaired, they have remained normal in some instances despite the presence of fibrosis or cirrhosis (Weinstein, ArchDermatol, 1973; 108:36; Shergy, AmJMed, 1988; 85:771).

Prevention is based on avoiding the drug in mild forms of psoriasis, or in patients with pre-existing liver lesions and those who cannot refrain from indulging in ethanol. Monitoring of liver tests every second month is recommended. Because liver tests may remain normal even in patients who develop fibrosis, serial liver biopsies at 2-yearly intervals, or after cumulative doses exceeding 2 to 4 g, have been recommended.[3]

Due to its more recent utilization in rheumatoid arthritis, the hepatotoxicity of methotrexate in this second condition is less extensively documented. Fibrosis and cirrhosis have also developed (Shergy, AmJMed, 1988; 85:771), but the general impression is that hepatotoxicity may be less of a problem (perhaps due a lower frequency of ethanol abuse) in this condition than in psoriasis. Monitoring of liver tests is nevertheless recommended.[162] Liver biopsies should be performed when liver tests abnormalities persist or fluctuate over three consecutive years of treatment.[162] Whether a liver biopsy should also be performed in patients with normal liver tests and prolonged treatments, remains unsettled at present.

An hepatoma has been observed in a child with methotrexate-induced hepatic fibrosis (Ruymann, JAMA, 1977; 238:2631).

Vitamin A

Perisinusoidal fibrosis also occurs in hypervitaminosis A.[163-168] Perisinusoidal fibrosis probably results from the increased synthesis of collagen by activated Ito cells (Kent, PNAS, 1976; 73:3719). The disease has occurred after a wide range of daily doses (20 000 to 1 200 000 units) and various lengths of treatment (7 weeks to 30 years).[165,167] Usually, however, the disease becomes symptomatic after several years of treatment and a cumulative dose exceeding 100×10^6 units.[167] Skin disorders, in particular alopecia, are frequently observed.[163] There is moderate elevation of both serum transaminase activity and alkaline phosphatase activity (Geubel, Gastro, 1991; 100:1701). Light and electron microscopy shows Ito cell hyperplasia, with vitamin A accumulation in large vesicles.[168] The concentration of vitamin A is markedly increased in hepatic tissue. In contrast, its level in the serum is often normal.[167]

Perisinusoidal fibrosis induced by hypervitaminosis A is frequently associated with sinusoidal dilation.[168] Portal and periportal fibrosis and even cirrhosis may develop if vitamin A administration is continued.[166,167]

Withdrawal of vitamin A results in the reduction of ALT activity, but the increased alkaline phosphatase activity is much more persistent, and, despite the withdrawal of the drug, cirrhotic lesions may develop (Geubel, Gastro, 1991; 100:1701). However, manifestations of portal hypertension may eventually improve after vitamin A withdrawal (Guarascio, JClinPath, 1983; 36:769).

Other drugs

Other drugs or chemicals known to cause this lesion include arsenical derivatives, azathioprine, 6-mercaptopurine, oral contraceptives, thorium dioxide, and, possibly, urethane.

Prolonged cholestasis

Two different types of drug-induced prolonged cholestasis may be distinguished, depending on the size of the injured bile ducts:[81]

1. A syndrome (resembling primary biliary cirrhosis) is associated with protracted lesions of ductules and/or small interlobular bile ducts. The interlobular bile ducts may progressively disappear, hence the term 'vanishing bile duct syndrome'.
2. A syndrome (resembling primary sclerosing cholangitis) is due to sclerosing lesions of the extrahepatic or large intrahepatic bile ducts.

Lesions of small bile ducts (vanishing bile duct syndrome)

Definition

Drug-induced prolonged cholestasis due to lesions of small bile ducts has been defined as either the persistence of jaundice for more than 6 months, or the persistence of high serum alkaline phosphatase and γ-glutamyl transferase activities for more than 1 year after the acute episode of drug-induced hepatitis and the withdrawal of the causative drug.[81] The definition excludes cases in which the initial, acute drug-induced episode is not well characterized and those in which asymptomatic, pre-existing liver disease cannot be ruled out.[81]

Liver lesions

Pathological lesions of drug-induced prolonged cholestasis are reminiscent of those observed in primary biliary cirrhosis. The characteristic portal tract lesion is the disappearance of interlobular bile ducts, with or without moderate polymorphous inflammatory infiltration and ductular proliferation. In severe icteric forms, liver lesions include cholestasis, occasionally associated with 'pseudo-xanthomatous' degeneration or necrosis of periportal hepatocytes. Lobular inflammatory infiltration is absent or mild.[4] Usually, the lobular architecture is preserved and portal fibrosis is moderate or absent.[169] Occasionally, secondary biliary cirrhosis can develop.

Clinical features

Drug-induced, prolonged cholestasis due to bile duct rarefaction may be subdivided into two clinical forms: a major, uncommon form and a minor, relatively frequent form.[81]

Major form

This severe form of the vanishing bile duct syndrome is characterized by the long persistence or even aggravation of jaundice despite interruption of the treatment. Xanthomata and xanthelasmata may develop.[170,171] In some cases, hepatomegaly, splenomegaly, and even symptoms related to malabsorption may appear. Serum alkaline phosphatase and γ-glutamyl transferase activities are very high, as are the serum concentrations of bilirubin, bile acids, and cholesterol.

Despite this impressive clinical presentation and the presence of histological features that resemble those of primary biliary cirrhosis, most patients with this severe form nevertheless progressively improve. Jaundice eventually subsides, although this may require several years.[171] The high alkaline phosphatase and γ-glutamyl transferase activities then decrease very slowly, although, in one patient, abnormalities still persisted 14 years after onset of the liver disease (Horst, Gastro, 1980; 79:550).

In a few patients, however, the syndrome seems to be irreversible. Jaundice persists unabated, and secondary biliary cirrhosis eventually develops, leading to death or liver transplantation.

Minor form

This minor form is much more common. The jaundice and pruritus that characterized the initial episode of acute cholestatic hepatitis both disappear rapidly after interruption of the treatment. However, the elevated levels of serum alkaline phosphatase and γ-glutamyl transferase nevertheless persist for more than 1 year. Liver lesions are less marked than in the major form, and consist of the partial disappearance of the interlobular bile ducts, mild inflammatory infiltration, and mild ductular proliferation. Portal fibrosis is absent or mild.

The prognosis of this minor form is good. Liver tests very slowly improve and can return to normal several years after the initial episode of acute hepatitis. The reversibility of cholestasis may depend upon the number of affected bile ducts.[172]

Mechanism(s)

The mechanism for the vanishing bile duct syndrome remains unknown, but tentative suggestions have been proposed. The features of the initial episode are usually consistent with an immunoallergic mechanism,[81] and early bile-duct lesions (cholangitis and cholangiolitis) can be disclosed at that time. These observations suggest that the initial destruction of bile ducts may be immunologically mediated.

Rarefaction of bile ducts progressively increases with time,[173] long after the drug and its metabolites have been cleared from the body. This has led to the hypothesis of a drug-triggered, autoimmune attack against small bile ducts.[81,172,173] Persisting blood eosinophilia (Dincsoy, Gastro, 1982; 83:694), circulating immune complexes (Horst, Gastro, 1980; 79:550), or both[173] were observed in some cases. As a hypothesis, it may be suggested that the causative drug (or one of its metabolites) may trigger an immune response directed against the normal biliary epithelium. However, a corticosteroid therapy has been attempted in a few patients without obvious benefit (Geubel, Liver, 1988; 8:350).[171]

A second hypothetical mechanism has been tentatively suggested,[174] and merits experimental testing. The MDR2 gene codes for a protein that may act as a phospholipid flippase, transferring phospholipids from the interior leaflet of the canalicular plasma membrane to its external leaflet, from which phospholipids are then removed by the solubilizing effects of bile acids. Bile phospholipids apparently exert an important protective action against the detergent effects of bile salts on bile duct cells. Indeed, animals whose MDR2 gene has been knocked out present a liver condition that resembles primary biliary cirrhosis. It will be interesting to determine whether drugs can actually repress the expression of the MDR2 gene in hepatocytes (and/or can lead to autoantibodies preventing the secondary access of this protein to the canalicular membrane).

Drugs causing prolonged cholestasis due to the vanishing bile duct syndrome

Chlorpromazine

This is the prototype for drug-induced prolonged cholestasis. Chlorpromazine has been involved in more than 30 cases of jaundice lasting for more than 1 year.[4,86,169,170] Prolonged cholestasis occurs in about 7 per cent of patients with chlorpromazine-induced acute hepatitis.[4] Despite an impressive clinical and histological picture, prolonged cholestasis caused by this drug often finally improved, with eventual disappearance of jaundice, sometimes several years after the onset of the disease.[4,169] However, irreversible biliary cirrhosis leading to death has been observed in some patients.[4] The main histological feature was the disappearance of interlobular bile ducts.[4] In one isolated case, however, histological lesions resembled those of chronic hepatitis (Russel, BMJ, 1973; 1:655).

Ajmaline derivatives

Many cases of prolonged cholestasis have been ascribed to ajmaline derivatives and these drugs are no longer used (Borsch, Klinwschr, 1984; 62:998; Knobler, ArchIntMed, 1986; 146:526).[171,173] Jaundice eventually subsided except in one patient in whom irreversible biliary cirrhosis developed.[171]

Arsenical derivatives

Prolonged cholestasis has been observed after the administration of arsenical derivatives (Stolzer, AmJMed, 1950; 9:124; Opolon, RevIntHep, 1964; 14:93).

Flucloxacillin

This penicillinase-resistant penicillin is widely used in several countries and is a frequent cause of the vanishing bile duct syndrome.[175,176] Treatment with ursodeoxycholic acid may be beneficial (Piotrowicz, JHepatol, 1995; 22:119).

Amoxacillin/clavulanic acid

One patient still exhibited increased serum alkaline phosphatase levels more than 1 year after an acute episode of focal destructive cholangiopathy due to this drug combination (Ryley, JHepatol, 1995; 23:278).

Tetracyclines

Two female patients with bile duct paucity due to tetracycline and doxycycline have been reported.[177]

Other drugs

Single cases of prolonged cholestasis have been reported with about 24 other drugs,[81,177–181] including several other phenothiazines and several tricyclic antidepressants (Table 10).

Lesions of large bile ducts (sclerosing cholangitis)

In this condition, one or multiple segmental strictures affect the large intrahepatic and extrahepatic bile ducts. This lesion is seen either after administration of floxuridine infused in the hepatic artery or after the intrakystic infusion of hypertonic saline or formaldehyde in hydatid cysts that communicate with intrahepatic bile ducts.

Floxuridine

Jaundice is a frequent complication of the infusion of floxuridine in the hepatic artery.[182,183] This treatment is used in patients with hepatic metastases from colorectal carcinoma. Jaundice is due either to drug-induced hepatitis or to sclerosing cholangitis.[182]

Sclerosing cholangitis may occur in 5 to 29 per cent of patients receiving this intra-arterial treatment. It usually develops several months (often 1 year) after starting this chemotherapy. It has been suggested that sclerosing cholangitis caused by floxuridine might be treated or prevented by intra-arterial dexamethasone (Paquette, ProcAmSocClinOncol, 1987; 6:89).

Sclerosing cholangitis is characterized by multiple segmental strictures of varying lengths as shown by cholangiography. The stictures taper smoothly both proximally and distally. In contrast to those seen in primary sclerosing cholangitis, the strictures observed after floxuridine infusions usually spare both the distal common bile duct and the smaller intrahepatic ducts. Instead, they occur almost exclusively in the region around the confluence of the left and right hepatic ducts and the proximal common bile duct (Shea, AmJRoent, 1986; 146:717). Because this region is selectively vascularized by the hepatic artery, it has been suggested that these strictures may be primitively due to arterial lesions that would then lead to the fibrosis of these ischaemic bile ducts.[183] Histological lesions resemble those found in primary sclerosing cholangitis.[183]

The outcome of the sclerosing cholangitis caused by the intra-arterial infusion of floxuridine is variable. In some patients, bile-duct strictures appear to be reversible (Botet, Radiol, 1985; 156:335). In most patients, however, they persist despite discontinuation of chemotherapy, and may require various types of biliary drainage (Botet, Radiol, 1985; 156:335). The condition may lead to death from progressive hepatic failure (Botet, Radiol, 1985; 156:335).

Scolicidal agents

Sclerosing cholangitis may also occur in the months following the intracystic administration of either 2 per cent formaldehyde or hypertonic saline in hydatid cysts that happen to communicate with the biliary tree.[184]

Other agents

Isolated cases of sclerosing cholangitis have been observed after the intra-arterial infusion of 5-fluorouracil, given either alone or in association with intravenous streptozotocin or mitomycin (Larrey, GastrClinBiol, 1993; 17:59). The lesion has also occurred after administration of a doxorubicin–mitomycin association (Larrey, GastrClinBiol, 1993; 17:59).

Vascular lesions

The liver receives blood through the portal vein and the hepatic artery. Both ramify into small intrahepatic branches located into the portal tracts. Blood then flows within the hepatic sinusoids, and is collected first into the centrilobular veins of the hepatic lobule, and then into small and large hepatic veins. Drugs and chemicals can cause lesions at all levels of this vascular system (Table 11). Often, the same drug can cause several of these vascular lesions, suggesting a basic, common mechanism (perhaps toxicity to endothelial cells).[185,186] The molecular or cellular mechanisms remain essentially unknown, however.

This section describes the various vascular lesions, with the exception of perisinusoidal fibrosis, which (albeit sometimes included among vascular lesions) has been described separately, and with the exception of tumours of vascular origin that are described in the context of hepatic tumours.

Table 10 Drugs causing prolonged cholestasis due to lesions of small intrahepatic bile ducts

Main causative drugs
    Ajmaline[173]
    Arsenical derivatives (Stolzer, AmJMed, 1950; 9:124)
    Chlorpromazine[4]
    Flucloxacillin[175,176]

Other drugs
    Acepromethazine (+meprobamate)[81]
    Amitriptyline[178]
    Amoxicillin/clavulanic acid (Ryley, JHepatol, 1995; 23:278)
    barbiturate (Pagliaro, Gastro, 1969; 56:938)
    Carbamazepine (Genève, GastrClinBiol, 1987; 11:242)
    Carbutamide (Fauvert, PressMed, 1963; 71:1287)
    Cimetidine (Clarke, DigDisSci, 1987; 32:333)
    Cyamemazine (Degott, Hepatol, 1992; 15:244)
    Cyproheptadine[180]
    Doxycycline[177]
    Erythromycin+chlorpropamide (Geubel, Liver, 1988; 8:350)
    Fenofibrate (Lepicard, GastrClinBiol, 1994; 18:350)
    Haloperidol[181]
    Imipramine (Horst, Gastro, 1980; 79:550)
    Methyltestosterone (Globert, JAMA, 1968; 204:170)
    Norandrostenolone (Gil, AnnIntMed, 1986; 104:135)
    Phenybutazone (Benjamin, Hepatol, 1981; 1:255)
    Phenytoin (Campbell, AmJDigDis, 1977; 22:255)
    Prochlorperazine (Lok, JHepatol, 1988; 6:369)
    Tetracycline (Hunt, Gastro, 1994; 107:1844)
    Thiabendazole (Manivel, Gastro, 1987; 93:245)
    Ticlopidine (Naschitz, ClinToxicol, 1995; 33:379)
    Tiopronin[4]
    Tolbutamide (Gregory, ArchPathol, 1967; 84:194)
    Trimethoprim-sulphamethoxazole (Kowdley, Gastro, 1992; 102:2148)
    Troleandomycin[179]
    Xenelamine (Hecht, ArchFrMalAppDig, 1965; 54:615)

Lesions of the portal vein and its branches

Thrombosis of the portal vein or its branches has been observed in a few women taking oral contraceptives (Rose, PostgradMedJ, 1972; 48:430) or in patients receiving arsenical derivatives.[186]

Lesions of the hepatic artery and its branches

Arterial intimal hyperplasia may occur in women taking oral contraceptives. The lesion may affect various arteries, including the hepatic one. Intimal hyperplasia of the hepatic artery usually remains silent (Irey, ArchPathLabMed, 1973; 96:227). Occasionally, however, it has led to multifocal haemorrhagic necrosis of the liver (Zafrani, Gastro, 1980; 79:1295; Jacobs, ArchIntMed, 1984; 144:642) or to spontaneous rupture of the liver (Frederick, ArchSurg, 1974; 108:93). This arterial intimal hyperplasia can be associated with the obstruction of large and/or small hepatic veins.[185]

Necrotizing angiitis of the hepatic artery has been observed in some subjects addicted to methamphetamine (Citron, NEJM, 1970; 283:1003).

Sinusoidal dilation

This lesion is characterized by the dilation of hepatic sinusoids in the absence of any structural (e.g. Budd–Chiari) or haemodynamic (e.g. cardiac failure) restriction to the outflow of blood from the liver.[185,186] Sinusoidal dilation is often asymptomatic. However, hepatomegaly, right upper quadrant abdominal pain, fever, and a raised erythrocyte sedimentation rate may be occasional features.[185,186] Liver tests are either normal or minimally disturbed.

Oral contraceptives

Oestrogen-containing oral contraceptives are the main cause of drug-induced sinusoidal dilation.[187] The lesion has been observed after several months to several years of oral contraception.[187] A peculiarity is that the sinusoidal dilation clearly predominates in periportal areas.[187] Recovery promptly occurs after withdrawal of the oral contraceptives, whereas their readministration may lead to relapse (Weinberger, ArchIntMed, 1985; 145:927). Occasionally, the sinusoidal dilation caused by oral contraceptives may lead to perisinusoidal fibrosis (Bretagne, SemHopPar, 1984; 60:3231).

Azathioprine

Sinusoidal dilation has been observed in several patients receiving azathioprine (Gerlag, JHepatol, 1985; 1:339). This vascular lesion disappeared after azathioprine withdrawal.

Peliosis hepatis

Peliosis hepatis is characterized by blood-filled cavities that are randomly distributed throughout the liver lobule. On electron microscopy, there are constant alterations of the endothelial lining

Table 11 Drugs reported to cause vascular lesions of the liver

Vascular lesions	Lesions possibly related to vascular injury
Thrombosis of the portal vein	Hepatoportal sclerosis
Arsenical derivatives	Arsenical derivatives
Oral contraceptives	Azathioprine
Intimal hyperplasia of the hepatic artery	Methotrexate
Oral contraceptives	Thorium dioxide
Necrotizing angiitis of the hepatic artery	Vitamin A
Methamphetamine[a]	Nodular regenerative hyperplasia
Sinusoidal dilation	Anabolic-androgenic steroids[a]
Azathioprine	Azathioprine
Chenodeoxycholic acid[a]	Corticosteroids[a]
Oral contraceptives	Oral contraceptives[a]
Peliosis hepatis	Perisinusoidal fibrosis
Anabolic-androgenic steroids	Methotrexate
Arsenical derivatives	Vitamin A
Azathioprine	Angiosarcoma
Corticosteroids[a]	Thorotrast
Medroxyprogesterone[a]	
Tamoxifen[a]	
Oestrone sulphate[a]	
Oral contraceptives[a]	
Thorium dioxide	
Veno-occlusive disease	
Azathioprine	
Carmustine (BCNU)[a]	
Cyclofenil[a]	
Cysteamine[a]	
Cytarabine	
Dacarbazine	
Doxorubicin (Adriamycin)[a]	
Indicine N-oxide[a]	
6-Mercaptopurine	
Mitomycin[a]	
Progestins[a]	
Pyrrolizidine alkaloids	
6-Thioguanine	
Urethane	
Vincristine[a]	
Vitamin E (intravenous)[a]	
Budd–Chiari syndrome	
Cyclosphosphamide[a]	
Dacarbazine	
Doxorubicin[a]	
Oral contraceptives	
Vincristine[a]	

[a] Drugs for which a causal relationship with the vascular disorder remains to be confirmed.

(Scoazec, GastrClinBiol, 1995; 19:505). In the less severe forms, endothelial cells are still present, but only in places. The gaps between endothelial cells allow the entry of red blood cells in the space of Disse. In the most severe forms, the endothelial lining is completely absent and the blood cavities are directly bordered by hepatocytes.

Most cases of peliosis hepatis are asymptomatic, and liver tests are either normal or minimally disturbed.[185,186] In some cases, however, the disease has been revealed by hepatomegaly, jaundice, portal hypertension, haemoperitoneum, and even hepatic failure.[185,186] Long-standing peliosis may lead either to perisinusoidal fibrosis or to nodular regenerative hyperplasia (Izumi, JHepatol, 1994; 20:129; Scoazec, GastrClinBiol, 1995; 19:505).

Anabolic steroids

Numerous cases of peliosis hepatis have been ascribed to anabolic–androgenic steroids, in particular, but not exclusively, 17-α-alkylated steroids.[107] Mild sinusoidal dilation may be concomitantly present. Many cases remain asymptomatic.

Other drugs

Other compounds responsible for peliosis hepatis include azathioprine,[188] 6-thioguanine,[189] vinyl chloride, and arsenical derivatives (Popper, AmJPath, 1978; 92:349). Despite several reports of peliosis hepatis occurring in users of oral contraceptives, the role of these compounds in this disease remains controversial.[187]

Considering the large number of women exposed and the low number of cases observed, this association might be fortuitous.[187]

Obstruction of the small hepatic veins (veno-occlusive disease)

Veno-occlusive disease is typically characterized by a non-thrombotic, concentric narrowing of the lumen of small centrilobular veins. Destruction of the vascular endothelium may lead to sub-intimal oedema, and a loose subintimal network of reticulin fibres in which red blood cells are often evident. Subsequent sclerosis of the vein wall may then produce the typical non-thrombotic narrowing of the vein lumen. An exception may be the veno-occlusive disease mediated by dacarbazine, which often involves thrombosis. Severe narrowing of the venous lumen blocks the outflow of blood from the hepatic sinusoids and thereby causes sinusoidal congestion and ischaemic necrosis of centrilobular area. This is followed, in chronic forms, by centrilobular scarring.

The clinical presentation of veno-occlusive disease may be either acute or chronic.[186] The acute form is characterized by the prompt onset of abdominal pain and ascites. Although recovery is possible, this acute form may lead to fatal hepatic failure.[186] Conversely, the disease may develop insidiously, leading to extensive central fibrosis and eventually to cirrhosis.[186]

Most cases of veno-occlusive disease occur as a complication of antimitotic agents, given either alone or in combination with radiotherapy.

Bone marrow transplantation

The irradiation and chemotherapy used in the preparation for bone marrow transplantation is a major cause of veno-occlusive disease, nowadays (Saint-Marc Girardin, JHepatol, 1985; 1:5323). Its incidence is estimated to be between 10 and 30 per cent. The risk of developing this complication is increased in patients with pre-existing liver disease, increased serum aminotransferase levels, intensive conditioning, or absence of a complete remission of the myeloproliferative syndrome before the bone marrow transplantation (Brodsky, AmJClinOnc, 1990; 13:221; McDonald, AnnIntMed, 1993; 118:255). The clinical course is frequently severe with a mortality rate of 50 per cent. Veno-occlusive disease is the third leading cause of death after bone marrow transplantation, with graft-versus-host disease and infection as the other major causes. Veno-occlusive disease usually occurs from 2 to 4 weeks after bone marrow transplantation. This early onset helps in the differential diagnosis from later complications such as graft-versus-host disease or viral hepatitis.

A non-controlled study suggested that prostaglandin E_1 may help prevent veno-occlusive disease in leukaemic patients treated by allogenic bone marrow transplantation (Gluckman, BrJHaemat, 1990; 74:277).

Immunosuppressive and antineoplastic agents

In the absence of any irradiation, veno-occlusive disease has also been ascribed to various immunosuppressive and antineoplastic agents, in particular thiopurine derivatives (azathioprine, 6-mercaptopurine, 6-thioguanine), and urethane (Table 11).[189] Veno-occlusive disease induced by thiopurines exhibits some particular features.[189] It occurs several months or years after the onset of therapy. Most patients are renal transplant recipients that are concomitantly treated with corticosteroids. Jaundice and/or hepatomegaly are frequently the first manifestations. The disease is often associated with peliosis and may be followed by nodular regenerative hyperplasia.

Pyrrolizidine alkaloids

Initial descriptions of veno-occlusive disease concerned patients poisoned by the pyrrolizidine alkaloids contained in some plants, in particular the *Heliotropium*, *Senecio*, and *Crotolaria* species. The disease mainly occurred in large outbreaks due to the consumption of wheat flour that was contaminated with these seeds (Tandon, AmJGastr, 1978; 70:607). It has also occurred as individual cases caused by decoctions or infusions prepared from these plants (Stillman, Gastro, 1977; 73:349; Ridker, Gastro, 1985; 88:1050).

Although the disease has been mainly observed in Jamaica, South Africa, Afghanistan, and India, a few cases are also seen in Western countries, following the ingestion of such herbal teas by recent immigrants (Stillman, Gastro, 1977; 73:349) or ill-advised adherents of herbal remedies (Ridker, Gastro, 1985; 88:1050). Pyrrolizine alkaloids undergo metabolic activation in the liver; the reactive pyrrole derivatives that are generated form adducts with DNA (Tomer, AnalChem, 1986; 58:2527).

Obstruction of large hepatic veins (Budd–Chiari syndrome)

The Budd–Chiari syndrome is characterized by the obstruction (generally thrombotic) of large hepatic veins. This lesion results in hepatic congestion, followed by necrosis of the ischaemic centrilobular hepatocytes. The Spiegel lobe, which is normally spared by the disease, undergoes compensatory hypertrophy.

The severity of the syndrome varies with the site and the extent of thrombosis. The clinical presentation may be acute, with abdominal pain or ascites, or chronic, mimicking decompensated cirrhosis.[185,186]

Oral contraceptives

The risk of developing a Budd–Chiari syndrome is 2.5 fold higher in women using oral contraceptive (Valla, AnnIntMed, 1985; 103:329). The thrombosis has been ascribed mostly to the oestrogenic component, which may act mainly by exacerbating an underlying thrombogenic condition, in particular a latent myeloproliferative disease (Valla, AnnIntMed, 1985; 103:329). Probably due to the lower oestrogen content of current pills, this complication is less frequently observed nowadays.

Other causes

Budd–Chiari syndromes have also been observed in patients receiving some antineoplastic agents. Dacarbazine has been responsible for several cases (Greenstone, BMJ, 1981; 282:1744). The course of the disease was fatal in all cases, within a few days after the onset of the first manifestations.

Other suspected agents include doxorubicin, vincristine, and cyclophosphamide (Lehrner, AnnIntMed, 1978; 88:575; Houghton,

Cancer, 1979; 44:2324). The role of the last compounds is questionable, however, since they were administered concurrently with dacarbazine.[186]

Lesions possibly related to vascular injury

Hepatoportal sclerosis

Hepatoportal sclerosis is characterized by portal and periportal fibrosis possibly caused by the obstruction of small portal venules, resulting in portal hypertension.

Hepatoportal sclerosis has been ascribed to various compounds, including vitamin A,[163] azathioprine (Zarday, JAMA, 1974; 222: 690), methotrexate (Podurgiel, MayoClinProc, 1973; 48:787), and arsenical derivatives (Huet, Gastro, 1975; 68:1270). It is noteworthy that most of these compounds may also cause perisinusoidal fibrosis (a lesion considered in a previous section, that may be related to adverse drug effects on sinusoidal Ito cells).

Nodular hyperplasia of the liver

Nodular hyperplasia of the liver is characterized by small nodules, that are made of hepatocytes, randomly distributed throughout the liver, and are seen in the absence of any marked fibrosis. The lesion has been ascribed to some heterogeneity in the liver vascularization (Rougier, Gastro, 1978; 75:169). Portal hypertension is its main manifestation. Nodular regenerative hyperplasia may be associated with peliosis hepatis[188] or sinusoidal dilation,[186] and may in some cases appear as a late sequel of these lesions.

Nodular hyperplasia has been observed after the administration of azathioprine, anabolic–androgenic steroids, oral contraceptives, and corticosteroids.[188,191]

Hepatic tumours

Mechanisms

Initiation and promotion

Tumour development is thought to require both initiation and promotion steps. The initiation stage probably involves some initial damage to DNA:[192]

1. This may be due to the drug itself when it is transformed into a reactive species which produces modified DNA bases that lead to misreadings during DNA replication, or when the drug produces free radicals, including the hydroxyl radical, that can cause DNA breaks, followed by rearrangements.[193]
2. The initial DNA damage may also be due to other causes, including viral infections, the endogenous production of reactive oxygen radicals by mitochondria, or the ingestion of environmental carcinogens, such as the aflatoxin contained in contaminated peanut products, the psoralens present in several comestible plants, the dimethylnitrosamine contained in beer, or the benzopyrene and other carcinogens that are found in barbecued meat and tobacco smoke (Shaw, TrendsPharmacolSci, 1994; 15:89).

Because most DNA damage is repaired quickly, and because the cellular turnover of hepatocytes is normally slow, the chances are that these hepatic DNA lesions will be repaired before a round of cell division occurs. Furthermore, cells possess mechanisms to prevent the replication of damaged DNA. Indeed, DNA damage leads to overexpression of $p53$ (Kuerbitz, PNAS, 1992; 89:7491). This cell cycle checkpoint protein transiently blocks the cell cycle in the G_1 phase, thus permitting the reparation of DNA lesions before the cell is allowed to proceed to the S phase of DNA replication (Kuerbitz, PNAS, 1992; 89:7491). When the DNA damage is even more extensive, expression of wild type $p53$ may also trigger apoptosis, thus destroying the damaged DNA together with the cell that harbours it (Symonds, Cell, 1994; 78:703). All these effects efficiently prevent the replication of damaged DNA.

All factors, however, that will tend to stimulate cell division may lead to the replication of a molecule of DNA which has not yet been repaired, leading to somatic mutations. Thus, 'promoting' events are mainly those which stimulate cell division.[193] This mitogenic response may be caused by hepatic regeneration after liver cell necrosis, direct growth effect of the promoter (for example a steroid hormone), modifications of endogenous growth factors, or interruption of cell–cell communications.[193]

Stepwise tumour development

Tumour development after exposure to chemicals is a long, stepwise process.[192] The initiated cells often exhibit changes in phenotype.[192] Transient elevation of serum α-fetoprotein, accompanied by the appearance of a new cell population with oval nuclei, the so-called 'oval cells', is often observed in the early stages of chemical hepatocarcinogenesis in the rat (Sell, Hepatol, 1982; 2:77). Oval cells may be derived from a stem cell compartment that has the potentiality of differentiating into either hepatocytes or ductal epithelium (Hsia, Hepatol, 1992; 16:1327). Oval cells have likewise been described in the regenerating nodules and the liver tissue surrounding the tumour in humans with hepatocellular carcinoma (Hsia, Hepatol, 1992; 16:1327).

At first, the initiated cells may have no autonomy of growth unless promoting events are continuously applied.[192] Further steps of proliferation produce increasingly abnormal progeny.[192] It is likely that there is stepwise acquisition of different mutations that eventually allow the cell to totally escape growth-controlling mechanisms. These diverse mutations may involve (among many others):

(1) the overexpression of receptors for growth stimuli, such as the hepatocyte growth factor receptor (c-*met* oncogen) (Boix, Hepatol, 1994; 19:88; Suzuki, Hepatol, 1994; 20:1231), or the epidermal growth factor receptor (*neu* oncogne, c-*erbB*-2) (Yu, CancerRes, 1994; 54:5106);

(2) a mutation in the gene encoding the cell cycle-blocking gene, $p53$ (Hsu, Hepatol, 1994; 19:122), or various mutations affecting the components of the cyclin system (Nobori, Nature, 1994; 368:753);

(3) mutant *ras* proteins that have lost the ability to become inactivated and will thus stimulate growth autonomously (Challen, JHepatol, 1992; 14:342), or multiplication of the alleles of the c-*myc* gene (Fujiwara, CancerRes, 1993; 53:857);

(4) overexpression of telomerase (Tahara, CancerRes, 1995; 55: 2734), which avoids the shortening of telomeres after each mitosis;

(5) mutations of β_2-microglobin that suppress the membrane expression of human leucocyte antigen class I molecules on the cell

surface and thus enable the cell to escape immune surveillance (Bicknel, PNAS, 1994; 91:4751);

(6) a variety of mutations involving cell–cell adhesion molecules (E-cadherin; CD44), that may allow the cell to metastasize (Oda, PNAS, 1994; 91:1858).

Tumourigenicity of sex hormones

In humans, sex hormones are the chief suspects for drug-induced tumourigenicity.[192] Accordingly, a vast body of literature has been devoted to the assessment of the experimental hepatotumourigenic effects of these hormones.[194] It is now well established that sex hormones can have tumour-promoting effects. In animals exposed initially to a potent carcinogen such as N-nitroso-morpholine or diethylnitrosamine, the secondary administration of ethinyl-oestradiol, mestranol, and, in some reports, oestradiol or testosterone, has enhanced the incidence of hepatic carcinomas.[194] The promoting effects of androgens and oestrogens are ascribed to their stimulating effect on liver-cell proliferation.[107,194] This effect is itself related to the presence of androgen and oestrogen receptors on hepatocytes.[107,194]

Not only do sex hormones promote hepatic carcinomas initiated by experimental carcinogens, but they can also increase the prevalence of hepatic tumours when given alone.[194] Indeed, a somewhat higher prevalence of hepatic carcinomas has been observed in animals after administration of diethylstilboestrol, ethinyloestradiol, norethisterone, norethinodrel, and methyltestosterone.[194] It must be realized, however, that such studies have usually been conducted at very high doses, 100 times or more of the human contraceptive dose.[194] These effects do not necessarily imply that sex hormones have initiating, genotoxic effects. Conceivably, they might act only by promoting the growth of cells initiated by spontaneous mutations, viruses, or food carcinogens. Nevertheless, some of these sex hormones, particularly oestrogens, may also be genotoxic. Indeed, both stilbene oestrogens and steroidal oestrogens, whether natural or synthetic, all form electrophilic metabolites, free radicals, and oxygen radicals, all of which can damage DNA (Metzler, ArchToxicol, 1984; 55:104).

Drug-induced tumours

Drugs may cause either benign or malignant hepatic tumours (Table 12).

Benign tumours

Benign tumours include adenomas, nodular focal hyperplasia, and benign haemangioma.

Hepatocellular adenoma

Hepatocellular adenoma is a benign tumour consisting of normal, tightly packed hepatocyte plates, often two to three cells thick, which are separated by compressed, slit-like sinusoids. In contrast to the normal parenchyma, adenomas contain no portal tract or centrilobular vein.[192]

Adenomas are frequently asymptomatic and are usually discovered incidentally by abdominal ultrasonography performed for unrelated complains. However, large tumours may be revealed by right upper quadrant abdominal pain or, uncommonly, by intra-peritoneal bleeding (Kerlin, Gastro, 1983; 84:994).

Tumours greater than 2 cm are easily detected by ultrasound as hyper- or hypoechogenic nodules without specific features. Computed tomography characteristically shows nodules of lower attenuation than the surrounding normal parenchyma, with early contrast enhancement. Magnetic resonance imaging provides similar features by showing a hypervascular, more or less homogeneous tumour. When the diagnosis remains unclear after these investigations, a liver biopsy guided by ultrasound is sometimes performed (Michel, GastrClinBiol, 1992; 16:35; Kerlin, Gastro, 1983; 84:994).

Hepatic resection is generally proposed, anyhow, because:

(1) large adenomas may be complicated by intratumoural or intraperitoneal bleeding;
(2) distinction from carcinoma may be difficult;
(3) the occasional degeneration of adenomas into well-differentiated hepatic carcinomas has been described (Gordon, AnnIntMed, 1986; 105:547; Janes, Hepatol, 1993; 17:583).

Oral contraceptives

At a time when high dosage contraceptives were still being used, or had been used recently, it was shown that women who had resorted to this oral contraception were more susceptible to develop hepatic adenomas than were non-users.[187,195-197] The relative risk of developing this tumour was practically unchanged after less than 1 year of oral contraception, was slightly increased from 1 to 3 years, but was 116-fold the normal risk after 5 years of oral contraception, and more than 500-fold the non-user risk after 7 years.[196] It was estimated that the annual incidence rate of hepatic adenomas was only 1 per million in females taking no oral contraceptive, but 34 per million in users of oral contraceptives.[196] It is important to realize, however, that these studies, which were performed in the 1970s, may not apply to the low-dosage pills which are used nowadays. Indeed, the general impression of hepatologists is that hepatic adenomas have become quite uncommon again.

The discontinuation of oral contraceptives has been occasionally followed by a slow decrease in the tumour size (Buhler, Gastro, 1982; 82:775) and even complete regression (Steinbrecher, DigDisSci, 1981; 26:1045). Adenomas can reoccur with the re-administration of oral contraceptives or with pregnancy.[195] However, as indicated above, it is now felt that adenomas should be surgically removed.

Other causes

The risk of developing a hepatic adenoma is also increased by prolonged administration of anabolic–androgenic steroids.[198,199] Most cases have occurred with 17-α-alkylated steroids.[198] One case, however, has been attributed to testosterone enanthate, a non-17-α-alkylated steroid.[199] Adenomas caused by anabolic–androgenic steroids may also evolve into hepatocellular carcinomas.[107,199] Isolated cases of adenoma have been observed after the administration of clomiphene (Carrasco, NEJM, 1984; 310:1120) or norethisterone, a progestin (Kalra, BMJ, 1987; 294: 808).

Table 12 Drugs reported to cause or to complicate hepatic tumours*

Benign tumours	Malignant tumours

Hepatocellular adenoma
    Anabolic-androgenic steroids
    Clofibrate[a]
    Clomiphene[a]
    Norethisterone[a]
    Methyldopa[a]
    Oral contraceptives
	Hepatocellular carcinoma
	    Anabolic-androgenic steroids
	    Cyproterone[a]
	    Methotrexate[a]
	    Oral hypoglycaemic agents[a]
	    Oral contraceptives
	    Phenelzine[a]

Nodular focal hyperplasia
    Anabolic-androgenic steroids[a]
    Chorionic gonadotrophins[a]
    Oral contraceptives[a] (increase the
    risk of complications)
	Angiosarcoma
	    Anabolic-androgenic steroids
	    Arsenical derivatives
	    Oral contraceptives[a]
	    Phenelzine[a]
	    Thorium dioxide

Benign haemangioma
    Oral contraceptives[a] (may increase size
    and the risk of complications)
	Cholangiocarcinoma
	    Anabolic-androgenic steroids[a]
	    Methyldopa[a]
	    Oral contraceptives[a]
	    Thorium dioxide

	Epithelioid haemangioendothelioma Oral contraceptives[a]

	Hepatoblastoma
	    Oral contraceptives[a]
	    Clomiphene[a]

	Lymphomas
	    Immunosuppressive therapy (cyclosporin
	      ± azathioprine and corticosteroids)

[a] Compounds for which a causal relationship remains to be confirmed.

Focal nodular hyperplasia

Focal nodular hyperplasia is a benign hepatic tumour (hamartoma) characterized by a central stellate scar surrounded by the liver cell nodule. The fibrous tissue septa contain blood vessels and bile ducts. Albeit uncommon, this tumour is now about 10 times more frequent than adenoma. In most cases, focal nodular hyperplasia is fortuitously discovered by ultrasonography performed for unrelated reasons. However, abdominal pain or the palpation of a liver mass may reveal the tumour.

Ultrasound examination discloses an hypo-, iso- or hyper-echogenic nodule. Computed tomography shows a slightly hypodense nodule, with a very hypodense central zone corresponding to the artery feeding the tumour, and the fibrotic scar. Computed tomography may also show an early and massive enhancement of the nodule with a central hypodense area. However, this central scar, which is characteristic of focal nodular hyperplasia, is observed in only 50 per cent of patients. Magnetic resonance imaging shows the central scar more easily, and is now the preferred, non-invasive method to ascertain the diagnosis. Liver biopsy may be resorted to in difficult cases. In a few cases, the distinction from an adenoma or a well differentiated hepatocellular carcinoma may be impossible (Kerlin, Gastro, 1983; 84:994; Michel, GastrClinBiol, 1992; 16:35).

Although oral contraceptives might not promote the *de novo* formation of focal nodular hyperplasia,[195] they certainly can increase the size of the tumour and the risk of developing intratumourous or intraperitoneal haemorrhage (Scott, JAMA, 1984; 251:1461). This has led some authors to propose the withdrawal of oral contraceptives in women affected by this tumour (Scott, JAMA, 1984; 252:1461; Stauffer, AnnIntMed, 1975; 83:301).

An isolated case of focal nodular hyperplasia has been attributed to chorionic gonadotrophins (Svastics, NEJM, 1985; 312:1259).

When the hepatic imaging is considered typical of this lesion, there is little risk that the tumour might be a hepatocarcinoma. Focal nodular hyperplasia does not evolve into cancer. It exceptionally leads to intratumoural or intraperitoneal bleeding. Therefore, small and asymptomatic forms of focal nodular hyperplasia can be left *in situ*, and just monitored by periodic ultrascans.

Benign haemangioma

This vascular tumour may not be induced by oral contraceptives, but these drugs may have a role in the enlargement of a pre-existing haemangioma and in the appearance of symptoms.[200]

Malignant tumours
Hepatocellular carcinoma

This is a malignant tumour developed from hepatocytes. The tumour may be discovered fortuitously or revealed by cholestasis, abdominal pain, weight loss, or asthenia.

Steroids

The risk of developing a hepatocellular carcinoma appears to be increased by prolonged administration of anabolic–androgenic steroids.[107] A mean delay of 72 months between the beginning of the anabolic–androgenic steroid therapy and the discovery of the tumour has been reported.[107] Similarly, much evidence suggests that prolonged administration of oral contraceptives also increases the risk of developing a hepatocellular carcinoma.[201,202] Indeed, the relative risk would be increased from 7 to 20 times, in women taking oral contraceptives for 8 years or more.[201,202]

The hepatocellular carcinomas that are associated with anabolic–androgenic steroids or oral contraceptives exhibit several features that distinguish them from the hepatocellular carcinomas complicating cirrhosis.[107,198] The cancer occurs in relatively young subjects (frequently less than 35 years old). There is no evidence of chronic liver disease or cirrhosis in the non-tumoural liver. The serum α-fetoprotein level is generally normal or moderately increased. Vascular extensions of the tumour and metastases are uncommon (but possible). Finally, the hepatocellular carcinomas induced by anabolic–androgenic steroids have sometimes receded after the discontinuation of these drugs.[198]

The role of steroids in the incidence of fibrolamellar carcinoma is still unknown but is thought unlikely (Goodman, Hepatol, 1982; 2:440).

Cyproterone

Three cases of hepatocellular carcinoma have been reported in children receiving high doses of cyproterone acetate, a synthetic progestagen that suppresses gonadotrophin secretion and blocks male hormone receptors (Watanabe, Lancet, 1994; 344:1567). A fourth case has been reported in an elderly male treated for prostate cancer (Ohri, BrJUrol, 1991; 67:213). Tumourigenicity may be explained by the genotoxic and growth-promoting effects of this drug (Neumann, Carcinogenesis, 1992; 13:373; Deml, Carcinogenesis, 1993; 14:1229).

Angiosarcoma

This is an uncommon, malignant tumour developed from the endothelial sinusoidal cells. This tumour may occur after exposure to several chemicals, in particular vinyl chloride and cupric sulphate, or after the administration of some drugs including arsenical derivatives and anabolic–androgenic steroids (Table 12).[200,203] Interestingly, several of these compounds are also able to cause sinusoidal dilation, peliosis hepatis, and perisinusoidal fibrosis.[200] This suggests some possible relationship between the mechanisms leading to these non-malignant diseases and the possible development of angiosarcoma.[200] Perhaps the common origin of these various lesions might be some initial toxic insult to sinusoidal endothelial cells.[200]

Other malignant tumours

Cholangiocarcinoma

Cholangiocarcinoma is a malignant tumour made up of cells resembling biliary epithelial cells. The serum level of α-fetoprotein is usually normal, whereas that of the carcinoembryonic antigen is frequently increased. This tumour has been observed in subjects exposed to thorium dioxide.[192] It has occasionally been reported in patients on long-term anabolic–androgenic steroid therapy,[107] in oral contraceptive users (Littlewood, Lancet, 1980; i:310), and in

a patient receiving methyldopa (Broden, ActaChirScand, 1980; 500: 7). However, the causal relationship between these treatments and the tumour remains to be confirmed.

Epithelioid haemangioendothelioma

A hypothetical link between this uncommon malignant tumour and the use of oral contraceptive has been suggested (Dean, AmJSurgPath, 1985; 9:695).

Hepatoblastoma

This tumour has been observed in two infants after maternal exposure to oral contraceptives or clomiphen,[192] but this association may be fortuitous.

Lymphomas

Prolonged administration of immunosuppressive drugs increase the incidence of lymphomas, which may affect the liver (Table 12).

Outlook

Looking back over the last two decades, it appears that considerable progress has been made in the field of drug-induced liver injury. The astonishing variety of drug-induced liver lesions has been recognized, and a main mechanism has been proposed for most of them. It is clear, however, that our present understanding represents, at best, a much simplified overview of the reality. Because there are so many hepatotoxic drugs, only a few mechanistic aspects, if any, have been investigated for any single drug. Reasons behind the susceptibility of a few patients remain largely unknown, and the possibility of preventive measures has been little explored.

Few young hepatologists are devoting themselves to this field nowadays, and this seriously limits the chances for quicker progress. Hopefully, this trend may be reversed in the near future. Indeed, recent advances in pharmacogenetics, molecular biology, immunology, and cell biology offer renewed opportunities for rapid and fascinating advances in this important field.

As drug-induced hepatotoxicity is relatively uncommon (when a single drug is concerned), large collaborative studies should be encouraged to define better the genetic background, acquired predisposing factors, frequency, early diagnosis, clinical characteristics, and outcome of these iatrogenic diseases. Improved understanding of the hepatotoxicity of drugs may hopefully lead to the safer use of current molecules and the development of safer alternatives in the future.

References

1. Benhamou JP. Drug-induced hepatitis. Clinical aspects. In Fillastre JP, ed. *Hepatotoxicity of drugs.* Rouen: Presses Universitaires de Rouen, 1986: 23–30.
2. Stricker BHC. *Drug-induced hepatic injury,* 2nd edn. Amsterdam: Elsevier, 1992.
3. Farrell GC. *Drug-induced liver injury.* New York: Churchill Livingstone, 1994.
4. Zimmerman HJ. *Hepatotoxicity. The adverse effects of drugs and other chemicals on the liver.* New York: Appleton-Century-Crofts, 1978.
5. Bernuau J, Rueff B, and Benhamou JP. Fulminant and subfulminant liver failure: definition and causes. *Seminars in Liver Disease,* 1986; **6**: 97–106.

6. Benichou C. Criteria for drug-induced hepatitis. Report of an international consensus meeting. *Journal of Hepatology*, 1990; **11**: 272–6.

7. Pessayre D. Role of reactive metabolites in drug-induced hepatitis. *Journal of Hepatology*, 1995; **23** (Suppl. 1): 16–24.

8. Gonzales FJ and Nebert DW. Evolution of the cytochrome P-450 gene superfamily: Animal-plant 'warfare', molecular drive and human genetic differences in drug oxidation. *Trends in Genetics*, 1990; **6**: 182–6.

9. Guengerich FP and Liebler DC. Enzymatic activation of chemicals to toxic metabolites. *CRC Critical Reviews in Toxicology*, 1985; **14**: 259–307.

10. Breen K, Wandscheer JC, Peignoux M, and Pessayre D. *In situ* formation of the acetaminophen metabolite covalently bound in kidney and lung. Supportive evidence provided by total hepatectomy. *Biochemical Pharmacology*, 1982; **31**: 115–16.

11. Esterbauer H, Schaur RJ, and Zollner H. Chemistry and biochemistry of 4-hydroxynonenal, malondialdehyde and related aldehydes. *Free Radical Biology and Medicine*, 1991; **11**: 81–128.

12. Mitchell JR and Jollow DJ. Metabolic activation of drugs to toxic substances. *Gastroenterology*, 1975; **68**: 392–410.

13. Mirabelli F, *et al.* Menadione-induced bleb formation in hepatocytes is associated with the oxidation of thiol groups in actin. *Archives of Biochemistry and Biophysics*, 1988; **264**: 261–9.

14. Bellomo G and Orrenius S. Altered thiol and calcium homeostasis in oxidative hepatocellular injury. *Hepatology*, 1985; **5**: 876–82.

15. Fagian MM, Pereire-Da-Silva L, Martins IS, and Vercesi AE. Membrane protein thiol cross-linking associated with the permeabilization of the inner membrane by Ca^{2+} plus prooxidants. *Journal of Biological Chemistry*, 1990; **32**: 19955–60.

16. Arends MJ and Wyllie AH. Apoptosis: mechanisms and roles in pathology. *International Review of Experimental Pathology*, 1991; **32**: 223–54.

17. Shen W, Kamendulis LM, Sidhartha DR, and Corcoran GB. Acetaminophen-induced cytotoxicity in cultured mouse hepatocytes: effects of Ca^{2+}-endonuclease, DNA repair, and glutathione depletion inhibitors on DNA fragmentation and cell death. *Toxicology and Applied Pharmacolcogy*, 1992; **112**: 32–40.

18. Fau D, *et al.* Diterpenoids from germander, a herbal medicine, induce apoptosis in isolated rat hepatocytes. *Gastroenterology*, 1997; **113** (in press).

19. Leist M, Single B, Castoldi AF, Kühnle S, and Nicotera P. Intracellular adenosine triphosphate (ATP) concentration: a switch in the decision between apoptosis and necrosis. *Journal of Experimental Medicine*, 1997; **185**: 1481–6.

20. Berson A, *et al.* Metabolic activation of the nitroaromatic antiandrogen flutamide by rat and human cytochromes P-450, including forms belonging to the 3A and 1A subfamilies. *Journal of Pharmacology and Experimental Therapeutics*, 1993; **265**: 366–72.

21. Larrey D, *et al.* Metabolic activation of the new tricyclic antidepressant tianeptine by human liver cytochrome P-450. *Biochemical Pharmacology*, 1990; **40**: 545–50.

22. Loeper J, *et al.* Hepatotoxicity of germander in mice. *Gastroenterology*, 1994; **106**: 464–72.

23. Larrey D, Distlerath LM, Dannan GA, Wilkinson GR, and Guengerich FP. Purification and characterization of the rat liver microsomal cytochrome P-450 involved in the 4-hydroxylation of debrisoquine, a prototype for genetic variation in oxidative drug metabolism. *Biochemistry*, 1984; **23**: 2787–95.

24. Jacqz E, Hall SD, and Branch RA. Genetically determined polymorphisms in drug oxidation. *Hepatology*, 1986; **6**: 1020–32.

25. Larrey D, *et al.* Genetically determined oxidation polymorphism and drug hepatotoxicity. Study of 51 patients. *Journal of Hepatology*, 1989; **8**: 158–64.

26. Spielberg S and Gordon GB. Glutathione synthetase-deficient lymphocytes and acetaminophen toxicity. *Clinical Pharmacology and Therapeutics*, 1981; **29**: 51–5.

27. Larrey D, *et al.* Effects of pregnancy on the toxicity and metabolism of acetaminophen in mice. *Journal of Pharmacology and Experimental Therapeutics*, 1986; **237**: 283–91.

28. Pessayre D, *et al.* Effect of fasting on metabolite-mediated hepatotoxicity in the rat. *Gastroenterology*, 1979; **77**: 264–71.

29. Pessayre D, *et al.* Isoniazid-rifampin fulminant hepatitis. A possible consequence of the enhancement of isoniazid hepatotoxicity by enzyme induction. *Gastroenterology*, 1977; **72**: 284–9.

30. Pessayre D, Allemand H, Benoist C, Afifi F, François M, and Benhamou JP. Effect of surgery under general anaesthesia on antipyrine clearance. *British Journal of Clinical Pharmacology*, 1978; **6**: 505–13.

31. Pessayre D, de Saint-Louvent P, Degott C, Bernuau J, Rueff B, and Benhamou JP. Iproclozide fulminant hepatitis. Possible role of enzyme induction. *Gastroenterology*, 1978; **75**: 492–6.

32. Seef LB, Cuccherini BA, Zimmerman HJ, Adler E, and Benjamin SB. Acetaminophen hepatotoxicity in alcoholics. A therapeutic misadventure. *Annals of Internal Medicine*, 1986; **104**: 399–404.

33. Pessayre D, *et al.* Additive effects of inducers and fasting on acetaminophen hepatotoxicity. *Biochemical Pharmacology*, 1980; **29**: 2219–23.

34. Germain RN. MHC-dependent antigen processing and peptide presentation: providing ligands for T lymphocyte activation. *Cell*, 1994; **76**: 287–99.

35. Gut J, Christen U, and Huwyler J. Mechanisms of halothane toxicity: novel insights. *Pharmacology and Therapeutics*, 1993; **58**: 133–55.

36. Kenna JG, Satoh H, Christ DD, and Pohl LR. Metabolic basis for a drug hypersensitivity: antibodies in sera from patients with halothane hepatitis recognize liver neoantigens that contain the trifluoroacetyl group derived from halothane. *Journal of Pharmacology and Experimental Therapeutics*, 1988; **245**: 1103–9.

37. Vergani D, *et al.* Antibodies to the surface of halothane-altered rabbit hepatocytes in patients with severe halothane-associated hepatitis. *New England Journal of Medicine*, 1980; **303**: 66–71.

38. Volpes R, van den Oord JJ, and Desmet VJ. Can hepatocytes serve as activated immunomodulating cells in the immune response? *Journal of Hepatology*, 1992; **16**: 228–40.

39. Satoh H, Fukuda Y, Anderson DK, Ferrans VJ, Gillette JR, and Pohl LR. Immunological studies on the mechanism of halothane-induced hepatotoxicity: immunohistochemical evidence of trifluoroacetylated hepatocytes. *Journal of Pharmacology and Experimental Therapeutics*, 1985; **233**: 857–62.

40. Loeper J, Descatoire V, Amouyal G, Lettéron P, Larrey D, and Pessayre D. Presence of covalently bound metabolites on rat hepatocyte plasma membrane proteins after administration of isaxonine, a drug leading to immunoallergic hepatitis in man. *Hepatology*, 1989; **9**: 675–8.

41. Neuberger J, Kenna JG, Aria KN, and Williams R. Antibody mediated hepatocyte injury in methyl-dopa induced hepatotoxicity. *Gut*, 1985; **26**: 1233–9.

42. Neuberger J and Williams R. Immune mechanisms in tienilic acid associated hepatotoxicity. *Gut*, 1989; **30**: 515–19.

43. Siprodhis L, Beaugrand M, Malledant Y, Brissot P, Guguen-Guillouzo C, and Guillouzo A. Use of adult human hepatocytes in primary culture for the study of clometacin-induced immunoallergic hepatitis. *Toxicity in Vitro*, 1991; **5**: 529–34.

44. Beaune P *et al.* Human anti-endoplasmic reticulum autoantibodies appearing in a drug-induced hepatitis are directed against a human liver cytochrome P-450 that hydroxylates the drug. *Proceedings of the National Academy of Sciences of the USA*, 1987; **84**: 551–5.

45. Bourdi M, *et al.* Anti-liver endoplasmic reticulum autoantibodies are directed against human liver cytochrome P-450 IA2. A specific marker of dihydralazine-induced hepatitis. *Journal of Clinical Investigation*, 1990; **85**: 1967–73.

46. Bourdi M, Tinel M, Beaune P, and Pessayre D. Interactions of dihydralazine with cytochromes P4501A: A possible explanation for the appearance of anti-P4501A2 autoantibodies. *Molecular Pharmacology*, 1994; **45**: 1287–95.

47. Robin AM, *et al.* Cytochrome P4502B follows a vesicular route to the plasma membrane in cultured rat hepatocytes. *Gastroenterology*, 1995; **108**: 1110–23.

48. Loeper J, *et al.* Presence of functional cytochrome P-450 on isolated rat hepatocyte plasma membrane. *Hepatology*, 1990; **11**: 850–8.

49. Loeper J, *et al.* Cytochrome P-450 on human hepatocyte plasma membrane. Recognition by several autoantibodies. *Gastroenterology*, 1993; **104**: 203–16.

50. Beaune P, Pessayre D, Dansette P, Mansuy D, and Manns M. Auto-antibodies against cytochromes P450: Role in human diseases. *Advances in Pharmacology*, 1994; **30**: 199–245.

51. Shear NH, Spielberg SP, Grant DM, Tang BK, and Kalow W. Differences in metabolism of sulfonamides predisposing to idiosyncratic drug reactions. *Annals of Internal Medicine*, 1986; **105**: 179–83.

52. Shear NH and Spielberg SP. Anticonvulsant hypersensitivity syndrome. In vitro assessment of risk. *Journal of Clinical Investigation*, 1988; **82**: 1826–32.

53. Farrell G, Prendergast D, and Murray M. Halothane hepatitis. Detection of a constitutional susceptibility factor. *New England Journal of Medicine*, 1985; **313**: 1310–14.

54. Larrey D, *et al.* Genetic predisposition to drug hepatotoxicity. Role in hepatitis caused by amineptine, a tricyclic antidepressant. *Hepatology*, 1989; **10**: 168–73.

55. Berson A, *et al.* Possible role of HLA in hepatotoxicity. An exploratory study in 71 patients with drug-induced idiosyncratic hepatitis. *Journal of Hepatology*, 1994; **20**: 336–42.

56. Prescott LF. Paracetamol overdosage. Pharmacological considerations and clinical management. *Drugs*, 1983; **25**: 290–314.

57. Rodman JS, Deutsch DJ, and Gutman SI. Methyldopa hepatitis. A report of six cases and review of the literature. *American Journal of Medicine*, 1976; **60**: 941–8.

58. Al-kawas FH, Seeff LB, Berendson RA, and Zimmerman HJ. Allopurinol hepatotoxicity. Report of two cases and review of the literature. *Annals of Internal Medicine*, 1981; **95**: 588–90.

59. Larrey D, *et al.* Amodiaquine-induced hepatitis. A report of seven cases. *Annals of Internal Medicine*, 1986; **104**: 801–3.

60. Zimmerman HJ. Effects of aspirin and acetaminophen on the liver. *Archives of Internal Medicine*, 1981; **141**: 333–42.

61. Waldman RJ, Hall WN, McGee H, and Amburg GV. Aspirin as a risk factor in Reye's syndrome. *Journal of the American Medical Association*, 1982; **247**: 3089–94.

62. Goldfarb G, Pessayre D, Boisseau C, Degott C, Béraud C, and Benhamou JP. Hépatite à la clométacine. *Gastroentérologie Clinique et Biologique*, 1979; **3**: 537–40.

63. Utili R, Boitnott JK, and Zimmerman HJ. Dantrolene-associated hepatic injury. Incidence and character. *Gastroenterology*, 1977; **72**: 610–16.

64. Banks AT, Zimmerman HJ, Ishak KG, and Harter JG. Diclofenac-associated hepatotoxicity. Analysis of 180 cases reported to the food and drug administration as adverse reactions. *Hepatology*, 1995; **22**: 820–7.

65. Pariente EA, Pessayre D, Bernuau J, Degott C, and Benhamou JP. Di-hydralazine hepatitis. Report of a case and review of the literature. *Digestion*, 1983; **27**: 47–52.

66. Lewis JH, Zimmerman HJ, Ishak KG, and Mullick FG. Enflurane hepatotoxicity. A clinico pathologic study of 24 cases. *Annals of Internal Medicine*, 1983; **98**: 984–92.

67. Larrey D, *et al.* Hepatitis after germander (*Teucrium chamaedris*) administration: another instance of herbal medicine hepatotoxicity. *Annals of Internal Medicine*, 1992; **117**: 129–32.

68. Davis P and Holdsworth CD. Jaundice after muliple halothane anaesthetics administered during the treatment of carcinoma of the uterus. *Gut*, 1973; **14**: 566–8.

69. Itoh S, Yamaba Y, Ichinoe A, and Tsukada Y. Hydralazine-induced liver injury. *Digestive Diseases and Sciences*, 1980; **25**: 884–7.

70. Black M, Mitchell JR, Zimmerman HJ, Ishak K, and Epler GR. Isoniazid-associated hepatitis in 114 patients. *Gastroenterology*, 1975; **69**: 289–302.

71. Rosenblum LE, Korn RJ, and Zimmerman HJ. Hepatocellular jaundice as a complication of iproniazid therapy. *Archives of Internal Medicine*, 1960; **105**: 583–93.

72. Homberg JC, Stelly M, Andreis, I, Abuaf N, Saadoun F, and André J. A new antimitochondrial antibody (anti-M6) in iproniazid-induced hepatitis. *Clinical and Experimental Immunology*, 1982; **47**: 93–103.

73. Danan G, Homberg JC, Bernuau J, Roche-Sicot J, and Pessayre D. Hépatite à l'iproniazide. Intérêt diagnostique d'un nouvel anticorps anti-mitochondrial, l'anti-M6. *Gastroentérologie Clinique et Biologique*, 1983; **7**: 529–32.

74. Lewis JH, Zimmerman HJ, Benson G, and Dandlshak KG. Hepatic injury associated with ketoconazole therapy. Analysis of 33 cases. *Gastroenterology*, 1984; **86**: 503–13.

75. Smilkstein MJ, Knapp GL, Fulig KW, and Rumack BH. Efficacy of oral *N*-acetylcysteine in the treatment of acetaminophen overdose. Analysis of the national multicenter study (1976 to 1985). *New England Journal of Medicine*, 1988; **319**: 1557–62.

76. De Herder WW, Schröder P, Purnode A, Van Vliet ACM, and Stricker BHC. Pirprofen-associated hepatic injury. *Journal of Hepatology*, 1987; **4**: 127–32.

77. Danan G, *et al.* Pirprofen-induced fulminant hepatitis. *Gastroenterology*, 1985; **89**: 210–13.

78. Durand F, *et al.* Deleterious influence of pyrazinamide on the outcome of patients with fulminant or subfulminant liver failure during anti-tuberculous treatment including isoniazid. *Hepatology*, 1995; **21**: 929–32.

79. Watkins PB, Zimmermann HJ, Knapp MJ, Gracon SI, and Lewis KW. Hepatotoxic effects of tacrine administration in patients with Alzheimer's disease. *Journal of the American Medical Asssociation*, 1994; **271**: 992–8.

80. Zimmerman HJ, Lewis JH, Ishak KG, and Maddrey WC. Ticrynafen associated hepatic injury: Analysis of 340 cases. *Hepatology*, 1984; **4**: 315–23.

81. Larrey D and Erlinger S. Drug-induced cholestasis. *Ballière's Clinical Gastroenterology*, 1988; **2**: 423–52.

82. Pariente EA, *et al.* Hépatite à l'ajmaline. Description de 4 observations et revue de la littérature. *Gastroentérologie Clinique et Biologique*, 1980; **4**: 240–5.

83. Larrey D, *et al.* Hepatitis associated with amoxycillin-clavulanic acid combination. Report of 15 cases. *Gut*, 1992; **33**: 368–71.

84. Hautekeete ML, *et al.* Liver injury related to amoxicillin-clavulanic acid: interlobular bile duct lesions and extrahepatic manifestations. *Journal of Hepatology*, 1995; **22**: 71–7.

85. Loiseau D, Degos F, Degott C, Carnot F, and Kreis H. Cholestasis after azathioprine administration in renal transplant recipients. *Clinical Transplantation*, 1987; **1**: 88–94.

86. Ishak KG and Irey NS. Hepatic injury associated with the phenothiazines. Clinico-pathologic and follow-up study of 36 patients. *Archives of Pathology*, 1972; **93**: 283–304.

87. Lunzer MR, Huang SN, Ward KM, and Sherlock S. Jaundice due to erythomycin estolate. *Gastroenterology*, 1975; **68**: 1284–91.

88. Funck-Brentano C, Pessayre D, and Benhamou JP. Hépatites dues à divers dérivés de l'érythromycine. *Gastroentérologie Clinique et Biologique*, 1983; **7**: 362–9.

89. Zafrani ES, Ishak KG, and Rudzki C. Cholestatic and hepatocellular injury associated with erythromycin esters. Report of nine cases. *American Journal of Digestive Diseases*, 1979; **24**: 385–96.

90. Pessayre D, Larrey D, Funck-Brentano C, and Benhamou JP. Drug interactions and hepatitis produced by some macrolide antibiotics. *Journal of Antimicrobial Chemotherapy*, 1985; **16**: 181–94.

91. Pessayre D, *et al.* Gold-salt induced cholestasis. *Digestion*, 1979; **19**: 57–74.

92. Favreau M, Tannenbaum H, and Lough J. Hepatotoxicity associated with gold therapy. *Annals of Internal Medicine*, 1977; **87**: 717–19.

93. Ticktin HE and Zimmermann HJ. Hepatic dysfunction and jaundice in patients receiving triacetyloleandomycin. *New England Journal of Medicine*, 1962; **267**: 964–8.

94. Danan G, Bernuau J, Moullot X, Degott C, and Pessayre D. Amitriptyline-induced fulminant hepatitis. *Digestion*, 1984; **30**: 179–84.

95. Johnson DA, Cattau EL, Kuritsky JN, and Zimmerman HJ. Liver involvement in the sulfone syndrome. *Archives of Internal Medicine*, 1986; **146**: 875–7.

96. Benjamin SB, Ishak KG, Zimmerman HJ, and Grushka A. Phenylbutazone liver injury: a clinical-pathologic survey of 23 cases and review of the literature. *Hepatology*, 1981; **1**: 255–63.

97. Koch MJ, Seeff LB, Crumley CE, Rabin L, and Burns WA. Quinidine hepatotoxicity. A report of a case and review of the literature. *Gastroenterology*, 1976; **70**: 1136–40.

98. Babany G and Pessayre D. Hépatites dues aux nouveaux antiinflammatoires non stéroïdiens. *Gastroentérologie Clinique et Biologique*, 1984; **8**: 523–9.

99. Dujovne CA, Char CH, and Zimmerman HJ. Sulfonamide hepatic injury. Review of the literature and report of a case due to sulfamethoxazole. *New England Journal of Medicine*, 1967; **277**: 785–8.

100. Ishak KG and Zimmerman HJ. Drug-induced and toxic granulomatous hepatitis. In Bircher J, ed. *Baillière's Clinical Gastroenterology*. London: Baillière Tindall, 1988: 463–80.

101. Forker EL. The effect of estrogen on bile formation in the rat. *Journal of Clinical Investigation*, 1969; **48**: 654–63.

102. Simon FR, Gonzalez M, Sutherland E, Accatino L, and Davis RA. Reversal of cthinyl estradiol-induced bile secretory failure with Triton WR-1339. *Journal of Clinical Investigation*, 1980; **65**: 851–60.

103. Vore M and Slikker W. Steroid D-ring glucuronides: a new class of cholestatic agents. *Trends in Pharmacological Sciences*, 1985; **6**: 256–9.

104. Métreaux JM, Dhumeaux D, and Berthelot P. Oral contraceptives and the liver. *Gut*, 1972; **7**: 318–35.

105. Miguet JP, *et al.* Jaundice from troleandomycin and oral contraceptives. *Annals of Internal Medicine*, 1980; **92**: 434.

106. Fisher D, *et al.* Inhibition of rat liver estrogen 2/4-hydroxylase activity by troleandomycin. Comparison with erythromycin and roxithromycin. *Journal of Pharmacology and Experimental Therapeutics*, 1990; **254**: 1120–7.

107. Ishak G and Zimmerman HJ. Hepatotoxic effects of the anabolic/androgenic steroids. *Seminars in Liver Disease*, 1987; **7**: 230–6.

108. Böhme M, Müller M, Leier I, Jedlitsky G, and Keppler D. Cholestasis caused by inhibition of the adenosine triphosphate-dependent bile salt transport in rat liver. *Gastroenterology*, 1994; **107**: 255–65.

109. Cadranel JF, Babany G, Oppolon P, and Erlinger S. Pharmacocinétique et effets hépatiques de la cyclosporine A. *Gastroentérologie Clinique et Biologique*, 1992; **16**: 314–21.

110. Lieber CS. Alcohol and the liver: 1994 update. *Gastroenterology*, 1994; **106**: 1085–105.

111. Fromenty B and Pessayre D. Inhibition of mitochondrial β-oxidation as a mechanism of hepatotoxicity. *Pharmacology and Therapeutics*, 1995; **67**: 101–54.

112. Dahl MGC, Gregory MM, and Scheuer PJ. Liver damage due to methotrexate in patients with psoriasis. *British Medical Journal*, 1971; **1**: 625–30.

113. Vockley J. The changing face of disorders of fatty acid oxidation. *Mayo Clinic Proceedings*, 1994; **69**: 249–57.

114. Schon EA, Hirano M, and DiMauro S. Mitochondrial encephalomyopathies: Clinical and molecular analysis. *Journal of Bioenergetics and Biomembranes*, 1994; **26**: 291–9.

115. Latipää PM, Kärki TT, Hiltunen JK, and Hassinen IE. Regulation of palmitoylcarnitine oxidation in isolated rat liver mitochondria. Role of the redox state of NAD(H). *Biochimica Biophysica Acta*, 1986; **875**: 293–300.

116. Maddaiah VT. Ammonium inhibition of fatty acid oxidation in rat liver mitochondria. A possible cause of fatty liver in Reye's syndrome and urea cycle defects. *Biochemical and Biophysical Research Communications*, 1985; **127**: 565–70.

117. Grimbert S, *et al.* Decreased mitochondrial oxidation of fatty acids in pregnant mice: Possible relevance to development of acute fatty liver of pregnancy. *Hepatology*, 1993; **17**: 628–37.

118. Grimbert S, *et al.* Effects of female sex hormones on liver mitochondria in non-pregnant female mice: possible role in acute fatty liver of pregnancy. *American Journal of Physiology*, 1995; **268**: G107–15.

119. Le Dinh T, *et al.* Amineptine, a tricyclic antidepressant, inhibits the mitochondrial oxidation of fatty acids and produces microvesicular steatosis of the liver in mice. *Journal of Pharmacology and Experimental Therapeutics*, 1988; **247**: 745–50.

120. Deschamps D, Fisch C, Fromenty B, Berson A, Degott C, and Pessayre D. Inhibition by salicylic acid of the activation and thus oxidation of long-chain fatty acids. Possible role in the development of Reye's syndrome. *Journal of Pharmacology and Experimental Therapeutics*, 1991; **259**: 894–904.

121. Shigenaga MK, Hagen TM, and Ames BN. Oxidative damage and mitochondrial decay in aging. *Proceedings of the National Academy of Sciences of the USA*, 1994; **91**: 1077–8.

122. Kukielka E, Dicker E, and Cederbaum AI. Increased production of reactive oxygen species by rat liver mitochondria after chronic ethanol treatment. *Archives of Biochemistry and Biophysics*, 1994; **309**: 377–86.

123. Fromenty B, *et al.* Hepatic mitochondrial DNA deletion in alcoholics. Association with microvesicular steatosis. *Gastroenterology*, 1995; **108**: 193–200.

124. Mitsuya H, *et al.* Long-term inhibition of human T-lymphotropic virus type III/lymphadenopathy-associated virus (human immunodeficiency virus) DNA synthesis and RNA expression in T cells protected by 2′,3′-dideoxynucleosides *in vitro*. *Proceedings of the National Academy of Sciences of the USA*, 1987; **84**: 2033–7.

125. Simpson MV, Chin CD, Keilbaugh SA, Lin TS, and Prusoff WH. Studies on the inhibition of mitochondrial DNA replication by 3′-azido-3′-deoxythymidine and other dideoxynucleoside analogs which inhibits HIV-1 replication. *Biochemical Pharmacology*, 1989; **38**: 1033–6.

126. Lai KK, Gang DL, Zawacki JK, and Cooley TP. Fulminant hepatic failure associated with 2′,3′-dideoxyinosine (ddI). *Annals of Internal Medecine*, 1991; **115**: 283–4.

127. Zoulim F and Trépo C. Nucleoside analogs in the treatment of chronic viral hepatitis. Efficiency and complications. *Journal of Hepatology*, 1994; **21**: 142–4.

128. Richardson FC, Engelhardt JA, and Bowsher RR. Fialuridine accumulates in DNA of dogs, monkeys and rats following long-term oral administration. *Proceedings of the National Academy of Sciences of the USA*, 1994; **91**: 12003–7.

129. Fréneaux E, *et al.* Stereoselective and non-stereoselective effects of ibuprofen enantiomers on the mitochondrial β-oxidation of fatty acids. *Journal of Pharmacology and Experimental Therapeutics*, 1990; **255**: 529–35.

130. Fréneaux E, *et al.* Inhibition of the mitochondrial oxidation of fatty acids by tetracycline in mice and in man: possible role in microvesicular steatosis induced by this antibiotic. *Hepatology*, 1988; **8**: 1056–62.

131. Labbe G, *et al.* Effects of various tetracycline derivatives on *in vitro* and *in vivo* β-oxidation of fatty acids, egress of triglycerides from the liver, accumulation of hepatic triglycerides, and mortality in mice. *Biochemical Pharmacology*, 1991; **41**: 638–41.

132. Deboyser D, Goethals F, Krack G, and Roberfroid M. Investigation into the mechanism of tetracycline-induced steatosis: study in isolated hepatocytes. *Toxicology and Applied Pharmacology*, 1989; **97**: 473–9.

133. Genève J, *et al.* Inhibition of mitochondrial β-oxidation of fatty acids by pirprofen. Role in microvesicular steatosis due to this nonsteroidal anti-inflammatory drug. *Journal of Pharmacology and Experimental Therapeutics*, 1987; **242**: 1133–7.

134. Zimmerman HJ and Ishak KG. Valproate-induced hepatic injury. Analysis of 23 fatal cases. *Hepatology*, 1982; **2**: 591–7.

135. Lüllman H, Lüllman-Rauch R, and Wassermann O. Drug-induced phospholipidoses. *CRC Critical Reviews in Toxicology*, 1975; **4**: 185–242.

136. Kodavanti UP and Mehendale HM. Cationic amphiphilic drugs and phospholipid storage disorder. *Pharmacological Reviews*, 1990; **42**: 327–54.

137. De La Inglesia FA, Feuer G, Takada A, and Matsuda Y. Morphologic studies on secondary phospholipidosis in humans. *Laboratory Investigation*, 1974; **4**: 539–49.

138. Shikata T, Kanetaka T, Endo Y, and Nagashima K. Drug-induced generalized phospholipidosis. *Acta Pathologica Japonica*, 1972; **22**: 517–31.

139. Beaugrand M, Chousterman M, Callard P, Camilleri JP, Petite JP, and Ferrier JP. Hépatites au maléate de Perhexiline (Pexid) évoluant vers la cirrhose malgré l'arrêt du traitement (2 cas). *Gastroentérologie Clinique et Biologique*, 1977; **1**: 745–50.

140. Paliard P, Vitrey D, Fournier G, Belhadjali J, Patricot L, and Berger F. Perhexiline maleate-induced hepatitis. *Digestion*, 1978; **17**: 419–27.

141. Pessayre D, Bichara M, Feldmann G, Degott C, Potet F, and Benhamou JP. Perhexiline maleate-induced cirrhosis. *Gastroenterology*, 1979; **76**: 170–7.

142. Poupon R, *et al.* Perhexiline maleate-associated hepatic injury. Prevalence and characteristics. *Digestion*, 1980; **20**: 145–50.

143. Simon JB, Manley PN, Brien JF, and Armstrong PW. Amiodarone hepato-toxicity simulating alcoholic liver disease. *New England Journal of Medicine*, 1984; **311**: 167–72.

144. Poucell S, *et al.* Amiodarone-associated phospholipidosis and fibrosis of the liver. Light, immunohistochemical, and electron microscopic studies. *Gastroenterology*, 1984; **86**: 926–36.

145. Lewis JH, *et al.* Amiodarone hepatotoxicity: prevalence and clinic-opathologic correlations among 104 patients. *Hepatology*, 1989; **9**: 679–85.

146. Adams PC, Bennett MK, and Holt DW. Hepatic effects of amiodarone. *British Journal of Clinical Practice*, 1986; **40**: 81–92.

147. Guigui B, *et al.* Amiodarone-induced hepatic phospholipidosis: a mor-phological alteration independent of pseudoalcoholic liver disease. *Hep-atology*, 1988; **8**: 1063–8.

148. Fromenty B, *et al.* Amiodarone inhibits the mitochondrial β-oxidation of fatty acids and produces microvesicular steatosis of the liver in mice. *Journal of Pharmacology and Experimental Therapeutics*, 1990; **255**: 1371–6.

149. Fromenty B, Fisch C, Berson A, Lettéron P, Larrey D, and Pessayre D. Dual effect of amiodarone on mitochondrial respiration. Initial pro-tonophoric uncoupling effect followed by inhibition of the respiratory chain at the levels of complex I and complex II. *Journal of Pharmacology and Experimental Therapeutics*, 1990; **255**: 1377–84.

150. Deschamps D, De Beco V, Fisch C, Fromenty B, Guillouzo A, and Pessayre D. Inhibition by perhexiline of oxidative phosphorylation and the β-oxidation of fatty acids: possible role in pseudoalcoholic liver lesions. *Hepatology*, 1994; **19**: 948–61.

151. Lettéron P, Fromenty B, Terris B, Degott C, and Pessayre D. Acute and chronic hepatic lipid steatosis leads to *in vivo* lipid peroxidation in mice. *Journal of Hepatology*, 1995; **24**: 200–8.

152. Zatloukal K, Böck G, Rainer I, Denk H, and Weber H. High molecular weight components are main constituents of Mallory bodies isolated with a fluorescence activated cell sorter. *Laboratory Investigation*, 1991; **64**: 200–6.

153. Morgan MY, Reshef R, Shah RR, Oates NS, Smith RL, and Sherlock S. Impaired oxidation of debrisoquine in patients with perhexiline liver injury. *Gut*, 1984; **10**: 1057–64.

154. Larrey D, *et al.* Polymorphism of dextrometorphan oxidation in a French population. *British Journal of Clinical Pharmacology*, 1987; **24**: 676–9.

155. Homberg JC, *et al.* Drug-induced hepatitis associated with anticytoplasmic organelle autoantibodies. *Hepatology*, 1985; **5**: 722–7.

156. Furet Y and Breteau M. Accidents hépatiques à la clométacine. *Thérapie*, 1984; **39**: 523–9.

157. Pessayre D, Degos F, Feldmann G, Degott C, Bernuau J, and Benhamou JP. Chronic active hepatitis and giant multinucleated hepatocytes in adults treated with clometacin. *Digestion*, 1981; **22**: 66–72.

158. Maddrey WC and Boitnott JK. Drug-induced chronic liver disease. *Gastro-enterology*, 1977; **72**: 1348–53.

159. Sharp JR, Ishak KG, and Zimmerman HJ. Chronic active hepatitis and severe hepatic necrosis associated with nitrofurantoin. *Annals of Internal Medicine*, 1982; **92**: 1419.

160. Stricker BHC, Blok APR, Claas FH, Van Parys GE, and Desmet VJ. Hepatic injury associated with the use of nitrofurans: a clinicopathological study of 52 reported cases. *Hepatology*, 1988; **8**: 599–606.

161. Sznol M, Ohnuma T, and Holland JF. Hepatotoxicity of drugs used for hematologic neoplasia. *Seminars in Liver Disease*, 1987; **7**: 237–56.

162. Kremer JM, Lee RG, and Tolman KG. Liver histology in rheumatoid arthritis patients receiving long-term methotrexate therapy. A prospective study with baseline and sequential biopsy samples. *Arthritis and Rheum-atism*, 1989; **32**: 121–7.

163. Muenter MD, Perry HO, and Ludwig J. Chronic vitamin A intoxication in adults. Hepatic, neurologic, and dermatologic complications. *American Journal of Medicine*, 1971; **50**: 129–36.

164. Hruban Z, Russell RM, Boyer JL, Glagov S, and Bagheri SA. Ultra-structural changes in livers of two patients with hypervitaminosis A. *American Journal of Pathology*, 1974; **76**: 451–61.

165. Minuk GY, Kelly JK, and Hwang WS. Vitamin A hepatotoxicity in multiple family members. *Hepatology*, 1988; **8**: 272–5.

166. Russell RM, Boyer IL, Bagheri SA, and Hruban Z. Hepatic injury from chronic hypervitaminosis A resulting in portal hypertension and ascites. *New England Journal of Medicine*, 1974; **291**: 435–40.

167. Rosenbaum J, Amédée-Manesme O, and Dhumeaux D. Le foie et la vitamine A. *Gastroentérologie Clinique et Biologique*, 1985; **9**; 255–62.

168. Zafrani ES, Bemuau D, and Feldmann G. Peliosis-like ultrastructural changes of the hepatic sinusoids in human chronic hypervitaminosis A: report of three cases. *Human Pathology*, 1984; **15**: 1166–70.

169. Read AE, Harrison CV, and Sherlock S. Chronic chlorpromazine jaundice. *American Journal of Medicine*, 1961; **31**: 249–58.

170. Walker CO and Combes B. Biliary cirrhosis induced by chlorpromazine. *Gastroenterology*, 1966; **51**: 631–40.

171. Beerman B, Ericsson JLE, Hellström K, Wengle B, and Werner B. Transient cholestasis during treatment with ajmaline, and chronic xantho-matous cholestasis after administration of ajmaline, methyltestosterone and ethinylestradiol. *Acta Medica Scandinavica*, 1971; **190**: 241–50.

172. Manivel JC, Bloomer JR, and Snover DC. Progressive bile duct injury after thiabendazole administration. *Gastroenterology*, 1987; **93**: 245–9.

173. Larrey D, *et al.* Prolonged cholestasis after ajmaline-induced acute hep-atitis. *Journal of Hepatology*, 1986; **2**: 81–7.

174. Leveille-Webster CR and Arias IM. Mdr2 knockout mice link biliary phospholipid deficiency with small bile duct destruction. *Hepatology*, 1994; **19**: 1528–30.

175. Olsson R, Wiholm BE, Sand C, Zettergen L, Hultzcrantz R, and Myrhed M. Liver damage from flucloxaxillin, cloxacillin and dicloxacillin. *Journal of Hepatology*, 1992; **15**: 154–61.

176. Davies MH, Harrison RF, Elias E, and Hübscher SG. Antibiotic-associated acute vanishing bile duct syndrome: a pattern associated with severe, prolonged cholestasis. *Journal of Hepatology*, 1994; **20**: 112–6.

177. Hunt CM and Washington K. Tetracycline-induced bile duct paucity and prolonged cholestasis. *Gastroenterology*, 1994; **107**: 1844–7.

178. Larrey D, *et al.* Amitriptyline-induced prolonged cholestasis. *Gastro-enterology*, 1988; **94**: 200–3.

179. Larrey D, Amouyal G, Danan G, Degott C, Pessayre D, and Benhamou JP. Prolonged cholestasis after troleandomycin-induced acute hepatitis. *Journal of Hepatology*, 1987; **4**: 327–9.

180. Larrey D, Genève J, Pessayre D, Machayekhi JP, Degott C, and Benhamou JP. Prolonged cholestasis after cyproheptadine-induced acute hepatitis. *Journal of Clinical Gastroenterology*, 1987; **9**: 102–4.

181. Dincsoy HP and Saelinger DA. Haloperidol-induced chronic cholestatic liver disease. *Gastroenterology*, 1982; **83**: 694–700.

182. Anderson SD, Holley HC, Berland LL, Van Dyke JJ, and Stanley RJ. Causes of jaundice during hepatic artery infusion chemotherapy. *Radiology*, 1986; **161**: 439–42.

183. Bognel C, *et al.* Etude anatomo-pathologique de la toxicité hépatique de la chimiothérapie intra-artérielle hépatique. *Gastroentérologie Clinique et Biologique*, 1989; **13**: 125–31.

184. Belghiti J, Benhamou JP, Houry H, Grenier P, Huguier M, and Fékété F. Caustic sclerosing cholangitis. A complication of the surgical treatment of hydatid disease of the liver. *Archives of Surgery*, 1986; **121**: 1162–5.

185. Zafrani ES, Pinaudeau Y, and Dhumeaux D. Drug-induced vascular lesions of the liver. *Archives of Internal Medicine*, 1983; **143**: 495–502.

186. Valla D and Benhamou JP. Drug-induced vascular and sinusoidal lesions of the liver. *Baillière's Clinical Gastroentrology*, 1988; **2**: 481–500.

187. Valla D and Benhamou JP. Liver diseases related to oral contraceptives. *Digestive Diseases*, 1988; **6**: 76–86.

188. Degott C, Rueff B, Kreis H, Duboust A, Potet F, and Benhamou JP. Peliosis hepatis in recipients of renal transplants. *Gut*, 1978; **19**: 748–53.

189. Larrey D, *et al.* Peliosis hepatis induced by 6-thioguanine administration. *Gut*, 1988; **29**: 1265–9.

190. Valla D, Le MG, Poynard T, Zucman N, Rueff, and Benhamou JP. Risk of hepatic vein thrombosis in relation to recent use of oral contraceptives. A case-control study. *Gastroenterology*, 1986; **90**: 807–11.

191. Stromeyer FW and Ishak KG. Nodular transformation (nodular 're-generative' hyperplasia) of the liver. A clinicopathological study of 30 cases. *Human Pathology*, 1981; **12**: 60–71.

192. Anthony PP. Liver tumours. *Baillière's Clinical Gastroenterology*, 1988; **2**: 501–22.

193. Lutz WK and Maier P. Genotoxic and epigenetic chemical carcinogenesis: one process, different mechanisms. *Trends in Pharmacological Sciences*, 1988; **9**: 322–6.

194. Metzler M and Degen GH. Sex hormones and neoplasia: liver tumours in rodents. *Archives of Toxicology*, 1987; Suppl. 10: 251–63.

195. Klatskin G. Hepatic tumors: possible relationship to use of oral contraceptives. *Gastroenterology*, 1977; **73**: 386–94.

196. Rocks JB, *et al.* Epidemiology of hepatocellular adenoma. The role of oral contraceptive use. *Journal of the American Medical Association*, 1979; **242**: 645–8.

197. Edmonson HA, Henderson B, and Benton B. Liver cell adenoma associated with use of oral contraceptives. *New England Journal of Medicine*, 1976; **294**: 470–2.

198. Ishak KG. Hepatic lesions caused by anabolic and contraceptive steroids. *Seminars in Liver Disease*, 1981; **1**: 116–28.

199. Carrasco D, *et al.* Multiple hepatic adenomas after long-term therapy with testosterone enanthate. Review of the literature. *Journal of Hepatology*, 1985; **1**: 573–8.

200. Zafrani ES. Update of vascular tumours of the liver. *Journal of Hepatology*, 1989; **8**: 125–30.

201. Forman D, Vincent TJ, and Doll R. Cancer of the liver and the use of oral contraceptives. *British Medical Journal*, 1986; **292**: 1357–61.

202. Neuberger J, Forman D, Doll R, and Williams R. Oral contraceptives and hepatocellular carcinoma. *British Medical Journal*, 1986; **291**: 1355–7.

203. Falk H, Herbert J, and Crowley S. Epidemiology of hepatic angiosarcoma in the United States: 1964–1974. *Environmental Health Perspectives*, 1981; **41**: 107–13.

18

Toxic liver injury

18.1 Toxic liver injury

Regine Kahl

Classification of toxic liver injury

A variety of classifications of hepatotoxic agents has been provided in the medical and toxicological literature.[1–3] Classification may focus on the source and chemical class of the toxicant, on the circumstances of exposure, on the type of lesion produced, on the cell structure predominantly damaged, or on the molecular or cellular mechanisms involved. Table 1 lists routes and circumstances of exposure to liver toxicants. This section will deal predominantly with group C and, less extensively, with group B; for group A exposure, see Section 17.

From the viewpoint of preventive medicine, it is obviously important to distinguish between intrinsic (true, obligatory, predictable) and idiosyncrasy-dependent (facultative, non-predictable) liver toxicity.[1,2] Theoretically, intrinsic liver toxicity is characterized by the following features: reproducibility in experimental animals; dose dependency; occurrence in every person exposed to a sufficient dose; and uniform latency period.

This type of hepatotoxicity is almost exclusively found among occupational, environmental, and household chemicals. For a drug, intrinsic liver toxicity, being a fundamental property of the molecule, will only be accepted under specific circumstances, such as the chemotherapy of cancer (e.g. methotrexate) or if the lesion only occurs above therapeutic dose levels (e.g. paracetamol). In contrast, many drugs produce unpredictable liver disease due to host idiosyncrasy, i.e. the inability of single individuals to tolerate the chemical. With this type of liver toxicity, characteristic features are: adequate animal models do not exist, dose dependency is not apparent, only members of a minor fraction of exposed persons develop the injury, and the latency period is highly variable.

The classical idiosyncratic reaction of the liver is accompanied by hypersensitivity phenomena (see Section 17). In such cases, the disease is often only seen at the second exposure and is associated with fever, eosinophilia, arthralgia, and exanthema. Notably, mixed-type liver toxicants do obviously exist. With a number of hypersensitivity-related drugs a considerable incidence of subclinical biochemical alterations is observed while clinically overt liver disease is extremely rare. The relation between the more or less 'predictable' subclinical signs and the clinical event is at present not fully understood. Examples of this type are halothane and chlorpromazine. Idiosyncratic liver toxicity may be due to pharmacogenetic differences between individuals, e.g. acetylation polymorphism (Weber, PharmRev, 1985; 37:25; May, JClinPharm, 1994; 34:881). In such cases, the disease is restricted to a minor fraction of exposed persons but is predictable once the metabolic deviation has been detected.

Morphological expression and clinical signs of toxic liver injury

Acute injury to liver parenchyma

A survey of morphological pictures encountered in liver toxicity is given in Table 2. Acute toxic injury of liver parenchyma is expressed either as structural changes of the hepatocyte (cytotoxic type) or as an impairment of bile formation (cholestatic type). Major elevation of serum transaminase activity, usually by a factor of between 10 and 500, with marginal elevation of alkaline phosphatase (for example, twofold) indicates cytotoxic injury. Cholestasis is recognized by a more distinct increase of alkaline phosphatase (threefold and more) while elevation of transaminase activity is less impressive with cholestatic injury than with cytotoxic injury (for example, five- to tenfold). Enzyme elevation may be the only indication of liver involvement in less severe intoxication. Liver enlargement is frequently present and, in older case reports, may be the only symptom described. Clinical signs of acute liver injury may be marginal or—in the other extreme—may resemble those of florid viral hepatitis. The course of the disease may be fulminant with hepatic encephalopathy, haemorrhage due to major deterioration of the coagulation status, and acute yellow dystrophy of the liver. No conclusion as to a specific liver toxicant can be drawn from the clinical or morphological picture, nor can a reliable discrimination between toxic

Table 1 Circumstances of exposure to liver toxicants

A. Drugs
    Treatment
    Abuse
    Self-poisoning
B. Natural toxicants
    Food
    Food contaminants
    Abuse
    Folk medicine
    Bacterial infection
    Insect and scorpion toxins
C. Industrial chemicals and pesticides
    Industrial accidents
    Household accidents with chemical products
    Self-poisoning with chemical products
    Low-level chronic exposure at the workplace
    Environmental pollution

Table 2 Morphological classification of toxic liver injury

Acute	Chronic
Liver parenchyma	
Cytotoxic type	Chronic–active hepatitis
Steatosis	Steatosis
Microvesicular	Fibrosis
Macrovesicular	Cirrhosis
Mixed micro/macrovesicular	Liver tumours
Necrosis	Focal nodular hyperplasia
Massive	Adenoma
Diffuse	Hepatocellular carcinoma
Focal	
Zonal	
Centrilobular	
Midzonal	
Peripheral	
Granuloma	
Cholestatic type	Vanishing bile ducts
Canalicular	Cholangiocellular carcinoma
Hepatocanalicular	
Vascular system	
Hepatic vein thrombosis	Portal hypertension
	Peliosis hepatis
	Veno-occlusive disease
	Angiosarcoma

liver injury and non-toxic liver disease be inferred with certainty from the type of damage. Drugs with unpredictable hepatotoxic properties are, however, more likely to cause inflammatory reactions ('drug hepatitis') and will more often induce cholestasis than intrinsic liver toxicants. Granuloma is also more often induced by drugs, but occasionally occurs upon exposure to chemicals such as copper sulphate (see Appendix 2).

Cytotoxic injury

In biopsies or autopsies, cytotoxic injury is visualized as ultrastructural changes and degeneration of hepatocytes, as abnormal accumulation of macromolecules, notably of fat (steatosis), or as cell death (necrosis). Steatosis and necrosis are often encountered together (for example, after intoxication with carbon tetrachloride or with yellow phosphorus); however, certain agents will produce necrosis preferentially without steatosis (for example, paracetamol) or steatosis without necrosis (for example, ethionine). Steatosis may be microvesicular, macrovesicular, or mixed; the type of steatosis is characteristic for a number of liver toxicants. For example, phosphorus will produce microvesicular steatosis while methotrexate will produce macrovesicular steatosis (for a detailed description of steatosis, see Section 17).

The histological injury can be classified according to its localization. For historical reasons the localization of toxic liver injury is commonly described in terms of the classical liver lobules and not of the physiologically more adequate acinar model. Zonal damage often occurs in parallel with the activity of enzymes which mediate the metabolic activation of the chemical to the ultimate toxic metabolite. Thus, carbon tetrachloride, paracetamol, and dimethylnitrosamine induce pericentral (centrilobular) necrosis because cytochrome P-450 is more abundant in the vicinity of the hepatic vein. Midzonal and periportal necrosis are less common.

In a case report, midzonal necrosis has been found after 1,2-dichloroethane intoxication (Yodaiken, ArchEnvironHlth, 1973; 26: 281); in an animal model, the plant toxin ngaione has been shown to induce midzonal necrosis at least in mice untreated with enzyme inhibitors or inducers (Seawright, BrJExpPath, 1972; 53:242). Yellow phosphorus has been a prominent example of agents inducing periportal necrosis; however, this has not been supported in a retrospective analysis of autopsies from patients poisoned by phosphorus (Salfelder, BeitrPath, 1972; 147:321). Allyl alcohol causes periportal necrosis, probably because its bioactivation to acrolein depends on oxygen supply (Badr, JPharmExpTher, 1986; 238:1138).

Cholestatic injury

Clinically overt cholestasis may be invisible to the pathologist. Morphological correlates are characterized by intracellular accumulation of bile or by canalicular bile deposits. Damage of microvilli in the canaliculi is detected by electron microscopy. Liver cells may exhibit yellow pigmentation. Cholestasis may be accompanied by portal inflammation and injury to parenchymal cells; this type has been named hepatocanalicular.[1] Clinically, cholestasis is indicated by jaundice, pruritus, and elevation of alkaline phosphatase.[4–6]

Chronic liver injury
Cirrhosis and chronic active hepatitis

Acute liver injury may result in hepatic failure and death. If this does not occur, prognosis is, in general, good: complete recovery from the morphological and functional disturbances is to be expected. Very rarely, long-term sequelae of acute intoxication result eventually in chronic liver disease; more frequently, chronic liver disease will result from repeated or long-term exposure. Chronic liver injury may be expressed as fatty degeneration or necrosis of single parenchymal cells. The necrotic process induces an increase in fibrous tissue. Transition from fibrosis to cirrhosis is characterized by nodular regeneration and alteration of the liver architecture. Excessive alcohol intake is the predominant toxic aetiology of human liver cirrhosis. However, prolonged exposure to industrial chemicals may also result in the development of cirrhosis. Thus, chronic exposure to arsenical pesticides among vintners has caused cirrhosis (see Appendix 2). Cirrhosis has also been claimed to have occurred as a long-term sequel of exposure to halogenated aliphatic hydrocarbons, e.g. tetrachloromethane (carbon tetrachloride) and trichloromethane (chloroform) (see Appendix 2).

Some drugs (for example, α-methyldopa, oxyphenisatin, sulphonamides, nitrofurantoin, phenylbutazone) have been shown to induce chronic active hepatitis which may present with signs resembling an autoimmune disease, including a positive lupus erythematosus phenomenon (see Section 17 for a detailed description of chronic hepatitis).

Tumours

In experimental animals, a large variety of chemicals has induced primary liver tumours.[7] In humans, a causal relationship between the occurrence of primary liver tumours and the exposure to a specific chemical has been shown convincingly for only a few compounds. Malignant tumours are caused by vinyl chloride, inorganic arsenicals, thorium dioxide (Thorotrast, a radiocontrast dye no longer used) and probably by aflatoxin B_1 (see below). Benign neoplasms (focal nodular hyperplasia and liver adenoma) have been ascribed to hormonal contraceptives (see Section 17).

Vascular lesions
Non-cirrhotic portal hypertension

A number of liver toxicants induce damage to the hepatic vascular system. The portal tracts may be affected, resulting in non-cirrhotic portal hypertension. The disease has been observed after exposure to vinyl chloride and to inorganic arsenicals (see Appendix 2) and has been described in depth for vinyl chloride intoxication.[8] Upper gastrointestinal bleeding from oesophageal varices is frequently the first symptom of the disease; liver function tests for hepatocyte integrity will yield erratic results, at least in the early stage, because parenchymal cells are not primarily affected. Splenomegaly and raised intrasplenic pressure are generally present; on peritoneoscopy, conspicuous focal capsular fibrosis is found. Biopsy specimens reveal enlargement and thickening of portal vein branches, intralobular perisinusoidal fibrosis, and collagenization of sinusoidal walls. Activation and proliferation of sinusoidal cells are present. It has been stated that vinyl chloride-induced and arsenical-induced portal hypertension closely resemble idiopathic portal hypertension (Banti's syndrome), suggesting that the latter disease may at times result from hitherto unknown toxic chemicals (Thomas, NEJM, 1975; 292:17). Clinical consequences from chemically induced portal hypertension do not only result from gastrointestinal haemorrhage but also from transition from the fibrotic state to multicentric angiosarcoma (Thomas, NEJM, 1975; 292:17; Jones, BrJIndMed, 1982; 39:306).

Peliosis hepatis

A second chemically induced vascular lesion, peliosis hepatis, has also been claimed to be a precursor of hepatic angiosarcoma (Popper, Internist, 1977; 18:182). Peliosis hepatis is characterized by massively enlarged, blood-filled sinusoids. These 'lacunae' are induced by the destruction of sinusoidal supporting membranes; the condition is frequently accompanied by hepatocyte injury (Yanoff, ArchPathol, 1964; 77:159). Hyperplasia of the hepatocytes leads to the formation of trabeculae invading the lumen of the peliosis cyst. These trabeculae are surrounded by inflammatory cell infiltration. Upon transition to malignancy, this will eventually result in a nodular type of angiosarcoma. Peliosis hepatis has been associated with vinyl chloride (Popper, Internist, 1977; 18:182) and with steroid therapy (Bagheri, AnnIntMed, 1974; 81:610; Nadell, ArchPathLabMed, 1977; 101:405).

Veno–occlusive disease

Veno–occlusive disease (endophlebitis obliterans; a lesion characterized by occlusion of hepatic venules and centrilobular necrosis) has been ascribed to pyrrolizidine alkaloids, plant toxins from various genera (for example, *Crotolaria*, *Senecio*, *Heliotropium*) which are widely used as herbal folk medicine in certain parts of the world. Clinically, veno–occlusive disease leads to hepatomegaly and ascites. Venous collaterals dilated by the stagnant blood may be seen on the abdomen. Vomiting and severe abdominal pain are the predominant symptoms of the acute form of the disease, jaundice is rarely seen. Liver function tests are abnormal, indicating damage to parenchymal cells. An epidemic outbreak of the intoxication was observed in South Africa in 1951; this outbreak has been traced back to the ingestion of *Senecio* alkaloids from ragwort (Selzer, BrJExpPath, 1951; 32:14). Another episode of pyrrolizidine alkaloid poisoning has occurred in Jamaica as a consequence of the intake of bush tea containing fulvine from *Crotolaria fulva* (Bras, ArchPathol, 1954; 57:285). In 1992 to 1993, about 4000 cases of pyrrolizidine intoxication due to the ingestion of wheat contaminated with *Heliotropium lasocarpium* occurred in Southern Tadjikistan during the course of a famine (Chauvin, Sante, 1994; 4:263). The natural history of the disease is characterized by progression from an acute stage to chronic liver damage with fibrosis proceeding from the centrilobular to the periportal area (Stuart, QJMed, 1957; 26:291). The prognosis of the disease is relatively poor: in a group of 64 persons who had consumed a pyrrolizidine-containing herbal tea, only 50 per cent recovered completely; 25 per cent died during the acute phase, and 10 per cent proceeded to cirrhosis. In an epidemic outbreak in India 1975–77, the 5-year survival rate was 50 per cent.

Mechanisms of liver toxicity

The primary mechanisms most often involved in liver toxicity are:

(1) lipid peroxidation;
(2) formation of reactive oxygen species;
(3) covalent binding to proteins;
(4) glutathione depletion;
(5) peroxisome proliferation;
(6) interference with protein synthesis;
(7) damage to the plasma membrane;

(8) interference with bile secretion;

(9) disturbance of haem synthesis;

(10) covalent binding to DNA (somatic mutation).

The injury may result in liver cell necrosis or in apoptosis; the ultimate biochemical processes involved, for example disturbance of ion homeostasis, damage of the cytoskeleton, mitochondrial dysfunction, ATP depletion, and activation of degradative enzyme activities, are uniform and will also occur in liver injury due to non-toxic origin.[9] Secondary events such as neutrophil invasion, decrease of gap junctional communication by downregulation of connexins, and stimulation or inhibition of tissue repair will modulate the outcome of the intoxication.[10] Interaction between sinusoidal cells, most notably Kupffer cells, and hepatocytes can aggravate the primary lesion in the hepatocytes, as shown for paracetamol,[11] carbon tetrachloride (Edwards, ToxAppl-Pharmacol, 1993; 119:275) or ethanol (Zhong, TransplProc, 1995; 27:528). Table 3 provides a list of methods used for the study of mechanisms of liver toxicity in experimental models. A comprehensive review of the detection and evaluation of chemically induced liver injury has been published.[12] It should be noted that many liver toxicants will also induce damage to other tissues. Their organotropic action is due to the presence of high hepatic activities of the enzymes responsible for metabolic activation to the ultimate toxicant. Section 17 contains a description of the main hepatotoxic mechanisms with respect to drug-induced liver injury, which is also pertinent to chemically induced liver injury. Below, some of the mechanisms listed above will be explained in connection with a number of prototype hepatotoxicants.

Lipid peroxidation

The prototype chemical inducing lipid peroxidation is carbon tetrachloride (tetrachloromethane, CCl_4).[13–15] CCl_4 is metabolically activated by cytochrome P-450 to the trichloromethyl radical, $CCl_3\bullet$ (Fig. 1). As a consequence, necrosis due to CCl_4 is predominantly centrilobular. In contrast to most reactions mediated by cytochrome P-450, $CCl_3\bullet$ radical formation does not proceed via mono-oxygenation but via reduction. The reaction is therefore more rapid in nitrogen than in air or oxygen atmospheres. Enzyme inducers such as phenobarbital stimulate the formation of $CCl_3\bullet$ radicals and aggravate toxicity in experimental animals. The cytochrome P-450 isoforms involved in CCl_4 reductions are cytochrome P-450IIB1 and cytochrome P-450IIE1—the latter can be induced by ethanol. This provides an explanation for the aggravation of CCl_4 toxicity in long-term ethanol consumers. However, acute ethanol administration may also potentiate CCl_4 toxicity. Cytochrome P-450IIE1 is predominantly located in zone 3 of the acinus. Consequently, necrosis and steatosis due to CCl_4 are predominantly found in zone 3.

CCl_4 initiates lipid peroxidation in experimental animals within a few minutes of administration. This effect is interpreted to be a primary toxic lesion since lipid peroxidation precedes other morphological and functional changes following CCl_4 administration. The $CCl_3\bullet$ radical is oxidized to the trichloromethylperoxy radical $CCl_3O_2\bullet$ in the presence of molecular oxygen (Packer, LifeSci, 1978; 23:2617). The free radicals derived from CCl_4 initiate lipid peroxidation within the endoplasmic reticulum by hydrogen abstraction from unsaturated fatty acids (LH) (McCay, JBC, 1984; 259:2135). $CCl_3\bullet$ is thereby reduced to

trichloromethane (chloroform). Lipid peroxidation is a chain reaction (Fig. 1): oxidation of the carbon-centred lipid radical, $L\bullet$, yields the hydroperoxy radical $LOO\bullet$ which, in turn, abstracts a hydrogen atom from another intact molecule of unsaturated fatty acid (for a detailed description of lipid peroxidation, see Section 17).

Figure 1 lists some of the most common detection methods for lipid peroxidation: resonance within the lipid radicals, $L\bullet$, yields conjugated dienes which exhibit a characteristic absorption at 233 nm. This absorption can therefore be used as a quantitative measure of lipid peroxidation. The breakdown of the lipid hydroperoxides, LOOH, yields low molecular weight compounds which may also be used for quantitation of lipid peroxidation; malondialdehyde concentration can be determined spectrophotometrically in blood and in tissues following reaction with thiobarbituric acid. Other aldehydes are also formed, some of which (for example, 4-hydroxynonenal) have been assumed to be stable cytotoxic factors capable of migrating to other cell compartments and able to initiate macromolecular damage distant from the primary site of CCl_4 action via covalent binding to critical proteins (Poli, BiochemJ, 1985; 227:629). The volatile alkanes formed, ethane and pentane, can be measured by gas chromatography in the head space of an incubation vessel or in exhaled air.

The $CCl_3\bullet$ radical also binds covalently to proteins, DNA, and lipids.[13] The onset of haloalkylation of lipids and proteins occurs simultaneously with the onset of lipid peroxidation.[14] The relative importance of haloalkylation of cellular macromolecules has therefore been a matter of debate.[14,15]

Concomitant with and/or subsequent to lipid peroxidation, other destructive processes take place in the endoplasmic reticulum. CCl_4 acts as a suicide substrate for cytochrome P-450, leading to rapid loss of enzyme activity. Activity of glucose 6-phosphatase, a marker enzyme for the endoplasmic reticulum, is also rapidly lost. Protein synthesis slows down, and ribosomal structures are lost from the membrane. Microsomal Ca^{2+}-ATPase, the pump responsible for sequestration of Ca^{2+} into the endoplasmic reticulum, is oxidatively damaged by the $CCl_3\bullet$ radical (Srivastava, JBC, 1990; 265:8392). Consequently, the intracellular free Ca^{2+} concentration is raised. This will activate a number of proteolytic enzymes capable of propagating membrane disturbance at distant sites.[16] Eventually, a complex pattern of hepatocyte damage is observed:

(1) accumulation of triglycerides;

(2) mitochondrial damage (decreased ATP concentration);

(3) damage to the plasma membrane (enzyme and potassium leakage); and

(4) cell death.

It is not possible at present to determine definitely the sequence of events leading to these biological end points. However, it is likely that at least a significant proportion of the toxic effects is due to the distortion of Ca^{2+} distribution within the cell. Calcium-channel blockers are capable of protecting experimental animals against some of the biochemical alterations caused by CCl_4 (Romero, LifeSci, 1994; 55:981).

Fat accumulation is not due to increased synthesis of triglycerides or decreased metabolism of fatty acids but to inhibition of protein synthesis, more specifically, to synthesis of the protein component of the very low density lipoproteins (VLDLs). VLDLs are required for triglyceride transport, and therefore inhibition

Table 3 Methods used in the study of hepatotoxic mechanisms

In whole animals
1. *In vivo*
   Lethality (if hepatotoxicity is already established)
   Liver function tests
     For the integrity of the plasma membrane:
       Increase of liver enzyme activities in serum
         liver specificity low: glutamate oxaloacetate transaminase (aspartate aminotransferase; GOT), lactate
           dehydrogenase (LDH)[a]
         liver specificity intermediate: glutamate pyruvate transaminase (alanine aminotransferase; GPT), glutamate
           dehydrogenase (GlDH)
         liver specificity high: sorbitol dehydrogenase (SDH); ornithine carbamoyl transferase (OCT)
     For the integrity of carbohydrate metabolism:
       Galactose elimination
     For the integrity of protein metabolism:
       Decrease of hepatogenic proteins in serum (albumin, clotting factors, serum cholinesterase)
     For the integrity of fat metabolism:
       Quotient cholesterin esters/free cholesterin
     For the integrity of biliary excretion:
       Increase of bilirubin and/or bile acids in serum
       Dye excretion (BSP)
       Increase of the activity in serum of enzymes normally excreted with the bile:
         Alkaline phosphatase (ALP), γ-glutamyl transpeptidase (GGT), leucine aminopeptidase, 5′-nucleotidase
     For the integrity of liver blood flow:
       Indocyanine green (ICG) clearance, sorbitol clearance[b]
   Tests for integrity of drug metabolism
     Metabolite(s) of a test drug in blood/urine
     Exhalation of labelled CO_2 formed from drugs to be demethylated (e.g. aminopyrine breath test)
     Pentobarbital sleeping time; zoxazolamine paralysis time
   Test for lipid peroxidation: exhalation of ethane and pentane
2. At necropsy
   Liver enlargement
   Histology
   Preneoplastic foci
     Electron microscopy (e.g. proliferation of endoplasmic reticulum; peroxisome proliferation; lysosome damage)
     Tissue analysis
       Changes in fat composition
       Glutathione content
       Cytochrome P-450 content; pattern of cytochrome P-450; activity of drug-metabolizing enzymes
       Concentration of malondialdehyde or conjugated dienes (lipid peroxidation)
     Damage to nucleic acids and proteins: covalent binding of toxicant; DNA stand breaks, etc.

In intact organ and intact cells
1. Isolated perfused liver
   Oxygen consumption, NAD(P)/NAD(P)H quotient
   Synthetic activity (e.g. leucine incorporation, thymidine incorporation, lipoprotein secretion)
   Drug metabolism
   Tissue analysis
   Damage to nucleic acids and proteins
   Enzyme leakage into the medium (damage to the plasma membrane)
   Excretory function (bile flow, bile acid excretion, bilirubin excretion, dye excretion)
2. Hepatocytes (freshly isolated single hepatocytes/hepatocyte couplets[c]/primary culture)
   As for isolated perfused liver, without excretory function
   Cytotoxicity, mutagenicity, malignant transformation

In subcellulcar fractions
Nuclei (covalent binding, DNA strand breaks, thymidine incorporation)
Ribosomes (protein synthesis)
Microsomes (drug metabolism, lipid peroxidation)
Mitochondria (respiration, oxidative phosphorylation)
Peroxisomes (H_2O_2 production)
Lysosomes (enzyme leakage)
Plasma membrane (carrier and receptor proteins; fluidity)

[a] Isoenzyme LDH-5 specific for liver.
[b] New method (Zeeh, Gastro, 1988; 95:749).
[c] New method (Gantam, Hepatol, 1987; 7:216).

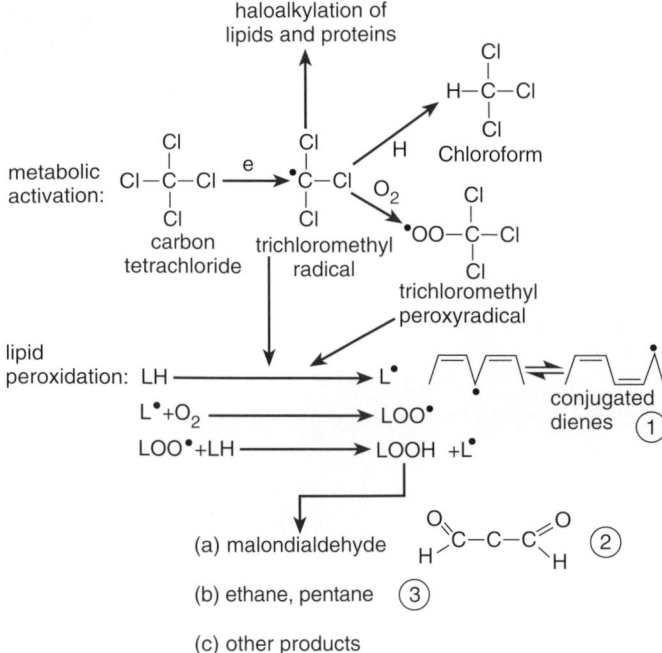

Fig. 1. Hepatotoxic mechanism of carbon tetrachloride (tetrachloromethane). Numbers (1)–(3) indicate lipid degradation products conventionally used for quantitation of lipid peroxidation.

of their synthesis will cause inhibition of triglyceride secretion. Alternatively, haloalkylation of the apolipoprotein may induce blocking of lipoprotein secretion.

In earlier decades, CCl$_4$ intoxications were frequently encountered both in the chemical industry and in households, since CCl$_4$ was widely used as a solvent, as a flame retardant, and even as a vermicide, but its use has been markedly reduced in the past 20 years. When the agent is inhaled the depressive effect on the central nervous system characteristic for haloalkane solvents may be predominant during the acute phase of the intoxication: the patient will experience headache and somnolence and may eventually become unconscious. Gastrointestinal intoxication signs with nausea, vomiting, pain, and diarrhoea may occur in the early phase, not only after oral uptake but also after inhalation or transdermal exposure. Liver injury occurs with a latency of 1 to 3 days. Initial symptoms are hepatomegaly, jaundice, decrease of clotting factors, and massive elevation of serum transaminases. The highest aspartate aminotransferase value so far reported (27 840 units) was observed in the course of a CCl$_4$ intoxication (Wroblewski, AnnIntMed, 1955; 43:345). Generally, hepatic failure dominates the course of the disease; however, toxic damage of the proximal tubules leading to uraemic coma may also cause fatalities. An analysis of 128 intoxications which had occurred between 1953 and 1965 demonstrated renal symptoms in 94 per cent of the patients. No established therapy of the liver injury exists; when renal injury is present haemodialysis or peritoneal dialysis may save the life of the patient. In experimental animals, a prophylactic action of chain-breaking antioxidants, such as vitamin E, has been described; a therapeutic action in man has not been established. A possible therapeutic role of *N*-acetylcysteine has been discussed (Flanagan, AmJMed, 1991; 91:131S). In some cases cardial manifestations

may occur: similar to other halogenated molecules, carbon tetrachloride may lead to a sensitization of the myocardium against noradrenaline and adrenaline, giving rise to arrhythmias and sudden death. Notably, chronic lesions such as fibrosis and cirrhosis can occur in subjects repeatedly exposed to CCl$_4$ (Hall, Hepatol, 1991; 13:815).

Covalent binding to cellular macromolecules is also involved in the hepatotoxicity of other haloalkanes, including halothane (2-bromo-2-chloro-1,1,1-trifluoroethane).[17] In animal experiments, liver necrosis can be caused reproducibly by halothane. Obviously, this experimental liver injury must be classified as intrinsic and predictable using the categories given above. This is not true for the human liver disease caused by halothane (see Section 17) which is characterized by hypersensitivity phenomena. However, subclinical disturbance of liver function is found in about 20 per cent of persons exposed. The immunological character of halothane hepatitis in humans may well be due to oxidative halothane metabolism. Covalent binding of the oxidatively formed trifluoroacetyl group to cytochrome P-450-related protein in the endoplasmic reticulum and in the plasma membrane has been described (Satoh, MolPharm, 1985; 28:468). In the serum of patients with halothane hepatitis, antibodies have been detected against a number of trifluoroacetyl-protein adducts, including protein disulphide isomerase, microsomal carboxylesterase, calreticulin, and ERp72. The fact that most exposed persons are not immunologically responsive may be due to tolerance induced by self-peptides which function as a molecular mimicry of the trifluoroacetyl adducts (Gut, PharmTher, 1993; 58:133). These findings demonstrate that alkylation hypothesis and hypersensitivity hypothesis need not necessarily be contradictory.

Oxidative stress, glutathione depletion, and covalent binding to cellular macromolecules

In experimental liver toxicology, formation of the O$_2$ radical from quinoid systems plays a major role.[18,19] Redox cycling between a quinone and the corresponding semiquinone radical is accompanied by univalent oxygen reduction of the semiquinone radical to yield O$_2$:

$$\text{flavoenzyme}$$

$$Q \rightarrow Q^\bullet$$

$$Q^\bullet + O_2 \rightarrow Q + O^{\bullet-}_2$$

This process has been studied in detail with menadione as a prototype quinone, and basic insights into the events preceding cell death, most notably the disruption of intracellular Ca^{2+} homeostasis, have been elaborated by use of hepatic quinone toxicity.[16] The increase in formation of O$^{\bullet}_2$ and of the reactive oxygen species derived from O$^{\bullet-}_2$ has been named oxidative stress.

Oxidative stress can be initiated in the hepatocyte by a number of foreign compounds capable of redox cycling. The radical O$^{\bullet-}_2$ is, however, also a normal byproduct of oxygen-consuming processes in various cell compartments. It is rapidly converted into H$_2$O$_2$ by the action of superoxide dismutase. In mitochondria, the reduction of oxygen to water with four electrons which takes place at the cytochrome oxidase does not allow for O$^{\bullet-}_2$ leakage and subsequent

H_2O_2 formation. However, $O^{\bullet-}_2$ leakage may occur at the ubisemiquinone site if the transmembrane proton gradient is disturbed (Nohl, FreeRadicResComm, 1993; 18:127). In the cytosol, flavoprotein enzymes are present which are capable of univalent oxygen reduction. One of them, xanthine oxidase, is assumed to play a critical role in hepatic ischaemia–reperfusion injury (Arthur, JHepatol, 1988; 6:125; Metzger, Hepatol, 1988; 8:580). In the endoplasmic reticulum, $O^{\bullet-}_2$ leaks from the cytochrome P-450 cycle and from the action of the flavoproteins involved in the mono-oxygenase reaction (Loida, Biochem, 1993; 32:11530).

Neither $O^{\bullet-}_2$ radicals nor H_2O_2 are highly damaging to the cell integrity. However, in the presence of reduced transition metals the highly reactive hydroxyl radical $OH^{\bullet}$ is formed from H_2O_2 and $O^{\bullet-}_2$ via the so-called Haber–Weiss reaction (Haber, ProcRoySocA, 1934; 147:332). The $OH^{\bullet}$ radical will attack virtually all molecules within its vicinity and may lead to lipid peroxidation and to functional disturbance of proteins. When H_2O_2 invades the nucleus and reaches a site where ferrous iron is present close to DNA, damage to the genetic material resulting in strand breaks may also occur.

A variety of antioxidative defence systems is available to the cell. These include the low molecular weight radical scavenger, vitamin E, and a number of enzymes involved in $O^{\bullet-}_2$ and H_2O_2 detoxication. The enzyme responsible for H_2O_2 detoxication in the cytosol and in mitochondria, glutathione peroxidase, is dependent on glutathione supply. Therefore, glutathione depletion will aggravate the injury induced by redox cycling compounds.

Liver damage due to the analgesic drug paracetamol is described in detail in Section 17. A short discussion of this lesion is given here because it is a useful model of a complex type of liver toxicity characterized by chemical modification of critical cellular macromolecules, oxidative stress, and glutathione depletion.[20,21] A large body of evidence suggests that N-acetyl-benzoquinone imine (NABQI, Fig. 2), formed by the action of cytochromes P-450IA, IIIA, or IIE, is the active metabolite covalently binding to proteins. Attempts to identify the critical target molecules have only recently started; an example is the finding of paracetamol adducts with the glycolytic enzyme, glyceraldehyde 3-phosphate dehydrogenase.[21] It is assumed that protein thiol arylation is a major modification type (Streeter, ChemBiolInteract, 1984; 48:349). Recently, DNA damage has also been observed in mouse liver (Hongslo, Mutagenesis, 1994; 9:93). NABQI is converted by a μ class glutathione transferase to a glutathione conjugate which is excreted as the respective mercapturic acid via the kidneys. Massive protein modification will only take place after glutathione is depleted.

Glutathione is required for maintaining cellular protein thiols in a reduced state. The loss of free protein thiol groups following both glutathione depletion and protein thiol arylation leads to a disturbance of intracellular calcium homeostasis due to functional impairment of Ca^{2+}-ATPases. Calcium accumulation in the cytosol and its consequences are similar to those described for CCl_4 and menadione toxicity. Inhibition of mitochondrial respiration appears to be an early event in the course of cellular damage (Donnelly, ArchToxicol, 1994; 68:110). Since glutathione is required for cellular H_2O_2 and lipid hydroperoxide detoxication by the enzyme glutathione peroxidase, paracetamol-induced glutathione depletion will lead to oxidative stress and lipid peroxidation in the hepatocyte.

The literature is replete with arguments about the relative importance of the necrosis pathways A, B, and C in Fig. 2. The older literature favours the covalent binding hypothesis (pathway A in Fig. 2), while more recently damage by covalent binding is thought not to be sufficient to induce cell death.[21] Loss of protein thiols is assumed to be critical, but it is an unsettled question whether thiol arylation (pathway A in Fig. 2) or thiol oxidation (pathway B in Fig. 2) is more important. Authors assuming that lipid peroxidation (pathway C in Fig. 2) is the main hepatotoxic mechanism refer to the complete protection that can be achieved by chain-breaking antioxidants. Others argue that lipid peroxidation is the result rather than the cause of necrosis.

The clinical course of paracetamol intoxication is similar to that of carbon tetrachloride intoxication. As with CCl_4 intoxication, the liver damage in most cases will only be diagnosed after a latency period which may be dominated by nausea and vomiting. An increase of transaminase activities will first become apparent after 12 to 24 h and is maximal after 3 or 4 days. Liver enlargement and icterus will occur at day 2 to day 4. Acute renal insufficiency may complicate the clinical situation. This occurs less frequently than with CCl_4 poisoning, in about 10 per cent of the patients.

Paracetamol is a safe analgesic in therapeutic doses of 0.5 to 3.0 g/day. With 4 to 10 g/day a few cases of liver damage in persons with pre-existing chronic alcohol abuse or low glutathione content due to malnutrition have been described. For healthy adults the toxic dose is 10 to 15 g/day (Brotodihardjo, MedJAust, 1992; 157: 382). The course of the plasma concentration versus time curve can be used to predict, during the early stage of the intoxication, the probability of liver necrosis in the later stages. Significant damage is likely with paracetamol concentrations greater than 200 µg/l at 4 h and greater than 50 µg/l at 12 h after ingestion; nomograms have been constructed to facilitate prognosis (Rumack, ArchIntMed, 1981; 141:380). Routine procedures include evacuation of the stomach, adsorption to charcoal, and administration of laxatives. If the prognostic data require pharmacological intervention N-acetylcysteine or, less frequently, methionine is given as an antidote. N-Acetylcysteine is protective mostly when given within the first 10 h after intoxication. The predominant protective mechanism of N-acetylcysteine is to provide the cysteine precursor for the *de novo* synthesis of glutathione (Nagasawa, JMedChem, 1984; 27:591). Anaphylactic reactions may occur infrequently, especially with parenteral administration of the antidote. In a total of 306 cases, 11 per cent experienced non-fatal allergic reactions (Brotodihardjo, MedJAust, 1992; 157:382).

Peroxisome proliferation

Peroxisomes are cytoplasmic organelles possessing a primitive electron transport system which uses molecular oxygen for the oxidation of a few types of substrates (predominantly fatty acids) and in turn produces H_2O_2. This implies that an efficient H_2O_2 detoxifying system must be present. This role is fulfilled by catalase which can be used as a marker enzyme of peroxisomes. Certain chemicals, including phthalate esters and lipid-lowering drugs belonging to the clofibrate group, can induce peroxisome proliferation and concomitant induction of peroxisomal enzymes.[22] Proliferation of peroxisomes may disturb the balance between H_2O_2 formation and H_2O_2 detoxication and may thus result in oxidative stress to the peroxisomes and to the cell (Reddy, CritRevTox, 1983; 12:1). In rodents, peroxisome proliferators induce hepatocarcinogenesis.[23]

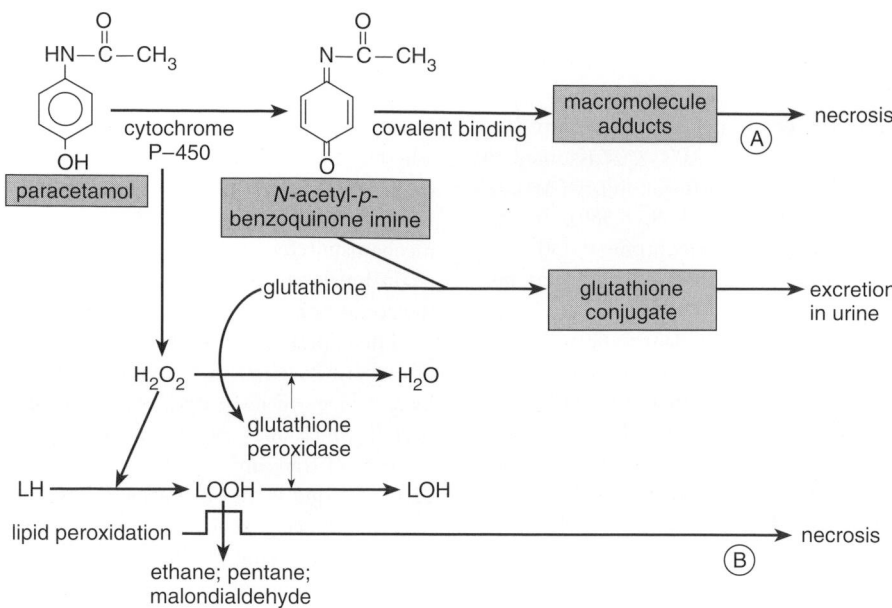

Fig. 2. Mechanisms involved in the hepatotoxic action of paracetamol.

It has been argued that the carcinogenic action is due to oxidative stress. However, lipid peroxidation, DNA single-strand breaks (Elliott, Carcinogenesis, 1987; 8:1213), and mutagenic action in the reactive oxygen-sensitive *Salmonella* strain TA102 and in eukaryotic test systems (Schmezer, Carcinogenesis, 1988; 9:37) have not been detected with the plasticizer di(2-ethylhexyl)phthalate (**DEHP**), a potent peroxisome proliferator, or its metabolite, mono-ethylhexylphthalate. DEHP is a rodent hepatic tumour promoter (Oesterle, JCancResClinOnc, 1988; 114:133), and it is likely that it acts as an epigenetic carcinogen.

Exposure of dialysis patients to DEHP from poly(vinyl chloride) (**PVC**) tubes and bags can be 3 mg/kg body weight/day (Nässberger, Nephron, 1987; 45:286); in the general population, exposure is estimated to be approximately 0.03 mg/kg body weight/day (IPCS/WHO, Environmental Health Criteria, 1992; 131). With a unit risk of 84 to 144×10^4 at 1 mg/kg body weight/day calculated from rodent experiments (Beliles, DrugsMetabolRev, 1989; 21:3), this would appear to be a high exposure. However, many regulatory agencies assume at present that hepatocarcinogenesis by peroxisome proliferators is a species-specific event which has no impact in humans. No excess of liver tumours was reported in epidemiological studies on phthalate exposure or long-term fibrate administration. While peroxisome proliferation has been observed in primates,[22] it has not yet been demonstrated unequivocally in human liver. Recently, however, a peroxisome proliferator activated receptor (**PPAR**) has been cloned from human liver and shown to be activated by the peroxisome proliferator WY-14 643 *in vitro* (Sher, Biochem, 1993; 32:5598). PPARs act—in the form of a heterodimer with the retinoid activated receptor RXR (Gearing, PNAS, 1993; 90:1440)—as transactivators at PPAR-responsive elements in the promoter region of the acyl CoA oxidase (rate-limiting enzyme of the peroxisomal β-oxidation pathway) gene (Tugwood, EMBOJ, 1992; 11:433). It remains to be elucidated whether the human PPAR has an impact on growth regulation, and possibly carcinogenesis, in humans.

Inhibition of protein synthesis

Mushroom poisoning due to the ingestion of the green or white *Amanita* species causes severe liver necrosis due to inhibition of protein synthesis.[24] Two types of poison are present in the *Amanita* species, the amatoxins and the phallotoxins, and both are hepatotoxic. However, the amatoxins are 10 to 20 times more potent and are assumed to play a critical role in the induction of liver injury. The prototype of the amatoxins is α-amanitin. This compound is a potent inhibitor of RNA polymerase II with a K_i of about 10^{-8} M. The toxin forms a 1 : 1 complex with an enzyme subunit (Cochet-Meilhac, BBActa, 1974; 353:160). RNA polymerase II is required for the synthesis of mRNA (Fig. 3). At concentrations of about 10^{-5} M RNA polymerase III (the enzyme mediating the synthesis of tRNA) is also inhibited. As a consequence of the inhibition of mRNA synthesis, enzymes, structural proteins, and the apoproteins for lipoprotein synthesis are no longer supplied. This results in fat accumulation and necrosis. α-Amanitin is a prototype of an indirect hepatotoxicant as defined by Zimmerman,[1] in that it causes liver injury by interference with a specific metabolic pathway. Gross structural damage to the cell ensues only secondarily. Toxicity occurs in all tissues, including the kidney and the pancreas; however, its consequences are most dramatic in the liver because of the high rate of hepatic protein synthesis and also because α-amanitin is subject to enterohepatic circulation.

Amanita poisoning is characterized by a progression through various clinical stages. Cholera-like gastrointestinal intoxication symptoms, with watery diarrhoea which may cause death due to exsiccosis, are thought to be due to phalloidin. They will only start after a latency period of some hours and will last for one to several days. After this period, clinical improvement is often seen but clinically silent organ damage is already occurring. Toxic liver injury becomes apparent by elevation of transaminase and bilirubin levels and by prolongation of prothrombin time. Progression into the final stage is characterized by severe coagulation disturbances and

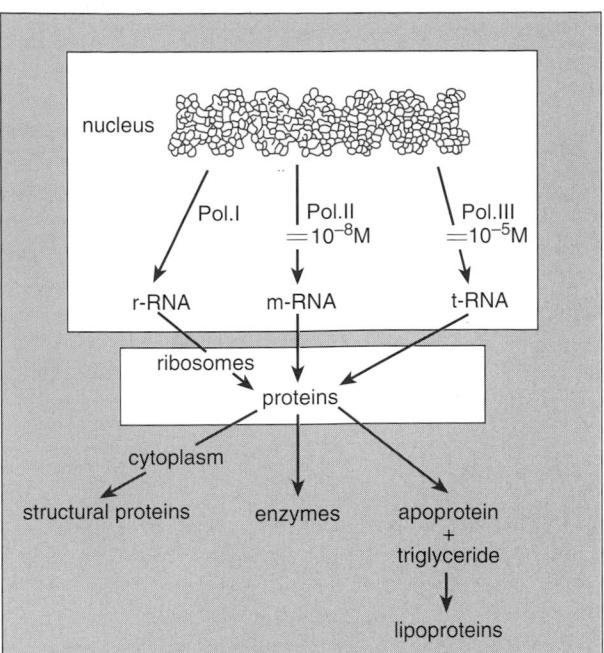

Fig. 3. Hepatotoxic mechanism of α-amanitin; Pol. I, II, III, RNA polymerases.

advancing hepatic encephalopathy. As little as 30 g of the fresh mushroom have been described to cause fatalities.

No generally accepted treatment protocol for *Amanita* poisoning is available (Klein, AmJMed, 1989; 86:187). Evacuation of the stomach, administration of charcoal, adjustment of fluid and electrolytes, substitution of clotting factors, and treatment of septic complications are recommended (Beer, SchMedWoch, 1993; 123: 892). Amatoxins are excreted via the kidneys and can be reabsorbed in the renal tubules. Therefore forced diuresis may be efficient in preventing fatal liver injury (Vesconi, CritCareMed, 1985; 13:402). Haemoperfusion is recommended by some authors, especially in the early phase after ingestion, but it is not generally accepted that this procedure is clinically efficient. Among the 'antitoxins' which have been claimed to be therapeutically efficient, benzylpenicillin and silibinin are routinely administered in many centres (Beer, SchMedWoch, 1993; 123:892); benzylpenicillin is assumed to decrease the uptake of the toxin into the hepatocyte, while the mechanism of action of the antioxidant silibinin is unclear. A retrospective investigation of the efficacy of various therapeutic regimens based on 205 cases has been published (Floersheim, SchMedWoch, 1982; 112:1164). Orthotopic liver transplantation may eventually be performed as the last resort to prevent fatality (Klein, AmJMed, 1989; 86:187). Death rates have been 50 to 90 per cent in the past (Piering, ClinChem, 1990; 36:571) and are now reported to range from 10 to 50 per cent (Parish, VetHumTox, 1986; 28:318). Mushroom poisoning exhibiting a similar clinical course as that seen with *Amanita phalloides* can also occur with *Lepiota helveola*; survival rate is low in patients in which coma develops (Larrey, SemLivDis, 1995; 15:183).

Intrahepatic cholestasis

More than 100 drugs are capable of inducing intrahepatic cholestasis.[5] A prototype is chlorpromazine. Among non-drug hepatotoxicants, few are encountered which primarily produce intrahepatic cholestasis. Methylene dianiline (4,4′-diamino-diphenylmethane) appears to be one example (see Appendix 2). This agent was first identified as a liver toxicant during an epidemic outbreak of jaundice in the population of the English town of Epping which had ingested bread baked with contaminated flour (Kopelman, PostgradMedJ, 1968; 44:78). In this incident 84 persons developed jaundice accompanied by elevation of serum alkaline phosphatase and of serum transaminases. Needle biopsies invariably showed cholestasis and hepatocellular damage; indications as to cholangitis existed in a number of specimens. Recovery was rapid in most patients, and none died. A 24-year follow-up did not reveal evidence of long-term health sequelae (Hall, JEpidCommHlth, 1992; 46:327).

In industry, methylene dianiline is used as an epoxy resin hardener, in the preparation of isocyanates, in the production of polyurethane and polychloroprene, and as an antioxidant in latex rubber. Consequently, intoxications have also been observed in these industries, usually when the agent was used as an epoxy resin hardener (see Appendix 2).

The mechanism of action of methylene dianiline has not been studied extensively. The literature is replete with mechanistical studies on α-naphthylisothiocyanate, a favourite experimental tool in cholestasis research. Research has also been performed on the mechanism by which chlorpromazine induces cholestasis. The biochemical–pathological mechanisms of intrahepatic cholestasis have recently been reviewed.[6,25] Figure 4 provides a survey of some of the target molecules discussed. Mechanism 1 applies to the formation of insoluble complexes between the chemical and bile acids (discussed for chlorpromazine) or bilirubin (discussed for manganese salts) and to the interference with micelle formation. Mechanism 2 refers to disturbance of membrane fluidity and its influence on sinusoidal uptake (discussed for contraceptive steroids). Mechanism 3 is the inhibition of the Na^+, K^+-ATPase of the sinusoidal membrane which is dependent on alterations of membrane fluidity (Davis, PNAS, 1978; 75:4130). However, the role of this enzyme in bile production is equivocal. Mechanism 4 is by inhibition of the Mg^{2+}-ATPase located in the canalicular membrane. This pump is functionally connected to the pericanalicular microfilament system. The mushroom poison phalloidin causes cholestasis because it induces polymerization of actin and thus disturbs the function of the microfilament apparatus (Dubin, Gastro, 1980; 79:646). Mechanism 5 is altered bile acid metabolism due to 'hypoactive hypertrophic smooth endoplasmic reticulum', [25] and mechanism 6 refers to disturbance of bile formation by the diffusion of solutes through leaky tight junctions; this mechanism has been described for α-naphthylisothiocyanate (Krell, Arch-Toxicol, 1987; 60:124).

Disturbance of haem synthesis

Chemicals may interfere with hepatic porphyrin synthesis.[26] Hexachlorobenzene, as a prototype chemical, inhibits hepatic coproporphyrinogen oxidase and uroporphyrinogen decarboxylase (Fig. 5) and causes secondary coproporphyrinuria which may progress to uroporphyrinuria and porphyria cutanea tarda. It has been suggested that oxidative metabolism of hexachlorobenzene is required for this effect (Van Ommen, ToxApplPharmacol, 1989;

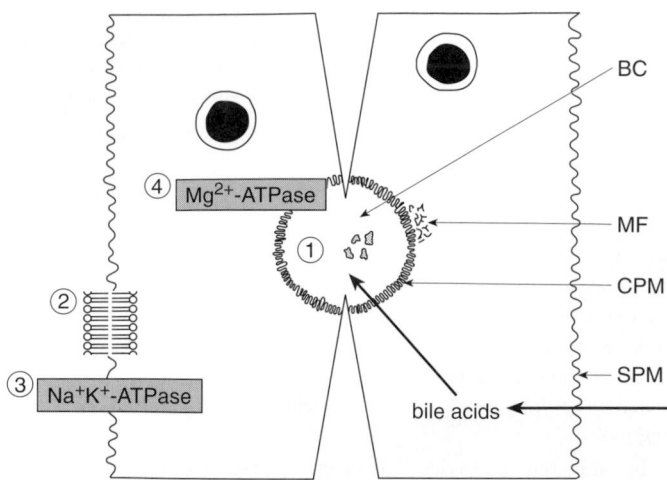

Fig. 4. Some targets discussed for the cholestatic action of hepatotoxicants. BC, bile canaliculus; MF, microfilament system; CPM, canalicular plasma membrane; SPM, sinusoidal plasma membrane. (1) Formation of insoluble complex with bile components. (2) Interference with bile acid transport by decrease of membrane fluidity. (3) Interference with bile acid transport by inhibition of NA$^+$K$^+$-ATPase. (4) Interference with bile secretion by inhibition of Mg^{2+}-ATPase and microfilament system.

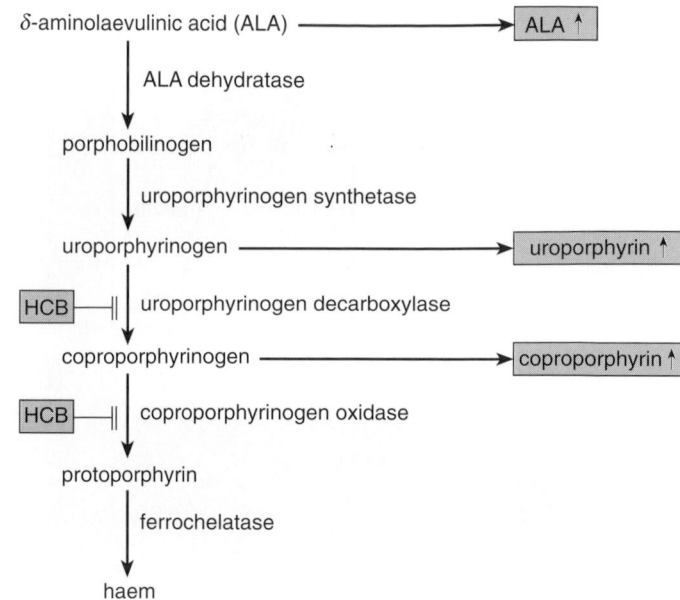

Fig. 5. Target enzymes of hexachlorobenzene (HCB) in porphyrin synthesis.

100:517) and that O$^{\bullet-}_2$ radicals are involved in inhibition of uroporphyrinogen decarboxylase (DeMatteis, SemHepatol, 1988; 25: 321). Genetic disposition for a defect in activity of uroporphyrinogen decarboxylase supports transition of toxic coproporphyrinuria to the clinically overt disease. This is illustrated by a number of cases observed after the Seveso accident in whom the manifestation of porphyria cutanea tarda was obviously triggered by trichlorodibenzodioxin on the basis of an inherited deficiency of uroporphyrinogen decarboxylase as determined by erythrocyte concentrations.[26]

A report of toxic porphyrinuria due to methyl chloride poisoning was published as early as 1940 (Chalmers, Lancet, 1940; ii:806). Attention was drawn to chemically induced porphyria cutanea tarda in 1956 when in three Turkish provinces an outbreak of the disease could finally be traced to the ingestion of wheat treated with the fungicide hexachlorobenzene (Schmid, NEJM, 1960; 263:397). Subsequently, the disease has been ascribed to trichlorodibenzodioxin, polychlorinated and polybrominated biphenyls, pentachlorophenol, 2,4,6-trichlorophenol, vinyl chloride, and silicium dioxide (see Appendix 2).

Covalent binding to DNA: somatic mutation

When a chemical is highly reactive, or can be metabolically activated to a species capable of forming a DNA adduct, a somatic mutation may result. The latent tumour cell formed by the genotoxic action of the mutagen may, under certain conditions, proliferate and eventually become a manifest tumour. The most potent hepatocarcinogen hitherto detected is a natural compound: aflatoxin B$_1$. Aflatoxin B$_1$ is a mycotoxin produced by *Aspergillus flavus*. In rats, it induces hepatocellular carcinomas at a daily uptake of 1 p.p.b. (1 mg/kg) in the diet. In rainbow trout, the daily intake required is even lower: 0.1 p.p.b.[27]

Aflatoxin B$_1$, like most other chemical carcinogens, is a precarcinogen which will bind to DNA only after metabolic activation. For aflatoxin B$_1$, the ultimate carcinogenic metabolite has been identified as the 8,9-epoxide (also named 2,3-epoxide). This epoxide forms an adduct with guanine-N^7.[27] The structure of the adduct is shown in Fig. 6. The steps between adduct and tumour are largely unknown; recently a mutational hot spot at the third base of codon 249 (a G:C to T:A transition, leading to an arginine to serine change) of the *p53* tumour suppressor gene was detected in hepatocellular carcinomas in patients in the Qi-Dong area in China, a region with high aflatoxin B$_1$ exposure (Li, Carcinogenesis, 1993; 14:169). Whether this mutation is causally related to aflatoxin B$_1$–induced carcinogenesis is at present unclear; this type of mutation has also been found in hepatocellular carcinoma of other origin. The DNA modification by the aflatoxin B$_1$–guanine adduct is relatively short-lived: it is cleared with a half-life of 7.5 h from rat liver DNA.[27] The adduct is eliminated by renal excretion and can be detected in human urine. Thus, it has been measured in the urine of inhabitants of the Murang'a district, a region in Kenya characterized by both high aflatoxin B$_1$ contamination of food and high incidence of hepatocellular carcinoma (Autrup, Carcinogenesis, 1983; 4:1193; Autrup, CancerRes, 1987; 47:3430). Biomonitoring of aflatoxin B$_1$ exposure can be based on the detection of the guanine N^7-adduct.[28,29] Renal excretion of the adduct reflects closely the amount of DNA adducts formed in the liver.[29] A sizeable part of the adduct is transformed into a secondary adduct *in vivo* by opening the imidazole ring (Fig. 6). This secondary adduct has a much longer half-life in the DNA than the primary adduct.[27] In addition to the guanine adduct, serum albumin adducts involving the lysine site of albumin can also be used for molecular dosimetry (Gan, Carcinogenesis, 1988; 9:1323).

Notably, aflatoxin B$_1$ will also induce acute hepatotoxicity. In an epidemic outbreak of acute aflatoxicosis in Taiwan and India due to the ingestion of mouldy rice or corn, respectively, over a period

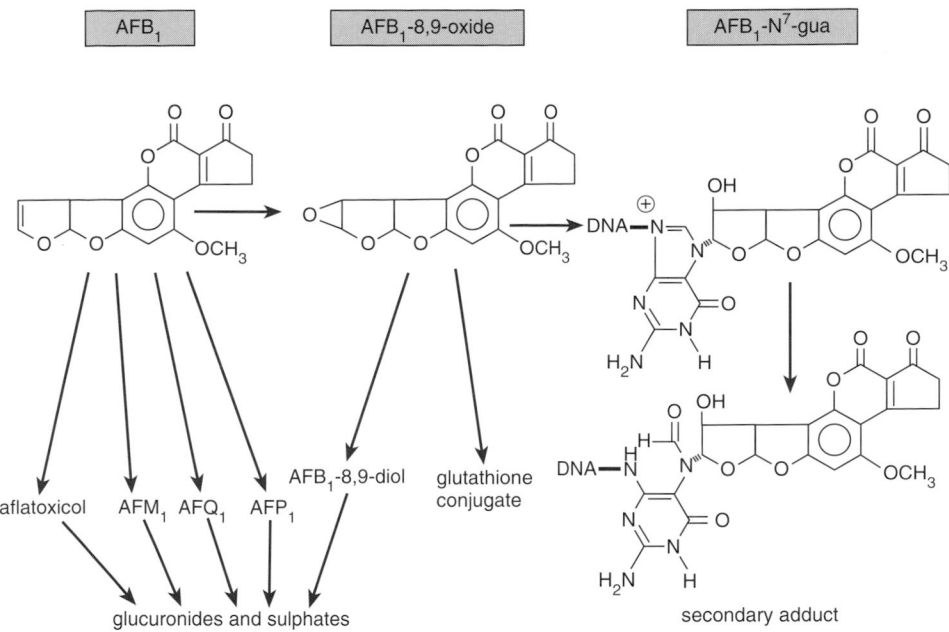

Fig. 6. Metabolic activation of aflatoxin B₁ and covalent binding of the reactive metabolite to DNA.

of some weeks, liver injury was a characteristic feature (Ling, JFormosanMedAss, 1967; 66:517; Krishnamachari, Lancet 1975; 1: 1061). Reye's syndrome in children has been connected with the ingestion of aflatoxin B₁-contaminated food in Thailand (see Chapter 32.2) and also in New Zealand (Becroft, BMJ, 1972; 4:117), Canada (Harwig, JCanMedAss, 1975; 113:281), the United States (Chaves-Carballo, MayoClinProc, 1976; 51:48; Ryan, Pediat, 1979; 64:71), and Czechoslovakia (Dvorackov, AnnNutrAliment, 1977; 31:977). However, in the United States it has been demonstrated that aflatoxin B₁ also occurs in blood and urine of control subjects not suffering from Reye's syndrome (Nelson, Pediat, 1980; 66:865).

Vinyl chloride, the monomer of poly(vinyl chloride) (PVC), causes angiosarcoma, a malignant liver tumour which is otherwise very rare in humans. Vinyl chloride, similar to aflatoxin B₁, is active as a mutagen and carcinogen only after metabolic activation to an electrophilic epoxide capable of forming DNA adducts (Fig. 7). The main site of formation of the reactive metabolites is the liver cell. In the newborn rat, exposure to vinyl chloride leads to hepatocellular carcinoma. This allows for evaluation of the action of vinyl chloride in a short-term test in which preneoplastic foci are used as the biological end point. *In vivo*, the adduct formed between the epoxide (chloroethylene oxide) and guanine-N⁷ in the DNA is thought to be the most important one, at least in rodent hepatocellular carcinoma. Whether the induction of angiosarcoma in humans is also related to this DNA modification is not clear. *p53* suppressor gene mutations (Hollstein, Carcinogenesis, 1994; 15:1) and serum anti-p53 antibodies (Trivers, JNCI, 1995; 87:1400) have been detected in vinyl chloride-associated angiosarcoma. At codon 13 of the c-Ki-*ras*-2 gene, a G:C to A:T transition leading to a defect in the gene product p21 was detected in five of six angiosarcomas due to vinyl chloride (Marion, MolCarcinog, 1991; 4:450). In RNA, etheno derivatives are found.[30] The epoxide is detoxified by conjugation with glutathione.

Chemically induced primary liver tumours

Primary liver tumours are rare in Western countries. However, they are among the most common tumours in parts of Africa (south of the Sahara) and in parts of Asia, thus indicating that environmental factors may be involved. This assumption is supported by the observation that immigrants from African and Asian countries with a high incidence of liver tumours do not exhibit an increased risk of liver malignancies in the United States (Alpert, AmJMed, 1969; 46: 325).

The liver tumour most often encountered is hepatocellular carcinoma. In high-incidence areas, a high incidence of hepatitis B virus infection is also present, and it is assumed that viral hepatitis is a predisposing factor (Popper, JHepatol, 1988; 6:229). However, chemical carcinogens may also contribute to the high incidence of hepatocellular carcinoma in African and Asian countries. In tropical regions, where humidity and heat favour the growth of moulds, humans may take up large quantities of aflatoxin B₁ with food. A daily intake as high as 220 ng aflatoxin B₁/kg body weight has been observed in Mozambique.[28] The causal relationship between aflatoxin B₁ intake and hepatocellular carcinoma in humans has not been proven; however, epidemiological data from a variety of countries (Swaziland, Kenya, Mozambique, Uganda, Thailand, and the Philippines) exist which indicate a close correlation between aflatoxin B₁ intake and primary liver cancer (refs[28,31]; see also Appendix 2). Thus, an extraordinarily high incidence of primary liver cancer is found in Mozambique, exceeding that in the United States by a factor of 500 (Higginson, CancerRes, 1963; 23:1624). This does not exclude the concomitant influence of other factors with a high prevalence in these countries, especially hepatitis B virus infection (Peers, IntJCanc, 1987; 39:545).[28,31,32] In a study of 18 244 male inhabitants of Shanghai, it was shown that subjects with liver cancer were more likely than were controls to excrete the N⁷-adduct and/or other products of aflatoxin B₁ metabolism.

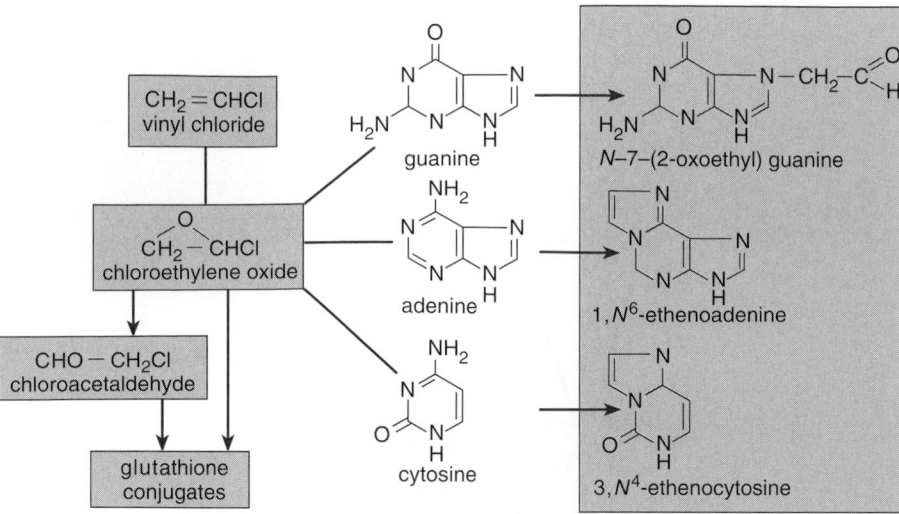

Fig. 7. Metabolic activation of vinyl chloride and covalent binding of the reactive metabolite to DNA.

HBsAg-positive subjects also had an elevated risk of liver cancer, both factors together increased the relative risk from about 2 for aflatoxin B_1 positivity to 60 (Ross, Lancet, 1992; 339:943). In Europe, high exposure to aflatoxin B_1 can occur in the food industry. In Danish animal-feed production-plant workers, an estimated daily intake of 64 ng/kg body weight was determined via serum albumin adduct dosimetry, which may partly explain the increased risk of liver cancer in this branch of industry (Autrup, Environ-HlthPerspect, 1993; 99:195).

Hepatocellular carcinoma is occasionally also found among the long-term sequelae of exposure to vinyl chloride and inorganic arsenicals (see Appendix 2). However, the predominant liver malignancy induced by these two industrial chemicals is angiosarcoma.[33] A register of 118 cases of angiosarcoma in vinyl chloride workers was held by the Vinyl Chloride Monomer Committee of the Association of Plastic Manufacturers in Europe in 1985 (Forman, BrJIndMed, 1985; 42:750). A review written in 1987 lists 20 epidemiological studies of cancer associated with exposure to vinyl chloride monomer.[34] This number has been extended since then (for example, Simonato, ScaJWorkEnvirHlth, 1991; 17:159; Wong, AmJIndMed, 1991; 20:317). Exposure most often occurred during production, especially in those workers who, upon cleaning of the autoclave vessels in which the polymerization process took place, were exposed to high concentrations of the monomer. However, angiosarcomas have also been described in persons employed in PVC processing since residual monomer concentrations were frequently very high during these operations.

The recognition of the tumour-producing potential of vinyl chloride came only after about 30 years of extensive PVC production. Health hazards from vinyl chloride had been known but the main attention had been paid to vinyl chloride-induced acro-osteolysis, a disease characterized by dissolution of the bones of fingers and toes and by signs of Raynaud's disease. Liver injury had been described in the USSR as early as 1949 (Tribukh, cited in ref.[25]) but appears to have received no specific attention during the following years. This is probably due to the fact that hepatocyte damage as recognized by serum enzyme tests is, in general, not an early prominent feature of chronic liver disease due to vinyl chloride,

while morphological changes may be more prominent.[8] Animal experiments in the early 1970s revealed the carcinogenic properties of vinyl chloride (Viola, MedLav, 1970; 61:174; Maltoni, EnvirRes, 1974; 16:19 and 150); angiosarcomas were observed among the tumours induced. In 1974, Creech and Johnson (JOccMed 1974; 16:150) reported on three cases of angiosarcoma in vinyl chloride workers. Angiosarcoma is a rare event in the general population. It was only because of the background of this very low incidence that the observation of angiosarcoma in workers employed in PVC production could rapidly be ascribed to the chemical. This is a most uncommon condition for statisticians involved in the epidemiological analysis of cancer-causing agents. A steadily increasing number of cases has since been observed. Workplace hygiene has been greatly improved since the association between exposure and angiosarcoma has been recognized, and exposure to high vinyl chloride monomer concentration is now very unlikely. However, due to the long latency of the disease, further cases must still be expected in the next decade. The association between the DNA modifications initiated by vinyl chloride (see above) and the development of angiosarcoma is not completely understood. It has been claimed that vinyl chloride-induced non-cirrhotic portal fibrosis is a precursor stage to angiosarcoma (Jones, BrJIndMed, 1982; 39:306).

It is as yet undetermined whether residents in areas near PVC plants may also have been exposed to tumour-inducing concentrations. There have been negative findings;[33] however, a case-control study indicated that environmental pollution may also cause the disease. The study identified five female patients with angiosarcoma for whom direct contact with vinyl chloride could be excluded but who lived in the near vicinity of vinyl chloride plants. None of the matched controls lived near a plant (Brady, JNCI, 1977; 59:1388). Doll (ScaJWorkEnvirHlth, 1988; 14:61) has stated that a very small risk may indeed have existed.

In addition to the more or less established human liver carcinogens, aflatoxin B_1, vinyl chloride, arsenicals,[35] and thorium dioxide,[36] further industrial chemicals and/or environmental pollutants have been suspected of inducing liver cancer. Support of such claims is given by the increase in hepatocellular carcinoma observed in industrialized countries during the past few decades. Thus, in Sweden the incidence of primary liver cancer in males increased from 3/100 000 in 1960 to 7/100 000 in 1980 (Hardell, BrJCanc, 1984; 50:389). Similarly, in Finland the number of new cases reported to the Cancer Registry was 87 in 1970 but increased to 196 in 1979 (Hernberg, IntArchOccupEnvirHlth, 1984; 54:147). One group of chemicals for which an association with hepatocellular carcinoma has repeatedly been suggested are solvents. A number of epidemiological studies is available to give some credence to the claim, but it is unproven. Data from the Danish Cancer Registry show a statistically significant excess risk of liver cancer (observed, 14; expected, 5.2; standardized ratio, 2.7) in women working in dry cleaning and exposed to tetrachloroethylene (Lynge, JOccMed, 1994; 36:1169). In the United States, a retrospective cohort mortality study in 1979 found four cases of liver cancer against 1.7 expected in laundry and dry-cleaning workers, but the result was not statistically significant. (Blair, AmJPublHlth, 1979; 69:508). Also in the United States, a case-control study in 1983 showed a statistical association between liver cancer and work in laundries and dry-cleaning establishments in which chlorinated hydrocarbons are used (Stemhagen, AmJEpid, 1983; 117:443). In Finland in 1984, an association between exposure to solvents and primary liver cancer was found for females only; the six female cases, but none of the matched controls, had a history of exposure (Hernberg, IntArchOccupEnvirHlth, 1984; 54:147). Also in 1984, a Swedish case-control study revealed a twofold increase in the risk of hepatocellular carcinoma by a history of occupational solvent exposure; the increase by alcohol was three- to fourfold (Hardell, BrJCanc, 1984; 50:389). On the other hand, a recent review of studies on cancer occurrence in the dry-cleaning industry does not confirm an excess risk of liver cancer (Weiss, CancerCauseContr, 1995; 6:257). Negative studies have been published (Malek, PracovLek, 1979; 31:124; Tola, JOccMed, 1980; 22:737; Katz, AmJPublHlth, 1981; 71:305; Paddle, BMJ, 1983; 286:846).

In addition to dry cleaning, other occupational fields have also been associated with liver and biliary cancer, such as the non-electrical machinery and primary metal industry (Houten, ArchEnvironHlth, 1980; 35:51), aircraft maintenance (Spirtas, BrJIndMed, 1991; 48:515), farming occupations (Stemhagen, AmJEpid, 1983; 35:51; Austin, JOccMed, 1987; 29:665; Kauppinen, ScaJWorkEnvirHlth, 1992; 18:18), sewage-plant work (Lafleur, AmJIndMed, 1991; 19:75), highway construction work (Austin, JOccMed, 1987; 29:665), petroleum refinery work (Marsh, AmJInd-Med, 1991; 19:29), gasoline service station work, restaurant work (Stemhagen AmJEpid, 1983; 117:443; Reviere, AmJIndMed, 1995; 27:195), breweries, bookbinding, sanitary services and repair, and household services (Olson, ScaJWorkEnvirHlth, 1987; 13 (suppl.); 1:91). For highway construction work, the relative rate of hepatocellular carcinoma was 5.0 and for asphalt exposure 3.2; in farming occupations the relative rate was 1.4 but for pesticide exposure it was 2.4 (Austin, JOccMed, 1987; 29:665). In an Italian study, the standardized mortality ratio for liver and bile duct cancer among pesticide applicators was 5.71 (Figa, IntJEpid, 1993; 22:674). Angiosarcomas have also been ascribed to pesticide exposure (El Zayadi, Hepatogastr, 1986; 33:148). Negative findings on pesticides (Wang, JOccMed, 1979; 21:741; Blair, JNCI, 1983; 71:31) and farming occupation in general (Blair, AmJIndMed, 1993; 23:729)

do exist. An excess mortality for liver cancer was reported for long-term exposure to polychlorinated biphenyls in the manufacture of electrical capacitors (Brown, ArchEnvironHlth, 1981; 36:120) and in the nickel alloy industry (Cragle, IARCSciPubl, 1984; 53:57; Redmond, IARCSciPubl, 1984; 53:73). Chronic exposure to benzidine plus β-naphthylamine resulted in an excess risk for cancer of liver, gallbladder, and bile ducts, in addition to the more common tumour sites, especially the bladder (Morinaga, AmJIndMed, 1982; 3:243). An excess in biliary and liver cancer was also observed in the rubber industry (Delzell, JOccMed, 1981; 23:677). A recent evaluation of 3400 primary liver cancer diagnoses reported to the Shanghai Cancer Registry found excess numbers of cases for chemical processors, textile workers, wood workers, blacksmiths and machine-tool operators, material handlers and dock workers, and female transport equipment operators (Chow, AmJIndMed, 1993; 24:93). Single observations of angiosarcomas have been ascribed to arsenic salts (Salgado, GastroHepato, 1995; 18:132), copper sulphate (Pimentel, Gastro, 1977; 72:275), and polychloroprene (Infante, EnvirHlthPerspect, 1977; 21:251).

In the Yusho incident, the inadvertent ingestion of contaminated rice oil caused exposure of nearly 2000 persons to polychlorinated biphenyls and polychlorinated dibenzofurans (reviewed by Kimbrough, AnnRevPharmTox, 1987; 27:87). A follow-up mortality study of this population indicates that the risk of liver cancer may have been increased. For males, 9 observed versus 1.61 expected liver cancers were seen; in females, observed cases were 2 against 0.66 expected. Only the finding for males was statistically significant (Kuratsune, Chemosphere, 1987; 16:2085).

Plausibility for associations between occupational exposure to certain chemicals and liver cancer is derived from animal experiments. Some of the most common solvents have caused liver cancer in rodents. Thus, tetrachloroethylene, a solvent frequently used in dry cleaning, has caused hepatocellular carcinoma in mice (NTP TechRepCase No.127–18–4, NIH Publication No.86–2567, 1986) Trichloroethylene has also induced liver tumours in mice (NTPTechBull, 1983; 9:9). Several organochlorine pesticides have caused liver tumours in mice, e.g. DDT, chlordane, heptachlor, dieldrin, and toxaphen (IARCEvalCarcinogRiskChemHumMonogr, 1979; 20:45, 129, and 327; IARCEvalCarcinogRiskChemHumMonogr, 1982; Suppl. 4:80 and 105). Polychlorinated biphenyls (Schaeffer, Tox ApplPharmacol, 1984; 75:278) and 2,3,7,8-tetrachlorodibenzo-p-dioxin (Kociba, ToxApplPharmacol, 1978; 46:279) are also liver carcinogens in rodents. However, a note of caution is required.[37, 38] Certain strains of mice are preferentially sensitive to chemically induced liver cancer, among them the B6C3F1 mouse. Such strains are characterized by a high incidence of spontaneous liver tumours (Tarone, JNCI, 1981; 66:1175). Activation of oncogenes by chemical carcinogens appears to be easily induced in the B6C3F1 mouse (Reynolds, Science, 1987; 237:1309). In rats, most carcinogenesis studies have been performed with the Fischer F344 rat which is more sensitive to chemical carcinogens than other rat strains. While the use of such sensitive strains may be looked upon as an efficient tool for detecting the carcinogenic potential of a chemical, it has also been claimed that extrapolation to humans from animals exhibiting high spontaneous incidence of liver cancer is not justified. This means that the impact of a major fraction of animal studies on hepatocarcinogenesis is at present subject to widespread criticism.

A number of agents which are positive in animal carcinogenesis tests lack a genotoxic potential. Probably such agents act by tumour promotion. They cause latent tumour cells (which have been initiated by an unknown mutagen) to express the transformed phenotype and to be subject to uncontrolled growth. It is at present not known whether agents identified as liver tumour promoters by animal experiments will also exhibit tumour promoting properties in humans. An increase of liver tumours due to exposure to chemicals known to be tumour promoters in rodents, such as DDT, polychlorinated biphenyls, 2,3,7,8-tetrachlorodibenzo-*p*-dioxin, or phenobarbital, has not definitely been shown in humans. However, the data on occupational pesticide exposure cited above have been interpreted in this way, and populations previously exposed to polychlorinated biphenyls or 2,3,7,8-tetrachlorodibenzodioxin are carefully observed for the development of liver cancer. For 2,3,7,8-tetrachlorodibenzodioxin, a large retrospective study in 5172 exposed chemical workers has not revealed an increased risk of liver cancer; however, the mortality due to all cancers and, in a subpopulation, due to soft tissue sarcomas and carcinomas of the respiratory tract was increased (Fingerhut, NEJM, 1991; 324:212). This may mean that the tumour promoting potential of the agent can be expressed in different tissues, depending on the species exposed. The argument most often put forward against a role of liver tumour promotion in humans is derived from the negative findings in the large population of epileptic patients treated with the prototype liver promoter in rodents, phenobarbital, for the major part of their lives (Clemmesen, EcotoxEnvirSafety, 1978; 1: 457; Olsen, CancerRes, 1995; 55:294).

In animal experiments, liver enlargement is often due to the proliferation of endoplasmic reticulum and the concomitant induction of drug-metabolizing enzymes. Enzyme induction by potential liver toxicants is also known in humans: pesticide handlers (Kolmodin, ClinPharmTher, 1969; 10:638), capacitor manufacturers (Alvares, ClinPharmTher, 1977; 22:140), and spray painters (Døssing, ClinPharmTher, 1982; 32:340) exhibited shortening of antipyrine half-life, reflecting enzyme induction. Enzyme induction is, by itself, not a sign of toxicity. However, depending on the inducer, specific isoenzymes may be induced which are capable of metabolizing precarcinogens to their ultimate carcinogenic metabolite. This may increase acute toxicity as well as hepatocarcinogenicity. It is at present unknown whether enzyme induction in humans may also have this consequence. Most liver tumour promotors also act to induce drug-metabolizing enzymes; whether a causal relation between both phenomena exists is at present unresolved.

Evaluation of reports on chemically induced liver injury in humans

A number of difficulties occur in the evaluation of reports on liver injury presumably due to chronic exposure to a toxic chemical. In an incident of acute disease characterized by signs of intoxication, workplace history will often indicate the responsible agent, but even in acute poisoning the causal relationship between the disease and a specific agent may remain equivocal. In reports, the argument is often based on tentative exclusion of other causes. More reliably, a causal link is supported by normalization of liver function after cessation of exposure. Inadvertent re-exposure can provide the strongest evidence but is rarely available. The problems most often encountered in establishing a causal link include the following:

Lack of exposure data

Dose dependency can, in most instances, hardly be assessed since reliable exposure data are lacking. Data on chronic industrial and environmental liver toxicity are almost exclusively derived from case reports or cross-sectional studies of a limited population in which biomonitoring by the determination of individual plasma or tissue content of the chemical in question has not been performed during exposure. Measurement of individual exposure can be partially substituted by postexposure measurements only in the case of persistent molecules such as polychlorinated biphenyls or dibenzodioxins. Retrospective quantitation of individual exposure is at best approximate. Prospective studies at different dose levels are unethical. This leads to the notorious problems of establishing upper limits of acceptable workplace concentrations.

Multiple exposure

In the workplace exposure to several chemicals is common. Døssing (JHepatol, 1986; 3:131) has cited a list comprising 29 chemicals used and generated as by-products or intermediates at a specific chemical plant in which toxic liver injury was observed in the employees. At least six of these chemicals had previously been shown to cause liver injury in humans. For 13 chemicals, no toxicological information was available. Such a situation probably pertains to many case reports and retrospective studies on industrial liver toxicity. Moreover, combination of hepatotoxicants will vary between specific operations within a plant. The situation is likely to be even more obscure with environmental liver toxicity. Apart from rendering causal analysis difficult, multiple exposure also poses the problem of synergistic effects. Examples are isopropanol and halogenated organic solvents (Folland, JAMA, 1976; 236:1853; Charbonneau, FundApplTox, 1988; 10:431) and tetrachloromethane and trichloroethylene (Pessayre, Gastro, 1982; 83:761).

Individual disposition

At long-term, low-dose exposure individual disposition appears to play an important role in the development of hepatotoxicity. This may reflect genetic polymorphism of toxicant metabolism or pre-existing liver injury due to a history of viral hepatitis or to alcohol and/or drug intake. In cross-sectional studies aimed at the detection of a chemically mediated effect on liver function, the percentage of abnormal results is often the same in the exposed group and the control group when body weight, dietary habits, and alcohol intake are taken into account (for example Hanusch, ZGesHyg, 1978; 24:544; Waldron, Lancet, 1982; ii:1276; Boewer, IntArchOccupEnvirHlth, 1988; 60:181). Excessive alcohol consumption, in addition to causing alcoholic liver disease, may interfere with hepatotoxicant elimination. Enhancement by ethanol of trichloroethylene metabolism and hepatotoxicity has been described in experimental animals (Nakajima, ToxApplPharmacol, 1988; 94:227).

Predominant toxic effect in other tissues

Liver injury may be part of a toxic syndrome dominated by extrahepatic manifestations or presenting as multiorgan failure.

With most solvents, neurotoxicity predominates in the early phase of acute intoxication; however, liver injury may well be the decisive factor for a fatal outcome of the disease. Liver damage is a minor event in aniline intoxication which is dominated by methaemoglobinaemia; in carbonyl nickel, hexafluorodichlorobutene, or ethylene chlorohydrin intoxication which is dominated by respiratory failure; or in dioxan, diethylene glycol, or petrol intoxication which may be dominated by renal insufficiency.

An example: the solvent debate

Undoubtedly, a number of commonly used solvents will cause liver damage at high concentrations, but sophisticated study protocols are required to prove such effects at workplace concentrations within or close to regulatory limits.[39] This can only be achieved by proper case-control studies which take into account not only the prevalent confounding factor of increased alcohol intake but also exposure to other hepatotoxicants which might occur at the workplace (Axelson, EurJClinInv, 1983; 13:109). These requirements have not been met completely by a number of studies. In 1982, Sotaniemi et al. (ActaMedScand, 1982; 212:207) reported that 23 exposed persons (15 chemical industry workers and eight painters) out of a cohort of 800 consecutive cases of diagnostic liver biopsies exhibited a two- to fourfold increase in serum transaminases, and the majority (19) also had histological signs of liver injury, including moderately fatty liver in six cases. The design of this study did not allow for adequate controls, and has therefore been heavily criticized (Kurppa, Lancet, 1983; 1:129). However, the return to normal of enzyme values after cessation of exposure gives some credit to the claims of the authors. In 1983, Døssing and co-workers (EurJClinInv, 1983; 13:151) reported that among 156 patients admitted to hospital because of suspected solvent intoxication (including a number of house painters), 23 had elevated serum transaminases. On biopsy, 11 had pathological findings, including steatosis, focal necrosis, and enlarged portal tracts with fibrosis. This study was also uncontrolled and has been criticized (Axelson, EurJClinInv, 1983; 13:109; Kurppa, EurJClinInv, 1983; 13:113) because of the lack of a suitable reference group and of possible bias due to the fact that the patients were primarily admitted to hospital because of alleged solvent neurotoxicity. Among a group of 206 house painters and house carpenters, the prevalence of biochemical findings pointing to liver dysfunction correlated with lifetime exposure (Lundberg, OccupEnvirMed, 1994; 51:347). It has also been pointed out that the extent of solvent exposure may be different in different occupational operations. Thus, the particular working conditions of housepainters in small, unventilated rooms and, in general, without any protective equipment, may predispose to heavier exposure than in other workplaces with solvent exposure. Notably, a number of studies, some of them well controlled by a case-reference design, have been carried out, and these could not find a causal relationship between mixed solvent exposure and elevation of serum enzymes (Hane, ScaJWorkEnvirHlth, 1977; 3:91; Kurppa, ScaJWorkEnvirHlth, 1982; 8:137; Lundberg, BrJIndMed, 1985; 42:596; Triebig, FortschrMed, 1985; 103:271; Nasterlack, IntArchOccupEnvirHlth, 1994; 66:161; Ukai, OccupEnvirMed, 1994; 51:523). In a number of studies, adjustment for confounding by alcohol consumption eliminated the increased risk due to occupational solvent exposure (Rasmussen, IntArchOccupEnvirHlth, 1993; 64:445; Rees,

ScaJWorkEnvirHlth, 1993; 19:236). A recent study shows, however, increased levels of γ-glutamyltransferase activity in a group of 180 workers in paint manufacture and spray-painting, which correlated with exposure levels even after adjustment for alcohol consumption (Chen, BrJIndMed, 1991; 48:696).

Data collection: Appendix 2

Appendix 2 is a data list for a number of hepatotoxicants for which the original case reports or epidemiological studies were available to the author. Only positive findings are included in the list; if negative findings for the compound listed also exist, these are mentioned in a footnote. For some compounds, all reports available are included in the list. This was not practicable for a number of notorious liver toxicants, such as carbon tetrachloride, for which there is extensive documentation. Only a few typical reports are given for such compounds. The quality of the data is highly variable. Few studies are epidemiologically well designed. In older reports, information is often not available regarding contamination of the product to which exposure had occurred. Typical cases are chlorinated compounds such as hexachloronaphthalene (the alleged cause of the so-called perna disease, or halowax chloracne) or chlorophenols, for which contamination with polychlorinated dibenzodioxins must be inferred in view of later findings using more sophisticated analytical methods. If this is known for a specific compound, an account of the contamination is given in a footnote. An additional problem encountered in the interpretation of older reports is that they rely on outdated diagnostic methods, making comparison with more recent papers difficult. Recognizing these and other problems in the evaluation of the original literature, Appendix 2 does not generally exclude equivocal findings, or those which are difficult to interpret; it gives, however, an indication of the data upon which a causal link between exposure and chemical has been based. Moreover, it includes an abbreviated description of the type and size of study, of the conditions of exposure, and of the clinical and pathological findings. It was not possible to include quantitative exposure data; the reader is referred to the original papers for this information.

References

1. Zimmerman HJ. Chemical hepatic injury and its detection. In Plaa G and Hewitt WR, eds. *Toxicology of the liver*. New York: Raven Press, 1982: 1–45.
2. Treinen Moslen M. Toxic responses of the liver. In Doull J, Klaassen CD, Amdur MO, eds. *Casarett and Doull's toxicology*. New York: Macmillan Publishing, 1996: 403–16.
3. Zimmerman HJ. Hepatotoxicity. *Disease-A-Month Series*, 1993; **39**: 675–787.
4. Klaassen CD and Watkins JB, III. Mechanisms of bile formation, hepatic uptake, and biliary excretion. *Pharmacological Reviews*, 1984; **36**: 1–67.
5. Zimmerman HJ and Lewis JH. Drug-induced cholestasis. *Medical Toxicology*, 1987; **2**: 112–60.
6. Reichen J. Mechanisms of cholestasis. In Travoloni N and Berk PG, eds. *Hepatic transport and bile secretion: physiology and pathophysiology*. New York: Raven Press, 1993: 665–72.
7. Remmer H, Bolt HM, Bannasch P, and Popper H. *Primary liver tumours*. Falk Symposium 25. Lancaster: MTP Press, 1978.
8. Marsteller HJ, Lelbach WK, Müller R, and Gedigk P. Unusual splenomegalic liver disease as evidenced by peritoneoscopy and guided liver biopsy among polyvinyl chloride production workers. *Annals of the New York Academy of Sciences*, 1975; **246**: 95–134.
9. Rosser BG and Gores GJ. Liver cell necrosis: cellular mechanisms and clinical implications. *Gastroenterology*, 1995; **108**: 252–75.

10. Mehendale HM, Roth RA, Gandolfi AJ, Klaunig JE, Lemasters JJ, and Curtis LR. Novel mechanisms in chemically induced hepatotoxicity. *FASEB Journal*, 1994; **8**: 1285–95.

11. Laskin DL. Role of macrophages and endothelial cells in hepatotoxicity. In Bilar TR and Curran RD, eds. *Hepatocyte and Kupffer cell interactions*. Boca Raton: CRC Press, 1992: 147.

12. Plaa GL and Charbonneau M. Detection and evaluation of chemically induced liver injury. In Hayes AW, ed. *Principles and methods of toxicology*. New York: Raven Press, 1994: 839–70.

13. Sipes IG and Gandolfi AJ. Bioactivation of aliphatic organohalogens: formation, detection, and relevance. In Plaa G and Hewitt WR, eds. *Toxicology of the liver*. New York: Raven Press, 1982: 181–212.

14. Dianzani MU. The role of free radicals in liver damage. *Proceedings of the Nutrition Society*, 1987; **46**: 43–52.

15. Williams AT and Burk RF. Carbon tetrachloride hepatotoxicity: An example of free-radical-mediated injury. *Seminars in Liver Disease*, 1990; **10**: 279–84.

16. Orrenius S. Mechanisms of oxidative cell damage. In Poli G, Albano E, and Dianzani MU, eds. *Free radicals: from basic science to medicine*. Basel: Birkhäuser, 1993: 47–64.

17. Bird GLA and Williams R. Anaesthesia-related liver disease. In Assem Esk, ed. *Allergic reactions to anaesthetics. Clinical and basic aspects*. Basel: Karger, 1992: 174–91.

18. Smith MT, Evans CG, Thor H, and Orrenius S. Quinone-induced oxidative injury to cells and tissues. In Sies H, ed. *Oxidative stress*. London: Academic Press, 1985: 91–113.

19. Cadenas E. One- and two-electron activation of quinonoid compounds. Oxidant and antioxidant aspects. In Nohl H, Esterbauer H, and Rice-Evans C, eds. *Free radicals in the environment, medicine and toxicology*. London: Richelieu Press, 1994: 119–35.

20. Vermeulen NPE, Bessems JGM, and Van de Straat R. Molecular aspects of paracetamol-induced hepatotoxicity and its mechanism-based prevention. *Drug Metabolism Reviews*, 1992; **24**: 367–407.

21. Nelson SD. Mechanisms of the formation and disposition of reactive metabolites that can cause acute liver injury. *Drug Metabolism Reviews*, 1995; **27**: 147–77.

22. Reddy JK, Usuda N, and Rao MS. Hepatic peroxisome proliferation: an overview. *Archives of Toxicology*, 1988; Suppl.12: 207–16.

23. Rao MS and Reddy JK. Peroxisome proliferation and hepatocarcinogenesis. *Carcinogenesis*, 1987; **8**: 631–6.

24. Faulstich H. New aspects of amanita poisoning. *Klinische Wochenschrift*, 1979; **57**: 1143–52.

25. Feuer G and DiFonzo CJ. Intrahepatic cholestasis: A review of biochemical-pathological mechanisms. *Drug Metabolism and Drug Interactions*, 1992; **10**: 1–161.

26. Doss MO. Porphyrinurias and occupational disease. *Annals of the New York Academy of Sciences*, 1987; **514**: 204–18.

27. Essigmann JM, Croy RG, Bennett RA, and Wogan GN. Metabolic activation of aflatoxin B_1: patterns of DNA adduct formation, removal, and excretion in relation to carcinogenesis. *Drug Metabolism Reviews*, 1982; **13**: 581–602.

28. Groopman JD, Busby WF Jr, Donahue PR, and Wogan GN. Aflatoxins as risk factors for liver cancer: an application of monoclonal antibodies to monitor human exposure. In Harris CC, ed. *Biochemical and molecular epidemiology of cancer*. New York: Alan R. Liss, 1986: 233–56.

29. Groopman JD, Zhu J, Donahue PR, Pikul A, Zhang L-S, and Wogan GN. Molecular dosimetry of urinary aflatoxin DNA adducts in people living in Guangxi Autonomous Region, People's Republic of China. *Cancer Research*, 1992; **52**: 45–51.

30. Laib RJ. Specific covalent binding and toxicity of aliphatic halogenated xenobiotics. *Reviews on Drug Metabolism and Drug Interactions*, 1982; **IV**: 1–48.

31. Reiss J, ed. *Mykotoxine in Lebensmitteln*. Stuttgart: Gustav Fischer Verlag, 1981.

32. Newberne PM. Chemical carcinogenesis: mycotoxins and other chemicals to which humans are exposed. *Seminars in Liver Disease*, 1984; **4**: 122–35.

33. Tamburro CH. Relationship of vinyl monomers and liver cancers: angiosarcoma and hepatocellular carcinoma. *Seminars in Liver Disease*, 1984; **4**: 158–69.

34. Purchase IFH, Stafford J, and Paddle GM. Vinyl chloride: an assessment of the risk of occupational exposure. *Food and Chemical Toxicology*, 1987; **25**: 187–202.

35. Bates MN, Smith AH, and Hopenhayn-Rich C. Arsenic ingestion and internal cancers: A review. *American Journal of Epidemiology*, 1992; **135**: 462–76.

36. Andersson M, Vyberg M, Visfeldt J, Carstensen B, and Storm HH. Primary liver tumors among Danish patients exposed to Thorotrast. *Radiation Research*, 1994; **137**: 262–73.

37. ECETOC. Hepatocarcinogenesis in laboratory rodents: Relevance for man. *ECETOC Monograph*, 1982; 4.

38. Goldsworthy TL, Hanigan ML, and Pitot HC. Models of hepatocarcinogenesis in the rat: Contrasts and comparisons. *Critical Reviews in Toxicology*, 1986; **17**: 61–89.

39. Klockars M. Solvents and the liver. *Progress in Clinical and Biological Research*, 1986; **220**: 139–54.

18.2 Hepatic injury due to physical agents

Antoni Mas and Juan Rodés

Although hepatic trauma is the most common physical agent causing hepatic injury (see Chapter 30.4), other factors, such as radiation, major burns, and heat stroke, may occasionally produce hepatic disturbances. These uncommon hepatic lesions are frequently associated with dramatic systemic manifestations, overshadowing hepatic histological and clinical features.

Radiation

Hepatic lesions are uncommon after abdominal radiotherapy since the liver is a relatively radioresistant organ. In 1986, Schacter *et al.* reviewed 32 patients from the medical literature who had hepatitis caused by radiation.[1] Most of these patients were women submitted to radiotherapy for ovarian tumours. In this series of patients there were other tumours such as lymphomas, hypernephromas, or intestinal neoplasms. Hepatic lesions have also been described in patients with primary liver carcinoma treated with radiotherapy.[2] The hepatic lesions appear to be dose-related and generally occur in patients receiving 3000 to 3500 cGy or more. Occasionally, fatal hepatic lesions in patients who received 2200 cGy have been described.[1] In addition to the dosage and the duration of radiation, other factors may be involved in the development and severity of hepatic lesions; for example, previous chemotherapy may facilitate, through a sensitizing mechanism, the hepatic toxicity induced by radiation.

The clinical picture may be initiated in an acute form (4–24 weeks after radiotherapy), in a subacute form (after 8–24 weeks), or chronically (after 2 or more years).[3] Other authors consider that there are two forms of presentation, acute (2 weeks to 6 months after radiotherapy) and chronic (6 months or more).[2] Patients develop ascites, hepatomegaly, and a slight increase in transaminases and hyperbilirubinaemia. Occasionally, these clinical features are similar to those observed in the Budd–Chiari syndrome, and some of these patients have been erroneously submitted to laparotomy. The mortality of patients with postradiotherapy hepatic lesions is very high; 15 out of the 32 patients reviewed by Schacter *et al.* died.[1] The cause of death in most patients was hepatic failure. One patient was reported as showing ascites refractory to diuretic treatment, in whom the insertion of a LeVeen shunt had been indicated. The procedure failed and the patient died because of hepatic and functional renal failure.

A more recent analysis of the incidence and relevance of radiationhepatitis indicates that although 44 per cent of patients treated with abdomino-pelvic radiation therapy for ovarian carcinoma developed liver enzyme elevations, these changes were transient in most cases; the authors concluded that there is a low risk of serious late toxicity, especially when a moving-strip technique of radiation is used (Fyles, Int JRadiatOncolBiolPhys, 1992; 22: 847).

The hepatic lesions are similar to those described in venoocclusive hepatic disease, with congestion and fibrosis in the perivenular regions. The portal tracts and biliary ducts are normal[2]. However, experimental studies in dogs submitted to radiotherapy have demonstrated that ductal fibrosis, partial biliary obstruction, and development of secondary biliary cirrhosis may be observed (Sindelar, Surgery, 1982; 92:533). In humans, two cases of common bile duct stricture 10 years after upper abdominal radiotherapy for malignant lymphoma have been reported (Cherqui, JHepatol, 1994; 20:693). In the acute form it is common to find sinusoidal congestion and haemorrhage in the central areas, while in the chronic form there is sclerosis and narrowing of the hepatic veins, together with portal fibrosis and arteriolar lesions.[2] Patients with these hepatic lesions show the same clinical picture as that of hepatic cirrhosis, with oesophageal varices, hypersplenism, and ascites.

Liver scans may show hepatomegaly and suggest the presence of space-occupying lesions. Furthermore, they may indicate that Kupffer cell alterations are more severe than those observed in hepatocytes.[1]

Changes in abdominal CT scan in cases of radiation hepatitis have been described as sharply defined bands of low density, with straight borders in the radiated area (Kolbenstvedt, Radiol, 1980; 135:391). These bands are seen to disappear on follow-up. This lesion may be confused with hepatic metastases (Brooke, AJR, 1980; 135:445). In contrast, the CT appearance of high-dose localized radiotherapy of the liver did not exhibit the sharp interfaces with the non-irradiated parenchyma (Yamasaki, AJR, 1995; 165:79). Other types of lesions, such as oval-shaped lesions, have been found in liver CT scans after phototherapy (Okumura, JComputAssist-Tomogr, 1994; 18:821).

The pathogenesis of hepatic changes is not clear-cut and could be a direct effect of radiotherapy on the hepatocytes and Kupffer cells or an indirect effect secondary to changes in blood vessels.

Although the mortality rate of postradiation hepatitis is very high, some patients may show a transient form with a good prognosis. A recent review of radiation-induced liver disease suggests that steroid therapy should be considered in severe cases.[4]

Burns

Patients with major burns usually show a slight increase in transaminases, while the development of jaundice is less common.[5] Some degree of liver involvement was found in 15/40 (37.5 per cent) cases of burned patients submitted to autopsy (Iliopoulou, ArchAnatCytolPath, 1993; 41:5).

Hypertransaminasaemia in such patients may be due to extrahepatic mechanisms. Three different chronological peak levels of transaminases have been described: (1) a few hours after the burns; (2) 2 to 4 days thereafter; and (3) 2 to 3 weeks later.[6] It is obvious that the cause of precocious hyertransaminasaemia is related to the skin and muscle lesions produced by the burns, while the increased levels of transaminases detected in later stages may be explained by other mechanisms such as arterial hypotension, shock, infection of the injured tissue, absorption of toxins from the burn areas, malnutrition, sepsis, and drugs. However, in spite of these possibilities, a specific hepatic lesion may exist in patients with major burns. Chiarelli et al. showed that the development of hypertransaminasaemia occurred in 60 per cent of patients in the second week after the burns, and that the enzymes were of hepatic origin.[6] They found no correlation between the extent of the burns and the plasma levels of transaminases. Moreover, they suggested that the increased levels of transaminases in patients with burns of moderate extent indicate the excellent capacity of the body to respond metabolically to the lesion.

The absence of histological hepatic lesions in most patients suggests that the hepatic changes in burns are functional.[5] Increases of lipid peroxidation products (malondialdehyde) in the early postburn period may affect the liver and other organs, resulting in release of enzymes into the bloodstream (Kumar, Burns, 1995; 21:96). In some patients there are non-specific hepatic lesions: these include hydropic degeneration in the hepatocytes, hepatic steatosis, and disappearance of hepatic glycogen,[5-7] together with ultrastructural alterations, such as dilatation of the endoplasmic reticulum, small biliary ducts, and mitochondrial lesions.[7]

Acalculous cholecystitis has been well described in adults following major burns (Alawneh, BrJSurg, 1978; 65:243).

Heat stroke

In a large series of 244 patients with heat stroke studied in 1959 only 10 had jaundice and 17 showed some abnormalities in hepatic function.[8] However, more recent studies produced evidence that hepatic lesions in such patients are much more frequent.[9,10]

Usually, patients with heat stroke show moderate hepatic changes, revealed only by a slight increase of transaminases with levels less than six to eight times normal values. Jaundice is very uncommon. Occasionally, hepatic failure may appear and may be the cause of death in these patients.[9]

Hepatic failure is associated with very high plasma levels of bilirubin (30 times greater than normal values) and transaminases (150 times greater than normal values), with a marked decrease of prothrombin time (less than 20 per cent).[11] Neurological disturbances may be due to heat stroke itself or secondary to hepatic failure. The development of these alterations may be precocious, appearing 2 to 3 days after hyperpyrexia. The clinical evolution of the patients submitted to conventional therapy for acute hepatic failure may be favourable.[12] Some patients have been referred for emergency liver transplantation.[10]

Hepatic lesions found in those patients who die after heat stroke include sinusoidal congestion, steatosis (microvesicular type), and increased blood cells in the sinusoid.[12] In patients who survive longer, liver biopsy, in addition to the lesions mentioned above, reveals perivenular zonal necrosis with hydropic degeneration and cholestasis with cholangiolitis.[12,13] Occasionally, confluent necrosis may be seen in some patients, similar to that observed in acute viral hepatitis. Sequential liver biopsies show that these lesions disappear within a few months.[13]

The pathogenesis of liver abnormalities is unknown. However, it is probable that hypoxic hypovolaemia and hyperpyrexia are important factors.[11,12] The use of neuroleptic or anticholinergic drugs may favour the risk of severe liver damage in heat stroke, by disturbing thermoregulation and increasing hyperthermia (Dohin-Caplanne, GastrClinBiol, 1995; 19:637; Finjheer, NedTGeneesk, 1995; 139:1391). The development of centroacinar necrosis suggests that the hepatic lesions may be due to hypoxia, secondary, presumably, to a reduced cardiac output. Obesity may be another factor favouring hepatic lesions.[11,12] In some patients with perivenular zonal necrosis the lack of evidence for systemic haemodynamic alterations suggests that the increased oxygen consumption in periportal areas induced by hyperthermia might reduce the oxygen content in blood reaching the central areas, this mechanism thereby causing centrizonal necrosis.[11] If this hypothesis is true, hyperoxygenation may be useful in these patients. Prevention, prompt diagnosis and immediate cooling and hydration, along with early recognition and management of complications, are the main strategy for the care of patients with heat stroke.

References

1. Schacter L, Crum E, Spitzer T, Maksem J, Diwan V, and Kolli S. Fatal radiation hepatitis: a case report and review of the literature. *Gynecologic Oncology*, 1986; **24**: 373–80.
2. Moorthy C, Kaul R, and Nori D. Role of radiation therapy in primary and metastatic liver malignancies. In Hodgson WJB, ed. *Liver tumours: multidisciplinary management*. St. Louis: Warren H Green, 1988: 272–301.
3. Wharton JT, Delclos L, Gallager S, and Smith JP. Radiation hepatitis induced by abdominal irradiation with cobalt 60 moving strip technique. *American Journal of Roentgenology*, 1973; **117**: 73–80.
4. Lawrence TS, Robertson JM, Anscher MS, Jirtle RL, Ensminger WD, and Fajardo LF. Hepatic toxicity resulting from cancer treatment. *International Journal of Radiation Oncology, Biology, Physics*, 1995; **31**: 1237–48.
5. Chlumsky J, Dobias J, Vrabec R, Marecek B, Chlumska A, and Matejicek V. Liver changes in burns, as seen in the clinical morphologic picture. *Acta Hepatologica-Gastroenterologica*, 1976; **23**: 118–24.
6. Chiarelli A, Siliprandi L, Casadei A, Schiavon M, and Mazzoleni F. Aminotransferase changes in burn patients. *Intensive Care Medicine*, 1987; **13**: 199–202.
7. Angela GC, Ambroggio G, Bréan L, Marino M, and Bormioli M. Istopatologia del fegato nei grandi ustionati. Studio bioptico preliminare. *Minerva Medica*, 1975; **66**: 2200–11.
8. Herman RH and Sullivan BH. Heatstroke and jaundice. *American Journal of Medicine*, 1959; **27**: 154–66.

9. Kew M, Bersohn I, Seftel H, and Kent G. Liver damage in heatstroke. *American Journal of Medicine*, 1970; **49**: 192–202.

10. Hassanein T, Razack A, Gavaler JS, and Van Thiel DH. Heatstroke: its clinical and pathological presentation, with particular attention to the liver. *American Journal of Gastroenterology*, 1992; **87**: 1382–97.

11. Chavoutier-Uzzan F, Bernuau J, Degott C, Rueff B, and Benhamou JP. Le coup de chaleur: une cause rare de nécrose hépatique massive d'origine hypoxique. *Gastroenterologie Clinique et Biologique*, 1988; **12**: 668–9.

12. Rubel LR and Ishak KG. The liver in fatal exertional heatstroke. *Liver*, 1983; **3**: 249–60.

13. Bianchi L, Ohnacker H, Beck K, and Zimmerli-Ning M. Liver damage in heatstroke and its regression. A biopsy study. *Human Pathology*, 1972; **3**: 237–48.

19

Fulminant and subfulminant liver failure

19 Fulminant and subfulminant liver failure

Jacques Bernuau and Jean-Pierre Benhamou

Fulminant and subfulminant hepatic failure is a complex and devastating syndrome resulting from the severe impairment of vital functions of the normal liver. Hepatotropic viruses, drugs, poisoning, and liver cell hypoxia are the most common causes.[1,2] Despite improvements in the medical management, only 5 to 60 per cent of the patients survive spontaneously.[1,2] In these patients, full recovery is the rule: that spontaneous survival—sometimes unexpected—may occur is a key feature of the syndrome. Introduced in the early 1980s, emergency total liver transplantation has improved the overall survival rate[3,4] but is associated with an operative risk of 10 to 30 per cent, a risk of overindication of at least 10 per cent,[5,6] and the still ill-defined consequences of lifelong immunosuppression. In the early 1990s, auxiliary partial liver transplantation was shown to be feasible,[5,7] allowing the patient to avoid lifelong immunosuppression.

Spontaneous full recovery remains the goal for all therapeutic modalities. To lower the incidence, overall fatality rate, and morbidity of the syndrome, early diagnosis, and, even better, lack of aggravation of any acute liver disease are important. To achieve these aims it is important to improve the education of non-specialist physicians who usually see these patients first, so that they may more readily detect the pre-encephalopathic stage of the syndrome. Two recent books provide comprehensive information.[1,2]

Definitions[1,2]

It is now more than 25 years after the initial definition of the syndrome (Trey, ProgLivDis, 1970; 3:282), but the vocabulary of fulminant and subfulminant hepatic failure remains controversial.[8] Originally, fulminant liver failure was defined as an acute liver disease complicated by hepatic encephalopathy within 8 weeks after the onset of symptoms. This definition remains widely used but does not reflect the clinical heterogeneity of the syndrome and delays diagnosis and referral to a specialized liver unit.

The first controversial issue is the requirement of clinical encephalopathy. Although it is regarded as mandatory for defining fulminant and subfulminant hepatic failure in North America[8] and the United Kingdom,[9] several authors do not share this view. Since 1982, Indian hepatologists have used the term 'subacute hepatic failure' in patients with acute liver disease, jaundice for more than 4 weeks, and clinically detectable ascites: in these Indian patients, the outcome is often fatal without encephalopathy.[10] In 1986, French hepatologists put forward the concept of the pre-encephalopathy stage of fulminant and subfulminant hepatic failure. This stage should be diagnosed as soon as the prothrombin ratio (or proaccelerin concentration) falls below 50 per cent of normal during the course of an acute liver disease.[11] At this stage (depending on the possible development of clinical encephalopathy and the geographical area), outcome will fall into one of four subgroups (Table 1). The term coined for this pre-encephalopathy (early) stage of fulminant and subfulminant hepatic failure was 'severe' acute hepatic failure,[10] although 'impending' (Ranek, Gut, 1976; 17: 959) or 'incipient' may be preferable. Although this terminology may include patients who eventually will not deteriorate, using it will enable anticipation or very early detection of encephalopathy, thus allowing the earliest possible referral to a specialized liver unit (Bernuau, Lancet, 1993; 342:252).

The second difficulty is to define the most critical interval between the clinical onset of liver disease and the onset of encephalopathy. Durations from 3 to 8 weeks have been proposed (Rueff, Gut, 1973; 14:805; European Association for the Study of the Liver, Gut, 1979; 20:620; Mathiesen, Gut, 1980; 21:72; Gimson, Gut, 1983; 24:1983). Most authors now agree that the onset of jaundice should be the starting point[9,11] but several definitions have been proposed for the interval between the onset of jaundice and the onset of encephalopathy. They include the terms fulminant (interval shorter than 2 weeks) and subfulminant (interval between 2 weeks and 3 months) hepatic failure,[11] and a classification of hyperacute, acute, and subacute liver failure.[9] In 1993, Indian hepatologists (Acharya, Lancet 1993; 342:1422) diagnosed fulminant hepatic failure when clinical encephalopathy occurs within 4 weeks of the clinical onset of acute hepatitis[12] and confirmed their previous criteria for subacute hepatic failure.[10] These various definitions reflect, at least in part, local observations and make overall comparisons between series of patients from different countries hazardous (Lee, Hepatol, 1996; 24:270).

The third controversial issue is that posed by the generic term. Although restrictive definitions have been proposed for 'fulminant' hepatic failure[11] and 'acute' liver failure,[9] both terms are routinely used as generic terms to encompass all clinical conditions including an acute liver disease with marked decrease in coagulation factors and hepatic encephalopathy.[2,11]

In this section, we will use the definitions we proposed previously. Severe acute hepatic failure will refer to any clinical

Table 1 The four possible outcomes of patients with severe acute hepatic failure

No occurrence of clinical encephalopathy	
Europe, North America	
South Asia (India, Bangladesh)[a]	1. Spontaneous survival (>98%)
	2. Death (50%)[b]
Occurrence of clinical encephalopathy	3. Death (40–95%)[c]
	4. Spontaneous survival (5–60%)[c]

[a] Tandon, JClinGastr, 1986; 8:664.
[b] If ascites for more than 4 weeks after the onset of jaundice.
[c] According to the patient's age and the cause of hepatic injury.

condition, including an acute liver disease with coagulation factors below 50 per cent of normal without clinical encephalopathy. Fulminant and subfulminant hepatic failure will be used to describe cases with similar coagulopathy and clinical encephalopathy.[11]. It is now accepted[9,11] that these definitions allow inclusion of patients in whom an acute liver disease with severe breakdown of liver function is the first manifestation of a previously asymptomatic chronic liver lesion.

Severe acute hepatic failure

As previously defined and despite its heterogeneous outcomes (Table 1), severe acute liver failure is a clinical continuum between acute liver diseases without serious coagulopathy (prothrombin > 50 per cent) and, in a few cases, acute liver diseases complicated by clinical encephalopathy. Jaundice is not always present but serum aminotransferase activity is increased. In the less severe and most common cases, the prothrombin ratio decreases below 50 per cent for only a short period (less than 1–7 days) and clinical symptoms of acute liver disease resolve rapidly. On the other hand, prothrombin ratio may remain below 50 per cent, and asthenia and jaundice may persist for more than 2 to 4 weeks before recovery. Ascites may develop within 2 to 4 weeks after the onset of jaundice, although this is uncommon in Western countries. Ascites may develop or persist 4 weeks after the onset of jaundice, particularly in south Asia and death may occur without encephalopathy (Tandon, JClinGastro, 1986; 8:664). Finally, in the most severe cases, severe acute hepatic failure is a transient, but mandatory, stage preceding clinical encephalopathy, thus giving early warning of fulminant or subfulminant hepatic failure. Its recognition is of major importance, since it allows adequate specific and unspecific measures to be taken at maximal efficacy (see under Prevention and curative treatment). Table 2 shows a set of 15 features which require immediate (even nocturnal) consultation with a hepatologist, if they are associated with severe acute hepatic failure.

The syndrome of fulminant and subfulminant hepatic failure

This is the ultimate and more severe stage of acute deterioration of liver function. The main clinical features are hepatic encephalopathy together with direct symptoms of liver cell damage, mainly jaundice, and coagulation disorders. Additional clinical features of varying severity include portal hypertension, respiratory and cardiovascular disorders, renal failure, metabolic abnormalities, and an increased incidence of bacterial and fungal infections. None of them, including encephalopathy, is specific with respect to hepatic failure. Another feature of the syndrome is a decrease in hepatic metabolism of drugs: this is an important aspect as drugs can be aggravating factors of the other components of the syndrome.

Hepatic encephalopathy[2,13-26]

Hepatic encephalopathy is a syndrome of impaired mental status and abnormal neuromuscular function resulting from a major breakdown of liver function. Its clinical and electroencephalographic manifestations are not specific: they may be influenced by extrahepatic factors and similarly occur in other metabolic encephalopathies (Bihari, UpdateIntensCareEmergMed, 1989; 9:1).

Clinical manifestations

Although the course of hepatic encephalopathy may be described in three stages of increasing severity (asterixis, confusion, and coma) (Rueff, Gut, 1973; 14:805), a four-grade classification is most commonly used (Trey, ProgLivDis, 1970; 3:282). Grade 1 is characterized by asterixis, a failure to sustain a fixed posture (the arms extended with dorsiflexion of the wrist and full extension of the fingers). Asterixis is usually bilateral, variable in intensity, and may be found intermittently at sequential examinations. The patient is fully alert but inversion of the sleep rhythm with diurnal somnolence is common. Grade 2 is characterized by confusion responsible for increased drowsiness, agitation, and inappropriate behaviour. Disorientation with respect to space and time, and palilalia are often seen. Asterixis is common and co-ordination is severely impaired. Grade 3 is characterized by the aggravation of grade 2. The patient looks stuporous and often asleep, and phases of restlessness with piercing cries occur spontaneously or are elicited by noises or other physical stimulation. No person-to-person communication is possible when the patient is awake. Grade 4 is characterized by coma. The term 'hepatic coma' should be applied only to this stage. Muscle tone is usually increased, with cogwheel rigidity and some degree of nuchal rigidity. It may be difficult to open the mouth. Myoclonic twitchings are frequent. Deep tendon reflexes may be exaggerated. There may be uni- or bilateral extensor plantar response. The pupils may be in the intermediate position, or slightly dilated or constricted. At least at the onset of coma, the respiratory rate is regular and often above 20/min. Increased levels of plasma benzodiazepine receptor ligands were found in patients with fulminant hepatic failure and grade 4 encephalopathy (Basile, Hepatol, 1994; 19:112) but a causal relationship remains unclear (Rothstein, Hepatol, 1994; 19:248).

Table 2 The 15 features requiring urgent consultation with hepatologist when prothombin ratio decreases below 50 per cent in patients with an acute liver disease (severe acute hepatic failure)

Patient's age <15 or >40 years

Fever >38°C for more than 24 h (risk of herpes simplex hepatitis)

Fever within 2 months after travelling overseas in malaria endemic areas (risk of associated falciparum malaria)

Cutaneous or mucosal haemorrhage

Persistent abdominal pain, clinical ascites

Recent (within a week) ingestion of paracetamol (therapeutic doses) for more than 2 days, especially when associated with fasting or alcohol ingestion

Prothrombin ratio <40% of normal

Serum bilirubin >150 μmol/l

Anaemia or leucopenia

Serum creatinine >100 μmol/l

Pregnancy or postpartum

Surgery within the past 4 weeks

Associated liver cirrhosis, cardiac disease, or chronic renal failure

Human immunodeficiency virus infection

Drug treatment, recently prescribed or changed (especially, anticoagulant therapy, antituberculous drugs, anticonvulsants, antidepressants, non-steroidal anti-inflammatory drugs, immunosuppressive drugs)[a]

[a] The administration of drugs must be interrupted.

Electroencephalographic (EEG) changes

EEG changes are universal in patients with fulminant or subfulminant hepatic failure. They always develop before the onset of clinical encephalopathy. Initial EEG changes include a progressive slowing together with an increased amplitude of the cerebral electrical activity (Kennedy, QJMed, 1973; 167:549). In comatose patients, triphasic waves are common. Further neurological deterioration is associated with a decrease in amplitude and paroxysmal bursts of non-specific triphasic waves. Intermittent flattening of the EEG precedes disparate cerebral activity.

Somatosensory evoked potentials (SSEP)

Median nerve-stimulated evoked potentials have been recorded in Austrian patients with fulminant and subfulminant hepatic failure. The loss of the N70 peak was reported to predict death if emergency liver transplantation was not performed (sedation was used in 56 per cent of patients after the loss of the N70 peak).[13] This finding was not confirmed in France (personal experience).

Extrahepatic factors of encephalopathy

Many extrahepatic factors may contribute to encephalopathy. Inappropriate administration of sedative drugs, or drugs with a sedative side-effect (such as metoclopramide), is one of the most common. These drugs may have been administered before transfer to the liver unit, shortly before the onset of jaundice, or early in its course. Sedative-induced encephalopathy should be suspected particularly when coma is associated with decreased muscle tone of the limbs, rapid frequency waves on EEG, and coagulation factor activity between 30 and 50 per cent (see below). The clinical efficacy of the intravenous administration of flumazenil, a specific antagonist of central receptors to benzodiazepine that allows the rapid reversal of coma secondary to a hitherto unrecognized benzodiazepine administration (Höjer, BMJ, 1990; 301:1308), suggests a recent ingestion of benzodiazepine. The sedative effect of other drugs, such as barbiturates or metoclopramide, is not reversed by flumazenil.

Metabolic factors may also contribute to encephalopathy. One of the most critical is acute renal failure. It may be due to, or aggravated by, causes other than liver failure itself, such as tissue ischaemia or toxicity due to a recent inappropriate ingestion of nephrotoxic drugs. Renal failure may contribute to encephalopathy by decreasing the excretion of endogenous substances, drugs such as ranitidine (Slugg, ArchIntMed, 1992; 152:2325), or drug metabolites with sedative activity such as conjugate metabolites of midazolam (Bauer, Lancet, 1995; 346:145). Hypoglycaemia, hypoxia,[14] hyponatraemia, and associated sepsis (Mizock, ArchIntMed, 1990; 150:443) may also contribute to coma. The existence of all these extrahepatic factors disposing to encephalopathy is a likely explanation of the repeated finding that the grade of encephalopathy is a poorly reliable prognostic factor (see below).

Cerebral oedema, cerebral blood flow, and intracranial pressure[15–26]

Cerebral oedema is a major complication contributing to intracranial hypertension in patients with fulminant or subfulminant hepatic failure.[15] It is not always demonstrable by cerebral computed tomography.[16] Clinically significant cerebral oedema develops in 15[9] to 85 per cent (Ede, SemLivDis, 1986; 6:107) of the patients, but is more frequent in those with a short interval between the onset of jaundice and the onset of clinical encephalopathy.[9,11] During severe bouts of intracranial hypertension, clinical manifestations may include profuse sweating, tachycardia (often above 150/min), cardiac arrhythmias (Jachuk, BMJ, 1975; 1:242; Weston, BrHeartJ, 1976; 38:1179), systemic hypertension, increased hyperventilation with bursts of tachypnoea, and high-grade fever. A more or less permanent decerebration posture may be observed (Conomy, NEJM, 1968; 278:876). Even in these cases, papilloedema is often absent (Hanid, Gut, 1980; 21:866). Sluggish mydriasis, sometimes unilateral, indicates a high risk of brain coning. Cerebral oedema is not prevented by hyperventilation (Ede, JHepatol, 1986; 2:43) and may be aggravated by hypercapnia, hyponatraemia, hypoglycaemia, and hypoxia. The last may be a deleterious consequence of a severe systemic hypotension secondary to untimely administration of sedative drugs with vasodilator properties (unpublished observations).

Cerebral blood flow, as measured by various techniques based on brain clearance of Xenon-133, was reported to be increased, normal, or decreased in patients with grades 3–4 encephalopathy.[17,18] Autoregulation of cerebral blood flow is impaired.[19] In one study, increased cerebral blood flow (suggesting hyperaemia) had a prognostic value and correlated significantly with brain swelling, depth of coma, and fatal outcome.[17] In another study, cerebral blood flow and depressed cerebral metabolic rate of oxygen both increased significantly after mannitol and N-acetylcysteine intravenous infusions, but cerebral blood flow had no prognostic value.[18] Prostaglandin I_2 increases the cerebral metabolic rate of oxygen without modifying the cerebral blood flow.[18]

Cerebral perfusion pressure was found to be related to the mean arterial blood pressure in one study (Munoz, TransplProc, 1993; 25:1776) but not in another (Wendon, Transpl, 1994; 57:165). Cerebral CO_2 reactivity was found to be preserved in hypocapnia, but reduced in hypercapnia, a feature often associated with cerebral vasodilatation and favouring hyperaemia and cerebral oedema.[20]

Intracranial hypertension is a life-threatening complication in patients with fulminant or subfulminant hepatic failure, especially when acute renal failure is present.[16] A CT scan of the brain may be normal.[16] In some patients with paracetamol overdose, full neurological recovery was observed after protracted (24–38 h) periods of refractory severe intracranial hypertension with reduced cerebral perfusion pressure (<50 mmHg).[21] Although invasive monitoring of intracranial pressure has not been shown to improve survival by any controlled trial,[22] its use was advocated (Donovan, Hepatol, 1992; 16:26) and it is now commonly performed in many liver units. Subarachnoid monitors were associated with high rates of fatal intracerebral haemorrhage.[23,24] Epidural transducers are preferable: their complication rate was said to be 3.8 per cent, with a 1 per cent rate of fatal haemorrhage,[23] but a 25 per cent incidence of haemorrhage was also reported (Aldersley, JHepatol, 1994; 21:S52). The benefit of this risky technique remains questionable. In an uncontrolled study, a significant increase in the duration of survival from the onset of grade 4 encephalopathy without change in overall survival was the only encouraging result in patients monitored with an epidural transducer.[25] The overall death rate of 71 French patients managed without intracranial pressure monitoring is in the same range as the rates obtained in centres using the technique (Bernuau, JHepatol, 1996; 25, Suppl. 1:63) (Table 3).

Outcome

Encephalopathy improves clinically at first and this improvement is preceded by the increase in activity of coagulation factors (Bernuau,

JHepatol, 1996; 25, suppl. 1:63). Slowing of the EEG may persist for several days even when the patient is awake (Kennedy, QJMed, 1973; 42:549). Full recovery is usual and has occurred in patients with cerebral oedema documented by cerebral computed tomography (personal experience) and in others with sustained phases of decerebrate posturing (Davis, NEJM, 1968; 278:1248; Hanid, Gut, 1980; 21:866) or protracted phases of flat EEG (Tanaka, Lancet, 1980; ii:1379). Permanent neurological sequelae were observed in a few patients surviving severe encephalopathy after respiratory arrest (O'Brien, Gut, 1987; 28:93) or after invasive monitoring of intracranial pressure[26] and in a few others who survived emergency orthotopic (either total[26] or auxiliary partial (Bismuth, AnnSurg, 1996; 224:712)) liver transplantation.

In non-ventilated patients, sudden respiratory arrest may occur. In patients on mechanical ventilation, bilateral areactive mydriasis, occurrence of polyuria, sudden reduction in the high rate tachycardia, and diffuse decrease in muscle tone are the common manifestations of irreversible damage to the brainstem. Brain death is thought to be the direct cause of death in 35 to 50 per cent of fatal cases, especially in hyperacute[9] or fulminant[11] hepatic failure. In such cases, postmortem examination of the brain shows flattening of the cortical gyri and, sometimes, anatomical aspects of cingulate, uncal, or cerebellar herniation (Gazzard, QJMed, 1975; 44:615). Fatal acute cerebral oedema during a conventional haemodialysis session was observed in patients recovering after paracetamol overdose, not given thiopental for several days, but still receiving a H_2-receptor antagonist (Schiodt, ScaJGastr, 1995; 30:927).

Symptoms of liver cell damage

Jaundice is almost universal. It usually develops before encephalopathy and deepens markedly within a few days. In a small minority of patients, it is still clinically undetectable when early encephalopathy occurs. In these patients, a diagnosis of psychiatric disorder may be made erroneously and potent sedative drugs may be inappropriately administered. In jaundiced patients, foetor hepaticus is often pronounced. The liver is variable in size; it may be normal, small, and not palpable, or may be increased in size, either transiently at the onset of the disease or permanently because of a peculiar aetiology. At autopsy or in patients undergoing liver transplantation, the liver weight is commonly lower than 800 g. The liver is not usually painful, especially in viral fulminant hepatic failure. However, abdominal pain, referred to the right upper or lower abdominal quadrant, may be a symptom in some aetiologies such as poisoning or acute hepatic vein thrombosis. Liver ultrasonography, which allows more accurate evaluation of liver size, may show subclinical ascites, heterogeneous liver echogenicity, and, in patients with subfulminant liver failure, regenerative nodules of 2 to 5 cm in diameter.

Serum aminotransferases are consistently, but unevenly, increased. Values above 50 times the upper limit of normal are common in patients with fulminant hepatic failure, especially at the onset of encephalopathy, or when the liver lesion is acute microvesicular steatosis (personal experience). Values below 30 times the upper limit of normal value are common in patients with subfulminant hepatic failure. Hyperbilirubinaemia, with conjugated bilirubin predominating in a ratio of more than 3:1, is the rule. Serum alkaline phosphatase activity is normal or moderately raised.

Table 3 Influence of invasive intracranial pressure monitoring on the outcome in patients with fulminant and subfulminant hepatic failure

Reference	Total number of patients	Paracetamol hepatitis (%)	Intracranial pressure monitoring (% of total)	Documented intracranial bleeding	Overall death rate (%)	Overall rate of brain death (%)
Ede, JHepatol, 1986; 2:43[1]	55	63	36 (65)	1/36	60[2]	
Vickers, JHepatol, 1988; 7:143	73	45	0 (0)	0	28	9
Sheil, MedJAust, 1991; 154:724	27	7	0 (0)	0	48	?
Lidofsky, Hepatol, 1992; 16:1	60	?	23 (38)[3]	5/23	31[4]	10[5]
Keays, JHepatol, 1993; 18:205	68	64	36 (53)	1/36	60[2]	40
Aggarwal, Hepatol, 1994; 20:1487	34	23	8 (23)	0/8	17[6]	3
Madl, Hepatol, 1994; 20:1487	25	0	7 (28)	0/0	40	32
Bismuth, AnnSurg, 1995; 222:109	139	2	43 (30)	4/43	40[4]	20
Philips, LiverTransplSurg, 1995; 1:436(abstr.)	51	?	51 (100)	4/51	70[4]	23
Bernuau, JHepatol, 1996; 25, suppl. 1:63(abstr.)	71	11	0 (0)	0	32[4]	19

[1] Controlled trial; [2] emergency liver transplantation not available; [3] 3 children; [4] prior to, and within 3 months after, emergency liver transplantation; [5] the cause of death was not provided in 12/19 patients; [6] post-transplantation survival is provided with no indication of the delay.

γ-Glutamyl transpeptidase activity is also increased non-specifically. Serum albumin levels are usually normal but may fall in patients affected by subfulminant hepatic failure. Arterial blood ammonia concentrations are elevated, although values close to normal have been observed.

Portal hypertension and ascites[27]

Portal hypertension documented by a hepatic venous pressure gradient above 5 mmHg is a constant finding in patients with fulminant or subfulminant liver failure (Lebrec, Gut, 1980; 21:962; Navasa, Gut, 1992; 33:965). Increased hepatic venous pressure gradient is related to the severity of liver failure, and is thought to be a consequence of the reduction of the intrahepatic vascular space secondary to the collapse of sinusoids (Navasa, Gut, 1992; 33:965).[27]

Ascites may be clinically detectable in up to 50 per cent of patients affected by acute hepatitis with factor V lower than 50 per cent of normal, with or without clinical encephalopathy.[27] Detection rates are increased by ultrasonography and direct observation by laparotomy when emergency liver transplantation is performed. Ascites is especially common in patients with subfulminant hepatic failure and is associated with more severe liver failure and a higher hepatic venous pressure gradient than those observed in patients without ascites.[27] Both portal hypertension and ascites regress fully in patients who recover spontaneously.

Renal disorders[28]

Renal disorders are common in patients with fulminant or subfulminant hepatic failure. Oliguria is a routine finding. Anuria may occur. Acute renal failure was recorded in 41 (Ritt, Medicine, 1969; 48:151) to 79 per cent (Wilkinson, BMJ, 1974; 1:186) of patients, using increased serum creatinine concentration as criterion. However, normal serum creatinine concentration does not exclude acute

renal failure.[29]. Small variations in normal serum creatinine values may result from large variations in glomerular filtration rate.[29] Among the many factors influencing serum creatinine measurement (hyperbilirubinaemia is a cause of artefactually lowered values when serum creatinine is measured by methods based on the Jaffé reaction (Takabatake, ArchIntMed, 1988; 148:1313; Weber, ClinChem, 1991; 37:695)).[29] In patients with serum bilirubin higher than 200 μmol/l, precipitation or oxidation (O'Leary, ClinChem, 1992; 38:1749) of bilirubin prior to creatinine measurement is useful to eliminate negative interference. Moreover, extracellular volume expansion may also lower serum creatinine (Takabatake, ArchIntMed, 1988; 148:1313). It is likely therefore that the true incidence of acute renal failure in patients with fulminant or subfulminant hepatic failure is being underestimated. It is useful and prudent to consider these patients, even those with normal serum creatinine levels, as being affected by impending acute renal failure, especially when clinically detectable ascites is present.

Various causes of overt acute renal failure may be recognized. As in patients with terminal cirrhosis (Ring-Larsen, Gut, 1981; 22:585), acute renal failure is most often functional in origin and marked renal vasoconstriction with increased plasma renin activity and reduced renal prostaglandin excretion are common (Guarner, Gut, 1987; 28:1643). However, acute tubular necrosis was diagnosed in 22 to 50 per cent of patients with fulminant or subfulminant liver failure (Wilkinson, BMJ, 1974; 1:186; Ring-Larsen, Gut, 1981; 22:585) and acute glomerulonephritis occurred in a few patients older than 60 with fatal fulminant or subfulminant hepatitis B (Oren, AnnIntMed, 1989; 110:691). In one series, the cause of acute renal failure remained undetermined in 18 per cent of patients (Ring-Larsen, Gut, 1981; 22:585). Extrahepatic causes of acute renal failure must be checked and, better still, prevented. Recent ingestion of nephrotoxic drugs (paracetamol (acetaminophen), analgesics, or aminoglycosides) or inappropriate injection of contrast media (Berns, KidneyInt, 1989; 36:730), superimposed bacterial or fungal sepsis with systemic hypotension, or excessive doses of mannitol can be precipitating factors.

The deterioration of renal function often parallels that of liver function and the development or the aggravation of encephalopathy. Severe intracranial hypertension and haemodynamic instability may occur. Continuous haemofiltration, either arteriovenous (Davenport, BMJ, 1987; 295:1028) or venovenous (Hammer, Transpl, 1996; 62:130), may be helpful in some of these patients prior to emergency liver transplantation. As shown experimentally in rats, acute renal failure can impair liver regeneration (Chen, BrJExpPath, 1973; 54:591). The mortality rate of patients with fulminant or subfulminant hepatic failure complicated by increased serum creatinine concentrations is close to 100 per cent (Wilkinson, BMJ, 1974; 1:186; Ring-Larsen, Gut, 1981; 22;585; Nusinovici, Gastr-ClinBiol, 1977; 1:861).

Respiratory and pulmonary disorders[30]

Respiratory condition and chest radiograph are usually normal at the onset of encephalopathy in most patients with fulminant or subfulminant hepatic failure. However, a raised respiratory rate, the first respiratory symptom to appear, often develops as encephalopathy worsens with aggravation of liver failure. This hyperventilation is central in origin. When brain oedema and intracranial hypertension develop, episodes of marked hyperventilation are a symptom of sudden increase in intracranial pressure. In unventilated patients, respiratory arrest may occur at the end of these episodes.

In addition to non-specific pulmonary complications associated with coma (Warren, ClinRadiol, 1978; 29:363), pulmonary oedema may affect up to 37 per cent of patients (Trewby, Gastro, 1978; 74:859) It is associated with an increased incidence of brain oedema and, at least in part, related to the severity of liver failure. Contributing factors can be intrapulmonary vasodilatation and an increase in pulmonary extravascular water. Left heart failure is usually not associated and no significant relation is shared with acute renal failure. Assisted ventilation is required in more than 80 per cent of patients with pulmonary oedema (Trewby, Gastro, 1978; 74:859).

Cardiovascular disorders[31]

Generalized vasodilatation and a hyperdynamic circulation are the characteristic cardiovascular features of fulminant and subfulminant hepatic failure. Generalized vasodilatation results in increased vascular capacitance and in relative hypovolaemia.[31] Central venous pressure is low in most, if not all, patients (Trewby, Gastro, 1978; 74:859). Arterial blood pressure is usually normal during the early stages of encephalopathy but tends to become lower as liver failure progresses (Trewby, ClinSciMolMed, 1977; 52:305). Although several endogenous substances could mediate generalized vasodilatation nitric oxide appears to play a central role (Groszmann, Hepatol, 1994; 20:1359).[32] Any drug with vasodilator activity, no matter how low, may induce severe hypotension and is contraindicated.

The hyperdynamic state which may be present at the very onset of, or even before, encephalopathy, parallels the severity of liver failure. Cardiac output is frequently high, averaging 7 l/min in a series of 100 patients (Trewby, Gastro, 1978; 74:859). Tachycardia is common and has some prognostic value (Rueff, AnnMedInt,

1971; 122:373): its absence in a comatose, normotensive patient with factor V below 50 per cent suggests either acute hepatic failure of moderate severity with sedative-induced encephalopathy or the recent administration of a chronotrope negative drug.

The development of cerebral oedema and intracranial hypertension may aggravate these cardiocirculatory disturbances further. Paroxysmal arterial hypertension, sudden severe systemic hypotension, and bursts of tachycardia over 150 beats/min may occur as well as various cardiac arrhythmias including sinus bradycardia (Weston, BrHeartJ, 1976; 38:1179).

Coagulation disorders[33-38] and bleeding tendency

Coagulation disorders are universal in fulminant and subfulminant hepatic failure. Plasma fibrinogen may not be reduced at the onset of clinical encephalopathy, but lower levels are common in comatose patients. Increased fibrinogen catabolism was reported (Clark, BrJHaemat, 1975; 30:95) and there may be low levels of fibrinogen degradation products.

Activities of factors II, V, VII, IX, and X are commonly less than 30 per cent of normal in comatose patients. Although disseminated intravascular coagulation may be a contributing factor, the decreases are mainly ascribed to reduced synthesis by the damaged liver (Pereira, Gut, 1992; 33:98) and almost always attest a 'true' hepatic encephalopathy (see Chapter 25.4). A less severe decrease (i.e. between 30 and 50 per cent of normal) in coagulation factors indicates a lower grade of liver insufficiency and suggests a predominantly non-hepatic cause of encephalopathy. Plasma factor VIII activity is increased in fulminant hepatic failure of various causes,[35] but is normal or moderately decreased when phalloidin poisoning is the cause (Meili, HelvMedActa, 1970; 35:304; Rueff, Gut, 1973; 14:805).

Evaluation of coagulation factor activity in patients with fulminant or subfulminant hepatic failure has special technical requirements. Assays for factor V activity should be carried out on fresh plasma samples because freezing–thawing of plasma induces a significant additional decrease when factor V is lower than 70 per cent (Denninger, Hepatol, 1992; 16:277A), although this has been disputed (Izumi, Hepatol, 1996; 23:1507). The decrease in factors II, V, VII, and X activities as well as low fibrinogen level are reflected by the protracted prothrombin time (Roberts, Gastro, 1972; 63: 297). The international normalized ratio (INR) (a standardized calculated value of prothrombin time in patients receiving anticoagulants) (Chapter 25.4) was advocated and routinely used in several liver units in order to standardize prothrombin time among patients with fulminant or subfulminant hepatic failure (Munoz, Gastro, 1991; 100:1480; O'Grady, Gastro, 1991; 100:1480).[36] However, it has been established that INR is not valid in patients with liver disease, especially in those with fulminant hepatic failure (personal experience).[37] It was also shown that prothrombin time, expressed as an activity percentage, is a better way to provide a common international scale allowing comparison from different centres.[37]

Coagulation inhibitors, such as antithrombin III, are manufactured by the liver. They are usually decreased, because of decreased synthesis and increased consumption (Langley, EurJClinInv, 1990; 20:627).

Platelet count is often normal when the patient is admitted to the liver unit, but decreases below 100 000/ml within 2 to 5 days while encephalopathy is progressing (see Chapter 25.4). When there is thrombopenia, the capillary bleeding time may be increased (Weston, Gut, 1977; 18:897) or normal (Guillin, AnnMédInt, 1971; 122:605). Protracted capillary bleeding time is often associated with renal failure. Platelet size is often reduced (Weston, Gut, 1977; 18: 897). Platelet dysfunction with deficient aggregation and adhesion has been reported (Rubin, QJMed, 1977; 183:339).

The hypothesis that disseminated intravascular coagulation is an important feature in patients with fulminant or subfulminant hepatic failure, a view apparently supported by several lines of evidence, [38] was put forward in 1970 (Rake, Lancet, 1970; i:533). However, its diagnosis is always debatable when acute hepatic failure is present (see Chapter 25.4). Factor VIII which should be decreased by disseminated intravascular coagulation is increased in most patients with fulminant or subfulminant hepatic failure.[35] Decreased clearance by the acutely injured liver may, at least in part, be responsible for some of the abnormalities underlying the diagnosis of disseminated intravascular coagulation, such as high plasma concentrations of D-dimer.[38] Moreover, heparin therapy does not improve survival (Gazzard, Gut, 1974; 15:9), may be dangerous (personal experience), and is not indicated in supportive management (Hillenbrand, Gut, 1974; 15:83). Thus, even if disseminated intravascular coagulation does occur in patients with fulminant or subfulminant hepatic failure, it plays only a minor role in overall coagulation disorders (Hillenbrand, Gut, 1974; 15:83).

Despite the coagulation defects, spontaneous bleeding tendency is not often life-threatening (Gazzard, Gut, 1974; 15:89). A high incidence of severe haemorrhage was reported in the early 1970s by some authors (Williams, BrMedBull, 1972; 28:114), but not by others (Rueff, Gut, 1973; 14:805). Among 400 patients with fulminant or subfulminant liver failure, clinically significant gastrointestinal bleeding occurred in less than 6 per cent and spontaneous intracranial bleeding in less than 1 per cent (personal experience). Postpartum genital bleeding may remain within normal limits or be life-threatening (Rueff, Gut, 1973; 14:805).

Acid–base disturbances and tissue oxygenation[30,40,41]

Hypocapnia is common and arterial pH is raised above 7.42 in more than 50 per cent of of patients with fulminant or subfulminant hepatic failure. Respiratory alkalosis reflects primary central hyperventilation. Normocapnia or hypercapnia may also be observed. In comatose patients, normocapnia may reflect either respiratory exhaustion when the patient was previously hypocapnic or the relative preservation of the liver function when factor V is above 30 per cent and encephalopathy was preceded by, and due to, inappropriate administration of sedative drugs. Causes of hypercapnia include obstruction of the respiratory passage in a comatose patient, depression of respiratory centres, or exhaustion of respiratory muscles. Arterial oxygen content may be normal or decreased (Bihari, CritCareMed 1985; 13:1034). Blood lactate is usually only moderately elevated, but has been observed above 5 mmol/l in 10 to 50 per cent of patients (Record, Gut, 1975; 16: 144; Bihari, JHepatol, 1985; 1:405). Such severe hyperlactataemia

has a dire prognostic value (Bihari, JHepatol, 1985; 1:405). Blood lactate and arterial pH share only a weak relationship.

Since respiratory alkalosis is the most common acid–base disturbance, any other acid–base disturbance suggests additional contributing factors. Metabolic alkalosis may be due to vomiting, abundant gastric aspiration, bicarbonate therapy, hypokalaemia, and hypovolaemia. Metabolic acidosis may reflect severe acute renal failure, severe diarrhoea, or severe hyperlactataemia; mechanisms may be diverse and may include tissue hypoxia-induced anaerobic metabolism and decreased hepatic clearance.[30,39]

Covert tissue hypoxia, characterized by abnormal dependency of the oxygen uptake upon oxygen supply, is considered to be important at the tissue level in patients with fulminant or subfulminant hepatic failure (Bihari, CritCareMed 1985; 13:1034).[30] Tissue hypoxia and the ensuing hyperlactataemia are thought to result from arteriovenous shunting of the blood, and hence oxygen, at the microcirculatory level (Bihari, JHepatol, 1985; 1:405). Oxygen delivery and tissue oxygen uptake, both of which have some prognostic value (Bihari, CritCareMed, 1985; 13:1034), increased after the infusion of prostacycline (epoprostenol),[30,40] a microcirculatory vasodilator, but also after the infusion of N-acetylcysteine.[40] Epoprostenol also reverses the decrease of oxygen consumption after the administration of vasopressor agents, adrenaline, or noradrenaline.[41]

Disorders of fluids and electrolytes

Water retention is common in patients with fulminant or subfulminant liver failure. The development of electrolyte disorders is governed by the deterioration of liver function, water and electrolyte supplies, the use of drugs such as diuretics and mannitol, and the progression of renal failure. Hypokalaemia due to potassium depletion may occur early in the disease whereas hyperkalaemia may complicate renal failure.

Urinary sodium output lower than 5 mmol/l and urinary sodium/potassium ratio below 1 are common in patients with encephalopathy, with or without ascites. The incidence of hyponatraemia, a marker of excessive free water retention, increases as soon as liver failure deepens. Hyponatraemia lower than 120 mmol/l may contribute to encephalopathy.[4] A shift of sodium into the intracellular compartment (Alam, Gastro, 1977; 72:914) could be an additional factor contributing to hyponatraemia. Overt acute renal failure may aggravate hyponatraemia and renal replacement therapy may be required especially during the waiting period for a liver graft (Larner, BMJ, 1988; 297:1514).

Hypophosphataemia

Hypophosphataemia is common, especially in patients with fulminant hepatic failure due to paracetamol (acetaminophen) overdose. Respiratory alkalosis and mandatory dextrose infusions contribute to hypophosphataemia which may coexist with hypercreatininaemia (Davenport, BMJ, 1988; 296:131). Severe hypophosphataemia is a recognized factor of respiratory failure, but whether it could be an aggravating factor of encephalopathy is unproved (Knochel, Hepatol, 1989; 9:504).

Metabolism
Glucose

Blood glucose is often in the lower range of normal. Hypoglycaemia, which may be a symptom of bacterial sepsis and suggests failure of gluconeogenesis, may occur and, sometimes recurs (Samson, Gastro, 1967; 53:291). Asymptomatic hypoglycaemia may be an unexpected aggravating factor of encephalopathy. In comatose patients, blood glucose should be monitored every 2 h.

Lipids and ketone bodies

Low plasma cholesterol is common in patients with fulminant and subfulminant liver failure. Plasma free fatty acids are increased (Record, Gut, 1975; 16:144) but do not contribute to encephalopathy.

Arterial ketone bodies are altered in patients with severe acute hepatic failure. The arterial ketone body ratio (KBR) (acetoacetate / 3β-hydroxybutyrate), possibly reflecting hepatic mitochondrial redox potential, is decreased, especially in patients with a fatal outcome (Scaiola, Hepatogast, 1990; 37:413), and this decrease was found to precede by 3 days or more the appearance of clinical encephalopathy (Saibara, Liver, 1992; 12:392) (see under Prognosis). However, whether KBR adequately reflects the mitochondrial energy charge is controversial (Matsushita, Hepatol, 1994; 20:331; Shimahara, Transpl, 1996; 61:1664; Kawasaki, Transpl, 1996; 61:666).

Nitrogen

Hyperammonaemia is very common (Opolon, AnnMedInt, 1970; 121:1) but is not useful in prognosis. It reflects renal failure, at least in part. Azotaemia, usually low, increases with renal failure. Plasma concentrations of most amino acids are increased but those of branched chain amino acids are normal. Increased concentrations of plasma amino acids are not related to the grade of encephalopathy (Record, EurJClinInv, 1976; 6:387).

Vitamins

Plasma concentrations of pyridoxal-5'-phosphate, the biologically active coenzyme form of vitamin B_6, are increased within a week of the onset of symptoms and are not returned to normal by the administration of pyridoxine hydrochloride (Rossouw, ScaJGast, 1977; 12:123).

Miscellaneous
Pancreatitis

Acute pancreatitis occurred in a few patients (Parbhoo, Gut, 1973; 14:428). The P3 isoenzyme of amylase and pancreatic lipase were increased in one-third of patients (Ede, Gut, 1988; 29:778). Various pancreatic enzymes are unrelated to prognosis.

Blood cells

Red blood cell and platelet counts are usually normal at the onset of encephalopathy. As soon as liver function declines further, progressive non-regenerative anaemia and thrombopenia below 100 000/ml develop. Aplastic anaemia was observed in several cases

of fatal severe acute hepatitis of undetermined origin (Watananukul, ArchIntMed, 1977; 137:898) and may develop after emergency liver transplantation (Cattral, Hepatol, 1994; 20:813). The association of haemolysis with severe acute, fulminant, or subfulminant hepatic failure strongly suggests Wilson's disease.[42] The frequent increase in leucocyte count (Opolon, AnnMedInt, 1971; 122:701) reflects hypovolaemia, bacterial infection, or both.

Bacterial and fungal infections[43]

Bacterial infections are both frequent events and aggravating factors in patients with fulminant or subfulminant hepatic failure. Spontaneous bacterial peritonitis is a risk when ascites is present (Chu, Hepatol, 1992; 15:799). Daily and standardized microbiological monitoring is recommended in these patients, especially when invasive procedures are used. Severity of liver failure itself is the main factor contributing to deleterious infections.

A variety of disorders including defective opsonization and complement deficiency (Wyke, Gut, 1980; 21:643), reduced neutrophil adherence (Altin, Gut, 1983; 24:746), decrease in the plasma levels of the opsonic glycoprotein fibronectin (Acharya, JHepatol, 1995; 23:8), reduced Kupffer cell function (Canalese, Gut, 1982; 23:265), and decreased hepatic production of hepatocyte-growth-factor-like/macrophage-stimulating protein (Harrison, Lancet, 1994; 344:27), have been documented and may well contribute to the altered antimicrobial host defences *in vivo*.

The overall incidence of proven bacterial infections was 80 per cent in a prospective study of 50 patients (Rolando, Hepatol, 1990; 11:49). Empirical antibiotic therapy in 90 per cent of them did not obviate a 25 per cent rate of positive cultures and a 20 per cent rate of bacteraemia. Each of the following was present in 50 per cent of the cases with bacterial infection: absence of fever or raised peripheral white cell count; infection of the respiratory tract, usually in mechanically ventilated patients; *Staphylococcus aureus* as the responsible bacterium. In a controlled trial of 104 patients with at least grade 2 encephalopathy, early administration of a selective parenteral and enteral antimicrobial regimen did not improve survival rate despite reducing the incidence of bacterial infections.[43]

Fungal infections, often disseminated, may also occur. Their overall, prospectively evaluated, incidence was 32 per cent in one study (Rolando, JHepatol, 1991; 12:1). *Candida albicans* and *Aspergillus fumigatus* (Walsh, ArchIntMed, 1983; 143:1189) were the fungi most frequently isolated. Markedly raised leucocytosis and fungal infection were always associated. Fungal infections clearly aggravate both encephalopathy and renal failure and death rate was 100 per cent when they remained untreated.

Cytokines

The cytokine pattern is seriously altered in patients with fulminant and subfulminant hepatic failure. Production of both tumour necrosis factor and interleukin-1 by circulating monocytes is enhanced together with decreased production of interleukin-2 (Muto, Lancet, 1998; ii:72). Increased plasma levels of tumour necrosis factor and interleukin-6 correlate with various features of terminal multiple organ failure but not with endotoxaemia (Sheron, Hepatol, 1990; 12:939). Plasma capacity to inhibit tumour necrosis factor *in vitro* is significantly lowered (Keane, ClinSci, 1996; 90:77). Whether this cytokine pattern is deleterious for liver tissue regeneration is unknown.

Drug metabolism and pharmacokinetics[44]

As in cirrhosis, sensitivity to either normal or toxic effects of drugs in various organs such as brain and kidney is increased.[44] Thus, any deleterious influence of a drug may mimick actual aggravation of liver failure and alter the accuracy of prognostic evaluation.

Numerous studies of drug metabolism and pharmacokinetics performed in cirrhotic patients appear to show that the metabolism of drugs and their pharmacokinetics are markedly altered in patients with fulminant or subfulminant liver failure. These changes in both the distribution and the elimination of drugs[44] result from the decrease in the capacity of the failing liver to metabolize drugs adequately. In 90 per cent of hepatectomized rats, the drug metabolizing system CYPIIB1/2 is reduced by 50 per cent (Tygstrup, JHepatol, 1996; 25:72). Moreover, because of the frequent association with renal failure, metabolism and elimination of water-soluble drugs or their metabolites, such as conjugate metabolites of midazolam (Bauer, Lancet, 1995; 346:145), are also often markedly altered.

It is recommended that drug use in patients with fulminant or subfulminant liver failure be severely restricted, and similar restriction is advocated in patients with severe acute liver failure. In the latter, any hepatotoxic drug and any sedative must be avoided.

Diagnosis

The combination of hepatic symptoms of acute non-alcoholic liver disease with jaundice, decrease in prothrombin and factor V activities, and encephalopathy usually make the diagnosis of fulminant or subfulminant liver failure easy. Difficulties may arise when abnormal behaviour heralding encephalopathy develops before jaundice (see above).

Various clinical situations may lead to an incorrect diagnosis. In a few patients with severe sepsis (usually intra-abdominal and associated with symptoms of septic shock) liver features may closely mimic fulminant hepatic failure (Dirix, QJMed, 1989; 73:1037). In a febrile patient living in, or recently returned from, developing countries in the tropics, the association of jaundice, encephalopathy, and prolonged prothrombin time may mimic fulminant hepatic failure although the patient is in fact suffering from falciparum malaria. These patients recover with specific antimalarial treatment (Joshi, Liver, 1986; 6:357). In a febrile patient at risk of having contracted malaria, urgent administration of quinine is never contra-indicated by hepatic symptoms or an associated acute liver disease such as hepatitis A (Bernuau, JHepatol, 1994; 21:S137).

In any patient with fulminant or subfulminant hepatic failure, the lack of specificity of the symptoms raises diagnostic questions. It must always be determined whether the symptoms were aggravated, or even fully induced, by factors other than hepatic failure alone. For example, inappropriately ingested or injected drugs may be such a factor. Answering these questions will allow a better understanding of the complex syndrome of the patient and, in some, may obviate an inappropriate decision for emergency liver transplantation.

Spontaneous survival rate (Table 4)

The spontaneous (without liver transplantation) overall survival rate of patients affected by fulminant or subfulminant hepatic failure is about 50 per cent[36] in patients with paracetamol overdose, but lower than 50 per cent when the cause is not paracetamol poisoning. Differences in spontaneous survival rates from different centres reflect variations in aetiology, age of patients, treatment modalities, and also the number of patients reported. The survival rate may be erroneously high in small series,[45] but ranges between 8 and 37 per cent when only the series including more than 40 patients are considered (Table 4). Twenty to 25 per cent is a reasonable estimate of the average spontaneous recovery rate of patients affected by fulminant or subfulminant hepatic failure of various causes, except paracetamol overdose. Data from multicentre studies including more than 100 patients (Table 5) do not differ significantly from those of single-centre series.

Overall course

The outcome will depend on several variables. The cause of the liver disease, the extent of liver cell destruction, the regenerative capacity of the uninjured liver parenchyma, the resistance of the patient (bearing in mind pre-existing extrahepatic visceral dysfunction), and ultimately therapeutic and iatrogenic factors are all important.

Cessation and extent of liver cell destruction

The cessation of liver cell destruction and its extent, rather than liver regeneration, appear to be the most critical variables governing outcome. Liver specimens obtained by biopsy during encephalopathy show that survival rate is significantly increased in patients with a hepatocyte volume of more than 35 per cent (Scotto, Gut, 1973; 14:927) as well as in those with less than 70 per cent necrosis (Donaldson, Hepatol, 1993; 18:1370). Markers of liver regeneration in liver tissue are not more abundant in patients with fulminant rather than those with acute non-fulminant hepatitis (Milandri, Gut, 1980; 21:423).[46] These important findings indicate that the survival of patients affected by acute hepatic injury is closely linked to the speed and efficacy of preventive and, when possible, curative measures aimed at limiting the destruction of liver parenchyma[46] (see below under Treatment). In patients with subfulminant (or late-onset) hepatic failure, the protracted course is associated with a persistently high serum aminotransferase activity probably indicating that liver tissue is still being destroyed.

Liver regeneration[47,48]

This is a highly complex process influenced by many subtances, some distributed systemically and others of local importance. In diseased liver tissue, human hepatocyte growth factor (hHGF), a polyvalent cytokine with a potent mitogenic effect on hepatocytes (Boros, Lancet, 1995; 345:293), was shown to be located in polymorphonuclear cells and in biliary epithelial cells (Sakaguchi, Hepatol, 1994; 19:1157). hHGF can play a central role as a trigger of liver regeneration. In patients with fulminant hepatic failure, plasma hHGF is closely related to the grade of coma (Tsubouchi, Hepatol, 1989; 9:875) and is higher in those who die (Hughes, JHepatol,

Table 4 Overall spontaneous[1] survival in patients affected by fulminant or subfulminant hepatic failure (paracetamol poisoning excluded): series including more than 40 patients managed in a single centre and reported after 1970

Reference	Number of patients	Acute hepatitis B (%)	Overall survival (%)	Country	Dates of the study
Caroli, PresseMed, 1971; 79:463	61	—	22	France	1965–70
Rueff, AnnMedInt, 1971; 122:373	77	—	17	France	1952–69
Gazzard, QJMed, 1975; 176:615	86	—	20	England	1967–74
Nusinovici, GastrClinBiol, 1977; 1:875	137	—	17	France	1965–75
Gimson, Gut, 1983; 24:1194	73	25	22	England	1977–81
Govindarajan, Gastro, 1984; 86:1417	71	100	35	USA	1969–83
Papaevangelou, Hepatol, 1984; 4:369	65	74	14	Greece	1981–83
Gimson, Hepatol, 1986; 6:288[2]	47	4	19	England	1972–84
Bernuau, Hepatol, 1986; 6:648	115	100	23	France	1972–81
Tandon, JClinGastro, 1986; 8:664	145	36	29	India	1976–81
Sheen, JFormosanMedAss, 1986; 85:679	62	34	8	Taiwan	1980–82
O'Grady, Gastro, 1989; 97:439[3]	240	28	19	England	1973–85
O'Grady, Gastro, 1989; 97:439[4]	42	18	23	England	1986–87
Rassam, AnnSaudiMed, 1991; 11:167	47	30	26	Iraq	1984–85
Ellis, JHepatol, 1995; 23:363[5]	41	0	12	England	1986–92
Huo, JGastrHepatol, 1996; 11:560	61	10	15	Taiwan	1982–94
Schiodt, Hepatol, 1996; 23:713	59	31	37	Denmark	1978–93
Acharya, Hepatol, 1996; 23:1448	423	28	34	India	1987–93

[1] Without emergency liver transplantation; [2] late-onset hepatic failure (one patient transplanted) probably includes some of the patients studied by Gimson (1983); [3] includes most of the patients studied by Gimson (1986); [4] 12 patients transplanted; [5] late-onset hepatic failure (21 patients transplanted) probably includes some of the patients studied by O'Grady (1989) (to compare with Gimson (1986)).

1994; 20:106). Moreover, hHGF can express an antihepatitis effect *in vivo* (Ishiki, Hepatol, 1992; 16:1227).

Plasma from patients with fulminant hepatic failure has been shown to contain an inhibitor of hepatic DNA synthesis in regenerating rat hepatocytes, and this could be a factor in delaying liver regeneration in these patients (Yamada, Hepatol, 1994; 19:133). Liver regeneration can be depressed by interferon (Frayssinet, Nature, 1973; 245:146) or glucocorticoids (Tsukamoto, Gut, 1989; 30:387) and can be increased by the immunostimulant OK-432 (Kato, Hepatol, 1994; 19:1241) or granulocyte colony-stimulating factor (Theocharis, EurJGastrHepatol, 1996; 8:805).

Clinical evaluation of liver regeneration is still difficult. Increased serum α-fetoprotein, a recognized marker of liver regeneration, although common in fulminant viral hepatitis, is not always associated with survival (Bloomer, Gastro, 1975; 68:342; Murray-Lyon, Gut, 1976; 17:76).[14] Moreover, in non-viral fulminant liver failure, recovery may occur with no increase in serum α-fetoprotein.

Spontaneous recovery

Spontaneous recovery is heralded hours or days before neurological improvement by a progressive increase in coagulation factor activity up to 50 per cent (Bernuau, JHepatol, 1996; 25). Factor V activity increases first and most rapidly (personal experience). The simultaneous decrease in serum aminotransferase activity probably reflects the end of parenchymal destruction.

Spontaneous recovery most often occurs in patients younger than 30 years affected by fulminant liver failure. The following features are common: acute viral hepatitis or paracetamol overdose; pre-encephalopathic consumption of sedative or antiemetic drugs; early admission to a liver unit before, or at the very onset of, encephalopathy; factor V level uncommonly decreased below 15 per cent of normal; absence of severe renal failure and deep coma. However, in these young patients with fulminant viral hepatitis or paracetamol overdose, spontaneous recovery may occur despite the presence of aggravating factors, such as deep coma and decerebrate rigidity, for one or several days (Davis, NEJM, 1968; 278:1248; Hanid, Gut, 1980; 21:866). Full recovery of the liver is the rule in patients surviving fulminant viral hepatitis (Karvountzis, Gastro, 1974; 67:870).

Downhill course and fatal outcome

An unfavourable course is usually characterized by the persistence of decreased (lower than 30 per cent of normal) coagulation factor activity, especially factor V, and the persistence or the short-term recurrence of grade 3 to 4 encephalopathy.

When the disease follows a fulminant course, deep coma is present. Often the patient was admitted to the liver unit more than 24 h after the onset of encephalopathy or even after the onset of coma. Acute renal failure is common and brain death is the major lethal factor. In a few cases, brain death occurs while liver function is improving (Gazzard, QJMed, 1975; 44:615).

Table 5 Overall spontaneous survival in patients affected by fulminant or subfulminant hepatic failure (paracetamol poisoning excluded): multicentre series including more than 100 patients reported after 1970

Reference	Number of patients	Overall survival (%)	Country	Dates of the study
Trey, CanMedAssJ, 1972; 106:525	284	18	USA	1968–70
Acute Hepatic Failure Study Group, Gastro, 1979; 77:A33	188	26	USA	
Smedile, In: Verme, Bonino, Rizzetto, eds. *Viral hepatitis and delta infection*. New York: Alan R Liss, 1983; 237	102	21	Europe	
Saracco, AnnIntMed, 1988; 108:380	377	41	Worldwide	
Takahashi, JGastroHepatol, 1991; 6:159	236	30	Japan	1983–87

When the disease follows a subfulminant course, a protracted phase of normal consciousness with abnormal EEG is common, even when prothrombin or factor V is lower than 20 per cent of normal. Serum aminotransferases decrease progressively and serum α-fetoprotein remains low or decreasing. A small nodular liver is usually found by ultrasonography. Large volume ascites is frequent after the fourth or fifth week of jaundice.[10] Temporary improvement of clinical encephalopathy may still occur (personal experience). Brain death is uncommon, but bacterial sepsis is the major risk. The incidence of death caused by fulminant and subfulminant hepatic failure has been calculated and reaches 3.5 per million in the United States[8] but only 1.7 per million in France (personal evaluation).

Pathology and pathogenesis

Massive liver cell necrosis is the most frequent liver lesion in patients affected by fulminant and subfulminant hepatic failure. Ultrastructural pathological examination does not allow the identification of minor ischaemic lesions or differentiation between viral and non-viral causes (McCaul, JHepatol, 1986; 276).

The pathogenesis of fulminant and subfulminant hepatic failure is poorly understood. The key question is why liver cell necrosis becomes so widespread and massive so quickly. It is possible that the process is multifactorial. In patients with fulminant or subfulminant hepatic failure in Taiwan, either multiple viral infections[49] or hepatotoxic drugs such as isoniazid and rifampicin in HBsAg carriers,[50] were found. HCV-RNA was found in several HBsAg positive patients with fulminant hepatitis in Paris.[51] Drugs may be associated with viral infections: recent ingestion of paracetamol and/or non-steroidal anti-inflammatory drugs was found to be common in severe infections due to viral hepatitis type A (Bernuau, Hepatol, 1988; 8:1428). Recent use of steroids or non-steroidal anti-inflammatory drugs commonly precedes fulminant Herpes simplex hepatitis (Bernuau, Hepatol, 1988; 8:1428). Infections combined with the acquired immune deficiency syndrome are not contributing factors for fulminant viral hepatitis in drug addicts (Amoroso, BMJ, 1986; 292).

Several mechanisms lead to liver cell death. Hypoxia or toxins may cause liver cell necrosis and an excess of hepatotoxins such as amanitin may have a massive effect. However, virus infection (usually not cytopathogenic), hepatotoxic parenteral drugs, and hepatotoxic drug metabolites (such as in paracetamol hepatototxicity), generally cause limited rather than massive liver cell necrosis, and there must, therefore, be some additional and still unrecognized factors to explain the unrestricted spread of liver tissue destruction.

Apoptosis, although a frequent finding in liver diseases (Patel, Hepatol, 1995; 21:1725), could play a role in massive liver cell necrosis. In mice, Fas-mediated apoptosis may occur when Fas antigen, a transmembrane protein expressed in liver tissue, interacts with its ligand or an anti-Fas antibody.[52] Administration of anti-Fas agonist antibody induced widespread hepatic apoptosis and fatal fulminant hepatic failure (Ogasarawa, Nature, 1993; 364:806) while the anti-apoptotic protein Bcl-2 protects transgenic mice against fatal hepatic Fas-mediated apoptosis.[52] Cocaine, the main component of 'crack', induces apoptotic death of hepatocytes in mice (Cascales, Hepatol, 1994; 20:992) and an unusual cluster of fatal fulminant hepatitis B was observed in 'crack' users (Comer, AmJGastr, 1991; 86:331).

Complement is an important effector of the immune response. Following its activation, it may form a cytolytic membrane attack complex (MAC) at cell membranes. This MAC was shown to be present only on hepatocytes surrounding necrotic areas in patients with fulminant or acute non-fulminant hepatitis[53] and thus may have a role in the pathogenesis of liver cell necrosis.

Causes (Table 6)
General epidemiology

No study evaluating the true incidence of fulminant and subfulminant hepatic failure is available. A case-fatality rate of 0.8 to 0.9 per cent for symptomatic, icteric acute hepatitis was found in Australia (McNeil, MedJAust 1984;141:637) and in the United States.[8] Assuming the generally agreed spontaneous survival rate of 20 to 25 per cent in patients with fulminant and subfulminant hepatic failure, its incidence would range between 1 and 1.2 per cent of the icteric cases of acute hepatitis.

Distribution of the causes throughout the world is inhomogeneous. Viral hepatitis, especially that due to hepatitis B, is more prevalent in developing than in developed countries.[12,54] The opposite is true for drug-induced hepatitis but this will be modified as health care level improves in, and drugs and medicines reach, developing countries. The incidence of toxic liver injury is influenced by the use of herbal medicines and the worldwide spread of illicit substances.

Table 6 Causes of fulminant or subfulminant hepatic failure

Acute viral hepatitis
Hepatitis A virus
Hepatitis B virus
    (primary infection, reactivation, other causes in chronic HBV carriers)
Hepatitis D virus (coinfection, superinfection)
Hepatitis C virus
Hepatitis E virus (epidemic non-A, non-B virus)
Hepatitis G virus
Acute infections with herpes viruses
    Herpes simplex viruses (types I and II)
    Varicelle-zoster virus
    Cytomegalovirus
    Epstein–Barr virus
    Human herpesvirus 6
Acute infections with other viruses
    Human parvovirus B19
    Adenovirus
    Viral haemorrhagic fever
    Coxsackie B virus

Acute poisoning
Paracetamol hepatotoxicity (overdose, therapeutic misadventure)
Amanita phalloides
Illicit substances
Atractylis gummifera L
Pennaroia
Acute drug-induced hepatitis

Other causes
Hypoxic liver cell necrosis
    (ischaemia, severe hypoxia, hyperthermia, heat stroke)
Autoimmune chronic active hepatitis
Syncytial giant-cell hepatitis
Wilson's disease
Microvesicular steatosis (drugs, Reye's syndrome, acute fatty liver of pregnancy,
    actractylis gummifera L)
Obstruction of the hepatic veins (Budd–Chiari syndrome, veno-occlusive disease
    of the liver)
Massive malignant infiltration of the liver
Complications of liver transplantation
Partial hepatectomy

Acute viral hepatitis

The incidence of serologically demonstrated acute viral hepatitis as a cause of fulminant or subfulminant hepatic failure varies from 13 per cent in London to 50 per cent in France (Tibbs, JHepatol 1995; 22 (Suppl. 1): 8) and 90 per cent in India.[12]

Acute hepatitis A

The presense of immunoglobulin M (IgM) antibody to hepatitis A virus (HAV) is diagnostic. Between 0.05 and 0.01 per cent of patients with symptoms are at risk of developing fulminant or subfulminant hepatic failure (Editorial, Lancet, 1990; 336:1158). Table 7 shows the prevalence of patients affected by hepatitis A among patients with fulminant viral hepatitis. The course of the illness is much more often fulminant than subfulminant (Tibbs, JHepatol, 1995; 22, suppl. 1:68). Recent ingestion of antiemetic drugs is common (J. Bernuau, personal experience). The overall survival rate ranges between 33 and 62 per cent (Table 7) (Bernuau, Hepatol, 1983; 3: 821). Death will usually result when encephalopathy develops during a short-term (within 3 months) recurrence of the disease (Ritt, Medicine, 1969; 48:151; personal experience) and emergency liver transplantation is indicated (Boudjema, Lancet, 1993; 342: 778).

Acute hepatitis associated with hepatitis B virus infection

Hepatitis B virus (HBV) infection is a major contributing factor to fulminant and subfulminant hepatic failure worldwide.[54] However, acute hepatitis type B, acute HBV reactivation, and chronic HBV carriage without HBV replication must be distinguished in order to clarify the variety of associated factors which actually trigger fulminant or subfulminant hepatic failure; these include hepatitis D virus (HDV) and drugs.

Acute hepatitis B

The presence of antibody to hepatitis B core antigen type IgM (IgM anti-HBc) is diagnostic. Close to 1 per cent of symptomatic patients with the disease are at risk of developing fulminant or subfulminant liver failure (Lettau, NEJM, 1987; 317:1256).[8] A fulminant course is much more common. Females are at increased risk (Woolf, BMJ, 1976; 2:669; Gimson, Gut, 1983; 24:615).[55] The prevalence of

Table 7 Fulminant viral hepatitis: worldwide prevalences of aetiologies and survival rates among all cases of fulminant and subfulminant hepatic failure

	Athens[a]	London[b]	Paris[c]	Delhi[d]	USA[e]	Japan[f]
HAV prevalence (%)	1.5	5	4	1.7	3	7.6
Survival (%)		63	50	43	33	61
HBV prevalence (%)	70	8	35	28	60	47
Survival (%)	12	41	22	33	33	36
HDV prevalence (%)	3		11	4		
Survival (%)			45	31		
NANB prevalence (%)	24.5	16	17	62	34	45
Survival (%)	19	26	18	33	13	19

[a] Papaevangelou, Hepatol, 1984; 4:369.
[b] Tibbs, JHepatol, 1995; 22 (Suppl. 1):68.
[c] Bernuau, Benhamou, personal data.
[d] Acharya, Hepatol, 1996; 23:1448.
[e] Acute Hepatic Failure Study Group, Gastro, 1979; 77:A33.
[f] Takahashi, JGastroHepatol, 1991; 6:159.

acute hepatitis B compared with other causes of fulminant viral hepatitis is shown in Table 7.

Fulminant hepatitis B more usually occurs in young adults, often drug addicts or their sexual partners, and in female sexual partners of asymptomatic male HBV chronic carriers (Fagan, Lancet 1986; ii:538), but also older patients may be affected when unexpectedly contaminated in a hospital (Oren, AnnIntMed,1989; 110:691). In patients older than 60, mortality of acute hepatitis B is between 5 and 8 per cent (Oren, AnnIntMed,1989; 110:691). In some countries, the disease was reported to follow recent blood tranfusions in 30 to 40 per cent of cases (Papaevangelou, Hepatol, 1984; 4:369; Takahashi, J GastrHepatol, 1991; 6:159) and, in some others result from injections of traditional medicines (Boxall, BMJ, 1987; 295:760).

Serum hepatitis B surface antigen (HBsAg) was shown by radioimmunoassay to be lacking in 15 to 21 per cent of patients (Papaevangelou, Hepatol, 1984; 4:369).[55] In one French study, the survival rate in HBsAg-negative patients (47 per cent) was considerably higher than that in HBsAg-positive patients (17 per cent).[55] Irreversible cerebral oedema was the main cause of death in 50 per cent of those who died. Intravenous anti-HBs immunoglobulins had no beneficial effect (Acute Hepatic Failure Study Group, AnnIntMed, 1977; 86:272).

The pathogenesis of the fulminant course of acute HBV infection is poorly understood. Early disappearance of HBsAg, early appearance of anti-HBs antibody (Trepo, Gut, 1976; 17:10; Woolfe, BMJ, 1976; 2:669), and the low detection rate (0 to 35 per cent) of serum HBV genome (HBV-DNA) in patients with fulminant hepatitis type B (Bréchot, BMJ, 1984; 288:270; De Cock, AnnIntMed,1986; 105:546; Tassopoulos, JHepatol,1986; 2:410; Mas, Hepatol, 1990; 11:1062) support the concept that rapid viral elimination occurs earlier and faster in fulminant than in non-fulminant cases of acute hepatitis type B (Trepo, Gut, 1976; 17:10; Woolfe, BMJ, 1976; 2:669). The rate of recurrent HBV infection in the graft after emergency liver transplantation is low in these patients (Samuel, Lancet, 1991; 337:813). A high survival rate was found in French patients with HBsAg-negative fulminant hepatitis B[55] as well as in English patients with early disappearance of pre-S2 antigen and early appearance of anti-HBs antibody (Brahm, JHepatol, 1991; 13:49). Thus, early HBV clearance seems to have a favourable prognostic influence and other factors must be involved in massive liver necrosis, liver recovery, and the outcome of patients with fulminant hepatitis B.

Seronegative acute hepatitis B

Detection of HBV-DNA liver tissue by the polymerase chain reaction was reported in some American patients with fulminant or subfulminant hepatic failure without any serological markers of HBV infection (Mason, Hepatol, 1996; 24:1361.[56] Isolated serum HBV-DNA was found in 8 otherwise seronegative Japanese patients (Inokuchi, JHepatol, 1996; 24:258).

Reactivation of HBV infection[57]

Reactivation of HBV infection is characterized by the reappearance of serum HBV-DNA, indicating a rather high level of HBV replication, in patients previously affected by chronic HBV infection with no, or low level of, viral replication.[57] It may be asymptomatic or induce acute hepatitis or, in some cases, massive liver cell necrosis. When severe acute liver failure develops during HBV reactivation, low levels of IgM anti-HBc antibody are commonly detected, but serum HBV-DNA and serum HBeAg may, or may not, be detectable.

Reactivation of HBV infection complicated by encephalopathy usually follows a subfulminant course. It may occur spontaneously, especially in male subjects with cirrhosis.[57] Recognized causes include recent withdrawal of antineoplastic or immunosuppressive chemotherapy (Galbraith, Lancet, 1975; ii:528; Flowers, AnnIntMed, 1990; 112:381), recent bone marrow allotransplantation (Pariente, DigDisSci, 1988; 33:1185), or cytotoxic therapy (Lok, Gastro, 1991; 100:182). Recent infection with human immunodeficiency virus-1 (HIV-1) may induce HBV reactivation[57] and also, in a few previously anti-HBs antibody positive patients, IgM anti-HBc positive fulminant hepatitis B (personal experience).

Therapeutic strategies in HBV reactivation include antiviral chemotherapy and, in a few HIV-negative and HBV-DNA-negative patients, emergency liver transplantation (see below).

Infection with HBV mutants[58-60]

Several cases of fulminant hepatitis were shown to be caused by recent infection with HBV mutants defective in the pre-core region and thus unable to encode HBe antigen (Kosaka, Gastro, 1991; 100: 1087).

The incidence of mutations in the pre-core or core region of the HBV genome isolated from patients with fulminant hepatitis B varies according to the geographical area. Most cases were found in patients in their fifties from Japan (Kosaka, Gastro, 1991; 100:1087; Ehata, JCI, 1993; 91:206; Aye, DigDisSci, 1994; 39:1281),[58] , [59]but also from Greece (Carman, Hepatol, 1991; 14:219) and Israël (Liang, NEJM, 1991; 324:1705), but the mutations were uncommon in France (Feray, JHepatol, 1993; 18:119), in the United States (Laskus, Gastro, 1993; 105:1173), and in children from Taiwan (Hsu, JInfDis, 1995; 171:776). A causal role of these hepatitis B virus mutants in fulminant hepatitis B is suggested by the development of sometimes fatal anti-HBe positive fulminant hepatitis B in patients previously contaminated by anti-HBe positive HBsAg chronic carriers in whom the viral mutants were found (Fagan, Lancet, 1986; ii:538; Liang, NEJM, 1991; 324:1705; Yotsumoto, Hepatol, 1992; 16:31). An enhanced replication of the mutants could be a contributing factor in the development of fulminant hepatitis (Hasegawa, JVirol, 1994; 68:651). However, in some patients, the similarity of the pre-core mutant genome between the patient source and the subject who developed fulminant hepatitis suggests that the acute liver disease is more dependent on host factors than on viral variations.[61] No specific mutation of the HBV genome was found in European patients with fulminant hepatitis B (Sterneck, Hepatol, 1996; 24:300). An HBsAg mutant was associated with a fatal case of reactivation (Carman, Lancet, 1995; 345:1406).

Multiple viral infections

Multiple viral infection with other hepatotropic viruses is the most common cause of fulminant and subfulminant hepatitis in areas endemic for hepatitis B virus such as Taiwan.[49] A double acute infection with hepatitis B virus and hepatitis A virus may be observed, with or without fulminant hepatic failure (Grijm, JHepatol, 1985, suppl. 1:S60). Concurrent infections with delta virus or hepatitis C virus may occur and are detailed below.

Causal factors of fulminant and subfulminant hepatic failure in HBV chronic carriers

HBV chronic carriage is a key factor predisposing to fulminant or subfulminant hepatic failure if an additional liver injury occurs.[54] Recognized causes triggering fulminant or subfulminant hepatic failure in HBV chronic carriers include acute viral hepatitis due to HAV (Tassopoulos, Gastro, 1987; 92:1844) or to a non-A, non-B virus[54] and drug-induced hepatitis. In Taiwan, fatal cases of isoniazid-induced hepatitis were observed, predominantly in

HBsAg chronic carriers (Wu, Gastro, 1990; 98:502). Superinfection with delta virus or hepatitis C virus are detailed below.

Acute infection with hepatitis D virus[62,63]

Acute infection with HDV, a defective virus which requires the presence of HBV for multiplication, can develop as either a coinfection with HBV or a superinfection in chronic HBV carriers. HBV replication is often, but not always, interrupted. Parenteral drug abusers are frequently affected (Lettau, NEJM, 1987; 317: 1256). The diagnosis of acute infection with HDV is established by the presence of HDV antigen, anti-HDV antibody of IgM type, or HDV-RNA (Di Bisceglie, Hepatol, 1989; 6:1014). The last may be detected in 15 per cent of patients with fulminant hepatitis D (Mas, Hepatol, 1990; 11:1062).

Coinfection with HBV and HDV (HDV coinfection)

Fulminant HDV coinfection is either clinically similar to fulminant hepatitis due to HBV alone or develops as a short-term relapse of an otherwise common acute hepatitis B (Govindarajan, Gut, 1986; 27:19). Serum HBsAg may be lacking (Caredda, JInfDis, 1989; 159: 977). In patients with fulminant hepatitis D, the incidence of HDV coinfection which was more than 50 per cent in the early eighties, [61,62] is sharply decreasing since the early nineties, at least in Western Europe.

Among patients with IgM anti-HBc positive acute hepatitis B, the incidence of HDV infection in those with fulminant hepatitis (30 per cent in two series)[61,62] was higher than that in patients with non-fulminant hepatitis. However, the mortality rate of patients with fulminant hepatitis due to HDV coinfection was not significantly higher than that of patients with fulminant hepatitis type B alone.[54,62]

Superinfection with HDV (HDV superinfection)

HDV superinfection threatens chronic HBV carriers and may unmask a hitherto asymptomatic HBV chronic carriage (Farci, Gastro, 1983; 85:669). The diagnosis is also based on HDV serum markers but the polymerase chain reaction allows diagnosis of seronegative cases (Wu, Hepatol, 1994; 19:836). HDV superinfection affects especially intravenous drug addicts (Lettau, NEJM, 1987; 317:1256) and HBV chronic carriers in developing countries.[54] Cases were observed in HBsAg-positive renal transplant recipients (Kharsa, Transpl, 1987; 44:221). Subfulminant hepatic failure is more frequent than a fulminant course and genotype I is predominant (Wu, Lancet, 1995; 346:939). The mortality rate of fulminant hepatitis due to HDV superinfection is higher than that of fulminant hepatitis due to HDV coinfection.[54] In patients surviving fulminant hepatitis due to HDV superinfection, development of severe chronic active hepatitis D and cirrhosis is common (Colombo, Gastro, 1983; 85:235).

Acute infection with hepatitis C virus

The actual role of HCV in the pathogenesis of fulminant hepatitis is still uncertain. The prevalence of serum HCV-RNA in patients with fulminant hepatitis is clearly related to the geographic area. In patients with HBV seronegative fulminant hepatitis, this prevalence was 45 per cent in Taiwan (Chu, Gastro, 1994; 107:189), 9 to 52 per cent in Japan (Inokuchi, JHepatol, 1996; 24:58; Yoshiba, Hepatol, 1994; 19:829), 19 per cent in India,[12] up to 12 per cent in the United States (Wright, AnnIntMed, 1991; 115:111; Liang, Gastro, 1993; 104:56), and zero in France[51] and in the United Kingdom (Sallie, JHepatol, 1994; 20:580; Mutimer, Gut, 1995; 36:433). In patients with HBsAg-positive fulminant hepatitis, the prevalence of serum HCV-RNA was 48 per cent in France,[51] 30 per cent in Taiwan (Chu, Gastro, 1994; 107:189), and up to 33 per cent in Japan (Inokuchi, JHepatol, 1996; 24:258; Ohnishi, IntHepatol-Comm, 1994; 2:347). In liver tissue, the prevalence of HCV-RNA was 40 per cent in HBsAg-positive patients in France,[51] 20 per cent in Germany (Sergi, Gastro, 1996; 110:A1319), and zero in the United Kingdom (Fagan, JHepatol, 1994; 21:587).

Fulminant hepatitis was associated with acute coinfection with HBV and HCV (Chu, JInfDis, 1995; 20:703)[51] and followed withdrawal of chemotherapy in chronic carriers of hepatitis C virus (Vento, Gut, 1995; 36:A949). In Japanese patients who developed subfulminant hepatitis after transfusion therapy and immuno-suppression, the acute exacerbation of a hitherto unrecognized chronic HCV infection could not be excluded (Yoshiba, Hepatol, 1994; 19:829).

Acute hepatitis E[63-66]

Hepatitis E virus (HEV) is the viral agent responsible for the waterborne, enterically transmitted non-A, non-B hepatitis (EN-ANB) (Reyes, Science, 1990; 247:1335). HEV is a non-enveloped, single-stranded, positive-sense RNA virus, present in water or food contaminated by faeces. There is only one serotype. The mode of transmission is exclusively faecal–oral. The average incubation period is 40 days. During acute hepatitis E, viraemia may be protracted for 112 days and faecal shedding may persist up to the seventh week of the illness (Nanda, Gastro, 1995; 108:225). Chronic hepatitis does not occur.

Enzyme immunoassays for detection of anti-HEV antibodies have become available recently, but need improvement (Lok, JHepatol, 1994; 20:567). The polymerase chain reaction allows detection of HEVp-RNA in blood, stools, and in liver tissue. Viral replication occurs in the cytoplasm of hepatocytes.[63] No important inflammatory infiltrate is associated with the degenerative lesions of liver tissue, suggesting that HEV is likely to be a cytopathic virus.[63]

Acute hepatitis E affects the population of several south-east Asian and African countries, such as India, Pakistan, Lebanon, Libya, Ghana, and Algeria.[64] Cases have, in addition, been reported from Mexico. Large epidemics have occurred in India and China,[64], but clusters of a few cases may also be encountered. In India, 30 per cent of the patients affected by acute hepatitis E are HBsAg chronic carriers (Tandon, BullWHO, 1985; 63:931). Although infection with HEV cannot yet be contracted in western Europe and North America, acute or fulminant hepatitis due to this virus may be observed in these areas in patients returning from an endemic zone in the developing world (De Cock, AnnIntMed, 1987; 106:227; Margulies, DigDisSci, 1987; 32:1151; Roberts, AnnInt-Med, 1992; 117:93).[63]

The risk of fulminant and subfulminant hepatic failure is relatively high, particularly during the third trimester of pregnancy[64] and acute fatty liver of pregnancy may occur.[65] The disease follows a fulminant course.[65] Acute hepatitis E is responsible for 60 per cent of the cases of fulminant non-A, non-B hepatitis in India.[12] In an outbreak in Khashmir, fulminant hepatic failure developed in 22 per cent of pregnant women suffering from NANB hepatitis (Khuroo, AmJMed, 1981; 70:252). The maternal mortality rate of fulminant hepatitis E in pregnant women ranges between 15 and 20 per cent.[65] Mother-to-fetus intrauterine transmission is common and severe liver necrosis may affect the infant.[66]

Acute hepatitis G

The RNA genome of hepatitis G virus (HGV), a recently cloned flaviviridae member (Linnen, Science, 1996; 271:505), was found in serum of some patients with fulminant hepatitis in Japan (Yoshiba, Lancet, 1995; 346:1131; Tameda, JHepatol,1996; 25:842) and in Germany (Heringlake, Lancet, 1996; 338:1626), but neither in the livers of British patients (Sallie, Lancet; 1996; 347:1552) nor in early sampled sera of other Japanese patients (Kuroki, Lancet, 1996; 347:908), with fulminant hepatitis. The role of HGV in fulminant hepatitis, if any, is still unknown.

Acute hepatitis due to infection with herpes viruses

Although acute hepatitis caused by herpes viruses is usually asymptomatic or benign, uncommon severe, sometimes fulminant, hepatitis due to these viruses may occur.

Herpes simplex viruses 1 and 2

Herpes simplex viruses 1 and 2 are highly cytopathic. Benign liver lesions include foci of liver cell necrosis surrounded by dense inflammatory cell infiltrates and hepatocytes with intranuclear inclusions. Multifocal (often haemorrhagic) cell necrosis, due to the unrestrained cytopathic effect, may develop in liver tissue. The lack of inflammatory infiltrate is noteworthy (Bernuau, Liver, 1981; 1: 244). Multifocal liver cell necrosis is a constant, diagnostic lesion in disseminated infections due to herpes simplex viruses (Rose, JClinPath, 1972; 25:79; Sutton, AmJMed, 1974; 56:545). These life-threatening infections most often affect patients on immuno-suppressive therapy (Elliott, ArchIntMed, 1980; 140:1656), neonates (Becker, AmJDisChild, 1968; 115:1), pregnant women in their third trimester,[67] individuals who have recently undergone surgery, and, a in few cases, apparently healthy adults (Abraham, ArchIntMed, 1977; 137:1198; Conner, Gastro, 1979; 76:590). Drug-induced immunosuppression due to either steroids (Fink, J Clin Pathol, 1993; 46:968) or non-steroidal anti-inflammatory drugs (Bernuau, Hepatol, 1988; 8:1428) is common. Antipyretic-resistant high-grade fever, profound asthenia, leucopenia, and serum amino-transferases above 30 times normal, are the usual presenting features. Herpetic cutaneous or mucosal (either oropharyngeal or genital) necrotic lesions and jaundice are frequently absent (Shlien, Gut, 1988; 29:257). Leucopenia may not be present. Coma may occur. Depressed coagulation factor activity and thrombocytopenia are common. Some patients die without developing cerebral dysfunction or with nervous disorders not typical of hepatic encephalopathy. Moreover, extrahepatic herpetic lesions such as adrenal necrosis (Joseph, AmJMed, 1974; 56:35) and disseminated intravascular coagulation may contribute to death. Herpes simplex virus may be isolated from blood and virus-infected tissues. Transjugular liver biopsy allows early sampling of liver tissue for histology and viral culture. The administration of acyclovir, a specific inhibitor of herpes simplex virus multiplication (Strauss, AnnIntMed, 1985; 103:404), is indicated even on a clinical basis (Glorioso, DigDisSci, 1996; 41:1273). The drug, which is nephrotoxic, must be administered intravenously (5–8 mg/kg, 3 times daily for 8–10 days). Several cases of full recovery after acyclovir have been reported (Bernuau, Hepatol, 1988; 8:1428).[67]

Varicella–zoster virus

Massive liver cell necrosis due to varicella-zoster virus is quite uncommon but may be observed in immunosuppressed patients (Ross, AmJGastr, 1980; 74:423) and following bone marrow transplantation (Morishita, JAMA, 1985; 253 511) or liver transplantation (Esquivel, SemLivDis, 1985; 5:369). Associated varicella pneumonia is frequent. Antiviral therapy with acyclovir is recommended (Strauss, AnnIntMed, 1988; 108:221). A successful liver transplantation was performed in an asthmatic 7-year-old boy who developed fulminant hepatic failure secondary to severe varicella-zoster hepatitis (Tojimbara, Transpl; 1995; 60:1052).

Cytomegalovirus

Cytomegalovirus (CMV) is a weakly cytopathic herpesvirus and may induce benign liver lesions which are usually not diagnostic for the virus. Severe liver cell necrosis is quite uncommonly associated with cytomegalovirus infection. At least three cases of CMV infection with acute hepatitis and encephalopathy have been reported (De Saint Florent G, AnnChirThoracCardiovasc, 1976; 15:77; Greydanus, Infection, 1977; 5:255; Shusterman, AnnIntMed, 1978; 88:810). In all of them, associated infection with other hepatotropic viruses cannot be excluded since sensitive serological tests for HBV and HCV were not available at that time.

Active infection with CMV may be associated with fatal HBsAg-positive chronic active hepatitis in patients with cirrhosis (Vandelli, JHepatol 1987; 4:343) and with fulminant hepatic failure (Harbison, Transpl, 1988; 46:82; personal experience). Patients with fulminant or subfulminant hepatic failure seem to be at especially high risk of post-tranplantation CMV infection (Paya, JHepatol, 1993; 18:185).

Epstein–Barr virus[68]

Epstein-Barr virus is a non-cytopathic herpesvirus which does not usually infect hepatocytes.[68] Nevertheless, in fatal cases of infectious mononucleosis, either sporadic or complicating the X-linked lymphoproliferative syndrome in males, hepatomegaly is present in 80 per cent ([68]; Allen, JClinPath, 1963; 16:337; Chang, ArchPathol, 1975; 99:185; Adkins, NZMedJ, 1977; 85:6; Hart, MedJAust, 1984; 141:112) and various liver lesions, sometimes associated in one patient, may be observed. Severe liver cell necrosis was observed in 22 per cent of these fatal cases.[68] Although encephalopathy was neither a constant symptom (Davies, PostgradMedJ, 1980; 56:794) nor always due to liver dysfunction (Jain, BMJ, 1975; 3:38), liver failure is considered to be the predominant cause of death in 50 per cent of fatal cases (Risdall, Cancer, 1979; 44:993; Deutsch, EurJPaediatr, 1986; 145:94).[68] EBV was reported to be the only cause of fulminant hepatitis after cardiac surgery in a 62-year-old man (Papatheodoridis, JHepatol, 1995; 23:348).

Mechanisms responsible for EBV-associated massive liver cell necrosis are controversial. It has been suggested that mononuclear cells infiltrating the liver parenchyma are important (Tazawa, HumPathol, 1993; 24:1135) but, in most cases, associated infections with other hepatotropic viruses were not excluded.[68] A haemophagocytic syndrome may be present (Posthuma, Gut, 1995; 36:311). Hepatotoxic drugs such as paracetamol (Rosenberg, SouthMedJ, 1977; 70:660) may also be contributing factors.

Human herpesvirus-6

Human herpesvirus-6 (HHV-6) is a lymphotropic virus discovered in cultured primary lymphocytes (Salahuddin, Science, 1986; 234:596). Two cases of fulminant hepatitis were associated with primary HHV-6 infection in Japan; one 3-month-old boy died (Asano, Lancet, 1990; 335:862) and a 29-year-old man survived (Sobue, NEJM, 1991; 324:1290). Pathogenicity of HHV-6 is not fully established (Agut, NEJM, 1993; 329:203).

Acute infection with other viruses
Human parvovirus B19

Human parvovirus B19 (HPVB19) may be responsible for a variety of clinical manifestations including bone marrow failure. The presence of the P antigen, the cellular receptor of the virus, on erythroid progenitor cells (Brown, Science, 1993; 262:114), explains the HPVB19 tropism for erythroid precursors. Erythrocyte P antigen is also present on fetal hepatocytes. HPVB19 infection has been shown to be associated with acute hepatitis (Yoto, Lancet, 1996; 347:868). HPVB19 genome was detected in liver tissue of several patients with fulminant hepatic failure, both associated and unassociated with aplastic anaemia (Langnas, Hepatol, 1995; 22:1661).

Adenovirus

Severe, often disseminated, infections due to adenovirus may develop in immunocompromised patients (Zahradnik, AmJMed, 1980; 68:725). High-grade fever, pneumonia, and liver dysfunction are the main features. Several cases of fulminant hepatitis have been reported (Carmichael, AmJClinPath, 1979; 71:52; Purtilo, NEJM, 1985; 312:1707; Koneru, JAMA, 1987; 258:489; Bouabdallah, AnnMédIntern, 1990; 141:81), some of them after liver transplantation (Koneru, JAMA, 1987; 258:489). Adenovirus may be cultured from blood, liver, and various other tissues. The presence of intranuclear inclusions in still viable hepatocytes (Zahradnik, AmJMed, 1980; 68:725; Purtilo, NEJM, 1985; 312:1707) suggests that the virus may have a role in liver cell necrosis but associated cofactors cannot be excluded.

Viral haemorrhagic fevers

Liver cell necrosis and features of hepatic failure, disseminated intravascular coagulation, and multiple organ failure occur in patients severely and often fatally infected with RNA viruses responsible for viral haemorrhagic fevers (Poinsot, Hepato-Gast, 1996; 3:265).[69,70] Patients with viral haemorrhagic fevers are more often encountered in Asia and Africa, but some cases may be imported into Western countries. Renal failure and coagulation disorders are the main factors contributing to death. Causal RNA viruses are classified into four families.

Flaviridae include yellow fever, absent in Asia and Oceania, and Dengue viruses, prevalent in south-east Asia (Monath, SemVirol, 1994; 5:133). Several fatal cases of yellow fever in persons returning from Senegal have been observed in France (Belaïche, GastrClinBiol, 1980; 4:799). Liver lesions include acidophilic liver cell necrosis and steatosis. Dengue haemorrhagic fever may be complicated, particularly in young children, by the fatal dengue shock syndrome (Gubler, EmergingInfectDis, 1995; 1:55; Lam, RevMedMicrobiol, 1995; 6:39).

Bunyaviridae include Rift Valley fever, prevalent in Africa,[69] Congo-Crimean haemorrhagic fever (Swanepoel, AmJTropMedHyg, 1987; 36:120) which can be treated by ribavirine and Korean haemorrhagic fever caused by Hantaviruses and associated with severe renal failure (Elisaf, JClinGastr, 1993; 17:33).

Arenaviridae are mainly represented by Lassa fever virus, a cytopathic virus prevalent in West Africa. Eighth-nerve deafness may occur. Increased serum aminotransferase activity and high-grade viraemia are associated with a mortality rate of more than 50 per cent (Johnson, JInfDis, 1987; 155:456). Ribavirin is effective (McCormick, NEJM, 1986; 304:20).

Filoviridae include Marburg virus and Ebola virus (Peters, SemVirol, 1994; 5:147). Both are highly virulent RNA viruses that may infect health-care workers. Mortality rate is over 50 per cent. Marburg virus infection may cause conjunctivitis and fatal hepatic failure (Gear, BMJ, 1975; 4:489). Ebola virus outbreaks have occurred in Africa, most recently in Zaire; supportive treatment only can be recommended and external protection of health-care workers must be in place (Bennett, BMJ, 1995; 310:1344).

Coxsackie B virus

Microabscesses were found in the liver of a patient who was given steroids and died from diffuse Coxsackie B virus infection (Gregor, MtSinaiMedJ, 1975; 42:575). It is not known whether fatal hepatic failure was solely due to the viral disease.

Acute hepatitis due to poisoning

The main causal agents of this type of liver damage are paracetamol (acetaminophen), especially in England and the United States,[71] Amanita mushrooms, and industrial solvents. Acute hepatitis due to poisoning from agents other than paracetamol is the cause of only 1 to 2 per cent of cases of fulminant and subfulminant liver failure.[11]

Parcetamol overdose

Paracetamol is responsible for 50 to 60 per cent of cases of fulminant liver failure in the United Kingdom.[72] Although it is now available worldwide,[71] paracetamol induced-fulminant hepatic failure is not observed to such an extent in other countries. Usually, and particularly in the United Kingdom, paracetamol is ingested in a suicide attempt.[36] However, cases of accidental, severe, acute, or fulminant hepatic failure are increasingly reported in patients given therapeutic doses of the drug (see under Acute drug-induced hepatitis) and also when amounts ingested are only just above the recommended therapeutic daily dose (Whitcomb, AASLD, 1992; A909). Fulminant hepatic failure can occur after a daily intake of 3 to 10 g for several days or weeks in association with alcohol (Seeff, AnnIntMed, 1986; 104:399) or drugs known to accelerate

paracetamol-induced liver cell necrosis such as phenobarbitone (Black, DigDisSci, 1982; 27:370). Isoniazid pretreatment potentiates paracetamol hepatotoxicity (Murphy, AnnIntMed 1991; 113:799) (Table 8).

Particularly noticeable features of paracetamol-induced fulminant hepatic failure include acute renal failure, hyperlactataemia with metabolic acidosis, and also hypophosphataemia (Dawson, BMJ, 1987; 295:1312). However, all of these may occur in the absence of liver failure (Cobden, BMJ, 1982; 284:21; Gray, QJMed, 1987; 246:811; Jones, Lancet, 1989; ii:608) and, thus, may interfere with the natural course of the paracetamol-induced fulminant hepatic failure (Record, Gut, 1975; 16:44; Bihari, SemLivDis, 1986; 6: 119). Myocardial lesions were reported in a few patients with fatal paracetamol poisoning (Mann, AmJCardiol, 1989; 63:1018) and, in some of them, may have been a key factor contributing to death (Wakeel, BMJ, 1987; 295:1097). Paracetamol may interfere with blood glucose analysis; glucose over-estimation may then lead to erroneous and potentially fatal administration of insulin (Farah, BMJ, 1982; 285:172).

Accurate individual prognosis of paracetamol-induced fulminant hepatic failure is exceedingly difficult to achieve because the survival rate ranges between 35 and 65 per cent.[72] The daily monitoring of prothrombin time seems effective in early identification of patients with a risk of fatal outcome of more than 90 per cent (Harrison, BMJ, 1990; 301:964) (see under Emergency liver transplantation). Paracetamol-induced acute renal failure aggravates encephalopathy and serum creatinine has some weak prognostic value in these patients.[72]

Oral *N*-acetylcysteine is effective in preventing paracetamol-induced severe acute liver damage (Smilkstein, NEJM, 1988; 319: 1557) (Table 9). However, in Europe, intravenous *N*-acetylcysteine is recommended to obviate inefficacy due to vomiting or insufficient absorption of the antidote. Intravenous infusion of *N*-acetylcysteine initiated up to 80 h after the overdose and continued until recovery from encephalopathy was shown to improve the survival rate significantly.[73]

Criteria for emergency liver transplantation for these patients were defined by the King's College group (see under Emergency liver transplantation) and applied prospectively for 4 years in London. Only 20 per cent of patients fulfilling the criteria for emergency liver transplantation were ultimately transplanted and the risk of overtransplantation ranges between 10 and 15 per cent.[36]

Amanita mushroom poisoning

Amanita mushroom poisoning is a relatively common accident in continental Europe and in the United States. *Amanita phalloides* is the cause of most of the fatal cases in Europe while *Amanita verna* is more often involved in the United States. *Amanita virosa* is responsible for a few cases and *Lepiota species* may also cause a phalloidin syndrome. The lethal dose is generally considered to be about 50 g, which corresponds to three middle-sized mushrooms. *Amanita phalloides* causes hepatotoxicity with amatoxins, primarily alpha amanitin (Faulstich, KlinWschr, 1979; 57:1143). These toxins are heat-stable and, therefore, not destroyed by cooking. They follow an enterohepatic cycle.

Liver damage is a late complication in the course of amatoxin intoxication (Faulstich, KlinWschr, 1979; 57:1143). After the 6 to

Table 8 Factors with an increased risk of severe hepatotoxicity after therapeutic doses of paracetamol

Factor	Reference
Starvation	Whitcomb, AASLD, 1992; April: A909
Malnutrition	Barker, AnnIntMed, 1977; 87:299
Alcoholism	Kaysen, ArchIntMed, 1985; 145:2019; Kumar, ArchIntMed, 1991; 151:1189; Eriksson, JInternMed, 1992; 231:567
Enzyme inducers	Black, DigDisSci, 1982; 27:370; Wootton, SouthMedJ, 1990; 83:1047; Hastier, GastrClinBiol, 1995; 19:446
Cardiopulmonary and renal insufficiency	Bonkovsky, Hepatol, 1994; 19:1141
Associated treatment with isoniazid	Moulding, AnnIntMed, 1991; 114:431; Bernuau, personal experience

Table 9 Recommended dosage of *N*-acetylcysteine for intravenous administration

Loading dose	150 mg/kg	15 min
Second dose	50 mg/kg	4 h
Third dose	100 mg/kg	16 h

From Vale, Lancet, 1995; 346:547.

12 h asymptomatic phase following ingestion, a second phase of 1 to 4 days occurs, characterized by severe vomiting and diarrhoea. Supportive care, in particular correction of hydroelectrolytic disorders resulting from vomiting and diarrhoea, are essential at this stage (Floersheim, MedToxAdvDrugExp, 1987; 2:1). Serum aminotransferases and coagulation factor activities must be monitored early during this second phase although liver symptoms usually coincide with the recovery of digestive symptoms. Patients in whom serum aminotransferases are higher than 100 times normal are especially at risk of hepatic encephalopathy which develops 2 to 4 days after the onset of hepatitis, i.e. 4 to 8 days after mushroom ingestion.

Prognosis in these patients is exceedingly difficult. In a series of 205 patients, overall mortality rate was 22 per cent but 84 per cent of patients with a prothrombin time below 10 per cent died (Floersheim, SchMedWoch, 1982; 112:1164). Although all patients who died went into coma, some comatose patients survived spontaneously (Trad, SemHôpParis, 1970; 46:2163; Teutsch, Ann-Neurol, 1978; 3:177). Of 8 patients who underwent emergency liver transplantation for fulminant liver failure due to Amanita intoxication, 7 were not in coma (encephalopathy grade 4) before surgery (Woodle, JAMA, 1985; 253:69; Klein, AmJMed, 1989; 86: 187; Boudjema, PresseMed, 1989; 18:937; Wright Pinson, AmJSurg, 1990; 159:493). One patient in coma and prothrombin time lower than 10 per cent survived spontaneously while awaiting a suitable graft for liver transplantation for a week (Langer, UpdateIntensCareEmergMed, 1990; 10:482).

Industrial solvents

Several industrial solvents, mainly chlorinated hydrocarbons, are highly toxic to the liver. Acute carbon tetrachloride poisoning which occurs after occupational inhalation or accidental ingestion is now very uncommon since the industrial use of this compound was prohibited. Acute carbon tetrachloride poisoning may induce fulminant liver failure which is frequently associated with acute renal failure due to acute tubular necrosis. Liver lesions are centrilobular necrosis and steatosis. Metabolism of carbon tetrachloride occurs in liver microsomes and increased activity of the microsomal mixed-function oxidase system increases carbon tetrachloride hepatotoxicity. Early treatment with *N*-acetylcysteine may thus minimize liver lesions (Ruprah, Lancet, 1985; i:1027).

Although intrinsic hepatotoxicity of trichloroethylene is low, severe liver injury was reported in sniffers of solvents containing trichloroethylene (Baerg, AnnIntMed, 1970; 73:713; Conso, GastrClinBiol, 1982; 6:539). In these patients, liver injury was probably related to fraudulent mixing of carbon tetrachloride with trichloroethylene (Conso, GastrClinBiol, 1982; 6:39) which potentiates carbon tetrachloride hepatotoxicity (Pessayre, Gastro, 1982; 83:761).

A non-fatal case of acute liver damage with coma was observed in an adult after the ingestion of both alcohol and chloroform (Storms, JAMA, 1973; 225:160).

Several cases of fulminant liver failure have been reported after massive inhalation of 2-nitropropane, a non-chlorinated industrial solvent (Harrison, AnnIntMed, 1987; 107:466) and after oral ingestion of a veterinary euthanasia drug containing dimethylformamide, an organic hepatotoxic solvent (Rodineau, RéaSoins-IntensMedUrg, 1989; 5:203). Severe, non-fatal acute hepatitis was observed after ingestion of a large amount of chlorobenzene (Babany, Gastro, 1991; 101:1734).

Illicit substances

Cases of severe hepatotoxicity caused by illicit substances may occur in any urban area with the constant progression of drug-addiction.

Cocaine-induced hepatotoxicity may be fatal. Liver lesions include periportal necrosis and diffuse micro- and macrovesicular fatty infiltration (Perino, Gastro, 1987; 93:176). Aggravation of subcapsular ischaemic liver cell necrosis before death may be evaluated by computed tomography (Radin, J ComputAssistTomogr, 1992; 16:155). Fulminant hepatitis B may be observed in drug-addicts using 'crack', a non-parenteral form of cocaine without hydrochloride (Comer, AmJGastr, 1991; 86:331).

'Ecstasy', or 3,4-methylenedioxymetamphetamine, was first used as an appetite suppressant but is neurotoxic. It is now used as an illicit drug and allows young people to dance tirelessly for protracted periods. Several cases of fulminant hepatic failure have been observed in western Europe (Ellis, Gut, 1996; 38:454).[5,74] The spontaneous fatality rate is high but at least three patients have survived after emergency liver transplantation including two after successful auxiliary liver transplantation.[5] The diagnosis of non-fatal acute hepatitis due to 'ecstasy' in young adults is important for alerting habitual users of the drug to the risks of continuing (Deltenre, ActaGastroBelg, 1994; LVII: 41; Fidler, JHepatol, 1996; 25:563).

Acute lead poisoning may cause acute haemolysis, acute hepatitis, and death. Lead levels in liver tissue are increased (Beattie, QJMed, 1975; 44:275).

Herbal medicines

In Western countries, several cases of severe acute fulminant and subfulminant hepatic failure have been observed after ingestion of herbal medicines available without medical prescription in health-food stores (MacGregor, BMJ, 1989; 299:1156; Katz, JClinGastr, 1990; 12:203). Herbal teas may cause fatal fulminant hepatic failure (Ridker, ArchEnvironHlth, 1987; 42:133).

Germander (*Teucrium chamaedrys*) is hepatotoxic (Larrey, Ann-IntMed, 1992; 117:29). Fulminant hepatic failure may occur (Mostefa-Kara, Lancet, 1992; 340:674; Diaz, GastrClinBiol, 1992; 16: 1006) and emergency liver transplantation may be necessary (Mattéi, JHepatol, 1995; 22:597).

Chinese herbal medicine may cause toxic hepatitis (Woolf, Ann-IntMed, 1994; 121:729; Itoh, DigDisSci, 1995; 40:1845).[75] Indian herbal medicine may cause lead poisoning (Dunbabin, Med-JAust, 1992; 157:835).

Pennyroyal oil has caused several cases of fulminant hepatic failure in California (Anderson, AnnIntMed, 1996; 124:726; Baker-ink, Pediatrics, 1996; 98:944). *N*-Acetylcysteine may be useful (Anderson, AnnIntMed, 1996; 124:726).

Roots of *Atractylis gummifera* L., a plant common in Mediterranean countries, may induce fatal hepatotoxicity, especially in children (Georgiou, ClinToxicol, 1988; 26:487; Ben Lakhal, RéanimUrg, 1993; 2:313). Symptoms develop within 1 day of ingestion. Hypoglycaemia may occur and liver cell necrosis is associated with microvesicular steatosis (Lemaigre, NouvPresse-Med, 1975; 4:2865).

Other hepatotoxic substances

Fulminant hepatic failure is a recognized complication of acute poisoning by yellow phosphorus (Diaz-Rivera, Medicine, 1950; 29: 269). Several cases of fulminant or subfulminant hepatitis have been reported in developing countries after ingestion of food containing aflatoxin and various, often unidentified, herbs prescribed by witch-doctors (Ngindu, Lancet, 1982; i:1346; Wainwright, SAfrMed, 1977; 51:571).

Acute drug-induced hepatitis[76,77]

Many drugs may induce massive liver cell necrosis and fulminant or subfulminant liver failure. In Western countries, drug-induced hepatitis causes between 10 and 15 per cent of cases of fulminant or subfulminant liver failure.

Drug-induced fulminant or subfulminant liver failure has two important characteristics with respect to aetiology. First, massive

liver cell necrosis is caused only by drugs which are known to induce limited liver cell necrosis in most patients; drugs inducing purely cholestatic liver disease do not cause massive liver cell necrosis.[76] Second, the risk of fulminant or subfulminant liver failure is seriously increased when administration of the hepatotoxic drug is maintained after the first symptoms of liver disease. Accordingly, administration of any drug must be interrupted in any patient, of whatever age, with jaundice or any other clinical manifestation suggesting acute hepatitis. This very simple preventive measure is most useful before the development of jaundice. Recognition of drug-induced hepatitis can be particularly difficult in patients with encephalopathy and often needs prompt information from the physicians who saw the patient and from the pharmacists who provided drugs.

The risk of fulminant or subfulminant liver failure in patients suffering drug-induced hepatitis with jaundice is about 20 per cent, i.e. considerably greater than that of patients suffering acute viral hepatitis with jaundice (1 per cent or less). Finally, in 70 per cent of patients with drug-induced hepatitis complicated by encephalopathy, the disease has a subfulminant course which is much less common for acute viral hepatitis.

More than 130 drugs can cause liver cell necrosis.[34,76] Most belong to the therapeutic armamentarium against neuropsychiatric, infectious and parasitic, rheumatic and muscular, cardiovascular, and malignant diseases. The drugs most commonly incriminated are antidepressants, non-steroidal anti-inflammatory drugs and paracetamol, isoniazid, pyrazinamide, and halothane and derivatives.

Among the antidepressants, monoamine oxidase inhibitors are the most hepatotoxic compounds, especially when associated with enzyme inducers (Pessayre, Gastro, 1978; 75:492; Capron, Gastr-ClinBiol, 1980; 4:123). A few cases of fulminant hepatitis have been reported in patients treated with tricyclic antidepressants (Powell, JAMA, 1968; 205:642; Danan, Digestion, 1984; 30:179). Alpidem, a new imidazopyridine derivative with anxiolytic properties, has caused several cases of subfulminant hepatitis (Baty, GastrClinBiol, 1994; 18:1129).

Fulminant hepatitis has been reported in patients taking non-steroidal anti-inflammatory drugs (Boelsterli, CritRevToxicol, 1995; 25:07). Piroxicam was the cause of several fatal cases (Paterson, Gut, 1992; 33:1436).

Cases of accidental, severe acute or fulminant, hepatic failure are increasingly observed in patients given therapeutic doses of paracetamol in the United Kingdom,[36] United States (Bonkovsky, Hepatol, 1994; 19:1141), and France (Bernuau, GastrClinBiol, 1996; 20:A188). Jaundice is absent or moderate. Paracetamol may be hepatotoxic in patients with low hepatic glutathione stores and is hepatotoxic in regular drinkers of alcohol (Zimmerman, Hepatol, 1995; 22:767). Factors for increased risk of severe paracetamol hepatotoxicity are listed in Table 8. Combination of these factors is common (Bernuau, personal experience). Liver dysfunction, sometimes severe, was also observed after the ingestion of low amounts of paracetamol at the onset of a febrile infectious disease (Rosenberg, SouthMedJ, 1977; 70:660; Davis, AmJMed, 1983; 74:349; Ackerman, Hepatol 1989; 10:203), including acute viral hepatitis (Bernuau, personal experience). It is highly probable that therapeutic doses of paracetamol were a causal factor in several cases of fulminant hepatic failure without jaundice in young children shortly after a febrile illness associated with fasting (Robberecht,

JHepatol 1994; 21:S137; Alonso, JPediatr 1995; 127:88; Conway, JPediatr 1996; 129:317).

In patients receiving isoniazid without pyrazinamide, fulminant hepatic failure may be due to excessive dosage of the drug or its association with several enzyme inducers but the mortality rate is low (Pessayre, Gastro, 1977; 72:284). However, the fatality rate of hepatitis due to antituberculous treatment is dramatically increased when pyrazinamide is used.[78] Adequate monitoring of liver status as well as information from general practitionners and patients should reduce the rate of life-threatening hepatitis due to antituberculous therapy.[79]

Halothane and its derivatives, such as enflurane (Lewis, AnnIntMed, 1983; 98:984), are the major cause of fulminant hepatic failure occurring 5 to 15 days after general anaesthesia. Fever is the most frequent inaugural symptom. Repeated administration of halothane or its derivatives reduces the interval between anaesthesia and the onset of symptoms and sharply increases the risk of fulminant hepatitis (Carney, AnesthAnalg, 1972; 51:135; Lewis, AnnIntMed, 1983; 98:984). The mortality rate of halothane-(or derivatives)-induced fulminant hepatitis is 90 per cent or more.

Sulphonamides, especially sulphasalazine, may cause immunoallergic fulminant hepatic failure (Ribe, AmJ Gastr, 1986; 81: 205; Marinos G, JClinGastro, 1992; 14:132). Severe hepatotoxicity due to mesalazine was described after hypersensitivity to sulphasalazine (Hautekeete, Gastro, 1992; 103:1925). The readministration of both drugs is contraindicated after an immunoalllergic accident with sulphasalazine.

Cases of fulminant or subfulminant hepatic failure have recently been ascribed to amiodarone (Lewis, Hepatol, 1989; 9:679; Kalantzis, HepatoGast, 1991; 38:71), linisopril (Larrey, Gastro, 1990; 99:1832), recombinant α-interferon (Durand, Lancet, 1991; 338: 1268; Wandl, Lancet, 1992; 339:123), chlormezanone (Bourlière, JGastrHepatol, 1992; 7:339), hydroxychloroquine (Makin, Gut, 1994; 35:569), ecarazine (Tameda, Hepatol, 1996; 23:465), erythromycin (Gholson, ArchIntMed, 1990; 150:215), flutamide (Dourakis, JHepatol, 1994; 20:350), nilutamide (Hammel, GastrClinBiol, 1993; 17:499), cyclophosphamide (JIntMed, 1996; 240:311), omeprazole (Jochem, AmJGastr, 1992; 87:523), and paroxetine (DeutschApothekZeit, 1996; 136:2356).

Several nucleoside analogues can cause fulminant hepatic failure because of microvesicular fatty infiltration of the liver: fialuridine in chronic hepatitis B patients (NEJM, 1995; 333:1099) and 2′,3′-dideoxyinosine (ddI) in HIV-positive patients (Lai, AnnIntMed, 1991; 115:283; Bissuel, JIntMed, 1994; 235:367).

Other causes (Table 10)

Between 5 and 10 per cent of cases of fulminant or subfulminant hepatic failure are due to causes other than viral hepatitis, hepatitis due to poisoning, or drug-induced hepatitis.

Hypoxic liver cell necrosis[80]

Hypoxic liver cell necrosis is characterized by predominantly centrilobular liver cell necrosis, without inflammatory cell infiltration. Hepatic vein enlargement and congestion are usually, but not always, associated. Acute renal failure, also hypoxic in origin, is common.

In a small number of patients, hypoxic liver cell necrosis results in fulminant liver failure with a high mortality rate (Nouel, DigDisSci, 1980; 25:49), especially when prothrombin time is lower than 20 per cent and encephalopathy is present.[80] Fulminant hepatic failure due to hypoxic liver cell necrosis is usually considered as a contraindication to liver transplantation. In patients recovering from hypoxic liver cell necrosis, serum aminotransferases which may be 200 times above normal return to normal within a few days.[80]

Hypoxic hepatitis was shown prospectively to occur in 20 per cent of patients with low cardiac output admitted to a coronary care unit.[81] Hypoxic liver cell necrosis is usually ischaemic in origin and results from an acute reduction in liver blood flow. In 9 out of 10 cases, this reduction in liver blood flow occurs in patients suffering from chronic congestive heart failure and is due to an acute and transient reduction in cardiac output. This acute cardiac decompensation occurs after a recent deterioration of the cardiorespiratory condition and the precipitating event is usually cardiac arrhythmia and, less often, myocardial infarction.[80] In 10 per cent of cases, the acute reduction in liver blood flow results from acute heart failure due to pulmonary embolism, acute cardiac tamponade, myocardial infarction, or severe arrhythmia.[80] Because the acute reduction in cardiac output has often subsided when clinical manifestations of liver cell necrosis develop, ischaemic liver cell necrosis can be confused with other causes of liver cell necrosis, in particular viral hepatitis (Cohen, Gastro, 1978; 74:583; Nouel, DigDisSci, 1980; 25:49). Acute reduction in cardiac output alone may be the only causal factor of hypoxic liver cell necrosis in some cases of protracted shock (Nunes, ArchSurg, 1970; 100:546; Larcan, GastrClinBiol, 1979; 3:105) or in patients with hepatic artery thrombosis (Dammann, DigDisSci, 1982; 27:73). However, hypoxic liver cell necrosis usually results from the association of ischaemia, induced by the acute reduction in cardiac output, with hepatic venous congestion (Arcidi, AmJPath, 1981; 104:159).[80,81]

In a small number of patients, hypoxic liver cell necrosis is due to profound hypoxaemia without ischaemia (Watson, BMJ, 1984; 289:1113; Zwaveling, Lancet, 1985; ii:388). In a patient with chronic respiratory failure, severe acute liver failure developed after an episode of deep hypoxaemia with raised central venous pressure and increased cardiac output.[80]

Obstructive sleep apnoea was the cause of severe acute hepatitis in an obese woman with severe arterial hypoxaemia (Mathurin, Gastro, 1995; 109:1682).

Hyperthermia

Massive liver cell necrosis has been reported in patients who died of heatstroke (Kew, AmJMed, 1970; 49:192; Rubel, Liver, 1983; 3: 249). It is probable that both liver failure and various extrahepatic factors contribute to the fatal outcome. Two patients with fulminant liver failure were transplanted after heatstroke and died later (Hassanein, Gastro, 1991; 100:1442; Saïssy, PresseMéd, 1996; 25:977). Survival after 6 days of coma with factor V lower than 10 per cent of normal has been reported (Chavoutier-Uzzan, GastrClinBiol, 1988; 12:668).

Liver cell necrosis can result from direct thermal injury (Kew, AmJMed, 1970; 49:192) or from hepatic ischaemia due to circulatory disorders or disseminated intravascular coagulation. In one patient who survived, the absence of hepatic vein congestion suggested that relative liver cell hypoxia was the main causal factor of liver cell necrosis (Chavoutier-Uzzan, GastrClinBiol, 1988; 12:668).

Table 10 Previously silent chronic liver diseases that may become clinically apparent by causing fulminant or subfulminant hepatic failure

Disease	Chronic liver lesion	Medical treatment when prothrombin <50% without clinical encephalopathy	Cases with successful emergency liver transplantation
Hepatitis B virus (HBV) reactivation	Absence of chronic hepatitis, cirrhosis	Antiviral therapy (famciclovir, lamivudine)	Yes[1] (after cessation of HBV replication)
Wilson's disease	Chronic hepatitis, cirrhosis	D-Penicillamine (high doses)	Yes[2]
Autoimmune hepatitis	Chronic hepatitis, cirrhosis	Corticosteroids (1–3 mg/kg per day) (+ azathioprine)	Yes
Erythropoietic protoporphyria	Cirrhosis	None	Yes[3]

[1] Bain, Transpl, 1996; 62:1456.
[2] Bellary, JHepatol, 1995; 23:373.
[3] Lock, Liver, 1996; 16:211.

Obstruction of the hepatic veins

Obstruction of the hepatic veins induces sinusoidal dilatation and reduced hepatic blood flow. Compression of the hepatic cords and ischaemia result in liver cell necrosis which predominates in the centrilobular area. In a small number of patients, liver cell necrosis is massive and fulminant hepatic failure develops (Berthelot, RevMedChirMalFoie, 1969; 44:25; Sandle, Lancet, 1980; i:1199; McClure, AmJClinPath, 1982; 78:236; Powell-Jackson, Gut, 1986; 27:1101; Bourlière, Gut, 1990; 31:949). Ascites is common. The most common cause is thrombosis secondary to a patent or latent primary myeloproliferative disorder (Valla, AnnIntMed, 1985; 103:329). Other causes include deficiency in coagulation inhibitors such as antithrombin III (McClure, AmJClinPath, 1982; 78:236) and protein C (Bourlière, Gut, 1990; 31:949). Fulminant hepatic failure due to Budd–Chiari syndrome is uncommon and always fatal. Early diagnosis at the stage of severe acute failure, before the development of clinical encephalopathy, may allow emergency mesocaval or mesoatrial shunt procedures to be performed successfully (Bourlière, Gut, 1990; 31:949). When encephalopathy is present, emergency liver transplantation followed by long-term anticoagulation (Campbell Jr, SGO, 1988; 166:511) may be successful in some patients.

In veno-occlusive disease of the liver, vascular obstruction affects the centrilobular veins. Pyrrolizidine alkaloids are a classical causal agent. Two causes often occurring together are antineoplastic chemotherapy (Zafrani, ArchIntMed, 1983; 143:495) and irradiation (Reed, AmJPath, 1966; 48:597). After bone marrow transplantation, veno-occlusive disease of the liver can be related to a graft-versus-host reaction as well as to irradiation and chemotherapy (Woods, AmJMed, 1980; 68:285; McDonald, Hepatoly, 1984; 4:116). Fulminant liver failure has been reported in patients with veno-occlusive disease of the liver induced by chemotherapy alone (Griner, AnnIntMed, 1976; 85:578; Weitz, VirchArchA, 1982; 395:245).

Massive malignant infiltration of the liver

Fulminant or, more often, subfulminant hepatic failure can develop in some patients with hepatic metastases (Eras, AnnIntMed, 1971; 74:581; Nouel, GastrClinBiol, 1979; 3:135; Myszor, JClinGastro, 1990; 12:441). Hepatomegaly and ascites are always found. The history of the causal carcinoma and liver imaging indicates liver metastases in most cases. However, when the causal carcinoma is latent, fulminant hepatic failure may be the first clinical manifestation of hepatic metastases. Furthermore, ultrasonography or computed tomography often show apparently homogeneous liver enlargement because the patient has diffusely distributed small liver metastases. In these patients, fulminant hepatic failure has been ascribed to hepatic ischaemia due to massive, intrasinusoidal invasion of the liver by the tumourous cells (Harrison, Gastro, 1981; 80:820; Henrion, GastrClinBiol, 1996; 20:535). Widespread infarction of the liver may occur (Harrison, Gastro, 1981; 80:820). The primary tumour is often a breast carcinoma, but melanoma (Bouloux, JRSocMed, 1986; 79:302), malignant haemoangio-endothelioma (Stein, AmJGastr, 1977; 67:370), or nasopharyngeal carcinoma (Hwang, Liver, 1996; 16:283) have also been reported.

Fulminant and subfulminant hepatic failure have also been observed in a few patients with massive liver infiltration by leukaemic cells (Zafrani, Hepatol, 1983; 3:428), Hodgkin's and non-Hodgkin's lymphoma (Zafrani, Hepatol, 1983; 3:428; Braude, PostgradMedJ, 1982; 58:301), and malignant histiocytosis (Colby, Gastro, 1982; 82:339). Again hepatomegaly is almost always present. Severe lactic acidosis is common (Zafrani, Hepatol, 1983; 3:428). In a few patients with acute leukaemia, intensive chemotherapy may allow fulminant hepatic failure to regress (Zafrani, Hepatol, 1983; 3:428).

Massive malignant infiltration of the liver is an absolute contraindication to liver transplantation.

Wilson's disease (see Table 10)

Severe acute hepatic failure associated with acute intravascular haemolysis and complicated within days or weeks by clinical encephalopathy may be the first clinical manifestation of so-called fulminant Wilson's disease (Roche-Sicot, AnnIntMed, 1977; 86:301; McCullough, Gastro, 1983; 84:161). In a few patients who have been on D-penicillamine therapy for several years this presentation may follow interruption of the treatment (Rector Jr, Liver,

1984; 4:341). The syndrome usually draws attention to the disease in young adults (often females younger than 30 years without wilsonian nervous manifestations). Most of them already have cirrhosis. The course is usually subfulminant.

Although fulminant and subfulminant hepatic failure due to Wilson's disease has several distinctive features (Roche-Sicot, AnnIntMed, 1977; 86:301; McCullough, Gastro, 1983; 84:161) diagnosis may be difficult. Information about liver or nervous disease in older siblings may be lacking. Kayser–Fleischer rings and diminished serum caeruloplasmin may also be absent. Caeruloplasmin can be within the normal range in a few cases of Wilson's disease (Scott, Gastro, 1978; 74:645) and may be decreased in non-wilsonian liver failure. However, serum aminotransferases are not usually increased above 10 times normal and, thus are much lower than the values commonly recorded in fulminant hepatitis. Intravascular haemolysis is due to increased ionic copper in the plasma. Its association with severe acute, fulminant or subfulminant, hepatic failure is noteworthy and, although not specific, is very suggestive of Wilson's disease. The alkaline phosphatase–total bilirubin ratio is significantly lower than in fulminant hepatic failure of non-wilsonian origin (Sallie, Hepatol, 1992; 16:1206) but does not allow by itself the specific diagnosis of wilsonian fulminant hepatic failure although this has been suggested (Berman, Gastro, 1991; 100:129).

Untreated fulminant hepatic failure due to Wilson's disease is consistently fatal within a few days or weeks. It has been claimed that a prognostic index, including serum aspartate aminotransferase, bilirubin, and prothrombin time, indicated early wilsonian patients with a rapidly fatal outcome and those who will survive with D-penicillamine (Nazer, Gut, 1986; 27:1377). Liver transplantation is now recommended for fulminant liver failure due to Wilson's disease (Sternlieb, Hepatol, 1984; 4:15S) and several patients have been successfully treated (Sokol, JPediatr, 1985; 107:549; Rakela, Gastro, 1986; 90:2004; Stampfl, Gastro, 1990; 99:1834).[82] However, in 9 out of 10 young adults with symptoms for less than 2 months and with haemoglobin levels still above 8 g/dl, early treatment with high doses of D-penicillamine was successful and emergency liver transplantation was not required (Durand, JHepatol, 1990; 11:S20).

Autoimmune chronic active hepatitis (see Table 10)

The clinical onset of autoimmune chronic active hepatitis often mimics acute hepatitis (Mistilis, AmJMed, 1970; 48:484). In a few of these patients, subfulminant liver failure develops 1 to 3 months after the clinical onset (Bernuau, JHepatol, 1985; 2:S193). In such patients, antibodies to smooth muscle are absent whereas type 1 antibodies to liver and kidney microsomes are present (Homberg, Hepatol, 1987; 7:1333). Emergency liver transplantation is usually indicated.

Syncytial giant-cell hepatitis (postinfantile giant-cell hepatitis)

Syncytial giant cell hepatitis appears to be secondary to a variety of causes such as autoimmunity (Devaney, Hepatol, 1992; 16:327; Lau, JHepatol, 1992; 15:216; Johnson, JClinPath, 1994; 47:1022; Protzer, Liver; 1996: 16:274), viruses (Lau, JHepatol, 1992; 15:216), and even drug exposure. In cases without a recognized origin, patients may develop fulminant hepatic failure: the outcome was fatal in three of these without corticosteroids (Lau, JHepatol, 1992; 15: 216), but was favourable in two others who were given steroids (Tordjmann, GastrClinBiol, 1993; 17:A292). Among 10 Canadian patients with severe hepatitis, bridging necrosis, and large syncytial giant cells, a paramyxoviral infection was suspected to be the cause; subfulminant hepatic failure developed in four patients, three died and one was transplanted (Phillips, NEJM, 1991; 324:455). In a French patient with syncytial giant cell hepatitis of unknown origin, subfulminant hepatic failure also developed; emergency liver transplantation was performed but was followed by recurrence of the same liver lesions. Early treatment with ribavirin was successful.[83]

Microvesicular steatosis

Microvesicular steatosis, a lesion characterized by hepatocytes with the nucleus in a central position and with cytoplasm containing numerous, small, fat-filled inclusions, is a recognized cause of fulminant and subfulminant hepatic failure. Serum aminotransferases may be mildly or sharply increased (up to 1300 times the normal value; personal experience). Main causes are acute fatty liver of pregnancy and Reye's syndrome.

Acute fatty liver of pregnancy which is characterized by a centrilobular distribution of microvesicular steatosis is now readily curable (Bernuau, GastrClinBiol, 1987; 11:128) because it is usually diagnosed early (polydipsia preceding nausea and vomiting is of high diagnostic value) and the disease is now an uncommon cause of fulminant hepatic failure. Early interruption of pregnancy allows regression of liver lesions long before the appearance of encephalopathy. Only when the diagnosis is ignored and the interruption of pregnancy delayed does fulminant liver failure develop and emergency liver transplantation become justified (Ockner, Hepatol, 1990; 11:59) (see Section 28).

Reye's syndrome is a rare condition, affecting children and rarely adults after various viral infections and/or salicylate ingestion. Fulminant liver failure develops in the major form of the syndrome. Cerebral oedema has an important role in the mechanism of brain disorders in these patients (Croker, SemLivDis, 1982; 2:340). Prognosis is difficult. Recovery of comatose patients with clinical features of decerebration may occur (personal experience), but in others, emergency liver transplantation may be justified.

Fulminant hepatic failure due to drug-induced microvesicular steatosis has been described in patients given high doses of intravenously administered tetracycline and in others receiving valproic acid, a drug used in the treatment of petit mal (Zimmerman, Hepatol, 1982; 2:591). Microvesicular steatosis associated with liver cell necrosis has also been reported in patients receiving pirprofen (Danan, Gastro, 1985, 89:210) and in others given certain nucleoside analogues (see above).

Liver transplantation

Fulminant hepatic failure may develop early after liver transplantation. The main causes are the association of pre-existing unrecognized lesions of the graft (mainly widespread steatosis), poor preservation of the graft, and protracted ischaemia. In such cases, awakening is delayed, oliguria is common, serum aminotransferases are high, and prothrombin ratio remains low. Lactic acidosis may develop. Emergency liver retransplantation is usually required (McCaughan, TransplInt 1995; 8:20).

Hyperacute graft rejection and liver ischaemia due to hepatic artery thrombosis, with or without associated portal vein or hepatic vein thrombosis (Starzl, NEJM, 1989; 321:1014), may also be the cause of early postoperative hepatic failure. In several cases, the liver lesion was a massive haemorrhagic necrosis (Hubscher, JClinPath, 1989; 42:360). These vascular complications are now usually prevented by early anticoagulant therapy and early postoperative monitoring of the hepatic vessels by Doppler ultrasonography. When these lesions are associated with features of fulminant liver failure, urgent retransplantation is usually required.

Fulminant hepatic failure later after liver transplantation may be caused by acute viral hepatitis due to infection of the graft by HBV, herpes simplex virus, or adenovirus.

Partial hepatectomy

Fulminant hepatic failure can develop in non-cirrhotic patients when 80 per cent or more of functional hepatic parenchyma is removed (Bismuth, WorldJSurg, 1983; 7:505; Yamanaka, AnnSurg, 1984; 200:653). In cirrhotic patients, the risk of postoperative fulminant hepatic failure after partial hepatectomy is present as soon as 50 per cent, or even less, of hepatic parenchyma was removed. The risk is dependent upon several, factors including the preoperative level of hepatic function (Bismuth, WorldJSurg, 1983; 7:505), the presence of an active parenchymal disease, the extent of liver resection, and the occurence of severe postoperative infections (Takenaka, WorldJSurg, 1990; 14:123).

Immediate postoperative fulminant hepatic failure is an important risk after *ex-vivo* surgery, especially in patients older than 50 years (personal experience). Contributing factors are extensive resection of liver parenchyma, hypothermia-associated ischaemia of liver tissue, and decreased oxygen supply because of impaired systemic haemodynamics.

Undetermined causes

Despite improved investigative methods aimed at elucidating the causes of fulminant and subfulminant hepatic failure, cases remain in which no aetiology can be identified. At present, these cases are considered to be caused by non-A to G hepatitis, although several groups have failed to identify markers of viral infection in such patients (Liang, Gastro, 1993; 104:556; Sallie, JHepatol, 1994; 20: 80; Porte, JHepatol, 1994; 21:592; Mutimer, Gut, 1995; 36:433; Mason, Hepatol, 1996; 24:1361). The outcome generally is poor and emergency liver transplantation is often required.

Prognosis[12,50,55,84,85]

The following prognostic features refer exclusively to patients with clinical encephalopathy: when this is absent during the course of an acute hepatitis, the risk of a fatal outcome is between 0 and 5 per cent (at least in Europe and in the United States).

Trey (CanMedAssJ, 1972; 106:525) first showed that the outcome of patients with fulminant or subfulminant hepatic failure is affected by many factors including the cause of the disease, the patient's age, and the severity of encephalopathy. However, accurate prognosis, especially early prediction of death, is exceedingly difficult. Although loss of the oculovestibular reflex was associated with death in 20 comatose patients in London (Hanid, BMJ, 1978; 1:

1029), a single clinical or biochemical feature is unlikely to predict fatal outcome accurately in all patients (Rueff, Gut, 1973; 14:805).

Unexpected recovery was observed in young patients with decerebrate rigidity or convulsions (Davis, NEJM, 1968; 278:1248; Hanid, Gut, 1980; 21:866), in at least one patient with a prolonged flat EEG (Tanaka, Lancet, 1980; ii:1379), and in a 21-year-old Indian girl after 26 days of deep coma (Antia, Gastro, 1980; 79:1098). Several patients in whom transplantation was decided survived unexpectedly before a liver graft became available (Langer, UpdateIntensCareEmergMed, 1990; 10:482; Bernuau, JHepatol, 1996; 25, suppl. 1:63).[36]

Coagulation factor activities are among the most striking indicators of prognosis in patients with clinical encephalopathy. This was reported in early studies (Ritt, Medicine, 1969; 48:151)[86] and has been confirmed more recently by multivariate analysis. Prothrombin time was the best prognostic indicator in fulminant and subfulminant hepatic failure not caused by paracetamol poisoning in London,[84] Taiwan,[50] and Delhi[12] and, to a lesser degree, in HBsAg-positive patients with fulminant hepatitis in Japan.[85] Factor V activity, measured on freshly sampled plasma, was the most effective independent predictor of survival in 115 patients with fulminant hepatitis B in Paris.[55] Serial evaluation of prothrombin time was also of great prognostic value within 4 days of paracetamol overdose complicated by fulminant hepatic failure in London (Harrison, BMJ, 1990; 301:964) (see below).

The prognostic value of the cause was also confirmed by multivariate analysis.[84] Even in patients affected by fulminant viral hepatitis, the survival rate is influenced by the causal virus (Table 8). The spontaneous survival rate, close to or even above 50 per cent in fulminant hepatic failure due to paracetamol overdose (Harrison, BMJ, 1990; 301:964),[84] is still consistently lower by 10 or even 20 per cent in patients affected by fulminant and subfulminant hepatic failure due to hepatitis of undetermined aetiology (non-A to G hepatitis),[11,84] or to halothane or drug reactions,[84] or to acute Wilson's disease (McCullough, Gastro, 1983; 84:161).

The patient's age usually has a strong prognostic influence although this is not true in halothane-induced fulminant and subfulminant hepatic failure (Trey, CanMedAssJ, 1972; 106:525). It is, however, an independent predictor of survival in fulminant hepatitis B[55] and correlates inversely with the survival rate in fulminant hepatic failure due to paracetamol overdose.[84] Overall survival rate is usually higher in adult patients younger than 40 and in children younger than 11 years.[84]

The maximal grade of encephalopathy also has prognostic value. The overall survival rate is lower in patients who developed coma (Trey, CanMedAssJ, 1972; 106:525) than in those who did not (Nusinovici, GastrClinBiol, 1977; 1:875).[55] Overall survival rate is also lower in patients admitted with coma.[84] However, coma by itself was not an independent predictor of death among 115 patients with fulminant hepatitis B in Paris,[55] while, in London, the survival rate of patients with fulminant or subfulminant hepatic failure not due to paracetamol overdose was lower in those admitted with grade 0-2, than in those admitted with grade 3-4, encephalopathy.[84]

The prognostic value of the interval between the onset of jaundice and that of clinical encephalopathy is controversial: it was found helpful for patients with non-paracetamol hepatitis in London,[84] unlike the experience in Paris[55] and India.[12]

Serum Gc protein, a member of the extracellular actin scavenger system which is synthesized in the liver,[87] was shown to be sharply decreased and to correlate with poor survival in patients with fulminant hepatic failure.[88] Its prognostic value, although imperfect, was confirmed by a retrospective study and shown to be of similar value to that of the King's College Hospital criteria for emergency liver transplantation[89] (see below).

Detectable liver atrophy and tachycardia over 100 beats/min are other clinical symptoms associated with poor prognosis (Rueff, AnnMedIntern, 1971; 122:373). Other routinely-monitored parameters which correlate with the outcome are serum bilirubin (Christensen, ScaJGastro, 1984; 19:90)[84] and, in patients with paracetamol overdose, admission serum creatinine and arterial pH.[84] Survival does not correlate with serum albumin, but does correlate with increased serum α-fetoprotein (Murray-Lyon, Gut, 1976; 17:576), especially in patients with fulminant hepatitis B.[55] Survival correlates with serum aminotransferases,[85] but neither with their rate of daily decline (Sawhney, NEJM, 1980; 302:970) nor with their absolute value.[55,84] Galactose elimination capacity (Ranek, Gut, 1976; 17:959), antipyrine clearance,[22] and the clearance of microaggregated albumin (Canalese, Gut, 1982; 23:265) correlate with survival but are not routinely performed. Plasma ammonia correlates poorly with survival.[22] Evaluation of the functional reserve of the liver by computed tomography (Kumahara, GastrJap, 1989; 24:290) and determination of the liver volume by ultrasonography were also proposed as valuable prognostic tools, but we could not confirm these results.

Prevention

Although it is the most cost-effective measure against fulminant and subfulminant hepatic failure, prevention is sadly often neglected. Preventive measures should target the cause of the acute liver disease as well as all stages of the established causal illness.

Prevention of the cause

Viral hepatitis

Vaccination against HBV is a cost-effective method of preventing infection with HBV and, therefore, fulminant hepatitis B.[90] Ideally, vaccination should be universal in all newborns or very young children. Vaccination associated with the injection of anti-HBs immunoglobulins (serovaccination) is indicated at birth in newborns where one of the parents or another family member living in the same home is, or is at high risk to be, a HBV carrier. Vaccination is strongly recommended in all non-immunized subjects at high risk of HBV infection, i.e. physicians, surgeons, nurses and other health-care workers, intravenous drug-addicts and their sexual partners, patients with multiple sexual partners, homosexual men, patients affected by sexually transmitted diseases, and sexual partners of recognized HBV chronic carriers. A greater use of vaccination against HBV requires considerable funding, but there is also a need for more education of general practitioners and medical students.

Acupuncture is a recognized mode of transmission of HBV infection, and acupuncture needles must be used once only.

Vaccination against HAV is effective and recommended in all non-immunized individuals at high risk of infection during trips in areas with relatively poor hygiene, in children living in such areas, and in patients with chronic liver disease and those older than 50 years in whom the risk of fulminant hepatitis is increased.[91]

Early studies with combined hepatitis A and hepatitis B vaccines indicated they were safe and effective (Leroux-Roels, ScaJGastro, 1996; 31:1027; Kallinowski, Liver, 1996; 16:271).

Drug-induced acute hepatitis

The first rule for prevention of severe drug-induced side-effects is to instruct the patient to stop using any drug as soon as any abnormal and previously absent symptom appears.

Several other rules are important. The readministration of some drugs with a high potential for immunogenicity, such as halothane or enflurane, must be avoided. The same is true when a drug, such as these or sulphonamides (Hautekeete, Gastro, 1992; 103:1925) has been responsible for a first bout of hepatitis. Drug doses must be adapted to the patient's weight and renal function. Prevention of the severe hepatotoxic effects of drug combinations, such as isoniazid and enzyme inducers (Pessayre, Gastro, 1977; 72:284) or isoniazid and pyrazinamide,[78] requires awareness from the physician, education of the patient, and monitoring of liver status.[79] Paracetamol is dangerous in patients given isoniazid (Murphy, AnnIntMed, 1990; 113:799).

Miscellaneous

Prevention of severe liver damage after an overdose of paracetamol is best achieved by giving N-acetylcysteine, a non-toxic glutathione precursor, as early as possible (Smilkstein, NEJM, 1988; 319:1557). Intravenous use of N-acetylcysteine is not yet permitted in the United States.

Prevention of recurrent cardiac arrhythmias and heat stroke will avoid fulminant hypoxic hepatitis. Limitation of excessive extension of hepatic resection, especially in patients with preoperative liver dysfunction, will prevent undue postoperative catastrophic fulminant liver failure.

Extreme care must be taken to identify a wild fungus as harmless before eating.

Prevention of the fulminant and subfulminant course of established acute liver diseases

Immediate (even nocturnal) advice by a hepatologist is recommended for any patient affected by acute liver disease with a 50 per cent or more decrease in coagulation factor activity. Those patients with overt or deep jaundice, even when present for a few days, and coagulation factors lower than 50 per cent, should be immediately admitted to a liver unit. This is a critical step for prognosis since early admission, before encephalopathy, correlates with an increased survival in patients with fulminant or subfulminant hepatic failure. It is also the most suitable time for aetiological liver treatment to be administered.

Drugs and herbal medicines

For two reasons, the administration of drugs or herbal medicines must be stopped immediately in any patient with early symptoms of acute liver disease, with the exception of insulin (at lowered doses) in insulin-dependent diabetic patients and quinine in those suffering, or at risk of developing, falciparum malaria. First, the drug(s) could be the cause of the acute hepatitis. Second, the drug(s) (mainly sedative, hepatotoxic, and nephrotoxic drugs) could be an aggravating factor for an otherwise common acute viral hepatitis. Full restriction of potentially nephrotoxic drugs is crucial for preventing superimposed drug-induced renal failure. The latter increases the risk of severe intracranial hypertension and is associated with a very poor prognosis (see above). In sexually active women, the administration of oral contraceptives should be interrupted.

Hepatitis due to paracetamol overdose

Intravenous administration of N-acetylcysteine, initiated 36 to 80 h after paracetamol overdose, was shown by a prospective controlled trial to improve the survival rate of patients with established fulminant hepatic failure.[73] Moreover, N-acetylcysteine can improve haemodynamics and oxygen delivery in the most severe forms of fulminant hepatic failure.[40]

Acute fatty liver of pregnancy

Early diagnosis, primarily based on the immediate identification of polydipsia (Kennedy, BrJObsGyn, 1994; 101:387), nausea, and vomiting in the third trimester, and early termination of pregnancy allows a 100 per cent maternal survival rate and stops the otherwise unavoidable descent towards fulminant liver failure (see Section 28).

Wilson's disease

In most (often young) patients with the acute form of Wilson's disease, early administration of high doses of D-penicillamine must be started on clinical grounds (Durand, JHepatol, 1990; 11, Suppl. 2:S20) and may obviate, or at least reduce, the requirement for emergency liver transplantation.

Hypoxic hepatitis

In patients with ischaemic liver cell necrosis, the cause of the transient reduction in cardiac output should be determined and treated early to avoid short-term recurrence which could aggravate the liver lesions.

Herpes simplex hepatitis

The specific treatment for herpes simplex hepatitis, acyclovir, must be started early, even on a clinical basis (Glorioso, DigDisSci, 1996; 41:1273) after sampling for blood and, if possible, liver, for virological studies, especially in immunocompromised patients.

Hepatitis B virus acute reactivation

Severe acute hepatitis due to HBV reactivation is commonly associated with the presence of HBV-DNA in plasma. This finding, a marker of viral replication, suggests that antiviral therapy directed against HBV could be valuable in protecting still uninfected hepatocytes. No data are currently available, but it is interesting to note that, in several transplanted patients, HBV replication was stopped

by using ganciclovir (Mertens, JHepatol, 1996; 25:968), famciclovir (Böker, Transpl, 1994; 57:706), or lamivudine (Bain, Transpl, 1996; 62:1462).

Prevention of further aggravation in patients with severe and fulminant or subfulminant hepatic failure

All previous measures discussed must still be applied. Rapid transfer to a liver unit is mandatory as soon as clinical encephalopathy is present. Patients must be cared for by an intensive care specialist. Early intubation is required in stuporous or comatose patients. Our policy is still to recommend a minimal use of drugs (especially those potentially sedative, hypotensive, hepatotoxic, or nephrotoxic) in order to avoid adding their effects, therapeutic or deleterious, to the natural course of the syndrome. Restraint may be needed in restless patients,. Although transfer by helicopter appears most suitable for long distances (Ede, SemLivDis, 1986; 6:107), overseas transfer by plane may be safe (personal experience).

Management of patients with clinical encephalopathy

The management of patients affected by fulminant or subfulminant hepatic failure includes the specific liver treatment if any, supportive management, and emergency liver transplantation if necessary.

A treatment strategy should take into account that (a) spontaneous recovery without sequellae, obviously the best outcome, is possible in some patients; (b) risky treatment modalities, especially drugs, may unexpectedly aggravate the patient's condition; and (c) emergency liver transplantation may be life-saving in patients who will otherwise die.

Specific liver treatments

Although specific treatment for the liver is effective only in a minority of causes, it is a crucial aspect of the management since it aims at reducing the aggravation of liver lesions. It is most suitable and effective at an earlier stage of the disease, before encephalopathy develops (see under Prevention of the fulminant and subfulminant course of established acute liver diseases and Table 11).

Medical supportive management (Tables 12 and 13)[6]

Medical supportive management aims to support the patient's life without iatrogenic deterioration up to a spontaneous recovery or emergency liver transplantation. It should be targeted with the following considerations in mind: (a) liver regeneration, the cornerstone process of recovery after destruction of a large amount of liver tissue, must be fully preserved; (b) the natural course of the disease should be preserved as much as possible in order to be able to obtain repeated information about the actual severity of the disease; (c) acute liver lesions and their extrahepatic consequences greatly affect normal hepatic and renal disposition of drugs and make their use very hazardous.

It is important to emphasize that many aspects of the medical management presented in Tables 12 and 13 are not supported by

Table 11 Specific liver treatments in patients with severe acute, fulminant, and subfulminant hepatic failure

A. Antidotes
1. *N*-Acetycysteine* (preferentially intravenously) in case of
   (a) Paracetamol overdose
   (b) Recent ingestion of therapeutic doses of paracetamol in patients at increased risk of hepatotoxicity
   (c) Carbon tetrachloride poisoning
   (d) Penaroia poisoning
2. Antidotes to *Amanita phalloides* poisoning

B. Antiviral therapy in fulminant viral hepatitis
1. Herpes simplex, varicella-zoster viruses (acyclovir)
2. HBV-DNA positive hepatitis B virus reactivation (ganciclovir?, famciclovir?, lamivudine?)
3. Crimean–Congo haemorrhagic fever and Lassa fever (ribavirin)

C. Specific measure for other causes of acute liver failure
1. Hypoxic hepatitis (oxygen, treatment of heart failure)
2. Autoimmune hepatitis (corticosteroids)
3. Giant-cell hepatitis (corticosteroids)
4. Wilson's disease (high doses of D-penicillamine)
5. Acute fatty liver of pregnancy (early delivery)
6. Malignant infiltration (urgent antineoplastic chemotherapy)

D. Special measures after emergency liver transplantation
1. Prevention of thrombosis of hepatic vessels
2. Early immunosuppressive therapy

* *N*-Acetylcysteine may also be used as a non-specific treatment.

Table 12 Theoretical aims of liver treatments in acute liver failure

1. To preserve the uninjured liver parenchyma
2. To eliminate the cause of the disease
3. To encourage liver regeneration

Table 13 Treatments that must be continued in patients with acute liver failure

Treatment	Associated disorder
Intravenous quinine	Falciparum malaria
Insulin	Insulin-dependent diabetes
Hormonal therapy	Adrenal or thyroid insufficiency

controlled trials.[6] Many teams use an aggressive intensive care strategy and only a few,[12] including ours, advocate a less invasive strategy. It is still unclear whether the results presented by the former are significantly better than those reported by the latter (Bernuau, JHepatol, 1996; 25, suppl. 1:63).[12,92]

Specialized intensive care liver unit

Admission to an intensive care liver unit with clinical expertise in the overall care of mutiple organ failure is highly recommended in patients affected by fulminant or subfulminant hepatic failure,[6, 92] particularly because prognostic evaluation will benefit from the database compiled from experience with previous patients.

Vascular accesses

Some authors use a pulmonary artery flotation catheter and a radial arterial line in all patients with severe acute hepatitis (without encephalopathy) or with fulminant hepatic failure admitted to their liver unit.[36] We recommend the use of one, or two, peripheral short venous catheter(s) for solute infusions and volume expanders in all non-comatose patients and in some of those with low-grade coma. Since a pulmonary artery catheter carries iatrogenic risks of bacterial superinfection and cardiac arrhythmias (O'Grady, Clin-Gastro, 1989; 3:75), we use it only when it is imperative. We routinely catheterize the jugular vein (Goldfarb, Anesthesiol; 56: 321) which is safer than the subclavian vein because an increased risk of haemopneumothorax is associated with the latter. The arterial catheter is useful for frequent blood sampling and control of arterial blood gases in comatose patients.

Nutritional support

Adequate caloric intake requires intravenous hypertonic (usually 10 per cent) dextrose on a daily basis (200 to 300 g). The use of insulin (usually at a reduced dose) should be restricted to patients previously affected by insulin-dependent diabetes. Daily supplementation with polyvitamins (particularly group B vitamins), potassium, and phosphorus supplementation is required. Daily sodium intake and water volume are modulated according to neurological, haemodynamic, and renal conditions and the daily results of plasma electrolyte assays. Magnesium supplementation may be needed. Amino acids and lipid solutions, the therapeutic efficacy of which has not been demonstrated, are not recommended.

Cardiovascular condition

Non-invasive cardiac monitoring is routine. We do not support systematic use of the pulmonary artery flotation catheter in any patient with fulminant or subfulminant hepatic failure.[36] A prospective study in five United States teaching hospitals found that right heart catheterization in critically-ill patients was associated with increased mortality,[93] and whether this invasive procedure benefits all critically-ill patients is now seriously questioned (Dalen, JAMA, 1996; 276:916). We restrict the use of intravascular haemodynamic monitoring to patients with a rapidly developing or already established major complication and those for whom renal replacement therapy or emergency liver transplantation has been decided.

Relative hypovolaemia with low central venous pressure is common. Blood volume expansion may be achieved with saline or a human albumin solution. Fresh frozen plasma should not be used as a volume expander since it would artificially modify coagulation factors, the best prognostic indicators, and thereby obscure prognostic evaluation. Blood units will maintain haematocrit above 30 per cent.

Administration of inotropes, noradrenaline, or adrenaline, is indicated when hypotension occurs and persists despite satisfactory blood volume repletion. Because of the reduction in oxygen delivery to tissues induced by these drugs, the use of vasodilators such as prostacycline[41] and N-acetylcysteine[40] has been recommended even in cases not due to paracetamol hepatotoxicity. We have used intravenous N-acetylcysteine for several years in all patients with fulminant or subfulminant hepatic failure.

Drugs with vasodilator or hypotensive activity are contraindicated if there is systemic hypertension because of the risk of further increasing brain tissue ischaemia (Overgaard, Stroke, 1975; 6:402).

Respiratory assistance

External monitoring of blood oxygen saturation is routine. Assisted mechanical ventilation is required if decrease in blood oxygen saturation persists despite nasal oxygen, or if there is respiratory failure as indicated by either the rapid correction of hypocapnia toward normocapnia or the abrupt occurrence of hypercapnia. Tracheal intubation may be extremely difficult because of a frequent trismus and the risk of mucosal haemorrhage from the mouth or the nasopharynx. A short half-life curare may be helpful. We recommend administration of low doses of penicillin (or penicillin derivatives) for 2 days to prevent pneumococcal bactaeremia associated with intubation. Reduction in hepatic blood flow may be a deleterious consequence of positive end-expiratory pressure (Bonnet, CritCareMed,1982; 10:703).

Renal failure

Oliguria attests to relative hypovolaemia and systematic blood volume expansion is recommended by some authors.[36] We do not use it in all patients. Blood volume expansion becomes less effective as the liver fails and may be a contributing factor to rising intracranial pressure without benefit to renal function.

Dopamine (2–4 μg/kg/min) may be of some value but may also be deleterious when high-rate tachycardia is present. Potentially nephrotoxic drugs such as aminoglycosides and iodine-derived opacifying agents must be avoided. Frusemide would be indicated in patients with high blood volume and pulmonary oedema, an uncommon condition in patients with fulminant hepatic failure and without congestive heart failure. High doses of mannitol alone may also aggravate deterioration of renal function (Dorman, Medicine, 1990; 69:153).

Renal replacement therapy may be indicated while waiting for a liver graft (Larner, BMJ, 1988; 297:1514) or during emergency liver transplantation because of severe renal failure associated with severe brain oedema. Haemodialysis may be used in haemodynamically stable patients but haemofiltration is better tolerated neurologically (Davenport, BMJ, 1987; 295:1028; Larner, BMJ, 1988; 297:1514). Sudden accidents of fatal decerebration have occurred during haemodialysis sessions (Schiodt, ScaJGastr, 1995; 30:927).

Encephalopathy and cerebral oedema

Metabolic disorders potentially deleterious for the brain, including hypoxaemia, hypoglycaemia, hypophosphataemia, and metabolic acidosis, must be corrected or, preferably, prevented. Correction of hyponatraemia may not be required and should be kept below 10 mmol/l daily to reduce the risk of central pontine myelinolysis (Karp, Medicine, 1993; 72:359; Abbasoglu, Hepatol, 1996; 24:427 A); haemofiltration could be useful.

Sedation is frequently used, especially in patients with psychomotor agitation before tracheal intubation and during mechanical ventilation (Munoz, SemLivDis, 1993; 13:395). We believe that sedative and antiemetic drugs should be avoided as much as possible, even after emergency liver transplantation has been decided upon: by altering the spontaneous neurological status, they interfere with the natural course of the disease and obscure prognosis. Restless patients may rather be restrained.

No specific treatment of hepatic encephalopathy is available. Intravenous administration of flumazenil, a benzodiazepine receptor antagonist, has been reported to be associated with awakening in a few comatose patients (Grimm, Lancet, 1988; ii:1392). Flumazenil can be useful in those with superimposed benzodiazepine-induced encephalopathy (personal experience).

Comatose patients often have cerebral oedema. They should be placed in a quiet room, and kept with the trunk and the head at 20 to 30° from the horizontal while avoiding any jugular vein compression. Severe cerebral oedema is improved neither by corticosteroids[94] nor by controlled hyperventilation although the onset of coning may be delayed.[22] The first and main treatment of severe (i.e. clinically symptomatic) cerebral oedema is mannitol (bolus infusion of 0.5 g/kg) which can be repeated every 4 h as necessary.[94] Renal function must be carefully monitored since renal failure makes mannitol infusions ineffective and dangerous and may indicate the need for renal replacement therapy.

Administration of sodium thiopentone (185–500 mg over 15 min for 1 h, followed by continuous infusion) was reported to control otherwise mannitol-resistant intracranial hypertension in patients with renal failure.[95] However, thiopental administration leads to barbiturate coma and invasive haemodynamic monitoring is required because of a high risk of hypotension. Inotropic catecholamines may be needed to maintain adequate cerebral perfusion pressure.

Invasive intracranial pressure monitoring, although unsupported by any controlled trial, is used in many centres especially in patients listed for emergency liver transplantation (Munoz, SemLivDis, 1993; 13:395; Riegler, MedClinNAm, 1993; 77:057; Ellis, SemLivDis, 1996; 16:379). Subdural transducers are usually used.

Although some authors claim the technique to be safe,[25] severe complications do occur, especially in those patients with a high intracranial pressure (Aldersley, JHepatol, 1994; 21:S52). Monitoring of the intracranial pressure by itself neither improves survival (Ede, JHepatol, 1986; 2:3) nor changes the indication for emergency liver transplantation. However, in one Spanish prospective study, the absence or the definitive control of significant intracranial hypertension (30 mmHg) was associated with a higher survival rate (Salmeron, JHepatol, 1991; 13, Suppl 2:S67). Our policy is not to use invasive intracranial pressure monitoring (Bernuau, JHepatol, 1996; 25, Suppl. 1:63).

Metabolic disorders

Hypoglycaemia requires additional dextrose bolus as well as meticulous monitoring aimed at detecting asymptomatic recurrences. Alkalosis should not be treated. Metabolic acidosis requires both the diagnosis and treatment of contributing factors (such as bacterial superinfection) as well as sodium bicarbonate infusion or even haemodialysis (see also under Encephalopathy and cerebral oedema above).

Coagulopathy and bleeding tendency

Because coagulation disorders are one of the most accurate prognostic factors (see above), any attempt to correct them in the absence of overt bleeding will decrease the accuracy of prognostic evaluation. Administration of fresh frozen plasma does not improve survival (Gazzard, Gut, 1975; 16:617), but does increase the risk of inappropriate indication for emergency liver transplantation (Langer, UpdateIntensCareEmergMed, 1990; 10:482) by modifying the patient's coagulation.

Spontaneous bleeding tendency is rare but skin puncture sites do require protracted compression. Thrombopenia occasionally requires platelet administration associated with small amounts of heparin in order to prevent exacerbation of disseminated intravascular coagulation. Prevention of gastrointestinal haemorrhage by cimetidine has been recommended (MacDougall, Gastro, 1978; 74: 464). However, we never use H_2-receptor antagonists in patients with fulminant or subfulminant hepatic failure, because their neurological side-effects are often seen (up to 80 per cent) in patients in hospital with liver failure and in those with renal failure.[96,97] Sucralfate or omeprazole are as effective as H_2-receptor antagonists for preventing stress-associated gastrointestinal haemorrhage.

Sepsis

Preventive administration of selective parenteral and enteral antibiotics does not improve survival rate.[98] Bacteraemia and parenchymal bacterial infections should be treated with appropriate antibiotics. Aminoglycosides are contraindicated because their nephrotoxicity is increased by liver failure (Moore, AmJMed, 1986; 80:1093). Fungal infections, the incidence of which can be increased by H_2-receptor antagonists (Triger, Lancet, 1981;ii:837), require antifungal therapy in patients with positive cultures from a significant site (Rolando, JHepatol, 1991; 12:1). Intrauterine devices must be extracted.

Liver regeneration

No effective treatment for initiation or acceleration of liver regeneration is currently known. Corticosteroids can be deleterious (Tsukamoto, Gut, 1989; 30:387). Several randomized and non-randomized trials have demonstrated that the combination of insulin and glucagon which probably plays a role in liver regeneration[40] has no beneficial effect in patients affected by fulminant liver failure (Van Severen, GastrClinBiol, 1987; 11:79A ; Harrison, JHepatol, 1990; 10:332)[99] and may cause fatal hypoglycaemia (Oka, GastrJap, 1989; 24:332).

Miscellaneous treatments

Several treatments were shown to be ineffective when they were evaluated by randomized trials. They include human cross-circulation (Sicot, AnnMédIntern, 1971; 122:381), extracorporeal liver perfusion (Parbhoo, Lancet, 1971; i:659), exchange-transfusion therapy (Redeker, Lancet, 1973; i:3), heparin (Gazzard, Gut, 1974; 15:89), corticosteroids (EASL Trial Committee, Gut, 1979; 20:620), haemodialysis (Denis, Gut, 1978; 19:787), and charcoal haemoperfusion (O'Grady, Gastro, 1988;94:1186). The beneficial effect of intravenous prostaglandin E_1 reported in an uncontrolled study (Sinclair, JCI, 1989; 84:1063) was not confirmed by others (Bernuau, Hepatol, 1990; 12:373A) and after a controlled trial by the same Canadian team (Sheiner, Hepatol, 1992; 16:88A).

Plasmapheresis (Lepore, AnnIntMed, 1970; 72:165) also did not improve survival but could be a temporary support while awaiting emergency liver transplantation (Winikoff, JPediatr, 1985; 107:547 ; Munoz, TransplProc, 1989; 21:3535). In a non-randomized trial by the Copenhagen group, high volume plasmapheresis was shown to improve cerebral haemodynamics and to allow a spontaneous survival rate of 35 per cent.[100]

Emergency total liver transplantation

Emergency liver transplantation is currently the only curative treatment for patients with fulminant or subfulminant hepatic failure in whom short-term prognosis is presumed to be fatal.

Orthotopic total liver transplantation is most often performed; because of the emergency conditions, ABO incompatible grafts may be used (Gugenheim, Lancet, 1990; 336:519). Full preservation of portal and caval flows is almost always feasible.[101,102] In most centres, emergency total liver transplantation is associated with a 50 to 70 per cent survival rate for adult patients who theoretically should all have died (Table 4). Survival in children is in the same range.[103] Per- or postoperative brain death is an important factor in mortality and threatens primarily patients with high-grade coma.[26] Preoperative acute renal failure is the most important component of the postoperative prognosis (Devlin, Hepatol, 1995; 21:1018). Survivors must receive lifelong immunosuppression. The actuarial 5-year survival rate in adults has been shown to be 61 per cent,[3] but the long-term future of these often young patients is still unknown.

In eight American patients, the operation was performed after extracorporeal liver support for several hours, using either an unwanted human liver (Fox, AmJGastr, 1993; 88:1876) or a porcine liver (Fair, Gastro, 1993; 104:899A; Chari, NEJM, 1994; 331:234). The survival rate was 50 per cent.

Table 14 Paracetamol-induced fulminant hepatic failure and emergency liver transplantation (King's College Hospital, London, 1987–93)[1]

Patients	*n*	Dead	Survivors	Emergency liver transplantation
Candidates[2]	112			
Not listed	62	52[3]	10	0
Listed	50	21	6	23
Total		73	16	23
Total (%)	100	65	14	20

[1] From Makin, Gastro, 1995; 109:1907.
[2] Fulfilling King's College transplantation criteria specific to patients with paracetamol-induced fulminant hepatic failure (8 per cent of those not fulfilling the criteria died).
[3] Among these 52 patients, 28 were in critical condition and emergency liver transplantation was contraindicated in 24 because of their history.

In other patients, the operation was performed as a two-stage procedure with an anhepatic time ranging from 6 to 74 h. In two series of patients, 32 with 5 patients with fulminant hepatitis in Hannover (Ringe, AnnSurg, 1993; 218:3) and 8 with fulminant hepatitis in London (Ellis, Gut, 1995; 36, Suppl. 1:A32), transplantation rates were 60 per cent and 63 per cent and survival rates 22 per cent and 25 per cent, respectively. Accordingly, we do not support this strategy. A bioartificial liver device was used during the anhepatic time in an American woman with paracetamol overdose who survived (Rozga, Lancet, 1993; 342:898).

Emergency auxiliary partial liver transplantation

Emergency auxiliary partial liver transplantation has been performed since 1991 (Gubernatis, WorldJSurg, 1991; 15:660). Its main advantage is that it allows, at least in 50 to 60 per cent of survivors, full regeneration of the native liver and the withdrawal of immunosuppression.[5] Disadvantages are somewhat increased operative and postoperative risks and, in some survivors, impaired regeneration of the native liver which does not allow the withdrawal of immunosuppression.[5] The best results are obtained in patients younger than 40 years affected by viral or paracetamol-associated hepatitis.[5] At Hôpital Beaujon,France, the operation was feasible in only one-third of candidates (Belghiti, Hepatol, 1995; 22:153A).

Emergency living-related partial liver transplantation

Emergency living-related partial liver transplantation has been performed since 1990 in a few children for whom no allograft from a cadaveric donor was available. At least 12 cases have been reported in Japan (Matsunami, Lancet, 1992; 340:1411; Tanaka, TransplInt, 1994; 7, Suppl. 1:S108), Belgium (Otte, personal communication), Germany (Broelsch, personal communication), Denmark (Ejlersen, TransplProc, 1994; 26:1794) and France (Bismuth, AnnSurg, 1996; 224:712; Valayer, personal communication). Overall short-term (1 month to 1 year) survival rate is 50 per cent.

Criteria for emergency liver transplantation

The major prerequisite for, and certainly one of the major difficulties of, emergency liver transplantation is to make an accurate individual prognosis. The ideal aim would be to transplant, as early as possible, the patients who otherwise would die from fulminant or subfulminant hepatic failure and not to transplant those who will either survive spontaneously or die from multiple organ failure. Our experience of 200 patients evaluated for emergency liver transplantation in the past 10 years has taught us that the decision is rarely straightforward.

From a retrospective study based on 763 patients with fulminant or subfulminant hepatic failure, the King's College Hospital group in London[72] established two different sets of criteria based on a fatal risk above 80 per cent for deciding emergency liver transplantation. The first set refers to 431 patients with paracetamol hepatotoxicity (more than 6 per cent did not develop encephalopathy) (Table 14). In other patients with fulminant hepatic failure also due to paracetamol overdose, the same group reported different criteria based on sequential assays of prothrombin time (Harrison, BMJ, 1990; 301:964) and modified one of the initial criteria, namely admission pH < 7.3.[36] During a 7-year experience in London, 23 to 42 per cent of patients fulfilling the criteria survived spontaneously.[36] The second set of King's criteria refers to 332 patients with fulminant or subfulminant hepatic failure not due to paracetamol. According to these criteria, clinical encephalopathy is not an absolute requirement and several patients were transplanted without encephalopathy (O'Grady, Lancet, 1986; ii:1227; Ellis, JHepatol, 1995; 23:363).

In the prospective study initiated in 1986 at Hôpital Beaujon, the presence of at least grade 3 (severe confusion) or 4 encephalopathy (coma) is an absolute requirement for emergency liver transplantation (the rationale is that the survival rate of patients who never develop clinical encephalopathy is close to 100 per cent). Among these patients with encephalopathy, we select the candidates for emergency liver transplantation according to two key independent prognostic factors, the patient's age and factor V activity, with the risk of death being above 85 per cent. With this strategy, 11 per cent of the patients fulfilling the criteria survive spontaneously, the brain death rate is 19 per cent, and the early survival rate 68 per cent (Bernuau, JHepatol, 1996; 25, Suppl. 1: 63).

Despite the remarkable early results obtained with emergency liver transplantation, we fully endorse Sherlock's statement that 'liver transplantation cannot be accepted as the perfect and ideal treatment for fulminant hepatic failure'.[104] We believe in caution for at least three important reasons. The most important is the now recognized risk of overtransplantation which ranges between 10 and 30 per cent. This risk is unavoidable since criteria were not calculated for a 100 per cent risk of death. Accordingly, an as yet unnoticed consequence of emergency liver transplantation is to reduce the overall spontaneous survival rate: in patients affected by late-onset hepatic failure, the spontaneous survival rate decreased from 19 to 12 per cent and simultaneously the transplantation rate increased from 2 to 50 per cent. The second risk is the postoperative mortality, which ranges between 15 and 30 per cent. The third risk is the requirement for lifelong immunosuppression making a previously normal individual into a permanent patient. In 1990, a controlled trial of emergency liver transplantation was proposed, [105] but several hepatologists, including ourselves, argued against it.

Actual improvement of the irreducible difficulties associated with the decision for emergency liver transplantation may only come from an improvement of prevention of fulminant and subfulminant hepatic failure. This requires raising the diagnostic awareness of general physicians so that earlier recognition of patients with severe acute hepatic failure and their earlier referral to liver units for urgent diagnosis and treatment prior to clinical encephalopathy can be achieved. Towards this aim we feel that the current definition of fulminant and subfulminant hepatic failure should be extended to the concept of acute hepatic failure before clinical encephalopathy.[11]

References

1. Hawker F, ed. *The liver.* London: Saunders, 1993.
2. Lee WM and Williams R, eds. *Acute liver failure.* Cambridge: Cambridge University Press, 1997.
3. Samuel D and Bismuth H. Liver transplantation in patients with acute liver failure: the European experience. In Lee WM and Williams R, eds. *Acute liver failure.* Cambridge: Cambridge University Press, 1997 .
4. Shaw BW Jr. Transplantation for acute liver failure: the American experience. In Lee WM and Williams R, eds. *Acute liver failure.* Cambridge: Cambridge University Press 1997.
5. Chenard-Neu MP, Boudjema K, Bernuau J, *et al.* Auxiliary liver transplantation: regeneration of the native liver and outcome in 30 patients with fulminant hepatic failure. A multicenter European study. *Hepatology,* 1996; **23**: 1119–27.
6. Carceni P and Van Thiel DH. Acute liver failure. *Lancet,* 1995; **345**: 163–69.
7. Boudjema K, Chenard-Neu MP, and Jaeck D. Auxiliary liver transplantation. In Lee WM and Williams R, eds. *Acute liver failure.* Cambridge: Cambridge University Press 1997: 211–21 .
8. Hoofnagle JH, Carithers RL, Shapiro C, and Ascher N. Fulminant hepatic failure: summary of a workshop. *Hepatology,* 1995; **21**: 240–52.
9. O'Grady JG, Schalm S, and Williams R. Acute liver failure: redefining the syndromes. *Lancet,* 1993; **342**: 273–75.
10. Tandon BN, Joshi YK, Krishnamurthy L, and Tandon HD. Subacute hepatic failure: is it a distinct entity? *Journal of Clinical Gastroenterology,* 1982; **4**: 343–46.
11. Bernuau J, Rueff B, Benhamou JP. Fulminant and subfulminant liver failure: definitions and causes. *Seminars in Liver Diseases,* 1986; **6**: 97–106.
12. Acharya SK, Dasarathy S, Kumer TL, *et al.* Fulminant hepatitis in a tropical population : clinical course, cause, and early predictors of outcome. *Hepatology,* 1996; **23**: 1448–55.
13. Madl C, Grimm G, Ferenci P, Kramer L, *et al.* Serial recording of sensory evoked potentials: a noninvasive prognostic indicator in fulminant liver failure. *Hepatology,* 1994; **20**: 1487–94.
14. Vexler ZS, Ayus JC, Roberts PL, Fraser CL, Kucharczyk J, and Arieff AI. Hypoxic and ischemic hypoxia exacerbate brain injury associated with metabolic encephalopathy in laboratory animals. *Journal of Clinical Investigation,* 1994; **93**: 256–64.
15. Munoz SJ, Robinson M, Northrup B, *et al.* Elevated intracranial pressure and computed tomography of the brain in fulminant hepatic failure. *Hepatology,* 1991; **13**: 209–12.
16. Blei A. Brain oedema and intracranial hypertension in acute liver failure. In Lee WM and Williams R, eds. *Acute liver failure.* Cambridge: Cambridge University Press 1997: 144–57 .
17. Aggarwal S , Kramer D, Yonas H, *et al.* Cerebral hemodynamic and metabolic changes in fulminant hepatic failure: a retrospective study. *Hepatology,* 1994; **19**: 80–7.
18. Wendon JA, Harrison PM, Keays R, and Williams R. Cerebral blood flow and metabolism in fulminant liver failure. *Hepatology,* 1994; **19**: 1407–13.
19. Larsen FS, Ejlersen E, Hansen BA, Knudsen GM, Tygstrup N, and Secher NH. Functional loss of cerebral blood flow autoregulation in patients with fulminant hepatic failure. *Journal of Hepatology,* 1995; **23**: 212–17.
20. Larsen FS, Hansen BA, Pott F, *et al.* Dissociated cerebral vasoparalysis in acute liver failure. A hypothesis of gradual cerebral hyperaemia. *Journal of Hepatology,* 1996; **25**: 145–51.
21. Davies MH, Mutimer D, Lowes J, Elias E, and Neuberger J. Recovery despite impaired cerebral perfusion in fulminant hepatic failure. *Lancet,* 1994; **343**: 1329–30.
22. Ede RJ, Gimson AES, Bihari D, and Williams R. Controlled hyperventilation in the prevention of cerebral oedema in fulminant hepatic failure. *Journal of Hepatology,* 1986; **2**: 43–51.
23. Blei AT, Olafsson S, Webster S, and Levy R. Complications of intracranial pressure monitoring in fulminant hepatic failure. *Lancet,* 1993; **341**: 157–8.
24. Lidofsky SD, *et al.* Intracranial pressure monitoring and liver transplantation for fulminant hepatic failure. *Hepatology,* 1992; **16**: 1–7.
25. Keays RT, Alexander GJM, and Williams R. The safety and value of extradural intracranial pressure monitors in fulminant hepatic failure. *Journal of Hepatology,* 1993; **18**: 205–9.
26. Bismuth H, Samuel D, Castaing D, *et al.* Orthotopic liver transplantation in fulminant and subfulminant hepatitis. The Paul-Brousse experience. *Annals of Surgery,* 1995; **222**: 109–19.
27. Valla D, Flejou JF, Lebrec D, Bernuau J, Salzmann JL, and Benhamou JP. Portal hypertension and ascites in acute hepatitis: clinical, hemodynamic and histological correlations. *Hepatology,* 1989; **10**: 482–7.
28. Ring-Larsen H. Associated renal failure. In Williams R, ed. *Liver failure.* Edinburgh: Churchill Livingstone, 1986; 72–92.
29. Perrone RD, Madias NE, and Levey AS. Serum creatinine as an index of renal function: new insights into old concepts. *Clinical Chemistry,* 1992; **38**: 1933–53.
30. Bihari DJ, Gimson AES, and Williams R. Cardiovascular, pulmonary and renal complications of fulminant hepatic failure. *Seminars in Liver Diseases,* 1986; **6**: 119–28.
31. Sherlock S. Vasodilatation associated with hepatocellular disease: relation to functional organ failure. *Gut,* 1990; **31**: 365–7.
32. Schneider F, Lutun P, Boudjema K, Wolf P, and Tempe JD. *In vivo* evidence of enhanced guanylyl cyclase activation during the hyperdynamic circulation of acute liver failure. *Hepatology,* 1994; **19**: 38–44.
33. O'Grady JG, Langley PG, Isola LM, Aledort LM, and Williams R. Coagulopathy and fulminant hepatic failure. *Seminars in Liver Diseases.* 1986; **6**: 159–63.

34. Langley PG, Hughes RD, and Williams R. Increased factor VIII complex in fulminant hepatic failure. *Thrombosis and Haemostasis*, 1985; **54**: 693–6.

35. Makin AJ, Wendon J, and Williams R. A 7-year experience of severe acetaminophen-induced hepatotoxicity (1987–1993). *Gastroenterology*, 1995; **109**: 1907–16.

36. Robert A and Chazouilleres O. Prothrombin time in liver failure: time, ratio, activity percentage, or international normalized ratio? *Hepatology*, 1996; **24**: 1392–4.

37. Pernambuco JRB, Langley PG, Hughes RD, Izumi S, and Williams R. Activation of the fibrinolytic system in patients with fulminant liver failure. *Hepatology*, 1993; **18**: 1350–6.

38. Consensus Conference. Tissue hypoxia. How to detect, how to correct, how to prevent? *American Journal of Respiratory and Critical Care Medicine*, 1996; **154**: 1573–8.

39. Harrison PM, Wendon JA, Gimson AES, Alexander GJM, and Williams R. Improvement by acetylcysteine of hemodynamics and oxygen transport in fulminant hepatic failure. *New England Journal of Medicine*, 1991; **324**: 1852–7.

40. Wendon JA, Harrison PM, Keays R, Gimson AES, Alexander GJM, and Williams R. Effects of vasopressor agents and epoprostenol on systemic hemodynamics and oxygen transport in fulminant hepatic failure. *Hepatology*, 1992; **15**: 1067–71.

41. Roche-Sicot J and Benhamou JP. Acute intravascular hemolysis and acute liver failure associated as a first manifestation of Wilson's disease. *Annals of Internal Medicine*, 1977; **86**: 301–3.

42. Rolando N, Gimson A, Wade J, Philpott-Howard J, Casewell M, and Williams R. Prospective controlled trial of selective parenteral and enteral antimicrobial regimen in fulminant hepatic failure. *Hepatology*, 1993; **17**: 196–201.

43. Arns PA and Branch RA. Prescribing for patients with liver disease. *Baillière's Clinical Gastroenterology*, 1989; **3**: 109–30.

44. Benhamou JP, Rueff B, and Sicot C. Severe hepatic failure: a critical study of current therapy. In: Orlandi F and Jezequel AM, eds. *Liver and drugs*. London: Academic Press, 1972; 213–28.

45. Wolf HK and Michalopoulos GK. Hepatocyte regeneration in acute fulminant hepatic and nonfulminant hepatitis: a study of proliferating cell nuclear antigen expression. *Hepatology*, 1992; **15**: 707–13.

46. Gove CD and Hughes RD. Liver regeneration in relationship to acute liver failure. *Gut Supplement*, 1991; S92–S96.

47. Hoffman AL, Rosen HR, Ljubimova JU, *et al*. Hepatic regeneration. Current concepts and clinical implications. *Seminars in Liver Diseases*, 1994; **14**: 190–210.

48. Wu JC, Chen CL, Hou MC, Chen TZ, Lee SD, Lo KJ. Multiple viral infection as the most comon cause of fulminant and subfulminant viral hepatitis in an area endemic for hepatitis B: application and limitations of the polymerase chain reaction. *Hepatology* 1994; **19**: 836–40.

49. Huo TI, Wu JC, Sheng WY, *et al*. Prognostic factor analysis of fulminant and subfulminant hepatic failure in an area endemic for hepatitis B. *Journal of Gastroenterology and Hepatology*, 1996; **11**: 560–5.

50. Feray C, Gigou M, Samuel D, *et al*. Hepatitis C virus RNA and hepatitis B virus DNA in serum and liver of patients with fulminant hepatitis. *Gastroenterology*, 1993; **104**: 549–55.

51. Lacronique V, Mignon A, Fabre M, *et al*. Bcl-2 protects from lethal hepatic apoptosis induced by an anti-Fas antibody in mice. *Nature Medicine*, 1996; **2**: 80–6.

52. Pham BN, Mosnier JF, Durand F, *et al*. Immunostaining for membrane attack complex of complement is related to cell necrosis in fulminant and acute hepatitis. *Gastroenterology*, 1995; **108**: 495–504.

53. Sarraco G, Macagno S, Rosina F, Caredda F, Antinori S, and Rizzetto M. Serologic markers with fulminant hepatitis in persons positive for hepatitis B surface antigen. A worlwide epidemiology and clinical survey. *Annals of Internal Medicine*, 1988; **108**: 380–3.

54. Bernuau J, Goudeau A, Poynard T, *et al*. Multivariate analysis of prognostic factors in fulminant hepatitis B. *Hepatology*, 1986; **6**: 648–51.

55. Wright TL, Mamish D, Combs C, *et al*. Hepatitis B virus and apparent fulminant non-A, non-B hepatitis. *Lancet*, 1992; **339**: 952–5.

56. Levy P, Marcellin P, Martinot-Peignou X, Degott C, Nataf J, and Benhamou JP. Clinical course of spontaneous reactivation of hepatitis B virus in patients with chronic hepatitis B. *Hepatology*, 1990; **12**: 570–4.

57. Omata M, Ehata T, Yokosuka O, Hosoda K, and Ohto M. Mutations in the precore region of hepatitis B virus DNA in patients with fulminant and severe hepatitis. *New England Journal of Medicine*, 1991; **324**: 1699–704.

58. Sato S, Suzuki K, Akahane Y, *et al*. *Annals of Internal Medicine*, 1995; **122**: 241–8.

59. Karayiannis P, Alexopoulou A, Hadziyannis S, *et al*. Fulminant hepatitis associated with hepatitis B virus e antigen-negative infection : importance of host factors. *Hepatology*, 1995; **22**: 1628–34.

60. Smedile A, Farci P, Verme G, *et al*. Influence of delta infection on severity of hepatitis B. *Lancet*, 1982; **ii**: 945–7.

61. Govindarajan S, Chin KP, Redeker AG, and Peters RL. Fulminant B viral hepatitis: role of delta agent. *Gastroenterology*, 1984; **86**: 1417–20.

62. Lau JYN, Sallie R, Fang JWS, *et al*. Detection of hepatitis E virus genome and gene products in two patients with fulminant hepatitis. *European Journal of Hepatology*, 1995; **22**: 605–10.

63. Krawczynski K. Hepatitis E. *Hepatology*, 1993; **17**: 932–41.

64. Hamid SS, Jafri SMW, Khan H, Shah H, Abbas Z, and Fields H. Fulminant hepatic failure in pregnant women : acute fatty liver or acute viral hepatitis? *Journal of Hepatology*, 1996; **25**: 20–7.

65. Khuroo MS, Kamili S, and Jameel S. Vertical transmission of hepatitis E virus. *Lancet*, 1995; **345**: 1025–6.

66. Klein N, Mabie W, Shaver DC, *et al*. Herpes simplex virus hepatitis in pregnancy. Two patients successfully treated with acyclovir. *Gastroenterology*, 1991; **100**: 239–44.

67. Markin RS, Linder J, Zuerlein K, *et al*. Hepatitis in fatal infectious mononucleosis. *Gastroenterology*, 1987; **93**: 1210–17.

68. Ishak K, Walker D, Coetzer J, Gardner J, and Gorelkin L. Viral haemorrhagic fevers with hepatic involvement: pathologic aspects with clinical correlations. *Progress in Liver Diseases*, 1982; **7**: 495–515.

69. Howard CR. Viral haemorrhagic fevers: properties and prospects for treatment and prevention. *Antiviral Research*, 1984; **4**: 169–86.

70. Makin AJ and Williams R. Acetaminophen-induced acute liver failure. In: Lee WM and Williams R, eds. *Acute liver failure*. Cambridge: Cambridge University Press, 1997: 32–42.

71. O'Grady JG, Alexander GJM, Hayllar KM, and Williams R. Early indicators of prognosis in fulminant hepatic failure. *Gastroenterology*, 1989; **97**: 439–45.

72. Keays R, Harrison PM, Wendon JA, *et al*. Intravenous acetylcysteine in paracetamol induced fulminant hepatic failure: a prospectivve controlled trial. *British Medical Journal*, 1991; **303**: 1026–9.

73. Henry JA, Jeffreys KJ, and Dawling S. Toxicity and deaths from 3,4-methylenedioxymetamphetamine ('ecstasy'). *Lancet*, 1992; **340**: 384–7.

74. Chan TYK, Chan JCN, Tomlinson B, and Critchley JAJH. Chinese herbal medicines revisited: a Hong-Kong perspective. *Lancet*, 1993; **342**: 1532–4.

75. Lee WM. Drug-induced hepatotoxicity. *New England Journal of Medicine*, 1995; **333**: 1118–27.

76. Durand F, Bernuau J, Pessayre D, *et al*. Deleterious influence of pyrazinamide on the outcome of patients with fulminant or subfulminant liver failure during antituberculous treatment including isoniazid. *Hepatology*, 1995; **21**: 929–32.

77. Durand F, Jebrak G, Pessayre D, Fournier M, and Bernuau J. Hepatotoxicity of antitubercular treatments. Rationale for monitoring liver status. *Drug Safety*, 1996; **15**: 394–405.

78. Henrion J, Luwaert R, Colin L, Schmitz A, Schapira M, and Heller FR. Hépatite hypoxique. Etude prospective, clinique et hémodynamique de 45 épisodes. *Gastroentérologie Clinique et Biologique*, 1990; **14**: 836–41.

79. Henrion J, Descamps O, Luwaert R, Schapira M, Parfonry A, and Heller FR. Hypoxic hepatitis in patients with cardiac failure: incidence in a coronary care unit and measurement of hepatic blood flow. *Journal of Hepatology*, 1994; **21**: 696.

80. Bellary S, Hassanein T, and Van Thiel D. Liver transplantation in Wilson's disease. *Journal of Hepatology*, 1995; **23**: 373–81.

81. Durand F, Degott C, Sauvanet A, *et al*. Subfulminant syncytial giant cell hepatitis: recurrence after liver transplantation treated with ribavirin. *Journal of Hepatology*, 1997; **26**: 722–6.

82. O'Grady JG, Alexander GJM, Hayllar KM, and Williams R. Early indicators of prognosis in fulminant hepatic failure. *Gastroenterology*, 1989; **97**: 439–45.

83. Takahashi Y, Kumada H, Shimizu M, *et al*. A multicenter study on the prognosis of fulminant viral hepatitis: early prediction for liver transplantation. *Hepatology*, 1994; **19**: 1065–71.

84. Tygstrup N and Ranek L. Assessment of prognosis in fulminant hepatic failure. *Seminars in Liver Diseases*, 1986; **6**: 129–37.

85. Lee WM and Galbraith RM. The extracellular actin-scavenger system and actin toxicity. *New England Journal of Medicine*, 1992; **326**: 1335–41.

86. Lee WM, Galbraith RM, Watt GH, *et al*. Predicting survival in fulminant hepatic failure using serum Gc protein concentrations. *Hepatology*, 1995; **21**: 101–5.

87. Schiodt FV, Bondesen S, Petersen I, Dalhoff K, Ott P, and Tygstrup N. Admission levels of serum Gc-globulin : predictive value in fulminant hepatic failure. *Hepatology*, 1996; **23**: 713–18.

88. Strader DB and Seeff LB . Immunization for viral hepatitis. *Current Opinion in Gastroenterology*, 1996; **12** : 224–30.

89. Lemon SM and Shapiro CN. The value of immunization against hepatitis A. *Infective Agents and Diseases*, 1994; **3**: 38–49.

90. Tandon BN, Joshi YK, and Tandon M. Acute liver failure. Experience with 145 patients. *Journal of Clinical Gastroenterology*, 1986; **8**: 664–8.

91. Connors AF, Speroff T, Dawson NV, *et al*. The effectiveness of right heart catheterization in the initial care of critically ill patients. *Journal of the American Medical Association*, 1996; **276**: 889–97.

92. Canalese J, Gimson AES, Davis C, Mellon PJ, Davis M, and Williams R. Controlled trial of dexamethasone and mannitol for the cerebral oedema of fulminant hepatic failure. *Gut*, 1982; **23**: 625–29.

93. Forbes A, Alexander GJM, O'Grady JG, *et al*. Thiopental infusion in the treatment of intracranial hypertension complicating fulminant hepatic failure. *Hepatology*, 1989; **10**: 306–10.

94. Cantu TG and Korek JS. Central nervous system reactions to histamine-2 receptor blockers. *Annals of Internal Medicine*, 1991; **114**: 1027–34.

95. Freston JW. Perspectives on safety issues and drug interactions with H_2-receptor antagonists. *Journal of Drug Developments*, 1989; **2** (Suppl. 3): 61–70.

96. Rolando N, Gimson A, Philpott-Howard J, Casewell M, and Williams R. Prospective controlled trial of selective parenteral and enteral antimicrobial regimen in fulminant liver failure. *Hepatology*, 1993; **17**: 196–201.

97. Woolf GM and Redeker AG. Treatment of fulminant hepatic failure with insulin and glucagon. A randomized, controlled trial. *Digestive Diseases and Sciences*, 1991; **36**: 92–6.

98. Tygstrup N, Larsen FS, and Hansen BA. Treatment of acute liver failure by high volume plasmapheresis. In Lee WM and Williams R, eds. *Acute liver failure*. Cambridge: Cambridge University Press, 1997 .

99. Belghiti J, Panis Y, Sauvanet A, Gayet B, and Fekete F. A new technique of side to side caval anastomosis during orthotopic hepatic transplantation without inferior vena caval occlusion. *Surgery, Gynecology, Obstetrics*, 1992; **175**: 270–2.

100. Belghiti J, Noun R, Sauvanet A, *et al*. Transplantation for fulminant and subfulminant hepatic failure with preservation of portal and caval flow. *British Journal of Surgery*, 1995; **82**: 986–9.

101. Devictor D, Desplanques L, Debray D, *et al*. Emergency liver transplantation for fulminant liver failure in infants and children. *Hepatology*, 1992; **16**: 1156–62.

102. Sherlock S. Fulminant hepatic failure. *Advances in Internal Medicine*, 1993; **38**: 245–67.

103. Chapman RW, Forman D, Peto R, and Smallwood R. Liver transplantation for acute hepatic failure? *Lancet*, 1990; **335**: 32–5.

20

Inherited metabolic disorders

20.1 Wilson's disease

Irene Hung and Jonathan D. Gitlin

Introduction

Wilson's disease is an autosomal-recessive disorder of copper metabolism due to the absence or dysfunction of a copper-transporting, P-type ATPase encoded on the long arm of chromosome 13. This ATPase is essential for the transport of copper[1] into the bile and affected patients accumulate excessive copper within the liver as well as the brain and other tissues. Wilson's disease commonly presents in childhood but the correct diagnosis may be delayed for many years. If diagnosed early and properly managed, this disease is one of the more easily treated inborn errors of metabolism.

Wilson's disease was recognized as a distinct clinical entity in 1912 by Samuel Alexander Kinnier Wilson, who reported several cases of a new familial disorder resulting in progressive degeneration of the lenticular nuclei. Wilson observed that hepatic cirrhosis was an invariable feature of the disease and he speculated that a toxin was the cause of the hepatic and neurological degeneration (Wilson, Brain, 1912; 34:295). During a study of metal chelation in neurological patients, excess urinary copper excretion was noted in a patient with Wilson's disease and following up on this observation Cummings ascertained that copper was the aetiological agent of this disease (Cummings, Brain, 1948; 71:410). In this same year, Laurell identified caeruloplasmin as the major copper-binding protein of plasma and subsequently Scheinberg and Gitlin demonstrated a marked decrease in the concentration of this protein in the serum of patients with Wilson's disease (Scheinberg, Science, 1952; 116: 484).

The recognition of caeruloplasmin deficiency in Wilson's disease greatly facilitated diagnosis by providing a reliable biochemical marker for this disorder. Not long after, Walshe (AmJMed, 1956; 21:48) introduced penicillamine chelation therapy as the first effective long-term oral treatment. Subsequently, Bearn (AnnHumGen, 1960; 24:33) defined the autosomal-recessive inheritance by analysis of multiple affected kindreds, and careful studies by Cox and Sass-Kortsak (AmJHumGen, 1972; 24:646) detailed the specific heterogeneous clinical presentations. In 1985 the Wilson's disease gene was linked to the esterase D locus on chromosome 13 and further studies utilizing polymorphic minisatellite probes refined this localization to 13q14.3 (Frydman, PNAS, 1985; 82:1819; White, PNAS, 1993;90:10 105). In 1993 the Wilson's disease gene was independently cloned in the laboratories of Cox, Tanzi and Gilliam, and Gitlin (Bull, NatGen, 1993; 5:327; Tanzi, NatGen, 1993; 5: 344; Yamaguchi, BBResComm, 1993; 197:271).

Pathogenesis and pathology

The Wilson's disease gene[2] encodes a 1466 amino-acid protein that is a novel member of the cation-transport, P-type ATPase family. This ATPase is a polytopic membrane protein that transfers copper to the secretory pathway of the hepatocyte in an ATP-dependent manner (Fig. 1). Characteristic features of this protein include six CXXC copper-binding motifs in the aminoterminus that sense the copper concentration in the cytosol and modulate copper transport accordingly, a CPC motif within the transport channel essential for metal transfer, a DKTGT region that mediates formation of the aspartyl-phosphate intermediate essential for energy transduction, and an ATP-binding domain GDGVND. In addition to these recognized functional motifs, the sequence SEHPL located between the phosphorylation and ATP-binding domains is present in all copper-transport ATPases identified thus far in prokaryotic and eukaryotic organisms (Solioz, FEBSLett, 1994; 346:44). This region is the site of the most common mutation (H1070Q) in patients with Wilson's disease, and it has been proposed that conformational changes at this site may regulate transport activity analogous to that observed in other cation-transporting, P-type ATPases (Petrukhin, HumMolGenet, 1994; 3:1647).

The Wilson's ATPase is localized to the *trans*-Golgi and late endosomal compartments of hepatocytes, where it functions to transfer copper into a common pool for holocaeruloplasmin biosynthesis and biliary copper excretion (Fig. 2; see Chapter 2.16.2). More than 25 distinct functional mutations consisting of small insertions, deletions or missense mutations have thus far been characterized in patients with Wilson's disease (Thomas, NatGen, 1995; 9:210). Biliary excretion is the primary determinant of copper homeostasis, and the absence of ATPase function results in progressive accumulation of copper in the cytosol of the hepatocyte eventually leading to cell injury and death, with release of copper to the plasma and subsequent copper deposition in other tissues. The Wilson's ATPase is expressed in other tissues including the kidney and brain, and it is possible that loss of function of this protein in these organs directly contributes to extrahepatic copper accumulation. Extrahepatic symptoms may also arise as a result of cell-specific impairment of Wilson's ATPase-dependent synthesis of essential copper proteins such as those involved in neurotransmitter biosynthesis within regions of the central nervous system.

The decreased serum caeruloplasmin concentration in patients with Wilson's disease is also due to the loss of ATPase activity. The impairment of copper transport into the hepatocyte secretory

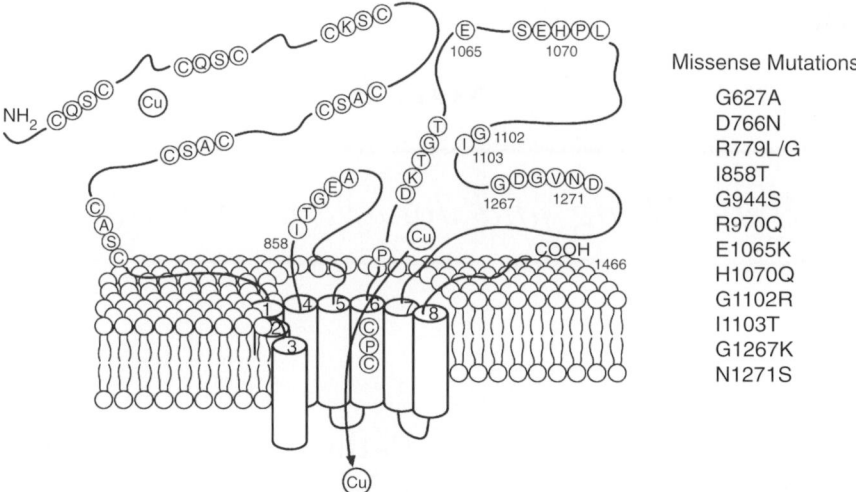

Fig. 1. Schematic of the Wilson's disease P-type ATPase with recognized protein motifs. Numbers indicate amino acids where missense mutations have thus far been identified (references in text). The function of this protein in the ATP-mediated transport of copper across the secretory membrane is illustrated.

pathway leads to an inability to provide copper for incorporation into newly synthesized apocaeruloplasmin, with resulting secretion of the apoprotein, which is rapidly degraded in the plasma. This explains why the serum caeruloplasmin concentration is decreased even in presymptomatic patients since the failure to synthesize holocaeruloplasmin is not related to the degree of cytosolic copper accumulation. The biosynthesis and secretion of apocaeruloplasmin is independent of copper availability and thus patients with Wilson's disease may at any given point in time have a normal serum caeruloplasmin if the rate of biosynthesis of this protein is increased. In all cases, however, an assay for caeruloplasmin oxidase activity

will confirm that the circulating protein is the apoprotein devoid of copper. Caeruloplasmin is not a copper-transport protein and the decreased serum concentration in patients with Wilson's disease plays no part in the pathogenesis of the copper accumulation observed in this disease. Consistent with this concept, patients with acaeruloplasminaemia have normal copper homeostasis and normal concentrations of hepatic copper (see Chapter 2.16.2).

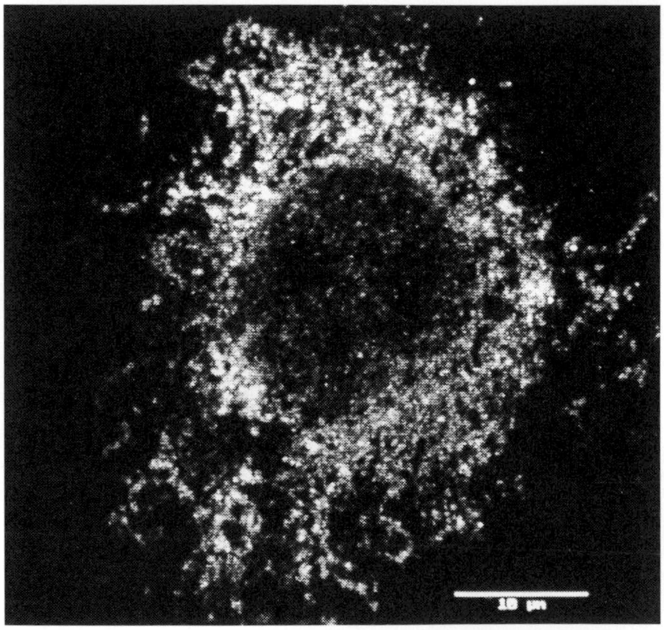

All patients with Wilson's disease, regardless of the clinical manifestations, will have pathological evidence of liver disease. The earliest change observed in liver biopsy specimens from such patients is fatty deposition, which eventual progresses to hepatic steatosis. In this early stage, microscopic studies reveal increased vacuolization of the mitochondria and other cellular organelles with preservation of the hepatic architecture. As the liver disease progresses there is an interstitial deposition of collagen and other matrix proteins characteristic of hepatic fibrosis. At this stage, the biopsy picture may be indistinguishable from that of chronic active hepatitis, with interspersed areas of hepatic necrosis and regenerating nodules. In the later stages of the disease, rubeanic acid staining will reveal excessive granular accumulations of copper in the lysosomes of hepatocytes. The rate of progression of hepatic disease varies considerably among patients and this is reflected in the appearances of biopsy specimens, which can range from a picture of chronic hepatitis with lymphocytic infiltration and piecemeal necrosis to that of multinucleated giant cells and coagulative hepatic necrosis observed in patients with sudden hepatic failure.

Clinical features and diagnosis

Wilson's disease is most frequently recognized as a triad of liver disease, neurological symptoms, and Kayser–Fleischer rings.[3] Nevertheless, because multiple organ systems can be affected by excessive copper accumulation, Wilson's disease is remarkable for clinical heterogeneity and patients may present in a number of different ways. In any given patient one or more of the classic triad of signs and symptoms may be absent and therefore the cornerstone of diagnosis in Wilson's disease is clinical suspicion. As noted above,

Fig. 2. Confocal immunofluorescent micrograph of the Wilson's disease P-type ATPase localized to the *trans*-Golgi network and endosomal compartment of a hepatoma cell. No specific signal for this protein is observed in the plasma membrane or nucleus.

liver disease in patients with Wilson's disease can have a markedly variable appearance. Symptoms of liver dysfunction account for the presenting feature in 50 per cent of patients and these individuals are generally diagnosed early in the second decade of life. Such patients may present with malaise and hepatosplenomegaly associated with biochemical markers of liver injury including an increase in serum transaminases and hypoalbuminaemia. Alternatively, patients may present with acute hepatitis that is either self-limited, leading to recovery without a diagnosis, or with rapidly progressive hepatic necrosis with a sudden release of copper into the plasma and an associated haemolytic anaemia and jaundice. Without a known family history of Wilson's disease or of a previous family member with hepatic or neurological symptoms, this latter presentation may be difficult to differentiate from other causes of acute hepatic failure. The aetiology of acute fulminant hepatic failure in Wilson's disease is unknown but may result from an intercurrent viral infection leading to hepatitis in a liver that is already decompensated by excessive hepatic storage. Diagnosis may be delayed in patients who present at an early age with chronic active hepatitis, as neurological symptoms and Kayser–Fleischer rings will be absent and the serum caeruloplasmin can be near normal due to inflammatory elevation of apocaeruloplasmin biosynthesis.

Neurological signs and symptoms account for the presenting features in about 35 per cent of patients with Wilson's disease. Such patients usually are diagnosed in their third or fourth decade and present with movement disorders that can be misdiagnosed as parkinsonism or multiple sclerosis. Although basal-ganglia symptoms such as tremor, drooling, dysphagia, and dysarthria are the most common symptoms, central nervous involvement can be much more extensive and a wide spectrum of features has been reported. Most typically, neurological involvement in Wilson's disease is associated with significant copper deposition elsewhere and patients will demonstrate associated features including the presence of Kayser–Fleischer rings. Neurological symptoms progress gradually with a relative sparing of the sensory system. Some patients will present with psychiatric symptoms and may be misdiagnosed as having primary psychosis or schizophrenia. In one study, more than 20 per cent of patients with Wilson's disease were found to have sought psychiatric evaluation before the diagnosis (Walshe, JNeurolNeurosurgPsych, 1992; 52:692). Radiographic imaging of the central nervous system by computed tomography or magnetic resonance imaging can be useful in revealing early signs of oedema and tissue atrophy attributable to copper deposition.

In addition to these hepatic and neurological presentations, excess free copper in the blood plasma of patients with Wilson's disease can result in haemolytic anaemia, and copper deposition in Descemet's membrane at the limbus of the cornea will result in Kayser–Fleischer rings. Cardiac copper deposition can result in dysrhythmias and excess copper in the hypothalamus, parathyroid, and adrenal glands can lead to amenorrhea, hypocalcaemia, and hypoglycaemia. A Fanconi syndrome with aminoaciduria and glycosuria may result from prolonged copper-mediated injury to the renal tubular epithelium. The long-term complications observed in patients with Wilson's disease are generally those related to hepatic failure, and include varices, bleeding, and encephalopathy. Hepatic carcinoma secondary to excessive copper storage is a rare complication in these patients, in contrast to the marked increased incidence of this malignancy in patients with hepatic iron overload from haemochromatosis.

None of the clinical signs and symptoms observed in patients with Wilson's disease is specific and thus confirmation of the diagnosis relies on laboratory investigation. Almost all patients will have a decrease in the serum caeruloplasmin below 20 mg/dl and in a patient with liver or neurological disease this finding is strongly suggestive of the diagnosis. Although severe malnutrition, protein-losing enteropathy or nephrotic syndrome can also decrease the serum caeruloplasmin, these are usually clinically distinguishable conditions. Patients with acaeruloplasminaemia will have no detectable serum caeruloplasmin and diagnostic confusion may arise due to the presence of basal-ganglia symptoms in such individuals (see Chapter 2.16.2). Ten per cent of individuals heterozygous for the Wilson's allele will also have a decreased caeruloplasmin and for this reason the serum caeruloplasmin concentration alone should never be used to make the diagnosis of Wilson's disease. Concomitant measurement of urinary copper excretion is a useful, safe, and inexpensive adjunct to routine laboratory investigation for the diagnosis of Wilson's disease. Urinary copper excretion is normally less than 30 µmol/24 h and this may be increased more than 100-fold in patients with significant hepatic involvement. A slitlamp ophthalmological examination for the presence of Kayser–Fleischer rings is similarly a useful component of the diagnostic evaluation and is positive in more than 90 per cent of patients who present with neurological symptoms.

In all cases where it is possible a liver biopsy should be performed for accurate quantitative measurement of the hepatic copper concentration. Liver biopsy specimens from patients with Wilson's disease reveal an increase in the amount of copper, often before signs or symptoms of the disease are present. The normal concentration of copper is 0.5 µmol/g of dry liver and in affected patients this is often increased 30- or 40-fold. Hepatic copper concentration will be increased even in the young child with Wilson's disease, and thus this evaluation can be very useful in establishing the diagnosis. Hepatic copper concentration will be elevated in any condition in which biliary copper excretion is impaired, including biliary cirrhosis, chronic cholestasis and idiopathic childhood cirrhosis, and this diagnostic test should always be correlated with the signs and symptoms present in the patient. Oral radiocopper has been used diagnostically, in patients who are unable to undergo liver biopsy, to detect a failure of copper incorporation into newly synthesized caeruloplasmin.

Asymptomatic siblings and first-degree relatives should always be screened for Wilson's disease by careful history and physical examination, ophthalmological studies, and measurements of serum caeruloplasmin, liver transaminases, and quantitative urinary copper excretion. If this evaluation is abnormal a liver biopsy should be performed for the quantitation of copper. A similar diagnostic evaluation should be done in any case of isolated elevation of serum transaminases or chronic active hepatitis of undetermined aetiology. This evaluation will be abnormal even in presymptomatic patients, but, with the exception of the serum caeruloplasmin, such an analysis will always be normal in heterozygous individuals, all of whom have normal copper homeostasis and should not receive treatment.

Molecular genetic analysis in patients with Wilson's disease has thus far identified more than 25 distinct mutations (Fig. 1). To add to this complexity a specific mutation has yet to be identified in at least 25 per cent of patients with Wilson's disease in whom linkage studies clearly identify 13q14.1 as the disease locus. For these reasons, routine DNA-based genetic screening for the diagnosis of Wilson's disease is not feasible. Nevertheless, several common disease-specific mutations have been identified and can be sought in any individual patient. DNA-based diagnosis is also possible within families where affected kindred have been identified. This may take the form of linkage analysis if informative polymorphisms are present (Naieraobersverger, Gastro, 1995; 109:2015) or may involve direct screening for a specific mutation previously identified in an affected family member. Molecular genetic analysis in patients with Wilson's disease should currently be viewed as a laboratory investigation that may, in select cases, accompany the diagnostic studies indicated above. Although it has been suggested that allelic heterogeneity may contribute to the clinical heterogeneity in patient's with Wilson's disease, the observation of such hetero-geneity, even within families sharing identical alleles, indicates that other genetic and environmental factors must play a dominant part in this process.[4]

Therapy and prognosis

The goal of treatment in Wilson's disease is to restore the patient to a state of normal copper homeostasis. This is accomplished by providing systemic chelation therapy to detoxify accumulated cop-per and increase urinary copper excretion. Persistent copper ac-cumulation is further prevented by dietary restriction of foods rich in copper, such as nuts, liver and chocolate, and by chelation within the gastrointestinal tract to impair copper absorption. Standard medical management of psychiatric symptoms, hepatic cirrhosis, and other underlying problems is also essential in individual patients.

D-Penicillamine is the treatment of choice for systemic chelation therapy of patients with symptoms of Wilson's disease. Although the precise mechanisms by which this drug results in detoxification remain unclear, long-term treatment with penicillamine promotes the urinary excretion of copper and has been shown to be effective in presymptomatic patients (Sternlieb, NEJM, 1968; 278:352). Therapy should be initiated with a small test dose, which, if tolerated, is gradually increased to 1 g/day administered orally in four divided doses. Penicillamine should be taken at least 1 h before eating to prevent chelation with food. A gradual but dramatic response in symptomatic patients will occur within the first 3 months of therapy. If no improvement occurs the dose may be increased up to twofold. Most patients become asymptomatic within 4 months of therapy but on occasion the neurological symptoms in such patients may worsen as a result of increased deposition of mobilized hepatic copper within the basal ganglia (Walshe, QJMed, 1993; 86:197). Once significant improvement and decreased total body copper has been achieved, patients may be placed on a half the initial dose for long-term maintenance therapy. Clinical follow-up to monitor serum factors and ensure compliance with therapy is important as a rapid demise can occur following discontinuation of penicillamine, presumably due to the sudden release of copper from sequestered 'non-toxic' sites.

Penicillamine is a toxic drug and more than 25 per cent of patients experience hypersensitivity reactions within the first several weeks of treatment. These include fever, erythematous dermatitis, urticaria, lymphadenopathy, leucopenia, thrombocytopenia, and proteinuria. These symptoms subside with stopping the drug and may be counteracted by the administration of prednisone for several weeks during re-initiation of penicillamine therapy. Once the drug is tolerated the prednisone therapy may be stopped. Autoimmune syndromes resembling systemic lupus erythematosus and Good-pasture syndrome may also develop and are an indication to dis-continue penicillamine therapy.

Triethylene tetramine dihydrochloride (trientiene) is an al-ternative systemic chelating agent that may be utilized in patients who are either unresponsive to penicillamine or who cannot tolerate the toxic side-effects of the drug. This drug is taken orally at a dose of 1 to 2 g divided before meals, and, although it is a less effective copper-chelating agent, significant improvement has been reported in a number of patients. Ammonium tetrathiomolybdate may also prove a useful adjunct in the treatment of Wilson's disease, although the results of long-term clinical trials have not been reported. Oral administration of this drug results in both the chelation of ingested copper, preventing absorption, and the impairment of uptake of absorbed copper into the liver from the blood plasma. Safe and effective treatment of patients with Wilson's disease using oral zinc has also been reported, but the long-term side-effects of this medication are unknown (Brewer, JLabClinMed, 1994; 123:849). The proposed mechanism of action of zinc is induction of enterocyte metallothionein resulting in impairment of copper absorption.

In patients with fulminant hepatitis or progressive hepatic in-sufficiency that is unresponsive to therapy, liver transplantation has been used (Schilsky, Hepatol, 1994; 19:583). The results of this approach are often good, with complete restoration of normal copper homeostasis within 6 months of transplantation and sustained im-provement in neurological symptoms. As such patients are es-sentially cured by liver transplantation, these observations support the concept that the primary defect in Wilson's disease is impairment of copper transfer into bile.

A rodent model of Wilson's disease has been identified in the Long–Evans cinnamon rat, which has been shown to have an inherited deletion in the rat homologue of the Wilson's disease ATPase (Li, JCI, 1991; 87:1858; Yamaguchi, BiochemJ, 1994; 301:1; Wu, NatGen, 1994; 7:541). The hepatic copper toxicosis in the Long–Evans cinnamon rat is responsive to penicillamine therapy, making it likely that this rodent model will permit further under-standing of the pathogenesis of this disorder as well as the de-velopment of novel therapeutic approaches to prevent or ameliorate tissue injury in this disease (Jong-Hon, Hepatol, 1993; 18:614).

References

1. Danks DM. Disorders of copper transport. In *The metabolic and molecular basis of inherited disease*. New York: McGraw-Hill, 1995: 2211–35.
2. Cuthbert JA. Wilson's disease: a new gene and an animal model for an old disease. *Journal of Investigative Medicine*, 1995; **43**: 323–36.
3. Brewer GJ and Yuzdasiyan-Gurkan V. Wilson disease. *Medicine*, 1992; **71**: 139–64.
4. Harris LH and Gitlin JD. Genetic and molecular basis of copper toxicity. *American Journal of Clinical Nutrition*, 1996; **63**: 836–41S.

20.2 Haemochromatosis

Pierre Brissot and Yves Deugnier

Introduction
Definition

Haemochromatosis (previously called idiopathic, primary, hereditary, or genetic) is a disease characterized by progressive iron deposition, especially in the liver, which is genetically transmitted as an autosomal recessive trait and principally determined by a gene situated on the short arm of the sixth chromosome. This definition, which does not imply substantial iron overload and even less the existence of organ damage, covers all the territory between the unexpressed and the advanced forms of the disease; it does not exclude the influence of possible accessory genetic factors or environmental factors.

Historical background

The clinical and pathological entity corresponding to haemochromatosis was first described by Trousseau (1865) and Troisier (1871) and the term haemochromatosis was later proposed by Von Recklinghausen. Sheldon, in 1935, proposed that haemochromatosis was due to an inborn error of iron metabolism. This concept was disputed by some authors, especially McDonald, but the discovery in 1975 by Simon et al. of an association between some HLA antigens and haemochromatosis, and the demonstration of a genetic linkage between the haemochromatosis locus and the HLA loci, definitively demonstrated the hereditary nature of the disease (Simon, JHepatol, 1988; 6:116).

Genetics
HLA linkage

The association between haemochromatosis and HLA antigen A3 described by Simon et al. (Simon, Gut, 1976; 17:332; Simon, NEJM, 1977; 297:1017) has been confirmed and extended by a large body of studies:

1. HLA A3 is increased in all series (55 to 100 per cent of patients, average 73) compared with 19 to 31 per cent in controls.
2. HLA A11 is relatively increased in so far as it does not undergo the decrease in frequency observed in other locus A alleles due to the extra space taken up by A3.
3. A significant association with HLA B7 is found in most of the series; B14 prevalence is increased in only half of the reported series but very significantly in some. It should be emphasized that these associations occur through a privileged linkage of the B alleles with the HLA A3 allele, realizing haplotypic associations such as A3–B7 (21.2 per cent versus 6.1 in controls, $p < 10^{-10}$), A3–B14 (13.8 per cent versus 1.5, $p < 10^{-10}$), A11–B5, or A11–B35.

Location of the haemochromatosis gene (HFE locus according to the human gene mapping workshop)

The proposal of haemochromatosis-specific genotypes, such as the haplotype D6S248-D6S265-HLAA-HLAF-D6S105 (Jazwinska, AmJHumGen, 1995;56:428) or homozygosity for the haplotype D6S265-1:D6S105-8 (Worwood, BrJHaemat, 1994; 86:863) indicated the likelihood of a predominant ancestral haplotype pointing to a common mutation. An important step has been the description of a strong linkage between the haemochromatosis gene and the D6S1260 locus, a DNA marker situated approximately 3 megabases telomeric of HLA-A (Raha-Chowdhury, HumMolGenet, 1995;4: 1869; Burt, Genomics, 1996;33:153-8). But the major breakthrough has been the recent report (Feder, NatureGenet, 1996;13:399) of the mutation of a novel MHC (major histocompatibility complex) class I-like gene in patients with haemochromatosis. This gene, located 4.5 megabases telomeric of HLA-A, has been initially termed HLA-H, and then HFE. It contains two missense alterations. The major mutation Cys282Tyr (or C282Y) was present in 85 per cent of the chromosomes of the 178 patients studied (versus 3.2 per cent of control chromosomes), and was found homozygous in 83 per cent. The prevalence of C282Y homozygosity in haemochromatosis patients throughout the world is between 69 and 100 per cent (Fig. 1). This gene is very likely to be the causative locus of haemochromatosis. The high degree of conservation of the ancestral chromosome, reflected by the low level of recombination in this disease, probably accounts for the paradoxical situation in which the candidate gene is physically distant from HLA-A while remaining in high linkage disequilibrium with it (physical distance is much larger than genetic distance).

Mode of transmission

Genotypic studies (i.e. based on HLA typing within families as well as in unrelated patients) have confirmed phenotypic investigations (based upon the presence or absence of symptoms of the disease). Haemochromatosis is a recessively transmitted disease.

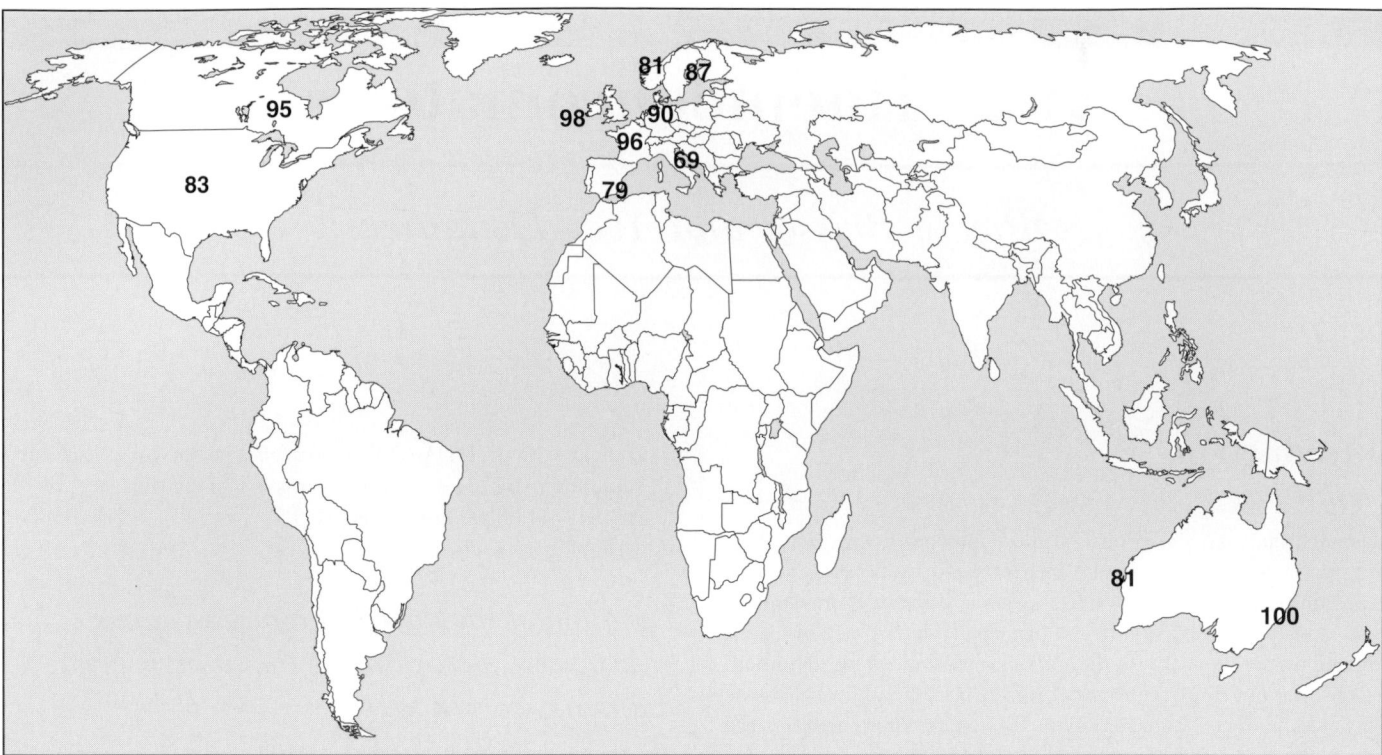

Fig. 1. Prevalence of C282Y homozygosity (percentage) in haemochromatosis patients

1. In families, haplotyping is in agreement with recessive transmission—siblings who have the same two haplotypes as the proband have homozygous genetic haemochromatosis and those with only one haplotypes are heterozygous. An exception occurs with heterozygous–homozygous matings where the three genetic haemochromatosis alleles, each with its own haplotype marker, can yield two types of HLA pairs reflecting the homozygous state with only one haplotype marker in common (see under preventive treatment and Fig. 3).

2. In unrelated subjects, the distribution of A3 (i.e. whether this marker is homozygous A3–A3 or heterozygous A3–AX) is dependent on whether or not it is necessary for the gene marked by A3 to be itself homozygous (recessive transmission) or heterozygous (dominant transmission) for disease expression; the observed distribution is exactly that expected for recessive transmission.

Prevalence of the haemochromatosis gene

The main gene prevalences, published to date, are summarized in Table 1.

These data must be interpreted with caution for the following reasons:

1. With the exception of family studies, there were at the time of these studies no reliable means of detecting a heterozygous state.

2. The various tests proposed as characteristic of a homozygous state (for example an increased transferrin saturation above 0.62) (Dadone, AmJClinPath, 1982; 78:196), an elevated serum ferritin, at least in subjects under 35 (Bassett, Gastro, 1984; 87:

628), or an hepatic iron index (ratio of liver iron concentration (μmol/g) to age (years) greater than 2) (Bassett, Hepatol, 1986; 6:24) are essentially valid in the population in which the threshold value was defined. Applying them to other populations may not be valid, especially when there are differences in disease prevalence (the lower the prevalence, the lower the predictive value). For example a positive test for iron overload, particularly if indirect (i.e. based on serum biochemical parameters) (Brissot, Gastro, 1981; 80:557), has a higher probability of revealing a homozygous state in the relatives of a proband than in the general population.

3. Numerous studies have been carried out in populations where the prevalence was assumed to be high; two studies, however, avoid this bias, one based on a population where autopsies were routinely performed (Lindmark, ActaMedScand, 1985; 218:299) and the other consisting of a screening for iron deficiency (Group, AmJClinNut, 1985; 42:1318).

On the whole, it is possible to conclude that the homozygous state affects approximately three to five per 1000 in white populations. Therefore, haemochromatosis is one of the most common autosomal recessive diseases. In a region such as Brittany (France) it is estimated that up to 16 per cent of the population are heterozygous for the disease.

Phenotypic expression of the haemochromatosis gene

In the homozygous state, phenotypic expression of the haemochromatosis gene was previously thought to be nearly constant, and

Table 1 Prevalence of haemochromatosis

Method	Country	Reference	Prevalences		
			Gene (%)	Heterozygotes (%)	Homozygotes (‰)
Autopsy	United States	MacDonald, AmJMedSci, 1965; 249:36	4.2	8.1	1.8
	Scotland	MacSween, JClinPath, 1973; 26:936	4.5	8.5	2
	Sweden (southern)	Lindmark, ActaMedScand, 1985; 218:299	3	5.8	9
Biochemical tests and family studies	United States	Dadone, AmJClinPath, 1982; 78:196	6.9	12.8	5
	Australia	Bassett, HumGenet, 1982; 60:352	8.8	16	7.7
	France (Brittany)	Simon, JHepatol, 1988; 6:116	6.4	12	4
Biochemical tests	Australia	Leggett, BrJHaemat, 1990; 74:525	5.9	—	3.6
	Sweden (central)	Olsson, ActaMedScand, 1982; 213:145	7	13.2	5
	United States	Edwards, NEJM, 1988; 318:1355	6.7	12.5	4.5
		Balan, Gastro, 1994; 105:453	—	—	0.3
		MacLaren, Blood, 1995; 86:2021	8.1 (M) 7 (F)	—	6.6 (M) 4.8 (F)
		Baer, AmJMed, 1995; 98:464	—	—	4

milder or delayed in women. However, neonatal screening for the C282Y mutation (Cullen, Blood, 1997; 90:4236) suggests that phenotypic expression may be prevented in one-third of individual homozygotes; moreover a study on 176 women indicated that the age at presentation and the hepatic iron index were similar between males and females, cirrhosis and diabetes being more common in men and fatigue more common in women (Moirand, AnnIntMed, 1997; 127:105).

In the heterozygous state, clinical expression is usually absent: a moderate biochemical expression (especially an increased transferrin saturation) is found in about 25 per cent of cases. A slight hepatic iron overload is observed in one-third of heterozygotes. There is no increase of iron overload with time, as shown in a series of 44 heterozygotes followed for 1 to 16 years (Bassett, Hepatol, 1981; 1: 120).

Haemochromatosis gene specificity

The evolution of the concepts regarding haemochromatosis is peculiar since, after a phase where the genetic nature of the disorder was disputed, it is today the non-genetic nature of the so-called 'secondary' iron overload states which is debated. This question can be approached by the search for an increased HLA A3 prevalence in the cases of secondary iron overload, provided a rigorous methodology is adopted. Moreover, evaluating the prevalence of the mutation C282Y has become essential.

1. The occasional occurrence of the haemochromatosis gene has been shown by family studies in idiopathic sideroblastic anaemia, hereditary spherocytosis, and β-thalassaemia trait.
2. A systematic or major implication of the haemochromatosis gene can probably be excluded for sideroblastic anaemia (Simon, BrJHaemat, 1985; 60:75) as well as for alcoholic liver disease. In the latter condition, when iron excess is moderate (by far the most frequent situation), it has been clearly demonstrated that HLA A3 prevalence is identical to controls and significantly

inferior to that of homozygous or heterozygous haemochromatosis populations (Simon, Gastro, 1977; 73:655); whenever iron overload is major, most of these alcoholic patients should be considered as homozygous haemochromatosis carriers (Lesage, Gastro, 1983; 84:1471)—thus the classical concept of 'haemochromatosis secondary to alcoholism' is no longer tenable.

3. With regard to porphyria cutanea tarda, systematic involvement of the haemochromatosis gene can be excluded (Beaumont, Gastro, 1987; 92:1833); nevertheless, family studies, which are increasing in number, favour frequent involvement of the gene in some regions (Edwards, Gastro, 1989; 97:972). These differences may result from selection bias—sporadic porphyria cutanea tarda probably needs complementary factors for expression; this may be alcohol in certain areas and the haemochromatosis gene in other regions. An increased frequency of the C282Y mutation in sporadic cutanea tarda has been reported by Roberts *et al.* (Lancet, 1997; 349:321).

Clinical features
Visceral and metabolic manifestations

The following signs correspond to the full-blown form of the disease. Early diagnosis reduces both their frequency and their intensity.

Liver involvement

The liver may be considerably increased in overall volume with a predominant left-lobe enlargement. The liver is firm to palpation and its inferior edge is sharp. This hepatomegaly is rarely associated with clinical symptoms of hepatic dysfunction (such as portal hypertension and/or hepatocellular insufficiency). Liver function tests are nearly normal, except for a slight increase in aminotransferase (usually less than three times the upper reference limit) (Brissot, Digestion, 1978; 17:479; Deugnier, Gut, 1994; 35:1107). The major complication of this liver disease is the development of hepatocellular carcinoma. This underlines the necessary screening for hepatocellular carcinoma in patients presenting the following risk factors; male sex, age over 50, liver fibrosis (even at a precirrhotic stage), alcoholism, tobacco, or previous contact with HBV or HCV (Deugnier, Gastro, 1993; 104:228; Fargion, Hepatol, 1994; 20:1426). Moreover, a systematic search for the presence of histological iron-free foci must be carried out, as they have been shown to have a preneoplastic significance (Deugnier, Hepatol, 1993; 18: 1363).

Skin and nails signs

Excessive skin pigmentation, more often greyish than brown ('bronzed' coloration), is frequently observed, especially in areas exposed to the sun, over the genital organs, and in scars. It is attributed to melanin deposition but evolves in tandem with iron deposits in the skin, which are preferentially found around sweat glands. Melanin pigmentation is absent in red-haired people. Other possible signs are ichthyosis, flattened or even spoon nails, and reduced body hair.

Joint and bone signs

Arthropathy (Schumacher, AnnNYAcadMed, 1988; 256:224) is a common manifestation of haemochromatosis, sometimes as a presenting feature, but it is often misdiagnosed; the diagnostic delay being estimated at between 4 and 10 years (Aellen, SchMedWoch, 1992; 122:842). Clinically, the most characteristic feature is chronic arthritis in the second and third metacarpophalangeal joints, which results in a 'painful handshake', a symptom suggestive of the disease in regions where haemochromatosis is highly prevalent. The proximal interphalangeal joints may also be affected, as well as the knees, wrists, and hips. Patients can also suffer acute attacks of pyrophosphate arthropathy (pseudogout). Radiologically, the most common changes are subchondral arthropathy (joint space narrowing, sclerosis, and subchondral cyst formation) and chondrocalcinosis (especially in the knees). Arthritis is a prominent clinical factor affecting quality of life in haemochromatosis (Adams, JRheum, 1996; 23:707).

Bone demineralization is frequent. Usually clinically asymptomatic, it may (rarely) lead to fractures (in particular in the spinal column). In addition to hypogonadism (Diamond, AnnIntMed, 1989; 110:430), ascorbic acid deficiency and/or vitamin D deficiency (Pawlotsky, PressMed, 1993; 22:1988) may contribute to bone demineralization.

Cardiac disease

Electrocardiographic abnormalities, in decreasing order of frequency, are T-wave flattening and inversion, low-voltage, and rhythm disturbances (atrial tachyarrhythmia and, less frequently, ventricular premature beats and tachycardia) (Mattheyses, ArchMalCoeur, 1978; 71:371). Cardiomyopathy, as assessed by echocardiography, is more often of the dilated type (increase in ventricular size and mass with reduction in systolic function) than restrictive (normal ventricular size but with impaired filling) (Dabestani, AnnNYAcadMed, 1988; 526:234). Cardiac magnetic

resonance imaging can be helpful (Liu, CardvascDrugTher, 1994; 8:101). Endomyocardial biopsy is a valuable technique for confirmation of the diagnosis (Olson, JAmCollCard, 1989; 13:116). Iron overload within myocardial cells can occur with minimal fibrosis or inflammation. The risk of death from cardiomyopathy is more than 300 times that expected for the normal population (Strohmeyer, AnnNYAcadMed, 1988; 526:245). Congestive heart failure may be especially fatal in young subjects.

The risk of coronary heart disease in haemochromatosis is not increased (Brock et al. pp. 255–7),[2] in keeping with several reports (Sempos, NEJM, 1994; 330:1119; Baer, Circul, 1994; 89:2915) which do not confirm the study by Salonen et al. (Circul, 1992; 86: 803) suggesting that high stored iron levels are associated with excess risk of myocardial infarction.

Diabetes and other endocrine abnormalities
Diabetes

The prevalence of diabetes in haemochromatosis is reported to be between 50 and 60 per cent. In a series of 163 patients (Niederau, NEJM, 1985; 313:1256), 55 per cent had overt diabetes and 10 per cent presented an abnormal glucose tolerance test. The degenerative complications of diabetes are observed in haemochromatosis with the same frequency as in ordinary diabetes but with less severity. Two main pathogenetic factors contribute to carbohydrate intolerance (Stremmel, AnnNYAcadMed, 1988; 526:209):

(1) impaired insulin secretion caused by selective deposition of iron within the β-cells of the pancreas;
(2) insulin resistance due to iron-related hepatocellular dysfunction.

Other endocrine disorders

The clinical picture is dominated by hypogonadism. It is expressed in men by loss of libido, sexual impotence, and testicular atrophy accompanied by a significant decrease in plasma testosterone levels. A decrease in plasma follicle-stimulating hormone and luteinizing hormone levels with little or no response to clomiphene or luteinizing hormone releasing hormone, together with an impaired prolactin response to thyrotrophin-releasing hormone, point to a predominant impairment in gonadotropin secretion. Iron deposition occurs preferentially within the gonadotrophic cells.

General and miscellaneous symptoms

Weakness is present in the majority of patients at the time of diagnosis.

A relationship has been suggested between iron overload and the occurrence of bacterial infections, particularly by *Yersinia enterocolitica* (Cover, NEJM, 1989; 321:16); however, the overall frequency of these infections in haemochromatosis seems limited. An increased prevalence of B and C viral markers has also been reported (Deugnier, JHepatol, 1991; 13:286; Piperno, JHepatol, 1992;16: 364).

Vitamin deficiencies, especially C and A (Brissot, Digestion, 1978; 17:479), have been reported in this disease.

Iron overload assessment
Indirect methods
Classical parameters
Serum iron

Normal serum iron levels are about 20 µmol/l and are slightly higher in males than in females. The range of normal values is large (in one of our series of 66 men it was 8.1 to 37.6, mean 21.5, and in 75 women 6.3 to 39.4, mean 19.7); furthermore, serum iron concentrations exhibit important circadian fluctuations (the levels are maximal in the morning, minimal in the afternoon) and there are marked day-to-day variations (≥ 30 per cent). In advanced haemochromatosis, values greater than 36 µmol/l are the rule.

Transferrin saturation

Normally the iron transport protein (transferrin) is on average 30 per cent saturated, slightly more in men than in women (32 and 26 per cent respectively; unpublished data). Above 45 per cent, iron overload should be evoked. In full-blown genetic haemochromatosis, transferrin is often totally saturated.

Serum ferritin

Normal ferritin levels, which fluctuate less than those of serum iron, approximate 100 µg/l in adult men, and 30 in females until menopause (after which values rise to about 80) (Custer, JLabClinMed, 1995; 126:88). Ferritin increase is proportional to the degree of iron excess. In fully expressed haemochromatosis, ferritin values above 1000 µg/l are common.

Overall interpretation of these parameters

In haemochromatosis, transferrin saturation is the best screening test in homozygotes—in a series of 537 subjects belonging to 18 families with haemochromatosis, transferrin saturation above 62 per cent diagnosed 92 per cent of the homozygous siblings (Dadone, AmJClinPath, 1982; 78:196); however, its 'ceiling' (100 per cent) is reached with relatively moderate iron overload, which accounts for its failure to predict the degree of iron excess (the same holds true for serum iron). Ferritinaemia is not subject to this limitation and is valuable for quantitative assessment of iron overload. It should be noted, however, that all three parameters can underestimate massive iron overload, due to the development of ascorbic acid deficiency. Liver dysfunction, either acute or chronic, of whatever origin (but particularly alcoholic) can lead to an increase of these various serum parameters and therefore to overestimation of iron load (Brissot, Gastro, 1981; 80:557).

Other parameters
Erythrocyte ferritin determination

This has been claimed to provide a better estimate of iron overload by avoiding the interfering effect of hepatic dysfunction and inflammatory syndromes (Guillemin, AnnBiolClin, 1993; 51:605).

Non-transferrin-bound iron

The presence of such iron has been demonstrated in secondary iron overload (Hershko, BrJHaemat, 1978; 50:255) as well as in haemochromatosis (Batey, DigDisSci, 1980; 25:340). Its potential pathogenic importance for the constitution of liver iron overload (Brissot, JCI, 1985; 76:1463) and of liver damage (in view of its ability to generate reactive oxygen species) accounts for the interest in determination of non-transferrin-bound iron levels in serum (Gutteridge, ClinSci, 1985; 68:463). However, a reliable and simple method for determining serum non-transferrin-bound iron is still needed.

Direct methods

These comprise invasive methods (liver biopsy, quantitative phlebotomy) and several non-invasive techniques.

Liver biopsy

This is essential for histological examination and biochemical assessment.

Histological examination

Using Perls technique, this establishes iron overload, identifies its predominantly periportal and hepatocytic distribution, and provides a semiquantitative evaluation of iron excess using a special grading system (Deugnier, Gastro, 1992; 92:2050) which permits the calculation of the histological hepatic iron index (ratio of total iron score to age) (Deugnier, Hepatol, 1993; 17:30); moreover, it gives information on the degree of tissue injury (existence and degree of fibrosis), on the presence of iron-free foci (Deugnier, Hepatol, 1993; 18:1363), and on associated lesions (e.g. alcoholism).

Biochemical assessment

Liver biopsy permits the determination of liver iron concentration, which correlates closely with the degree of iron stores, and has become a key method for assessing iron overload (the upper normal value is about 36 µmol/g dry liver weight) (Brissot, Gastro, 1981; 80: 557). It can be performed on deparaffinized liver biopsy specimens (Olynick, Gastro, 1994; 106:674), which saves the totality of the initial material for histological examination. It enables the calculation of the biochemical hepatic iron index (ratio of hepatic iron concentration to age), which has been, before the discovery of the C282Y mutation, the most reliable means, in a given individual (and after exclusion of an iron-loading anaemia), for establishing homozygosity for haemochromatosis (biochemical hepatic iron index >2).

Quantitative phlebotomy

This provides an accurate determination of the degree of storage iron and serves as a reference for other methods, provided that venesections are carried out according to a strict protocol (400–500 ml/week). With good record keeping the degree of storage iron is easily obtained by adding the number of phlebotomies (knowing that 500 ml are equivalent to 250 mg of iron) and correcting the data for the alimentary iron input (i.e. by adding about 2 mg/day of iron during the venesection programme).

Magnetic resonance imaging

Magnetic resonance imaging provides a non-invasive assessment of hepatic iron by detecting a specific reduction in signal intensity related to a decrease in T2 relaxation time. It is a promising technique, whose sensitivity will be improved, especially by using high-field-strength systems (Guyader, JHepatol, 1992; 16:756; Gandon, Radiol, 1994; 193:533).

Computed tomography

Computed tomography is able to detect a specific increase in X-ray density (equivalent to increased liver attenuation). However, computed tomography is insensitive—liver attenuation values may be in the normal range for liver iron content up to 150 µmol/g dry weight (Guyader, Gastro, 1989; 97:737), which limits considerably its clinical usefulness.

Magnetic susceptibility measurement

Based on the paramagnetic properties of ferritin and haemosiderin, this technique provides a rapid, safe, reliable, and quantitative measurement of liver iron load. However, the instrumentation for this technique is limited to a few centres in the world.

Genetic markers

Diagnostic value of HLA typing

The practical diagnostic value of HLA typing was dependent on the clinical situation.

1. In a given individual when iron overload was diagnosed, the presence of HLA A3 had no diagnostic value since about 25 per cent of normal subjects are 'A3 carriers'; likewise, the absence of A3 was meaningless to exclude haemochromatosis, since 25 per cent of authentic cases are 'devoid' of A3.
2. Within a family in whom an affected individual has been diagnosed (proband), HLA typing permitted identification of subjects at risk (especially the HLA-identical siblings).
3. The prevalence of HLA A3 within a population has been used as a marker for the genetic status of this population with respect to the *HFE* gene (Simon, JHepatol, 1988; 6:116).

Direct analysis of genomic DNA

A blood test for the C282Y mutation represents today the ideal means of identifying affected subjects. Patients with iron overload and who are homozygous for this mutation are homozygous for the disease. However, it should be kept in mind that (i) this test can occasionally be negative despite a phenotypic picture compatible with haemochromatosis and (ii) some individuals who are homozygous for the mutation do not develop damaging iron overload during their lives.

Varying pictures and general course of the disease

Typical expression of haemochromatosis

Until the 1960s, diagnosis was generally made at an advanced stage when complications occurred, usually in the fifth decade in males and later for females. The clinical picture of the disease has changed considerably due to an active diagnostic approach, based on the greater attention paid by physicians to minimal symptoms and on the wider use of HLA typing in family screening programmes.

Thus, haemochromatosis is recognized sooner, before complications occur, and more often in women.

Special forms

Usually a disease of middle age, haemochromatosis can be clinically manifest in a number of patients less than 20 years old. Unlike the adult form, 'juvenile haemochromatosis' has been claimed to affect males and females equally, to cause essentially cardiac dysfunction and hypogonadotropic hypogonadism, and to be of particular severity. Whether juvenile haemochromatosis represents a separate entity or only a more severe form of the adult disorder remains to be elucidated.

General course of the disease

A study of 163 patients (Strohmeyer, AnnNYAcadMed, 1988; 526: 245) followed for a mean period of 10.5 ± 5.6 years ($\pm$ SD) provided the following data. Cumulative survival was 76 per cent at 10 years and 49 per cent at 20 years. Patients without cirrhosis or diabetes had a nearly normal life expectancy. Analysis of the causes of death in 53 patients showed that liver cancer, cardiomyopathy, liver cirrhosis, and diabetes were respectively 219, 306, 13, and 7 times more frequent compared to death rates expected for an age-matched normal population. The risk of death from other causes did not differ from expected rates in normal subjects, especially from extrahepatic cancer (Bradbear, JNCI, 1985; 75:81).

Overall diagnostic strategy

1. Classically diagnosis involves the following steps:

(1) Consider the disease even in women and in 'non-specific' geographic areas;
(2) Consider the diagnosis in monosymptomatic forms of the disease;
(3) Check suspected iron overload disorder by checking serum iron load parameters, especially transferrin saturation, while being aware of possible false positive and negative results;
(4) Confirm hepatic iron overload by magnetic resonance imaging and liver biopsy;
(5) Confirm its gastrointestinal origin by checking lobular (periportal) and cellular (hepatocytic) distribution;
(6) Relate iron intensity to age, using two indexes (the biochemical hepatic iron index and the histological hepatic iron index) which suggest haemochromatotic homozygosity when their respective values are over 2 and 0.2 (provided an iron-loading anaemia has been excluded);
(7) Search for hepatic lesions (fibrosis, iron-free foci) and extrahepatic symptoms.

2. Up-to-date strategy requires a search for the C282Y mutation:

(1) Suspected iron overload as shown by clinical and biochemical data, and possibly confirmed by MRI, requires a search for the C282Y mutation;
(2) Homozygosity for the mutation (C282Y+/+) confirms haemochromatosis and a liver biopsy will be required only if there is a high degree of iron overload, making development of fibrosis or cirrhosis possible. The deciding criteria for performing a liver biopsy are yet to be determined, but will

probably take into account ferritinaemia levels (>1500 ?), presence of hypertransaminasaemia and/or MRI data;

(3) Heterozygosity for mutation (C282Y + /−) or the absence of mutation (C282Y − / −) excludes 'HFE related haemochromatosis'. However, a liver biopsy will be necessary where there are strong clinical and/or biochemical indications of iron overload with a 'negative' (i.e. non-homozygote) result for the genetic test.

Differential diagnosis: non-haemochromatotic iron overload

Iron-loading anaemias

Nature of the anaemias, routes, and toxicity of iron overload

Various haematological disorders are of relevance; these include congenital disorders (thalassaemia major and, to a lesser degree, thalassaemia intermedia, sickle cell disease, red cell dysplasia, and congenital sideroblastic anaemia) or acquired disorders (acquired refractory sideroblastic anaemia and hypoplastic or myelodysplatic disorders). In these conditions, iron accumulation is related:

(1) mainly to transfusions (e.g. aplastic anaemias);
(2) to increased iron absorption due to increased erythroid activity (e.g. thalassaemia intermedia);
(3) to both mechanisms (e.g. thalassaemia major or sideroblastic anaemias).

The excess absorbed iron is mainly deposited in parenchymal sites (i.e. in hepatocytes but also in the pancreas and the heart) in a similar fashion to haemochromatosis. Transfused iron is initially deposited within macrophages in the mononuclear phagocytic system but subsequently iron redistribution occurs, leading to parenchymal deposition and damage so that finally the pattern of organ involvement resembles that encountered in haemochromatosis (Schafer, NEJM, 1981; 304:319). In the case of thalassaemia major, most patients require 200 to 300 ml/kg per year of blood which corresponds to between 0.25 and 0.40 mg/kg per day of iron.

Clinical picture

Only thalassaemia major, which represents the most frequent cause of major iron excess, will be considered here. Hepatomegaly (with fibrosis) occurs during the first decade of life. The second decade is marked by lack of sexual development and the appearance of cardiac dysfunction, which is a major cause of death. Serum parameters (ferritin, transferrin saturation, iron as well as non-transferrin-bound iron) are markedly increased. As for haemochromatosis, liver biopsy is of major importance to assess iron overload and to evaluate liver damage (fibrosis).

Treatment of thalassaemia and other iron-loading anaemias

Classical therapy

The goal is to reduce iron overload. Dietary measures, such as tea taken with meals, can contribute to reduce iron absorption. Iron removal by phlebotomy is not feasible in the severely anaemic patient so that chelation constitutes the essential therapeutic means. At present, desferrioxamine, which is a naturally occurring trihydroxamic acid produced by *Streptomyces pilosus*, is the main clinical agent. Due to its poor intestinal absorption, desferrioxamine must be given parenterally and, since the half-life of circulating desferrioxamine is only 5 to 10 min, it must be administered by continuous (subcutaneous) infusion to be effective. A dose of 2 to 4 g of desferrioxamine is usually given, for 12 h each day, using a small portable infusion pump. Desferrioxamine, provided its use is early and regular, has been demonstrated to decrease hepatic iron, to improve cardiac and pancreas dysfunction, to ameliorate growth and sexual maturation, and to increase survival (Brittenham, NEJM, 1994; 331:567; Olivieri, NEJM, 1994; 331:574). However, desferrioxamine can cause to several side-effects, including cataracts and retinopathy, sensorineural hearing loss, and renal failure. In addition, long-term compliance of nightly infusions is problematic for many young patients and the cost of the treatment renders this procedure unaffordable for most areas of the world where thalassaemia is common.

New therapeutic approaches

The orally active, iron-chelating agent, under current clinical investigation, is 1,2-dimethyl-3-hydroxypyridin-4-one, or deferiprone (also known as CP20 and L1). Patented by Hider *et al.* in 1982, it appears a promising candidate in terms of efficacy (Kontoghiorghes, BMJ, 1987; 295:150; Al-Refaie, Blood, 1992; 80: 593; Olivieri, NEJM, 1995; 332:918). Further clinical studies are, however, needed in order to evaluate its safety, since adverse effects, especially arthropathy and severe neutropenia (corresponding in some cases to reversible agranulocytosis), have been reported.

Other approaches consist, in thalassaemia major, of bone marrow transplantation (Walters, AmJPedHemOnc, 1994; 16:11), prenatal screening, and genetic counselling, and will hopefully, in the future, be based on gene therapy.

Chronic alcoholic liver disease

Iron overload is found in about 30 per cent of chronic alcoholics (Chapman, DigDisSci, 1982; 27:909) and is usually mild to moderate. The mechanism(s) of this slight increase is (are) unclear:

1. The systematic involvement of haemochromatotic heterozygosity has been ruled out (Simon, Gastro, 1977; 73:655; Bassett, Hepatol, 1981; 2:120).
2. A direct favouring effect of alcohol on iron absorption has not been conclusively shown.
3. Indirect effects of alcohol are possible through:

(a) the iron content of alcoholic beverages, particularly red wines;
(b) folic acid deficiency which may increase iron absorption;
(c) transferrin desialylation which could account for an increase in parenchymal cell iron.

Clinically, the picture may involve some degree of skin pigmentation associated with hypogonadism, glucose intolerance, marked increase in serum iron load parameters, especially ferritin (Moirand, JHepatol, 1995; 23:431), so that the diagnosis of 'haemochromatosis' can be evoked. It is then of utmost importance to resort to direct iron-load parameters, especially liver biopsy (if necessary via the transjugular route), in order to visualize and quantify hepatic iron. In the case of alcoholic siderosis, iron deposition is mild and found primarily within Kupffer cells rather than hepatocytes. Furthermore, the ratio of liver iron concentration to age is below 2 (Bassett, Hepatol, 1986; 6:24; Sallie, Gut, 1991; 32:207), which helps to separate alcoholic siderosis from iron overload in young alcoholic haemochromatosis homozygotes. One should be aware, however, that cirrhosis *per se* can be responsible for heterogeneous iron deposition in the liver, which may fortuitously provide a biochemical hepatic iron index over 2, especially in endstage cirrhosis (Ludwig, Gastro, 1997; 112:882; Villeneuve, JHepatol, 1996; 25:172; Deugnier, AmJSurgPath, 1997; 21:669). On the other hand, when major hepatic iron excess is certified in an alcoholic patient, the diagnosis of homozygous haemochromatosis associated with alcoholism must be adopted; this event is relatively frequent since alcoholism aggravates the hepatic expression of haemochromatosis (Loréal, JHepatol, 1992; 16:122; Adams, Hepatol, 1996; 23:724).

Porphyria cutanea tarda

This is a chronic hepatic porphyria due to deficient activity of uroporphyrinogen decarboxylase. Two main forms of the disease have been described—in the sporadic form, uroporphyrinogen decarboxylase deficiency is restricted to the liver (erythrocyte activity is normal), whereas in the familial form the genetic deficiency (ascribed to mutations at the urodecarboxylase locus on chromosome 1) is found in all tissues (particularly the red cells) and is transmitted in the autosomal dominant mode. The excessive amount of porphyrins in blood and skin accounts for the characteristic cutaneous photosensitivity (with skin fragility and bullas). Clinical expression of both forms of the disease usually requires exogenous factors such as alcohol, oestrogen intake, liver disease, and iron. Iron overload is frequently observed in porphyria cutanea tarda but remains of moderate intensity (it does not exceed four times the normal values); its origin is controversial (see haemochromatosis gene specificity above) but its effect on disease expression is certain. Oral or parenteral iron administration is followed by relapse of porphyria cutanea tarda whereas phlebotomies lead to clinical and biochemical remission of the disease with a return to normal of hepatic uroporphyrinogen decarboxylase activity. The mechanisms whereby iron interferes with porphyria cutanea tarda expression remain poorly understood. *In vitro*, iron may inhibit uroporphyrinogen carboxylase activity by direct competitive inhibition, and by indirect action through the generation of free radicals altering the enzyme (Mukerji, Gastro, 1984; 87:1248). *In vivo*, however, activity is not decreased either in rat experimental iron overload or in haemochromatosis. Moreover, phlebotomy is efficient even in the absence of iron overload, indicating that iron removal may not be the sole factor in the beneficial effect of venesections.

Chronic viral C hepatitis and iron overload

Moderate iron excess is frequent in chronic viral C hepatitis (Farinati, JHepatol, 1995; 22:429). Hyperferritinaemia is recognized as a factor of lesser response to interferon. The decrease in iron load by venesections causes a decrease in serum transaminase activity (Hayashi, JHepatol, 1995; 22:268). Ribavirin increases hepatic iron load (Di Bisceglie, JHepatol, 1994; 21:1109), whereas interferon

decreases hepatic iron (Boucher, Gut, 1997; 41:115). In contrast with these accepted data, the following are still under debate: the mechanism of hepatic iron excess in this disease; the influence of hepatic iron concentration on the response to interferon (Olynyk, Gastro, 1995; 108:1104; Piperno, Liver, 1996; 16:248); the effect of decreasing iron load by venesections on the response to interferon.

Neonatal iron overload

Neonatal (or perinatal) 'haemochromatosis'

This is a generally fatal disease characterized by severe liver failure of intrauterine onset and by massive hepatocytic iron deposition with cirrhosis. Iron overload is present, to a lesser extent, in parenchymal cells of endocrine organs, the heart, and kidney. Little iron is found in the mononuclear phagocytic system. The overall pattern of iron excess recalls that of haemochromatosis. Neonatal 'haemochromatosis' is likely not to represent a single entity—a genetic (non-HLA related) factor may be involved, as well as environmental or immune components (Knisely, AdvPediat, 1992; 39:383; Schoenlebe, AmJDisChild, 1993; 147:1072).

Cerebrohepatorenal syndrome (Zellweger's syndrome)

This is a fatal autosomal recessive disorder, characterized clinically by hypotonia, abnormal facies, and polycystic kidneys. In some cases, increased parenchymal iron is found in the liver (with fibrosis), spleen, kidneys, and lungs.

Hereditary tyrosinaemia

Hepatic iron overload is inconstant and moderate in this disease, in which there is a peculiar fishy odour, cirrhosis, and renal abnormalities.

Congenital atransferrinaemia

Due to the absence of transferrin (the plasma iron transport protein) this rare disorder is characterized by microcytic hypochromic anaemia, associated with iron overload in the liver (within the hepatocytes) and also in the heart, kidneys, thyroid, and pancreas. Anaemia is improved by transferrin infusion.

Acaeruloplasminaemia

This new disease entity is due to a mutation in the caeruloplasmin gene (Yoshida, NatureGen, 1995; 9:267). It mimics haemochromatosis in that it is a family disease, responsible for massive hepatocytic iron overload, and diabetes mellitus. The differences are represented by the coexistence of neurological (extrapyramidal and cerebellous) and ocular symptoms, due to iron deposition in the central nervous system. No serum caeruloplasmin is detectable. This disease does not present copper accumulation and further illustrates the connection between copper and iron metabolisms (see Chapter 2.16.1).

African iron overload

This is found in sub-Saharan Africa and is likely to result from the combination of two factors (Gordeuk, NEJM, 1992; 326:95).

(1) excess dietary iron related to a traditional maize beverage, fermented in iron pots at a low pH which enhances intestinal iron absorption;

(2) a non-HLA-related gene.

Iron deposition is found in the mononuclear phagocytic system throughout the body as well as in parenchymal cells. African iron overload may present clinical manifestations similar to haemochromatosis, but differs in its good correlation between bone marrow iron stores and total body iron.

Hyperferritinaemia, normal transferrin saturation, and iron overload

Despite normal transferrin saturation, hyperferritinaemia may be associated with hepatic iron excess. The excess is often moderate, but can be pronounced (hepatic iron index >2) in one-third of cases. It is non-HLA-A related and is most often observed in patients presenting a special metabolic profile: 95 per cent are overweight, with increased blood pressure, hyperlipidaemia, or glucose intolerance. This 'dysmetabolic' hepatosiderosis seems to correspond to a novel entity, whose mechanism is not yet established (Moirand, Lancet, 1997; 349:95).

Pathogenesis
Mechanisms of hepatic iron toxicity
Models of liver iron toxicity

For the clinician, the hepatic toxicity of iron is illustrated by:

(1) the correlation between the intensity (and the duration) of iron excess and the development of hepatic fibrosis;

(2) the regression of hepatomegaly with disappearance of the slight initial hypertransaminasaemia by venesections.

However, experimental models of iron overload producing hepatic damage are difficult to obtain. Interesting data were obtained *in vivo* with:

(1) baboon overloaded with parenteral iron (Brissot, DigDisSci, 1983; 28:616; Brissot, DigDisSci, 1987; 32:620);

(2) gerbil submitted to parenteral iron–dextran (Carthew, Hepatol, 1991; 13:534);

(3) rat fed with carbonyl iron.

In the rat model, the distribution pattern of iron resembles that of haemochromatosis and, by 8 months of iron overloading, periportal fibrous tissue was reported, which became more pronounced at 12 months (Park, Hepatol, 1987; 57:555); however this fibrogenic effect seems inconstant (Iancu, VirchArchCP, 1987; 53: 208) and no cirrhosis was produced.

In vitro, liver cell cultures exposed to iron load also represent interesting experimental models (Desvergne, EurJCellBiol, 1989; 49:162).

Cellular targets for iron toxicity

Iron-related hepatocyte damage is illustrated, in haemochromatosis, by the recently characterized features of sideronecrosis (Deugnier, Gastro, 1992; 102:2050). In 135 patients, sideronecrosis was absent in moderate iron overload and present in increasing proportion from important to massive haemochromatosis. It was associated with a slight but highly significant increase of serum transaminase activity and with the development of fibrosis. Experimentally (Morel, BiochemPharm, 1990; 39:1647), adult rat hepatocyte cultures supplemented with ferric nitrilotriacetate released higher levels of LDH and transaminases in the culture medium as compared with controls.

The plasma membrane as well as the membranes of the various intrahepatocytic organelles represent the major target of iron toxicity. Iron-induced lipid peroxidation represents the main mechanism accounting for membrane damage (Bacon, JCI, 1983; 71: 429):

1. An increase of free malondialdehyde recovery in the cells and in the culture medium of rat hepatocytes cultures supplemented with ferric nitrilotriacetate reflected the pro-oxidant activity of ferric iron (Morel, BiochemPharm, 1990; 39:1647).

2. In carbonyl iron fed rats, the presence of aldehyde–protein adducts in the cytosol of periportal hepatocytes which colocalized with iron overload provided strong evidence for the occurrence of iron-catalysed lipid peroxidation *in vivo* (Houglum, JCI, 1990; 86:1991).

As to the intrahepatocytic organelles involved in this peroxidative process, mitochondria are a major target whereas microsomes are affected at a lesser degree. Impairment in mitochondrial functions (Bacon, Gastro, 1993; 105:1134) could represent functional consequences of these organelle injuries. Peroxidative injury has been demonstrated in iron-loaded lysosomes (Mak, JCI, 1985; 75:58).

Nature of the toxic iron

Non-transferrin-bound iron is increasingly considered as the potentially damaging form of iron. Often found in the serum of haemochromatotic patients, it is likely to represent complexes of iron ions with low molecular weight organic ligands, especially with citrate and acetate (Grootfeld, JBC, 1989; 264:4417). Non-transferrin-bound iron has been shown, in the isolated perfused rat liver, to be avidly taken up by hepatocytes (Brissot, JCI, 1985; 76: 1463). This efficient uptake is not reduced by iron loading (Wright, JBC, 1986; 263:1842) and can even be increased (Kaplan, JBC, 1991; 26:2997; Randell, JBC, 1994; 269:16046). Therefore, non-transferrin-bound iron which is capable of stimulating the formation of hydroxyl radicals and lipid peroxidation (Gutteridge, ClinSci, 1985; 68:463) could play an important, harmful role towards the liver (as well as for other targets, such as pancreas and joints).

Mechanisms of hepatic fibrosis

In the carbonyl iron rat model, enhanced hepatic collagen type 1 mRNA expression has been found within acinar zone 1 (Houglum, AmJPhysiol, 1994; 267:G908) and in stellate cells (Pietrangelo, Hepatol, 1994; 19:714). There was also stimulation, in acinar zone 1, of reactive aldehydes and transforming growth factor-β, both known as inducers of collagen gene expression. These mechanisms could be a link between iron overload and fibrosis in haemochromatosis.

Whatever the precise mechanisms involved, the fibrogenic effect of iron *per se* is probably weak, when taking into account the

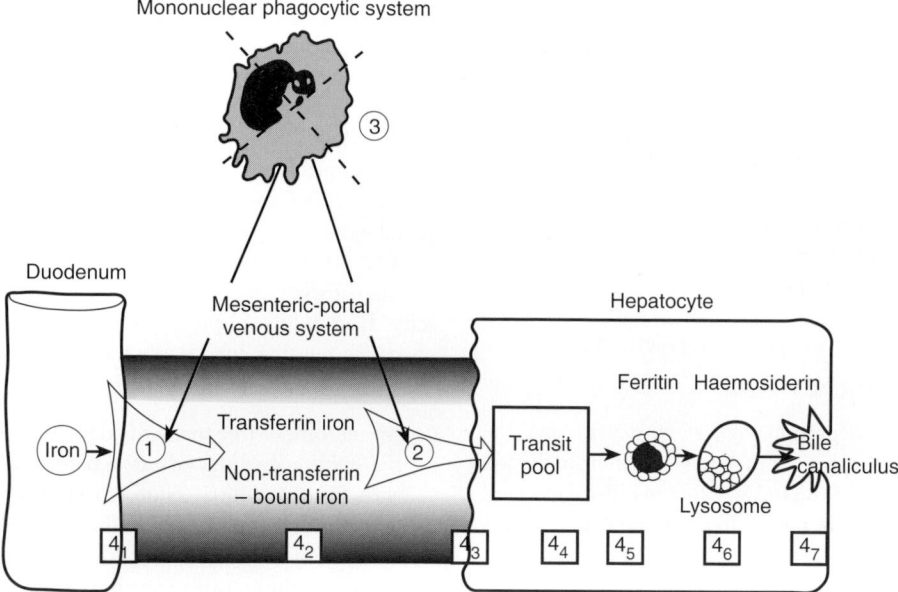

Fig. 2. Hypothetical mechanisms of iron overload in haemochromatosis. Now agreed—intestinal hyperavidity for iron (1); hepatic hyperavidity for iron (2). Under discussion—failure of the mononuclear phagocytic system (3) responsible for (1) and (2); possible targets (4) if there is integrity of the mononuclear phagocytic system: 4_1 (disturbance of intestinal absorption), 4_2 (abnormal linkage of iron to transferrin), 4_3 (abnormal hepatocytic uptake), 4_4 ('transit pool' disturbance), 4_5 (abnormal ferritin synthesis), 4_6 (lysosomal abnormality), 4_7 (disturbed biliary excretion).

difficulties of finding an adequate animal model of iron-related fibrosis, and, in haemochromatosis, the high critical liver iron levels associated with fibrosis (Bassett, Hepatol, 1986; 6:24; Loréal, JHepatol, 1992; 16:122). It is likely that, in order to become fibrogenic, iron requires high concentrations, long-standing exposure, and cofactors such as alcohol or viral infection.

Pathogenesis of iron overload (Fig. 2)

The precise factors accounting for iron overload in haemochromatosis remain poorly understood. There are three main questions.

Is intestinal and hepatic hyperavidity for iron solely responsible?

Intestinal involvement is certain, as demonstrated by radioactive studies in haemochromatosis patients showing iron hyperabsorption, involving both non-haem and haem iron (Lynch, Blood, 1989; 74:2187); moreover, the isolated duodenal mucosa has been shown to exhibit high iron uptake in haemochromatosis compared with secondary iron overload (Cox, Lancet, 1978; i:123), and McLaren *et al.* (McLaren, JLabClinMed, 1991; 117:390) reported an enhanced mucosal transfer of iron in haemochromatosis. An increased iron uptake by the liver has also been reported for both transferrin and non-transferrin-bound iron. However, beside this hyperavidity mechanism, the role of an associated decrease in iron biliary excretion cannot be excluded. The importance of biliary iron excretion in the iron overloaded rat has been emphasized (Lesage, JCI, 1986; 77:90), and ferritin-iron biliary excretion has been shown in

haemochromatosis (Cleton, Hepatol, 1986; 6:30; Hultcrantz, Gastro, 1989; 96:1539). These biliary data could of course indicate a relative compensatory mechanism to liver iron excess but, conversely, an alteration of this iron elimination route could play some role in the production of iron overload, especially through (primary or secondary) lysosomal functional impairment.

Is this intestinal (and hepatic) iron hyperavidity secondary to dysfunction of the mononuclear phagocytic system or primary?

The iron level in the mononuclear phagocytic system is known to be a major regulating factor for iron intestinal absorption. Several arguments favour deficiency of the system in haemochromatosis:

(1) low iron concentration in the macrophages of intestinal villi, bone marrow, and the liver (Kupffer cells);
(2) poor capacity of the system to retain iron coming from erythrocyte dysfunction (Fillet, Blood, 1975; 46:1007);
(3) decrease of ferritin secretion by monocytes in HLA A3 compared with non-A3 subjects (Pollack, ClinImmunPath, 1983; 27:124);
(4) data from Flanagan *et al.* (Flanagan, JLabClinMed, 1989; 113:145) indicating that mononuclear cell ferritin release in haemochromatosis is increased compared with that of controls.

However, other data tend to militate against such dysfunction of the mononuclear phagocytic system:

(1) there is no confirmation of the failure of the system to retain iron (Stefanelli, AmJPhysiol, 1984; 247:842);

(2) absence of monocyte abnormalities, in haemochromatosis, in both ferritin synthesis and transferrin iron uptake (Sizemore, AmJHemat, 1984; 16:347);

(3) it is possible to explain the poor involvement of the mononuclear phagocytic system (in terms of iron overload) by the intestinal source of iron (in contrast to the predominant deposition in the system of iron produced by blood transfusions), and/or by the biochemical nature of the implicated iron—non-transferrin-bound iron, which is very efficiently taken up by hepatocytes, and could be responsible for the preferential periportal and hepatocytic iron distribution in haemochromatosis (Brissot, JCI, 1985; 76:1463).

Regardless of the initial cellular target, what is the nature of the basic metabolic defect making the link between the abnormal gene located on chromosome 6 and the development of iron overload ?

Only incomplete data are available:

1. The involvement of the main proteins of iron metabolism can be ruled out on the following arguments:

(a) the corresponding genes have been cloned and ascribed to chromosomes other than chromosome 6: chromosome 3 for the iron transport protein, transferrin, and for the iron uptake protein, the transferrin receptor; chromosomes 11 and 19 for the iron storage protein, ferritin; chromosome 9 for the iron regulatory protein.

(b) the co-ordinate regulation of transferrin receptor and ferritin is preserved in haemochromatotic duodenum (Pietrangelo, Gastro, 1992; 102:802).

(c) the low accumulation of duodenum ferritin in haemochromatosis is not caused by a defective control of ferritin synthesis but by low expression of ferritin mRNA and sustained activity of iron regulatory protein
(Pietrangelo, Gastro, 1995; 108:208).

2. The major protein candidate is the protein encoded by the HFE gene. This 343 amino-acid protein represents a novel MHC class I-like molecule sharing significant features with that family, among which are the number and spacing of the cysteine residues involved in disulphide bridges. One hypothesis suggests that the C282Y mutation disrupts the formation of a disulphide bridge, therefore compromising the association of this protein with β_2-microglobulin. This process might affect iron metabolism in a way similar to that of β_2-microglobulin deficient mice which develop a type of iron excess resembling that of haemochromatosis (De Souza, Immunolett, 1994; 39:105; Rothenberg, PNAS, 1996; 93:1529). However, the mechanisms whereby such a protein would influence transmembrane iron transport remain to be determined. Indeed, it is likely that, in this disease, the primary defect is an increased flux of NTBI through the intestine resulting, at the duodenal level, in a 'paradoxical' cellular iron deficiency which, in turn, would explain the observed variations of the transferrin receptor and ferritin transcripts.

Treatment

The therapeutic management of haemochromatosis comprises both curative and preventive measures.

Curative treatment
Modalities
Symptomatic treatment of visceral and metabolic complications

Against asthenia, vitamin C should be avoided since it is potentially deleterious especially towards the heart. For the liver, alcohol consumption should be suppressed in case of fibrosis. For heart failure, digitalis should be used with caution since it may precipitate rhythm disturbances. Diabetes requires adequate diet and, when overt, most often insulin. Joint inflammation responds (partially) to salicylates and non-steroidal anti-inflammatory drugs, but systemic corticosteroid therapy should not be given due to the risk of diabetes.

Elimination of iron overload

Low iron diet is useless since a 1-year diet is equivalent to only two or three venesections. Chelation therapy is reserved for the rare contraindications to venesection such as anaemia, hepatocellular insufficiency, or associated general disease (e.g. arteriosclerosis). It is then based on prolonged subcutaneous desferrioxamine infusion and hopefully in the near future on oral chelators such as hydroxypyridinones (see above). Erythrocytapheresis may be an interesting method in those cases contraindicating venesections (Conte, IntJArtifOrg, 1989; 12:59).

Venesection therapy represents, of course, the ideal means to eliminate iron overload, according to a two-phase protocol:

1. The initial phase consists of one 400 to 500 ml venesection per week (corresponding to the removal of 200 to 250 mg of iron); follow-up is based on haemoglobin values for tolerance and on serum ferritin levels for efficacy. The duration of this phase depends on the degree of iron overload. The initial schedule is stopped as soon as the various serum iron load parameters reach the appropriate levels (<50 µg/l for ferritin, ~10 µmol/l for iron, ~20 per cent for transferrin saturation). For heavily iron-loaded patients a period of 2 years of weekly venesections may be necessary, but more and more, due to moderately iron overloaded forms, several weeks or a few months are sufficient.

2. Maintenance therapy consists of 400 to 500 ml venesection every 1 to 3 months. Its goal is to keep serum iron parameters within the normal range (in practice, serum ferritin ≤ 50 µg/l and transferrin saturation ≤ 50 per cent).

Results

They are good for general health, skin pigmentation, liver, and heart symptoms, but moderate for diabetes. Insulin dependence is not reversible but insulin dose can be reduced in about one-third of patients, and, in those with glucose intolerance, carbohydrate metabolism is improved in about 50 per cent of cases (Stremmel, AnnNYAcadMed, 1988; 526:209). The results are poor for joint symptoms (which may worsen despite phlebotomies) and for gonadal insufficiency. Moreover, with respect to the liver, when cirrhosis is present at the time of starting phlebotomies, the risk of hepatocellular carcinoma remains, despite adequate depletive therapy. On the whole, curative treatment of haemochromatosis results in a significant improvement in life expectancy which may even be

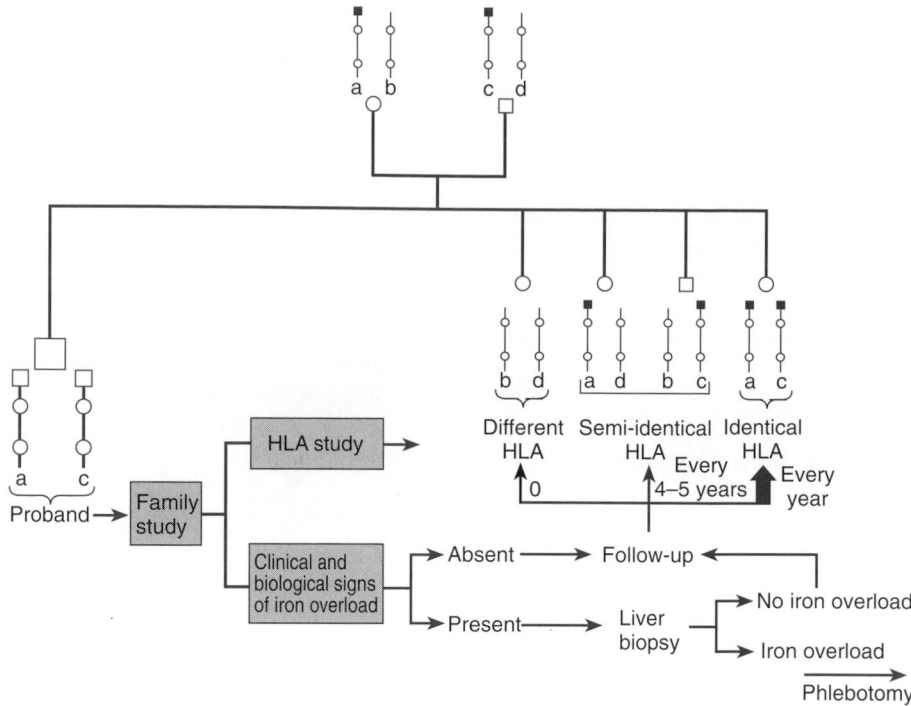

Fig. 3. Organigram of classical family screening and management in haemochromatosis (heterozygous–heterozygous marriage); a, b, c, d = HLA haplotypes, –O– = HLA A and B loci, ■ = haemochromatosis gene.

normal in patients who present without cirrhosis or diabetes at the time of diagnosis (Niederau, Gastro, 1996; 110:1107); this underlines the importance of an early diagnosis.

Preventive treatment
Family screening (Fig. 3)

This is of paramount importance.

1. Classical strategy

Family members to be screened

Screening must be proposed to all the proband's siblings. Whenever possible, the parents, spouse, and children (over 10 years old) should be included.

Data to be collected are of two types

1. Signs of iron overload, clinical and/or biochemical—this search should not forget factors susceptible to modify the expression of the disease including: overexpression factors such as associated liver disease (especially of alcoholic origin) or consumption of iron tablets; underexpression factors such as blood donations, menses, pregnancies. This implies careful clinical examination and several blood tests (transferrin saturation, serum iron, ferritin, transaminases, γ-glutamyl transpeptidase, blood cell count with mean corpuscular volume, etc.).
2. HLA typing was essential for this classical screening approach. The key point was that when the diagnosis of homozygous haemochromatosis had been established in a given individual (on the non-HLA basis above-mentioned), the HLA group (whatever its nature) of this proband became a diagnostic marker

of the haemochromatosis gene not only for the patient but also for other family members. Complete A and B HLA typing (i.e. testing all known A and B antigens) was required to be carried out; testing only for A3, B7, or B14 was meaningless.

Interpretation of the data The prerequisite for this interpretation was to reconstitute the HLA haplotypes (i.e. the HLA 'couples' A–B) of the proband; this was only possible by taking into account the HLA groups of the various family members tested. Both proband haplotypes were markers for the haemochromatosis gene. The conclusions were then deduced from the combination of iron overload and HLA data obtained from the family:

1. In siblings (brothers and sisters) each HLA-identical subject (i.e. sharing the same haplotypes as the proband) is homozygous for the disease (i.e. carrier of the haemochromatosis gene at double dose). Most often, iron overload is present at the time of the screening; it can however be absent or only moderate due to young age and/or underexpression factors of the disease (blood donations, pregnancies, etc.). HLA semi-identical siblings (i.e. sharing only one haplotype with the proband) are usually heterozygous and therefore will not develop the disease. Two notions should, however, be kept in mind concerning HLA semi-identical siblings:
   (a) if they are heterozygous, they will be able to transmit the gene to their children;
   (b) they can in fact be homozygous if one of their parents was heterozygous and the other one homozygous. This heterozygous–homozygous parental mating (instead of the usual heterozygous–heterozygous mating) is far from exceptional

since it concerns more than 10 per cent of the probands. HLA-different siblings are usually free of the gene; they can however be heterozygous in case of a heterozygous–homozygous parental mating.

2. In parents (mother and father), provided they are still alive, it is usually easy to define their genetic status since homozygosity is expected to be obviously expressed at this advanced age (with always the reserve of possible interfering factors of underexpression).

3. In children—all the children of a proband are at least heterozygous. The real concern is to know whether they are 'only' heterozygous or in fact 'young homozygous' due to the fact that, by chance, the proband's spouse was also heterozygous. The dilemma remained difficult to solve in this classical strategy because expression of homozygosity is usually absent in young children and expression of heterozygosity is absent (or quite mild) in adults. In practice, careful follow-up (every 2 years) of children (aged over 10) was the only way to avoid misdiagnosis of homozygosity in this young population.

Therapeutic consequences

In certified homozygotes, the detection of iron excess (subsequently quantified by MRI and/or liver biopsy) will lead to venesection therapy. In the absence of iron overload, a preventive venesection programme (for instance four phlebotomies a year) is engaged, with careful follow-up of serum ferritin. In certified heterozygotes, subjects without suspicion of iron overload are merely advised to undergo venesections two to three times a year in order to prevent a putative slight iron overload; in case of moderate iron excess, a weekly venesection programme is prescribed in order to lower serum iron load parameters to normal values (a few phlebotomies usually suffice to reach this goal). Subjects free of the haemochromatosis gene do not require any follow-up. For children aged over 10 (born from either certified homozygotes or known heterozygotes) a follow-up every 2 years is generally advised.

2. Up-to-date screening strategy

This strategy requires blood HFE genetic testing (Fig. 4), which must now replace HLA-A testing. This new approach permits immediate evaluation risks of haemochromatosis among siblings and children of a typical C282Y + / + proband, remembering, however, that the penetrance of the disease is not yet established.

The best way to perform family screening

Experience shows that performing such screening is difficult for reasons which are both practical (scattering of the subjects) and theoretical (problems of interpretation). It is essential to avoid the

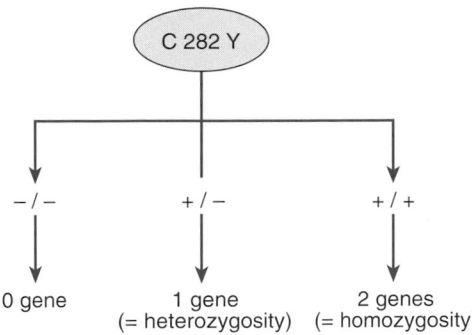

Fig. 4. New screening strategy based on the search for the C282Y mutation

'pseudo-screening', still too often performed, based exclusively on testing serum iron (and/or ferritin) and which, in case of normal or 'almost normal' results, may unduly reassure and stop any follow-up. Taking into account the combined data provided by clinical examination, biochemical blood testing (including transferrin saturation), and genotypic testing is the only informative and reliable procedure. For performing such studies, haemochromatosis family screening centres can be very useful, allowing studies of the family members from every proband to be carried out in close collaboration with their own physicians.

Mass screening

As a frequent, severe, and treatable disease, haemochromatosis meets fully the criteria for a beneficial screening. Three main studies (Edwards, NEJM, 1993; 328:1616; Balan, Gastro, 1994; 107:453; Adams, Gastro, 1995; 109:177) conclude that large screenings are cost effective and advocate 'universal' screening for presymptomatic haemochromatosis. This should certainly remain the final goal; meanwhile, it is of utmost importance to extend the indications of checking serum iron load parameters (especially transferrin saturation) in various clinical situations (asthenia, arthropathy, etc.), and also to modify the perception of homozygosity by the institutions, especially insurance companies, in order to avoid adverse genetic discrimination (Billings, AmJHumGen, 1992; 50:476).

References

1. Weintraub LR, Edwards CQ, and Crikker M (eds). Hemochromatosis. Proceedings of the First International Conference. *Annals of the New York Academy of Sciences*, 1988; 526.
2. Brock JH, Halliday, JW, Pippard MJ, and Powell LW (eds). *Iron Metabolism in Health and Disease*. London: WB Saunders, 1994.
3. Brissot P, Moirand R, Guyader D, and Deugnier Y. Surcharges en fer. In *Encyclopédie médico-chirurgicale hépatologie*. Paris, 1995: 7–200–A–10.

20.3. α_1-Antitrypsin deficiency and related disorders

Sten Eriksson and Joyce Carlson

Definition

The classical α_1-antitrypsin deficiency, **PI** (protease inhibitor) ZZ, is a codominantly inherited disease characterized by concentrations of 10 to 15 per cent of normal in circulating α_1-antitrypsin. An amino-acid substitution in the molecule is responsible for a secretory defect, with accumulation of the protein in the endoplasmic reticulum. The clinical expression of this abnormality is variable, but is dominated by emphysema and liver disease, and, rarely, by vasculitic syndromes.

Introduction

A deficiency of α_1-antitrypsin and its association with obstructive lung disease were first described in 1963.[1] The hereditary nature of the defect, the identification of homo- and heterozygotes, and the predisposition of primarily tobacco-smoking homozygotes to develop early panlobular emphysema were further described in 1964–5.[2–4]

Juvenile cirrhosis was first observed in 1969 in seven children with α_1-antitrypsin deficiency.[5] Two years later came the description of the presence of diastase-resistant, periodic acid–Schiff (**PAS-D**)-positive inclusions in hepatocytes, corresponding to immunoreactive α_1-antitrypsin, and of distension of the endoplasmic reticulum seen by electron microscopy.[6] From these findings came the suggestion that the circulating deficiency of α_1-antitrypsin was secondary to a secretory defect. Isolation and partial characterization of the PAS-D inclusions verified the presence of α_1-antitrypsin in 1975, and an abnormal carbohydrate structure was proposed.[7] This was supported by the demonstration of excess mannose in the accumulated α_1-antitrypsin in 1978, corresponding to core-glycosylated oligosaccharide side-chains.[8] The ultrastructural characteristics of the accumulation of this abnormal α_1-antitrypsin in the endoplasmic reticulum were confirmed in 1974.[9] In 1972, the genetic α_1-antitrypsin deficiency causing both lung and liver disease was identified.[10] In the early 1970s, cases of adult cirrhosis and complicating hepatoma were published,[10,11] but a causal relation between the deficiency state and adult cirrhosis/hepatoma was not demonstrated until 1986.[12] A prospective investigation of α_1-antitrypsin deficiency in new-borns was initiated by Laurell and Sveger in 1972,[13] and the natural history of the deficiency state has been followed and reported up to the age of 18 years.[14]

In parallel with these clinical observations, the biochemistry of the α_1-antitrypsin molecule has been clarified. An amino-acid substitution from Glu342–Lys in the PI Z protein was identified in 1976.[15] Purification permitting reliable immunochemical quantitation of plasma α_1-antitrypsin was described in 1978.[16] The entire amino-acid sequence of the 52-kDa protein was published in 1982,[17] and confirmed by the cDNA sequence published 2 years later.[18] α_1-Antitrypsin is the major extracellular proteinase inhibitor,[19] and the central role of the Met–Ser residues at its reactive centre was described in 1978.[20] The importance of neutrophil elastase as primary target enzyme then became evident; this topic was reviewed in 1985.[21]

The genetic polymorphism for α_1-antitrypsin was first defined in 1967[22] and the symbol PI was chosen to denote the phenotypes. The PI system has been expanded to include more than 75 variants.[23] The microheterogeneity of the molecule and its numerous genetic variants have been extensively reviewed by Cox.[24] Recent reviews cover the early history of α_1-antitrypsin deficiency,[25] its molecular pathology,[26] analytical methods for α_1-antitrypsin,[27] as well as the molecular genetics of the protein.[28] Carrell has discussed serine-proteinase inhibitors (serpins) in a broad context,[29] and the function of α_1-antitrypsin has been generally reviewed.[30] The clinical association of α_1-antitrypsin deficiency with juvenile[31,32] and adult[33] liver disease has also been reviewed.

The structure and function of α_1-antitrypsin

From gene to protein

The human genes for α_1-antitrypsin and α_1-antichymotrypsin are localized to chromosome 14 (Darlington, PNAS, 1982; 79:870) in close linkage with the immunoglobulin heavy-chain cluster (G_M) (Bissbort, HumGenet, 1988; 79:289). Complementary DNAs (cDNA) synthesized from mRNAs immunoprecipitated from human liver (Leicht, Nature, 1982; 297:655) and monocytes (Perlino, EMBOJ, 1987; 6:2767) have been used as probes to clone genomic DNA.[18] The structural gene and some aspects of its 5′ regulatory region (*cis*-acting elements) are shown in Fig. 1. Alternative splicing of exons IA, IB, and IC occurs, with all three or A and C being present in gene transcripts from macrophages; only

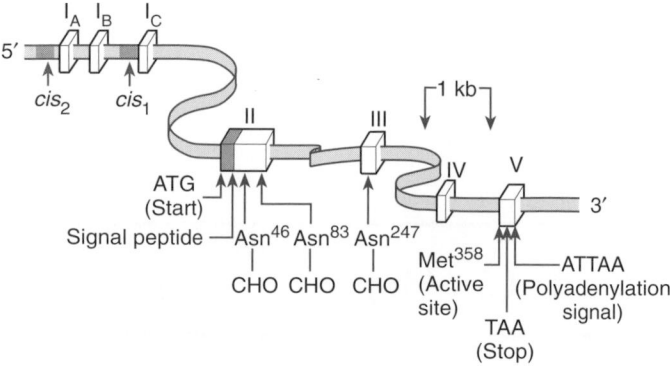

Fig. 1. Schematic structure of the human α_1-antitrypsin gene. Exons IA and IB are expressed in monocytes and macrophages. This expression is probably regulated by elements marked cis_2. Exon IC is the transcription initiation site for liver α_1-antitrypsin. Its expression is regulated by sequences marked cis_1. Translation starts at ATG in exon II. Oligosaccharide side-chains are attached to appropriate Asn residues. The active site Met358 and the PI Z mutation site Glu342 are found in exon V. Modified from ref. 28 with permission.

C is found in liver α_1-antitrypsin transcripts (Perlino, EMBOJ, 1987; 6:2767). The signal ATG for the start of translation is found in exon II (Fig. 1). This initiates the sequence for an aminoterminal, 24-residue signal peptide that locates the nascent protein in the endoplasmic reticulum. During protein elongation, three carbohydrate side-chains in a high-mannose (core-glycosylated) form are attached to appropriate asparagine residues. The signal peptide is removed, and post-translational modifications of the side-chains occur in the Golgi (Carlson, JBC, 1982;257:12 987). This results in secretion of a 52-kDa plasma glycoprotein containing 394 amino acids and three terminally glycosylated carbohydrate side-chains.[17]

α_1-Antitrypsin contains a single cysteine, which is available for participation in thiol–disulphide interchanges (Laurell, JChromatogr, 1978; 159:25). A small fraction of plasma α_1-antitrypsin is normally found in a disulphide bond with the IgA heavy chain.

The active site of α_1-antitrypsin is a Met residue at position 358 followed by a Ser.[17] This site mimics the substrate sequence for serine proteases (such as neutrophil elastase, trypsin, chymotrypsin, kallikrein) and is cleaved with varying rate constants by such enzymes, effecting their inactivation. This characteristic is common for all members of the serpin (serine protease inhibitor) family, of which α_1-antitrypsin is the best-studied example.[26] Other members of this protein and gene superfamily include α_1-antichymotrypsin, antithrombin III, protein C inhibitor, thyroxine-binding globulin, corticosteroid-binding globulin, and angiotensinogen. These proteins display significant homology in protein and gene structures. Most serpins effect amidolytic inactivation of their target proteases as the carboxyterminal of the serpin is cleaved and translocated.[26] Target enzyme specificity is determined by the amino-acid sequence at the active site. Oxidation of the active-site methionine of α_1-antitrypsin by cigarette smoke, or by oxidative enzymes released from neutrophils, inactivates the inhibitor.[30]

α_1-Antitrypsin as an acute-phase protein—regulation of biosynthesis

The plasma concentration of α_1-antitrypsin increases three- to fourfold in inflammation and as a response to tissue injury [Aronsen, ScaJCLI, 1972; 29(Suppl. 124):127], and approximately twofold as a response to oestrogens (Laurell, ScaJCLI, 1967; 21:337). A selective increase in plasma α_1-antitrypsin is often found in liver disease and correlates directly with the degree of inflammation seen in liver biopsies (Carlson, ActaMedScand, 1980; 207:79). During acute-phase conditions, qualitative differences in circulating α_1-antitrypsin are frequently observed. Changes in its electrophoretic mobility are noted and correspond to increased branching of carbohydrate side-chains (Vaughan, BBActa, 1982; 701:339). Other alterations appear to be responsible for functionally inert forms in advanced cancer (Chawla, CancRes, 1987; 47:1179) and active liver disease (Miszczul-Jamska, FolHistochemCytol, 1986; 24:173). These inactive forms cannot be differentiated from normal forms by immunochemical methods alone and are not due to oxidation or complex formation. A common serpin receptor has been identified that mediates catabolism of α_1-antitrypsin, α_1-antichymotrypsin, antithrombin III, and other serpins (Pizzo, BBActa, 1988; 967:158). Shorter half-lives for complex bound serpins than native serpins, and competition for binding the serpin receptor in the presence of other serpin complexes, have been demonstrated.

Biosynthesis of acute-phase reactant proteins has been studied in sections of rat liver after the induction of inflammation; sequential recruitment of cells is seen across the hepatic lobule (Lamri, CellMolecBiol, 1986; 32:691). Derivatives from stimulated monocytes, such as interleukin I and tumour necrosis factor, stimulate the biosynthesis of most acute-phase proteins in cultures of human hepatoma cells, but not α_1-antitrypsin (Darlington, JCellBiol, 1986; 103:787; Perlmutter, Science, 1986; 232:850). Interleukin 6 (Castell, Hepatol, 1990; 12:1179), transforming growth factor-β_1 (Mackiewicz, PNAS, 1990; 87:1491), endotoxin (Ganter, EurJBioch, 1987; 169:13) and C5a anaphylatoxin (Buchner, JImmunol, 1995; 155:308) specifically induce α_1-antitrypsin biosynthesis in cell culture.

The α_1-antitrypsin gene is expressed in many extrahepatic tissues (Carlson, JCI, 1988; 82:26). Monocytes and bronchoalveolar macrophages in primary culture synthesize and secrete α_1-antitrypsin, and have been useful in studies of regulation of biosynthesis. The addition of neutrophil elastase increases the biosynthesis of α_1-antitrypsin. This effect is probably mediated by the 4-kDa C-terminal α_1-antitrypsin fragment, which is cleaved during complex formation (Perlmutter, JCI, 1988; 81:1774; JBC, 1988; 263:16499). Similar mechanisms may operate in hepatocytes and explain the 'positive feed-back induction' of α_1-antitrypsin biosynthesis observed in human fetal liver explants (Eriksson, BBActa, 1978; 542: 496). Thus the rate of protease–antiprotease complex formation may regulate the expression of the α_1-antitrypsin gene in macrophages at the microenvironmental level, and in hepatocytes, providing increased circulating α_1-antitrypsin.

The genetic polymorphism of α_1-antitrypsin

More than 75 phenotypes of α_1-antitrypsin have now been identified on the basis of charge differences in the circulating protein.[23]

Table 1 α₁-Antitrypsin allele frequencies in selected populations

Reference	Population tested	n	PI*M[a]	PI*S	PI*Z	Other
3	Swedish adults	6995			0.024	
13	Swedish infants	200 000			0.026	
23	Norway	2830	0.946	0.023	0.016	0.015
24	Denmark	909	0.946	0.022	0.023	0.009
24	England	926	0.924	0.048	0.022	0.006
b	Netherlands	357	0.955	0.029	0.013	0.003
24	Portugal	900	0.823	0.150	0.009	0.018
24	United States (white)	904	0.956	0.023	0.014	0.007
24	United States (black)	549	0.982	0.015	0.004	0.0
24	China	1010	0.988	0.0	0.0	0.012
24	Japan	746	1.00	0.0	0.0	0.0

[a] Includes PI*M1, PI*M2, PI*M3, PI*M4.
[b] Arnaud, ClinGenet, 1979; 15: 406.

Phenotypes were initially designated according to their electrophoretic mobility in a starch–agarose gel system. PI (protease inhibitor) M is the most common, with medium mobility, PI F is fast, PI S is slow, and PI Z is even slower (Fagerhol, SemHemat, 1968; 1:153). Phenotypes are currently determined by isoelectric focusing.[27] Within each phenotype a microheterogeneity is apparent (Fig. 2), due to variable degrees of branching of the three carbohydrate chains and to the presence or absence of an N-terminal pentapeptide (Jeppsson, JChromatogr, 1985; 327:173). Inheritance of the α₁-antitrypsin phenotype is autosomal-codominant, with equal contributions to the phenotype from both alleles. Phenotypes are designated PI M, PI MZ, etc., and alleles are designated PI*M, PI*S, etc. Common PI variants associated with a decreased plasma concentration of α₁-antitrypsin are PI S at 60 per cent, and the classical deficiency phenotype PI Z at 10 to 15 per cent of normal. The rare alleles PI*I, PI*P, PI*Mmalton, PI*Mduarte, PI*Mheerlen, and PI*Mprocida also produce low plasma concentrations. Several other rare gene mutations have been identified that give rise to PI null (PI 0 or PI –) phenotypes with no detectable circulating α₁-antitrypsin.[28] PI*S is relatively common in Spain and Portugal. PI*Z, although common in Scandinavia, has the highest reported frequency in South Tyrol with one per 981 inhabitants [Pittschieler, ActaPaedScand, 1994; 393(Suppl.):21]. Gene frequencies in some populations are summarized in Table 1.

Specific DNA or amino-acid substitutions are known for multiple variants.[24] The classical deficiency allele PI*Z results from a single base-pair substitution in exon V corresponding to the Glu342–Lys substitution (Sifers, NucAcidRes, 1987; 15:1459) (see Fig. 1). In addition, a Val213–Ala substitution has been found in nearly all PI*Z alleles studied and in the PI*M1 background population.[28] The rare Pi*Z Augsburg variant has 342Lys on a Pi*M2 background. PI*Mduarte and Mmalton have nearly normal electrophoretic mobilities, but are also associated with low plasma concentrations, intracellular aggregates, and lung and liver disease (Crowley, Gastro, 1987; 93:242; Reid, Gastro, 1987; 93:181).

PI*S has a substitution in exon III[18] resulting in Glu264–Val. This protein and other rare deficiency variants presumably undergo abnormal folding with subsequent decreased stability and degradation rather than accumulation in liver cells. Once in plasma,

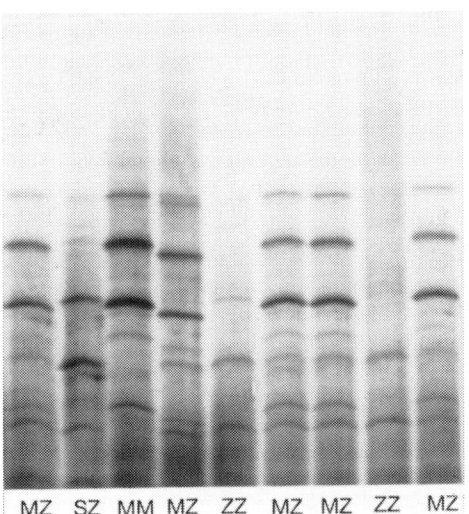

Fig. 2. Isoelectric focusing patterns at pH 4.2–4.9 of some PI variants (Jeppsson, ClinChem, 1982; 28:219). (By courtesy of Dr J-O Jeppsson.)

PI S α₁-antitrypsin has a normal half-life, and a nearly normal affinity for leucocyte elastase. The PI*O alleles that have been sequenced all have mutations resulting in premature termination, presumably leading to intracellular degradation of α₁-antitrypsin and related abnormal protein translation products.[28] These variants are not associated with liver disease.

α₁-Antitrypsin Pittsburgh (Met358–Arg) has an interesting mutation at the active site of the protease inhibitor, changing its enzyme specificity from neutrophil elastase to thrombin. This dysfunctional variant resulted in a fatal bleeding disorder in a young heterozygous patient (Owen, NEJM, 1983; 309:694).

The secretory defect and liver-cell injury

The hallmark of the PI Z α₁-antitrypsin deficiency is the accumulation of PI Z α₁-antitrypsin in the endoplasmic reticulum of hepatocytes (Fig. 3). This prototype of a protein secretory defect has stimulated research into the mechanisms of protein biosynthesis

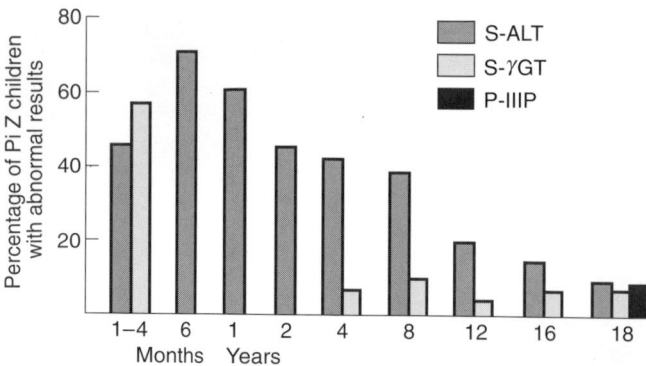

Fig. 3. Prevalence of abnormal liver function tests with increasing age during prospective monitoring of PI ZZ children.[14] S-ALT, alanine aminotransferase; S-γGT, γ-glutamyl transpeptidase; P-PIIIP, plasma precollagen III propeptide. P-PIIIP was analysed only at the 18-year check-up.

at the gene and protein levels (e.g. Derman, Cell, 1981; 23:731; Lodish, JCellBiol, 1987; 104:221). Comparisons of total DNA and α_1-antitrypsin mRNA in cirrhotic PI M, cirrhotic PI Z, and normal human liver have verified normal rates of transcription of the α_1-antitrypsin gene and normal amounts of α_1-antitrypsin mRNA in PI Z livers (Schwarzenberg, Hepatol, 1986; 6:1252). Experimental systems have further demonstrated similar rates of mRNA translation (protein biosynthesis) of *PI M* and *PI Z* mRNA (Foreman, FEBSLett, 1984; 168:84). The typical PAS-D-positive globular inclusions, isolated and purified from a PI Z cirrhotic liver (Jeppsson, NEJM, 1975; 293:576), consist of α_1-antitrypsin containing excess mannose.[8] Furthermore, there are insignificant differences in the rates of catabolism of PI M and PI Z α_1-antitrypsin (Laurell, ClinSciMolMed, 1978; 55:103). Thus the PI Z-deficiency state is clearly the result of blocked protein transport from the endoplasmic reticulum to the Golgi. X-ray crystallographic studies of the structure of α_1-antitrypsin show that Glu342 normally participates in a central salt bridge with Lys290, and suggest a conformational change in PI Z α_1-antitrypsin due to disruption of that bridge (Loebermann, JMolBiol, 1984; 177:531). This conformational change leads to a temperature- and concentration-dependent polymerization of the PI Z protein *in vitro* (Lomas, Nature, 1992; 357:605). However, recent data suggest that the polymerization process, which may be accelerated by bouts of pyrexia, is more complex than this model predicts.[26]

Mechanisms for liver-cell injury

Whereas emphysema is inversely related to plasma α_1-antitrypsin concentrations, liver disease correlates with the extent of intracellular accumulation of α_1-antitrypsin. Liver injury occurs in α_1-antitrypsin phenotypes associated with intracellular protein accumulation (PI Z, PI Mmalton, PI Mduarte). In contrast, no liver disease is seen in deficiency phenotypes due to intracellular protein degradation (PI S, PI Null).[24,28]

The microenvironment of PI Z hepatocytes is deficient in protease inhibitory activity. It has been shown that activated polymorphonuclear neutrophils exhibit hepatotoxicity that can be reproduced by pancreatic elastase and cathepsin G and prevented by serine protease inhibitors (Mavier, Hepatol, 1988; 8:254).

Immunological mechanisms may participate in the development of PI Z-related liver disease. Breit and others (ClinImmunPath, 1985; 35:363) have reviewed the role of α_1-antitrypsin deficiency in immune disorders. Increased phythaemagglutin responses of lymphocytes cultured with PI Z serum as compared to control serum, and enhanced activation of monocytes and polymorphonuclear neutrophils from PI Z as compared to PI M individuals, have been seen. It is thought that this activation is mediated by membrane-bound serine esterases and is dependent on the circulating protease inhibitor.

The putative pathogenetic importance of intracellular accumulation has been investigated in an experimental animal model. Cloned human *PI*M* and *PI*Z* structural genes have been introduced into mouse embryos to create transgenic mice (Sifers, NucAcidRes, 1987; 15:1459; Kelsey, GenesDevelop, 1987; 1:161). These mice have normal synthesis of endogenous mouse α_1-antitrypsin as well as enhanced biosynthesis of the human gene product. PI Z mice bearing exons Ic–V of the α_1-antitrypsin gene develop more histological signs of liver disease than PI M or control mice (Carlson, JCI, 1989; 83:1183), but no liver cirrhosis or hepatomas. Although signs of liver damage occur in young mice bearing exons IABC–V, no clear case of neonatal hepatitis or juvenile cirrhosis has been seen (Dycaico, Science, 1988; 242:1409). The presence of this DNA construct has, however, led to dysplasia, adenomas, and possibly invasive hepatocellular carcinoma in these mice at 16 to 20 months of age (Geller, Hepatol, 1994; 19:389). Different mouse species as well as different DNA constructs may explain the discrepancies between these findings.

Concomitant infection with hepatitis B or C virus has recently been suggested as a major pathogenetic mechanism for liver disease in PI Z patients (Propst, AnnIntMed, 1992; 117:641; JHepatol, 1994; 21:1006). We and others have been unable to confirm those results. Differences in the incidence of viral hepatitis, in diagnostic methods, or in the background population may explain the conflicting findings.

Phenotypic expression of PI Z α_1-antitrypsin deficiency

As in most hereditary diseases, the clinical expression of α_1-antitrypsin deficiency is highly heterogeneous. Clinical manifestations vary from predominant emphysema in adults to the syndrome of cholestasis in neonates. These disease entities are primarily associated with the homozygous deficiency state, although heterozygotes may be affected. Homozygotes are sufficiently rare that any individual physician, even at large referral centres, will personally treat only a small number of patients. Clinical case studies are therefore often subject to ascertainment bias resulting in inaccurate prognostic estimates. Presentation of liver disease in α_1-antitrypsin deficiency varies extensively with respect to age at onset, rate of progression, and stage at diagnosis. None the less, a composite of several epidemiological studies allows a fairly realistic analysis of the natural history of the disease.

Neonatal hepatitis and childhood cirrhosis

α_1-Antitrypsin deficiency in childhood is described in detail in Section 26. As a background for understanding liver disease in adults, it is helpful to review the continuing prospective study of

Sveger in which 200 000 consecutive Swedish new-borns were screened for α_1-antitrypsin deficiency (NEJM, 1976; 294:1316). Among the PI*Z homozygotes identified, neonatal cholestasis was seen in 10 per cent, non-cholestatic liver disease in 6 per cent, and abnormal values for alanine aminotransferase in 73 per cent at 6 months of age. At 18-year follow-up,[14] three children have died with liver cirrhosis, and one had fibrosis at death. Figure 3 illustrates the prevalence of abnormal liver function tests in both PI Z and PI SZ children through adolescence.[14] Although these prognostic data are considerably more optimistic than those obtained in retrospective, case-oriented studies [Ibarguen, JPediat, 1990; 117:865; Mowat, ActaPaedScand, 1994; 393 (Suppl.):13], they may identify PI Z and PI SZ adolescents at risk of developing cirrhosis as adults. No common predisposing genetic or exogenous factors have been identified to explain the severe outcome in the minority of PI Z children, but there is a 2:1 male predominance in children with liver disease. Despite normal liver function tests, slow-rate fibrogenesis may be present in PI Z and PI SZ children, but is not reflected in elevated serum concentrations of N-terminal procollagen III peptide.[14]

Phenotypic expression in homozygous adults

Obstructive lung disease, in particular basal panlobular emphysema, is the predominant clinical manifestation of homozygous α_1-antitrypsin deficiency in adults. Nonetheless, many individuals have mild or subclinical signs of pulmonary disease, and 30 to 50 per cent are expected to develop liver disease during their lifespan.[12] In adults, as in children, males are twice as likely to develop liver disease as females. No other predisposing factors for liver disease in homozygotes are known. Coexisting alcoholism, viral hepatitis, or autoimmune markers are rare. Some families with both haemochromatosis and α_1-antitrypsin deficiency have been reported (Anand, Hepatol, 1983; 3:714; Eriksson, JHepatol, 1986; 2:65), but there is no systematic linkage between these two genetic traits (Lindmark, ActaMedScand, 1987; 218:299), although three PI Z homozygotes were identified in a Swedish case series of 67 patients with genetic haemochromatosis (Elzouki, Gut, 1995; 36:922).

Cases of cirrhosis and hepatoma in PI Z adults were first reported in the early 1970s.[10,11] Larsson found definite signs of liver cirrhosis in only 2 per cent of 104 PI*Z homozygotes between 20 and 50 years of age, and in 19 per cent of 142 homozygotes over the age of 50.[4] Numerous other cases of fibrosis or non-specific hepatopathy were seen.

The frequency of cirrhosis in Canadian PI Z men between 50 and 60 years of age was estimated at 15 per cent (Cox, AmJMed, 1983; 74:221). The risks for cirrhosis and hepatoma have recently been evaluated in a retrospective case-control study based on all PI Z cases examined at autopsy in Malmö, Sweden, over a 20-year period.[12] The frequency of autopsy was 70 per cent and nearly all PI Z cases identified had been examined at autopsy. This study demonstrated a 47 per cent risk for cirrhosis and 29 per cent risk for hepatoma, but the odds ratio was significant only for males. A similar predominance of elderly males was noted in the United States (Rakela, DigDisSci, 1987; 32:1358). Male predominance and a high incidence of hepatoma were confirmed in a large retrospective study based on 94 PI Z cases diagnosed and examined at autopsy in Sweden (Eriksson, ActaMedScand, 1987; 221:461). Cirrhosis was

present in 37 per cent and hepatoma was found in 15 per cent, with a mean age at death of 66 years compared to 54 years in the remaining non-cirrhotic patients ($p<0.001$). These data suggest that lung disease, the major cause of premature mortality, was considerably less pronounced in the cirrhotics than in the remaining homozygotes. Thus smoking habits may indirectly influence the risk for cirrhosis/hepatoma by accelerating the progress of pulmonary disease.[4]

The clinical presentation of α_1-antitrypsin-deficient patients is similar to that of others with cryptogenic liver disease. The majority have some form of obstructive respiratory disorder, but it may be mild and overlooked. Presentation is frequently with ascites and/or other signs of portal hypertension. A past history of neonatal or viral hepatitis, evidence of excessive alcohol intake, and the presence of autoimmune markers are rare. Apart from the low plasma α_1-antitrypsin, other clinical and laboratory features are indistinguishable from those found in cirrhosis of other aetiologies. Laboratory findings at the time of diagnosis in one series of such patients are shown in Table 2. Cholestatic features are not prominent, although alkaline phosphatase and IgA are moderately raised (Eriksson, ActaMedScand, 1987; 221:461). The prognosis is generally grave, with a mean survival of 2 years after diagnosis. Cirrhosis in PI Z adults appears to represent the final stage of a constant, low-grade increase in hepatocyte turnover. The diagnosis of cirrhosis is therefore rarely made before the age of 50 years unless portal hypertension or hepatoma have become clinically manifest. These adults represent one end of a clinical spectrum. At the other are the children with neonatal cholestasis and abnormal results from liver function tests. It is probable that the predominantly male subgroup of clinically healthy children who have had elevated serum enzymes will continue to exhibit a low-grade necrosis of liver cells and increased fibrogenesis.

Risk for liver disease in PI*MZ and PI*SZ heterozygotes

The accumulation of PI Z α_1-antitrypsin in hepatocytes is seen as PAS-D inclusions in individuals with intermediate deficiency (PI MZ, SZ), although less abundantly than in homozygotes. The accumulation increases with age and in the presence of active disease. Inflammatory activity enhances the biosynthesis of both normal (PI M) and abnormal (PI Z) α_1-antitrypsin. A normal plasma concentration is therefore often found in the presence of active disease at any site (Carlson, ScaJGastr, 1985; 20:835).

In a northern Italian screening programme, 833 PI MZ newborns were identified by isoelectric focusing and randomly selected to either prospective treatment with vitamin E supplements to reduce a putative excess of free radicals and oxidants or to control observation (Pittschieler, ActaPaedScand, 1994; 393:21). At 2 months of age, subclinical liver involvement was present in 19 per cent of all 833 PI MZ infants, but in only 7.5 per cent of the 400 supplemented with vitamin E ($p<0.01$); these differences were not significant at 5 months of age. This study suggests that subclinical liver involvement is common in heterozygous infants, with spontaneous resolution by 5 to 6 months, and that oxidative stress may be a major mechanism of injury.

Screening of about 1000 liver biopsy specimens with PAS-D staining resulted in the detection of globules and the identification

Table 2 Laboratory findings at diagnosis in adult cirrhosis related to α_1-antitrypsin deficiency

	n	Range	Mean	SD
Aspartate aminotransferase (μkat/l)	25	<0.7	1.2	0.5
Alanine aminotransferase (μkat/l)	25	<0.7	0.8	0.3
γ-Glutamyl transpeptidase (μkat/l)	12	<1.0	1.2	1.0
Alkaline phosphatase (μkat/l)	22	<4.6	10.0	16.5
Bilirubin (mmol/l)	24	<22	43.3	43.6
Albumin (g/l)	21	40–50	28.3	6.4
Prothrombin (%)	21	80–120	49	13
IgA (g/l)	10	0.5–3.0	3.1	1.4

Reproduced with permission from Eriksson, ActaMedScand, 1987; 221: 461.

of PI MZ or PI SZ phenotypes in 21 per cent of biopsies with non-B chronic active hepatitis and cryptogenic cirrhosis (Hodges, NEJM, 1981; 304:557). In another retrospective screening of 857 consecutive adult Swedish patients evaluated for liver disease, the *PI Z* allele was identified by a PI Z-specific monoclonal antibody using an enzyme immunosorbent technique, and phenotypes were verified by isoelectric focusing. PI MZ and PI SZ phenotypes were significantly more frequent than in the general population (Carlson, ScaJGastr, 1985; 20:835). Two-thirds of the heterozygotes were males. Heterozygotes had significantly less alcohol-related disease, no increase in viral causes, and more 'cryptogenic' disease than controls with liver disease. The relative risk for cirrhosis in heterozygotes was 1.8 and for hepatoma 5.7, compared with other patients investigated for liver disease.

Several other investigators have found no increase in the number of heterozygotes among their patients with liver disease (Kueppers, MayoClinProc, 1976; 51:286; Vecchio, Digestion, 1983; 27:100). In two large series, the prevalence of heterozygotes among patients with alcoholic liver disease did not differ from that in control populations (Morin, Lancet, 1975; i:250; Roberts, AmJClinPath, 1984; 82:424).

In general, the Swedish studies cited above indicate a greater risk for adult liver disease and hepatoma, in both homo- and heterozygotes, than do studies from other centres. Perhaps a different epidemiological approach, a higher index of suspicion, routine α_1-antitrypsin determinations in the diagnostic evaluation of patients with liver disease, and a high frequency of biopsy/autopsy explain the discrepancy.

Diagnosis

α_1-Antitrypsin deficiency may be screened for by extremely inexpensive and readily accessible methods. The diagnosis of α_1-antitrypsin deficiency should therefore be considered early in the evaluation of neonatal or juvenile liver disease, and in Caucasian and particularly northern European adults with chronic liver disease (Table 1). It should also be considered in the initial evaluation of all patients with chronic obstructive lung disease, and in all family members of known patients with the deficiency. The probability of α_1-antitrypsin deficiency as a cause of liver disease increases in patients with a family history of liver or obstructive lung disease, and in patients in whom alcohol or viral hepatitis may be excluded.

Children with neonatal hepatitis, giant-cell hepatitis, juvenile cirrhosis, or chronically abnormal liver function tests should be further investigated for α_1- antitrypsin phenotype.

Biochemical studies

In most routine clinical laboratories the plasma α_1-antitrypsin may be determined by automated immunoturbidimetry or immunonephelometry.[27] Most commercial protein calibrators are now standardized against CRM 470, a protein standard approved by the International Federation of Clinical Chemists (Whicher, AnnBiolClin, 1993; 51:358). The normal plasma concentration of α_1-antitrypsin is 1.35 g/l (range 0.97–1.68) for PI M, with increases during inflammation, pregnancy, or with the use of oral contraceptives. Subnormal concentrations suggest a genetic α_1-antitrypsin variant and are only rarely secondary to a disease process. Low concentrations have, however, been described in the infant respiratory distress syndrome (Evans, AmRevRespDis, 1970; 101: 359), in protein-losing states, and in terminal liver failure (Talamo, Pediat, 1975; 56:91). Concentrations below 0.4 g/l suggest the homozygous deficiencies *PI*Z*, *PI*Mmalton*, *PI*Mduarte* or *PI-*Null*, or heterozygous combinations of these alleles. Concentrations in the range 0.4 to 1.2 g/l are compatible with heterozygous deficiency (*PI*MO*, **SZ*, **MZ*, etc.). As discussed above, heterozygotes with liver disease or active inflammation may well exhibit normal to elevated concentrations. The variable quantitative expression of the *PI* gene in response to different stimuli prohibits phenotype determination by plasma concentrations alone. For further characterization, isoelectric focusing of plasma or DNA analysis is mandatory.

Determination of phenotype

Isoelectric focusing is the method of choice for phenotyping.[24] Interpretation of the band pattern (Fig. 2) requires considerable experience and may be difficult on aged or lipaemic samples. The microheterogeneity reflects not only charge differences due to amino-acid substitutions, but also variable branching of the oligosaccharide side-chains and loss of an N-terminal pentapeptide. New variants discovered at the protein level are characterized by their electrophoretic mobilities in isoelectric focusing.

A monoclonal antibody specific for PI Z α_1-antitrypsin has been developed and is useful in detecting the presence of the *PI*Z* allele.

It has been used for mass population screening in an enzyme-linked immunosorbent assay (Wallmark, PNAS, 1984; 81:5690). Such antibodies may also be used for specific staining of histological material (Callea, JHepatol, 1991; 12:372).

Most phenotypes can also be specifically diagnosed at the DNA level. Some genetic mutations may be identified by Southern blotting due to their fortuitous localization at a restriction endonuclease site (restriction fragment length polymorphism). A single DNA haplotype defined by several endonucleases appears common for $PI*Z$ alleles (Cox, Nature, 1985; 316:79). When looking for a specific known mutation, the method may be simplified by using ^{32}P-labelled synthetic oligonucleotide probes on a DNA segment after amplification by the polymerase chain reaction (Landegren, Science, 1988; 241:1077; Newton, NucAcidRes, 1988; 16:352; Dahlén, ClinChem, 1993; 39:1626). These methods may be used on DNA purified from very few cells and are therefore ideally suited to prenatal diagnosis (see Section 26).

Morphology

Liver inclusions

α₁-Antitrypsin globular inclusions are localized predominantly in periportal hepatocytes, are weakly acidophilic, and may be easily overlooked on routine haematoxylin-and-eosin sections. After diastase treatment to remove glycogen, the remaining immature glycoprotein is strongly PAS-positive, reflecting a high mannose content (Fig. 4). In general, the number and size of globules increase with age and disease activity, with recruitment of hepatocytes across the lobule (Callea, Liver, 1984; 4:325). Thus, globules may be missed entirely in liver biopsies from heterozygotes due to sampling error.

Immunofluorescence and immunoperoxidase staining with monospecific antisera against α₁-antitrypsin are more sensitive than PAS-D staining for the detection of intrahepatocellular aggregates. These techniques, which can be applied to both frozen and formalin-fixed tissue, stain the rim of globules more intensely than the centre. Pretreatment of sections with trypsin or pepsin increases the intensity of staining. In addition, the selective accumulation of α₁-antitrypsin in PI Z hepatocytes may be demonstrated by immunohistochemical methods using primary antisera against other plasma proteins.

Retained α₁-antitrypsin is seen as an electron-dense amorphous material in dilated cisternae of the endoplasmic reticulum (Fig. 5), but the Golgi remains unaffected (Feldman, Gastro, 1974; 67:1214). Electron microscopy has demonstrated dilatation of the endoplasmic reticulum in periportal hepatocytes, where biosynthesis generally predominates, in both hetero- and homozygotes with minimal disease (Hultcrantz, Hepatol, 1984; 4:937).

The specificity of PAS-D-positive inclusions as markers of the $PI*Z$ allele was 0.94 when globules were 3 mm or more in diameter and 0.77 for globules more than 1 mm in diameter, although the large globules were found in less than half of the PI Z patients (Clausen, Liver, 1984; 4:353). Other inclusions such as Mallory bodies, Councilman bodies, and fibrinogen (Callea, Histopath, 1986; 10:65) are PAS-D negative. 'Congestive globules' are PAS-D positive, but are easily distinguished from true α₁-antitrypsin globules by their centrilobular localization (Qizilbash, AmJClinPath, 1983; 79:697) and non-selective accumulation of plasma proteins. Further,

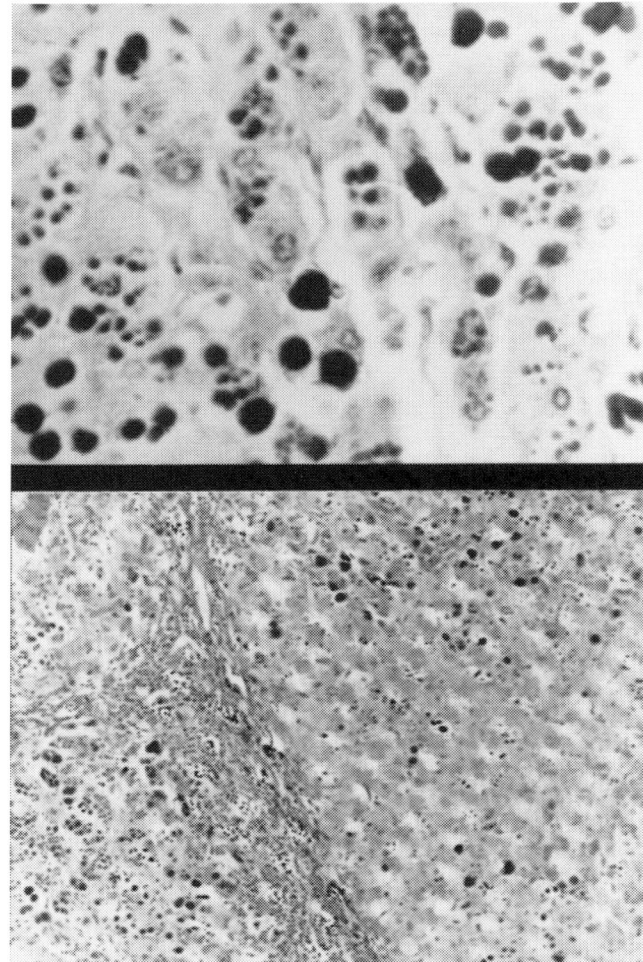

Fig. 4. (a) Periportal area from a PI ZZ liver stained by periodic acid–Schiff after diastase digestion (PAS-D) (× 416). (b) A cirrhotic PI ZZ liver with focal accumulation of large amounts of PAS-D material (× 96).

true α₁-antitrypsin globules may be seen in normal phenotypes during extreme acute-phase conditions (Carlson, JClinPath, 1981; 34:1020) or in homo- or heterozygotes for such rare phenotypes as Mduarte or Mmalton (Reid, Gastro, 1987; 93:181; 242). Therefore it must be emphasized that phenotype can never be determined on the basis of histology alone. Isoelectric focusing of serum samples or DNA studies are always required.

Histopathological changes

The pathology of neonatal and juvenile liver disease is described in Section 26. Adult liver disease in α₁-antitrypsin deficiency is usually characterized by relatively low-grade inflammation radiating from portal tracts. Inflammatory cells (primarily lymphocytes) are distributed in close proximity to areas of abundant PAS-D globules. As the disease slowly progresses, the liver becomes more fibrotic and occasionally displays piecemeal necrosis. Bile-duct proliferation is often seen in fibrotic portal tracts as in other forms of cirrhosis (Triger, QJMed, 1976; 45:351). Cirrhosis is generally of a macronodular type. Hepatoma is a frequent complication of this form of cirrhosis and is usually of hepatocellular, and occasionally cholangiocellular type (Eriksson, ActaMedScand, 1987; 221:461).

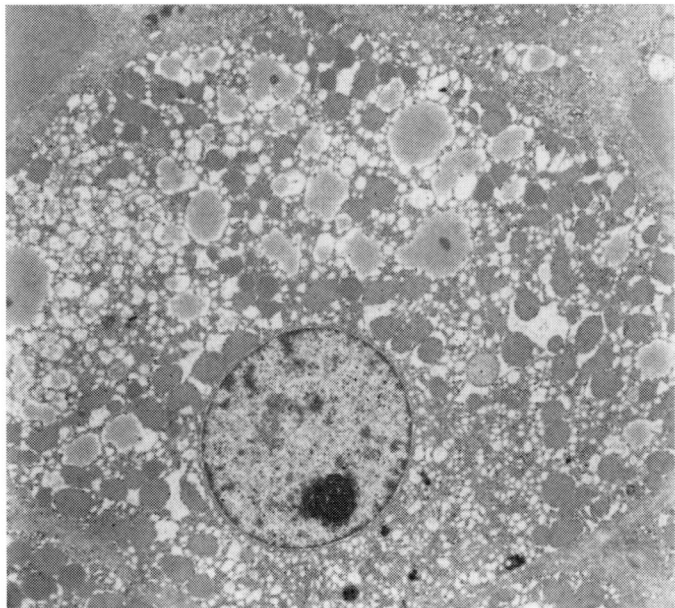

Fig. 5. Electron micrograph of a PI ZZ hepatocyte containing α_1-antitrypsin-immunoreactive material in dilated cisternae of the endoplasmic reticulum ($\times$ 4324). (By courtesy of Dr F. Callea.)

Malignant cells are usually devoid of PAS-D globules, but globules are frequently abundant in non-malignant tissue bordering the tumour.

Management and treatment
General considerations

As in other genetic diseases, the diagnosis of α_1-antitrypsin deficiency in a patient, irrespective of the mode of clinical presentation (lung, liver, or other symptoms), should lead to family investigations. It is desirable to identify homozygotes in an asymptomatic stage. Advice against smoking is at present the only preventive measure likely to prolong survival. Genetic counselling in families with one or more child affected by juvenile disease is discussed in Section 26.

Although emphysema is the basic defect in α_1-antitrypsin deficiency-related lung disease, a reversible bronchospastic component due to bronchial hyper-reactivity may be amenable to treatment. Asymptomatic individuals with severe α_1-antitrypsin deficiency should therefore undergo occasional lung function studies, even if they are non-smokers. In those with manifest liver disease, lung function abnormalities are often overlooked, and evaluation of lung function is also indicated. Physicians should also be alert to the possible presence of renal disease, particularly in children and adolescents with homozygous deficiency (Ibarguen, JPediat, 1990; 117:864) and vasculitic complications in both homo- and heterozygous deficiency (Segelmark, KidneyInt, 1995; 48:844).

A regular assessment of liver function is appropriate for patients with α_1-antitrypsin deficiency. The indolent nature of the process should be remembered. Tests reflecting a decline in total hepatocellular function are the most useful in monitoring. Aminotransferase and bilirubin may be normal at any given time. Therefore testing should be done regularly. The significant risk of malignant

transformation developing in a cirrhotic liver should also be considered. The value of α-fetoprotein analyses is uncertain. Ultrasonography is a preferable form of surveillance in high-risk patients.

Specific therapy

At present, three therapeutic approaches are available for α_1-antitrypsin deficiency. Several drugs increase the biosynthesis of α_1-antitrypsin, resulting in increased plasma concentrations. Intravenous augmentation therapy results in intermittent elevations of plasma concentrations and orthotopic liver transplantation provides a more definitive alternative. A potential distant therapeutic goal is somatic gene therapy.

The weak androgen danazol and the oestrogen antagonist tamoxifen have been used to stimulate synthesis of α_1-antitrypsin in homozygous patients with deteriorating lung function. Whereas such drugs cause increased plasma concentrations in *PI*SZ* heterozygous deficiency (Eriksson, AnnClinRes, 1983; 15:95), the response in homozygotes is too small and variable to be clinically significant. Increased biosynthesis of PI Z α_1-antitrypsin may increase intracellular accumulation and liver-cell injury (see above). In one study, danazol produced a mean increase in plasma α_1-antitrypsin of 28 per cent over baseline, and liver function abnormalities were noted in 19 per cent of PI Z patients so treated (Wewers, AmRevRespDis, 1986; 134:476). Similar results were obtained with tamoxifen (Wewers, AmRevRespDis, 1987; 135:401). Such treatment can therefore not be advised in PI Z patients with liver disease.

Human α_1-antitrypsin purified from plasma is available for weekly intravenous infusion in patients with deteriorating lung function (Wewers, NEJM, 1987; 316:1055; Hubbard, JAMA, 1988; 260:1259). Intravenous administration results in plasma concentrations that are 'protective' and hopefully will inhibit further alveolar destruction. No side-effects have been reported. At present there is no evidence that such augmentation therapy is beneficial in α_1-antitrypsin-related liver disease. For several reasons it should probably be avoided. Whereas the severity of emphysema is inversely related to the plasma concentration of α_1-antitrypsin, liver disease correlates primarily with its endoplasmic accumulation. Furthermore, as discussed above (acute-phase reactant), the carboxyterminal fragment of α_1-antitrypsin has biological effects that theoretically may provoke liver-cell injury: it acts as a neutrophilic attractant (Banda, JExpMed, 1988; 167:1608) and is a putative mediator of feedback induction of biosynthesis (Perlmutter, JCI, 1988; 81:1774). This effect may result in an increased accumulation of variant α_1-antitrypsin in the endoplasmic reticulum and potentiate liver-cell injury.

Orthotopic liver transplantation provides a new source of plasma α_1-antitrypsin, so that the recipient assumes the donor's phenotype and approximate concentration of plasma α_1-antitrypsin. Transplantation does not, however, completely reverse the metabolic defect. The α_1-antitrypsin gene is expressed in several extrahepatic tissues, in particular monocytes and macrophages. Whether continuous PI Z α_1-antitrypsin biosynthesis in these cells may contribute to immunological or other abnormalities remains unknown. At present, considerable experience of liver transplantation for juvenile cirrhosis in α_1-antitrypsin deficiency has shown a 5-year survival of 83 per cent, with about 17 per cent of chronic complications (Belle, ClinTranspl, 1992; 17:32).

Experience of liver transplantation for cirrhosis in PI Z adults is limited (Belle, ClinTranspl, 1992; 17:32). Rapidly progressive decompensation of liver disease is frequent. In the absence of serious pulmonary manifestations, indications for liver transplantation are essentially those for decompensation due to chronic liver disease of any type. Careful preoperative evaluation, of lung function and for the presence of hepatoma, is mandatory.

Gene replacement therapy

Somatic gene therapy has been attempted in cell culture and in animal models with liver resection, hepatocellular transformation *in vitro*, and reimplantation or hepatocellular transplantation (Kay, PNAS, 1992; 89:89). Retro- or adenoviral vector-mediated transformation of hepatocytes has been performed *in vivo* (Rettinger, PNAS, 1994; 91:1460). Various approaches have been summarized.[34] In short, single-stranded retroviral vectors have a high transfection efficiency, but require dividing cells for stable incorporation into the host genome, which involves the risk of damage or oncogenesis at the site of incorporation. In contrast, double-stranded DNA adenoviral vectors can infect non-dividing cells, may be expressed in an episomal fashion, decreasing the risk for host DNA damage, but are often extruded from the cell upon division, and often elicit an immune response. Further attempts using a polycationic delivery system avoid the problems of viral mediators, but lack the biological ability of selected targeting. Finally, the highly specific technique of homologous recombination (Savransky, LabInvest, 1994; 70:676) allows specific targeting with a low risk for oncogenic injury, and may be a promising solution. At present, gene therapy directed toward the lungs seems more plausible than to the liver, but all systems have considerable drawbacks. Pulmonary delivery systems are unstable; before becoming a realistic option, repeated gene administration must demonstrate competitive cost and safety compared with existing augmentation therapy. To have a significant effect, hepatic gene therapy must ideally result in correction of the genetic defect in a majority of cells. Increased synthesis of normal α₁-antitrypsin in the presence of residual *Pi*Z genes may possibly have a hepatotoxic effect via feedback induction of the aberrant PI Z protein.

Other endoplasmic-reticulum storage diseases

Hereditary fibrinogen deficiency

α₁-Antitrypsin deficiency, PI Z, is the prototype of an endoplasmic-reticulum storage diseases, with significant distension of the endoplasmic reticulum by abnormally glycosylated α₁-antitrypsin. Lysosomes and the Golgi remain unaffected. Familial fibrinogen storage associated with plasma deficiency and with autosomal-dominant inheritance was first described in 1981 (Pfeifer, Virch-ArchCP, 1981; 36:247). Since then, several families from Germany (Wehinger, EurJPed, 1983; 141:109), Italy (Callea. In Lowe, ed. *Fibrinogen 2. Biochemistry, physiology and clinical relevance.* Amsterdam: Elsevier, 1987; 75), and Japan (Callea, JHepatol, 1988; 7: 516) have been described. The condition is associated with chronic liver disease varying from modest biochemical abnormalities to established cirrhosis. Despite the low plasma fibrinogen (20–40 mg/ 100 ml), no marked bleeding tendency has been noted. In some affected individuals, immunoreactive fibrinogen has been two to three times higher than thrombin-clottable fibrinogen, suggesting a dysfunctional molecule.

Light microscopy reveals pale, faintly eosinophilic inclusions in the hepatocytes. The inclusions are weakly PAS-positive. Peroxidase staining has demonstrated a selective storage of fibrinogen, which on ultrastructural examination is confined to dilated cisternae of the rough endoplasmic reticulum. The molecular basis for the secretory defect(s) in the reported families has not yet been characterized.

α₁-Antichymotrypsin deficiency

α₁-Antichymotrypsin is a member of the serine protease inhibitor (serpin) family. It is strongly homologous with α₁-antitrypsin, and its major target enzyme is neutrophil cathepsin G. In liver disease, the plasma α₁-antichymotrypsin varies in parallel with α₁-antitrypsin. A familial heterozygous deficiency has been described (Lindmark, CCActa, 1985; 152:261; Eriksson, ActaMedScand, 1986; 220:447), and specific mutations associated with a decreased plasma α₁-antichymotrypsin have been identified (Faber, JHepatol, 1992; 18:313). Some of these patients have liver disease of variable clinical severity. Hepatocytes may exhibit immunoreactive α₁-antichymotrypsin inclusions (Lindmark, Histopath, 1990; 16:221). Their exact subcellular localization is at present unknown. The clinical significance of heterozygous as well as homozygous α₁-antichymotrypsin deficiency requires further investigation.

References

1. Laurell C-B and Eriksson S. The electrophoretic α₁-globulin pattern of serum in α₁-antitrypsin deficiency. *Scandinavian Journal of Clinical and Laboratory Investigation*, 1963; **15**: 132–40.
2. Eriksson S. Pulmonary emphysema and α₁-antitrypsin deficiency. *Acta Medica Scandinavica*, 1964; **175**: 197–205.
3. Eriksson S. Studies in α₁-antitrypsin deficiency. *Acta Medica Scandinavica*, 1965; **177** (Suppl. 432):1–85.
4. Larsson C. Natural history and life expectancy in severe α₁-antitrypsin deficiency, PI Z. *Acta Medica Scandinavica*, 1978; **204**: 345–51.
5. Sharp HL, Bridges RA, and Krivit W. Cirrhosis associated with alpha-1-antitrypsin deficiency: a previously unrecognized inherited disorder. *Journal of Laboratory and Clinical Medicine*, 1969; **73**: 934–9.
6. Sharp HL. Alpha-1-antitrypsin deficiency. *Hospital Practice*, 1971; **5**: 83–96.
7. Eriksson S and Larsson C. Purification and partial characterization of PAS-positive inclusion bodies from the liver in α₁-antitrypsin deficiency. *New England Journal of Medicine*, 1975; **292**: 176–80.
8. Hercz A, Katona E, Cutz E, Wilson JR, and Barton M. α₁-Antitrypsin: the presence of excess mannose in the Z variant isolated from liver. *Science*, 1978; **201**: 1229–32.
9. Feldmann G, *et al.* Hepatocyte ultrastructure changes in α₁-antitrypsin deficiency. *Gastroenterology*, 1974; **67**: 1214–24.
10. Berg NO and Eriksson S. Liver disease in adults with α₁-antitrypsin deficiency. *New England Journal of Medicine*, 1972; **287**: 1264–7.
11. Gherardi GJ. α₁-Antitrypsin deficiency and its effect on the liver. *Human Pathology*, 1971; **2**: 173–5.
12. Eriksson S, Carlsson J, and Velez R. Risk of cirrhosis and primary liver cancer in α₁-antitrypsin deficiency. *New England Journal of Medicine*, 1986; **314**: 736–9.
13. Laurell C-B and Sveger T. Mass screening of newborn Swedish infants for α₁-antitrypsin deficiency. *American Journal of Human Genetics*, 1975; **27**: 213–17.
14. Sveger T and Eriksson S. The liver in adolescents with α₁-antitrypsin deficiency. *Hepatology*, 1995; **22**: 514–17.

15. Jeppsson J-O. Amino acid substitution Glu–Lys in α_1-antitrypsin PiZ. *FEBS Letters*, 1976; **65**: 195–7.

16. Jeppsson J-O, Laurell C-B, and Fagerhol MK. Properties of isolated α_1-antitrypsin of Pi types M, S and Z. *European Journal of Biochemistry*, 1978; **83**: 143–53.

17. Carrell RW, *et al*. Structure and variation of human α_1-antitrypsin. *Nature*, 1982; **298**: 329–34.

18. Long GL, Chandra T, Woo SLC, Davie E, and Kurachi K. Complete sequence of the cDNA for human α_1-antitrypsin and the gene for the S variant. *Biochemistry*, 1984; **23**: 4828–37.

19. Jacobsson K. Studies on trypsin and plasma inhibitors in human blood serum. *Scandinavian Journal of Clinical and Laboratory Investigation*, 1955; **14** (Suppl.): 57–63.

20. Johnson D and Travis J. Structural evidence for methionine at the reactive site of human α_1-proteinase inhibitor. *Journal of Biological Chemistry*, 1978; **253**: 7142–7.

21. Janoff A. Elastases and emphysema. Current assessment of the protease-antiprotease hypothesis. *American Review of Respiratory Disease*, 1985; **132**: 417–33.

22. Fagerhol MK and Laurell C-B. The polymorphism of 'pre-albumins' α_1-antitrypsin in human sera. *Clinica Chimica Acta*, 1967; **16**: 199–203.

23. Fagerhol MK and Cox DW. The Pi polymorphism: genetic, biochemical and clinical aspects of human α_1-antitrypsin. *Advances in Human Genetics*, 1981; **11**: 1–62, 371–2.

24. Cox DW. α_1-Antitrypsin deficiency. In Scriver CR. Beaudet AL, Sly WS, and Valle D, eds. *The metabolic basis of inherited disease*. 6th edn. New York: McGraw-Hill, 1989: 2409–37.

25. Eriksson S. α_1-Antitrypsin deficiency: lessons learned from the bedside to the gene and back again. Historic perspectives. *Chest*, 1989; **95**: 181–9.

26. Stein PE and Carrell RW. What do dysfunctional serpins tell us about molecular mobility and disease? *Structural Biology*, 1995; **2**: 96–101.

27. Arnaud P and Chapius-Cellier C. α_1-Antitrypsin. In Colowick SP and Kaplan NO, eds. *Methods in enzymology 163*. New York: Academic Press, 1988: 400–18.

28. Crystal RG, Brantley ML, Hubbard RC, Curiel DT, States DJ, and Holmes MD. The α_1-antitrypsin gene and its mutations. *Chest*, 1989; **95**: 196–208.

29. Carrell RW, Pemberton PA, and Boswell DR. The serpins: evolution and adaptation in a family of protease inhibitors. In *Cold Spring Harbor symposia on quantitative biology*, LII. Cold Spring Harbor Laboratory, 1987: 527–35.

30. Heidtmann H and Travis J. Human α_1-proteinase inhibitor. In Barrett AJ and Salvesen G, eds. *Proteinase inhibitors*. Amsterdam: Elsevier, 1986: 441–56.

31. Mowat AP. α_1-Antitrypsin deficiency (PiZZ): features of liver involvement in childhood. *Acta Paediatrica Scandinavica*, 1994; **393** (Suppl.): 13–17.

32. Sharp HL. Alpha-1-antitrypsin: an ignored protein in understanding liver disease. *Seminars in Liver Disease*, 1982; **2**: 314–28.

33. Carlson J. Diagnosis, clinical course and therapy of α_1-antitrypsin deficiency. In Schmid R, Bianchi L, Blum HE, Gerok W, Maier KP, and Stalder GA, eds. *Acute and chronic liver diseases: molecular biology and clinics*. Dordrecht: Kluwer, 1996: 231–48.

34. Knoell DL and Wewers, MD. Clinical implications of gene therapy for α_1-antitrypsin deficiency. *Chest*, 1995; 107: 535–45.

20.4 The liver in cystic fibrosis

Gianni Mastella and Marco Cipolli

Cystic fibrosis: an introduction

Definition

Cystic fibrosis is the most common autosomal-recessive genetic disorder with a severe prognosis in the population of Caucasian origin. It is a complex disease that involves many organ systems, which are essentially affected by an alteration of their exocrine secretions chronically and progressively compromising their function and structure. Involvement of the respiratory system is life-threatening for most affected individuals.

Genetics and epidemiology

The gene involved is located on the long arm of the chromosome 7 and encoded for a protein named cystic fibrosis transmembrane conductance regulator (**CFTR**) and composed of 1480 amino acids. It is a large gene, spanning more than 250 000 bp.[1] More than 700 mutations of this gene are known to date, some very common but most very rare. They are scattered along the codifying portion of its 27 exons, and also along the large intron segments.

The frequency of the disease is estimated to be, on average, 1 in 2500 live births in the Caucasian population: it is lower in the African and even lower in the Asiatic populations.[2] Therefore, it calculates to a carrier frequency of approximately 1 in 25 and a coupling probability for two carriers of 1 in 600: a couple of carrier parents has a 25 per cent risk of an affected child at any pregnancy.

Although the most affected individuals present the classic manifestations of the disease (exocrine pancreatic insufficiency, chronic lung disease, high concentration of electrolytes in sweat), a growing number with atypical or monosymptomatic manifestations is now being detected: a typical example is the not uncommon congenital absence of the vas deferens, which is now regarded as a monosymptomatic form of cystic fibrosis disease carrying some CFTR mutations (Chillon, NEJM, 1995; 332:1475). This fact is widening the clinical spectrum of the disease, which includes, at one extreme, severe and precociously lethal forms, and at the other, mild forms that can allow a long survival.[3] The spreading of the diagnosis to mild and monosymptomatic expressions of disease, often associated with particular CFTR genotypes, suggests that the gene frequency is rather higher than usually estimated.

Physiological defects

Cystic fibrosis is characterized by two fundamental peculiarities: on the one hand, serous secretions (typically the sweat) have a very high concentration of sodium chloride, on the other, the mucous secretions (typically the intestinal and bronchial mucus) are thick, hyperviscous, and poorly flowing, and tend to obstruct ducts and cavities.

Electrophysiological studies conducted in the 1980s (Knowles, Science, 1983; 221:1067; Quinton, Nature, 1983; 301:421; Frizzel, Science, 1986; 233:558) led to the notion of cystic fibrosis as a disease that primarily affects epithelia: in each of the organs affected the chief site of involvement is epithelium. Currently, there is a unifying hypothesis about the basic defect: it has been identified in a relative impermeability to chloride of the apical membrane of the epithelial cells. In fact, we know that the CFTR is a Cl^- channel, which is a complex molecule in the cell membrane that acts as a gate for anions.[4] Cl^- ions can move easily through it only when it is open and functioning normally, but not when it is closed, altered, or absent. This channel is regulated through a phosphorylation process in response to an increase in cellular levels of cAMP. The direction of ion movements depends on the function of the particular epithelium: in the excretory duct of sweat glands the direction is from the lumen to the inside of cells; in the respiratory and intestinal epithelia it is from inside the cell to the mucosa surface.

Parallel to the movements of Cl^- ions there is absorption or secretion of Na^+ ions, promoted by a favourable electrochemical gradient, and of water, resulting in dehydration of secretions at the surface of the airways or other secretory organs, with adverse effects on their rheological properties (defective clearance) and defence against micro-organisms (colonization and infection).

More complex aspects of the function and involvement of CFTR in cystic fibrosis are known.[5] Alternative chloride channels are present in the epithelial cells. There is defective activation of outwardly rectifying chloride channels (**ORCCs**) by cAMP-dependent protein kinase A, while Ca^{2+}-dependent Cl^- secretion is enhanced (Schwiebert, Cell, 1995; 81:1063). Remarkably, CFTR, when activated by cAMP, moves ATP in addition to Cl^- to the mucosal surface. ATP would seem to activate, by an autocrine mechanism, a series of Cl^- secretory pathways, including ORCCs and Ca^{2+}-dependent chloride channels. The airway epithelia of patients with cystic fibrosis also show a great increase of sodium and fluid absorption, suggesting that CFTR can interact with Na^+-reabsorptive pathways. There is now evidence that a salt-sensitive natural antibiotic (β-defensin 1) in lung mucosa is compromised because of a defective chloride channel, thus leading to lung infection (Wine, NatureMed, 1997; 3:494). However, despite some

Table 1 The most common clinical features of cystic fibrosis

CFTR gene mutation

↓

Abnormal CFTR protein

↓

Organs	Abnormal function/structure	Clinical implications
Serous secreting:		
Lacrimal glands	Salt hyperconcentration	
Parotid glands	Salt hyperconcentration	
Sweat glands	Salt hyperconcentration	Salt loss syndrome
Mucous secreting:		
Mouth	Cystic and fibrotic alterations in mucous salivary glands	Defective salivation (80%)
Intestine	Mucus inspissation/obstruction	Meconium ileus (10–12%)
		Meconium ileus equivalents (10%)
Pancreas	Ductular obstruction with fibrocystic transformation	Maldigestion–malnutrition (85–87%)
Hepatobiliary system	Bile inspissation	Microgallbladder (15–30%)
		Gallstones (10–15%)
		Biliary cirrhosis (10–20%)
Nose and paranasal sinuses	Mucus stagnation/infection	Pansinusitis (95%)
		Nasal polyposis
Lower airways	Defective mucus clearance–obstruction–infection–inflammation	Chronic progressive lung disease (97%)
Vas deferens	Aplasia/azoospermia	Male infertility (97%)
Uterine cervix	Mucus abnormalities	Reduced female fertility

attractive suggestions and hypotheses about how cystic fibrosis-associated mutations cause CFTR dysfunction (Welsh, *Molecular biological membrane transplantation disorders*. New York: Plenum Press, 1996:605),[5] our understanding remains superficial.

Clinical manifestations

An outline of the clinical manifestations of cystic fibrosis is given in Table 1. The salty sweat can lead to severe salt loss, with metabolic alkalosis during hot seasons or fevers.

In the pancreas, the ductular obstruction and precocious activation of enzymes, due to defective HCO_3^- secretion (defective Cl^- exchange with HCO_3^-), lead to destruction and atrophy of the organ, and hence exocrine insufficiency and maldigestion, in approximately 85 per cent of patients. In the long run, progressive fibrosis involves also the islets of Langerhans, with consequent glucose intolerance and in some cases, during adolescent or adulthood, diabetes mellitus.

Ten to 15 per cent of patients are born with meconium ileus, a complication that usually requires surgical intervention by ileal resection. Intestinal obstructions, mainly at the level of ileum and caecum, are frequent also in the postneonatal period and particularly in adolescence (distal intestine obstruction syndrome).

In all patients affected by the classic form of the disease, alterations of both the upper and lower airways sooner or later become apparent. Chronic sinusitis, radiologically demonstrable, is the rule; nasal polyposis is frequent, relapsing despite surgical treatment. Lung disease begins in the small airways, which are obstructed by thick and stagnant secretions, with progressive colonization by pathogenic organisms, mainly *Haemophilus influenzae*, *Staphylococcus aureus*, *Pseudomonas aeruginosa*, and *Burkholderia cepacia*.

Lung disease develops with episodes of acute infection at the beginning but persistent infection later on. A chronic inflammatory response usually follows the chronic infection and eventually this becomes almost invariably the predominant and poorly controllable feature of the progressive lung devastation.

Several pathological alterations follow one another, such as atelectasis, obstructive emphysema, bronchiectasis, and fibrosis. The profile of lung function is that of a progressive obstruction, ultimately combined with restriction. Pneumothorax and haemoptysis are common complications of advanced disease. Hypoxaemia, pulmonary hypertension with cor pulmonale, and finally hypercapnic respiratory failure represent the typical sequence of events that leads to death.

Some 95 to 97 per cent of male patients show infertility due to azoospermia from bilateral absence of the vas deferens. This condition, as mentioned above, can also occur as an isolated manifestation of the disease. Reduced fertility may also occur in female patients, due to abnormalities of the cervical mucus.

Complications involving the liver and biliary tree are common.

Diagnosis

In the person presenting symptoms consistent with cystic fibrosis, the diagnosis is usually confirmed when chloride and sodium concentrations in sweat, collected twice from the skin surface of a forearm after pilocarpine iontophoresis, exceed 60 mEq/l. In a few cases the sweat test may result in normal or borderline values, due to some mild CFTR mutations (Stewart, AmJRespCritCareMed, 1995; 151:899). Mutation analysis and measurement of the potential difference in nasal secretions can then often, but not always, resolve a doubtful diagnosis.

In the neonate, cystic fibrosis may be suspected after a screening test for elevated blood immunoreactive trypsin, but only a positive sweat test or mutation analysis can provide confirmation of the diagnosis (Pederzini, Screening, 1995; 3:172).

Treatment and prognosis

With early treatment and continuous follow-up with timely management of any complications, the mean life expectancy for patients with cystic fibrosis currently tends to exceed 30 years. The two main points of treatment for the classic forms of disease involve, on the one hand, the pancreatic maldigestion and malnutrition, and on the other, the respiratory disease.[6] Exocrine pancreatic insufficiency is compensated by a large supplementation of pancreatic enzymes, while special attention is given to high-energy intake, which is required because of an energy expenditure that is, on average, higher than normal. Nutritional strategy also includes supplementation with fat-soluble vitamins, particularly A and E.

The treatment of respiratory disease includes daily respiratory physiotherapy, mainly aimed at removing bronchial secretions. This is aided by mucolytic drugs; currently the use of recombinant dornase-α is widespread. Respiratory infections are treated with antibiotics, which are chosen on the basis of deep sputum cultures: strategies range from the treatment of exacerbations to chronic treatment by daily antibiotic aerosol and periodic cycles of antibiotics in chronic infection by *Pseudomonas aeruginosa*.

Specific treatments are considered for problems such as diabetes (usually insulin), nasal polyposis (often repeated surgical interventions), pulmonary complications (pneumothorax, haemoptysis, irreversible atelectasis) that can require surgical procedures, respiratory failure, and intestinal obstructions.

For the endstage lung disease a double lung transplantation can be considered, with an expected survival rate at 4 to 5 years of approximately 60 per cent (Hosenpud, JHeartLungTranspl, 1994; 13:361).

Epidemiology of liver and biliary-tract disorders in cystic fibrosis

Even the earliest reports of the disease indicate that liver and biliary-tract complications were well-recognized features of cystic fibrosis (Farber, ArchPathol, 1944; 37:238; di Sant'Agnese, Pediat, 1956; 18:387).[7] The range of hepatobiliary disorders is wide, as summarized in Table 2.

Prolonged neonatal jaundice

Some infants with prolonged neonatal jaundice, probably due to a temporary plugging of intrahepatic bile ducts, may have cystic fibrosis; this is recognized as a rare complication of the disease (Psacharopoulos, Lancet, 1981; ii:78; Perkins, ClinPediat, 1985; 24:107).[8] Cholestasis with or without jaundice can be associated with meconium ileus (Fig. 1), whose incidence in infants with cystic fibrosis with neonatal cholestasis is estimated to be more frequent than expected (Valman, ArchDisChild, 1971; 4:805).

Table 2 Liver and biliary-tract disorders in cystic fibrosis
Liver
Prolonged neonatal jaundice
Liver steatosis
Chronic liver disease:
Focal biliary cirrhosis
Multilobular cirrhosis
Portal hypertension
Oesophageal and gastric varices
Hypersplenism
Ascites
Hepatocellular failure
Cardiac liver
Hepatitis
Gallbladder and biliary tree
Microgallbladder
Cholelithiasis
Cholangitis/cholecystitis
Biliary-duct anomalies

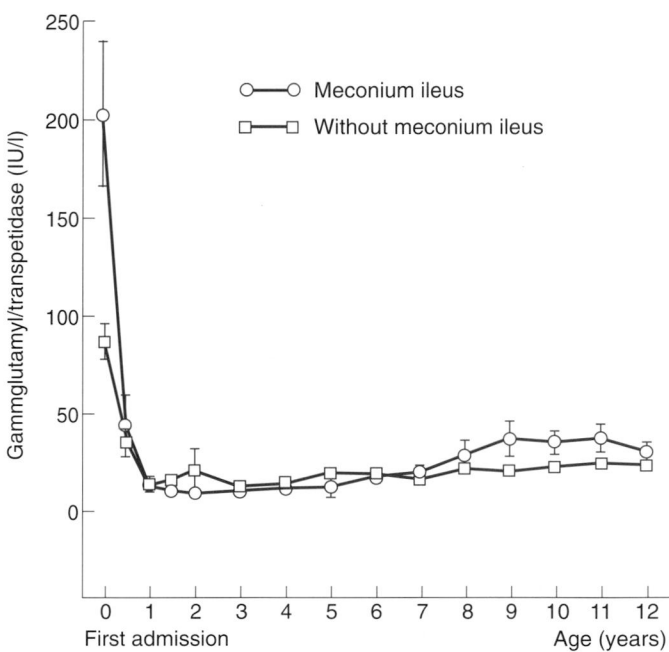

Fig. 1. γ-Glutamyl-transpeptidase in cystic fibrosis patients with (40) and without (138) meconium ileus (diagnosed within 6 months of birth).

There is no evidence of a correlation between neonatal jaundice and subsequent development of biliary cirrhosis (Valman, ArchDisChild, 1971; 4:805), even though there is a case reported of neonatal cirrhosis presenting prolonged neonatal jaundice (Feigelson, ArchDisChild, 1993; 68:653).

Liver steatosis

Liver steatosis is a very common disorder in cystic fibrosis: 65 per cent of cases in an old autopsy study (Craig, AmJDisChild, 1957; 93:357) and 30 per cent in a study on liver biopsies (Dietzch, Proc. 8th Int Congr CF, Toronto: Canadian CF Foundation, 1980: 220). It is mainly due to fat malabsorption and particularly to essential fatty-acid deficiency (Strandvik, ScaJGastr, 1988; 23 (Suppl. 143):

1). The disorder is suspected when, on palpation, the liver appears enlarged and soft. It is usually reversible after adequate pancreatic enzyme supplementation. There is no evidence that steatosis adversely influences the development of liver disease in cystic fibrosis.[9]

Chronic liver disease (biliary cirrhosis)

Focal biliary cirrhosis[7] is considered pathognomonic of the disease: it can remain completely asymptomatic or progress to the more severe, multilobular biliary cirrhosis with portal hypertension (di Sant'Agnese, Pediat, 1956; 18:387).[7]

Estimates of the prevalence of chronic liver disease in cystic fibrosis vary according to the diagnostic criteria used. In autopsy studies, histological features of liver cirrhosis were observed in 20 to 40 per cent of patients (di Sant'Agnese, Pediat, 1956; 18:387; Oppenheimer, JPediat, 1975; 86:683),[10,11] and if cross-sectional data from autopsy studies are combined it appears that its prevalence rises steadily with age. Actually, the improved survival of patients with cystic fibrosis has led to an increased recognition of the impact of associated liver disease on morbidity and mortality: liver disease is now considered the second most common cause of death in cystic fibrosis, with an estimated rate of 3.4 per cent.[12] However, the natural history of the liver disease is not well elucidated and the prevalence of symptomatic disease is, on average, much lower than that of liver involvement observed at autopsy (Stern, Gastro, 1976; 70:645), being considered to be around 4 to 5 per cent. Homogeneous criteria for assessing the clinical status of the liver in cystic fibrosis are still lacking, and the published autopsy studies do not relate histopathological findings to the clinical conditions or biochemical abnormalities.

The most recent clinical studies give an idea of the differences in evaluation:

- 15 patients with symptomatic liver disease in a population of 693 (2.2 per cent) (Stern, Gastro, 1976; 70:645)
- nine cases of 'overt liver disease' among 204 patients with cystic fibrosis less than 13 years old (4.4 per cent)[8]
- biochemical alterations or 'overt liver disease' in 57 of 233 patients over 15 years old (24.5 per cent) (Nagel, Lancet, 1989; ii:1422)
- an overall prevalence of 'overt liver disease', as indicated by the presence of an enlarged liver and/or spleen, of 4.2 per cent in a cystic fibrosis population of 1100 (Scott-Jupp, ArchDisChild, 1991; 66:698)
- multilobular cirrhosis reported in 31 of 450 patients with cystic fibrosis (6.9 per cent), almost all diagnosed before 14 years of age in a French study (Feigelson, ArchDisChild, 1993; 68:653).

Those studies were mainly retrospective. Two prospective clinical studies of liver disease in cystic fibrosis have been published (Colombo, JPediat, 1994; 124:393; Cipolli, ItalJPediat, 1995; 21:58). In both, screening for liver disease was by clinical (liver and/or spleen enlargement), biochemical (classic markers of liver function), and echographic assessments. In the first study, 189 patients over 3 years old, and in the second, 231 consecutive patients over the age of 1 year, were screened: 18 per cent in the former and 20.8 per cent in the latter were classified as having liver disease (Table 3).

These figures are consistent with those from autopsy studies (di Sant'Agnese, Pediat, 1956; 18:387; Oppenheimer, JPediat, 1975; 86: 683).[13] The latest prospective study (Cipolli, ItalJPediat, 1995; 21: 58–62) was performed in accordance with the definition of chronic liver disease by Gaskin (NEJM, 1988; 318:340) and Nagel (Lancet, 1989; ii:1422), i.e. that clinical hepatomegaly is present for more than 6 months (liver edge more than 2 cm below the right costal margin and increased liver span), and/or splenomegaly (palpation of an enlarged spleen), and/or a significant increase of a least one of the following biochemical markers: aspartate aminotransferase, alanine aminotransferase, γ-glutamyl transferase. Rather similar criteria were adopted in the earlier prospective study (Colombo, JPediat, 1994; 124:393). A prevalence of overt liver disease of 16 per cent and 12 per cent was reported in two series of Swedish patients with cystic fibrosis observed longitudinally (Lindblad, JPediat, 1995; 126). In another prospective study (O'Brien, Gut, 1992; 33:387), in 104 adult patients, 19 per cent presented chronic liver disease.

Chronic liver disease was once considered to occur exclusively in patients with pancreatic insufficiency (Scott-Jupp, ArchDisChild, 1991; 66:698; Colombo, JPediat, 1994; 124:393).[14] However, in the recent Cipolli series (ItalJPediat, 1995; 21:58–62), 4 out of 48 patients with chronic liver disease were pancreatic-sufficient, and three patients with biliary-tract anomalies and liver disease have recently been described as pancreatic-sufficient (Waters, Hepatol, 1995; 21:963). Some cases of liver cirrhosis without pancreatic insufficiency were occasionally reported also in the older literature (di Sant'Agnese, Pediat, 1956; 18:387; Stern, AnnIntMed, 1977; 87:188).

To establish the prevalence of portal hypertension in cystic fibrosis is even more difficult, and again depends on the diagnostic criteria used. There are very few published data. If we consider palpable enlargement of the spleen associated with hepatomegaly as a diagnostic criterion, then in our experience 60 per cent of patients with cystic fibrosis and chronic liver disease had portal hypertension. If we combine splenomegaly with ultrasonographic features of portal hypertension, such as increased portal diameter and portosystemic venous collaterals, some 75 per cent of those with chronic liver disease had to be considered as having portal hypertension. Thirty-two per cent of those with suspected portal hypertension had oesophageal varices and some of them also gastric varices (Cipolli, ItalJPediat, 1995; 21:58–62). Oesophageal varices were detected in 11 out of 23 (Scott-Jupp, ArchDisChild, 1991; 66:698) and in 20 out of 31 (Feigelson, ArchDisChild, 1993; 68:653) patients with liver disease. The general estimate of oesophageal varices in adolescents and adults with cystic fibrosis is about 1 per cent (Oppenheimer, JPediat, 1975; 86:683; Stern, Gastro, 1976; 70:64; Penketh, Thorax, 1987; 42:526). Ascites is a late complication of portal hypertension. Hypersplenism, mainly characterized by thrombocytopenia and neutropenia, is frequently associated with portal hypertension: 25 per cent of those with portal hypertension in our series (Cipolli, ItalJPediat, 1995; 21:58–62). Hepatocellular failure is usually a very late complication of cystic fibrosis-associated liver disease, but a fatal liver insufficiency is still a very rare condition.

The age of onset of the liver complications is difficult to estimate, but it seems that the prevalence of clinically overt liver disease does not rise progressively but peaks in adolescence (Scott-Jupp,

Table 3 Data from two prospective studies on cystic fibrosis liver disease

	Colombo *et al.* (1994)	Cipolli *et al.* (1995)
Patients screened (*n*)	189	231
Age considered (year)	>3	>1
Age observed (mean ± SD) (year)	15.1 ± 7.4	15.2 ± 7.1
Gender (M/F)	90/99	113/118
Pancreatic insufficiency (*n*)	165 (87.3%)	188 (81.4%)
Meconium ileus (*n*)	17 (9%)	23 (10%)
Hepatomegaly (*n*)	57 (30.2%)	45 (19.5%)
Splenomegaly (*n*)	11 (5.8%)	27 (11.2%)
Biochemical abnormalities (*n*)	32 (16.9%)	22 (9.6%)
Ultrasonography suggesting cirrhosis (*n*)	20 (10.6%)	29 (12.5%)
Chronic liver disease	34 (18%)	48 (20.8%)

ArchDisChild, 1991; 66:698; Feigelson, ArchDisChild, 1993; 68: 653; Tanner, ArchDisChild, 1995; 72:281), even if some cross-sectional studies detect that the disease is apparently more prevalent in adults (Cipolli, ItalJPediat, 1995; 21:58–62). Data from follow-up studies show that almost all those with cirrhosis were diagnosed before 14 years of age, including one case of neonatal cirrhosis (Psacharopoulos, Lancet, 1981; ii:78; Feigelson, ArchDisChild, 1993; 68:653). The incidence of focal biliary cirrhosis in an autopsy study (Maurage, JPediatGastrNutr, 1989; 9:17) was 30 per cent in those who died in the first year of life.

Risk factors for the development of liver disease have been considered. There are several reports of familial concordance for clinical liver disease (Shuster, JPediatSurg, 1977; 12:201; Duthie, Hepatol, 1992; 15:660), but this is not the rule. No genotypic difference between patients with and without liver disease with respect to ΔF508 or other cystic fibrosis mutations has thus far emerged in published data (Ferrari, AmJHumGen, 1991; 48:815; Johansen, Lancet, 1991; 337:631; De Arce, ClinGenet, 1992; 42: 271; Duthie, Hepatol, 1992; 15:660; Colombo, JPediat, 1994; 124: 393; 48). Information from an unpublished study of histo-compatibility antigens by Duthie *et al.* suggests that a genetic predisposition for liver disease in cystic fibrosis is linked with the *A2-B7-DR2-DQW6* haplotype. Pancreatic insufficiency cannot be considered a predisposing factor (Cipolli, ItalJPediat, 1995; 21:58; Tanner, ArchDisChild, 1995; 72:281; Waters, Hepatol, 1995; 21: 963). The male gender seems more predisposed to liver disease (Craig, AmJDisChild, 1957; 93:357; Feigelson, ArchDisChild, 1993; 68:653; Colombo, JPediat, 1994; 124:393; Cipolli, ItalJPediat, 1995; 21:58; Tanner, ArchDisChild, 1995; 72:281). Autopsy findings suggest that meconium ileus or its equivalents may predispose to liver disease (Maurage, JPediatGastrNutr, 1989; 9:17). In a recent study (Colombo, JPediat, 1994; 124:393; 48) the frequency of meconium ileus or its equivalents was significantly higher in patients with cystic fibrosis and liver disease (35.3 per cent) than in those without liver disease (12.3 per cent); this might be due to a combination of inspissated gut contents with inspissated bile-duct contents. However, that association was not confirmed by other studies if meconium ileus is considered separately (Scott-Jupp, ArchDisChild, 1991; Feigelson, ArchDisChild, 1993; 68:653; Lindblad, JPediat, 1995; 126). The prevalence of meconium ileus was similar in the two groups of our series, with and without liver

disease: 10.4 and 9.9 per cent, respectively (Cipolli, ItalJPediat, 1995; 21: 58–62).

Gallbladder disease

Anatomical abnormalities of the gallbladder are very common in cystic fibrosis, even though symptomatic gallbladder disease is relatively uncommon.

Microgallbladder is the most common abnormality: about 30 per cent seen at autopsy (Stern, JPediatGastrNutr, 1986; 5:35; Maurage, JPediatGastrNutr, 1989; 9:17) and about 15 per cent suspected by radiological or ultrasonographic studies (Rovsing, ActaRadiol, 1973; 14:588; Willi, AmJRoent, 1980; 134:1005).[10] Microgallbladder can also be detected by ultrasound investigation in the fetus: no sonographic evidence of a gallbladder was found in 9 of 12 fetuses affected by cystic fibrosis (Duchatel, FetDiagTher, 1993; 8:28). Microgallbladder may contain thick material and the cystic duct can often be occluded and sometimes atretic (Stern, JPediatGastrNutr, 1986).

Macrogallbladder also occurs: an enlarged gallbladder with a delay in emptying was found through hepatobiliary scintigraphy in 31 of 45 patients with clinical liver disease (Gaskin, NEJM, 1988; 318:340).

Cholelithiasis is detectable in at least 10 per cent of patients with cystic fibrosis (L'Hereux, AmJRoent, 1977; 128:953). Routine echographic screening shows that the incidence of gallstones is much higher than expected because most patients remain asymptomatic. The risk of developing gallstones probably increases with age. At autopsy, 24 per cent of adults with cystic fibrosis were found to have gallstones.[11] From a clinical survey of 815 patients with cystic fibrosis currently being followed at our centre, gallstones have been recorded in 1.8 per cent of those under 12 years of age, in 6.4 per cent between 12 and 18 years, and in 15.4 per cent over 18 years. Chronic cholecystitis is commonly seen when the gallbladder is removed at surgery.[15]

Biliary duct anomalies

An important observation, made by hepatobiliary scintigraphy in 48 of 50 patients with clinical liver disease, is that distal obstruction of the common bile duct is commonly associated with liver disease in cystic fibrosis (Gaskin, NEJM, 1988; 318:340). The findings were confirmed in 27 out of 28 of those patients who underwent percutaneous cholangiography and were interpreted as a consequence of pancreatic fibrosis. It was suggested that multilobular cirrhosis in cystic fibrosis might be the consequence of an extrahepatic obstruction.

Different results were obtained in another study (Nagel, Lancet, 1989; ii:1422). Hepatobiliary scintigraphy showed delayed excretion of radionuclide in 13 out of 20 patients with liver disease but the site of the delay was scattered along the biliary tree, both extra- and intrahepatic. Fifteen out of 17 of those patients showed intrahepatic biliary abnormalities, but only two had a lower obstruction of the common bile duct. In a series of 14 patients with liver disease (O'Brien, Gut, 1992; 33:387), endoscopic retrograde cholangiopancreatography failed to show abnormality of the common bile duct, while intrahepatic changes consistent with sclerosing cholangitis were seen. The controversy has not yet been resolved, but the typical extrahepatic biliary lesion is probably multiple constrictions/dilatations more or less combined with beading and strictures involving the intrahepatic ducts (Nagel, Lancet, 1989; ii:1422; Bilton, Gut, 1990; 31:236; Bilton, Lancet, 1990; 335:357; O'Brien, Gut, 1992; 33:387), resembling the picture of sclerosing cholangitis described in four patients with cystic fibrosis (Strandvik, Sca JGastr, 1988; 23(Suppl. 143):121).

In Gaskin's experience (Gaskin, NEJM, 1988; 318:340; Gaskin, PediatrPulmonol, 1992; (Suppl. 8):128), a large proportion of patients with liver disease had abdominal pain, which almost invariably was relieved by surgical intervention after cholangiographic demonstration of common bile-duct strictures.

Adenocarcinoma of the extrahepatic biliary tree was reported in two adult patients with cystic fibrosis (Abdul-Karim, Gastro, 1982; 82:758),[16] with involvement of the neck of the gallbladder in one of them.

Pathology and pathogenesis of hepatobiliary disorders

The apparent pathogenesis of neonatal cholestasis and jaundice is an obstruction of intra- and extrahepatic biliary ducts by inspissated secretions and hyaline concretions (Valman, ArchDisChild, 1971; 4:805; Oppenheimer, JPediat, 1975; 86:683). However, other factors may be associated with neonatal jaundice in cystic fibrosis, such as cytomegalovirus or giant-cell hepatitis and also biliary atresia (Rosenstein, JPediat, 1977; 91:1022).

The pathogenesis of the macroglobular fatty metamorphosis of the hepatocytes in cystic fibrosis remains obscure. It seems mainly correlated with untreated pancreatic insufficiency; the low concentrations of lipoproteins reported in cystic fibrosis (Vaughan, Science, 1989; 199:783), and the deficiency of essential fatty acids in this disease (Chase, JPediat, 1979; 95:337; Strandvik, ScaJGastr, 1988; 23(Suppl. 143):1) could play a part. Liver steatosis was reduced in patients with cystic fibrosis treated by intravenous lipids as compared with untreated ones (Strandvik, ScaJGastr, 1988; 23 (Suppl. 143):1). Malnutrition has been recognized as a common cause of liver steatosis (Chase, JPediat, 1979; 95:337). No correlation between steatosis and the development of biliary disease has been shown.

Unexplained features of hypoxic liver disease, with centrizonal necrosis and some degree of phlebosclerosis, have also been found frequently at autopsy (Maurage, JPediatGastrNutr, 1989; 9:17).

Recently, a 'nodular regenerative hyperplasia', a liver lesion not previously described in cystic fibrosis, was found in cystic fibrosis-associated colitis and fibrosing colonopathy (Schwarzenberg, JPediat, 1995; 127:565). Such a lesion has been associated with vascular insufficiency of the liver.

The most characteristic liver lesion in cystic fibrosis is focal biliary cirrhosis, defined by the presence of enlarged portal triads with bile-duct proliferation, a variable degree of fibrosis, and chronic inflammation (Maurage, JPediatGastrNutr, 1989; 9:17). When such a lesion involves adjacent lobules, which become stranded in fibrous tissue with destruction of their architecture and the appearance of regenerative nodules, a picture of multilobular biliary cirrhosis is recognizable (di Sant'Agnese, Pediat, 1956; 18:387).[7,13] With the progression of the disease we can see severely damaged liver zones beside undamaged ones: this is a distinctive type of biliary cirrhosis, the classic cholestatic cirrhosis being characterized by diffuse perilobular fibrosis.[13]

The pathogenesis of liver disease in cystic fibrosis is believed to be related to obstruction of intrahepatic bile ducts by plugs, which are usually seen as eosinophilic material in the portal bile ducts only, not in the canaliculi. There is evidence that the abnormally concentrated bile in the bile ducts is related to the basic defect of the disease. In fact, in both humans and rats the CFTR is located at the apical membrane of epithelial cells lining the branching intrahepatic bile ducts, as shown by *in situ* hybridization and immunostaining studies (Nguyen, PediatPulmonol, 1992; 14 (Suppl. 8):261; Basavappa, Gastro, 1993; 104:1796; Cohn, Gastro, 1993; 105:1857; Fitz, JCI, 1993; 91:319). There is no evidence to date of CFTR expression on hepatocyte membranes (including the bile canaliculi).

It follows that the primary abnormality is in biliary cells rather than in hepatocytes. This can also explain why the liver has a relatively normal parenchyma in contrast to the grossly expanded and fibrotic portal tracts, while portal hypertension and biliary symptoms are prominent but jaundice and hepatocellular failure are rare (Tanner, ArchDisChild, 1995; 72:281).

In bile secretion the liver functions as an exocrine gland, in that it contains distinct acinar and ductular structures: hepatocytes and bile-duct cells. The canalicular secretion represents the primary bile, which is partly bile acid-dependent, being the water flow probably effected through an osmotic mechanism, and partly dependent on electrolyte transport. Reabsorption and secretion of fluid and inorganic electrolytes occur through the intrahepatic duct system: in the bile-duct cells, secretin increases cAMP (McGill, GastrLiverPhysiol, 1994; 29:G731), which stimulates the opening of Cl^- channels (Fitz, JCI, 1993; 91:319) and Cl^-/HCO_3 exchange (Strazzabosco, JCI, 1991; 87:1503). A HCO_3^-/Cl^- exchanger has been localized to the apical membrane of the biliary cells. The bile ducts resemble intralobular pancreatic ducts, in which CFTR-associated Cl^- channels have an important role in the regulation of ductular secretion. In cystic fibrosis, failure of the apical chloride channel to open could account for the obstruction of intrahepatic ducts with inspissation of secretions (Cohn, Gastro, 1993; 105:1857), as the paracellular movement of Na^+ and water for the dilution of bile is prevented. This is consistent with the pathological data suggesting that obstruction of the intrahepatic ducts is the earliest feature of cystic fibrosis in the liver (Oppenheimer, JPediat, 1975; 86:683).

Focal biliary fibrosis with ductular proliferation represents a reactive process that is secondary to a long-standing sedimentation involving a growing obstruction of the ductular network.

Why not all children with cystic fibrosis develop liver fibrosis may depend on several risk factors variously combined with the primary defect. One of these factors was suggested to be an obstruction at the lower end of the common bile duct (Gaskin, NEJM, 1988; 318:340). As mentioned above, that lesion is not so common as originally claimed, while a more typical extrahepatic biliary lesion seems to be that of multiple constrictions and dilatations resembling a fibrosing cholangitis. Those lesions are accompanied by epithelial loss and mural fibrosis throughout the biliary tree (Bilton, Gut, 1990; 31:236; Bilton, Lancet, 1990; 335:357). Similar lesions were also found in biopsy specimens of patients without evidence of liver disease (Lindblad, Hepatol, 1992; 16:372). They could be the consequence of inflammatory processes due to inspissation and stasis of bile within the biliary system.

Obstruction of the bile ducts may induce retention of hepatotoxic bile acids, production of inflammatory cytokines and free radicals, and lipid peroxidation. The toxicity of bile acids seems mainly attributable to the net predominance of the more hydrophobic glycoconjugated over tauroconjugated bile acids,[13] as a consequence of malabsorption of bile acids, which causes increased faecal loss of taurine (Thompson, PediatRes, 1988; 23:323). However, the bile-acid factor cannot be important for patients with hepatobiliary disease and normal pancreatic function (Waters, Hepatol, 1995; 21: 963).

The role of the cellular immune response to liver membrane antigens in the progression of liver damage (Mieli-Vergani, 1980; 55:696) is no longer considered important.

An association of hyperimmune vasculitis with advanced liver disease has been occasionally reported (Soter, JPediat, 1979; 95:197; Finnegan, QJMed, New Series 72, 1989; 267:609) and also observed by ourselves and D Katznelson (personal communication): we wonder whether this is only a chance association.

Portal hypertension develops gradually in few patients with liver disease, due to extensive diffusion of portal fibrosis. The common complication of portal hypertension is the development not only of oesophageal varices but also gastric varices (Cipolli, ItalJPediat, 1995; 21:58–62), always associated with enlargement of the spleen and in the long run with hypersplenism. Variceal bleeding can be precipitated by aspirin (Psacharopoulos, Lancet, 1981; ii:78). Ascites is a very late event in our experience. It can be combined with massive pleural effusion, as observed in one of our cirrhotic patients, probably due to shunting between portal and pleural vessels. Intestinal malabsorption can be worsened by portal hypertension.

Liver disease in cystic fibrosis can have some as yet unexplained implications with regard to lung disease, as shown by the improvement in pulmonary symptoms and function reported after isolated liver transplantation in children with cystic fibrosis (Cox, PediatPulmonol, 1990; (Suppl. 5):78; Mieles, PediatPulmonol, 1991; (Suppl. 6):130; Noble-Jamieson, ArchDisChild, 1994; 71: 349; Mack, JPediat, 1995; 127:881). A hepatopulmonary syndrome, characterized by the development of shunting between pulmonary arteries and veins (Lange, AnnIntMed, 1995; 122:521), was reported

by Couetil et al. (JThoracCardiovascSurg, 1995; 110:1415). Moreover, there is some convincing in vivo evidence that abnormal dilatation of interalveolar vessels, which has been documented in a non-cystic fibrosis cirrhosis, may result in a significant diffusion impairment for O_2 (Crawford, EurRespirJ, 1995; 3:2015).

Organomegaly, ascites, leucopenia, and malnutrition may all contribute to the lung functional involvement (Sharp, JPediat, 1995; 127:944).

The rarity of hepatocellular failure as a cause of death may be explained by the histopathology of biliary cirrhosis, in which the hepatic parenchyma is left largely intact (Webster, ArchDisChild, 1953; 28:343).

Microgallbladder, so commonly documented in cystic fibrosis, can be a very early consequence of reduced bile flow and viscous bile secretion leading to fetal hypoplasia of the gallbladder or morphological changes of its wall (Oppenheimer, JPediat, 1975; 86: 683),[17] even though there is some evidence that increased plasma cholecystokinin in cystic fibrosis can be correlated with a reduced gallbladder volume (Van Haren, ClinSci, 1991; 81:85).

The higher incidence of gallstones in patients with cystic fibrosis had been attributed to an increased biliary cholesterol saturation.[13] However, those original findings were not confirmed by more recent studies (Kattwinkel, JPediat, 1973; 82:234; Weizman, Gut, 1986; 27:1043; Becker, JPediatGastrNutr, 1989; 8:308; Strandvik, JHepatol, 1996; 25:43). At stone analysis, cholesterol was often little represented, calcium bilirubinate and proteins being the major components.[18] The formation of gallstones in cystic fibrosis does not seem to be a result of a primary abnormality of biliary lipid metabolism but rather might be related to a variety of hepatobiliary disturbances, among which bile stasis and hyperconcentration involving some kind of 'nucleation factor' could play a fundamental part.

Clinical aspects

Liver disease

Cholestasis and neonatal jaundice

Jaundice may appear either during the neonatal period or even several weeks after birth.[19] When this condition is present, occasionally the liver can be slightly enlarged. Faeces are acholic, and serum conjugated bilirubin and alkaline phosphatase are increased. The other liver function tests are not particularly useful at this early stage of liver involvement (Valman, ArchDisChild, 1971; 4:805).[13] This type of cholestasis is not permanent and tends to spontaneous regression. So, it would seem that there are no irreversible anatomical lesions and obstructive jaundice disappears without any residual liver damage (Valman, ArchDisChild, 1971; 4:805; Oppenheimer, JPediat, 1975; 86:683).[13]

While obstructive jaundice is rare, neonatal cholestasis without jaundice is a more common occurrence and it may be present during the first few months of life, with elevated serum alkaline phosphatase and γ-glutamyl transpeptidase. This condition appears to occur particularly in infants with meconium ileus, as shown in Fig. 1 by the results of cholestasis tests carried out over a period of 12 years on two groups of patients with cystic fibrosis (with and without meconium ileus) diagnosed in the first months of life at the cystic fibrosis centre, Verona.

Fatty liver

Massive hepatic steatosis was frequently described in cystic fibrosis before the need for adequate pancreatic supplementation was recognized (Turla, B, RivClinPediat, 1966; 78:485).[8,19]

Histological examination of liver biopsies showed a massive fatty infiltration of the parenchyma, but no focal biliary cirrhosis. Although liver steatosis is usually asymptomatic, some patients show hepatomegaly (Stern, Gastro, 1976; 70:645), and oedema with hypoalbuminaemia may be present at diagnosis. There is no clear correlation with nutritional and pulmonary status, and splenomegaly is usually absent. In some individuals, liver function tests are slightly abnormal, while jaundice is never present. On clinical examination the liver can appear enlarged and smooth, with or without a sharp edge. Hypoglycaemia may be present (Balistreri, JPediat, 1980; 97: 689), and a patient with symptoms resembling those of the Reye's syndrome, combined with secondary carnitine deficiency, has also been reported (Treem, Pediat, 1989; 83:993).

Cirrhosis

Clinical and biochemical manifestations of chronic hepatitis in cystic fibrosis are few or completely absent at the focal cirrhosis stage, even when widespread hepatic damage is present. Jaundice is usually absent and one-third of patients only have abnormal test results for hepatic function (Kattwinkel, JPediat, 1973; 82:234; Feigelson, ActaPaedScand, 1975; 64:337; Davidson, JClinPath, 1980; 33: 390).[20] These results vary greatly, even when clinical overt cirrhosis is present. The most reliable biochemical tests would seem to be γ-glutamyl transpeptidase, transaminases (aspartate and alanine aminotransferases), and alkaline phosphatase.[2,8,10,15]

On clinical examination, moderate hepatomegaly can be found. The liver is not tender and has a sharp edge. Hepatic nodules may be palpable, particularly over the epigastrium. When multilobular cirrhosis is present, with diffuse changes in the hepatic parenchyma, there is a reduction of volume in the right lobe. At this point there can be clinical and biochemical evidence of parenchymal involvement, while signs and symptoms of hepatic failure become apparent at very advanced stages of liver disease.

Many patients develop splenomegaly as a result of increased portal pressure due to abnormal intrahepatic venous circulation. The spleen feels hard and smooth, and, in advanced cases, can become enormous. The presence of hepatosplenomegaly in patients with cystic fibrosis renders the diagnosis of cirrhosis with portal hypertension practically certain.

Portal hypertension and its complications

Portal hypertension in patients with cystic fibrosis who have cirrhosis is of intrahepatic and postsinusoidal type.[19] It becomes clinically evident, with hepatomegaly, splenomegaly, and hypersplenism. Other signs of portal hypertension, such as the presence of venous collateral circles, abdominal distension and ascites, generally appear later on. The main complications of portal hypertension are oesophageal and gastric varices, and hypertensive gastropathy. Hypersplenism, the result of portal hypertension, is characterized by thrombocytopenia and varying degrees of granulocytopenia. Thrombocytopenia can become very serious and cause bruising, spontaneous ecchymoses, and different types of haemorrhaging such as epistaxis.

It should be remembered, when dealing with patients with cystic fibrosis, that the first sign of hepatic disease may be bleeding from oesophageal varices, without any previous relevant manifestation. Recently, a 26-year-old woman who came to our attention was diagnosed as having cystic fibrosis with pancreatic sufficiency.[21] The only evidence to suggest cystic fibrosis was a severe liver disease characterized by cirrhosis with portal hypertension complicated by oesophageal varices and hypersplenism. The above signs were noticed the year before the diagnosis of cystic fibrosis was made, because of a chance test that showed the presence of thrombocytopenia. This may lead to the consideration that a sweat test and a genetic study should be compulsory when faced with liver disease and portal hypertension of unknown aetiology.

Clinical or echographic splenomegaly (Willi, AmJRoent, 1980; 134:1005; Wilson-Sharp, ArchDisChild, 1984; 59:923; Cipolli, ItalJPediat, 1995; 21:58) are considered more reliable markers of portal hypertension than the sonographic findings of increased diameter of the portal veins or the presence of portosystemic venous collaterals. Moreover, splenomegaly appears the most predictive marker of oesophageal varices; indeed, it is always present in those with varices (Cipolli, ItalJPediat, 1995; 21:58).[20]

As regards the natural history of varices, between 30 per cent and 40 per cent of patients with overt liver cirrhosis will have bleeding within 2 years of diagnosis (Sauerbruch, NEJM, 1988; 319:8). Although bleeding from oesophageal varices is the most serious manifestation of portal hypertension, the possibility of bleeding from the gastric mucosa as a complication of portal hypertensive gastropathy (Editorial, Lancet, 1991; 338:1045) should not be underestimated . This condition is characterized by diffuse and pronounced dilatation of mucosal capillaries and mucosal oedema. The gastric mucosal bleeding may be insidious, manifesting itself with an iron-deficiency anaemia, haematemesis, and melaena. Haemorrhagic risk is higher in patients with varices than in those with hypertensive gastropathy, but the latter are more prone to further deterioration of liver function (Editorial, Lancet, 1991; 338: 1045). The bleeding from gastric varices at times present in these patients is most dangerous as it is difficult to treat.

Hepatic failure

In the liver disease of cystic fibrosis, portal hypertension and its consequences are common whereas hepatic failure is less so (Stern, Gastro, 1976; 70:645; Psacharopoulos, Lancet, 1981; ii:78; Berkin, EurJRespDis, 1985; 67:103; Noble-Jamieson, ArchDisChild, 1994; 71:349).[13] The major problems are: deterioration of quality of life, poor nutritional status, abdominal distension with diaphragmatic splinting from organomegaly or ascites or both, pancytopenia from hypersplenism, and large varices. Ascites appears as a consequence of splanchnic and renal haemodynamic alterations in the presence of severe portal hypertension and hepatic failure. Hepatic encephalopathy is a rare complication and occurs only in the most serious and advanced cases.

Signs and symptoms of liver disease with hepatic failure will probably develop slowly and for most sufferers death is due to respiratory rather than hepatocellular failure.

Other clinical manifestations correlated with liver disease in cystic fibrosis

Steatorrhoea and fat-soluble vitamin deficiency

Steatorrhoea is a symptom of pancreatic insufficiency and is also associated with malabsorbtion of fat-soluble vitamins. It is argued (Noble-Jamieson, ArchDisChild, 1996; 74:88) that steatorrhoea may be a symptom of both hepatic disease and pancreatic insufficiency. Indeed, 6 out of 13 patients with cystic fibrosis and cirrhosis assessed for liver transplantation had steatorrhoea and a high daily intake of pancreatic enzymes. After transplantation, fat absorbtion improved and steatorrhoea disappeared.

All patients with pancreatic insufficiency malabsorb fat-soluble vitamins and risk developing clinical signs and symptoms of vitamin deficiency. Liver disease may further compromise the absorption of fat-soluble vitamins when cholestasis is present. Symptoms linked to these deficiencies are rarely seen, but they have been reported in cystic fibrosis (Keating, Pediat, 1970; 46:41; Friedman, Gastro, 1985; 88:808; Willison, JNeurolNeurosurgPsych, 1985; 48:1097). One of our patients who had severe hepatic disease, with portal hypertension, from an early age developed a complex neuromuscular syndrome as a result of serious vitamin E deficiency.

Inadequate caloric intake

Patients with cystic fibrosis require increased energy intakes because of faecal losses, pulmonary infections, and respiratory insufficiency. Cirrhosis is often associated with metabolic disorder and decreased dietary intake, and can cause or worsen malnutrition.

Pulmonary effects

Impaired hepatic metabolism may alter drug pharmacokinetics (Williams, NEJM, 1983; 309:1616) and this condition should be considered in choosing drugs and their dosage in the treatment of pulmonary infections. However, there are few studies of these problems in cystic fibrosis. As mentioned above, another complication is the appearance of shunts between pulmonary arteries and veins, with the possibility of cyanosis.[15]

The development of pulmonary hypertension in those with cirrhosis has been reported (Williams, NEJM, 1983; 309:1616), but at the moment the relevance of this finding in cystic fibrosis is unclear.

Gallbladder and biliary-tract disease

Clinical manifestations of gallbladder and biliary-tract disease are less common in patients with cystic fibrosis than other gastro-intestinal problems, despite the high prevalence of abnormalities involving those organs.

Gallstones and microgallbladder

In most patients the gallstones are silent. Occasionally, some patients develop symptoms of cholelithiasis before the diagnosis of cystic fibrosis is made (Goriup, HelvPaedActa, 1980; 35:177; Stern, JPediatGastrNutr, 1986; 5:35). Cholelithiasis is generally a problem in adult patients with cystic fibrosis, while children and adolescents are less commonly affected (Scott, Surgery, 1989; 195:671).

In Stern's study (JPediatGastrNutr, 1986; 5:35), 20 patients between the age of 4 and 34 years were diagnosed as having symptomatic cholelithiasis; only six of them were below 16 years of age; there was no gender difference; all but one had clinically apparent exocrine pancreatic insufficiency. Only one patient had evident cirrhosis (portal hypertension and hypersplenism), while in the others the alkaline phosphatase was normal or only slightly elevated.

When symptomatic cholelithiasis is present, classic biliary colic with acute pain in the right upper quadrant of the abdomen, often with vomiting, is a possible manifestation. Jaundice is generally absent, as are abnormal results from liver function tests. Physical examination reveals tenderness and involuntary guarding in the right upper quadrant. Frequently there is only a non-specific abdominal pain, which renders the diagnosis of symptomatic cholelithiasis more problematic.

In patients with cystic fibrosis, abdominal pain is, in fact, common and in differential diagnosis some other typical manifestations of cystic fibrosis should be considered. A common cause of abdominal pain is distal intestinal obstruction syndrome, while pancreatic insufficiency inadequately corrected by supplementation with pancreatic enzymes may cause abdominal pain in both children and adults. Also, other cystic fibrosis-related and unrelated causes of pain should be considered, such as reflux oesophagitis, ulcer and bile gastritis, kidney abnormalities, and inflammatory bowel disease. An upper abdominal pain could suggest also the presence of bile-duct strictures (Gaskin, NEJM, 1988; 318:340; Connon, Pediat-Pulmonol, 1989; 7(Suppl. 4):41; Gaskin, PediatrPulmonol, 1992; (Suppl. 8):128) whereas the presence of jaundice might be secondary to intrahepatic cholestasis, just as the presence of an increased serum alkaline phosphatase may be secondary to focal hepatic lesions (Kattwinkel, JPediat, 1973; 82:234; Stern, JPediatGastrNutr, 1986; 5:35).

Microgallbladder is usually asymptomatic. Either gallstones or sludge may be present, while intrahepatic stones were generally not found in association with microgallbladder (Stern, JPediatGastrNutr, 1986; 5:35).[22]

Common bile-duct abnormalities

As said before, Gaskin (NEJM, 1988; 318:340) described strictures of the distal common bile duct in patients with abnormal liver tests or hepatomegaly. The common sign was upper abdominal pain, usually in the right hypochondrium. The pain was colicky, usually centred in the right upper quadrant but radiating to the back or around the right costal margin. It could be precipitated by meals, but was controlled by avoiding fatty foods. Where symptoms persisted over a 6-month period, cholecysto- or choledochojejunostomy was performed; all patients had either multilobular biliary cirrhosis or focal hepatic fibrosis. After invasive intervention the pain was almost invariably relieved (Gaskin, NEJM, 1988; 318:340; Gaskin, PediatrPulmonol, 1992; (Suppl. 8):128). In those patients with cholestasis before surgery, the serum conjugated bilirubin and fasting bile acids returned to normal within 2 months. The cause of pain from the biliary tract is not clear but we suggest that it might result from increased pressure within the biliary tree, cholangitis or both.

Cholangitis/cholecystitis

Superimposed infection may produce further damage to extra-hepatic biliary ducts and cholecystitis, leading to frank clinical cholangitis. Smouldering or subclinical infection may contribute to bile stasis and subsequent liver injury. The frequent need of anti-biotic treatment for respiratory infections might explain the rare appearance of symptomatic cholangitis–cholecystitis.

Furthermore, there are some descriptions of sclerosing chol-angitis in patients with cystic fibrosis who presented typical symp-toms and signs: pain in the right upper quadrant, weight loss, intermittent jaundice, and persistently elevated alkaline phosphatase (Strandvik, ScaJGastr, 1988; 23(Suppl. 143):121). At diagnosis, made by endoscopic retrograde cholangiography showing beading and strictures, especially in the intrahepatic ducts, all patients had elevated serum concentrations of liver enzymes.

Diagnostic approach
Liver function tests

It is unusual to find biochemical evidence of fatty liver, even when the steathosis is associated with clinical manifestations such as massive hepatomegaly and failure to thrive in malnourished infants.

The results of laboratory tests for liver function vary con-siderably when biliary cirrhosis is diagnosed; the biochemical pat-tern does not correlate well with the extent of liver damage and it is not particularly useful in follow-up.[15] Like others,[19,23] we found an inconsistent relation between hepatosplenomegaly and abnormal liver enzyme activities (Cipolli, ItalJPediat, 1995; 21:58). Hepatic-derived alkaline phosphatase and γ-glutamyl trans-peptidase are considered the most reliable, even though inconstant, indicators of biliary cirrhosis, after drug toxicity and heart failure secondary to cor pulmonale have been excluded (Kattwinkel, JPediat, 1973; 82:234; Boat, ClinPediat, 1974; 13:505). In our study, 22 out of 48 patients with cystic fibrosis who had one or more signs of chronic liver disease showed biochemical evidence of it as well. γ-Glutamyl transpeptidase and alanine aminotransferase were the enzymes most frequently raised. We also found that patients with splenomegaly had higher concentrations of γ-glutamyl trans-peptidase than those with normal-sized spleens. Serum collagen VI levels have been found significantly elevated in patients with cystic fibrosis and fibrotic liver disease (Gerling NEJM, 1997; 22:1611), and it thus seems to be a good marker of liver fibrosis in cystic fibrosis; if found to correlate with the degree of hepatic involvement its use could be even more intriguing.

Concentrations of bilirubin are usually low, even in patients with life-threatening complications of portal hypertension (Stern, Gastro, 1976; 70:645). Davidson et al. (JClinPath, 1980; 33:390) suggested that elevated serum conjugates of cholic acid are a more sensitive finding in diagnosing the liver disease of cystic fibrosis, but this assertion has not been confirmed.[13] The albumin con-centrations do not correlate well with the condition of the liver. Strober's findings (Pediat, 1969; 43:416) highlight that the most frequent cause of hypoalbuminaemia in cystic fibrosis is the hypervolaemia secondary to cor pulmonale. However, hypo-albuminaemia is generally present in those with overt cirrhosis and hepatic insufficiency. Hypoprothrombinaemia is more often due to steatorrhoea and malabsorption of vitamin K, but when a large involvement of the liver parenchyma has developed it can be secondary to hepatic disease.

Haematological findings of hypersplenism are leucopenia and thrombocytopenia, but frequently these features do not give rise to clinical symptoms.

Hepatobiliary scintigraphy

Hepatobiliary scintigraphy is performed with [^{99}Tc^m]diiso-propyliminodiacetic acid (**DISIDA**) or trimethylbromo-iminodiacetic acid (**TMBIDA**). In the evaluation of patients with cystic fibrosis by this technique, delayed clearance of [^{99}Tc^m] DIS-IDA or TMBIDA from the liver parenchyma and biliary tree, in the presence of liver disease, has been shown (O'Brien, Gut, 1992; 33:387; Degan, JNuclMed, 1994; 35:432; O'Connor, Hepatol, 1996; 23:281). In addition, some other hepatobiliary scintigraphic findings on liver disease in cystic fibrosis are recognized: non-visualization of the gallbladder and dilated intrahepatic ducts with a predilection for the left lobe of the liver; only one out of 12 patients with cystic fibrosis studied had completely normal hepatobiliary scintigraphy (Degan, JNuclMed, 1994; 35:432). Non-visualization of the gall-bladder could be related to inspissated bile in the cystic duct and might be one of the earliest manifestations of liver disease in cystic fibrosis. The dilated intrahepatic ducts may be a result of repetitive injury to intra- and/or extrahepatic ducts. As mentioned above, Gaskin (NEJM, 1988; 318:340) found distal obstruction of the common bile duct in over 90 per cent of patients with cystic fibrosis and liver disease by DISIDA scanning. Nagel et al. (Lancet, 1989; ii:1422) showed delayed excretion of TMBIDA in 65 per cent of patients with cystic fibrosis and hepatic disease, even though at endoscopic cholangiography only two had obstruction of the lower common bile. Colombo et al. (Hepatol, 1992; 15:677) showed, by hepatobiliary scintigraphy, an improvement in hepatobiliary excretory function after a 1-year treatment with ursodeoxycholic acid.

These observations indicate that hepatobiliary scintigraphy may be valuable in differentiating between intra- and extrahepatic in-volvement of the biliary tract in cystic fibrosis and, in addition, may be useful in following patients undergoing therapy with urso-deoxycholic acid.

Ultrasonography

Ultrasound scanning is a safe, non-invasive, and relatively in-expensive investigation, particularly useful in assessing abdominal complications in patients with cystic fibrosis. The ultrasonographic abnormalities of the liver in cystic fibrosis are well described (Wilson-Sharp, ArchDisChild, 1984; 59:923; McHugo, BrJRadiol, 1987; 60:137; Dobson, JCanAssocRadiol, 1988; 39:257). Hetero-geneously increased hepatic echogenicity and periportal hyper-echogenicity are the more frequent findings. Diffuse hyperechogenicity is common in younger children, while diffuse heterogeneity or periportal hyperechogenicity are more common in older children and adolescents. These changes may reflect the histopathological progression from fatty infiltration to periportal fibrosis and overt biliary cirrhosis. The inferior edge of the liver can be irregular until becoming grossly irregular in appearance. The ultrasonographic modification of the liver edge may precede clinical and biochemical evidence of liver disease and might reflect the developing hepatic fibrosis.

A good correlation between increased echogenicity and histological fatty infiltration has been recorded (Quillin, PediatRadiol, 1993; 23:533). In the presence of heterogeneously increased echogenicity, Willi *et al.* (AmJRoent, 1980; 134:1005) showed a variety of biopsy patterns, including cholestasis, cholangitis, biliary cirrhosis, focal periportal fibrosis, and fatty changes. However, other studies have shown a poor correlation between liver function tests and echographic abnormalities.

Ultrasound scanning can be used to detect signs of portal hypertension with varices, and splenomegaly seems the most useful finding in assessing the presence of varices. The size of the portal vein and its collaterals was poorly correlated with portal hypertension and varices (Kumari-Subaiya, JPediatGastrNutr, 1987; 6: 71; Goyal, JUSMed, 1990; 9:45). Some (Brunelle, AnnRadiol, 1981: 24:121; De Giacomo, JPediatGastrNutr, 1989; 9:431) considered the thickening of the lesser omentum as a good predictive marker of portal hypertension and oesophageal varices in children with various chronic liver diseases . However, other studies on adolescent patients with portal hypertension in cystic fibrosis did not find any evidence of this condition on sonography (Kumari-Subaiya, JPediatGastrNutr, 1987; 6:71; Cipolli, ItalJPediat, 1995; 21:58).

Ultrasonography is also reliable for detecting gallbladder disease. The typical findings include stones and sludge, small gallbladder, and obstruction of the cystic duct. The presence of echogenic sludge indicates the risk of progressive stone formation. Thickening of the gallbladder walls is another echographic aspect, but the differential diagnosis between chronic cholecystitis and hypertrophy related to chronic mucous inspissation is difficult to resolve by ultrasound.

Duplex Doppler ultrasound has been proposed as a useful, noninvasive method in the monitoring and management of portal hypertension in children (Zoli, JClinUltrasound, 1986; 14:429; Burns, Gastro 1987; 92:824; Kozaiwa, JPediatGastrNutr, 1995; 21: 215). However, some publications point out that this technique is subject to many errors and therefore its clinical use should be limited (Vergesslich, PediatRadiol, 1989; 19:371; Hasmann, PediatPulmonol, 1990; (Suppl. 5): 270A). We recently suggested that duplex Doppler ultrasound was an unreliable tool in the management of young patients with cystic fibrosis and portal hypertension at risk of oesophageal varices (Valletta, ScaJGastr, 1993; 28: 1042; Cipolli, JPediatGastrNutr, 1996; 23:510). The most evident critical points were (i) the wide overlapping of haemodynamic measurements between those with portal hypertension and oesophageal varices and those without varices or even without liver disease, (ii) the high intraobserver variability of repeated Doppler evaluations, and (iii) the difficulty of obtaining good-quality measurements because of meteorism or poor cooperation.

Therefore, at the moment, it is difficult to imagine how duplex Doppler ultrasound can modify the clinical approach to children with portal hypertension, or how the need for more invasive procedures could be avoided by using this technique. There is no doubt that in the evaluation of splanchnic circulation, duplex Doppler ultrasound may theoretically offer important advantages over conventional ultrasound. Nevertheless, its reliability, actual clinical role, and practical implications for children with portal hypertension are still critical points.

Computed tomography

CT adds little to the ultrasound examination. However, Schwartz *et al.* (JComputAssistTomogr, 1983; 7:530) found that it may show a distinctive pattern of low-density areas representing fatty infiltration, and fibrotic bands of cirrhosis forming the walls of cyst-like areas.

Endoscopy

Upper gastrointestinal endoscopy provides information about the presence, the degree, and, when indicated, the sclerosis of oesophageal varices, and also indicates the presence of oesophagitis, gastric varices, gastropathy, ulcers, which are all conditions potentially associated with liver disease.

Endoscopic retrograde cholangiography

Endoscopic retrograde cholangiography might be helpful in showing possible strictures of the distal common bile duct in patients with cystic fibrosis who experience recurrent abdominal pain. Also, percutaneous transhepatic cholangiography has been used to show the same bile-duct abnormality (Gaskin, NEJM, 1988; 318:340), and its utilization in the liver disease of cystic fibrosis is linked to this aspect.

Liver biopsy

Needle biopsy of the liver may give information on liver disease and cholestasis, particularly in infants, to distinguish between a neonatal hepatitis and biliary obstruction. In younger adults it is possible to distinguish the liver disease of cystic fibrosis from parenchymal disease that is caused by viruses, drugs or alcohol. Also, in the presence of serological evidence of chronic aggressive hepatitis, liver biopsy is indicated. However, it is important to remember that in biliary fibrosis the hepatic lesion is focal so a liver biopsy may miss this change. We cannot justify a biopsy when trying to identify subclinical liver disease or when following the course of hepatic involvement in cystic fibrosis, in the absence of any specific treatment.

Treatment of hepatobiliary problems
Fatty liver

Steathosis, when present at the diagnosis of cystic fibrosis, usually regresses on correct supplementation with pancreatic enzymes. Massive steathosis responded well in the majority of individuals to a low-fat, high-carbohydrate and high-protein diet supplemented with pancreatic enzymes,[8,19] but we do not now believe that a low-fat diet is really necessary for this purpose.

Prevention and treatment of liver disease

There is no specific or definitely effective therapeutical strategy for the prevention and treatment of liver disease in cystic fibrosis. Over the last few years, ursodeoxycholic acid has been introduced as a therapeutic option for chronic liver disease, and it has been relatively efficient when cholestasis was present (de Caestecker, Gut, 1991; 32:1061). Also, in the liver disease of cystic fibrosis, ursodeoxycholic acid showed beneficial effects by improving liver function tests

(Cotting, Gut, 1990; 31:918; Colombo, Hepatol, 1992; 15:677; Colombo, Hepatol, 1992; 16:924).

Ursodeoxycholic acid (UDCA) is a hydrophilic, non-toxic, exogenous bile acid, and the rationale suggested for its use in liver disease of cystic fibrosis includes: its capacity to displace detergent endogenous bile acids from the enterohepatic circulation (Hofmann, Lancet, 1987; ii:398), the cytoprotective effect at the level of the canalicular membrane,[24] and the possibility of a choleretic effect (Anonymous, Lancet, 1992; 340:1260). Some controlled trials (O'Brien, EurJGastroHepatol, 1992; 4:857) have confirmed that giving ursodeoxycholic acid in cystic fibrosis improves the serum liver enzymes.[25] An Italian multicentre double-blind trial (Colombo, Hepatol, 1993; 18:142A) showed a significant improvement in liver function tests (cytolysis and cholestasis functions) in the group treated with ursodeoxycholic acid. These effects tended to decrease when the therapy was stopped, and the biochemical response was dose-dependent, requiring a higher dosage in patients with cystic fibrosis than in those affected by other cholestatic liver diseases (Galabert, JPediat, 1992; 121:138). A dose of at least 20 mg/kg per day has been considered as necessary in cystic fibrosis (Colombo, Hepatol, 1992; 16:924; Van de Meeberg, ScaJGastr, 1997; 32:369). However, long-term therapy with ursodeoxycholic acid may increase faecal loss of taurine, and taurine supplementation becomes necessary during this treatment (Colombo, Hepatol, 1996; 23:1484). It has also been suggested that patients with cystic fibrosis and meconium ileus or its equivalents might benefit from prophylactic treatment with ursodeoxycholic acid (Colombo, JPediat, 1994; 124:393; Tanner, ArchDisChild, 1995; 72:281).

The long-term effectiveness of ursodeoxycholic acid therapy in modifying the course of liver disease, or preventing serious conditions linked to chronic cholestatic liver involvement, has not yet been proven. Progress from the early focal hepatic lesion to overt biliary cirrhosis appears to have been arrested or at least slowed down in 14 patients with cystic fibrosis treated over a 2-year period with ursodeoxycholic acid.[26] However, individuals with other forms of biliary cirrhosis whose livers deteriorated during treatment with ursodeoxycholic acid have been reported (Vogel, Lancet, 1988; i:1163; Perdigoto, Gastro, 1992; 102:1389).

To summarize, we can say that ursodeoxycholic acid may improve biochemical abnormalities associated with liver disease in cystic fibrosis and scintigraphic biliary flow, but none of the studies has demonstrated that it prevents progression of cirrhosis in established cystic fibrosis-associated liver disease or its onset. We therefore conclude, as have others (Durie, PediatrPulmonol, 1997; S14:144), that existing studies of ursodeoxycholic acid in cystic fibrosis-associated liver disease provide no clinical or scientific justification for its routine use .

Cholestasis and neonatal jaundice

A conservative approach to the prolonged neonatal jaundice is recommended, even if a long period of recovery is required (up to 6 months) (Valman, ArchDisChild, 1971; 4:805). However, there have been cases where surgery has proved necessary (Festen, ZKinderchir, 1988; 43:106). Evans et al. (JPediatGastrNutr, 1991; 12:131) reported a severe case of neonatal cholestasis that was successfully treated by infusing N-acetylcysteine into the biliary tree, together with intravenous injections of synthetic cholecystokinin.

Gallstones

Ursodeoxycholic acid is well known as an agent for dissolving cholesterol gallstones and it may also be used in patients with cystic fibrosis who have cholelithiasis,[23] even if no favourable results have been reported as regards its capacity to dissolve gallstones in cystic fibrosis (Colombo, ActaPaed, 1993; 82:562). Cholecystectomy is the appropriate treatment when symptomatic gallstones are present and it offers total pain relief. When surgery is considered, it is mandatory to evaluate the pulmonary status. The advent of laparoscopic cholecystectomy, allowing the use of epidural anaesthesia, has decreased the risks involved in surgical intervention.

Common bile-duct stenosis

For isolated strictures and pain in the common bile duct, surgical correction may be appropriate (either cholecystojejunostomy or choledochojejunostomy) for the relief of symptoms (Patrick, JPediat, 1986; 108:101; Gaskin, NEJM, 1988; 318:340).

Portal hypertension and its complications

Apart from the hepatocellular failure, acute bleeding from oesophageal or gastric varices is the most serious condition for the management of portal hypertension in cystic fibrosis.

Acute variceal bleeding

This manifestation is frequent in the presence of portal hypertension and varices. Bleeding may stop spontaneously; if so, an elective endoscopy with injection of sclerosant into the varices can be done within a few days of the episode. In the presence of active bleeding it is necessary: to prepare a blood transfusion or its equivalent, to monitor vital functions, to introduce a nasogastric tube, and to perform an emergency endoscopy to sclerose the bleeding varices. This last manoeuvre requires a skilled operator and, when difficult, the use of splanchnic vasoconstrictor drugs (e.g. vasopressin or glipressin) and balloon tamponade should also be considered.

Variceal sclerotherapy

Injection sclerotherapy has been used satisfactorily in children with bleeding oesophageal varices in cystic fibrosis (Howard, BrJSurg, 1988; 75:404; Feigelson, ArchDisChild, 1993; 68:653; Stringer, ArchDisChild, 1993; 69:407), with a high rate of success in controlling the haemorrhage. Moreover, variceal obliteration is achieved in an average of four to six sessions over a period of about 6 months (Stringer, ArchDisChild, 1993; 69:407).[20] Sclerotherapy is by combined intravariceal and paravariceal injection. Different sclerosants have been used, most commonly sodium morrhuate and polidocanol (Sauerbruch, NEJM, 1988; 319:8; Proujansky, JPediatGastrNutr, 1991; 12:33). Known complications of sclerotherapy include oesophagitis, necrosis, ulcerations, perforation of the oesophagus, fistula formation, and mediastinitis. There is nothing to suggest the need for injecting varices before the first episode of haemorrhage (Cello, NEJM, 1984; 311:1589; Anonymous, Lancet, 1988; 1369; Sauerbruch, NEJM, 1988; 319:8).[23]

The obliteration of varices with the prevention of rebleeding is an effective and safe method in the management of this problem and appears more satisfactory than portosystemic shunt surgery

(Shuster, JPediatSurg, 1977; 12:201; Sauerbruch, NEJM, 1988; 319:8).[20]

Our population of patients with oesophageal varices (unpublished data) comprises 18 individuals. Among these, 11 underwent sclerosis for bleeding with a mean follow-up of 5.7 years (range 3–7 years). Complete eradication was achieved in 9 out of 11 patients. One bled again after eradication; varices reappeared in two cases. Submucosal haematoma was the only side-effect observed. Four out of 11 patients died a long time after sclerotherapy: two because of respiratory insufficiency and two after liver transplantation.

Shunt surgery

Shunt surgery (splenorenal or portocaval) has all the disadvantages of major surgery, and anaesthesia is a risk condition for patients with cystic fibrosis who have pulmonary deterioration. These shunts can be complicated by hepatic encephalopathy, even though this does not appear so frequently in cystic fibrosis. However, the shunting can aggravate a pre-existent hepatic failure; Alagille et al.[27] reported that a patient with cystic fibrosis died of an unexpected rapid deterioration of liver function 3 months after shunt surgery.

β-Blockade

To prevent variceal bleeding, long-term pharmacological therapy with this class of drugs, particularly propranolol, has been considered. However, there are conflicting results from different trials (Burroughs, NEJM, 1983; 309:1539; Groszmann, Gastro, 1990; 99:1401; Bendtsen, ScaJGastr, 1991; 26:933), suggesting that we should remain cautious about this treatment. Indeed, bronchospasm is a side-effect that often contraindicates the use of propranolol in cystic fibrosis.[20]

Transjugular intrahepatic portosystemic shunt (TIPS)

Transjugular placement of an intrahepatic stent is a new technique for establishing a portosystemic shunt for the treatment of portal hypertension and variceal bleeding in patients with cirrhosis (Richter, BailClinGastr, 1992; 6:402; Rossle, NEJM, 1994; 330:165). TIPS might also represent a satisfactory alternative to surgical shunting in patients with cystic fibrosis when sclerotherapy fails to stop variceal bleeding.

Kerns et al. (AmJRadiol, 1992; 159:1277) reported a case of a 13-year-old with cystic fibrosis who had overt cirrhosis and variceal bleeding in which TIPS was performed. Through 6 months of follow-up the shunt remained widely patent and no further bleeding occurred. A single episode of encephalopathy was recorded, with rapid resolution. A more recent case is described by Berger et al. (JPediatGastrNutr, 1994; 19:322). A 14-year-old boy with cystic fibrosis, cirrhosis, hepatosplenomegaly, mild ascites, and oesophageal varices not controlled by sclerotherapy underwent a TIPS procedure. Eleven months later he had had no recurrent bleeding or signs of encephalopathy. Ascites was resolved and splenomegaly was clearly decreased. TIPS may present some complications: stent stenosis (treated by balloon expansion of the stent), embolization of the stent to the pulmonary artery, intraperitoneal bleeding, and

bacteraemia (Zemel, JAMA, 1991; 266:390). However, TIPS appears a promising procedure for children or adolescents with variceal bleeding refractory to sclerotherapy.

Partial splenectomy

The presence of a voluminous splenomegaly and hypersplenism is a serious problem, particularly as regards quality of life, the risk of splenic rupture, and the risk of haemorrhage from thrombocytopenia. Splenectomy could be a treatment for hypersplenism but increases the risk of overwhelming infection (Dickerman, Pediat, 1979; 63:938). In order to reduce the volume of the spleen in cystic fibrosis, while maintaining its function, partial splenectomy with conservation of the upper pole has been proposed (Louis, EurJPediatSurg, 1993; 3:22). Twelve patients with cystic fibrosis who had major splenomegaly, hypersplenism, and oesophageal varices and with FEV_1 above 70 per cent of that expected have undergone this partial splenectomy. The spleen became clinically impalpable and hypersplenism was corrected (improving platelet and white-cell counts) in all patients; a reduction of varices was also observed in all but one (Chazalette, IsrJMedSci, 1996 (Suppl.); 32:S83). The technique appears promising, but needs further evaluation before being considered reliable; moreover, it appears contraindicated in the presence of significant hepatocellular failure.

Partial splenic embolization

As an alternative, in the presence of splenomegaly and hypersplenism, partial splenic embolization has been performed. Israel et al. (JPediat, 1994; 124:95) described the outcome of this in seven children who did not have cystic fibrosis but suffered splenomegaly and hypersplenism (varices were present in six of them). Six of these patients had extrahepatic causes of portal hypertension, and one had autoimmune liver disease. The spleen was partially infarcted, preserving about 25 per cent of functional tissue. Hypersplenism improved, with an increase of platelet and leucocyte counts. The size of the spleen was significantly reduced over a period of a few months. During the period soon after partial splenic embolization, all but one child reported significant pain and tenderness localized in the left upper quadrant. In one child a pulmonary complication (atelectasis) was observed.

At present, there is no published experience of partial splenic embolization in patients with cystic fibrosis, but it should be considered that abdominal pain could cause restricted chest motion in these individuals, with increased risk of atelectasis and/or infection.

Liver transplantation

For the endstage liver disease of cystic fibrosis, liver transplantation should be considered as a therapeutic option that is beginning to have an encouraging outcome. The first liver transplantation in cystic fibrosis was attempted in 1985 (Cox, Pediat, 1987; 80:571) and was unsuccessful because of early death caused by an *Aspergillus* brain abscess. Transplantation has seldom been attempted because it is difficult to judge the best time for the procedure and there was concern with the lung problems that might increase the immediate risk of the operation. In addition, it was feared that postoperative pulmonary infection might progress rapidly on immunosuppression (Cox, PediatrPulmonol, 1990; (Suppl. 5):78).

Table 4 Summary of experiences on liver transplantation in cystic fibrosis

Authors	No. of subjects	Age (years)	Survival (1 year)	Late survival	Procedures
Cox (1990)	10	2.3–30	70%	?	Liver
Mieles *et al.* (1991)	14	6–31	78%	68% (5 years)	Liver
Stern *et al.* (1994)	1	21	1/1	1/1 (2 years)	Pancreas, kidney
Mack *et al.* (1995)	8	0.7–23	75%	62% (4 years)	
Noble Jamieson *et al.* (1996)	12	5–14	11/12	?	Liver
Thevenot *et al.* (1996)	1	15	1/1	1/1 (3 years)	Liver
Dennis *et al.* (1996)	3	21–27	2/3	2/2 (2–4 years)	Heart–lung–liver
Couetil *et al.* (1997)	11	10–18	85%	85% (3 years)	Heart–lung–liver (4) Double lung–liver (2) Bilateral lobar lung-liver (1) Liver (4)

To date, we can do a first balance on liver transplantation in cystic fibrosis based upon a published experience of almost 60 patients (Cox, PediatrPulmonol, 1990; (Suppl. 5):78; Mieles, PediatrPulmonol, 1991; (Suppl. 6): 130; Noble-Jamieson, JRSoc-Med, 1996; 89 (Suppl.) 27:31, JPediat, 1996; 129:314; Stern, Clin-Transpl, 1994; 8:1; Couetil, TransplInt, 1997; 10:33; Lange, AnnIntMed, 1995; 122:521; Mack, JPediat, 1995; 127:881; Thevenot, ArchPediat, 1996; 3:1248) (see Table 4).

Forty-nine patients underwent isolated liver transplantation (Cox, PediatrPulmonol, 1990; (Suppl. 5):78; Noble-Jamieson, JRSocMed, 1996; 89 (Suppl.) 27:31; Mack, JPediat, 1995; 127: 881), one patient a combined pancreas–liver–kidney transplantation (Stern, ClinTranspl, 1994; 8:1), and 7 others had combined heart–lung–liver or lung–liver transplantation (Couetil, TransplInt, 1997; 10:33). In the series of isolated transplants the main indication was severe portal hypertension judged as life-threatening after failure of palliative procedures, sometimes combined with hepatic decompensation. Those patients were selected for transplantation because they also presented only mild or mild/moderate lung involvement. Remarkably, both the immediate (70–5 per cent) and the long-term survival rates (60–85 per cent) are similar to those reported for other established indications for liver transplantation (Gordon, TransplProc, 1991; 23:1393). Another important finding after transplantation was an improvement in the lung function, or the absence of pulmonary complications or deterioration. These effects have been attributed to several factors: relief of diaphragmatic splinting with organs enlarged by pulmonary oedema and pulmonary arteriovenous shunts, nutritional improvement and inhibition of inflammatory processes in the lung by the immunosuppressive medication employed (prednisone, cyclosporin, tacrolimus) (Noble-Jamieson, ArchDisChild, 1994; 71:349; Mack, JPediat, 1995; 127:881; Sharp, JPediat, 1995; 127:944). Also, fat absorption was improved after liver transplantation (Noble-Jamieson, ArchDisChild, 1996; 74:88).

The most recent reports of combined lung–liver or heart–lung–liver transplantation (Couetil, JThoracCardiovascSurg, 1995; 110:1415; Couetil, TransplInt, 1997; 10:33; Dennis, JHeart-LungTranspl, 1996; 15:536) have opened the hope of a prolonged survival for patients with cystic fibrosis who have endstage lung and liver disease. The reported morbidity and mortality for such interventions is equalling that for separate replacements. The report in one case of a successful bilateral lobar lung transplant from a split left lung, together with a reduced liver lobe transplant, is remarkable. Unpublished data from three Italian centres give a current experience of 11 cystic fibrosis patients treated by liver transplantation (one with a heart–lung–liver procedure): eight of them are alive 5 to 96 months after operation (S. Quattrucci, personal communication).

In conclusion, liver transplantation in cystic fibrosis should be considered for life-threatening hepatocellular failure or uncontrollable variceal bleeding. Advanced lung disease is no longer a contraindication provided that a combined lung–liver transplantation is possible.

Perspectives of gene therapy

Cystic fibrosis is now considered one of the diseases for which a somatic gene transfer could provide a chance of treatment or prevention of liver disease (Chang, Gastro, 1994; 106:1076; Tanner, ArchDisChild, 1995; 72:281).[28] As the expression of CFTR is limited to the epithelial cells lining the intrahepatic bile ducts, somatic gene transfer must clearly be directed at the biliary cell, not the hepatocyte.

Initial attempts have been made to transfer the human *CFTR* gene into biliary epithelium of rats by using recombinant adenovirus as vector (Yang, PNAS, 1993; 90:4601). Retrograde injection of the vector into the common bile duct resulted in gene expression in almost all epithelial cells of the intrahepatic bile duct. Expression remained stable in those cells after 21 days, while it diminished in the large biliary ducts.

A more recent study has succeeded in correcting *in vitro* the cystic fibrosis defect by gene complementation in human intrahepatic epithelial cell lines (Grubman, Gastro, 1995; 108:584). Following infection with the adenovirus vector Ad2/CFTR2, a cAMP-induced chloride efflux was observed for 31 days, although the number of responsive cells decreased with time.

These results are attractive because they suggest that it may be possible to deliver by endoscopy *CFTR* gene vectors to human patients with liver problems in cystic fibrosis.

An outline of management of liver disorders

No special intervention is usually required for the neonatal cholestasis or the rare prolonged neonatal jaundice. An early pancreatic enzyme supplementation, with adequate nutritional support, can prevent liver steatosis. The liver condition should be periodically assessed and monitored over the entire lifespan of the patient with cystic fibrosis. Clinical examination to detect hepatomegaly and splenomegaly is more important than tests measuring liver function. In patients with hepatomegaly an ultrasonographic assessment, aimed at the evaluation of portal vasculature, should be done by an experienced radiologist.

Quantitative hepatobiliary scintigraphy may be useful to demonstrate delayed clearance of liver and dilated intra- or extrahepatic ducts, but it does not seem to be routinely indispensable.

When the ultrasonogram demonstrates portal hypertension, oesophageal and gastric varices should be assessed by endoscopy. Varices need to be injected with sclerosant drugs only if they have bled. Usually repeated sessions of sclerotherapy are necessary, depending on the size and severity of the varices. Caution is indicated with gastric varices, which are more difficult to treat. An acute severe variceal haemorrhage should prompt the use of vasoconstrictors. When varices are present, the faeces should be periodically monitored for occult blood.

When portal hypertension is established, liver function tests are necessary to detect and monitor the presence of hepatocellular insufficiency: they should include prothrombin, albumin, cholinesterase, and plasma ammonium. If splenomegaly is evident, white blood cells and platelets should be counted periodically.

With bleeding varices refractory to sclerotherapy, partial splenectomy or partial splenic embolization or transjugular intrahepatic portosystemic shunt can be considered, even though experience of these procedures is lacking experience in cystic fibrosis. Portosystemic shunt surgery could be considered if liver function is normal

At present, ursodeoxycholic acid seems to be indicated in the treatment of selected cases of liver disease when cholestasis or cytolysis markers are increased. A trial with ursodeoxycholic acid may be also proposed to treat small gallstones or biliary sludge, even though a limited outcome is to be expected.

Recurrence of abdominal pain, especially if localized to the right upper quadrant, renders compulsory a differential diagnosis among several causes of abdominal pain in cystic fibrosis, including gallstones and obstruction of the extrahepatic biliary duct, for which a surgical solution may be considered; percutaneous transhepatic or endoscopic retrograde cholangiography are necessary to demonstrate bile-duct obstructions.

For the endstage liver disease (severe portal hypertension with ascites and/or intractable variceal bleeding, and hepatocellular failure), liver transplantation now appears as a promising option. Combined double lung–liver transplantation could also include patients with endstage liver and lung disease.

References

1. Tsui L-Ch. The cystic fibrosis transmembrane conductance regulator gene. *American Journal of Respiratory and Critical Care Medicine*, 1995; 151: 547–53.
2. Boat TF, *et al.* Cystic fibrosis. In Scriver A, Sly WS, and Valle D, eds. *The metabolic basis of inherited disease.* New York: McGraw-Hill, 1989: 2649–80.
3. Zielenski J and Tsui L-CH. Cystic fibrosis: genotypic and phenotypic variations. *Annual Review of Genetics*, 1995; 29: 777–807.
4. Welsh MJ. The path of discovery in understanding the biology of cystic fibrosis and approaches to therapy. *American Journal of Gastroenterology*, 1994; 89: S97–105.
5. Wine JJ. How do CFTR mutations cause cystic fibrosis? *Current Biology*, 1995; 5: 1357–9.
6. Davis PB, Drumm M, and Konstan HW. State of the art. Cystic fibrosis. *American Journal of Respiratory and Critical Care Medicine*, 1996; 154: 1229–56.
7. Bodian M. *Fibrocystic disease of the pancreas.* London: Heinemann Medical, 1952.
8. Schwartz HP, Kraemer R, Thurneer U, and Rossi E. Liver involvement in cystic fibrosis. *Helvetica Paediatrica Acta*, 1978; 33: 351–64.
9. Sinaasappel M. Hepatobiliary pathology in patients with cystic fibrosis. *Acta Paediatrica Scandinavica*, 1989; Suppl. 363: 45–51.
10. Isenberg JN, L'Hereux P, Warwick WJ, and Sharp HL. Clinical observations on the biliary system in cystic fibrosis. *American Journal of Gastroenterology*, 1976; 65: 134–41.
11. Vawter GF and Schwachman H. Cystic fibrosis in adults: an autopsy study. *Pathology Annual*, 1979; 14: 357–82.
12. Fitzsimmons SC. The changing epidemiology of cystic fibrosis. *Journal of Pediatrics*, 1993; 122: 1–9.
13. Roy CC, Weber AM, Morin CL, Lepage G, Brisson G, Yousef I, and Lasalle R. Hepatobiliary disease in cystic fibrosis: a survey of current issues and concepts. *Journal of Pediatric Gastroenterology and Nutrition*, 1982; 1: 469–78.
14. Shwachman H. Gastrointestinal manifestations of cystic fibrosis. *Pediatric Clinics of North America*, 1975; 22: 787–805.
15. Stern RC. Cystic fibrosis and the gastrointestinal tract. In Davis PB, ed. *Cystic fibrosis.* New York: Marcel Dekker, 1993: 417–19.
16. Tesluk, H, McCaulex K, Kurland G, and Reubner BH. Cholangiocarcinoma in an adult with cystic fibrosis. Preprint (Department of Pathology. University of California, Davis CA), 1991.
17. Isenberg JN. Cystic fibrosis: its influence on the liver, biliary tree and bile salt metabolism. *Seminars in Liver Disease*, 1982; 2: 302–13.
18. Angelico M, *et al.* Gallstones in cystic fibrosis: a critical reappraisal. *Hepatology*, 1991; 14: 768–75.
19. di Sant'Agnese PA and Von Hubbard S. The hepatobiliary system. In Taussig LM, ed. *Cystic fibrosis.* New York: Thieme-Stratton, 1984; 296–322.
20. Tanner MS. Current clinical management of hepatic problems in cystic fibrosis. *Journal of the Royal Society of Medicine*, 1986; 79: 38–43.
21. Castellani, C, Cipolli M, Cazzola G, d'Orazio C, Bonizzato A, and Mastella G. An unusual event: pancreatic sufficiency in three cystic fibrosis patients with biliary cirrhosis. (Abstr.) Proceedings: 20th European Cystic Fibrosis Conference, Brussels, 1995: 64.
22. Park RW and Grand RJ. Gastrointestinal manifestations of cystic fibrosis: a review. *Gastroenterology*, 1981; 81: 1143–61.
23. Tanner MS. Liver and biliary problems in cystic fibrosis. *Journal of the Royal Society of Medicine*, 1992; 85 (Suppl. 19): 20–4.
24. Hofmann AF. Bile acid hepatotoxicity and the rationale for UDCA therapy in chronic cholestatic liver disease: some hypotheses. In Paumgartner G, Stiehl A, Barbara L, and Roda E, eds. *Strategies for the treatment of hepatobiliary diseases.* Dordrecht: Kluwer, 1990: 13–33.
25. Bittner P, *et al.* The effect of treatment with ursodeoxycholic acid in cystic fibrosis and hepatopathy; results of a placebo controlled study. In Paumgartner G, Stiehl A, and Gerok W, eds. *Bile acids as therapeutic agents: from basic science to clinical practice* (Proceedings of the 58th Falk Symposium, Freiburg, Germany, 1990). Dordrecht: Kluwer, 1991: 345–8.
26. Nousia-Arvanitakis S, Fotoulaki M, Rafailides D, Economou I, and Makedou A. Early detection and therapy of biliary cirrhosis in cystic fibrosis. In Escobar H, Baquero F, and Suarez L, eds. *Clinical ecology of cystic fibrosis.* Amsterdam: Elsevier Science, 1993: 285–9
27. Alagille D. Portal hypertension. In *Liver and biliary tract disease in children.* Paris, New York; Wiley-Flammarion, 1979: 262–95.
28. Kormis KK and Wu GY. Prospects of therapy of liver diseases with foreign genes. *Seminars in Liver Disease*, 1995; 15: 257–67.

20.5 Human hereditary porphyrias

Yves Nordmann

Introduction

The porphyrias are a group of disorders of haem biosynthesis in which specific patterns of overproduction of haem precursors are associated with characteristic clinical features. Each type of porphyria is the result of a specific decrease in the activity of one of the enzymes of haem biosynthesis.

Porphyrias as clinical entities were recognized and described at the end of the nineteenth and the beginning of the twentieth centuries. This recognition was linked to the appearance on the market of hypnotics such as sulphonemethane and barbiturates. The history of porphyrias cannot be dissociated from the evolution of knowledge of the biochemistry of porphyrins and the haem biosynthesis pathway. In 1968, Levin demonstrated that the primary mechanism of the bovine and human congenital erythropoietic porphyrias depends on a deficiency of the activity of the uroporphyrinogen III cosynthetase. Between 1969 and 1980, enzymatic deficiencies were described for all the porphyrias (see below). In 1986, the nature of the genic mutation of a porphyria was described for the first time (de Verneuil, Science, 1986; 234:732). cDNAs and genes have now (1995) been isolated and characterized for all the enzymes of human porphyrias. These advances have been quickly followed by identification of mutations in the corresponding diseases.

Full coverage of every aspect of this large area of research is not possible here; reference will mostly be made to review articles.

Classification and inheritance

Porphyrias are at present classified as erythropoietic or hepatic in type, depending on the primary organ in which excess production of porphyrins or precursors takes place (Table 1).

Hepatic porphyrias[1-5]

Acute hepatic porphyrias

Acute attacks are identical in four of the hepatic porphyrias—acute intermittent porphyria, hereditary coproporphyria, variegate porphyria, and Doss porphyria.

Clinical features

All the clinical features of an acute attack can be explained by lesions in various areas and components of the nervous system. Attacks usually begin with abdominal pain (more generalized than localized); constipation, nausea, and vomiting may precede and accompany an abdominal crisis. Examination does not reveal abdominal tenderness or signs of peritoneal irritation; radiographic films of the abdomen usually show a normal pattern of bowel gas. Tachycardia, excess sweating, hypertension (or unstable blood pressure), and insomnia are often associated with the abdominal pain. Acute attacks occur more commonly in females (aged 18–40 years) and exacerbations of the disease may recur periodically (mostly during the week preceding the menses). Occasionally, the finding of red or dark-coloured urine (usually after its exposure to light and air) may help the physician in the diagnosis.

In 20 to 30 per cent of patients, there are signs of mental disturbance, such as anxiety, depression, disorientation, hallucinations or confusional states.

Abdominal pain may disappear within a few days, generally when no harmful drug has been used. When acute attacks last several days, the gastrointestinal manifestations frequently lead to weight loss and sometimes to emaciation, while prolonged vomiting may cause oliguria and hyperazotaemia.

Porphyric neuropathy often occurs when harmful drugs have not been avoided during an acute attack. Neurological manifestations are also a problem in differential diagnosis and treatment when the type of porphyria is not known (for instance, an acute attack of porphyria may begin with seizures and all antiseizure drugs have the potential to affect this disease adversely).

Neuropathy is primarily motor: in the early stages, pain in the extremities is very common (described as 'muscle pain'); weakness often begins in the proximal muscles, and more commonly in the arms than in the legs. Symmetrical or asymmetrical paresis may occur in the extremities and can also be strikingly local. Muscle weakness may progress to tetraplegia with respiratory and bulbar paralysis and death. Cranial nerves can be affected (mostly the Xth and VIIth). Seizures are not uncommon; sometimes the intervals between individual convulsions may be so short that they are virtually continuous. The central nervous system is seldom involved; pyramidal signs, cerebellar syndrome, transitory blindness, or abnormalities of consciousness can occur. The cerebrospinal fluid is usually normal.

After a severe attack, complete or partial improvement in muscle function can follow over a period of months. Recovery from paralysis may be incomplete, with sequelae mostly in the extremities. It is very difficult to foresee the long-term outcome in acute crisis with neuropathy.

Table 1 Classification of the inherited human porphyrias

Classification	Inheritance	Deficient enzyme
Hepatic porphyrias		
Acute porphyrias		
Acute intermittent porphyria	Autosomal dominant	Porphobilinogen deaminase
Hereditary coproporphyria*	Autosomal dominant	Coproporphyrinogen oxidase
Variegate porphyria*	Autosomal dominant	Protoporphyrinogen oxidase
Doss porphyria	Autosomal recessive	ALA dehydrase
Porphyria cutanea symptomatica* (familial type)	Autosomal dominant	Uroporphyrinogen decarboxylase
Erythropoietic porphyrias		
Congenital erythropoietic porphyria (Günther disease)	Autosomal recessive	Uroporphyrinogen III cosynthetase
Erythropoietic protoporphyria*	Autosomal dominant	Ferrochelatase

* A homozygous variant has been described (see text).

During acute attacks, severe hyponatraemia may become alarming: many mechanisms have been suggested, such as gastrointestinal loss of sodium, imprudent fluid therapy, inappropriate ADH secretion, or sodium-losing nephropathy possibly related to a toxic effect of δ-aminolaevulinic acid (**ALA**).

It is often very hard for even a well-trained physician to distinguish acute intermittent porphyria from hereditary coproporphyria or variegate porphyria. Sometimes, in the variegate type, neuropsychiatric and cutaneous lesions (similar to those of porphyria cutanea tarda) occur simultaneously and the diagnosis is easy, because in acute intermittent porphyria there are no cutaneous lesions. However, cutaneous lesions may precede or follow the acute attacks in variegate porphyria and it is then confused with porphyria cutanea tarda. In hereditary coproporphyria, cutaneous lesions (similar to those of porphyria cutanea or milder) are rarer than in variegate porphyria; usually hereditary coproporphyria is not distinguishable clinically from acute intermittent porphyria. Often only biochemical data allow precise diagnosis of the type of acute hepatic porphyria.

Classical biochemical features

An increase in the intracellular concentration of the substrate of each defective enzyme gives rise to a characteristic pattern of tissue accumulation and excretion of haem precursors. Table 2 summarizes these patterns.

Acute intermittent porphyria

During acute attacks, patients with acute intermittent porphyria excrete large amounts of porphobilinogen and ALA (20–200-fold more than normal). Uro- and coproporphyrin are usually moderately increased (uroporphyrin is often the result of a non-enzymatic reaction favoured by light and/or heat). High concentrations of precursors (mostly porphobilinogen) are an important diagnostic feature; urinary porphyrin can be increased in several other conditions and therefore lacks diagnostic specificity.

About one-third of clinically asymptomatic carriers excrete abnormal amounts of porphobilinogen (two- to fivefold above normal); others show normal excretion of this precursor.

Stool porphyrins are normal or moderately increased in this porphyria. Excess porphobilinogen and ALA has been found in liver and kidney after death. During an acute attack, concentrations of porphobilinogen are much higher in plasma than are those of ALA.

Hereditary coproporphyria

During acute attacks of hereditary coproporphyria the profile of urine porphyrins and precursors is similar to that in acute intermittent porphyria, although coproporphyrin is sometimes dramatically increased. Examination of stool porphyrins usually allows the type of porphyria to be established, the characteristic

Table 2 Acute hepatic porphyrias: biochemical features

	Urine			Faeces		
	Precursors	Uroporphyrin	Coproporphyrin	Uroporphyrin	Coproporphyrin	Protoporphyrin
Acute intermittent porphyria	1 +++	++	++	++	+	
	2 ++		±			
Hereditary coproporphyria	1 +++	++	+++	++	++++	+
	2 +		+		+++	
Variegate porphyria	1 +++	++	+++	+	++	+++
	2 +		+		+	++

1 = during attack, 2 = during remission.

abnormality being a huge excess of coproporphyrin compared with normal protoporphyrin. Some 20 to 30 per cent of asymptomatic carriers show this typical faecal profile (and often a normal urinary profile) after puberty.

Variegate porphyria

During acute attacks of variegate porphyria the urinary findings are identical to those in acute intermittent porphyria and hereditary coproporphyria. Carriers with only chronic cutaneous manifestations or even those without symptoms often show a slight increase of precursors.

The characteristic finding is elevated faecal protoporphyrin and to a lesser degree (at least when measurement is carried out using the differential extraction method) coproporphyrin; high-performance liquid chromatography of faecal porphyrins usually shows only an isolated peak of protoporphyrin. A heterogeneous group of porphyrin-peptide conjugates called X porphyrins (ether-insoluble porphyrins) is also increased in variegate porphyria. A plasma fluorescence emission maximal at 626 nm has been described as a diagnostic marker for this type.

Doss porphyria (ALA-dehydrase deficiency)

Doss et al. (KlinWschr, 1979; 57:1123) described two young adults with a new acute hepatic porphyria, characterized by hugely increased excretion of ALA and coproporphyrin (mainly isomer type III) in urine. Porphobilinogen was only moderately elevated; faecal excretion of porphyrins was normal, but erythrocyte protoporphyrin was slightly increased (three times normal). Thunell (JClin-ChemClinBioch, 1987; 25:5) has also described a case of this new porphyria; the only differences were the age of the patient (a very young child with several attacks including nervous palsy during the first 2 years of life) and a moderate increase of faecal porphyrins (mainly harderoporphyrin, i.e., a tricarboxyporphyrin, which is an intermediate step between coproporphyrin and protoporphyrin). In Doss porphyria, the pattern of overproduction of haem precursors closely resembles that of severe lead poisoning. However, certain features allow rejection of this diagnosis: these include normal urinary and blood concentrations of lead, or the activity of ALA dehydrase, which is not restored by dithiothreitol.

Enzymatic abnormalities and genetic defects (Fig. 1)

Increased hepatic ALA synthase activity is described during acute attacks in patients with acute intermittent porphyria, hereditary coproporphyria, and variegate porphyria. It was initially postulated that induction of ALA synthase might represent the primary enzyme abnormality in all these diseases, notwithstanding the differences between patterns of porphyrin excretion (or the absence of cutaneous features in acute intermittent porphyria, compared with variegate porphyria or hereditary coproporphyria). As will be discussed later in connection with the mechanism of acute attacks, it is now accepted that the induction of ALA synthase is a secondary phenomenon; it is the result of exposure to several factors (such as drugs, hormones) that act on an enzyme more or less derepressed by haem deficiency. Haem deficiency itself is the consequence of an enzyme defect specific for each porphyria.

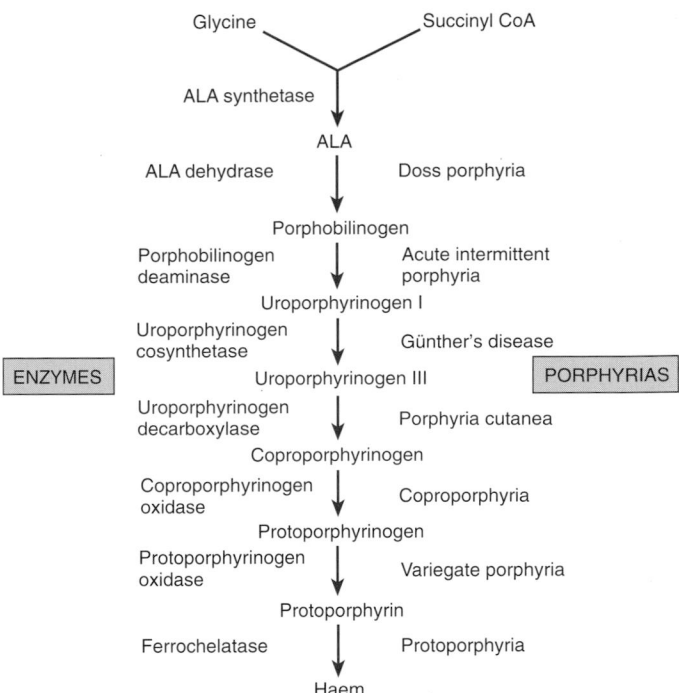

Fig. 1. Inherited enzyme deficiencies in the porphyrias.

Acute intermittent porphyria

Porphobilinogen deaminase deficiency (50 per cent of normal activity) has been demonstrated in all tissues examined. Measurement in erythrocytes is now widely used, not only to confirm the type of porphyria but also to detect clinically latent individuals, who often do not show evidence of overproduction of haem precursors (Fig. 2).

The genetic heterogeneity of acute intermittent porphyria is well known. Mustajoki (AnnIntMed, 1981; 95:162) and later Wilson (NethJMed, 1986; 29:393) describe families that each contain individuals with the usual phenotypic expression of the disease but with normal activity of porphobilinogen deaminase in erythrocytes.

More recently, it has been shown (Grandchamp, EurJBioch, 1987; 162:105) that porphobilinogen deaminase from human non-erythropoietic sources (i.e., liver, lymphocytes) differs in molecular mass (39 220 Da) from its erythropoietic counterpart (37 627 Da). The protein sequence of both isoforms is identical, except for an additional stretch of 17 amino acids at the NH₂ terminus of the non-erythropoietic enzyme. This difference is due to the existence of two distinct, tissue-specific mRNAs differing by their 5′ extremity: both mRNAs are generated from a single gene through alternative splicing of two primary transcripts arising from two promoters separated by 3 kb. If, as in some families with acute intermittent porphyria, the porphobilinogen deaminase deficiency appeared to be restricted to non-erythropoietic tissues, it seemed logical to look for a molecular defect lying within sequences of the porphobilinogen deaminase gene that are specifically expressed in non-erythropoietic cells. Grandchamp et al. (PNAS, 1989; 86: 661) investigated one Dutch family with this subtype of acute intermittent porphyria. Using the recently described restriction fragment length polymorphisms of the human porphobilinogen deaminase gene they found a strong linkage (Lod score 3.2) between one haplotype and the phenotype for acute intermittent porphyria.

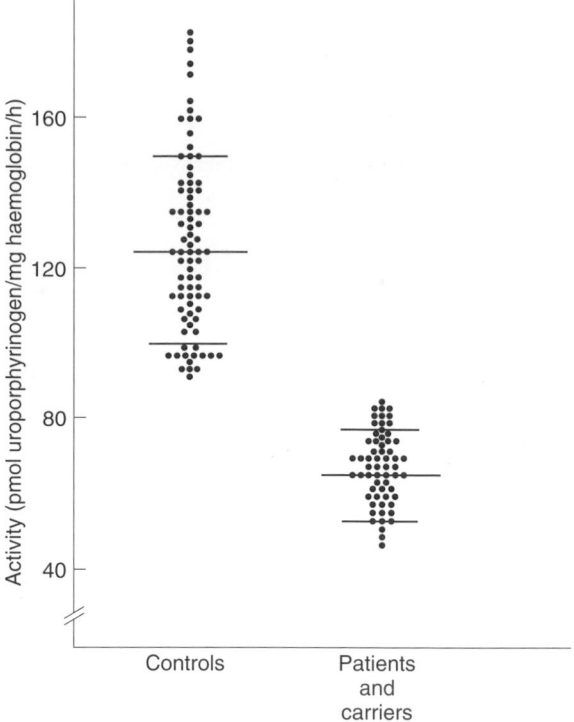

Fig. 2. Erythrocyte porphobilinogen deaminase activity in acute intermittent porphyria.

This finding suggested that the mutation lay within the gene and involved its non-erythropoietic-specific sequence, remembering that the porphobilinogen deaminase activity of these patients' erythrocytes was normal. Cloning and sequencing of the non-erythropoietic part of the porphobilinogen deaminase gene from an affected individual revealed a G → A transition at the first position of the first intron. Similar mutations had been shown to abolish normal splicing completely. Normal porphobilinogen deaminase activity is expected in these patients' erythrocytes, since transcription in erythropoietic cells starts 2.8 kb downstream from the identified mutation.

The other acute intermittent porphyrias (and later, porphobilinogen deaminase gene mutations) were initially classified according to the cross-reacting immunological material (**CRIM**) status of the patients. In the CRIM-positive subtypes (about 15 per cent of patients) the heterogeneity of the mutation is rather limited: several patients (around 75 per cent) have mutations that lead to replacement of either of two conserved arginine residues in exon 10 by glutamine or tryptophan (many of the substitutions occur at sites that are generally well conserved as polar residues close to the active site).

The most common subtype (CRIM-negative) is much more heterogeneous: the base substitutions, insertions or deletions have been found in only one or two families (see Table 3); however, in Sweden and in Holland a few mutations were found with a high prevalence, suggesting a founder effect (Elder, JClinPath, 1993; 46: 977; Lee, PNAS, 1991; 88: 10 912).

Over the past 50 years, only three unrelated homozygous cases of acute intermittent porphyria have been described. Most of the children were severely ill (neurological defects, cataract, psychomotor retardation): the first two cases reported were both compound heterozygotes for three of the CRIM-positive, exon 10 mutations (Picat, JInherMetDis, 1990; 13:684; Llewellyn, HumGenet, 1992; 89:97); the third one was homozygous for one of these mutations (arginine replaced by a tryptophan).

Hereditary coproporphyria

In coproporphyria, coproporphyrinogen oxidase is decreased to around 50 per cent of normal in liver, fibroblasts, lymphocytes, and leucocytes. Two different types of homozygous cases have been described, both with a deficiency of coproporphyrinogen oxidase activity to about 90 per cent of normal. In the first type, the patient was very small (height 140 cm at 20 years), showed skin photosensitivity, and had had several acute attacks since the age of 5 years. Her faeces and urine contained a huge amount of coproporphyrin. The residual lymphocyte coproporphyrinogen oxidase showed a normal K_m for coproporphyrinogen and normal thermosensitivity (Grandchamp, Lancet, 1977; i:1348). The other type of homozygous coproporphyria was found in children with intense jaundice and haemolytic anaemia at birth (Nordmann, JCI, 1983; 72:1139). The pattern of faecal porphyrin excretion was atypical for coproporphyria because the major porphyrin was harderoporphyrin (> 60 per cent; normal < 20 per cent): this variant was called 'harderoporphyria'. Harderoporphyrin is the natural intermediate between copro- and protoporphyrinogen. Kinetic variables of coproporphyrinogen oxidase were clearly modified, with a K_m 15 times normal and a maximal velocity of half normal; a marked sensitivity to thermal denaturation was also observed. The distinct difference between the mutations again underlines the heterogeneity among these inherited diseases.

The recent cloning of human cDNAs and of the gene encoding coproporphyrinogen oxidase permitted deduction of the primary structure of the protein and elucidation of the molecular basis of hereditary coproporphyria, not only in the homozygous cases described above but also in some usual heterozygous cases. All the known mutations were searched for and not detected in other patients with coproporphyria, suggesting that there is a high degree of allelic heterogeneity, as has been documented in other porphyrias (Grandchamp, JBioenergBiomembr, 1995; 27:215).

Variegate porphyria

Several studies have shown a 50 per cent deficiency in the activity of protoporphyrinogen oxidase in variegate porphyria; data from homozygous cases (see below) with more than 90 per cent deficiency of protoporphyrinogen oxidase show that the mutation depends on the protoporphyrinogen oxidase gene.

Four homozygous cases of variegate porphyria have been described. All had severe, life-long photosensitivity, a more or less decreased growth rate, and an increased erythrocyte protoporphyrin. Both patients of Kordac et al. (Lancet, 1984; i:851) showed neurological symptoms; onset was in childhood in all cases. All the parents were apparently healthy in spite of a 50 per cent decrease of protoporphyrinogen oxidase. The mechanism underlying the accumulation of protoporphyrin in the red cells of these patients is still unexplained, but it seems to be common to all homozygous cases of hepatic porphyrias.

Table 3 Mutations in the *PBGD* gene

	Position	Mutation	Sequence modification
Exon 1	3	ATG→ATA	Initiation codon:translation impairment
	33	GCG→GCT	SD
Intron 1	33+1	gtg→atg	SD
	33+3	gtg→atg	SD
Exon 3	64	CGC→TGC	R22C
	76	CGC→TGC	R26C
	77	CGC→CAC	R26H
	86	CAG→CTG	Q29L
Exon 4	91	CGCT→CACT	A31T
	97	Del A	Frameshift (stop→cod+10)
	100	CAG→AAG	Q34K
	100	CAG→TAG	Q34X
Exon 5	163	GCT→TCT	A55S
	168–169	Del GT	Frameshift (stop→cod+9)
	174	Del C	Frameshift (stop→cod+40)
	182	Ins G	Frameshift (stop→cod+5)
Intron 5	210+1	gta→ata	SD (Del exon 5)
Exon 6	218–219	Del AG	Frameshift (stop→cod+9)
Exon 7	277	GTT→TTT	V93F
	287	TCC→TTC	S96F
	293	AAG→AGG	K98R
	314	Ins C	Frameshift (stop→cod+16)
	295	GAC→CAC	D99H
	331	CGGA→CAGA	G111R
Intron 7	345−1	cag→caa	SA (Del exon 8)
Exon 8	346	CGG→TGG	R116W
	347	CGG→CAG	R116Q
	417	Ins CA	Frameshift
Exon 9	445	CGA→TGA	R149X
	446	CGA→CAA	R149Q
	446	CGA→CTA	R149L
	463	CAG→TAG	Q155X
	470	Ins A	Frameshift (stop→cod+37)
Intron 9	499−1	cag→caa	SA (Del exon 10)
Exon 10	499	CGG→TGG	R167W
	500	CGG→CAG	R167Q
	517	CGG→TGG	R173W
	518	CGG→CAG	R173Q
	530	CTG→CGG	L177R
	583	GCGC→TGC	R195C
	593	TGG→TAG	W198X
	601	CGG→TGG	R201W
	604	Del G	Frameshift (stop→cod+53)
	610	CAG→TAG	Q204X
	612	CAG→CAT	SD (Del 9 bp exon 10)
Exon 11	625	GAG→AAG	E209K
Intron 11	652−3	cag→gag	SA (Del exon 12)
Exon 12	664	CGTG→ATG	V222M
	667	GAA→AAA	E223K
	673	CGA→GGA	R225G
	673	CGA→TGA	R225X
	713	CTG→CGG	L238R
	730–731	Del CT	Frameshift (stop→cod+6)
	734	CTT→CGT	L245R
	739	TGC→CGC	C247R
	740	TGC→TTC	C247F
	742	s 8 bp: (TTCGCTG)	Frameshift (stop→cod+10)
	748	GAA→AAA	E250K
	754	GCC→ACC	A252T
	755	GCC→GTC	A252V
	766	CAC→AAC	H256N
	771	CTG→CTA	SD (Del exon 12)
	771	CTG→CTC	SD (Del exon 12)
Exon 13	806	ACA→ATA	T269I
	820	GGG→AGG	G274R
Intron 13	825+1	gta→ata	SD (Del exon 13)
	826−2	cag→cgg	SA (Del exon 14)

Table 3 continued

	Position	Mutation	Sequence modification
Exon 14	833	CTG→CCG	L278P
	838	GGA→AGA	G280R
	848	TGG→TAG	W283X
	849	TGG→TGA	W283X
	886	CAG→TAG	Q296X
	900	Del T	Frameshift (stop→cod+15)
Intron 14	912+1	gta→ata	SD (Del exon 14)
Exon 15	973	CGA→TGA	R325X
	1062	Ins C	Frameshift (stop→cod+4)
	1073	Del A	Frameshift

R. Enz., restriction enzyme (mutation-specific); SD, splice donor-site mutation; SA, splice acceptor-site mutation.
Del, deletion; ins, insertion; (stop→cod+X): stop codon occurs X codons downstream, mutated bases are in bold.
Mutations occurring at CpG dinucleotide are underlined.

Other variants have been described, such as 'dual' porphyrias: some workers have found cases of variegate porphyria and of porphyria cutanea, or cases of acute intermittent porphyria in the same family; further studies are clearly needed to confirm these data.

Recently, human cDNA encoding protoporphyrinogen oxidase has been sequenced (Nishimura, JBC, 1995; 270:8076) and this human gene has been cloned and assigned to chromosome 1 (Taketani, Genomics, 1995; 29:698; Roberts, HumMolGenet, 1995; 4: 2387) in contrast to a previous report on chromosome 14 (Bissport, HumGenet, 1988; 79:289). Deybach *et al.* (HumMolGenet, 1996; 5:407) described the first mutations in patients with variegate porphyria and supported the conclusion that protoporphyrinogen oxidase gene defects are disease-causing mutations in human variegate porphyria.

Doss porphyria

This porphyria has an autosomal-recessive pattern of inheritance and ALA dehydrase activity is dramatically decreased in erythrocytes and bone marrow cells, as would be expected for homozygotes (1 per cent of mean control values), with a decrease of approximately 50 per cent from the activities found in parents. The same decrease was also found in erythrocytes of a heterozygous case (Bird, AmJHumGen, 1979; 31:662). All cases of Doss porphyria have been CRIM-positive, suggesting that there is a structural mutation in a coding sequence of the ALA dehydrase gene (de Verneuil, HumGenet, 1985; 69:175).

The human ALA dehydratase gene (located on chromosome 9) contains two promoter regions that generate housekeeping and erythroid-specific transcripts by alternative splicing (Kaya, Genomics, 1994; 19:242), analogous to the expression of the human porphobilinogen deaminase. The molecular nature of the lesions causing severe ALA dehydratase deficiency were recently described (Plewinska, AmJHumGen, 1991; 49:167; Ishida, JCI, 1992; 89: 1431): most of the patients were compound heterozygotes for four different missense mutations in the ALA dehydrase gene.

Prevalence of acute hepatic porphyrias

The high incidence of latent cases of acute intermittent porphyria, hereditary coproporphyria, and variegate porphyria gives a very rough approximation of the prevalence of these autosomal-dominant diseases. Most of the estimates of acute intermittent porphyria were established by screening populations for urinary porphyrin precursors and are therefore underestimates; they ranged from 1 to 8 per 100 000. The incidence of variegate porphyria in South Africa (3/1000) is higher than elsewhere; in Finland, it is 1.3/100 000. The estimated incidence of hereditary coproporphyria is 2/million. Tishler *et al.* (AmJPsychiat, 1985; 142:1430) measured porphobilinogen deaminase activity in a psychiatric patient population and found an overall prevalence of 2 per cent. Recently, an epidemiological study of a healthy population was made in France (Paris): erythrocyte porphobilinogen deaminase activity was measured in blood samples of 3305 blood donors; when the enzyme deficiency was confirmed, other members of the family were also tested and the type of mutation was studied using molecular biological techniques. Two individuals were found to be carriers of the acute intermittent porphyria trait (prevalence 0.06 per cent); each of these asymptomatic carriers has a specific mutation of the porphobilinogen deaminase gene. Similar results (prevalence 2 per cent) have also been obtained in Finland (Mustajoki, JIntMed, 1992; 231:389; Nordmann, JIntMed, 1997;242:213).

The onset of all acute porphyrias is usually delayed until after infancy, except in homozygous cases. Furthermore, at least 80 per cent of individuals who inherit a gene for one of the autosomal-dominant porphyrias probably remain asymptomatic throughout life; 66 per cent of latent porphyrics have normal precursors and excretion of porphyrins (almost 100 per cent before puberty). Among 301 acute attacks studied in our laboratory, 200 (66 per cent) were acute intermittent porphyria, 41 (14 per cent) hereditary coproporphyria, and 60 (20 per cent) variegate porphyria. In acute intermittent porphyria, acute attacks are more common in women than in men; the important role of endocrine factors will be discussed later.

Pathogenesis of the acute attack
Neuropathy[6]

It is generally accepted that the symptoms of acute attacks of porphyria are due to the effect of the disease on the nervous system. There are excellent reviews on this subject, describing histological changes in peripheral and autonomic nerves as well as changes in central nervous system or electrodiagnostic findings.[1-6] Several hypotheses for the precise mechanism of the neurological lesions have been put forward and two are presently favoured: one involves the deficiency of haem synthesis in neural tissues; the other involves the neurotoxicity of the precursors of haem, chiefly ALA (mainly synthesized in the liver).

The second hypothesis is more favoured for the following reasons. Symptoms of acute attacks never occur when excretion of porphyrin precursors is normal. Typical neurological manifestations have been observed in patients who overproduce ALA but not porphobilinogen, such as in Doss porphyria, lead intoxication, or tyrosinaemia. Unfortunately, the results of *in vivo* or *in vitro* experimental assays of ALA toxicity are unimpressive, mostly because variables such as species used or ALA concentration differ too greatly from the human case.

Precipitating factors

Individuals with latent or clinically expressed acute porphyria may be precipitated into an acute attack by several factors such as steroid sex hormones, drugs, alcohol, stress, infectious diseases, and dieting. Only drugs and steroid sex hormones will be discussed here.

Endocrine

The major role of endocrine factors is very well known: 80 per cent of patients with acute attacks are women between puberty and the menopause, and the attacks occur especially during the week preceding the menses; synthetic oestrogens and progesterone of oral contraceptives have been clearly implicated in inducing acute attacks. Surprisingly, most women with acute porphyria have a normal gestation when untreated with porphyrinogenic drugs; however, mild attacks have been observed in early pregnancy. The 5β epimers are more porphyrinogenic than the 5α epimers. There is an impaired (and acquired) reduction of 5α steroid hormones in the group of patients with clinical expression of the disorder.

Drugs[2,7,8]

Before describing the role of drugs as precipitating factors, it is useful to consider the regulation of the haem biosynthesis pathway. The rate of flux through the pathway is under the control of its end-product, haem, which exerts a negative feedback effect on the limiting enzyme, ALA synthetase.

The haem concentration of the so-called regulatory haem pool may decrease as a result of (a) increased breakdown, (b) decreased production, or (c) increased utilization. Impaired haem synthesis may occur when the activity of one of the enzymes along the pathway is decreased either genetically (in the porphyrias) or by external factors (e.g. lead intoxication); the partial defect in haem synthesis in acute hepatic porphyrias results in increased ALA synthetase activity. The resulting increase in porphobilinogen production may be sufficient to compensate for the defect in haem synthesis. Such compensation may explain the situation in patients with 'latent' porphyria. Drugs may upset this balance at several stages.

A very few chemicals are known to be porphyrinogenic in normal individuals. Allyl-containing acetamides (e.g. allylisopropylacetamide) cause massive degradation of the haem moiety of cytochrome P450 and a resulting disturbance of haem synthesis.

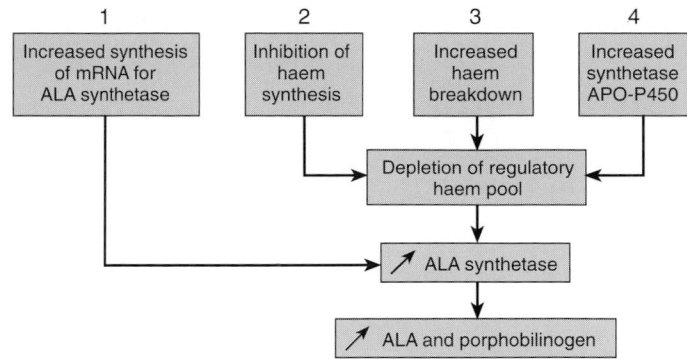

Fig. 3. Mechanisms by which a drug may reduce the feedback control exercised by haem at the level of ALA synthetase (in hepatocyte). Depletion of the regulatory haem pool is the main point.

Diethoxydicarbethoxycollidine and griseofulvin both decrease haem synthesis through specific inhibition of ferrochelatase. Hexachlorobenzene, well known for its role in epidemic porphyria cutanea tarda in Turkey, inhibits uroporphyrinogen decarboxylase. However, numerous drugs, such as barbiturates and sulphonamides, are porphyrinogenic only if a genetic (or acquired) defect in porphyrin metabolism is already present. The heterogeneity of these compounds should be emphasized, since they share few chemical features apart from lipid solubility. There is evidence that lipid-soluble drugs induce a further depletion of the hepatic haem pool by stimulating synthesis of cytochrome P450 apoprotein, thereby increasing the demand for haem from a pathway whose capacity is already limited by the inherited enzymatic defect. Different ways of stimulating ALA and porphobilinogen accumulation are summarized in Fig. 3.

Drugs that are unable to induce the enzymes of the haem biosynthesis pathway should be selected for the treatment of porphyric individuals. This is generally achieved through the prior testing of drugs in animal models either *in vivo* (rats, mice, chicken embryos) or *in vitro* (chick embryo liver cells in culture).

Observed inducing effects of drugs on haem synthesis are usually followed by measurements of ALA synthetase activity, concentrations of porphyrins, and/or cytochrome P450. In the most sensitive models, partial blocks in the haem pathway are first produced by appropriate chemical means in order to mimic the hereditary enzymatic defects found in hepatic porphyrias: for instance, diethoxydicarbethoxycollidine produces a rapid and effective inhibition of ferrochelatase activity. The use of a small 'priming' dose of diethoxydicarbethoxycollidine in the chick embryo *in ovo* allows testing of porphyrinogenicity under the conditions of an experimental block in haem synthesis (i.e., a porphyria-like situation) and simplifies drug testing. As a high correlation was found between ALA synthetase induction and liver porphyrins, the accumulation-inducing effects of drugs can be detected only by measurement of the accumulation of liver porphyrins.

Because of its good predictive value and ease of handling, we have used the diethoxydicarbethoxycollidine-primed chick embryo system to test a large number of drugs. For easier clinical use the drugs have been classified as non-porphyrinogenic (safe) and porphyrinogenic (unsafe) (Table 4). These drugs are in addition

Table 4 Drug porphyrinogenicity (DDC-primed chicken embryo liver system *in ovo*)

Non-porphyrinogenic		Porphyrinogenic	
Acetylsalicylic acid	Ciprofloxacin	Mefenamic acid	Danazol
Clavulanic acid	Cisapride	Nalidixic acid	Dapsone
Fusidic acid	Clarythromycin	Pipemidic acid	Dexfenfluramine
Niflumic acid	Clidinium	Priomidic acid	Dextromoramide
Oxolinic acid	Clobenzorex	Acitretine	Dextropropoxyphene
Tiaprofenic acid	Clomipramine	Alcool	Diazepam
Tienilic acid	Clonazepam	Alizapride	Dihydralazine
Tranexamiic acid	Clozapine	Allopurinol	Dimenhydrinate
Acamprosate	Codeine	Alminoprofen	Disopyramide
Acebutolol	*Corticoids*	Alprazolam	Dosulepine
Acetazolamide	Cyamemazine	Alverine	Doxepin
Aciclovir	Cyproheptadine	Amidopyrine	Econazole
ACTH	Dexchlorpheniramine	Amineptine	Enalapril
Adrenaline	Diacerein	Amiodarone	Enflurane
Alfentanil	Diazoxide	Amisulpride	*Ergotamine* (+derivatives)
Alfuzosine	Dibekacine	Amobarbital	Erythromycin
Alimemazine	Diclofenac	*Androgens*	Etamsylate
Amfepramone	Diflunisal	Articaine	Ethenzamide
Amiloride	Digitoxin	Astemizole	Ethosuximide
Amitriptyline	Digoxin	Baclofen	Etidocaine
Amlodipine	Diltiazem	*Barbiturates*	Etomidate
Amoxapine	Diphenhydramine	Benfluorex	Famotidine
Amoxicillin	Diphenoxylate	Benzbromarone	Fenfluramine
Amphotericin B	Dipyridamole	Benzylthiouracil	Fenofibrate
Aptocaine	Dobutamine	Bepridil	Fenoprofen
Atenolol	Domperidone	β-histine	Fenoverine
Atracurium	Doxorubicin	Biperidene	Fenspiride
Atropine	Doxycycline	Bisoprolol	Floctafenine
Azathioprine	Doxylamine	Bromocriptine	Fluconazole
β-Alanine	Droperidol	Bupivacaine	Flumequine
Betaxolol	EDTA	Busipirone	Flunarizine
Bezafibrate	Enoxacin	Captopril	Flurbiprofen
Bleomycin	Estazolam	Carbamazepine	Fluvoxamine
Bromazepam	Ethambutol	Cefaclor	Gemfibrozil
Bromure	Ether	Cefuroxime	Griseofulvin
Buflomedil	Etidronate	Chloramphenicol	Halofantrine
Buprenorphine	Fentanyl	Chlormezanone	Halothane
Butacaine	Ferrous*	Chloroquine*	Hydantoins
Butylhyoscine	Finasteride	Cibenzoline	Hydralazine
Carbimazole	Flecainide	Cicletanine	Hydroxyzine
Carpipramine	Flucytosine	Ciprofibrate	Ibuprofen
Cefixime	Flumazenil	Clobazam	Ifosfamide
Cefotaxime	Flunitrazepam	Clofibrate	*MOAI*
Celiprolol	Fluorouracil	Clomethiazole	Isoniazid
Cetirizine	Fluoxetine	Clomifene	Isradipine
Chloral hydrate	Fluphenazine	Clonidine	Ketamine
Chlordiazepoxide	Flutamide	Clorazepate	Ketoconazole
Chlorpromazine	Fosfomycin	Clotiazepam	Lignocaine
Cyclosporin	Frusemide	Cyclophosphamide	Loflazepate
Cimetidine	Gallamine	Cyproterone	Loprazolam

to those already well known as inducers, such as barbiturates, sulphonamides, or antiepileptic drugs.

The danger for porphyric patients of any untested medication is obvious and cannot be easily predicted. Clinicians must base their treatment of affected individuals on drugs whose porphyrinogenicity has been established in several ways on different animal models. At the time of writing, all drugs clearly involved in the induction of acute attacks in humans were porphyrinogenic in the chicken embryo system *in ovo*.

Treatment of acute attacks

Before the so-called 'specific' therapies (acting on the biosynthetic pathway) are discussed, a few general points must be made. As soon as an attack has been diagnosed, a careful search should be made for any precipitating factor, especially drugs (including oral contraceptives), underlying infection, and hypocaloric diet. Agitation and other psychiatric manifestations are usually controlled with chlorpromazine. Treatment of severe pain requires morphine-like drugs such as pethidine, but the danger of addiction (in patients who experience frequent attacks) must always be remembered. We usually combine chlorpromazine with pethidine and keep the patient in a quiet room.

Specific therapies are now superseded by glucose and haematin: the 'glucose effect' frequently leads to a reduction in excretion of urinary porphyrin precursors by a mechanism that is not certain. It is well known that poor carbohydrate intake aggravates the attack

Table 4 continued

Non-porphyrinogenic		Porphyrinogenic	
Gancyclovir	Oxybate (sodium)	Loxapine	Tetrazepam
Gentamicin	Oxybuprocaine	Mebeverine	Theophylline
Glafenine	Oxytocin	Medifoxamine	Thioridazine
Glucagon	Pancuronium	Mefloquine*	Tiadenol
Granisetron	Paroxetine	Mephenesine	Tiapride
Guanethidine	Pefloxacin	Mepivacaine	Ticlopidine
Guanfacine	Penicillin	Meprobamate	Tilbroquinol
Haloperidol	Perhexiline	Methyldopa	Tiliquinol
Heparin	Perindopril	Methylergometrine	Tinidazole
Heptaminol	Perphenazine	Metronidazole	Tolbutamide
Hydrochlorothiazide	Pethidine	Mexiletine	Toloxatone
Imipramine	Phenoperidine	Mianserine	Trazodone
Indomethacin	Phloroglucinol	Miconazole	Triazolam
Indoramine	Pinaverium	Moclobemide	Trimethadione
Insulin	Pipotiazine	Nifedipine	Trimipramine
Isosorbide	Piracetam	Nitrazepam	Tritoqualine
Josamycine	Piroxicam	Nitrendipine	Urapidil
Ketoprofen	Pivampicillin	Nizatidine	Valproate (sodium)
Ketotifen	Pizotifen	Noramydopyrine	Valpromide
Labetalol	Prazosin	Nordazepam	Veralipride
Latamoxef	Prifinium	*Oestrogens*	Vigabatrin
Levomepromazine	Probucol	*Oestro-progestatives*	Viloxazine
Lisinopril	Procaine	Ornidazole	Vinburnine
Loperamide	Promethazine	Oxetorone	Zolpidem
Loratadine	Propericiazine	Oxybutynine	
Lorazepam	Propofol	Paracetamol	
Maprotiline	Propranolol	Pentamidine	
Meclofenoxate	Proxymetacaine	Pentazocine	
Melatonin	*Pygenum Africanum*	Pentoxifylline	
Mequitazine	Pyrimethamine	Periciazine	
Mesna	Reserpine	Phenacetine	
Metformin	Rifampicin	Phenazone	
Methotrexate	Salbutamol	Phenobarbital	
Metoclopramide	Selegiline	Phenylbutazone	
Metopimazine	Sennoside	Phenytoin	
Metoprolol	*Serenoa repens*	Pipamperone	
Midazolam	Sulbutiamine	Piribedil	
Minaprine	Sulindac	Pravastatine	
Minocycline	Teicoplanin	Prazepam	
Minoxidil	Tenoxicam	Prilocaine	
Misoprostol	Terbutaline	Primidone	
Molsidomine	Terfenadine	Probenecide	
Morphine	Tetracaine	Progabide	
Moxisylyte	Thiocolchicoside	*Progestins (and progesterone)*	
Naftazone	Thioproperazine	Propafenone	
Naftidrofuryl	Thyroxine	Propantheline	
Nalbuphine	Tianeptine	Pyrazinamide	
Naloxone	Timolol	Pyrrocaine	
Naproxen	α-Tocopherol	Quinapril	
Nefopam	Triamterene	*Quinine* (+derivatives)	
Netilmicin	Trihexyphenidyl	Ramipril	
Nicardipine	Trimebutine	Ranitidine	
Nicergoline	Trimetazidine	Rilmenidine	
Nifuroxazide	Trinitrine	Roxithromycin	
Nilutamide	Tropatepine	Simvastatin	
Nitroprussiate	*Vaccines*	Sotalol	
Noradrenaline	Vancomycin	Spironolactone	
Norfloxacine	Vecuronium (bromide)	*Succinimides*	
Nystatin	Verapamil	*Sulphamides*	
Ofloxacine	*Vitamins*	Sulpiride	
Omeprazole	Yohimbine	Sultopride	
Ondansetron	Zopiclone	Sumatriptan	
Organon		Tamoxifen	
Oxazepam		Terbinafine	

* Allowed at low doses in the treatment of porphyria cutanea tarda.
DDC, diethoxycarbethoxycollidine.

and an adequate supplement (300–400 g/day) should be administered, usually by slow intravenous perfusion.

Treatment of a porphyric attack has been greatly improved by the introduction of haematin. Earlier observations showed its superiority over glucose: most patients responded favourably to haematin, whereas many were recalcitrant to glucose. Haematin is given intravenously in doses up to 3 to 4 mg/kg body wt per 24 h, usually over 4 days. Haem gains access to the hepatocyte and probably replenishes the depleted haem pool; urinary ALA (and porphobilinogen) decreases dramatically in 2 to 3 days, showing that feedback control of ALA synthase has become efficient. Side-effects of haematin, such as coagulopathy or phlebitis, have never been associated with real haemorrhage; however, haematin should not be used in conjunction with anticoagulant therapy, and it is necessary to change the vein for infusion each day. Stable preparations of haematin are now available (e.g. Haem-arginate, Medica, Finland) and side-effects have been practically excluded. All the types of treatment described must be used early in the attack, before any nervous or respiratory complication develops, or a biochemical response without concomitant clinical benefit may occur.

Porphyria cutanea symptomatica (syn: porphyria cutanea tarda) and hepatoerythropoietic porphyria
Porphyria cutanea symptomatica

Porphyria cutanea symptomatica is the most common form of porphyria. Cutaneous photosensitivity is the predominating clinical feature; acute attacks with abdominal pain, psychiatric and/or neurological manifestations are never observed. Porphyria cutanea symptomatica is a heterogeneous group including at least two types.

1. The sporadic type (or type I) more often observed in male patients (aged 40–50 years) without a family history of the disease; its development appears related to some inducing compound such as alcohol.
2. The familial type (less common) has an earlier onset (sometimes before puberty) and is observed equally in both sexes; other members of the kindred may have overt porphyria cutanea symptomatica.

In the sporadic type, uroporphyrinogen decarboxylase activity is deficient only in liver (50 per cent reduction); in familial porphyria cutanea symptomatica there is a 50 per cent reduction of activity in all tissues and this defect is inherited in an autosomal-dominant pattern.

The incidence of porphyria cutanea symptomatica is uncertain: it has been found in all parts of the world, with perhaps a higher frequency among the Bantu in South Africa. Our records show that among 681 patients, 576 (85 per cent) have a sporadic type and 105 (15 per cent) a familial type with a 50 per cent decrease of uroporphyrinogen decarboxylase activity in erythrocytes. In the United States the familial type seems more prevalent.

Clinical features

The lesions of photosensitivity affect areas exposed to light, such as the backs of the hands, the face, neck and also in women the legs and backs of the feet. Skin fragility is perhaps the most specific feature: minimal injury is followed by a superficial erosion soon covered by a crust. Bullae or vesicles usually appear after exposure to sun and take several weeks to heal, leaving hypo- or hyperpigmented atrophic scars. White papules (milia) may develop in areas of bullae, particularly on the backs of the hands. Hypertrichosis is often found in the upper part of the cheeks (malar area) and sometimes also in ears and arms. Increased uniform pigmentation of sun-exposed areas is common. Alopecia and hypopigmented, scleroderma-like lesions of the skin are less common. All these skin lesions are similar to those seen in variegate porphyria and hereditary coproporphyria.

Variable degrees of liver dysfunction are common among patients with porphyria cutanea symptomatica, particularly in association with excessive alcoholic intake. However, it is unclear to what extent liver cell injury is important in the expression of the syndrome. It is well known that in patients with typical cirrhosis, porphyria cutanea symptomatica is very rare; in patients with porphyria cutanea symptomatica there could be an underlying constitutional abnormality that may predispose the liver to the development of porphyria cutanea symptomatica (Taddeini, SemHemat, 1968; 5: 335). Needle-like inclusions have been found in the cytoplasm of hepatocytes; these are probably composed of uroporphyrin, which could promote progressive liver damage.

The incidence of hepatic cancer among patients with porphyria cutanea symptomatica seems to be greater than in the general population, but published results differ greatly, from 47 per cent in a Czechoslovakian series (Kordac, Neoplasma, 1972; 19:135) to none in an Italian series (Topi, BrJDermatol, 1984; 111:75).

Precipitating factors

Among the possible precipitating factors, alcohol, oestrogens, iron, and hepatitis C virus are most frequently incriminated. Although consumption of alcohol is often acknowledged, the mechanisms by which it exacerbates the disease are unclear: uroporphyrinogen decarboxylase and ALA dehydrase are decreased by alcohol, whereas ALA synthase is stimulated in the patients' livers. Ethanol increases cytochrome P450, and also the higher-chain (three to five carbon atoms) alcohols influence the induction of ALA synthase and cytochrome P450 in primary cultures of chick embryonic hepatocytes (Sinclair, BiochemPharm, 1981; 30:2805).

Oestrogen-containing oral contraceptives have increased the prevalence of porphyria cutanea symptomatica in women; the role of oestrogen was already well known in male patients treated with stilboestrol for prostatic cancer.

We have found in our patients that nearly all the drugs classified as porphyrinogenic (i.e., unsafe for use in acute porphyrias) (Table 4) will precipitate or exacerbate porphyria cutanea symptomatica. As in any hepatic porphyria, most patients may receive toxic drugs (or alcohol) over several years before developing porphyria cutanea symptomatica.

Abnormal iron metabolism appears to be another precipitating factor of the clinical onset: serum iron is frequently 60 per cent above normal in patients with porphyria cutanea symptomatica. A mild hepatic siderosis is described in at least 80 per cent of patients, but some have found a normal total-body iron store in most of their patients. Iron removal by phlebotomy is a highly effective treatment. At the time of writing, iron-mediated induction of free radicals seems to be the most popular explanation of the effect of iron on the uroporphyrinogen metabolism in porphyria cutanea symptomatica. Mice given both iron and hexachlorabenzene readily became porphyric: iron exerted its synergistic action through the formation of highly reactive hydroxyl radicals, which in turn caused site-selective damage to uroporphyrinogen decarboxylase without a fall in the concentration of immunoreactive enzyme (Smith, BiochemJ, 1983; 214:909).

The cause of the iron overload is still unknown. It is suggested (Kushner, Gastro, 1985; 88:1232) that patients with porphyria cutanea symptomatica are heterozygous for the haemochromatosis allele. However, a study (Beaumont, Gastro, 1987; 92:1833) of 69 patients (42 with the sporadic, and 27 unrelated with the familial type) found the same incidence (24 per cent) of HLA-A3 (the best marker of haemochromatosis) in each type of porphyria cutanea symptomatica and in controls. If there is no systematic association between haemochromatosis and porphyria cutanea symptomatica, some random association, which would probably favour the clinical manifestations of porphyria cutanea symptomatica, must occur (Roberts, Lancet, 1997; 349:321).

Polyhalogenated hydrocarbons are porphyrinogenic in man and in animals (rodents); the first identified was hexachlorobenzene, which precipitated a massive outbreak of about 4000 cases of porphyria cutanea symptomatica in Turkey (between 1956 and 1961) following the ingestion of treated wheat. Slight abnormalities in urinary porphyrin excretion were found among 13 workers exposed to tetrachlorodibenzodioxin (**TCDD**) in an Italian industrial plant; two siblings with a familial type developed a clinically manifest porphyria cutanea symptomatica (Doss, IntJBiochem, 1984; 16:369). TCDD is highly porphyrinogenic, but, if uroporphyrinogen decarboxylase activity is strongly decreased the immunoreactive protein is unchanged, suggesting that only the catalytic site of the enzyme has been modified.

A strong association has been found between hepatitis C virus and porphyria cutanea (Fargion, Hepatol, 1992; 16:1322; Lacour, BrJDermatol, 1993; 128:121) in several countries. Hepatitis B virus is not as closely associated with porphyria cutanea as is hepatitis C virus. Hepatitis C virus infection may be an important trigger factor (acting alone or in combination with others) for the development of porphyria cutanea. Antibodies to hepatitis C virus should be evaluated in each patient with this porphyria at the time of diagnosis.

Biochemical findings

Urine contains increased concentrations of uroporphyrin (mainly isomer I) and 7-carboxy-porphyrin (mainly isomer III); coproporphyrin, 5-, and 6-carboxylic-porphyrins are moderately increased. Both precursors are usually normal but the accompanying liver disease may cause a minor increase in the excretion of ALA.

In the faeces, the dominant porphyrin excreted is often isocoproporphyrin. However, concentrations of coproporphyrin, 7-carboxy-porphyrin, uroporphyrin, and X-porphyrin (ether-insoluble fraction) may all be enhanced in porphyria cutanea symptomatica. During clinical remission, total porphyrin excretion decreases progressively and measurement of urinary porphyrins is one of the best methods for following the effects of treatment (usually repeated phlebotomy). After a few months, urinary porphyrin concentrations appear normal, but in the faeces copro- and

isocoproporphyrin may remain increased for a long period. An additional characteristic of porphyria cutanea symptomatica is the accumulation of large quantities of porphyrin in liver, mostly uroporphyrinogen and 7-carboxy-porphyrin (hydrophilic porphyrins). The same porphyrins are also found in plasma. Serum iron and ferritin are frequently increased (see above).

Enzymatic abnormalities

Uroporphyrinogen decarboxylase is decreased in the liver of all patients with porphyria cutanea symptomatica. In the familial type it was decreased by 50 per cent in all tissues, including erythrocytes. Kindred studies of uroporphyrinogen decarboxylase deficiency in erythrocytes have demonstrated the autosomal-dominant pattern of inheritance and allowed detection of latent carriers without biochemical abnormalities. Familial porphyria cutanea symptomatica is not rare (15 to 20 per cent of all cases of porphyria cutanea symptomatica), but it is uncommon to find several patients in the same family, the latent carriers being predominant. Using specific antibodies, Elder (Lancet, 1983; i:1301) and de Verneuil (AmJHumGen, 1984; 36:613) showed that in patients with familial porphyria cutanea symptomatica, the erythrocyte immunoreactive uroporphyrinogen decarboxylase protein was decreased to the same extent as catalytic activity (CRIM-negative), whereas in sporadic porphyria cutanea symptomatica both were normal. Later studies (Elder, Lancet, 1985; ii:22) measured both catalytic and immunoreactive uroporphyrinogen decarboxylase protein in the liver of sporadic patients: the ratio of catalytic activity to immunoreactive protein was lower in those with active disease; during remissions following venesection, enzyme activity and immunoreactive enzyme concentration were normal. These findings were consistent with the view that sporadic porphyria cutanea symptomatica is an acquired disorder. In our patients, two brothers both had overt porphyria cutanea symptomatica (clinical features and biochemical data were typical), but uroporphyrinogen decarboxylase activity in erythrocytes was normal. These patients were therefore indistinguishable from sporadic cases. Activities were normal in erythrocytes, fibroblasts and, after prolonged remission, in liver. Similar cases have also been described in England (by the Elder group) and Italy (by the Topi group). A liver-specific mutation for this form of porphyria cutanea symptomatica therefore seems implausible, and a mutation at some other locus predisposing individuals to develop porphyria cutanea symptomatica in response to acquired factors (such as alcohol, or drugs) is likely.

Treatment

All patients with porphyria cutanea symptomatica should first be advised to avoid precipitating factors (e.g. alcohol, drugs) and also exposure to sunlight until clinical and biological remission has been obtained by treatment. Phlebotomy is at present the treatment of choice, even when the serum iron or ferritin are not increased. Venesections of 300 ml at 10- to 12-day intervals are continued for 2 months until the serum iron falls to 60 to 70 per cent of its original value. Urine porphyrin concentrations are monitored each month: clinical and biological remissions are usually obtained within 6 months.

When phlebotomy is contraindicated (anaemia, cardiac or pulmonary disorders, age), low-dose chloroquine therapy (250 mg weekly) is the favoured alternative. Duration of treatment and relapse rate are only marginally greater than with venesection. High-dose treatment must be avoided because it causes a hepatitis-like syndrome in patients with porphyria cutanea symptomatica.

Topi (BrJDermatol, 1984; 111:75) reported 16 cases of porphyria cutanea symptomatica treated successfully by avoidance of hepatic toxins only. Rocchi (BrJDermatol, 1986; 114:621) tested the efficacy of long-term subcutaneous infusion of desferrioxamine; they were able to recommend it when severe associated diseases contraindicate venesection.

Recent molecular biological findings will be described with hepatoerythropoietic porphyria.

Hepatoerythropoietic porphyria

This is a very rare porphyria resulting from a homozygous defect in uroporphyrinogen decarboxylase activity; clinically it is very similar to congenital erythropoietic porphyria, with a severe photosensitivity usually beginning in early infancy.

Clinical findings

These will be described under 'congenital erythropoietic porphyria' below, from which it differs by the absence of erythrodontia and, usually, of haemolytic anaemia.

Biochemical findings

Patterns of excretion of porphyrins in the urine and faeces excretions are similar to those found in porphyria cutanea symptomatica (see above). As in other homozygous cases of porphyria, increased zinc protoporphyrin is found in erythrocytes.

Enzymatic features and molecular biology

Elder (Lancet, 1981; i:916) described a severely deficient (7 per cent of normal) activity of uroporphyrinogen decarboxylase in these patients, suggesting that they are homozygous for the gene that causes porphyria cutanea symptomatica. Several other studies have confirmed the homozygous inheritance of a defect of the uroporphyrinogen decarboxylase gene and showed a 50 per cent reduction of activity also in parents and in children of the patient (parents and children being asymptomatic).

Immunological studies on uroporphyrinogen decarboxylase in patients with hepatoerythropoietic porphyria showed that there were two groups, one displaying the enzyme deficiency with a CRIM-positive mutation and the other with a CRIM-negative mutation. Molecular heterogeneity of uroporphyrinogen decarboxylase deficiency was also described in these patients (e.g. varying enzyme half-life among families; varying molecular weight).

Cloning and sequencing of a cDNA for the mutated gene in a patient from one family has revealed the nature of the mutation, which consists of a G–A change at nucleotide 860 in the cDNA sequence leading to a Gly (GGG)–Glu (GAG) change in the amino-acid sequence at position 281 (de Verneuil, Science, 1986; 234:732). *In vitro* experiments revealed that the cDNA with this mutation encoded a polypeptide product that was very rapidly degraded (compared with the polypeptide encoded by the normal cDNA) in the presence of cell lysate. This observation was consistent with the decreased stability of the mutant protein *in vivo*.

The prevalence of the 281(Gly→Glu) mutation in hepatoerythropoietic porphyria was investigated by hybridization with a synthetic oligonucleotide probe. The mutation was found in affected members of two unrelated families from Spain, but was absent in two other patients from Italy and Portugal; moreover, it was not detected in 13 unrelated cases of familial porphyria cutanea symptomatica. A few mutations have been described in familial porphyria cutanea (exon 6 deletion was found five times out of 22 different families). Until very recently, the mutations identified in patients with hepatoerythropoietic porphyria were not found in those presenting with familial porphyria cutanea. It was concluded that in porphyria cutanea the causative mutations were too severe for homozygotes to survive. In 1995, a mutation causing (in the same family) both hepatoerythropoietic porphyria and familial porphyria cutanea was described (Roberts, JInvDermatol, 1995; 104:500). This paper confirmed that hepatoerythropoietic porphyria is undoubtedly a homozygous case of porphyria cutanea.

Erythropoietic porphyrias

Erythropoietic porphyrias have few features in common other than solar photosensitivity. Congenital erythropoietic porphyria is very rare and follows an autosomal-recessive mode of inheritance; clinical manifestations are usually very spectacular. Erythropoietic protoporphyria is more frequent and follows an autosomal-dominant mode of inheritance. Clinical manifestations are usually modest. In these forms of porphyria, patients do not experience acute attacks and a list of porphyrinogenic agents is not required.

Congenital erythropoietic porphyria[9]

Fewer than 200 cases of this disease have been published in the world literature. Congenital erythropoietic porphyria was, however, the first porphyria described and the first porphyria in which a specific enzyme defect was demonstrated (uroporphyrinogen III cosynthetase).

Clinical features

The predominant site of metabolic expression is the erythropoietic system. The highly abnormal accumulation of porphyrins in bone marrow, peripheral blood, and other organs leads to the three main manifestations: chronic photodermatitis with photosensitivity, massive porphyrinuria, and haematological alterations (see references for detailed descriptions). In infants, the first symptom is usually the excretion of red urine with staining of the diapers (from pink to dark reddish brown). Photosensitivity is manifested when the child is in sunlight. A vesicular or bullous eruption may follow exposure, with effects on the face and the back of the hands. The repetition of bullous eruptions, minor injuries, and infections may lead to severe mutilation of ears, nose cartilage, and digits. Hypertrichosis appears in most patients; it also affects the exposed areas, especially the upper arm and the temple and malar region on the face. The additional hair is typically blond, downy, and of lanugo type, but may be coarse and dark.

Erythrodontia is reported in almost all cases and, if present, is pathognomonic of congenital erythropoietic porphyria. The teeth, deciduous and/or permanent, may exhibit a red, or more usually, dirty brown discoloration under normal light and a red fluorescence under ultraviolet light, due to large deposits of porphyrins in the dentine. Splenomegaly is another feature commonly reported in patients. It has been found at birth or soon after in a few cases, but more usually appears as the disease progresses and in most cases is related to the haemolytic activity. The eyes may be afflicted by severe ulcerations, ectropion, or cataract, with ensuing blindness.

Haematological findings

Increased haemolytic activity was found in the majority of previously reported cases and also in all our seven patients. The intermittent nature of the course of the haemolytic process is a striking and specific feature. At times a patient may manifest an obvious haemolytic anaemia; at other times only slight, subdetectable haemolysis may occur. Early death due to anaemia has been reported.

Fluorescence of a large proportion of the normoblasts is readily demonstrable in the bone marrow of all patients with congenital erythropoietic porphyria. Fluorescence is principally localized in the nuclei of the cells and is bright red under ultraviolet light.

Biochemical findings

Urine

This always contains large amounts of uroporphyrin and to a lesser extent coproporphyrin, but with daily and seasonal fluctuations. Smaller amounts of 7-, 6-, and 5-carboxy-porphyrins are also present, but their pattern of excretion is quite different from that found in porphyria cutanea symptomatica. The major fraction of urinary uroporphyrin and coproporphyrin is of isomeric series I (> 80 per cent), but there is an absolute increase in uroporphyrin III in all patients. ALA is usually within normal limits or only slightly increased in some cases. Porphobilinogen is normal in most cases.

Faeces

These contain large amounts of coproporphyrin, but little uroporphyrin. Most faecal porphyrins belong to isomeric series I as in urine. The protoporphyrin concentrations are usually within the normal range.

Plasma and erythrocytes

These contain large amounts of uroporphyrin and (less) coproporphyrin, both of isomeric series I. The values for protoporphyrin in erythrocytes are usually no higher than those found in other haemolytic conditions.

Porphyria overproduction and enzyme defect

A genetic defect resulting in a primary deficiency of the activity of uroporphyrinogen III cosynthetase is now widely accepted and documented: a residual cosynthetase activity of 10 to 30 per cent has been demonstrated in bovine erythrocytes and in those of human patients, and in cultured skin fibroblasts from these patients.

Several family studies (cattle and human beings) have shown that presumed heterozygotes have a cosynthetase activity in erythrocytes between that of porphyrics and controls.

Among the practical implications of a defective cosynthetase activity as the primary defect, the possibility of prenatal diagnosis

is of interest. Congenital erythropoietic porphyria has already been excluded prenatally in a fetus at risk (Deybach, HumGenet, 1980; 53:217). Cosynthetase was measured in amniotic cells and found to be normal compared with control cells. These data were confirmed by the normal amount of porphyrins in amniotic fluid: coproporphyrin only was detected and no uroporphyrin type I was found.

Variants

Late-onset disease

Since 1965, five cases of late-onset disease have been described with clinical features similar to sporadic porphyria cutanea occurring in adulthood. However, biological data have confirmed that these cases were congenital erythropoietic porphyria. Some have suggested that late manifestation may represent the heterozygous state, but Deybach (JLabClinMed, 1981; 97:551) showed that the blood cosynthetase of two patients was very low compared with the enzyme activity of presumed heterozygotes and not significantly different from the activity in homozygous patients. Furthermore, familial studies of cosynthetase activity showed that all the children of one patient were heterozygous; although the mechanism of late onset is presently unknown, the mild cases demonstrate the heterogeneity of congenital erythropoietic porphyria.

Therapy

No important advances have been made in the treatment of congenital erythropoietic porphyria. Packed erythrocyte transfusions markedly reduce excessive haemolysis and its stimulation of erythropoiesis. They also decrease porphyrin excretion, but, as is well known, multiple transfusions can be harmful. Continuous medical care is required to maintain the iron load of the patients at a sufficiently low level to prevent serious damage to the heart, liver, and endocrine organs.

Splenectomy is not necessarily recommended. The decision for or against splenectomy would seem to depend on an evaluation of the degree of hypersplenism. In 1991 (Kauffman, Lancet, 1991; 337:1510), a girl (10 years old) received a bone-marrow graft from an HLA-identical sibling: uroporphyrin overproduction was greatly reduced and skin changes reversed. Unfortunately, the patient died 11 months after transplantation from a cytomegalovirus infection associated with pneumonitis and encephalopathy. Two other bone-marrow transplantations have recently been carried out in France with a very encouraging response (Thomas, JPediat, 1996;129:453).

Ten mutations have been identified in the cosynthetase gene (Deybach, Blood, 1990; 75:1763; Bensidhoum, EurJHumGenet, 1995; 3:102). One of these (Cys73 replaced by Arg) accounts for about 20 per cent of congenital erythropoietic porphyria alleles. The individuals homoallelic for this mutation have a very severe disease.

Erythropoietic protoporphyria[10]

Erythropoietic protoporphyria is a porphyria involving a partial defect of ferrochelatase activity; it is usually inherited in an autosomal-dominant manner and there is no racial or sexual predilection.

Clinical features

Photosensitivity is the major clinical manifestation: short exposures to sunlight induce painful, burning sensations in the exposed areas of the skin; these symptoms occur without any immediately observed change in the appearance of the skin but several hours later they are usually followed by oedema and erythema; vesicles, bullae, and crusting occasionally occur.

Chronic skin changes may develop, which consist of thickening of skin areas most exposed to sunlight (back of the hands, face). More typically, facial skin appears normal. However, it bears a few shallow, circular scars often scattered over the bridge of the nose, forehead, and cheeks.

Onset of cutaneous symptoms is usually in early childhood (3–5 years) but penetrance is variable: several individuals carrying the abnormal gene remain asymptomatic whereas a few others show only a mild photosensitivity and erythropoietic protoporphyria is sometimes detected in late adulthood. It is generally a benign disease, although a number of cases associated with abnormalities of the biliary tract and/or the liver have been reported: cholelithiasis often requires cholecystectomy; chemical analysis of the gallstones reveals high concentrations of protoporphyrin. In rare cases (one of 107 patients in our study), fatal liver disease with cirrhosis may develop; massive deposition of protoporphyrin was revealed by microscopic examination of liver biopsy specimens from these patients. However, protoporphyrin deposition has often been described in liver biopsy specimens from patients with erythropoietic protoporphyria and normal tests of liver function. The pathogenesis of the skin lesions relies on high concentrations of free protoporphyrin (and not zinc protoporphyrin) in erythrocytes and extracellular fluids (see reviews in reference list).

Biochemical findings

Erythropoietic protoporphyria is characterized by elevated protoporphyrin in erythrocytes and plasma. Faecal protoporphyrin is often (but not always) abnormally increased; urinary porphyrin excretion is normal, except in occasional cases with deteriorated hepatic function who show an increased porphyrinuria (mostly coproporphyrin) whereas baseline concentrations of protoporphyrin rise in erythrocytes and decrease in faeces. On the other hand, several asymptomatic patients have been detected only by measurement of ferrochelatase activity.

Enzymatic abnormalities

The primary defect is the deficiency of the mitochondrial enzyme ferrochelatase (haem synthetase). This defect has been found in all tissues studied.

For some reasons as yet unknown, the activity of ferrochelatase in patients with erythropoietic protoporphyria was less than 50 per cent of normal (usually between 20 and 30 per cent). In our records (33 patients and 60 asymptomatic carriers) we found a mean ferrochelatase defect of 44 per cent in carriers and 30 per cent in patients; this difference is highly significant ($p < 0.001$). Gouya et al. (AmJHumGenet, 1996; 58:292) have shown that a low expression of the normal ferrochelatase gene could explain the difference in activity between asymptomatic carriers and patients: the co-inheritance of a low-output normal allele and a deleterious mutant one would result in a more pronounced enzyme deficiency in patients than in carriers (who inherit the deleterious gene and the normal one without low output).

Recently, Deybach[11] described the first homozygous case of erythropoietic protoporphyria: the clinical features of the proband were similar to those of other patients with erythropoietic protoporphyria. However, the ferrochelatase activity of the patient's lymphocytes was only 6.5 per cent of the mean normal, whereas the activity in both parents was approximately 50 per cent. Cases with a similar defect were found in families of both parents. It is now obvious that this case is a variant with a recessive mode of inheritance, as has been described in cattle.

In most patients, erythropoietic tissue is the main source of the excess protoporphyrin. The rate of loss of protoporphyrin from erythrocytes can account for the amount of protoporphyrin excreted in faeces without invoking any additional contribution from a hepatic source of overproduction of protoporphyrin in these patients. On the other hand, Benhamou et al. have described a patient with erythropoietic protoporphyria complicated by severe cirrhosis in whom liver transplantation was successfully performed (Samuel, Gastro, 1988; 85:816): the concentration of protoporphyrin in erythrocytes decreased rapidly from 100 000 nmol/l to 20 000 nmol/l (normal, 750 $\pm$ 250 nmol/l) and remained constant (at least over 2 years) between 20 000 and 30 000 nmol/l which is the usual level in uncomplicated erythropoietic protoporphyria. This supports the view that in erythropoietic protoporphyria the part played by the liver in protoporphyrin overproduction is relatively very small, if it exists at all.

Molecular investigation of ferrochelatase cDNA in patients with erythropoietic protoporphyria has revealed various types of mutations. The apparently homozygous case described above was in fact a compound heterozygous with a Gly–Cys substitution on one chain and a Met–Ile substitution on the other (Lamoril, BBResComm, 1991; 18:281). At present, there is no evidence that particular genotypes are associated with the propensity to develop liver diseases.

Treatment

Oral administration of β-carotene may afford photoprotection, resulting in improved tolerance to the sun, but results are variable. Whereas several patients report increased tolerance to light, a few (approximately 20 per cent) seem to receive no improvement. β-carotene would prevent the photosensitivity reaction by quenching the singlet oxygen or the triplet states of protoporphyrin (porphyrin concentrations remain unchanged).

Treatment of liver disease in erythropoietic protoporphyria has included several trials, such as of ingestion of cholestyramine resin to try to interrupt the enterohepatic recirculation of protoporphyrin to the liver, or the administration of bile salts to mobilize protoporphyrin directly from the liver. Liver transplantation is the treatment of last resort in irreversible liver damage.

References

1. Kappas A, Sassa S, Galbraith RA, and Nordmann Y. The porphyrias. In Scriver CR, et al, eds. The metabolic basis of inherited disease. 7th edn. Vol. 2. New York: McGraw-Hill, 1995: 2103–59.

2. Nordmann Y and Deybach JC. Human hereditary porphyrias. In Dailey HA, ed. *Heme biosynthesis*. New York: Macmillan, 1990: 491–542.

3. Meyer UA, and Schmid R. The porphyrias. In Stanbury JB, Wyngaarden JB, and Fredrickson DS, eds. *The metabolic basis of inherited disease*. 4th edn. New York: McGraw-Hill, 1978: 1166–220.

4. Moore MR, McColl KE, Rimington C, and Goldberg A. *Disorders of Porphyrin Metabolism*. New York: Plenum Medical, 1987.

5. Elder GH. Metabolic abnormalities in the porphyrias. In Mascaro JM, ed. *Seminars in dermatology*. Orlando (FL): Grune and Stratton, 1986: 88–98.

6. Bonkowsky HL and Schady W. Neurologic manifestations of acute porphyria. In Schmid R, ed. *Seminars in liver disease*. New York: Thieme-Stratton, 1982: 108–24.

7. De Matteis F. Hepatic porphyrias caused by AIA, DDC, griseofulvin, and related compounds. In De Matteis F and Aldridge WN, eds. *Heme and hemoproteins*. Berlin: Springer-Verlag, 1978: 129–55.

8. Marks GS. The effects of chemicals on hepatic heme biosynthesis. In De Matteis F and Aldridge WN, eds. *Heme and hemoproteins*. Berlin: Springer-Verlag, 1978: 201–37.

9. Nordmann Y and Deybach JC. Congenital erythropoietic porphyria. In Mascaro JM, ed. *Seminars in dermatology*. Orlando (FL): Grune and Stratton, 1986: 106–14.

10. Poh-Fizpatrick MB. Erythropoietic porphyria. In Mascaro JM, ed. *Seminars in dermatology*. Orlando (FL): Grune and Stratton, 1986: 99–105.

11. Deybach JC *et al*. Ferrochelatase in human erythropoietic porphyria: the first case of a homozygous form. In Nordmann Y, ed. *Porphyrins and porphyrias*. Paris: John Libbey, 1986: 123.

20.6 Hyperbilirubinaemia

Johan Fevery·and Norbert Blanckaert

Bile pigment metabolism can be disturbed at several steps, and combinations of disorders occur frequently. Disturbances usually lead to enhanced serum bilirubin levels. The plasma level of unconjugated bilirubin depends directly on the production rate of bilirubin and inversely on the uptake and conjugation by the liver. From Fig. 1, it can be deduced that in patients with a low hepatic clearance (as is the case in Gilbert's syndrome, for example) a small increase in bilirubin production will markedly enhance plasma bilirubin concentration. Decreased biliary secretion will result in enhanced plasma concentrations of conjugates.

In general, diazo-reactions are used to quantitate serum bilirubin levels. Unconjugated bilirubin IXα only reacts after addition of accelerator substances (so-called 'indirect-reaction') whereas the polar non-α isomers and all conjugates react directly. However, the direct diazo-reaction is insufficiently specific for conjugated bilirubins. The ratio between direct- and indirect-reacting pigment gives only an indication of the proportion of conjugated and unconjugated bilirubin. The alkaline methanolysis procedure allows accurate determination of esterified bilirubins but is more time consuming. In this assay methyl esters are formed by trans-methylation of the glycoside esters; the former can be separated by thin layer chromatography or high-pressure liquid chromatography (**HPLC**) and are determined photometrically (Blanckaert, JLab-ClinMed, 1980; 96:1988; Muraca, Gastro, 1987; 92:309). Kodak introduced a slide test based on the diazo-procedure, it also separates albumin conjugates of bilirubin from the esterglycosides.

Values of plasma total bilirubin are between 2 and 10 mg/l in 95 per cent of a healthy population. In general, a value of 10 mg/l or 17 mmol/l is accepted as the upper limit of normal.

A useful clinical classification to describe the disordered bilirubin metabolism is based upon the predominance in serum of either the unconjugated or the conjugated pigment in cases of hyper-bilirubinaemia (Table 1). The most relevant clinical syndromes will be discussed below.

Overproduction

Overproduction of bilirubin is most often the result of haemolysis and, more rarely, of dyserythropoiesis. Breakdown of extravasated erythrocytes (e.g. in haematoma) or enhanced turnover of haemo-proteins are unusual causes of jaundice. Blood transfusions lead to marked bilirubin overproduction because transfused packed red cells have a greatly shortened lifespan (usually only 20–30 days). In most haemolytic disorders, destruction of defective or injured red cells occurs in mononuclear phagocyte cells of the spleen, liver, and bone marrow. In intravascular haemolysis, erythrocytes are destroyed within the circulation and haemoglobin is released directly into plasma.[1] Plasma haemoglobin binds to haptoglobin, and this complex is taken up and degraded principally by parenchymal cells. Haemolysis thus becomes apparent from the presence of unconjugated hyperbilirubinaemia, enhanced reticulocytosis (as an expression of enhanced red cell production in the bone marrow), decreased plasma levels of free haptoglobin or haemopexin, and increased urobilinuria. Anaemia will develop when the bone marrow cannot compensate for the increased loss of red cells. Serum iron levels are usually enhanced due to release of iron from the (dying) red cells. If large amounts of haemoglobin are released (haemoglobin in excess of 1–2 mg/ml plasma), haptoglobin may be depleted and unbound haemoglobin will appear in plasma, where it is oxidized to methaemoglobin. Oxidized haem dissociates more readily from

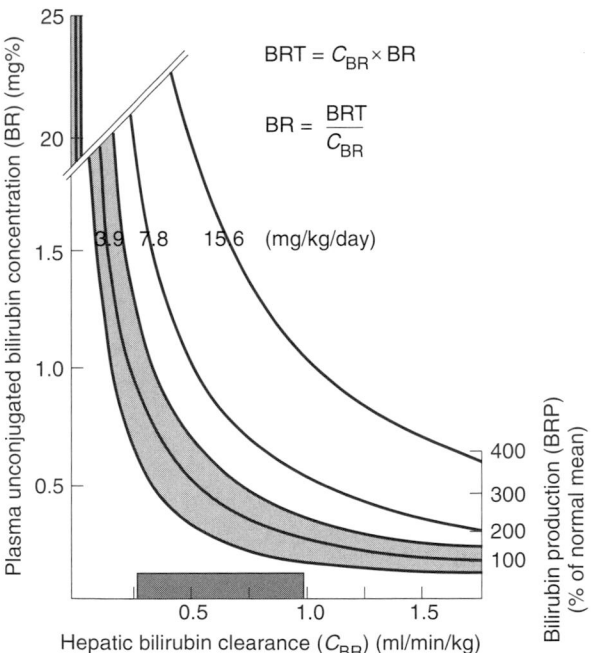

Fig. 1. Relationship between hepatic bilirubin clearance and plasma unconjugated bilirubin level. The bar on the abscissa represents the mean and 2 SD of the clearance (CBR) for normal healthy adults. The bilirubin production is given as 100 per cent ± 2 SD. (Taken from ref. [2] with permission.)

Table 1 Differential diagnosis of hyperbilirubinaemia

	Unconjugated bilirubin IXa[a]	BMC[a]	BDC[a]	EB/TB[a]
Unconjugated hyperbilirubinaemia				
1. Overproduction	↑	↑	↑	nl
Haemolysis (e.g. transfusion)				
Ineffective erythropoiesis				
2. Decreased hepatic uptake	↑			↑
Drugs? Some cases of Gilbert's syndrome				
3. Decreased glucuronidation	↑	nl	nl	↑
Gilbert's syndrome				
Crigler–Najjar disease				
Neonatal jaundice				
Inhibition by drugs (pregnanediol, chloramphenicol)				
Predominantly conjugated hyperbilirubinaemia	nl or −	↑	↑	↑
(bilirubinostasis, cholestasis)				
Hepatitis, cirrhosis				
Intrahepatic cholestasis				
Obstructive jaundice				
Dubin–Johnson syndrome				
Rotor syndrome				
Overloading syndrome				
Septicaemia				

[a] Refers to unconjugated, mono-, or diesterified bilirubin, and to the proportion of esterified to total bilirubin which is 4 to 10 per cent when assayed with alkaline methanolysis-HPLC, 10–25 per cent with alkaline methanolysis-TLC, and 15 to 25 per cent with a 10-min direct diazo-reaction.
nl, Normal.

globin and binds to haemopexin and albumin. The haem–haemopexin complex is taken up by the parenchymal cells where it is degraded to bilirubin. In addition, a major part of circulating unbound haemoglobin or methaemoglobin is cleared by the kidneys.

Megaloblastic and sideroblastic anaemias, erythroleukaemia, lead poisoning, and hereditary syndromes of unknown pathogenesis, called 'primary shunt hyperbilirubinaemia' and 'idiopathic dys-erythropoietic jaundice' are associated with ineffective erythropoiesis. In these cases abnormal haem molecules or abnormal erythrocyte precursors undergo premature catabolism in the bone marrow, as such the erythropoietic early labelled bile pigment fraction can raise to 30 to 80 per cent of all bile pigment. The bone marrow shows a marked erythroid hyperplasia, sometimes with active erythrophagocytosis. A greatly accelerated plasma iron turnover is present and a relatively low reticulocytosis when compared to the degree of anaemia. Plasma haptoglobin levels are usually normal.

Enhanced turnover of hepatic haem proteins (cytochromes P-450) has been documented in experimental conditions such as bile-duct obstruction in the rat (Robinson, JLabClinMed, 1969; 73: 668) and might be present in the mutant Southdown sheep (Mia, PSEBM, 1971; 136:227) an animal model resembling Rotor syndrome in humans (see below).

A small number of patients with Gilbert syndrome have a reduced uptake of bromsulphophthalein and indocyanine green (Martin, Gastro, 1976; 70:385). It is not clear whether this also holds for bilirubin as it is difficult to separate uptake rates from the effects of conjugation deficiency.

Bilirubin overproduction leads to enhanced serum levels of both unconjugated and conjugated pigments (Table 1) but the hyperbilirubinaemia remains predominantly of the unconjugated type. As can be deduced from Fig. 1, the plasma bilirubin concentration will rise linearly with increasing rates of pigment production until a new steady state is reached in which hepatic bilirubin removal equals pigment production. Since erythropoiesis can increase maximally eight to tenfold, the highest plasma bilirubin concentration in severe chronic haemolysis does not exceed 40 mg/l, provided that the hepatic bilirubin clearance is normal.[2] In acute haemolytic crises plasma bilirubin levels in excess of 40 mg/l are encountered, regardless of the prevailing hepatic bilirubin removal.

The increased production rate remains far below the maximal conjugating and secretory capacity. As such, a highly increased biliary excretion of bilirubin conjugates is present, leading to enhanced faecal and urinary urobilinogen excretion. If chronic, these enhanced biliary concentrations will lead to formation of pigment gallstones.

Decreased microsomal bilirubin glucuronidation[3]

Defective glucuronidation results in a rise of unconjugated bilirubin in plasma. A severe deficiency leads to Crigler–Najjar's disease type I, a less severe one to the type II disease, and a mild defect to the so-called Gilbert's syndrome (Table 2). The gene defects involved have recently been identified.

Crigler–Najjar disease type I

This rare disorder was first described by Crigler and Najjar (Pediat, 1952; 10:169) and investigated later on in more detail (Arias, AmJMed, 1969; 47:395). The underlying defect is a severely depressed glucuronidation of bilirubin due to the (near-?) absence of

Table 2 The inherited unconjugated hyperbilirubinaemias

	Crigler–Najjar disease, type I	Crigler–Najjar disease, type II	Gilbert's syndrome
Incidence	Rare	Uncommon	3–7% of adult population
Jaundice	Severe, beginning 3–4 days after birth	Usually beginning shortly after birth, but occasionally not recognized until childhood	Usually fluctuating slight scleral icterus recognized postpuberty, many instances remain undetected
Bilirubin encephalopathy	Developing within 18 months but occasionally delayed until early adulthood	Very rare	None
Plasma bilirubin concentration	17–50 mg/dl or 290–850 μM; usually >20 mg/dl or >390 μM	6–22 mg/dl 100–375 μM; usually <20 mg/dl <340 μM	<6 mg/dl <100 μM; usually <3 mg/dl <50 μM and fluctuating
Plasma bilirubin clearance	<50% of normal	<50% of normal	Approximately 30% of normal
Response to phenobarbital	Absent	Marked improvement of plasma bilirubin clearance and >30% decrease of hyperbilirubinaemia	Virtual normalization of plasma bilirubin clearance and concentration
Bile composition	Unconjugated bilirubin and trace amounts of bilirubin monoglucuronides	Mostly bilirubin monoglucuronides; some UCB and diglucuronide	Decreased proportion of bilirubin diconjugates (>50% instead of 70% in normal)
Hepatic bilirubin UDP-glucuronyl-transferase activity	Absent or near zero	Absent or near zero	About a third of normal; occasionally near zero
Mode of inheritance	Autosomal recessive	Autosomal recessive	Probably autosomal dominant; phenotypic expression more frequent in males
Gene defects described	In all 5 exons	In all 5 exons	Two extra TA in promotor region

UCB, Unconjugated bilirubin.

hepatic bilirubin UDP-glucuronyltransferase (**UGT**) activity. With current methods, transferase activity assayed in liver tissue is negligible. Serum bilirubin levels are usually in the range of 350 to 450 mmol/l. Analysis by alkaline methanolysis and HPLC showed that nearly all of the pigment in plasma is present as unconjugated bilirubin IXα. The bile is rather pale as only a minor fraction of the bilirubin produced reaches it. This is evident, for example, when comparing the molar ratio in bile of bilirubin to bile acids, which averages 0.021 in normal individuals, and 0.006 in patients with Crigler–Najjar type I. Small amounts (up to 0.3 per cent) are present as monoglucuronide in serum (Muraca, Gastro, 1987; 92: 309). Similarly, analysis of bile showed a markedly enhanced proportion of unconjugated bilirubin IXα (30–57 per cent) with greatly varying relative amounts of monoglucuronide (40–70 per cent of total pigment) and 0 to 10 per cent diglucuronide (Fevery, JCI, 1977; 60:970; Sinaasappel, Gastro, 1991; 100:783). Conventional liver tests, biliary secretion, and liver histology are normal. The high unconjugated bilirubin in plasma finally leads to kernicterus. This bilirubin encephalopathy is occasionally also seen in neonates or premature infants with erythroblastosis fetalis. Symptoms include hypertonicity, a high-pitched voice, opisthotonus, spastic paralysis, mental retardation, and eventually death if not treated by phototherapy or liver transplantation. Several of the children described were the offspring of related consanguinous parents. This led to the suggestion that the disease is inherited in an autosomal recessive mode. Recent molecular biology analysis has confirmed this inheritance. Indeed, the structure of the human liver UGT

gene complex encoding for the glucuronyltransferase has recently been identified at the telomeric end of chromosome 2 (locus 2937) (Ritter, JBC, 1991; 266:1043; Bosma, Hepatol, 1992; 15:941; Moghrabi, AnnHumGenet, 1992; 56:91; Ritter, JBC, 1992; 267:3257; Van Es, CytogenetCellGenet, 1993; 63:114). The UGT1A encodes for the bilirubin transferase (Bosma, JBC, 1994; 269:17960). It is composed of five exons, four of these at the 3′ end are identical and encode for the UDP-glycosyl binding site and the membrane-spanning domain consisting of 246 amino acids, common for all UDP-glycosyltransferase isoforms derived. Exon 1 at the 5′ end is specific for the various isoforms of UDP-glucuronyltransferase (see Chapter 2.9, Fig. 6).

Analysis of the UGT1A gene in patients with Crigler–Najjar type I has shown that a series of mutations are present, such as an homozygous A to C transition at nucleotide 1207, or C to G at nucleotide 1143 in exon 4, or G insertion after nucleotide 1223 (Labrune, HumGenet, 1994; 94:693). Mutations have been observed in all exons (Ritter, JBC, 1991; 269:23573; Bosma, Hepatol, 1992; 15:941; Moghrabi, AmJHumGenet, 1993; 53:722). As a result of these mutations, an active glucuronyltransferase is not formed.[3]

A mutant strain of Wistar rats characterized by severe non-haemolytic unconjugated hyperbilirubinaemia was described by Gunn (JHered, 1938; 29:137). These rats serve as model of Crigler–Najjar type I. Their bile is equally pale due to absence of conjugated bilirubins. Only small amounts of bilirubin IXα and its non-α isomers and some hydroxylated derivatives are present (Blanckaert, BiochemJ, 1977; 164:237). It is not clear how the unconjugated bilirubin IXα reaches the bile. Diffusion across the biliary ductules, or transhepatocellular secretion as photoisomers ZE, EZ, or EE and reformation to the natural ZZ configuration are possibilities. The mutation in the UGT1 gene in Gunn rats differs from those currently described in Crigler–Najjar disease. The conjugating defect in the Gunn rat arises from a -1 frameshift mutation that removes 115 amino acids at the COOH terminus in the domain shared by all members of the UGT1 gene family and results in formation of a truncated protein (Iyanagi, JBC, 1989; 264:21302; Iyanagi, JBC, 1991; 266:20048).

Crigler–Najjar disease should be recognized as soon as possible after birth and treated by phototherapy. Characteristically type I does not respond to phenobarbitone therapy. Serum bilirubin levels can be reduced rapidly by repeated plasmapheresis. Bilirubin, tightly bound to albumin, is removed and the replaced albumin mobilizes pigment from tissues back to plasma. Phototherapy constitutes a more chronic therapy. Bilirubin is partly photo-oxidized and degraded or undergoes photoisomerization to its water-soluble ZE, EZ, or EE geometrical isomers.[4] The latter can be excreted in bile without conjugation. To prevent intestinal reabsorption of unconjugated bilirubin IXα, it might be advisable to administer oral agar, charcoal, or cholestyramine. Phototherapy seems to become less effective when the child grows older because of skin thickening and pigmentation. Liver transplantation is therefore more effective (Sokal, Transpl, 1995; 60:1095; Van der Veere, Hepatol, 1996; 24:311). It should be proposed when phototherapy is no longer effective or practical (Pett, MolAspMed, 1987; 9:473). Transplantation of a normal kidney in the homozygous Gunn rat results in a mild decrease of serum bilirubin levels. However, in contrast to the situation in the rat, the human kidney does not conjugate bilirubin. In the Gunn rat, subcutaneous implants of hepatoma cells or intrasplenic implants of isolated hepatocytes also decrease plasma bilirubin levels. Administration of tin mesoporphyrin markedly decreases bilirubin production by competition with haem for the haem oxygenase. It has been administered with success to newborn rats and to human neonates and in Crigler–Najjar disease type I patients (Rubaltelli, Pediat, 1989; 84:728; Galbraith, Pediat, 1992; 89:175).

Crigler–Najjar disease type II

This syndrome represents a more benign condition with serum unconjugated bilirubin levels of 100 to 300 mmol/l, although these can increase due to infection, concurrent medication, anaesthesia, etc. Characteristically phenobarbitone therapy (5–10 mg/kg body weight in children) in type II patients decreases serum bilirubin levels by more than 30 per cent. A similar effect has been obtained with glutethimide, phenazone, and with chlorpromazine. These drugs enhance UDP-glucuronyltransferase activity in normal rat and humans and in heterozygous Gunn rats. The effect in type II patients is presumed to result from stimulation of the defective, residual enzyme. When measured with current assays, bilirubin UDP-glucuronyltransferase activity is, however, undetectable or minute in liver. Analysis of serum and bile shows markedly increased levels of unconjugated bilirubin IXα and monoglucuronidated bilirubin. Unlike the type I disease, diglucuronide can usually be demonstrated in type II patients (Fevery, JCI, 1977; 60:970;

Sinaasappel, Gastro, 1991; 100:783; Rubaltelli, Pediat, 1994; 94:553). However, in our experience differentiation of type I and II by analysis of serum and bile is not unequivocal. The response to phenobarbital has to be investigated. Most cases of type II disease remain asymptomatic except for jaundice. Some patients developed kernicterus in association with infections. Some family members seem to have Gilbert's syndrome and it was proposed that type II disease represents the homozygous form of Gilbert's syndrome. Until now, this has not been confirmed. Crigler–Najjar type II was shown also to be inherited as an autosomal recessive trait. A great variety of mutations have already been documented with single transitions in the unique exon 1 as well as in the shared exons 2 to 5 (Moghrabi, Genomics, 1993; 18:171; Bosma, Gastro, 1993; 105:216; Aono, BBResComm, 1993; 197:1239; Labrune, HumGenet, 1994; 94:693).

Gilbert's syndrome

Gilbert's syndrome or hereditary ('constitutional') non-haemolytic unconjugated hyperbilirubinaemia is most frequently recognized in adolescents and young adults. It occurs in 5 to 7 per cent of the overall population. It is more frequently detected in males, presumably because at puberty serum bilirubin levels increase in males and decrease in females; this gender difference may be related to hormonal effects on UDP-glucuronyltransferase activity (Muraca, Gastro, 1984; 87:308). Gilbert's syndrome is probably inherited as an autosomal dominant trait.

Serum bilirubin levels are usually 51 mmol/l but may be higher; indeed, they may overlap with levels seen in patients with Crigler–Najjar type II disease. Levels may fluctuate and are occasionally within the normal range. Patients with Gilbert's syndrome may complain of non-specific symptoms such as hyporexia, fatigue, nausea, and abdominal discomfort; these complaints were equally frequent in a control population (Olsson, ActaMedScand, 1989; 24:617). It is generally accepted that these symptoms are only an expression of anxiety when the individuals become aware of (intermittent) icterus. Frequently, they represent an intercurrent influenza-like disease which induces a rise in bilirubin level, leading to the detection of Gilbert's syndrome. Indeed, haemolysis or caloric deprivation may be associated with viral infections and thereby enhance the serum bilirubin levels, leading to overt jaundice.

Fasting or a low calorie intake (400 kcal over 24–48 h) induces a two- to threefold increase in plasma unconjugated bilirubin levels. A similar relative increase is seen in normal individuals; but in Gilbert's syndrome, the absolute values and increase are far more impressive. Addition of a small amount of lipids reverses this effect (Gollan, Gut, 1976; 17:335). The mechanisms involved in producing fasting hyperbilirubinaemia are complex but the pronounced decrease of intestinal motility during fasting allows enhanced intestinal absorption of unconjugated bilirubin; this represents a major pathway leading to fasting hyperbilirubinaemia (Kotal, Gastro, 1996; 111:217). Previously, the response to fasting was used as a test to diagnose Gilbert's syndrome, but the specificity of this test is low. A more rapid and possibly more sensitive test is the response to nicotinic acid (Gentile, JLabClinMed, 1986; 107:166). Structural liver disease is excluded by the finding of normal liver tests and normal serum bile acids; haemolysis must be excluded. In addition, the use of alkaline methanolysis with thin layer chromatography (Sieg, CCActa, 1986; 154:41) or HPLC (Muraca, Gastro, 1987; 92:309) permits diagnosis because the relative amount of unconjugated bilirubin IXα and monoglucuronide in serum and bile (Fevery, JCI, 1977; 60:970) are increased in combination with a decrease of the diconjugate.

Plasma clearance rate of an intravenously injected tracer dose of radiolabelled bilirubin is decreased in Gilbert's syndrome to approximately 30 per cent of the clearance rate in normal subjects. The fraction of pigment retained 4 h after injection averages 24 to 33 per cent of the dose in Gilbert's syndrome, compared with 10 per cent in healthy subjects. The major underlying mechanism is a decreased conjugation rate, supported by the finding that hepatic bilirubin UDP-glucuronyltransferase activity is significantly decreased in virtually all individuals with Gilbert's syndrome. The decreased amounts of bilirubin diglucuronide in serum and bile also point to a decreased conjugation rate. Enzyme-inducing agents such as phenobarbitone or glutethimide return serum bilirubin levels to normal. The heterozygous Gunn rat or the Bolivian squirrel monkey serve as a model for Gilbert's syndrome with a UDP-glucuronyltransferase activity reduced by 60 per cent and a decreased di- to monoglucuronide ratio in bile (Portman, Hepatol, 1984; 4: 175; Van Steenbergen, Gastro, 1990; 99:488). A recent study suggested that the genetic abnormality resulted from two extra bases (TA) in the 5′ promotor region of the UGT1A gene (Bosma, NEJM, 1995; 333:1171). This mutation seems necessary but it might not be sufficient to explain the syndrome since it was also present in homozygous form in some controls.

Reassurance that the disorder is benign and needs no treatment is necessary.

Bilirubinostasis and cholestasis

Decreased hepatobiliary secretion of bilirubin conjugates ('bilirubinostasis') and of bile acids, cholesterol, etc. ('cholestasis') is present in most cases of acquired liver diseases as biliary secretion represents the most vulnerable step. Several changes of bilirubin metabolism occur and can be useful for diagnosis.

Acyl shift

Enzymic esterification of bilirubin results in glycoside-conjugates in which the sugar moiety, glucuronic acid, glucose, or xylose, is bound at its carbon-1 atom in ester linkage with the propionic acid side-chain of bilirubin. In cholestasis, this ester linkage shifts from the original carbon-1 position to the carbon-2, carbon-3, or carbon-4 atom of the sugar (Compernolle, BiochemJ, 1978; 171:185). These non-C1 glucuronides are resistant to β-glucuronidase and are formed in a non-enzymic way during stasis in mild alkaline medium both *in vivo* and *in vitro*. It has been noted that this acyl shift also occurs with glucuronidated derivatives of frusemide, zomepirac, and tolmetin (Caldwell, BiochemPharm, 1982; 31:953; Hasegawa, DrugMetDisp, 1982; 10:469). Theoretically, formation of non-C1 glucuronides may constitute a protective mechanism since they do not undergo deconjugation by β-glucuronidase. As such, intestinal reabsorption of the resulting unconjugated bilirubin and transformation to glucuronides is limited. Indeed, glucuronides are not always harmless. For example, glucuronides of oestrogen at the C27 position have been shown to be cholestatic (Durham, JPharmExpTher, 1986; 237:490).

Formation of bilirubins covalently bound to albumin (bilirubin–protein conjugates)

During stasis in an albumin-containing environment, *in vivo* as well as *in vitro*, gradual formation of bilirubin conjugates linked irreversibly, and presumably covalently, to albumin occurs (McDonagh, JCI, 1984; 74:763). These bilirubin–albumin conjugates remain in plasma and do not undergo glomerular filtration. Their presence in plasma explains the absence of bilirubinuria despite a conjugated hyperbilirubinaemia as is the case, for example, when a mechanical bile-duct obstruction has been unblocked (Weiss, NEJM, 1983; 309:147; Van Hootegem, Hepatol, 1985; 5:112) or in the recovery phase of a cholestatic syndrome or hepatitis. After the obstruction is removed the bilirubin glucuronides and bile acids rapidly decrease in plasma but the bilirubin–albumin conjugates persist for a long time. This is consistent with the clinical observation that itching disappears usually within 1 or 2 days after removal of obstruction whereas jaundice persists. In the latter situation, almost all of the direct-reacting bilirubin in serum consists of bilirubin–protein conjugates. The *in vivo* relevance of formation of such bilirubin–albumin conjugates is unknown. Hypothetically it might constitute a mechanism to keep the glucuronides in plasma and to prevent them from entering tissues where they might possibly exert a toxic action.

They appear in serum in all conditions causing an accumulation of esterified bilirubin, such as biliary obstruction, hepatitis, cirrhosis, infiltrative liver disease, Dubin–Johnson syndrome, and in jaundice associated with sepsis (Weiss, NEJM, 1983; 309:147; Blanckaert, JLabClinMed, 1986; 108:77). The pigment's long half-life readily explains the persistence of high serum bilirubin levels in the absence of bilirubinuria during the resolution phase of liver disease.

Increase of plasma conjugated bilirubin

In cholestasis and bilirubinostasis an increase of the ratio of conjugated to total bilirubin as measured by alkaline methanolysis is an early and sensitive marker of hepatocellular damage yielding decreased secretion (Van Hootegem, Hepatol, 1985; 5:112).

The predominance of diconjugates

In conditions of bilirubinostasis bilirubin diconjugates will prevail above monoconjugates in bile as well as in serum. This has been observed during administration of ioglycamide (Mesa, Hepatol, 1985; 5:600; Mesa, JHepatol, 1990; 10:35), bromosulphophthalein (**BSP**), indocyanine green (**ICG**), or bromocresol green, or after temporary bile-duct obstruction; it is also present in a mutant Wistar rat strain with defective biliary secretion (Jansen, Hepatol, 1985; 5:573) and in the hypothyroid rat model (Van Steenbergen, JHepatol, 1988; 7:229). This predominance of diconjugates is presumably the result of a retarded elimination of the monoconjugates out of the cell; the latter thus remain available to the conjugating enzyme for a more prolonged time to serve as a substrate for further conjugation to diconjugates. In rat models of cholestasis, the ratio of di- to monoconjugates is also an early marker of disturbed biliary secretion of bilirubins.

Renal excretion of glucuronides

The enhanced reflux of bilirubin conjugates into plasma results in renal excretion of bilirubin conjugates. As mentioned above, only the non-covalently bound glucuronides are ultrafiltrable. From experiments in man and rats with chronic near-total biliary obstruction, it has been estimated that only approximately 0.6 to 1.6 per cent of the total bilirubin conjugates undergo glomerular filtration (Fulop, JCI, 1965; 44:666; Fevery, CCActa, 1967; 17:63). During total obstruction, the plasma level of conjugates will remain at levels between 510 and 680 mmol/l. Indeed, at that level the urinary excretion rate (0.006×400 mg/l × glomerular filtration rate (**GFR**)) will be equal to the daily bilirubin production rate (250–300 mg/day) in men. Higher plasma levels can only be obtained when a decrease of glomerular filtration or an increased bilirubin production such as haemolysis is associated with the cholestasis. Thus very high serum levels of bilirubin must lead to the suspicion of haemolysis or an associated decrease in renal function (Fulop, ArchIntMed, 1971; 127:254).

Dubin–Johnson's and Rotor's syndrome[5,6]

The Dubin–Johnson's syndrome represents an inherited defect of the biliary transport of conjugated bilirubin and BSP and an unexplained abnormality in coproporphyrin metabolism. The liver has a black appearance due to retention of a melanin-like pigment. Most of the patients are asymptomatic and the plasma bilirubin levels range between 20 and 50 mg/l (35–85 mmol/l). The hyperbilirubinaemia is direct-reacting with bilirubinuria. Non-C1 bilirubin glucuronides are present, as well as bilirubin–protein conjugates. The kinetics of injected BSP are highly characteristic: initial plasma disappearance rate is normal but a secondary rise due to reflux of conjugated BSP is observed after 45 to 90 min, suggesting that conjugation of BSP proceeds at a higher rate than biliary secretion. This secondary rise is not noted with dibromosulphophthalein (DBSP) or ICG, two substances that can be secreted without conjugation (Erlinger, Gastro, 1973; 64:106). The computed hepatic uptake and storage capacity are (near) normal, but the secretory maximum (Tm) is grossly impaired. In this syndrome urinary excretion of coproporphyrins is normal, but the excretion of isomer III is reduced, whereas that of the I isomer is enhanced to approximately 80 per cent of total coproporphyrins (in normal individuals, < 45 per cent). A recent study in the transport-deficient rat documented a single nucleotide deletion in the gene coding for the secretory carrier protein (*c moat*) (Paulusma, Science 1996; 27:1126). It is likely that a similar mutation is present in the Dubin–Johnson syndrome.

Rotor's syndrome seems to represent a decreased hepatic storage disease. This rare disorder is characterized by fluctuating direct-reacting hyperbilirubinaemia. In contrast to Dubin–Johnson's syndrome, coproporphyrin excretion in urine is enhanced and the ratio of I to III isomers is only mildly increased. Plasma BSP kinetics show a decreased disappearance rate, resulting in increased retention at 45 min. An autosomal recessive inheritance has been suggested.

Analysis of bilirubin conjugates in serum revealed a predominance of the diester conjugates in Dubin–Johnson syndrome, in agreement with data obtained in bilirubinostasis in the rat (Mesa, Hepatol, 1985; 5:600), and a predominance of the C-12 monoconjugate in Rotor's syndrome (Rosenthal, Hepatol, 1984; 4: 1026).

Differential diagnosis of jaundice based on analysis of plasma bilirubin pigments (Table 1)

Experiments in a series of animal models have greatly helped in understanding the altered bilirubin metabolism in disease states. To mimic bilirubin overproduction in the rat, unconjugated bilirubin has been infused intravenously or injected intraperitoneally; in other animals red cells haemolysed *in vitro* have been injected intravenously, or haemolysis was induced *in vivo* by injection of taurocholate. Results of serum and bile analysis are given in Table 3. Conditions of decreased bilirubin conjugation are present in the heterozygous Gunn rat; alternatively treatment with trijodothyronin can be used to decrease bilirubin UDP-glucuronyltransferase, whereas phenobarbitone, glutethimide, spironolactone, or clofibrate will enhance the transferase activity. Transferase activity correlated well with the biliary output of diglucuronide and inversely with the level of unconjugated bilirubin in plasma and bile. Decreased bilirubin secretion is present in the mutant TR rat or can be induced by infusion of ICG, BSP, bromocresol green, or ioglycamide (a cholangiographic substance), these agents compete with the biliary secretory process of bilirubin conjugates. During bilirubinostasis, plasma levels of bilirubin conjugates rise rapidly together with a predominance of bilirubin diconjugates in plasma and bile and a decrease of unconjugated bilirubin in bile (Table 3).

In general, three major fractions should be distinguished: unconjugated, esterified, and albumin-conjugated bilirubins. In healthy adults more than 95 per cent of bile pigment present in plasma is in the form of unconjugated bilirubin IXα (Muraca, Gastro, 1987; 92:309). In steady-state conditions, the concentration of unconjugated bilirubin IXα is directly related to the bilirubin production rate and inversely to the hepatic clearance rate. From Fig. 1, it can be deduced that a doubling of the bilirubin production rate will result in a twofold increase of serum unconjugated bilirubin. The relation between serum bilirubin and the conjugation rate is represented by an inverse hyperbola: decreases of the conjugation will at first be barely observed in serum, but at lower absolute conjugation rates a similar decrease will result in marked changes of the serum levels. Similarly, increased bilirubin production as, for example, produced by blood transfusion in Gilbert's syndrome, will lead to a rapid temporary increase of serum bilirubin levels. This suggests that small alterations in bilirubin production or conjugation occurring in individuals with Gilbert's syndrome (defective conjugation) will be expressed by great variations in serum levels. This situation resembles the relation between serum creatinine and the glomerular filtration rate. Very probably, the relation between serum concentration of esterified bilirubins and the biliary secretion rate is similar: as such, a marked decrease in biliary secretion is already present before serum bilirubin levels tend to go up (e.g. in primary biliary cirrhosis). However, once cholestasis is present, a further rather small decrease will produce a marked enhancement of serum bilirubin conjugates.

Usually, the upper limit of normal serum bilirubin values in adults is set at 1 mg/dl or 17 mmol/l, irrespective of gender.

Table 3 Experimental models of hyperbilirubinaemia in the rat

	Serum				Bile (nmol/min/kg)				GT activity (μg/h)	References
	UCB	MC	DC	MC:DC	UCB	MD	DC	MD:DC		
Normal rats	0.90	0.06	0.04	1.5	0.08	2.5	3.5	0.8	2.9	Muraca, Gastro, 1987; 92:309
Bilirubin overproduction										
UCB IP (34 μM/kg)	4.45	0.51	0.14	5						Muraca, Gastro, 1987; 92:309
IV (30 nmol/min/kg)	4.50	0.20	0.14	1.4	0.50	12	20			Mesa, JHepatol, 1989; 9:10
Haemolysis—red cells		nd			0.16	4.1	6.7			Mesa, JHepatol, 1989; 9:10
—due to TCA	2.76	0.18	0.13	1.4	0.21	5.2	8.5			Mesa, JHepatol, 1989; 9:10
Decreased glucuronidation										
Heterozygous Gunn rat	1.23	0.06	0.02	3	0.1	3.1	2.2	1.4	1.9	Van Steenbergen, Gastro, 1990; 99:488
Trijodothyronin (120 nmol/day/kg)	0.35	0.04	0.02	2	0.18	5.7	5.8	9.10	1.6	
Augmented glucuronidation due tophenobarbital, etc.	nd	nd	nd	nd	0.06	2.1	3.5	0.6	5.0	Van Steenbergen, Gastro, 1990; 99:488
Decreased bilirubin secretion										
TR rat		5.0	27	0.2	0.06	0.8	2.3	0.3		Jansen, Hepatol, 1985; 5:573
Competitive inhibition										
by BSP		1.1	1.5	0.7	0.02	0.6	1.8	0.4	2.7	Mesa, JHepatol, 1990; 10:35
Ioglycamide		0.5	0.6	0.8	0.01	0.4	1.8	0.3		Mesa, JHepatol, 1985; 5:600

BSP, bromosulphophthalein; DC, diconjugates; GT, glucuronyltransferase; IP, intraperitoneally; IV, intravenously; MC, monoconjugates; nd, not done; UCB, unconjugated bilirubin.

However, to define normal levels, one should also take into account that a sex difference in serum bilirubin concentration is well documented, adult males having significantly higher total bilirubin values than females (Werner, ZKlinChemKlinBiochem, 1970; 8:105; Owens, JMedGenet, 1975; 12:152). It is surprising that such a well-established observation has never been applied to clinical practice. It is not clear whether the lower total bilirubin values for serum in females are the result of a lower bilirubin production rate or of a higher hepatic clearance compared with males. The finding of a higher excretion of faecal urobilinogen in males (Bloomer, CCActa, 1970; 29:463) suggests a sex difference for bilirubin production rate, even if no difference is observed between males and females in plasma turnover studies with radiolabelled bilirubin (Berk, JCI, 1969; 48:2176). Experimental work in rats has demonstrated a more efficient hepatic conjugation and lower serum bilirubin values in female animals compared with males; progesterone enhances and testosterone decreases the glucuronyltransferase activity (Muraca, Gastro, 1984; 87:308; Muraca, ClinSci, 1983; 64:85).

Small amounts of bilirubin ester conjugates are found in the serum of normal healthy adults. Individual concentrations of mono- and diesterified bilirubins averaged 0.10 and 0.11 mmol/l, respectively, corresponding to 3.6 per cent of total bilirubin in a series of 43 healthy men and women (Muraca, ClinChem, 1983; 29:1767). The esterified pigments in normal serum have been identified as 1-O-acyl glucuronides, which most likely originate from hepatic reflux into plasma, since in man the liver seems to be the only organ that can esterify bilirubin to a significant extent and conjugates are not reabsorbed from the intestine (Lester, JCI, 1963; 42:736). Infusion of unconjugated bilirubin in rats leads to a parallel increase in the concentration of all bilirubin pigments in plasma, suggesting that an equilibrium exists between the amount of conjugates formed in the liver and their plasma concentrations (Muraca, Gastro, 1987; 92:309; Mesa, JHepatol, 1989; 9:10). In the absence of hepatobiliary disease, the concentration of esterified bilirubin in plasma seems to be determined principally by the rate of pigment production.

Differential diagnosis

With standardized diazo methods, it is of clinical interest at first to differentiate jaundice into a 'indirect', 'direct-reacting', or 'mixed' hyperbilirubinaemia on the basis of a total and a 10 min direct diazo-reaction (Fevery, CCActa, 1967; 17:73) (Fig. 2). Results can depend on the method used and may sometimes be difficult to interpret in patients with mild hyperbilirubinaemia (17–30 mmol/l) (Killenberg, Gastro, 1980; 78:1011). The alkaline methanolysis–HPLC method allows additional information: increased levels of esterified pigment can be demonstrated in patients with liver disease even at normal levels of total bilirubin, and the ratio of esterified to total bilirubin is specifically increased in hepatobiliary disorders. Moreover, it has been demonstrated that, unlike Gilbert's syndrome or Crigler–Najjar disease, patients with hyperbilirubinaemia due to bilirubin overproduction display a parallel increase of both unconjugated and conjugated bilirubins.

In summary, the three fundamentally different patterns of serum bilirubins can be differentiated by alkaline methanolysis–HPLC or –thin layer chromatography:

1. The purely unconjugated hyperbilirubinaemia associated with deficient hepatic conjugation (Gilbert's syndrome, Crigler–Najjar disease) is characterized by a selective increase of unconjugated bilirubin with normal or decreased absolute concentrations of the ester conjugates, resulting in a decreased percentage of esterified versus total bilirubin (Sieg, CCActa, 1986; 154:41; Muraca, Gastro, 1987; 92:309).

2. A parallel increase of both unconjugated and esterified bilirubins, with a normal ratio of esterified to total pigment, is characteristic

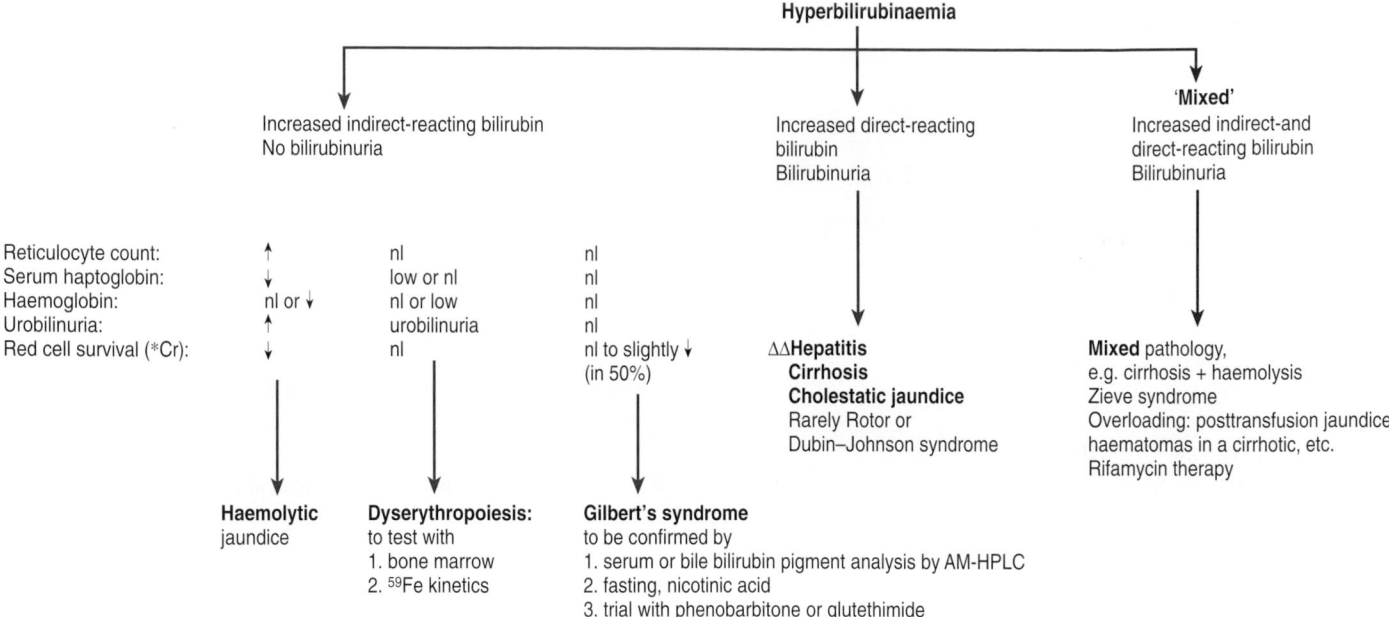

Fig. 2. Differential diagnosis of hyperbilirubinaemia by standardized diazo methods. nl, Normal level; AM-HPLC, alkaline methanolysis–HPLC; ΔΔ, differential diagnosis.

of increased pigment production (Muraca, Gastro, 1987; 92:309; Mesa, JHepatol, 1989; 9:10).

3. A normal or a moderately increased unconjugated bilirubin with a markedly increased concentration of esterified bilirubin, resulting in an increased percentage of esterified to total pigment, is found in hepatobiliary disease (Scharschmidt, Gut, 1982; 23: 643; Van Hootegem, Hepatol, 1985; 5:112).

Differentiation of esterified bilirubins into mono- and diesterconjugates rarely provides additional clinically useful information. The ratio of mono- to diester conjugates ratio is increased in both haemolytic jaundice and Gilbert's syndrome (Muraca, Gastro, 1987; 92:309).

Just as the other liver tests, serum bilirubin cannot discriminate between intrahepatic and extrahepatic causes of biliary obstruction. Total serum bilirubin is usually normal in the case of partial or incomplete biliary obstruction as can occur with intrahepatic gallstones or tumours or in sclerosing cholangitis or primary biliary cirrhosis (early phase); whereas serum bile acids and alkaline phosphatase are markedly elevated. Such a discrepancy reflects the large reserve capacity of the non-obstructed parenchyma to excrete bilirubin. Serum alkaline phosphatase and bile acids are elevated in such conditions, apparently as a result of enzymatic induction and altered permeability of the biliary tree (Wulkau, AnnClinBioch, 1986; 23:405). In alcoholic hepatitis, serum bilirubin is far in excess of the other liver tests, the reasons are not clear: a combination of haemolysis and cholestasis might be of importance in this situation.

The neonatal situation

Compared with the adult, bilirubin metabolism in the neonate is characterized by a higher pigment production and a lower conjugation rate. Unconjugated bilirubin accumulates in blood, with a

maximal level at day 4 or 5 after birth and declines afterwards. The presence of esterified bilirubins has previously been considered to result from an immaturity of the bile secretory process. However, in humans, using the sensitive alkaline methanolysis–HPLC procedures, accumulation of esterified bilirubin as seen in cholestasis could not be demonstrated since the ratio of esterified to total bilirubin in sera of 4-day-old neonates was only 0.5 to 1.5 per cent, [7] as compared to 3.6 ± 2.1 per cent in 42 healthy adults, and 40 to 80 per cent in cholestasis. The absolute concentration of bilirubin ester conjugates is higher in neonatal than in adult serum; nevertheless they constitute only 1 per cent of total pigment. This pattern seems to be the result of both an increased pigment production (leading to enhanced concentration of unconjugated and conjugated bilirubins) and of a decreased hepatic conjugation (resulting in a decrease of the ratio of conjugates to total). The situation was found to be quite different in newborn rats. In this species, the concentration of esterified bilirubin increases steeply at birth to account for approximately 40 per cent of total pigment (Muraca, BiolNeon, 1986; 49:90). This observation is in agreement with a neonatal immaturity of biliary secretion present in this species, as also evidenced by histochemistry and electron microscopy (De Wolf-Peeters, PediatRes, 1971; 5:704; ExpMolPath, 1974; 21:339). The enterohepatic circulation of unconjugated bilirubin IXα possibly represents a sizeable contribution to serum levels. Feeding agar decreased serum levels in some (Poland, NEJM, 1971; 284:1) but not in other studies. Recently, oral agar was found to be as effective as phototherapy in decreasing neonatal hyperbilirubinaemia, but the combination of both procedures was even more effective (Caglayen, Pediat, 1993; 92:86); similarly oral charcoal was found to be an effective adjunct to phototherapy (Amitai, JPerinatMed, 1993; 21:189).

Pigment gallstones

Black stones and brown stones constitute two greatly different types of pigmented gallstones (Trotman, Hepatol, 1982; 2:879). The brown stones are easily crushable, have a dull brown surface and alternating lighter and darker concentric layers on cross-section (Malet, Hepatol, 1984; 4:227). They contain mainly calcium palmitate, and frequently form in the bile ducts, presumably secondary to stasis and infection which might occur intermittently. Bacterial and leucocyte β-glucuronidase can induce deconjugation and thus augment concentrations of unconjugated pigment. Studies from Japan have demonstrated that bile of patients with brown pigment stones and cholangitis contains more unconjugated bilirubin in absolute and relative amounts in parallel to the bacterial cell count. In addition, infection lowers the pH of the bile from 8.0 ± 0.3 to 7.4 ± 0.4, thus promoting pigment precipitation (Nakano, Dig-DisSci, 1988; 33:1116). The black stones are hard and shiny; they occur mainly in the gallbladders of patients with haemolysis, hyperparathyroidism, or cirrhosis, and their incidence increases with age. They can be subdivided according to their predominant salt into calcium carbonate, calcium phosphate, or bilirubinate stones. All seem to have copper- and sulphur-containing proteins (Malet, Hepatol, 1984; 4:297). It has been suggested that mucin glycoproteins, presumably of gallbladder origin, form a protein network on to which bilirubins or cholesterol precipitate. On the other hand, bilirubin pigments seem to polymerize into a network which could initiate stone formation (Burnett, AnnSurg, 1981; 193: 331; Rege, BiochemJ, 1984; 224:871). It is not yet clear how and why bilirubin pigments precipitate. In haemolytic disorders, the amount of pigment in bile is enhanced tenfold or more (Fevery, EurJClinInv, 1980; 10:219) and the absolute concentration of unconjugated bilirubin may exceed the limits of solubility. Bile acids enhance the solubility of the bile pigments but calcium ions seem to lead to a decrease. Small amounts of monoconjugated bilirubins also occur in black pigment stones.

References

1. Bissell DM. Heme catabolism and bilirubin formation. In Ostrow JD, ed. *Bile pigments and jaundice*. New York: Marcel Dekker, 1986: 133–56.
2. Berk PD, Isola LM, and Jones EA. Specific defects in hepatic storage and clearance of bilirubin. In Ostrow JD, ed. *Bile pigments and jaundice*. New York: Marcel Dekker, 1986: 279–316.
3. Jansen PLM. Genetic diseases of bilirubin metabolism: the inherited unconjugated hyperbilirubinemias. *Journal of Hepatology*, 1996; **25**: 398.
4. Stoll MS. Phototherapy of jaundice. In Ostrow JD, ed. *Bile pigments and jaundice. Molecular, metabolic, and medical aspects*. New York: Marcel Dekker, 1986: 551–80.
5. Wolkoff AW, Cohen LE, and Arias IM. Inheritance of the Dubin–Johnson syndrome. *New England Journal of Medicine*, 1973; **288**: 113.
6. Wolkoff AW, *et al*. Rotor's syndrome: a distinct pathophysiologic entity. *American Journal of Medicine*, 1976; **60**: 173.
7. Muraca M, *et al*. In Rubaltelli F and Jori G, eds. *Neonatal jaundice*. New York: Plenum Press, 1984: 13.

20.7 The liver in intracellular and extracellular lipidosis

P. K. Mistry and A. V. Hoffbrand

The liver is commonly involved in many types of inherited lipidosis. Some of these conditions may not present until adult life when they are referred to the hepatologist because of an enlarged liver. The pattern of liver disease reflects the cell type involved in the lipidosis. Thus, Gaucher's disease and Niemann–Pick type A and B disease (Section 26) are primarily Kupffer cell lipidosis. In contrast, cholesterol ester storage disease and Niemann–Pick type type C disease (Section 26) affect hepatocytes as well as Kupffer cells. In extracellular lipidosis, a primary genetic defect in the hepatocytes leads to abnormal intravascular trafficking of lipids, causing extrahepatic disease which can be associated with hepatic steatosis. A large number of rare inherited diseases which may involve the liver are considered briefly in Appendix 3. Most of these abnormalities are discussed in detail in ref. [1] and their hepatological aspects are covered in ref. [2]. Recently, there have been major advances in the delineation and treatment of Gaucher's disease, the most common lysosomal storage disorder, affecting up to 20 000 individuals in the United States alone. This inborn error is widely regarded as a paradigm for the modern management of genetic diseases. Patients with Gaucher's disease commonly present to hepatologists, and therefore this topic will be covered in some depth in this chapter.

Gaucher's disease

Gaucher's disease is the most common lysosomal storage disorder. Deficient catalytic activity of glucocerebrosidase, caused by mutations in the structural gene encoding the enzyme, results in widespread accumulation of abnormal macrophages laden with glucosylceramide (Gaucher cells) that is derived from the degradation of membrane glycosphingolipids of effete cells.[3] Approximately 380 mg of glycolipid is turned over each day as a result of leucocytorrhexis and about 10 mg/day from erythrocytorrhexis but only 0.19 to 0.27 mg glucocerebroside accumulates daily in the liver of a typical patient with Gaucher's disease, suggesting that residual enzyme activity catabolizes most of the glucocerebroside (Kattlove, Blood, 1963; 33:379).

The clinical features include hepatosplenomegaly, marrow replacement, skeletal disease, lung infiltration, and a hypermetabolic state; rarely, neurological lesions occur. Three major phenotypes of Gaucher's disease are recognized based on the absence (type I) or the presence and severity (types II and III) of primary central nervous system involvement. The non-neuronopathic form of the

disease (type I) is the most common, and within this group there is wide interindividual variation in the rate of disease progression, which is only partly explained by the genotype at the glucocerebrosidase gene locus (Mistry, JMedGenet, 1993; 30:889). Patients may present in childhood with hepatosplenomegaly, pancytopenia, and crippling skeletal disease, or come to light in the ninth decade of life because of the incidental finding of splenomegaly. Type I Gaucher's disease occurs rarely in all ethnic groups but is more frequent in the Ashkenazi Jewish population. Type II (acute neuronopathic) disease is a rare disorder with no ethnic predilection. It causes a rapidly progressive neurovisceral storage disease and death in infancy. Type III (subacute neuronopathic) Gaucher's disease is a less rapidly progressive neurovisceral strorage disease, with death occurring in childhood or early adulthood. The prototype of type III is the genetic isolate of patients in the Norrbottnian region of northern Sweden. The patients are all descended from a common ancestor and are homozygous for the L444P mutation at the glucocerebrosidase gene locus. Three distinct subtypes of subacute neuronopathic form of the disease are now recognized: type IIIa describes progressive neurological involvement beginning in adolescence but mild visceral involvement; type IIIb describes severe systemic disease including massive hepatosplenomegaly and portal hypertension but mild neurological disease (Brady, ArchNeurol, 1993; 50:1212); and the recently discovered type IIIc Gaucher's disease describes a genetic isolate in Jenin. The patients are homozygous for the D409H mutation and exhibit a unique phenotype comprising corneal clouding, left–sided cardiac valvular calcification, and oculomotor apraxia but only mild visceral and skeletal disease (Abrahamov, Lancet, 1995; 346:1000).

Type I Gaucher's disease is frequent among the Jews of eastern European origin in whom the carrier frequency is 1 in 10 and disease frequency 1 in 855.[3] It is rare in non-Jewish people, with a disease frequency of approximately 1 in 60 000, similar to that of haemophilia. It appears that many affected patients of Ashkenazi origin, who are homozygous for the milder mutation (N370S, which accounts for 75 per cent of all disease alleles in this population), never come to medical attention. In contrast, type I Gaucher's disease in the non-Jewish population appears to be more aggressive. The usual presentation is with non-tender splenomegaly, often associated with cytopenia, although these features may be unrecognized for many years. The degree of splenomegaly is highly variable, ranging from five- to 75-fold when adjusted for body weight (a normal spleen is about 0.2 per cent of body weight). The absolute size can vary from 300 g to over 10 kg, accounting for 15 to 25 per cent of body weight. The glycolipid content of the spleen of a patient with Gaucher's disease is greatly increased, with values ranging from 3 to 40.5 mg/g wet weight, compared to 60 to 280 μg/g in the normal spleen (Kennaway, JLipRes, 1968; 9:755). The spleen appears to enlarge most rapidly in children. Rapid enlargement of the spleen in an adult patient should lead to suspicion of an associated disorder which could have resulted in increased glycolipid turnover, for example haematological malignancy, immune thrombocytopenia, or autoimmune haemolytic anaemia. Nodules on the suface of the spleen may represent regions of extramedullary haemopoiesis, collections of Gaucher's cells, or resolving infarcts. Evidence of old infarcts is common in spleens that are over twentyfold larger than normal. Most infarcts have been asymptomatic, but subcapsular infarcts can present as localized abdominal pain.

Hepatomegaly occurs in over 50 per cent of patients with Gaucher's disease type I. In a series of 88 patients, liver volumes ranged from 0.74 to 8.7 times the predicted normal (normal is about 2.5 per cent body weight) with a median of 1.75 (Sibille, AmJHumGen, 1993; 52:1094). Hepatic glucocerebroside levels are elevated from 23- to 389-fold above normal; that is, 702 μg/g to 17.9 mg/g wet weight compared to normal levels of 31 to 46 μg/g (Brady, NEJM, 1974; 291:989). The massively enlarged liver is usually hard to palpate, with an irregular surface. Cirrhosis and portal hypertension are uncommon but do occur in a small number of patients (Gall, AmJClinPath, 1956; 26:1398; James, Gastro, 1981; 80:126). Portal hypertension can be accentuated by compression of the sinusoids by Gaucher's cells. Death from variceal haemorrhage has been reported (Fellows, JPediat, 1975; 87:739). Minor elevations of liver enzymes are common, even in mildly affected patients, but the presence of jaundice appears to be a poor prognostic sign. Jaundice in a patient with Gaucher's disease is usually a result of infection, the development of chronic hepatitis, or, rarely, due to hepatic decompensation in the late stages (Patel, AmJMed, 1986; 80:523). Haemolysis should be considered in the presence of unconjugated hyperbilirubinaemia. There may be prolonged prothrombin, partial thromboplastin, and bleeding times because of hepatic involvement (Boklan, ArchIntMed, 1976; 136:489). The level of serum ferritin may be very high although transferrin saturation is normal (Morgan, BMJ, 1983; 286:1864). Hepatic involvement in Gaucher's disease is always evident on biopsy by the presence of glycolipid-laden Kupffer cells in liver sinusoids. Hepatocytes do not manifest overt glycolipid storage, presumably because there is substantial excretion of glucocerebroside in the bile and because the bulk of glycolipid turnover from effete cells is handled by mononuclear phagocytes (Tokoro, JLipRes, 1987; 28:968). This sparing of the hepatocytes is in keeping with a low incidence of severe liver failure. On liver biopsy, Gaucher's cells are diastase–periodic acid–Schiff reagent positive, and have a finely striated appearance due to the presence of glycolipid-engorged lysosomes (James, Gastro, 1981; 80:126). Gaucher's cells are autofluorescent, and intense acid phosphatase activity can be demonstrated by enzymic histochemical methods. Some patients may have only scattered foci of Gaucher's cells in the liver. Most patients have more extensive involvement with zonal distribution; the central zones are more commonly involved. This is in keeping with the

liver as the major organ harbouring tissue macrophages. There is usually pericellular fibrosis and a small number of patients have established cirrhosis. The liver may exhibit extramedullary haemopoiesis.

Haematological manifestations include cytopenia and acquired coagulopathy due to deficiency of factor XI. However, there is a high incidence of genetic deficiency of factor XI among the Ashkenazim, who are also at high risk of Gaucher's disease. When cytopenia occurs in splenectomized patients it reflects advanced marrow infiltration by Gaucher's cells. Bone marrow failure and myelofibrosis occur in a small number of these patients (Mistry, QJMed,1992; 84:541). T-lymphocyte deficiency in spleen and blood, as well as decreased natural killer cells and impaired neutrophil chemotaxis, have been demonstrated but there are no compelling data to show that Gaucher's patients are more susceptible to infections. There appears to be a higher incidence of polyclonal hypergammaglobulinaemia, benign paraproteinaemia, and multiple myeloma in Gaucher's disease.[3]

The skeletal manifestations of Gaucher's disease are protean, ranging from asymptomatic 'Erlenmeyer flask deformity' of the distal femur to pathological fractures, vertebral collapse, and acute bone crises. Fever is common during episodes of bone crises, raising suspicion of osteomyelitis.[4]

Rarely, cardiopulmonary involvement may occur in Gaucher's disease. Pulmonary hypertension due to infiltration of lung parenchyma and alveolar spaces by glycolipid-laden macrophages has been described. Some patients with pulmonary hypertension do not have such infiltrative disease; these patients appear to have intrapulmonary shunting secondary to liver disease. Cardiac abnormalities include pericarditis and interstitial infiltration of the myocardium, resulting in impaired left ventricular function. More recently valvular abnormalities have been described in the newly designated type IIIc Gaucher's disease (Mistry, Lancet, 1995; 346: 982).

Other manifestations of Gaucher's disease include yellow-brown cutaneous pigmentation and much-cited ocular manifestation of pingueculas. The resting energy expenditure in Gaucher's disease is increased by about 25 per cent and this is associated with increased basal glucose production (Corssmit, JEndocrMetab, 1995; 80:2653).

The diagnosis is often made by the finding of classical glycolipid-laden macrophages (Gaucher's cells) in bone-marrow aspirate carried out because of haematological abnormalities, or in liver biopsy performed to explain hepatosplenomegaly. However, similar pseudo-Gaucher's cells have been described in a variety of other disorders, including chronic granulocytic leukaemia, thalassaemia, multiple myeloma, Hodgkin's disease, plasmacytoid lymphomas, and in AIDS patients with *Mycobacterium avium* infection (Beutler, Medicine, 1995; 74:305). Thus, measurement of acid β–glucosidase activity of peripheral blood leucocytes remains the investigation of choice to establish the diagnosis of Gaucher's disease. A finding of less than 15 per cent of mean normal activity is diagnostic of the disease. Generally, heterozygotes have half the enzyme activity, but there is up to 20 per cent overlap with controls. Genetic diagnosis can be helpful, especially in Ashkenazi patients in whom four mutations at the glucocerebrosidase gene locus (N370S, L444P, 84GG, and IVS2 + 1) account for about 97 per cent of disease alleles. However, in non-Jewish patients these mutations account for about 75 per cent of disease alleles (Mistry, JMedGenet, 1993;

30:889). Thus, if Gaucher's disease is suspected clinically in a Jewish patient, there is an excellent chance of being able to confirm the diagnosis by DNA analysis. Among non-Jewish patients there is also a good chance of being able to do so, but there are many 'private' mutations and therefore a negative result does not exclude the diagnosis. Mutation analysis for Gaucher's disease in routine clinical practice can be complicated because the structural gene for glucocerebrosidase is closely linked to a highly homologous pseudogene which harbours many of the causal mutations and, unusually, this pseudogene is transcribed at high level. However, several polymerase chain reaction (**PCR**)-based techniques have overcome many of these difficulties (Mistry, Lancet, 1992; 339: 889). An important advantage of mutation analysis is that it has considerable predictive value with respect to disease progression and may thus identify patients who will derive significant benefit if enzyme therapy is initiated during the presymptomatic stage of the disease and before onset of irreversible tissue damage (Zimran, Lancet, 1989; ii:349).

Therapy
Splenectomy

With the availability of enzyme therapy, there are now very few indications for splenectomy. Rapid development of splenomegaly in an adult patient should raise the suspicion of increased glycolipid turnover due to development of an associated disorder, for example haemolytic anaemia or onset of malignancy. A massively enlarged spleen associated with severe hypersplenism can itself result in rapid progression of Gaucher's disease due to increased glycolipid turnover and can also make the patient refractory to enzyme treatment by acting as a sink, thus diverting enzyme molecules from other sites affected by the disease.[5] Such patients may be transfusion dependent, which will further accentuate cellular glycolipid overload. Occasionally, the spleen is greatly increased in size as well as severely fibrotic. In this setting, enzyme therapy is unlikely to cause a significant reduction of spleen size.[5] Fortunately, such patients are rare, but when splenectomy is undertaken prophylaxis with Pneumovax® and *Haemophilus influenzae* type b vaccine (**Hib**) followed by oral penicillin is essential to protect against infections by encapsulated organisms. There is a theoretical risk of rapid progression of Gaucher's disease at other sites following splenectomy, especially with regard to skeletal complications in type I disease and neurological disease in type III. This is controversial, but carefully planned enzyme therapy after splenectomy should obviate these problems. When splenectomy is indicated some physicians recommend partial splenectomy to avoid the risks of an asplenic state as well as the risk of rapid disease progression in extrasplenic tissues (Ber-Maor, JPediatSurg, 1993; 28:686).

Skeletal disease

The quality of life of patients with Gaucher's disease may be greatly enhanced by appropriate surgical intervention. It is important to exclude vitamin D deficiency. The use of phosphonates has produced encouraging results.[3] To help prevent skeletal complications, patients should be advised to avoid activities that put sudden stress on the skeleton.

Liver transplantation

It has been claimed that orthotopic liver transplantation can cure Gaucher's disease through microchimerism between donor macrophages and lymphocytes in extrahepatic tissues of the recipient, where these donor-derived cells produce normal enzyme for uptake by deficient cells (Starzl, NEJM, 1993; 328:745). However, unlike other lysosomal enzymes, endogenous glucocerebrosidase does not undergo secretion-recapture and therefore, as expected, Gaucher's disease progresses rapidly following transplantation if enzyme therapy is not administered (Carlson, Transpl, 1990; 49:1192). Thus, the only indication for liver transplantation in Gaucher's disease is the rare patient with cirrhosis and hepatic decompensation. Such patients also respond poorly to enzyme therapy, presumably because mannose receptors are downregulated in cirrhosis (Toth, Hepatol, 1992; 16:255) and thus liver transplantation will not only replace the failing liver, it will also restore responsiveness to enzyme therapy.

Enzyme therapy

For the treatment of Gaucher's disease, industrial-scale preparations of glucocerebrosidase are purified from human placentas or from recombinant Chinese hamster ovary cells and sequentially deglycosylated to expose core mannose residues (Ceredase® and Cerezyme®, respectively: Genzyme Corp.) in order to render the exogenous enzyme molecule a putative ligand for the mannose receptors which are selectively expressed on macrophages and sinusoidal endothelial cells. Macrophage-targeted glucocerebrosidase is highly effective in reversing the visceral and haematological manifestations of Gaucher's disease, but skeletal disease is slower to respond (Barton, NEJM, 1991; 324:1464). The treatment is costly at the recommended initial dose of 60 U/kg administered intravenously once every fortnight. However, comparable responses have been reported at doses of 1.15 U/kg thrice weekly (Hollak, Lancet, 1995; 345:1474) or 2.5 U/kg thrice weekly (Zimran, AmJMed, 1994; 97:3), as well as 5 U/kg twice weekly (Mistry, QJMed, 1992; 84:541). Recent studies on *in vivo* tissue pharmacokinetics of mannose-terminated glucocerebrosidase in patients with Gaucher's disease show that it is possible to achieve consistent restitution of cellular enzyme activity when the enzyme is administered at doses which are subsaturating for the mannose receptors (<5 U/kg) and when it is given up to twice weekly to take account of the intracellular half-life of the enzyme.[5] Thus a strong case can be made in favour of frequent administration of low doses, which is economical and may also be safer because such a regimen permits very rapid clearance of contaminating mannose-terminated proteins in Ceredase® from the blood.[5] The issue of enzyme dosage and frequency is highly controversial (Beutler, AmJMed, 1994; 97:1). In adult patients the authors start Ceredase® at 2 U/kg body weight twice or thrice weekly and have observed satisfactory responses. Individualized stepwise increase of dose as well as frequency of enzyme infusion is undertaken when patients show a poor response to enzyme therapy. Children affected by Gaucher's disease have, in general, more rapidly progressive disease which merits higher-dose therapy, preferably with the recombinant enzyme.

Enzyme therapy with macrophage-targeted glucocerebrosidase (Ceredase® or Cerezyme®) is indicated for patients with type I

Gaucher's disease who exhibit severe clinical symptoms of the disease due to anaemia, thrombocytopenia, skeletal disease, or visceromegaly. In the future, patients harbouring genotypes at the glucocerebrosidase gene locus which predict poor prognosis may also qualify for enzyme therapy before the onset of symptoms and irreversible tissue damage. However, before the indications for enzyme therapy are broadened in this way it is desirable that recombinant enzyme (Cerezyme®) is universally available. Overall, there is about a 25 per cent decrease in liver and spleen volumes after 6 months of therapy. In anaemic patients the haemoglobin rises by about 1.5 g/dl during the first 4 to 6 months of therapy. An additional 1 g/dl increase is observed in the subsequent 9 to 18 months in persistently anaemic patients. The platelet count increases more slowly and requires at least 1 year to double. Skeletal disease is the slowest to respond, with significant symptomatic improvement within the first year of treatment, although a much longer period of enzyme therapy is required to achieve a radiological response (Rosenthal, Pediat, 1995; 96:629; Elstein, BloodCellsMol Dis, 1996; 22:101).

The response to enzyme therapy should be monitored by following symptoms, radiology, and laboratory markers of Gaucher's disease. Six- to nine-monthly magnetic resonance imaging (**MRI**) scans of the abdomen, femora, and tibia allow the most accurate staging of the disease, including precise assessment of skeletal involvement. A number of serum markers of macrophage activation provide a useful indication of response; these include tartarate-resistant acid phosphatase, chitotriosidase (Hollak, JCI, 1994; 93: 1288), and angiotensin-converting enzyme activity. In addition, the authors have found immunoglobulins, ferritin, and serum lipoprotein levels helpful for monitoring the response.

There is wide interindividual variation in responsiveness to enzyme therapy. This does not correlate with genotype at the glucocerebrosidase gene locus, disease severity, splenectomy, age, or enzyme dosage (Zimran, AmJMed, 1994; 97:3). However, a number a factors portend a poor response to enzyme therapy. These include severe hypersplenism resulting in transfusion dependency, pulmonary disease, cirrhosis of the liver with portal hypertension, and those with underlying haematological malignancy. Increased frequency of enzyme infusion may be required for patients who show a poor response to treatment to compensate for a reduced intracellular half-life of the enzyme.[5] In patients with advanced cirrhosis, intensive enzyme therapy, whatever the regimen, fails to ameliorate portal hypertension and the risk of life-threatening variceal haemorrhage (R. O. Brady and P. K. Mistry, personal communication).

Some 2000 patients are receiving enzyme therapy. Generally it is extremely well tolerated. About 10 to 15 per cent of patients develop antibodies against enzyme protein. A few of these develop pruritus during enzyme infusion, but it has been possible to continue therapy in such patients without the occurrence of serious reactions. Only one patient has had an anaphylactic reaction with complement activation. All antibodies reported to date have been IgG, mostly of the IgG1 subclass. The processing of placental extract destroys known viruses, including human immunodeficiency virus, hepatitis B, and hepatitis C. It is expected that the recombinant enzyme will become widely available over the next 2 to 3 years.

Marrow transplantation

Macrophages are the progeny of haematopoietic stem cells. The Gaucher phenotype is attributable largely to changes in the macrophages, although deficiency of glucocerebrosidase is present in all cell types. Therefore, marrow transplantation should be curative, and so it is (Erikson, ActaPaedScand, 1990; 79:680). However, the risks of transplantation are prohibitive in those most severely affected by the disease. Thus with the availability of enzyme therapy, it is difficult to justify marrow transplantation as a treatment modality for type I Gaucher's disease. This form of treatment has been advocated for type III patients in the expectation that wild-type donor macrophages will populate the brain (a site which is inaccessible through systemic enzyme infusions) to reverse neurological damage. However, the pathophysiology of brain disease in type III is complex, with good evidence for the extraneurological origin of brain glucocerebroside and, in keeping with this, a satisfactory response to systemic enzyme administration (Erikson, Neuropediatrics, 1995; 26:203).

Gene therapy

Because the disease can be corrected by transplantation of allogeneic haematopoietic stem cells, the introduction of a wild-type cDNA encoding glucocerebrosidase into autologous haematopoietic stem cells and infusion of these genetically engineered cells into the patient is an attractive prospect for management of Gaucher's disease in the future. Development of such a strategy is hampered by the fact that the genetically corrected cells do not enjoy a selective advantage over those that have not received the wild-type glucocerebrosidase gene, and the former do not secrete the enzyme for uptake by the latter cell type. Thus the prerequisites of successful gene therapy will be to achieve a high-frequency transformation of the cells that have been removed from the body, as well as to destroy the endogenous cells of the patient.[3]

Wolman's disease and cholesterol ester storage disease

Cholesterol ester storage disease (**CESD**) and Wolman's disease are autosomal recessive disorders associated with reduced activity of lysosomal acid lipase due to mutations in the gene encoding this enzyme (Anderson, PNAS, 1994; 91:2718). Deficient activity of lysosomal acid lipase results in massive accumulation of cholesteryl esters and triglycerides in most tissues of the body. Wolman's disease occurs in infancy and is nearly always fatal before the age of 1 year. Hepatosplenomegaly, steatorrhoea, adrenal calcification, and failure to thrive are observed in first weeks of life.[6] CESD is less severe, being caused by milder mutations in the lysosomal acid lipase gene which are associated with higher residual enzyme activity (Aslanidis, Genomics, 1996; 33:85). CESD may not be detected until adulthood. Lipid deposition is widespread, although hepatomegaly may be the only clinical abnormality. Hyperlipidaemia (type IIa or IIb) is common and premature atherosclerosis may be severe. Adrenal calcification is rare in CESD.

Hepatomegaly is a constant feature of Wolman's disease and CESD. The liver function tests, and other routine laboratory investigations, are usually normal, but serum bile acids were very high in one patient (Schiff, AmJMed, 1968; 44:538). The normal architecture of the liver is sometimes preserved but may be severely distorted. The heptocytes appear hypertrophied and vacuolated. The Kupffer cells are prominent with large numbers of foamy histiocytes. Portal and periportal fibrosis may be marked, and there may be frank cirrhosis. The liver in CESD has an extraordinary orange or butter-yellow appearance. Microscopic examination of the CESD liver reveals many of the same abnormalities as in Wolman's disease. There are lipid droplets in hepatic parenchymal cells resembling those in ordinary fatty infiltration and enlargement of Kupffer cells by smaller vacuoles and by periodic acid–Schiff-positive granules. This is accompanied by variable amounts of septal fibrosis, which has progressed in some patients to micronodular cirrhosis with oesophageal varices. There is massive storage of birefringent material in hepatocytes. Birefringence under polarized light disappears on heating to between 50 and 60 °C and returns on cooling, a feature not seen in other lysosomal deficiency states.

The diagnosis is often made after a liver biopsy, as the sample has a characteristic orange appearance to the naked eye and there are typical abnormalities on light and electron microscopy. The cholesterol ester content of the biopsy is very high: levels from 95 to 244 mg/g wet weight have been described. Samples should be taken for electron microscopy in all young patients who might have a metabolic cause for hepatomegaly, and measurement of cholesteryl ester or lysosomal acid lipase activity should be undertaken if the person doing the biopsy appreciates the significance of the appearance of the biopsy sample. However, the liver biopsy is not necessary if the condition is suspected on clinical grounds as the diagnosis can be made by measuring lysosomal acid lipase activity in peripheral blood leucocytes or in cultured skin fibroblasts; patients with CESD (or Wolman's disease) will have an activity which is only 1 to 10 per cent of that found in normal subjects. Routine genotyping at the lysosomal acid lipase gene locus for diagnosis of CESD is not feasible at the present time, due to the heterogeneity of mutations.

Lipoprotein disorders
Hypolipoproteinaemias
Abetalipoproteinaemia

Abetaliporoteinaemia is an autosomal recessive disorder characterized by the virtual absence of apolipoprotein B-containing lipoproteins (chylomicrons, very low density lipoprotein (VLDL), and low density lipoprotein (LDL)) from plasma.[7] However, there is intracellular accumulation of apolipoprotein B associated with triglyceride accumulation in enterocytes and hepatocytes. Fat malabsorption is severe. Acanthocytes and echinocytes are seen in peripheral blood, and red cell membrane phospholipids contain much more sphingomyelin than normal. There is usually a shortened red cell half-life, with reticulocytosis, hyperbilirubinaemia, and marrow hyperplasia. The prothrombin time is prolonged due to vitamin K deficiency, but this corrects with treatment. Deficits in transport of tocopherol in blood leads to spinocerebellar ataxia with degeneration of fasciculus gracilis, peripheral neuropathy, degenerative pigmentary retinopathy, and ceroid myopathy. The metabolic defect in abetalipoproteinaemia is the absence of activity of microsomal triglyceride transfer protein, a

factor critical to the intracellular lipidation of apolipoprotein B (Wetterau, Science, 1992; 258:999). There is an unexplained excess of males (2 : 1). The gene encoding microsomal triglyceride transfer protein has been assigned to chromosome 4q22–24, and thus the role of gender in disease expression is not understood.

Despite the inability of the liver to secrete VLDL, abnormalities of liver function are uncommon in abetalipoproteinaemia. Several patients have had abnormal levels of transaminases in serum and three have had cirrhosis. However, two of these cases had been treated with medium-chain triglycerides. The third case did not receive medium-chain triglycerides but had micronodular cirrhosis without inflammation but with a large-droplet hepatocellular steatosis (Black, Gastro, 1991; 101:520). In this patient there was no history of blood transfusion or of exposure to hepatotoxic drugs, although she had been given large doses of vitamin A. This patient went on to have liver transplantation but there was no follow-up.

Tangier disease

Tangier disease is characterized by severe deficiency or absence of normal high density lipoprotein (HDL) in plasma and results in accumulation of cholesteryl esters in many tissues of the body. [1] These include tonsils, liver, spleen, lymph nodes, thymus, intestinal mucosa, and peripheral nerves. The major signs are hyperplastic orange tonsils, splenomegaly, and relapsing splenomegaly. Hepatomegaly has been reported in about one-third of the patients, but liver function tests are usually normal. The plasma apolipoprotein A1 level is extremely low and turnover studies suggest that it is due to hypercatabolism. The genetic defect underlying this disorder has not yet been worked out.

Hyperlipoproteinaemia
Types I, IV, and V

Three inherited disorders have been described in which chylomicrons accumulate in plasma (type I hyperlipidaemia): familial lipoprotein lipase deficiency, familial apolipoprotein C II deficiency, and familial inhibitor to lipoprotein lipase. Patients suffer recurrent abdominal pain due to acute pancreatitis triggered by massively elevated triglycerides in plasma, which may reach 50 to 100 mmol/l. Classically, patients present with eruptive cutaneous xanthomas and lipaemia retinalis. Familial type IV hyperlipidaemia is rare as most patients with this phenotype have an acquired abnormality. The nature of the genetic abnormality is not known, nor is the mechanism of hypertriglyceridaemia, but some patients may have excess VLDL secretion and others impaired VLDL catabolism. Familial type V hyperlipidaemia is the result of the presence in fasting plasma of large amounts of both chylomicrons and VLDL.

In each of these types of hyperlipoproteinaemia an enlarged and easily palpable liver is commonly found when there is severe hypertriglyceridaemia. Splenomegaly is less common but it also occurs in patients with hyperchylomicronaemia syndrome (types I and IV). The size of the organ decreases when when plasma triglyceride falls. Presumably, there is reversible accumulation of triglyceride within these organs; they show lipid-laden macrophages (foam cells) which are also present in bone marrow. The hepatocytes may also show vacuolation.

Familial hypercholesterolaemia

Familial hypercholesterolaemia is an autosomal dominant disease with a gene dosage effect that results in elevation of LDL and widespread accumulation of cholesterol ester-laden macrophages, resulting in severe coronary atherosclerosis and tendon xanthomas. The defect in familial hypercholesterolaemia is a mutation in the gene encoding the receptor for LDL. Located on the cell surface of liver and other organs, this receptor binds LDL with high affinity to mediate endocytosis and its delivery to lysosomes, where the ligand is degraded and its cholesterol released (Brown and Goldstein, Science, 1986; 232:34). When LDL receptors are deficient, the rate of removal of LDL from blood is markedly slowed, leading to elevation of LDL in inverse proportion to the receptor number. The excess plasma LDL is deposited in macrophages and other cell types, producing xanthomas and atheromas. More than 150 mutations in the gene encoding the LDL receptor have been reported to impair receptor function.[8] The prevalence of heterozygotes is about 1 in 500 and that of homozygotes is estimated to be 1 in one million people. Heterozygotes have a mean twofold elevation of plasma LDL (total serum cholesterol 9–15 mmol/l) from birth. Tendon xanthomas and coronary atherosclerosis develop after the mid-twenties. Homozygotes have severe hypercholesterolaemia (serum cholesterol 20–30 mmol/l) and have cutaneous xanthomas by 4 years of age. Coronary heart disease begins in childhood and frequently causes death from myocardial infarction before age 20.

In homozygous familial hypercholesterolaemia, there is little or no response to dietary modification, bile-acid-binding resins, ileal bypass, or to HMG CoA reductase inhibitors, which all act through inducing the normal LDL receptor gene. The main interest of this condition for hepatologists lies in the surgical treatments that have been employed in this life-threatening condition. In 1973, Starzl (Lancet, 1973; ii:940) observed that intravenous hyperalimentation reduced the plasma cholesterol of one homozygote and, stimulated by this observation, he went on to create an end-to-side portacaval shunt. The level of plasma cholesterol fell from 20 mmol/l to 6.5 mmol/l. Since then, at least 45 homozygotes, from 2.5 to 35 years of age, have undergone portacaval shunt surgery, and in most of them the plasma cholesterol was reduced by 25 to 50 per cent (Bilheimer, Artscler (Suppl.), 1989; 9:1158). Metabolic studies suggested that diversion of portal blood away from the liver reduced total body cholesterol synthesis, LDL synthesis as well as bile-acid synthesis, through an unknown mechanism. Portacaval shunt surgery, although well tolerated, is not associated with sufficient reduction of cholesterol levels to be used as the sole therapy in familial hypercholesterolaemia homozygotes.

The rationale for liver transplantation in homozygous familial hypercholesterolaemia is based on experimental data in animals showing that more than 70 per cent of the body's LDL receptors are in the liver. In the published literature there are five cases of patients with homozygous familial hypercholesterolaemia who have undergone liver transplantation (Bilheimer, Artscler (Suppl.), 1989; 9:1158). The authors have knowledge of a further three cases (Mistry, unpublished). There was a dramatic reduction of LDL cholesterol to near-normal levels in all patients; liver transplantation conferrred responsiveness to HMG CoA reductase inhibitors and these agents resulted in a further reduction of LDL levels. There was concomitant regression of xanthomatous deposits. However, the risk of transplantation in the presence of severe atherosclerosis, as well as the risks of long-term immunosuppression, have to be weighed carefully against the likely prognosis without transplantation.

The response to liver transplantation in homozygous familial hypercholesterolaemia underscores the importance of hepatic LDL receptors *in vivo*, paving the way for liver-targeted somatic cell gene therapy. However, preliminary attempts at *ex vivo* gene therapy have been disappointing. Five patients were treated using an *ex vivo* strategy in which the patients underwent partial hepatic lobectomy, followed by primary culture of hepatocytes, retroviral-mediated transduction of wild-type cDNA for the LDL receptor, and finally infusion of genetically engineered hepatocytes back into the patient via an indwelling cannula into the superior mesenteric vein (Grossman, NatureMed, 1995; 1:1137). Overall, a minor reduction of LDL levels was achieved and this proved to be transient. Further developments in this area will require *in vivo* hepatocyte-targeted gene therapy strategies with appropriate vectors that achieve a markedly higher efficiency of gene transduction and longer-term transgene expression.

References

1. Scriver CR, Beaud AL, Sly WS, and Valle D, eds. *The metabolic and molecular basis of inherited disease*, 7th edn. New York: McGraw Hill, 1995.
2. Ishak KG and Sharp HL. Metabolic errors and liver disease. In MacSween RMN, Anthony PP, and Scheuer P, eds. *Pathology of the liver*, 2nd edn. Edinburgh: Churchill Livingstone, 1987: 99–180.
3. Zimran A and Beutler E. Gaucher disease. In Brenner MK and Hoffbrand AV, eds. *Recent advances in haematology*. Edinburgh: Churchill Livingstone, 1996: Vol. 8, 83–117.
4. Mankin. Metabolic bone disease in Gaucher's disease. In Avioli, ed. in *Metabolic bone disease*. W. B. Saunders, 1990.
5. Mistry PK, Wraight EP, and Cox TM. Therapeutic delivery of proteins to macrophages: implications for treatment of Gaucher's disease. *Lancet*, 1996; **348**.
6. Assman G and Seedorf U. Acid lipase deficiency: Wolman disease and cholesteryl ester storage disease. In Scriver CR, Beaud AL, Sly WS, and Valle D, eds. *The metabolic and molecular basis of inherited disease*, 7th edn.: McGraw Hill, 1995.
7. Sharp D, *et al*. Cloning and gene defects in microsomal triglyceride transfer protein associated with abetalipoproteinaemia. *Nature*, 1993; **365**: 65.
8. Goldstein JL, Hobbs HH, and Brown MS. Familial hypercholesterolaemia. In Scriver CR, Beaud AL, Sly WS, and Valle D, eds. *The metabolic and molecular basis of inherited disease*, 7th edn. New York: McGraw Hill, 1995.

20.8 Glycogen storage diseases

P. K. Mistry

Glycogen storage diseases are inherited disorders characterized by an abnormal accumulation of glycogen. Most proteins involved in the metabolism of glycogen or its regulation have been found to cause some form of glycogen storage disease. The glycogen that accumulates in these disorders is abnormal either in quantity or quality. The disorders are numbered I to VI, in the order in which the enzymatic defects were discovered. Liver and muscle have abundant glycogen stores and are the most seriously affected tissues. Because carbohydrate metabolism in the liver ensures plasma glucose homeostasis, glycogen storage diseases that mainly affect the liver have hepatomegaly and hypoglycaemia as the usual presenting features; they are type I (glucose 6-phosphatase deficiency), type III (debrancher), type IV (brancher), and type VI (liver phosphorylase and phosphorylase kinase deficiency). The hepatic glycogen storage diseases show striking variation in age of onset, rate of progression, severity, and extrahepatic organ involvement. In contrast, the role of glycogen in muscle is to provide substrates which enable the ATP generation necessary for muscle contraction. The predominant features of glycogen storage diseases that affect the muscle are muscle cramps, exercise tolerance, suceptibility to fatigue, and progressive weakness. Glycogen storage diseases that affect the muscle predominantly are type II (α-glucosidase deficiency), type V (muscle phosphorylase deficiency; McArdel's disease), and type VII (phosphofructokinase deficiency). The overall frequency of all forms of glycogen storage diseases is approximately 1 in 20 000 to 25 000 live births. Types I, II, III, and VI are the most common and account for more than 90 per cent of all cases.[1]

The first clinical and pathological description was by von Gierke in 1929 (BietrPatholAnat; 82:497). Enzymatic classification commenced with the Cori's discovery of glucose 6-phosphatase deficiency (JBC, 1952; 199:661). Twelve types of glycogen storage disease, each with a different enzymatic defect in glycogen metabolism, have been defined. Table 1 lists hepatic forms of the disease. Subtypes have been assigned to some major groups of glycogen storage disease according to differences in the distribution of enzyme activity as well as different mechanisms causing diminished enzymatic activity. For example, the common defect in the type I form is failure of hydrolysis of glucose 6-phosphate for release out of the cell; type Ia results from a defect in glucose 6-phosphatase enzyme protein, type Ib results from impaired activity of endoplasmic reticulum glucose 6-phosphate transport protein, type Ic is due to reduced activity of endoplasmic reticulum phosphate/pyrophosphate transport proteins, and type Id results from defective endoplasmic reticulum glucose transport protein (GLUT 7).

Table 1 Hepatic forms of glycogen storage diseases

Type	Enzyme deficiency	Tissue diagnosis
Ia	Glucose 6-phosphatase	Liver
Ib	Endoplasmic reticulum glucose 6-phosphate transport protein	Fresh unfrozen liver
Ic	Endoplasmic reticulum phosphate/pyrophosphate transport proteins	Fresh liver
Id	Endoplasmic reticulum glucose transport protein	Fresh liver
IIIa	Debranching enzyme	Liver/muscle
IIIb	Debranching enzyme	Liver
IV	Branching enzyme	Liver
VI	Liver phosphorylase	Liver
	Liver phosphorylase kinase (X-linked and autosomal)	

Glycogen structure, function, and metabolism

Although glucose is the primary energy source for cells, most tissues cannot synthesize glucose *de novo*. Therefore, blood glucose levels have to be maintained within a narrow range to support normal metabolic function in the brain and other tissues. This is achieved by storage of glucose in the liver and muscle in a compact, macro-molecular form as glycogen, which can be mobilized rapidly. In addition to producing glucose in this way, the hepatocyte has a large capacity for gluoconeogenesis. The latter pathway has a significant impact on the phenotypic expression of glycogen storage diseases which do not involve the glucose 6-phosphatase enzyme complex.

There are α- and β-forms of glycogen. Both forms have polymers of glucose linked to the 37-kDa protein glycogenin at tyrosine-194.[2] Glycogen β-particles are spherical and contain up to 60 000 glucose residues. The hepatocytes also contain α-particles, which are large aggregates of β-particles. The glucose residues in glycogen are α-1–4 linked, branching at intervals of 6 to 10 residues via an α-1–6 linkage. If phosphorylase or debranching enzyme is deficient, glycogen can be synthesized normally but it cannot be broken down, leading to intracellular accumulation in the liver and muscle. In branching enzyme deficiency, glycogen with an abnormal structure is synthesized and this insoluble material accumulates in the hepatocytes. The phosphorylase enzyme is activated by phosphorylase kinase and glycogen storage also occurs if phosphorylase kinase is deficient. In these types of glycogen storage disease, hypoglycaemia may occur, but this is often abrogated by the capacity of liver to engage in gluconeogenesis. In contrast, glucose 6-phosphatase mediates the last step of glycogenolysis as well as gluoconeogenesis; thus, when glucose 6-phosphatase is deficient, both pathways are impaired and fasting hypoglycaemia is more common.[1]

The enzymes of glycogen metabolism are notable for their complexity and this undoubtedly contributes to the phenotypic diversity seen in glycogen storage diseases. Liver branching enzyme is a monomeric protein with a molecular mass of approximately 70 kDa. In contrast, the liver debranching enzyme is a large monomeric protein of 160 to 170 kDa that, uniquely, has two independent catalytic activities at separate sites on a single polypeptide chain. Phosphorylase kinase is a complex enzyme with four different subunits (α, β, δ, and γ, with a molecular mass of 1300 kDa); in response to hormonal stimulation it activates phosphorylase which mediates glycogen breakdown. The catalytic subunit is γ, but the rest (α, β, and δ) have regulatory functions. This complex subunit structure is responsible for the broad spectrum of phenotypic expression as well as inheritance (X-linked and autosomal) that characterize type VI glycogen storage disease.

Glucose 6-phosphatase is a multicomponent complex.[2] The active site of the 38-kDa glucose 6-phosphatase enzyme is located in the lumen of the endoplasmic reticulum. Thus, substrates and products must cross the endoplasmic reticulum membrane via transport proteins for glucose 6-phosphate (T1), phosphate (T2a), pyrophosphate (T2b), and glucose (T3). There is also an associated calcium-binding protein (SP). Defects in any of these components will impair the production of free glucose from glucose 6-phosphate, resulting in the phenotype of type I glycogen storage disease.

Type 1 glycogen storage disease

The deficiency of glucose 6-phosphatase enzyme activity (type Ia disease) or the associated microsomal transport systems for glucose 6-phosphate (type Ib disease), phosphate (type Ic), and glucose (type Id) results in abnormal hepatic storage of glycogen as well as fat.[2] Hypoglycaemia is a prominent feature because the failure to release glucose from glucose 6-phosphate in these disorders is also associated with impaired hepatic production of glucose via gluconeogenesis.

Typically, patients with type I disease present in the neonatal period with hypoglycaemia and lactic acidosis or later at 3 to 4 months of age with hepatomegaly and/or hypoglycaemic seizures. These children often have doll-like fascies due to excess adipose tissue in cheeks, a protruberant abdomen, thin extremities, and a short stature. The patient may exhibit stigmas of severe hyperlipidaemia as cutaneous xanthomas and lipaemia retinalis. Commonly, the liver is massively enlarged, but the liver enzymes are minimally deranged. The kidneys are often symmetrically enlarged. There is no splenomegaly nor any cardiac abnormalities.

The clinical presentation of type Ib disease is similar to that of type Ia but, in addition, there is characteristic neutrophil dysfunction resulting in recurrent bacterial infections. Ulceration of the oral and intestinal mucosa commonly occur, and cases of inflammatory bowel disease have been reported. Too few cases of type Ic disease have been described to determine if there are any distinguishing clinical features. There has been one case report of

type Id disease and the clinical features were similar to that of type Ia.[2]

Hypoglycaemia and lactic acidosis can occur after a short fast. Blood glucose does not rise with administration of glucagon. Hyperuricaemia is common. The bleeding time is prolonged and associated with bruising and epistaxis. The basis of platelet dysfunction, despite normal or high platelet count, is not understood. The plasma is frequently lipaemic due to a striking elevation of very low density lipoproteins and low density lipoproteins manifesting as type IIb hyperlipidaemia. Characteristically, the apolipoprotein profile reveals elevation of apolipoproteins B, C, and E, but not of A or D.

In the past, many patients with unrecognized and/or untreated type I disease died during infancy from profound hypoglycaemia and lactic acidosis. Some patients do not show classic symptoms and have relatively mild manifestations of the disease. Many of these patients are not diagnosed until adulthood. They may have escaped detection through subconscious adjustment of diet to reduce the frequency of hypoglycaemic episodes. Rarely, type I disease can be entirely asymptomatic. In the majority of patients, administration of glucagon results at best in a feeble rise of blood glucose. Histology of the liver is characterized by universal distension of hepatocytes by glycogen and fat. Steatosis is of macrovesicular type. There is no associated fibrosis.

Growth retardation is prominent in childhood and adolescence. Puberty is frequently delayed. Fertility appears to be normal, but symptoms of type I disease may be exacerbated by pregnancy. Symptoms of gout usually start around puberty associated with long-term hyperuricaemia. Severe hyperlipidaemia may result in pancreatitis. Hepatic adenomas develop in most patients by the age of 20 to 30 years. Haemorrhage into adenomas has been described (Fink, Surgery, 1985; 97:117). However, the most serious complication is transformation of these premalignant lesions to hepatocellular carcinoma (Bianchi, EurJPed, 1993; 152:S63). The mechanism underlying increased propensity for hepatocarcinogenesis in type I disease is not understood, but it has been suggested that the greatly increased availability of free fatty acids in hepatocytes in this condition promotes extramitochondrial fatty acid oxidation, thus increasing oxidant stress and DNA damage (Ockner, Hepatol, 1993; 18:673).

Although type I disease primarily affects the liver, multiple organ systems are also involved. Renal disease is common, manifesting as glomerular hyperfiltration as the sole abnormality in younger patients (Chen, NEJM, 1988; 318:7). In adults, proteinuria accompanied by falling glomerular filtration rate is evident. Renal stones and nephrocalcinosis have also been described. With advanced renal disease, focal segmental glomerulosclerosis and interstitial fibrosis typically are seen on renal biopsy. Progression to renal failure requiring dialysis and transplantation has been described. Other renal abnormalities include amyloidosis, a Fanconi-like syndrome, distal renal tubular acidosis, and hypercalciuria. Secondary to lipid abnormalities, there is an increased risk of pancreatitis and possibly of premature atherosclerosis, but this is controversial.[1] It is likely that platelet dysfunction abrogates the risk of atherosclerosis. Three teenage patients have died from right heart failure secondary to pulmonary hypertension. Evidence for early onset of osteoporosis has been found in some patients (Lee, EurJPed, 1995; 154:483).

Diagnosis of type I glycogen storage disease

The diagnosis of type I glycogen storage disease should be considered in a patient with hepatomegaly and episodes of hypoglycaemia associated with the characteristic laboratory abnormalities. Administration of glucagon or adrenaline results in little or no rise in blood glucose, but the lactate levels rise significantly. A number of mutations have been described in the gene encoding glucose 6-phosphatase which cause type I disease.[3] However, the definitive diagnosis requires a liver biopsy to demonstrate either a deficiency of glucose 6-phosphatase activity or in one of the three microsomal translocase systems. Skin fibroblasts and leucocytes do not have glucose 6-phosphatase activity and therefore cannot be used for enzymatic diagnosis. The complexity of the glucose 6-phosphatase system is such that DNA-based molecular diagnosis is not likely to have a significant impact on routine clinical practice.

Treatment of type I glycogen storage disease

The aim of treatment of type I glycogen storage disease is to maintain euglycaemia.[4] Normoglycaemia corrects most of the associated metabolic abnormalities and morbidity. Normoglycaemia can be achieved through nocturnal nasogastric drip feeding of glucose or orally administered uncooked cornstarch. These measures have dramatically improved the outlook for these patients. Nocturnal nasogastric drip feeding is usually introduced in early infancy at the time of diagnosis. The requirements for glucose in an infant are 8 to10 mg/kg per min and in an older child 5 to 7 mg/kg per min, usually given as elemental enteral formula or as glucose or glucose polymer. Frequent feedings with high carbohydrate content are given during the day. The distribution of calories should be 65 to 70 per cent carbohydrate, 10 to 15 per cent protein, and 20 to 25 per cent fat with one-third of the total caloric intake given with nocturnal feeds. Care should be taken with nasogastric drip feeds as hypoglycaemia and deaths have resulted from mechanical problems with the pump or dislodgement of the tube. Uncooked cornstarch acts as a slow-release form of glucose and can be introduced at a dose of 1.6 g/kg every 4 h for infants under 2 years. The response of the older child is variable. As the child grows older, the cornstarch regimen can be changed to every 6 h. Dietary intake of fructose and galactose should be restricted as it cannot be converted to glucose. Additional therapies include vitamin supplements, calcium, and allopurinol. In type Ib glycogen storage disease, granulocyte colony-stimulating factor and granulocyte/monocyte colony-stimulating factor have been used successfully to correct neutropenia and reduce the frequency of bacterial infections, as well as ameliorate inflammatory bowel disease.[1]

Portocaval shunts have been performed in patients with type I disease; it had no effect on glucose homeostasis but, interestingly, it corrected the hyperlipidaemia (Starzl, CibaSymp, 1977; 55:311). Liver transplantation has been performed successfully in several patients with type I disease (Malatack, Lancet, 1983; i:1073). The hypoglycaemia and other metabolic abnormalities were corrected and normal growth parameters were achieved. Liver transplantation is indicated when uncooked cornstarch feeds and other measures have failed to achieve metabolic control or if the patient is especially intolerant of these regimens. An important new indication is emerging for liver transplantation in type I glycogen storage disease: development of symptomatic, multifocal, hepatocellular adenoma. This is an especially challenging problem for the clinician because all standard investigations (i.e. targeted biopsy, angiography, and α-fetoprotein) to detect malignant transformation in these premalignant lesions are unreliable and once such a change has occurred the outcome of liver transplantation is poor due to tumour recurrence. We recommend liver transplantation when the adenomas show progressive enlargement and become symptomatic. It is not advisable to wait until there is definite evidence for malignant transformation. Unfortunately, after resection of adenoma, there remains a high risk of recurrence despite good metabolic control (Bianchi, EurJPed, 1993; 152:S63).

Kidney transplantation has been performed for renal failure complicating type I disease.[1] The renal allografts do not correct hypoglycaemia and the metabolic abnormalities can be exaggerated as a result of corticosteroid therapy for immunosuppression. Candidates for kidney transplantation should be considered for combined liver–kidney transplantation. The merit for such an approach is that the metabolic disorder is cured, risk of malignant transformation in hepatic adenomas is removed, and immunological outcome for combined liver–kidney transplantation is significantly better than single organ transplantation (Gonwa, Transpl, 1988; 46:690).

Surgery in patients with type I disease should not be undertaken without a formal evaluation of haemostatic factors and establishment of good metabolic control. Prolonged bleeding time can be minimized by intensive intravenous glucose infusion for 24 to 48 h prior to surgery. Lactated Ringer's solution should be avoided because it contains lactate but no glucose. Glucose levels should be maintained in the normal range throughout surgery with 10 per cent dextrose.

Prognosis of type I glycogen storage disease

In the past, many patients died and prognosis was guarded in those who survived. During the last 15 years the introduction of nocturnal nasogastric glucose infusions and oral administration of uncooked cornstarch has dramatically changed the outlook for these patients (Smit, EurJPed, 1993; 152:S52). Both are effective in preventing hypoglycaemic attacks and ameliorating hyperlipidaemia, lactic acidosis, and hyperuricaemia. Early diagnosis and initiation of treatment has improved the prognosis, with normal growth and development in children, as well as reduced risk of gout in adult patients. Unfortunately, it now appears that hepatic adenoma, hepatocellular carcinoma, and renal dysfunction can not be prevented entirely by optimal metabolic control. Regression of hepatic adenomas after the initiation of optimal dietary therapy has been reported (Bianchi, EurJPed, 1993; 152:S63), but this is not a universal experience (Limmer, Hepatol, 1988; 8:531). Dietary therapy has been found to be effective in improving proximal renal tubular dysfunction. However, it is unknown if renal disease can be avoided completely by optimal metabolic control alone; even with good treatment, glomerular hyperfiltration is still seen.[1] Thus the success of medical therapy has ensured the survival of these patients into adulthood, unmasking a further dimension of the natural history of this disease—the development of hepatocellular adenoma/carcinoma and renal disease.

Type III glycogen storage disease

There is marked diversity in enzymatic defects as well as in clinical expression of the disease in debranching enzyme deficiency. The majority of patients express the type IIIa pattern with both hepatic and muscle involvement. About 15 per cent of the patients exhibit the type IIIb pattern characterized by mainly hepatic involvement. During childhood it can be difficult to distinguish the type III disease from type I because the patients present with hypoglycaemia, hepatomegaly, hyperlipidaemia, and growth retardation. The distinguishing features of type III disease are that blood lactate levels are normal and it is common to find elevated aminotransferases and fasting ketosis. The liver-related symptoms improve with age and disappear after puberty. Overt cirrhosis can occur but this is rare; however, it seems to be common among Japanese patients. In type IIIa disease, muscle symptoms are minimal in childhood but can become prominent in adults, with signs of neuromuscular involvement, slowly progressive weakness, and distal muscle wasting. Cardiac muscle disease manifests as abnormal ECGs and evidence of left ventricular hypertrophy. In contrast, hepatic symptoms in some patients are so mild that the diagnosis is not made until adulthood, when the patients present with neuromuscular disease. Liver histology typically shows distended glycogen-laden hepatocytes and the presence of fibrosis evolving into cirrhosis.[1]

Glucagon administered 2 h after a carbohydrate meal provokes a normal rise of blood glucose; after an overnight fast, glucagon may provoke no rise of blood glucose. Treatment is symptomatic: if hypoglycaemia is present, frequent meals high in carbohydrates, with cornstarch supplements or nocturnal nasogastric drip feeding, constitute effective therapy. Currently, there is no effective therapy for progressive myopathy or cardiomyopathy.

Type IV glycogen storage disease

Type IV glycogen storage disease (also known as Anderson's disease or amylopectinosis) is caused by a deficiency of branching enzyme activity, which results in the accumulation of abnormal glycogen in the tissues. The disease was first described by Anderson in a patient who had hepatosplenomegaly with hepatocyte storage of abnormal polysaccharide with poor solubility (Anderson, LabInvest, 1956; 5: 11). The abnormal glycogen had fewer branch points, more α-1–4-linked glucose units, and longer outer chains than normal glycogen, resulting in a structure resembling amylopectin.

Type IV disease typically presents in the first year of life, with hepatosplenomegaly and failure to thrive. Progressive liver cirrhosis with portal hypertension, ascites, oesophageal varices, and death usually occur before the age of 5 years. Hypoglycaemia is rarely seen but can occur when cirrhosis progresses, as few hepatocytes are available for glucose mobilization. The neuromuscular manifestations include hypotonia, muscle weakness, muscle atrophy, and attenuated deep tendon reflexes. Severe cardiomyopathy can be a predominant feature of clinical presentation.

Tissue deposition of an amylopectin-like material is widespread, including in the liver, heart, muscle, skin, intestine, brain, spinal cord, and peripheral nerves. Liver histology shows distorted architecture with diffuse interstitial fibrosis and wide fibrous septa surrounding micronodular areas of parenchyma. [1] The hepatocytes are enlarged to two or three times their normal size and contain faintly stained, basophilic, cytoplasmic inclusions. These inclusions consist of coarsely clumped, stored material that is periodic acid–Schiff positive and partially resistant to diastase digestion. Electron microscopy shows, in additon to α- and β-glycogen particles, accumulation of fibrillar aggregations that are typical of amylopectin. The electron microscopic appearance and distinct staining characteristics of cytoplasmic inclusions can be diagnostic. The pathogenesis of liver injury is not understood but the stored material is probably toxic to the hepatocytes. Although liver involvement occurs in most patients, rarely, patients have survived without evidence of progressive liver disease.[1]

Treatment of type IV disease involves maintenance of euglycaemia and adequate nutrient intake. For progressive liver failure, orthotopic liver transplantation has been performed in eight patients (Selby, NEJM, 1991; 324:M39). Five surviving patients have not had neuromuscular or cardiac complications for up to a 7-year follow-up period. Remarkably, in some patients, reduction in the amylopectin content of myocardial biopsies has been demonstrated. It has been suggested that this therapeutic benefit derives from microchimerism established by donor cells in extrahepatic tissues which act as enzyme couriers.[5] However, the role of liver transplantation for this multisystem disease in the long term remains to be evaluated.

Type VI glycogen storage disease

Of the type VI glycogen storage diseases, the X-linked phosphorylase kinase deficiency is the most common accounting for approximately 75 per cent of all cases. Besides the liver, enzyme activity may also be deficient in erythrocytes, leucocytes, and fibroblasts. The classic presentation at age 1 to 5 years is a protuberant abdomen due to hepatomegaly, mild hyperlipidaemia, mildly elevated liver enzymes, and fasting ketosis. These abnormalities gradually disappear with age and most adults are essentially asymptomatic. Growth retardation is a concern for most patients but eventually most achieve normal parameters. Hypoglycaemia if present is usually mild. Patients respond normally to glucagon. The deficiency is generally considered a benign condition, although there is wide phenotypic diversity. Asymptomatic hemizygous males as well as mildly symptomatic female carriers have been described. Some patients have phosphorylase kinase deficiency in the liver and blood cells with autosomal inheritance; hepatomegaly and growth retardation in early childhood are predominant symptoms. Liver histology shows glycogen-laden hepatocytes. The accumulated glycogen (α-particles, rosette form) is less compact than glycogen seen in the type I or III forms of disease. Liver histology may also reveal fibrous septa formation and low-level inflammatory change. Patients with liver phosphorylase deficiency appear to have a benign course very similar to liver phosphorylase kinase deficiency. Hypoglycaemia and hyperlipidaemia if present are usually mild.

References

1. Chen Y-T and Burchell A. Glycogen storage diseases. In: Scriver CR, Beaudet AL, Sly WS and Valle D, eds. *The metabolic and molecular bases of inherited disease*. New York: McGraw-Hill, 1995: 935–65

2. Burchell A. Molecular pathology of glucose 6-phosphatase. *FASEB Journal*, 1990; **4**: 2978–88.

3. Lei K-J, Shelly LL, Pau C-J, Sidbury JB, and Chou JY. Mutations in glucose 6-phosphatase gene that cause glycogen storage disease type 1a. *Science*, 1993; **262**: 580–3.

4. Sidbury JB, Chen Y-T, and Roe CR. The role of raw starches in the treatment of type 1 glycogenosis. *Archives of Internal Medicine*, 1986; **46**: 370–3.

5. Strazl TE, *et al.* Chimerism after liver transplantation for type IV glycogen storage disease and type 1 Gaucher's disease. *New England Journal of Medicine*, 1993; **328**: 745–9.

21

Vascular abnormalities

21.1 Hepatic arteries

Josep Terés

Anatomy and physiology

The common hepatic artery usually emerges from the coeliac axis as well as the left gastric and splenic arteries. However, this anatomical appearance is only observed in 55 to 65 per cent of subjects.[1] In the most common distribution, the hepatic artery becomes the proper hepatic artery after the branching of the gastroduodenal artery and sometimes the dorsal pancreatic artery. The hepatic artery enters the porta hepatis, together with the portal vein and the common bile duct and divides into a right, left, and occasionally middle hepatic branch. The middle hepatic branch emerges from the left hepatic branch in 45 per cent of patients; it is the main supply of the quadrate lobe and may supply the caudate lobe and the gallbladder. The gallbladder, however, is usually supplied by the cystic artery which emerges from the right hepatic branch before it enters the right hepatic lobe. The most frequent variations of this anatomical distribution are the left hepatic artery emerging from the left gastric artery (25 per cent), the right hepatic artery emerging from the superior mesentery artery (14 per cent), the right hepatic artery partially replaced by the superior mesentery artery (8 per cent), the entire hepatic artery or one of its branches emerging from the aorta, and the entire hepatic artery emerging from the mesentery artery (rare).

The hepatic artery supplies 35 per cent of the hepatic blood flow (800 to 1200 ml/min) and 50 per cent of the oxygen supply to the liver (Tygstrup, JCI, 1962; 41:447), with the remaining requirements of the liver being supplied by the portal vein. The regulation of the blood flow of the hepatic artery is not well understood. There is a compensatory mechanism between the hepatic artery and the portal vein called 'reciprocity' (Richardson, Gastro, 1981; 8:159) or the 'hepatic artery buffer response'[2] such that a decrease in the blood flow through one circuit leads to a decreased inflow resistance in the other circuit. This mechanism allows the maintenance of a constant blood flow through the liver. Recently, it was suggested that this response, as well as pressure-flow autoregulation, are mediated by adenosine, which acts as a dilator when locally accumulated after a reduction in the blood flow (Ezzat, AmJPhysiol, 1987; 252:H836).

Hepatic artery aneurysms

Hepatic artery aneurysms are the fourth most common abdominal aneurysms (20 per cent). However, it is a rare condition and no more than 400 cases have been reported (Cooper, JClinGastro, 1988; 10:104). Aneurysms may be intra- or extrahepatic; the latter

is four times more frequent with the main hepatic artery being the most common site. The size is seldom less than 2 cm and, only on rare occasions, greater than 10 cm.

The aetiologies of hepatic artery aneurysms are arteriosclerosis, systemic infections (mainly bacterial endocarditis), trauma (including liver biopsy and other procedures), syphilis, tuberculosis, intra-abdominal septic conditions (cholecystitis, liver abscess, and appendicitis), and congenital conditions (Stack, BMJ, 1968; 3:659; Porter, AmJMed, 1979; 67:697). Hepatic artery aneurysms have also been described in systemic diseases which may be associated with diffuse vascular abnormalities and multiple aneurysms (Marfan syndrome, Ehlers–Danlos syndrome, Osler–Weber–Rendu disease, and fibromuscular hyperplasia). The liver is involved in 66 per cent of the cases of polyarteritis nodosa, the typical angiographic findings being multiple fusiform or sacular aneurysms associated with an irregular calibre of the medium and small arteries, the aneurysms may become thrombosed and cause peripheral infarction or may rupture causing haemorrhage, the number of intrahepatic arteries may be decreased, [4]and nodular regenerative hyperplasia may be a complication of this disease. Hepatic artery dissections are rare and have been described in association with abdominal surgery, peritonitis (Larson, ArchPathLabMed, 1987; 111:300), arterial hypertension, pre-existing arterial disease, and trauma (Bushkin, SurgGynecolObstet, 1972; 135:721).

Hepatic artery aneurysms are usually discovered in middle age (mean 38 years and range 10 to 80 years) and the male:female ratio is 4:1. Patients with aneurysmatic dilatation may remain asymptomatic for long periods of time. Upper abdominal pain is the first symptom in 75 per cent of cases.[5] The pain is acute and severe (dissection) or vague (compression) and is often misinterpreted as biliary or pancreatic pain. Rupture occurs in up to 80 per cent of the cases and produces intraperitoneal haemorrhage (extrahepatic aneurysms) or massive haemobilia associated with gastrointestinal bleeding and jaundice (intrahepatic aneurysms) (Chen, ArchSurg, 1983; 118:759). A less common mechanism of jaundice is extrinsic compression of the biliary tree (Shultz, AJR, 1985; 144:1287). This triad of abdominal pain, jaundice, and gastrointestinal bleeding is present in approximately one-third of cases and should lead to a diagnosis of hepatic artery aneurysms.

Unfortunately, hepatic artery aneurysms are usually fatal since, if untreated or treated after rupture, only one patient in five survives (Kibbler, Gut, 1985; 26:752). In most patients, the diagnosis is made only after rupture. This diagnosis may also be suspected when a ring-like calcification not involving the gallbladder or kidney is seen by X-ray in the upper right quadrant.[1] Ultrasonography (Stokland, JClinUltrasound, 1985; 13:369), a computed tomography (**CT**) scan with intravenous contrast injection (Kibbler, Gut, 1985; 26:752), radionuclide imaging (Sukerkard, Radiol, 1977; 124:444), angiography, and magnetic resonance imaging (**MRI**) have been used for the diagnosis of hepatic artery aneurysms.

The treatment of a ruptured aneurysm is emergency surgery. In asymptomatic patients, the diagnosis of a hepatic artery aneurysm implies surgery with excision or obliteration of all the aneurysm.[5] An aneurysm in the common hepatic artery, proximal to the gastroduodenal artery, can be safely ligated. If the aneurysm is located distal to the gastroduodenal artery, ligation interrupts the collateral circulation through the gastroduodenal and right gastric arteries and may produce hepatic ischaemia; hence aneurysms in this area should be treated with resection and reconstruction. Intrahepatic aneurysms may be treated by resecting the part of the liver involved or ligating the specific feeding vessel. Transcatheter embolization using gel foam or cyanocrylate may be an alternative treatment for this condition because of its high efficacy and low morbidity. Coil occlusion (Nosher, AmJSurg, 1986; 152:326) and percutaneous thrombin injection (Cope, AJR, 1986; 147:383) have also been proposed.

Hepatic arterioportal fistulas

Arteriovenous fistulas in the portal circulation are rare but of great clinical interest since they are a potentially curable cause of portal hypertension. The aetiology includes blunt trauma, erosion of aneurysms into the portal system, iatrogenic complications of diagnostic or therapeutic procedures, congenital lesions, and neoplasms. Fistulas between the hepatic artery and the portal vein are usually caused by rupture of a hepatic artery aneurysm or trauma. Fistulas within the liver are usually iatrogenic in origin (needle biopsy and percutaneous cholangiography) or neoplastic (hepatocellular carcinoma). Rendu–Osler–Weber syndrome may also cause hepatic arteriovenous fistulas (Lumsden, AmSurg, 1993; 59:722).

Arterioportal fistulas may be asymptomatic or may cause abdominal pain, intestinal ischaemia, portal hypertension with gastrointestinal bleeding, ascites, and, in a few patients, congestive heart failure. Abdominal bruit is present in 80 per cent of patients (Strodel, ArchSurg, 1987; 112:563), while portal hypertension develops in approximately 40 per cent, in particular in those fistulas involving large vessels.

A CT scan and Doppler ultrasound examination may detect the presence of arterioportal fistulas, with angiography providing the best information about the anatomic configuration of the fistula (Fig. 1).

The treatment depends on the size and location of the fistula and on the presence of portal hypertension or other symptoms. Since small intrahepatic fistulas without portal hypertension remain fairly constant in size and may even close spontaneously, the patients should be kept under observation. In contrast, extrahepatic fistulas have a tendency to increase in size with time and, consequently, the patient should be treated, even when asymptomatic, by surgery or transcatheter embolization (Uflacker, AJR, 1982; 139:1212).

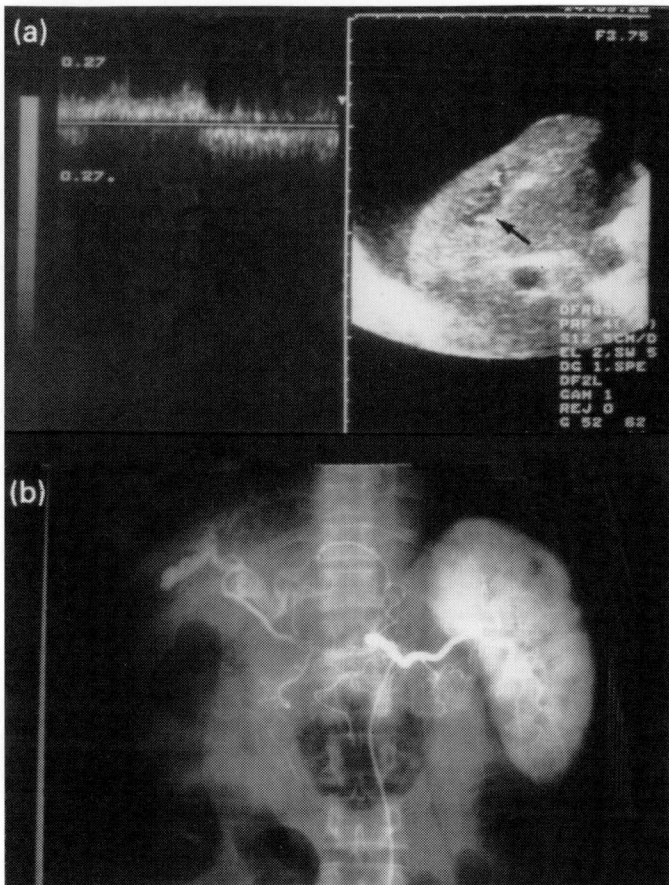

Fig. 1. Duplex Doppler exploration of an arteriovenous hepatic fistula in a patient with cirrhosis. (a) Right hepatic lobe surrounded by ascites showing a tubular image in the middle corresponding to an arteriovenous fistula. The Doppler signal is a mixture of the arterial and venous patterns. (b) Arteriographic demonstration of the fistula in the same patient. (By courtesy of Dr C. Bru.)

Hepatic artery occlusion and ischaemia

The common causes of hepatic artery obstruction are arterosclerosis, thrombosis, embolism, aneurysms, polyarteritis nodosa, neoplastic encasement, polycythaemia vera, oral contraceptives,[1] and complications of transcatheter therapeutic procedures (Trjanowski, AmJSurg, 1980; 139:272). On the other hand, ligation of the hepatic artery is a procedure widely used for bleeding control of incisive hepatic wounds and the treatment of liver tumours.

The consequences of hepatic artery occlusion depend on the site, time of occlusion, and state of the portal circulation (Bechtein, TransplProc, 1987; 19:3830). When occlusion of the hepatic artery occurs above the branching of the gastric and gastroduodenal arteries, development of the collateral circulation does not occur. Slow thrombosis is better tolerated than sudden occlusion. Simultaneous occlusion of the hepatic artery and portal vein is nearly always fatal. Hepatic infarction usually follows hepatic arterial occlusion although it may also occur with low cardiac output states and diabetic ketosis. Hepatic infarction may occur after surgical ligation of the hepatic artery (Lucas, ArchSurg, 1978; 113:1107);

thus, this procedure should be reserved for selected patients or when other therapeutic procedures have failed. Hepatic artery embolization with particulate materials is, in general, a safe therapeutic method for liver cancer. Although mild hepatic functional abnormalities may follow embolization, clinically significant hepatic infarction and abscesses rarely develop. The placement of a hepatic artery infusion catheter for chemotherapy, another widely used procedure for the treatment of hepatic tumours, rarely results in hepatic artery thrombosis.[4]

Experimental models of hepatic ischaemia–reperfusion in rats and pigs have shown that hepatic injury, liver cell necrosis, and microvascular injury correlate with enhanced Kupffer cell activity and neutrophil activation and infiltration. Both types of cells, as well as endothelial cells, generate a variety of inflammatory and cytotoxic mediators and superoxide anion release which lead to a self-aggravating injury mechanism (Jaeschke, ZblChir, 1994; 119: 309; Liu, Shock, 1995; 3:56). The inhibition of Kupffer cells by gadolinium chloride or latex results in reduced hepatic injury and an improved survival rate in a rat model (Shiratori, DigDisSci, 1994; 39:1265; Suzuki, CircShock, 1994; 42:204). Albumin, prostaglandin E$_1$, and misoprostol have been shown to protect against ischaemia–reperfusion injury in different experimental models. Inflammatory and cytotoxic mediators, mainly the platelet activating factor (**PFA**), have been suspected of being the cause of the systemic microcirculatory abnormalities and shock that often accompanies ischaemic liver failure (Fukuoca, SurgToday, 1995; 25:351).

Initially, patients with hepatic artery occlusion tend to have sharp, severe abdominal or back pain, arterial hypotension, and, eventually, shock. Signs of severe acute hepatic failure develop and progress rapidly. Serum aminotransferases (**AST**, **ALT**), lactate dehydrogenase (**LD**), and bilirubin rise, the prothrombin activity falls, and hepatic encephalopathy appears. The ALT–LD ratio is significantly lower in ischaemic hepatitis and acetaminophen injury than in viral hepatitis; ratios of 1:5 or lower rule out viral hepatitis with a sensitivity of 94 per cent and a specificity of 84 per cent (Cassidy, JClinGastro, 1994; 19:118). Fever and leucocytosis are frequently present. The prognosis of this condition is very poor. A CT scan and ultrasonography show a circumscribed lesion, often wedge-shaped extending to the periphery. However, the image may be similar to other lesions (tumours or abscesses). Scintigraphy shows peripheral, wedge-shaped, sharply defined defects and may be more sensitive than ultrasonography and CT scans. The treatment of this condition depends on its cause. In addition, these patients should be treated the same as those with acute hepatic failure.

Hepatic artery lesions following orthotopic liver transplantation

Hepatic artery lesions are a common and serious complication of orthotopic liver transplantation (**OLT**) (7 to 36 per cent) (Hesselink, TransplProc, 1986; 18:1205; Wozney, AJR, 1986; 147:657; Tzakis, Transpl, 1985; 40:667). Hepatic artery occlusion, stenosis, and, less

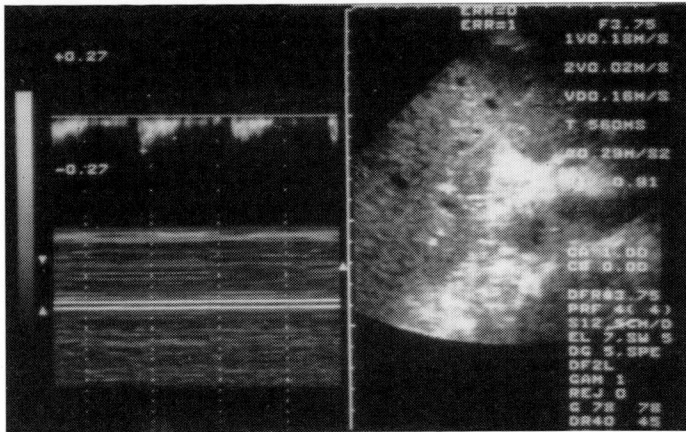

Fig. 2. Duplex Doppler exploration of a patient 5 days after OLT. The Doppler plot of the hepatic artery shows a decrease in the systolic and diastolic signals, corresponding to a partial thrombosis of the arterial lumen assessed by arteriography. (By courtesy of Dr C. Bru.)

frequently, anastomotic aneurysm are the main arterial complications of OLT. Hepatic arterial thrombosis is more frequent in children than in adults; the clinical features are fulminant hepatic necrosis, delayed biliary leak, or relapsing bacteraemia as a consequence of graft necrosis, graft bile duct necrosis, or abcesses within the necrosed areas of the liver, respectively. Hepatic necrosis may not develop when arterial thrombosis is gradual allowing collateral formation.

The diagnosis of hepatic artery lesions after OLT requires hepatic arteriography. However, a pulsed Doppler examination of the hepatic artery combined with real-time ultrasonography of the liver parenchyma (Fig. 2) is a good selection procedure for patients requiring hepatic angiography when thrombosis is suspected: patients with a Doppler arterial patency and normal liver ultrasonic architecture do not require angiography (Segel, AJR, 1986; 146: 137). The treatment of hepatic artery thrombosis after OLT is retransplantation.

References

1. Friedman AC. *Radiology of the liver, biliary tract, pancreas and spleen.* Baltimore: Williams and Wilkins, 1987.
2. Lautt WW. Role and control of hepatic artery. In: *Hepatic circulation in health and disease.* New York: Raven Press, 1981: 203–6.
3. Sherlock S and Dooley T. *Diseases of the liver and biliary system.* Oxford: Blackwell Scientific Publications, 1997.
4. Reuter SR, Redman HC, and Cho KJ. *Gastrointestinal angiography.* Philadelphia: W.B. Saunders Co., 1986.
5. Busuttil RW and Brin BJ. The diagnosis and management of visceral artery aneurysms. *Surgery,* 1980; 88: 619–24.
6. Goldblatt M, Rad FF, Goldin AR, and Shaff MI. Percutaneous embolization for the management of hepatic artery aneurysms. *Gastroenterology,* 1977; 73: 1142–6.
7. Kadir S, Athanasoulis ChA, Ring EJ, and Greenfield A. Transcatheter embolization of intrahepatic arterial aneurysms. *Radiology,* 1980; 134: 335–9.
8. Baker KS, Tisnado J, Cho SR, and Beachley MC. Splanchnic artery aneurysms and pseudoaneurysms. Transcatheter embolization. *Radiology,* 1987; 163: 135–9.

21.2 Obstruction of the portal vein

Juan Carlos García-Pagán and Jaime Bosch

Definition, aetiology, and diagnosis

Prehepatic portal hypertension is an infrequent condition in which increased portal pressure is due to obstruction of the portal venous tree prior to entering the liver (Groszmann, SemLivDis, 1982; 2: 177). The site of the obstruction may be limited at the splenic or mesenteric veins, but most commonly involves the portal vein. It may be caused by congenital abnormalities or, more usually, is related to several underlying diseases that favour the obstruction of part or all the vessels of the portal venous system. The causes of prehepatic portal hypertension are listed in Table 1.

In patients with an overt underlying disease such as blood dyscrasias or acute pancreatitis, the manifestations of portal hypertension may be obscured by the main illness. Portal vein obstruction may be suggested by the appearance of spleen enlargement or, more frequently, be detected by abdominal ultrasonography or computed tomography (**CT**) or by the onset of gastrointestinal bleeding due to ruptured gastroesophageal varices in the absence of demonstrable chronic liver disease. These cases usually exhibit prominent (or exclusively) gastric varices, which represent hepatoportal collaterals 'bridging' the obstruction in the portal vein and carrying portal blood to the liver. Only a minor proportion (less than 10 per cent) of patients admitted to hospital because of variceal bleeding will ultimately be diagnosed as having prehepatic portal hypertension, the main proportion of cases being attributable to hepatic cirrhosis. More than 50 per cent of cases of prehepatic portal hypertension are diagnosed after a bleeding episode. Nevertheless, the suspicion of portal hypertension must be followed up by the use of several diagnostic techniques aimed at assessing and classifying its presence and type.

The patency of the portal venous system should be established by ultrasound using pulsed Doppler equipment (Fig. 1).[1] This imaging technique offers reliable information and in some cases may be preferable to arteriography of the coeliac trunk and of the mesenteric artery with delayed visualization of the portal vein. The absence of an underlying liver disease with sinusoidal portal hypertension can be ruled out by liver biopsy and the measurement of hepatic venous pressures (Groszmann, Gastro, 1979; 76:253). Magnetic resonance imaging (**MRI**) of the portal venous system appears to be even more reliable than duplex Doppler sonography for evaluating the portal venous patency (Rodgers, Radiol, 1994; 191:741; Finn, AJR, 1993; 161:989). For exceptional cases where these techniques do not lead to a definite diagnosis, transhepatic catheterization of the portal vein may be the only way to demonstrate portal hypertension clearly and to localize the exact point of the

Table 1 Aetiology of prehepatic portal hypertension
Portal vein thrombosis
Omphalitis
Trauma and liver biopsy
Pancreatitis
Intra-abdominal sepsis
Blood dyscrasias
Polycythaemia vera
Essential thrombocytosis
Myelofibrosis
Acute and chronic leukaemia
Ulcerative colitis
Antithrombin III deficiency
Antiphospholipid antibodies (lupus anticoagulant)
Protein C deficiency and protein S deficiency
Endoscopic sclerotherapy
Retroperitoneal fibrosis
Following splenectomy or splenorenal shunt
Cirrhosis of the liver
Hepatocellular carcinoma
Idiopathic
Splenic vein thrombosis
Acute pancreatitis
Chronic pancreatitis
Carcinoma of the pancreas
Retroperitoneal infection
Renal neoplasms
Retroperitoneal fibrosis
Congenital stenosis of the portal vein
Aneurysms of the portal vein
Extrinsic compression of the portal vein
Partial nodular transformation
Retroperitoneal fibrosis
Arteriovenous fistula
Rendu–Osler–Weber syndrome
Trauma
Liver biopsy
Rupture of an arterial aneurysm
Hepatocellular carcinoma

obstruction. Splenoportography, a technique frequently employed in the past to measure intrasplenic pressure and to visualize the splenic vein, is considered too risky to be performed routinely and should be reserved for special cases as a last resort.

Portal vein thrombosis

This is the most frequent cause of prehepatic portal hypertension and is mainly observed in children, in whom a history consistent with omphalitis and/or umbilical catheterization can often be obtained from their parents. In these cases, the infection passes from

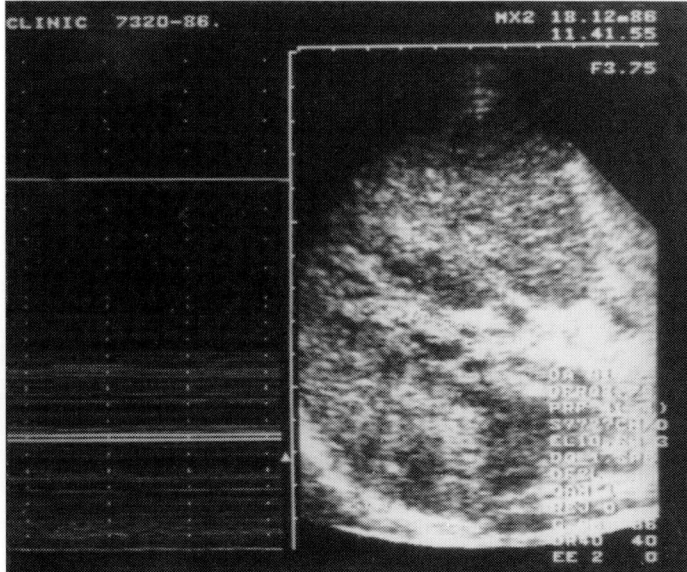

Fig. 1. Thrombosis of the portal vein. Doppler ultrasound shows echoes within the lumen of the portal vein, there being no signals of flow.

the umbilical vein into the left branch of the portal vein and afterwards into the main portal trunk, thus inducing complete venous obstruction. In adults, the cause of portal thrombosis is less frequently identified. The more common causes in adults are intra-abdominal infections,[4] oral contraceptives (Nesbitt, SouthMedJ, 1977; 70:360), abdominal trauma (Ivatury, AnnSurg, 1987; 206: 733), pancreatitis (Zalcman, GastrRad, 1987; 12:114), pregnancy (Chambers, BMJ, 1983; 2:1104), or underlying disorders favouring a hypercoagulative state, such as blood dyscrasias,[6] antithrombin III deficiency (Winter, QJMed, 1982; 51:373; Editorial, Lancet, 1983; i:1021), the presence of antiphospholipid antibodies (Love, AnnIntMed, 1990; 112:682), protein C deficiency (Orozco, Hepatol, 1988; 8:1110), protein S deficiency (Seifert, Chirurgie, 1994; 65: 1143), as a complication of transjugular liver biopsy (Spahr, JHepatol, 1996; 24:246), or autoimmune diseases.[5] Recent investigations have shown that 48 per cent of patients with portal thrombosis, in whom no disposing factor can be identified, suffer from a primary myeloproliferative disorder (mostly polycythaemia vera) which cannot be detected by conventional criteria.[6] The most useful technique for confirming the presence of a latent myeloproliferative disease is to assess the formation of erythroid colonies in a culture of bone marrow cells with and without the addition of erythropoietin (McLeod, Blood, 1974; 44:517).

Portal vein thrombosis may be a complication of cirrhosis. In these patients, portal vein thrombosis may induce a further increase in portal pressure and perhaps precipitate variceal bleeding. However, the prevalence of portal thrombosis in cirrhotics is low (0.6 per cent) (Okuda, Gastro, 1985; 89:279), whereas it is a frequent event after splenectomy and in patients with hepatocellular carcinoma (approximately 25 per cent) (Okuda, Gastro, 1985; 89:279), there being a clear relationship between tumour size and the prevalence of portal thrombosis (Calvet, JHepatol, 1990; 10:311). Several authors have pointed out that endoscopic sclerosis of the varices may promote portal vein thrombosis (Leach, JVascSurg, 1989; 10:9;

Terada, JClinGastro, 1990; 12:238), a risk that should be taken into account in patients who could eventually benefit from liver transplantation; this may constitute a major drawback for sclerotherapy. Splenectomy carries the same risk since it is recognized as an important favouring factor for portal thrombosis (Okuda, Gastro, 1985; 89:279).

In most adult cases, portal vein thrombosis is diagnosed after a bleeding episode due to ruptured oesophageal varices, while in children it is more frequently diagnosed after detecting splenomegaly. The tolerance of bleeding is much higher than in cirrhotic patients because liver function has not failed.[4] In some rare cases, the diagnosis is made in the acute phase of the disease and the manifestations of acute portal vein obstruction are mixed with those of the favouring factor such as recent surgery or abdominal infection. Patients complain of abdominal pain, ileus, fever, liver failure, and gastrointestinal bleeding due to intestinal infarction. The degree of these symptoms is variable.

Clinical suspicion of portal hypertension should prompt an ultrasound examination of the portal system. The identification of solid echoes within the portal vein (Van Gansbeke, AJR, 1985; 144: 749) and the absence of flow signals when using pulsed Doppler equipment (Fig. 1)[1] confirms the diagnosis. MRI may also be useful although not essential. There is then no need for more invasive diagnostic tools, such as angiography or splenoportography, although angiography may be used as a confirmatory tool in selected cases, in particular in those in whom a surgical approach is required. In the chronic phase, the obstruction is associated with the development of new vascular channels aimed at bypassing the vascular stop and giving a cavernomatous appearance to the portal vein (Fig. 2) (Weltin, AJR, 1985; 144:999). This is best shown on angiography.

Patients with portal vein obstruction exhibit the same haemodynamic abnormalities as in any other type of portal hypertension (Braillon, JHepatol, 1989; 9:312). Thus, the systemic circulation is characterized by a hyperdynamic state with an increased blood volume and cardiac output and reduced arterial pressure and peripheral vascular resistance (Braillon, JHepatol, 1989; 9:312). The splanchnic circulation is also hyperdynamic with an increased inflow of blood into the portal venous system. Studies of experimental models of prehepatic portal hypertension indicate that in these cases the increased portal pressure is related not only to the increased resistance offered to blood flow by the vascular obstruction, but also to the increased blood flow entering the portal venous system (Vorobioff, AmJPhysiol, 1983; 244:G52; Benoit, Gastro, 1985; 89: 1092). Serum biochemistry will show either no abnormalities or a mild elevation of globulins and haematological examination may disclose a variable degree of hypersplenism as evidenced by leucopenia, thrombocytopenia, and reduced haemoglobinaemia.[4]

Treatment

The diagnosis of portal vein thrombosis does not *per se* indicate the need for treatment. The underlying condition potentially responsible for the vascular occlusion should be treated if possible; only those cases who have suffered bleeding related to portal hypertension should be considered for treatment aimed at the prevention of rebleeding. The acute episode of gastrointestinal haemorrhage is treated as is any variceal bleeding from other causes;

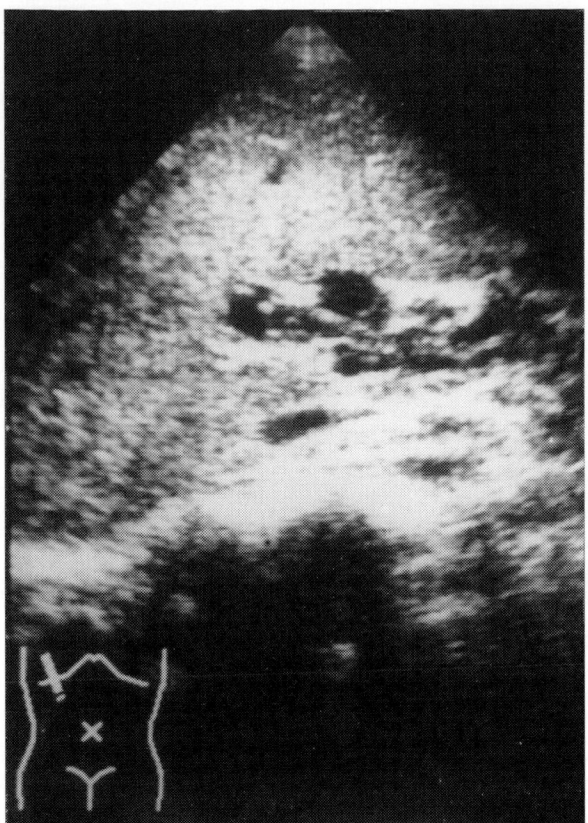

Fig. 2. Ultrasound imaging of new vascular channels in a patient with cavernomatosis of the portal vein.

after achieving haemostasis, elective treatment must be indicated. The role of pharmacological therapy with propranolol has not yet been adequately explored but propranolol could be used in the primary prophylaxis of patients who have never bled. Endoscopic variceal sclerotheropy or ligation of the varices may reduce the proportion of patients needing surgery (Kahn, AnnSurg, 1994; 219: 34). The most useful operation is splenorenal anastomosis, but this is possible only when the splenic vein is patent. Other portosystemic anastomoses, such as portocaval or mesocaval, are frequently precluded by the extended thrombosis of all the portal bed. In addition, the splenorenal shunt is less frequently seen to be thrombosed during follow-up,[8] a complication that may promote new episodes of variceal bleeding. Other procedures, such as oesophageal transection or splenectomy and ligation of the varices, are less useful because of the high frequency of gastric varices and the high index of late rebleeding due to the reappearance of the varices.

In cases of recent thrombosis, without bleeding varices, thrombolitic therapy through a catheter introduced into the portal vein either percutaneously or through the transjugular approach may be useful (Rehan, EurJPed, 1994; 153:456). Spontaneous recanalization after recent thrombosis has also been observed (Spahr, JHepatol, 1996; 24:246).

Transjugular intrahepatic portosystemic shunt is a new non-surgical approach to portal hypertension that has also been shown to be useful in the recanalization of chronic non-cavernomatous portal thrombosis (Radosevich, Radiol, 1993; 186:523; Blum, Radiol, 1995; 195: 153).

Splenic vein thrombosis

The main causes of isolated splenic vein thrombosis are chronic pancreatitis and carcinoma of the pancreas (Table 1) (Sutton, ArchSurg, 1970; 100:623; Muhletaler, Radiol, 1979; 132:593; Johnston, AnnSurg, 1973; 177:736; Moosa, WorldJSurg, 1985; 9:384; Nishiyama, AmJGastr, 1986; 81:1193). Occasionally, splenic vein thrombosis has been described in relation to retroperitoneal infections (Gea, GastroHepato, 1986; 9:294), renal neoplasms (Ginés, GastroHepato, 1982; 5:27), or retroperitoneal fibrosis (Lavender, BMJ, 1970; 3:627). Usually, splenic vein obstruction is diagnosed after a bleeding episode related to gastric varices; the development of oesophageal varices is less common because of possible drainage through the left coronary vein. Diagnosis is established by ultrasound and by radiological visualization in the venous phase of splenic artery angiography, although non-visualization of the splenic vein is not unequivocal evidence of splenic vein thrombosis. In some patients with cirrhosis and severe portal hypertension, the presence of an extensive network of collaterals arising from the spleen and a slow-retrograde portal blood flow may impede the filling of the vein, thus creating false-positive results. In some cases, MRI may be of help. It is very unlikely to require the use of splenoportography, transhepatic catheterization of the portal vein, or even perioperative measurement of the pressures along the portal bed with a simultaneous perioperative ultrasound examination of the splenic vein (Vanwaeyenbergh, Hepatogast, 1989; 36:376) to achieve the definite diagnosis. However, the finding of an increased pressure in the splenic pulp or in the splenic vein with normal pressure in the portal and mesenteric veins indicates that the cause of the portal hypertension is located in the splenic vein.

Physical examination reveals an enlarged spleen; biochemical determinations are usually normal, while the haematological parameters may show signs of hypersplenism. As discussed above, gastric varices are a prominent (if not the only) endoscopic finding in these patients.

Unlike subjects with portal thrombosis, patients diagnosed with splenic vein obstruction do not need to wait for a bleeding episode to receive treatment. Since splenectomy is a curative operation and is not associated with high morbidity and mortality, surgical treatment is clearly justified. However, patients submitted to splenectomy without prior bleeding must be informed in detail of the risks and long-term care that will be needed afterwards.

Congenital stenosis of the portal vein

It is important to consider this aetiology in children with prehepatic portal hypertension. The stenosis may be located at any point along the portal vein, but it is particularly common at the hepatic hilus or in the middle of the portal vein (Odievre, ArchDisChild, 1977; 52: 383). The mechanism of the stenosis is not fully understood, but is thought to be related to the circulatory changes that occur early after birth. Before birth, the umbilical vein carries blood flow into the umbilical portion of the portal vein; after passing through the Arancius duct, blood flow drains into the inferior vena cava or the hepatic vein. Just after birth, the umbilical vein and the Arancius duct occlude and undergo a progressive fibrosis, thus forming the ligamentum teres and the ligamentum venosum. If the fibrotic process is exceedingly intense the portal vein may become stenosed at the hepatic hilium.

As in other patients with prehepatic portal hypertension, the disease is usually diagnosed after the patient suffers gastrointestinal bleeding due to ruptured gastroesophageal varices. Physical examination may show splenomegaly and subcutaneous collateral vessels. The liver function parameters remain within the normal range and ultrasound shows the patency of the portal vein, thus making a false diagnosis of intrahepatic portal hypertension. However, the liver histology is normal, as is the measurement of hepatic venous pressures. Careful ultrasound examination of the portal vein and an analysis of the venous phase of splanchnic angiography may reveal the stenosis, which can thereafter be confirmed by measuring the venous pressure along the portal vein and showing a pressure gradient just at the location of the stenosis. These children can be managed surgically, although some cases may be corrected by transluminal angioplasty.

Aneurysms of the portal vein

Abnormal, aneurysm-like dilatations of the portal vein are infrequent and, in most cases, appear to be associated with portal hypertension (Planas, GastroHepato, 1986; 9:129). However, there are reports suggesting that such dilatation may occur in subjects with normal portal pressure (Thomas, Surgery, 1967; 61:550; Liebowitz, NYStateJMed, 1967; 67:1443). It is usually diagnosed by chance during an ultrasound examination in a patient known or suspected to have portal hypertension. The most frequent location of these aneurysms is at the junction of the splenic and mesenteric veins, although there have been cases with other locations (even intrahepatic) (Ohnishi, Gastro, 1984; 86:169). The mechanism of the abnormal portal vein dilation is not known, but there is evidence of both a congenital and an acquired origin (Ohnishi, Gastro, 1984; 86:169). The identification of a marked enlargement of the diameter of the portal vein suggests the diagnosis, but in some cases it may be difficult to differentiate an aneurysm with partial thrombosis from a leiomioma of the portal vein. CT shows the enlarged diameter of the portal vein, filled after contrast enhancement, except in those cases with partial thrombosis. Venous phase angiography (Fig. 3) confirms the diagnosis and may sometimes reveal aneurysms or congenital malformations in other locations, thus favouring the suggestion of congenital origin. Cirrhosis with portal hypertension should always be considered in patients with portal aneurysms, even in the absence of overt liver disease. This may require an ultrasound-guided liver biopsy and portal pressure measurements.

Unlike arterial aneurysms, the risk of spontaneous rupture of an aneurysm of the portal vein appears to be minimal. There are only two reports of such cases: one bled into the biliary tree (Barzilai, ArchSurg, 1950; 72:725) and another into the retroperitoneum (Thomas, Surgery, 1967; 61:550). This is probably due to the fact that rupture is related to the force exerted on the wall of the aneurysm; according to Laplace's law this can be calculated as the product of the transmural pressure and the radius of the vessel. Obviously, the force on the wall of venous as opposed to arterial aneurysms is much lower. It is likely that rupture occurs only when there is portal hypertension in patients with very large aneurysms of the portal vein (that is, greater than 50 mm in diameter). Perhaps the major clinical relevance of these vascular abnormalities is that they reinforce the need for ultrasound control in patients submitted to a liver biopsy, to avoid the risk of puncturing the aneurysm.

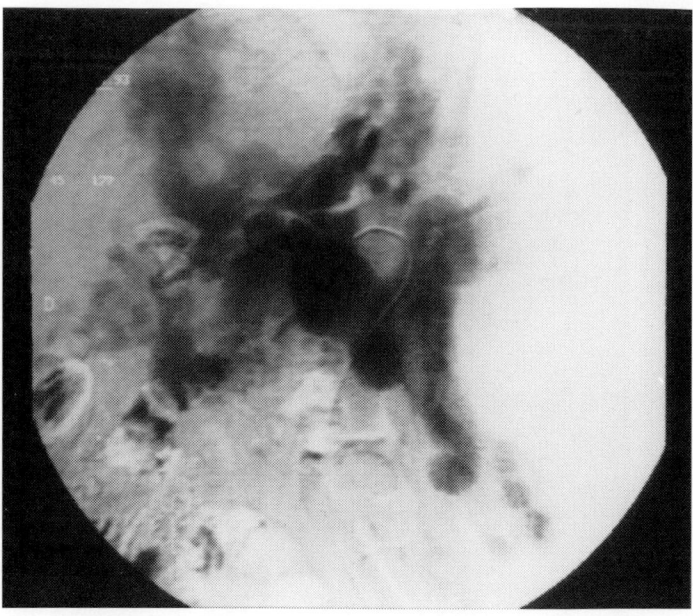

Fig. 3. Venous phase angiography in a patient with extra- and intrahepatic aneurysms of the portal vein.

Several cases of portal hepatic venous shunt via an intrahepatic portal vein aneurysm, in patients with or without portal hypertension, have recently been described in the literature (Kudo, AmJGastr, 1993; 88:723; Saka, IntMed, 1992; 31:899). This situation is easily diagnosed by colour Doppler ultrasonography.

Extrinsic compression of the portal vein

Portal hypertension due to stenosis of the portal vein induced by a mass or a process located at some point in the portal vein is an unusual condition. However, as already discussed, the splenic vein may be compressed by benign or malignant disease of the pancreas.

Partial nodular transformation of the liver is an infrequent disease of unknown origin characterized by the appearance of large nodules (up to 8 cm) located in the hilar area of the liver (Nakanuma, JClinGastro, 1990; 12:460).[10] Liver function tests are usually normal and patients are diagnosed either after bleeding from oesophageal varices or during the diagnostic work-up of an enlarged spleen. Pathological examination shows the hilar nodules, composed of normal hepatocytes with minimal fibrosis, while the surrounding liver has a normal appearance (Nakanuma, JClinGastro, 1990; 12: 460). The nodules compress the portal vein, which on portography shows a characteristic smooth narrowing at the hepatic hilum.

Retroperitoneal fibrosis is a chronic inflammation of the cellular tissue of the lower lumbar area. This inflammatory process may constrict the vessels. There is only one case report of a patient with portal hypertension secondary to the severe constriction of the portal vein due to retroperitoneal fibrosis (Mosimann, BrJSurg, 1980; 67:804).

Arteriovenous fistulas in the portal venous system

Portal pressure is the result of the relationship between portal blood flow and the vascular resistance offered to that flow (Groszmann,

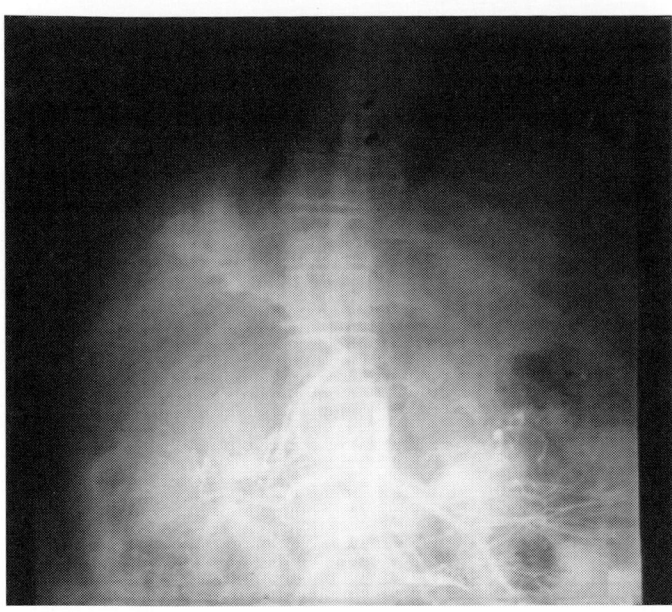

Fig. 4. Intrahepatic arteriovenous fistula. The hepatic artery is filled through the pancreatic vessels and immediately after reaching the fistula the portal vein becomes apparent showing a retrograde flow.

SemLivDis, 1982; 2:177). It is possible, therefore, that portal hypertension could be related to a greatly increased blood flow, which cannot be counteracted by a large enough decrease in the vascular resistance. This may be the mechanism of increased portal pressure in patients with arteriovenous fistulas (Martin, AnnSurg, 1965; 161:209; Foster, AnnSurg, 1961; 154:300; Ponsky, Surgery, 1979; 85:408) in whom no evidence of liver disease can be demonstrated. However, it should be stressed that in some patients portal hypertension is not entirely corrected despite the surgical closure of the fistula (Donovan, Surgery, 1969; 66:474), thus indicating that increased portal pressure was, at least in part, related to the increased vascular resistance.

Arteriovenous fistulas may be located intra- or extrahepatically (Fig. 4). They may have a congenital origin (Martin, AnnSurg, 1965; 161:209), be associated with Rendu–Osler–Weber syndrome, or be due to trauma. Intrahepatic arterioportal fistulas may be due to liver biopsy or other invasive procedures (Donovan, Surgery, 1969; 66:474; Danchin, AmHeartJ, 1983; 105:856; Strodel, ArchSurg, 1987; 122:563; Van Way, Surgery, 1971; 70:876). In other cases, the fistula is observed within a hepatocellular carcinoma (Nagasue, SGO, 1977; 145:504). In patients with cirrhosis the development of an intrahepatic arteriovenous fistula may markedly aggravate portal hypertension. In rare cases, an aneurysm of the hepatic artery may rupture into the portal vein and give rise to a fistula and portal hypertension. Approximately one-third of patients complain of abdominal pain and in some of these it is possible to hear an abdominal bruit. The treatment of these patients by arterial embolization (Redmond, CardiovascIntRadiol, 1988; 11:274) or surgical ligation of the fistula should be followed by a return to normal of the portal pressure.

References

1. Lafortune M, Patriquin H, and Burns P. Doppler ultrasound in the evaluation of portal and splanchnic blood flow. In Ferrucci JT and Mathieu DG, eds. *Advances in hepatobiliary imaging*. St Louis: CV Mosby, 1990: 29–180.
2. Raffensperger JG, Shkolnik AA, Boggs DD, and Swensson O. Portal hypertension in children. *Archives of Surgery*, 1972; 105: 249–54.
3. Mikkelsen W. Extrahepatic portal hypertension in children. *American Journal of Surgery*, 1966; 111: 333–40.
4. Webb LJ and Sherlock S. The aetiology, presentation and natural history of extrahepatic portal venous obstruction. *Quarterly Journal of Medicine*, 1979; 48: 627–39.
5. Sherlock S. Extrahepatic portal hypertension in adults. *Clinical Gastroenterology*, 1985; 14: 1–19.
6. Valla D, Casadevall N, Huisse M, *et al.* Etiology of portal vein thrombosis in adults. A prospective evaluation of primary myeloproliferative disorders. *Gastroenterology*, 1988; 94: 1063–9.
7. Bismuth H, Franco D, and Alagille D. Portal diversion for portal hypertension. The first ninety patients. *Annals of Surgery*, 1980; 192: 18–24.
8. Warren WD, Henderson JM, Millikan WJ, Galambos JT, and Bryan FC. Management of variceal bleeding in patients with non-cirrhotic portal vein thrombosis. *Annals of Surgery*, 1988; 207: 623–34.
9. Pedro-Botet J and Pedro-Pons A. Bloqueos portales prehepáticos. In Pedro-Pons A and Pedro-Botet J, eds. *Enfermedades de la circulación portal*. Barcelona: Ediciones Toray SA, 1966: 151–98.
10. Goodman ZD. Benign tumors of the liver. In Okuda K and Ishak KG, eds. *Neoplasms of the liver*. Tokyo: Springer-Verlag, 1987:105–25.

21.3 Obstruction of the hepatic venous system

Dominique Valla and Jean-Pierre Benhamou

Introduction

There are two types of hepatic venous outflow block. The predominant type is characterized by the obstruction of the main hepatic veins or suprahepatic inferior vena cava. The other type of hepatic venous outflow block is diffuse obstruction of the hepatic venules without involvement of the main hepatic veins. This last entity is usually, but not always, due to a peculiar type of non-thrombotic lesions of the hepatic venules called veno-occlusive disease.[1] The terms 'Chiari's disease' and 'Budd–Chiari syndrome' have been used with various and sometimes confusing meanings and should be avoided (Ludwig, MayoClinProc, 1990; 65:51).

Physiopathological and histopathological consequences of hepatic venous outflow block

A large part of the hepatic venous outflow tract must be occluded before clinical manifestations develop. The obstruction of a single main hepatic vein is clinically silent and only recognized at necropsy.[2] The obstruction of the venous drainage of a region corresponding to two or to the three main hepatic veins has two main effects:

(1) blood pressure increases in the corresponding sinusoids;
(2) blood flow through these sinusoids drops (Widmann, AmJ-Pathol, 1962; 41:439).

Raised sinusoidal pressure has several consequences. First, it induces sinusoidal dilatation and congestion, predominating in the central area of the hepatic lobules.[2] The corresponding clinical feature is enlargement of the liver. Increased sinusoidal pressure enhances the filtration of interstitial fluid. When the drainage capacity of hepatic lymphatics is exceeded, filtration of fluid through the liver capsule occurs (Henriksen, Liver, 1984; 4:221). The filtrated fluid has a high protein content, due to the high permeability to proteins of the sinusoidal wall. However, in most patients with hepatic venous outflow block, the protein content of ascitic fluid is often less than 2.5 g/100 ml. This relatively low protein concentration may be attributed to two factors:

(1) a progressive decrease in permeability of the sinusoidal wall;

(2) admixture of a protein-poor fluid originating from the mesentery (Witte, Gastro, 1980; 78:1059).

Rapid, massive production of ascitic fluid can induce:

(1) effective hypovolaemia and subsequent functional renal failure;
(2) raised sinusoidal pressure which is transmitted to the portal vein and results in portal hypertension;
(3) raised sinusoidal pressure in the obstructed areas of the liver which induces the development of gross and microscopic collateral venous channels between the obstructed areas and the contiguous patent areas of the liver or the contiguous parietal or diaphragmatic veins.

The 'spider-web network', a pattern visible at angiography, corresponds to these intrahepatic and extrahepatic collaterals (Cho, AJR, 1982; 139:703). The collateral channels can ultimately diminish the sinusoidal pressure and thus prevent the development of clinical manifestations.[3]

Ischaemia, due to the reduced sinusoidal perfusion, is not always present. The more sudden the obstruction, the more marked is the ischaemia. Ischaemic liver cell necrosis is visible as a loss of centrilobular hepatocytes.[2] Liver failure resulting from ischaemic liver cell necrosis is rarely fulminant. The consequences of ischaemia are usually transient. Reversibility may be explained by the development of collaterals between the obstructed areas and the neighbouring patent areas. The development of collateral circulation is a major determinant of prognosis[3] (Gupta, QJMed, 1986; 60: 781).

Within a few weeks of obstruction of the hepatic veins, centrilobular fibrosis develops, as a consequence of sinusoidal hypertension and ischaemia. Within a few months, nodular regeneration may take place, predominantly in the periportal area[2] (Castellano, JClinGastro, 1989; 11:698). Moderate portal fibrosis can be present. Cirrhosis can eventually develop.[2] These lesions (fibrosis, nodular regeneration) can develop in the absence of hepatic vein thrombosis in various thrombogenic disorders (Wanless, Medicine, 1980; 59: 367). Therefore, it is difficult to identify them as the consequence of hepatic vein obstruction alone. Regenerative hyperplasia is one of the mechanisms explaining liver enlargement.

In approximately half of the cases of obstruction of the main hepatic veins, the caudate lobe is hypertrophic (Tavill, Gastro, 1975; 68:509). Hypertrophy can be marked, resulting in compression of the inferior vena cava. Hypertrophy of the caudate lobe is explained by the anatomy of its outflow tract: several veins draining the caudate lobe terminate directly in the inferior vena cava caudal to the ostia of the main hepatic veins. Thus, in patients with obstruction of the main hepatic veins, the venous outflow of the caudate lobe is preserved, which allows compensatory hypertrophy. In addition, the veins of the caudate lobe can serve as intrahepatic collateral channels. When the obstruction of the hepatic veins is asynchronous, atrophy of the liver segments affected early may coexist with the congestive enlargement of the areas of the liver that were affected later.

Obstruction of the main hepatic veins or suprahepatic inferior vena cava

Causes

Compression by space occupying lesions

Obstruction is more likely to complicate compression by infectious space-occupying lesions than by benign or malignant neoplastic tumours. In amoebic (Aikat, IndJMedRes, 1978; 67:128) and pyogenic liver abscess (McCarthy, ArchSurg, 1985; 120:657), the systemic and local inflammatory changes may contribute to the formation of hepatic vein thrombosis. In hydatid disease due to *Echinococcus granulosus* (Aikat, IndJMedRes, 1978; 67:128), there is compression by the large-sized and/or the multiple parasitic cysts. In alveolar hydatid disease due to *Echinococcus multilocularis*, direct invasion of the hepatic veins by *Echinococcus multilocularis* also contributes to hepatic vein obstruction (Khuroo, PostgradMedJ, 1980; 56:197).

Secondary liver cancer, the most common cause of malignant liver tumour, is an uncommon cause of hepatic venous outflow block.[2]

Compression by aortic aneurysm has been reported (Sigal, Gastro, 1984; 87:1367). In polycystic dominant kidney disease, compression of the hepatic veins by large-sized or infected liver cysts is the cause of the portal hypertension occasionally found in this disease (Uddin, Gut, 1995; 36:142).

Hepatic veins can be compressed by an intrahepatic haematoma following blunt abdominal trauma (Nicoloff, JThoracCardiovasc-Surg, 1964; 47:225). Hepatic vein ligation during hepatic resection can be followed by hepatic decompensation when asymptomatic obstruction of the remaining veins is overlooked (Ambrosetti, GastrClinBiol, 1992; 16:894).

Endoluminal invasion by a tumour

This complication is specific to those malignant tumours which tend to progress inside the lumen of their venous outflow tract, toward the inferior vena cava, up to the point where they obstruct the hepatic vein ostia, producing an acute or fulminant variant of hepatic outflow block. These malignant tumours include: Wilms' tumour (Nakayama, AnnSurg, 1986; 204:683) and renal cell carcinoma (Beaugrand, ArchFrMalAppDig, 1975; 64:331), hepatocellular carcinoma (Kato, AnnIntMed, 1983; 99; 472), adrenocortical carcinoma (Carbonnel, JClinGastro, 1988; 10:441), and leiomyosarcoma of the inferior vena cava (Taylor, Liver, 1987; 7:201). Myosarcoma of the right atrium can

obstruct the inferior vena cava by a similar but retrograde mechanism (Theodossi, JPath, 1979; 128:159).

The endoluminal tumour can usually be cleaved from the venous walls; thus emergency treatment may be performed to relieve the obstruction. However, prognosis is dismal because lung metastasis is almost always present. Protracted remission or cure has only been recorded when an efficient chemotherapy–radiation therapy was available (Schraut, Gastro, 1985; 88:576).

Thrombosis

Table 1 lists the thrombogenic conditions reported in association with obstruction of the main hepatic veins or suprahepatic inferior vena cava. Their relative prevalence, which is presented in Table 1, is derived from our experience but does not markedly differ from that of several series published in the last 25 years.[4,5] Our experience, and these other series, are based on patients observed in Western countries; the aetiology of occlusion of the main hepatic veins may be different in other parts of the world.

Primary myeloproliferative disorders

Hepatic venous outflow block can complicate (and can be the presenting manifestation of) primary myeloproliferative disorders. In a necropsic study, thrombosis of large hepatic veins was found in eight of 137 patients with polycythaemia vera or agnogenic myeloid metaplasia (Wanless, Hepatol, 1990; 12:1166). Indeed, primary myeloproliferative disorders of any type are the cause of about two-thirds of the cases of hepatic vein thrombosis in recent prospective studies (Levy, Hepatol, 1985; 5:858; Muller, ScaJGastr, 1993; 28 Suppl. 200:74; Pagliuca, QJMed, 1990; 76:981; Teofili, Thromb-Haem, 1992; 67:297) but this high prevalence has only been recognized since the identification of occult myeloproliferative disorders.[4] Overt myeloproliferative disorders are characterized by changes in peripheral blood: conventionally, diagnosis requires that several criteria are met (Berlin, SemHemat, 1975; 12:339), in particular, an increase in red cell and/or platelet count. In patients with occult primary myeloproliferative disorders, peripheral blood changes are not characteristic but a specific abnormality of bone marrow progenitor cells can be demonstrated—a spontaneous formation of erythroid colonies occurs when progenitor cells are cultured in an appropriate, erythropoietin-poor medium (Reid, Lancet, 1982; i:14). The sensitivity of this test is probably not 100 per cent; the specificity is regarded as excellent.[4] Several factors may explain the absence of peripheral blood changes in occult myeloproliferative disorders when hepatic vein thrombosis is present:

(1) an increase in red cell volume can be masked by a parallel increase in plasma volume;
(2) iron deficiency of unclear origin can interfere with erythropoiesis.

However, in most patients with occult myeloproliferative disorders demonstrated by spontaneous formation of erythroid colonies, there are various suggestive abnormalities: bone marrow biopsy showing dystrophic megacaryocytes or hyperplasia of bone marrow cells, liver biopsy or histological examination of a splenectomy specimen showing myeloid metaplasia.[4] Whereas primary myeloproliferative disorders affect mainly men over 50, primary

Table 1 Causes of obstruction of the hepatic veins

Condition	Relative prevalence[a]	Specific diagnostic test
Primary myeloproliferative disorders		
full-blown form	36%	Set of conventional criteria
occult form	36%	Culture of bone marrow cells
Paroxysmal nocturnal haemoglobinuria	10%	Depletion of CD55 and CD59 positive blood cells (flow cytometry)
Lupus anticoagulant and anticardiolipin antibodies	15%	Activated partial thromboplastin time. Specific radio- or enzyme-linked immunoassay
Disorders of coagulation or fibrinolysis	rare	Specific measurements
Drugs		
dacarbazine	rare	Clinical history
oral contraceptives	30%[b]	Clinical history
Pregnancy	4%[b]	Clinical history
Miscellaneous conditions		
Behçet's disease	6%	Set of conventional criteria
sarcoidosis	rare	Tissue biopsy
ulcerative colitis	rare	Endoscopy
connective tissue diseases	rare	Serological tests
immunoallergic vasculitis	rare	Biopsy of skin lesions

[a] In 50 patients admitted to Hôpital Beaujon in whom systematic appropriate investigations for detecting a thrombogenic condition were performed (including bone marrow culture for demonstrating a latent primary myeloproliferative disorder).
[b] In most of the patients, oral contraceptives and pregnancy act in exacerbating a pre-existing thrombogenic conditions.

myeloproliferative disorders complicated by obstruction of hepatic veins affect mainly women below 40.[4]

Paroxysmal nocturnal haemoglobinuria

This is an acquired clonal disorder of the blood cells characterized by a deficiency in the glycosyl-phosphatidyl-inositol residue through which various surface proteins are anchored in the plasma membrane (Yet, JCI, 1994; 93:2305). For unknown reasons, hepatic vein thrombosis is a very common complication of this rare disease (Hartman, JohnsHopkMedJ, 1980; 146:247). The blood changes characteristic of paroxysmal nocturnal haemoglobinuria may be absent when hepatic vein obstruction occurs or is recognized. Manifestations and prognosis are related to the extent of hepatic vein obstruction: manifestations are absent or transient when thrombosis is limited to a few small hepatic veins; chronic ascites results from partial occlusion of the main hepatic veins; a fatal course is a consequence of complete obstruction of the main hepatic veins.[5]

The antiphospholipid syndrome

This entity is characterized by the presence of various antiphospholipid autoantibodies, and by an increased risk of arterial or venous thrombosis and spontaneous abortion. This entity was initially described in patients suffering from systemic lupus erythematosus, connective tissue disease, or malignancy, but it can be also found in the absence of these conditions (Love, AnnIntMed, 1992; 112:682). The antiphospholipid syndrome was recently reported to rank as the second cause of hepatic vein thrombosis, accounting for almost 20 per cent of cases (Pelletier, JHepatol, 1994; 21:76). In most of the reported cases, the American Rheumatism Association criteria for the diagnosis of systemic lupus were not fulfilled. Frequently, interruption of anticoagulant therapy is followed by the development or the exacerbation of manifestations of hepatic venous outflow obstruction (Owendijk, Gut, 1994; 35:1004).

Disorders of coagulation and fibrinolysis

Several disorders of the coagulation and fibrolysis system are common in patients with thrombosis. However, surprisingly, deficiency of antithrombin III, protein C, or protein S are uncommon causes of hepatic vein obstruction: questionable cases in patients with antithrombin III deficiency (Das, Surgery, 1985; 97:242) and a well documented case of protein C deficiency (Bourlière, Gut, 1990; 31: 949) have been reported. It should be emphasized that liver failure *per se* induces a non-specific decrease in the serum level of these factors, which must be distinguished from a primary anomaly. The newly identified resistance to activated protein C (factor V Leiden) (Vorberg, Lancet, 1994; 343:1535) may well prove to be a common cause of hepatic vein thrombosis (Denninger, Lancet, 1995; 345: 525).

Drugs

Dacarbazine may cause fulminant hepatic vein occlusion. The mechanism of the vascular lesion may be an immunoallergic injury affecting the small- and medium-sized hepatic veins (Ceci, Cancer, 1988; 61:1988). Extension of thrombosis to the main hepatic vein has been reported (Runne, DMedWoch, 1980; 105:230).

Use of oral contraceptives increases the risk of hepatic vein occlusion approximately by two. Circumstantial evidence suggests that oral contraceptives act by exacerbating the thrombogenic potential of an underlying thrombogenic disorder (Valla, Gastro, 1986; 90:807).

Pregnancy and postpartum

Several cases of hepatic vein occlusion have been reported during pregnancy or in the postpartum period.[6] In several instances, an associated thrombogenic condition was also present such as paroxysmal nocturnal haemoglobinuria (Spencer, BrJObsGyn, 1980; 87:246) or primary myeloproliferative disorder.[4] Thus, in pregnant women as well as in women taking oral contraceptives affected by hepatic vein occlusion, an underlying thrombogenic condition must be suspected.

Miscellaneous systemic thrombogenic conditions

Behçet's disease, a recognized cause of inferior vena cava thrombosis, can be complicated by hepatic vein occlusion (Bismuth, Hepatol, 1990; 11:969); in most patients, hepatic vein occlusion is associated with, and probably secondary to, thrombosis of the inferior vena cava.

Ulcerative colitis can be complicated by hepatic vein thrombosis due to the hypercoagulability resulting from high fibrinogen level, decreased antithrombin III, raised factor VIII activity, and thrombocytosis (Chesner, Gut, 1986; 27:1096).

The association of hepatic vein thrombosis and celiac disease has been reported recently (Marteau, JHepatol, 1994; 20:650). This association is not well explained at present. There was no evidence for hyposplenism or anticardiolipin antibodies or lupus anticoagulant in the reported cases.

Sarcoidosis is a very uncommon cause of obstruction of the main hepatic veins (Russi, AmJGastr, 1986; 81:71); however, granulomatous invasion of small-sized hepatic veins in the absence of significant main hepatic vein obstruction is more common (Nakanuma, ArchPathLabMed, 1989; 104:406). Some of these cases may be responsive to steroid treatment (Young, Gastro, 1988; 94:503).

In a few patients with connective tissue disease, hepatic vein occlusion seems to have developed in the absence of lupus anticoagulant or antiphospholipid autoantibodies (Disney, JClinGastro, 1984; 6:253). Immunoallergic vasculitis without obvious cause deserves comment: this type of vasculitis can precede the development of overt primary myeloproliferative disorders by several months or years (Longley, AmJMed, 1986; 80:1027).

Idiopathic hypereosinophilic syndrome was associated with a few cases of idiopathic hepatic vein obstruction (Ito, AmJGastr, 1988; 83:316). The endothelial toxicity of certain eosinophil constituents has been incriminated (Elouaer-Blanc, ArchIntMed, 1985; 145:751).

Association of thrombogenic conditions

It is increasingly recognized that the association of two thrombogenic conditions and a triggering factor might be necessary for thrombosis to develop (Shafer, Lancet, 1994, 344:1739). This possibility has not yet been appropriately evaluated in patients with hepatic vein obstruction. However, there are isolated cases of such an association (Denninger, Lancet, 1995; 345:525). Therefore, a systematic investigation of all the recognizable thrombogenic conditions should be performed in any patients with hepatic or inferior vena cava obstruction.

Hepatic and inferior vena cava obstruction of unknown cause

In most retrospective studies, this category accounts for 25 to 50 per cent of cases of hepatic venous outflow block.[6] However, when all the tests listed in Table 1 are performed, the proportion of idiopathic cases falls to less than 20 per cent. This is mainly due to the identification of occult myeloproliferative disorders.[4]

Membranous obstruction of inferior vena cava

Membranous obstruction of the inferior vena cava is the major cause of hepatic venous outflow block in South Africa (Simson, Gastro, 1982; 82:171), Japan[7] (Hirooka, ArchSurg, 1970; 100: 656), and, to a lesser extent, in India.[6] The inferior vena cava is obstructed at or above the level of hepatic vein ostia. One of the main hepatic veins usually remains patent and drains into the caudal portion of the inferior vena cava. Inferior vena cava blood is returned to the right atrium through large lumbar and azygous collateral veins. The other main hepatic veins are usually obstructed.

This lesion has long been considered of congenital origin because of its regular shape and because the embryonic development of the terminal portion of inferior vena cava is highly complex.[6] However, there are several lines of circumstantial evidence suggesting the acquired nature of membranous obstruction of the inferior vena cava:

1. The prominent caval–caval collateral circulation usually develops in adulthood which is not consistent with a congenital malformation (Takaishi, GastrInternat, 1990; 3:70).
2. When systematically investigated, a associated thrombogenic disorder is usually found (Terabayashi, Gastro, 1986; 91:219; Mion, EurJGastroHepatol, 1994; 6:363). In most of the other reported cases of membranous obstruction, investigation for an underlying thrombogenic condition had not been systematically carried out.
3. In a patient with lupus anticoagulant, inferior vena cava thrombosis was showed to transform into membranous obstruction (Terabayashi, Gastro, 1986; 91:219).
4. Histopathology of membranous obstruction strongly suggests a thrombotic origin (see below).
5. Associated obstruction of the hepatic vein is of various types:

    (a) the termination of one, two, or three hepatic veins may be obliterated;
    (b) the hepatic vein opening can be located below or above the membranous obstruction (Takeushi, AmJMed, 1971; 51: 11).

Such a variety is less compatible with a congenital malformation than with an acquired origin.

Manifestations

The prevalence of the main manifestations of hepatic venous outflow block in a series of 87 patients admitted to Hôpital Beaujon is set out in Table 2. Manifestations differ according to the date at which patients were seen because recent, non-invasive imaging procedures have allowed easy recognition of previously overlooked cases. Patients can be ascribed to one of four main clinical variants.

Table 2 Clinical manifestations of hepatic venous outflow block due to hepatic vein or inferior vena cava thrombosis in 1970–1987 and 1987–1991*		
Signs and symptoms	1970–1987 (%, n = 47)	1987–1991 (%, n = 34)
Ascites	95	65
Liver enlargement	95	76
Abdominal pain	80	53
Leg oedema	47	15
Jaundice	43	21
Fever	40	18
Hepatic encephalopathy	20	3
Gastrointestinal bleeding	16	6
None of the above symptoms	0	24

Asymptomatic variant

This entity was recently identified.[3] These patients have no ascites, hepatomegaly, or abdominal pain. Hepatic outflow obstruction is either fortuitously discovered by imaging investigation of other complaints or documented by the investigation for abnormal liver tests. Persistent patency of one large hepatic vein or development of a large venous collateral probably explains the absence of clinical manifestations in these patients. Approximately 20 per cent of patients with hepatic venous outflow block seen since 1990 fall into this category.

Fulminant variant

This entity is characterized by the development of fulminant liver failure within a few days, with renal failure and marked increase in serum aminotransferase (Powell-Jackson, Gut, 1986; 27:1101). This entity is very uncommon in patients with hepatic venous outflow block.

Acute/subacute variants

This entity is characterized by the rapid development of ascites, with hepatomegaly, functional renal failure, and jaundice.[3,6] Serum aminotransferase is greater than five times the upper limit of the normal range. Prothrombin level is less than 40 per cent of normal. This syndrome develops within a month. Approximately 20 per cent of patients with hepatic outflow block fall into this group. Prognosis is good in the short term but it could be worse than in the chronic variant in the long term (Denié, Hepatol, 1995; 22: 253A).

Chronic variants

This entity is characterized by a progressive formation of ascites over 2 months or more. Serum aminotransferase is slightly increased or normal. Jaundice is absent. Prothrombin level is higher than 40 per cent of normal. A functional renal failure is present only in half of the cases. Approximately 60 per cent of the patients with hepatic outflow block can be ascribed to this group.

Complications

The spontaneous outcome is not well known because many patients undergo surgery. There have been reports of spontaneous regression of severe acute manifestations (Brinson, DigDis, 1988; 33:1615). Three major complications may occur:

1. Rapidly developing liver failure is uncommon (Powell-Jackson, 1986, Gut; 27:1101).
2. Gastrointestinal bleeding occurs in approximately 15 per cent of patients and was responsible for most of the fatalities observed before the introduction of portal–systemic shunt in the therapy of hepatic venous outflow block.
3. Ascites is the main complication.[3,6] It is our experience that, in one-third of the patients ascites is resistant to medical therapy at the time of presentation or is associated with functional renal failure; in one-third of the patients, ascites can initially be controlled by medical therapy but within 6 months becomes resistant; in the remaining one-third of the patients, ascites is and remains easily controlled by medical therapy. When ascites is controlled by medical therapy, prolonged survival can be observed. In recent series including unoperated and operated patients, mortality was about 50 per cent after 3 years; very few deaths were noted thereafter (Powel-Jackson, QJMed, 1982; 51: 79; Gupta, QJMed, 1986; 60:781; Zeitoun, Hepatol, 1995; 22: 144A).

Several features of membranous obstruction of inferior vena cava are distinct from those of hepatic vein obstruction:[7]

1. The clinical manifestations develop much more insidiously; ascites is usually absent; prominent subcutaneous thoracic, lumbar, and abdominal collaterals are common; all these manifestations have been present for several years before patients seek medical attention.
2. Centrilobular congestion is not as marked as in cases of primary lesions of the hepatic veins; portal fibrosis and cirrhosis are more common.
3. Chronic infection with hepatitis B virus is common; the nature of this association is unclear.
4. Hepatocellular carcinoma develops in 6 to 50 per cent of these patients. The mechanism of this association has not been clarified; hepatocellular carcinoma might result from the malignant transformation of an originally benign regenerative nodule, a transformation facilitated by the protracted course of the disease.

Pathology of the lesions of hepatic veins and inferior vena cava

The lesions of the hepatic veins have been well documented in necropsy studies[2] (Aikat, IndJMedRes, 1978; 67:128). In patients with non-tumorous obstruction, the commonest lesion is a concentric thickening of the vein wall by non-inflammatory, subintimal fibrosis. As a result, the lumen of the hepatic vein is greatly reduced or obliterated. This lesion can involve the whole length of a main hepatic vein, which appears as a fibrous cord remnant. In other cases, fibrous thickening is limited to the terminal, juxtaostial portion of the main hepatic vein, forming short-length stenoses[2] (Valla, Hepatol, 1994; 20:103A) or hepatic vein webs (Tavill, Gastro, 1975; 68:509; Vickers, JHepatol, 1989; 8:287). Finally, in a small number of cases, only the ostium of the hepatic veins is occluded, a condition sometimes called Chiari's disease (Gagné, CanMedAssJ, 1963; 88:155). In patients with short-length stenoses, the disease follows a more indolent course and survival is better than in other types of primary venous lesions (Valla, Hepatol, 1994; 20:103A).

Recent and old (i.e. organized and recanallized) thrombi are superimposed on fibrous lesions. Pure thrombosis is uncommon. There has been debate as to whether the primary event is thrombosis or fibrosis of the venous wall[1] (Takaishi, GastrInternat, 1990; 3: 70). The discussion has been obscured as the cause of hepatic vein occlusion has not been identified in most of the necropsy cases. In our experience, short-length stenoses affecting the terminal portion of the hepatic veins is as commonly associated with thrombogenic disorders as other types of hepatic vein obstruction (Valla, Hepatol, 1997; 25:814). The release of fibrosing agents by platelets, such as platelet-derived growth factor, is known to occur in the primary myeloproliferative disorders and may account for the development of myelofibrosis. Subendothelial fibrosis in atheromatous lesions has been attributed to the release of platelet-derived growth factor from platelets adhering to the damaged endothelial surface (Ross, NEJM, 1986; 314:488). Therefore, it is tempting to hypothesize that the adherence of abnormal platelets to areas of damaged endothelium in the terminal portion of the hepatic veins might be responsible for the fibrous lesions; a possible cause of damaged endothelium might be the mechanical distortion of the terminal portion of the hepatic veins by the diaphragm during the respiratory movements (Gayet, personal communication).

Lesions of the small-sized hepatic veins are various. There is either no lesion or dilatation, thrombosis, fibrosis, endophlebitis, and/or disappearance of the small hepatic veins.[2]

Histopathology of membranous obstruction of the inferior vena cava shows that the basic structure of the venous wall is maintained with transformation of the intima into a fibrous laminar structure, organized thrombi of various ages, recanallization, and calcifications (Kage, Gastro, 1992; 102:2081). As mentioned above, this is strong evidence for the acquired, thrombotic origin of this fibrous or membranous lesion.

Obstruction of the hepatic venules

Obstruction of hepatic venules without involvement of large-sized hepatic veins may be observed in some of the conditions already mentioned; for example paroxysmal nocturnal haemoglobinuria and treatment with dacarbazine. In addition, various lesions of the hepatic venules have been described in alcoholic liver disease: lymphocytic phlebitis, perivenular fibrosis, and veno-occlusive changes (Goodman, Gastro, 1982; 83:786). In hepatic sarcoidosis, granulomas can be found within the wall of hepatic venules (Nakanuma, ArchPathLabMed, 1980; 104:456). In alcoholic liver disease and in hepatic sarcoidosis, these lesions are likely to participate in the mechanism of portal hypertension.

Veno-occlusive disease of the liver must be distinguished from the lesions mentioned above and is characterized by a non-thrombotic, concentric, luminal narrowing of the central or intercalated (sublobular) veins by loose connective tissue, without obstruction of large-sized hepatic veins.[1] This definition can be extended to include earlier stage of the lesion (subendothelial oedema with entrapped blood cells) as well as the later stage (perivenular fibrosis and dense fibrous scar replacing the central vein). The venular lesions are always associated with severe haemorrhagic congestion and hepatic cell necrosis affecting the central area of the lobules.

The disease can progress to an extensive central fibrosis with central-to-central or central-to-portal bridging, nodular regeneration, and, ultimately, cirrhosis.

Acute, subacute, and chronic clinical types of veno-occlusive disease have been recognized.[1] In the acute type, there is sudden abdominal distension due to enlargement of the liver and ascites; complete recovery can occur or the clinical course can be fulminant with early death from liver failure. The subacute type results from incomplete recovery of the acute type. The chronic type is clinically indistinguishable from cirrhosis of any cause.

Pyrrolizidine alkaloids, irradiation, antineoplastic drugs, and conditioning for bone marrow transplantation are the main causes of veno-occlusive disease.

Veno-occlusive disease due to pyrrolizidine alkaloids

These alkaloids are found in as many as 352 plant species belonging to 10 families (Smith, JNatProd, 1981; 44:129). Toxicity results most commonly from ingestion of plants belonging to the species *Heliotropium*, *Crotolaria*, and *Senecio*, which have a worldwide distribution. Other species have also been incriminated. When poisoning is due to ingestion of flour contaminated with alkaloid-containing plants, the disease may be epidemic (Tandon, AmJGastr, 1978; 70:607). Ingestion of an alkaloid-containing plant infusion or decoction (as a herbal tea or an enema) is responsible for most endemic[1] and sporadic cases (Lyford, Gastro, 1976; 70:105). The unsaturated pyrrolizidine alkaloids are toxic because they are dehydrogenated by the liver microsomes; the pyrrolic derivatives are reactive compounds that damage hepatocyte DNA and proteins (Huxtable, GenPharmacol, 1979; 10:159). Experimental hepato-toxicity is dose dependent . This is relevant to the natural history of the human disease. The acute form results from recent ingestion of large amounts of pyrrolizidine alkaloids whereas chronic disease results from prolonged ingestion of small amounts of these toxins.

The term 'veno-occlusive' might be inappropriate to describe the early lesions caused by pyrrolizidine alkaloids. Injury to the perivenular hepatic cells and sinusoids may actually be the initial lesion in the absence of central vein occlusion (Tandon, Lancet, 1976; ii:271). A specific toxic action of pyrrolic derivatives released by the liver on the cardiac and pulmonary arterial endothelium has been found in animal experiments (Bruner, ToxApplPharmacol, 1986; 85:416).

Veno-occlusive disease due to irradiation

Liver irradiation is the second main cause of veno-occlusive disease. Clinical onset take place 2 to 5 weeks after liver irradiation. The severity ranges from asymptomatic to a fatal course. Although sensitivity to liver irradiation varies from patients to patients, a direct relationship is suggested by the limitation of the lesion to the irradiated part of the liver and by the dose-dependant prevalence of the lesion (Ingold, AJR, 1965; 93:200; Lansing, ArchSurg, 1968; 96:878). Veno-occlusive disease rarely occurs below 30 cGy, if irradiation is not associated with administration of antineoplastic drugs. Veno-occlusive disease can take place with 10 cGy if irradiation is combined with chemotherapy (Fajardo, ArchPathLabMed, 1980; 104:584), as in conditioning for bone marrow transplantation (see below).

Veno-occlusive disease due to antineoplastic drugs

Several antineoplastic drugs have been reported to cause veno-occlusive disease. At a cumulative dose ranging from 150 to 2500 g, urethane (ethyl carbamate) induced either an acute or a subacute type of veno-occlusive disease (Weiss, AmJMed, 1960; 28:476; Brodsky, AmJMed, 1961; 30:976). Most cases were fatal. The drug is no longer used but a case resulting from surreptitious administration has recently been reported (Cadranel, JClinGastro, 1993; 17:52).

Azathioprine and the closely related compounds 6-mercaptopurine and 6-thioguanine have been implicated in several cases of centrilobular haemorrhagic necrosis attributed to veno-occlusive disease.[8] Several features distinguish veno-occlusive disease due to azathioprine from veno-occlusive disease due to other causes.[8] The clinical onset takes place after 6 to 108 months of continuous administration. Most patients are renal transplant recipients also receiving corticosteroids. The initial manifestations are jaundice and/or liver enlargement rather than ascites. Serum alkaline phosphatase is often increased. Perivenular and perisinusoidal fibrosis are prominent. Veno-occlusive lesions are often associated with peliosis and nodular regenerative hyperplasia.

Several other antineoplastic drugs have been implicated such as mitomycin C, carmustine, indicine-N-oxide, mustinehydrochloride, vincristine, and doxorubicin; however, their role has not always been clearly established.[8]

Veno-occlusive disease due to conditioning for bone marrow transplantation

Conditioning for bone marrow transplantation has become the major cause of veno-occlusive disease. Conditioning usually includes the administration of cyclophosphamide with or without other alkylating agents, together with total body irradiation. The features of the disease have been reviewed[9] (Shulman, Hepatol, 1994; 19: 1171). The clinical onset takes place within 4 weeks after transplantation, with rapidly rising serum bilirubin, upper abdominal pain, liver enlargement, ascites, and weight gain. Liver failure causes or contributes to death in nearly half of the patients. When the diagnosis is based on clinical criteria including hepatomegaly, weight gain, and jaundice, the prevalence of veno-occlusive disease after bone marrow transplantation reached 54 per cent in recent series.[9] The prevalence of veno-occlusive disease after bone marrow transplantation ranged from 13 to 20 per cent in older series. Clinical criteria tend to overestimate the prevalence of histologically documented criteria (Carreras, BoneMTrans, 1993; 11:21). There is a good clinicopathological correlation when the definition of veno-occlusive disease is extended to include fibrosis and necrosis in acinar zone 3 (Shulman, Hepatol, 1994; 19:1171). The prevalence of veno-occlusive disease is related to elevated transaminases value before transplantation, cytoreductive therapy with high-dose regimen, and previous therapy to the abdomen[9] (Ganem, IntJRadiatOncolBiolPhys, 1988; 14:879). This finding may indicate that chronic viral hepatitis would be a predisposing factor; alternatively, the increased aminotransferases would reflect an individual sensitivity to prior radiochemotherapy. The latter interpretation is consistent with the low prevalence of veno-occlusive disease in patient suffering from bone marrow aplasia (who therefore did not receive previous antineoplastic chemotherapy) and the high prevalence of veno-occlusive disease in recipients of second transplantation, or after cytoreductive therapy with a high-dose regimen, or after previous radiation therapy to the abdomen.[9]

Diagnosis

The diagnosis of hepatic venous outflow block should be suspected in the following circumstances:

(1) whenever ascites and liver enlargement and upper abdominal pain are simultaneously present;
(2) in patient with signs of chronic liver disease, whenever intractable ascites contrasts with mildly altered liver function tests;
(3) whenever liver disease is documented in a patient with known thrombogenic disorder;
(4) whenever fulminant hepatic failure is associated with liver enlargement and ascites;
(5) whenever chronic liver disease remains unexplained after alcoholism, chronic viral hepatitis, autoimmunity, iron overload, Wilson's disease, and α-1-antitrypsin deficiency have been excluded.

In the majority of cases, non-invasive imaging procedures give evidence of obstruction of the hepatic outflow. In patients in whom the non-invasive imaging procedures fail to establish the diagnosis, liver biopsy should be performed. Rarely, opacification of the hepatic veins is needed.

Ultrasonography

In 75 per cent of the patients with obstruction of the main hepatic veins, diagnosis can be based simply on ultrasonography. The specific features (Menu, Radiol, 1985; 157:761; Gupta, Gut, 1987; 28:242) are:

(1) echogenic material in the lumen of the main hepatic veins or inferior vena cava;
(2) stenosis on inferior vena cava and/or main hepatic veins with upstream dilatation;
(3) hyperechogenic cord replacing one of the main hepatic veins;
(4) intrahepatic venous collaterals.

The concordance between ultrasound abnormalities and findings at necropsy or venography is excellent, except when occlusion is limited to a hepatic vein ostium and then may give a false normal aspect of that vein. Non-visualization, tortuosity, and reduced diameter of the main hepatic veins are frequently noted; however, these abnormalities are also present in cirrhosis in the absence of obstruction of the main hepatic veins. Ultrasonography usually allows recognition of intraluminal tumourous invasion and compression of the hepatic veins.

The patency of the portal vein and superior mesenteric vein can be well evaluated by ultrasonography. This information is essential for the choice of therapeutic options.

Pulsed Doppler and colour Doppler imaging improve the diagnostic accuracy of ultrasound (Bolondi, Gastro, 1991; 100:1324).

Computed tomography

In general, information provided by computed tomography simply confirms information provided by ultrasonography. However, in patients in whom ultrasound findings are compatible with, but not specific for, the diagnosis, results of computed tomography can be very useful. Contrast infusion produces characteristic images: in the early phase, there is a mottling and enhancement of the liver, predominating in the peripheral and perihilar regions; in the late phase, opacification of the liver becomes homogeneous (Baert, Gastro, 1983; 84:587; Gupta, Gut, 1987; 28:242). Tumours invading or compressing the hepatic veins are well delineated by computed tomography.

Magnetic resonance imaging

The main hepatic veins are well recognized by magnetic resonance imaging. Small series have suggested that magnetic resonance imaging is as efficacious as ultrasonography for recognizing hepatic vein obstruction and intrahepatic collateral circulation; it might be better than ultrasonography for studying the inferior vena cava (Menu, DiagIntervRadiol, 1990; 2:23). The ability of magnetic resonance imaging to differentiate stagnant flow from thrombosis needs further evaluation.

Liver biopsy

According to our experience, in about half of the cases of hepatic vein occlusion, coagulation disorders preclude percutaneous needle biopsy of the liver; however, in 90 per cent of our patients, non-invasive imaging procedures render liver biopsy unnecessary. The characteristic histological lesions, that is centrilobular congestion, may not be obvious in a needle biopsy specimen, especially in patients with long-standing hepatic venous outflow block and cirrhosis.[7]

Angiography

Opacification of the hepatic veins can be obtained using transhepatic thin needle punction of a hepatic vein radicle (Rector, Gastro, 1984; 86:1395) or by retrograde cannulation of the hepatic veins via the superior or inferior vena cava (Kreel, BrJRadiol, 1967; 40:755). The former procedure is preferred to the latter because it gives better delineation of hepatic vein lesions. When severe coagulation disorders or massive ascites are present, the only feasible procedure is retrograde cannulation. Angiographic abnormalities indicating hepatic vein occlusion are:

(1) segmental obliteration or stenosis of a main hepatic vein;
(2) luminal filling defects;
(3) opacification of a collateral network.

Failure to cannulate the hepatic vein ostia is only a presumptive evidence for hepatic vein occlusion. A drawback of retrograde cannulation is the risk of aggravating thrombosis or dislodging a recent thrombus.

Patency of the inferior vena cava is a major determinant of the treatment. Inferior vena cavography must be performed whenever patency cannot be clearly demonstrated by non-invasive imaging procedures. Inferior vena cavography must be coupled with a measurement of inferior vena cava pressure to assess the haemodynamic consequences of compression by an hypertrophied caudal lobe.

Prevention of renal failure induced by a contrast agent is essential in patients with hepatic venous outflow block. Whenever pharmacological thrombolysis is envisaged, the invasive angiographic procedures should not be performed.

Treatment

Treatment aims at four goals: eradication or control of the cause, prevention of venous thromboses, control of manifestations with non-specific measures, and restoration of the hepatic venous outflow with the hope that this is associated with a better survival.

Treatment of the cause

This essential part of the therapeutic strategy is beyond the scope of this review.

Prevention of other venous thromboses

Prevention of the development of thrombosis in still patent hepatic veins, inferior vena cava, portal vein, as well as in other venous territories is of utmost importance. It is justified in the patients with a documented thrombogenic condition. It is also justified when no cause has been identified, on the assumption that a thrombogenic condition is probably present but has been overlooked. In our experience, heparin in the early phase and a vitamin K antagonist in the long term can be used safely. Overt, primary myeloproliferative disorders must be treated urgently.

An additional justification of anticoagulation is the observation that treatment with heparin alone has allowed repermeation of thrombosed hepatic veins (Schmets, GastrClinBiol, 1993; 17:955) and of thrombosed portal vein associated with thrombosed hepatic veins (Marteau, JHepatol, 1994; 20:650) to take place without the need for an operation.

Control of manifestations with non-specific measures

Treatment of ascites

Control of ascites is usually achieved with diuretics. When diuretics are inefficient, paracentesis with infusion of albumin is indicated. Peritoneovenous shunting should only be performed when ascites is resistant to medical therapy and portosystemic shunting is not feasible; obstruction of the valve and thrombosis of the recipient vein are common, due to the protein-rich ascitic fluid and to the frequently associated thrombogenic condition. When control of ascites requires permanent diuretic therapy, an operation aiming at restoration of hepatic blood outflow must be considered.

Treatment of gastrointestinal bleeding due to portal hypertension

The procedures which have proved to be efficient in cirrhosis can be employed in patients with hepatic vein thrombosis with the following particularities. During active bleeding, balloon tamponade or endoscopic sclerotherapy should be preferred to vasoconstrictor agents because the reduction in splanchnic blood flow might precipitate mesenteric or portal vein thrombosis and intestinal infarction in patients with a thrombogenic disorder. Prevention of first or recurrent bleeding should rely first on β-adrenergic blocking agents because the associated anticoagulant therapy may make sclerotherapy difficult. When bleeding recurs or is difficult to control, an operation aimed at hepatic blood outflow must be considered.

Restoration of hepatic blood outflow

This aspect of the treatment aims to correct sinusoidal and portal venous hypertension, thereby controlling ascites and preventing gastrointestinal bleeding. Another theoretical goal is to reduce hepatic ischaemia and therefore the severity of liver failure. There are three ways to restore hepatic blood outflow: repermeation of obstructed hepatic venous outflow, portal–systemic shunting, and transplantation.

Repermeation of obstructed hepatic venous outflow

Thrombolytic therapy

Thrombolytic therapy has achieved good results in selected cases of hepatic vein or inferior vena cava thrombosis (Sholar, AnnIntMed, 1985; 103:359). However, failure has also been reported (Thompson, EurJGastroHepatol, 1994; 6:835). Series of consecutive cases are awaited. This therapy should be used early and only when recent thrombosis can be clearly documented. The criteria for recent thrombosis could be an increase in serum transaminases activity to values higher than five fold the upper limit of normal values (Valla D, unpublished observations). When thrombolytic therapy is considered, no invasive diagnostic procedure should be performed.

Angioplasty

Angioplasty has been attempted in patients with a short-length stenosis of the hepatic veins, usually using the percutaneous endoluminal route. Although an immediate relief of obstruction was obtained in most reported cases, recurrence was common (Martin, AJR, 1990; 154:1007). Insertion of metallic stents may prevent restenosis (Lopez, Gastro, 1991; 100:1435). Several procedures have been used for direct treatment of membranous obstruction of inferior vena cava: transcardiac membranotomy (Kimura, Surgery, 1972; 72:551), percutaneous transluminal angioplasty using dilatation balloons (Martin, AJR, 1990; 154:1007) or laser (Furui, Radiol, 1988; 166:673). Recurrence of stenosis can occur (Sarfati, GastrClinBiol, 1993; 17:223), but may be prevented by the insertion of an expandable metallic stent (Gillams, JHepatol, 1991; 13:149). Various reconstructive or caval–atrial bypass operations have also been used associated with extracorporeal circulation[7] (Wang, JVascSurg, 1989; 10:149), but preference is now given to percutaneous angioplasty (Kohli, Lancet, 1993; 342:718). These procedures are justified only when at least one main hepatic vein remains patent and drains into the caudal segment of the inferior vena cava.[7] Mortality can be high, up to 20 per cent; nevertheless the overall survival rate in operated patients seems to be better than the spontaneous outcome.[7]

Dorsocranial liver resection with direct hepatoatrial anastomosis

Dorsocranial liver resection with direct hepatoatrial anastomosis was proposed on the basis of the observation that hepatic veins are usually occluded in their terminal portion (Bansky, JHepatol, 1986; 2:101). Recent results do suggest that it is as good an operation as portosystemic shunting in patients with patent portal vein and compressed or occluded inferior vena cava (Pasic, JThoracCardiovascSurg, 1993; 106: 275). The results in patients with thrombosed portal vein are less impressive (Sauvannet, Hepatogast, 1974; 41:174).

Portal–systemic shunting

Transformation of the portal vein into an outflow tract is the rationale for portosystemic shunting.

Side-to-side portacaval shunt and mesocaval shunt

Side-to-side portacaval shunt and mesocaval shunt have given the best results (Bismuth, AnnSurg, 1991; 214, 581; Henderson, AmJSurg, 1990; 159:41; Kholi, Lancet, 1993; 342:718; Orloff, ArchSurg, 1992; 127:1182; Panis, Surgery, 1994; 115:276; Shaked, SGO, 1992; 174:453). Interposition of a venous graft is usually necessary. Inhospital mortality ranges from 0 to 30 per cent. Most of the patients have no ascites at 1 year of follow-up. Shunt thrombosis occurs in approximately 25 per cent of patients (Panis, Surgery, 1994; 115:276), and is usually an early complication. The postoperative period is uneventful if liver fibrosis is mild or moderate; however, massive ascites may develop if extensive fibrosis or cirrhosis is present (Belghiti, GastrClinBiol, 1988; 12:A9). The high cardiac output and low resistance haemodynamic state that follows the opening of the portosystemic shunts may be poorly tolerated (Beattie, Surgery, 1988; 104:1). Ascites and heart failure have been responsible, directly or indirectly, for postoperative death in some series. Preoperative liver tests and the level of pressure in the inferior vena cava are of no value in predicting the outcome of surgery; however, it is usually accepted that a pressure in the inferior vena cava exceeding 20 mmHg precludes portacaval or mesocaval shunting (Cameron, AnnSurg, 1983; 198:335).

Portoatrial and mesoatrial shunts

Portoatrial and mesoatrial shunts using a long prosthetic graft are a logical solution to cope with simultaneous occlusion of the hepatic veins and occlusion of the inferior vena cava, when the portal vein is patent (Franco, Surgery, 1986; 99:378; Ahn, JVascSurg, 1987; 5: 28; Stringer, BrJSurg, 1989; 76:474; Wang, JVascSurg, 1989; 10: 149). Initial results have been disappointing—the mortality was close to 60 per cent at 1 year of follow-up and the risk of thrombosis of the long prosthetic graft ranges from 30 to 40 per cent—but recent series have achieved results similar to those of portacaval or mesocaval shunts. Anastomosis of the portal vein to the innominate vein has been proposed to avoid the opening of the pericardium and the ensuing risk of tamponade (Hay, GastrClinBiol, 1988; 12:755).

Liver transplantation

Liver transplantation has been used as an alternative to portacaval and mesocaval shunt[10] (Campbell, SGO, 1988; 166:511; Halff,

AnnSurg, 1990; 211:43; Shaked, SGO, 1992; 174:453). Overall results are similar to those of portosystemic shunting. There are three critical issues in the debate whether or not to perform a transplantation in patients with hepatic venous outflow block. The first issue pertains to the risk of thromboses of the vascular anastomoses and of recurrent thrombosis of the hepatic veins. This risk has been controlled with systematic, early postoperative anticoagulation. The second issue relates to the risk that immunosuppression exacerbates the myeloproliferative disorder which is commonly associated. At present, there are no data to substantiate this fear. The third issue, still unresolved, is to determine whether hepatic transplantation is an alternative to portal–systemic shunting, a rescue operation after a failing portal–systemic shunt, or a primary operation in patients with predictably bad results after portal–systemic shunting.[10] Since portacaval and mesocaval shunting has achieved good results in patients without severe liver lesions, hepatic transplantation should be reserved for patients with severe cirrhosis or with fulminant liver failure.[10]

Indications

The indications for the currently available procedures mainly depends on three conditions: the presence or the absence of manifestations, the patency of the inferior vena cava and portal vein, and the presence or the absence of severe liver failure.

For asymptomatic patients and patients in whom manifestations have been easily controlled, no operation is justified. When permanent treatment is necessary for ascites or when gastrointestinal bleeding recurs, an operation should be considered. However, current evidence suggest that no global improvement in survival has yet been obtained with decompressive surgery. Therefore these operations should be envisaged mainly for the control of symptoms (Zeitoun, Hepatol, 1995; 22:144A).

Patent inferior vena cava

Patent portal vein

In patients without severe liver failure, a portacaval or a mesocaval shunt can be constructed. Hepatoatrial anastomosis, hepatic vein angioplasty, and thrombolytic therapy have been used in patients with a patent portal vein. However, the superiority of these procedures over portacaval or mesocaval shunt has not yet been established.

In patients with severe liver failure, transplantation should be envisaged. In fulminant variants, the development of encephalopathy should indicate emergency transplantation (Powell-Jackson, Gut, 1986; 27:1101). In acute/subacute variants, reversibility of the signs of liver failure can generally be expected. In chronic variants, signs of severe liver failure justify inscription on the waiting list.

Thrombosed portal vein

When the portal vein is extensively thrombosed, neither portal–systemic shunting nor liver transplantation can be performed. One of the various repermeation procedures can be attempted. However, the experience with each of them is limited and a clear evaluation cannot be made.

Obstructed hepatic veins with obstructed inferior vena cava

Patent portal vein

In patients without severe liver failure, percutaneous angioplasty procedures should first be attempted when feasible.[6] Such procedures cannot be carried out in patients with long-length stenoses and in patients in whom no main hepatic vein drains into the inferior vena cava caudal to the obstruction. When percutaneous angioplasty is impossible, mesoatrial shunt, mesoinnominate shunt, or mesocaval shunt after reconstruction or bypass of the stenosed portion of inferior vena cava can be performed.

In patients with severe liver failure, occlusion limited to the suprahepatic portion of inferior vena cava does not preclude liver transplantation.

Thrombosed portal vein

The therapeutic choice is reduced in this situation. Percutaneous or surgical angioplasty, and dorsocranial resection with hepatoatrial anastomosis can be performed when obstruction of the suprahepatic portion of inferior vena cava is limited. Caval–caval bypass operation may be of benefit in some patients by allowing more efficient portal–caval circulation to develop.

References

1. Stuart KL and Bras G. Veno-occlusive disease of the liver. *Quarterly Journal of Medicine*, 1957; **26**: 291–315.
2. Parker RGF. Occlusion of the hepatic veins in man. *Medicine* (Baltimore), 1959; **38**: 369–402.
3. Hadengue A, Poliquin M, Vilgrain V, *et al.* The changing scene of hepatic vein thrombosis: recognition of asymptomatic cases. *Gastroenterology*, 1994; **106**: 1042–7.
4. Valla D, Casadevall N, Lacombe C, *et al.* Primary myeloproliferative disorders and hepatic vein thrombosis. A prospective study of erythroid colony formation *in vitro* in 20 patients with Budd-Chiari syndrome. *Annals of Internal Medicine*, 1985; **103**: 325–34.
5. Valla D, Dhumeaux D, Babany G, *et al.* Hepatic vein thrombosis in paroxysmal nocturnal hemoglobinuria. A spectrum from asymptomatic occlusion of hepatic venules to fatal Budd-Chiari syndrome. *Gastroenterology*, 1987; **93**: 569–75.
6. Dilawari JB, Bambery P, Chawla Y, *et al.* Hepatic outflow obstruction (Budd-Chiari syndrome). Experience with 177 patients and review of the literature. *Medicine*, 1994; **73**: 21–36.
7. Rector WG, Xu Y, Goldstein L, Peters RL, and Reynolds TB. Membranous obstruction of inferior vena cava in the United States. *Medicine*, 1985; **64**: 134–43.
8. Valla D and Benhamou JP. Drug-induced vascular and sinusoidal lesions of the liver. *Baillière's Clinical Gastroenterology*, 1988; **2**: 481–500.
9. McDonald GB, Hinds MS, Fisher LD, *et al.* Veno-occlusive disease of the liver and multiorgan failure after bone marrow transplantation: A cohort study of 355 patients. *Annals of Internal Medicine*, 1993; **118**: 255–67.
10. Ringe B, Lang H, Oldhafer KJ, *et al.* Which is the best surgery for Budd-Chiari syndrome: venous decompression or liver transplantation? A single-center experience with 50 patients. *Hepatology*, 1995; **21**: 1337–44.

21.4 Vascular malformations

Jean-Pierre Benhamou

Congenital hepatic artery aneurysm

In a small number of cases, hepatic artery aneurysm results from a vascular malformation. It can be isolated or associated with Rendu–Osler–Weber disease or Ehlers–Danlos syndrome (Nosher, AmJSurg, 1986; 152:326). The aneurysm is located on the common hepatic artery or, more rarely, on the intrahepatic branches of this artery. It can be diagnosed easily by ultrasonography and demonstrates an anechoic, well-circumscribed mass, which may or may not be pulsatile (Athey, AJR, 1986; 147:725). Calcifications of the wall of the aneurysm are common. CT scanning and MRI are useful for confirming the diagnosis (Zalcman, GastrRad,1987; 12: 203). Hepatic artery aneurysm can be complicated by rupture, occlusion, arterioportal fistula, compression of the common bile duct, and haemobilia.

Congenital portal vein aneurysm

Congenital portal vein aneurysm, in the absence of portal hypertension, is a very rare malformation that may be isolated or is less commonly associated with other vascular malformations (Dorval, GastrClinBiol, 1994; 18:520; Ito, JGastro, 1994; 29:776; Brock, Surgery, 1997; 121:105). The condition is usually asymptomatic. Diagnosis is based on information provided by ultrasonography, CT scanning, and MRI. Congenital portal vein aneurysm can be complicated by thrombosis and rupture (Thomas, Surgery, 1967; 61:550).

Congenital absence of the portal vein

Congenital absence of the portal vein has been described in 10 patients (Matsuoka, GastrRad, 1992; 17:31): venous blood flow from the intestines returns to the inferior vena cava either directly or through the left renal vein.

Ductus venosus: congenital intrahepatic portosystemic venous shunt

The ductus venosus, or Arantius duct, connects the umbilical vein and inferior vena cava during fetal life and closes after birth (Rudolph, Hepatol, 1983; 3:254). Patent ductus venosus in adults is usually asymptomatic. In a few patients, the condition results in fatty liver and in hepatic encephalopathy (Uchimo, Gastro, 1996; 110:1964).

Intrahepatic portosystemic venous shunts through pathways other than the ductus venosus have been reported (Kudo, AmJGastr, 1993; 88:723).

Rendu–Osler–Weber disease or hereditary haemorrhagic telangiectasia

Rendu–Osler–Weber disease or hereditary haemorrhagic telangiectasia is an autosomal dominant vascular dysplasia. Its prevalence ranges from 1/10 000 to 1/100 000.[1-3] Mutations have been shown in the genes encoding for a transforming-growth factor receptor, endoglin, which are located on chromosomes 9, 3, and 12. Hepatic lesions are present in 25 to 50 per cent of the patients. These lesions consist mainly of arteriovenous fistulas and strips of connective tissue containing dilated vessels. Hepatic arterial aneurysms and angiomas have been observed. Intrahepatic lithiasis has been described (Ball, ArchPathLabMed, 1990; 114:423). The hepatic lesions seem to be more severe in women than in men and are usually asymptomatic.[3] In a few patients, portal hypertension develops due to the hepatic fibrotic strips, and/or associated regenerative nodular hyperplasia (Wanless, ArchPathLabMed, 1986; 110:331), and/or increased hepatic blood flow through arteriovenous fistulas. Rarely, cholestasis (usually anicteric), heart failure (due to arteriovenous fistulas), cholangitis (due to intrahepatic lithiasis), and secondary biliary cirrhosis (Mendoza, JGastHepatol, 1995; 7:999) have been reported. Liver transplantation may be envisaged in patients with life-threatening liver lesions (Bauer, JHepatol, 1995; 22:586).

References

1. Guttmacher AE, Marchuk DA, and White RJ, Jr. Hereditary hemorrhagic telangiectasia. *New England Journal of Medicine*, 1995; **333**: 918–24.
2. Haitjema T, *et al.* Hereditary hemorrhagic telangiectasia (Osler–Weber–Rendu disease). *Archives of Internal Medicine*, 1996; **156**: 714–9.
3. Buscarini E *et al.* Hepatic vascular malformations in hereditary hemorrhagic telangiectasia: Doppler sonographic screening in a large family. *Journal of Hepatology*, 1997; **26**: 111–18.

22

Tumours of the liver and bile duct

22.1 Benign hepatic and biliary tumours

22.1.1 Liver haemangioma

Jean-Pierre Benhamou

Haemangioma is the most common benign tumour of the liver. At autopsy, the prevalence of liver haemangioma is 2 to 5 per cent. The male and female prevalence is the same, but lesions are larger in women than men.

Pathology

The size of liver haemangiomas varies from a few millimetres to between 10 and 15 cm (giant haemangioma). They may be single or multiple and may be located at the surface or inside the liver. On macroscopic examination, liver haemangiomas have a soft, spongy consistency and contain dark blood and occasionally thrombi. On microscopic examination, these haemangiomas are composed of large vascular channels lined by mature, flattened endothelial cells, enclosed in a loose fibroblastic stroma with various amounts of connective tissue.

In the majority of cases, liver haemangiomas are isolated. In a few cases, they are associated with focal nodular hyperplasia of the liver (Mathieu, Gastro, 1989; 97:154), extrahepatic haemangioma, or Rendu–Osler–Weber disease (Buscarini, JHepatol, 1997; 26:111)

Presentation and diagnosis

In most cases, liver haemangioma is asymptomatic and is recognized fortuitously on ultrasonography performed for symptoms that are either non-specific or unrelated to haemangioma. In a few patients, liver haemangioma is recognized because of abdominal pain which is often due to associated irritable colon.

Clinical examination is normal in most cases except in the few patients in whom a large haemangioma produces a palpable tumour. Liver tests are normal, except in patients in whom haemangioma is associated with an unrelated diffuse liver disease.

Diagnosis of liver haemangioma is based on ultrasonography: the lesion appears as a well-defined hyperechoic area. On CT scan without contrast, liver haemangioma appears as a hypodense area. On CT scan after intravenous injection of a contrast bolus, there is first an irregular enhancement in the periphery of the lesion and then, after several minutes, the area of enhancement increases towards the centre of the lesion (Itai, Radiol, 1980; 137:149). The most sensitive and specific procedure for diagnosing hepatic haemangioma is MRI: the lesion appears as a well-defined, very high intensity area on T_2 sequences (Itai, AJR, 1985; 145:1195). In a few patients, the haemangioma appears as a hypervascular area and/or is associated with an arterioportal shunt (Ando, JClinGastro, 1984; 6:365; Shimada, Cancer, 1994; 73:304). Arteriography or scanning with $^{99}Tc^m$-labelled human red cells are techniques no longer used for the diagnosis of haemangioma.

It is generally admitted that liver biopsy may be dangerous because of the risk of haemoperitoneum, but it has been performed in some patients without being complicated by intraperitoneal bleeding (Cronan, Radiol, 1988; 166:135). However, because liver haemangioma is soft, the tumour is pushed by the liver biopsy needle, often resulting in no fragment of the tumour being collected.

Natural history and treatment

Usually, liver haemangioma does not increase in size with time. However, it has been reported that during pregnancy or oestrogen therapy the tumour may grow (Reading, QJMed, 1988; 67:431). In a small number of patients, in the absence of pregnancy and oestrogen therapy, the tumour may increase in size (Trastek, AmJSurg, 1983; 145:49; Conter, AnnSurg; 1988, 207:115).

Spontaneous rupture of liver haemangioma is very rare (Aiura, JHepatBilPancrSurg, 1996; 3:308). Large haemangiomas can be complicated by thrombosis, with a triad of symptoms consisting of fever, right upper quadrant abdominal pain, and normal white cell count (Borman, Surg, 1987; 101:445; Pateron, DigDisSci, 1991; 36:524). Large haemangiomas can be complicated by thrombocytopenia, consumptive coagulopathy, and microangiopathic anaemia (Kasabach–Merritt syndrome) (Watzke, JClinGastro, 1989; 11:347). In the few cases with an arterioportal shunt, heart failure can develop. Large haemangiomas can result in abdominal discomfort.

In most patients, liver haemangioma needs no treatment (Farge, WorldJSurg, 1995; 19:19). Complicated liver haemangioma must be treated by surgical resection (Schwartz, AnnSurg, 1987; 205:456) or enucleation (Alper, ArchSurg, 1988; 113:660; Baer, AnnSurg, 1992; 216:673). Spontaneous rupture of liver haemangioma can be treated by transcatheter hepatic arterial embolization, which can be followed by surgical resection (Iamamoto, AmJGastr, 1991; 86:1645).

Hepatic haemangiomatosis

Hepatic haemangiomatosis—haemangioma involving the entire liver in a diffuse manner—is very rare. It can be isolated or associated with extrahepatic haemangioma or with Rendu–Osler–Weber disease. A case has been reported in a patient receiving metoclopramide (Furle, Gastro, 1990; 99:258). Heart failure (Vorse, AmJDisChild, 1983; 137:672), intraperitoneal bleeding (Painter, BrJSurg, 1961; 59:8), and Kasabach–Merritt syndrome are common.

22.1.2 Hepatobiliary and hepatocellular tumours

22.1.2.1 Benign biliary tumours

Miguel Bruguera

Bile duct adenoma

Bile duct adenoma, also termed cholangioadenoma and benign cholangioma in earlier literature, is a tumour-like lesion, small in size (1 to 22 mm in diameter), usually solitary, and subcapsular in location, found incidentally at laparotomy or autopsy in adults older than 40 years of age.[1]

Macroscopically, it is a firm, grey-white, well circumscribed, uncapsulated nodule. Histologically, bile duct adenomas are formed by a compact proliferation of narrow duct-like structures containing mucine, but no bile, with tubular or tortuous appearance. They are included in a fibrous stroma containing inflammatory cells, typically lymphocytes, which allows their differentiation from von Meyemburg complexes formed by dilated bile ducts containing bile and included in a mature connective stroma. Bile duct adenomas may be confounded macroscopically with metastatic carcinoma, but histologically they may be distinguished by the absence of nuclear hyperchromatism, mitotic activity, and vascular invasion. During their evolution the inflammatory component surrounding the bile ducts decreases and the fibrous stroma increases, giving the aspect of a subcapsular scar (Govindarajan, ArchPathLabMed, 1984; 108:922).

The pathogenesis of bile duct adenoma is obscure, but it has been suggested that it may be secondary to a focal, ichaemic, or traumatic injury (Nakanuma, PathInt, 1955; 45:703). Unlike von Meyemburg complexes, malignant transformation has not been documented.

Biliary papillomatosis

Biliary papillomatosis is an extremely uncommon condition, characterized by multiple polypoid masses growing in the intra- or extrahepatic biliary tract (Veloso, AmJGastr, 1983; 78:645). Less than 50 cases have been reported up to 1995, most being in middle-aged or elderly people, with a slightly higher incidence in men.

It presents clinically with recurrent bouts of obstructive jaundice, which may be complicated by bacterial cholangitis. Patients die within a few years of diagnosis as a result of recurrent cholangitis, liver failure, or malignant transformation.[2]

Histologically, this tumour is a papillary adenoma composed of mucus-secreting columnar epithelial cells supported by a delicate, branching, fibrovascular core (Padfield, Histopath, 1988; 13:687).

Hepatic lobectomy may be useful for the rare patients in whom biliary papilloma is restricted to one hepatic lobe (Gouma, BrJSurg, 1984; 71:72). When the common bile duct is affected, curettage and drainage may temporarily relieve bile obstruction. Hepatic transplantation should be considered in these patients (Rambaud, AmJGastr, 1989; 4:448).

Biliary hamartoma (microhamartoma, von Meyemburg complex)

Biliary hamartoma represents a developmental malformation consisting of an anomalous collection of small bile ducts surrounded by abundant fibrous stroma; it falls into the spectrum of fibropolycystic diseases of the liver resulting from ductal plate malformation (Summerfield, JHepatol, 1986; 2:141).

Occurrence

It is usually an incidental finding of laparotomy (0.6 per cent of cases; Thommesen, ActaPMIScand, 1978; 86:93), autopsy (0.7 per cent of cases; Chung, Cancer, 1970; 26:287), or needle liver biopsies.

Pathology

On gross examination, biliary hamartomas appear as small grey-white nodules (less than 0.5 cm in diameter). They may be single, but they are more often multiple. Microscopically, they consist of small, irregular, bile ducts, sometimes dilated with a branching configuration, lined by cuboidal or flattened epithelial cells that are embedded in a hyalinous fibrous stroma. Some bile ducts contain proteinaceous or bile-stained secretions. Microhamartomas develop at the border of hepatic parenchyma and the portal tracts.

Biliary hamartoma should be differentiated from well-differentiated cholangiocarcinoma and from bile duct adenoma.

Clinical features

Microhamartomas are asymptomatic. A slight elevation of γ-glutamyl transferase activity is seen in cases with multiple lesions (Saló, AmJGastr, 1992; 87:221). They may be found associated with other polycystic diseases of the liver, congenital hepatic fibrosis, Caroli's disease, or adult polycystic liver disease.

On ultrasound examination these lesions can mimic metastatic disease because they are seen as multiple anechoic, hypoechoic, or hyperechoic nodules, uniformly or non-uniformly distributed throughout the liver (Tan, JClinUltrasound, 1989; 17:667). On CT scans, biliary hamartomas are hypodense without evidence of contrast enhancement (Lev-Toaff, AJR, 1955; 165:309). On MRI they are slightly hypodense with respect to liver on T_1-weighted images and hyperintense on T_2-weighted images (Slone, AJR, 1993; 161:581). Guided biopsy of the liver with a large-gauge needle is needed whenever hamartomas must be distinguished from metastases, since imaging methods cannot differentiate these conditions. However, multiple bile-duct hamartomas should be suspected when multiple small-sized nodules are found on ultrasound examination in a patient with otherwise good health and with normal liver tests.

Four patients have been reported in whom malignant transformation from a microhamartoma to a cholangiocarcinoma was thought to occur (Honda, HumPath, 1986; 17:1287; Dekker, DigDisSci, 1989; 34:952; Burns, ArchPathLabMed, 1990; 114: 1287).

References

1. Allaire GS, Rabin L, Ishak KG, and Sesterhenn IA. Bile duct adenoma. A study of 152 cases. *American Journal of Surgical Pathology*, 1988; **12**: 708–15.

2. Colombari R and Tsui WMS. Biliary tumours of the liver. *Seminars in Liver Disease*, 1995; **15**: 402–13.

22.1.2.2 Benign hepatocellular tumours

Jean-François Fléjou, Yves Menu, and Jean-Pierre Benhamou

Hepatic benign tumours can develop from all types of cells present in the liver. The most common type is haemangioma, but many other rare benign mesenchymal tumours have been described.[1] Epithelial benign tumours developed from biliary cells include bile duct adenoma, biliary cystadenoma, and biliary papillomatosis. Only two benign tumours originate from hepatocytes, namely hepatocellular adenoma and focal nodular hyperplasia. Although both of these are rare tumours, they have received considerable interest for many years because of their association with contraceptive steroids—a link that has only been demonstrated clearly for hepatocellular adenoma.[2]

Hepatocellular adenoma
Definition

Hepatocellular adenoma is a benign neoplasm composed of hepatocytes occurring in a liver that is otherwise histologically normal or nearly normal.[3] The terms benign hepatoma and minimal deviation hepatoma should be discontinued.

Pathology

Hepatocellular adenoma is usually a solitary nodule, although multiple lesions are present in 10 to 20 per cent of patients. Cases of multiple adenomas have been reported, and the term 'adenomatosis' has been proposed when more than 10 tumours are present (Fléjou, Gastro, 1985; 89:1132). The relationship of this rare form of adenomatosis with either nodular regenerative hyperplasia or well-differentiated hepatocellular carcinoma is still debated. Adenomas are usually large (1 to 20 cm or more in diameter), soft, and sharply demarcated from the adjacent liver, although a capsule is present only in one-third of the cases. One-fifth of the tumours are pediculated. Hepatocellular adenoma always occurs within parenchyma that has a normal architecture. Cut sections show a tumour that may be lobulated, but that has neither the stellate scar nor the radiating fibrous septa seen in focal nodular hyperplasia (Fig. 1). The colour varies from yellow to brown, sometimes with green areas due to cholestasis. Haemorrhage is present in the majority of cases.[4]

On microscopy, hepatocellular adenomas are composed of liver cell plates of one or two cells in width, underlined by an abundant, well-defined, reticulin framework. There are no portal tracts. Sinusoidal dilatation or peliosis are frequently present, and areas of recent and old haemorrhage and, less often, infarction can be observed. When these lesions are marked, it can be difficult to recognize the adenoma, which then presents as a liver haematoma. The neoplastic cells are usually larger than hepatocytes in the non-neoplastic parenchyma. In most cases, these cells are uniform in

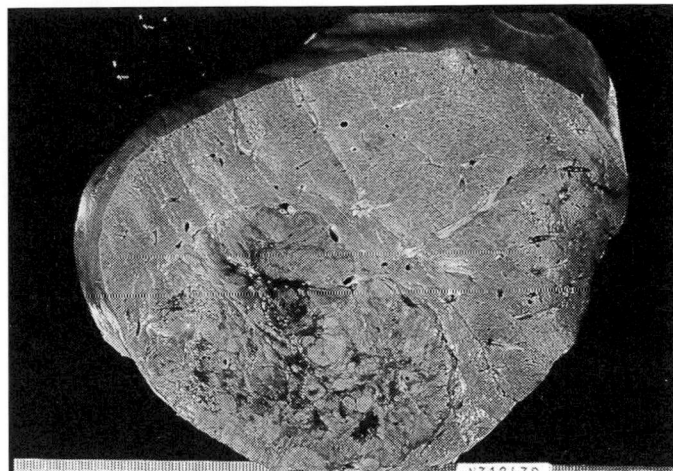

Fig. 1. Hepatocellular adenoma, presenting macroscopically as a large unencapsulated tumour with haemorrhage.

nuclear and cytoplasmic details with a normal nuclear–cytoplasmic ratio. Mitosis is not seen. Occasional atypia can be seen, especially in hepatocellular adenomas associated with anabolic steroids. The cytoplasm may be fatty, or may contain lipofuschin. Mallory bodies are very uncommon. In some cases, bile is present, and may be responsible for the pseudoglandular pattern around dilated canaliculi. Occasional tumours may contain haematopoietic cells in the sinusoids. Thin-walled vessels are scattered throughout the tumour. In rare cases, non-caseating granulomas are present in the tumour.

Pathogenesis

Although hepatocellular adenoma occurs less frequently than haemangioma and focal nodular hyperplasia, there has been a marked increase in its incidence since 1970.[2] Hepatocellular adenoma is very uncommon in children except when associated with some rare metabolic diseases. In adults there is a marked female predominance (9:1). Most of the cases occur in women aged 15 to 45 years, with an annual incidence of $1/10^6$ and a prevalence of 0.001 per cent when there is no oral contraception (Rooks, JAMA, 1979; 242:644). Two case–control studies have demonstrated the role of oral contraceptives as well as the influence of their duration of treatment and oestrogen content on the development of hepatocellular adenoma (Edmondson, NEJM, 1976; 294:470; Rooks, JAMA, 1979; 242:644). In these two studies, there was an increased risk of hepatocellular adenoma when an oral contraception was taken for more than 1 year, and after 5 years, the risk was increased by 20 to 100 times. However, it must be pointed out that there has been no recent study reassessing the risk of hepatocellular adenoma in women taking oral contraceptives with a much lower content of oestrogen. The risk is probably far less than with the drugs used initially. The precise mechanism by which oral contraceptives increase the risk of hepatocellular adenoma has not been established.[5] As it has been shown that oestrogen receptors are present within the tumour, oestrogens could probably act as a tumour-promoting agent.

The other circumstances that increase the risk of hepatocellular adenoma are much less common than oral contraception. They include anabolic and androgenic drugs (Carrasco, JHepatol, 1985; 1:573), type I glycogenesis (Kharsa, GastrClinBiol, 1990; 14:84), galactosaemia (Edmonds, Pediat, 1952; 10:40), and diabetes mellitus (Forster, NEJM, 1978; 299:239).

Clinical features

A large proportion of patients is asymptomatic, especially for small-sized tumours, and the lesion is discovered incidentally by ultrasonography or computed tomography (**CT**). In some cases, abdominal pain reveals the tumour; pain is due to intratumorous haemorrhage. The largest tumours can be revealed as abdominal masses. Some cases are revealed by a spontaneous acute haemoperitoneum due to tumour rupture. In 20 per cent of patients, abdominal palpation discloses a firm liver enlargement. In most cases, standard liver tests are normal, although γ-glutamyl transferase and alkaline phosphatase can be mildly increased, especially when the tumours are large. The level of α-fetoprotein is normal. Blood cell counts and the erythrocyte sedimentation rate are usually within the normal range. However, in rare cases with extensive tumour necrosis, hyperleucocytosis and increased erythrocyte sedimentation rate can be present.

Imaging

Imaging of hepatocellular adenoma is very disappointing. The lesion can be detected in most cases, but characterization is seldom possible, as the morphological appearance is very similar to that of nodular hepatocellular carcinoma (for figures, see Chapter 5.5).

Ultrasonography shows a nodular lesion, sometimes hypoechoic but more often hyperechoic, which is usually heterogeneous. Necrosis is possible. Tumour haemorrhage, with intratumorous haematoma or subcapsular haemorrhage is possible, and may even reveal the lesion in up to one-third of cases. Doppler studies may reveal tumoural vascularization, but this is not specific (Golli, Radiol, 1994; 190:741).

At CT, the lesion is hypodense on plain films and is enhanced after injection of contrast medium, although contrast uptake is less dramatic than in the case of focal nodular hyperplasia. Enhancement is heterogeneous in necrotic cases (Small, JComputAssistTomogr, 1994; 18:266). In some instances, no enhancement is seen, as the tumour can be hypovascular. In cases of haemorrhage, the lesion can be hyperdense on parts of plain films (due to blood clots) and does not enhance after injection. On late films, the tumour appearance is hypodense.

Magnetic resonance imaging (**MRI**) may show the appearance of a hyperintense tumour on T_1 images, which is related to tumour fatty infiltration, and/or peliosis (Chung, AJR, 1995; 165:303). This is different to the appearance of focal nodular hyperplasia, but similar to that of hepatocellular carcinoma.

In summary, imaging methods are able to detect the lesion, to give some suspicion for the diagnosis of hepatocellular adenoma, and to differentiate it from focal nodular hyperplasia, but not from hepatocellular carcinoma (Arrive, Radiol, 1994; 193:507).

Natural history and complications

In the rare cases without predisposing factors, the volume of the tumour remains unchanged or grows very slowly.[2] When hepatocellular adenoma is associated with oral contraceptives, the size of the tumour may decrease when oral contraceptives are withdrawn (Bühler, Gastro, 1982; 82:775; Edmonson, AnnIntMed, 1997; 86:180). However, this diminution occurs only in 20 per cent of cases and is usually a slow process. When oral contraception is maintained, or pregnancy occurs, the tumour often increases in size (Klastkin, Gastro, 1997; 73:386). The most serious complication is haemorrhage, either intratumorous or intraperitoneal. The risk of haemorrhage is high in large tumours and when oral contraceptives are not discontinued. Much rarer complications include biliary or venous compression by a large hepatocellular adenoma (Meirowitz, Gastro, 1990; 99:1502) and systemic AA amyloidosis induced by the tumour (Fievet, Gut, 1990; 31:361).

The magnitude of the risk of malignant transformation of hepatocellular adenoma into hepatocellular carcinoma is difficult to assess, although it is probably very low. Very few cases of hepatocellular adenoma either associated with, or transforming into, a hepatocellular carcinoma have been published (Tesluk, ArchPathLabMed, 1981; 105:296; Gyorffy, AnnIntMed, 1989; 110:489). Several case–control studies have demonstrated a moderately increased risk of hepatocellular carcinoma in women taking oral contraceptives (Forman, BMJ, 1986; 292:1357; Neuberger, BMJ, 1986; 292:1355; Palmer, AmJEpid, 1989; 130:878). However, it has not been demonstrated that in those cases the hepatocellular carcinoma was preceded by a stage of hepatocellular adenoma. The risk of malignancy is higher in hepatocellular adenoma associated with anabolic or androgenic steroids or complicating type I glycogenesis.

Treatment

Due to the risk of haemorrhage and the possibility of malignant transformation, hepatocellular adenomas have to be surgically resected whether they are symptomatic or not (Benhamou, GastrClinBiol, 1989; 13:277). Only in small-sized (less than 3 cm in diameter) asymptomatic tumours can surveillance be proposed, with surgery indicated if the size of the lesion does not decrease. In large tumours with a major surgical risk, a close ultrasonographic surveillance is also indicated, with surgery when the size of the tumour increases even after oral contraceptives are withdrawn. In such cases, arterial embolization may facilitate surgical resection (Derby, GastrClinBiol, 1991; 15:424). The use of oestrogen must be discouraged after surgery. A postoperative surveillance is necessary, with ultrasonographic examination every 2 years, to detect a recurrence or the development of a new tumour.

Focal nodular hyperplasia
Definition

Focal nodular hyperplasia is a nodule composed of normal hepatocytes occurring in a liver that is otherwise histologically normal or nearly normal. It is supplied by large arteries accompanied by a fibrous stroma containing biliary ductules. The stroma is usually prominent and forms a stellate 'scar'.[3]

This lesion has also been referred to as focal cirrhosis, hepatic pseudotumour, solitary hyperplastic nodule, hepatic hamartoma, mixed adenoma, and, unfortunately, adenoma and benign hepatoma. All these terms should be discontinued.

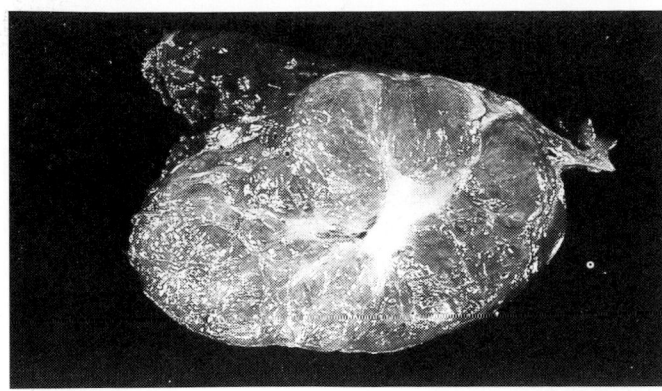

Fig. 2. Focal nodular hyperplasia, presenting macroscopically with a typical stellate central scar.

Pathology

Focal nodular hyperplasia is a solitary lesion in two-thirds of cases. A form of multiple focal nodular hyperplasia of the liver has been described, frequently associated with vascular malformations of various organs and neoplasms of the brain (Wanless, ModPathol, 1989; 2:456). The size of focal nodular hyperplasia is usually less than 5 cm in diameter, but varies from less than 1 cm to more than 20 cm. The lesions are firm and well circumscribed but not encapsulated. In some cases, they appear umbilicated on the surface of the liver. The cut surface is usually lighter than the surrounding liver, yellow to light brown in colour. In two-thirds of cases there is a typical central stellate scar prolonged with fibrous septa (Fig. 2), giving a nodular appearance on liver imaging techniques. This scar is easily recognized by these techniques, and cases lacking the typical radiological aspect correspond to those lacking a well-defined scar.[6] Areas of haemorrhage, necrosis, or infarction are not seen. Rare cases with calcification in the scar have been described, which can be difficult to distinguish preoperatively from other calcified tumours (Caseiro Alves, Radiol, 1996; 198:889).

On histology, a fibrous scar is usually present even when not evidenced macroscopically and this contains one or more large arteries with intimal and medial fibromuscular proliferation. The fibrous scar also contains an inflammatory cell infiltrate, predominantly lymphocytic, and biliary ductules at the interface with the liver cell plates.[2] These plates are one or two cells in width with normal hepatocytes. There is no normal lobular architecture, but a well-developed reticulin framework is always present on silver preparation.

Cases of atypical focal nodular hyperplasia have been described, which include cholestatic and telangiectatic forms. Cholestasis induces feathery degeneration, bile plugs, copper-associated protein, Mallory bodies, and some degree of nuclear pleomorphism (Butron Villa, Liver, 1984; 4:387). The telangiectatic type of focal nodular hyperplasia has multiple dilated blood spaces near the centre of the lesion, which may grossly resemble haemangioma or peliosis.[7] These telangiectatic lesions are frequent in the multiple focal nodular hyperplasia syndrome (Wanless, ModPathol, 1989; 2:456).

Pathogenesis

Focal nodular hyperplasia has variously been considered as a neoplasm, a hamartoma, or a reaction to focal injury. Although this latter hypothesis is now favoured by most authors, the demonstration that a majority of focal nodular hyperplasias are monoclonal may be considered as an argument for a true neoplastic origin (Gaffey, AmJPath, 1996; 148:1089). From the histological study of 51 cases, Wanless *et al.*[7] concluded that focal nodular hyperplasia is a hyperplastic response of the liver parenchyma to the presence of a pre-existing vascular malformation. The frequent coexistence of focal nodular hyperplasia with other vascular (haemangioma) (Mathieu, Gastro, 1989; 97:154) and neuroendocrine anomalies suggests that the malformations are developmental in origin. A role for oestrogens in the pathogenesis of focal nodular hyperplasia is suggested by the marked female predominance. However, most authors consider that oral contraceptive use does not increase the risk of focal nodular hyperplasia by itself, but that those lesions occurring in women on oral contraceptives may be larger and more symptomatic.

Clinical and biochemical features

Focal nodular hyperplasia is not as rare as hepatocellular adenoma. Its prevalence in the general population is estimated at 0.01 per cent. Most of the lesions are asymptomatic, and are discovered fortuitously on ultrasonography, CT scan, laparotomy for an irrelevant lesion, or even autopsy (Belghiti, BrJSurg, 1993; 80:380; Cherqui, Hepatol, 1995; 22:1674). When symptoms are present, they are similar to those observed in hepatocellular adenoma, except that haemoperitoneum secondary to rupture is very uncommon, if it even exists. Liver tests are normal except for γ-glutamyl transferase, which can be raised in rare cases.

Imaging

Different methods have merit for detection and characterization of focal nodular hyperplasia. Ultrasonography, CT, and MRI are the preferred methods, but scintigraphy and angiography have been claimed to be relevant (for figures, see Chapter 5.5).

Ultrasonography

At ultrasonography, focal nodular hyperplasia is mildly hyperechoic or, rarely, faintly hypoechoic (Shirkhoda, AbdomImag, 1994; 19:34). In rare instances, the contrast with the liver is high, but it would be very unusual for focal nodular hyperplasia to appear similar to a haemangioma. The lesion is homogeneous and the central scar is not seen, except in rare cases where there is a faint hypoechoic central area. The tumour can be lobulated and there is no capsule. The lesion is very similar to the normal liver and, therefore, it can be detected only when it is large, with distortion of the liver contour or vessels. It is very likely that many small nodules of focal nodular hyperplasia are overlooked as they do not differ from the liver parenchyma.

Recent work has stressed that Doppler ultrasonography and especially power Doppler could be capable of identifying central vascular activity and the wheel-like disposition of tumoural vessels (Golli, Radiol, 1993; 187:113). On pulsed Doppler, only the arterial signal is registered, although at the periphery of the lesion, the venous signal can be recorded. So far, it is not clear whether these findings are characteristic for focal nodular hyperplasia, and one should consider these records as suggestive for the diagnosis, but not precluding the need for other examinations.

Computed tomography

CT should be performed with the helical technique in order to examine the entire liver within the arterial phase and parenchymal phase after contrast medium injection. On plain films, the lesion is faintly hypodense or sometimes isodense. If the lesion is small in size, it should be stressed that the exact location of the tumour should be recorded by ultrasonography before CT is performed. In arterial phase slices, 20 to 40 s after intravenous injection of contrast medium, there is a dramatic uptake of contrast medium, with homogeneous distribution in the whole lesion, except the central scar which remains hypointense. In very rare instances, a central artery can be identified within the scar, and this would be the most characteristic sign for focal nodular hyperplasia. In the parenchymal phase, the contrast vanishes and the lesion returns to a faint hyperdensity; when delayed films are taken, 5 min or more after injection, the central scar can be identified as a hyperdense area, as the fibrous tissue shows a progressive contrast uptake. Despite the numerous abnormalities that can be seen on CT, MRI should be preferred as a characterization test.

Magnetic resonance imaging

MRI is the most recent imaging method to be utilized in the diagnosis of focal nodular hyperplasia and has been claimed to be the most specific.[6] On T_1-weighted images, the lesion is isointense or faintly hypointense. In some instances, the central scar can be seen as a darker (hypointense) area. On T_2-weighted images, the lesion is faintly hyperintense, sometimes markedly brighter than normal liver. The central scar is very intense, which is probably linked to the amount of water and bile within the central scar. The appearance of the scar is different from one patient to another. Sometimes it is a stellate thick area, but it can be a very thin linear image. The central scar is not visible in all cases, but it is necessary for MR characterization of the focal nodular hyperplasia. On dynamic T_1-weighted images, shortly after gadolinium chelate injection and during a single breath hold, the lesion has a similar appearance to that observed on CT—a strong early uptake of contrast medium, promptly released. The most significant feature is the uptake of contrast by the central scar on late slices (5 min or more). When all the signs are present, MRI allows a specific diagnosis for focal nodular hyperplasia, which precludes the need for other investigations or treatment, as long as the patient is not symptomatic. Specificity of MRI for the diagnosis has been reported to be 50 to 75 per cent. When the MR scan is not specific, additional examinations could be considered (Cherqui, Hepatol, 1995; 22: 1674).

Other examinations

Scintigraphy has been claimed to be specific for focal nodular hyperplasia in the case of colloid uptake by the tumour, due to Kupffer cells. In fact, uptake can also be observed in hepatocellular adenoma and scintigraphy should not remain a diagnostic test for focal nodular hyperplasia.

Angiography may show a wheel appearance of tumour arteries, but this is not absolutely specific either. Moreover, angiography is an invasive test, and it appears that power Doppler ultrasonography is able to provide the same image. Angiography is no longer performed as a routine evaluation for focal nodular hyperplasia,

although some surgeons would feel more secure when surgical resection of the liver is considered, for instance in large tumours or symptomatic lesions.

Biopsy is a useful tool and various methods are considered. Percutaneous biopsy is performed in most centres. It is an easy method, with a very low rate of complications, but the interpretation of the tissue core can be difficult as it can be very similar to the normal liver. It is very helpful for the pathologist to take a concomitant biopsy of the normal liver in order to compare the different areas in this same patient. Other authors favour surgical biopsy, arguing that a larger tissue core helps in the identification of the lesion, and that immediate surgical resection could be done if necessary. However, frozen sections can be very difficult to assess and diagnostic errors may occur in this situation.

All authors agree that when the imaging appearance of the lesion is typical for focal nodular hyperplasia on MRI, no other examination or treatment is necessary (Cherqui, Hepatol, 1995; 22: 1674).

Natural history and complications

Focal nodular hyperplasia is an entirely benign lesion. Ultrasonography and CT surveillance usually does not show any change in the size of the nodule. In rare cases, an increase in size has been reported during oral contraceptive use or pregnancy (Scott, JAMA, 1984; 251:1461). A case characterized by multiple tumours and recurrence after surgical resection has been published (Sadowski, Hepatol, 1995; 21:970). Haemorrhage does not occur, except in some cases with a questionable diagnosis (Stauffer, AnnIntMed, 1975; 83:301; Grangé, Gastro, 1987; 93:1409). Rare cases have been reported in association with hepatocellular adenoma, hepatocellular carcinoma, and fibrolamellar carcinoma (Saul, Cancer, 1987; 60: 3049), but no case of malignant transformation has been reported.

Treatment

As it is a benign condition and usually asymptomatic, focal nodular hyperplasia has to be managed conservatively. Such typical cases represent about two-thirds of those in recent series (Belghiti, BrJSurg, 1993; 80:380; Cherqui, Hepatol, 1995; 22:1674). Some authors consider that oral contraceptives must be discontinued and the lesion can be followed-up by serial ultrasonographic examinations. In cases of tumour enlargement or occurrence of symptoms, a surgical approach must be considered. In atypical cases at liver imaging, a diagnosis of hepatocellular adenoma or hepatocellular carcinoma cannot be ruled out, and the lesion must be surgically removed. A guided percutaneous biopsy can be useful, by demonstrating a typical histological lesion; however, if the tumour is malignant, there is a risk of dissemination. Some authors have proposed that, during surgery, a decision not to resect (if the lesion is histologically proven to be focal nodular hyperplasia) or to resect can be efficiently assisted by frozen-section diagnosis (Cherqui, 1995). This policy could be envisaged if surgical resection represents a risk (when the lesion is located in the vicinity of the hepatic veins).

References

1. Goodman ZD. Benign tumors of the liver. In Okuda K and Ishak KG, eds. *Neoplasms of the liver.* Tokyo: Springer-Verlag, 1987:105–25.
2. Ishak KG. Hepatic neoplasms associated with contraceptive and anabolic steroids. *Recent Results in Cancer Research*, 1979; **66**: 73–128.
3. International Working Party. Terminology of nodular hepatocellular lesions. *Hepatology*, 1995; **22**: 983–93.
4. Kerlin P, Davis GL, McGill DB, Weiland DH, Adson MA, and Sheedy II PF. Hepatic adenoma and focal nodular hyperplasia: clinical, pathologic, and radiologic features. *Gastroenterology*, 1983; **84**: 994–1002.
5. Porter LE, Van Thiel DH, and Eagon PK. Estrogens and progestin as tumor inducers. *Seminars in Liver Disease*, 1987; 7: 24–31.
6. Vilgrain V *et al.* Focal nodular hyperplasia of the liver: MR imaging and pathologic correlation in 37 patients. *Radiology*, 1992; **184**: 699–703.
7. Wanless IR, Mawdsley C, and Adams R. On the pathogenesis of focal nodular hyperplasia of the liver. *Hepatology*, 1985, **5**: 1194–200.

22.2.1 Primary liver cell carcinoma

Kunio Okuda and Hiroaki Okuda

Definition

Primary liver cell carcinoma is a malignant epithelial tumour arising from the parenchymal liver cell; hence its cells show histological features resembling those of hepatocytes. It is also called 'hepatocellular carcinoma' in order to distinguish it from other histological types of liver cancer. Of the several varieties of primary malignant neoplasm of the liver, hepatocellular carcinoma is by far the most common. Because of the frequent coexistence of cirrhosis of the liver, and difficulty in early diagnosis, the prognosis remains poor.

Introduction

The pathology and clinical features of hepatocellular carcinoma were well understood by the end of the last century. In 1901, Eggel analysed the pathological features of hepatocellular carcinoma in more than 200 autopsies described in the literature, and proposed a gross anatomical classification of hepatocellular carcinoma.[1] His classification was used widely until Japanese pathologists proposed a better one about 10 years later. Yamagiwa (VirchArch, 1911; 206: 437) characterized liver tumours histologically and distinguished between hepatocellular carcinoma and intrahepatic bile duct carcinoma, using the terms 'hepatom' and 'cholangiom' which were subsequently adopted throughout the world. The meaning of the word 'hepatoma', which was based on the origin of the tumour cells, was ambiguous and led to the use of the terms 'benign hepatoma' and 'malignant hepatoma'. For this reason, the International Association for the Study of the Liver recommended the terms 'hepatocellular carcinoma' and 'cholangiocellular carcinoma (cholangiocarcinoma)'.[2]

Berman's monograph *Primary Carcinoma of the Liver*, published in 1951, noted the peculiar epidemiology of hepatocellular carcinoma; it was far more common among South African black people than populations from other countries for which crude incidence rates were available in the literature. Berman deserves credit for his detailed clinical description of the disease. He worked in a dispensary attached to gold mines around Johannesburg, where many youths from Mozambique were employed; a large number of them suffered from liver cancer soon after their arrival (Fig. 1). He studied 75 patients and described the clinical features using a

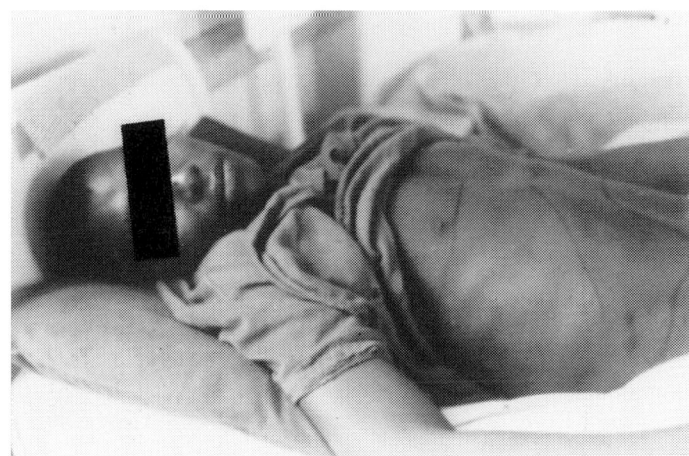

Fig. 1. A young Mozambican boy coming down with hepatocellular carcinoma while working in a gold mine near Johannesburg.

classification based on the major presenting symptoms (see below); he also documented the autopsy findings in 51 cases.[3] It was in the late 1970s that the author (KO) recognized clinical and histopathological differences between the Bantu patients described by Berman and patients seen in Japan. An expanding hepatocellular carcinoma, which acquires a fibrous capsule, is the predominant histopathological type in Japan (Okuda, Cancer, 1977; 40:1240), whereas in the United States of America an infiltrating (spreading) type is much more common, and coexistent cirrhosis is much less common and less advanced among the Bantu black population.[4] It was also realized recently that fibrolamellar hepatocellular carcinoma (Craig, Cancer, 1980; 46:372) is more frequent among Caucasians and extremely rare in the Far East.

The close association between hepatocellular carcinoma and cirrhosis had long been an enigma. The discovery that hepatitis B virus (**HBV**) caused chronic liver disease, and the subsequent demonstration of the role of HBV infection in hepatocarcinogenesis, have been important in our understanding of the aetiology. More recently, hepatitis C virus (**HCV**) was discovered; this virus is more frequently associated with hepatocellular carcinoma than HBV in certain countries. Before the recognition of the close relationship of HBV to hepatocellular carcinoma, experimental chemical carcinogenesis was the main tool for studying the mechanism of malignant transformation. The first experimental carcinoma was produced in 1915 by the same Yamagiwa (MittMedFakTokio, 1915; 15:295) who coined the term 'hepatoma'. He repeatedly painted coal tar on the ears of rabbits which eventually developed skin cancer. Experimental liver cancer was also produced by Japanese investigators 20 years later (Yoshida, TransJpnPathSoc, 1933; 23: 636). From studies using chemical carcinogens in animals, it has been established that carcinogenesis (in the liver and other tissues) involves a first step called 'initiation', and a subsequent process generally called 'promotion'. It is still unclear whether carcinogenetic processes triggered by a virus and a carcinogen differ, and if so, how they are different in molecular terms.

The liver is a deep-seated organ, difficult to access, and malignant cells easily spread within it because of its unique portal circulation, in which flow is often to and fro in cirrhosis. Thus, early detection is difficult and prognosis is very poor; patients with advanced hepatocellular carcinoma seldom live more than 2 months after diagnosis. The discovery of α-fetoprotein by Abelev in 1963 (Transpl, 1963; 1:174) was a major advance in diagnosis. However, early attempts in Africa to use it in mass screening for early detection failed (Masseyeff, CancerRes, 1973; 14:3). The advent of real-time ultrasonography changed the diagnostic approach completely, and the current strategy for early detection was established by Japanese gastroenterologists in the late 1970s. They began following patients with cirrhosis by measuring serum α-fetoprotein levels and using abdominal ultrasonography at regular intervals.[5] The same strategy was soon adopted in Taiwan and other countries where hepatocellular carcinoma is prevalent. As a result, increasing numbers of small hepatocellular carcinomas were detected. However, new problems have emerged because of the high sensitivity of ultrasonography; small benign lesions, such as haemangiomas and large regenerative nodules, are also picked up by ultrasonography. The former have to be identified and the latter assessed for the potential of transforming into hepatocellular carcinoma.

Although hepatic resection has been the treatment of choice, experience has shown that postoperative recurrence of hepatocellular carcinoma is frequent. Despite the development of various recent therapeutic modalities, the overall prognosis remains poor, and room for further improvement in therapy seems limited. Three lines of effort are required world-wide: to curtail virus infection with vaccination; to cure chronic liver disease; and to prevent malignant transformation of cirrhotic livers, perhaps by the use of chemopreventive agents.

Prevalence and epidemiology
Prevalence

Berman,[3] and later Higginson (CancerRes, 1963; 23:1624), called world attention to the extremely high incidence rate of hepatocellular carcinoma among the male black population in Mozambique. According to the figures of Higginson, and Munoz and Linsell,[6] the crude incidence among Mozambican males aged 25 to 34 years is over 500 times that among comparable white males in the United Kingdom and the United States. The relative importance of this particular type of cancer among all malignancies may be appreciated from the age-standardized cancer rates. Table 1 was taken from the paper of Munoz and Bosch[7] and Table 2 from the statistics compiled by the Ministry of Health and Welfare of Japan.[8] Although epidemiological data are not entirely accurate, because of infrequent histological diagnosis, the misdiagnosis of metastatic liver cancer for a primary cancer is probably uncommon in areas where the latter is prevalent. Furthermore, cholangiocarcinoma, the second most frequent primary cancer, is much less common in such areas; the current ratio of hepatocellular carcinoma

Table 1 Age-standardized cancer ratios of primary liver cancer*

Country (Registry)	Males (%)	Females (%)
Uganda, West Nile	21.0	9.2
Zambia, Kuska	15.9	17.0
Kenya, National Registry	8.8	4.7
Sudan	6.4	2.6
Tunisia	0.6	0.2
Malaysia, Kuala Lumpur		
Malaysians	13.8	0.4
Chinese	12.9	3.6
Indian	6.0	0
Iraq, Baghdad	2.1	1.1
Bangladesh	1.3	1.3
Sri Lanka, Colombo	0.8	0.5
Argentina, Santa F	1.3	1.3
Uruguay, Montevideo	0.2	0.2

Types of registry are not the same.
* Taken from Munoz and Bosch.[7]

to cholangiocarcinoma in Japan is 24.2:1.[9] Table 3 gives the incidence rates in selected areas of the world.

It is clear from these figures that hepatocellular carcinoma is a common and important malignant neoplasm in tropical and subtropical regions of the world, particularly among the sub-Saharan African black population and ethnic Chinese. Even in the same region, the incidence rate varies significantly with the ethnic group as well as the tribe. Chinese people carry a very high risk of developing hepatocellular carcinoma wherever they live. In Transvaal and Mozambique, the Shangan tribe has the highest incidence, followed by the Xhosa, Ndebele, Zulu, Sotho, Tswana, and Swazi, the differences being quite large (Robertson, BrJCanc, 1971; 25:30).

From these statistical data from various geographical locations, it seems that the greater the incidence rate, the younger the peak age. Among Mozambican males, the peak age is between 25 and 34 years (Fig. 2); the average age in Japan is 61.0 years in males and 64.9 years in females (Table 4), but both were 5 years younger 10 years earlier. The change in average age perhaps reflects increasing HCV-related hepatocellular carcinoma relative to HBV-related hepatocellular carcinoma. The latter occurs at younger ages (Shiratori, Hepatol 1995; 22:1027). Although the majority of liver cancers occurring below the age of 5 years are hepatoblastoma, a histologically distinct variety, there are occasional young cases of hepatocellular carcinoma, and conversely there are rare cases of hepatoblastoma in adults. In most types of primary liver cancer, the age-adjusted incidence rate increases continually with advancing age, but it is not established whether this rule applies to hepatocellular carcinoma (Beasley, Hepatol, 1982; 2:21S); it is possible that those who are destined to develop hepatocellular carcinoma will die out before certain ages, resulting in a decline in the age–incidence rate curve after a certain age is reached. It is also evident that the incidence is lower in females than in males, regardless of population, perhaps in part because chronic liver disease is less common in the former. Among the developed countries, Japan is the only country where hepatocellular carcinoma is very common.

Studies on trends over time are subject to large errors because of changing diagnostic capability and classification, as exemplified

Table 2 Relative frequency (percentage) of primary liver cancer among all malignancies in developed countries

	Males			Females		
Organ	Japan	USA	England and Wales	Japan	USA	England and Wales
Stomach	27.2	3.5	8.5	24.3	2.7	6.1
Liver	12.9 (3rd)	1.6 (16th)	0.9 (16th)	7.2 (9th)	1.2 (16th)	0.8 (18th)
Lung	18.8	34.0	35.4	10.1	17.2	14.8

Taken from the following sources: Japan, Vital Statistics 1985 Japan; USA, Vital Statistics of the United States, Vol II, Part A, 1984; England and Wales, Mortality Statistics Cause 1985.

Table 3 Age-adjusted incidence rates of liver cancer*

	Incidence rate (per 100 000/year)	
Country (Registry)	Males	Females
Mozambique, Lourenco Marques	112.9	30.8
Zimbabwe, Bulawayo	64.6	25.4
Cape		
Bantu	26.3	8.4
Coloured	1.5	0.7
White	1.2	0.6
Algeria	1.6	1.4
Argentina, Tandil	9.9	5.8
Brazil, Fortaleza	3.8	3.8
Jamaica	6.1	2.1
USA, San Francisco		
Chinese	19.1	3.6
Black	3.9	1.8
Japanese	3.0	0.4
White	2.9	1.1
Canada		
Eskimos	6.9	3.7
Alberta	1.3	0.5
Switzerland, Geneva	9.7	1.3
Spain, Zaragoza	6.9	5.1
France, Doubs	1.9	1.1
West Germany, Hamburg	3.6	1.6
Denmark	2.9	2.6
Yugoslavia, Slovenia	2.0	0.9
United Kingdom, Oxford	1.1	0.4
China, Shanghai	31.7	9.1
Singapore		
Chinese	32.2	7.1
Malay	17.1	3.1
Indian	14.0	4.8
Korea	13.8	3.2
Japan, Nagasaki	11.9	2.9
India, Bombay	2.7	1.0
Pakistan	0.7	0.8
New Zealand, Maori	8.7	2.5
Australia, South	1.3	0.4

* Taken from Munoz and Bosch. [7]

by the repeated revisions in the International Classification of Diseases, and because of registration artefacts. Autopsy records and registrations are much more accurate in diagnosis, but are also subject to biases due to the socioeconomic state of the society and changing interest on the part of physicians. Therefore, well-established regional cancer registry figures are perhaps more reliable. In the study of Saracci and Repetto (JNCI, 1980; 65:241), which may be subject to similar errors, primary liver cancer increased in 24 out of 37 countries among males, and in 26 of 37 countries among females. According to a more recent study,[6,10] populations with low incidence rates show an increasing trend in males; only 5 of 13 populations show the same trends in females. In sub-Saharan Africa, some studies suggest decreasing trends (Harington, BrJCanc, 1975; 31:665), but others dispute this (Kew,

Age (years)	HCC	CCC	HCC+CCC	Hepatoblastoma
0–4	4	0	0	7
5–0	1	0	0	0
10–14	2	0	0	1
15–19	6	0	0	0
20–24	14	0	0	0
25–29	9	1	0	0
30–34	35	1	0	0
35–39	110	5	2	0
40–44	277	11	1	0
45–49	536	21	5	0
50–54	1127	28	5	0
55–59	2426	37	3	0
60–64	2525	62	2	0
65–69	1863	61	5	0
70–74	1156	29	1	0
75–79	665	30	1	0
80–84	186	10	0	0
85–89	37	3	1	0
90+	9	1	1	0
Total	10 988 (36.6:1)	300	26	8
Mean age				
Men	61.0	61.8	56.7	3.8
Women	64.9	64.9	56.9	2.8

Table 4 Age distribution of patients with hepatocellular carcinoma (HCC), cholangiocarcinoma (CCC), and hepatoblastoma in Japan (1990 to 1991)[9]

HCC+CCC, combined type.

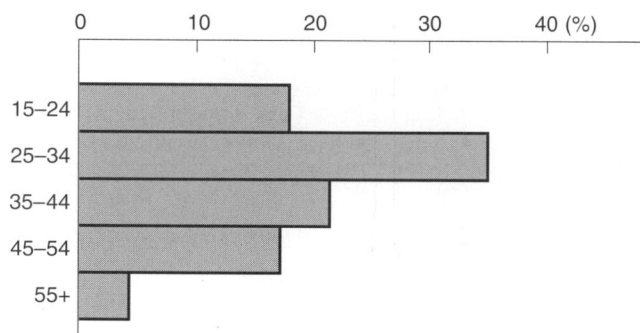

Fig. 2. Estimated ages of patients who were diagnosed as having hepatocellular carcinoma in Mozambique according to Harington (BrJCanc, 1975; 31:665). Note the age peak at 25 to 34 years (vertical axis, years).

personal communication). In the United States, autopsy records both in Boston and Los Angeles showed an increase up to 1973. Peters suggested that the sudden increase after 1964 could have been a sequel to yellow fever vaccination during the Second World War.[11] One remarkable trend is the sharp rise in incidence of hepatocellular carcinoma among Japanese men in recent years (Okuda, CancerRes, 1987; 47:4967). It has more than doubled in the past 15 years, whereas no such changes have been noted in other Asian countries such as Hong Kong and Singapore (Fig. 3); the suggestion was made that this new trend is due to increased chronic hepatitis C virus (HCV) disease in Japan.

The great majority of patients with hepatocellular carcinoma have underlying cirrhosis, most commonly non-alcoholic post-hepatitic cirrhosis. In a study from London, there was a very high

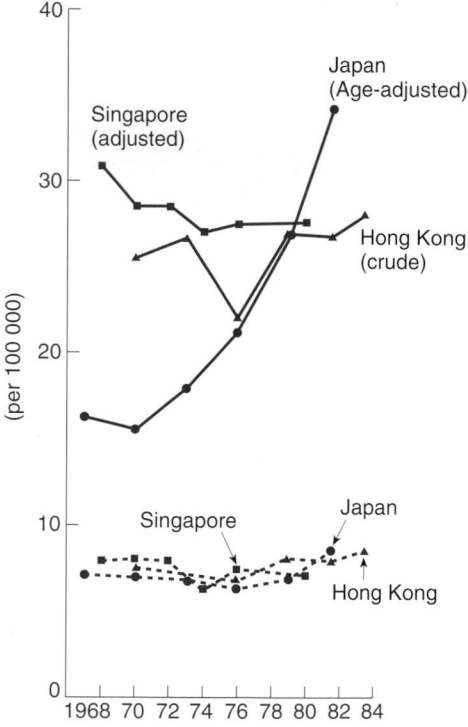

Fig. 3. The recent rise in incidence of hepatocellular carcinoma among Japanese men based on the Osaka Cancer Registry (adapted from Okuda, CancerRes, 1987; 47:4967). Solid line, males; interrupted line, females (ordinate, incidence rate).

incidence of hepatocellular carcinoma in patients with alcoholic cirrhosis who had abstained, and whose micronodular cirrhosis had become macronodular (Lee, Gut, 1966; 7:77). Table 5 gives the frequency of associated hepatocellular carcinoma in different morphological types of cirrhosis in Japan. Clearly, cirrhotic livers with relatively large nodules and medium to thin stromas, mainly representing HBV and HCV associated cirrhosis (Shimamatsu, JGastrHepatol, 1994; 9:624), are more commonly associated with hepatocellular carcinoma than livers with small nodules (alcoholic) and thick stromas.

It is generally thought that cirrhosis itself is preneoplastic because synthesis of DNA is accelerated in regenerative nodules, and hence rearrangements of DNA sequences in the chromosomes occur more frequently. The livers with micronodular cirrhosis typically seen in alcoholic patients have much less regenerative activity. With abstinence, there is a surge in regenerative activity, transforming small nodules to large ones. Alcoholic micronodular cirrhosis is much more common in Western countries compared with those of the Far East. This has been noted in a comparative study between northern Italy (Trieste) where micronodular cirrhosis predominates, and Japan where posthepatitic cirrhosis is far more common; hepatocellular carcinoma developed in livers with micronodular cirrhosis at a significantly later age, reflecting a low carcinogenic propensity (Fig. 4) (Tiribelli, Hepatol, 1989; 10:998). It is also the experience of hepatologists in Western countries that hepatocellular carcinoma very seldom emerges in patients with active alcoholic liver disease while they are imbibing.

There are areas where the association between cirrhosis and hepatocellular carcinoma is not very strong. In our study in which Los Angeles, Pretoria, and Japan were compared for gross pathology of hepatocellular carcinoma, less than 60 per cent of cases in South Africa had associated cirrhosis and the cirrhosis itself was very mild.[4] This raises the question of whether hepatocellular carcinoma arising in a cirrhotic liver is virus induced, while chemical carcinogens may play a more important role in a non-cirrhotic liver bearing hepatocellular carcinoma (Okuda, Gastro, 1989; 97:140). Aflatoxin is commonly detected in foods eaten by the black population in Mozambique, where hepatocellular carcinoma frequently arises in non-cirrhotic livers. According to van Renzburg et al. (BrJCanc, 1985; 51:713), there is a close correlation between hepatocellular carcinoma incidence and aflatoxin B_1 levels in food (Table 6). Within Mozambique, there is a ninefold difference in the incidence rate between the inland area and the coastal region where hepatocellular carcinoma is more prevalent; the method of storing staple foods varies between the two locations and contamination by

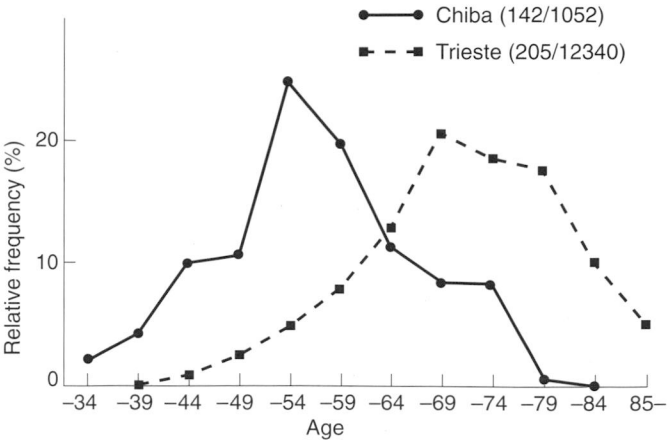

Fig. 4. Age distribution of autopsy cases of hepatocellular carcinoma—comparison of Chiba City, Japan and Trieste, Northern Italy. Note that the major type of underlying liver disease is posthepatitic cirrhosis in Chiba and alcoholic cirrhosis in Trieste. Hepatocellular carcinoma occurs in more advanced ages in alcoholic cirrhosis.

moulds is more common along the coast (Harington, BrJCanc, 1975; 31:665).

In Qidong County, north of Shanghai across the Yangtse River (People's Republic of China), the HBsAg carrier rate is about the same throughout the county, but the incidence rate of hepatocellular carcinoma along the coast is several-fold that in the interior. The hepatocellular carcinoma incidence is extremely high, even higher than that among Mozambican males, particularly in the farmers who cannot afford a well and drink stagnant ditch water; those drinking well water have a much lower incidence rate (Yu, JGastroHepatol, 1995; 10:674). The coastal area is newly claimed land, and to get drinkable water, it is necessary to dig a well 200 m deep. With an increase in the number of wells (built with government aid) the incidence has clearly declined. Contamination of ditch water with farmland pesticides was first thought to be responsible, but subsequent studies in which the pesticide content of cadaver fat tissue was quantified failed to confirm the suspicion. It now seems that microcystins elborated by green algae are aetiologically involved (Ueno, Carcinogenesis, 1996; 17:1317). In this region the epidemiological data are highly reliable; community doctors frequently visit all families within the brigade, and file with the central health office a complete list of patients and follow-up data. Our survey in

Table 5 Frequency of hepatocellular carcinoma in various types of cirrhosis in Japan			
	Thickness of stroma		
Size of nodules	Broad (>2 mm) (thick stromal)	Medium	Narrow (<1 mm) (thin stromal)
<3 mm (micronodular)	0/16 (0)	5/27 (19)	6/29 (21)
3–4 mm	1/11 (9)	10/40 (25)	54/93 (58)
>4 mm (macronodular)	4/12 (33)	10/20 (50)	39/59 (67)

Data by courtesy of Dr Toru Miyaji.
Percentages in parentheses.

Table 6 Relationship between crude hepatocellular carcinoma (HCC) rate and aflatoxin intake according to Van Rensburg et al. (BrJCanc, 1985; 51:713)

Location	HCC rate (100 000/year)	Aflatoxin B₁ intake (ng/kg per day)
Kenya, high altitude	1.2	3.5
Thailand, Songkhla	2.0	5.0
Swaziland, highveld	2.2	5.1
Kenya, low altitude	4.0	10.0
Transkei	6.9	16.5
Mozambique, Manhica-Magude	5.9	20.3
Swaziland, lowveld	9.2	43.1
Mozambique		
Massinga	5.0	38.6
Inharrime	9.0	86.9
Morrumbene	17.7	131.5
Zavala	14.0	183.7

Qidong showed slight contamination by aflatoxin of cereal fed to ducks.

Aetiological factors—hepatitis viruses

Hepatitis B virus infection

Several epidemiological observations suggest an important role of HBV infection in hepatocarcinogenesis. HBV seromarkers are more frequently positive in patients with hepatocellular carcinoma compared with controls, as shown in Table 7. In Taiwan, more than 90 per cent of hepatocellular carcinoma cases are positive for HB surface antigen. There is a crude parallelism between the rate of HBsAg carriage in a given population and that in patients with hepatocellular carcinoma in the same population: both are high among the sub-Saharan African black population and the Chinese, and are low in Northern Europe and the United States of America. The other global areas fall more or less in between. There is also a parallel relationship between the rate of HBsAg carriage and hepatocellular carcinoma prevalence on a global scale as shown in Fig. 5. There are several regions in which the same parallel does not hold, such as Sri Lanka and South American countries, but it is not clear how reliable the epidemiological data are in these areas. Another important clue to the role of HBV is the familial clustering of hepatocellular carcinoma patients and HBsAg carriers, first demonstrated in 1972 by Ohbayashi (Gastro, 1972; 62:618). In a national study of liver cancer in Japan (1968 to 1977), 48 out of 150 families in whom there was a patient with hepatocellular carcinoma had one or more family members who were carriers.[10] In Africa, more than 70 per cent of patients with hepatocellular carcinoma have HBsAg-positive mothers, in contrast to 14 per cent positivity in the

Table 7 HBsAg and anti-HCV positivity in patients with hepatocellular carcinoma (HCC) and controls in selected countries

Country	HBsAg positivity (%)		Anti-HCV positivity (%)	
	HCC	Controls	HCC	Controls
Finland[1]	4	0.2		
France[2]	9	2.2	58	0.68
Japan[3]	12	1.8	75	1.15
Spain[4]	17		75	0.5
USA[5]	18	0	29	0.7
Italy[6]	21		76	0.87
Greece[7]	46	7.3	39	0.6
South Africa[8]	61	11.3	29	0.7
Hong Kong[9]	82	18.0	7	0.64
China[10]	86	22.0	25	
Taiwan[11]	91	15–22	33	0.95

Data taken from:
[1] Rouslahti, ScaJGastr, 1973; 8:197.
[2] Nalpas, JHepatol, 1991; 12:70; Poynard, Hepatol, 1991; 13:896.
[3] Kiyosawa, Hepatol, 1990; 12:671; Shiratori, Hepatol, 1995; 22:1027.
[4] Bruix, Lancet, 1989; ii:1004; Ruiz, Hepatol, 1992; 16:637.
[5] Yu, JNCI, 1990; 82:1038; Austin, Cancer, 1985; 47:962.
[6] Simonetti, Lancet, 1989; ii:1338; Sirchia, Lancet, 1989; ii:797; Benvegnu, Cancer, 1994; 74:2442.
[7] Tricjopoulos, IntJCanc, 1987; 39:45; Kaklamani, JAMA, 1991; 265:1974.
[8] Kew, JNCI, 1979; 62:517; Kew, Lancet, 1990; i:873.
[9] Lam, CancerRes, 1982; 42:5246; Ieung, Cancer, 1992; 70:40.
[10] Yeh, CancerRes, 1985; 45:872; Ito, JGastroHepatol, 1993; 8:232.
[11] Sung, ProcNatlSciCouncRepubChina, 1981; 5:384; Chen, JInfDis, 1990; 162:817.

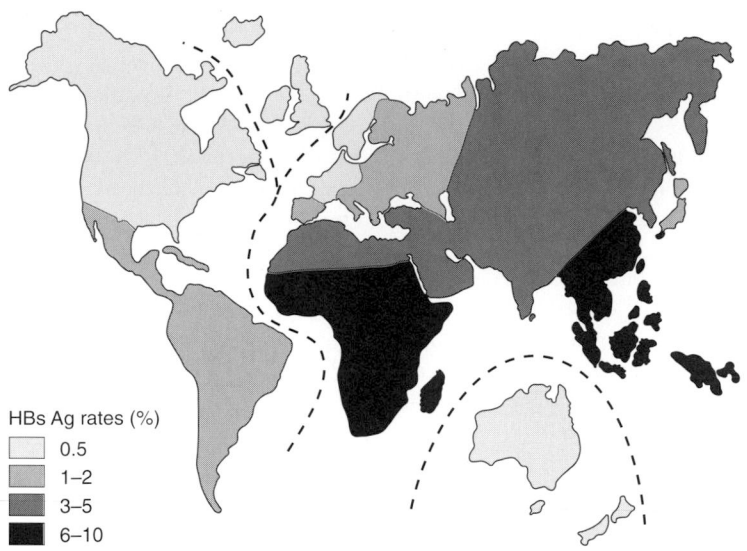

Fig. 5. World map based on HBsAg carrier rate. The populations in the black areas have carrier rates greater than 6 per cent and also have the highest incidence rates of hepatocellular carcinoma (Szmuness, ProgMedVirol, 1978; 24:40, reproduced with permission from S. Karger Verlag).

mothers of controls (Larouze, Lancet, 1976; ii:534). Two prospective studies, one by Beasley *et al.* in Taiwan (Lancet, 1981; ii: 1129) and the other by Sakuma *et al.* in Tokyo (Gastro, 1982; 83:114), have clearly demonstrated that hepatocellular carcinoma incidence is much higher among HBsAg carriers, with a relative risk of more than 100 compared with non-carriers. The age at which hepatocellular carcinoma is diagnosed is significantly lower in patients positive for HBsAg than negative for it (Okuda, Hepatogast, 1984; 31:64; Shiratori, Hepatol 1995; 22:1027).

Hepatitis C virus infection

In 1982, one of the authors (Okuda, Hepatol, 1982; 2:117) suggested a possible aetiological role of non-A, non-B virus in hepato-carcinogenesis based on a recent acute increase in HBV-unrelated hepatocellular carcinoma in Japan. Subsequent identification of hepatitis C virus (HCV) and development of antibody testing systems for its diagnosis prompted elucidation of a close association of HCV infection and hepatocellular carcinoma throughout the world. In countries like Italy, Japan, and Spain, more than 70 per cent of hepatocellular carcinoma cases were found to be associated with chronic hepatitis C and C cirrhosis. Even in countries where HBV infection is present in the majority of cases, if HBV-negative cases are studied, HCV antibody positivity is high (Chen, JInfDis, 1990; 162:817). Excluding areas such sub-Saharan Africa, where aflatoxin is presumed to be the leading aetiological factor, the world may be divided into areas where either HBV or HVC is the dominant factor. Table 7 lists some reported figures on HCV positivity in patients with hepatocellular carcinoma. HCV is not reverse transcribed to DNA, hence not integrated into the host genome. At the moment, the exact aetiological role this virus plays in hepatocarcinogenesis is unclear, but it is possible that an expressed protein has a function similar to that of an oncogene protein, or a capability of transactivating certain areas along the host chromosome. There has been a rapid change in the prevalence of HCV infection, which occurs mainly through the skin, and the age distribution of antibodies in Japan; anti-HCV positivity is very high in people over 50 years of age and practically nil in those below age 16, suggesting iatrogenic spread of HCV through vaccination in children in the past. There was a period after the Second World War in Japan when post-transfusion non-A, non-B hepatitis (mostly HCV) infection was rampant. The rate of HCV prevalence reflects the quality of medical practice in the past and present in each country.

Unlike HBV-associated cirrhosis, which is usually macronodular with a thin stroma and minimal inflammation, cirrhosis associated with HCV is mesonodular with a wider stroma and active inflammation at the time of hepatocellular carcinoma development (Shimamatsu, JGastHepatol, 1994; 9:624). Acute hepatitis C develops into chronic hepatitis in more than one-half of patients, frequently progressing into cirrhosis (Alter, NEJM, 1992; 327: 1899), and it takes about 30 years from acute HCV infection to the evolution of hepatocellular carcinoma (Kiyosawa, Hepatol, 1990; 12:671; Tong, NEJM, 1995; 332:463). Most studies in Japan showed a significantly more frequent development of hepatocellular carcinoma in patients with HCV-positive cirrhosis than in HBV-positive counterparts (Ikeda, Hepatol, 1993; 18:47). The frequency with which hepatocellular carcinoma occurs among patients with cirrhosis varies from 3 per cent per year in Italy (Colombo, NEJM, 1991; 325:675), 5.8 per cent in France (Paterson, JHepatol, 1994; 20:65), and up to 8 per cent in Japan (Kaneko, Intervirology, 1994; 20:65; Okuda, Cancer, 1995; 76:743).

The involvement of the newly found hepatitis G virus in hepato-carcinogenesis is unknown at the time of writing this revision, but it is perhaps less important than HBV and HCV (Kanda, JHepatol, 1997; 27:464); coinfection of HCV and HGV is rather common, however (Linnen, Science, 1996; 271:505).

Other aetiologically related factors
Chemical carcinogens

As already discussed, aflatoxin is one of the established hepato-carcinogenic mycotoxins. It is produced by *Aspergillus flavus* and *A.*

parasiticus. It was discovered in England when turkeys died after being fed contaminated peanut meal. Of various analogues, aflatoxin B₁ is the most toxic. Its role has been suggested from epidemiological studies, but direct evidence that it causes hepatocellular carcinoma in humans is lacking. There was a large outbreak of acute intoxication caused by aflatoxin or related toxins in northern India in 1974. About 1000 villagers came down with acute toxic liver injury with a 10 per cent mortality (Tandon, Gastro, 1977; 72:488). These people have since been followed, but none has developed hepatocellular carcinoma as yet. Aflatoxin caused hepatocellular carcinoma in all animals tested, but chronic exposure was required, and the Indian incidence does not necessarily contradict its carcinogenic property in humans. Reports abound that a point mutation occurs at codon 249 of p53 in patients with hepatocellular carcinoma in aflatoxin areas (Breszac, Nature, 1991; 350:429; Hsu, Nature, 1991; 350:427), but it is also refuted (Oda, CancerRes, 1992; 52: 6358).

Other chemicals known to cause hepatocellular carcinoma in animals are mycotoxins, such as luteoskyrin, cyclochlorotine, and sterigmatocystin; plant carcinogens, such as pyrrolizidine alkaloids, cycasin, and safrole; and synthetic carcinogens, including azo dyes, aromatic amines, nitrosamines, nitrosamides, chlorinated hydrocarbons, and organochlorine pesticides. However, at the time of writing, their contribution to human hepatocarcinogenesis is not known.

Oral contraceptives

The role of contraceptives in hepatocarcinogenesis in women is not altogether clear. It is established that both hepatic adenoma and focal nodular hyperplasia are associated with the use of contraceptives, but whether the hepatocellular carcinoma which develops in women using contraceptives is the same as that seen in non-users is disputed. Goodman and Ishak (Hepatol, 1982; 2:440) studied 128 cases of hepatocellular carcinoma in women; 48 were under age 40 and 12 (27 per cent) had used contraceptives. However, 62 per cent of the hepatocellular carcinoma associated with contraceptives, and 58 per cent of that in women under age 40 not using contraceptives, was found histologically to be fibrolamellar carcinoma, a relatively benign lesion. They concluded that the apparent association of hepatocellular carcinoma with contraceptives is coincidental. Attempts to produce hepatocellular carcinoma in animals with the same steroids have mostly failed.

Androgen-anabolic steroids

In 1971, Bernstein *et al.* (NEJM, 1971; 284:1135) described a male patient with Fanconi anaemia who had been on a C17-alkylated testosterone derivative and developed hepatocellular carcinoma. Several similar cases have since been documented. The tumours in such cases are androgenic steroid dependent.

Alcohol

There is no clear experimental evidence that ethanol is carcinogenic, but there are a number of reports suggesting its indirect promotive effects. A rare case of hepatocellular carcinoma in an alcoholic man which regressed with abstinence has been described (Gottfried, Hepatol, 1982; 2:770). Ohnishi *et al.* (Cancer, 1982; 49:672) studied 158 patients with cirrhosis and 79 with hepatocellular carcinoma,

and found that the mean age of HBsAg-positive patients with hepatocellular carcinoma with a drinking habit was 48.9 years, 9 years younger than the mean age of those without a drinking habit. The reason why habitual drinking apparently hastens hepatocarcinogenesis is not clear, but it could be due to early development of cirrhosis, a preneoplastic state, or increased biotransformation of carcinogens by the mixed-function oxidase and microsomal ethanol-oxidizing systems activated by ethanol intake.

Thorotrast (ThO₂)

This is the best-documented hepatocarcinogen in man; it emits α-radiation with a very slow decay (half-life 1.4×10^{10} years). It was used intravenously as an angiographic agent from 1930 to 1945, particularly in soldiers in whom vascular injury was suspected. It is deposited in the reticuloendothelial system in the liver, spleen, and bone marrow. Due to α-ray bombardment, the liver undergoes fibrosis; the main late effect of thorotrast is malignant transformation of the liver.[12] Many patients have died from hepatic malignancies in Portugal, Germany, and Japan. In 1972, Smoron and Battifora (Cancer, 1972; 10:1252) collated, from the literature, 41 cases of sarcoma, 42 cases of cholangiocarcinoma, and 24 cases of hepatocellular carcinoma due to thorotrast. A governmental committee in Japan followed those who received thorotrast angiography during the Second World War. The diagnosis of hepatic thorotrastosis is easy from a plain abdominal film. Initially, there were 200 such ex-soldiers throughout the country. Within 10 years, 116 had died; autopsy was performed on 47, and 33 of them had hepatic malignancies (13 were hepatocellular carcinoma, 14 cholangiocarcinoma, and 6 were angiosarcoma).

Smoking

In 1966, Hammond (NatlCancerInstMonogr, 1966; 19:127) reported a higher mortality from cancers of the liver and biliary tract among smokers than among non-smokers. In another study, mortality among habitual smokers was more than twice that among non-smokers, and the risk went up when smoking was combined with drinking; the effect of the former was stronger than the latter.[13] Trichopoulos *et al.* (JNCI, 1980; 65:111) studied Greek patients with hepatocellular carcinoma and demonstrated a highly significant association between smoking and hepatocellular carcinoma in patients negative for HBsAg; the risk ratio was 8.4 among those who smoked more than 30 cigarettes a day.

Parasites

The parasites implicated in hepatocarcinogenesis include *Echinococcus* sp., *Schistosoma japonicum*, *Schistosoma mansoni*, and *Clonorchis sinensis*, but evidence for aetiological association of these parasites with hepatocellular carcinoma is not strong.

α₁-Antitrypsin deficiency (see Chapter 20.3)

Deficiency of α₁-antitrypsin occurs in subjects homozygous for the *Z* allele. Severe deficiency occurs in 0.1 to 0.2 per cent of the general Caucasian population with intermediate levels in approximately 5 per cent. The *ZZ* or *MZ* phenotype is frequently associated with hepatocellular carcinoma. The tumour cells frequently contain α₁-antitrypsin in a globular pattern. The α₁-antitrypsin globules were found in 7 of 78 cases of primary liver cancer in the series of Berg and Erickson (NEJM, 1972; 287:1264) and in 5 of 21 in the series of Palmer and Wolfe (ArchPathLabMed, 1976; 100:232).

Disease associated with hepatocellular carcinoma

Any liver disease in which liver cell regeneration occurs seems to predispose to hepatocarcinogenesis. Haemochromatosis is long known for its frequent association with hepatocellular carcinoma, the reported rate ranging from 8.1 (Berk, AmJMedSci, 1941; 202: 780) to 18.9 per cent (Warren, AmJPath, 1951; 27:573). It may develop at any stage of the disease after cirrhotic changes have developed. In the past, it was thought that primary biliary cirrhosis would not be complicated by hepatocellular carcinoma, but several recent reports suggest that it too is associated with hepatocellular carcinoma (Krasner, Gut, 1979; 20:255); however, the incidence is still low, perhaps due to female predominance and low regenerative activities in the liver. Membranous Budd–Chiari syndrome, in which the inferior vena cava is occluded at the level of the diaphragm, is rare in Western countries, but is more common in India and Japan, and very common in the South African black population. The hepatic changes are those of congestion which will result in congestive cirrhosis. This condition is frequently complicated by hepatocellular carcinoma. In Simson's series of 101 cases in Pretoria, South Africa, 47.5 per cent had complicating hepatocellular carcinoma (Gastro, 1982; 82:171). In a Japanese survey, 29 out of 71 cases (41 per cent) had developed hepatocellular carcinoma (Nakamura, Angiol, 1968; 19:479). The reason for the high rate of association is not clear, because the regenerative activity in the liver is generally thought to be low in chronic congestion. A more recent national study in Japan showed a hepatocellular carcinoma incidence of 6.4 per cent in a 15-year period (Okuda, JHepatol, 1995; 22:1). Frequent association of porphyria cutanea tarda and hepatocellular carcinoma has been reported in European countries along the Mediterranean Sea (Salata, JHepatol, 1985; 1:477), but it may be due to HCV infection in such patients (Hepatol, 1992; 16:956).

Pathogenesis and pathophysiology
Mechanism of carcinogenesis

The mechanism for hepatocarcinogenesis, which involves a number of molecular or genetic alterations, is no better understood than that for other types of cancer. Attempts to identify a particular oncogene, which is activated or inactivated in the hepatocytes in the process of malignant transformation, have not yet yielded consistent results, and more information on the role of oncogenes and suppressor oncogenes and their expression is needed. The non-cancerous area of the liver bearing hepatocellular carcinoma in an HBsAg-positive patient often contains stainable HBsAg in the cytoplasm of the hepatocyte (Fig. 6), and cell lines derived from human hepatocellular carcinoma such as the Alexander cell line (MacNab, BrJ-Canc, 1976; 34:509) often shed HBsAg into the culture medium. With molecular biological techniques it has been repeatedly demonstrated that the chromosomal DNA of hepatocellular carcinoma cells frequently contains integrated HBV DNA (Fig. 7). It is now understood that HBsAg seen in the cytoplasm is a product of

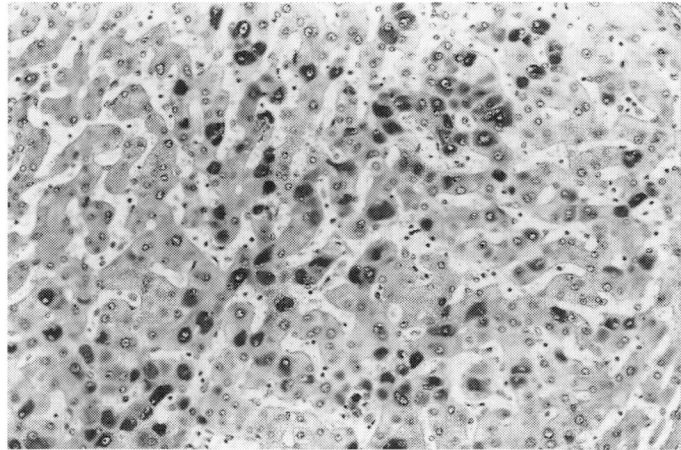

Fig. 6. Cytoplasmic inclusions of stainable HBsAg in hepatocytes in the non-cancerous parenchyma of a liver bearing hepatocellular carcinoma. The patient is an HBsAg carrier.

integrated *S*-gene, a part of the HBV genome. It is also known that enhancer sequences are present in the HBV genome and that integration of HBV DNA occurs at random sites. The *X*-gene of the HBV genome is suspected of its role in carcinogenesis through its transactivating potential, but more proof is still needed. Claims have been made that even patients with alcoholic cirrhosis, with no seromarkers of HBV, have HBV DNA integration in hepatocellular carcinoma cells (Brechot, Hepatol, 1982; 2:22S). There are no consistent chromosomal changes in human hepatocellular carcinoma tissue, loss of allelic heterozygocity being demonstrated in various chromosomes (Okuda, Hepatol, 1992; 15:948). A number of transgenic mouse systems have been developed for the study of the mechanism of HBV-induced carcinogenesis (Chisari, Cell, 1989; 59: 1145; Koike, Hepatol, 1994; 18:810), but as yet they have not provided a clear-cut understanding.

A number of animal hepatitis viruses have been identified recently, and they are collectively called **HEPADNA** viruses (Summers, Hepatol, 1981; 1:179). These viruses are similar to human hepatitis virus in many aspects. The HEPADNA viruses indigenous to the woodchuck, Pekin duck, and ground squirrel have been studied extensively. About one-third of woodchucks with woodchuck hepatitis virus infection develop hepatocellular carcinoma, beginning in the first year while the histological changes in the liver are still those of acute hepatitis (Popper, Hepatol, 1982; 2: 1S). The oncogenicity of duck B hepatitis virus is less strong. In our study, Pekin ducks that were made chronic carriers of virus, by inoculation immediately after hatching, spontaneously developed hepatocellular carcinoma after a lapse of a couple of years in a clean laboratory cage. In Qidong County north of Shanghai, the major cause of natural deaths among domestic ducks older than 5 years is hepatocellular carcinoma. In this region, human hepatocellular carcinoma is prevalent as discussed above and duck hepatocellular carcinoma is also very common. More than one-half of the domestic ducks in this region are carriers of duck B hepatitis (Omata, Gastro, 1983; 85:260), and we have been able to demonstrate integration of duck B hepatitis virus DNA in the chromosomal DNA of hepatocellular carcinoma cells (Yokosuka, PNAS, 1985; 82:6180).

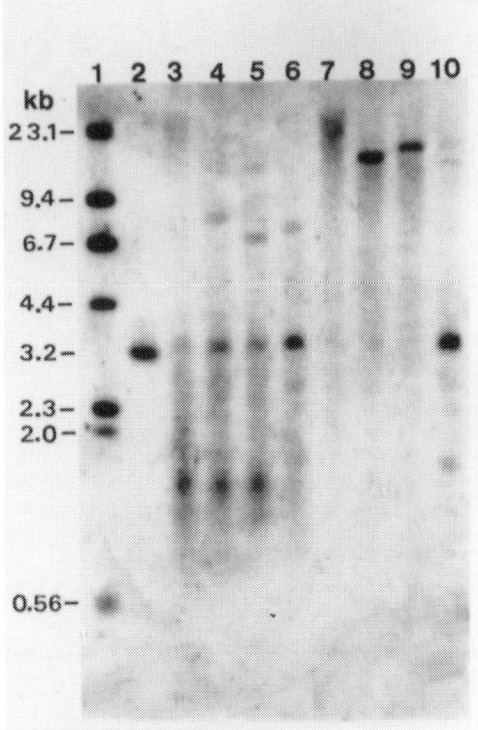

Fig. 7. Southern blot of DNA extracts from cancerous and non-cancerous portions of the liver from an HBsAg-positive patient. Lanes 3 to 6, non-cancer tissue; lane 3, undigested; lanes 4 to 6, digested with endonucleases; lanes 7 to 10, cancer tissue: lane 7 undigested, lanes 8 to 10 digested. Stains above 3.2 kb in size are DNA containing integrated HBV DNA. Cancer and non-cancer tissues have HBV DNA integrated at different sites (reproduced from Imazeki, Cancer, 1986; 58:1055 with permission from JB Lippincott, publishers).

Pathology

Hepatocellular carcinoma by definition is a malignant tumour composed of cells resembling hepatocytes. The vascular anatomy is characteristic in that typical hepatocellular carcinoma is highly arterialized, and the cancer tissue is solely supplied by arterial blood for growth. This cancer has a propensity to grow into the portal and hepatic vein systems, and occasionally into the biliary system. By contrast, intravascular invasion is very uncommon in cholangiocarcinoma. The liver in which hepatocellular carcinoma has developed is usually cirrhotic and intrahepatic spread occurs readily because blood flow in the portal branches within the liver changes direction under various conditions, and cancer cells in the portal branches may float back towards the hilum and then go into other branches, even from the right lobe to the left. Similarly, cancer cells frequently go into the hepatic vein and form metastatic lesions in the lung.

There is a general trend for a hepatocellular carcinoma arising in a highly cirrhotic liver to be well differentiated, whereas one arising in a non-cirrhotic liver is poorly differentiated (Okuda, Cancer, 1982; 49:450). Steiner's observations in Africa (Cancer, 1960; 13:1085) that poorly differentiated hepatocellular carcinoma is more frequent and cirrhosis less frequent among the black population, compared with the Cape coloured and white populations, fit with such a trend.

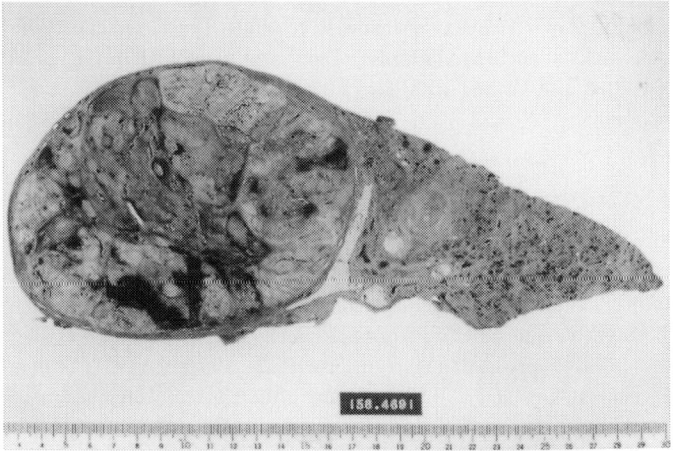

Fig. 8. An encapsulated hepatocellular carcinoma of an expanding growth type. The large main mass occupying the right lobe consists of several tumours of differing textures and colours. Note also fibrous septation at the boundaries between differing tumour tissues.

Gross pathology

The liver bearing hepatocellular carcinoma is often cirrhotic, and the surface nodular with irregular bosselations due to hepatocellular carcinoma, depending upon the growth type. The tumour may or may not be exposed directly on the surface. Adhesion of the liver to the neighbouring tissues is uncommon and so is direct invasion into them, except for the diaphragm. Rarely, the tumour grows mainly outside the liver in a pedunculated form; it may be a metastatic hepatocellular carcinoma fused with the liver. The cancer tissue is soft, whitish or brown in colour, with a yellow to green tinge when hepatocellular carcinoma cells are producing bilirubin (this is called 'green hepatoma'). The yellow colour turns green in formalin. The cancer tissue is not necessarily uniform in the same liver and various tumour nodules may have differing colours and textures. If the mass is large and growing in an expanding fashion, there are several different textures within the single mass (Fig. 8), suggesting changes in phenotypic expression or evolution of new cancer cell clones. Analysis of various mass lesions within the same liver with the Southern blot technique may show the same or differing integration patterns for HBV DNA, and there is no consistent trend—some may be intrahepatic metastases and others may be newly evolved tumours. If there is a more fibrous stroma, the tumour is whitish and firm. Hepatocellular carcinoma and cholangiocarcinoma are grossly distinguishable, because the former is soft and brownish compared with the whitish and firmer appearance of the latter except when there is a whitish sclerosing or fibrosing hepatocellular carcinoma.

Several gross anatomical classifications were proposed in the past, such as that by Eggel,[1] but these classifications were based on advanced hepatocellular carcinoma and are no longer applicable to the small tumours currently diagnosed and resected. In the 1970s, Nakashima *et al.*[14] and Peters[11] proposed new classifications, which were subsequently refined: in the Okuda–Peters–Simson classification,[4] hepatocellular carcinomas are grossly divided into the expanding, spreading (infiltrating), multifocal, and indeterminate types; and in the Nakashima–Kojiro classification,[15] they are divided into the expansive, infiltrative, mixed infiltrative and expansive, diffuse, and special types; special types include small hepatocellular carcinoma (less than 2 cm) and pedunculated hepatocellular carcinoma. The classification should not vary with the size, but should consider the mode of growth, its boundary with the parenchyma, and the number of masses.

Expanding type

This type has a discrete boundary with the non-cancerous portion and the mass grows in an expanding manner, distorting the surrounding parenchyma and frequently forming a fibrous capsule. Large vessels are displaced curvilinearly and come to lie on the surface of the capsule. It starts as a single mass, but during its growth secondary tumours form in its immediate vicinity, in continuity with the primary tumour, or in distant areas. At autopsy, the primary expanding lesion is often identifiable among many secondary lesions. The mechanism for acquisition of the capsule has been disputed. Some believe that liver cells drop out by the pressure from the growing mass, leaving behind reticulin fibres which condense and become collagenized. We suspect that procollagen is elaborated where tumour cells meet a different type of cell; this is based on the observation that within the same mass one often sees the formation of fibrous septa between secondary tumours of differing textures (different clones), as illustrated in Fig. 8. Furthermore, an expanding mass originating immediately beneath the liver surface also acquires a thick capsule on the protruding surface where there were no hepatocytes to drop out. A recent study in France based on resected hepatocellular carcinoma also indicated that encapsulated hepatocellular carcinoma is common in Europe (Kemeney, Hepatol, 1989; 9:253).

Spreading type (Fig. 9)

This type of hepatocellular carcinoma is less well differentiated and tumour nodules of irregular size interdigitate with the parenchyma in such a fashion that, unlike the encapsulated hepatocellular carcinoma, visible vessels come to lie in the tumour mass rather than being displaced. Such a relationship between the mass and blood vessels can be discerned by coeliac arteriography (Okuda, Radiol, 1977; 123:21).

Multifocal type

In this type, several tumours of similar sizes are seen at multiple sites and the primary-to-secondary relationship is not clear (Fig. 10). If there are numerous small-sized tumours scattered throughout the liver, it is called the 'diffuse type' (Fig. 11). This type of hepatocellular carcinoma seldom occurs in non-cirrhotic livers; since the definition is not strict, some pathologists classify multifocal hepatocellular carcinoma with many small lesions as 'diffuse'. Thus, the reported relative frequency of this type varies from zero (Schupbach, ArchIntMed, 1952; 89:436; MacDonald, ArchIntMed, 1957; 99:532) to 15 per cent (Liu, ChinMedJ, 1953; 71:183). In most diffuse-type hepatocellular carcinoma, there are portal tumour thrombi, and intraportal spread occurring within a short period of time is the likely cause of diffuse spread. The clinical course of the patient with this type of hepatocellular carcinoma is rapidly downhill (Okuda, Liver, 1981; 1:280).

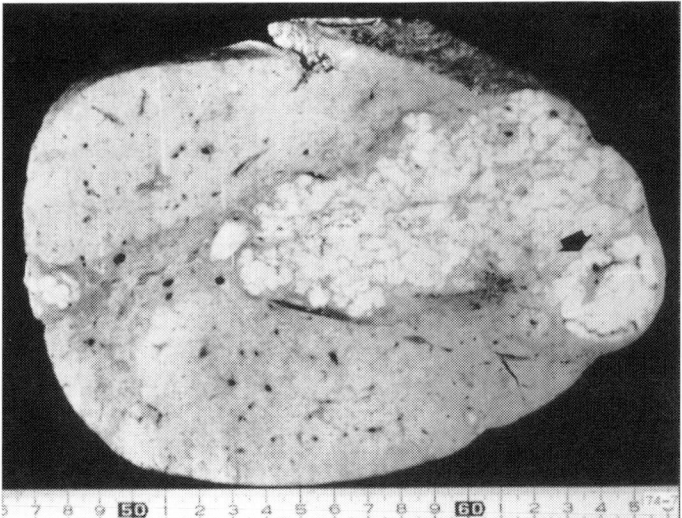

Fig. 9. Tumour growing in an infiltrating fashion (spreading type). A small, partially encapsulated, primary lesion is recognizable (arrow).

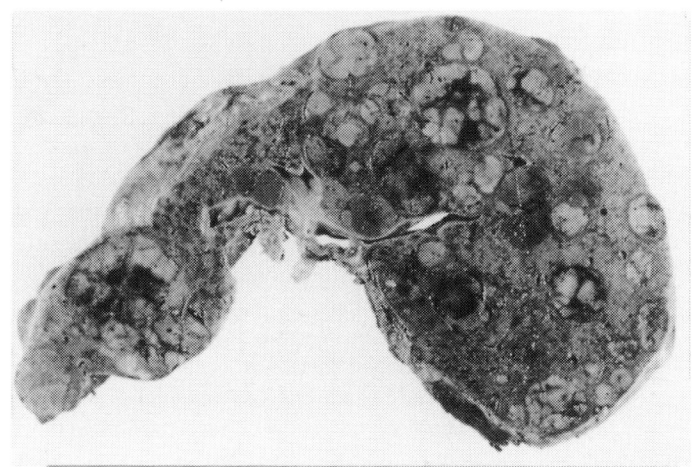

Fig. 10. Multifocal type of hepatocellular carcinoma. A number of discrete masses of expanding growth can be seen. Some are whitish; others are dark, perhaps producing bilirubin.

Small (minute)

Hepatocellular carcinomas classified as small or early are not synonymous in the strict sense of word, because if a cancer grows very slowly, even a small mass at detection is not early, and vice versa. Before the advent of real-time ultrasonography, detection of very small hepatocellular carcinoma was not possible and an arbitrary size for being called 'minute' was 4.5 cm (Okuda, Gastro, 1977; 73: 109); the current definition set by the Japan Liver Cancer Study Group is a single hepatocellular carcinoma smaller than 2 cm. Malignant transformation occurs within adenomatous hyperplastic nodules in posthepatitic cirrhosis when they are smaller than 2 cm (Arakawa, JGastHepatol, 1986; 1:3; Arakawa, Gastro, 1986; 91:198). For reasons which are unclear, small hepatocellular carcinoma is mostly found in patients with advanced cirrhosis, and hepatic resection is seldom indicated because of the poor liver function. The tumour is usually well differentiated. Perhaps poorly differentiated

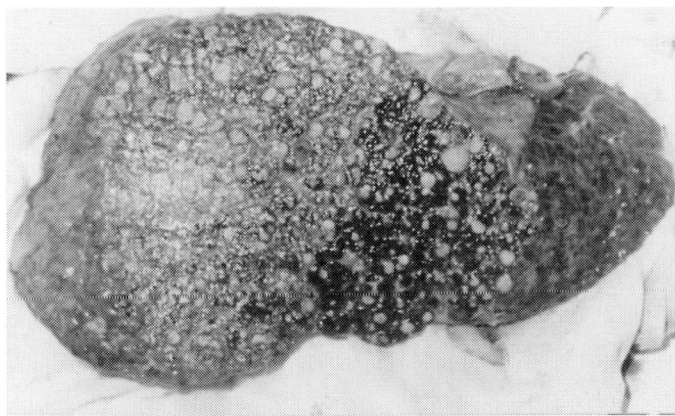

Fig. 11. Diffuse-type hepatocellular carcinoma in a liver with advanced cirrhosis. Many cirrhotic nodules are replaced by whitish tumour nodules. Unless the colour of the tumour is white, hepatocellular carcinoma nodules cannot be clearly distinguished from cirrhotic nodules.

hepatocellular carcinoma escapes detection while it is still small because it grows fast.

Intravascular and intraductal growth

In our study based on 232 autopsy cases of hepatocellular carcinoma, [16] about 65 per cent of the livers bearing hepatocellular carcinoma had tumour growths in the portal trunk and/or major portal vein branches, and there was tumour growth in the major hepatic vein in 23 per cent. When there was tumour growth in the major hepatic vein, portal tumour invasion was invariably present. Other reported figures vary from 10.9 to 85 per cent for portal invasion and from 3.7 to 14.7 per cent for intravenous invasion. Intrabile-duct invasion is less common, and in Kojiro's series it occurred in 9.2 per cent (Cancer, 1982; 99:2144). Intraductal invasion mimics gallstone disease in clinical presentation. Extrahepatic metastases are either haematogenous, lymphogenous, infiltrative, or disseminated within the abdominal cavity. Since tumour invasion into the hepatic vein is common, the lung is the organ where metastasis occurs most frequently. In our study of patients with cirrhosis and hepatocellular carcinoma, 23.6 per cent of the cases had histologically demonstrable tumour cells in the oesophageal varices, and 12 of 13 cases of intravariceal tumour thrombi had lung metastases, suggesting a portal vein–varices–lung route for cancer cell transport (Arakawa, Hepatol, 1986; 6:419). Some of the tumour thrombi in the portal trunk are highly arterialized, and contrast medium injected into the hepatic artery delineates the tumour thrombi on angiography, during the late arterial phase, as a structure resembling a bundle of thread, radiologically called the 'thread and streaks sign', a term coined by one of us (Okuda, Radiol, 1975; 117:303). When this sign is demonstrable, arterial blood is flowing in a retrograde fashion in the portal axis, pushing cancer cells back through the varices into the superior vena cava. Not all portal tumour thrombi have an ample arterial supply, and some undergo necrosis, whereas tumour thrombi in the hepatic vein always grow actively, and often invade the right atrium; such growth occasionally crosses the tricuspid valves and expands further into the pulmonary arteries.[17] Tumour growths in large bile ducts are less viable, and are frequently seen as a mixture of necrotized tumour tissue and blood clot. Fragments

are detached and become stuck at the papilla of Vater, eliciting symptoms similar to those of stone incarceration. Bleeding into the biliary system also occurs, causing right upper quadrant pain.

Metastases

The lung was involved most frequently by haematogenous metastases in our series (51.6 per cent), being followed in decreasing order of frequency by the adrenal tissue (8.4 per cent), bone (5.8 per cent), meninges (5.4 per cent), pancreas (3.1 per cent), brain (2.7 per cent), and kidney (2.2 per cent). Lymphogenous metastases were seen in the lymph nodes in the area of the hepatic hilum (14.1 per cent), head of the pancreas (10.7 per cent), aorta (7.0 per cent), retroperitoneum (5.8 per cent), stomach (5.3 per cent), mediastinum (4.9 per cent), trachea (4.9 per cent), carina (4.0 per cent), neck (3.1 per cent), and in Virchow's node (2.2 per cent). Direct infiltration into the diaphragm was seen in 10.2 per cent, dissemination in the Douglas' pouch in 6.2 per cent, invasion of the gallbladder in 5.8 per cent, and dissemination over the peritoneum in 4.0 per cent. Peritoneal dissemination of hepatocellular carcinoma is rather infrequent; small peritoneal lesions are covered by endothelium and look shiny, and such dissemination is quite different from that of adenocarcinomas originating from the stomach and pancreas in that it does not produce an adhesive mass involving intra-abdominal organs and lymph nodes.

Histopathology

The most important criterion in histological diagnosis is similarity of the cancer cells to normal hepatocytes, namely, relatively large acidophilic cytoplasm. The degree of cancer cell differentiation varies from case to case, and from area to area in the same liver. Extremely well differentiated hepatocellular carcinoma cells are indistinguishable from normal liver cells without recognition of subtle structural changes. Except for poorly differentiated hepatocellular carcinoma, cancer cells are arranged in thick cell cords or plates, in a trabecular arrangement lined by endothelial cells which form blood sinuses (Fig. 12). It is expected that if the blood sinuses are wide, the blood flow into the mass is large in quantity. Occasionally, cancer cells are arranged in an acinar fashion assuming a picture which may be called 'pseudoglandular'.

In less well differentiated hepatocellular carcinoma, large multinucleated cells are often present (Fig. 13) and, in an anaplastic hepatocellular carcinoma, the trabecular arrangement is lost and the cancer cells may resemble sarcoma cells growing in a solid or compact arrangement (Fig. 14). Edmondson and Steiner[18] attempted to classify hepatocellular carcinoma cells into four grades according to the degree of cell differentiation, but their material did not contain cases of extremely well differentiated hepatocellular carcinoma. Without illustrative cases, they defined grade I as cancer cells indistinguishable from normal hepatocytes, seen in a liver which has overt hepatocellular carcinoma elsewhere. Although grade I was hypothetical, their classification has been generally accepted and is currently used in many countries including Japan. Well-differentiated cancer cells have a strong cell-to-cell cohesiveness and tend to grow in an expanding fashion, not infiltrating into the parenchyma, and poorly differentiated cells have least cohesiveness with a tendency to grow in an infiltrative fashion.

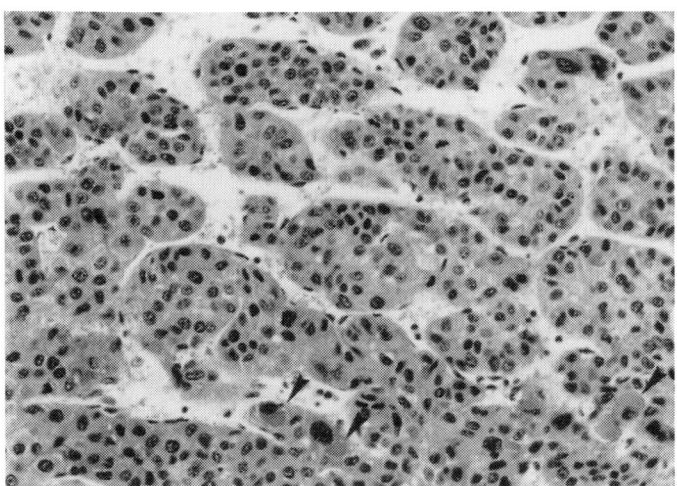

Fig. 12. Typical trabecular arrangement of relatively well-differentiated hepatocellular carcinoma cells. Note the wide blood sinuses between the tumour cell nests, and also cytoplasmic inclusions (arrowheads). These cells are classified as Edmondson–Steiner's grade II (haematoxylin and eosin, 170 ×).

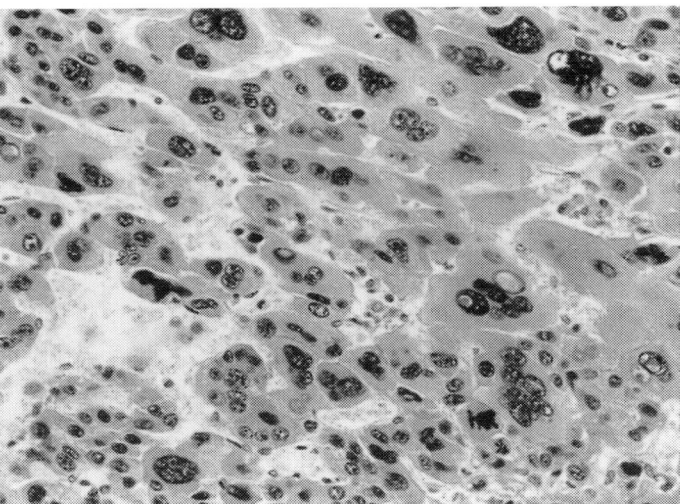

Fig. 13. Multinucleated giant tumour cells which are interpreted as less well differentiated and may be classified as Edmondson–Steiner's grade III (haematoxylin and eosin, 170 ×).

Nakashima and Kojiro divided the growth patterns into pseudo-capsular (expanding), replacing, and sinusoidal.[15] In the replacing growth pattern, hepatocytes are replaced by cancer cells within an intact reticulin frame that holds the muralium; in the sinusoidal growth pattern, cancer cells are floating in the sinusoids. The latter is associated with early haematogenous metastases. Some of the well-differentiated hepatocellular carcinoma cells produce bilirubin, and bile plugs appear within the cancer tissue because it does not have a bile duct system. Hepatocellular carcinoma cells often contain cytoplasmic inclusion bodies such as globules, Mallory hyalin bodies, spherical inclusions, and ground-glass cytoplasm (Fig. 12). These cytoplasmic inclusion bodies represent accumulation of certain proteins that are normally secreted by the cell. In some cases, cancer cells in a macrotrabecular arrangement look like the clear cells of renal cancer (Fig. 15). According to Buchanan and Huvos (AmJClinPath, 1974; 61:529) such cells constituted 30 to 100 per cent of tumour cells in 13 per cent of their 150 cases. The earlier suggestion by Edmondson[19] that patients with clear-cell type hepatocellular carcinoma have a longer survival has been disputed (El-Domeiri, Cancer, 1971; 27:7), but these cells are usually very well differentiated.

Scirrhous or sclerosing hepatocellular carcinoma

Abundant fibrous stromas separating tumour cells are commonly seen following chemotherapy, radiotherapy, and arterial embolization, but there are occasional cases of hepatocellular carcinoma that contain more fibrous tissue than cancer cells without treatment. Such hepatocellular carcinoma may be called scirrhous or sclerosing hepatocellular carcinoma (Fig. 16), and may pose problems in differential diagnosis from cholangiocarcinoma. Omata *et al.* (Liver, 1981; 1:33) described 30 cases of scirrhous primary liver carcinoma and demonstrated frequent association with hypercalcaemia. They called them sclerosing hepatic carcinoma. Histopathologically, the tumour resembles peripheral-type cholangiocarcinoma with abundant stromas interspersed with tubular neoplastic structures. The

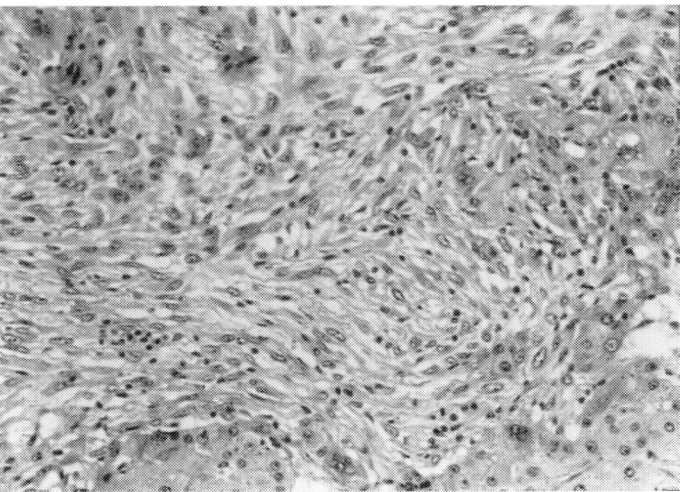

Fig. 14. Anaplastic hepatocellular carcinoma which has sarcomatous features mixed with areas of epithelial cell tumour and may be classified as Edmondson–Steiner's grade IV (haematoxylin and eosin, 170 ×).

tumour cells were thought to be of apparent hepatocytic origin in 63 per cent, apparent ductal in 20 per cent, and mixed or indistinguishable in 17 per cent. Cirrhosis coexisted in only 30 per cent.

Fibrolamellar carcinoma

Craig *et al.* in 1980 described 23 cases of hepatocellular carcinoma characterized by deeply eosinophilic neoplastic hepatocytes and fibrosis arranged in a lamellar fashion (Craig, Cancer, 1980; 46:372) (Fig. 17). Grossly, the mass was sharply demarcated and contained fibrous septa mimicking focal nodular hyperplasia. In their series, this type constituted about 7 per cent of all cases of primary liver cancer. Most patients with this type of hepatocellular carcinoma are young, operability is high, and survival period is significantly longer than that of patients with ordinary hepatocellular carcinoma. Table 8

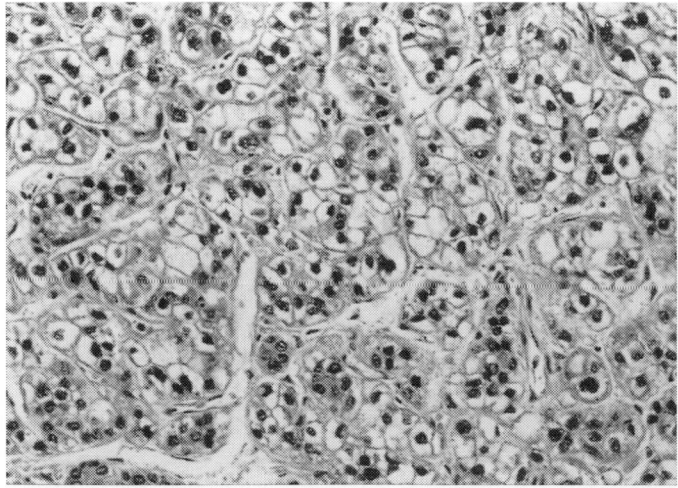

Fig. 15. Well-differentiated, clear cell-like, hepatocellular carcinoma (haematoxylin and eosin, 166 ×).

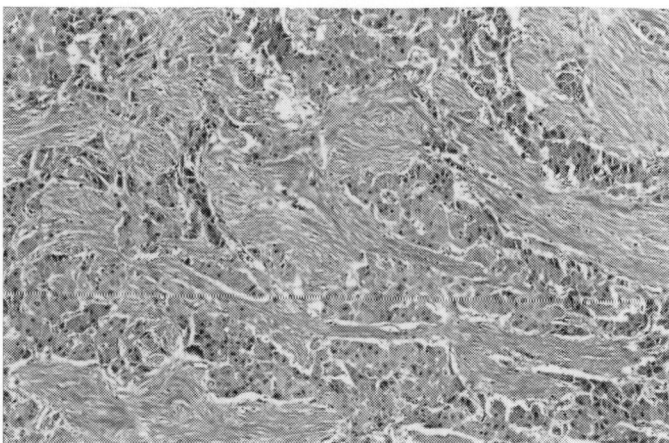

Fig. 17. Fibrolamellar carcinoma of the liver. Eosinophilic cancer cells in cords are buried in abundant fibres of lamellar arrangement (haematoxylin and eosin, 116 ×).

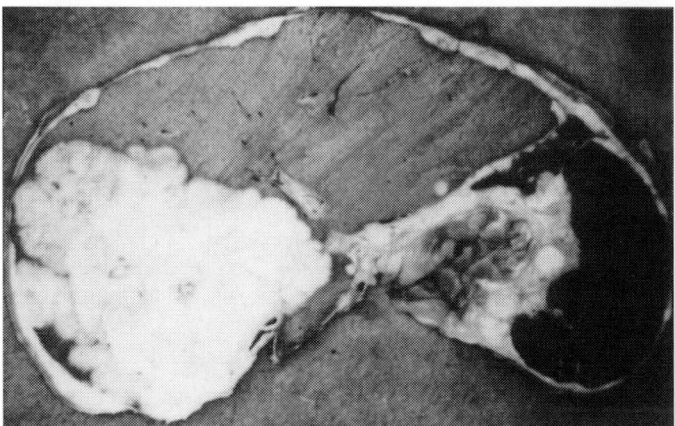

Fig. 16. Scirrhous hepatocellular carcinoma in a non-cirrhotic liver. Note that the mass is white and firm, resembling cholangioma. This patient, who had an exploratory laparotomy, lived for more than 3 years. At autopsy, the liver was covered by firm, whitish, cancer tissue and was adherent to the surrounding organs, perhaps as a result of laparotomy.

compares fibrolamellar carcinoma and conventional hepatocellular carcinoma.

Cholangiolocellular carcinoma

The tumour cells in this type of primary liver cancer, first described by Steiner (ActaUnioIntContraCancerum, 1957; 13:268), are fairly uniform and retain the configuration associated with cholangioles, forming double-layered cuboidal epithelial cell cords that have a tiny lumen. The cytoplasm is scanty. The tumour structures resemble the proliferating pseudoductules or cholangioles seen in areas of hepatic fibrosis. This type occurred in 1.1 per cent of the series of Steiner and Higginson (Cancer, 1979; 12:753), and in 0.8 per cent in the series of Peters.[11]

Hepatocholangiocarcinoma

This cancer is also called combined (mixed) hepatocellular and cholangiocellular carcinoma. Hepatocellular carcinoma with areas of ductal or glandular changes is fairly common and should not be referred to as 'combined'. Hepatocholangiocellular carcinoma contains unequivocal elements of both hepatocellular and cholangiocellular carcinomas. According to Allen (AmJPath, 1949; 25: 647), there are three subtypes depending upon the relation between hepatocellular and cholangiocellular elements: (1) hepatocellular carcinoma and cholangiocarcinoma are present at different sites in the same liver, each composed of a single cell type; (2) hepatocellular carcinoma and cholangiocarcinoma are present at adjacent sites, each composed of a different cell type, but becoming intermingled as they develop; and (3) histologically, hepatocellular carcinoma and cholangiocarcinoma are mixed within the same tumour, combined in a manner suggesting that they have developed at the same site.

Clinically, this type presents features more similar to hepatocellular carcinoma than to cholangiocarcinoma.

Hepatoblastoma

This occurs mainly in the non-cirrhotic liver in the postnatal period and early childhood (Table 4), and is the single most common liver tumour in children. Although it occurs mostly before the age of 3 years, in a Japanese series,[10] 20 per cent of the patients were older than 5 years, and there were occasional adult cases. The tumour is usually a single mass, and about one-half of them are encapsulated. The presenting symptom is an enlarging abdomen. Ishak and Glunz (Cancer, 1967; 20:396) studied 35 cases of hepatoblastoma and divided them into an epithelial type and a mixed epithelial and mesenchymal type. The Japanese Pathological Society has classified this carcinoma histologically into: (1) highly differentiated hepatoblastoma (fetal hepatoblastoma) in which cells with a high degree of differentiation are predominant; (2) poorly differentiated hepatoblastoma (also known as embryonal hepatoblastoma) in which cells of a low degree of differentiation are predominant; and (3) immature hepatoblastoma (also known as undifferentiated hepatoblastoma) in which small cells shaped like discs or short spindles are predominant. For more details of the histology, readers are referred to the review of hepatoblastoma by Stocker and Ishak.[21]

Table 8 Comparison of fibrolamellar carcinoma and typical hepatocellular carcinoma

	Fibrolamellar carcinoma	Hepatocellular carcinoma
Age (years)	5–35	40–75
Sex, M/F	Equal	4–8/1
Liver parenchyma	Normal	Cirrhosis (80%)
α-Fetoprotein	Normal	Elevated (85%)
HBsAg in serum	Negative	Positive (30–90%)
Biochemical change	Increased transcobalamin I	No increase
Surgical resectability (%)	50–75	10–20
Survival from diagnosis (months)	32–68	<6

Adapted from Roles.[20]

Serum α-fetoprotein is elevated in the majority of patients and urinary excretion of cystathionine is increased in nearly 50 per cent. Some boys may present initially with signs of precocious puberty. The prognosis depends largely on the resectability of the tumour, which also varies with the histological type.

Clinical features and diagnosis
Patients' histories

Many patients with hepatocellular carcinoma have a past or current history of chronic liver disease. Table 9 lists the major histories elicited from about 2000 patients with hepatocellular carcinoma in a national survey conducted by the Japan Liver Cancer Study Group in the period 1982 to 1983.[22] Note that 23 per cent of the cases had received a blood transfusion in the past, and 29 per cent were habitual drinkers. Sixty-one per cent of them were aware of having cirrhosis, and about 50 per cent had past or ongoing chronic hepatitis. The past diagnosis of acute hepatitis in some of the patients could have been due to acute exacerbation of chronic hepatitis. The frequent past history of blood transfusion in this table is peculiar to Japanese patients (see above), because of the increasing incidence of HCV-associated hepatocellular carcinoma in this country. The awareness of the ongoing chronic liver disease is important for the patient in any country if emergence of hepatocellular carcinoma is to be detected early.

Presenting symptoms

These include general malaise, abdominal pain, full sensation of the abdomen, anorexia, a palpable mass, weight loss, ascites, oedema of the lower extremities, jaundice, fever, nausea, haematemesis, or melaena. Table 10 gives the frequency of these symptoms in the 1984 to 1985 survey conducted by the Japan Liver Cancer Study Group in comparison with the earlier data among the Bantu black population.[3] These symptoms are either due to the underlying disease, cirrhosis, or to hepatocellular carcinoma. However, if a patient with established cirrhosis under observation develops abdominal pain, a palpable liver mass, or fever, hepatocellular carcinoma should be clinically suspected. In an earlier survey in Japan,[23] the symptoms of hepatocellular carcinoma associated with cirrhosis were compared with those in hepatocellular carcinoma not associated with cirrhosis: it was found that abdominal pain and a palpable mass were more frequent in patients without cirrhosis. Such differences are more obvious from Table 10; abdominal pain, weight loss, a palpable mass, jaundice, and fever were more frequent among the Bantu black population. These differences are due in part to late diagnosis, and also to frequent absence of associated cirrhosis among the black patients. In other words, in the absence of underlying cirrhosis, cancer-associated symptoms are more common. In our study of 37 patients with a hepatocellular carcinoma smaller than 3 cm, abdominal pain was noted in only one. In the

Table 9 Past histories in patients with hepatocellular carcinoma

History	No. of cases[+] Yes/no	Percentage
Acute hepatitis		
Confirmed	214/1378	15.5
Suspected	71/1378	5.2
Chronic hepatitis	678/1365	49.7
Liver cirrhosis	906/1485	61.0
Blood transfusion*	373/1623	23.0
Alcohol (more than 0.5 litre of sake/day for more than 10 years)	510/1749	29.2
Drug-induced liver disease	8/1646	0.5
Prolonged use of medicines	102/1700	6.0

[+] The denominators vary because not all questionnaires were answered.
* Blood transfusion in the majority was more than 10 years previously.
Data based on Okuda and Nakashima. [23]

Table 10 Early symptoms in patients with hepatocellular carcinoma. Comparison of recent Japanese data and early data in South Africa

Symptom	Japan (1984–1985)*	South Africa (1951)+
General malaise	60.5	86
Abdominal pain	46.2	90
Full sensation in abdomen	44.9	
Anorexia	44.7	
Weight loss	28.9	83
Ascites	26.5	45
Palpable mass	23.3	100 (90%, tender)
Oedema of the legs	16.8	30
Jaundice	16.7	45
Fever	16.7	38
Nausea, vomiting	15.6	
Haematemesis, melaena	7.6	
Dyspnoea		25
Anaemia		34

Numbers are percentages.
* Taken from the Eighth Report of the Japan Liver Cancer Study Group (2300 cases).
+ Taken from Berman [3] (75 cases).

Table 11 Clinical types of hepatocellular carcinoma. Comparison of South African cases and Japanese cases seen before 1970

Clinical type	Japan* (n=376)	South Africa+ (n=75)
Frank	229 (60.9)	47 (62.7)
Cirrhotic	87 (23.1)	
Occult	14 (3.7)	12 (16.2)
Febrile	8 (2.1)	6 (8.0)
Acute abdominal	11 (2.9)	6 (8.0)
Metastatic	11 (2.9)	4 (5.3)
Cholestatic	7 (1.9)	
Others	9 (2.4)	
Total	376 (100)	75 (100)

Percentages in parentheses.
* Seen before 1970, not including small hepatocellular carcinoma.
+ According to the data of Berman. [3]

Hong Kong series (Lai, Cancer, 1981; 47:2746), the presenting symptoms included (beside the symptoms listed) hypoglycaemia (2 per cent), diarrhoea (2 per cent), encephalopathy, and dyspnoea due to pleural effusion.

Clinical manifestation

In countries where there is no screening programme for early detection of hepatocellular carcinoma, most patients at the time of diagnosis describe malaise, loss of appetite and weight, abdominal fullness, right upper quadrant pain, and often a palpable mass or enlarged liver. Anaemia is unusual in the Far East unlike Berman's experience in the South African black population. The size of the liver tends to be large in the absence of cirrhosis, because the general status of the patient remains good till the tumour becomes visible. A large palpable liver distorts the symmetry of the upper abdomen and the right costal margin may protrude due to compression from below. On auscultation, an arterial bruit is frequently heard, particularly in African black patients. In such patients, a highly vascularized hepatocellular carcinoma should be suspected. The right liver sometimes enlarges caudally, without appreciable elevation of the diaphragm, or enlarges upwards, raising the level of the right diaphragm without existing much below the costal margin. Elevation of the right diaphragm can be diagnosed by percussion and from diminished breath sounds in the right lower lung. Sometimes, only the left side of the liver is palpably enlarged. Berman called these cases with classical signs of advanced hepatocellular carcinoma 'frank cancer'. He grouped clinical manifestations into five types based on his experience with African black patients. He used the term 'occult cancer' for those in whom physical examination (done for reasons unrelated to liver cancer) has disclosed liver tumour. Some patients are rushed to hospital because of abdominal pain and symptoms mimicking an acute abdomen; he called this 'acute abdominal cancer'. The sudden onset of these signs is due to rupture of the mass, and emergency management is required. If a frail hepatocellular carcinoma mass protrudes from

the liver surface, even a slight external force could cause damage and lead to continuous and profuse bleeding. Forceful palpation of the liver in such patients is very dangerous. We have seen two cases of iatrogenically induced rupture of tumour. Without an acute episode, bleeding into ascites can occur, and at autopsy more than 50 per cent of patients with advanced hepatocellular carcinoma have bloody ascites.

Some patients present with a high remittent fever; Berman called this 'febrile cancer'. Such patients usually have leucocytosis and, in the presence of hepatomegaly, liver abscess is a likely diagnosis. Histologically, the cancer cells are very poorly differentiated, often appearing sarcomatous. Our experience includes two such patients in whom differential diagnosis of hepatocellular carcinoma and abscess was impossible and laparotomy was necessary (Okuda, Hepatol, 1991; 13:695). This type occurred in 8 per cent of Berman's series, but in Japan it is much less common. In others, the first presentation may be a metastasis, such as a lump on the head (bone metastasis), or neurological signs due to a spinal metastasis. In one unusual case, our patient suddenly coughed up soft material with sputum, which was shown to be hepatocellular carcinoma on histological examination; chest radiography disclosed a small coin lesion in the lung.

Table 11 compares the relative frequency of the different clinical types in Berman's series, and in ours in Japan. In the Far East, particularly in Japan, the majority of patients have advanced underlying cirrhosis, and clinical signs may be the same as, or masked by, those of cirrhosis itself, namely ascites, dilated abdominal wall veins, encephalopathy, ankle oedema, and variceal bleeding. Without palpable hepatic enlargement, the patient will be treated as for cirrhosis. Such cases may be classified as a cirrhotic type.

Growth of hepatocellular carcinoma into the biliary tract causes obstructive jaundice and we have called such patients, presenting with jaundice, 'the cholestatic type'. Some of them have complaints typical of gallstone disease. Haemobilia can also occur with a sudden onset of colicky pain. Direct cholangiography is required to make the diagnosis. The frequency of the cholestatic type was 1.9 per cent in our series and in a French series was 2.1 per cent (Carella, Liver, 1981; 1:251). At autopsy, intraductal growth is found more frequently (9.2 per cent, Kojiro, see above).

Small hepatocellular carcinoma is usually found in patients with cirrhosis as a result of clinical follow-up by ultrasonography and serum α-fetoprotein measurement, and such patients usually do not have signs attributable to hepatocellular carcinoma.

Analysis of 2380 cases of hepatocellular carcinoma seen in Japan during the 10-year period from 1968 to 1977, when there were more classic cases, showed that the most common physical findings were hepatomegaly (67.2 per cent), ascites (43.6 per cent), jaundice (30.6 per cent), and splenomegaly (14.4 per cent). In our series of 258 cases during the same period, the liver was not palpable in 19.8 per cent, was slightly palpable in 20.2 per cent, was two to three finger breadths below the costal margin in 32.6 per cent, and was more than four finger breadths in 27.5 per cent. Dilated abdominal veins were noted in 32.9 per cent, vascular spiders in 34.5 per cent, tenderness in the right upper quadrant in 32.9 per cent, and palmar erythema in 19.0 per cent. These features have changed after the early detection programme was initiated in Japan, because the diagnosis is made before hepatocellular carcinoma becomes 5 cm in size in the majority of patients who have no tumour-related symptoms. In Berman's series from the African black population, hepatomegaly was found in 100 per cent, ascites in 55 per cent, and jaundice in 45 per cent.

On palpation, the tumour itself is seldom palpable as a discrete mass; an enlarged, irregularly surfaced liver is the usual finding. In rare instances, a pedunculated mass is palpated outside the liver. Ascites is usually due to cirrhosis; the conglomeration of adherent bowel and nodes, frequently seen in advanced cancer of the pancreas and stomach, is extremely rare. At autopsy, peritoneal metastases are common, more often seen in the Douglas pouch, but disseminated carcinomatosis is very rare. We have seen one patient in whom attempted resection failed and perihepatic tumour invasion, with adhesion, occurred after laparotomy. This was shown to be a sclerosing hepatocellular carcinoma in a non-cirrhotic liver, and the patient lived for more than 3 years. We have also encountered three cases in which detection of hepatocellular carcinoma was preceded by an acute hepatitis-like episode. In retrospect, these patients had chronic active hepatitis and cirrhosis, and the former was exacerbated with an acute bout of inflammation. Cancer was already present but unnoticed at the time of exacerbation and the patients were treated as having severe hepatitis. Cooney et al. (AmJGastr, 1980; 74:436) described a patient without cirrhosis who developed portal hypertension as a result of microscopic tumour invasion in the central vein and small portal radicles. In a series of 918 autopsies for hepatocellular carcinoma without cirrhosis, oesophageal varices were found in 8.2 per cent, most likely due to intraportal invasion.[24] The literature abounds with various presentations of metastases that are not peculiar to hepatocellular carcinoma.

Diagnostic criteria

To demonstrate histological similarity of the neoplastic cells to hepatocytes, tissue must be taken either by biopsy or at surgery. However, in the countries where hepatocellular carcinoma is prevalent, a space-occupying lesion seen by imaging in a cirrhotic liver almost invariably represents hepatocellular carcinoma (Melato, Cancer, 1989; 64:455). In such patients the diagnosis is almost always correct, if malignancy in other organs can be excluded by a complete work-up. In the presence of high serum α-fetoprotein levels, biopsy is not required. In Western countries where hepatocellular carcinoma is uncommon, tissue diagnosis is necessary.

Investigations and other diagnostic considerations

Laboratory findings

Haematology

Blood counts and haemoglobin are unchanged in the early stage of the disease, in the absence of bleeding episodes, or there may be mild pancytopenia due to splenomegaly (hypersplenism) secondary to cirrhosis. Leucoytosis is not uncommon, but it is not clear whether such leucocytosis is a result of production of granulopoietin, or similar substances, by neoplastic cells. Erythrocytosis occurs in a small proportion of patients as a paraneoplastic syndrome (see below).

Blood chemistry

This depends on the stage of hepatocellular carcinoma and the underlying disease. In patients with advanced cirrhosis, serum albumin, prothrombin, and other proteins made in the liver are reduced, plasma clearance of bromosulphthalein and indocyanine green (ICG) is delayed, and there may be mild hyperbilirubinaemia; in the presence of active hepatitis, serum aminotransferase levels are elevated. These changes are difficult to separate from the biochemical changes induced by hepatocellular carcinoma. In advanced hepatocellular carcinoma, there will be elevation of aspartate aminotransferase (AST), alanine aminotransferase (ALT), lactate dehydrogenase (LDH), and alkaline phosphatase (AP). One of the important biochemical features of hepatocellular carcinoma is the difference between AST and ALT levels, the former being invariably higher and the difference becoming greater with the progression of the disease (Shimokawa, Cancer, 1977; 40:319). The concentration of AST in cancer tissue is lower than that in noncancerous parenchyma, and it seems that cancer tissue releases AST into the circulation at a faster rate. In isolated cases, AP is extremely high, and it is possible that the elevation is due to tumour-specific AP (Warnock, CCActa, 1969; 24:5). The LDH levels are usually not very high, and are not necessarily proportional to the size of tumour. Isoenzyme LDH_5 is almost always higher than LDH_4 in hepatocellular carcinoma, whereas the reverse is true with metastatic liver cancer.[17] Occasionally, hypercholesterolaemia occurs in patients with hepatocellular carcinoma. Alpert et al. (AmJMed, 1969; 46:794) studied Ugandan patients with hepatocellular carcinoma and found elevation of serum cholesterol in 33 per cent. However, hypercholesterolaemia is generally less common elsewhere. There is no in vitro evidence that hepatocellular carcinoma tissue synthesizes more cholesterol than does normal liver tissue, and the exact mechanism for hypercholesterolaemia remains to be determined.

Tumour-specific proteins

Neoplastic cells produce certain embryonic proteins as a result of dedifferentiation of the chromosomes. Some of these carcinoembryonic proteins are utilized for diagnosis.

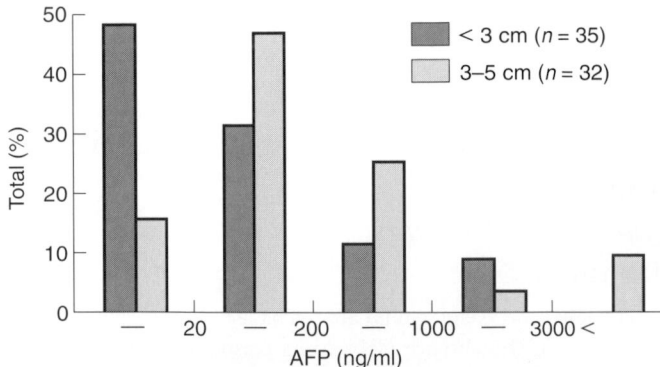

Fig. 18. Serum α-fetoprotein levels in small hepatocellular carcinoma (less than 5 cm). About 50 per cent of hepatocellular carcinomas smaller than 3 cm show normal α-fetoprotein levels (less than 20 ng/ml), and very few more than 1000 ng/ml.

α-Fetoprotein

This is an α_1-globulin produced in fetal yolk sac, liver, and intestine, and is present in serum only during fetal life and in the immediate postnatal period. This protein is the most important diagnostic marker for hepatocellular carcinoma. A number of methods have been used, and are currently available, but the radioimmunoassay is the most sensitive and perhaps most expensive. The reported positivity rates vary with the method used and with the population studied. It is not established whether the differences among the positivity rates are attributable solely to ethnic differences, since the methods used were different, the stage of disease was not uniform, and although the figures obtained in Western countries were generally low, the clinical material could have included fibrolamellar carcinoma which does not elaborate α-fetoprotein. The normal level of α-fetoprotein in adults is below 20 ng/ml and values above 1000 ng/ml are highly suggestive of hepatocellular carcinoma.

The pitfall with the use of α-fetoprotein in diagnosis is the non-specific elevation in patients with various liver diseases. It increases with the active cell regeneration that follows massive or submassive hepatic necrosis (Karvountzis, AnnIntMed, 1974; 80:156). In patients with chronic hepatitis and cirrhosis, serum α-fetoprotein often fluctuates between 20 and 1000 ng/ml reflecting necrosis and compensatory regeneration of liver cells. One point value in this range of levels is not reliable and follow-up α-fetoprotein measurements are required. Furthermore, α-fetoprotein levels in patients with small hepatocellular carcinoma are mostly in this equivocal value range (Fig. 18). When α-fetoprotein rises continuously at an 'exponential' rate (Fig. 19), the diagnosis is almost certain. According to Kojiro et al. (Cancer, 1982; 99:2144), the number of carcinoma cells with stainable α-fetoprotein is roughly proportional to the serum levels of α-fetoprotein, but some of the other hepatocytes in cancer-bearing livers may also contain stainable α-fetoprotein, particularly proliferating oval cells (Sakamoto, AnnNY-AcadMed, 1975; 259:253).

More recently, Kobata's group in Japan determined the sugar structure of the α-fetoprotein molecule and demonstrated that α-fetoprotein derived from hepatocellular carcinoma is fucosylated at N-acetyl-glucosamine; α-fetoprotein derived from yolk sac is not

(CancerRes, 1980; 40:4276; 1983; 43:4791). Based on such differences which are reflected in the binding to lentil lectin, α-fetoprotein associated with hepatocellular carcinoma and α-fetoprotein derived from the liver in benign diseases can be differentiated (Aoyagi, BBActa, 1985; 830:217).

Recently, determination of lectin-reactive fractions of α-fetoprotein became possible using lectin–affinity electrophoresis coupled with antibody–affinity blotting (Taketa, Electrophoresis, 1985; 6: 492), and α-Fetoprotein Differentiation Kits L and P (Shimizu, CCActa, 1993; 214:3) (Wako Pure Chem Ind, Ltd, Osaka, Japan) have been developed. Kit L measures the proportion of α-fetoprotein present as lens culnaris agglutinin-A-reactive α-fetoprotein (α-fetoprotein-L3) and Kit P measures that of α-fetoprotein present as erythroagglutinating phytohaemagglutinin-reactive α-fetoprotein (α-fetoprotein-P4+P5). From the maximum Youden indices determined, the cut-off level was set at 15 per cent for both α-fetoprotein-L3 and α-fetoprotein-P4+P5. α-Fetoprotein-L3 exceeded the cut-off level of 15 per cent at 4.0 ± 4.9 months before detection of hepatocellular carcinoma by imaging with a sensitivity of 48 per cent and a specificity of 81 per cent (Taketa, CancerRes, 1993; 53:5419). Twenty-four of the 33 patients (73 per cent) with cirrhosis and hepatocellular carcinoma had higher percentages of α-fetoprotein-L3, α-fetoprotein-P4+P5, or both than the 32 patients with cirrhosis but no hepatocellular carcinoma. In 24 patients, one or both of these markers were first elevated 3 to 18 months before the detection of hepatocellular carcinoma by imaging (Sato, NEJM, 1993; 328:1802). Thus, measurements of α-fetoprotein-L3 and α-fetoprotein-P4+P5 permit the differentiation of hepatocellular carcinoma from cirrhosis or chronic hepatitis, serve as predictive markers for the development of hepatocellular carcinoma during the follow-up of patients with cirrhosis, and are useful for the early detection of hepatocellular carcinoma.

α-Fetoprotein mRNA was detectable in the blood of all 6 patients with hepatocellular carcinoma having metastasis at extrahepatic organs (100 per cent), whereas only 11 of 27 hepatocellular carcinoma cases without metastasis (41 per cent) had demonstrable mRNA (Matsumura, Hepatol, 1994; 20:148). The presence of α-fetoprotein mRNA in peripheral blood may be an indicator of circulating malignant or benign hepatocytes, but whether it predicts haematogenous metastasis or tumour cells in hepatocellular carcinoma remains to be seen. An allelic loss in chromosome 4q was significantly associated with hepatocellular carcinoma when there were elevated levels of serum α-fetoprotein, but not when α-fetoprotein was normal (Yeh, Gastro, 1996; 110:184)

Des-γ-carboxy prothrombin (DCP; PIVKA-II)

In 1984, Liebman et al. (NEJM, 1984; 310:427) detected elevated DCP levels in serum in 67 per cent of patients with hepatocellular carcinoma from Taiwan and the United States. This abnormal prothrombin occurs in vitamin K deficiency because carboxylation in the γ-position of the prothrombin structure requires vitamin K. Vitamin K deficiency causes similar structural abnormalities in several other coagulation factors. In the paediatric field, determination of protein induced by vitamin K absence or by antagonist-II (PIVKA-II) had been used for the diagnosis of vitamin K deficiency, and Motohara et al. (PediatRes, 1985; 19:354) developed an enzyme-linked immunosorbent assay (**ELISA**) for vitamin K

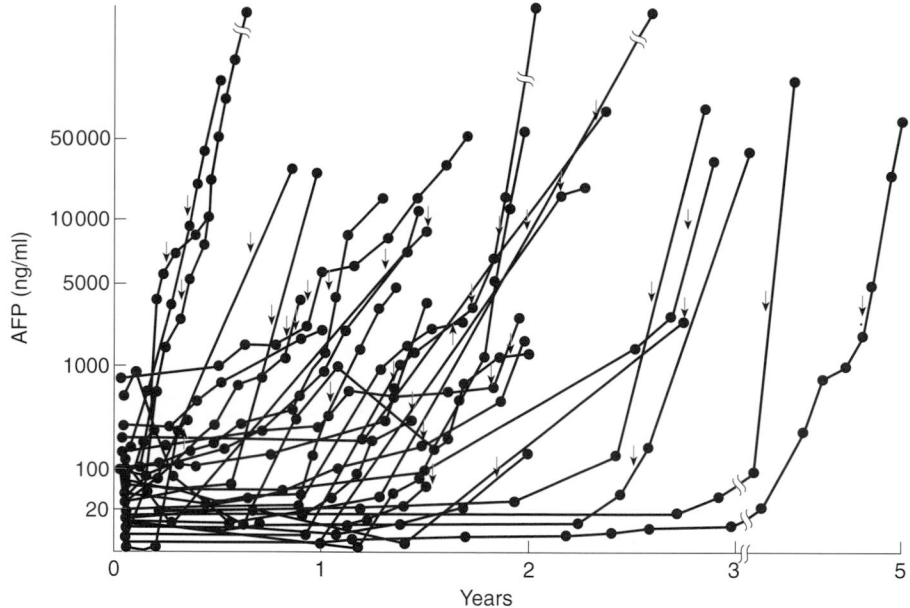

Fig. 19. Sharp rises in serum α-fetoprotein levels in patients with hepatocellular carcinoma. Arrows indicate the time when diagnosis was made. The size of the mass was invariably larger than 4 cm in these patients, and α-fetoprotein measurement alone did not serve the purpose of early detection. Very sharp rises suggest multiple intrahepatic spreads.

deficiency using a monoclonal antibody raised against PIVKA-II. PIVKA-II measured by this method was positive in about 60 per cent of Japanese patients with hepatocellular carcinoma.[25] Soulier *et al.* (Gastro, 1986; 91:1258) developed a method for measurement in which staphylocoagulase is used, and found that 74 per cent of French patients with hepatocellular carcinoma were positive. Hepatoma cells in culture produce PIVKA-II in the absence of vitamin K, but its production ceases upon addition of the vitamin (Okuda, Hepatol, 1991; 6:392). Plasma PIVKA-II also declines upon administration of vitamin K to patients with hepatocellular carcinoma positive for DCP (Okuda, JGastHepatol, 1991; 6:392). The specificity of DCP for hepatocellular carcinoma seems better than that of α-fetoprotein (Fig. 20), but it is not as sensitive as α-fetoprotein. PIVKA-II was not correlated with α-fetoprotein and was positive in 50 per cent of patients with normal α-fetoprotein levels (Fig. 21). Thus, if both α-fetoprotein and DCP were measured, the diagnosis would be improved.

The exact mechanism whereby PIVKA-II or DCP is increased in plasma in hepatocellular carcinoma is not known, but some studies suggested an imbalance between the overproduction of prothrombin precursors and the supply of vitamin K with a relative vitamin K deficiency (Okuda, ActaHepatolJpn, 1988; 29:47). There is no abnormality of prothrombin DNA (Tagawa, Cancer, 1992; 69:643), nor is there overexpression of prothrombin mRNA in hepatocellular carcinoma (Okuda, Hepatol, 1996; 23:I-66).

To overcome the inadequate sensitivity of the present ELISA method for DCP measurement in the detection of small hepatocellular carcinomas, the avidin–biotin complex method, which is rather cumbersome, was developed. It was further revised, and the new kit can now handle many samples. When the cut-off level was set at 40 mAU/ml, the positivity rates with this new kit were 60, 8, and 7 per cent in patients with hepatocellular carcinoma, cirrhosis, and chronic hepatitis, respectively. The positivity rates were 42 and

50 per cent in patients with small hepatocellular carcinomas less than 2 cm and 3 cm, respectively. Eightly-seven per cent of the patients with hepatocellular carcinoma were positive for either DCP with this new kit or α-fetoprotein (at 20 ng/ml or more). Thus, the measurement of serum DCP levels with this new revised kit in combination with either α-fetoprotein or α-fetoprotein-L3 and α-fetoprotein-P4 + P5 is useful not only for the diagnosis of hepatocellular carcinoma but also for the early diagnosis and monitoring of small hepatocellular carcinoma (Okuda, Hepatol, 1996; 24:473A).

γ-Glutamyl transferase

This enzyme increases in the preneoplastic nodules in the liver during experimental hepatocarcinogenesis in animals. It is in the form of carcinofetal γ-glutamyl transferase. Sawabu *et al.* (JpnJCancerRes, 1983; 51:327) using a polyacrylamide slab gel found three, hepatoma-specific, novel, γ-glutamyl transferase isoenzymes in sera from patients with hepatocellular carcinoma. These tumour-specific, γ-glutamyl transferase isoenzymes were present in 53 per cent of patients with hepatocellular carcinoma in contrast to a near zero positivity in other liver diseases. Some patients negative for α-fetoprotein had tumour-specific γ-glutamyl transferase in their serum. However, the activities of tumour-specific γ-glutamyl transferase are very low in serum, and a diagnostic kit has not been produced commercially.

Variant alkaline phosphatase

The alkaline phosphatase isoenzymes which occur in patients with cancer include Regan isoenzyme, Nagao isoenzyme, and the variant isoenzyme of Warnock and Reisman (CCActa, 1969; 24:5) (see above). Of these, only the variant alkaline phosphatase isoenzyme occurs in the serum in hepatocellular carcinoma. The reported frequency with which this enzyme was demonstrated in sera of

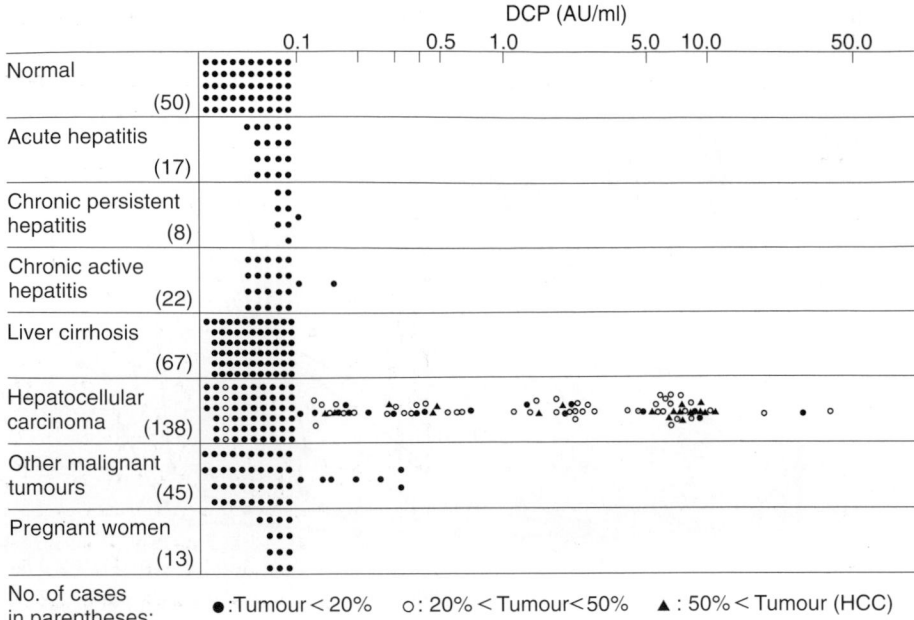

Fig. 20. Plasma des-γ-carboxy prothrombin (DCP) levels in various diseases. This marker is much more specific than α-fetoprotein with very few false positives. However, the levels are more or less proportional to the tumour size, and 51 of 68 cases with small hepatocellular carcinoma (two-dimensional area less than 20 per cent of that of whole liver) showed normal DCP levels.

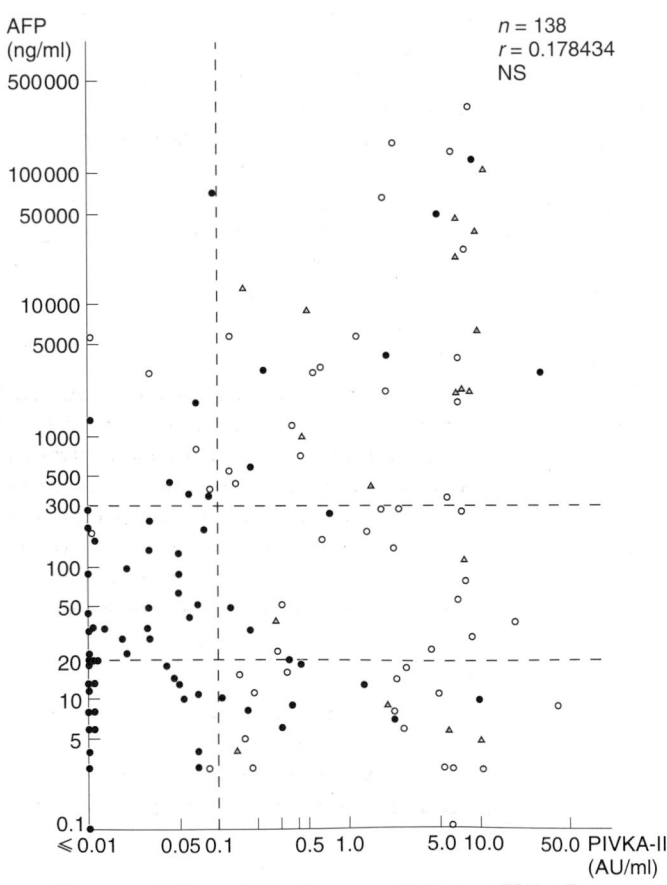

● : Tumour < 20%,   ○ : 20% < Tumour < 50%,   △ : 50% < Tumour

Fig. 21. DCP (PIVKA-II) levels were not at all correlated with α-fetoprotein values. Fifty per cent of patients with normal α-fetoprotein levels (less than 20 ng/ml) were positive for DCP (more than 0.1 AU/ml).

patients with hepatocellular carcinoma varies, has been generally low, and this enzyme is of little diagnostic value.

Carcinoembryonic antigen

This glycoprotein increases in advanced digestive tract cancers, particularly colonic, and in extensive metastatic liver cancer. In hepatocellular carcinoma, carcinoembryonic antigen is usually not elevated, and if both α-fetoprotein and carcinoembryonic antigen are measured in serum, differential diagnosis of hepatocellular carcinoma and metastatic liver cancer becomes more accurate. According to Aburano et al. (EurJNucMed, 1980; 5:373), the predictive value for hepatocellular carcinoma with positive α-fetoprotein alone was 80 per cent, and when negative carcinoembryonic antigen was combined with positive α-fetoprotein, the predictive value increased to 91 per cent.

α-L-Fucosidase

A number of isomers of this enzyme have been identified in human tissues. Deugnier et al. (CCActa, 1980; 108:385) first noted raised α-L-fucosidase levels in patients with hepatocellular carcinoma and later reported a sensitivity of 75 per cent, and a specificity of 90 per cent, in European patients with hepatocellular carcinoma. The enzyme also increases in serum in benign liver diseases. This test is less specific in African black patients, and less sensitive compared with α-fetoprotein, but the number of false-negative α-fetoprotein results was reduced from 13 to 5.5 per cent when the two markers were used together (Bukofzer, BrJCanc, 1989; 59:417). Thus, α-L-fucosidase may be useful in regions with a low hepatocellular carcinoma incidence, if used together with α-fetoprotein.

Other biochemical markers suggested as being diagnostic in patients with hepatocellular carcinoma include ferritin, isoferritin, tissue polypeptide antigen, carbohydrate antigen 19–9, calcitonin, and the tumour-associated isoenzyme of 5′-nucleotide phospho-diesterase. All these markers are inferior to α-fetoprotein and do not seem to be of practical significance in the diagnosis of hepatocellular carcinoma.

Transcobalamin I

In 1973, Waxman and Gilbert (NEJM, 1973; 282:1053) noted a marked elevation of vitamin B_{12} levels in serum in adolescent patients with primary liver cancer. This was due to elevation of transcobalamin I, a vitamin B_{12}-binding protein in serum. Subsequent studies suggested that these young patients with increased serum transcobalamin I had fibrolamellar carcinoma of the liver and that transcobalamin I was produced by fibrolamellar cancer cells (Paradinas, BMJ, 1982; 285:840). This type of cancer also seems to be associated with increased levels of neurotensin, a gut hormone (Collier, Lancet, 1984; i:538)

Systemic manifestations related to humoral effects of the tumour

In patients with hepatocellular carcinoma, an unusual syndrome (paraneoplastic syndrome), or a generalized systemic effect, is sometimes the presenting symptom and may even dominate the clinical picture. The underlying mechanism for these clinical manifestations is thought to be either synthesis by the tumour of proteins, hormones, and hormone-like substances; altered metabolism as a result of loss of regulatory mechanisms; increased utilization of normal constituents of serum by the massive tumour tissue; or a decrease in their production due to insufficient liver tissue remaining.

Erythrocytosis

The frequency of erythrocytosis in patients with hepatocellular carcinoma varies with the report; the highest incidence is 10 per cent, recorded from Hong Kong (McFadzean, Blood, 1967; 29:808), but it is much lower elsewhere. Practically all such patients have cirrhosis, and due to the expanded plasma volume in cirrhosis, haematocrit values as low as 48 per cent can occur with a significantly increased red cell mass. In about 50 per cent of reported cases, erythropoietin assays were positive, but there is no clear evidence that hepatocellular carcinoma tissue produces erythropoietin. Suggestions have been made that production of erythropoietin is a result of an enzymatic interaction between a renal erythropoietic factor and globulin substrate secreted by the tumour, or that inactivation of erythropoietin by normal liver tissue is reduced because normal liver tissue is markedly decreased by extensive tumour invasion. Tumour regression is followed by reduction in the red blood cell count.

Hypoglycaemia

Low blood glucose levels are common in patients with large tumours, but hypoglycaemia does not occur if the tumour is small. The reported prevalence varies, and is up to 30 per cent. It is sometimes associated with other abnormalities such as erythrocytosis, hypercalcaemia, and hypercholesterolaemia. McFadzean and Yeung (AmJMed, 1969; 47:220) divided hypoglycaemia into two types. In type A, which constitutes about 87 per cent of the cases, the tumour is poorly differentiated and fast growing. Patients with type A hypoglycaemia rapidly develop wasting and profound muscle weakness, and hypoglycaemia occurs only in the preterminal stage. In type B, the tumour is well differentiated and grows slowly, with little weight loss or muscle weakness until late in the disease. Hypoglycaemia develops 2 to 10 months before death, and is characterized by a precipitous fall in glucose level on fasting which is very difficult to control.

The exact mechanism for tumour-associated hypoglycaemia is not understood. Explanations that have been offered include: (i) increased utilization of glucose by the tumour; (ii) decreased production of glucose by the liver tissue; and (iii) production of insulin or insulin-like substance by the tumour. Evidence for insulin production is lacking, and some observations do not support this theory, such as slow disappearance of intravenously administered glucose and a less than normal decrease of serum inorganic phosphorus following intravenous glucose. It may be that type A is due to an increased requirement for glucose by a massive tumour, which exceeds the gluconeogenetic capability of the non-cancer liver, and that type B is secondary to an abnormal enzymatic pattern which results in glycogen storage with defective glycogenolysis.[23]

Hypercalcaemia

Hypercalcaemia, also called pseudohyperparathyroidism, occurs in hepatocellular carcinoma, particularly in sclerosing hepatocellular carcinoma (see above). Cochrane and Williams measured blood levels of parathyroid hormone in the hepatic and portal veins in one patient and demonstrated a large gradient, suggesting its production by the liver or tumour; after liver transplantation, blood calcium and parathyroid hormone levels were reduced dramatically.[26] Tashijan et al. (JExpMed, 1964; 119:467) demonstrated an immunological cross-reactivity between bovine parathyroid hormone and an antigenic extract from 6 of 12 tumours. Other immunological studies of sera from patients with pseudohyperparathyroidism suggested heterogeneity of immunoreactive parathyroid hormone associated with neoplasms.

Sexual precocity and gonadotrophin secretion

Sexual precocity associated with liver carcinoma is attributable to the secretion of ectopic gonadotrophin by the tumour, with positive biological tests for chorionic gonadotrophin in serum and liver extract. In one study (Braunstein, AnnIntMed, 1973; 78:857), 15 of 81 patients with hepatocellular carcinoma or hepatoblastoma were positive for chorionic gonadotrophin assays. This syndrome occurs exclusively in young boys having hepatocellular carcinoma or hepatoblastoma of a histologically well-differentiated type.

Other tumour-associated syndromes

Other syndromes reported include dysfibrinogenaemia, increased fibrinolytic activity in plasma, cryofibrinogenaemia, porphyria cutanea tarda with increased uroporphyrin, hypertrophic pulmonary osteoarthropathy, and carcinoid syndrome.

Diagnosis

Although definitive diagnosis depends on histological examination, this is not crucial in regions where the incidence of hepatocellular carcinoma is high. Diagnosis seems unequivocal in patients with established cirrhosis if serum α-fetoprotein is above 1000 ng/ml or rising sharply, and a mass lesion is found by ultrasonography and computed tomography (**CT**). Diagnosis becomes more definite if it is hypervascular on dynamic CT or angiography. Careful physical examination often suffices for diagnosing advanced hepatocellular carcinoma when a large hepatic mass with vascular murmurs is found in a patient living in a highly endemic area such as sub-Saharan Africa and China. In less obvious cases, laboratory tests that include HBsAg, anti-HCV, aminotransferase, albumin, gamma-globulin (for the diagnosis of chronic liver disease), α-fetoprotein and DCP, and imaging should be carried out. The imaging study includes plain chest and abdominal films, real-time ultrasonography, CT with dynamic enhancement or magnetic resonance imaging (**MRI**), radiocolloid scintigraphy, and coeliac angiography.

Plain radiography

Chest radiological examination may demonstrate coin lesions or elevation of the right hemidiaphragm or both. The whole right diaphragm may be elevated owing to a liver mass, or elevation may be localized. In such patients, a lateral view is indispensable. Localized elevation of the diaphragm must be differentiated from partial eventration of the diaphragm, which increases in incidence with advancing age (Okuda, BrJRadiol, 1979; 52:870). According to Levin *et al.* (SAMedJ 1976; 50:1323), only 36 per cent of 449 patients in South Africa showed normal chest films on admission. In the remainder, there were pulmonary metastases and/or elevation of the diaphragm. All these patients had advanced hepatocellular carcinoma and these figures do not apply to many other countries (definitely not to Japan). Abdominal films may demonstrate hepatomegaly and caudal displacement of the duodenal gas by an enlarged liver.

Radionuclide scanning

Despite improved instrumentation, the sensitivity of colloid scans for determining the size and location of a mass in the liver leaves much to be desired. Using $^{99}Tc^m$-labelled colloids, the smallest detectable superficial mass is 2 to 3 cm, and the sensitivity sharply drops for deep-seated lesions. Colloid uptake by a cirrhotic liver is irregular, particularly if the patient has been drinking heavily, and delineation of a small mass is unreliable (Fig. 22). Single photon emission CT (SPECT) and positron emission CT (PET) are slightly more sensitive than plain γ-camera imaging, but less so than other imaging modalities. Gallium-67 citrate, a carcinophilic agent, is taken up by hepatocellular carcinomas, but its uptake varies and is unpredictable. As hepatocellular carcinoma cells have biochemical functions similar to normal hepatocytes they may take up biliary imaging agents such as $^{99}Tc^m$-pyridoxyl-5-methyltryptophan (**PMT**). When scanned 3 to 8 h later, the tumour may still retain the agent because bile ducts are lacking, but the liver parenchyma has already cleared it; thus the mass is seen as a positive image against the liver silhouette (Fig. 23) (Hasegawa, Cancer, 1986; 57:230). This phenomenon is seen in more than one-half of Japanese patients but not in black African patients (Savitch, JNucMed, 1983; 24: 1119).

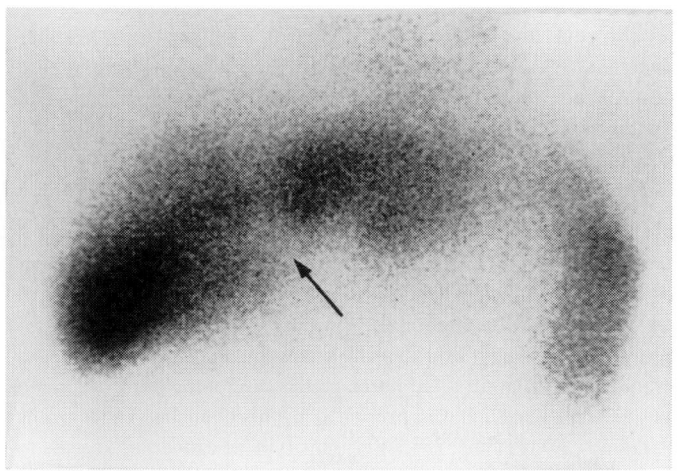

Fig. 22. Small hepatocellular carcinoma in a highly cirrhotic liver is difficult to detect by colloid scintigraphy. This patient had a 4 × 4-cm hepatocellular carcinoma near the hilum (at arrow), but on this scan the interpretation of this defect could be a normal hilum indented by dilated major portal branches.

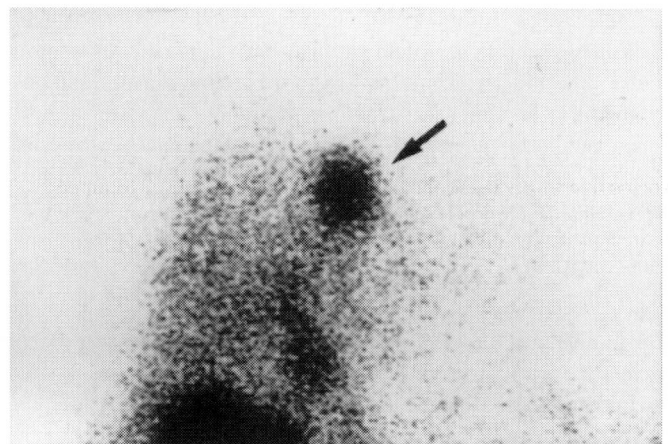

Fig. 23. Liver scan using a biliary imaging agent (PMT). This scan made 5 h later shows a small positive lesion (at arrow). Well-differentiated hepatocellular carcinoma cells take up the agent but cannot excrete it into bile.

Computed tomography

Most mass lesions including hepatocellular carcinomas larger than 2 cm are seen as areas of decreased attenuation. Occasionally, iso-dense tumours present problems in diagnosis if contrast enhancement is not used. The reported accuracy of CT for detecting metastatic liver tumours has been about 90 per cent. In Kunstlinger's series of 16 cases of hepatocellular carcinoma (AJR, 1980; 134:431), the detection rate was 94 per cent, and in Itai's series of 47 cases (Radiol, 1979; 131:165), 11 per cent gave a negative image. In our own experience with 116 cases of hepatocellular carcinoma, the tumour was hypodense in 87 per cent, isodense in 9.5 per cent, and hyperdense in none. The contrast between the tumour and surrounding parenchyma is usually enhanced by intravenous injection of iodinated contrast medium. A solitary or expanding hepatocellular carcinoma is usually hypodense, but in a liver with diffuse cirrhotic nodules, CT images are frequently

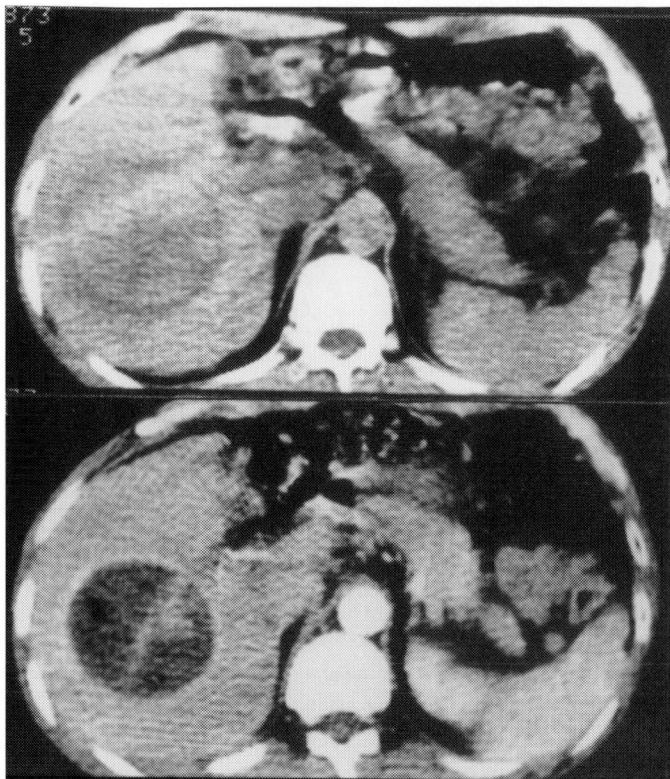

Fig. 24. Encapsulated hepatocellular carcinoma. The thick capsule is seen as a thin low-density rim around the mass on plain CT (upper), and by dynamic CT (lower) the capsule is enhanced. The interior of the mass shows a low density area (necrosis) as well as a high density area (actively growing with arterialization).

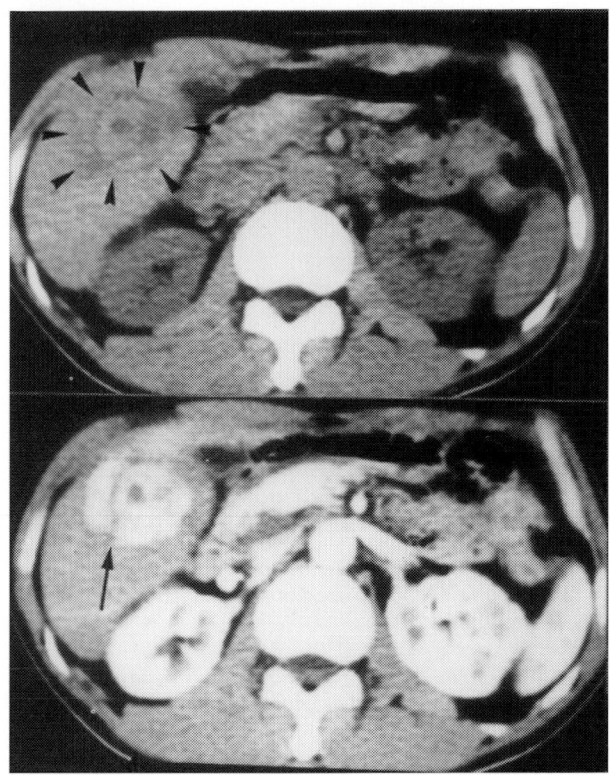

Fig. 25. A round, mixed low and isodense mass was seen in the right lobe inferiorly (segment V to VI) (at arrowheads, upper CT). On dynamic enhanced CT (lower), a thin non-enhanced septum became apparent as the mass itself was enhanced (arrow).

isodense with poor or no recognizable contrasts. If the mass is solitary and large, the interior often exhibits a non-homogeneous texture with varying densities, the hypodense areas perhaps representing necrosis. A thick capsule around the mass is suggested by a thin hypodense rim which is enhanced upon dynamic enhancement (Fig. 24), with bolus intravenous injection of contrast medium. Sometimes, septa may be discerned within such a mass (Fig. 25).

Bolus (dynamic) enhancement is also important for delineating an isodense lesion and differentiating it from haemangiomas. Following dynamic enhancement, a haemangioma is enhanced slowly from the periphery of the mass and increased contrast remains for a considerable period of time, whereas a hepatocellular carcinoma is enhanced immediately and uniformly (Fig. 26), and de-enhanced quickly. Dynamic CT also demonstrates arterioportal shunts (Nakayama, AJR, 1983; 140:953), a pathognomonic feature of hepatocellular carcinoma. Small lesions are difficult to delineate even with dynamic CT. Table 12 shows the sensitivity of CT examination (plain and dynamic combined) in hepatocellular carcinoma smaller than 5 cm.

One of the merits of CT is its diagnostic accuracy for underlying cirrhosis which exhibits irregularity of the surface, splenomegaly, collateral veins, and ascites. If one of the major portal branches is occluded by a tumour thrombus, the lobe of that particular side shows decreased density due to metabolic changes (Nishikawa, Radiol, 1981; 141:725). Dynamic CT is also useful in making the diagnosis of a tumour thrombus growing in the portal vein and

Table 12 Sensitivity of CT in the detection of small hepatocellular carcinoma (HCC)

Tumour size (cm)	No. of cases	No. of patients with detected HCC
<1	1	0
1–2	19	10 (53)
2–3	23	21 (91)
3–4	18	18 (100)
4–5	21	21 (100)

Data from Tsunetomi, JGastHepatol, 1989; 4:395.
Percentages in parentheses.
* Plain CT and dynamic CT combined.

inferior vena cava; a hyperdense peripheral ring is seen around the tumour thrombus. With the new helical (spiral) CT machine, one can carry out dynamic CT without knowledge of tumour location; the whole liver is sectioned within one breath hold. Detection of small hepatocellular carcinoma is further facilitated if CT is combined with hepatic anteriography (CTA) and anterial portography (CTAP).

Lipiodol CT

This modality was developed by Japanese surgeons (Konno, EurJCanClinOnc, 1983; 19:1053), and is the most sensitive technique for the detection of small hepatocellular carcinoma lesions. It

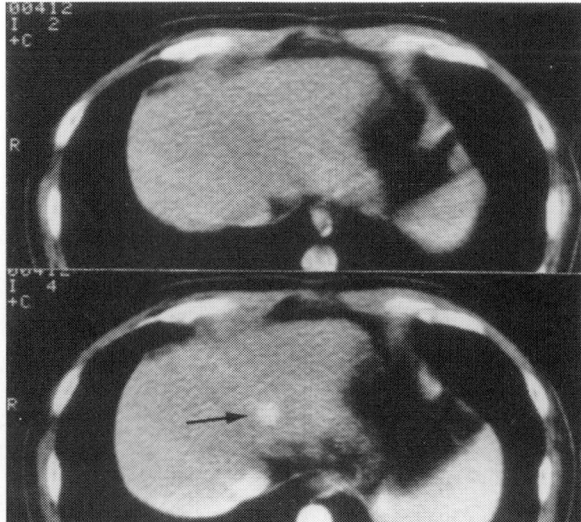

Fig. 26. This small hepatocellular carcinoma was isodense on plain CT (upper), and became enhanced upon bolus injection of contrast medium (at arrow, lower CT).

is based on the phenomenon that hepatocellular carcinoma is highly arterialized, and that Lipiodol, an oily contrast medium which is distributed throughout the liver parenchyma following arterial injection, is cleared by hepatocytes but not by hepatocellular carcinoma. After coeliac arteriography, a small amount of Lipiodol is injected into the hepatic artery and a CT scan is made 2 weeks later; hepatocellular carcinoma is clearly seen as a very dense lesion (Fig. 27), and a lesion as small as 3 mm may be discerned despite the partial volume phenomenon (Yumoto, Radiol, 1985; 154:19).

Magnetic resonance imaging

This modality is relatively new and is still progressing in instrumentation together with development of contrast media. At high magnetic fields of 1.5 to 2.0 T, scan time is shortened and with restricted respiratory movements and cardiac gating, the current images are much improved. At the moment, the diagnostic accuracy

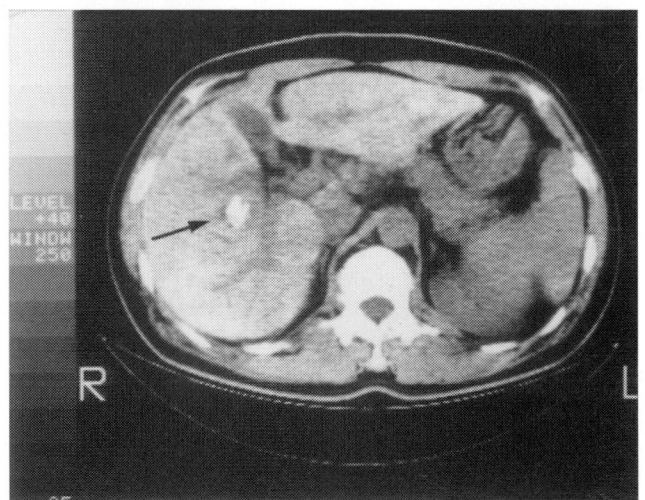

Fig. 27. Lipiodol CT clearly delineates this 1.5 × 2-cm hepatocellular carcinoma near the hilum; this was not discerned on plain CT.

Table 13 Detection of relatively small hepatocellular carcinomas (HCC) by MRI

Tumour size (cm)	No. of cases	No. of patients with detected HCC	Detectability (%)
<1.9	3	1	33.3
2.0–2.9	9	8	88.9
3.0–3.9	8	8	100
4.0–4.9	8	8	100
5.0+	15	15	100

Data from Ebara, Radiol, 1986; 159:371.

for hepatic neoplasms is about the same as that with CT, but MRI has several advantages over CT such as blood-flow study and tissue diagnosis. Itai *et al.* (JComputAssistTomogr, 1986; 10:963) studied 42 cases of hepatocellular carcinoma; the presence of tumour was suggested in 41 by a high intensity area on T_2-weighted spin-echo images with a repetition time of 1.6 s. Specific findings of hepatocellular carcinoma such as a capsule (Fig. 28), mosaic interior, and tumour thrombus in major veins were noted in 10, 7, and 7 cases, respectively. The same author (Radiol, 1987; 164:21) compared MRI (at 1.5 T) and CT in the diagnosis of hepatocellular carcinoma in 60 patients. MRI was superior to CT in demonstrating the details of tumours, especially pseudocapsules. In 58, main tumours were detected by T_1-weighted spin-echo (600 ms/25 ms), and the tumour was hyperintense in 18 (Fig. 29(a)), isointense in 10, and hypointense in 30. On 2000/60 ms sequences, all but 2 had high signal intensity. Ebara *et al.* (Radiol, 1986; 159:371) studied relatively small hepatocellular carcinoma lesions in 43 patients and demonstrated that the detection rate depended on tumour size, being 97.5 per cent for hepatocellular carcinomas larger than 2 cm (Table 13). They also found that MRI closely reflected tissue changes within the tumour, and found increased copper content in small hyperintense hepatocellular carcinomas on T_1-weighted images (Ebara, Radiol, 1991; 180:617). One other advantage of MRI is its capability to differentiate hepatocellular carcinoma from haemangioma, a benign lesion frequently detected by ultrasonography, which is not to be confused with hepatocellular carcinoma. In their study with a 0.26-T system, the average T_2 value of hepatocellular carcinoma was 80.8 ± 92 ms, whereas that of haemangioma was 139.4 ± 59.7 ms. Ohtomo *et al.* (Radiol, 1988; 168:621) also found significant differences in T_2 values at 1.5 T in 72 cases of hepatocellular carcinoma and 56 of haemangioma (Table 14).

Table 14 Differences in T_2 values between hepatocellular carcinoma (HCC) and benign haemangioma

MRI system (T)	Tumour size (cm)	HCC (ms)	Haemangioma (ms)
0.26*		80.8 ± 9.2	139.4 ± 59.7
1.5+	<2	46.1 ± 9.8	85.3 ± 21.2
	>2		97.0 ± 15.9

* Data taken from Ebara, Radiol, 1986; 159:371.
+ Data taken from Ohtomo, Radiol, 1988; 168:621.

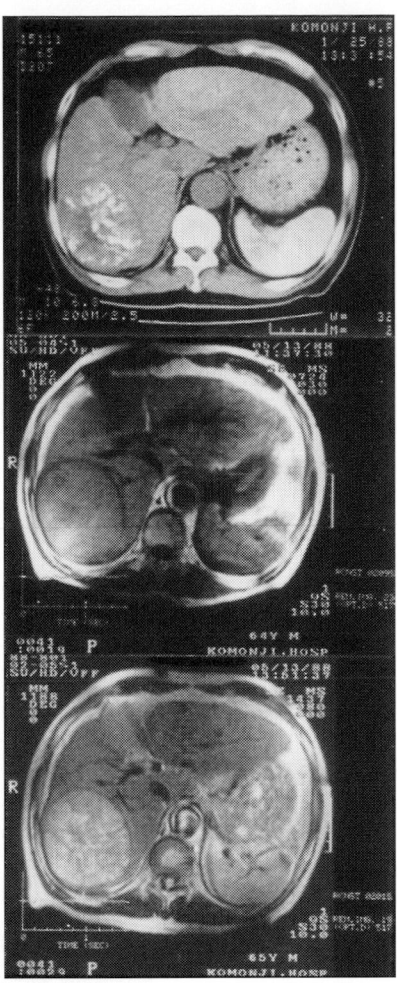

Fig. 28. A large expanding mass, with previously injected Lipiodol deposited, is seen in the right lobe posteriorly (segments VI to VII) on CT (top). The capsule is recognized more clearly on MR images. Middle, T_1-weighted image (SE 724/30). Bottom, T_2-weighted image (SE 1437/80). The capsule is also clearly seen.

With enhancement agents as in CT, dynamic imaging using a high tesla system can be carried out. Ohtomo *et al.* (Radiol, 1987; 163:27) used gadolinium diethylenetriaminepentaacetate, a paramagnetic complex, in 36 patients with hepatocellular carcinoma, and demonstrated that degree of contrast enhancement corresponded to tumour vascularity and that the peripheral halo in the delayed phase corresponded to a fibrous capsule. Several other contrast agents have been developed, such as superparamagnetic iron oxide particles (ferrite), which are not taken up by hepatocellular carcinoma (Stark, Radiol, 1988; 168:297; Hahn, Radiol, 1990; 174:361) (Fig. 29(b)).

Ultrasonography

Real-time ultrasonography using a linear, convex, or sector transducer is a most practical and useful method for the detection of space-occupying lesions in the liver. Not only are localized lesions and vascular and ductal structures seen, but with these scans splenomegaly, ascites, and even large collateral veins are recognized easily (Okuda, Hepatol, 1981; 1:662). If irregularity of the hepatic surface can be identified, diagnosis of coexistent cirrhosis becomes more definite. A tumour is seen as a round lesion having echo patterns different from the surrounding homogeneous parenchyma, but its organ of origin cannot be specifically defined. The interior echo of a mass, determined perhaps by its histological composition, may vary from case to case, even among the same kind of carcinoma. In a metastatic carcinoma, the interior is often hyperechoic, less often mixed hyper- and hypoechoic with or without central or peripheral sonolucency, or diffusely hypoechoic (Kamin, Radiol, 1979; 131:459). A large hepatocellular carcinoma may exhibit similar echo patterns and is not distinguishable from a metastatic carcinoma, but the coexisting cirrhotic changes assist in differential diagnosis. A diffuse hepatocellular carcinoma displays an irregular parenchymal echogenicity without a distinct tumour echo, and is sometimes difficult to identify.

A small hepatocellular carcinoma, particularly when smaller than 3 cm, more often shows a hypoechoic interior or a rim (Fig. 30), in contrast to a more frequent hyperechoic pattern in a metastatic carcinoma of comparable size (Shinagawa, JpnJGastro, 1981; 78: 2402). It is now known that very small hepatocellular carcinoma lesions often undergo fatty change and are seen as hyperechoic lesions; such lesions resemble small haemangiomas (Fig. 31). The current problem facing hepatologists and radiologists in the Far East is the differential diagnosis between small hepatocellular carcinoma and haemangioma, and ultrasonography alone may not be able to distinguish the two. For more definitive differentiation, dynamic CT and MRI, and sometimes angiography are required. If the diagnosis is still equivocal, the patient can be followed for 6 months or so to see if the lesion is growing.[23] A haemangioma seldom grows (Gibney, AJR, 1987; 149:953).

An important merit of real-time ultrasonography is its ability to demonstrate major portal and hepatic veins, and intravascular tumour thrombi (Fig. 32). Complete occlusion of the portal vein is followed by cavernomatous transformation at the porta hepatis (Ohnishi, Gastro, 1985; 88:1034), readily seen by ultrasonography. For the detection of a lesion in the right lobe immediately below the diaphragm, the convex transducer excels other types of transducer. As discussed below, ultrasonography is indispensable in early detection of hepatocellular carcinoma among patients with chronic liver disease. It also assists in aimed biopsy. Doppler ultrasonography, particularly colour Doppler, is being used more frequently in the diagnosis of hepatocellular carcinoma. It can differentiate blood-clot and tumour thrombi in the portal vein. Contrast agents that augment echogenicity of blood are being developed, but it remains to be seen how much blood flow measurement contributes to the early diagnosis of hepatocellular carcinoma.

Angiography

Although invasive coeliac angiography is valuable in the diagnosis of hepatocellular carcinoma and other space-occupying lesions of the liver. This and other modalities frequently prove complementary. It is indispensable in differential diagnosis between hepatocellular carcinoma and other less vascular lesions such as cholangiocarcinoma and haemangioma. Coeliac angiography also provides information about the gross anatomical features of the tumour (Okuda, Radiol, 1977; 123:21), presence of tumour thrombus in the portal vein (Okuda, Radiol, 1975; 117:303) and hepatic vein (Okuda, Radiol, 1977; 124:33), and existence of a fibrous capsule (Okuda,

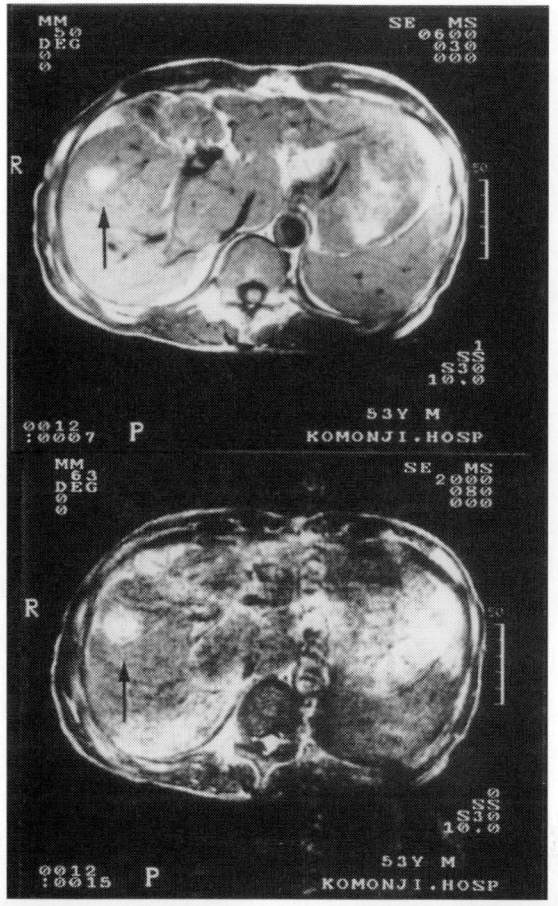

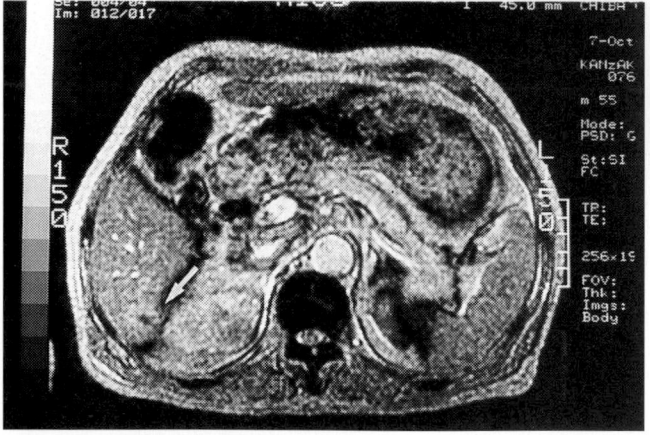
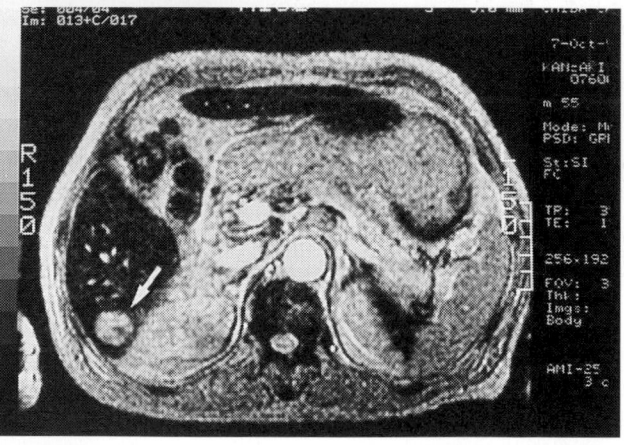

Fig. 29. (a) MR image of a small hepatocellular carcinoma (arrow). It is a high intensity mass on a T_1-weighted image (above, SE 600/30) and is also of high intensity on a T_2-weighted image (below, SE 2000/80) (by courtesy of Dr Iwamoto). (b) Enhanced MR image of a small hepatocellular carcinoma. Plain gradient echo image (left) and after administration of ferrite (right) (by courtesy of Dr Ebara).

Cancer, 1977; 40:1240). For the delineation of a small hepatocellular carcinoma, infusion arteriography is perhaps the most effective (Takashima, Radiol, 1980; 136:321) but superselective catheterization is required. A lesion lying over the spinal column, and hence obscure on angiography, may be better recognized by digital subtraction angiography (Okuda, SemLivDis, 1989; 9:50).

Well-differentiated hepatocellular carcinoma has abundant blood sinuses with increased arterial supply, and therefore the lesion displays hypervascularity, neovasculature, and tumour stains (Fig. 33) in which contrast medium temporarily remains on the surface of the endothelial lining. In contrast, poorly differentiated hepatocellular carcinoma may be hypovascular. In our series of 170 advanced cases of hepatocellular carcinoma, lack of hypervascularity occurred in only 4.1 per cent (Table 15). However, small hepatocellular carcinoma seldom demonstrates hypervascularity; it is recognized from a stain, and increased or displaced arteries around it (Fig. 34). If the lesions are very small, stains are the only abnormal findings (Fig. 35) (Table 16) (Sumida, AJR, 1986; 147:531).

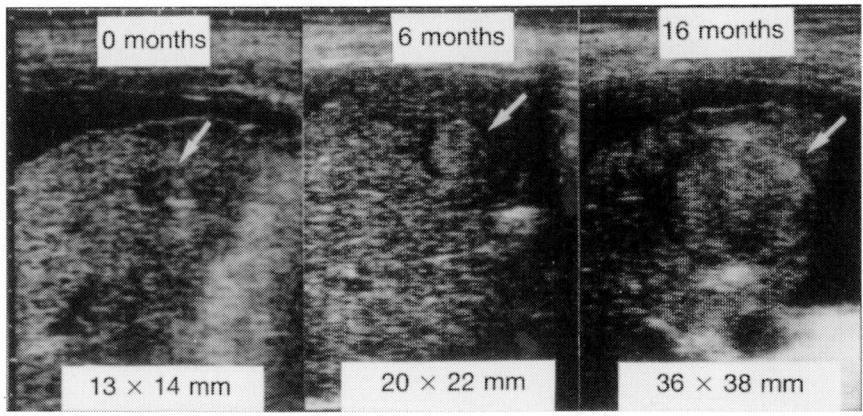

Fig. 30. Small hepatocellular carcinoma followed for 16 months. At detection, the mass was hypoechoic measuring 13 × 14 mm (arrow). At 6 months, it had a hypoechoic periphery and an isoechoic interior (arrow), and at 16 months it measured 36 × 38 mm with a mixed echo interior. The doubling time was 3 months.

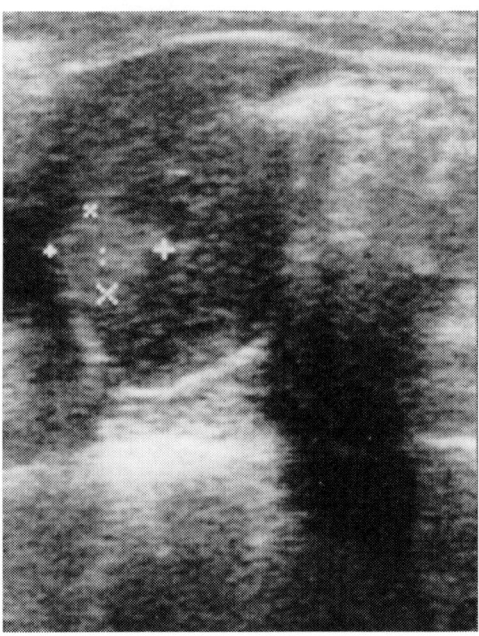

Fig. 31. A haemangioma is seen as a homogeneously hyperechoic mass by ultrasonography.

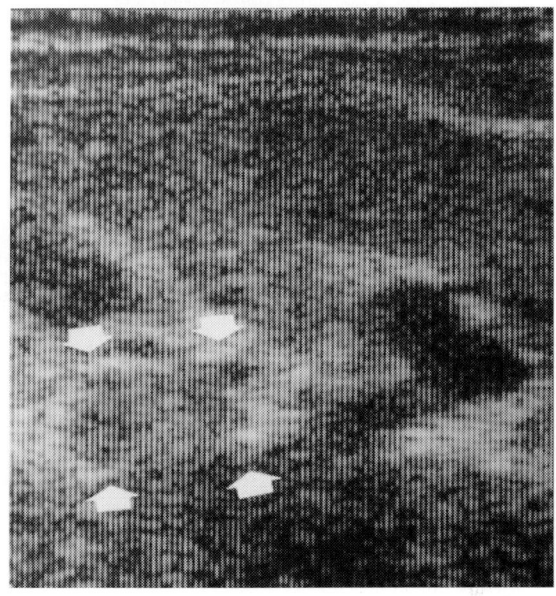

Fig. 32. Portal vein tumour thrombus (at arrows) seen by ultrasonography. The lumen of the portal vein, which is normally anechoic, is echogenic in this case.

One important piece of information provided by angiography is whether there is an actively growing tumour thrombus in the portal vein or its major branch. Such a thrombus receives ample arterial supply and is seen as bundle of threads (thread and streaks sign, Fig. 33), as demonstrated by postmortem arteriography (Fig. 36). Through the tumour thrombus, contrast medium injected into the hepatic artery may flow longitudinally and retrogradely into the splenic vein. Small portal branches are frequently opacified during the arterial phase of angiography indicating the presence of arterioportal communications. Such communications occur through intraportal tumour thrombi (Okuda, Radiol, 1977; 122:53). Benign haemangiomas exhibit stains resembling cotton wool on hepatic arteriography, and the stain remains for a much longer period compared with hepatocellular carcinoma.

Catheterization of the hepatic (coeliac) artery is a necessary procedure for Lipiodol CT (see above). With the same technique,

Table 15 Angiographic changes and their frequencies in advanced hepatocellular carcinoma (170 cases)

Findings	No. positive (%)
Hypervascularity	163 (95.9)
Tumour stain	160 (95.2)
Displaced large arteries	121 (71.6)
Arterial tumour vessels	112 (65.9)
Encasement of arteries	92 (54.1)
Arterioportal shunts	88 (53.4)
Portal regurgitation	45 (26.6)
Radiolucent rim (capsule)	23 (13.5)

All tumours were greater than 5 cm.

Table 16 Angiographic changes and their frequency in small hepatocellular carcinoma (51 cases)				
	No. positive (%)			
	1–2 cm (n = 9)	2–3 cm (n = 26)	3–4 cm (n = 7)	4–5 cm (n = 9)
Increased vascularity	1	9	2	6
Displacement	0	5	3	8
Encasement	0	1	0	0
Dilated artery	0	0	0	0
Arterioportal shunt	0	0	0	0
Tumour stain	7	22	5	8
Portal thrombi	0	0	0	0

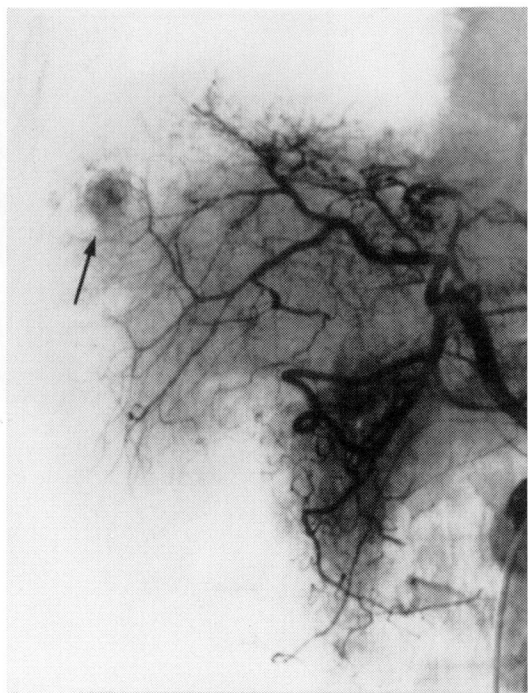

Fig. 34. This 2-cm hepatocellular carcinoma is not only showing a tumour stain, but also has some hypervascularity. Arterial branches near the mass are displaced curvilinearly.

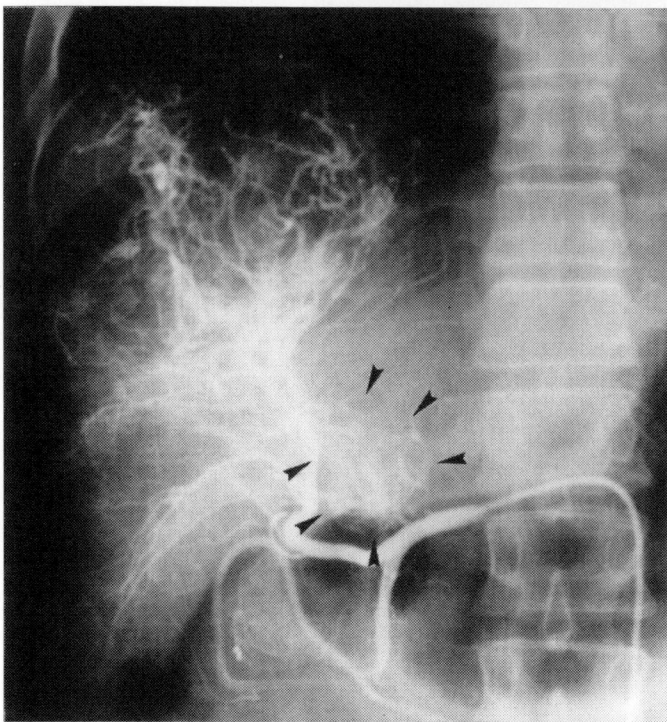

Fig. 33. Hypervascular hepatocellular carcinoma occupies the cranial half of the right lobe. There are very thin thread-like densities (arrowheads) in the hilar area. They represent a large growing tumour thrombus in the portal vein (thread and streaks sign).

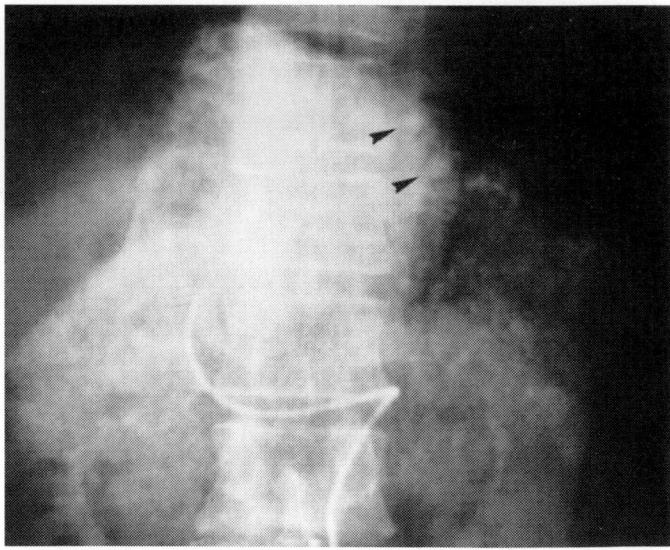

Fig. 35. Infusion hepatic arteriography demonstrating two 1-cm tumour stains (arrowheads). Note that the catheter tip is in the proper hepatic artery past the gastroduodenal.

the superior mesenteric artery may also be catheterized for arteriography. This procedure permits opacification of the portal vein in the venous phase and this postarteriographic (arterial) portography is important in the detection of portal tumour thrombosis which will contraindicate surgery (Fig. 37); it can also be combined with CT (see above).

Liver biopsy

Blind needle biopsy is not recommended in the diagnosis of hepatocellular carcinoma, or of any tumour suspected as being hepatocellular carcinoma, because of the risk of bleeding. If the tumour is on the surface of the liver, bleeding may never cease. It is less hazardous if there is sufficient parenchyma between the mass and the liver capsule. With the current imaging modalities available,

aimed biopsy is a necessity. For aimed biopsy, ultrasonography is superior to CT; several ultrasonography transducers are available, one aiming straight (Ohto, Radiol, 1980; 136:171) and the other at an angle (Makuuchi, Radiol, 1980; 136:165). To prevent seeding of cancer cells along the needle path, the thinnest possible needle is desirable, such as the 22-gauge needle developed in our department which has a Menghini device in it. Aspiration cytology is much less diagnostic, particularly when cancer cells are well differentiated,

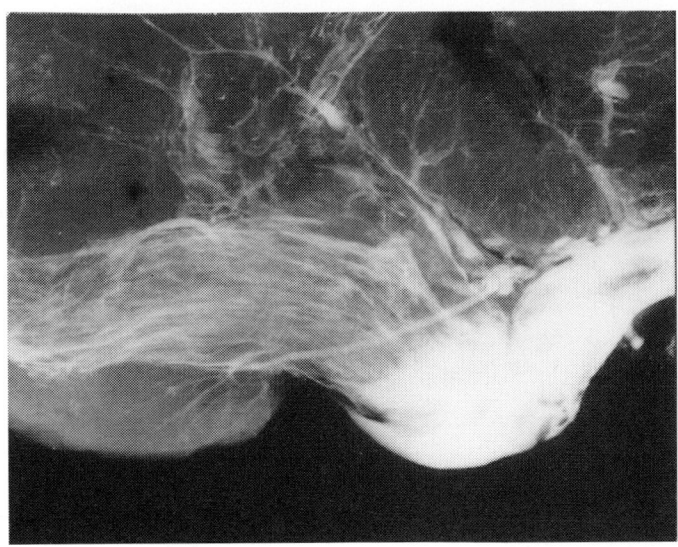

Fig. 36. Postmortem angiography. The portal tumour thrombus is seen as a bundle of threads (arterially supplied).

since they resemble normal hepatocytes if smeared on glass slides and stained.

Early detection and mass screening

In the early 1970s, Masseyeff and his group attempted to detect hepatocellular carcinoma by screening normal people in Senegal

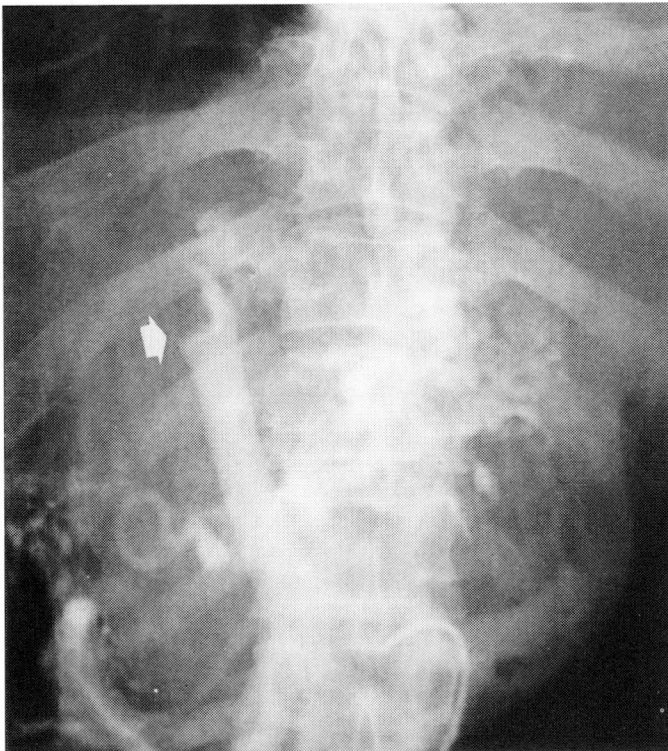

Fig. 37. Postsuperior mesenteric arteriographic portogram. Sudden cut-off of the portal vein (at arrow) is apparent, suggesting occlusion by a tumour thrombus.

using the Ouchterlony method for α-fetoprotein; they found hepatocellular carcinoma in three individuals, but only one was small enough to permit resection (Gann, MonogrCancerRes, 1973; 14:3). A similar attempt in South Africa failed. Much better results were obtained in the People's Republic of China where mass screening for hepatocellular carcinoma was first launched in 1971, during the Cultural Revolution, as part of the national campaign for cancer control. Later, a more concentrated screening programme was carried out using a technique more sensitive than the Ouchterlony method, where 48 patients with asymptomatic hepatocellular carcinoma were found in a 5-year period from 1972 to 1976; the tumour was resectable in 68.6 per cent of them. Subsequently, similar programmes have been rewarding in Shanghai City and Qidong, and α-fetoprotein measurement is now generally used for identifying patients with asymptomatic hepatocellular carcinoma in these areas.

In Japan, Okuda *et al.* first studied patients with hepatocellular carcinoma smaller than 4.5 cm and found all had cirrhosis, and that α-fetoprotein values were generally low, with only a few exceptions (Gastro, 1977; 73:109); they suggested that a very close follow-up with scintigraphy and α-fetoprotein measurement was necessary for early diagnosis. Subsequent studies by the same (Kubo, Gastro, 1978; 74:578), and other groups (Obata, IntJCanc, 1980; 25:741), found that the size of hepatocellular carcinoma detected from a sudden sharp rise of α-fetoprotein was larger than 4 cm, just detectable by scintigraphy. The introduction of real-time ultrasonography into clinical medicine totally changed the approach of physicians to the early detection of hepatocellular carcinoma, since abdominal ultrasonography is much more sensitive than scintigraphy, can be performed on outpatients, and takes little time. It was also learned subsequently, that some patients with small hepatocellular carcinomas show diagnostically high levels of α-fetoprotein, and that a slight but continuous elevation of serum α-fetoprotein levels, measured by radioimmunoassay, is suggestive of small hepatocellular carcinoma. In other words, α-fetoprotein is still useful and should be measured at regular intervals for the detection of small hepatocellular carcinomas. The interval with which patients with chronic liver disease are followed should vary with the degree of risk of developing hepatocellular carcinoma. Our study with ultrasonography in which the speed of growth of small hepatocellular carcinoma was measured (Ebara, Gastro, 1986; 90: 289) showed that on average it took 3 months for a hepatocellular carcinoma of 2 cm to expand by 1 cm (Fig. 38). A study in Taiwan (Sheu, Gastro, 1985; 89:259) analysed the growth speed differently but produced a similar figure. In their observation with ultrasonography, the most rapidly growing hepatocellular carcinoma of 1 cm took 4.6 months to reach 3 cm, and an interval of 4 to 5 months was suggested as practical. This policy for early detection depends on the cost. Radioimmunoassay of α-fetoprotein is expensive and, unless the national health insurance policy permits frequent α-fetoprotein measurements in patients with cirrhosis, this strategy is difficult to execute. Recent studies in Japan all showed figures between 4 and 10 per cent for the annual rate of hepatocellular carcinoma detection in patients with cirrhosis by a regular follow-up, and the calculated cost for detecting hepatocellular carcinoma in one patient with ultrasonography carried out four times per year, α-fetoprotein measurement four times per year, and CT every 8 months is US$4115 (10 per cent detection rate/year) to $8230 (5 per

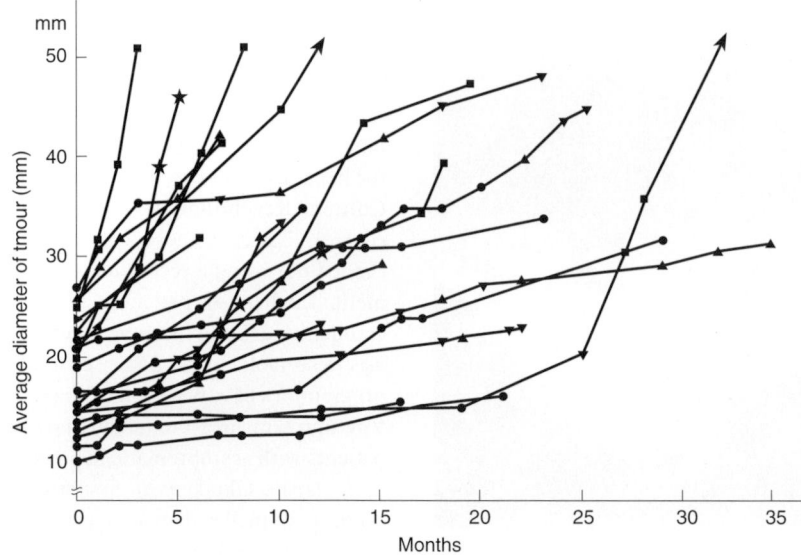

Fig. 38. Measurement of tumour growth speed in 22 patients with hepatocellular carcinoma smaller than 3 cm. The growth speed varies a great deal in individual cases and it may also change suddenly (tumour spread within liver).

cent detection rate). In countries where hepatocellular carcinoma is less prevalent, this early detection strategy is too costly.

Currently, most Japanese gastroenterologists follow patients with cirrhosis at intervals of 3 to 4 months, and in Italy every 6 months (Colombo, NEJM, 1991; 325:675).

Some centres do not depend totally on ultrasonography, and carry out CT scans at an interval of 6 to 10 months. Sometimes CT identifies a small lesion not detected by ultrasonography. With this strategy, small hepatocellular carcinoma is found in patients with cirrhosis, and occasionally in patients with chronic hepatitis. The results of this strategy have been remarkable; when we analysed 300 consecutive hepatocellular carcinoma cases seen during the period from January 1980 to October 1985, hepatocellular carcinomas were smaller than 5 cm at the time of diagnosis in 57.3 per cent, and smaller than 2 cm in 14.6 per cent. More recent corresponding figures are 80 and 20 per cent.

With increasing use of ultrasonography, several problems have arisen. One is the differential diagnosis from benign lesions, particularly haemangioma, which occurs at a rate of several per cent among the Japanese adult population. For this differential diagnosis, dynamic CT, coeliac angiography, and MRI are useful (see above). Large benign regenerative nodules are also picked up by ultrasonography. Biopsy is interpreted as a non-malignant nodule. However, such lesions, which have a differing sonographic texture, should be suspected as being histologically different from the surrounding parenchyma; close follow-up is required.

Histological characteristics of early hepatocellular carcinoma

With rapidly increasing numbers of resected specimens of hepatocellular carcinoma and similar lesions, and of patients followed after resection, it is now generally accepted in Japan that large hyperplastic nodules recognized by imaging, and interpreted histologically as non-malignant, are frequently premalignant or very early hepatocellular carcinoma. The conventional histological criteria for

malignant cells such as large nuclei, increased nucleus/cytoplasm ratio, and mitosis are not present in an extremely well-differentiated hepatocellular carcinoma.[27] Such lesions, if left alone, start growing and exhibit typical histological features of hepatocellular carcinoma within a year or two (Arakawa, JGastHepatol, 1986; 1:3). Careful examination of a large hyperplastic nodule often demonstrates nodules within nodules (Arakawa, Gastro, 1986; 91:198), the smaller nodules originating within a large older nodule. The smaller newer ones are clearly malignant. The cells in the larger nodule, or the older clone of cells, often exhibit subtle features of malignant transformation, such as nuclear crowding (Fig. 39(a)), acinar formation (Fig. 39(b)), and basophilia while the normal cell thickness is kept (normotrabecular) (Kondo, Hepatol, 1989; 9:751). It has also been found that within such an early hepatocellular carcinoma there occur changes of cell clones; early changes are usually extremely well differentiated, and later clones less well differentiated.[28] However, most imaging techniques are incapable of differentiating benign hyperplastic nodules and those that are destined to turn malignant (Takayama, Lancet, 1990; 336:1150). A key feature for differentiating preneoplastic and early cancer lesions is to identify the blood supply, whether portal or arterial. Attempts have been made with techniques using contrast agent in ultrasonography (Kudo, Radiol, 1992; 182:155). No similar studies have been done with alcoholic cirrhotic livers which, according to Peters, [11] may exhibit paraneoplastic changes within micronodules. Malignant transformation may also occur *de novo* unrelated to nodular lesions.

Differential diagnosis (Table 17)

Any mass lesion in the liver has to be differentiated from hepatocellular carcinoma. Cystic lesions are very unlikely to be hepatocellular carcinoma, but in rare cases the interior of hepatocellular carcinoma is necrotized and liquefied, giving an appearance of an abscess on imaging.[17] We.have seen a lesion on CT with a density index lower than water and similar to that of fat. It was necessary to

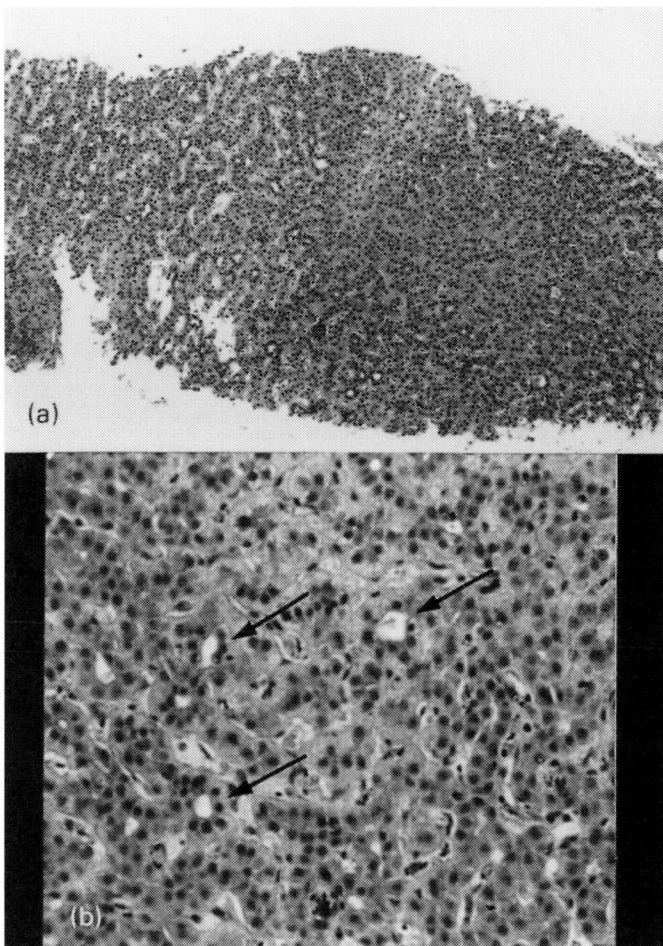

Fig. 39. Extremely well-differentiated hepatocellular carcinoma from a biopsy of a small lesion found by ultrasonography. (a) Nuclear crowding is apparent (haematoxylin and eosin, 40 ×). (b) Within the same section, there are acinar formations (at arrows) mixed with cords of two or three cell thickness which may be called 'normotrabecular' hepatocellular carcinoma (by courtesy of Dr F. Kondo).

change the tentative diagnosis of lipoma to hepatocellular carcinoma when biopsy disclosed fatty changes of hepatocellular carcinoma tissue with deposition of cholesterol crystals.

Metastatic carcinoma

This is usually, but not always, multiple—occurring in a non-cirrhotic liver. Serum α-fetoprotein is not elevated and, if the origin of the tumour is the digestive tract or pancreas, other tumour markers such as carcinoembryonic antigen, carbohydrate antigen 19–9, and tissue polypeptide antigen may be elevated. It is necessary to exclude all the possible primary cancers before the diagnosis of hepatocellular carcinoma is made; therefore, the stomach, colon, pancreas, lung, and kidney must be carefully examined radiologically, and by various types of imaging. Dynamic CT and coeliac angiography demonstrate peripheral enhancement, compared with the homogeneous enhancement and neovascularization in the case

of hepatocellular carcinoma. However, some metastatic sarcomas exhibit hypervascularity (Okuda, SemLivDis, 1989; 9:50).

Cholangiocarcinoma

This occurs usually in non-cirrhotic liver, and without elevated α-fetoprotein. Occasional cases show mild α-fetoprotein elevation, however. Obstructive jaundice is frequently the presenting symptom. Angiographically, it is hypo- or normovascular, and seldom hypervascular. Even if vascularity is increased, there is not the bizarre neovasculature often seen in hepatocellular carcinoma. In cholangiocarcinoma of the peripheral type[29] there is dilatation of the intrahepatic bile duct radiating from the lesion, demonstrable with CT and ultrasonography (Okuda, WorldJSurg, 1988; 12:18).

Angiosarcoma

There may be an aetiological factor such as exposure to thorotrast, vinyl chloride monomer, or other known carcinogenic chemicals. This occurs in a non-cirrhotic liver with multiple lesions and early extrahepatic metastases. Serum α-fetoprotein is not elevated. Angiographically, multiple poolings of contrast medium are seen (Okuda, Liver, 1981; 1:110). Final diagnosis is possible only with biopsy.

Adenoma and focal nodular hyperplasia

These lesions, particularly the former, occur mostly in women taking contraceptive drugs, whereas hepatocellular carcinoma is seen predominantly in males. The liver is not cirrhotic. Serum α-fetoprotein is not elevated. Angiographically, focal nodular hyperplasia and most adenomas show hypervascularity, arteries entering the mass from the periphery; in focal nodular hyperplasia it is supplied from the centre. Imaging with CT and MRI will delineate a central radiating scar in the case of focal nodular hyperplasia. Arterial flow radiating from the centre may be recognized with the new ultrasonography technique in which CO_2 microbubbles are used (Kudo, AJR, 1992; 158:65). There is no portal invasion or arteriovenous shunt. Oncofetal seromarkers do not rise.

Benign haemangioma

Small haemangiomas are difficult to distinguish from small hyperechoic hepatocellular carcinoma (see above). There are characteristic features of haemangioma such as slow enhancement of the mass from the periphery, and a longer retention of contrast medium, compared with rapid enhancement of the entire mass and rapid disappearance of the contrast in the case of hepatocellular carcinoma. In a large haemangioma, angiography will prove diagnostic as many vascular lakes resembling cotton wool are seen in the periphery. Most small haemangiomas remain unchanged in size during clinical follow-up (Gibney, AJR, 1987; 149:953), while there is demonstrable growth of small hepatocellular carcinoma.[30] However, we have seen one small haemangioma which increased in size during a 3-year follow-up; a diagnosis of hepatocellular carcinoma was made and an unnecessary resection was carried out.

Liver abscess

Occasionally, very poorly differentiated hepatocellular carcinoma presents with high fever, and a space-occupying lesion on imaging.

Table 17 Differential diagnosis

Disease	Diagnostic features	Investigations
Metastatic cancer	Multiple lesions, no cirrhosis, negative α-fetoprotein, no portal invasion	Oncofetal seromarkers, biopsy, CT, angiography
Cholangiocarcinoma	No cirrhosis, hypovascular mass, negative α-fetoprotein, no portal invasion	Oncofetal seromarkers, biopsy, CT, angiography
Angiosarcoma	Exposure to thorotrast, vinyl chloride, etc.; no cirrhosis, negative α-fetoprotein, multiple contrast pooling, early extrahepatic metastases	Oncofetal seromarkers, CT, angiography, biopsy
Adenoma, focal nodular hyperplasia	Use of contraceptives, no cirrhosis, negative α-fetoprotein, hypervascular, no portal invasion	Oncofetal seromarkers, biopsy, CT, angiography
Haemangioma	Negative α-fetoprotein, no portal invasion, slow peripheral enhancement	Oncofetal seromarkers, dynamic CT, MRI, angiography
Liver abscess	High fever, leucocytosis, negative α-fetoprotein, no portal invasion, low density interior, purulent content	Oncofetal seromarkers, CT, ultrasonography, aspiration

There is leucocytosis and severe prostration. The interior of the mass may be necrotic, giving an imaging feature similar to that of abscess (Okuda, Hepatol, 1991; 13:695). Only biopsy can provide the differential diagnosis.

Therapy

Complete cure can only be expected if the cancer tissue is totally removed. However, most patients who develop hepatocellular carcinoma have underlying cirrhosis which makes surgery difficult; furthermore, cirrhosis itself is a preneoplastic state, and new cancer lesions may arise after surgery. At the National Cancer Center Hospital, Tokyo, the recurrence rate after resection for small (less than 5 cm) hepatocellular carcinoma has been 74 per cent at 5 years (Takayasu, Hepatol, 1992; 16:906), and in a series of 28 resections of tumour in non-cirrhotic livers, the recurrence rate was 39 per cent in 2 years (Okuda, JGastHepatol, 1986; 1:129). Some liver surgeons now question whether surgery is indicated. However in most studies, the survival curves for those who undergo surgery are better than for those treated non-surgically, even if both groups were at a comparable stage of the disease. This is in part due to selection of patients for surgery; among patients at the same stage, those who have better liver function tests, and hence better hepatic reserve, tend to be chosen for surgery. We have observed (Ebara, Gastro, 1986; 90:289) that patients with small hepatocellular carcinoma (less than 3 cm), who received no specific treatment, did fairly well with a 1-year survival rate close to 90 per cent. In such patients with cirrhosis, operative death is not uncommon due to postoperative hepatic failure, and the 1-year postoperative survival is invariably lower than that of untreated patients. However, at 3 years, the majority of untreated patients have died and the survival rate for patients treated with surgery is always better.

We are of the opinion that if transplantation is carried out in an early stage of hepatocellular carcinoma without extrahepatic metastasis, it will afford a complete cure.

It is useful to remember the chronological development of the therapy of hepatocellular carcinoma. In the early days, systemic chemotherapy was the only available treatment; the response rate was very low, although occasionally a partial response was obtained.

In Japan, bolus injection of chemotherapeutic agents into the hepatic artery (one-shot chemotherapy) became popular in the 1960s, and remained the major method of treatment until 1977 when Yamada and his colleagues[31] began embolizing the hepatic artery, a procedure developed in the United States for treating renal cancer. This technique was quickly adopted by others in the late 1970s, because the results with one-shot chemotherapy had not been satisfactory; in the early 1980s one-shot chemotherapy was totally replaced by transcatheter arterial embolization. This proved better than one-shot therapy,[32] but the overall results were still unsatisfactory. Then came targeted chemotherapy and chemo-embolization. This trend was initiated by the development of a chemotherapeutic agent called SMANCS (styrene–maleic acid-conjugated neocarzinostatin) (Konno, EurJCanClinOnc, 1983; 19: 1053). This was mixed with Lipiodol and administered into the hepatic artery, with the rationale that Lipiodol would remain in cancer tissue and effect a slow release of the chemotherapeutic agent. Lipiodol suddenly became very popular following the development of the imaging technique called 'Lipiodol CT' (see above). It is now believed that the therapeutic effect is enhanced if cancer tissue receives a chemotherapeutic agent in a targeted fashion, followed by blockage of the arterial flow by embolization, so that the agent is not readily washed away. At about the same time, our group developed the technique of intratumour injection of ethanol for the treatment of small hepatocellular carcinoma found in a cirrhotic liver.[33] There have been a number of other approaches in recent years, but their efficacy remains to be determined.

Surgical treatment

Operative techniques have vastly improved over the years (Fortner, Cancer, 1981; 47:2162; Iwatsuki, AnnSurg, 1983; 197:247). Originally, bleeding during hepatectomy was such a problem that Professor Lin's finger fracture method[34] was adopted by many surgeons because of the demand for a quick operation. At present, several cutting instruments which minimize bleeding are available. The improvement is particularly significant if past and present rates of operative death are compared; Table 18 tabulates the relevant figures on surgical treatment for hepatocellular carcinoma compiled

Table 18 Trends in surgery for hepatocellular carcinoma (HCC) in Japan (Japan Liver Cancer Study Group)

Period	No. of HCC cases registered	No. of resections*	No. of exploratory laparotomies (%)	Operative deaths (%)	Reference
1968–1977	2 014	288	409 (20.3)	27.5 (died within 1 month)	10
1978–1979	1 047	279	111 (10.5)		Cancer, 1984; 54:1747
1980–1981	2 038	619	60 (2.9)	4.2	Cancer, 1987; 60:1411
1982–1983	2 054	888	59 (2.8)	3.9	ActaHepatolJpn, 1986; 27:1161
1984–1985	2 300	1286	0	3.4	ActaHepatolJpn, 1988; 29:1619
1986–1987	2 982	1839	0	3.1	ActaHepatolJpn, 1991; 32:1138
1988–1989	10 082	2990	0	1.9	ActaHepatolJpn, 1993; 34:805
1990–1991	10 988	3734	0	2.7	ActaHepatolJpn, 1995; 36:208

* Resection rates range from 14 to 20 per cent of all cases with and without tissue diagnosis.

by the Japan Liver Cancer Study Group in the past 24 years. From 1968 to 1977, operative death (within 1 month of operation) occurred in 27.5 per cent of patients undergoing laparotomy; after 1988, this rate was below 3 per cent, a remarkable reduction. In the early period, 20.3 per cent of the patients underwent only exploratory laparotomy, because on opening the abdomen, it was seen that nothing could be done; the preoperative diagnosis was inaccurate and failed to predict the state of the liver. After 1984, there were no simple laparotomies. The steady increase in the rate of hepatic resection reflects the positive policy on the part of the surgeon but, due to the method of recording, relative percentages are not accurate. Another important progress in hepatic surgery is intraoperative ultrasonography, which allows very accurate determination of the position of the tumour and detection of lesions not seen by preoperative imaging (Makuuchi, JpnJClinOncol, 1981; 11:367).

Hepatic resection

A healthy liver can tolerate three-quarters resection (extended lobectomy), with rapid regeneration of the residual liver tissue; within 3 months or so, hepatic mass returns to the previous size. Unfortunately, the liver is cirrhotic in most patients with hepatocellular carcinoma. The surgeons must decide whether or not the tumour is resectable and, if so, how much to resect—a decision based on liver function tests. Standard reference tests, including serum albumin, bilirubin, aminotransferase, and organic anion clearance (ICG, bromosulphthalein), or simply Child's classification, are used as guidelines. The mass is easy or difficult to resect depending on its location, and the amount of blood lost during the operation also depends on this factor. Some patients with large oesophageal varices may bleed during the immediate postoperative period because hepatic resection elevates portal venous pressure; for that reason some surgeons recommend sclerotherapy prior to hepatic resection. The survival rate after operation depends on whether the resection was curative or non-curative (cancer cells positive at the surgical margin), whether the liver was cirrhotic or not, and whether recurrence occurs in the residual liver. The survival rate is clearly lower in patients with cirrhosis than those without (Fig. 40).

With hepatic resection, the ideal is to have sufficient surgical margin so that no cancer cells remain in the residual parenchyma; this ideal is not often achieved because of the cirrhotic changes, the small volume of the residual liver, and poor liver function. Initially,

Japanese surgeons carried out prior hepatic arterial embolization, with the hope that it would prevent spread of cancer cells during the operation, but this is no longer practised because embolization reduces liver function. The functional (not anatomical) right and left lobes of the liver are divided by the line connecting the inferior vena cava at the cranial level of the liver and the gallbladder fossa, the so-called Cantlie line. Segmentectomy or subsegmentectomy should be carried out without cutting the major arteries and portal branches supplying other segments, and our understanding of the anatomy of the segments and subsegments is important (see Chapter 1.1). A number of studies have analysed the predictive factors for tumour recurrence, hence the prognosis. Most of them agree that tumour size, number of tumours, cancer cell infiltration of the fibrous capsule, portal invasion, and stage of the tumour are important factors (Arii, Cancer, 1992; 69:913).

Currently, eight segments are considered based on the study of Couinaud (PressMed, 1954; 62:709), and these segments are identified by modern imaging, particularly CT, because hepatic veins are seen between these segments supplied by the hepatic artery and portal vein. Until 1984, the relationship between the anterior and posterior vessels and bile ducts was described incorrectly in textbooks, because the corrosion studies had been misinterpreted (Healey, ArchSurg, 1953; 66:599); the anterior was described as the posterior and vice versa. Takayasu recognized this error while studying biplane portograms (Radiol, 1984; 154:31). In current surgical anatomy, eight segments are identified: caudate lobe (SI), left lateral posterior (SII), left lateral anterior (SIII), and left medial (SIV) segments, and four segments in the right lobe, anterior inferior (SV), posterior inferior (SVI), posterior superior (SVII), and anterior superior (SVIII) segments. These segments and their subsegments can be clearly identified by injecting a dye into the feeding portal branch (Tobe, SurgAnnu, 1984; 16:177).

Staging of patients

When we compared the survival curves for 157 patients who underwent hepatic resection and those from 464 patients who were treated medically, there was a considerable difference; the median survival in the former group was 21.6 months, but 3.1 months in the latter. The Japan Liver Cancer Study Group obtained similar results. However, surgery was done only in highly selected patients, and such a comparison is of little significance. It is necessary to compare patients in a similar disease state. For that reason, several

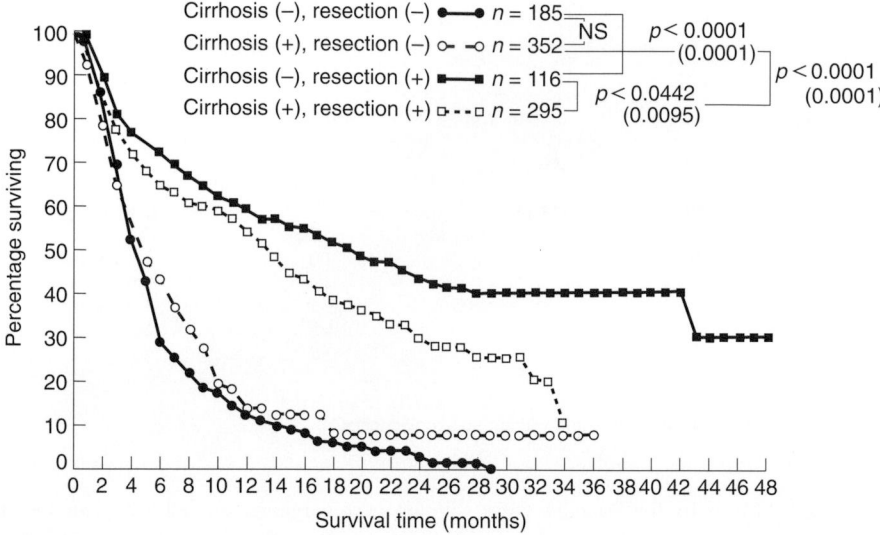

Fig. 40. Comparison of survival curves for patients with and without cirrhosis in whom resection was or was not carried out (Japan National Study). Resection in a non-cirrhotic liver gave the best results (from Cancer, 1987; 60:1400, with permission from JB Lippincott, publishers).

staging schemes have been proposed. Primack *et al.* (Cancer, 1975; 35:1357) considered ascites, weight loss, portal hypertension, and serum bilirubin; weight loss was the only indicator of cancer size. There was no imaging done in the Ugandan patients on whom this scheme was based. The median survival of their stage I (least advanced) patient was 3 months and that of stage III patients only 2 weeks. Such results are far from those seen elsewhere, particularly in Asia, where many patients are diagnosed long before cancer becomes massive. Therefore, we have proposed a new scheme based on 850 patients in which the size of cancer and severity of cirrhosis are considered, as shown in Table 19.[31] Patients in stage III had a median survival of less than 2 months as shown in Fig. 41. Without treatment, all died within 3 months; the Ugandan patients studied by Primack *et al.* all seem to belong to stage III by our criteria, as judged from the prognosis. Figure 42 compares 115 patients treated by surgery in stage I and 157 patients in the same stage treated non-surgically. The median survival in the surgical group was more than 2 years whereas in the non-surgical group it was only 9 months. Again, even among these stage I patients, surgical cases had been highly selected and were in better condition than non-surgical cases. Some reports from China give very high resection rates and high survival rates with subclinical cases.[35] However, these figures are not comparable with other studies because of the difference in the selection criteria. The TNM classification proposed by UICC has been expanded to apply to hepatocellular carcinoma.[36] This classification was primarily developed for tumour surgery, and now may be used in hepatic resection for hepatocellular carcinoma.

Other surgical treatments

Before transcatheter arterial embolization became popular, surgeons frequently ligated the hepatic artery when the cancer was deemed unresectable upon opening the abdomen. However, operative ligation of the hepatic artery was found to be ineffective in the Japan National Study, with a short survival time.[10] Some surgeons even ligated the portal vein instead of the artery, but the rationale was not clear and the results were equivocal. Tang and his group in

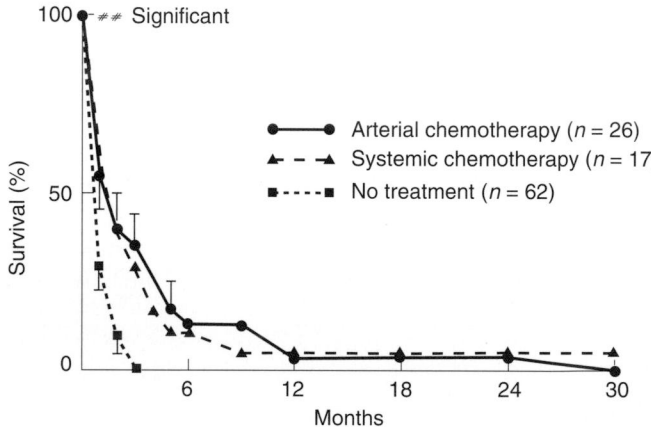

Fig. 41. Survival curves for stage III patients treated and not treated by anticancer chemotherapy. Note that those without treatment all died within 3 months. With either intravenous or intra-arterial chemotherapy, percentage survival was significantly better after 2 months; a small number of patients lived more than 1 year (Okuda, Cancer, 1985; 56: 918, with permission from JB Lippincott, publishers).

Shanghai advocate cryosurgery,[37] but this method has not been widely used.

Liver transplantation

In the early days of liver transplantation, it was favoured for primary liver cancer at Cambridge; there were fewer postoperative complications than when transplantation was carried out for advanced cirrhosis, but it was soon realized that there was frequent recurrence. Starzl in Denver (and later in Pittsburgh) had a similar experience. A patient with a hilar carcinoma was transplanted and the new liver developed carcinoma at the same site, the hilum. It was suspected that cancer cells floating in blood during the operation had settled back where they had resided; this was not the case, and the recurrence was most probably due to lymphatic spread down

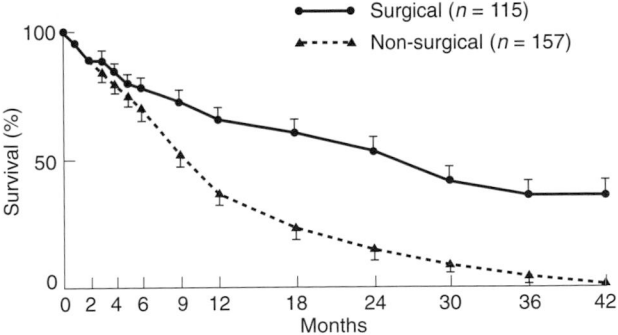

Fig. 42. Comparison of stage I patients treated surgically and non-surgically. Whereas all of the non-surgical group died within 3.5 years, about 40 per cent of the surgically treated group lived more than 3 years (Okuda, Cancer, 1985; 56:918, with permission from JB Lippincott, publishers).

toward the pancreas along the biliary tract. Therefore, transplantation should be carried out before extrahepatic spread occurs. Although transplant surgeons are not enthusiastic about transplanting for liver cancer at the moment, observations in Pittsburgh are very encouraging. Seventeen livers were removed, for other diseases such as tyrosinaemia, in which a small hepatocellular carcinoma was found on examination of the specimen; 90 per cent of the patients were still alive after 5 years (Iwatsuki, TransplProc, 1988; 20:498). Although the overall results with hepatocellular carcinoma have been rather poor (Scharschmidt, Hepatol, 1984; 4: 95S), patients with fibrolamellar carcinoma do very well, with a 5-year survival rate of more than 50 per cent (O'Gray, AnnSurg, 1988; 207:373). In our opinion, a patient with a small hepatocellular carcinoma in a liver with advanced cirrhosis is a good candidate for transplantation; extrahepatic metastasis is unlikely and the patient will otherwise die either from cirrhosis or cancer spread. A recent study in Milan confirms this view (Mazzaferro, NEJM, 1996; 334:683).

Non-surgical treatment
Systemic chemotherapy

This modality is generally not very efficacious and the reported response rates, particularly with a single agent, are very low.[38,39] The agents studied are: alkylating agents such as cyclophosphamide, triethyleneglycol diglycidyl ether, alanine mustard, DL-serine bis(2-chloropropyl)carbamate ester, bischloroethylnitrosourea,

chloroethylcyclohexylnitrosourea, chloroethylmethylcyclohexyl-nitrosourea; antimetabolites such as methotrexate, 6-mer-captopurine, 5-fluorouracil hydroxyurea, 1- hexylcarbamoyl-5-fluorouracil, cytosine arabinoside, dichloromethotrexate, tegafur; plant alkaloids such as vincristine, vinblastine; antibiotics andrelated substances such as mitomycin-C, carzinophyllin, actinomycin-D, chromomycin-A3, neocarzinostatin, doxorubicin; and others such as bisdiaminodichloroplatinum, dehydroemetine, procarbazine, butyryloxyglyoxal, dithiosemicarbazone. Of these, mitomycin-C, doxorubicin, tegafur, and mitoxantrone are among those reported with inconsistent but somewhat high response rates (Table 20). The extremely high response rate described by Olweny (Cancer, 1980; 46:2717) has not been reproducible elsewhere. The route of administration is either oral or intravenous; tegafur is available in suppository form, and can be given to patients with anorexia and stomach troubles.

Various combination chemotherapies have been tried but the results are no more encouraging because little is gained by adding ineffective cytotoxic agents which cause increased toxicity and necessitate reduced dosage.[39] As yet, no reliable *in vitro* assay is available for testing the drug sensitivity of particular cancer cells taken from the patient to be treated. Sugimachi and his group have developed an assay system with resected specimens in which succinate dehydrogenase inhibition is measured as an indicator of cancer cell viability (Anai, Oncol, 1987; 44:115). Using this system, Kanematsu et al. (EurJCanClinOnc, 1988; 24:1511) tested 29 resected hepatocellular carcinoma and 12 metastatic cancer specimens for sensitivity to adriamycin, mitomycin-C, 5-fluorouracil, cisplatin, aclacino-mycin A, and carboquone, and demonstrated that hepatocellular carcinoma responded much better than did metastatic cancers. Such results suggest that if these cytotoxic agents were used at high concentration in cancer tissue, they should prove effective, and encourage development of techniques to achieve higher tissue concentrations.

Although the reported response rates are low, a remarkable regression of mass is occasionally achieved in response to systemic chemotherapy.[38] There have been sporadic reports of complete remission with various agents (Harada, Cancer, 1978; 42:67), and it seems that at the moment response is totally unpredictable. Our study in stage III patients showed that chemotherapy had a significant effect on the survival of patients (Fig. 41),[31] that is, chemotherapy is indicated even in patients with advanced hepatocellular carcinoma. In 1981, Novi (Science, 1981; 212:251) observed

	Tumour size (%)		Ascites		Albumin (g/dl)		Bilirubin (mg/dl)	
Table 19 Staging for the patients with hepatocellular carcinoma based on imaging*								
State	>50 (+)	<50 (−)	(+)	(−)	<3 (+)	>3 (−)	>3 (+)	<3 (−)
I		(−)		(−)		(−)		(−)
II			1 or 2 (+)					
III			3 or 4 (+)					

(+) Sign of advanced disease.
* Data taken from Okuda, Cancer, 1985; 56:918–28.

Table 20 Systemic chemotherapy and reported response rates

Agent	Response rate	Author	Year
Doxorubicin	22/50	Olweny	1980
	8/28	Melia	1983
	5/43	Falkson	1984
	6/52	Chlobowski	1984
Epiriubicin	3/18	Hochster	1985
	0/14	Shiu	1986
Mitoxantrone	2/34	Falkson	1985
	6/22	Dunk	1985
	2/33	Davis	1986
Tegafur	1/15	Ohya	1982
HCFU	3/18	Kubo	1986
Cisplatin	1/13	Melia	1981
	1/20	Ravry	1986
Neocarzinostatin	1/18	Falkson	1984
VP-16	2/24	Cavalli	1981
	4/22	Melia	1983

Supplied by courtesy of Dr Nobou Okazaki.

regression of aflatoxin B_1-induced hepatocellular carcinoma in rats by administration of reduced glutathione, and Kawano et al. (Acta-HepatolJpn, 1984; 25:1468) reported a remarkable response obtained with a large dose of glutathione in one patient with advanced hepatocellular carcinoma. The exact mechanism is not clear. Some hepatoma cells are hormone dependent in vitro (Mishkin, Gastro, 1979; 77: 547), but attempts to exploit such characteristics of cancer cells in human cases have been unsuccessful. The effects of tamoxifen are equivocal.

Intra-arterial chemotherapy

In order to deliver cytotoxic agents directly to cancer tissue in higher local concentrations, intra-arterial administration was used either in a bolus dose or by infusion through a catheter placed in the hepatic artery (inserted surgically via the gastroduodenal artery). More recently, the catheter has been introduced from the subclavian or femoral artery, thus circumventing laparotomy, but without fixation of the tip it may slip off the coeliac artery. An alternative is to connect the catheter to an infusion port implanted subcutaneously, and anticancer agents are injected periodically through the port (Yoshikawa, AJR, 1992; 158:885). There was a time when intra-arterial bolus-dose chemotherapy was popular, but the results in Japan were generally unexciting; our comparison of 141 cases of arterial bolus chemotherapy and 82 cases of systemic chemotherapy showed the former to be only marginally more effective (Fig. 43).[31] Continuous or intermittent arterial infusion chemotherapy through a chronic infusion pump, whether implantable (Daly, ArchSurg, 1984; 119:936) or non-implantable (Cady, SGO, 1974; 138:381), is reportedly more effective. However, the benefit seems to be cancelled by frequent complications, such as peptic ulcer, gastritis (Chuang, AJR, 1981; 137:347), and infection; some of the infused cytotoxic agent perfuses through the stomach wall and exerts deleterious effects.

Arterial embolization

This technique, called transcatheter arterial embolization, in which small gel-foam particles are injected into an artery to occlude the branches supplying a cancer, was first used for the treatment of renal cancer in the United States (Lang, Radiol, 1971; 98:391; Goldstein, Radiol, 1976; 120:539), and was introduced to Japan by Yamada (Radiol, 1983; 148:397). It rapidly gained popularity among Japanese hepatologists/radiologists and was soon adopted by other countries. The rationale is to interrupt the arterial blood supply to a hepatocellular carcinoma, which is totally dependent on arteries.[24] The effect is dramatic as assessed by ultrasonography and CT. Immediate induction of tissue necrosis (Hsu, Cancer, 1986; 57: 1184) is evident from the changes in ultrasonography image, and the gas formation that occurs quickly in the mass (Furui, Radiol, 1984; 150:773) (Fig. 44). The effect is more apparent if the mass is expanding and encapusulated because the cancer tissue then receives no portal blood at all. However, it soon became clear that the fibrous capsule has a blood supply also from the portal vein, and that viable hepatocellular carcinoma cells remain undamaged in the capsule. Although the interior of the mass liquefies in due course, the viable cancer cells in the capsule will cause late spread.[30] Lin et al. (Gastro, 1988; 94:453) carried out a randomized controlled study comparing this technique with high-dose 5-fluorouracil in unresectable patients, and demonstrated greater efficacy with the former.

The technique is not always possible and it is not without complications. If a patient with portal tumour thrombosis receives this treatment, the blood supply to the liver is cut off, and he will die from anoxic hepatic necrosis. Thus, assessment of the patency of the portal vein and its major branches by ultrasonography is imperative. Arterial embolization is contraindicated in patients with tumour thrombosis in the major portal branches. During the procedure, some of the gel-foam particles already clogging arterial branches may bounce back into the coeliac trunk and further into the splenic artery when the second arteriography is carried out to confirm blockade of arterial branches. This causes splenic infarction (Takayasu, Radiol, 1984; 151:371). Some of the injected particles may go into the cystic artery, and aseptic cholecystitis may result (Kuroda, Radiol, 1983; 149:85). An infiltrative type of hepatocellular carcinoma is exposed to portal blood at its expanding periphery and therefore does not respond as well as an expanding hepatocellular carcinoma. Following embolization, arterial neovasculature soon develops to feed the cancer tissue and the primary effect does not last very long. Repeated arterial embolizations or infusion chemotherapy are required through another artery (Soo, Radiol, 1983; 147:45).

Our own results indicate a greater efficacy of embolization compared with intra-arterial bolus chemotherapy in stage II patients (Fig. 43), but not in those in stage I. Blockade of arterial blood flow not only kills hepatocellular carcinoma cells but also induces an anoxic state in the parenchyma which results in considerable functional damage. Thus, if transcatheter arterial embolization is done in patients with a small hepatocellular carcinoma found in a liver with advanced cirrhosis, the advantage of the the tumour-suppressing effect may be negated by the parenchymal damage. This was our experience with such patients. However, in the series of Takayasu et al. (CancChemoPharm, 1989; 23:S123) all patients with a hepatocellular carcinoma smaller than 2 cm lived for 3 years, and the survival rate for patients with a hepatocellular carcinoma of 2 to 5 cm was 81, 33, and 16 per cent at 1, 2, and 3 years, respectively. They analysed various factors and showed that the size of tumour

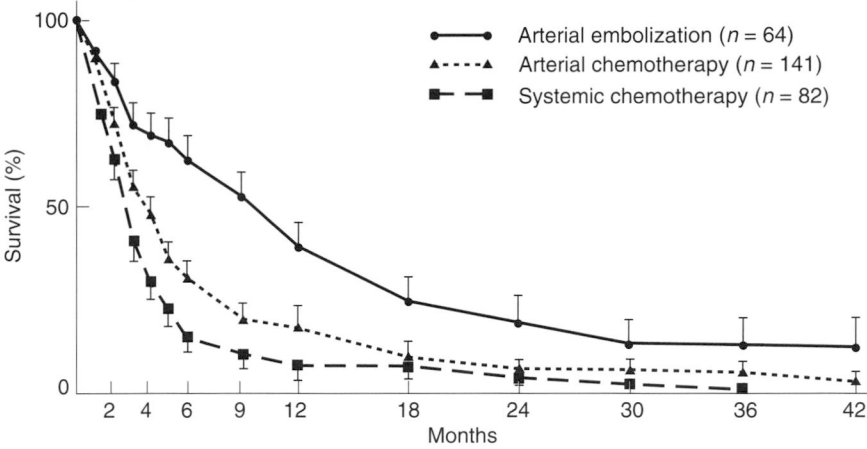

Fig. 43. Comparison of survival curves for stage II patients treated by arterial embolization, intra-arterial chemotherapy, and systemic chemotherapy. Arterial embolization gave a significantly better survival curve. Patients treated by intra-arterial chemotherapy did slightly better than those receiving systemic chemotherapy (Okuda, Cancer, 1985; 56:918, with permission from JB Lippincott, publishers).

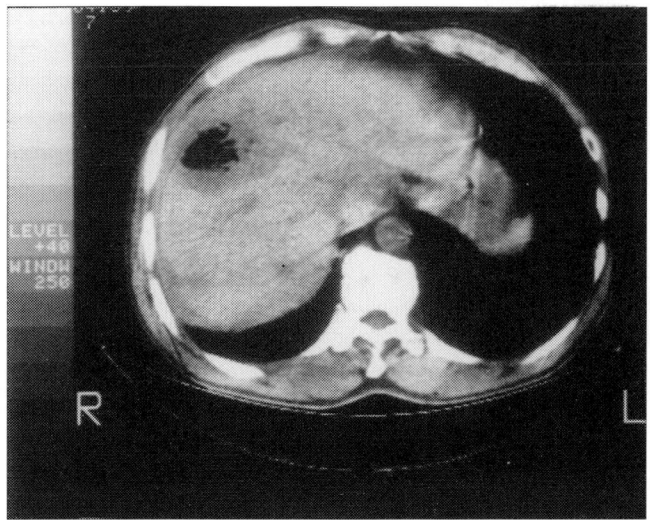

Fig. 44. Marked gas formation following arterial embolization, suggesting necrosis of the mass.

significantly influenced the prognosis, provided that there was no severe liver dysfunction nor portal thrombosis.

Since the capsule of a hepatocellular carcinoma, and the expanding tumour front, receive portal blood, there have been attempts in Japan to occlude the portal branch going to the tumour following transcatheter arterial embolization (Nakao, Radiol, 1986; 161:303), but whether portal embolization further prolongs survival remains to be determined.

Chemoembolization, targeting chemotherapy, and lipiodolization

After the introduction of arterial embolization, various related therapeutic modalities have been developed. Since transcatheter arterial embolization occludes large feeding arteries and invites formation of new arteries within the liver, some investigators felt

that feeding arteries could be occluded more peripherally with smaller particles; if they contained a chemotherapeutic agent, the cell killing effects might be augmented. Kato *et al.* (JAMA, 1981; 245:1123) prepared 0.2-mm sized microencapsulated mitomycin C using cellulose, and injected it into arteries for the treatment of various cancers. Our results with this technique were similar to those with transcatheter arterial embolization (Ohnishi, Radiol, 1984; 152:51). In 1979, Maeda synthesized a polystyrene–maleic acid conjugated with neocarzinostatin (**SMANCS**) and administered it mixed with Lipiodol, an oil-contrast medium, into the hepatic artery, with the rationale that this lipophilic anticancer agent would remain in the cancer tissue (Fig. 45) and effect a slow release (Konno, EurJCanClinOnc, 1983; 19:1053). This so-called targeted chemotherapy proved very effective, as evident from the decline of serum α-fetoprotein levels.[40] Since SMANCS was not generally available, attempts were also made to mix an anticancer agent directly with Lipiodol and to inject the mixture intra-arterially. Kanematsu *et al.* (JSurgOncol, 1984; 25:218) found that if a hydrophilic agent was first mixed with Urografin, an iodized contrast medium with a specific gravity similar to Lipiodol, it was readily emulsified with Lipiodol. They called this procedure 'lipiodolization' of antitumour agents. The results were almost as good as with SMANCS. Arterial Lipiodol injection serves another purpose, that is, detection of small lesions not detected by ultrasonography and chemotherapy; currently, most hepatologists throughout the world use lipiodolized anticancer agents intra-arterially followed by transcatheter arterial embolization. The rationale is that lipiodolized agents would not be washed away from cancer tissue so quickly if arterial blood flow is blocked by the latter. Lipiodol alone has no therapeutic effect, although this oil agent causes fat embolism within the cancer tissue (Takayasu, Radiol, 1987; 162:345).

Radiotherapy

In the past, radiotherapy was thought to be useless unless combined with immunotherapy (Balasegaram, AmJSurg, 1975; 130:33) or chemotherapy (Cochrane, Cancer, 1977; 40:609). More recently, we have found that irradiation with a linear accelerator killed or

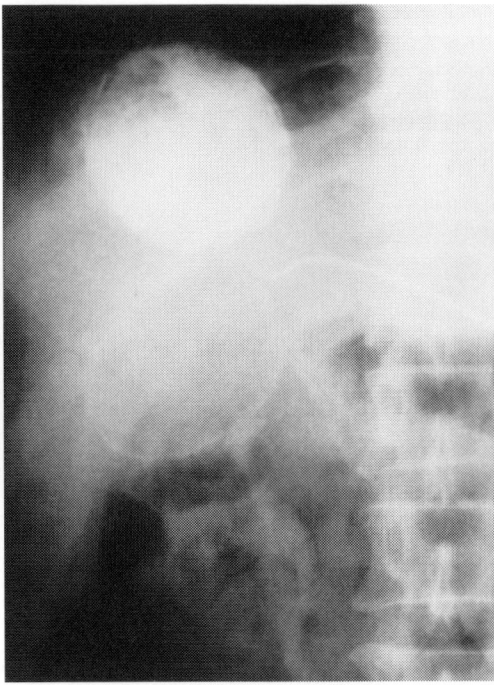

Fig. 45. Retention of Lipiodol by hepatocellular carcinoma. Lipiodol mixed with an anticancer agent (lipiodolization) was injected into the hepatic artery several months earlier. The mass is clearly seen by the contrast given by deposited Lipiodol on this hepatogram.

suppressed hepatocellular carcinoma cells very effectively as shown by the reduction of tumour size.[33] However, it was also learnt that irradiation induces slowly progressive atrophy of the liver parenchyma and, in Child's C patients, eventually causes hepatic failure. In our experience, tumour never grew further from the primary site to which radiotherapy was directed. Irradiation over the stomach causes radiation ulcer which is difficult to cure, but hepatocellular carcinoma located laterally in a liver with mild cirrhosis (Child A) is a good candidate for irradiation. Several attempts have been made in which antibody to α-fetoprotein labelled with radioactive iodine was administered intravenously, with the expectation that it would attach to hepatocellular carcinoma cells and irradiate them. Although α-fetoprotein is a secretory protein, some remains on the cancer cell surface and hepatocellular carcinoma is visualized several days later, following administration of radiolabelled anti-α-fetoprotein antibody, as a positive image. Using a higher dose of radioactivity, the same procedure can be used for irradiation. However, antibody injected will combine with circulating α-fetoprotein and the amount going to the cancer itself is much reduced. If radiolabelled antibody is given repeatedly, it is necessary to change the source of antibody each time, because the patient develops antibody to the previous radiolabelled antibody given. Thus, it is necessary to change animal species to be immunized for antibody production in sequence, and the number of animal species available is limited (Order, NatlCancerInstMonogr, 1987; 3:7). More recently, powerful heavy-particle bombardment has been used for the treatment of hepatocellular carcinoma. The particle beams have the Bragg peak which limits the beam distribution and minimizes the damage to liver parenchym. The reported results for proton irradiation are remarkable (Matsuzaki, Gastro, 1994; 106:1032).

Percutaneous intratumour injection

With the improved aiming achieved by using an ultrasonography puncture transducer (Ohto, Radiol, 1980; 136:171; Makuuchi, Radiol, 1980; 136:165), it has become possible to inject a solution containing an antitumour agent directly into the mass. However, an aqueous solution will be quickly washed away by increased arterial flow within the mass. Ethanol is an innocuous and useful substance that will coagulate the tissue as it diffuses through it. We developed this modality in 1983 (Sugiura, ActaHepatolJpn, 1983; 24:920) out of necessity because of the frequent detection of a small hepatocellular carcinoma in a liver with advanced cirrhosis which cannot tolerate major surgery. In this technique, a thin Chiba needle is inserted into the mass under ultrasonography guidance; absolute ethanol is injected while the needle is slowly withdrawn from the deepest end of the mass. In one session several millilitres of ethanol are used, and sessions are repeated at least five times at intervals of several days until the whole mass is considered to have been coagulated. This technique is best indicated in patients with one to three small (less than 3 cm) lesions. There is pain during the procedure, followed by slight fever, but the procedure is safe and well tolerated.[33] Under ultrasonography, there is an immediate change to a very high echo pattern and on CT some gas formation may be seen in time (Shiina, AJR, 1987; 149:1495). The injected lesion slowly shrinks or disappears (Livraghi, Radiol, 1986; 161: 309). Some hepatologists in Taiwan inject a steel coil into the centre of the lesion and follow the change in the size of the mass. In our experience, the primary lesion never grows further after ethanol coagulation, but recurrence of new lesions in other parts of the liver is just as common as postoperative recurrence (see above). However, there is no immediate death (unlike hepatic resection), and the overall survival is just as good as that after hepatic resection for small hepatocellular carcinomas in cirrhotic livers. Acetic acid instead of ethanol has been used with similar results (Ohnishi, Radiol, 1994; 193:747). Various other agents such as immunostimulants and hot water have also been used in Japan.

Other treatment modalities

Immunotherapy

A number of immunomodulating and immunostimulant agents have been used, but the results have not been very satisfactory except for occasional responses. The agents tried include BCG (Hahn, VerDschGesInnMed, 1977; 83:1205; Minden, CancerRes, 1980; 40: 3214), OK-432, a streptococcal preparation (Sakurai, CancChemo-Rep, 1972; 56:9), interferon (Forbes, JRSM, 1985; 78:826), interleukin 2, and lymphokine activated killer cells (LAK, adoptive immunotherapy) (Okuno, Cancer, 1986; 58:1001; Ohnishi, Hepatol, 1989; 10:349; Komatsu, JClinImmunol, 1990; 10:167). Several reports on the effects of LAK are forthcoming but, as far as we are aware, they are no more exciting than the other therapies already discussed.

Gene therapy

This is still in an experimental stage.

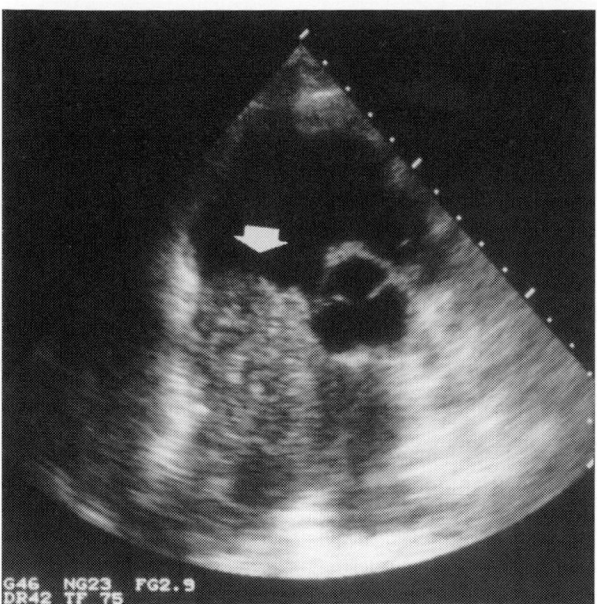

Fig. 46. A mass is growing into the right atrium in continuity from the inferior vena cava (at arrow) seen by sector ultrasonography scanning.

submassive localized necrosis of the parenchyma (Okuda, Cancer, 1976; 37:1965). The major portal venous branches and hepatic veins should be monitored regularly with ultrasonography to assess whether the tumour is invading the venous system. Tumour thrombus growing into the inferior vena cava, and further into the right atrium, may be seen, and this can be studied by a sector-type ultrasonography probe (Fig. 46). Such patients may develop sudden dyspnoea with changes in posture (Kato, AnnIntMed, 1983; 99: 472), but otherwise the diagnosis of an inferior vena cava tumour thrombus is difficult clinically. If the patient develops jaundice, this could be a terminal event or an intraductal tumour growth; these two different events have to be differentiated by imaging. The most serious complication is intra-abdominal bleeding from a lesion on the liver surface. The patient complains of abdominal pain of varying degree, and anaemia and increasing abdominal girth are recognized. When an abdominal tap demonstrates blood, immediate coeliac arteriography is required. Although determination of the bleeding site is not easy, if the approximate area of bleeding is identified, arterial embolization should be carried out as is done for the transcatheter arterial embolization technique.

Multidisciplinary treatment

The current practice is to employ more than one therapeutic modality, such as ethanol injection followed by arterial embolization.

Prevention of hepatocellular carcinoma

There are three steps by which hepatocellular carcinoma may be prevented: prevention of viral hepatitis B and C, prevention of chronic viral liver disease from progressing toward cirrhosis, and chemoprevention in which development of hepatocellular carcinoma in a cirrhotic liver is prevented with a chemical agent. Vaccination, personal hygiene, and treatment of chronic hepatitis are the realistic and possible practices. Recently, several studies in Japan have shown significant reduction in the incidence of hepatocellular carcinoma among patients with cirrhosis and chronic hepatitis after treatment (Nishiguchi, Lancet, 1995; 346:1051; Oka, Cancer, 1995; 76:743).

Monitoring of condition

Progress of the disease can be most accurately assessed by imaging, particularly with ultrasonography for small lesions, and with CT. In patients with an elevated serum α-fetoprotein, this is the most important marker. However, a clonal change of hepatocellular carcinoma cells may occur during chemotherapy; the previously α-fetoprotein-producing hepatocellular carcinoma may give way to a new clone which does not produce α-fetoprotein, and vice versa; α-fetoprotein may not prove diagnostic of tumour growth. Other biochemical markers are less accurate, except for the AST/ALT ratio which steadily increases as the mass enlarges (Shimokawa, Cancer, 1977; 40:319). A sudden sharp rise in AST, ALT, and LDH may occur in a terminal stage, due to a temporary drop in blood pressure in patients with portal tumour thrombosis, and resulting

References

1. Eggel H. Ueber das primäre Carcinoma der Leber. *Beiträge zur Pathologischen Anatomie und Allgemeinen Pathologie*, 1901; **30**: 506–604.
2. *Fogarty International Center Proceedings No. 22*. Diseases of the liver and biliary tract. Standardization of nomenclature, diagnostic criteria, and diagnostic methodology. Washington DC: NIR, 1976: 79–81.
3. Berman C. *Primary carcinoma of the liver*. London: Lewis, 1951: 19–36.
4. Okuda K, Peters RL, and Simson IA. Gross anatomical features of hepatocellular carcinoma from three disparate geographic areas. Proposal of new classification. *Cancer*, 1984; **54**: 2165–73.
5. Okuda K. Early recognition of hepatocellular carcinoma. *Hepatology*, 1986; **6**: 729–38.
6. Munoz N and Linsell A. Epidemiology of primary liver cancer. In Correa P and Haenszel W, eds. *Epidemiology of cancer of the digestive tract*. The Hague: Martinus Nijhoff, 1982: 161–95.
7. Munoz N and Bosch X. Epidemiology of hepatocellular carcinoma. In Okuda K and Ishak KG, eds. *Neoplasms of the liver*. Tokyo: Springer-Verlag, 1987: 3–19.
8. Health and Welfare Statistics Association. Trends in the health of nation. *Kosei no Shihyo*, 1988; **35**: 53–6 (in Japanese).
9. Liver Cancer Study Group of Japan. Survey and follow-up of primary liver cancer in Japan—Report 11. *Acta Hepatologica Japonica*, 1995; **36**: 208–17.
10. Okuda and the Liver Cancer Study Group of Japan. Primary liver cancers in Japan. *Cancer*, 1980; **45**: 2663–9.
11. Peters RL. Pathology of hepatocellular carcinoma. In Okuda K and Peters RL, eds. *Hepatocellular carcinoma*. New York: Wiley, 1976: 107–68.
12. Van Kaick G, *et al*. Late effects and tissue dose in Thorotrast patients. Recent results of the German Thorotrast study. In IAEA, ed. *Late biological effects of ionizing radiation*. Vienna: IAEA, 1976; 1: 263–76.
13. Hirayama T. A large-scale cohort study on the relationship between diet and selected cancers of digestive organs. In *Banburg Report 7. Gastrointestinal cancer. Endogenous factors*. Cold Spring Harbor Laboratories, 1981; 65: 111–14.
14. Nakashima T, Kojiro M, Sakamoto K, Okuda K, Shimokawa Y, and Kubo Y. Studies of primary liver carcinoma. I. Proposal of new gross anatomical classification of primary liver cell carcinoma. *Acta Hepatologica Japonica*, 1974; **15**: 279–90.
15. Nakashima T and Kojiro M. *Hepatocellular carcinoma. An atlas of its pathology*. Tokyo: Springer-Verlag, 1987: 4–8.

16. Nakashima T, *et al.* Pathology of hepatocellular carcinoma in Japan. 232 consecutive cases autopsied in ten years. *Cancer*, 1983; **51**: 863–77.

17. Okuda K. Clinical aspects of hepatocellular carcinoma—analysis of 134 cases. In Okuda K and Peters RL, eds. *Hepatocellular carcinoma*. New York: Wiley, 1976: 387–436.

18. Edmondson HA and Steiner PE. Primary carcinoma of the liver. A study of 100 cases among 48 900 necropsies. *Cancer*, 1954; **7**: 462–503.

19. Edmondson HA. *Tumours of the liver and intrahepatic bile ducts.* Section VII Fascicle 25. Washington DC: Armed Forces Institute of Pathology, 1958.

20. Roles DB. Fibrolamellar carcinoma of the liver. In Okuda K and Ishak KG, eds. *Neoplasms of the liver*. Tokyo: Springer-Verlag, 1987: 137–42.

21. Stocker JT and Ishak KG. Hepatoblastoma. In Okuda K and Ishak KG, eds. *Neoplasms of the liver*. Tokyo: Springer-Verlag, 1987: 127–36.

22. Japan Liver Cancer Study Group. Primary liver cancer in Japan. Report 7. *Acta Hepatologica Japonica*, 1986; **27**: 1161–9.

23. Okuda K and Nakashima T. Primary carcinomas of the liver. In Berk JE *et al.*, eds. *Bockus—Gastroenterology*. 4th edn. Philadelphia: Saunders, 1984; **5**: 3315–76.

24. Nakashima T. Vascular changes and hemodynamics in hepatocellular carcinoma. In Okuda K and Peters RL, eds. *Hepatocellular carcinoma*. New York: Wiley, 1976: 169–204.

25. Okuda H, Obata H, Nakanishi T, Furukawa R, and Hashimoto E. Production of abnormal prothrombin (des- carboxy prothrombin) by hepatocellular carcinoma. A clinical and experimental study. *Journal of Hepatology*, 1987; **4**: 357–63.

26. Cochrane M and Williams R. Humoral effects of hepatocellular carcinoma. In Okuda K and Peters RL, eds. *Hepatocellular carcinoma*. New York: Wiley, 1976: 333–52.

27. Okuda K. What is the precancerous lesion for hepatocellular carcinoma in man? *Journal of Gastroenterology and Hepatology*, 1986; **1**: 79–85.

28. Okuda K and Kojiro M. Small hepatocellular carcinoma. In Okuda K and Ishak KG, eds. *Neoplasms of the liver*. Tokyo: Springer-Verlag, 1987: 215–26.

29. Okuda K, *et al.* Clinical aspects of intrahepatic bile duct carcinoma including hilar carcinoma. *Cancer*, 1977; **39**: 232–46.

30. Okuda K. Primary liver cancer. Quadrennial review lecture. *Digestive Diseases and Sciences*, 1986; **31**: 113S–46S.

31. Yamada R, Sato M, Kawabata M, Nakatsuka H, Nakamura K, and Takashima S. Hepatic artery embolization in 120 patients with unresectable hepatoma. *Radiology*, 1983; **148**: 397–401.

32. Okuda K, *et al.* Natural history of hepatocellular carcinoma in relation to treatment. Study of 850 patients. *Cancer*, 1985; **56**: 918–28.

33. Ohto M, Ebara M, Yoshikawa M, and Okuda K. Radiation therapy and percutaneous ethanol injection for the treatment of hepatocellular carcinoma. In Okuda K and Ishak KG, eds. *Neoplasms of the liver*. Tokyo: Springer-Verlag, 1987: 335–42.

34. Lin TY. Surgical treatment of primary liver cell carcinoma. In Okuda K and Peters RL, eds. *Hepatocellular carcinoma*. New York: Wiley, 1976: 449–68.

35. Tang ZY. Surgical treatment of subclinical hepatocellular carcinoma. In Okuda K and Ishak KG, eds. *Neoplasms of the liver*. Tokyo: Springer-Verlag, 1987: 67–73.

36. International Union Against Cancer. *TNM Classification of malignant tumours*. 4th Rev. Edn. Genova: Springer, 1987.

37. Zhou XD, Tang ZY, and Yu YQ. Cryosurgery for hepatocellular carcinoma—experimental and clinical study. In Tang ZY, ed. *Subclinical hepatocellular carcinoma*. Beijing: China Academic Publishers, 1985: 107–19.

38. Okazaki N. Systemic chemotherapy of hepatocellular carcinoma. In Okuda K and Peters RL, eds. *Hepatocellular carcinoma*. New York: Wiley, 1976: 469–75.

39. Falkson G and Coetzer B. Chemotherapy of primary liver cancer. In Okuda K and Ishak KG, eds. *Neoplasms of the liver*. Tokyo: Springer-Verlag, 1987: 320–6.

40. Konno T and Maeda H. Targeting chemotherapy of hepatocellular carcinoma: arterial administration of SMANCS/Lipiodol. In Okuda K and Ishak KG, eds. *Neoplasms of the liver*. Tokyo: Springer-Verlag, 1987: 343–52.

22.2.2 Malignant biliary obstruction

Pietro E. Majno, Daniel Azoulay, and Henri Bismuth

Introduction

Malignancy is second only to gallstones as a cause of obstruction of the biliary tree. The obstruction can be caused by:

(1) primary tumours of the biliary epithelium of the ducts or of the gallbladder;
(2) compression of the biliary system from lymphatic or haematogenous metastases from other tumours;
(3) invasion of the bile duct from tumours of the pancreas or the periampullary region.

In the management of malignant biliary obstruction it is important (i) to differentiate between the different causative factors and (ii) to establish the anatomical level of the obstruction. Primary tumours of the biliary epithelium, whether originating from the extrahepatic biliary tree or the gallbladder, have special clinical and pathological features that make them a group apart from other intra-abdominal malignancies. They are a major challenge in modern hepatobiliary surgery: curative treatment, once exceptional, is now possible in many cases, and palliation can be rewarded by long, symptom-free survival. The lessons learned in the palliation of malignant biliary tumours can be applied to biliary obstruction caused by compression from other tumours, generally occurring in the presence of advanced disease in the liver or elsewhere in the body, where the aim is the effective relief of symptoms rather than the surgical removal of the neoplasm. Tumours of the ampulla and the head of the pancreas belong to the field of pancreatic surgery and will not be discussed here.

Malignant tumours of the extrahepatic bile ducts

For reasons of surgical approach, tumours of the extrahepatic bile ducts are classified into tumours of the upper third in the region of the hepatic hilum (defined by the portal bifurcation), the middle third in the hepatoduodenal ligament, and the lower third within the head of the pancreas. A definition of tumours of the upper third according to the insertion of the cystic duct is impractical as this point is variable. Primary biliary tumours of the upper third are the most common (56 per cent) (Reding, AnnSurg, 1991; 213:236) and when they involve the confluence of the hepatic ducts they are called Klatskin tumours from the original description (Klatskin, AmJMed, 1965; 38:241)

Incidence and epidemiology

As a group, primary tumours of the extrahepatic bile ducts are relatively rare, with an annual incidence in the United States of 1.2/100 000, equally distributed between males and females.[1] The median age of the population affected is 69 years but tumours in younger patients have been described, bearing a stronger relation to the causative factors that will be discussed below.

Aetiology

Several causative factors have been implicated in the origin of primary biliary tumours through mechanisms of chronic inflammation, genetic instability of the biliary epithelium, or chemical damage. A progression from benign papilloma to adenoma to malignant tumour has been postulated (Henson, Cancer, 1992; 70:1498), and some studies underline the link between chronic inflammation, dysplasia, and carcinoma *in situ* (Duarte, Cancer, 1993; 72:1878). The molecular equivalent of these changes has recently been investigated, with findings of increased immunoreactivity for p53 protein in biliary tumours (Diamantis, Hepatol, 1995; 22:774; Soon Lee, Pathology, 1995; 27:117) and of mutations in the *ras* oncogene family (Watanabe, Gastro, 1994; 107: 1147).

An increased incidence of cholangiocarcinoma is observed in the presence of intrahepatic stones, especially when causing recurrent pyogenic cholangitis as seen in infestation with the parasite *Chlonorchis siniensis* in the Far East. It is not known, however, whether the stones are responsible for the preneoplastic changes or whether dilatation of the bile ducts forms first, with both the stones and the preneoplastic changes being a secondary effect. Indeed the risk of cholangiocarcinoma probably remains increased for some years after the treatment of intrahepatic stones. (Chijiiwa, SGO, 1993; 177:279). Whether the presence of stones in the gallbladder is associated with an increased incidence of bile-duct carcinoma is still an issue of debate (Eckborn, Lancet, 1993; 177:279).

Bile stasis in choledochal cysts is accompanied by an increased risk of cholangiocarcinoma at a young age (10 per cent for patients older than 20 years), and surgical treatment of this condition is advocated (Chijiiwa, AmJSurg, 1993; 165:238). Patients with an anomalous junction of the pancreaticobiliary duct, favouring reflux of pancreatic juice into the biliary tree and the gallbladder, are at risk of malignant transformation; resection of the bile duct with cholecystectomy is advocated for this condition (Tanaka, BrJSurg, 1993; 80:622).

Cholangiocarcinoma has been reported with a frequency of 9 to 20 per cent in patients with sclerosing cholangitis (Rosen, AnnSurg, 1991; 213:21)[2,3] associated or not with inflammatory bowel disease, and ulcerative colitis in itself may be associated with an increased incidence of cholangiocarcinoma (Haworth, ArchPathLabMed, 1989; 113:434). A recent change in symptoms in a patient with known sclerosing cholangitis should be taken seriously and may reveal an associated cholangiocarcinoma. Monitoring of tumour markers is indicated: a value of (CA19.9 + CEA × 40) higher than 400 had a 100 per cent positive predictive value for the presence of malignant transformation in one study (Ramage, Gastro, 1995; 108:865). The application of the Mayo model designed for liver transplantation in primary biliary cirrhosis (Nashan, Hepatol, 1996; 23:1105) may allow prediction of the occurrence of a tumour in these patients.

It is suggested that some forms of cholangiocarcinoma develop from the degeneration of benign biliary adenomas, and this may be particularly true for the papillary histological variant of cholangiocaracinoma more commonly found in the lower biliary tract

(Kozuka, Cancer, 1984; 54:65). Adenomas do indeed develop in 50 per cent of dogs submitted to a choledocopancreatic anastomosis, an experimental model for an abnormal pancreaticobiliary junction that is associated with biliary tumours (Miyano, JPediatSurg, 1989; 24:539). Multiple biliary papillomatosis is a rare disease in which there are several polyps of premalignant potential in the bile ducts, sometimes sparing the gallbladder (Gouma, BrJSurg, 1984; 71:72).

Histopathology, mode of spread, and staging

The great majority of primary tumours of the biliary tract are adenocarcinomas.[1] Three macroscopic forms are recognized: nodular, sclerosing, and papillary variants. There appears to be a characteristic distribution in frequency, with the nodular and sclerosing types being more common for proximal tumours, and the papillary type more common for distal tumours. It is useful to distinguish three microscopic types with different invasiveness and prognoses: the most common is adenocarcinoma without specific features, accounting for 70 per cent of all cancers; next in frequency is the papillary variant (10 per cent), which is less invasive and has a better prognosis; and the third is the mucin-producing (5 per cent), associated with a poorer prognosis.[1]

The particular feature of cholangiocarcinoma is slow growth and longitudinal spread along the bile ducts and the perineural tissues (Ogura, WorldJSurg, 1994; 18:778). This explains the characteristic pattern of proximal and distal progression of the tumour along the biliary tree, and, for hilar tumours, the early invasion of the small branches of the caudate lobe that originate directly from the biliary confluence. Vascular and lymph-node invasion, particularly of the hepatoduodenal and retropancreatic nodes, is a later occurrence, and is found in 13 to 50 per cent of patients undergoing surgery (Nakeeb, AnnSurg, 1996; 224:463; Kurosaki, AmJSurg, 1996; 172: 239).[4] Distant spread, usually in the form of peritoneal rather than of other types of intra- or extra-abdominal metastasis, is a late manifestation and is present in half of the patients at the time of death.

The accepted staging for tumours of the extrahepatic biliary tract is the UICC TNM (Table 1).

Clinical presentation

Cholangiocarcinoma is a slow-growing tumour, remaining silent for a long time before causing a complete obstruction of the bile flow. The presenting symptom in the majority of patients is obstructive jaundice, with clear stools and dark urine, often preceded or accompanied by pruritus. Jaundice is typically progressive and painless, but may sometimes be intermittent in patients with tumours of the papillary type. Rarely, more proximal tumours, causing obstruction of only part of the biliary system, may be discovered in a patient without jaundice because of fever with altered liver function tests suggesting cholangitis or in the investigation of a nonspecific complaint such as fatigue, weight loss, or abdominal pain.

Clinical examination will show the characteristic yellow discoloration of the skin and of the mucosae, and scratching marks, in the absence of general signs of liver disease. Hepatomegaly is sometimes present and the gallbladder may be palpable (Courvoisier's sign) if the tumour is located below the insertion of the cystic duct. Physical examination will otherwise be normal or show non-specific signs of malignant disease such as wasting and

Table 1 TNM staging of cholangiocarcinoma

UICC stage	T	N	M
0	Tis	N0	M0
I	T1	N0	M0
II	T2	N0	M0
III	T1	N1,N2	M0
	T2	N1,N2	M0
IV A	T3	any N	M0
IV B	any T	any N	M1

From Bahars OH, Henson DE, Hutter RPV and Kennedy BJ. *AJCC manual for staging of cancer.* 4th edn. Philadelphia: Lippincott, 1992.
Tis, carcinoma *in situ*.
T1a, tumour invades the mucosa.
T1b, tumour invades the muscle layer.
T2, tumour invades the perimuscular connective tissue.
T3, tumour invades adjacent structures (liver, pancreas, duodenum, gallbladder, colon, stomach).
N1, metastasis in the cystic duct nodes, percholedochal and/or hilar lymph nodes (i.e., in the hepatoduodenal ligament).
N2, metastasis in the peripancreatic (head only), periduodenal, periportal, coeliac and/or superior mesenteric lymph nodes.
M0, no distant metastases.
M1, distant metastases present.

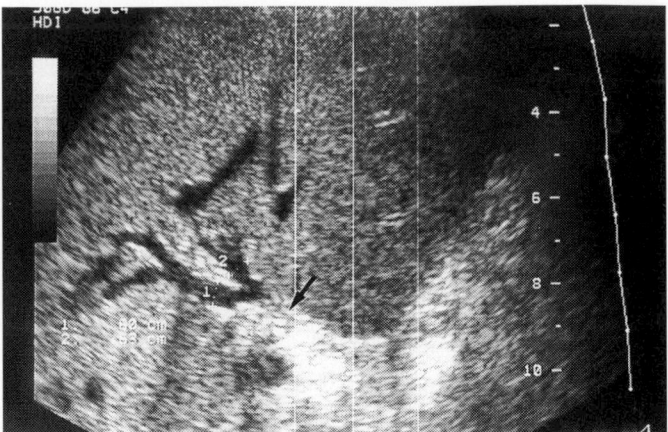

Fig. 1. Ultrasonographic examination of a patient with hilar cholangiocarcinoma. Note the dilatation of the bile ducts at the level of the right secondary biliary confluence (+). The primary biliary confluence is interrupted by the tumour, showing as hyperechoic material within the lumen of the right duct (arrow).

weight loss. The finding of a mass in the right hypochondrium is unusual and should alert to the possibility of gallbladder or pancreatic cancer.

Blood tests will show a variably increased conjugated and non-conjugated bilirubin, alkaline phosphatase, and γ-glutamyl transferase, according to the pattern and the duration of the obstruction. An increase in transaminase above four to five times the normal suggests parenchymal damage from associated factors such as cholangitis. Blood clotting may be deranged by impaired vitamin K absorption and should be corrected with parenteral vitamin K. Tumour markers such as CEA and CA 19–9 may be increased, the latter non-specifically so, as it also increases with cholestasis.

Diagnosis, staging, and assessment of resectability

Radiological examinations establish the diagnosis of the obstruction, demonstrate its level, and give information on the extent of the local spread that is needed to classify the disease in terms of resectability and surgical strategy.

Alternative causes of obstructive jaundice, such as tumours in the pancreatic head or chronic pancreatitis, can generally be ruled out easily. Obstruction from metastatic disease involving the hepatic pedicle is generally obvious from evidence of tumour dissemination elsewhere in the abdominal cavity and in the body. Stones in the gallbladder may cause a difficult diagnostic problem because of their high prevalence in the general population and their association with primary biliary malignancies. It is, in fact, rather common to see patients with cholangiocarcinoma referred after an operation performed for a mistaken diagnosis of obstructive gallstones, and the possibility of a tumour should always be considered in the management of biliary obstruction believed to be secondary to cholelithiasis. Alternative and rarer differential diagnoses, such as benign idiopathic strictures, probably a form of isolated sclerosing cholangitis, are diagnosed at surgery or on histological examination of

the specimen, and represented some 10 per cent of the cases in series of patients with a preoperative diagnosis of malignant biliary obstruction (Verbeek, Surgery, 1992; 112:866).

Radiological examination
Ultrasonography

Ultrasound is the first and most important diagnostic procedure in the investigation of biliary obstruction. It will show dilatation of the intrahepatic biliary channels down to the level of the blockage, where the lumen is lost, the walls are thickened, and/or contain hyperechoic or heterogeneous neoplastic tissue (Fig. 1). It is also useful in showing enlarged lymph nodes in the hepatic pedicle and, with the help of Doppler techniques, in demonstrating arterial and portal venous invasion that can contraindicate surgical resection.

Endoscopic ultrasonography

Endoscopic ultrasound is particularly useful in the investigation of the causes of obstruction in the biliary tree as it can explore the middle and distal bile duct better than conventional ultrasound (Fig. 2). Its usefulness in the investigation of tumours of the biliary confluence is, however, limited to the assessment of lymph-node invasion. In the preoperative staging of hepatic-duct tumours the accuracy was 70 per cent for T2 and 91 per cent for T3 tumours, while the incidence of positive lymph nodes may be overestimated (29 per cent and 94 per cent accuracy for N0 and N1 nodes, respectively) (Tio, Endoscopy, 1993; 25:81).

CT scanning

The CT scan shows dilatation of the bile ducts, generally in the absence of a visible tissue mass responsible for the obstruction. Atrophy of one sector or hemiliver and hypertrophy of the contralateral side suggest long-standing obstruction of one duct before extension of the tumour to the biliary confluence has caused jaundice and rendered the tumour clinically obvious (Fig. 3). CT scanning

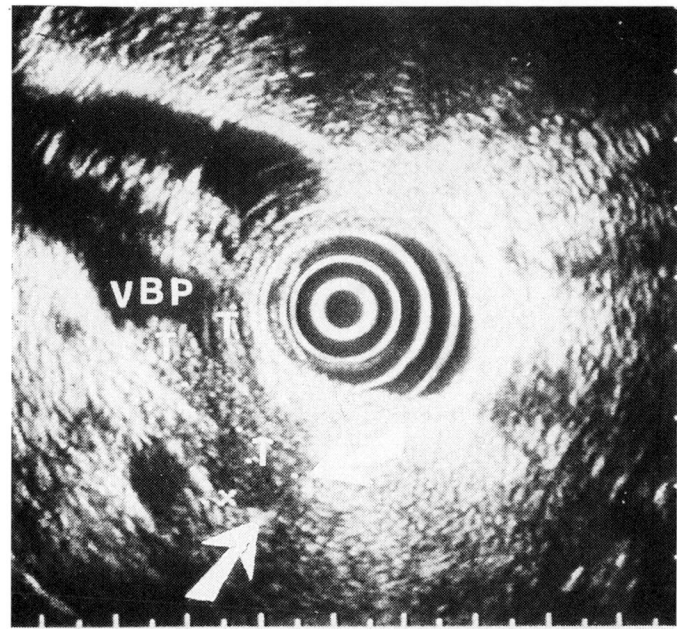

(a)

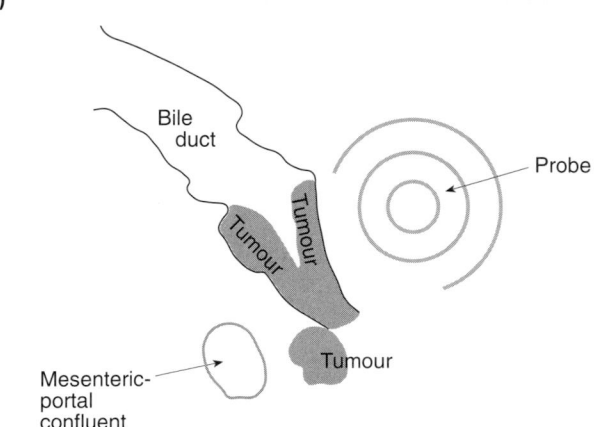

(b)

Fig. 2. Endoluminal ultrasonography in a patient with a cholangiocharcinoma of the middle bile duct. The tumour (T) can be clearly seen within the lumen of the bile duct (VBP). The white arrows demonstrate invasion by the tumour outside the wall of the bile duct at the level of the head of the pancreas. The black hypoechoic structure above and to the left of the lower arrow is the confluent of the mesenteric and portal vein, which is spared by the tumour (stage T2 of the TNM classification). (By courtesy of Dr Laurent Palazzo, Paris, France.)

offers a visual depiction of the amount of liver tissue that needs to be resected for radical treatment, which can be completed by precise volumetric measurements (see Chapter 29.1).

MRI

MRI with special acquisition procedures may provide a picture of the biliary tree similar to that of a cholangiogram, with the advantage of being non-invasive (Fig. 4). Although it is not certain that the information on the spread of the tumour is better than with conventional or endoscopic ultrasonography, MRI technique is

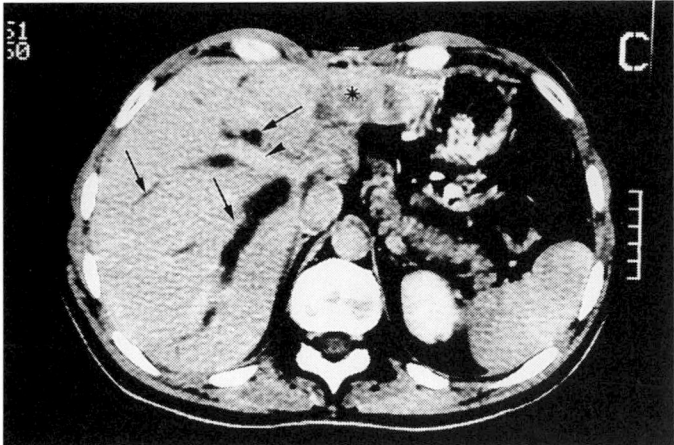

Fig. 3. CT scan of a patient with hilar cholangiocarcinoma (Klatskin tumour). Dilatation of the bile ducts (arrows) next to the branches of the portal vein (arrowhead). Note the marked atrophy of the left liver (*), suggesting long-standing obstruction of the left hepatic duct before further growth of the tumour obstructed the primary biliary confluence, causing jaundice and making the tumour clinically manifest.

evolving rapidly and it is possible that it will replace preoperative cholangiography (Becker, Radiol, 1997; 205:523).

Angiography

Angiography is useful in evaluating the extent of malignant invasion of the hepatic artery and portal vein, and aids in orientating the operative dissection of the hilar region, where abnormalities of the vascular anatomy are common. Tumour invasion showing as stenosis or occlusion of the portal vein or the hepatic artery that may contraindicate resection can be identified (Fig. 5).

Radiographic imaging, drainage, and instrumentation of the bile ducts

Percutaneous transhepatic cholangiography (PTC)

PTC can depict the exact anatomy of the obstruction and the pattern of invasion of the biliary tree. Several punctures may be needed to opacify all the sectors of the liver in tumours with proximal invasion. The cholangiogram shows dilatation of the bile ducts proximal to the obstruction. The pattern of the stenosis may provide important information on the spread of the tumour: a V-shaped termination suggests lack of compliance of the duct from duct-wall or periductal infiltration by the tumour, as opposed to a U-shaped pattern, showing that the bile-duct wall is still pliable (Fig. 6).

Endoscopic retrograde cholangiopancreatography (ERCP) (Fig. 4)

This procedure, although often used in the investigation of the jaundiced patient, is of limited utility in cases of complete occlusion of the bile ducts as it shows only the distal level of the obstruction, which is of little relevance for treatment. In cases of incomplete occlusion it exposes the patient to a greater risk of septic complications than does PTC.

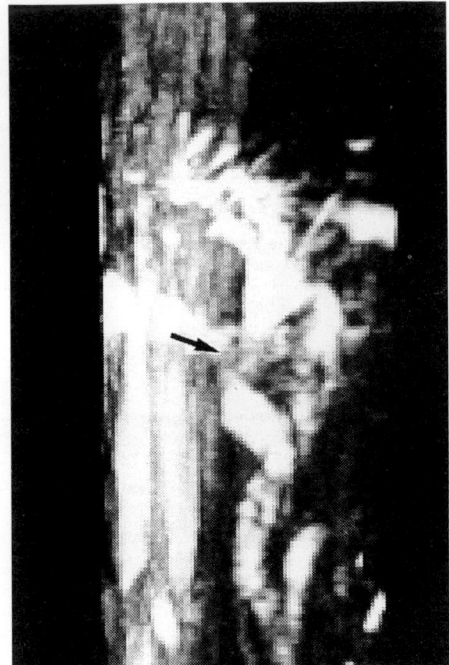

(a)

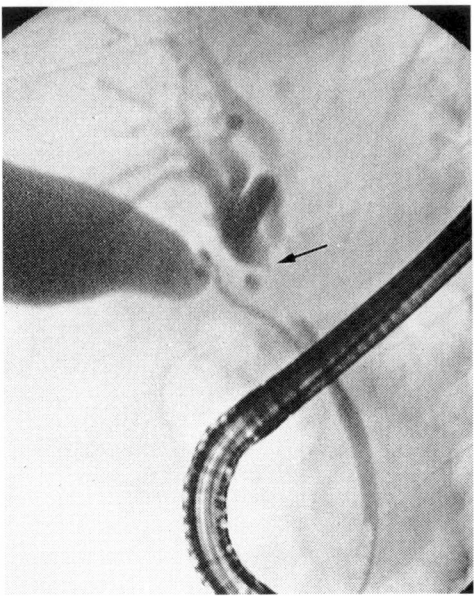

(b)

Fig. 4. (a) MRI scan: coronal reconstruction of the biliary tree in a patient with obstruction of the upper hepatic duct (arrow). (b) Endoscopic retrograde cholangiography in the same patient. The stenosis, with characteristic features of malignant obstruction (V-shaped ending, arrow), proved in fact to be a localized form of sclerosing cholangitis.

Other methods

Percutaneous cholangioscopy has been used in specialized units to map the intraluminal extension of tumour in the bile ducts (Nimura, Endoscopy, 1993; 25:76), and intraluminal ultrasonography inside the ducts (Tamada, AmJGastr, 1995; 90:239) may prove to be the most accurate tool for preoperative evaluation of the extent of tumour invasion along the ductal walls.

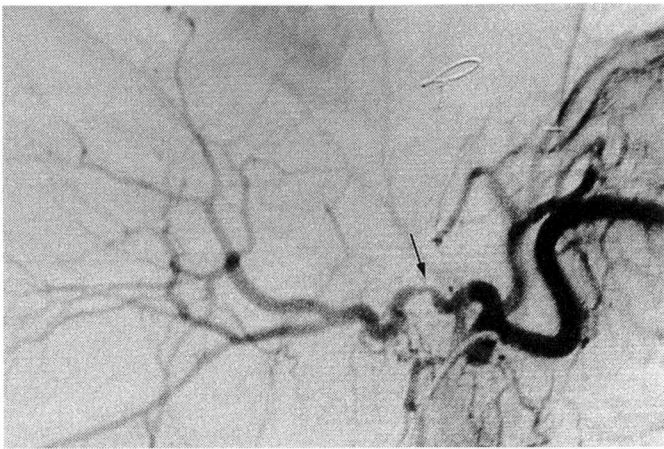

(a)

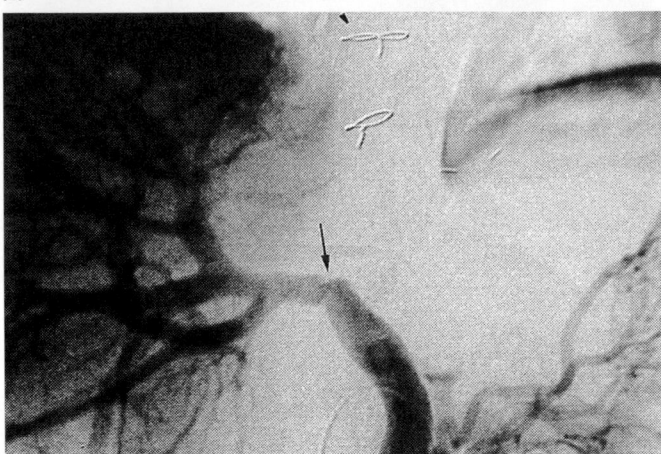

(b)

Fig. 5. Angiography in a patient with hilar cholangiocarcinoma (Klatskin tumour). Note the stenoses localized at the level of the hepatic artery (a) and the portal vein (b) (arrows), and the absence of a left branch of the portal vein, suggesting compression or infiltration of the vessel wall by the neoplasm or by metastatic lymph nodes.

Bile cytology and brush cytology, either by PTC or ERCP, can provide the definitive diagnosis of a malignant disease involving the biliary tree in 30 per cent of the patients. This figure rises to 60 per cent when both bile and brush cytology are combined (Kurzawinski, Hepatol, 1993; 18:1399).

Comment

Controversy still exists on the best timing for contrast imaging of the bile duct above the obstruction. The traditional view is that this should be postponed until all other preoperative investigations have been completed, or until the operation itself, because of the risk of inducing infection (with ERCP) or (rarely) a biliary leak by PTC. This may render preoperative drainage necessary, with consequent loss of the dilatation of the bile ducts, making the construction of a bilioenteric anastomosis more difficult and an anastomosis on the smaller intrahepatic ducts impossible. While there is no doubt that hasty drainage, intubation, or prosthetic stenting of a malignant biliary obstruction before full assessment of the disease in a specialized hepatobiliary unit must be condemned, many arguments

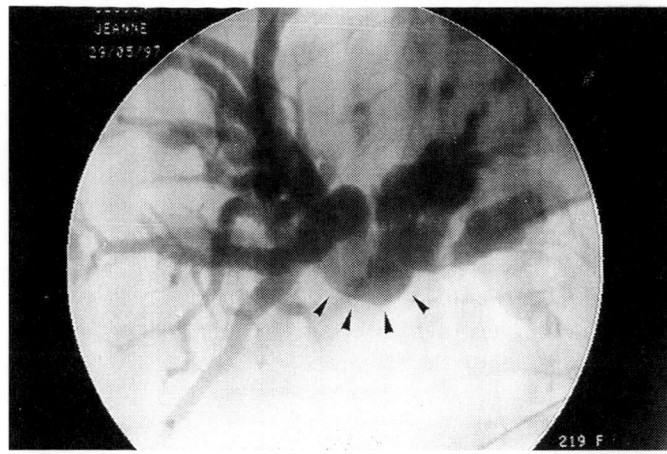

(a)

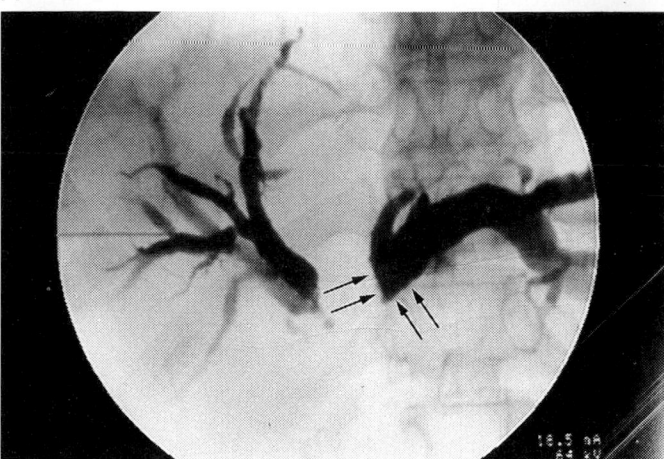

(b)

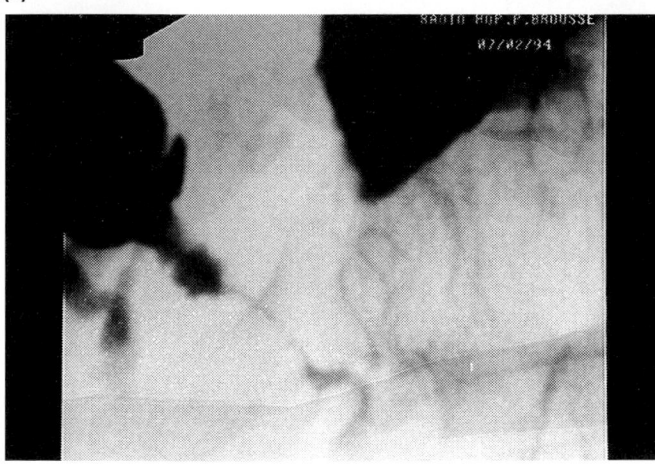

(c)

Fig. 6. PTC in two patients with hilar cholangiocarcinoma (Klatskin tumour). (a) The tumour spares the biliary confluence (type I); note the dilatation of the bile ducts, and the smooth, U-shaped contour of the obstruction (arrowheads), suggesting that the duct wall is still pliable and not infiltrated by tumour. (b) The tumour interrupts the biliary confluence and the secondary confluence on the right (type III). Near total interruption of the secondary confluence is suggested by the different densities of contrast in the ducts of the anterior sector (darker) and posterior sector (lighter). Note the sharp, V-shaped ending of the left duct, suggesting tumour infiltration of its wall (arrows). (c) Enlarged view.

are emerging in favour of preoperative instrumentation of the bile ducts. It has, in fact, been demonstrated that meticulous cholangiographic mapping of the extent of the disease, obtained by PTC, cholangioscopy, and endobiliary ultrasonography, allows excellent rates of curative resection and survival.[5] Furthermore, the resectability of the most extensive tumours can be increased by techniques such as portal venous embolization, which are effective only on liver tissue that is unobstructed,[6] and that preoperative drainage decreases the morbidity and mortality of surgery in the presence of segmental cholangitis.[7] These findings, together with better methods for controlling infection, improvements in surgical technique, and the availability of effective non-surgical palliation, have mitigated the arguments against preoperative cholangiographic imaging and drainage, leaving the issue open.

Treatment: resectional surgery and palliative procedures
Principles and classification

The most important step in the treatment of primary tumours of the bile ducts is the decision whether curative surgery is feasible or a palliative procedure only is possible. This involves:

(1) evaluating the location and regional spread of the disease;
(2) planning the resection to be performed;
(3) estimating the functional capacity of the residual liver in cases where a liver resection is needed.

As noted above, tumours are classified into lower-third tumours, amenable to a pancreatic resection, middle-third tumours, which can be treated by resection of the bile duct, and tumours of the hilar region. Tumours of the hilar region (Klatskin tumours) are further divided according to the classification represented in Fig. 7: the rationale of this classification is the tendency to periductal spread of cholangiocarcinoma and the extent of resection needed for curative surgery. Type I tumours can generally be treated by resection of the bile duct only; type II tumours require at least resection of segment 1 because of the early involvement of the biliary branches draining this segment directly into the hepatic confluence. Type III tumours require resection of segment 1 and a right or left hepatectomy and type IV tumours can rarely be removed unless a total hepatectomy (with liver transplantation) is performed.[8] Involvement of the trunk of the portal vein or of the hepatic artery proper, or bilateral invasion of either the portal, arterial, or biliary branches, generally indicate that resection is impossible. Lymph-node metastases beyond the hepatic pedicle (N2) and evidence of peritoneal dissemination are signs of unresectable disease.

The function of the liver remaining after the operation will have to be sufficient to support the patient until parenchymal regeneration takes place. Radical removal of hilar cholangiocarcinomas type III and IV generally requires a major liver resection, and, although this may involve a part of the liver that is already atrophic due to the long-standing obstruction, severe cholestasis in the residual liver may depress its function in the postoperative period. Hypertrophy of the part of the liver spared from the resection and more radical surgery may be permitted by ipsilateral biliary drainage (Kawasaki, JAmCollSurg, 1994, 178:480) or cholangioenteric anastomosis followed by contralateral portal

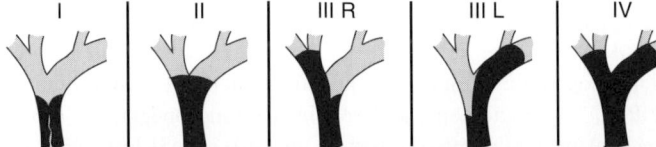

Fig. 7. Classification of hilar cholangiocarcinoma (Klatskin tumour). The rationale for this classification is the extent of the surgical resection theoretically needed for curative removal of the tumour. Type I, resection of the biliary confluence only; type II, resection of the confluence and of segment 1; type III right or left, resection of the confluence, segment 1, and right or left hepatectomy; type IV, total hepatectomy and liver transplantation, with the exception of cases with particularly favourable anatomy). (By courtesy of Prof. D. Castaing, Hepatobiliary Foundation, Hôpital Paul Brousse, Villejuif, Paris.)

venous embolization. Wider use of these procedures, together with improved surgical technique, has increased the resectability and the curative resection rate (R0) above 50 per cent in many recent series (Table 2).

Resectional surgery: procedures and results

The aim of the procedure is resection of the bile duct with all the surrounding connective tissue and lymph nodes in the hepatic pedicle associated, for hilar tumours, with resection of the liver parenchyma in close contact with the involved ducts. Because of the infiltrative pattern of growth of these tumours along the walls of the bile ducts and the perineural tissues, a clear margin of at least 5 mm is needed and has to be confirmed at surgery by frozen-section examination of the resected specimen. A Whipple pancreaticoduodenectomy is performed for tumours of the intrapancreatic portion of the bile duct. A resection of the bile duct, gallbladder, and a radical lymph-node dissection of the hepatic pedicle and the retropancreatic and coeliac nodes is done for tumours of the middle third of the bile duct. The extent of resection for curative removal of cholangiocarcinoma at the hepatic confluence (Klatskin tumour) varies according to the level in the classification and has been mentioned above. Details of the procedure, including resection of the caudate lobe, can be found in specialized articles.[9] Although in type IV tumours it is rarely possible to perform the

Table 2 Results of surgical resection for malignant biliary tumours (series with more than 40 patients since 1990)

Study (reference)	Period	Patients No.	Resectability (% of patients in the study)	R0 (% of patients resected)	Morbidity/ mortality (% of patients resected)	Survival of patients resected (%)		
						1 year	3 years	5 years
Nimura* (9)	1979–89	66	55 (83%)	46 (70%)	41*/6*		51†	38†
Reding (17)	1955	552/307*	98 (32%)*	na/16*	70*	30*	11*
Bismuth* (8)	1960–90	136	23 (17%)	9 (39%)	9/0	87	25	
						100†	50†	
Ogura* (18)	1976–91	65	55 (85%)	28 (51%)	21/2	63	31	23
						83†	46†	29†
Tashiro* (19)	1975–90	46	34 (74%)	18 (53%)	27/3	62	47	25
						75†	59†	30†
Buhya* (20)	1979–90	70	‡					25
Gazzaniga* (21)	1970–90	100	43 (43%)	25 (58%)	na/10	70†	20†	20†
Nagorney (22)	1976–85	79*		12 (15%)	24/5	51§		13§
Sugiura* (23)	1973–91	158	83 (53%)	47 (57%)	na/8		30	20
								33†
								46¶
Washburn (24)	1985–94	88	59 (67%)	29 (49%)	35/11	75	38	10
Miyagawa* (25)	1989–94	53	24 (45%)		25/0**	79**	56**	
Pichlmayr* (2)	1975–93	249	125 (50%)	91 (73%)	52–65/ 3–13††	69†	41†	31†
						53‡‡	10‡‡	10‡‡
Nimura* (5)	1977–93	127	100 (79%)	82 (82%)	51/10			31†
								43§§
Nakeeb (26)	1973–95	196	109 (56%)	28 (26%)	47/4	68	30	11
								19†
Su* (27)	1983–95	49	‡	24 (49%)	47/10	80†	30†	15
								30†

R0, curative resection (negative histological margins).
na, not available.
, series concerns only hilar cholangiocarcinoma (Klatskin tumour), or figure concerns hilar cholangiocarcinoma.
†, concerns patients after curative resection (R0).
‡, study comprising only patients undergoing resection.
§, survival is given for all patients whether resected or not.
¶, survival after associated caudate-lobe resection (47 patients).
**, on 24 patients undergoing extended right hepatectomy; survival is disease-free.
††, morbidity: preoperatively drained–undrained patients; mortality, hilar resection–hepatectomy.
‡‡, survival after palliative resection; positive histological margins (R1).
§§, survival after R0 resection in patients without portal vein resection; this study includes patients from ref. 20.

extensive bilateral resection needed for radical removal, and liver transplantation represents the most satisfactory procedure from a theoretical point of view, some cases of curative resection of type IV tumours (either deep hilar or liver resections) are reported, with long-term survival probably reflecting a particularly favourable local anatomy.[4]

Biliary continuity is re-established with a hepaticojejunal anastomosis on a roux-en-Y loop at a level determined by the extent of the biliary and hepatic resection.

The postoperative care does not generally differ from what is usual in patients after major hepatobiliary surgery. Liver insufficiency is minor and short-lived if the resection has been correctly planned and performed.

In spite of the very poor figures reported in the past, the results for surgical resection of cholangiocarcinoma have markedly improved in recent years: in some centres an approach including systematic resection of the caudate lobe and a right or left hepatectomy, as appropriate, resulted in resectability and curative resection (R0) rates in over 75 per cent of the patients and 5-year survival rates of 30 per cent or higher (Table 2). An example of the modern treatment of these tumours is shown in Fig. 8. Complications are frequent, depending to some extent on the aggressiveness with which curative resection is pursued. Surgical resection with macroscopically negative but histologically positive margins (R1) still affords good palliation in specialized centres.[4] Resection leaving gross tumour in place (R2) significantly increases morbidity and mortality and should not be done.

Adjuvant chemotherapy for complete resection (R0) is still of unproved benefit, although tumours are sometimes responsive to platinum salts and 5-fluorouracil, and in our centre some excellent responses have been recorded for both recurrence after surgery and preoperative down-staging of the tumour. External or intracavitary radiotherapy have been used with success in selected cases of R0 and R1 resection as well as in cases of tumour recurrence after surgery (Koyama, SGO, 1993; 176:239; Kraybill, JSurgOncol, 1994; 55:239; Shoenthaler, AnnSurg, 1994, 19:267).

Transplantation

Liver transplantation for cholangiocarcinoma had raised hopes mainly for unresectable tumours. Unfortunately the frequency of positive lymph nodes in these patients is responsible for the high recurrence rate, with a 3- and 5-year survival of 21 and 17 per cent in the largest reported series of 25 patients.[4] Patients with unresectable, early-stage disease, however, have a 5-year survival as high as 41 per cent, substantiating the conclusion that liver transplantation can be considered in these cases as well as for patients with R1 resections and provenly negative lymph nodes. Although the results for incidental tumours in patients with sclerosing cholangitis could logically be expected to be better, the majority of these patients have stage IV disease and their survival is poor.

Palliative surgical and non-surgical approaches for malignant biliary obstruction

Introduction

For patients with malignant biliary obstruction in whom curative surgery cannot be performed (or after recurrence of a resected tumour), the most distressing symptoms are itching, which responds poorly to medical treatment, and jaundice, which is often accompanied by severe anorexia and nausea. Cholangitis from bacterial infection of the obstructed biliary system is rare in the absence of previous instrumentation or surgery on the biliary tract, but may be life-threatening and should be treated as a medical emergency. Duodenal obstruction is uncommon in high bile-duct tumours but occurs in up to 30 to 50 per cent of lower bile-duct and pancreatic tumours (Bakkevold, AnnSurg, 1993, 217:356). Variceal bleeding from portal venous obstruction is rare because of the rapid formation of an hepatopetal collateral circulation in the absence of an intrahepatic block to portal flow, unless previous surgery (such as pancreaticodoudenectomy) has interrupted the pericholedocal venous network.

Jaundice and pruritus can be relieved by:

(1) percutaneous external tube drainage;
(2) an intraluminal tube (Fig. 9) or stent (Fig. 10) forcing a path through the obstruction, placed either at surgery, endoscopically, or percutaneously;
(3) a surgical anastomosis between the dilated biliary tree and the gastrointestinal tract below the obstruction (bypass) (Figs 11 and 12).

Three important considerations apply to all forms of treatment, as follows.

1. A palliative procedure for malignant biliary obstruction never has to be performed as an emergency, with the exception of overt cholangitis, which is rare in the absence of previous surgery or instrumentation of the biliary tract. The indications for palliation and choice of the best method to achieve it need to be established in close collaboration with a hepatobiliary surgeon. Resectability is sometimes difficult to appreciate, and even the surgeon may be in doubt until laparotomy. Hasty drainage of the biliary tract as a complement to a diagnostic procedure such as PTC or ERCP may render an intrahepatic cholangioenteric anastomosis, often the best option for slow-growing unresectable cholangiocarcinomas, impossible to perform.
2. Ideally all the liver should be drained, which is rarely possible in cases of hilar or intrahepatic obstruction. While only one-quarter of functional liver tissue is enough to relieve jaundice, the effect on itching is less constant. The bypass or drainage should be done on the largest part of the liver that is functional and should not be done on a part that is atrophic from long-standing obstruction.

With incomplete drainage of the biliary tree the patient is at increased risk of cholangitis, owing to the communication between the biliary system and the external environment or the gastrointestinal tract. Generally the cholangitis responds to antibiotic treatment but further drainage should be considered if there is a poor response or worsening clinical condition.

External drainage

External drainage by the percutaneous–transhepatic route, often under local anaesthesia, is the simplest method for relieving jaundice. It transforms the obstruction into an external biliary fistula that can be equipped with a bag to collect the bile. The main disadvantages are the inconvenience caused by the collecting system, the bacterial contamination of the biliary tract, which may cause cholangitis if drainage is incomplete, and the loss of fluids and electrolytes, which need replacing by enteral or parenteral adjustment. For these reasons, external drainage alone is not generally used as a form of palliation but rather as a preliminary to internal tube drainage or stenting.

Internal drainage and prosthetic stenting

The principle is to re-establish a communication between the two sides of the tumour with a guide wire on which either a multiperforated external drain can be threaded or a prosthesis inserted. Prostheses can be placed by the endoscopic or the percutaneous routes according to the preference and the expertise of

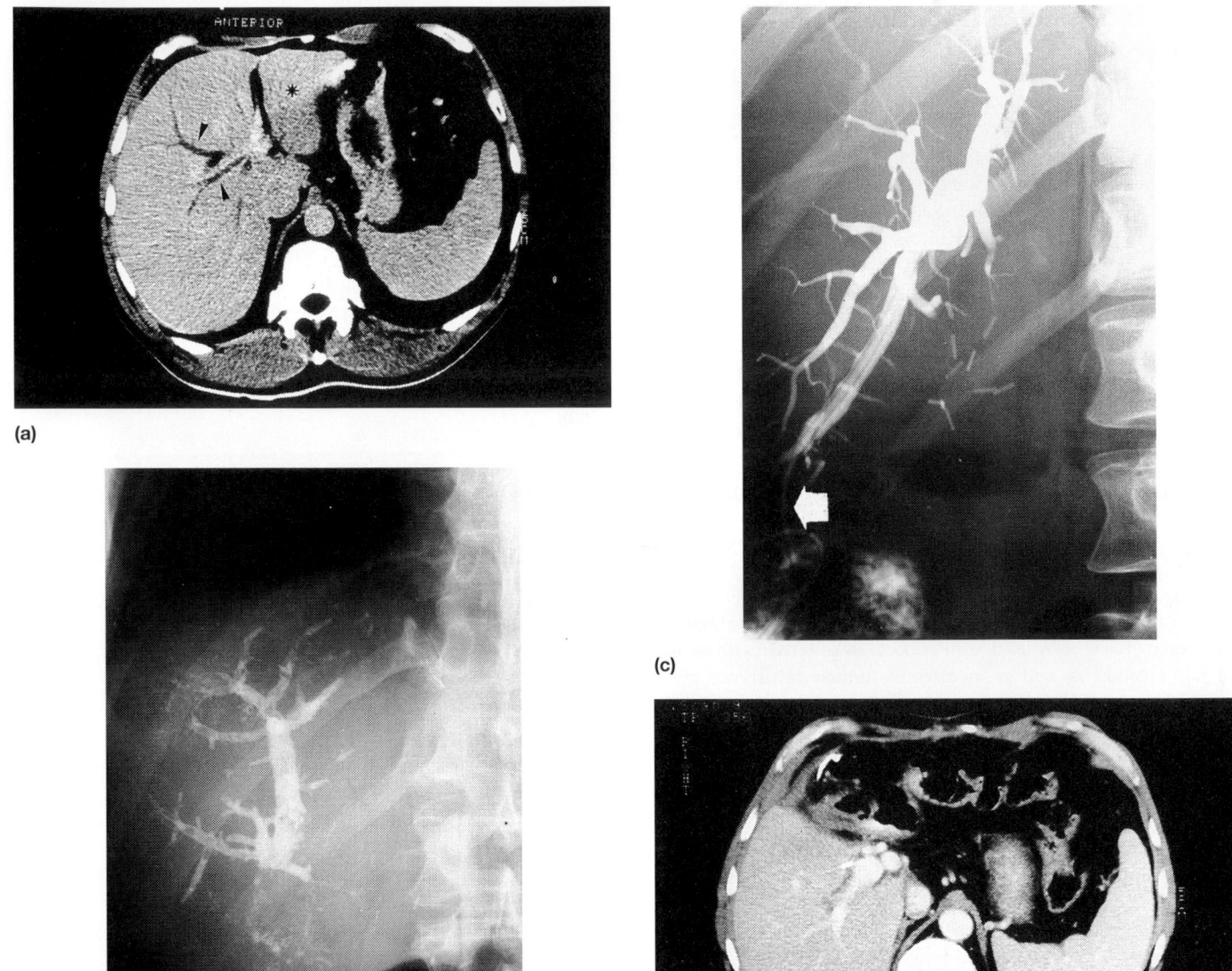

Fig. 8. Radical management of a Klatskin tumour (type IV) in a 50-year-old patient. (a) Preoperative CT scan: note dilatation of the bile ducts on the right side (arrowheads) and atrophy of the left lobe (*), suggesting that the tumour originated in the left ductal system. (b) The largest portion of functioning liver parenchyma was chosen for a cholangioenteric bypass and an anastomosis was made on the duct of segment 6 draining the channels of segments 6 and 7 (arrow, silicone drain stenting the anastomosis between a channel of segment 6 and the roux-en-Y bowel loop). (c) After recovery from surgery, portal venous embolization of the branch to the anterior sector (segments 5 and 8) was done to induce hypertrophy of segments 6 and 7. A left hepatectomy extended to segments 1, 5, and 8 was performed 2 months later with no complications. (d) Postoperative CT scan: note hypertrophy of the residual liver. The patient is well without recurrence 3 years after the operation.

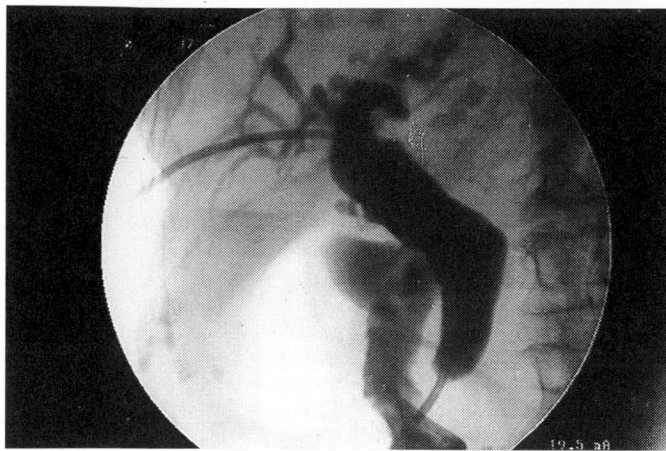

Fig. 9. Internal tube drainage in a patient with lower bile-duct obstruction from pancreatic cancer. The tube is multiperforated allowing bile flow across the obstruction. A prosthesis was eventually inserted.

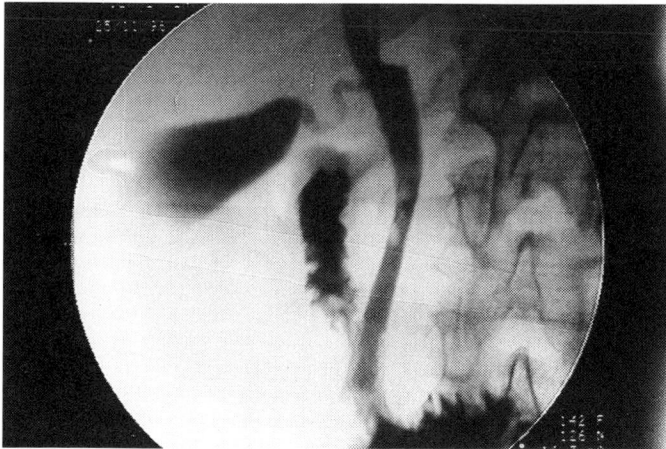

Fig. 10. Prosthetic stenting of a low bile-duct obstruction in a patient with a tumour of the head of the pancreas and liver metastases. An expandable metal prosthesis (Wallstent) across the papilla allowed satisfactory relief of jaundice and itching for 6 months.

the operator, although in general the percutaneous route offers a better angle to negotiate the obstruction. Intubation of the obstruction at laparotomy performed for unresectable tumours (Praderi technique) is infrequently done at present (Millikan, AnnSurg, 1993; 218:621), owing to the remarkable technical progress in radiological and endoscopic interventions, and because it is probably associated with higher morbidity than the percutaneous route or a cholangioenteric anastomosis. Prostheses can be made either of an inert plastic material (polyethylene) or of an expandable metal mesh that can be dilated by a pneumatic balloon, resulting in a large passage through the obstruction (Wallstent). Plastic stents have a higher propensity for obstruction, and may require frequent replacement. Expandable metal stents have a higher patency rate (Davids, Lancet, 1992; 340:1488), but the tumour may regrow through the mesh, a disadvantage that may have been solved in the newer prostheses by a layer of inert tissue covering the metal frame. According to the level of the blockage, the drain or the prosthesis can be placed with the distal end above the papilla [with the

theoretical advantage of preserving the function of the sphincter of Oddi (decreasing the risk of cholangitis or pancreatitis)] or beyond it. With regard to the advantages and disadvantages of the multiperforated drain and the prosthesis, the drain has the drawback of an external device that needs care and dressings. Although more prone to obstruction, it is easily accessible for imaging and replacement, and more than one tube can be accommodated in the biliary tree, offering the possibility of more complete drainage when there is separation of the biliary ducts. Prostheses have the advantage of freeing the patient from the hindrance of external appliances. The problem is that they tend to become blocked either by biliary sludge and encrustations or by the tumour, with a median patency of 6 months and the need for repeat procedures in most series. Either method is acceptable, and the choice will in part depend on the personal preference of the surgeon and patient.

Surgical bypass

The biliary obstruction can be bypassed by a surgical anastomosis between the biliary channels above the occlusion and the digestive system below it. According to the level of the obstruction, two operations are commonly performed, as follows.

If the obstruction is in the lower bile duct, the operation is the same as with pancreatic cancer: the dilated main hepatic duct can be anastomosed side-to-side to a loop of jejunum. The operation preferred in our unit is shown in Fig. 11(a), linking the biliary drainage to a gastroenterostomy (Bismuth, *Enciclopédie médico-chirurgicale*. Paris: Editions Techniques, 1981: 40 940). If the obstruction is higher in the hepatic duct or at the hilum, an anastomosis is performed on the dilated channel of segment 3, approached through the round ligament on the inferior surface of the liver where the duct can be localized more constantly, as originally described by Soupault and Couinaud (Figs 11(b,c) and 12(a,b)) (Traynor, BrJSurg, 1987; 74:952). This procedure is particularly effective for hilar cholangiocarcinomas. It will drain all sectors of the liver if the confluence is not interrupted, but only the left liver otherwise. An alternative, technically more demanding procedure is an anastomosis on the dilated duct of segment 6, as shown in Figs 8(b) and 12(c,d). A gastroenterostomy is added according to the pattern of spread of the tumour and the threat of duodenal obstruction. Other types of biliodigestive bypass, such as choledocoduodenostomy or using the gallbladder as a conduit, have shown poor results, owing to the anatomical proximity and predisposition to recurrent obstruction by the tumour, and have been abandoned in most centres.

The choice of procedure

Three factors should be considered, as follows.

The stage and the likely evolution of the malignant disease

Palliative treatment must be tailored to the life expectancy of the patient, taking into account the possibility that this may be modified by treatment such as chemotherapy or radiotherapy. Biliary cancers are slow-growing and it is not uncommon to see patients with unresectable tumours to survive for more than 1 or 2 years. Surgical palliation therefore appears more appropriate in these patients. At

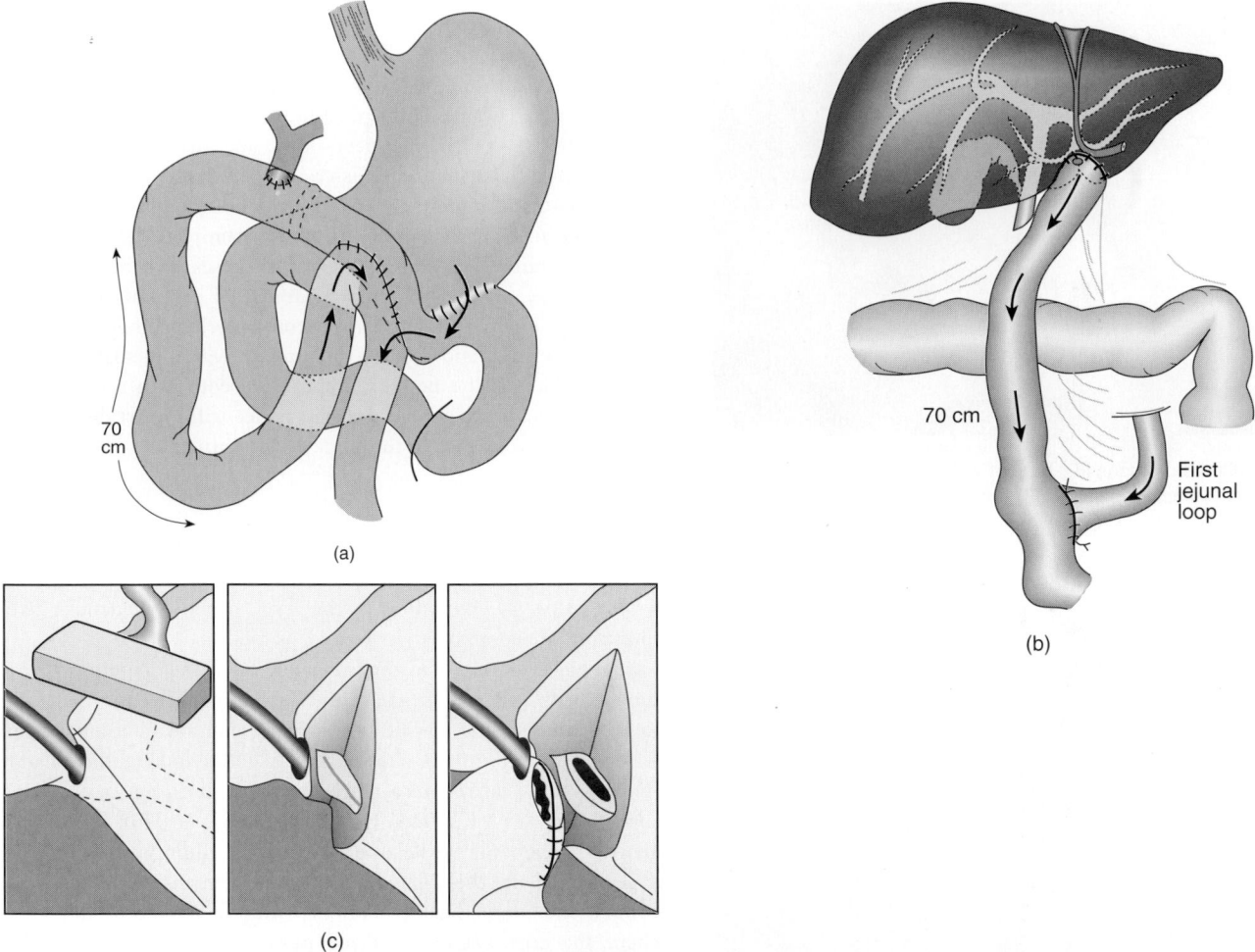

Fig. 11. Schematic representation of two types of surgical anastomoses used for palliative treatment of malignant biliary obstruction. (a) 'Asymmetric omega loop' with anastomosis on the dilated bile duct and gastrointestinal bypass to prevent symptoms of duodenal obstruction. Note the staple line (*) to prevent passage of food into the biliary anastomosis. The biliary loop is 70 cm long to avoid alimentary reflux into the biliary tree. This operation is used mainly for pancreatic or lower bile-duct cancers, where a relatively long stump of the hepatic duct is available. The advantage over a roux-en-Y loop is that it avoids transection of the bowel and mesentery. (b) Intrahepatic cholangioenteric anastomosis on the dilated duct of segment 3; this type of bypass is used mainly for hilar tumours. A gastroenterostomy can be added if the duodenum is threatened by the tumour. (c) The duct of segment 3 is found, by intraoperative ultrasonography, superior to the insertion of the round ligament on the inferior aspect of the left lobe of the liver. (By courtesy of Professor D. Castaing, Hepatobiliary Foundation, Hôpital Paul Brousse, Villejuif, Paris.)

the opposite end of the spectrum a patient with jaundice from an exocrine pancreatic tumour with liver metastases has a life expectancy shorter than 6 months and a prosthesis represents a wiser choice.

The clinical condition of the patient

Elderly and frail patients may tolerate surgery poorly and a prosthesis may be indicated in this context, even in the presence of a slow-growing tumour.

The anatomical pattern of the obstruction

A solitary lesion obstructing the hepatic duct below the confluence can be managed either by a surgical bypass or a prosthesis, on the criteria mentioned above. For tumours interrupting the primary or secondary biliary confluences a prosthesis in a duct may in fact occlude other ducts along its path, with no gain in liver function and exposing the patient to the risk of cholangitis. Drainage with multiple internal or external tubes may be required, but is rarely indicated unless the obstruction is caused by tumours for which an excellent response to chemotherapy is anticipated, and for which jaundice represents the main contraindication for starting treatment (Fig. 13).

Results

Surgical bypass, stent, or percutaneous internal-tube placement are all effective in relieving symptoms of biliary obstruction. As the indications for each depend to a large extent on the clinical condition, the results of the series on each type of treatment cannot readily be compared. Surgical bypass is preferably done for patients in better general condition, and it is not surprising that in uncontrolled series survival is longer than with stenting. Controlled studies, too, are biased, mainly because of poor standardization or

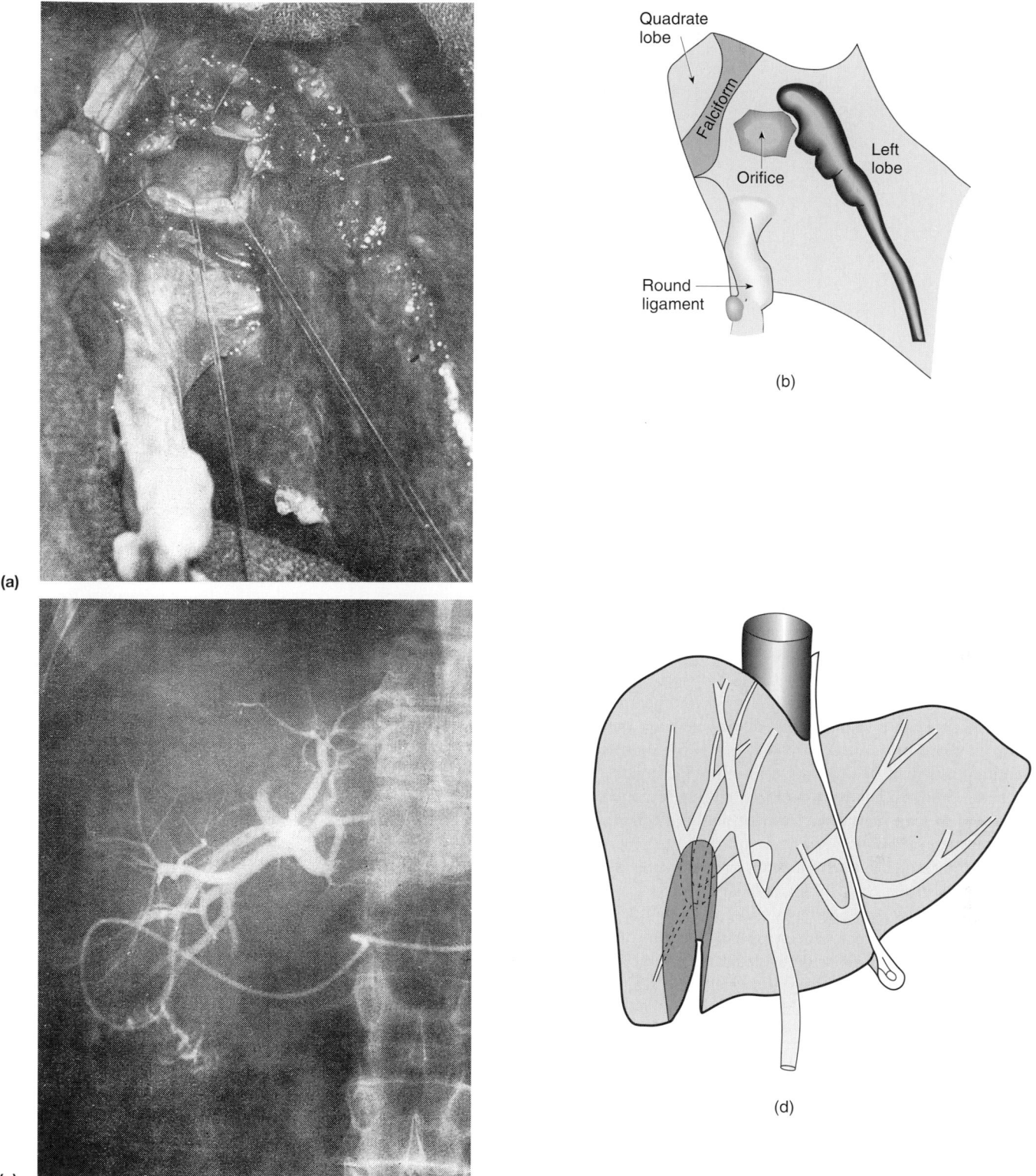

Fig. 12. Intrahepatic biliary anastomoses: operative view (a) and schematic representation (b) of a cholangioenteric anastomosis on the channel of segment 3. The same concept can be applied to anastomosis on the channel of segment 5. Postoperative cholangiogram (c) and schematic representation (d).

suboptimal surgical procedures such as using the gallbladder as a conduit.[10,11] The results for surgical bypass in specialized centres are excellent, several series reporting a mortality of less than 10 per cent and a mean survival ranging from 8 to 15 months for segment

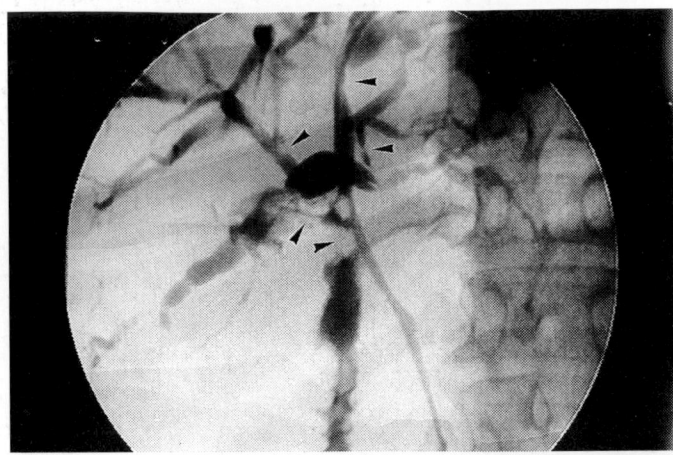

Fig. 13. Malignant obstruction at multiple levels caused by diffuse infiltration of the hepatic pedicle by metastatic disease from cancer of the pancreas. Note the multiple irregularities of the bile ducts signalling compression and infiltration by tumour (triangular arrows). Drainage is contraindicated unless a rapid response to anticancer treatment is anticipated.

3 hepaticojejunostomies.[12] In our institution, in a series of 160 palliative procedures for hilar cancer, although survival was similar to that with intubation (9 months), the length of time the patient was free of symptoms was significantly longer with a cholangioenteric segment-3 bypass than with intubation (8 as compared to 2–4 months) (Bismuth, WorldJSurg, 1988, 12:39). This bypass is the preferred treatment for patients with slowly evolving, unresectable tumours or when a favourable response to chemotherapy is anticipated. The procedure is adequately effective even if only one-half of the liver can be drained, provided that this is not atrophic (representing more than 30 to 40 per cent of the liver mass) (Baer, HPBSurgery, 1994; 8:27), that its ducts are not threatened by metastases, and that the undrained liver has not been contaminated by previous instrumentation.

Similarly, the results for percutaneous or endoscopic stents in hilar tumours or obstruction of the lower biliary tract have improved since expandable stents have been used as opposed to polyethylene prostheses. Figures of 78 per cent symptom-free after a median follow-up of 14 months are reported by dedicated units[13] and are similar to those obtained with surgery. Even in these cases, however, further reintervention is required in 24 per cent of the patients (Glättli, HPBSurgery, 1993; 6:175).

Gallbladder carcinoma

Epidemiology

Gallbladder carcinoma has an incidence of 1 to 1.5/100 000. The prevalence in different populations parallels the prevalence of gallstones, with peaks in some ethnic groups or countries such as native Americans and Chile (Morris, Cancer, 1978; 42:2472). The median age for invasive carcinoma is 73 years and for carcinoma *in situ* 69 years. A male:female ratio of approx 1:3 also probably corresponds to the increased prevalence of gallstones in women.[1] Gallbladder carcinoma is an incidental finding in approx 1 per cent of patients undergoing cholecystectomy for gallstones (Yamaguchi, ArchSurg, 1996, 131:981).

Causative factors

A strong association exists between cholelithiasis and carcinoma of the gallbladder, and stones are present in 75 to 90 per cent of cases (Cubertafond, AnnSurg, 1994; 219:275). It is estimated that the risk of developing gallbladder cancer is 1 per cent after 20 years from the original diagnosis of gallstones (Maringhini, AnnInternMed, 1987; 107:30), and the risk increases with calcified (porcelain) gallbladder, which is associated with cancer in 13 to 22 per cent of patients (Fig. 13) (Ashur, Arch Surg, 1978; 113:594). The proposed mechanism is, sequentially, chronic inflammation, dysplasia, carcinoma *in situ*, invasive carcinoma, and it would apply particularly to large stones (Lowenfels, IntJEpid, 1989; 18:50). A similar mechanism is probably responsible for the association between gallbladder carcinoma and chronic salmonella infection (Caygill, Lancet, 1994, 343:83). The progression from gallbladder polyps to adenomas to carcinoma is well documented and cholecystectomy is indicated for polyps larger than 10 mm (Aldrige, Surgery, 1991; 109:107).

Pathology, mode of spread, and staging

Three histological types are described, the most common being adenocarcinoma with no specific features (74 per cent), followed by the papillary (6 per cent), and the mucinous (5 per cent) variants. The papillary type is associated with a lesser propensity for distal spread and a better prognosis. A squamous type of carcinoma represents 1 to 5 per cent of cases.[1]

The pattern of spread of gallbladder carcinomas has been studied. The main lymphatic route goes along the common bile duct to the paraortic nodes, other routes travel on the left of the hepatoduodenal ligament to the posterior common hepatic node, and another ascends toward the hilum (Uesaka, JAmCollSurg, 1996; 183:345). Lymph-node metastases are common and are found in 48 per cent of patients with tumours reaching the muscle layer (T1b + T2).[14] Three patterns of intrahepatic spread are recognized: direct invasion through the gallbladder bed, angiolymphatic invasion of the portal tracts, and intrahepatic metastatic nodules. A correlation between the extent of direct penetration into the liver and of angiolymphatic invasion is described, and may guide the extent of the liver resection needed for radical excision (Shirai, Cancer, 1995; 75:2062). The disease eventually extends by contiguity to the hepatic pedicle producing obstruction of the bile duct first, then of the portal and arterial blood vessels, and eventually spreading to the duodenum. Distant haematogenous metastases are rare.

The TNM staging classification for gallbladder carcinoma is shown in Table 3.

Clinical presentation

Gallbladder carcinoma may present in four ways with different clinical implications.

Inapparent carcinoma

The existence of the tumour is first discovered by the pathologist after the operation. Hopefully this is a very small tumour missed by the surgeon, who should always open the gallbladder and examine it on its removal from the patient. It is suggested that no further

Table 3 TNM staging of gallbladder cancer

UICC stage	T	N	M
0	Tis	N0	M0
I	T1	N0	M0
II	T2	N0	M0
III	T1	N1	M0
	T2	N1	M0
	T3	any N	M0
IV	T4	any N	M0
	any T	any N	M1

From Bahars OH, Henson DE, Hutter RPV and Kennedy BJ. *AJCC manual for staging of cancer.* 4th edn. Philadelphia: Lippincott, 1992.
Tis, carcinoma *in situ.*
T1a, mucosal invasion.
T1b, tumour invades into the muscular layer.
T2, tumour invades into the perimuscular connective tissue, no extension beyond the serosa or into the liver.
T3, invasion beyond the serosa or into an adjacent organ or both (invasion into the liver ≤2 cm).
T4, invasion into the liver 2 cm or invasion into two or more adjacent organs.
N1, invasion into the cystic duct, pericholedochal, perihilar lymph nodes (into the hepatoduodenal ligament).
N2, invasion into the peripancreatic, periduodenal, periportal, coeliac and/or superior mesenteric lymph nodes.
M0, no distant metastases.
M1, distant metastases present.

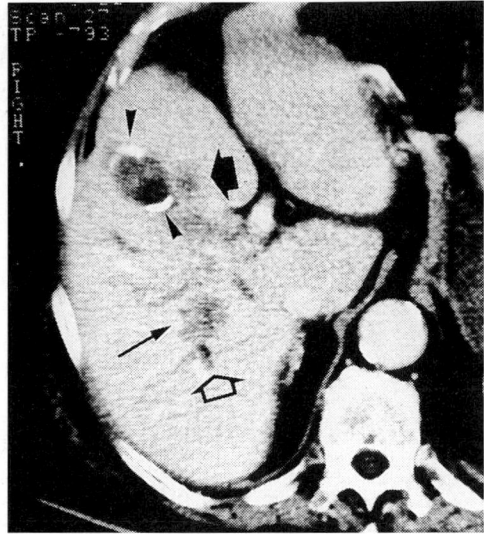

Fig. 14. Gallbladder carcinoma in an 89-year-old patient. Note calcifications in the gallbladder wall (small triangular arrows), a tumour nodule infiltrating segment 4 (wide arrow), a distant liver metastasis more posterior in segment 5 (arrow), and early dilatation of the bile ducts (empty arrow).

action is needed for tumours Tis or T1a. Patients with T1b or T2 tumours, and the rare patient in whom the presence of a T3 tumour has not been recognized, should undergo a formal reoperation removing the bed and the lymph nodes of the gallbladder.[15]

During cholecystectomy

The surgeon discovers the existence of the tumour on opening the specimen. It is uncommon for the facilities or the expertise to carry out a satisfactory radical resection to be immediately available locally. The patient is best referred in the postoperative period to a centre used to performing major liver resections where definitive surgery can be done. The same applies if the tumour is discovered before the removal of the gallbladder, as generally the tumour is more advanced in these cases.

In a patient with symptoms of gallstones

The ultrasonogram reveals a mass in the gallbladder, with variable penetration into the liver. A full preoperative evaluation is carried out to investigate the local extent of the disease.

As a liver mass in a patient with jaundice

In this case, obstruction of the bile duct has occurred due to progression of the tumour along the cystic duct or to the hepatic hilum, or because of compression from extensive lymph-node metastases. Generally it is too late for curative surgery and the patient has to be evaluated for the best possible form of palliation, the principles of which are the same as for other forms of malignant biliary obstruction, as discussed above.

Management

Preoperative investigations aim at defining the extent of the disease and the resectability.

Ultrasonography

Ultrasound gives an accurate depiction of the tumour in the gallbladder, which may be replaced by a mass containing a stone. It will also show the presence and level of any biliary obstruction and of lymph-node metastases. This information may be completed, as in the case of bile-duct tumours, by Doppler examination to assess the permeability of the arterial supply and the portal vein, and by the use of endoscopic ultrasonography.

CT scan (Fig. 14)

This completes the information provided by ultrasonography, especially in relation to intrahepatic and lymph-node metastases, and on the presence of peritoneal or pulmonary metastases, which are infrequent.

Arteriography

Arteriography is helpful in detecting involvement of the hepatic artery and the portal vein by the tumour, which are generally considered as a contraindication to surgical resection. Portal hypertension from compression or thrombosis of the portal vein may complicate the surgical access to the region, and may influence the choice between operative and non-operative palliation.

Operative treatment

It is now generally accepted that the best operation for gallbladder cancer of stages more advanced than Tis and T1a, that is, for tumours invading the muscularis, is *en bloc* resection of the gallbladder with segments 4 and 5 (Bismuth, WorldJSurg, 1982; 6: 10), the bile duct, and the lymphatic tissues extending to the peripancreatic and paraortic lymph nodes.[14] A schematic representation of the liver resection performed in radical surgery for gallbladder cancer is shown in Fig. 15. Although more extensive

Table 4 Results of resection for gallbladder carcinoma (series with more than 40 patients, from single institutions, since 1990)

Study (reference)	Period	Patients No.	Resected (% of patients in the study)	R0 (% of patients resected)	Morbidity/ mortality (% of patients resected)	Survival (%) 3 years	5 years
Shirai (15) (inapparent carcinoma)	1981–89	98			na/7*		100† 40‡
Chijiiwa (28)	1982–92	73	32 (44%)	50	na/3	75§	75§
Onoyama (29)	1971–93	227	158 (70%) 66*		na/0*		79 (stage I)* 64 (stage II)* 44 (stage III)* 8 (stage IV)*
Bloechle (30)	1984–93	66	38 (58%)	29 (74%)	20/2	22§	3§
Tsukada (14)	1981–94	142	106 (75%) 15 (stage I)¶ 24 (stage II) 28 (stage III) 8 (stage IVa) 31 (stage IVb)	74 (70%) 15 (100%) 24 (100%) 23 (82%) 6 (75%) 6 (19%)	21/1	100 (stage I) 92 (stage II) 67 (stage III) 29 (stage IV)	91 (stage I) 85 (stage II) 40 (stage III) 19 (stage IV)
Bartlett (16)	1985–93	58**	23 (40%)		26/0	66*	58*

R0, curative resection (negative histological margins).
na, not available.
*, extended cholecystectomy (segmentectomy 4–5 and lymph-node dissection).
†, survival for patients with pT1 tumours (35 patients PT1a and 4 patients PT1b); one patient underwent reoperation.
‡, survival for patients with pT2 tumours (35 patients, 10 patients underwent reoperation).
§, survival for patients after R0 resection.
¶, repartition according to tumour stage of 106 patients undergoing radical surgery.
**, figures concern patients undergoing surgical exploration (58/149); the series does not distinguish between R0 and R1 resection.

procedures involving pancreaticoduodenectomy and portal venous resection have been described for gallbladder as well as bile-duct cancers (Nakamura, ArchSurg, 1994; 129:625; Tsukada, BrJSurg, 1994; 81:108), the high rate of complications (7/9 patients in one series) and the short median survival (1 year) do not appear to offer arguments in favour of such extensive procedures.

Adjuvant treatment by chemotherapy with platinum salts and radiotherapy is currently under evaluation, with promising results in some centres.

In cases where curative surgery cannot be performed, the principles and procedures for palliative treatment of malignant biliary obstruction given above for cholangiocarcinoma are applied.

Results

While the outcome for stage I and stage II gallbladder cancer, generally found incidentally at cholecystectomy, is good (over 90 and 80 per cent survival at 5 years, respectively), the overall prognosis is poor, with, in a modern, multi-institutional French survey, a 5-year survival as low as 5 per cent with no survivors for stage III and IV (Cubertafond, AnnSurg, 1994; 219:275). Results from specialized institutions, however, report survival rates of 40 per cent for 28 patients with stage III tumours and 19 per cent for 39 patients with stage IV tumours.[14] Good results are correlated with extensive lymphadenectomy and being able to remove all microscopic evidence of tumour (R0 resection). These results show the importance of specialized care in the management of this challenging condition. Lymph-node status was said to be the most powerful predictor of survival in a recent Western series (Table 4).[16]

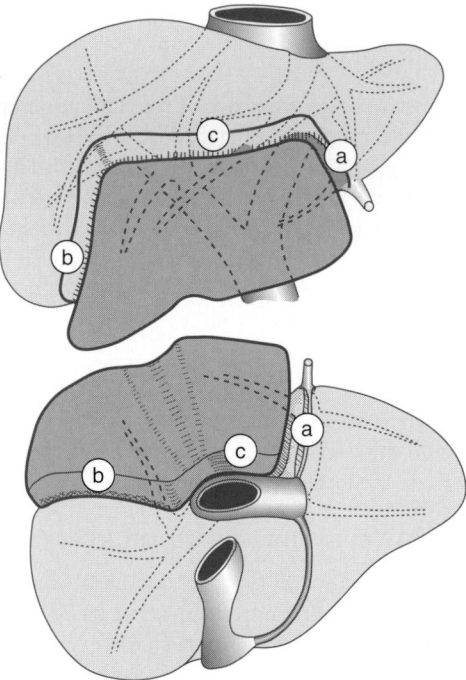

Fig. 15. Schematic representation of the resection of segments 4 and 5 for radical surgery of gallbladder carcinoma: (a) dissection along the plane of the round ligament, ligating the branches to segment 4; (b) hepatic resection along the plane of the right hepatic vein; (c) dissection on the plane of the biliary confluence ligating the terminal branches of the middle hepatic vein. Resection of the bile duct and lymph-node dissection extending to the coeliac and retropancreatic nodes are added to this procedure.

Metastases have been reported at the site of trocar insertion after laparoscopic removal of gallbladders with early tumours, as a consequence of the implantation of neoplastic cells at the time of the delivery of the specimen or of blowing, by the CO_2, of neoplastic cells spilled after accidental operative opening of the gallbladder. For this reason, caution in using laparoscopy on patients at risk for gallbladder carcinoma, the extraction of all gallbladder specimens through a nylon bag, and the removal of the trocar site if a tumour is present are all recommended (Zucker, JAmCollSurg, 1995; 181: 561).

Conclusions

The management of malignant biliary obstruction is changing rapidly: curative resection is increasingly possible, even in patients with advanced disease, and palliative treatment can result in good-quality survival in many patients, sometimes for prolonged periods of time. These advances have been made possible by better understanding of the principles of major hepatic surgery, the remarkable developments in interventional and endoscopic techniques, and careful adaptation of treatment to each individual case. The management of these patients in units where the full range of surgical, radiological, and endoscopic approaches for hepatobiliary disease is available is the best guarantee of a successful outcome.

References

1. Carriaga MT and Henson DE. Liver, gallbladder, extrahepatic bile ducts and pancreas. *Cancer*, 1995; **75**: 171–90.
2. Lee YM and Kaplan MM. Primary sclerosing cholangitis. *New England Journal of Medicine*, 1995; **332**: 924–33.
3. Farges O, Malassagne B, Sebagh M, and Bismuth H. Primary sclerosing cholangitis: liver transplantation or biliary surgery. *Surgery*, 1995; **117**: 146–55.
4. Pichlmayr R, *et al.* Surgical treatment in proximal bile duct cancer. A single-center experience. *Annals of Surgery*, 1996; **224**: 628–38.
5. Nimura Y, Hayakawa N, Kamiya J, Kondo S, Nagino M, and Kanai M. Hepatectomy for bile duct cancer. *Asian Journal of Surgery*, 1996; **19**: 94–100.
6. Makuuchi M, Thai BL, and Takayasu K. Preoperative portal vein embolization increases the safety of major hepatectomy for hilar bile duct carcinoma. *Surgery*, 1990; **107**: 521–7.
7. Kanai M, Nimura Y, and Kamiya J. Preoperative intrahepatic segmental cholangitis in patients with advanced carcinoma involving the hepatic hilus. *Surgery*, 1996; **119**: 498–504.
8. Bismuth H, Nackache R, and Diamond T. Management strategies in resection for hilar cholangiocarcinoma. *Annals of Surgery*, 1992; **215**: 31–8.
9. Nimura Y, Hayakawa N, Kamiya J, Kondo S, and Shionoya S. Hepatic segmentectomy with caudate lobe resection for bile duct carcinoma of the hepatic hilus. *World Journal of Surgery*, 1990; **14**: 535–44.
10. Smith AC, Dowsett JF, Russell RCG, Hatfield ARW, and Cotton PB. Randomised trial of endoscopic stenting versus surgical bypass in malignant low bile duct obstruction. *Lancet*, 1994; **344**: 1655–60.
11. Pasricha PJ. Stent or surgery for the palliation of malignant biliary obstruction. Is the choice clear now? *Gastroenterology*, 1995; **109**: 1398–400.
12. Bismuth H and Castaing D. Surgical bypass of malignant tumours of the bile duct. In Terblanche J, ed. *Hepatobiliary malignancy*. London: Edward Arnold, 1994: 416–23.
13. O'Brien S, Hatfield ARW, Craig PI, and Williams SP. A three year follow up of self expanding metal stents in the endoscopic palliation of long term survivors with malignant biliary obstruction. *Gut*, 1995; **36**: 618–21.
14. Tsukada K, *et al.* Outcome of radical surgery for carcinoma of the gallbladder according to the TNM stage. *Surgery*, 1996; **120**: 816–22.
15. Shirai Y, Yoshida K, Tsukada K, and Muto T. Inapparent carcinoma of the gallbladder. *Annals of Surgery*, 1992; **215**: 326–31.
16. Bartlett DL, Fong Y, Fortner Jg, Brennan MF, and Blumgart LH. Long term results after resection for gallbladder cancer. *Annals of Surgery*, 1996; **224**: 639–46.
17. Reding R, Buard JL, Lebeau G, and Launois B. Surgical management of 522 carcinomas of the extrahepatic bile ducts (gallbladder and periampullary tumours excluded: results of the French Surgical Association survey). *Annals of Surgery*, 1991; **213**: 236–41.
18. Ogura Y, Mizumoto R, Tabata M, Matsuda S, and Kusuda T. Surgical treatment of carcinoma of the hepatic duct confluence: analyisis of 55 resected carcinomas. *World Journal of Surgery*, 1993; **17**: 85–93.
19. Tashiro S, Tsuji T, Kanenemitsu K, Kamimoto Y, Hiraoka T, and Miyauchi Y. Prolongation of survival for carcinoma at the hepatic duct confluence. *Surgery*, 1993; **113**: 270–8.
20. Buhiya MMR, Nimura Y, Kamiya J, Kondo S, Nagino M, and Hayakawa N. Clinicopathologic factors influencing survival of patients with bile duct carcinoma : multivariate statistical analysis. *World Journal of Surgery*, 1993; **17**: 653–7.
21. Gazzaniga GM, Flauro M, Bagarolo C, Ciferri E, and Bondanza G. Neoplasm of the hepatic hilum: the role of resection. *Hepatogastroenterology*, 1993; **40**: 244–8.
22. Nagorney DM, Donohue GH, Farnell MB, Schleck CD, and Ilstrup LS. Outcomes after curative resection for cholangiocarcinoma. *Archives of Surgery*, 1993; **128**: 871–9.
23. Suguira Y, Nakamura S, and Iida S. Extensive resection of bile ducts combined with liver resection for cancer of the main hepatic duct junction: a cooperative study of the Keio Bile Duct Cancer Study Group. *Surgery*, 1994; **115**: 445–51.
24. Washburn KW, Lewis D, and Jenkins RL. Aggressive surgical resection for cholangiocarcinoma. *Archives of Surgery*, 1995; **130**: 270–6.
25. Miyagawa S, Makuuchi M, and Kawasaki S. Outcome of extended right hepatectomy after biliary drainage in hilar bile duct cancer. *Archives of Surgery*, 1995; **130**: 759–63.
26. Nakeeb A, *et al.* Cholangiocarcinoma. A spectrum of intrahepatic, perihilar and distal tumours. *Annals of Surgery*, 1996; **224**: 463–75.
27. Su CH, *et al.* Factors influencing postoperative morbidity, mortality and survival after resection for hilar cholangiocarcinoma. *Annals of Surgery*, 1996; **223**: 384–94.
28. Chijiiwa K and Tanaka M. Carcinoma of the gallbladder: an appraisal of surgical resection. Surgery, 1994: **115**: 751–6.
29. Onoyama H, Yamamoto M, Tseng A, Ajiki T, and Saitoh Y. Extended cholecystectomy for carcinoma of the gallbladder. *World Journal of Surgery*, 1995; **19**: 758–63.
30. Bloechle C, *et al.* Is radical surgery in locally advanced gallbladder carcinoma justified? *American Journal of Gastroenterology*, 1994; **91**: 2195–200.

22.2.3 Malignant mesenchymal tumours of the liver

Miguel Bruguera and Juan Rodés

Primary mesenchymal tumours of the liver are much less common than tumours of epithelial origin. Angiosarcoma, epithelioid haemangioendothelioma, and undifferentiated embryonal sarcoma are those most frequently observed. Others, such as rhabdomyosarcoma, fibrosarcoma, leiomyosarcoma, and malignant fibrotic histicytoma, are exceedingly rare.

In general the aetiology of these tumours is unknown, although nowadays the cause of angiosarcoma is recognized in some patients. The clinical course depends on the type of tumour, very aggressive in

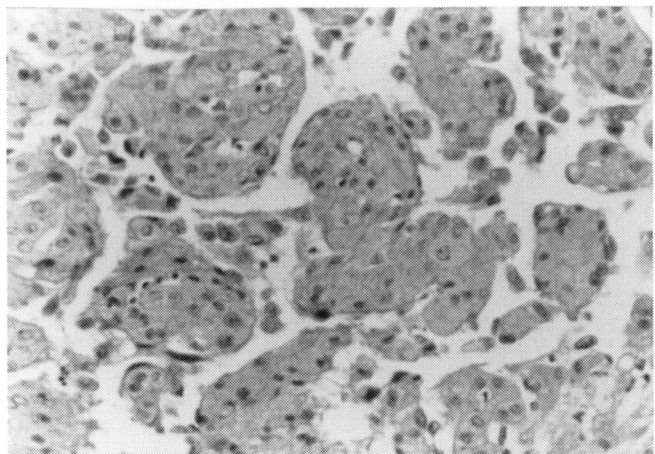

Fig. 1. Angiosarcoma. Large malignant endothelial cells cover thick hepatic cords and are present in the lumen of dilated sinusoids (HE × 175).

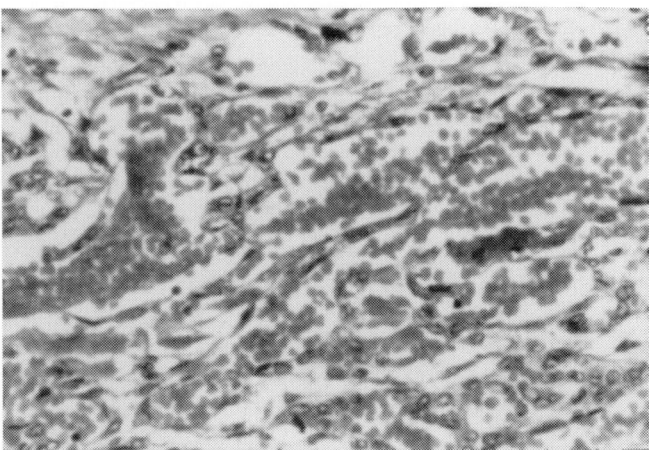

Fig. 2. Angiosarcoma. The hepatic structure has been replaced by vascular spaces lined by spindle-shaped cells (HE × 245).

angiosarcoma and relatively benign in haemangioendothelioma. Diagnosis is based on morphological examination of the tumour.

Several excellent reviews of this topic have been published.[1-4] The most outstanding clinical and morphological characteristics are described in this chapter.

Angiosarcoma

Occurrence

Angiosarcoma, also termed haemangiosarcoma or malignant haemangioendothelioma, is the most frequent mesenchymal primary malignant tumour affecting the liver (Zafrani, JHepatol, 1989; 8: 125). It accounts for 2 per cent of all malignant tumours seen at autopsy, with an estimated 25 cases occurring annually in the United States (Falk, EnvironHlthPerspect, 1981; 41:107) and one or two in Great Britain (Baxter, BrJIndMed, 1980; 37:213).

Angiosarcoma originates from the endothelial cells of the sinusoidal lining (Fortwengler, Gastro, 1981; 80:1415). It generally appears in adults, although it has been recognized in some children, mostly in association with infantile haemangioendothelioma (Noronha, AmJSurgPath, 1984; 8:863).

Pathology

The tumour affects both lobes and appears as multiple nodules of varied size which have ill-defined borders, are greyish-white in colour, and have haemorrhagic foci which occasionally produce a blood-filled cavity. The uninvolved liver is often normal.

The tumour cells are spindle-shaped or irregular in outline and have elongated and hyperchromatic nuclei with prominent nucleoli. Other cells are polyhedric or irregular with conspicuous cytoplasm and rounded nuclei (Fig. 1).

The tumour cells infiltrate sinusoids, hepatic and portal veins, and finally, substitute the hepatic parenchyma. Three histological patterns, which may coexist in the same patient, may be seen: (i) a sinusoidal pattern in which proliferating cells are within the sinusoids and induce sinusoidal dilatation and atrophy of hepatic plates (Fig. 2), (ii) a solid pattern characterized by a dense proliferation of sarcomatous cells which replace large areas of hepatic parenchyma, and (iii) a cavernomatous pattern consisting of large vascular spaces surrounded by thick fibrotic cords lined by multilayered tumour cells (Fig. 2).

Staining of tumour cells with antibodies to the factor VII-related antigen and *Ulex europeus* I lectin is positive in most cases (Miettinen, AmJClinPath, 1983; 79:332). Extramedullary haematopoiesis within the tumour is often present.

In angiosarcomas associated with thorotrast, this material may be identified in the form of refractile granules of brown colour. Its nature is confirmed by autoradiography or by X-ray dispersive energy microanalysis (Bowen, ArchPathLabMed, 1980; 104:459; Landas, ArchPathLabMed, 1984; 108:231).

Non-tumoural hepatic tissue is usually not cirrhotic, but may show several morphological changes, particularly in patients exposed to vinyl chloride, such as increased thickness of Glisson's capsule, portal and periportal fibrosis, deposition of collagen in Disse's space, proliferation and activation of sinusoidal cell lining, and hypertrophic hepatocytes with abnormal and double nuclei (Delorme, UnionMedCan, 1975; 104:1836; Thomas, NEJM, 1975; 299:17; Tamburro, Hepatol, 1984; 4:413).

Clinical features

Angiosarcoma usually develops in the sixth and seventh decades of life, and is more frequent in males than in females (ratio 3:1). The clinical presentation is variable.[4] Two-thirds of the patients have symptoms and signs mimicking chronic liver disease, such as malaise, anorexia, weight loss, right upper quadrant pain, and ascites, often serohaematic. Occasionally, abdominal pain is intense and may be the first symptom. In approximately 15 per cent of patients the initial complaint is an acute spontaneous haemoperitoneum secondary to the rupture of a nodule on the surface of the liver. In other patients clinical manifestaions are related to the presence of pulmonary or skeletal metastases.

Physical examination reveals liver enlargement, which is often painful, or a palpable abdominal mass. Splenomegaly is greatly accentuated in patients with angiosarcoma associated with exposure to vinyl chloride monomer. At diagnosis, metastases are common.

There are no specific biochemical changes. Standard liver function tests are abnormal in more than two-thirds of cases. High serum alkaline phosphatase activity is the most frequent alteration. Microangiopathic haemolytic anaemia and thrombocytopenia secondary to blood cell damage by passing through the tumoural vascular channels may be observed (Neshiwat, AmJMed, 1992; 93:219). Intravascular disseminated coagulation is detected very occasionally (Trull, Gastro, 1973; 65:936). Plasma levels of α-fetoprotein are not elevated.

Imaging techniques show non-specific changes. Ultrasonography and CT scans reveal hepatic areas of dense heterogeneity, while hepatic arteriography shows a peripheral hypervascularity with an avascular central area. False-negative imaging with CT and ultrasound scans may occur when the tumour infiltrates hepatic sinusoids.

When the tumour is associated with previous thorotrast administration, storage of radiopaque material in the liver, spleen, and lymph nodes is seen on abdominal radiography (Levy, AJR, 1986; 14F:997).

Liver biopsy is required for histological diagnosis. Needle biopsy is hazardous because it may be complicated by uncontrollable bleeding.[4]

Natural history

The prognosis of angiosarcoma is dismal. Most patients die within 6 months of diagnosis. The most frequent causes of death are hepatic failure and intra-abdominal bleeding. Fifty per cent of the patients develop metastases before death.[3] Very few patients have limited tumour at the time of diagnosis to allow surgical resection.

Pathogenesis

In more than 70 per cent of patients the pathogenesis is unknown. In the remainder, the development of angiosarcoma has been found associated with the following agents: (i) exposure to thorotrast (Falk, AmJMed, 1981; 2:43; Kojiro, ArchPathLabMed, 1985; 109:853); (ii) continuous exposure to arsenic in insecticides used by vineyard sprayers (Roth, GerMedMon, 1957; 2:172), following prolonged treatment for psoriasis with Fowler liquor (potassium arsenite) (Lauder, Gastro, 1975; 68:1582), or due to consumption of water contaminated with arsenic (Rennks, RevMedChile, 1971; 99 664); (iii) prolonged industrial exposure to vinyl chloride monomer (Berk, AnnIntMed, 1976; 84:1120; Dannaher, AmJMed, 1981; 70:279; Lee, Gut, 1996; 39:312); and (iv) treatment with anabolic drugs (Falk, Lancet, 1979; ii:1120).

Single cases of angiosarcoma have been reported in a patient with primary haemochromatosis (Sussman, ArchPathLabMed, 1974; 97: 39), in patients treated with phenelzine (a monoaminocyclase inhibitor) (Dashmend, BMJ, 1979; ii:1679), diethylstilboestrol (Hoch-Ligeti, JAMA, 1978; 240:1510), and urethane (Cadranel, JClin-Gastro, 1993, 17:52), and in association with von Recklinghausen's disease (Lederman, Gastro, 1987; 92:234).

Thorotrast is a 20 per cent colloidal solution of thorium dioxide which was used as a radiological contrast medium between 1930 and 1953. It accumulates in the reticuloendothelial system, particularly in the liver, emitting α-radiation for a long period. The biological half-life of thorotrast is 400 years. The time required for development of the tumour is between 12 and 40 years (Selinger, Gastro, 1975; 68:799). In addition to angiosarcoma, patients who received thorotrast may develop other malignant tumours, such as hepatocellular carcinoma and cholangiocarcinoma, which may present simultaneously (Kojiro, Cancer, 1982; 49:2161).

Angiosarcoma has been reported in males working in contact with vinyl chloride monomer. This chemical is polymerized to polyvinyl chloride on autoclaving, and residual deposits were removed manually from the walls of the autoclaves. During this procedure large amounts of trapped gaseous vinyl chloride monomer are released and, in the past, were inhaled by the cleaners. Although the frequency of angiosarcoma associated with vinyl chloride is diminishing due to technological changes and to strict programmes applied to plastic factories (Dannhaer, AmJMed, 1981; 70:279), it is calculated that new cases will still appear in Western Europe and in the United States in the following years, since there is a latency period of 12 to 29 years between first exposure to the chemical to the development of angiosarcoma (Forman, BrJIndMed, 1985; 42: 750).

Treatment

Surgical removal of the tumour or liver transplantation are rarely possible as the tumours are large and multifocal at the time of diagnosis. Radiotherapy and chemotherapy are ineffective.

Epithelioid haemangioendothelioma
Occurrence

This tumour was described initially in the lungs, and later identified in soft tissue and bone. In 1984, Ishak et al. reported 32 patients with epithelioid haemangioendothelioma primarily affecting the liver.[5] The tumour may be found at any age and is more frequent among women. It has been reported particularly in Caucasian patients.

Pathology

On gross examination, it consists of multiple nodules of variable size (0.5 to 12 cm diameter) which at times form confluent masses, of grey-white colour and firm consistency, distributed diffusely throughout the liver. The uninvolved liver is usually normal, although cases with cirrhosis have been recorded.

Histologically, it comprises two types of cells, epithelioid and dendritic, surrounded by a myxoid stroma which becomes sclerotic and may occasionally be calcified (Dietze, Histopath, 1989; 15:225). Epithelioid cells are rounded, display abundant cytoplasm, and have hyperchromatic nuclei with prominent nucleoli. They grow in cohesive groups on the periphery of the nodules infiltrating the sinusoids, producing atrophy and eventually disappearance of the hepatic plates. Dendritic cells are irregular in shape with interdigitating processes and are embedded singly in the central stromal matrix, many have cytoplasmic vacuoles that represent intracellular vascular lumina which may contain erythrocytes (Fig. 3). Recognition of these vacuoles facilitates diagnosis of the tumour.[6]

Two features of epithelioid haemangioendothelioma are: (i) the tendency for invasion by blood vessels, portal vein branches, and central veins, and (ii) a peripherally active growth, with the central part of the tumour becoming sclerotic.

Immunohistochemical techniques may help in the diagnosis. Cells of epithelioid haemangioendothelioma are immunoreactive for

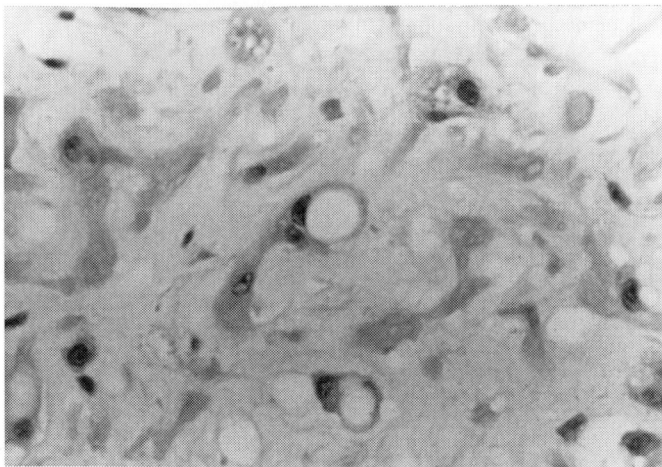

Fig. 3. Epithelioid haemangioendothelioma. Isolated epithelioid neoplastic cells are intermingled with spindle-shaped cells in a fibromyxoid stroma. Some cells contain large intracytoplasmic vacuoles (HE × 280).

vimentin and factor VII-related antigen, negative for cytokeratins, and positive for *Ulex europeus* I lectin (Fig. 4).

Clinical features

The most common clinical manifestations of the tumour (in 45 per cent of patients) are weakness, anorexia, pain in the right upper abdominal quadrant, and loss of body weight. The clinical presentation occasionally mimics decompensated chronic liver disease, and patients present with ascites and gastrointestinal bleeding related to the intravascular growth of the tumour (Rojter, LiverTransplSurg, 1996; 2:156). A single patient has presented with veno-occlusive liver disease (Eckstein, Pathology, 1986; 18:459). In some patients the tumour is discovered by chance as a consequence of ultrasound or CT examination.

Physical examination reveals liver enlargement in all patients. Splenomegaly rarely develops. Liver function tests may be normal,

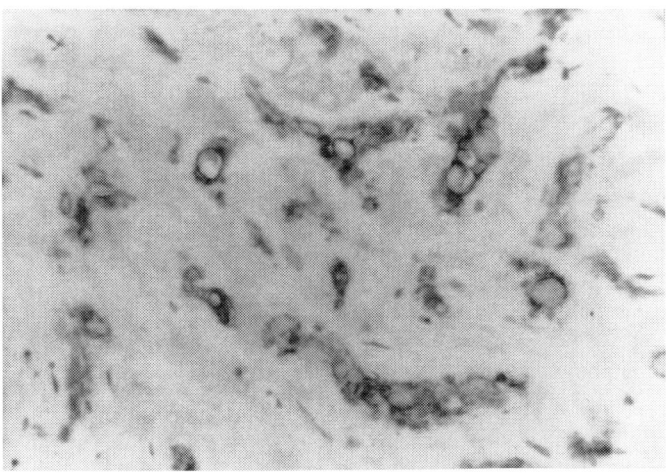

Fig. 4. Epithelioid haemangioendothelioma. Factor VIII-related antigen is present in the cytoplasm of the neoplastic cells (avidin-biotin-peroxidase technique × 245).

except for an increased serum alkaline phosphatase activity. α-Fetoprotein is negative.

Imaging methods allow recognition of the tumour, but do not permit its distinction from metastatic tumours. Abdominal ultrasound shows hypoechogenic nodules with a centre of variable echogenicity. CT scan reveals nodules of low density with an undefined periphery (Radin, Radiol, 1988; 169:145; Furui, Radiol, 1989; 171:63; Van Beers, JComputAssistTomogr, 1992; 16:420). Abdominal plain films may reveal calcifications. On hepatic arteriography the tumour appears as an avascular mass (Clements, JHepatol, 1986; 2:441).

Natural history

The evolution of epithelioid haemangioendothelioma is unpredictable. In some patients the clinical course is long and apparently benign, without affecting the general health status for many years, whereas in others it is rapidly progressive with the development of hepatic failure causing death within a few months.[7,8] Twenty per cent of the patients reported by Ishak *et al.* had died within 2 years of diagnosis, while another 20 per cent had a survival rate of over 5 years.[5] The presence of metastases at diagnosis of the tumour does not represent a worse prognosis compared with those patients without metastases (Kelleher, AmJSurgPath, 1989; 13:999). About 40 per cent of patients have metastases at diagnosis or during follow-up, although distinction between metastases and multicentric disease is not easy.

Pathogenesis

The pathogenesis is unknown. Some authors have suggested a relationship with oral contraceptives (Dean, AmJSurgPath, 1985; 9: 695; Kelleher, AmJSurgPath, 1989; 13:999), but this has not been confirmed by others. In one patient, epithelioid haemangioendothelioma developed after exposure to vinyl chloride (Gelin, JHepatol, 1989; 8:99), and in another it was associated with primary biliary cirrhosis (Terada, Gastro, 1989; 97:810)

Treatment

Surgical removal is not feasible since the tumour is multifocal and chemotherapy is not effective. Successful transplantation has been performed in several patients (Kelleher, AmJSurgPath, 1989; 13: 999; Bancel, HumPath, 1993; 13:23; Vernon, ItalJGastr, 1996; 28: 28). Such treatment could be performed even when metastases are present, as the survival expectancy of these patients may be prolonged (Marino, Cancer, 1988; 61:1079). However, it is possible that the survival rates are not influenced by hepatic transplantation as this tumour has a relatively good prognosis. Gelin *et al.* (JHepatol, 1989; 8:99) have proposed liver transplantation only in patients with a rapidly progressive course. Tumour recurrence after liver transplantation has been reported.

Undifferentiated (embryonal) sarcoma

Undifferentiated sarcoma, also termed primary sarcoma, embryonal sarcoma, mesenchymal sarcoma, fibromyxosarcoma, or malignant mesenchymoma, is a very uncommon tumour that appears in older children, aged between 6 and 10 years; more than 95 per cent of cases develop in patients under 20 years of age. The sexes are equally affected.[9]

Pathology

The tumour appears as a single, large, globular mass (10 to 20 cm in diameter), usually in the right lobe of the liver. It is soft or gelatinous and of variable colour. A thick fibrous pseudocapsule is usually present. Cystic areas containing blood and necrotic tissue may exist within the tumour.

Histologically, it is composed of fusiform or stellate cells, of ill-defined outline, with rounded or elongated nuclei, inconspicuous nucleoli, and eosinophilic cytoplasm. Mitoses are abundant. The neoplastic cells are compactly or loosely arranged in a myxoid stroma that contains trapped bile ducts. Occasionally, this matrix has collagenous or reticulin fibres. The tumour is vascularized and usually contains extramedullary haematopoietic foci. Sarcomatous cells have no histological element of differentiation, rhabdomyoblast or fibroblast. Most tumours contain large cells with cytoplasmic globular inclusions positive for periodic acid–Schiff stain (Walker, Cancer, 1992; 69:52). The nature of these inclusions is unknown, but in one case they reacted with α_1-antitrypsin serum antibody (Abramowsky, Cancer, 1980; 45:3108).

Clinical features

The most frequent clinical manifestations are abdominal pain, the presence of a mass in the upper right abdominal quadrant, or both. Fever and weight loss may be present. In one patient, the invasion of the inferior vena cava and right atrium produced clinical manifestations of a cardiac tumour (Gallivan, PediatPath, 1983; 1:281).

Ultrasonography demonstrates a large solid mass, with hypoechoic areas due to intratumoural necrosis.[10] CT scans show a hypodense mass with a dense peripheral ring corresponding to the pseudocapsule. Arteriography reveals an avascular mass.

Treatment

The prognosis for undifferentiated sarcoma is very poor and most patients die within the first year after diagnosis due to liver failure.[10] Usually the tumour cannot be removed surgically, but those patients in whom surgery was feasible have survived for several years. Promising results have been obtained by using aggressive therapy combining radiotherapy, chemotherapy, and ligation of the hepatic artery (Horowitz, Cancer, 1987; 59:396; Lack, AmJSurgPath, 1991; 15:1; Walker, Cancer, 1992; 69:52).

Fibrosarcoma

Fibrosarcoma is a very uncommon tumour; less than 25 cases have been reported. It develops in middle-aged or elderly adults, and is more frequent in males (85 per cent of cases).

Pathology

Usually, it consists of a single, large, well-circumscribed, greyish-white, non-encapsulated mass. Histologically, it is composed of spindle cells with hyperchromatic and pleomorphic nuclei arranged in interlacing bundles. Mitoses are not prominent. Among the tumour cells there is a high number of collagen fibres.

Clinical features and treatment

An abdominal mass and hepatic enlargement are the most common clinical features. Acute spontaneous haemoperitoneum may occur as a consequence of the rupture of the tumour. Their association with recurrent hypoglycaemia has been documented.

Survival of patients with hepatic fibrosarcoma is very short, although some have survived several years following surgical resection or radiotherapy.

Leiomyosarcoma

This is another very rare tumour. Cases have been observed in middle-aged and elderly people, with both sexes being equally affected. This tumour may be primarily hepatic (Fong, HumPath, 1974; 5:115), or may arise in the ligamentum teres (Tomaszewski, PediatPath, 1986; 5:147), or in the wall of the suprahepatic veins (MacMehne, Gastro, 1971; 61:139). One case was associated with cirrhosis (Ruiz Valverde, MedicinaClin, 1991; 97:783).

Pathology

Leiomyosarcoma is a large, greyish-white, solitary, non-encapsulated mass formed by spindle cells with slightly eosinophilic cytoplasm, which display longitudinal striations. The nuclei are hyperchromatic and elongated with abundant mitoses. Vimentin reaction is often diffusely positive. Desmin and myosin are positive only in some cases.

Clinical features

The tumour presents as an abdominal mass, sometimes associated with pain in the right upper abdominal quadrant, weakness, anorexia, and weight loss. A Budd–Chiari syndrome may develop secondary to hepatic vein obstruction. Hepatic arteriography detects an avascular lesion.

Treatment

Surgical removal, when possible, is indicated since it is followed by prolonged survival. When resection is not feasible, because of a massive tumour, the patient survives only a few months (Masur, Gastro, 1975; 69:994; Chen, JSurgOncol, 1983; 24:325). The prognosis is worse in tumours that arise in the hepatic veins or in the ligamentum teres than in those that develop in the liver.

Malignant fibrous histiocytoma

The liver is very rarely the primary location for this tumour (Katsuda, AmJGastr, 1988; 83:1278). It may appear as either a solitary mass or multiple nodules. Histologically, it is formed by fibrohistiocytic pleomorphic cells with numerous atypical mitoses disposed in a fascicular or storiform pattern, admixed with collagen bundles and with inflammatory cells, lymphocytes, and plasma cells (Fukayama, ArchPathLabMed, 1986; 110:203). A moderate number of giant cells is common.

Neoplastic cells are positive for vimentin and negative for cytokeratin and desmin. Ultrastructural examination shows that tumour cells share features of fibroblasts and histiocytes.

Clinically, the tumour is revealed as a palpable abdominal mass. Metastatic malignant fibrous histiocytoma from soft tissue (retroperitoneum or extremities) must be considered. Surgical removal is indicated (McGrady, Histopath, 1992; 21:290).

Embryonal rhabdomyosarcoma

This is an extrahepatic biliary tract tumour growing towards the liver. In general, it occurs in children (most patients are under 5 years of age; Ruyman, Cancer, 1985, 56:575), but it has been documented in adults (Aldabagh, ArchPathLabMed, 1986; 110: 547).

Clinically, this tumour causes obstructive jaundice. Imaging techniques may reveal a hilar mass. Histologically, there is a proliferation of rounded, spindle- or strap-shaped cells, with numerous mitoses and cross-striations in the cytoplasm, set in a loose myxoid stroma. Immunohistochemistry demonstrates myoglobin, myosin, and desmin in liver cells.

Malignant rhabdoid tumour

This is an infantile tumour which usually arises in the kidneys. Three primarily hepatic cases with a very aggressive clinical course not responding to chemotherapy have been reported (Gonzalez-Crusi, Cancer, 1982; 49:2365; Parham, ArchPathLabMed, 1988; 112:61). Tumour cells are polygonal with eccentric and vesicular nuclei, prominent nucleoli, and eosinophilic globular inclusions in the cytoplasm. They react with antibodies to cytokeratins, epithelial antigen membranes, and vimentin.

References

1. Ishak KG. Malignant tumours of the liver. In Okuda K and Ishak KG, eds. *Neoplasms of the liver*. Berlin: Springer-Verlag, 1988: 160–76.
2. Craig JR, Peters RL, and Edmonson HA. *Tumors of the liver and intrahepatic bile ducts*. Washington: Armed Forces Institute of Pathology, 1988.
3. Zafrani ES. Update on vascular tumors of the liver. *Journal of Hepatology*, 1989; 8: 125–30.
4. Locker GY, Doroshow JH, Zwelling LA, and Chabner BA. The clinical features of hepatic angiosarcoma: a report of four cases and review of English literature. *Medicine*, 1979; 58: 48–64.
5. Ishak KG, Sesterhenn IA, Goodman ZD, Rabin L, and Stromeyer FW. Epithelioid hemangioendothelioma of the liver: a clinicopathological and follow-up study of 32 cases. *Human Pathology*, 1984; 15: 839–52.
6. Weiss SW, Ishak KG, Dail DH, Sweet DE, and Enzinger FM. Epithelioid hemangioendothelioma. *Diagnostic Histopathology*, 1986; 3: 259–87.
7. Scoazec JY, *et al*. Epithelioid hemangioendothelioma of the liver. Diagnostic features and role of liver transplantation. *Gastroenterology*, 1988; 94: 1447–53.
8. Terg R, Bruguera M, Campo E, Hojman R, Levi D, and Podest A. Epithelioid hemangioendothelioma of the liver: report of two cases. *Liver*, 1988; 8: 105–10.
9. Stocker JT and Ishak KG. Undifferentiated embryonal sarcoma of the liver. *Cancer*, 1978; 42: 336–48.
10. Ros PR, Olmstead WW, Dachman AH, Goodman ZD, Ishak KG, and Harman DS. Undifferentiated (embryonal) sarcoma of the liver: radiologic–pathologic correlation. *Radiology*, 1986; 161: 1410–5.

22.3 Metastatic tumours

22.3.1 Metastatic liver disease

Josep M. Llovet, Antoni Castells, and Jordi Bruix

The liver is frequently affected by the spread of tumour cells originated in other organs. However, while some neoplasms almost never metastatize into the liver, other tumours, principally those in the abdominal cavity, are responsible for most of the metastatic lesions[1] (Table 1). This chapter focuses mainly on the diagnosis, prognosis, and treatment of patients with liver metastases from colorectal cancer, since they constitute a specific group that should be differentiated from the patients with metastatic liver involvement of other origin. However, the diagnostic management of patients with suspected metastatic liver involvement is common to all patients, the main differences relying on the prognosis and the potential therapeutic approaches.

Biology of cancer metastases

The development of metastasis may be seen clinically as a simple, mechanic event merely involving the release of neoplastic cells from the primary tumour and their subsequent seeding and growth into the new organ. However, the path between the appearance of the primary tumour and the recognition of a metastatic nest is a complex process regulated at a molecular level and involving the activation–inactivation of several genes.[2] It has been proposed that only one out of 100 000 cells released from primary tumour turns into a clinically recognizable metastasis.

The replication of normal cells and the progressive growth or regeneration of an organ is based on the adequate attachment of the

Table 1 Primary sites for metastatic cancer to the liver

Primary tumour	Percentage with liver metastases
Gallbladder	78
Pancreas	70
Colorectal	56
Breast	53
Skin	50
Stomach	44
Lung	42
Urinary bladder	38
Uterus	32
Oesophagus	30
Kidney	24
Prostate	13

Data from ref. 1.

new cells to the neighbour cells and to the basement membrane of the tissue (Frenette, NEJM, 1996; 334:1526). Thus, if a malignant cell is to invade and disseminate, it must be able to detach from these structures and migrate in the proper direction (Weiss, InvasMetast, 1995; 14:192). In addition, the surrounding extracellular matrix has to be degraded to allow the cell to penetrate and reach a vascular or lymphatic vessel. The basement membrane is formed by a dense net of collagen, fibronectin, laminin, entactin, and heparan sulphate proteoglycans, while the cell–cell and cell–basement connections are controlled by several cell adhesion molecules, such as the laminin binding protein, the catherins, the integrins, the CD44, and the immunoglobulin superfamily. The degradation of the surrounding extracellular matrix is tightly regulated by proteases, with most of the available knowledge involving serine proteases and metalloproteases (Stetler-Stevenson, FASEBJ, 1993; 7:1434). This last group are produced as proenzymes requiring proteolytic conversion, and are inhibited by chelating agents and by the so-called tissue inhibitors of the metalloproteases (**TIMPs**). The metalloproteases family comprises seven members with known activity: intestinal collagenase, neutrophil collagenase, stromelysin-1, stromelysin-2, matrilsyn, gelatinase A, and gelatinase B. The timing and degree of activation of these different agents, which may have tissue specificity both in terms of expression and effects, determines the invasive potential of malignant cell. Furthermore, it must be taken into account that until being released into a vessel, the invasive displacement of the cell requires the proteolytic or adhesive activity to be differentially expressed along the cell surface: the invading protrusion of the cell should exhibit proteolytic activity, while the remaining surface of the cell remains attached to the matrix by the expression of adhesion molecules.[2] After successfully degrading part of the matrix and the displacement of the cell into the tract created by the proteases, the adhesion molecules are expressed in the front part of the cell while the previously adherent part is freed from the matrix, thus allowing the displacement of the cell body.[2] Upon arriving at a vessel, the wall of the vessel is destroyed to permit the passage of the cell into the bloodstream. At this stage, the moving cell is completely detached from the matrix and other invading cells, with which it forms a 'cluster', and enters the circulation. While being displaced by the blood flow the neoplastic cell must survive the deleterious effects of turbulent flow and the action of the immune system (Bayon, Hepatol, 1996; 23:1224). Thereby, the risk of an organ suffering metastatic invasion is related not only to the organ blood flow, but also to the specific characteristics of the tissue favouring the growth of a metastatic colony of a given organ; this ability to host a metastatic nest being quantitated by the so-called metastatic efficiency index. The seeding of the cell into a new organ requires cell attachment to the vessel wall, which is then perforated to allow the escape of the cell into the matrix. In addition, the successful growth after leaving the vessel depends on the creation of a new vascular supply, this new vascularization also being regulated by a complex angiogenic process, which has also occurred during the growth of the main tumour[2,3]. At any point during this sequential chain of molecular events the cell may receive different signals or sense the presence of an adverse environment and this can prompt the activation of apoptotic cell death, which is supposed to be the main factor in determining the non-viability of most of the cells released from the main tumour. The very active research in cancer development and progression will allow a complete understanding of the previously depicted process and it is expected that in the future the prevention and treatment of metastasis will be based on the modulation of one or more of the steps.

Diagnostic approach to patients with liver metastases

The search for the primary tumour in most patients with hepatic metastases is justified not only to obtain the definitive diagnosis of the disease, but also because of the therapeutic possibilities which may be derived from it. In general, the prognosis of patients presenting hepatic metastasis is poor. However, survival of patients with colorectal metastatic disease may be increased by surgical resection in selected cases. Likewise, neuroendocrine tumours should be differentially evaluated since they present a more benign course (48 per cent survival rate of carcinoid tumours at 5 years) and may respond to surgery with intention to cure. Therefore, the aetiological diagnosis of the tumour allows the use of curative approaches in selected cases of colorectal and neuroendocrine metastatic disease or, in some of the remaining cases, the use of more individualized palliative treatments (chemotherapy and radiotherapy).

The strategy of the aetiological diagnosis of hepatic metastases is based on the form of clinical presentation and, overall, on the anatomopathological properties of the tumour (Wood, NEJM, 1993; 329:257). Ultrasonography-guided fine-needle aspiration biopsy has shown to be a safe and accurate procedure that has assumed a primary diagnostic role in the evaluation of hepatic masses, significantly increasing the diagnostic sensitivity (85 per cent) and specificity (93–100 per cent) of malignant lesions.[4] Three different situations may be considered.

Patients with a known primary tumour

Patients with a known primary tumour presenting hepatic metastasis in the context of tumoral stratification or after treatment of the primary tumour. In this case only the identity of either histology must be verified when the nature of the focal hepatic lesion is uncertain.

Patients with an unknown primary tumour, asymptomatic or symptomatic with slight involvement of the general state

The search for the tumour is mainly based on the pathological study. The most frequent hepatic metastases are as follows:

Well or moderately differentiated neoplasms
Adenocarcinoma

Histopathology allows the distinction between digestive tumours or those of another origin. If adenocarcinoma is of intestinal origin, colorectal, stomach, and pancreatic primaries must be discarded. Otherwise, if the tumour is extradigestive, lung and prostatic cancer in men and breast and ovarian cancer in women must be discarded.

Non-adenocarcinoma

Among the squamous carcinomas, the lung, oesophageal, laryngeal, and squamous neoplasms of the perineal zone must be discarded. Finally, lymphomas, sarcomas, and melanomas may, when well differentiated, be diagnosed by optical microscopy and may be confirmed by immunohistochemistry.

Poorly differentiated neoplasms

In this group of neoplasms the immunohistochemical techniques, and in a few cases, electronic microscopy are of great clinical usefulness in the search for the primary tumour. First, carcinomas can be distinguished from the remaining tumours by means of anti-cytokeratin Ac immunohistochemistry. With regard to carcinomas, primaries from the lung, breast, pancreas, urological tract, or thyroid must be ruled out. Given their differential features, the neuroendocrine tumours make up a separate subgroup. The diagnosis of these tumours requires a high degree of clinical suspicion, and can be confirmed by immunohistochemistry with chromogranin or neural enolase. The visualization of secretion granules on electronic microscopy is of additional help. Secondly, among the non-carcinomatous tumours, the most frequently found are lymphomas, sarcomas, melanomas and, very rarely, germinal tumours.

Patients with an unknown primary tumour, with severe illness

The patients who make up this group are those who appear very ill, presenting symptoms of infiltration and hepatic insufficiency, such as jaundice and ascites. Usually, important analytical alterations and multiple metastatic images are present. In these cases, the value of a search for the primary tumour is unclear since the characteristics of the patient limit certain explorations and the therapeutic usefulness is null. The prognosis of these patients is very poor.

Liver metastases from colorectal cancer
Incidence

The incidence of colorectal cancer in Western countries ranges from 20 to 47 cases per 100 000 (Waterhouse, LyonIntAgResCancer, 1982; 4:42; NIH Consensus Conference, JAMA, 1990; 264:1444). Despite the high resectability rate and a general improvement in therapy, nearly half of all patients with colorectal cancer still die of metastatic tumours. Colorectal carcinoma metastasizes to the liver in about 35 to 50 per cent of patients. Many authors have noted a high rate (up to 20 per cent) of liver involvement at the time of diagnosis (Saenz, SurgClinNAm, 1989; 69:361; Foster, Hepatogast,

Table 2 Survival of patients with untreated liver metastases from colorectal cancer: natural history		
Authors	Number of patients	Median survival (months)
Jaffe, 1968[18]	73	6–10
Bengmark, 1970[32]	38	6 (mean)
Cady, 1970[33]	241	13
Abrams, 1971[34]	58	7
Baden, 1975[35]	105	10
Wood, 1976[5]	113	3–17
Bengtsson, 1981[12]	25	3–6
Boey, 1981[36]	73	6–9
Goslin, 1982[16]	125	10–24
Lahr, 1983[10]	147	4.5–12
Wagner, 1984[17]	252	11–21
Finan, 1986[9]	86	8–15.5
Scheele, 1990[7]	983	6.9–14.2
Steele, 1991[11]	47	16.5
Stangl, 1994[6]	484	7.5

1990; 37:182). Another 20 to 30 per cent will develop metastatic disease subsequent to resection of their primary tumours[5] (Asbun, SurgClinNAm, 1993; 73:145).[5] From autopsy series, liver involvement can be observed in 60 to 70 per cent of patients who die of colorectal carcinomas, with solitary liver metastases present in up to 12 to 17 per cent of the cases.[1]

Natural history

Metastatic cancer to the liver still carries a dismal prognosis for most patients. The accurate evaluation and choice of therapy of liver metastases from colorectal cancer can only be based upon the knowledge of the natural history of untreated metastases and determinants of prognosis derived from treated and untreated patients. However, the natural history of colorectal liver metastases has varied with time because certain factors such as diagnostic techniques and follow-up programmes have changed, even though the main biological properties remain unchanged. In fact, recent reports have shown that survival without treatment may be considerably better than previously [6]recognized[6] (Foster, Hepatogast, 1990; 37:182). This could be partially due to early diagnosis, since therapy has changed little in the past decades. Thus it would be of interest to know the current survival time of different subgroups of untreated patients diagnosed according to new imaging modalities and followed with aggressive monitoring after resection of the primary tumour.

The fact that surgical resection of liver metastases represents a potentially curative treatment in a selected subgroup of patients (applicable to only 10–20 per cent of all patients)[7] (Scheele, Surgery, 1991; 110:13) has precluded the inclusion of these patients in prospective randomized trials comparing natural history and resection. Therefore only retrospective studies have provided some insight into the natural history of liver metastases by analysing groups of patients with non-surgically resected tumours. Table 2 summarizes the median survival of patients reported in 15 retrospective studies of the natural history of untreated patients. Many factors, in particular a difference in diagnostic standards, small numbers of patients and the absence of categorization by extent of hepatic or extrahepatic involvement may have influenced survival in these studies, a belief that is reflected in the range of survival figures reported. In summary, median survival from the time of diagnosis found in these series ranges from 3 to 24 months. However, some of these patients showed solitary lesions (or a few lesions representing a minimal percentage of liver replacement) 'suitable' for surgical resection according to currently accepted criteria. Survival analyses of this subgroup of patients would improve our understanding of the natural progression of lesions that would no longer be left untreated. Using these data, and according to the extension of liver involvement, the 1-year survival for solitary or limited liver metastases varies from 38 to 83 per cent, whereas comparable figures for diffuse liver involvement range from 5.7 to 32 per cent. The 3-year survival for solitary or limited metastases extends from 0 to 33 per cent, and the figures for multiple and diffuse metastases fall between 0 and 4 per cent. Five-year survival is seldom reported in the absence of resection. In a review of world literature from 1952 Hugues et al. (Hughes, Surgery, 1988; 103:278) analysed 1650 cases of untreated patients; only 14 (0.8 per cent) of these patients survived for 5 years. Otherwise, anecdotal 5-year survival figures up to 16 per cent in the presence of solitary liver lesions have been documented.[8]

Diagnosis

Although definitive diagnosis of hepatic metastases requires pathological confirmation, there is controversy whether a definite tissue diagnosis should be obtained if one is considering further surgical or palliative treatment in controlled trials (Foster, Hepatogast, 1990; 37:182; Asbun, SurgClinNAm, 1993; 73:145). The combination of laboratory tests and imaging studies is probably enough to detect and stage most lesions.

Clinical presentation

Most patients with hepatic metastases are asymptomatic for a long period of time (Sugarbaker, AdvSurgery, 1989; 22:1). Clinical symptoms such as fatigue, weight loss, ascites, jaundice, and pain, associated with large or rapidly growing hepatic tumours, indicate a late sign of progressive liver failure and patient demise.[5,9] Jaundice may develop in association with occlusion of the common hepatic duct or with extensive hepatic replacement, usually upwards of 50 per cent. Ascites associated with liver metastases is also a severe sign. Thus, clinical presentation of the disease is essential for the management and outcome of these patients.

Usually, colorectal cancer metastases of the liver are presented in one of two ways.

Patients with known colorectal cancer

Liver metastases may appear as a finding during perioperative staging of the primary tumour (synchronous metastases) or during follow-up monitoring after resection (metachronous metastases). When metastatic disease is detected, an even more complete staging is of crucial importance in order to determine resectability after ruling out extrahepatic disease. This should include history and physical examination, assays of serum carcinoembryonic antigen, liver function test, ultrasound and computed tomography (**CT**) of the abdomen, chest radiology, and, when indicated, hepatic magnetic resonance imaging (**MRI**), chest CT and bone scintigraphy (Asbun, SurgClinNAm, 1993; 73:145; Bennet, Hepatol; 1990; 12: 761). Intraoperative ultrasonography should be performed when resection is proposed (Asbun, SurgClinNAm, 1993; 73:145).

Patients with unknown colorectal cancer

Liver metastases can be detected as a cause of symptoms due to liver replacement, altered liver tests and tumoral markers, or as a consequence of an imaging study. Once pathological confirmation of liver metastases has been established, accurate assessment of the primary tumour is mandatory, including colonoscopy and the complete work-up described above.

Laboratory tests

Laboratory measurements of liver enzymes and tumoral markers have been examined as a method of detecting hepatic metastases and as prognostic determinants. Patients with minute or solitary liver metastases may show a normal biochemical profile. When the disease progresses, the liver function parameters disclose cholestasis due to the space occupation by the neoplastic masses. On the other hand, some investigators have correlated abnormal liver function tests, such as bilirubin, alkaline phosphatase, and lactate dehydrogenase, with survival[10] (Kemeny, AmJMed, 1983; 1:720). In a multivariate analysis Lahr et al.[10] correlated hyperbilirubinaemia and elevated alkaline phosphatase with poor prognosis. Unfortunately, elevation of these parameters are non-specific and no definitive association with survival has been established.

Several authors have found that most patients with colorectal hepatic metastases (from 73 to 90 per cent) have elevated serum carcinoembryonic antigen levels (Wanebo, AnnSurg, 1978; 188: 481; Hohenberger, AnnSurg, 1994; 219:135). However, it is still controversial whether preoperative serum carcinoembryonic antigen levels are of prognostic value in regard to resectability[11] (Doci, BrJSurg, 1991; 78:797). Otherwise, carcinoembryonic antigen levels can be especially helpful when tracking patients after primary tumour resection and may be the first indication of potential recurrence of metastasis (Hohenberger, AnnSurg, 1994; 219:135).

Imaging studies

Imaging techniques have played an increasing role in the early detection and staging of liver metastases. Most studies are aimed at determining the accuracy of different imaging modalities to establish the extent of metastatic disease and help to plan surgical resection of potentially 'curable' lesions.

Ultrasound is a relatively economical non-invasive radiological test available for screening liver metastases. Ultrasound examination is highly dependent on equipment and sonographer expertise. Although the appearance of liver metastases on ultrasound may vary from discrete hypoechoic masses to mixed echo patterns, a highly echogenic lesion is usually suggestive of metastases from adenocarcinoma (Sheiner, SemLivDis, 1994; 14:169).

The introduction of intraoperative ultrasound has contributed to improving surgical hepatic resection (Igawa, Radiol, 1985; 156: 473; Makuuchi, SGO, 1985; 161:346). This technique can identify liver tumours located deep within the liver parenchyma and can define the relationship to vascular structures. In a study summarizing the results of a combined series for prospective evaluation of intraoperative ultrasound compared to preoperative ultrasound, arteriography, computed tomography, and surgeon palpation, intraoperative ultrasound showed the best sensitivity (78 per cent), specificity (100 per cent), and diagnostic accuracy (84 per cent) (Sheiner, SemLivDis, 1994; 14:169). Particularly, this technique allows the detection of 25 to 30 per cent of tumours less than 1 cm in diameter which are not found in routine preoperative imaging studies or palpation (Emre, AnnSurg, 1993; 217:15).

Abdominal CT enhanced with specific contrast agents is the recommended procedure of choice in evaluating liver metastases (Bennet, Hepatol, 1990; 12:761). This technique is highly accurate in defining the total number and anatomical position of liver tumours. In addition, extrahepatic abdominal spread is also well evaluated and is fairly reproducible worldwide. However, recent studies have proposed a variant of CT, arteriographically enhanced CT, as the standard radiological investigation that best defines hepatic tumours preoperatively (Sitzmann, AmJSurg, 1990; 159: 137; Asbun, SurgClinNAm, 1993; 73:145). This sophisticated technique is highly sensitive in detecting lesions less than or equal to 2 cm in diameter (Nelson, Radiol, 1989; 172:27). CT arterial portography has a sensitivity of 94 per cent in detecting liver metastases, compared with 70 per cent by hepatic MRI, with the former being significantly higher for lesions of less than 1 cm (Sitzmann, AmJSurg, 1990; 159:137). Although this technique is currently the most sensitive radiological preoperative test, its invasiveness and difficult logistics are limiting factors for its use worldwide.

In MRI, metastases are seen as low signal areas on T1-weighted images and high signal on T2-weighted images (Bennett, Hepatol, 1990; 12:761). MRI has a similar accuracy in the detection of liver metastases as compared to dynamic CT (Sark, Radiol, 1987; 165: 399). None the less, MRI has significantly greater accuracy than dynamic CT in demonstrating vascular involvement (Sitzmann, AmJSurg, 1990; 159:137). Otherwise, CT allows for assessment of abdominal metastases in a slightly more precise way than MRI. Further studies are necessary to determine the definitive role of MRI in the preoperative imaging assessment of liver metastases.

The role of other imaging techniques, such as hepatic scintigraphy and angiography, has decreased dramatically due to the

Table 3 Prognostic determinants in unresected colorectal liver metastases: multivariate analyses	
Authors	**Prognostic factors**
Lahr, 1983[10]	Bilobar metastatic disease
	Bilirubin; alkaline phosphatase
	Lymph node metastases
Fortner, 1984[14a]	LVRT
	Lymph node metastases
	Prior chemotherapy
Finan, 1986[b]	LVRT
	Albumin; alkaline phosphatase
	Histological grade of the primary
	Weight loss; liver enlargement
	Lymph node metastases
Ekberg, 1986[13a]	LVRT
	Lymph node metastases
	Elevated liver function tests
	Synchronous liver metastases
Stangl, 1994[6]	LVRT
	Histological grade of the primary
	Extrahepatic tumour
	Lymph node metastases
	Serum carcinoembryonic antigen
	Age

[a] Series of patients treated with palliative chemotherapy.
[b] Finan, BrJSurg, 1986; 72:373.
LVRT, percentage of liver volume replaced by tumour.

improvement in the imaging techniques described above. Finally, recent advances in radiolabeled monoclonal antibody scans for detection of hepatic metastases are still in investigative stages.

Prognostic factors and staging

The identification of prognostic factors related to survival of untreated metastatic liver of colorectal origin is of importance in defining risk categories and allowing adequate stratification within controlled trials. The natural progression of metastatic disease 'classically' depends on the extent of hepatic involvement, the primary histological type, the presence of coexisting extrahepatic disease or lymph node involvement, and the physiological status of the liver parenchyma. However, only prognostic determinants obtained in studies using the multivariate regression analysis technique are able to define the specific relevance of each variable. Among several prognostic factors analysed during the past decade, four variables were found to be widely related with outcome in multivariate analyses (Table 3): extent of liver replacement by tumour, extrahepatic disease, mesenteric lymph node involvement, and histological grade of primary tumour. Additional factors, such as the location or number of nodules, altered liver function test, alkaline phosphatase, bilirubin, weight loss, and liver enlargement, are probably related to the more important above-mentioned factors[3,9] (Sugarbaker, AdvSurg, 1989; 22:1). Finally, other variables have been related to survival in some studies, but not in others (age, sex, Dukes' staging of primary tumour, and preoperative serum carcinoembryonic antigen concentration[6]) (Hughes, Surgery, 1988; 103:278; Sugarbaker, AdvSurg, 1989; 22:1). Factors with prognostic significance after hepatic resection for colorectal metastases, such as stage of the primary tumour, involvement of lymph nodes, involvement of margin resection, and number of liver metastases, are discussed below.

Extent of liver replacement by tumour

This has been shown to be the most significant indicator of outcome.[5,6,9,12,13,14] Stangl et al. [6] recently reported that patients with less than 25 per cent of liver volume replaced by tumour (**LVRT**) had a clear outcome advantage (median survival 11.1 months) compared with patients with a LVRT greater than 25 per cent (median survival 6.3 months). Other authors stratified the volume of liver occupied into three groups with divisions at 25, 50 or 75 per cent, resulting in different survival data.[12,15] In Stangl's study[6] other variables somehow related to the extent of liver replacement with prognostic significance in univariate analyses, lost their predictive power in multivariate analyses. Thus, hepatomegaly, distribution, and/or number of liver metastases, maximum diameter of metastases, alkaline phosphatase, and bilirubin were not independently related with outcome.[6] Nevertheless, other authors have shown that altered liver function test have independent predictive value.[9,10,13,16] Lahr et al.[10] concluded that serum alkaline phosphatase and bilirubin were the two risk factors best able to predict survival, while Goslin[16] and Ekberg[13] established a relationship between the liver impairment tests and outcome.

Extrahepatic tumour

Colorectal cancer is a stepwise progressive disease, therefore it is not uncommon for the liver to be the only site of distant cancer deposits (Sugarbaker, AdvSurg, 1989; 22:1). When extrahepatic spread occurs, the prognosis becomes ominous, particularly in patients with low liver replacement. Accordingly, extrahepatic tumour allows an accurate prognostic discrimination in patients with less than 25 per cent of the liver replaced by tumour, while no predictive value is found among patients with more than 25 per cent of the liver occupied.[6] Therefore, extrahepatic disease constituted a determinant indicator of outcome in several studies (Petrelli, DisColonRectum, 1984; 27:249; Chang, JSurgOncol, 1989; 40:245), and has been included in some staging systems.[15]

Mesenteric lymph node involvement

The staging of the primary tumour at the time of colorectal resection has been found to be of prognostic value when metachronic liver metastases occur.[6,9,10,13,14,17] Mesenteric lymph node involvement (Dukes' C classification) has been significantly associated with outcome in those patients with minimal hepatic replacement, but loses significance as liver disease advances.[6,17]

Grade of malignancy of the primary tumour

The histological grades of the hepatic metastases or primary tumour have been established to be of prognostic significance in some studies[6,9,12,16,18] but not in others.[10] Some authors state that primary tumour grade is almost as important a prognosis determinant as the extent of liver replacement.[6] In the series by Finan[9] and Goslin[16] the median survival time for patients with well and moderately differentiated tumours was 13 to 30 months, but decreased to 6 to 7 months in poorly differentiated tumours. In contrast, other multivariate models show that the pathological grade loses its independent prognostic significance for survival.[10]

Finally, to better understand the natural history of different subgroups of patients with liver metastases from colorectal cancer, recently published data stratified survival of 417 untreated patients according to the prognostic factors obtained[6]. Estimations of the probable survival for each subgroup stated a median survival time of 21.3 months (range 5–68 months) for patients with the best prognostic factors—well-differentiated primary tumour with a liver replacement of less than 25 per cent without lymph or extrahepatic involvement. In contrast, patients presenting the worst prognostic categories showed a median survival time of 3.8 months (range 1–38 months).

The National Institutes of Health Consensus Conference recommended the TNM staging system to stratify colorectal cancers.[4] Stage IV (any T, any N, M1) accounts for liver metastases of colorectal cancer. However, TNM classifications for metastatic disease do not exist. In agreement with the prognostic factors described above, a specific staging system for liver involvement from colorectal cancer is advocated. Several staging systems for hepatic metastases have been proposed, but none are universally accepted (Gennari, Tumori, 1982: 68:443). Van del Velde[15] stated an international staging system for hepatic metastases which included three features: (a) extent of liver replacement (P_1 < 25 per cent; P_2, 25–75 per cent; P_3 > 75 per cent); (b) extrahepatic disease (E); and (c) symptoms attributable to metastases (S). Four stages are proposed: stage O, curatively resected metastases; stage I, P_1; stage II, P_2; stage III, P_3 or any P with E or S. Although this system takes into account some of prognostic factors described above, it must be prospectively validated.

Treatment

The therapeutic options for hepatic metastases from colorectal cancer include surgical resection, systemic chemotherapy, regional procedures, and other investigational treatments such as radiotherapy, immunotherapy, or liver transplantation[19,20] (Ridge, SGO, 1985; 101:597; Sheiner, SemLivDis, 1994; 14:169). However, up to now, the only treatment shown to improve survival in patients with liver metastases is surgical resection. Unfortunately, this procedure can be applied in less than 15 per cent of the patients with metastatic colorectal cancer (Ridge, SGO, 1985; 101:597; August, AnnSurg, 1985; 201:210). Thus, most of the patients must be considered for palliative options, which are designed to reduce the tumoral bulk and, consequently, to delay the appearance of symptoms related to tumour progression and the impairment of the patients' baseline physical condition[19,20] (Ridge, SGO, 1985; 101:597; Asbun, SurgClinNAm, 1993; 73:145; Sheiner, SemLivDis, 1994; 14:169).

Surgical resection

Liver resection has become a standard therapy for colorectal metastases. When metastases are confined to the liver, the 5-year probability of survival after surgery ranges from 20 to 40 per cent.[7,11, 14,21–25] Table 4 summarizes the results of some of the largest series published up to now. It is interesting to emphasize that these figures are much better than those previously reported.[7,11,14, 21–25] More accurate preoperative tumour staging allows earlier

Table 4 Survival after resection of hepatic metastases from colorectal cancer		
	Number of patients included	5-year probability of survival
Steele, 1991[11]	87	29 months (median)
Scheele, 1990[7]	183	40%
Iwatsuki, 1989[22]	86	38%
Hughes, 1989[23]	800	32%
Butler, 1986[21]	62	34%
Adson, 1984[24]	141	25%
Fortner, 1984[14]	65	40%
Foster, 1981[25]	231	23%

detection of metastases. In addition, improvement in surgical technique, including anatomical dissection and proper homeostasis, have reduced operative mortality to less than 2 per [11,21,22]cent (Gennari, AnnSurg, 1986; 203:49). This enhanced operative survival probably improves long-term prognosis. However, it is difficult to interpret these results because no uniform staging system is used and prospective controlled trials are lacking. Moreover, many series only reported the 2- or 3-year survival rates, while recent data suggest that patients with unresected hepatic metastases may live longer than previously reported. The median survival rates for patients with unresected solitary and multiple unilobar lesions are 21 and 15 months, respectively, and more than 20 per cent of patients with unresected solitary liver metastases live at least 3 years. Otherwise, in about 35 per cent of the patients whose tumours recur after hepatic resection, the liver is the initial site of recurrence. In selected cases, repeated hepatic resection for isolated metastases can result in long-term survival (Griffith, Surgery, 1990; 107:101; Stone, ArchSurg, 1990; 125:718).

Recent studies analysing the results of hepatic resection in patients with colorectal metastases in the liver have identified which factors determine their outcome. Among these, the parameters with a clear prognostic significance are the presence of extrahepatic disease, metastatic lymph nodes, positive margins, and more than three or four lesions. Other factors associated with a poor prognosis in some studies, but not universally accepted, are the stage of the primary lesion, preoperative carcinoembryonic antigen concentration, type of resection, and perioperative blood transfusions[7] (Ekberg, BrJSurg, 1986; 73:727; Sheiner, SemLivDis, 1994; 14: 169).

First of all, although extrahepatic disease is not an absolute contra-indication to resection when the patient could be made disease-free by surgery alone (Hughes, SurgClinNAm, 1989; 69: 339), the 5-year disease-free survival of these patients significantly decreases, compared with those without extrahepatic disease at the time of hepatic resection[7,24] (Nordlinger, AnnSurg, 1986; 305: 256; Murray, SemSurgOncol, 1991; 7:157).

Metastatic involvement of coeliac or hepatic lymph nodes results in a very grim prognosis, even when all the gross tumour is removed at the time of hepatic surgery (Adson, ArchSurg, 1984; 119:647). Therefore, most groups consider this situation as a contra-indication for surgical resection.

Adequate margins may also influence prognosis after metastases resection. Survival in patients with disease-free margins is significantly longer than in those with positive margins. Therefore, a margin of at least 1 cm of normal liver parenchyma should be excised with the specimen[23] (Cady, ArchSurg, 1992; 127:561).

Several data suggest that the number of nodules in the liver is associated with prognosis. It is well known that patients with bilobar involvement are at increased risk for recurrence of metastasis in the liver after resection (Hughes, Surgery, 1986; 100:2278), and most authors agree that resection should not be attempted when more than four hepatic lesions are present[14,23] (Ekberg, BrJSurg, 1986; 73:727; Cady, ArchSurg, 1992; 127:561). However, it is not so clear whether patients with a solitary lesion have a longer survival after resection than those who undergo resection of multiple nodules in the same lobe.[14,21,23] Similarly, data from the Registry of Hepatic Metastases shows that the overall 5-year survival is 37 per cent in patients with resected solitary lesions and 34 per cent in those with two resected nodules, there being no significant difference between the two groups.[23] In addition, survival may be even shorter in cases with true multiple nodules than in those who developed a single nodule with satellites (Cobourn, SGO, 1987; 165:239).

Although location of the primary colorectal tumour does not seem to have prognostic significance, the stage of the primary lesion has been correlated with prognosis in some studies[23] (Adson, AnnSurg, 1980; 191:563; Younes, AnnSurg, 1991; 214:107). Therefore, patients who develop a colorectal tumour without nodal involvement (stage B of Dukes' classification) have significantly better survival rates than those with colorectal cancer showing nodal involvement (stage C of Dukes' classification). In addition, in a large series of patients with hepatic metastases from colorectal cancer submitted to surgical resection, not only did Dukes' staging influence prognosis, but also the outcome of patients in whom liver metastases were completely removed was equivalent to that of patients with similar tumour stage without hepatic involvement.[23] However, this correlation has not always been observed, since some authors did not find any significant relationship between the stage of the primary lesion, the presence of mesenteric lymph nodes, and survival after resection of liver metastases (Cady, ArchSurg, 1992; 127:561).

The prognostic value of an elevated carcinoembryonic antigen concentration in the presence of recognized hepatic metastases is controversial. While some authors identify carcinoembryonic antigen concentration as one of the most significant preoperative prognostic factors[23] (Cady, ArchSurg, 1992; 127:561), thus likely to indicate the presence of subclinical disease dissemination in patients with high levels, other groups fail to demonstrate its predictive value.[14]

The type of resection has also been identified as a prognostic factor. Many authors report significantly better survival among patients undergoing wedge resections than in those requiring extended hepatectomies[14] (Cady, ArchSurg, 1992; 127:561). However, tumour removal by a limited resection most likely reflects a smaller tumour burden. Thus, tumoral volume may have a more important predictive value than the type of resection.

Finally, it has been suggested that perioperative blood transfusions may adversely affect patients undergoing hepatic resection for secondary neoplasms of the liver, in the same way as in surgically resected hepatocellular carcinoma (Stephenson, AnnSurg, 1988; 208:679). However, since this variable loses its predictive significance in multivariate analysis, it is likely that transfusional requirements were related with the type of resection and, consequently, with disease extension (Younes, AnnSurg, 1991; 214: 107).

In summary, most groups consider candidates for resection as those patients in whom the primary tumour could be resected with curative intention and in whom there is no evidence of extrahepatic disease. As explained above, the extension of liver involvement may influence recurrence and survival rates and thus, although it is not universally accepted, more than four lesions should preclude surgical treatment.

Systemic chemotherapy

The existing chemotherapy for disseminated colorectal cancer is disappointing, with only a modest efficacy reported for fluoro-pyrimidines (5-fluorouracil, 5-fluorodeoxyuridine), nitrosoureas, and mitomycin C. Among these drugs, 5-fluorouracil is the most commonly used, and has been administered as an oral agent, intravenously in bolus doses, or by continuous intravenous infusion[26–30]. The overall response rate to 5-fluorouracil in hepatic metastases from colorectal cancer is approximately 20 per cent in most studies. In addition, response is not maintained for a long period of time, and is not associated with an improvement in survival (Engstrom, Cancer, 1982; 49:1555). Finally, there is no rational basis for combining different chemotherapeutic drugs, considering both efficacy and toxicity[26–30]. Table 5 summarizes the results of systemic chemotherapy in the treatment of hepatic metastases from colorectal cancer.

Several prospective randomized trials have investigated the biochemical modulation of 5-fluorouracil with leucovorin (tetrahydrofolate).[28–30] At present, it seems clear that the combination of 5-fluorouracil and high-dose leucovorin is superior to 5-fluorouracil alone in terms of antitumoral effect (Table 5). However, the overall survival has not yet been demonstrated to be significantly increased.[28–30] The optimal doses of 5-fluorouracil and leucovorin, and the optimal mode of administration remain to be determined. Finally, modulation of 5-fluorouracil with recombinant alpha-2a interferon or interleukin-2 is being evaluated in several studies, but early results derived from prospectively randomized trials do not suggest a significant enhancement of the antitumour effectiveness with the addition of these drugs (Wadler, JClinOncol, 1991; 9:1806; Heys, EurJCan, 1995; 31A:19; Raderer, EurJCan, 1995; 31A:1002).

Regional chemotherapy

Regional chemotherapy following potentially curative hepatic resection has been used, but definitive results are not available. Some results suggest a small benefit of using direct hepatic artery infusion of 5-fluorouracil. Although the overall recurrence rate was not diminished, in most of the patients the liver was not the site of recurrence (Balch, AnnSurg, 1983; 198:567). In addition, many groups are studying the therapeutic effects of adjuvant portal vein infusion of 5-fluorodeoxyuridine combined with systemic 5-fluorouracil and leucovorin administration (Nagasue, BrJSurg, 1985; 72:565). However, up to now, there are no differences in either survival and recurrence rates between patients submitted to this intensive approach and the control group.

Table 5 Antitumoral effect of systemic chemotherapy in hepatic metastases from colorectal cancer

	Number of patients included	Drugs used	Response rate (%)
Moertel, 1969[26]	118	5-FU	24
Grage, 1979[27]	31	5-FU	23
Machover, 1986[28]	73	5-FU + LV	30
Petrelli, 1989[29]	85	5-FU + LV	27
Ardalan, 1991[30]	18	5-FU + LV	44

5-FU, 5-fluorouracil; LV, leucovorin.

Selective infusion of chemotherapy agents into the hepatic arterial system may be employed in the treatment of unresectable colorectal liver metastases (Kemeny, ProcAmSocClinOncol, 1982; 2:123; Balch, AmJSurg, 1983; 145:285; Balch, AnnSurg, 1983; 198: 567; Stagg, AnnIntMed, 1984; 100:736; Kemeny, AnnIntMed, 1987; 107:459; Ridge, Cancer, 1987; 59:1547). Fluoropyrimidines have high hepatic extraction and, consequently, this approach achieves higher drug concentration in the tumour with lower systemic exposure and, therefore, lower toxicity. In this technique, the infusion catheter is placed into the hepatic artery through the gastroduodenal artery at laparotomy, and chemotherapy is administered by means of an implantable infusion pump. Response rates using continuous hepatic arterial infusion of 5-fluorodeoxyuridine or 5-fluorouracil to treat hepatic metastases in unresectable colorectal cancer patients have ranged from 51 to 88 per cent (Table 6), these figures being greater than those obtained when these drugs are administered systemically (Reed, Cancer, 1981; 47: 402; Balch, AnnSurg, 1983; 198:567; Niederhuber, Cancer, 1984; 53:1336; Kemeny, Cancer, 1985; 55:1265; Patt, JClinOncol, 1986; 4:1356; Vaughn, Cancer, 1993; 71:4278; Sugihara, Surgery, 1995; 117:624). However, the criteria for evaluating response are not identical, and it is unclear whether this method increases survival. Randomized trials comparing systemic versus regional administration of 5-fluorodeoxyuridine in patients with liver metastases confirmed a significantly higher antitumoral effect for regional chemotherapy (Table 7), but the impact on survival remains unclear (Chang, AnnSurg, 1987; 206:685; Kemeny, AnnIntMed, 1987; 107; 459; Hohn, JClinOncol, 1989; 7:1646; Martin, ArchSurg, 1990; 125: 1022; Kemeny, Cancer, 1992; 69:327). This fact may be due to procedure complications, limitations imposed by toxicity and lack of control of extrahepatic tumour growth[19] (Stagg, AnnIntMed, 1984; 100:736; Hohn, Cancer, 1986; 57:465).

Hepatic arterial therapy has a number of complications not seen with conventional intravenous therapy. These include catheter displacement, kinking or thrombosis, local infection, partial or complete hepatic arterial thrombosis, and upper gastrointestinal haemorrhage (Stagg, AnnIntMed, 1984; 100:736; Hohn, Cancer, 1986; 57:465). Furthermore, toxicity of chronic hepatic arterial chemotherapy is related to the regionally high exposure to 5-fluorodeoxyuridine and may appear in up to 50 per cent of the patients. This includes gastric ulceration, diarrhoea, elevation of bilirubin and transaminases, and biliary sclerosis (Stagg, AnnIntMed, 1984; 100:736; Holin, Cancer; 1986; 57:465; Kemeny, AnnIntMed, 1987; 107:459; Hohn, JClinOncol, 1989; 7:1646). Nevertheless, gastrointestinal toxicity can be avoided or diminished by assuring proper placement of the catheter and by using fluorescein to confirm that delivery of the drug is targeted to the liver[31] (Hohn, Cancer, 1986; 57:465). Finally, the combination of systemic and intra-arterial therapy has been proposed to control extrahepatic neoplastic disease. With combined treatment, tumour spread occurred less frequently (33 per cent) than with hepatic arterial administration alone (61 per cent),. Survival was similar in both groups of patients (Safi, Cancer, 1989; 64:379).

Other treatments

Immunotherapy

In recent years, radiolabelled monoclonal antibodies against colorectal cancer cell-related antigens have been developed, either for radio-immunodetection of metastatic lesions or for immunotargeted therapy. Antibodies can be linked to cytotoxic agents such as biological toxins or chemotherapeutic drugs. To date, most patients treated with this therapy have advanced disease, and further studies using this approach are needed (Beatty, Cancer, 1992; 70:1425).

Table 6 Antitumoral effect of phase II trials employing hepatic arterial chemotherapy for hepatic metastases from unresectable colorectal cancer

	Number of patients included	Response rate (%)
Reed, Cancer, 1981; 47:402	77	83
Balch, AnnSurg, 1983; 198:567	81	88
Niederhuber, Cancer, 1984; 53:1336	93	78
Kemeny, Cancer, 1985; 55:1265	24	73
Patt, JClinOncol, 1986; 4:1356	29	52
Sugihara, Surgery, 1995; 117:624	53	51

Table 7 Randomized trials comparing systemic versus intrahepatic chemotherapy for the treatment of hepatic metastases from colorectal cancer

	Number of patients included	Response rate (%)		*p*
		Systemic	Intrahepatic	
Kemeny, AnnIntMed, 1987; 107:459	99	20	50	0.001
Hohn, JClinOncol, 1989; 7:1646	115	10	42	0.001
Chang, AnnSurg, 1987; 206:685	64	17	62	0.003
Martin, ArchSurg, 1990; 125:1022	60	21	48	0.02
Kemeny, Cancer, 1992; 69:327	79	22	46	0.04

Immunostimulant therapy using cytokines such as interleukin-2 or interferon remains experimental, the results being too preliminary to evaluate their efficacy.

Radiation therapy

At present, it seems clear that radiation therapy improves the prognosis of patients with rectal cancer whose lesions have penetrated the bowel wall or who have regional lymph nodes (Dukes' B2 and C tumours), not only decreasing local recurrence but also prolonging patients' survival (Krook, NEJM, 1991; 324:709). However, there is no evidence that this treatment modifies the appearance of distant metastases. Moreover, the usefulness of radiation therapy in the treatment of hepatic metastases has not been demonstrated.

Liver transplantation

Orthotopic liver transplantation has become a conventional treatment for chronic liver diseases, including hepatocellular carcinoma (Castells, Hepatol, 1993; 18:1121). However, the results of liver transplantation for metastatic disease are generally poor (Pichlmayr, TransplProc, 1988; 20:478; Penn, Surgery, 1991; 110:726). In fact, most patients submitted to this procedure due to metastatic colorectal cancer developed tumour recurrence, thus resulting in very short patient survival (Penn, Surgery, 1991; 110:726; Pichlmayr, TransplProc, 1988; 20:478). Furthermore, the results have not been modified after the combination of liver transplantation with systemic chemotherapy, total body irradiation, and bone marrow transplantation (Margreiter, TransplProc, 1986; 18:74). Therefore, taking the lack of liver donors into account, orthotopic liver transplantation should be restricted to patients with liver metastases in whom long-term survival may be possible, i.e. patients with symptomatic neuroendocrine hepatic tumours not suitable for surgical resection.

Non-colorectal hepatic metastases

Non-colorectal, non-neuroendocrine hepatic metastases

Excluding liver metastases from neuroendocrine or carcinoid tumours, surgical resection of hepatic metastases from other primary sites seems to play an irrelevant therapeutic role[19] (Wolf, SGO, 1991; 173:454; Sheiner, SemLivDis, 1994; 14:169). However, there are very few prospective controlled studies and, therefore, the conclusions obtained by comparing results of phase II trials with the natural history of the disease are unclear.

Overall, the mean survival after surgical resection of liver metastases from non-colorectal, non-neuroendocrine carcinomas is nearly 2 years (Wolf, SGO, 1991; 173:454; Sheiner, SemLivDis, 1994; 14:169). However, there are some exceptions. Liver metastases from primary renal carcinomas are associated with a better prognosis, there being a 5-year survival rate of 50 per cent, with no tumoral recurrence in patients who survived more than 5 years (Foster, Hepatogastr, 1990; 37:182). Similarly, a probability of survival higher than 40 per cent at 5 years after surgical resection of Wilms' tumour metastases has been reported. Finally, some selected patients with metastatic breast cancer or melanoma isolated in the liver may survive longer than 2 years after resection (Foster, Hepatogastr, 1990; 37:182; Wolf, SGO, 1991; 173:454; Sheiner, SemLivDis, 1994; 14:169).

Long-term survival after surgical resection of other metastastic non-colorectal, non-neuroendocrine tumours (stomach, pancreas, cervix, endometrium) are disappointing. Given these poor results, palliative intention for surgery becomes an issue. Unfortunately, most patients with symptomatic lesions have progressive endstage disease, and true palliation is unlikely. As reported by Foster *et al.* (Foster, Hepatogastr, 1990; 37:182), all patients who underwent palliative hepatic resection died of tumoral progression within 1 year.

Therefore, surgical resection of liver metastases should be considered an appropriate treatment for Wilms' tumour and primary renal carcinoma. Selected patients with metastatic melanoma or breast cancer may also benefit from surgery. In contrast, resection of liver metastases from other primary sites should be avoided (Sheiner, SemLivDis, 1994; 14:169).

Systemic chemotherapy constitutes the most frequently therapeutic option used in the treatment of hepatic metastases from non-colorectal cancer because the liver is rarely the only site of metastatic disease. For tumours responsive to chemotherapy, intravenous drug treatment represents the most efficient and cost-effective approach, only being limited by the systemic toxicities of the agents applied (mucositis, myelosuppression, diarrhoea).[19]

Finally, there are no randomized, controlled trials of hepatic arterial therapy in patients with hepatic metastases from non-colorectal cancer. Moreover, as mentioned above, almost all of these patients have extrahepatic disease and, consequently, there is no rationale to perform a regional procedure.

Carcinoid and neuroendocrine hepatic metastases

Carcinoid and other neuroendocrine tumours should be considered apart from other cancers. Their slow growth allows a better prognosis, with a mean survival ranging from 5 to 10 years after the onset of symptoms. Moreover, the introduction of a more generalized use of imaging techniques, such as ultrasonography, has changed the natural history of these tumours. Thus, many hepatic metastases from carcinoid and neuroendocrine tumours are discovered in an asymptomatic stage, and, thus, the survival of these patients might be considered even better than thought. Symptoms include both those related to functioning peptide hormone-release and those due to tumour growth. Thus, surgery and regional therapy may be considered as therapeutic options for radical and palliative intention (see Chapter 21.3.2).

References

1. Edmondson HA and Peters RL. Neoplasms of the liver. In Shiff L, Shiff EL, eds. *Diseases of the liver*, 6th edn. Philadelphia: JB Lippincott, 1987: 1109–58.
2. Kohn EC and Liotta LA. Molecular insights into cancer invasion: strategies for prevention and intervention. *Cancer Research*, 1995; **55**: 1856–62.
3. O'Reilly MS, *et al.* Angiostatin: a novel angiogenesis inhibitor that mediates the suppression of metastases by a Lewis lung carcinoma. *Cell*, 1994; **79**: 315–28.
4. Saul SH. Masses of the liver. In Sternberg S, ed. *Diagnostic surgical pathology*, 2nd edn. New York: Raven Press, 1994.
5. Wood CB, Gillis CR, and Blumgart LH. A retrospective study of the natural history of patients with liver metastases from colorectal cancer. *Clinical Oncology*, 1976; **2**: 285–8.
6. Stangl R, Altendorf-Hofmann A, Charnley R, and Scheele J. Factors influencing the natural history of colorectal liver metastases. *Lancet*, 1994; **343**: 1405–10.
7. Scheele J, Stangl R, and Altendorf-Hofmann A. Hepatic metastases from colorectal carcinoma: impact of surgical resection on natural history. *British Journal of Surgery*, 1990; **77**: 1241–6.
8. Wood CB. Natural history of liver metastases. In Van de Velde CJH, Sugarbaker PH, eds. *Liver metastases. Basic aspects, detection and management*. Amsterdam: Martinus Nijhoff, 1984: 47.
9. Finan PJ, Marshall RJ, Cooper EH, and Giles GR. Factors affecting survival in patients presenting with synchronous hepatic metastases from colorectal cancer: a clinical and computer analyses. *British Journal of Surgery*, 1986; **72**: 373–7.
10. Lahr CJ, Soong SJ, Cloud G, Smith J, Wrist MM, and Balch CM. A multifactorial analyses of prognostic factors in patients with liver metastases from colorectal carcinoma. *Journal of Clinical Oncology*, 1983; **1**: 720–6.
11. Steele G Jr, Bleday R, Mayer RJ, *et al.* A prospective evaluation of hepatic resection for colorectal carcinoma metastases to the liver: Gastrointestinal Tumour Study Group Protocol, 6584. *Journal of Clinical Oncology*, 1991; **9**: 1105–12.
12. Bengtsson G, Carlsson G, Hafström L, and Jönsson P. Natural history of patients with untreated liver metastases from colorectal cancer. *American Journal of Surgery*, 1981; **141**: 586–9.
13. Ekberg H, *et al.* Determinants of survival after intraarterial infusion of 5-fluorouracil for liver metastases from colorectal cancer: a multivariate analyses. *Journal of Surgical Oncology*, 1986; **31**: 246–54.
14. Fortner JG, Silva JS, Cox EB, Golbey RB, Gallowitz H, and MacLean BJ. Multivariate analyses of a personal series of 247 patients with liver metastases from colorectal cancer; II. Treatment by intrahepatic chemotherapy. *Annals of Surgery*, 1984; **199**: 317–24.
15. Van de Velde CJH. Methodology in the clinical study of hepatic metastases. In Van de Velde CJH, and Sugarbaker PH, eds. *Liver metastases. Basic aspects, detection and management*. Amsterdam: Martinus Nijhoff, 1984: 358.
16. Goslin R, Steele G, Zamcheck N, Mayer R, and MacIntyre J. Factors influencing survival in patients with hepatic metastases from adenocarcinoma of the colon and rectum. *Diseases of the Colon and Rectum*, 1982; **25**: 749–54.
17. Wagner J, Adson M, Van Heerden J, Adson M, and Ilstrup D. The natural history of hepatic metastases from colorectal cancer. A comparison with resective treatment. *Annals of Surgery*, 1984; **199**: 502–8.
18. Jaffe BM, Donegan WI, Watson F, and Spartt JS. Factors influencing survival in patients with untreated hepatic metastases. *Surgical Gynecology and Obstetrics*, 1968; **127**: 1–11.
19. Niederhuber JE and Ensminger WD. Treatment of metastatic cancer to the liver. In DeVita VT, Heman S, Rosenberg SA, eds. *Cancer: principles and practice of oncology*, 4th edn. Philadelphia: JB Lippincott, 1993: 2201–25.
20. Bresalier RS and Kim YS. Malignant neoplasms of the large intestine. In Sleisenger MH, and Fordtran JS, eds. *Gastrointestinal disease*, 5th edn. Philadelphia: WB Saunders, 1993: 1449–93.
21. Butler J, Attiyeh FF, and Daly JM. Hepatic resection for metastases of the colon and rectum. *Surgical Gynecology and Obstetrics*, 1986; **102**: 109–13.
22. Iwatsuki S, Sheahan DG, and Starzl TE. The changing face of hepatic resection. *Current Problems in Surgery*, 1989; **26**: 283–379.
23. Hughes H, Scheele J, and Sugarbaker PH. Surgery for colorectal cancer metastatic to the liver. *Surgical Clinics of North America*, 1989; **69**: 339–59.
24. Adson MA, Van Heerden JA, Adson MH, Wagner JS, and Ilstrup DM. Resection of hepatic metastases from colorectal cancer. *Archives of Surgery*, 1984; **119**: 647–53.
25. Foster JH and Lundy J. Pathology of liver metastasis. *Current Problems in Surgery*, 1981; **18**: 157–68.
26. Moertel CG, and Reitemeier RJ, eds. Advanced gastrointestinal cancer. *Clinical management and chemotherapy*. New York: Harper and Row, 1969.
27. Grage TG, *et al.* Results of a prospective randomized study of hepatic artery infusion with 5-fluorouracil vs intravenous 5-fluorouracil in patients with hepatic metastases from colorectal cancer. *Surgery*, 1979; **86**: 550–5.
28. Machover D, *et al.* Treatment of advanced colorectal and gastric adenocarcinoma with 5-fluorouracil and high-dose folinic acid. *Journal of Clinical Oncology*, 1986; **4**: 685–96.
29. Petrelli N, *et al.* The modulation of fluorouracil with leucovorin in metastatic colorectal carcinoma: a prospective randomized phase III trial. *Journal of Clinical Oncology*, 1989; **7**: 1419–26.
30. Ardalan B, *et al.* A phase II study of weekly 24–hour infusion with high-dose fluorouracil with leucovorin in colorectal carcinoma. *Journal of Clinical Oncology*, 1991; **9**: 625–30.
31. Niederhuber JE. Surgical aspects of intrahepatic artery therapy. In Bottino JC, Opfell RW, Muggia FM, eds. *Liver cancer*. Boston: Martinus Nijhoff, 1985: 179–94.
32. Bengmark S and Hofstrom L. The natural history of primary and secondary malignant tumours of the liver: I. The prognosis for patients with hepatic metastases from colonic and rectal carcinoma by laparotomy. *Cancer*, 1970; **23**: 198–202.
33. Cady B, Monson DO, and Swinton NW. Survival of patients after colonic resection for carcinoma with simultaneous liver metastases. *Surgical Gynecology and Obstetrics*, 1970; **131**: 697–700.
34. Abrams MS and Lerner HJ. Survival of patients at Pennsylvania Hospital with hepatic metastases from carcinoma of the colon and rectum. *Diseases of the Colon and Rectum*, 1971; **14**: 431–4.
35. Baden H and Anderson B. Survival of patients with untreated liver metastases from colorectal cancer. *Scandinavian Journal of Gastroenterology*, 1975; **10**: 221–3.
36. Boey J, *et al.* Carcinoma of the colon and rectum with liver involvement. *Surgical Gynecology and Obstetrics*, 1981; **153**: 864–8.

22.3.2 Carcinoid tumours

H. J. F. Hodgson

The term carcinoid was coined to describe tumours that differed from cancers in their more benign behaviour despite similarities in macroscopic and microscopic appearances.[1] Carcinoid tumours in the liver are usually secondary deposits from gastrointestinal primary carcinoids, less commonly from bronchial. The prognosis for patients with hepatic carcinoids is substantially better than for those with secondary adenocarcinomas in the liver. A substantial proportion of patients with hepatic carcinoid tumours come to medical attention because of the associated and sometimes dramatic features of the carcinoid syndrome—cutaneous flushing, diarrhoea, asthma, and cardiac disease.[2] Comprehensive reviews include those of Hodgson,[3] Kvols *et al.*,[4] Oberg,[5] and for the surgical aspects of this disease, Soreide *et al.*[6]

Cell of origin

Carcinoids are solid tumours arising from enterochromaffin or enterochromaffin-like cells, one constituent of the diffuse neuro-endocrine system scattered throughout the body. The cell types comprising this system share functional and anatomical characteristics, including the presence of neurosecretory granules, and the biochemical pathways for amine precursor uptake and decarboxylation (APUD). Carcinoids therefore have their origin in the cell types similar to those giving rise to islet-cell tumours of the pancreas and phaeochromocytomas (Stevens, Lancet, 1983; i: 118).

Enterochromaffin cells are scattered in the lamina propria of the gut, mainly near the base of intestinal crypts (the Kulchitsky cell) or in the submucosal layers of main bronchi. 'Enterochromaffin' reflects their ability to stain with potassium chromate. The cells are also 'argentaffin', taking up and spontaneously reducing silver salts. Other closely related cells may take up silver, but do not spontaneously reduce it ('argyrophilic' cells). These properties are variably present in carcinoid tumours originating in different sites, and the classification of carcinoids based on their origin in tissues of embryological fore-, mid- or hindgut origin is classical (Table 1).[7] The main product released from the oval or biconcave neurosecretory granules is serotonin (5-hydroxytryptamine), but other regulatory peptides have been demonstrated histochemically (substance P, encephalin, and motilin).[8] Enterochromaffin-like cells in the stomach are rich in histamine. The heterogeneity of the enterochromaffin cell population sets the scene for different histochemical reactions from carcinoid tumours in different sites, for the differing propensities of tumours in different sites to release active substances capable of inducing the carcinoid syndrome, and for the variety of symptoms occurring in the carcinoid syndrome if sufficient tumour product reaches the systemic circulation.

Macroscopic characteristics

Primary carcinoids are most common in the appendix, followed by the rectum, small intestine, stomach, and colon (Table 1).

Appendiceal and rectal carcinoids are generally insignificant. One-third of small-intestinal tumours are multiple, most occurring within 60 cm of the ileocaecal valve. Gastric carcinoids may be multiple, but a single antral tumour is more common. Bronchial carcinoids are usually solitary, arising in the main bronchi, although a minority are peripheral or multiple.

Primary carcinoids are usually spherical, submucosal, and yellow because of their high lipid content. In the gut, tumours rarely ulcerate but spread outwards. Carcinoids from all sites are potentially malignant, but there are marked differences in the likelihood of these tumours producing metastases, depending on their site. The majority from the colon, for example, metastasize (Table 1), whilst metastasis is extremely rare from appendiceal and rectal carcinoids. If invasive, the tumour spreads throughout the muscularis mucosa to the serosa, involving lymphatics. A dense, fibrotic reaction may occur around the tumour and extend into the mesentery, and it is this, rather than the tumour itself, that may cause local gastrointestinal symptoms. Local nodal involvement, which may be massive, precedes hepatic involvement. Rare sites of primary carcinoids include larynx, gallbladder, thymus, uterus, ovary, breast, kidney, and skin.

Hepatic carcinoids are usually multiple and secondary but, very occasionally, apparently solitary secondaries occur, and apparently primary hepatic carcinoids are occasionally reported. The pattern of deposits is variable, including either diffuse infiltration with multiple, small deposits or larger masses that may be 10 cm or more in diameter.

Microscopic appearances

These are usually characteristic. The tumours have no capsule, with uniform cells, polygonal in shape, with a centrally situated nucleus containing speckled chromatin and basal granules (Fig. 1). Differing patterns of cellular arrangements have been described—insular, trabecular, glandular, or mixed or undifferentiated (Soga, Cancer, 1971; 28:990)—and there are suggested correlations between these types and prognosis (Johnson, Cancer, 1983; 51:882). Occasionally, there is a scirrhous pattern. Electron-dense granules, which differ according to the site of the primary tumours, are seen on electron microscopy (Fig. 2).

The cells may stain red with eosin, brown with potassium chromate, black with iron haematoxylin, orange-red with Ehrlich's diazo reaction, and brownish black with silver nitrate. Carcinoid tumours arising in different sites may exhibit a variety of staining reactions to these and other agents. In addition to serotonin, a wide variety of biologically active products has been identified in carcinoid tumours (Leviston, JClinEndoc, 1981; 53:682; Sporrong, Cancer, 1982; 49:68) (see Table 2).[9] Neurone-specific enolase is a useful marker for all tumours of the carcinoid series, and neuroendocrine cells in general.[10]

Clinical features

Carcinoid tumours present over a wide range of ages, affecting both sexes, and often present in substantially younger individuals than do adenocarcinomas. Autopsy series indicate an incidence of about 1 per cent—overwhelmingly asymptomatic appendiceal tumours. There appears to be a rare association with neurofibromatosis.

Table 1 Carcinoid tumours: site of primary, and the presence of metastases and the carcinoid syndrome

	No. of cases	No. of cases with:		Silver stain characteristics
		metatases	syndrome	
Foregut				
Oesophagus	2	0		Argyrophil or negative
Stomach	84	23	8	
Duodenum	115	20	4	
Pancreas	5	20	1	
Gallbladder	18	30	1	
Bile duct	5	0		
Ampulla	7	14		
Larynx	4	50		
Bronchus	2% of lung tumours	5	66	
Thymus	74	25	0	
Midgut				
Jejunum	65	35		Argentaffin
Ileum	1013	35	91	
Meckel's diverticulum	44	19	6	
Appendix	1687	2	6	
Colon	89	60	5	
Liver	4			
Ovary	34	6	17	
Testis	2		2	
Cervix	33	25	0	
Hindgut				
Rectum	573	18	1	Negative

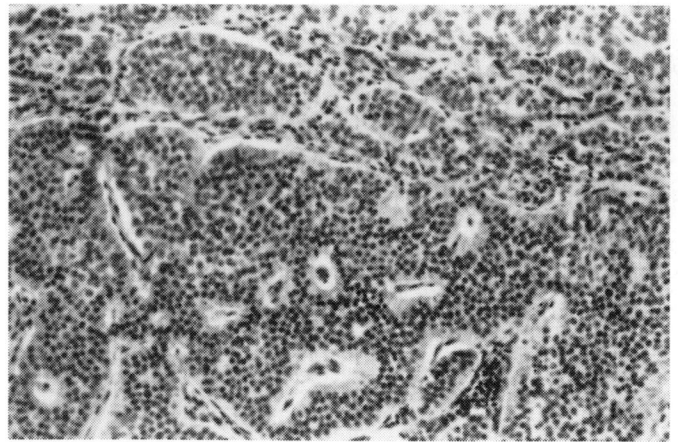

Fig. 1. A haematoxylin and eosin-stained section of an argentaffin (serotonin-producing) carcinoid tumour of the ileum. Uniform, polygonal cells with abundant cytoplasm are arranged in sheets and nests separated by fine, fibrovascular stroma. × 150.

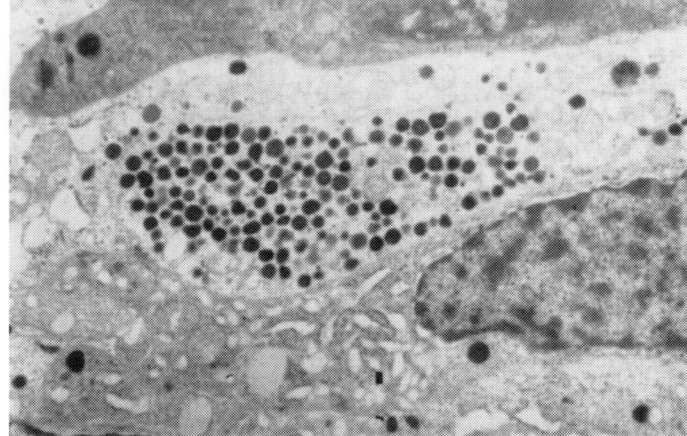

Fig. 2. An electron micrograph of an ileal carcinoid tumour showing abundant secretory granules that are typically electron-dense with an irregular shape. × 6000.

Multiple gastric carcinoids have been reported in patients with pernicious anaemia, probably representing the trophic effect of gastrin on enterochromaffin-like cells (Borch, Gastro, 1985; 888: 638). It appears that those cases of multiple gastric carcinoids that are induced by hypergastrinaemia do not metastasize, whereas those occurring without a background of high gastrin frequently do (Gough, WorldJSurg, 1994; 18:437).

Primary carcinoids normally present as mass lesions in the primary site with appropriate symptom patterns: obstruction or more rarely bleeding in the gastrointestinal tract, or particularly in the case of the appendix, coincidentally. Chest lesions may appear as coincidental coin lesions, or with haemoptysis, cough, wheezing, or segmental obstruction. Primary carcinoids present only very occasionally with features of the carcinoid syndrome in the absence of hepatic metastases (see below).

Hepatic carcinoids may be found on survey of patients presenting with primary lesions, may present with local symptoms of hepatomegaly or pain, or appear with one or more symptoms of the carcinoid syndrome. Local symptoms of hepatic carcinoids are relatively uncommon, except when spontaneous haemorrhage or tumour necrosis occurs. Occasionally, portal hypertension may follow pressure on the portal or hepatic veins.

Table 2 Substances identified in carcinoid tumours or in serum of patients with carcinoid syndrome
Serotonin
Kallikrein
Substance P
Neurokinin A
Neuropeptide K
Peptide YY
Prostaglandins
Insulin
Somatostatin
Glucagon
Chromogranin A
Cholecystokinin/procholecystokinin
Encephalins
Gastrin
Pancreatic polypeptide
ACTH
β-MSH
Calcitonin
Catecholamines
Chorionic gonadotrophin

Sporrong, Cancer, 1982; 49: 68; Leveston, JClinEndoc, 1981; 53: 682; Matsuyama, Cancer, 1979; 44: 1818; Goedert, Cancer, 1980; 45: 104; Grossman, EurJClinInv, 1994; 24: 131.
β-MSH, β-melanocyte stimulating hormone.

Diagnosis

The presentation and investigation of non-functioning hepatic carcinoid tumours differ little from those of other space-occupying lesions in the liver. However, as hepatic carcinoids are compatible with long survival, hepatomegaly may be huge. Local bruits, and occasionally hepatic rubs, are detectable. The presentation with features of the carcinoid syndrome is discussed below.

Laboratory investigations for hepatic carcinoid tumours

The diagnosis of non-functioning carcinoid tumours in the liver is established by imaging techniques followed by biopsy. Of the routine biochemical tests, the serum alkaline phosphatase is often abnormal, but confusingly it may be normal, even in the presence of large tumour deposits.

Screening for 5-hydroxyindoleacetic acid, the breakdown product of 5-hydroxytryptamine, in the urine is worthwhile, even if there are no symptoms suggestive of the carcinoid syndrome, as higher concentrations may precede this. Other tumour markers such as elevated circulating pancreatic polypeptide may be also detected in the absence of any obvious clinical correlate (see below). Other hepatic carcinoid deposits, particularly from hindgut primaries, are truly 'non-functioning', insofar as no secretory products can be detected in the circulation.

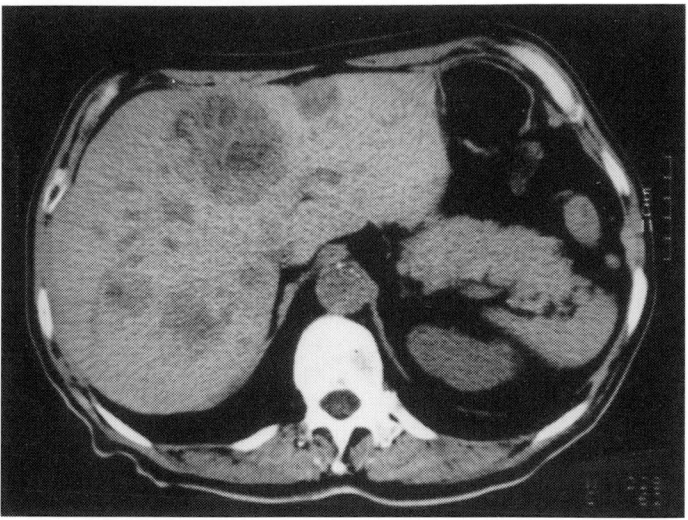

Fig. 3. CT scan (transverse section of abdomen at the level of liver) showing multiple deposits of carcinoid tumour.

Imaging techniques

Hepatic carcinoid deposits may be found at laparotomy for a primary carcinoid tumour of the gut. The indirect investigative techniques for imaging hepatic carcinoids have been reviewed (Adam, BrJ-HospMed, 1986; 35:154). Hepatic ultrasonography should reveal carcinoid deposits of 1 cm or greater, which may be varying in echogenicity, occasionally cystic with sometimes both hyper- and hypoechoic lesions being found in the same patient (Hemmingson, ActaRadiol, 1981; 22:657). CT scanning of the liver should reveal lesions of 0.5 cm or more, usually of low but occasionally of high attenuation (Fig. 3). Regional low-attenuation areas may be difficult to interpret, representing either diffuse tumour or fatty infiltration associated with local compromise of the portal circulation. The difference between carcinoid tissue and surrounding liver is usually diminished by giving a contrast medium. MRI of the liver can sometimes detect tumours with greater clarity than CT (Fig. 4). It may be preferred for long-term annual follow-up, because of the reduction in radiation. Angiography is currently the most sensitive indirect technique for demonstrating carcinoid lesions in the liver. There are four patterns corresponding to the macroscopic nature of the deposits: diffuse fine nodular, diffuse coarse nodular, single masses, or a combination of the last two (Sato, GastrRad, 1984; 9: 23). Most carcinoid deposits are extremely vascular and blush dramatically during the capillary phase. In the case of single mass lesions, angiography will be of value in investigating the feasibility of resection, in combination with CT scanning for extrahepatic spread (Fig. 5). A visceral angiogram may also detect a primary site within the territory of the superior mesenteric artery.

Isotope studies using radio-iodinated m-iodobenzyl guanidine (Kimming, Radiol, 1987; 164:199) or labelled somatostatin analogues can also visualize tumours (Kwekkeboom, EurJNuclMed, 1993; 20:283). The latter technique is, however, more effective for extrahepatic deposits (Fig. 6) and not all carcinoids express the full range of somatostatin receptors: there is selectivity in analogue binding to somatostatin receptors, and octreotide, for example binds only to subtype II.

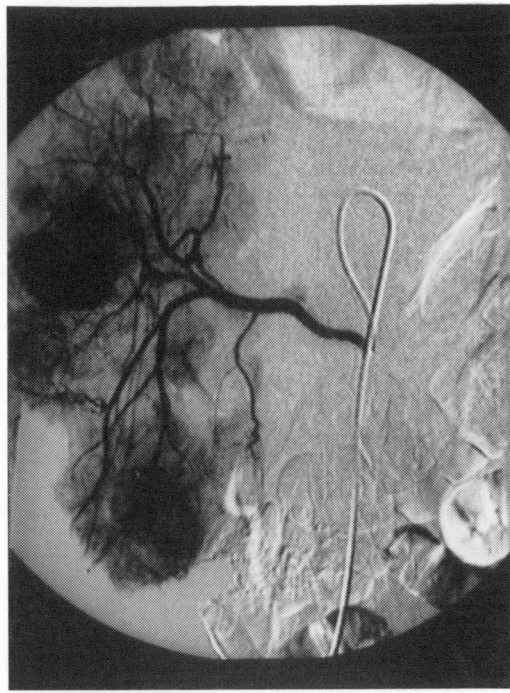

Fig. 4. Sagittal MRI scan of the liver, demonstrating a hepatic metastasis (white) against the dark background of the liver in a patient with carcinoid syndrome.

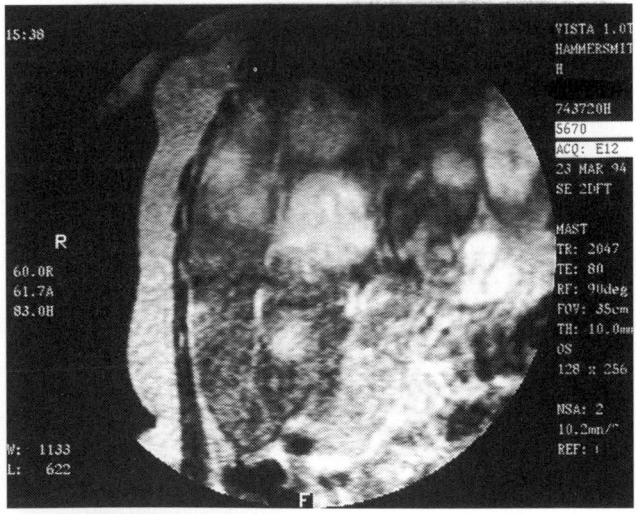

Fig. 5. Arterial phase of visceral arteriogram in a patient with carcinoid syndrome showing multiple, densely vascular deposits.

Hepatic carcinoid tumours with carcinoid syndrome

The carcinoid syndrome occurs when the tumour produces active substances, which reach the systemic circulation in adequate amounts, resulting in the characteristic symptoms of flushing, diarrhoea, and heart disease. With gastrointestinal carcinoids, the presence of the syndrome is associated with hepatic metastases in 95 per cent of cases (Davies, SGO, 1973; 137:637). Occasionally, primary tumours in the gut with extensive nodal involvement giving

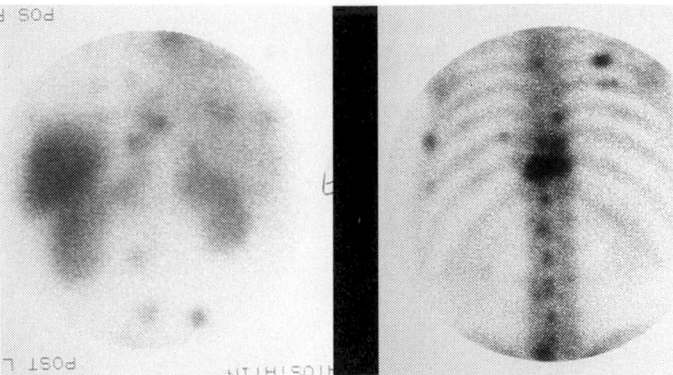

Fig. 6. Labelled octreotide scan (left) demonstrating uptake of octreotide into hepatic and bony metastases in a patient with carcinoid. The conventional bone scan (right) is also positive.

direct access to the systemic venous circulation will produce the syndrome without liver metastases (Feldman, AnnSurg, 1982; 196: 33). Also occasionally, primary ovarian (Waldenstrom, Gastro, 1958; 35:565) and bronchial carcinoids can give symptoms directly, though in fact metastases in the liver are usually present when the syndrome occurs. The classical manifestations of the carcinoid syndrome may on rare occasions be associated with other neuroendocrine tumours such as medullary carcinoid of the thyroid, and oat-cell carcinoma of the lung. Not all carcinoids metastatic to the liver will produce the carcinoid syndrome, and in particular hindgut carcinoids do so very rarely (Table 1) (Spread, DisColRec, 1994; 37:482). The majority of cases of the carcinoid syndrome are associated with metastasized ileal carcinoids.

Clinical features

Linell and Mansson (ActaMedScand, 1966; 179 (Suppl.): 377) indicate an annual incidence of about 1 per million. Both men and women are affected, the sixth decade being the most common time for presentation. The cardinal features of the syndrome are flushing, diarrhoea, and heart disease, with differing symptoms in individuals reflecting the origin and mass of the tumours, length of history, and qualitative and quantitative differences in the release of tumour products. Table 3 shows the presenting features in 63 patients with the carcinoid syndrome.

Cutaneous manifestations

Ninety per cent of patients experience flushing attacks, mainly affecting the upper part of the body. The attacks are highly variable, lasting from minutes to hours, often associated with sweating, lacrimation, itching, facial and conjunctival oedema, palpitations, hypotension (more rarely hypertension), and diarrhoea. Some patients remain entirely unaware of dramatic flushes. The episodes may be spontaneous or precipitated by stress, alcohol, exertion, or abdominal palpation. Gastric carcinoids that produce predominantly histamine may cause a specific pattern of bright red geographical flushing of the face and neck.[11] The long-term effects of the carcinoid syndrome in the skin include telangiectasia of the face, morphoea-like thickening of the skin, and occasionally pellagra (see below).

Feature	Number	%
Diarrhoea	14	22
Flushing	10	16
Diarrhoea and flushing	7	11
Hepatic enlargement	9	14
Bowel obstruction	5	8
Abdominal pain	7	10
Haemoptysis	2	3
Wheeze	1	1.5
Sweating	1	1.5
Palpitations	1	1.5
Geographical rash	1	1.5
Incidental during investigation for other cause	3	5
Incidental during laparotomy for other cause	2	3
TOTAL	63	

Table 3 Presenting features in 63 patients with the carcinoid syndrome

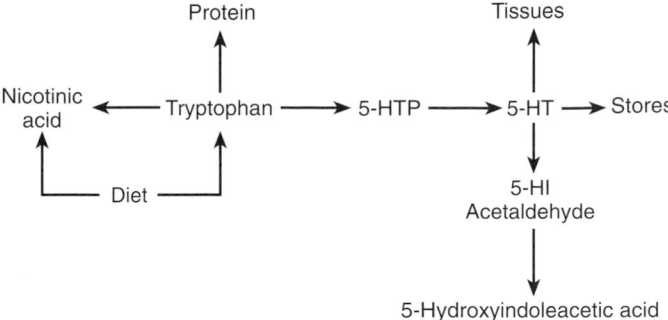

Fig. 7. Pathway of serotonin metabolism.

Gastrointestinal manifestations

Diarrhoea occurs in about 75 per cent of cases.[2] Although it is classically attributed to circulating hormone products, and associated with proven hypermotility (von der Ohe, NEJM, 1993; 329:1073), borborygmus, and a secretory state in the small intestine (Donowitz, AmJDigDis, 1975; 20:1115), abdominal symptoms and diarrhoea may often be due to other causes. These include subacute intestinal obstruction due to a primary tumour, the effects of previous intestinal resection, bile-salt spillage, bacterial overgrowth, and lymphatic obstruction. Abdominal pain may reflect intestinal obstruction, spontaneous necrosis of hepatic metastases, or rarely gut ischaemia due to fibrotic narrowing of mesenteric vessels.

Cardiac manifestations

Only a minority (approx. 40 per cent) of patients with malignant carcinoids and the syndrome have heart disease. Unlike the flushing and diarrhoea that appear as immediate responses to released tumour products, the cardiac disease is due to a slowly developing fibrosis, usually involving the endocardium of the right side of the heart, leading progressively to right-sided failure, with tricuspid regurgitation, and mixed pulmonary regurgitation and stenosis being the most common lesions (Pellikka, Circul, 1993; 87:1188).

Other manifestations

A similar fibrosis to that in the heart and around primary ileal tumours may occur in the intima of the great vessels, in the pleura and pericardium, and retroperitoneally. Wheezing occurs in about 10 per cent of patients and late-onset asthma may occasionally be a presenting feature. Pleural thickening may occur (Moss, QJMed, 1993; 86:49). Intrapulmonary shunting (as in the 'hepatopulmonary syndrome') has been reported (Hussain, ClinEndoc, 1994; 41:535). Confusional states may occur as part of prolonged flushing episodes, particularly in patients with gastric or bronchial carcinoids; they may be a feature of liver failure with advanced disease, or they may be a side-effect of therapy, particularly if p-chlorophenylalanine is used. Confusion may also be part of the pellagra syndrome. A rare peripheral arthropathy has been reported.

Pathogenesis of carcinoid syndrome

The syndrome represents the long- and short-term results of release of substances from the tumour into the systemic circulation.

5-hydroxytryptamine (5HT)

Midgut carcinoids secrete large amounts of 5HT (serotonin), which is responsible for many of the clinical features. 5HT markedly increases gut motility and probably induces secretion in the small intestine (Hendrix, AmJMed, 1957; 23:886). It may play a part in producing bronchoconstriction (Herxheimer, JPhysiol, 1953; 122:49P), and seems to be involved in fibrotic reactions that occur in the heart and elsewhere. The metabolic pathway is shown in Fig. 7, which also demonstrates how nicotinic acid (niacin) deficiency can occur in the carcinoid syndrome, as dietary nicotinic acid is side-tracked to synthesis of 5HT.

Foregut tumours lack the decarboxylase enzyme and thus may secrete 5-hydroxytryptophan, not 5HT. Other tissues, however, usually metabolize sufficient 5-hydroxytryptophan to 5HT and allow a diagnostic amount of 5-hydroxyindoleacetic acid to appear in the urine. The monoamine oxidase normally present in the liver is responsible for the fact that serotonin solely draining into the splanchnic circulation is not associated with systemic symptoms.

Histamine

Primary gastric carcinoids often produce predominantly histamine. This seems to be associated with the distinctive flush (Roberts, NEJM, 1979; 300:236).

Kinins

Carcinoids contain kallikrein, an enzyme that, when released into the blood, converts plasma kininogen to lysylbradykinin, and thence bradykinin (Mehmon, CCActa, 1965; 12:292). They are vasoactive, and probably play some part in initiating flushing (Oates, JCI, 1966; 45:173). Tachykinins have also been identified as potential mediators of flushing (Theodorsson–Norheim, BBResComm, 1985; 131:77).

Other substances

Prostaglandins E, F, and other unidentified prostaglandins have been extracted from carcinoid tumours (Sandler, Lancet, 1968; ii: 1053). However, the response to inhibitors of prostaglandin synthesis suggests that they are unlikely to be major mediators of flushing and diarrhoea (Metz, Metabolism, 1981; 30:299).

Although gastrointestinal peptides of many kinds can be identified in carcinoid tumours (Table 2), when symptoms of diarrhoea have been induced in patients with carcinoid syndrome, no changes in plasma concentrations of insulin, gastrin, pancreatic polypeptide, vasoactive intestinal polypeptide, gastric inhibitory polypeptide, somatostatin, or neurotensin have been found.

Diagnosis of carcinoid syndrome

Once the suspicion has been raised, making the diagnosis of carcinoid is not difficult. Urinary 5-hydroxyindoleacetic acid can be measured quantitatively in a 24-h sample. Levels of more than 30 mg (90 mmol)/24 h are usually diagnostic. Mild elevations may, however, be seen in the blind-loop syndrome, Whipple's disease, and coeliac disease. False-positive results can occur if patients are eating large amounts of food containing 5HT (bananas, pineapples, and walnuts), or taking reserpine, acetanilide, methysergide, or cough medicines containing glyceryl guaiacolate (Young, ClinChem, 1975; 21:3981). As already mentioned, foregut carcinoids may not be associated with elevated excretion of 5-hydroxyindoleacetic acid. Circulating concentrations of substance P are also substantially elevated in patients with carcinoid syndrome (Emson, Cancer, 1984; 54:715), and in some cases concentrations of human chorionic gonadotrophin or its subunits are elevated (Oberg, ActaEnd, 1981; 98:256).

Prognosis

Both primary carcinoid tumours and metastases may grow slowly. Trivial symptoms of occasional mild flushing or diarrhoea may persist for some years with no treatment. The survival may be relatively long. In one series the mean survival time of patients was 8 years, with some patients surviving up to 20 years (Peskin, SurgClinNAm, 1969; 49:137). In our own series the 5-year survival is 48 per cent.

Treatment of carcinoid tumours

The management of primary carcinoid tumours presenting without the syndrome is surgical, at least for disease that is not too advanced locally.

The optimal surgical policy for apparently solitary hepatic secondaries is unclear, but if metastases are readily amenable surgically then local hepatic resection may be appropriate, both to prevent local symptoms and to slow progression (Galland, BrJHospMed, 1986; 35:166). In most patients, in whom complete surgical resection is not possible, choices between conservative treatment, or palliative surgery, chemotherapy, or radiotherapy for the tumour may be difficult: these procedures reduce tumour mass, but it is not clear that this is associated with any prolongation of survival. The presence or absence of the carcinoid syndrome is obviously of major importance. For patients with these slowly progressive neoplasms, medical therapy aimed at controlling the synthesis, release, or peripheral effects of active substances from the tumour may provide extremely effective palliation, and induce a greater improvement in the quality of life than is obtained when partial reduction of tumour mass is produced by chemotherapy or radiotherapy.

Treatment of carcinoid syndrome
General measures

Factors known to precipitate carcinoid attacks such as alcohol, provocative foods, or marked physical activity may be avoided.

Sufficient nicotinamide should be included in the diet. Codeine phosphate may be used to control the diarrhoea, and potassium supplements may be necessary. In the presence of an ileal resection, cholestyramine may be helpful to prevent bile-salt induced colonic secretion. Asthmatic attacks should be treated with aminophylline or salbutamol. Prognosis is poor after heart failure has developed, unless cardiac surgery (valve surgery) can be performed, and patients with heart involvement should be formally assessed (Connolly, JAmCollCard, 1995; 25:410).

Specific pharmacological therapy

Many drugs have been used to modify the acute attacks of flushing and diarrhoea by inhibition or blocking of the synthesis of tumour products.

The receptors of 5HT have been subdivided into $5HT_1$-, $5HT_2$-, and $5HT_3$-receptors, present in different parts of the body in smooth muscle and neural tissue (Bradley, Neuropharmacol, 1986; 25:563). This has helped clarify the relative value of blockers in treating one or more symptoms.

The main drugs in use are as follows.

Inhibitors of 5HT synthesis

p-Chlorophenylalanine (500 mg, four times daily) may substantially reduce diarrhoea and abdominal pain, and also flushing episodes. Side-effects include headaches, dizziness, anxiety, depression and hallucination, and are frequent enough to restrict its use to severe cases or to cases prior to embolization or surgery; following the introduction of somatostatin analogues (see below), pharmaceutical-grade preparations have been difficult to obtain.

5HT antagonists

Methysergide

This $5HT_1$- and $5HT_2$-receptor antagonist, at doses of 3 to 8 mg/day, reduces diarrhoea but has no significant effect upon flushing. Numerous side-effects include nausea, heartburn, abdominal pain and vomiting, and even diarrhoea. Central effects including unsteadiness, drowsiness, confusion, and psychosis have been reported. The major drawback to the use of this drug is the occurrence of retroperitoneal fibrosis after as little as 3 months of continuous therapy. Carcinoids themselves may induce retroperitoneal fibrosis and so the use of this drug is severely limited.

Cyproheptadine

This drug is a $5HT_2$-receptor blocker on smooth muscle and is predominantly used in the treatment of diarrhoea. In addition it possesses weak anticholinergic activity and is a histamine H_1-blocker and a central depressant. This drug is one of the mainstays of medical therapy in the carcinoid syndrome. The usual dose is 4 mg four times daily (Moertel, Cancer, 1991; 67:33).

Ketanserin

Ketanserin is a $5HT_2$-antagonist, occasionally reducing diarrhoea but of more value in alleviating flushing (Gustafsen, ScaJGastr, 1986; 21:816). The usual dose is 20 mg three or four times daily.

Ondansetron

This $5HT_3$-antagonist may be helpful in reducing stool frequency (Schworer, AmJGastr, 1995; 90:645).

Inhibitors of kinin production

Aprotinin

This inhibits the action of tumour kallikrein and thus prevents generation of bradykinin. However, it does not seem to reduce flushing and also suffers from the disadvantage of having to be given intravenously. It is mainly used during the embolization of carcinoid tumours and in the rare spontaneous carcinoid crises, which are probably precipitated by spontaneous tumour necrosis.

Histamine antagonists

Combination therapy with the H_1-antagonist diphenhydramine (50 mg, four times daily) and the H_2- antagonist cimetidine (300 mg, four times daily) may be effective in reducing the flushing and hypotension associated with gastric carcinoids (Roberts, NEJM, 1979; 300:236).

Corticosteroids

Prednisolone in doses of 20 mg/day is said to reduce the facial oedema, diarrhoea, and hyperdynamic state associated with bronchial carcinoids. It has no effect on symptoms associated with a gastrointestinal carcinoid.

Somatostatin

Intravenous infusion of short-acting somatostatin was shown to abolish flushing caused by gastric or ileal carcinoids irrespective of the mode of provocation. On using long-acting analogues of somatostatin, diarrhoea, flushing, and other symptoms of the carcinoid syndrome were relieved in 75 to 80 per cent of patients (Kvols, NEJM, 1986; 315:633). Those that do not respond reflect in part low expression of tumour somatostatin receptors (Kvols, YaleJBiolMed, 1992; 65:505). With an initial dose of 50 µg three times daily, control is usually established for a few months but escalating doses are required over time. Eventually troublesome steatorrhoea may limit its usefulness, and the drug frequently induces the appearance of small cholesterol gallstones (Redfern, AmJGastr, 1995; 90:1042). Its mode of action is a combination of a reduction in output of serotonin and other substances, and peripheral inhibition of end-organ activity. In a small proportion of patients an action in reducing tumour mass is reported but this is in general temporary (Arnold, Metabolism, 1992; 41:116). As doses escalate (up to 500 µg, three times daily), continuous subcutaneous infusion may help reduce cost, and in the future longer-acting analogues will become available.

Other drugs

Calcitonin and clonidine (an α_2-receptor agonist) have each been said to be helpful in anecdotal reports.

Debulking

For the treatment of hepatic metastases, surgery has been advocated to reduce tumour mass, in particular if they are associated with local symptoms, and also as a means of reducing the release of 5HT and other substances. Both partial hepatectomy (when deposits are confined to one lobe) and the shelling out of metastases have been advocated (Foster, Cancer, 1970; 26:493; Strodel, ArchSurg, 1983; 118:391). Such operations will only be indicated occasionally, for example in fewer than 10 per cent of cases of carcinoid syndrome (Galland, BrJHospMed, 1986; 35:166), because the disease is almost always extensive in the liver. Liver transplantation can be performed but in general the identification of extrahepatic tumour dissemination prevents the procedure from being carried out (Frilling, Digestion, 1994; 55:104).

An alternative surgical approach is ligation of the hepatic artery, but this has probably now been superseded by devascularization by hepatic arterial embolization (see below). Extensive surgical devascularization of the liver except for the main hepatic artery, followed by intermittent occlusion of that artery via a percutaneous sling, has also been advocated (Soreide, Surgery, 1992; 111:48).

Surgery in patients with the carcinoid syndrome is potentially hazardous, due to rapid alterations in blood pressure, bronchial constriction, hyperpnoea, vomiting, diarrhoea, and hyperglycaemia (Dery, CanAnaesthSocJ, 1971; 18:245). Such patients should initially be blocked pharmacologically to prevent the action of released 5HT, using a regimen similar to that described below under hepatic embolization. Precipitators of flushing attacks should be avoided in anaesthesia, and nerve blockers, acetylcholine, and morphine all used with care. Hypotensive episodes should be treated with transfusion and angiotensin (not catecholamines). Hydralazine is recommended for hypertension.

Radiotherapy

There are reports of radiotherapy inducing prolonged disease-free remission of carcinoid tumours with metastases (Tochner, Cancer, 1985; 56:20), but others have been less enthusiastic (Keane, IntJRadiatOncolBiolPhys, 1981; 7:1519). The best established place for radiotherapy is in symptomatic relief from skin and bone metastases. In well-selected cases, local disease stabilization and local symptomatic relief are probably achievable in 50 per cent of cases (Chakravarthy, Cancer, 1995; 75:1386).

Chemotherapy

A variety of studies have suggested that single agents, or drug combinations, may produce a reduction in the size of liver metastases. The most generally used regimen recently has been a combination of streptozotocin and 5-fluorouracil, which produces partial response in approx. 30 per cent of patients treated, but with a considerable toxicity.[5]

Interferon

A study (Oberg, NEJM, 1983; 309:129) reports the effects of administering 3 to 6 million units of interferon intramuscularly

Table 4 Hepatic arterial embolization of carcinoid tumours (Hammersmith Hospital regimen)

Pre-embolization
Routine investigations, electrolytes, creatinine, liver function tests, and packed cell volume, urinary 5-hydroxyindoleacetic acid (three times then daily)

Medication before embolization and continued afterwards
(a) Cyproheptadine, 4 mg thrice daily oral—24 h before embolization and afterwards
(b) Nicotinamide, 250 mg four times daily
(c) Octreotide, 50 μg three times daily, subcutaneous for 2 days pre-embolization; 100 μg hourly for 48 h starting 2 h pre-embolization

Premedication
Omnopon (papaveretum), 15 mg IM
Atropine, 0.4 mg IM
Prochlorperazine, 12.5 mg IM
Gentamicin, 80 mg; flucloxacillin, 500 mg; metronidazole, 500 mg IV; give intravenously at same time as premedication, then continue for 10 days (N.B. facilities for monitoring gentamicin concentrations should be available)

During embolization
1. Antiemetics as necessary
2. Methylprednisolone 1 g IV at start
3. Trasylol (aprotinin) 50 000 units hourly (1 h before and 48 h after), IV infusion
4. Low-osmolality contrast medium to be used if possible
5. Experienced physician or anaesthetist should always be present during the procedure

To be available if needed
Hydralazine IV for hypertension (or nitroprusside), or labetalol
Albumin for hypotension (i.e., plasma)
Methylprednisolone

Monitoring
1. CVP line: insert before embolization (or good peripheral line)
2. Peripheral line (left arm easier for radiologist)
3. Blood pressure: measure very frequently during embolization and immediately afterwards (e.g. every 2–3 min; automatic non-invasive monitoring is useful if available)

Postembolization
1. Usual postangiogram observations
2. Close watch on blood pressure and urine output
3. Daily 5-hydroxyindoleacetic acid, full blood count, daily liver function tests
4. Adequate hydration throughout is very important

IV, intravenous; IM, intramuscular; CVP, central venous pressure.

thrice weekly for 3 months. Subsequently, partial remission was observed in 47 per cent of a group of patients treated with daily interferon, with remissions lasting for up to 3 years (Oberg, CancerTreatRep, 1986; 70:1267). The treatment may be symptomatically successful after long-acting somatostatin (octreotide) has failed, and the combination of the two reduced excretion of 5-hydroxyindoleacetic acid in 72 per cent of cases (Janson, ActaOncol, 1993; 32:225). The side-effects of interferon are predominantly transient malaise at the initiation of treatment, and mild pancytopenia.

Hepatic arterial embolization

This technique reduces the arterial blood flow to both tumour deposits and normal liver cells. The latter survive due to their simultaneous blood supply from the portal circulation, but the procedure can induce substantial necrosis of hepatic tumour deposits. As with chemotherapy, destruction of hepatic deposits may release large amounts of tumour-blocking agents causing severe symptoms, so blocking agents are used before and after the procedure. The protocol in current use at the Hammersmith Hospital, London, is shown in Table 4.[12]

The procedure involves selective cannulation of the coeliac axis and hepatic artery, and requires the portal blood supply to the liver to be intact. A variety of absorbable or non-absorbable embolic materials can be used. Usually, successful embolization is followed by fever, a leucocytosis, and hepatic pain, with a marked rise in serum hepatic enzymes.

The results of this procedure are variable, depending on the selection of patients. It has some effect in reducing the local symptoms of the tumour, but is most effective in control of distressing symptoms due to release of active substances. In a majority of patients, flushing and abdominal pain can be abolished, with improvement in diarrhoea and a significant reduction in urinary excretion of 5-hydroxyindoleacetic acid. Clinical remissions last from 1 to 18 months, and on a number of occasions successful re-embolization has been performed with further remissions. However, repeated embolization after this rarely produces substantial improvement. Whether long-term survival is affected by embolization is not yet clear (Martensson, JSurgOncol, 1984; 27:152; Mitty, Radiol, 1985; 155:623) and would be difficult to prove (Coupe, Gut, 1987; 28:1329). Chemoembolization combining transcatheter embolization with local chemotherapy (iodized oil plus deoxorubicin) has also been advocated (Therasse, Radiol, 1993; 189: 541), but evidence of enhanced effectiveness compared with simple embolization is only anecdotal.

Other treatments

Radioactive *m*-iodobenzyl guanidine injected intravenously will localize in carcinoid deposits. Introduced as an imaging agent, the feasibility of local radiotherapy by this means has been explored, but after initial enthusiasm follow-up reports have been less encouraging (Bestagno, JNuclBiolMed, 1991; 35:343).

Choosing the right therapy

In patients with hepatic metastases from carcinoid tumours without systemic symptoms, surgery is indicated for readily resectable tumours, in particular if the primary tumour is also resectable. Such a policy should prolong life. If the tumour is not readily resectable, and the patient is asymptomatic, many physicians will hesitate to recommend chemotherapy or radiotherapy, but may reserve such relatively ineffective but potentially distressing therapies until symptoms occur.

For the patients with carcinoid syndrome, the indications for surgery are as above. For patients with mild symptoms, no active treatment for the syndrome may be required other than avoidance of precipitating factors. As symptoms become more severe a reasonable approach is to use cyproheptadine and codeine phosphate to control diarrhoea, and subsequently most patients will respond to a long-acting somatostatin analogue given subcutaneously. An alternative approach at this juncture would be a trial of interferon therapy. When acceptable pharmacological therapies are no longer effective, we proceed to embolization of the hepatic artery as it seems effective and appears to carry a lower risk than surgical debulking. Though we are prepared to embolize on more than one occasion, this procedure should not be undertaken lightly as subsequent remissions are likely to be shorter than the first.

References

1. Obendorfer J. Karzinodie. Tumoren des Duenndarmes. *Frankfurter Zeitschrift fur Pathologie*, 1907; **1**: 426.
2. Thorson A. Studies on carcinoid disease. *Acta Medica Scandinavica*, 1958; **334** (Suppl.): 7–132.
3. Hodgson HJ. Carcinoid tumours and the carcinoid syndrome. In Bouchier IA, Allan RN, Hodgson HJF, and Keighley MRB, eds. *Gastroenterology clinical science and practice*, 2nd edn. London: WB Saunders, 1993: 643–66.
4. Kvols LK. Chemotherapy of metastatic carcinoid and islet cell tumours. *American Journal of Medicine*, 1987; **82** (5B): 77–83.
5. Oberg K. Chemotherapy and biotherapy in neuroendocrine tumours. *Current Opinion in Oncology*, 1993; **5**: 110–20.
6. Soreide O, *et al.* Surgical treatment as a principle in patients with advanced abdominal carcinoid tumours. *Surgery*, 1992; **111**: 48–54.
7. Soga J and Tazawa K. Pathologic analysis of carcinoids. *Cancer*, 1971; **28**: 990–8.
8. Solcia E, Capella C, and Buffa R. Endocrine cells of the digestive system. In Johnston LR, ed. *Physiology of the gastrointestinal tract*. New York: Raven, 1981: 39–58.
9. Falkmer S, Martensson H, Robin A, and Sundler F. Peptide hormones in various types of gastroentero/pancreatic tumours. In Bresciani F *et al.*, eds. *Progress in cancer research and therapeutics*. New York: Raven, 1984; **31**: 597–611.
10. Marangos PJ. Clinical utility of neuron-specific enolase as a neuroendocrine tumour marker. In Polak JM and Bloom SR, eds. *Endocrine tumours*. Edinburgh: Churchill Livingstone, 1985: 181–92.
11. Grahame-Smith DG. *The carcinoid syndrome*. London: Heinemann Medical, 1972.
12. Maton PN, Camilleri M, and Griffin G. The role of hepatic arterial embolisation in the carcinoid syndrome. *British Medical Journal*, 1984; **287**: 932–5.

23

Biliary tract diseases

23.1 Cholestasis

Neil McIntyre

'There's glory for you!' 'I don't know what you mean by "glory",' Alice said. 'I meant, "there's a nice knock-down argument for you!"' 'But "glory" doesn't mean "a nice knock-down argument",' Alice objected. 'When I use a word,' Humpty Dumpty said in a rather scornful tone, 'it means just what I choose it to mean—neither more nor less.'

Lewis Carroll, Through the Looking Glass.

In this book, and particularly this section, you will often meet the words cholestasis and cholestatic, derived from the Greek words 'χολη' ('chole', for bile) and 'στασις' ('stasis' or 'standstill').

According to Popper and Schaffner (HumPath, 1970; 1:1), Roessle coined the terms cholangiolitic and cholestatic in 1930.[1] In a discussion on the histology and pathogenesis of biliary cirrhosis, he used cholangiolitic as an adjective for cirrhosis caused by obstruction of the smallest biliary passages when inflammation was present, and cholestatic when such inflammation was absent.

The first appearance of cholestasis and cholestatic in Dorland's and Stedman's Medical Dictionaries was in 1932 (16th and 12th editions, respectively). In Dorland's, cholestasis was the 'stoppage or suppression of the flow of bile'; it has the same meaning in the 28th edition (1994), but with the phrase 'having intrahepatic or extrahepatic causes'. In both the 12th and 26th editions of Stedman's dictionary cholestasis is 'an arrest in the flow of bile', but the 26th edition (1995) has an additional statement—'c.[holestasis] due to obstruction of bile ducts is accompanied by formation of plugs of inspissated bile in the small ducts, canaliculi in the liver, and elevation of serum direct bilirubin and some enzymes'.

The term was rarely used but in 1952, Popper and Schaffner published their paper 'Laboratory diagnosis of liver disease: coordinated use of histological and biochemical observations'.[2] They wrote: 'Interference with the flow of bile after its formation is termed cholestasis ... [it] may be caused by extrahepatic or intrahepatic factors; however, laboratory tests do not differentiate between the two'. Tumours, gallstones, and strictures were extrahepatic causes of bile duct obstruction. The intrahepatic form (primary cholestasis) was thought to result either from rare mechanical factors (congenital atresias or inflammatory obliteration of the intrahepatic ducts) or from functional factors acting on small bile ducts or on cholangioles. Differentiation between intrahepatic and extrahepatic cholestasis was considered a major diagnostic problem.

The meaning of cholestasis, as used in this article, seemed quite clear. It meant the 'stoppage or suppression of the flow of bile' or 'arrest in the flow of bile' due to obstruction, whether this occurred in large bile ducts or in smaller biliary radicles. Obstruction caused histological changes, and if enough liver was involved there were clinical and biochemical consequences. The word cholestasis did not appear in the first edition of Sherlock's classic text *Diseases of the liver and biliary tract* in 1955;[3] it occurs only once in the second edition (1958), as an alternative term for the clinical syndrome of chronic obstructive jaundice; it first appeared in the index in the third edition (1963), where it had the same meaning.

Popper and Schaffner paid greater attention to what they called histological cholestasis, characterized by bile pigment in Kupffer cells and the presence of inspissated bile and bile plugs in dilated canaliculi (mainly in the centrilobular region in early cases). Sometimes, with extrahepatic block, changes suggesting extravasation of bile occur in the lobular parenchyma or portal triads—necrosis of surrounding cells causing 'bile infarcts'. Prolonged obstruction resulted in fibrosis in the portal triads, with little cellular infiltration in the absence of infection. Granular bile pigment in liver cells was considered evidence of liver cell degeneration concomitant with cholestasis, although in some cases of cholestasis liver cell degeneration was absent. In viral and toxic hepatitis, in which there was liver cell degeneration, intrahepatic cholestasis was often present in the form of cholangiolitis. Popper and Schaffner[2] thought that liver cell degeneration *per se* might interfere with bile flow at the source of bile, that is from the hepatocyte.

In a subsequent study of the light and electron microscopic features of cholestasis Schaffner and Popper (Schaffner, Gastro, 1959; 37:565) stressed the overall similarity in the histological features of intrahepatic cholestasis and those of extrahepatic obstruction. They argued that in extrahepatic obstruction a primary hydrostatic effect caused a secondary lesion involving the canaliculus and its microvilli. In intrahepatic cholestasis 'a similar membrane effect, possibly primary, is also associated with evidence of increased hydrostatic pressure, whereas the liver cell itself is uninvolved or only secondarily so'. In 1965 Albot and his colleagues (*Progress in Liver Diseases* II:26, Popper and Schaffner, eds) reaffirmed the definition of cholestasis as 'retention of bile in the blood resulting from mechanical impairment to flow in the bile ducts, ductules or canaliculi. In intrahepatic cholestasis, the obstruction is localized within the liver.'

The clinical syndrome of biliary obstruction consisted of jaundice, dark urine, pale stools, and itching; the accompanying biochemical changes in serum were the combination of hyperbilirubinaemia, an elevated level of alkaline phosphatase, and a

Table 1 Definitions of cholestasis

Dictionaries
1   i 'Stoppage or suppression of the flow of bile, having intrahepatic or extrahepatic causes' (Dorland)
    ii 'An arrest in the flow of bile' (Stedman)

Pathological
2   Macroscopic—green liver and hepatomegaly
3   Light microscopy—canalicular bile plugs and bile pigment in Kupffer cells and hepatocytes
4   Ultrastructural

Clinical and biochemical
5   Clinical—jaundice, dark urine, pale stools, and pruritus
6   Biochemical—raised conjugated bilirubin, akaline phosphatase, and cholesterol

Physiological
7   A primary hepatocellular alteration of secretion of micelles containing bile salts
8   Decrease in bile flow
9   'Diminution of the volume of that fraction of bile that is dependent on bile acids'
10 'A reduction of bile salt output into the bile (complete, incomplete, localized, and abortive forms) and into the intestine'
11 Failure of normal amounts of bile to reach the intestine

raised cholesterol. At this stage, cholestasis had already acquired at least four meanings (Table 1): 'stoppage or suppression of the flow of bile', or 'an arrest in the flow of bile', thought to be due to biliary obstruction; 'histological cholestasis'; 'clinical cholestasis'; and 'biochemical cholestasis'. The seeds for further confusion about the meaning of the word were sown by Schaffner and Popper in two articles published in 1969 and 1970—'Cholestasis is the result of hypoactive hypertrophic smooth endoplasmic reticulum in the hepatocyte'[4] and 'Pathophysiology of cholestasis'.[5]

In the *Lancet* paper[4] they pointed out that 'cholestasis, which implied the visible stagnation of bile in the liver, was originally ascribed to mechanical obstruction', and that 'the obvious obstacle in extrahepatic biliary obstruction fostered the belief that obstruction within the liver accounted for intrahepatic cholestasis.' However, they were concerned that there was no evidence of obstruction on light microscopy in the great majority of cases of intrahepatic cholestasis (Popper, Gastro, 1956; 31:683), even though their own studies had stressed the overall similarity in the histological features compared with those of extrahepatic obstruction.

Their concern about visible 'obstruction' is difficult to understand. Even with extrahepatic causes of jaundice due to tumours, stones, or strictures, a complete block is unusual. As flow through a tube is inversely related to the fourth power of the radius, relatively small changes in the diameter of the smallest biliary radicles would have a disproportionate effect on bile flow and/or the pressure drop along the biliary system. Clearly, there might be obstruction to bile flow in many types of intrahepatic liver damage if there were small but functionally significant changes in the radius of the biliary radicles, due to swelling of hepatocytes or biliary epithelium, but such small changes might well be histologically undetectable.

In the *Lancet* article,[4] which is not easy reading, they reviewed the findings of many studies under the following headings: electron microscopic observations, clinical pathological correlations, bile salt metabolism, physicochemical properties of bile, toxicological experiments, and physiological studies of the biliary tree. They pointed out that histological features of cholestasis were seen in animals with experimental choleperitoneum in which there was no reason to suspect mechanical obstruction to the flow of bile. Furthermore, in hamsters, intravenous administration of taurolithocholate, which does not form micelles at body temperature, caused electron microscopic and functional changes similar to those of cholestasis (Schaffner, LabInvest, 1966; 15;1783). It had been suggested that taurolithocholate might precipitate in newly formed bile (Javitt, JCI, 1968; 47:1002); this, of course, could have caused a localized obstruction to bile flow.

Although the amounts of monohydroxy bile acids necessary to induce experimental cholestasis were not found in human bile in cholestatic syndromes (Javitt, AmJMed, 1971; 51:637), Schaffner and Popper[4] hypothesized that cholestasis is a primary hepatocellular alteration of secretion of micelles that contain bile salts. They suggested that impaired bile salt production in hepatocytes, due to a 'hypoactive hypertrophic smooth endoplasmic reticulum', might result in excessive production of toxic monohydroxy bile acids, like lithocholate, which would create a vicious cycle enhancing the cholestatic injury. Such a change in the smooth endoplasmic reticulum also seemed to be a consequence of biliary obstruction but, if the 'vicious cycle' hypothesis was correct, it would be difficult to explain why relief of extrahepatic obstruction rapidly improves the clinical situation.

Schaffner and Popper[4] were led to assume that cholestasis must be a 'primary' effect on the secretion of micelles that contain bile salts, due either to an increased amount of monohydroxy bile salts or to a direct effect on the process of micelle formation. The logic behind this assumption is far from clear. In the *Human Pathology* article[4] they were more cautious about the term 'cholestasis', suggesting that it was a 'non-committal descriptive term … used to designate a lesion in which the initial alteration need not be mechanical and may reside in the liver'.

The choice of the word 'primary' in the above context was curious. Cholestasis was, and still is, considered to result from extrahepatic and intrahepatic causes. With extrahepatic biliary obstruction the primary event is clearly mechanical. One might expect secondary changes in hepatocytes as a result of hydrostatic pressure, intracanalicular accumulation of biliary materials which might damage the hepatocytes, impaired secretion into bile of substances which may then accumulate in hepatocytes (including bile acids), and/or reuptake by hepatocytes of biliary substances which have regurgitated into plasma. Resulting changes in bile salt handling and bile secretion, or in the biliary secretion of other compounds, would clearly have to be considered 'secondary' phenomena in the case of extrahepatic obstruction.

To avoid this issue, advocates of a primary role of secretory failure at the level of the hepatocyte have tended to use 'cholestasis' as if it referred only to intrahepatic cholestasis; this only causes further confusion. Furthermore, little attention has been paid to the fact that some forms of intrahepatic cholestasis do indeed result from obstruction to the smallest biliary passages, and to the probability that other forms might also be due to obstruction. Several workers had suggested that the serum biochemical changes in obstructive jaundice resulted because bile passed from canaliculi between the hepatocytes to the peris-inusoidal spaces (DePalma, JAMA, 1968; 204:534; Schatzki, LabInvest, 1969; 20:87), or that bile traversed the biliary ductules. Popper and Schaffner[5] accepted the presence of a 'ductular–hepatocyte circulation', but argued that the 'integrity of the junctional complex as long as the liver cell secretes bile' argued against the transport of bile between the hepatocytes. There is now good evidence that phospholipid can regurgitate from bile into plasma when the pressure in the biliary system rises (see Chapter 2.12), and Landmann and his colleagues found evidence of tight junctional impairment as a result of biliary ligation and also in ethinyloestradiol cholestasis.[6]

Javitt and Arias (Gastro, 1967; 53:171) had pointed out that there is no cholestasis in hereditary disorders of man and sheep in which there is impaired excretion of biliary anions other than bile acids. They wrote: 'Apparently bile secretory failure must involve the excretion of bile acids as well as other organic anions and perhaps cations in order to produce intrahepatic cholestasis'. The term 'cholestasis' was already confusing and imprecise; partly on the basis of the comments of Javitt and Arias, physiologists added to the confusion by rejecting definitions based on clinical features and morphology, requiring only that bile flow be decreased.[7] However, Javitt and Arias (Gastro, 1967; 53:171) had made it clear that intrahepatic cholestasis was a consequence of some types of biliary secretory failure; it could not therefore be equated with these forms of secretory failure.

Physiologists were concerned because morphological (and clinical) definitions did not meet requirements to explain the apparent functional impairment in bile flow.[7] However, this posed the wrong question. The questions which needed answering were implicit in the comments of Javitt and Arias. Why do some types of disturbance in bile flow, including extrahepatic obstruction, cause the clinical and morphologic features of 'cholestasis' as it had been defined by Popper and Schaffner[2] and why are these features seen when there is no obvious obstruction to the flow of bile, for example with a choleperitoneum, or possibly with the infusion of taurolithocholate? Some of the earlier definitions were at least based on observable variables (histological changes, and clinical and biochemical features). To replace them with one based on reduction of bile flow, which is essentially unmeasurable except as the final output of bile through the main bile ducts of experimental animals, seems to me to have been a retrograde step.

Physiologists added the definition that 'cholestasis' is a decrease in bile flow. In an article 'What is cholestasis?' Magnenat (HelvMedActa, 1973; 37:175) argued, somewhat illogically, that the 'non-hepatocytic fraction of bile is not bile', and also that 'hepatocytic bile flow independent of bile salt secretion is not bile'. He therefore defined cholestasis in two ways: first, as a 'diminution of the volume of that fraction of bile that is dependent on bile acids', and 'finally . . . [as] a reduction of bile salt output into the bile (complete, incomplete, localized, and abortive forms) and into the intestine'. His suggestion that cholestasis is a reduction of the flow of bile into the intestine persists today; it is the definition used in the latest (10th) edition of Sherlock and Dooley's *Diseases of the liver and biliary system*.[3] There have, therefore, been at least eleven definitions of cholestasis put forward (Table 1).

Problems with the definitions of cholestasis

Karl Popper pointed out that good definitions in science should be read from right to left, not left to right. The sentence 'A di-neutron is an unstable system comprising two neutrons' is the scientists' answer to the question 'What shall we call an unstable system comprising two neutrons?', not an answer to the question 'What is a di-neutron?'.[8] In this sense, words provide a form of shorthand for the ideas that they express. Had this principle been appreciated it is difficult to believe that so many 'definitions' would have resulted for the word 'cholestasis'. There is no 'essence' of cholestasis which requires definition. Hepatologists have simply used the same word, somewhat carelessly, to express many different ideas; when this is done confusion is inevitable, particularly if, as sometimes happens, the different meanings are used interchangeably within the same text, without clarification of the change in usage. This confusion has been recognized by a number of authors,[7,9,10] and as Javitt and Arias wrote 'it is not surprising that the promiscuous application of the term [cholestasis] has depreciated its usefulness' (Gastro, 1967; 53:171).

There are problems with all of the current definitions of the word 'cholestasis'. 'Stoppage or suppression of the flow of bile' in Dorland's dictionary is slightly ambiguous; 'stoppage' suggests obstruction to bile flow, but 'suppression' might be thought to include impairment of bile flow at the level of the hepatocyte. Stedman's 'an arrest in the flow of bile' is also open to interpretation, but the additional statement—'cholestasis due to obstruction of bile ducts . . .'— found in later editions, clearly indicates the emphasis placed on biliary obstruction.

Histological cholestasis

'Histological cholestasis' seems to be the most relevant of the other definitions. The light microscopic features were described above; they have been reviewed by Desmet[10] who accepted that the bile retention seen (in hepatocytes, Kupffer cells, and canaliculi) might be more correctly termed 'bilirubinostasis' (Bianchi, PatholResPract, 1983; 178:2). The intensity of bile staining varies from lobule to lobule, and does not appear related to the severity of the clinical picture. All the histological changes of intrahepatic cholestasis are seen in large bile duct obstruction. Features favouring the latter include bile plugging of the interlobular bile ducts, bile-stained 'infarcts', marked ductular proliferation, oedema, and a predominantly polymorphonuclear infiltration of the portal tracts. However, these features are often absent, and distinction from intrahepatic cholestasis may then be impossible on histological grounds. With many forms of chronic cholestasis, periportal fibrosis develops, with ultimate progression to portal–portal bridging and biliary cirrhosis.

The electron microscopic findings are also similar regardless of the cause of histological cholestasis; they have also been reviewed by Desmet.[10] Prominent features include dilated canaliculi, with fewer microvilli (which appear blunted), a reduction in the Golgi and rough endoplasmic reticulum, and changes in the smooth endoplasmic reticulum. Schaffner and Popper considered the smooth endoplasmic reticulum to be hypertrophic and hypoactive; [4] not all workers agree about the hypertrophy, and several studies suggest that the hypoactivity is not the cause but the result of cholestasis.[10] Although tight junctions are preserved they show changes on electron microscopy, and there is evidence that their permeability may be increased.[7,10]

In their early papers, Popper and Schaffner made a distinction between 'histological cholestasis' and 'cholestasis', and there was resulting confusion about the nature of intrahepatic cholestasis.[5] They wrote that in cholestasis 'all biliary substances besides direct and indirect bilirubin are increased in the serum'; to them, therefore, clinically evident jaundice appeared an essential aspect of cholestasis. They also wrote:

> Cholestasis as defined occurs in two forms. In one a mechanical obstruction encroaches upon the lumen of the extrahepatic biliary tract ... the same clinical and laboratory manifestations of cholestasis as well as the same histologic picture in the liver have been found in conditions in which surgical exploration, roentgenologic examination, or even autopsy failed to reveal a lesion of the extrahepatic biliary tract. This second form has been designated 'intrahepatic cholestasis'. In a few cases a mechanical cause is obvious radiologically. . . . Most mechanical intrahepatic lesions, however, do not lead to jaundice. A focal lesion may produce considerable morphologic cholestasis in the respective portion of the liver without causing jaundice. The uninvolved parts excrete bilirubin in a compensatory fashion.[5]

Thus, many causes of histological cholestasis were excluded from the classification of cholestasis, conditions which, if they had involved a greater proportion of the liver, and altered serum biochemistry, would obviously have been considered as causes of cholestasis. Continuing with their argument, Popper and Schaffner wrote 'it is clinically useful to reject mechanical obstruction in the intrahepatic bile duct system as the main mechanism [for intrahepatic cholestasis] and to accept damage of the hepatocytic bile secretory apparatus'. They even excluded early primary biliary cirrhosis, because it appeared to cause regurgitation of bile through altered ducts.

The rejection of mechanical obstruction as a cause of histological intrahepatic cholestasis is not soundly based, even though it may be absent in some cases. In 1952, Popper and Schaffner[2] noted that intrahepatic cholestasis occurred with conditions such as congenital atresias and inflammatory obliteration of the intrahepatic ducts. Furthermore, the two major chronic cholestatic conditions of adults, primary biliary cirrhosis and sclerosing cholangitis, cause damage to and loss of bile ducts, and bile duct lesions resembling those of primary biliary cirrhosis are found in sarcoidosis, acute and chronic rejection of liver allografts, Hodgkin's disease, and chronic viral hepatitis.[11] This clearly suggests that the effects of these disorders are caused by mechanical obstruction. Obstruction to bile flow would also seem to be an inevitable consequence of the paucity of intrahepatic bile ducts seen in many cholestatic syndromes.[11] Even without such obvious histological changes one cannot exclude the possibility that relatively small changes in the diameter of the smallest biliary radicles would cause obstruction to bile flow, while bile plugs *per se* would constitute a form of mechanical obstruction. Widespread acceptance of the idea that intrahepatic cholestasis is primarily due to a reduction in the secretion of bile

from hepatocytes is likely to minimize efforts to explore other mechanisms.

Clinical cholestasis

The original 'clinical definition' of cholestasis was the clinical syndrome of jaundice, dark urine, and pale stools, together with pruritus, usually accompanied by a number of biochemical abnormalities in serum. The first three features are easily explained as a result of biliary obstruction, at any level, but we still have no good explanation for the itching, which is often present in patients with primary biliary cirrhosis without hyperbilirubinaemia. Unfortunately, the classic clinical syndrome may be seen in many liver diseases which are not usually considered obstructive (see below), and patients with proven extrahepatic obstruction may present without jaundice, pale stools, pruritus, or hepatomegaly. The term 'clinical cholestasis' is therefore of doubtful value.

Biochemical cholestasis

Biochemical cholestasis was originally considered to be present when there was an elevation of serum bilirubin (and bilirubinuria), alkaline phosphatase, and cholesterol (Popper, JAMA, 1952; 150: 1367). Later, as they became available, other tests were added as markers of biliary obstruction/cholestasis (5-nucleotidase, γ-glutamyl transferase, and LP-X).

In a recent book on the standardization of nomenclature in liver disease[12] it is stated that 'The laboratory features common to all forms of cholestasis are a rise in serum bilirubin, an elevation of γ-glutamyl transpeptidase to levels more than twice normal, increased alkaline phosphatase, an increase in serum cholesterol and total bile salt concentration and the presence of bilirubin in the urine'. However, this statement is misleading. The total serum cholesterol is often normal, even with confirmed extrahepatic obstruction; and all of the other features are seen (like the clinical features) in patients whose diseases are not usually thought of as 'cholestatic' (see below). Furthermore, in many patients with 'cholestatic' conditions, bilirubin may be absent from the urine at some stage, jaundice being due to the presence of bili-alb (see Chapter 5.1). In some forms of intrahepatic cholestasis the γ-glutamyl transferase is normal or low (Chapter 5.1); even for liver disease in general, an increased γ-glutamyl transferase has low specificity.

The serum alkaline phosphatase activity has been considered of particular importance, ever since Roberts (BMJ, 1933; i:734) found high levels with bile duct obstruction (and lower but still high levels in 'toxic, infective, and catarrhal' jaundice); the increase was attributed to regurgitation of bile phosphatase, but this is probably an unimportant mechanism.

An alkaline phosphatase level of more than 30 King–Armstrong units (two and a half times the upper normal level of 13 **KA units**) became accepted as a diagnostic criterion for an extrahepatic block, even though early workers cast doubt on the value of phosphatase measurements in the differential diagnosis of jaundice (Morris, QJMed, 1937; 6:211); they did so because values above 30 KA units were sometimes found in hepatitis and cirrhosis, and because the plasma phosphatase rose in subjects with a bile fistula. We now know that serum alkaline phosphatase activity goes up in many types of liver disease (Chapter 5.1), and that obstructive jaundice does not always result in a high phosphatase, even when an extra-hepatic block is confirmed; the alkaline phosphatase may also be normal with primary biliary cirrhosis and primary sclerosing cholangitis.

The lipid changes in liver disease are complex (Chapter 2.12). It is mainly free cholesterol which rises with biliary obstruction (Widal, SemaineMed, 1912; 32:529); because cholesteryl ester may be high, normal, or low, the total cholesterol is quite variable. Nowadays, the serum cholesterol is rarely considered in the interpretation of serum liver tests unless it is obviously raised, when it is considered to support the diagnosis of obstructive jaundice.

Popper and Schaffner[5] thought that the rise in serum cholesterol might be related to hypertrophy of the smooth endoplasmic reticulum, with loss of the negative feedback control mechanism for cholesterol synthesis, and to increased solubility of lipids in serum because of increased serum bile acid levels. However, the total phospholipid also rises and there is a linear relationship between lecithin and free cholesterol. There is now good evidence that the hypercholesterolaemia sometimes seen with obstructive jaundice is due to accumulation in plasma of lecithin regurgitated from the biliary tree (see Chapter 2.12). When lecithin alone was infused into the obstructed biliary tree in dogs, almost all appeared in plasma; as plasma lecithin increased, so did plasma free cholesterol (Quarfordt, Lipids, 1973; 8:522). Hypercholesterolaemia also resulted when phospholipid was infused intravenously into animals after hepatectomy (Byers, JBC, 1962; 237:3375; Lipids, 1969; 4:123) suggesting that cholesterol came, at least partly, from pre-existing cholesterol in other tissues. As there was no increase in hepatic cholesterol synthesis with intravenous infusion of lecithin when an equimolar amount of cholesterol was also given (Quarfordt, Gastro, 1973; 65: 566), it would appear that the increase in hepatic cholesterol synthesis found when lecithin accumulates in plasma is simply a compensatory mechanism, triggered by removal of cholesterol from the liver.

In obstructive jaundice, another factor influencing the accumulation in plasma of lecithin and free cholesterol (which accounts for the appearance of LP-X, in which they are present in a 1:1 molar ratio) is a reduction in the activity of the plasma enzyme, lecithin cholesterol acyltransferase (**LCAT**), which removes lecithin and free cholesterol with the formation of cholesteryl ester. LCAT activity falls in many types of liver disease.

The concept of 'biochemical cholestasis', i.e. that there was a combination of test results indicating biliary obstruction, was incorporated in an early classification of jaundice—into haemolytic, hepatocellular, or obstructive (or cholestatic) jaundice. This classification is unsatisfactory for several reasons (Chapter 5.8) but it is still advocated by some authors. Obstructive or 'cholestatic' jaundice is considered to be present when most of the serum bilirubin is conjugated (although this is rarely determined), aminotransferase levels are only moderately elevated, and alkaline phosphatase activity is more than two and a half times the upper reference limit (but see above). Unfortunately, the classification of jaundice on this basis is unstisfactory.

Clearly, a sound diagnostic strategy should be based on a sound diagnostic classification, in which the classes should be collectively exhaustive, and ideally, mutually exclusive (i.e. all diagnostic possibilities should be included, but should not appear under more than one heading). With the above classification many conditions

Table 2 Parenchymal liver diseases which may present with biochemical (and clinical) features suggesting extrahepatic biliary obstruction
Acute viral hepatitis
Alcoholic liver disease
Chronic active hepatitis and cirrhosis
Syphilitic hepatitis
Graft-versus-host disease
α_1-Antitrypsin deficiency
Intrahepatic cholestasis of pregnancy
Benign recurrent intrahepatic cholestasis
Drug-induced hepatitis
Primary biliary cirrhosis
Postoperative jaundice
Sarcoidosis
Lymphoma
Cystic fibrosis
Amyloidosis

coming under the heading of 'hepatocellular' jaundice would also appear under the heading of obstructive or cholestatic jaundice: viral hepatitis, drug-induced hepatitis, alcoholic liver disease, chronic active hepatitis, and cirrhosis may all present with biochemical (and clinical) features considered 'typical' of biliary obstruction (Table 2). To overcome this problem it was suggested recently in a small text, widely used by students, that jaundice should be classified as haemolytic jaundice, congenital hyperbilirubinaemias, and cholestatic jaundice, 'because in hepatocellular jaundice there is invariably cholestasis';[13] all the important causes of jaundice were therefore considered as cholestatic jaundice, which was divided into intrahepatic and extrahepatic causes. This approach seems to stem directly from the confusion which has arisen about the meaning of 'clinical cholestasis'. It certainly ignores the criteria which have been used to define clinical and biochemical cholestasis in the past.

Undue emphasis on the results of biochemical tests, particularly alkaline phosphatase, is a common cause of diagnostic error (see Chapter 5.8). Indeed many clinicians appear to accept an increase in alkaline phosphatase alone as an indication of cholestasis, ignoring the possibility that it may be due to an increase in bone, intestinal, or placental phosphatase.

The physiologists' definition

Some have suggested that the best definition of 'cholestasis' is 'that of the physiologist who requires only that bile flow be decreased', [7] others that it is a reduction of bile salt output into the bile (and into the intestine). The possibility that clinical cholestasis might simply be related to problems of the secretion of bile and bile acids has undoubtedly been a stimulus to work in this area, and we now have a much greater understanding of events taking place in and around the canalicular membrane. However, reduction of bile flow and bile acid secretion do not equate with cholestasis. Both fall with external biliary diversion, clinical or experimental, which reduces serum bile acid levels. Few would consider this a form of cholestasis. Javitt (AmJMed, 51; 637:1971) pointed out that in the cholestatic syndrome the reduction in bile flow is also related to an elevation in serum bile acid levels. The retention of biliary substances was a key component of early ideas about cholestasis; if in experimental situations serum bile acids were not elevated it would have little meaning or relevance, certainly for clinicians, to consider that 'cholestasis' was present.

Unfortunately, bilirubin, bile acids, alkaline phosphatase, and free cholesterol and lecithin may accumulate in diseases of the liver which are not usually considered cholestatic; the mechanisms are complex, but it is hardly surprising that liver cell damage results in the retention of bilirubin and bile acids, even in the absence of a basic defect of bile acid excretion. Occasionally, the traditional clinical features of cholestasis may be present in these conditions, and the biochemical changes in serum liver tests may mimic those of extrahepatic obstruction. The reasons for the variation in the clinical picture are not understood; the task of the physiologist should be to explain these differences. One step in this process has come from the discovery of mice with a defect in the *mdr2* gene, which codes for a protein that transfers lecithin, and possibly other phospholipids, into bile across the canalicular membrane (Smit, Cell, 75; 451:1993).

In homozygous *mdr2* knockout mice (−/−) there is a striking reduction in the biliary output of phospholipid and cholesterol. There is no defect in bile salt excretion, and they have a high bile flow. They show damage to the biliary epithelium which is thought to be due to the toxicity of bile salts in the absence of the protective effect of phospholipids. They become jaundiced and have a high serum alkaline phosphatase. On electron microscopy their canaliculi remain wide, smooth, and tortuous, and they develop ductular proliferation, portal expansion, and inflammation with a mixed infiltrate on light microscopy (Mauad, AmJPathol, 145; 1237:1994). Presumably, physiologists would not consider these animals to be suffering from cholestasis. However, it is now thought that defective expression of the *MDR3* gene may explain some types of progressive familial intrahepatic cholestasis (Deleuze, Hepatol, 1996; 23:904).

Is there a place for the term 'cholestasis'

It may be asked whether the introduction of the word cholestasis has been helpful, and whether any real benefit will result from its continued use. Used in accordance with its dictionary definitions, it is certainly a useful shorthand to describe 'stoppage or arrest of the flow of bile' based on obstruction to the biliary tree. It might be better to use it to mean 'impairment of the flow of bile through the biliary tree as a result of obstruction (complete or incomplete) at any level from the extrahepatic bile ducts to the biliary canaliculi'.

As obstruction to the flow of bile also causes characteristic histological changes, on light and electron microscopy, it would also be useful to retain the term 'histological cholestasis' to mean 'the morphological changes seen in the liver, on light or electron microscopy, which result from impairment of bile flow as a result of obstruction to the biliary tree at any level'.

Because there is considerable variation in the clinical and biochemical consequences of biliary obstruction, even when there is a confirmed narrowing of the extrahepatic ducts, there seems little point in retaining the terms 'clinical' and 'biochemical' cholestasis. The task for the clinician is to explain the cause of the clinical symptoms and signs and abnormal test results which suggest the presence of liver or biliary tract disease. This task is not made easier

Table 3 Classification of hepatobiliary diseases
Unconjugated hyperbilirubinaemia
Large bile duct disease (identifiable by imaging)
Diffuse parenchymal liver disease
Space-occupying lesions and infiltrations
Disorders of the hepatic circulation (physiological)

by using a classification which pre-empts the diagnostic process, but rather by using one (which is collectively exhaustive, mutually exclusive, and useful) which reminds the clinician of the wide range of diagnostic possibilities. Such a classification (of liver disease, not of jaundice to which it is also applicable) is presented in Table 3 (see also Chapter 5.8.

The physiological 'definitions' of cholestasis seem to serve little purpose. 'Alteration of secretion of bile-salt containing micelles', 'decrease in bile flow', and 'diminution of the volume of that fraction of bile that is dependent on bile acids' seem to have been adopted as definitions because they were potential mechanisms to explain the basis of 'histological cholestasis'. The suggestion that they were primary mechanisms completely ignored the fact that 'histological cholestasis' results from extrahepatic biliary obstruction, and that obstruction to bile flow is a major factor in the pathogenesis of many disorders causing what we now call 'intrahepatic cholestasis'. The term 'intrahepatic cholestasis(es)' seems to be of value only if it is used to mean 'a condition(s) in which there are histological, and usually clinical and biochemical, features of biliary obstruction in the absence of obstruction to the extrahepatic ducts'. Intrahepatic disorders involving biliary obstruction at any level would be included. What is required from physiologists is the clear and rigorous demonstration that the above definition of 'intrahepatic cholestasis' is met by conditions in which there is no form of obstruction to the biliary tree, including a reduction in the radius of the smaller biliary radicles.

References

1. Roessle R. Entzeundungen der Leber. In Henke F and Lubarsch O, eds. *Handsbuch der speziellen Pathologischen Anatomie und Histologie*. Berlin: Springer-Verlag, 1930: Vol. 5, Part 1, pp. 434–52.
2. Popper H and Schaffner F. Laboratory diagnosis of liver disease: coordinated use of histological and biochemical observations. *Journal of the American Medical Association*, 1952; **150**: 1367–72.
3. Sherlock S. *Diseases of the liver and biliary system*. 1st edn, 1955; 2nd edn, 1958; 3rd edn, 1963; 10th edn (with Dooley JS), 1997. Oxford: Blackwell.
4. Schaffner F and Popper H. Cholestasis is the result of hypoactive hypertrophic smooth endoplasmic reticulum in the hepatocyte. *Lancet*, 1969; ii: 355–9.
5. Popper H and Schaffner F. Pathophysiology of cholestasis. *Human Pathology*, 1970; 1: 1–24.
6. Landmann L, Rahner C, and Steiger B. Morphological aspects of cholestasis. In Gentilini P, Arias IM, McIntyre N, and Rodes J, eds. *Cholestasis*. Amsterdam: Excerpta Medica, 1994.
7. Reichen J and Simon FR. Cholestasis. In Arias IM, Boyer JL, Fausto N, Jakoby WB, Schacter DA, and Shafritz DA, eds. *The liver: biology and pathobiology*. New York: Raven Press, 1994.
8. Magee B. *Popper*. London: Fontana/Collins, 1973.

9. Arias IM. Cholestasis: reflections backwards and forwards. In Gerok W, Loginov AS, and Pokrowskij VI, eds. *New trends in hepatology 1996.* Dordrecht: Kluwer Academic Publishers, 1997.

10. Desmet VJ. Cholestasis: extrahepatic obstruction and secondary biliary cirrhosis. In MacSween RN, Anthony PP, and Scheuer PJ, eds. *Pathology of the liver.* 2nd edn. Edinburgh: Churchill Livingstone, 1987.

11. Ishak KG. Hepatic histopathology. In Schiff L and Schiff ER, eds. *Diseases of the liver.* 7th edn. Philadelphia: JB Lippincott Co, 1993.

12. International Hepatology Informatics Group. Cholestasis and biliary tract disorders. In Leevy CM, Sherlock S, Tygstrup N, and Zetterman R, eds. *Diseases of the liver and biliary tract: standardization of nomenclature, diagnostic criteria, and prognosis.* New York: Raven Press, 1994.

13. Kumar P and Clark M. *Clinical medicine.* 3rd edn. London: WB Saunders, 1994.

23.2 Extrahepatic biliary obstruction: systemic effects, diagnosis, management

James S. Dooley

Definition

This chapter describes the hepatic and extrahepatic consequences of obstructive jaundice as well as the work-up and general management of biliary obstruction. For present purposes, extrahepatic biliary obstruction is anatomical obstruction to the common bile duct, common hepatic duct, and major intrahepatic bile ducts. Causes include calculi, malignant and benign tumours, and benign strictures including primary sclerosing cholangitis.

My aim is to encourage all those involved in the care of patients with obstructive jaundice to use optimal management based on available experimental and clinical data, and to develop new approaches to reduce postoperative and postprocedural complications based on knowledge of the underlying abnormalities present.

Pathophysiology of obstructive jaundice

Obstruction to bile flow increases biliary pressure with dilatation of the biliary tree. There is regurgitation of bile into the circulation, and hepatocellular damage. The degree of rise in biliary pressure depends upon the secretory capacity of the hepatocytes and ductular cells, and the distensibility of the biliary tract. It is difficult to study directly.

Bile reflux

Some bile reaches the circulation via the lymphatics. In the rat, lymph flow from the liver increases after bile duct ligation and approaches the normal bile flow of 0.5 to 1.0 ml/h (Bloom, JPhysiol, 1978; 281:88). Paracellular flow is another potential route (Desmet, ProgLivDis 1982; 7:31). There is also passage of bile across the hepatocyte in intracellular vacuoles (Raper, Surgery, 1989; 105:352). Only a small rise in biliary pressure is necessary for regurgitation of bile into the circulation (Huang, ArchSurg, 1969; 98:629).

Hepatocellular damage

Bile duct obstruction results in numerous changes in hepatic structure and function. Collagen content is increased. Glycogen content is reduced. Mitochondrial changes include loss of cristae and internal structure. Rough endoplasmic reticulum is reduced (Muriel,

JHepatol 1994; 21:95). The mitochondrial concentration of antioxidants (glutathione, ubiquinones) decreases while products of lipid peroxidation increase, changes that correlate with mitochondrial electron transport chain dysfunction (Krahenbuhl, Hepatol, 1995; 22:607). Mitochondrial fatty acid oxidation is also disturbed (Krahenbuhl, Hepatol, 1994; 19:1272). Vesicle transport to the canaliculus is inhibited and the integrity of tight junctions impaired (Stieger, Hepatol, 1994; 20:201). Interestingly, neither the trafficking of newly synthesized albumin and transferrin from endoplasmic reticulum to basolateral membrane and serum, nor receptor mediated endocytosis at the basolateral membrane is affected (Stieger, Hepatol, 1994; 20:201).

The cause of the hepatocellular injury is likely to be multifactorial, and is not well understood. However, retained bile salts have detergent properties and are cytotoxic *in vitro*. The toxicity increases with increasing relative hydrophobicity. This depends on the number of hydroxyl groups, the addition of which makes bile salts more hydrophilic (less hydrophobic). Thus, in general, monohydroxy bile salts such as lithocholate are more toxic than dihydroxy bile salts such as chenodeoxycholate or deoxycholate, which in turn are more toxic than trihydroxy bile acids such as cholate (Palmer, ProgLivDis, 1982; 7:221). Experimentally, the hydroxylation capacity of the liver is decreased 3 days after bile duct obstruction which may result in higher levels of more toxic bile salts (Vitale, JHepatol, 1992; 14:151). Copper, normally excreted in bile, is retained in cholestasis. High copper levels in the liver in Wilson's disease are associated with mitochondrial lipid peroxidation (Sokol, Gastro, 1994; 107:1788); whether the same process can be incriminated in cholestasis has not been studied.

Whatever the mechanism(s), mitochondrial respiratory enzyme activity and ketogenesis are impaired and take several weeks to recover after relief of obstruction (Koyama, AmJSurg, 1981; 142: 293). Antipyrine elimination is also impaired. Antipyrine, a minor analgesic, depends almost entirely on oxidation in the liver for its elimination which thus gives an indication of hepatic damage; in patients with obstructive jaundice its half-life is considerably prolonged compared with control patients (28.4 compared with 10.4 h) (McPherson, Gut, 1982; 23:734), and postoperative mortality is greater in those patients with an antipyrine half-life of greater than 20 h. The half-life improves with percutaneous biliary drainage. The hepatic mitochondrial response to oral glucose (redox tolerance test) is impaired in patients with obstructive jaundice and relates to survival (Tsubono, AmJSurg, 1995; 169:300).

Hepatic transport processes appear to remain intact. After relief of bile duct obstruction, bile acid transport into bile begins virtually immediately and the serum non-sulphated bile acid concentration falls rapidly to normal (Dooley, ClinSci, 1984; 67:61). Bilirubin excretion has a lower T_{max} and it is uncertain whether transport is impaired. In general, after relief of obstruction, serum bilirubin concentrations fall with a half-life of approximately 7 days (Little, AustNZJSurg, 1986; 56:35). Persistent hyperbilirubinaemia is seen when there is cholangitis, partial obstruction to drainage, or when there are hepatic metastases.

During prolonged obstruction serum albumin falls even in the absence of sepsis. Experimentally, this relates initially to increased capillary permeability and the lack of a compensatory increase in albumin synthesis; later there is an increased plasma volume and decreased albumin synthesis (Krahenbuhl, JHepatol, 1995; 23:79). The prothrombin time lengthens but this is due primarily to malabsorption of vitamin K, correcting rapidly after parenteral administration of vitamin K.

Systemic effects
General

The clinically apparent systemic effects of extrahepatic biliary obstruction are fatigue, jaundice, and itching. Cardiovascular effects are usually subclinical but become important after surgical and non-surgical intervention. Clinical risks include renal failure, sepsis, delayed wound healing, and gastrointestinal bleeding. The cause of these is likely to be multifactorial. Bilirubin, bile acids, lipids, and endotoxin have been implicated. Cytokines, prostaglandins, and nitric oxide may play a role. Plasma membrane and receptor characteristics are altered.

Bilirubin can be toxic to tissues. The kernicterus of the newborn, resulting from unconjugated hyperbilirubinaemia, is well known. High concentrations of unconjugated bilirubin have been shown to uncouple oxidative phosphorylation by brain mitochondria (Zetterstrom, Nature, 1956; 178:1335). Bilirubin also inhibits NADH reduction in mammalian cell cultures (Cowger, FedProc, 1964; 23:223A). However, whether such toxic effects have any relevance in the conjugated hyperbilirubinaemia of cholestasis is unknown.

Bile acids are detergents and in excess would be expected to interfere with lipid membranes. They inhibit ATPase activity and oxygen uptake in in vitro studies of rat jejunum (Parkinson, LifeSci, 1964; 3:107) and cause disruption of lysosomal membranes (Weissman, BiochemPharm, 1965; 14:525). Bile acids also increase intracellular ionized calcium in renal cell cultures (Montrose, PfleugersArchPhysiol, 1988; 412:164), and have a negative inotropic effect on isolated ventricular myocytes (Binah, ArchPharmacol, 1987; 335:160). At high concentrations they alter cell-mediated immune mechanisms.

Plasma free cholesterol, phospholipids, and triglycerides are elevated in obstructive jaundice and there are changes in lipoproteins and particles which depend in part on whether lecithin cholesterol acyltransferase (**LCAT**) activity falls (Chapter 2.12).[1] A change in cell membrane composition follows (Owen, JLipRes,

1982; 23:124) and there are changes in membrane fluidity and function (Owen, Drugs, 1990; 40(Suppl.3):73). There is inhibition of frusemide-sensitive sodium transport (Jackson, ClinSci, 1982; 62:101) and receptor-mediated uptake of ligands may also be altered (North, JBC, 1983; 258:1242).

Systemic endotoxaemia occurs in some patients with obstructive jaundice and experimentally has many effects (see below), such as those on kidney function and coagulation.

Fatigue

This is a common complaint in those with prolonged cholestasis, as well as with chronic hepatocellular disease. The mechanism is not well understood but a central neurotransmitter alteration seems likely (Jones, Hepatol, 1995; 22:1606). In experimental cholestasis, behavioural changes, which may be an equivalent to clinical fatigue, have been found in association with impaired corticotrophin-releasing hormone responses (Swain, Hepatol, 1995; 22:1560).

Itching

This may be the predominant symptom in obstructive jaundice. It disappears within a few days of biliary decompression. In the past, bile salts were suggested as the cause of itching but most of the evidence was circumstantial. Although cholestyramine relieves itching in patients with cholestasis, it binds many compounds other than bile salts and also relieves the itching of uraemia (Silverberg, BMJ, 1977; i:752) in which bile salts are not implicated. These data together with studies of the bile salt concentration and pattern in blister fluid (Bartholomew, ClinSci, 1982; 63:65) suggest that bile salts are not the cause of itching in cholestasis.

The focus has moved towards agents that may produce itching by a central neurotransmitter mechanism (Jones, Gut, 1996; 38: 644). Animal studies and therapeutic trials suggest that an endogenous opioid peptide may be responsible (Bergasa, Gastro, 1995; 108:1582). In experimental cholestasis, endogenous opioids accumulate and the animals are in a state of analgesia, reversible by naloxone. The perception of itching in cholestatic patients is less during naloxone treatment (Bergasa, AnnIntMed, 1995; 123:161). Serotonin may also have a central role. Ondansetron, a 5-hydroxytryptamine type 3 receptor antagonist, also ameliorates itching in cholestatic patients (Schworer, Pain, 1995; 61:33). These data hold promise for effective alternative therapies for patients with severe itching resistant to cholestyramine.

Cardiovascular effects[2] (Chapter 25.1)

The peripheral vascular resistance is reduced in both humans and animals with obstructive jaundice (Shasha, ClinSci, 1976; 50:533). Blood pressure is usually normal, but there is an exaggerated hypotensive response to volume depletion. The capacity for vasoconstriction is impaired as shown by the greater fall in blood pressure after venesection in jaundiced dogs compared with normal control animals (Williams, ArchSurg, 1960; 81:334). There is also a reduced responsiveness of skeletal muscle vasculature to noradrenaline in vitro (Bomzon, ClinSci, 1978; 55:109). This is associated with an enhanced pressor response in renal and cerebral vessels. There is evidence for a functional defect in the expression of α_1-adrenoreceptors (Jacob, AmJPhysiol, 1993; 265:G579). The mechanism of these changes, and whether nitric oxide is involved, is unknown. Data suggest a role for nitric oxide in the hyperdynamic circulation of cirrhosis (Vallance, Lancet, 1991; 337:776; Claria, Hepatol, 1992; 15:343).

Cardiac changes include bradycardia, an increase in PR–QT interval on electrocardiography, and the depletion of myocardial cell glycogen (Tajuddin, AdvMyocardiol, 1980; 2:209). At the cellular level there is mitochondrial swelling and a decrease in glycogen content in rat atria exposed to bile acids. Bile acids have a negative chronotropic effect at concentrations found in human serum in bile duct obstruction. They also have a concentration-dependent negative inotropic action on rat papillary muscle and isolated ventricular myocytes (Binah, ArchPharmacol, 1987; 335: 160).

Although reports on the changes in cardiac output in obstructive jaundice are conflicting, data suggest that there is a jaundice-induced cardiac myopathy. Thus there is a depressed response to isoproterenol in dogs after ligation of the common bile duct (Binah, ClinSci, 1985; 69:647). Left ventricular function is impaired (Green, Surgery, 1986; 100:14). Susceptibility to hypotension in obstructive jaundice has been attributed to a blunting of the myocardial contractile response to sympathomimetic stimulation.

These changes in both cardiac function and peripheral vascular resistance provide the basis for prerenal renal failure under hypovolaemic conditions in patients with obstructive jaundice.

Renal changes[2,3,4]

Renal failure (acute tubular necrosis) is the classic complication of obstructive jaundice after surgery or an invasive procedure.[4] Approximately 60 to 75 per cent of such patients have a fall in glomerular filtration rate after surgery. The overall incidence of acute renal failure is 8 per cent.

The mechanism is multifactorial. The changes in cardiovascular responses described above—reduced peripheral vasoconstriction under hypovolaemic circumstances with increased renal vasoconstriction, even in the apparently healthy patient or animal—will play a part. Other possible contributing factors are bile acids, bilirubin, and endotoxin.

Overall, the data on glomerular filtration rate and renal blood flow in obstructive jaundice are conflicting.[2] However, there is a shift in renal blood flow away from the outer cortex to the deep cortex and medulla. This may be related to the exaggerated response of the renal vasculature to α-adrenergic stimulation. The glomerular filtration rate is preserved, perhaps due to cholestatic effect on the efferent arteriole, or a compensatory vasodilation mediated by prostaglandins. Prostaglandins E_2 and I_2 are increased in obstructive jaundice (Zambraski, JLabClinMed, 1984; 103:549). Their involvement in renal function in liver disease is shown by the effect of indomethacin, which reduces renal blood flow and glomerular filtration rate (Levy, AmJPhysiol, 1983; 245:F521). Additionally, there is enhanced synthesis of renal glomerular thromboxane A_2, which suppresses glomerular filtration rate and predisposes to renal failure (Kramer, ClinSci, 1995; 88:39). Treatment with a receptor antagonist restores glomerular filtration rate to normal.

Bile components, bile acids, and conjugated bilirubin, seem to potentiate ischaemic injury, rather than being directly toxic themselves (Dawson, BMJ, 1964; 1:810; Dawson, ArchPathol, 1964;

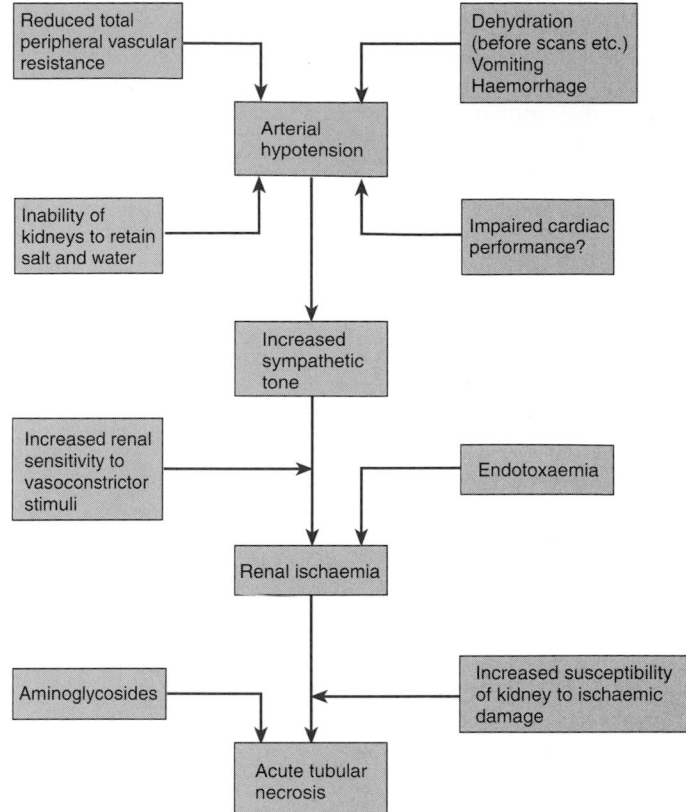

Fig. 1. Pathogenesis of renal failure in obstructive jaundice.

78:254; Baum, BMJ, 1969; ii:229). Thus infusion of bile acids into the renal artery does not affect total renal or renal cortical blood flow (Bomzon, IsraelJMedSci, 1979; 15:169). High concentrations of conjugated bilirubin (Baum, BMJ, 1969; ii:229) and bile acids (Aoyagi, JLabClinMed, 1968; 71:686) increase the susceptibility of renal tissue to ischaemic damage. Moreover, histological changes are seen in the kidney during obstructive jaundice. There are pigmented granules in the glomeruli and changes in the epithelial and endothelial cells and the basement membrane (Allison, ClinSci, 1978; 54:649). These changes may reduce glomerular filtration rate. Finally, there are data to suggest that hypercholesterolaemia (Bloom, BrJPharmacol, 1975; 54:421) and endotoxaemia (see section below) may be involved.

Whatever the mechanism, the combination of an impaired systemic vasoconstrictor response to hypotension and an increased renal vascular response to adrenergic stimuli favours the development of renal hypoperfusion when there is dehydration or haemorrhage (Fig. 1). Interestingly, there is evidence for renal tubular cell damage, based on greatly increased urinary N-acetylglucosaminidase excretion in patients with obstructive jaundice before any intervention, despite normal blood urea and creatinine levels (Dooley, Hepatol, 1983; 3:853A).

Apart from the effects of obstructive jaundice on cardiac and renovascular responses, and direct effects of biliary components amd endotoxin on the kidney, there are also changes in total body water, sodium, and potassium. Bile acids reduce sodium absorption from the proximal tubule (Topuzlu, NEJM, 1966; 274:760) and increase urine flow, fractional sodium excretion, and potassium excretion (Alon, ClinSci, 1982; 62:431; Finestone, CanJPhysPharm, 1984; 62:762), without changing inulin or *p*-aminohippurate (PAH) clearance. In microperfusion studies, bile acid reduced fluid absorption (Better, ClinSci, 1987; 72:139). The mechanism may be a non-specific detergent effect of bile acids, or it may depend upon changes in cyclo-oxygenase (prostaglandin E_2) (Alon, MinElecMetab, 1988; 14:338). Indomethacin abolishes the natriuresis. Other data have shown that sulphated bile acids (elevated in cholestasis) impair Na^+/H^+ antiporter function (Sellinger, AmJPhysiol, 1990; 258:F986).

These findings provide the basis for changes in experimental models. Body water compartments change following ligation of the common bile duct (Martinez-Rodenas, BrJSurg, 1989; 76:461). There is a significant decrease in water intake (60 per cent), creatinine clearance, total body water (15 per cent), extracellular water (24 per cent), and plasma volume (15 per cent), which persists for at least 12 days following duct ligation. In patients with cholangiocarcinoma and jaundice, urinary sodium excretion increases (Sitprija, KidneyInt, 1990; 38:948) and there is an inability to retain sodium. These changes will increase the risk of hypotension and renal failure associated with obstructive jaundice, and are the opposite of those seen with chronic hepatocellular disease and cirrhosis.

An additional iatrogenic factor which is potentially nephrotoxic is the use of aminoglycosides. A prospective study of renal failure in patients with obstructive jaundice found that 32 per cent of patients treated with gentamicin developed nephrotoxicity compared with 11 per cent in those treated with other antibiotics or no antibiotic (Lucena, JHepatol, 1995; 22:189). The most significant predictor for gentamicin toxicity was serum bilirubin level. Although a control trial of antibiotic treatment of acute cholangitis with and without tobramycin did not show increased renal damage in those treated with the aminoglycoside (Thompson, SGO, 1990; 171:275), the renal toxicity of gentamicin is increased in experimental studies of obstructive jaundice (Vakil, Hepatol, 1989; 9:519).

Endotoxaemia

In some patients with obstructive jaundice, endotoxaemia is present before surgery. This correlates with reduced pre- and postoperative creatinine clearance (Thompson, AmJSurg, 1988; 155:314). Postoperative systemic endotoxaemia can be detected in 50 per cent or more of patients with jaundice[4] and relates to outcome (Ingoldby, AmJSurg, 1984; 147:776). In these patients endotoxaemia is caused by increased intestinal absorption of endotoxin together with reduced clearance by reticuloendothelial cells, particularly in the liver.

In obstructive jaundice there is an increased passage of bacteria across the intestinal mucosa (Clements, AmJSurg, 1993; 165:749). There is also increased intestinal absorption of endotoxin, probably because of the decrease in luminal bile salts (Kocsar, JBacteriol, 1969; 100:220). Oral administration of bile salt reduces endotoxaemia in animal studies (Van Bossuyt, JHepatol, 1990; 10:274) and prevents renal dysfunction in patients with obstructive jaundice (Cahill, BrJSurg, 1983; 70:590).

Biliary micro-organisms are another source of systemic endotoxin. During percutaneous manipulation of the obstructed biliary tree, both the presence of infected bile and the serum bilirubin concentration before the procedure predict the development of endotoxaemia (Lumsden, AmJSurg, 1989; 158:21).

Clearance of endotoxin from the circulation depends upon the liver (Kupffer cells) and the reticuloendothelial system elsewhere (Drivas, BMJ, 1976; 1:1568). In both obstructive jaundice and liver disease *per se*, Kupffer cell clearance capacity is impaired (Clements, ArchSurg, 1993; 128:200). The important role of the liver in removing endotoxin is shown by the greater degree of endotoxaemia in patients with cirrhosis undergoing a portal systemic shunt than in patients with jaundice having surgery to relieve obstruction (Lumsden, Hepatol, 1988; 8:232).

Circulating endotoxin has many effects. Interaction with macrophages produces reactive oxygen molecules, bioactive lipids, and cytokines (e.g. interleukins 1 and 6, and tumour necrosis factor). Endotoxin stimulates the production of vasoactive compounds including prostaglandins, thromboxanes, leukotrienes, and platelet activation factor. Systemic effects include fever, metabolic acidosis, disseminated intravascular coagulation, haemodynamic instability, reduced cellular immunity (Greve, Gastro, 1990; 98:478), renal failure, and gastrointestinal haemorrhage. Excretion of bilirubin and taurocholate into bile is decreased by endotoxin (Roelofsen, Gastro, 1994; 107:1075).

Opinions vary as to the importance of endotoxin in the pathogenesis of renal failure in obstructive jaundice (Fogarty, BrJSurg, 1995; 82:877).[2] Administration of polymyxin B, a non-absorbable antibiotic active against endotoxin-producing bacteria, did not produce clinical benefit (Ingoldby, AmJSurg, 1984; 147:766). On the other hand, experimental infusion of endotoxin into the renal artery reduced renal blood flow (Cavanough, AmJObsGyn, 1970; 108:705) and glomerular filtration rate in animal studies. Electron microscopy shows abnormalities including endothelial swelling (Kikeri, AmJPhysiol, 1986; 250:F1098), and endotoxin can cause intracapillary thrombosis (Colucci, JCI, 1985; 75:818). Endotoxin appears to have a role that is difficult to define exactly because of the many other confounding changes.

Gastrointestinal changes

Haemorrhagic gastritis occurs in approximately 7 per cent of patients and is fatal in half (Dixon, Gut, 1983; 24:845; Dixon, AnnSurg, 1984; 199:271). The mechanism is not clear, but the role of noradrenaline and prostaglandin E_2 and the reduced mucosal blood flow have been studied in rat gastric mucosa (Urakawa, ScaJGastr, 1987; 22:634). Stress produced greater falls in gastric wall blood flow and in mucosal noradrenaline and prostaglandin E_2 content in animals with obstructive jaundice. In addition the degree of gastric damage (erosions predominantly) was greater. Administration of oral prostaglandin E_2 prevented the fall in mucosal blood flow after stress.

There are pancreatic changes in rats after 1 day of bile duct ligation, including an increase in volume, weight, protein content, and amylase (both basal and post-secretin stimulation) (Yoshida, BrJExpPath, 1988; 69:441). Bicarbonate secretion does not change. Microscopically there is an increase in acinar cell number, size, and number of zymogen granules, with dilatation of cisternae in the Golgi apparatus. The authors postulated that hyperbilirubinaemia and inhibition of normal mitochondrial function might inhibit granule discharge from the acinar cell.

Nutrition

Experimentally, there is anorexia, weight loss, and decreased nitrogen balance initially (Gouma, AmJClinNut, 1986; 44:362). Later, the appetite returns and nitrogen balance becomes normal. Hypoalbuminaemia in obstructive jaundice is related to decreased hepatic synthesis and increased capillary permeability. It correlates poorly with other changes in nutritional status such as weight loss and nitrogen balance. The plasma amino acid pattern in obstructive jaundice is essentially unchanged from normal. There are mild increases in levels of methionine, phenylalanine, aspartic acid, and glutamine, but these are minimal compared with the major increases seen in acute hepatitis (Freund, AmJSurg, 1980; 139:142). Total hepatic amino acid uptake is unaltered in experimental bile duct obstruction, but peripheral uptake by skeletal muscle is decreased (Starnes, JSurgRes, 1987; 42:383). Muscle protein is reduced.

Wound healing

Wound healing after surgery for obstructive jaundice is impaired (Ellis, BrJSurg, 1977; 64:733; Irvin, BrJSurg, 1978; 65:521; Armstrong, BrJSurg, 1984; 71:267). Some studies designed to test wound strength in jaundiced animals have demonstrated wound weakness (Bayer, BrJSurg, 1976; 63:392; Arnaud, AmJSurg, 1981; 141:593). Other studies did not confirm this (Greaney, BrJSurg, 1979; 66:478; Than Than, BrJExpPath, 1979; 60:107), but there are data showing that neovascularity (Bayer, BrJSurg, 1976; 63:392), polyhydroxylase activity (Than Than, PhD Thesis, University of Glasgow, 1976), and collagen production (Greaney, BrJSurg, 1979; 66:478) are all reduced in experimental wounds in the presence of obstructive jaundice. Moreover, fibroblast proliferation in tissue culture is reduced when bilirubin is added (Ellis, BrJSurg, 1977; 64:733).

The data available strongly suggest that in the presence of obstructive jaundice there is impaired wound healing. Analysis of various features in clinical studies have implicated poor nutritional status and malignancy rather than simply hyperbilirubinaemia *per se* in the pathogenesis of this problem (Armstrong, BrJSurg, 1984; 71:267).

Lipid metabolism[1] (Chapter 2.12)

The absence of bile acids in the intestinal lumen impairs the absorption of fat because of the lack of micelle formation. In addition, plasma free cholesterol, phospholipids, and triglycerides increase, and there are changes in lipoproteins.[1] Low-density lipoprotein has an abnormal composition and, if plasma LCAT activity is low, lipoprotein X appears. Very low-density lipoprotein has an altered lipid content and lipoprotein pattern. Changes in high-density lipoprotein are controversial but the normal pattern changes, especially in patients with a high serum bilirubin (Clifton, JLipRes, 1988; 29:121). The reason for the changes in plasma lipids is complex (Chapter 2.12). Four factors at least have been implicated including regurgitation of biliary cholesterol into the circulation, increased hepatic synthesis of cholesterol, reduced plasma LCAT activity, and finally, regurgitation of biliary lecithin, which produces a shift of cholesterol from pre-existing tissue cholesterol into the plasma. As a result of the changes in lipoprotein particle composition seen in chronic liver disease, there are rapid alterations in membrane

composition (Owen, JCI, 1985; 76:2275; Owen, Drugs, 1990; 40(Suppl3):73) which are likely to affect receptor function (Heron, ProcNatlAcadSciUSA, 1980; 77:7463; North, JBC, 1983; 258:1242). Similar changes in membrane function would be expected to occur in obstructive jaundice, but await study.

Bone disease[5]

In short-term obstructive jaundice, bone disease is not a clinical problem and has not been studied. With prolonged cholestasis, bone disease—so-called hepatic osteodystrophy—occurs as it does in chronic hepatocellular disease (see Chapter 25.10).

In prolonged cholestasis, bone pain and fractures occur. Although malabsorption of vitamin D will occur, depending on the degree of steatorrhoea, and osteomalacia is therefore a risk, the bone disease that occurs more frequently in patients with primary biliary cirrhosis and primary sclerosing cholangitis is osteoporosis. Bone mineral density is reduced in patients with advanced primary sclerosing cholangitis, particularly with a raised bilirubin (Hay, Hepatol, 1991; 14:257). The pathogenesis is complex. It has been suggested that reduced bone formation occurs in patients with precirrhosis, and increased resorption in those with advanced disease (Hay, Gastro, 1995; 108:276). Immobility, poor nutrition, and a reduced muscle mass probably play a role, as well as changes in vitamin D, calcitonin, parathyroid hormone, growth hormone, and sex steroids. Plasma from patients with jaundice inhibits osteoblast proliferation (Janes, JCI, 1995; 95:2581). Unconjugated bilirubin, but not bile salts, has an inhibitory effect.

Improvement in bone density is delayed for 1 to 5 years after liver transplantation for chronic cholestatic liver disease (Argao, Hepatol, 1994; 20:598). Spontaneous bone fractures are common before recovery (Eastell, Hepatol, 1991; 14:296). The delay in improvement is probably due to corticosteroids used for immunosuppression.

Resistance to infection[6]

Infection frequently causes morbidity and mortality after surgery for obstructive jaundice (Feduska, ArchSurg, 1971; 103:330). Postoperative septic complications are related not only to biliary bacteria but also defective host defence mechanisms. After 2 weeks of biliary obstruction, there is a decreased phagocytic capacity which correlates inversely with bilirubin levels (but not aminotransferase or bile salt concentration) (Pain, BrJSurg, 1987; 74:1091) and endotoxin and anticore glycolipid concentration (Clements, ArchSurg, 1993; 128:200). Changes in plasma membranes, in particular the phospholipid fatty acid profile (Scriven, Gut, 1994; 35:987), may affect cell function.

Experimentally administered bacteria are cleared slowly (Ding, BrJSurg, 1992; 79:648; Scott-Conner, AmJSurg, 1989; 157:210). This appears to be the result of reduced Kupffer cell function, as the number of Kupffer cells increases (St John Collier, JPath, 1986; 150:187). Other cellular responses, such as phagocytosis and cytokine production by extrahepatic phagocytes and polymorphonuclear cells, are impaired (Roughneen, AnnSurg, 1987; 206:578; Greve, Gastro, 1990; 98:478). Neutrophil adhesion is also impaired (Swain, Gastro, 1995; 109:923). Although some functions of polymorphonuclear cells are enhanced (Levy, Hepatol, 1993; 17:908), this is probably due to a proinflammatory state related to cytokines and/or endotoxaemia. The function of Kupffer cells is restored by a short period of internal bile drainage (Clements, Gut, 1996; 38:925).

Specific cell-mediated (T cell) immunity is impaired (Roughneen, JSurgRes, 1986; 41:113; Feduccia, AmJMedSci, 1988; 296:39) and is related to the duration of jaundice. There is prolonged allograft survival in hosts with obstructive jaundice (Beaudoin, Transpl, 1969; 7:576). B-cell function does not seem to be impaired (Roughneen, Transpl, 1986; 42:687). Studies suggest that impaired cellular immunity is related to endotoxin (Greve, Gastro, 1990; 98: 478) as well as other factors (Thompson, WorldJSurg, 1993; 17: 783), although endoscopic biliary drainage did not reverse T-lymphocyte dysfunction in a group of patients with malignant biliary obstruction (Fan, JGastroHepatol, 1994; 9:391).

Unconjugated bilirubin impairs many aspects of the host anti-bacterial defence mechanisms *in vitro*, for example phagocytosis (Thong, AustPaedJ, 1977; 13:287), movement of neutrophils in response to chemotactic agents (Thong, IRCSJMedSci, 1977; 5: 483), and lymphocyte responses to mitogens (Rola-Pieszcynski, JPediat, 1975; 86:690).

Anergy is well documented in jaundiced patients with biliary obstruction, but there is no difference between malignant and benign obstruction (Cainzos, BrJSurg, 1988; 75:147). A greater incidence of postoperative septic complications was found in the patients with anergy.

Circulating tumour necrosis factor (**TNF**) is increased in animal models of bile duct obstruction (Bemelmans, Hepatol, 1992; 15: 1132) and can be detected in patients with jaundice.[6] However, it is immunoreactive rather than biologically active, because of the presence of soluble TNF receptors (**TNFr**) which are shed or released from the cell membrane. TNFr are thought to play a role in the regulation of the effects of TNF and correlate with postoperative mortality (Bemelmans, Gut, 1996; 38:447). Experimental administration of TNF-α reduces bile flow and basal bile salt excretion (Whiting, Hepatol, 19; 22:1273). Interleukin 6 (Bemelmans, Hepatol, 1992; 15:1132) and intrahepatic platelet-activating factor (Zhou, AmJPhysiol, 1992; 263:G587) are increased in the presence of bile duct obstruction.

Finally, many studies have shown increased translocation of viable enteric bacteria across the mucosal barrier to lymph nodes and other tissues in obstructive jaundice (Deitch, AmJSurg, 1990; 159:79; Ding, JSurgRes, 1994; 57:238). This is related to lack of intraluminal bile (Slocum, AmSurg, 1992; 58:305) and endo-toxaemia (Deitch, JCI, 1989; 84:36; Deitch, Surgery, 1989; 106: 292). It may be inhibited by activating mucosal macrophages with liposomal muramyl tripeptide phosphatidylethanolamine (Ding, JHepatol, 1994; 20:720). The clinical significance of bacterial trans-location is uncertain. However, the absence of bile from the intestine is associated with a reduced mucous blanket over duodenal cells and an increase in coliform micro-organisms (Kalambaheti, Gut, 1994; 35:1047).

Coagulation

Although administration of vitamin K rapidly corrects the pro-longed prothrombin time in patients with obstructive jaundice, blood coagulation does not necessarily then return to normal. Bleeding sometimes still appears greater than expected at surgery,

though the cause is not established. Data have shown that there is a low-grade disseminated intravascular coagulation (**DIC**) in some patients (Hunt, AmJSurg, 1982; 144:325), and serum fibrin de-gradation products are often increased. Procoagulant production by mononuclear phagocytes is enhanced (Semeraro, Gastro, 1989; 96: 892), and fibrin degradation products may be increased in the serum. There is also inhibition of fibrinolysis (Jedrychowski, BMJ, 1973; i:640; Wardle, ArchSurg, 1974; 109:741) which, in com-bination with DIC, may result in fibrin thrombosis and subsequent tissue damage. It seems likely that DIC is caused by the presence of increased circulating levels of endotoxin and activated coagulation enzymes.

Platelet function may be impaired. *In vitro* platelet aggregation in response to adenosine diphosphate and collagen is decreased following bile duct ligation and this could be related to elevated bile acid concentrations or an as yet uncharacterized plasma inhibitor (Bowen, ThrombRes, 1988; 52:649).

Clinical features of biliary obstruction
History

Features in the presenting history cannot be taken as specific for a particular cause. Thus fever, jaundice, and right upper quadrant pain, although suggestive of cholangitis caused by a stone in the common duct, may occur with cholestatic hepatitis due to a drug (Nissan, ArchSurg, 1996; 131:670). In general, however, certain features linked with jaundice are associated with a particular cause.

Fever

Fever usually indicates choledocholithiasis. When common duct stones are present, bacteria are usually present in bile. Duct ob-struction raises biliary pressure, and infected bile enters the cir-culation with systemic signs of sepsis. Bile from patients with a malignant bile duct obstruction is usually sterile, so that fever in these cases is rare. This generalization is not true for patients who have had diagnostic or therapeutic cholangiography. Thus, in patients who have been treated with an endoscopic or surgical stent, bacteria adhere to the stent, bile is colonized, and stent blockage results in systemic sepsis ('cholangitis').

Pain

Pain should suggest calculous rather than malignant obstruction, the latter classically producing painless jaundice. However, there may be a preceding history of pain in some patients with carcinoma of the pancreas, bile duct, or ampulla.

Itching

Itching may occur with any cause of biliary obstruction, but tends to be more frequent with malignant obstruction or intrahepatic cholestasis. It is unusual for there to be itching in calculous ob-struction, perhaps because obstruction is rarely complete and may not be sufficiently prolonged to cause retention of the pruritic agent. Relief of obstruction is followed by loss of itching in a few days.

Weight loss

Weight loss occurs more often with malignant obstruction, although benign causes resulting in prolonged steatorrhoea will do the same.

Previous cholecystectomy

Previous cholecystectomy clearly arouses a suspicion of a retained common duct stone. If surgery is recent and followed by abnormal drainage of bile through the wound or drain, a traumatic bile duct stricture should be suspected.

Drugs

A complete list of previous medication is mandatory. Many drugs are capable of mimicking obstructive jaundice.

Ethnic origin

Any patient with jaundice and fever from the Far East may have recurrent pyogenic cholangitis.

Inflammatory bowel disease

A history of inflammatory bowel disease should raise the possibility of primary sclerosing cholangitis as a cause of jaundice and itching.

Previous malignancy

Previous malignancy, especially colonic, may indicate jaundice due to hepatic metastases, or bile duct obstruction from lymph node involvement.

Examination

Jaundice, scratch marks, and loss of body mass are clearly non-specific. Signs of chronic liver disease (spider naevi, palmar erythema) denote long-standing intrahepatic cholestasis (primary sclerosing cholangitis, primary biliary cirrhosis) rather than obstruction to the major bile ducts, although these signs may be seen in the now rare patient with secondary biliary cirrhosis.

The liver is usually palpable in patients with bile duct obstruction. This sign is again non-specific unless nodules are palpable due to tumour. Splenomegaly denotes hepatic rather than major bile duct disease, except in the case of splenic vein block due to carcinoma of the pancreas. A palpable gallbladder suggests malignant obstruction to the distal common bile duct (Courvoisier's law), but is only present in approximately half of such patients. A tender gallbladder (Murphy's sign) suggests cholecystitis.

Laboratory investigations

Full blood count, urea, electrolytes, serum creatinine, prothrombin time, and liver function tests should be done. There may be leucocytosis in cholangitis. It is essential to check the levels of urea, electrolytes, and serum creatinine. Impaired renal function is a complication of obstructive jaundice. Hyponatraemia and hypokalaemia are often found. The prothrombin time may be prolonged due to malabsorption of vitamin K. Liver tests characteristically show raised bilirubin (total and conjugated), alkaline phosphatase, and γ-glutamyl transpeptidase. When there is acute obstruction of the bile duct the levels of aspartate and alanine aminotransferases may be very high (Fortson, JClinGastro, 1985; 7:502), even reaching 50 times normal for a short time and causing confusion as to the cause of jaundice. There are changes in lipids, in particular lipoprotein X, but these are not of diagnostic value.

To assess liver function in more detail, tests such as galactose elimination are helpful, but are used at present only as research tools.

Liver function tests are not specific to any one diagnosis but are used in combination with clinical data (history and examination) to choose the next step in the diagnostic work-up. Imaging provides a further step along the route and in some cases the definitive diagnosis.

Imaging (Fig. 2) (Chapter 5.5)

The work-up for cholestatic jaundice uses non-invasive techniques first (ultrasonography or computed tomography (CT)).

Non-invasive techniques

These are to show whether the bile ducts are dilated thus differentiating between 'surgical' and 'medical' jaundice. Real-time ultrasonography is the technique of choice. Although static grey-scale ultrasound scanning may show the anatomy more clearly, real-time ultrasonography is more flexible and has practical advantages in very ill or uncooperative patients. Ultrasonography can demonstrate duct dilatation in 95 per cent of patients with bile duct obstruction (Taylor, ArchSurg, 1977; 112:820). In the small number of false-negative cases, either there is failure on the part of the radiologist or radiographer, or there is truly no duct dilatation, as may occur in calculous disease of the common duct. Ultrasonography and computed tomography show the level of obstruction in about two-thirds of patients, and can define the cause in only one-third (Baron, Radiol, 1982; 145:91). They should not therefore be used as diagnostic tests but as a guide to the next step in the work-up, that is, cholangiography or liver biopsy.

Ultrasonography or CT are not always necessary. If the clinical history is strongly suggestive of a common bile duct stone, endoscopic retrograde cholangiopancreatography (ERCP) is the next step as cholangiography is necessary whether or not ultrasonography shows bile duct pathology. Ultrasonography is still valuable, however, to show whether there are stones in the gallbladder. This may influence subsequent management.

The major application of radioisotopic imaging with an iminodiacetic acid derivative (IDA) as contrast is in the diagnosis of acute cholecystitis. It can differentiate between the obstructed and normal bile duct (O'Connor, Gastro, 1983; 84:1498), but ultrasonography is more appropriate. Biliary scintigraphy is valuable in demonstrating bile leaks after surgery such as cholecystectomy or liver transplantation, or after traumatic duct damage, for example with liver biopsy. Scintigraphy may not be able to differentiate partial bile duct obstruction from intrahepatic cholestasis in deeply jaundiced patients, although this is less of a problem with the third-generation agents such as bromotrimethyl or iododiethyl iminodiacetic acids.

When there is jaundice, intravenous cholangiography should not be performed. Even in the patient with normal liver function, visualization is inferior to that from direct cholangiography (Osnes, Lancet, 1978; ii:230) and tomography is needed for good definition of the anatomy.

Although cross-sectional magnetic resonance (MR) imaging adds little to ultrasonography or CT, MRI scans can be used to give two-

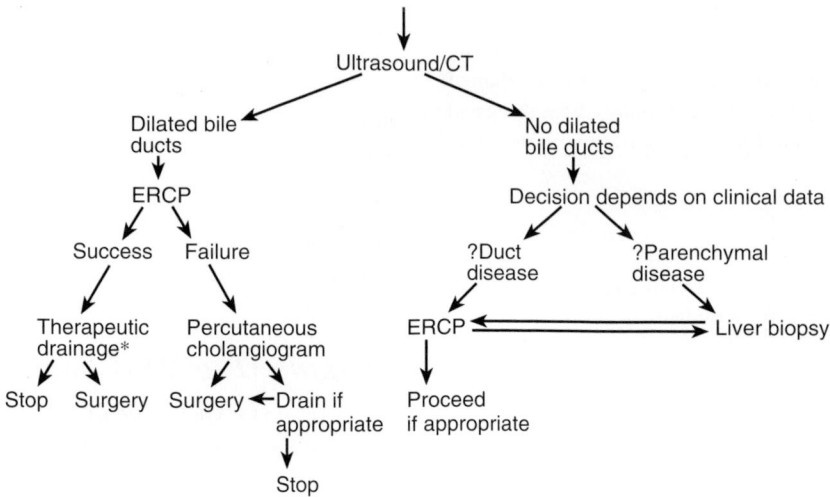

Fig. 2. Imaging in cholestatic jaundice.

or three-dimensional images of both biliary and pancreatic systems. Such MR cholangiopancreatography does not need any contrast material, biliary and pancreatic systems being visible because of the water content of bile and pancreatic juice. MR cholangiography is highly accurate in the diagnosis of bile duct obstruction and its cause (Guibaud, Radiol, 1995; 197:109; Soto, Gastro, 1996; 110: 589). Because of expense, this technique is likely to be restricted to complicated clinical problems. CT cholangiography by an equivalent reconstructive process is also possible (Van Beers, AJR, 1994; 162:1331) but, for best results, intravenous contrast material needs to be given, limiting the technique to patients with normal or near normal liver function.

Invasive techniques

Percutaneous transhepatic cholangiography (**PTC**) and ERCP provide direct cholangiography. PTC, the older procedure first described in the 1930s (Huard, BullSocMedChirIndochine, 1937; 62: 1090), was radically modified in the 1970s with the introduction of the fine gauge, Chiba or skinny needle, in Japan (Okuda, AmJDig-Dis, 1974; 19:21). This allowed bile ducts of any size to be punctured using a 22-, 23-, or even 25-gauge needle. Success rates approach 100 per cent and an accurate diagnosis can be made in 95 per cent of cases (Ferrucci, AJR, 1977; 129:11). The risk of bile leakage is reduced with the fine needle technique and the overall complication rate is less than 5 per cent (bleeding, peritonitis, and sepsis).

ERCP was first described in the early 1970s. The success rate is between 80 and 90 per cent depending on the experience of the endoscopist (Cotton, Gut, 1977; 18:316). Certain features make the procedure more difficult, including previous Billroth II gastrectomy, a periampullary diverticulum, papillary stenosis, or tumour. Complications occur in 2 to 3 per cent of examinations (sepsis, pancreatitis).

PTC and ERCP should be regarded as complementary. Both can be successful in demonstrating the biliary system in most patients. Unless certain factors make ERCP impossible or very difficult, this should be the approach chosen first. Both percutaneous and endoscopic techniques can be used to decompress the biliary

system when obstructed, but the endoscopic techniques carry a lower complication rate (Speer, Lancet, 1987; ii:57).

Thus, if dilated ducts are shown by ultrasonography or CT, the next step is to plan future management depending upon the clinical status of the patient (age, other medical diseases) and probable diagnosis. If the patient is under the care of physicians, liaison with surgeons is wise at this stage. Then ERCP is performed, the radiological diagnosis made, cytology performed, and drainage attempted. If ERCP fails, then the decision is made whether to repeat ERCP later (success is sometimes possible at a second session), or to refer for PTC, after appropriate discussion with the radiologist concerned. PTC should not be arranged in patients with obstructive jaundice without discussion of the plan of management with the radiologist, who will need to know whether bile duct catheterization and drainage is required.

If ultrasonography or CT do not show dilated bile ducts, the next procedure will depend upon the clinical picture. If a common duct stone or primary sclerosing cholangitis is suspected, then ERCP is done. If intrahepatic cholestasis is probable, for example a drug reaction, then liver biopsy is the next step. Some patients will need both procedures.

Management of the patient with obstructive jaundice
Fluid balance

The patient with obstruction jaundice must be kept well hydrated because of the increased susceptibility to acute renal failure (tubular necrosis). Fluid balance charts are essential to monitor input and output. Skin turgor is observed (Section 4); urea, electrolytes, and serum creatinine are monitored daily if necessary. Before a procedure such as ultrasonography, CT, or cholangiography when eating and drinking is forbidden, the jaundiced patient should have parenteral fluid replacement to avoid dehydration. Normal saline (0.9 per cent NaCl) is given to all but the elderly patient with cardiac disease, in whom heart failure is a concern.

Prophylactic measures against renal failure

Good hydration, as pointed out above, is central to the avoidance of renal problems. Other measures have been studied and some appear valuable. Pre- and perioperative intravenous mannitol, as an osmotic diuretic, has been advocated for many years since the key studies of Dawson (Dawson, BMJ, 1965; i:82). However, hydration with parenteral normal saline is essential in parallel to avoid dehydration caused by the diuretic response to mannitol. Recently, a controlled study of mannitol in the management of obstructive jaundice showed no beneficial effect on postoperative renal failure (Gubern, Surgery, 1988; 103:39). The question of its value has thus been challenged, hydration being the more important factor.

Endotoxaemia is implicated in many of the complications seen in association with obstructive jaundice (Pain, BrJSurg, 1985; 72: 942), and is thought to occur because of increased absorption of endotoxin from the intestine and a reduced clearance of endotoxin by the reticuloendothelial cells in the liver. Many experimental and clinical studies have attempted to identify the measures which might reduce endotoxaemia and thus the development of (in particular) renal dysfunction.

Bile acids have antiendotoxaemic effects. Experimentally, the absorption of endotoxin from the intestine is increased when there is no bile present (Kocsar, JBacteriol, 1969; 100:220) and absorption is prevented when oral bile acids are given (Bailey, BrJSurg, 1976; 63:774). Clinical studies show the same effect of oral sodium deoxycholate in patients with obstructive jaundice with protection of renal function (Cahill, SGO, 1987; 165:519). Chenodeoxycholic acid is less effective. A randomized controlled trial has shown a beneficial effect of preoperative sodium deoxycholate in preventing postoperative renal dysfunction, but only in those patients with normal preoperative renal function (Pain, BrJSurg, 1991; 78:467). In a study of ursodeoxycholic acid, portal venous endotoxaemia was reduced, but systemic endotoxaemia was not and there did not appear to be any protection of renal function (Thompson, BrJSurg, 1986; 73:634). It seems likely that this difference is due to the lower antiendotoxic effect of ursodeoxycholic acid than of sodium deoxycholate (Cahill, SGO, 1989; 105:239). Thus, the antiendotoxic activity of bile salts has been shown to be related to their known detergent activities; deoxycholate and its conjugates are the most effective both *in vitro* and *in vivo* (Pain, HPBSurgery, 1988; 1:21).

Lactulose, a synthetic disaccharide, also has an antiendotoxin effect and when given orally reduces systemic endotoxaemia (Liehr, Hepatogast, 1980; 27:356). This agent was initially evaluated in hepatocellular diseases and cirrhosis. Experimental studies in rats given lactulose orally have shown that it reduces endotoxin-related mortality, and in patients with obstructive jaundice, portal and systemic endotoxaemia was prevented, as well as renal dysfunction (Pain, BrJSurg, 1986; 73:775). The same randomized controlled trial mentioned above (Pain, BrJSurg, 1991; 78:467) showed that oral lactulose given preoperatively has the same protective effect on postoperative renal function as does sodium deoxycholate.

Polymyxin B and bowel preparations with antibiotics might be expected to reduce endotoxaemia, but have not been found to produce any benefit in patients with obstructive jaundice (Hunt, AustNZJMed, 1980; 50:476; Ingoldby, AmJSurg, 1984; 147:766).

Thus, at present, oral sodium deoxycholate (500 mg, 8 hourly) or lactulose (30 ml, 6 hourly: reduced if diarrhoea develops) given

before surgery for 48 or 72 h, respectively, appear to be logical additional measures which will protect against renal dysfunction and perhaps other complications in patients with obstructive jaundice. However, it should be emphasized that they will not reverse renal failure once present. Moreover, careful preoperative hydration remains the most important measure to reduce the risk of renal dysfunction/failure. Dopamine adds no protection (Parks, BrJSurg, 1994; 81:437).

Correction of coagulopathy

In some patients with obstructive jaundice, the prothrombin time is prolonged. Vitamin K given intramuscularly at a dose of 10 mg should be prescribed and continued for a few days—an empirical duration. In the majority of patients the prothrombin time returns to normal rapidly, sometimes overnight. If it does not, then underlying parenchymal liver disease or metastases should be suspected.

Prevention of infectious complications

Bacteria may be present in the obstructed bile duct without clinical symptoms or signs. Radiological, endoscopic, and surgical procedures may produce systemic sepsis in such cases, with resulting Gram-negative septicaemia, abscess formation, and wound infection. Premedication with a single dose of antibiotic reduces the risk of postsurgical sepsis. For the non-surgical procedures, a single dose of piperacillin is not effective (van den Hazel, AnnIntMed, 1996; 125:442). It is necessary to continue the antibiotic until biliary drainage is completely unobstructed (Byl, ClinInfDis, 1995; 20: 1236). Suitable antibiotics for such prophylaxis include ciprofloxacin (Mehal, EurJGastroHepatol, 1995; 7:841), cefuroxime, cefotaxime (Niederau, GastrEnd, 1994; 40:533), or piperacillin (Byl, ClinInfDis, 1995; 20:1236). Ciprofloxacin has the advantage of oral use. The choice should depend upon knowledge of the sensitivity of micro-organisms in the hospital, which will change with the use of selected antibiotics (Mohandas, GastrEnd, 1996; 43:175). It should be emphasized that successful biliary decompression is central to avoiding postprocedural sepsis.

Itching

Itching due to bile duct obstruction from a stricture or stone usually disappears within a few days of biliary decompression, whether surgical, endoscopic, or percutaneous. Before drainage, cholestyramine and antihistamines are generally ineffective. If the cholestasis is intrahepatic, cholestyramine is usually helpful. Antihistamines and ursodeoxycholic acid have a variable benefit. In patients resistant to these measures, rifampicin (Cynamon, Gastro, 1990; 98:1013) and ondansetron (Schworer, Pain, 1995; 61:33) may help, but should be used under careful supervision. Opiate antagonists remain experimental but show promise (Bergasa, AnnIntMed, 1995; 123:161).

Preoperative non-surgical biliary drainage

Early reports of preoperative, percutaneous transhepatic external bile drainage suggested that it was beneficial, reducing postoperative mortality and morbidity after surgery for the relief of malignant bile duct obstruction (Nakayama, Gastro, 1978; 74:554). However, subsequent randomized controlled trials showed no reduction of postoperative mortality (Hatfield, Lancet, 1982; ii:896; McPherson, BrJSurg, 1984; 71:371; Pitt, AnnSurg, 1985; 201:545). Thus, despite the theoretical benefit of a lower serum bilirubin concentration at the time of surgery, the complications associated with percutaneous drainage removed any advantage. Preoperative endoscopic drainage, although a safer approach than percutaneous drainage, showed no benefit on postoperative morbidity or mortality in a randomized controlled trial (Lai, BrJSurg, 1994; 81:1195).

Because of the risks of surgery in the patient with cholangitis, endoscopic biliary drainage is indicated (Lai, NEJM, 1992; 326: 1582). If obstruction is caused by a gallstone, then endoscopic sphincterotomy and stone removal, or drainage by nasobiliary tube, is necessary. If endoscopic access is not possible, percutaneous transhepatic bile drainage can be performed, and may be valuable (Kadir, AJR, 1982; 138:25). The problem of this approach, however, is the risk of bile reflux into the circulation because of vascular–biliary fistulas, frequently caused by percutaneous transhepatic catheterization (Hoevels, GastrRad, 1980; 5:127).

Prediction of risk

Several studies have analysed factors which may predict an increased mortality and morbidity after surgery for obstructive jaundice. In a study of 373 patients with obstructive jaundice (Dixon, Gut, 1983; 24:845), three independent risk factors were identified which were associated with a significantly increased risk of postoperative mortality. These were an initial haematocrit of 30 per cent or less, an initial plasma bilirubin of greater than 200 µmol/l (normally less than 17 µmol/l), and a diagnosis of malignant rather than benign obstruction. Patients with two or three of these risk factors had a 30 per cent risk of dying postoperatively. Despite correction of the low haematocrit by transfusion, this remained a risk factor. Clearly, the underlying cause of obstruction—malignant or benign—cannot be influenced by such therapy. Finally, although the serum bilirubin can be lowered by preoperative percutaneous biliary drainage, this procedure has not been found to be beneficial.

References

1. Harry DS and McIntyre N. Plasma lipoproteins and the liver. In Millward-Sadler GH, Wright R, and Arthur MJP, eds. *Liver and biliary disease*. 3rd edition. London: WB Saunders, 1992: 61–78.
2. Green J and Better OS. Systemic hypotension and renal failure in obstructive jaundice—mechanistic and therapeutic aspects. *Journal of the American Society of Nephrologists*, 1995; **5**: 1853–71.
3. Bomzon A, Jacob G, and Better OS. Jaundice in the kidney. In Epstein M, ed. *The kidney in liver disease*. Baltimore: Hanley & Belfus, 1996; 423–46.
4. Fogarty BJ, Parks RW, Rowlands BJ, and Diamon, T. Renal dysfunction in obstructive jaundice. *British Journal of Surgery*, 1995; **82**: 877–84.
5. Hay JE. Bone disease in cholestatic liver disease. *Gastroenterology*, 1995; **108**: 276–83.
6. Kimmings AN, van Deventer SJH, Obertop H, Rauws EAJ, and Gouma DJ. Inflammatory and immunologic effects of obstructive jaundice: pathogenesis and treatment. *Journal of the American College of Surgeons*, 1995; **181**: 567–81.

23.3　Intrahepatic cholestasis

Dermot Gleeson and James L. Boyer

Definition

'Cholestasis' is a clinical and biochemical syndrome usually characterized by pruritus, jaundice, and elevation of the serum alkaline phosphatase; it results from a generalized impairment in the secretion of bile. Intrahepatic cholestasis refers to all cholestatic disorders that impair bile secretion within the liver. The term cholestasis is derived from the morphological appearance of 'bile plugs' within the bile canaliculus of the hepatocyte. Ultrastructural findings usually include dilation of the canalicular lumen, loss of microvilli, and pericanalicular accumulation of microfilaments and small vesicles.

Introduction

Historically, mechanical obstruction of the large bile ducts was believed to account for cholestasis. Virchow thought that jaundice in viral hepatitis resulted from obstruction of the ampulla of Vater by a mucous plug.[1] However, when Eppinger[2] and Watson and Hoffbauer[3] described cases of viral hepatitis with prolonged cholestasis in the absence of apparent bile-duct obstruction, attention was directed to the liver. Intrahepatic cholestasis was first ascribed to obstruction of the small intrahepatic bile ducts, resulting from direct damage, periportal oedema, and/or inflammation. Such cases were labelled 'cholangiolitic hepatitis'. However, the degree of portal inflammation often failed to correlate with the severity of the cholestasis,[4] and when it was observed that steroid hormones caused canalicular cholestasis without portal inflammation it was recognized that hepatocyte dysfunction was of primary importance in the pathogenesis of many types of intrahepatic cholestasis. Several reviews of this subject have appeared recently.[1,5–13]

Aetiology and clinical manifestations

The syndrome of intrahepatic cholestasis results from many different forms of liver injury, as illustrated in Table 1. Jaundice and pruritus are often present whereas signs and symptoms of severe parenchymal cell injury, such as ascites, coagulation defects, and encephalopathy, are typically absent. The clinical presentations of certain common liver diseases, such as viral hepatitis and alcohol- and drug-induced liver injury, vary considerably and include features of cholestatic liver injury, as well as the well-recognized manifestations of hepatocellular dysfunction.

Table 1 Classification of intrahepatic cholestasis

Hepatitis
　Viral (A, B, C, Epstein–Barr, cytomegalovirus)
　Autoimmune
　Alcoholic
Drugs and hormones (see Table 4)
Diseases of intrahepatic bile ducts (vanishing bile-duct syndromes)
(see Table 5)
Liver infiltrations/storage disorders
　Lymphoma
　Idiopathic hypereosinophilic syndrome
　Systemic mastocytosis
　Amyloidosis
　Sickle cell crises
　Wilson's disease
　Haemochromatosis
　Protoporphyria
Systemic infection (endotoxins and cytokines)
Total parenteral nutrition
Postoperative intrahepatic cholestasis
Cholestasis of pregnancy
Benign recurrent intrahepatic cholestasis
Infantile cholestatic syndromes, including α_1-antitrypsin deficiency
(see Table 6)

Physiology of bile formation[5,14–20]

Mechanisms of bile formation are still incompletely understood. Therefore it is not surprising that the pathophysiology of many cholestatic disorders is not known. Nevertheless, progress is being made in understanding both processes. Hepatic bile is formed by the active transport of bile acids and other organic anions and electrolytes from the blood into the hepatocyte and then into the bile canaliculus, where osmotic gradients are formed that stimulate the flow of bile. The bile canaliculus is formed between adjacent hepatocytes and is sealed by specialized regions known as 'tight junctions', which form a diffusion barrier between the extracellular environment and the bile canalicular lumen. Tight junctions also divide the hepatocyte plasma membrane into canalicular (apical) and sinusoidal (basolateral) domains that define the cell's polarity. These membrane domains differ with respect to lipid composition and ion-transport proteins. Thus, like cells of other ion-transporting epithelia, hepatocytes are highly polarized. The tight junctions are more permeable to cations than to anions (Bradley, AmJPhysiol, 1978; 235:E570)[14] and thus limit back-diffusion of actively secreted anions from the bile canaliculus to the intercellular space, but they allow movement of water and small cations into bile, thereby preserving electroneutrality and osmotic equilibrium. Water also enters bile from the hepatocyte across the canalicular (apical) membrane, but the relative contributions of these transcellular and paracellular routes have not been defined (Tavoloni, Gastro, 1988; 94:217).

Canalicular bile secretion is normally determined by both bile-acid dependent and independent mechanisms. Bile acid secretion is the major driving force for bile flow. Hepatocytes take up conjugated bile acids via specific, saturable, carrier-mediated transporters localized on the basolateral membrane. These include a 50-kDa, sodium-coupled, cotransport polypeptide cloned from both rat (ntcp) and human (NTCP) liver (Hagenbuch, PNAS, 1991; 88:10629; Hagenbuch, JCI, 1994; 93:1326) and a 72-kDa, sodium-independent, organic anion, transport polypeptide cloned from both rat and human liver (Jacquemin, PNAS, 1994; 91:133; Kullack-Ublick, Gastro, 1995; 109:1274). Bile acid uptake via the 50-kDa carrier is driven by the out-to-in Na^+ gradient, which is maintained by the Na^+/K^+ATPase pump located on the sinusoidal membrane (Duffey, JCI, 1983; 72:470; Sellinger, Hepatol, 1990; 11:223).[5,18] Na^+/K^+ATPase also generates an in-to-out K^+ gradient. This gradient helps to maintain the negative intracellular potential (Graf, JMembrBiol, 1987; 95:241), which also functions as an electrogenic driving force.

After uptake into hepatocytes, transcellular transport of bile acids involves binding to 3-α-hydroxy steroid dehydrogenase, a cytoplasmic protein (Stolz, AnnRevPhysiol, 1989; 51:161), and rapid diffusion to the apical canalicular domain. Bile acids are then excreted across the canalicular membrane by a saturable ATP-dependent transporter that is distinct from the multispecific organic acid transporter that mediates excretion of bilirubin and other organic anions (Muller, JBC, 1991; 266:18920; Nishada, PNAS, 1991; 88:6590). Recently (Gerloff, Hepatol, 1997; 26:358A) a member of the P-glycoprotein family, termed sister of P-glycoprotein (SPGP) has been cloned from rat liver and shown to have several properties of the ATP-dependent canalicular bile acid transporter. The negative intracellular potential may also function as a driving force for bile acid excretion (Meier, JBC, 1984; 259:10614; Weinman, AmJPhysiol, 1989; 256:G826), although its role is controversial (Kast, JBC, 1994; 269:5179).

Approximately one-third of canalicular bile flow is formed independently of bile acid secretion; the osmotic driving forces for this component are derived in part from excretion of bicarbonate ions (Hardison, AmJPhysiol, 1978; 235:E158; Bruck, AmJPhysiol, 1993; 265:G347), which are transported via a chloride/bicarbonate exchange mechanism (Meier, JCI, 1985; 75:1256) in parallel with a chloride channel on the canalicular membrane (Sellinger, Hepatol, 1988; 8:1262). Bicarbonate secretion may also be involved in the 'hypercholeresis' produced by some bile acids, such as ursodeoxycholic acid, although the source of bicarbonate may be the bile ductules rather than the hepatocyte (Yoon, Gastro, 1986; 90:837; Gautam, JCI, 1989; 83:565; Strazzabosco, AmJPhysiol, 1991; 260:G658).

Another important driving force for bile-acid independent flow is biliary excretion of glutathione and its metabolites. Excretion of these anions correlates with bile flow under a variety of conditions (Ballatori, AmJPhysiol, 1989; G256:G22; Trauner, Hepatol, 1997; 25:263) and specific transport mechanisms have been demonstrated (Inoue, EurJBioch, 1983; 134:467) on canalicular plasma membranes

from rat liver. Some bile is also formed by exocytosis, when vesicles fuse with the canalicular membrane and discharge their contents, but the magnitude of this contribution is small. Regulation of canalicular excretory function is thought to occur by insertion and retrieval of canalicular transporters that reside on vesicles in the pericanalicular cytoplasm (Boyer, Gastro 1995; 109:1600). A bicarbonate-rich component of bile is also secreted from the bile ducts and this secretion is stimulated by the hormone secretin. In man this third component of bile accounts for approximately 20 per cent of total bile production (Boyer, JCI, 1974; 54:773).

Hepatocytes possess a dense array of actin microfilaments (Oda, LabInvest, 1974; 31:314);[8] they are concentrated in the pericanalicular region, and insert into the cores of canalicular microvilli and into specialized areas of the lateral cell plasma membrane adjacent to the tight junctions. Apart from maintaining cell shape, they play a role in maintaining the integrity of the tight junction. In addition, they may mediate canalicular contractions, which have been observed by time-lapse cinematography in isolated hepatocyte couplets (Oshio, LabInvest, 1985; 53:270) and whole liver preparations (Watanabe, JCellBiol 1995; 113:1069). Canalicular contractions, co-ordinated by calcium waves (Nathanson, AmJPhysiol, 1995; 269:G167), assist in canalicular bile flow by a peristaltic action.

Two components of tight junctions, occludin (which forms the junction seal) and ZO-1 have been cloned and are up-regulated during cholestasis (Fallon, AmJPhysiol, 1993; 264:G1439; Fallon, AmJPhysiol, 1995; 269:G1057).

A lobular gradient exists for bile secretion (Groothius, AmJPhysiol, 1982; 238:G233). Normally, bile acids are transported from blood predominantly by periportal hepatocytes (zone I). Perivenular (zone III) hepatocytes are located 'downstream' in the lobule and, because of efficient bile-acid clearance in zone I and the 'countercurrent' flow of canalicular bile in the opposite direction, zone III hepatocytes are normally exposed only to low concentrations of bile acids. Bile secretion in this region thus occurs mainly by bile-acid independent mechanisms (Gumucio, JLabClinMed, 1978; 91:350). The lobular gradient may explain why in cholestasis, of any cause, bile staining is most marked in zone III. When canalicular bile secretion is impaired, as in oestrogen-induced cholestasis (Buscher, Hepatol, 1993; 17:494), a greater proportion of bile acid bypasses zone I and is then transported by zone III hepatocytes at the 'blind end' of the canaliculus. Stagnation of bile flow occurs, presumably because of a parallel decrease in bile-acid independent flow. When the transport of bile acids is impaired throughout the lobule, they accumulate in the systemic circulation.

Mechanisms of cholestasis[5–13]

Bile formation is a complex multistep process, which requires distributed liver perfusion with an intact lobular gradient, normal hepatocyte uptake mechanisms, a rapid transcellular transport system, intact mechanisms for canalicular excretion of bile acids and other anions, co-ordinated microfilament-induced canalicular contractions, sealed tight junctions to retain the excreted products, and a patent biliary tree. In most forms of human intrahepatic cholestasis (Table 1) it is not known which of these steps in the bile secretory process is initially impaired, as all may ultimately be affected. Several animal models of cholestasis have been studied in an attempt to unravel the pathophysiological sequence of events.[9,10] The best studied experimental cholestatic models include the following:

1. Oestrogens may cause intrahepatic cholestasis of pregnancy and cholestasis may also occur after oral contraceptive use in humans. Oestrogens impair both bile-acid dependent and independent flow and excretion of bile acids and bilirubin in animals, but do not produce the ultrastructural changes in the canalicular membrane (dilatation and loss of microvilli) associated with most cholestatic agents.[21–24]

2. Endotoxins are a primary cause of cholestasis in sepsis and stimulate the release of cytokines (interleukin 1, interleukin 6, and tumour necrosis factor-α), which inhibit bile secretory function.

3. The monohydroxy bile acid, lithocholic acid, causes cholestasis and hepatocellular damage in rats (Layden, Gastro, 1975; 69: 724; Kakis, Gastro, 1978; 75:595). Lithocholic acid is formed in the ileum and colon by bacterial dehydroxylation of the primary bile acid chenodeoxycholic acid. Monohydroxy bile acids are found in small amounts in normal human bile, and increased levels in serum or bile have been found in patients with primary biliary cirrhosis (Murphy, Gut, 1972; 13:201), progressive familial intrahepatic cholestasis (Williams, JPediat, 1972; 81:493), and cholestasis associated with total parenteral nutrition (Fouin-Fortunet, Gastro, 1982; 82:932). Whatever the primary mechanism of cholestasis, retention of monohydroxy and other hydrophobic bile acids within the liver causes secondary hepatocellular damage by their detergent effects that may initiate a vicious cycle of cell injury (see section on ursodeoxycholic acid below).

4. Agents which disrupt microfilaments, such as phalloidin and cytochalasin B, produce cholestasis in rats (Phillips, Gastro, 1975; 69: 48; Dubin, Gastro, 1978; 75:450). Chlorpromazine, which also damages microfilaments, has caused cholestatic jaundice in as many as 5 per cent of patients, and a dose–dependent reduction in bile flow has been demonstrated in several species.[10]

5. Bile-duct ligation. Models of extrahepatic obstructive cholestasis have been useful in determining which of the morphological and functional changes seen in cholestatic livers are primary events and which can be attributed to secondary consequences of cholestasis.

Cellular and molecular mechanisms of cholestasis (Table 2)

Based on studies in experimental models, a number of defects in cell function have been described.[13]

Impairment of plasma membrane ion transporters

Oestrogen treatment is associated with a fall in the activity of several plasma membrane enzymes relevant to bile flow. On the basolateral membrane, these include $Na^+/K^+ATPase$ (van Dyke, AmJPhysiol, 1987; 253:G613), Na^+/H^+ exchange (Arias, Hepatol, 1983; 3:372), and the sodium-dependent, bile-acid uptake transporter (ntcp) (Simon, Hepatol, 1994; 19:1241). Oestrogens decrease the fluidity of the basolateral plasma membrane of rat hepatocytes (as measured by fluorescence polarization) by changing the lipid composition of the membrane (Davis, PNAS, 1978; 75:4130). Such changes are likely to impair spatial mobility and activity of several membrane enzymes and

transport systems (Schachter, Hepatol, 1984; 4:140).[5] This effect on fluidity probably explains the fall in $Na^+/K^+ATPase$ activities, since mRNA and protein concentrations relating to this transport system are little changed (Kupferschmidt, Hepatol, 1994; 20:175A; Simon, AmJPhysiol, 1994; 271:G1043). Changes in membrane fluidity and $Na^+/K^+ATPase$ activity are not seen following bile duct ligation (Fricker, JCI, 1988; 84:876), suggesting that they are not a non-specific consequence of oestrogen-induced cholestasis. Indeed, several agents, including triton-WR1339 (Simon, JCI, 1980; 65:851), S-adenosylmethionine (SAME) (Boelsterli, Hepatol, 1983; 3:12), and dietary modification (Storch, BBActa; 1984; 798:137) which reverse the fluidity changes, also reverse oestrogen-associated cholestasis.

In contrast, ntcp activity falls after oestrogen administration and is associated with a parallel decrease in ntcp mRNA and protein production (Simon, AmerJPhysiol, 1994; 271:G1043). These effects are probably a consequence rather than a cause of cholestasis since they are also observed in other forms of cholestasis, including those caused by bile duct ligation (Gartnung, Gastro, 1996; 110:199), cyclosporin (Moseley, JPharmExpTher, 1990; 253:974), and endotoxin (Green, AmJPhysiol, 1994; 30:1094; Moseley, AmJPhysiol, 1996; 271:G137). These changes at the molecular level may represent a compensatory mechanism to minimize bile acid accumulation and further injury to hepatocytes in any form of cholestasis.

Several other cholestatic agents and interventions, including chlorpromazine (Keefe, Gastro, 1980; 79:222; van Dyke, AmJPhysiol, 1987; 253:G613), thyroidectomy (Layden, JCI, 1976; 57:1009), lithocholic acid (Reichen, Experientia, 1979; 35:1186), and some volatile anaesthetics (Thalhammer, Hepatol, 1987; 7:1040), decrease membrane fluidity and also the activities of $Na^+/K^+ATPase$, hepatocyte bile acid uptake, and other membrane transport systems. Spironolactone decreases membrane fluidity, although bile flow actually increases; however, additional effects of this drug that are independent of changes in fluidity are possible (Smith, JHepatol, 1987; 6:362). Other interventions, including adrenalectomy (Miner, Gastro, 1980; 79:212), endotoxin (Utilli, JInfDis, 1977; 136:583), and protoporphyrin (Avner, Gastro, 1983; 85:700), also cause cholestasis and decrease $Na^+/K^+ATPase$ activity, although effects on plasma membrane fluidity have not been assessed. These widely documented changes in $Na^+/K^+ATPase$ activity, although a convenient marker of membrane dysfunction, may not be a primary cause of cholestasis since phenobarbital increases $Na^+/K^+ATPase$ activity but does not reverse oestrogen-induced cholestasis (Gumucio, Gastro, 1973; 65:651).

Despite the potentially important effects of oestrogens and other agents on transport function at the basolateral membrane, the striking intrahepatic bile staining in most forms of cholestasis, including that induced by oestrogens, suggests that there are additional effects on canalicular transport, the rate- limiting step in hepatobiliary excretion. Fewer studies have assessed the effects of cholestatic agents on canalicular membrane transport function. However, ATP-dependent bile acid and glutathione transport across the canalicular membrane, are major driving forces for bile-acid dependent and independent flow, respectively, and are decreased following oestrogen treatment (Bossard, JCI, 1993; 91:22714), cyclosporin (Bohme, Gastro, 1994; 107:255), and endotoxin (Moseley, AmJPhysiol, 1996; 271:G137). These effects are not associated

Table 2 Cellular mechanisms of cholestasis

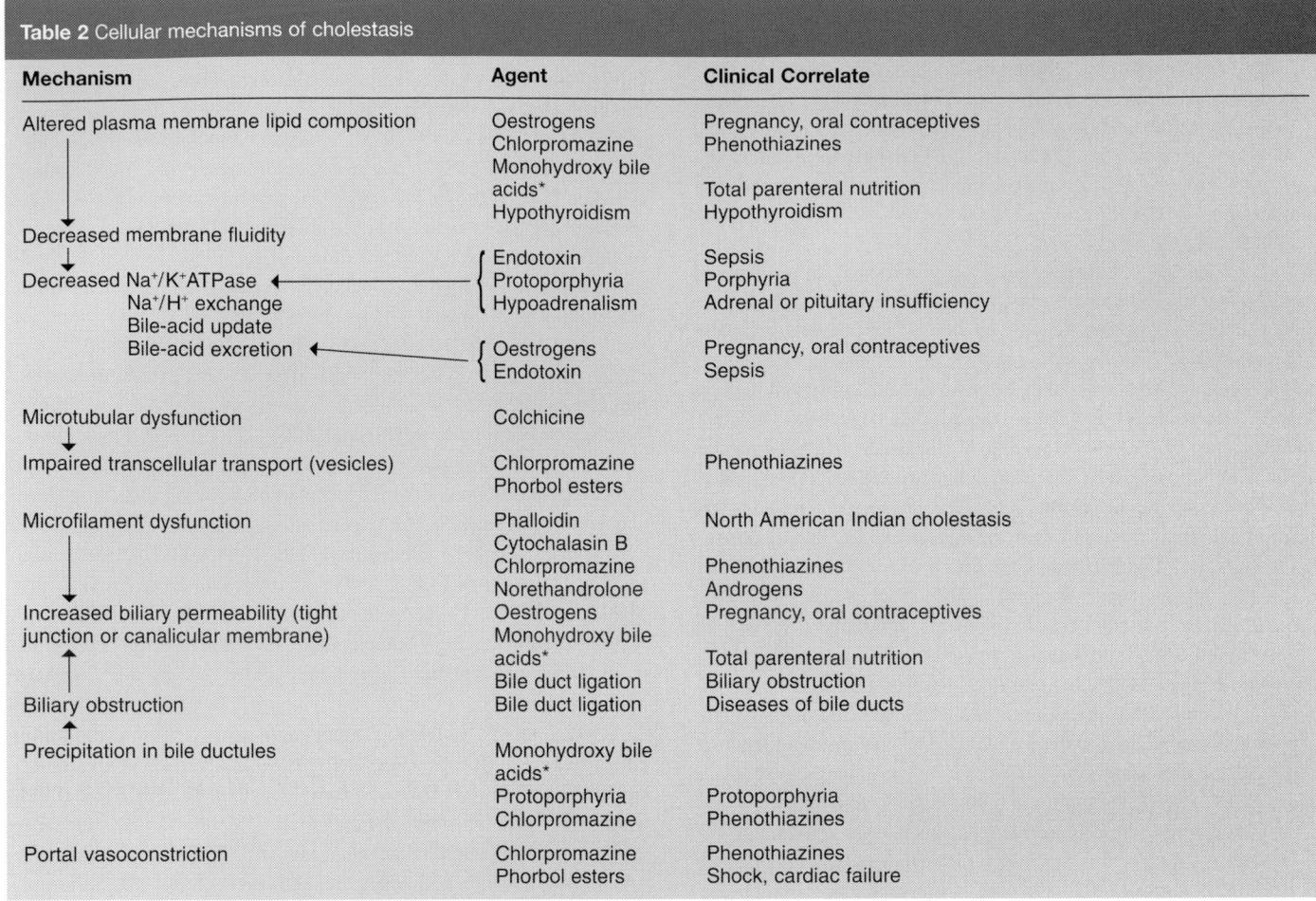

Mechanism	Agent	Clinical Correlate
Altered plasma membrane lipid composition	Oestrogens	Pregnancy, oral contraceptives
	Chlorpromazine	Phenothiazines
	Monohydroxy bile acids*	Total parenteral nutrition
	Hypothyroidism	Hypothyroidism
Decreased membrane fluidity		
Decreased Na⁺/K⁺ATPase	Endotoxin	Sepsis
	Protoporphyria	Porphyria
Na⁺/H⁺ exchange	Hypoadrenalism	Adrenal or pituitary insufficiency
Bile-acid update		
Bile-acid excretion	Oestrogens	Pregnancy, oral contraceptives
	Endotoxin	Sepsis
Microtubular dysfunction	Colchicine	
Impaired transcellular transport (vesicles)	Chlorpromazine	Phenothiazines
	Phorbol esters	
Microfilament dysfunction	Phalloidin	North American Indian cholestasis
	Cytochalasin B	
	Chlorpromazine	Phenothiazines
	Norethandrolone	Androgens
Increased biliary permeability (tight junction or canalicular membrane)	Oestrogens	Pregnancy, oral contraceptives
	Monohydroxy bile acids*	Total parenteral nutrition
	Bile duct ligation	Biliary obstruction
Biliary obstruction	Bile duct ligation	Diseases of bile ducts
Precipitation in bile ductules	Monohydroxy bile acids*	
	Protoporphyria	Protoporphyria
	Chlorpromazine	Phenothiazines
Portal vasoconstriction	Chlorpromazine	Phenothiazines
	Phorbol esters	Shock, cardiac failure

with demonstrable changes in canalicular membrane lipid composition or fluidity. Furthermore the effects may be selective since the activities of other canalicular membrane transport systems, such as electrogenic bile acid transport and the chloride/bicarbonate exchanger, are unchanged (Alvaro, JHepatol, 1997; 26:146). Recent studies indicate that the canalicular multispecific organic acid transporter (**cMOAT**) or multi-drug-resistance protein (**MRP2**) is down-regulated in several animal models of cholestasis (Arrese, Hepatol, 1996; 24:215A; Trauner, Gastro, 1997; 113:255).

Taken together, these findings suggest that during many forms of experimental cholestasis there is a widespread but selective impairment of ion and organic solute transport systems on both the basolateral and canalicular plasma membranes of the hepatocyte. Cholestasis is also associated with impaired transcytosis of vesicles which target canalicular transport proteins to the canalicular membrane. This process is dependent on microtubules, whose ATP-driven motors can be inhibited by bile acids (Marks, Gastro, 1995; 108:824). While some changes, such as the decrease in bile acid uptake by the basolateral membrane, appear to be secondary consequences of cholestasis, other effects, such as impaired vesicle transcytosis and canalicular membrane transport defects, may be primary causes. For example, several cases of progressive familial intrahepatic cholestasis have now been described with deficiencies of the canalicular phospholipid transporter, MDR3 (Dumoulin, Hepatol, 1997; 26:852; Deleuze, Hepatol, 1996; 23:904).

Cytoskeletal abnormalities

Phalloidin, which induces irreversible polymerization of actin filaments, produces cholestasis in rats, together with ultrastructural evidence of condensation of pericanalicular microfilaments (Dubin, Gastro, 1979; 75:450). A similar condensation of microfilaments is found in a familial cholestatic syndrome in North American Indians (Weber, Gastro, 1981; 81:653), progressive familial intrahepatic cholestasis (deVos, Gut, 1975; 16:943), and in some cases of cholestasis associated with hepatitis and with drugs (Adler, AmJPathol, 1980; 98:603; Kutty, DigDisSci, 1987; 32:933).

Cytochalasin B detaches actin filaments from the plasma membrane and is also cholestatic in animals (Phillips, Gastro, 1975; 69:724). On electron microscopy, the pericanalicular region has a granular appearance and microfilaments appear disrupted. Similar morphological changes can be induced by other cholestatic agents, including chlorpromazine (Miyai, LabInvest, 1977; 36:249) and androgens (Phillips, AmJPathol, 1978; 93:729), but not oestrogens. Chlorpromazine induces actin polymerization in vitro (Elias, Science, 1979; 206:1404).

Microfilament dysfunction may induce cholestasis by several mechanisms: (i) disrupting the tight junction (see under increased biliary permeability below), (ii) impairing transcellular transport of bile acids (Kacich, Gastro, 1983; 85:385), (iii) disrupting hepatocyte membrane polarity (Durand-Schneider, Hepatol, 1987; 7:1239), or (iv) impairing co-ordinated canalicular contractions, as can be demonstrated with phalloidin (Watanabe, Gastro, 1983; 85:245) or cytochalasin B (Phillips, LabInvest, 1983; 48:205).

However, it is not certain whether microfilament dysfunction is a primary or secondary event in many cholestatic disorders, because similar morphological changes may also be seen following bile duct ligation in animals (Jones, Gastro, 1976; 71:1050) as well as in human extrahepatic obstruction (Adler, AmJPathol, 1980; 98:603). Furthermore, phalloidin and chlorpromazine have other toxic effects on hepatocytes, including inhibition of bile acid uptake (Reichen, BBActa, 1981; 643:1216; Wieland, PNAS, 1984; 81:5232) and portal vein constriction (Tavoloni, JPharmExpTher, 1980; 214:269), which may also contribute to the decline in bile flow.

The hepatocyte tubulovesicular system mediates transcellular movement of macromolecules such as IgA (Renston, Science, 1980; 208:1276) and can affect the cellular transport of bilirubin, biliary lipids, and hydrophobic bile acids under certain circumstances (Crawford, AmJPhysiol, 1988; 255:G121). Colchicine, an inhibitor of microtubular function, is cholestatic when bile acid flux is increased (Crawford, JLipRes, 1988; 29:144), and also augments the cholestatic effects of phalloidin (Dubin, Gastro, 1980; 79:646). Chlorpromazine, cyclosporin, and oestrogens can also inhibit the transcellular transport of horseradish peroxidase, a marker of the vesicular pathway (Okanoue, Hepatol, 1984; 4:253).

Increased biliary permeability and tight junction disruption[26]

Many agents that produce cholestasis, including oestrogens (Forker, JCI, 1969; 48:654), phalloidin (Elias, PNAS, 1980; 77:2299), chlorpromazine (Strasberg, CanJPhysPharm, 1979; 57:1138), and lithocholic acid (Layden, Gastro, 1977; 73:120), accelerate the clearance of inert markers such as inulin and sucrose from blood to bile, and enhance their regurgitation from bile to blood following retrograde biliary injection. These findings suggest that these well-known cholestatic agents increase the permeability of the biliary tree. Oestrogens (deVos, PatholResPract, 1980; 171:381) and phalloidin (Elias, PNAS, 1980; 77:2299) disrupt tight junctions by decreasing the number and density of interconnecting strands, which lose their parallel orientation, suggesting that the increased biliary permeability resides at this paracellular barrier. Oestrogen treatment results in a more diffuse distribution of the major tight-junctional protein ZO-1 (Anderson, AmJPathol, 1989; 134:1055). In cholestasis induced by lithocholic acid the more striking morphological changes are at the canalicular plasma membrane (Layden, Gastro, 1975; 69:724). Inert markers also enter bile through routes mediated by transcellular vesicles (Lake, JCI, 1985; 76:676; Lorenzini, Gastro, 1986; 91:278), so that the increase in biliary permeability associated with lithocholic acid and other cholestatic agents may also involve vesicular events at the canalicular plasma membrane rather than an increase in paracellular permeability alone (Reichen, ClinRes, 1985; 33:97A). Whatever the exact site, an increase in biliary permeability may result in regurgitation of excreted bile acids and other anions from the canaliculus to the hepatocyte or to extracellular fluid, thereby dissipating the osmotic driving forces for bile flow. Other biliary constituents such as lipids and bilirubin may also reflux from bile to blood.

Disruption of the tight junctions may not always be a primary mechanism of cholestasis, since morphological (deVos, BrJExpPath,

1978; 59:220) and immunohistochemical (Fallon, AmJPhysiol, 1993; 264:1439) changes in junction structure and permeability (Accatino, JLabClinMed, 1981; 97:525) commonly follow duct ligation in animal models and extrahepatic bile-duct obstruction in man (Robenek, AmJPathol, 1980; 100:93). Furthermore, with some cholestatic agents, such as oestrogens, bile flow falls long before biliary permeability increases, suggesting that these changes are a secondary phenomenon (Jaeschke, Gastro, 1987; 93:533).

Nevertheless, disruption of the tight junctions is an important cause of loss or reversal of hepatocyte polarity in some forms of cholestasis. For example, in the rat with ligated bile ducts, not only is there a fall in basolateral ntcp activity (see above), but the canalicular enzyme alkaline phosphatase,[27] and the 100-kDa, bile-acid canalicular-transport protein (Fricker, JCI, 1989; 84:876) may partially relocate to the sinusoidal membrane. Loss of polarity is also induced by phalloidin and by colchicine (Durand-Schneider, Hepatol, 1987; 7:1239). Reversal of the polarity of membrane transport systems for bile acids may be a further hepatoprotective mechanism in cholestasis by also contributing to a reduction in the intracellular concentrations of these toxic anions.

Disorders of intracellular calcium release

Increases in cytosolic calcium have been implicated in the pathogenesis of some forms of experimental liver injury,[28] and may be a critical phenomenon leading to cell death (Lemasters, Nature, 1987; 325:78). The cholestatic bile acids lithocholic acid and chenodeoxycholic acid, but not the choleretic taurocholic acid, increase intracellular calcium levels in isolated hepatocytes (Combettes, JBC, 1988; 263:2299; Spivey, JCI, 1993; 92:17), either by releasing calcium from intracellular stores or by increasing cell membrane permeability to calcium. In contrast, bile duct ligation is associated with an impaired rise in intracellular calcium in response to the hormone phenylephrine (Beuers, JCI, 1993; 92:2984). Furthermore, propagation of the intracellular calcium release signal via the gap junctions is impaired. This may also contribute to impairment of canalicular contractions, which are calcium-dependent (Watanabe, Liver, 1988; 8:178; Nathanson, AmJPhysiol, 1995; 269:G167).

Intraluminal obstruction of small bile ducts

Lithocholic acid-induced cholestasis in rats is associated with concretions in the canaliculi and small bile ductules that are soluble in the calcium chelating agent EGTA and may represent precipitated calcium salts of lithocholic acid.[6] Some cholestatic diseases, such as protoporphyria (Bloomer, Gastro, 1982; 82:569), are associated with intraluminal precipitates.

Inadequate liver perfusion

Agents causing vasoconstriction in the isolated perfused rat liver, including α_1-agonists (Lenzen, Hepatol, 1986; 6:1133), phorbol esters (Corasanti, Hepatol, 1989; 10:8), and chlorpromazine (Tavoloni, JPharmExpTher, 1980; 214:269), also reduce bile flow. Inadequate or mismatched perfusion ('perfusion–secretion mismatch') may partly explain the cholestasis associated with shock, cardiac failure, sickle cell crises, or vasoactive agents.

In summary, experimental models of intrahepatic cholestasis are associated with multiple functional and morphological abnormalities, each of which may impair bile secretion. To complicate the picture even further, cholestasis results in the intrahepatic accumulation of mono- and dihydroxy bile acids which can also cause liver damage and cholestasis (Scholmench, Hepatol, 1984; 4: 661), thereby perpetuating a vicious cycle of cholestatic liver injury. For this reason, it is often difficult to clarify in full the sequence and relative importance of the individual cellular events that contribute to the development of cholestasis.

Pathology[27–29]

Light microscopic examination of liver biopsies from patients with intrahepatic cholestasis only occasionally suggests a definite aetiology. For example, there may be features suggestive of viral or alcoholic hepatitis or neoplastic infiltration. However, in most cases the histological changes are non-specific. Bile may accumulate in the hepatocytes, Kupffer cells, and bile canaliculi. Typically, retention of bile is most marked in the centrilobular regions (zone III), probably because of the lobular gradient that determines bile flow (see under physiology of bile formation above). The intensity of bile staining varies from lobule to lobule, and bears no relationship to the severity of the clinical picture. The liver cells may be swollen and show 'feathery' degeneration. If the cholestasis is severe, bile infarcts, although seen more commonly in extrahepatic obstruction, can be found. Mononuclear cell infiltration is usually minimal in the areas of cholestasis. At a later stage, bile ductular cells may proliferate and mononuclear inflammatory cells may infiltrate the portal tracts. As cholestasis becomes chronic, periportal fibrosis develops and ultimately there is progression to portal–portal bridging and biliary cirrhosis.

All of the histological changes associated with intrahepatic cholestasis may also be seen in patients with obstruction of the large bile duct. Features that favour extrahepatic obstruction include bile plugging of the interlobular bile ducts, bile-stained infarcts, marked ductular proliferation, oedema, and a predominantly polymorphonuclear infiltration of the portal tracts. Often these features are absent and a distinction from intrahepatic cholestasis may not be possible.

Electron microscopic findings are also very similar whatever the cause of the cholestasis (Layden, Gastro, 1975; 69:724; Jones, Gastro, 1976; 71:1050; Adler, AmJPathol, 1980; 98:603). Prominent features include dilated bile canaliculi with blunting and a reduction in number of microvilli; tight junctions are disrupted. Several intracellular organelles are reduced in number, including the Golgi regions, rough endoplasmic reticulum, mitochondria, and lysosomes. Accumulations of bile-stained vesicles are often observed in the pericanalicular (apical) cytoplasm of the cell.

Features of the cholestatic syndrome (Table 3)

The clinical and biochemical features of the cholestatic syndrome result from: (i) accumulation of substances in the liver, blood, and other tissues that are normally excreted in bile, including bile acids, bilirubin, biliary lipids, and several liver plasma membrane enzymes; and (ii) malabsorption of fat and fat-soluble vitamins A, D, E, and K as a result of inadequate postprandial bile-acid concentrations in the upper small intestine.

Table 3 Clinical features of the cholestatic syndrome

	Clinical consequence
A. *Primary: accumulation of biliary constituents*	
Bilirubin	Jaundice
Bile acids	
Pruritogenic substances	Pruritus
Lipids	Xanthomata, xanthelasmata
	Hypercholesterolaemia
	Abnormal red cell morphology
Copper	Kayser-Fleischer rings (rare)
Liver enzymes	Alkaline phosphatase
	5′-Nucleotidase
	γ-Glutamyl transpeptidase
B. *Secondary: decreased intestinal content of bile acids, causing malabsorption of*	
Dietary fat	Steatorrhoea
	Weight loss
	? Finger clubbing
Vitamin A	Night blindness
Vitamin D	Osteomalacia
Vitamin E	Neuromyelopathy
Vitamin K	Bleeding tendency

Primary features
Jaundice and hyperbilirubinaemia

Bilirubin is taken up by the hepatocyte by a multispecific, yet to be cloned sodium-independent, organic acid transport carrier mechanism on the basolateral membrane (Berk, ProgLivDis, 1986; 8:125; Jacquemin, PNAS, 1994; 91:133; Kullack-Ublick, Gastro, 1995; 109:1274). Bilirubin is transported to the smooth endoplasmic reticulum bound to two cytosolic proteins (Y and Z protein) (Levi, JCI, 1969; 48:2176), where it is conjugated to form mono- and diglucuronides. Maximum bilirubin uptake and conjugation rates greatly exceed maximum bilirubin excretory rates, suggesting that excretion of conjugated bilirubin is the rate-limiting step in bilirubin clearance. Transport of conjugated bilirubin to the canalicular membrane involves at least two pathways, including binding to other cytosolic proteins and a vesicular pathway that can be inhibited by colchicine (Crawford, AmJPhysiol, 1988; 255:G121). Canalicular excretion of bilirubin occurs by a multispecific, ATP-dependent, organic anion transport mechanism (cMOAT/cMRP/MRP2) (Bruchler, JBC, 1996; 271:15091; Paulusma, Science, 1996; 271: 1126), which also transports other organic anions including bromosulphthalein and glutathione conjugates, but not bile acids (Alpert, JGenPhysiol, 1969; 53:238; Boyer, JCI, 1971; 49:206). However, bile acids can increase maximum rates of excretion of organic anions like bromosulphthalein and bilirubin (Boyer, JCI, 1971; 49:206; Goersky, CanJPhysPharm, 1984; 52:389), possibly by stimulating the transcytotic vesicular pathway (Crawford, AmJPhysiol, 1988; 255:G121; Hayakowa, Gastro, 1990; 99:216). Bile acid micelles may also bind bilirubin in the bile canaliculus thus forming a 'micellar sink' (Scharschmidt, JCI, 1978; 68:1122; Hayakawa, Gastro, 1990; 99:216).

Jaundice is not an invariable feature of cholestasis, and typically follows the onset of symptoms such as pruritus and raised serum alkaline phosphatase by weeks or even years, as often occurs in patients with primary biliary cirrhosis. However, even when total serum bilirubin levels are normal, elevations in the conjugated bilirubin fraction, which is normally less than 4 per cent (Muraca, ClinChem, 1983; 29:1767), can be demonstrated using high-performance liquid chromatography (Jansen, EurJClinInv, 1984; 14: 295). Indeed, serum conjugated bilirubin, or the conjugated/total bilirubin ratio, may be a more sensitive index of cholestasis than either serum alkaline phosphatase or serum bile acids (van Hootegem, Hepatol, 1985; 5:112). In contrast, in patients with haemolysis, both conjugated and unconjugated fractions show a modest increase in serum; however, their ratio remains normal (Muraca, Gastro, 1987; 92:309).

In patients with extrahepatic biliary obstruction, about 80 per cent of the serum bilirubin is in the form of glucuronide conjugates. In patients with intrahepatic cholestasis, the proportion of glucuronide conjugates is less, averaging 50 per cent, although it can vary from 10 to 90 per cent (Scharschmidt, Gut, 1982; 23:643). In contrast to normal bile, most conjugated bilirubin in the serum of patients with intrahepatic cholestasis is bilirubin monoglucuronide, owing to inhibition of diglucuronide formation by the accumulation of bilirubin in the liver. Most serum conjugated bilirubin is unbound and is easily filtered by the glomeruli, causing the urine to darken.

A further portion of conjugated bilirubin in the serum of patients with cholestasis becomes tightly bound to serum albumin through a covalent linkage. Clinical studies (Weiss, NEJM, 1983; 309:147) demonstrate that this fraction constitutes 20 to 50 per cent of total bilirubin in patients with cholestatic jaundice, but it is not found in patients with unconjugated hyperbilirubinaemia. This bilirubin–albumin fraction can constitute up to 90 per cent of total serum bilirubin during resolution of jaundice, because the disappearance of the bilirubin–albumin complex is determined by the half-life of albumin (10 to13 days) rather than by the restoration of excretory function. This explains why during resolution of cholestasis, conjugated bilirubin disappears from the urine within hours, whereas total serum bilirubin falls slowly and disappearance of jaundice may take several days or weeks.

The rise in unconjugated, monoconjugated, and diconjugated bilirubin fractions in serum implicates abnormalities in both hepatic conjugation and excretion. In contrast, bilirubin uptake is normal in several types of intrahepatic cholestasis,[30,31] although oatp activity is reduced (Gartung, Hepatol, 1996; 24:369A). This suggests that there are other, as yet unidentified, mechanisms for bilirubin uptake. Reductions in cytosolic binding proteins may diminish hepatic clearance (Gartnung, Gastro, 1996; 110:199); however, bilirubin excretion is impaired primarily as a result of diminished cMOAT/cMRP/MRP2 transporters at the canalicular domain, as recently demonstrated in endotoxin-induced cholestasis (Trauner, Gastro, 1997; 113:255). Regurgitation via abnormally permeable paracellular pathways may also play a role.

Because many organic anions, including radiographic contrast media, share canalicular excretory mechanisms (oatp/cMOAT) with bilirubin, their excretion is also impaired in patients with cholestasis and, consequently, the biliary tree often cannot be visualized during oral or intravenous cholangiography.

Serum bile acids[32]

The bile acid pool (~3 to 4 g) in adults circulates in the enterohepatic circulation about six times a day, and must be transported by the liver into bile. Serum levels of bile acids normally range up to $10\ \mu M$; about 20 per cent is cholic acid and most of the remainder is chenodeoxycholic and deoxycholic acid. After a meal, the flux of bile acids returning to the liver via the portal vein increases several fold, which, given a constant hepatic extraction ratio, leads to a small but detectable increase in the serum level of bile acid.

During cholestasis, the total serum level of bile acid can rise to 100 to 200 μM. As cholestasis progresses, increased proportions (up to 50 per cent) are sulphated and filtered by the kidney (Summerfield, ClinSci, 1977; 52:51).[33] Thus, urinary excretion limits the rise in serum bile acids even when there is complete cessation of bile flow.

Serum levels of bile acid are a more sensitive index of impaired bile secretion than serum total bilirubin, because only about 250 mg of bilirubin is excreted each day in contrast to the larger flux of bile acids. However, serum levels of bile acid are not more sensitive than serum levels of alkaline phosphatase in detecting most cholestatic disorders. Moreover, levels of serum bile acids may be raised in many forms of liver disease, including all forms of cirrhosis (Festi, Hepatol, 1983; 3:707) and acute and chronic hepatitis (Mishler, JAMA, 1981; 246:2340; Monroe, Hepatol, 1982; 2:317). Thus, total serum levels of bile acid are a sensitive but non-specific index of cholestasis.

Pruritus[34–36]

Pruritus is a major but not invariable feature of cholestasis, occurring in 20 to 50 per cent of patients with jaundice and in most patients with primary biliary cirrhosis. It may result in significant sleep deprivation and depression and even suicide. The pruritus of cholestasis has been commonly assumed to result from the accumulation of unidentified pruritogenic agents normally excreted in bile. A causative role for bile acids has been postulated for decades but direct evidence is lacking. Application of bile acids to skin blisters causes pruritus but at higher concentrations than found in cholestatic patients with pruritus (Kirby, BMJ, 1974; 4:693). There appears to be no correlation between pruritus severity and total levels of bile acid in serum, skin, or interstitial fluid (Ghent, Gastro, 1977; 73:1125; Friedman, AmJMed 1981; 70:1011; Bartholomew, ClinSci, 1982; 63:65). Patterns of individual bile acids and bile-acid conjugation and sulphation patterns are also similar in cholestatic patients, whether or not pruritus is present. The bile-acid binding agent cholestyramine often relieves the pruritus of cholestasis, but it may also relieve the pruritus of uraemia (Silverberg, BMJ, 1977; i:752) and polycythaemia rubra vera (Chanaru, BrJHaemat, 1970; 29:669), where serum bile acids are not elevated. Relief of pruritus by several other agents does not correlate with lowering of serum bile acids (Hanid, Lancet, 1980; ii:530; Lauterberg, Lancet, 1980; ii:53).

The pruritus in patients with cholestasis might result from an unidentified component of the liver which is released by the detergent action of retained bile acids (Ghent, AmJGastr, 1987; 82: 117). Consistent with this, rifampicin, which inhibits bile acid uptake into hepatocytes (Galezzi, DigDisSci, 1980; 25:108), may be useful in treating pruritus (Ghent, Gastro, 1988; 94:488).

Recently, work by Bergasa and Jones[35,36] has suggested that increased endogenous opiate activity contributes to the pruritus of cholestasis. Supporting observations in both humans and animals include: (i) several opiate agonists cause pruritus, which can be reversed by naloxone; (ii) opiate 'tone', serum encephalin levels, and liver encephalin mRNA are increased in cholestasis; and (iii) opiate antagonists improve the pruritus of cholestasis in double-blind studies. However in another study, no correlation was found between between methionine–encephalin levels and pruritus in patients with primary biliary cirrhosis (Spivey, AmJGastr, 1994; 89: 2628).

Serum alkaline phosphatase

Elevations in serum alkaline phosphatase are the most characteristic liver function abnormalities in cholestasis and are often the first clinical sign. The rise in serum alkaline phosphatase consists mainly of the hepatic isoenzyme (Brensilver, Gastro, 1975; 68:1556). Following acute bile duct ligation in rats, alkaline phosphatase activity in liver tissue increases several fold in parallel with its rise in serum, and peaks after 24 h of obstruction (Kaplan, JCI, 1970; 49:508; Seetharam, Hepatol, 1986; 6:374). It is thus dissociated from bile duct hyperplasia, which reaches a peak 7 days after bile duct ligation (Kaplan, CCActa, 1979; 99:113). The increase in hepatocyte alkaline phosphatase greatly exceeds that observed in bile ductular cells (Wootton, CCActa, 1975; 61:183). There is also a temporary and lesser rise in alkaline phosphatase in intestinal tissue (Komoda, AmJPhysiol, 1984; 246:G393). Immunoreactive alkaline phosphatase, as measured by a specific antibody, increases in parallel with enzyme activity (Schlaeger, JClinChemClinBioch, 1975; 13: 277), and the rise can be blocked by cyclohexamide (Kaplan, JCI, 1970; 49:508), suggesting that the increased enzyme activity reflects increases in enzyme synthesis rather than activation. No increase in liver or intestinal alkaline phosphatase mRNA can be demonstrated (Sheetharam, Hepatol, 1986; 6:374), suggesting that the signal for increased synthesis occurs at the translational level. Impaired degradation of alkaline phosphatase does not contribute to the raised serum levels since the half-life of infused alkaline phosphatase is normal in patients with cholestasis (Clubb, JLabClinMed, 1965; 66: 493).

In normal rats, alkaline phosphatase is found in two forms: one in the cytosol and the other in the plasma membrane; following bile duct ligation the increase is in the plasma membrane fraction (Simon, JCI, 1973; 52:756), which expands from its normal canalicular location to involve the entire membrane (Komoda, AmJPhysiol, 1984; 256:G393).[27] Functional studies suggest that some canalicular membrane bile-acid transport activity is also translocated to the basolateral membrane (Fricker, JCI, 1989; 84:876), suggesting that hepatocyte secretory polarity is reversed, as occurs normally in the neonate. Interestingly, such reversed secretory polarity is not seen in experimental oestrogen-induced cholestasis (Fricker, Hepatol, 1988; 8:1224), which may explain why serum alkaline phosphatase is only mildly raised in clinical cholestasis associated with oestrogen use (Ockner, NEJM, 1967; 276:331).

The rise in serum alkaline phosphatase during cholestasis may be related in part to increased hepatic bile acid concentrations. Bile acids increase alkaline phosphatase synthesis in isolated hepatocytes (Hatoff, Gastro, 1979; 77:1062) and also increase biliary excretion of alkaline phosphatase (Hatoff, Hepatol, 1982; 2:433). Thus, the increase in serum levels of alkaline phosphatase that is observed following bile duct ligation (Hatoff, Gastro, 1981; 80:666) probably

results from the detergent action of bile acids on hepatocyte plasma membranes. Bile acids that have little or no detergent effects, such as ursodeoxycholic acid, release much less alkaline phosphatase in these experimental models, a phenomenon that may partly explain how ursodeoxycholic acid lowers serum alkaline phosphatase in patients with several cholestatic disorder (see section on urso-deoxycholic acid treatment below). Alkaline phosphatase in the serum of patients with cholestasis is also associated with plasma membrane vesicle fragments (De Brol, Hepatol, 1985; 5:118), a finding which is again consistent with a detergent effect of bile acids on plasma membrane. Finally, in rats with choledochocaval fistulas, where there is retention of biliary constituents without cholestasis, serum alkaline phosphatase levels are even higher than in animals with ligated bile ducts, as a result of increased rather than decreased transhepatic bile acid flux in this experimental model (Hardison, Hepatol, 1983; 3:383). In addition to bile acids, a heat-stable constituent of bile with a low molecular weight may play a role in inducing hepatocyte synthesis of alkaline phosphatase (Komoda, AmJPhysiol, 1984; 246:G393).

γ-Glutamyl transferase

This enzyme is found on the canalicular membrane of hepatocytes and the apical membrane of bile ductular cells. Following bile duct ligation in rats, liver γ-glutamyl transferase activity and mRNA increase progressively (Bulle, Hepatol, 1990; 11:545). The increase parallels the bile ductular proliferative response and most of the histochemically demonstrable γ-glutamyl transferase activity is in bile ductular cells, with relatively little in hepatocytes.

Serum γ-glutamyl transferase levels are increased in most liver diseases and in a variety of other situations (see Chapter 6.1). Levels are increased in most forms of cholestasis; exceptions include one form of progressive familial intrahepatic cholestasis (Byler's disease) and benign recurrent intrahepatic cholestasis, where levels are usually normal, despite (in the case of Byler's disease) high γ-glutamyl transferase activity in liver tissue (Chobert, JHepatol, 1989; 8:22). Biliary excretion of γ-glutamyl transferase in animals is dependent on bile acid secretion (Hirada, JBiochem(Tokyo) 1984; 96:289). The failure of serum γ-glutamyl transferase to increase in these two cholestatic diseases might thus result from a postulated primary failure of bile acid secretion (Jacquemin, EurJPed, 1994; 153:424).

Hyperlipidaemia[37,38]

Cholesterol and phospholipids are excreted in bile in the form of lipid vesicles[18] and are associated with bile acids in mixed micelles. Therefore, serum levels of total cholesterol and phospholipids are increased in patients with chronic cholestasis; serum triglycerides may also be raised. Several abnormalities of serum lipoproteins have been described and may in part result from an associated deficiency of serum lecithin cholesterol acyl transferase (Agorastos, ClinSci, 1978; 54:369). Some of the cholesterol is incorporated into an abnormal serum low-density lipoprotein termed lipoprotein X, which also contains phospholipid, albumin, and apolipoprotein C. When bile is incubated with albumin or serum, a complex is formed that is very similar to lipoprotein X, suggesting that this abnormal lipoprotein is formed from interaction of plasma with refluxed biliary constituents (Manzato, JCI, 1976; 57:1248). Serum levels of lipoprotein X tend to be higher in patients with extrahepatic obstruction than in those with intrahepatic cholestasis, but there is a large degree of overlap and the test is of little discriminatory value (Meredith, ArchPathLabMed, 1986; 110:1123). Bile duct ligated mdr2C(-/-) deficient mice fail to produce lipoprotein X, consistent with their inability to secrete phospholipids into bile (Oude-Elbenink, Hepatol, 1997; 26:369A).

Chronic hyperlipidaemia results in the formation of cholesterol deposits in the periorbital skin folds (xanthelasmas) and in tendon sheaths, bony prominences, and peripheral nerves (xanthomas). Cholesterol also accumulates in red cell membranes, resulting in diminished membrane fluidity (Owen, JLipRes, 1982; 23:124). The presence of deformed cells (echinocytes) on wet films in patients with cholestasis and other liver diseases has been ascribed to an abnormal high-density lipoprotein, enriched in apolipoprotein E (Owen, JCI, 1985; 76:2275). However, there is no evidence that cholestasis predisposes to atheroma or to coronary artery disease (Propst, DigDisSci, 1993; 38:379), perhaps because this abnormal high-density lipoprotein inhibits cellular uptake of low-density lipoprotein particles (Owen, JLipRes, 1984; 25:919).

Copper accumulation[39]

Bile is the major route for copper excretion. Thus, in long-standing cholestatic diseases, such as primary biliary cirrhosis (Fleming, Gastro, 1974; 67:1182), primary sclerosing cholangitis (Gross, Gastro, 1985; 89:272), and Byler's disease (Evans, Gastro, 1978; 75: 875), copper concentrations in the liver may approach those found in Wilson's disease. In contrast to Wilson's disease, however, serum copper and caeruloplasmin tend to be normal or high in patients with chronic cholestasis. Corneal deposition of copper may rarely give rise to Kayser–Fleischer rings in cholestasis (Jones, Gastro, 1976; 71:675; Fleming, AnnIntMed, 1977; 86:285), and copper deposition in the kidney has been implicated in the pathogenesis of the renal tubular acidosis associated with primary biliary cirrhosis (Pare, Gastro, 1981; 80:681). However, copper is no longer thought to make an important contribution to secondary liver damage in patients with cholestasis.

Secondary consequences of cholestasis
Fat malabsorption

Steatorrhoea is common in patients in advanced stages of chronic cholestatic liver disease and is due primarily to an inability to digest dietary lipids as a result of impaired intestinal bile-acid delivery and inadequate micelle formation (Ros, Gastro, 1984; 93:584). Coincidental pancreatic enzyme deficiency (Epstein, Gastro, 1982; 83:1177), small bowel disease (Logan, Lancet, 1978; ii:230), and cholestyramine therapy may also be contributing factors. Fat malabsorption often results in profound weight loss in patients with advanced chronic cholestasis (Beckett, Gut, 1980; 21:734). Patients with idiopathic cholestasis of pregnancy also may have biochemical evidence of steatorrhoea (Reyes, Gastro, 1987; 93:584), which can result in failure to gain weight normally during pregnancy. Steatorrhoea also results in decreased absorption of fat-soluble vitamins (see below), and impaired calcium absorption due to the formation of insoluble calcium–fatty acid complexes (soaps).

Bone disease[40,41]

The major bone disease in chronic cholestasis is osteoporosis. Between 10 and 40 per cent of patients have vertebral thinning and/or crush fractures on radiography (Stellon, QJMed, 1985; 223: 783; Compston, DigDisSci, 1989; 25:28). Bone mineral density, as measured by dual photon absorpiometry,[42] (van Berkum, Gastro, 1990; 98:1134; Hay, Hepatol, 1991; 14:257) and trabecular bone volume, measured by histomorphometry[44–46] (Diamond, Gastro, 1989; 96:213; Guanabens, AmJGastr, 1990; 85:1396), are lower in patients with chronic cholestasis than in age- and sex-matched controls, and in 10 to 40 per cent of cases are more than 2 standard deviations below the mean for age and sex.. In longitudinal studies, patients with primary biliary cirrhosis lose bone at double the normal rate.[42] Bone mineral density correlates inversely with severity and duration of cholestasis.

Some reports from the United Kingdom suggested a high (25 to 60 per cent) prevalence of osteomalacia in cholestatic liver disease (Atkinson, QJMed, 1956; 99:299; Long, Gut, 1978; 19:85); however, when defined by strict histological criteria, including measurement of calcification rate by tetracycline labelling, this lesion is observed in less than 15 per cent of patients (Stellon, Bone, 1986; 7:1181).[43–45]

Despite its relative rarity, the pathogenesis of the osteomalacia has been extensively studied. Vitamin D, whether synthesized in the skin or absorbed from the diet, is first hydroxylated at the C-25 position in liver microsomes, then at the C-1 position in the kidney to form the biologically active molecule 1,25-dihydroxy-cholecalciferol. In primary biliary cirrhosis, serum vitamin D and 25-hydroxyvitamin D levels tend to be low or low normal (Kaplan, Gastro, 1981; 81:681; Davies, DigDisSci, 1983; 28:145).[41,43–46] Reasons include inadequate intraluminal bile-salt concentrations, and ingestion of cholestyramine for pruritus (Thompson, Gut, 1969; 10:717), resulting in dietary vitamin D malabsorption (Compston, Lancet, 1977; i:721); however, a major additional factor in northern climates may be reduced exposure to sunlight. 25-Hydroxylation rates are well preserved in liver disease (Krawitt, Lancet, 1977; ii:1246; Skinner, Lancet, 1977; i:720), and serum levels of 25-hydroxyvitamin D can be returned to normal by parenteral or oral vitamin D or 25-hydroxyvitamin D supplementation.[46] Despite the low serum 25-hydroxyvitamin D, increased renal 1-hydroxylation usually maintains normal serum levels of 1,25-dihydroxyvitamin D (Davies, DigDisSci, 1983; 28:145), probably explaining the relative rarity of osteomalacia.

The pathogenesis of the osteoporosis is not understood. Bone mineral density is unrelated to vitamin D status and is unaffected by vitamion D supplementation (Kaplan, Gastro, 1981; 81:681).[44, 45] Most, although not all (Mitchison, Hepatol, 1989; 9:528), histological studies in patients with primary biliary cirrhosis have demonstrated reduced osteoid seam width and bone formation rates, suggestive of reduced osteoblast function (Stellon, Hepatol, 1987; 7:136; Guanabens, AmJGastr, 1990; 85:1396).[43,44] These patients also have low serum levels of osteocalcin or Gla protein, an index of osteoblast function.[43] Osteocalcin undergoes vitamin K-dependent carboxylation, like some plasma clotting factors (Hauschka, PhysiolRev, 1989; 69:990), but bone mineral density in patients with cholestasis appears unrelated to vitamin K status (Aguilar, Gastro, 1993; 1104:A868); therefore whether vitamin K deficiency contributes to the osteoporosis remains speculative. Some studies, (Cuthbert, Hepatol, 1984; 4:1; Stellon, Hepatol, 1987; 7:136) but not others,[43] have also demonstrated an increased surface area of bone resorption in patients with primary biliary cirrhosis. A direct effect of cholestasis on bone formation is suggested by recent experiments (Janes, JCI, 1995; 95:2581) in which serum from patients with cholestasis inhibited proliferation of cultured osteoblasts. The serum inhibitor seemed to be bilirubin because the effect was simulated by bilirubin but not by bile acids and was blocked by removal of bilirubin from serum by photobleaching.

Other likely contributing factors to the osteoporosis include malabsorption of calcium (Guanabens, AmJGastr, 1990; 85:1356),[44] steroid treatment of the underlying liver disease, immobility, generalized failure of protein synthesis, and malnutrition.

Vitamin A deficiency[47]

Low serum levels of vitamin A are commonly found in patients with primary biliary cirrhosis (Herlong, Hepatol, 1981; 1:348), and are occasionally associated with impairment of dark adaptation (Walt, BMJ, 1984; 288:1030; Shepherd, BMJ, 1984; 289:1484).

Vitamin E deficiency[47]

Clinical evidence of vitamin E deficiency develops by 4 years of age in 50 per cent of children who present with cholestasis at infancy (Sokol, GastrClinNAm, 1994; 23:673). Hyporeflexia is usually the initial manifestation, and the condition may gradually progress to include ataxia, loss of vibration and position sensation, peripheral neuropathy, gaze palsies, and quadriplegia (Guggenheim, JPediat, 1982; 100:51; Rosenblum, NEJM, 1985; 304:503). Nerve conduction velocities are preserved, suggesting an axonal type of neuropathy (Guggenheim, JPediat, 1982; 100:51). Vitamin E deficiency results from malabsorption of vitamin E due to low intraluminal bile-acid concentrations (Sokol, Gastro, 1983; 85:1172). Serum vitamin E levels are usually low but may be normal in cases of hyperlipidaemia. The serum vitamin E to total lipid ratio has been proposed as a more accurate index of vitamin E status (Sokol, NEJM, 1984; 310:1209). Vitamin E concentrations in muscle and fat are also low.

Low serum levels of vitamin E are also found in 20 to 60 per cent of adults with cholestasis, especially when long standing and severe (Sokol, AmJClinNut, 1985; 41:66; Jeffrey, JHepatol, 1987; 4:307). However, clinical evidence of neuropathy in adult patients is rare and when present cannot usually be ascribed to vitamin E deficiency.

Vitamin K deficiency[47]

Vitamin K is a cofactor in a post-translational modification of clotting factors II, VII, IX, and X (Stenflo, PNAS, 1974; 71:2730). Malabsorption of vitamin K results in prolongation of the prothrombin time (due to impaired activity of factors II, VII, and X) and a modest prolongation of the partial thromboplastin time (due to reduced factor IX activity). Because stores of vitamin K are limited, cholestasis, even of short duration, is associated with low serum levels of vitamin K (O'Brien, JRSM, 1994; 87:320) and often prolongation of the prothrombin time. In the absence of associated liver disease, serious haemorrhage is uncommon but it has been observed in infants (Bancroft, JPediatGastrNutr, 1993; 16:78) and

during treatment with cholestyramine (Gross, AnnIntMed, 1970; 72:95).

Specific intrahepatic cholestatic disorders
Hepatitis

Histological features of cholestasis are common in acute viral hepatitis (Section 12) and may be the dominant feature (Sciot, JHepatol, 1986; 3:172). Less commonly, the clinical picture of viral hepatitis is dominated by cholestasis, with prolonged jaundice and pruritus, lasting several months (Shaldon, BMJ, 1957; ii:734; Overholt, ArchIntMed, 1959; 103:859). Fever may be present and weight loss may occur, but patients usually otherwise feel well. Serum alkaline phosphatase is always raised, but serum aminotransferases are often minimally elevated, especially in the later stages of the disease. Distinction from extrahepatic obstruction may require endoscopic or percutaneous cholangiography. Prolonged cholestasis has been described in association with hepatitis A (Gordon, AnnIntMed, 1984; 101:635), hepatitis B (Laverdant, AnnMedIntern, 1973; 124:607), and cytomegalovirus infection (Takeuchi, IntMed, 1992; 312:1376). The pathogenesis of cholestatic viral hepatitis is not understood, but a factor has been isolated from patients' serum and lymphocytes that causes cholestasis in rats (Marbert, EurJClinInv, 1984; 14:346; Mizoguchi, AnnAllergy, 1986; 56:304), suggesting that the cholestasis may be an idiosyncratic immunologically mediated response. Release of cytokines (interleukin-1, tumour necrosis factor-α), which may mediate cholestasis of sepsis (see below), may also play a role in cholestatic hepatitis. Corticosteroids produce a rapid fall in serum bilirubin and relieve pruritus in about two-thirds of such patients (Summerskill, BMJ, 1958; ii:1499).

Cholestasis may be the major presenting feature in autoimmune chronic active hepatitis (Cooksley, AmJDigDis, 1972; 17:495; Krawitt, NEJM, 1995; 334:897) (Section 7). Alcoholic hepatitis and alcoholic fatty liver (Chapter 15.3) may also present with cholestatic jaundice, often in association with severe pain in the right upper quadrant, fever, and leucocytosis (Morgan, ScaJGastr, 1978; 13:299). Serum alkaline phosphatase is usually raised, but serum aminotransferases may be normal and rarely exceed 200 U/l. These findings may mimic acute cholangitis. The condition must be recognized in order to avoid the high mortality associated with unnecessary surgery. Sometimes the presenting feature of alcoholic liver disease is a marked elevation of serum alkaline phosphatase (Perillo, DigDisSci, 1978; 23:1061). Histological evidence of cholestasis is common in patients with alcoholic hepatitis. It is not always associated with jaundice but is of adverse prognostic significance (Nissenbaum, DigDisSci, 1990; 35:891).

About 20 per cent of patients who undergo liver transplantation for chronic hepatitis B develop cholestatic fibrosing hepatitis in the transplanted liver (Davies, Hepatol, 1991; 13:150; Benner, Gastro, 1992; 103:1307). Cholestasis is prominent with marked hyperbilirubinaemia but only mildly elevated aminotransferases. However, patients also develop progressive hepatocellular failure with encephalopathy and coagulopathy. Liver biopsy shows a characteristic histological pattern comprising cholestasis, periportal fibrosis, hepatocyte ballooning, and only mild inflammation. Hepatocytes contain large amounts of hepatitis B antigens (surface and core) (Lau, Gastro, 1992; 102:956) and also have high expression of hepatitis B DNA and RNA (Mason, Gastro, 1993; 105:237). The disease is thought to result from a direct cytopathic effect of uncontrolled hepatitis B replication and antigen production.

The development of fibrosing cholestatic hepatitis is more likely in patients infected with pre-core mutant forms of hepatitis B than with the 'wild' type (Angus, Hepatol, 1995; 21:14). The condition is not seen in uncomplicated hepatitis B but has developed in patients with hepatitis B if they undergo renal (Lam, Transpl, 1996; 61:378) or bone marrow (McIvor, AnnIntMed, 1993; 121:274) transplantation or if they also have HIV infection (Fang, Lancet, 1993; 342:1175), suggesting that immunosuppression may also be a predisposing factor.

The outlook is very poor. Liver transplantation or re-transplantation is usually followed by early and severe recurrence of the disease. Few patients survive more than a few months after diagnosis. Systemic antiviral agents such as ganciclovir may sometimes arrest progression of liver disease (Jinal, AmJGastr, 1996; 91:1027).

Recently, a similar progressive cholestatic syndrome with hepatocellular failure has been described in patients with hepatitis C infection following liver transplantation. (Dickson, Transpl, 1996; 61:701; Schluger, Hepatol, 1996; 23:973) and heart transplantation (Lim, Gastro, 1994; 106:248).

Drug-induced cholestasis (Table 4)[9,48–51]

Drug-induced cholestasis accounts for approximately 2 per cent of patients presenting with jaundice (Bjarnaboe, ActaMedScand, 1980; 182:491). Diagnostic criteria have recently been proposed by an international consensus group (Benichou, JHepatol, 1990; 11:272). Usually cholestasis develops between 1 week and 3 months after the drug is administered. However, several drugs have sometimes been associated with longer latency periods; examples include diclofenac, labetalol, methyltestosterone, amiodarone, captopril, and chinese herbs. Furthermore, the latency period may be as short as 24 h if the patient has been exposed to the drug previously. Importantly, the onset of cholestasis may also be as long as 1 month after cessation of drug administration. This phenomenon has been described with cholestasis following exposure to several antibiotics, including amoxycillin/clavulanic acid, flucloxacillin, thiabendazole, and clindamycin.

Clinical and laboratory features are non-specific. There is often a prodromal illness resembling viral hepatitis. There may be severe pain in the right upper quadrant and fever is found in about one-quarter of cases. Other features of a generalized hypersensitivity reaction are much rarer. For example, skin rash is a common feature with a small number of drugs, including allopurinol, sulindac, and thiabendazole. Peripheral blood eosinophilia is found in less than 10 per cent of cases, although it appears to be more common in cases related to certain drugs, including amoxycillin/clavulanic acid, erythromycin, captopril, carbamazepine, and flucloxacillin.

Serum aminotransferases are usually raised in drug-induced cholestasis, sometimes by more than 10-fold, even in cases where the histological abnormality is confined to the portal tracts. However, aminotransferase values over 1000 U/l are uncommon and are usually associated with prominent hepatocellular damage on liver biopsy, reflecting a mixed cholestatic and parenchymal cell pattern of injury (see below).

Usually, symptoms and liver enzymes resolve progressively following withdrawal of the drug. Prolonged cholestasis, including jaundice for more than 6 months and/or liver enzyme abnormalities lasting more than 12 months, has been observed following reactions to several drugs (see Table 4), although this is unusual. Such cases are usually associated with bile duct paucity on liver biopsy (DeGott, Hepatol, 1992; 15:244; Davies; JHepatol, 1994; 20:112).

Drugs which produce cholestasis may also be associated with a variety of liver biopsy abnormalities.[29] With some drugs, designated H in Table 4, the predominant lesion is hepatocellular degeneration and necrosis, often accompanied by a chronic inflammatory cell infiltrate of the lobules that mimics viral hepatitis. The cholestasis is often mild and the clinical picture is that of an acute systemic illness, associated with high serum aminotransferases and hepatocellular dysfunction, occasionally progressing to hepatic failure.

However, with most drugs, designated C in Table 4, clinical and histological features of cholestasis predominate. Liver biopsies show evidence of cholestasis and an inflammatory cell infiltrate, involving the portal tracts. Lymphocytes predominate and eosinophils may be present, but are inconsistently seen and are not specific for drug-related injury.[29] Indeed, like peripheral eosinophilia, a predominately eosinophilic portal infiltrate is rare. It is increasingly recognized that many drugs produce injury to the interlobular bile-duct epithelium, including ajmaline, amitriptyline, (DeGott, Hepatol, 1992; 15:244), amoxycillin/clavulanic acid (Hautekete, JHepatol, 1995; 22:71), clindamycin, flucloxacillin, carbamazepine (Larrey, DigDisSci, 1987; 32:554), azathioprine (Horsmans, Liver, 1991; 11:89), and phenytoin. Sometimes there is polymorphonucleocyte infiltration, mimicking acute bacterial cholangitis. In other cases, bile duct paucity is seen sometimes in the early stages and coexisting with evidence of acute bile duct injury, but more often as an accompanying feature of prolonged drug-induced cholestasis (see below). In addition to portal tract pathology, there are variable degrees of hepatocellular damage or necrosis, most commonly in the periportal region. Indeed, many drugs, designated CH in Table 4, are associated with a mixed histological pattern, with features of both cholestasis and hepatocellular injury of comparable severity.

In patients with prolonged drug-induced cholestasis, acute bile duct injury and a portal inflammatory infiltrate are seen in the early stages (Degott, Hepatol, 1992; 15:244). The predominant abnormality, especially in biopsies obtained where cholestasis has lasted more than 6 months, is bile duct paucity (see section below). In addition, there may be ductal oedema and fibrosis and, occasionally, cirrhosis. Such cases may closely resemble primary biliary cirrhosis, but antimitochondrial antibody is typically absent from serum.

Cholestasis resulting from steroid hormones such as oestrogens is characteristically manifested on light microscopy by centrilobular canalicular bile retention, and only minimal portal inflammation and necrosis. This histological picture is sometimes termed 'bland' cholestasis. Similar changes may be induced by cyclosporin.

Cholestasis associated with damage to the larger interlobular bile ducts is a special feature of diaminodiphenylethane poisoning, described in an epidemic in Epping in the 1960s (Koppelman, QJMed, 1966; 35:533). A condition resembling primary sclerosing

Table 4 Drugs in current usage reported as causing intrahepatic cholestasis

Hormone derivatives
C Oestrogens (Kreek, SemLivDis, 1987; 7:8, * Weden, JIntMed, 1992; 23:1561)
C Methyltestosterone (* Hartleb, AmJGastro, 1990; 85:766)
C Other C-17 anabolic steroids (Ishak, SemLivDis, 1981; 1:116)
C 19-Norandrostenolone (Garrigues Gil, AnnIntMed, 1986; 104:135)
C Megesterol (Forth, Cancer, 1989; 63:438)
C Danazol (Boue, AnnIntMed, 1986; 105:139)
CH Flutamide (Wysowski, AnnIntMed, 1993; 118:860)
C Stanozol (Evely, BMJ, 1987; 294:612).

Sedatives and relaxants
C Phenothiazines (general) (Ishak, ArchPath, 1972; 93:283)
H Chloroxazone (Powers, ArchIntMed, 1986; 146:1183)
C Chlorpromazine (* Moradpour, Hepatol, 1994; 20:437)
C Clozapine (Dorta, ZGastr, 1989; 27:388)
C Prochlorperazine (* Lok, JHepatol, 1988; 6:369)
C Fluphenazine (Snyder, AmJGastro, 1980; 73:336)
C Thoridiazine (Reinhart, JAMA, 1966; 197:113)
C Trifluperazine (Kohn, NEJM, 1961; 264:549)
C Haloperidol (* Dincsoy, Gastro, 1982; 83:694)
C Phenobarbitone (* Pagliaro, Gastro, 1969; 56:938)
C Potassium chlorazepate (Parker, PostMedJ, 1979; 55:908)
C Chlordiazepoxide (Abbruzzese, NEJM, 1965; 273:321)
C Flurazepam (Fang, AnnIntMed, 1978; 89:363)
C Triazolam (Cobden, PostgradMedJ, 1981; 57:730)

Anaesthetic agents
H Halothane (Thomas, AnnIntMed, 1974; 81:487)
CH Thiopentone (Hasselstrom, BrJAnaesth, 1979; 51:801)
CH Enfluorane (Foutch, CleveMedJ, 1982; 54:210)
C Enoxacin (Amitrano, JHepatol, 1993; 18:139)
C Propafenone (Konz, DrschMedWoch, 1984; 109:1525)

Hypoglycaemics
C Tolbutamide (* Gregory, ArchPath, 1967; 84:194)
CH Glibenclamide (Peres-Roldan, RevEspEnfDig, 1995; 87174)
H Chlorpropamide (Schneider, AmJGastro, 1984; 79:721, * Geubel, Liver, 1988; 8:350)
C Tolazamide (Bridges, SouthMedJ, 1980; 73:1072)

Antimicrobial drugs
C Amoxycillin (* Davies, JHepatol, 1992; 20:112)
C Amoxycillin clavulanic acid (Larrey, Gut, 1992; 36:368)
C Ampicillin (* Cavanzo, Gastro, 1990; 99:854)
C Azithromycin (Longo, AmJMed, 1997; 102:217)
C Cefaclor (Bosio, JToxicol, 1983; 20:79)
CH Ceftibuten (Combe, ZGastr, 1996; 34:434)
Chloramphenicol (48)
C Ciprofloxacin (Hautekete, JHepatol, 1995; 23:759)
C Clindamycin (Altraif, AmJGastro, 1994; 89:1230)
C Cloxacillin (Enat, BMJ, 1980; 280:482)
C Co-trimoxazole (Minoz, Hepatol, 1990; 12:342, *Knowdley, Gastro, 1992; 102:2148)
CH Dapsone (Johnson, ArchIntMed, 1986; 146:875)
C Dicloxacillin (Tauris, ActaMedScand, 1985; 217:567)
C Erythromycin estolate (Zafrani, DigDisSci, 1979; 24:385)
C Erythromycin ethylsuccinate (Diehl, AmJMed, 1984; 76:931, * 48b)
C Erythromycin stearate (Inman, BMJ, 1983; 286:1954)
C Ethambutol (Guillford, BMJ, 1986; 292:866)
C Flucloxacillin (Turner, MedJAust, 1989; 151:701, * Davies, JHepatol, 1994; 20:112)
CH Fusidic acid (Humble, BMJ, 1980; 280:1495)
C Griseofulvin (Chirput, Gastro, 1976; 70:1141)
H Isoniazid (Bistritzer, JPediatr, 1980; 97:480, Mitchell, AnnIntMed, 1986; 84:181)
CH Ketoconazole (Benson, DigDisSci, 1988; 35:240)
C Nafcillin (Presti, DigDisSci; 1996; 41:180)
CH Nitrofurantoin (Engel, ArchIntMed, 1975; 135:733)
C Oxacillin (Ten Pas, JAMA, 1965; 191:138)
Para-amino-salicylic acid (Simpson, AmJMed, 1960; 29:297)
CH Piperazine (Hamlyn, Gastro, 1976; 70:1144)
H Rifampicin (Bachs, Gastro, 1992; 102:2077)
C Spiramycin (Denie, JHepatol, 1992; 16:386)
CH Sulphamethoxazole (Steinbrecher, DigDisSci, 1981; 26:756)
C Terbinafine (* Mallat, DigDisSci, 1987; 42:1486)
C Tetracyclines (* Hunt, Gastro, 1994; 107:1844)
C Thiabendazole (Manival, Gastro, 1987; 93:245)
C Ticarcillin-clavulinic acid (Sweet, AmJGastro, 1995; 90:675)
C Trimethoprim (Tanner, BMJ, 1986; 293:1072)
C Troleandomycin (* Larrey, JHepatol, 1987; 4:327)

Table 4 *Continued*

Anti-inflammatory and immunosuppressive agents
H Aspirin (Benson, AmJMed, 1983; Suppl Nov 14:85)
CH Azathioprine (DePinho, Gastro, 1984; 86:162, Horsmans, Liver, 1991; 11:89)
C Cyclosporin (Kallinowski, Transplantation, 1991; 51:1128)
C Dextropropoxyphene (Bassendine, Gut, 1986; 27:644)
CH Diclofenac (Banks, Hepatol, 1995; 22:820)
C Diflunisal (Warren, BMJ, 1978; 2:736)
H Etodolac (Mabee, AmJGastro, 1995; 90:659)
FK-506 (Tacrolimus) (Fisher, Transplantation, 1995; 59:1631)
C Ibuprofen (Alam, AmJGastro, 1996; 91:1626)
C Gold (Favreau, AnnIntMed, 1977; 81:717)
CH Indomethacin (Fenech, BMJ, 1967; 3:155)
H Mesalazine (Hautekete, Gastro, 1992; 103:1925)
C Naproxen (Victorino, PostgradMedJ, 1980; 56:368)
H Penicillamine (Mutz, JAMA, 1981; 246:674)
CH Phenylbutazone (Benjamin, Hepatol, 1981; 1:255)
H Piroxicam (Planas, AmJGastro, 1990; 85:468)
H Sulphasalazine (Mihas, JAMA, 1979; 72:561)
CH Sulindac (Terazi, Gastro, 1993; 104:569)

Antidepressants
C Amitriptyline (* Larrey, Gastro, 1988; 94:200, 48b)
CH Imipramine (* Horst, Gastro, 1980; 79:550)
C Fluoxetine (Cosme, AmJGastro, 1996; 91:2449)
CH Mocobemide (Timmings, Lancet, 1996; 347:762)

Anticonvulsants
C Phenytoin (Spechler, AnnIntMed, 1981; 95:455, * Campbell, DigDisSci, 1977; 22:255)
C Carbamazapine (Larrey, DigDisSci, 1987; 32:554, * Forbes, Gastro, 1992; 102:1385)
H Sodium valproate (Zimmerman, Hepatol, 1982; 2:591)

Antimitotic agents
C Busulphan (Underwood, BMJ, 1971; 1:556)
CH Chlorambucil (Amronin, Gastro, 1962; 42:401)
Cisplatinum (Cavalli, CancerTreatRep, 1978; 62:2125)
C Cytosine arabinoside (George, Cancer, 1984; 54:2360)
CH Etoposide (Tran, JHepatol, 1991; 12:36)

Antacids
CH Cimetidine (van Steerbergen, JHepatol, 1985; 1:359)
H Ranitidine (Souza-Lima, AnnIntMed, 1986; 105:140)
CH Famotidine (Arrent, AnnPharmTher, 1994; 28:40)
H Nizatidine (Chey, JClinGastro, 1995; 20:164)
H Omeprazole (Jochem, AmJGastro, 1992; 87:523)

Antithyroid drugs
C Carbimazole (Blom, ArchIntMed, 1985; 145:1513)
H Propylthiouracil (Hanson, ArchIntMed, 1984; 144:994)
CH Methimazole (Schmidt, Hepatogast, 1986; 33:244)

Cardiovascular drugs
C Ajmaline (* Larrey, JHepatol, 1986; 2:81, 48b)
C Amiodarone (Macarri, ItalJGastro, 1995; 27:436)
C Atenolol (Schwartz, AmJGastro, 1989; 84:1084)
CH Captopril (Rahmat, AnnIntMed, 1985; 102:56)
H Disopyramide (Meinertz, Lancet, 1977; ii:828)
C Flecainide (Hopmann, DtschMedWoch, 1994; 109:1863)
CH Hydralazine (Itoh, DigDisSci, 1980; 25:884)
H Labetalol (Clarke, AnnIntMed, 1990; 113:210)
H Lisinopril (Larrey, Gastro, 1988; 99:1832)
H Methyldopa (Rodman, AmJMed, 1976; 60:941)
CH Nifedepine (Rotmench, BMJ, 1980; 281:976)
C Procainamide (Ahn, ArchIntMed, 1990; 150:2589)
C Quinidine (Hogan, CanMedAssJ, 1984; 130:973)
CH Chlorthiazide (Drerup, MEJM, 1958; 259:534)
C Verapamil (Guarascio, BMJ, 288:362)

Anticoagulants and antiplatelet agents
C Warfarin (Adler, ArchIntMed, 1985; 146:837)
CH Phenindione (Hargreaves, BrHeartJ, 1963; 27:932)
C Ticlodipine (Grimm, AmJGastro, 1994; 89:279)

Lipid-lowering drugs
C Clofibrate (Valdes, AmJGastr, 1976; 66:69)
C Fenofibrate (Lepicard, GastroClinBiol, 1994; 18:1033)
H Lovastatin (Hucherzermeyer, DtschMedWoch, 1995; 120:252)
C Nicotinic acid (Einstein, AmJDigDis, 1975; 20:282)

Table 4 *Continued*

Herbal preparations
Chaparral (Katz, JClinGastro, 1990; 12:203)
H Germander (Larrey, AnnIntMed, 1992; 117:129)
CH Jin bu huan (Woolf, AnnIntMed, 1994; 121:729)
H Valerian (McGreger, BMJ, 1989; 299;1156)
CH Xaio-chai-hu-tang (Itoh, DigDisSci, 1995; 40:1845)
C Ackee-fruit (Larson, AmJGastro, 1994; 898:577)

Miscellaneous
H Allopurinol (Al Kawas, AnnIntMed, 1981; 95:588)
C Cyproheptadine (* Larrey, JClinGastr, 1987; 9:102)
CH Dantrolene (Wilkinson, Gut, 1979; 220:33)
CH Disulfiram (Bartle, DigDisSci, 1985; 30:834)
CH Etretinate (Kano, JAmAcadDerm, 1994; 31:133)
H Nicotinamide (Winter, NEJM, 1973; 289:1180)
Danthron plus dioctyl calcium sulfosuccinate ('Doxidan') (Tolman, AnnIntMed, 1976; 84:290)
Senna (Beuers, Lancet, 1991; 337:372
C Tiopronin (Nada, JpnJGastro, 1996; 93:216)

Cholestasis is defined here as either jaundice or pruritus; drugs which induce only asymptomatic liver enzyme abnormalities are not included. Where possible, references are chosen which either describe series of several cases or include up to date literature reviews. C: cholestasis predominant; H: hepatocellular damage predominant; CH: mixed lesion; * may cause prolonged cholestasis, defined as jaundice for more than 6 months or abnormal liver enzymes for more than 12 months.

cholangitis has followed infusion of the anticancer agent floxuridine into the hepatic artery (Ludwig, Hepatol, 1989; 9:215).

A definite diagnosis of drug-induced cholestasis often cannot be made on liver biopsy alone and, thus, must usually rely on the time course of the hepatic injury and its resolution in relation to drug ingestion, using the diagnostic criteria recently agreed by international consensus (Benicchou, JHepatol, 1990; 11:272). Rechallenge with a suspected agent should never be undertaken deliberately because repeat cholestatic reactions tend to be more severe than the initial reaction and are occasionally fatal. However, a reaction to inadvertent rechallenge with a drug is occasionally a valuable pointer to its implication as the cause of a cholestatic illness.

The pathogenesis of drug-induced cholestasis is complex. Some drugs, such as oestrogens, androgens, and chlorpromazine, produce cholestasis in animals (see mechanisms of cholestasis above). However, these effects are predictable and usually dose dependent. Thus, they do not explain the idiosyncratic nature of drug-induced cholestasis in man. Less than 5 per cent of patients taking chlorpromazine and less than 1 per cent of those taking oestrogens develop jaundice. With most other drugs, the risk of jaundice is much less, and rarely exceeds 1 in 1000. The two most likely explanations for idiosynchratic drug reactions are immune-mediated reactions and cholestatic drug metabolites.

Immune-mediated reactions

The frequent portal inflammatory reaction, the occasional presence of fever, eosinophilia and autoantibodies, and the shorter latency period following drug re-exposure all suggest that the immune-mediated damage plays an important role in drug-induced cholestasis. Further evidence includes an association between certain HLA genotypes and cholestasis induced by several drugs (Berson, JHepatol, 1994; 20:336).

Both cell-mediated and antibody-mediated cytotoxicity may be involved. For example, diclofenac, when given to animals, combines with hepatic proteins to form adducts that are antigenic and can lead to activation of sensitized lymphocytes. These lymphocytes are cytotoxic for diclofenac-treated hepatocytes, which carry diclofenac-modified antigenic determinants in association with MHC type I complexes (Krentz-Rommel, Hepatol, 1995; 22:213). Serum from patients with hepatitis induced by halothane (Vergani, NEJM, 1980; 233:66), tienilic acid (Neuberger, Gut, 1989; 30:515), or methyldopa (Neuberger, Gut, 1985; 26:1233) contains antibodies which react against drug-modified antigens on the plasma membrane of rabbit hepatocytes. Although direct evidence is lacking, it seems likely that a similar immunoallergic reaction directed against drug-modified antigens on bile ductular cells, leading to bile duct damage and obstruction, is an important mechanism of drug-induced cholestasis.

Cholestatic drug metabolites

Altered metabolism of drugs may also be a factor in initiating liver and bile duct injury. In animals, metabolites of chlorpromazine inhibit Na^+/K^+ ATPase more than the parent drug (Samuels, Gastro, 1978; 74:1183) and some oestrogen metabolites are more cholestatic than others (Meyers, JPharmExpTher, 1980; 214:87). [22] Patients with a history of chlorpromazine-induced jaundice had impaired mechanisms of hepatic sulphoxidation (Watson, JHepatol, 1988; 7:72) and patients with hepatotoxicity due to perhexiline (Morgan, Gut, 1984; 25:1057) and isoniazid (Mitchell, AnnIntMed, 1976; 84:181) had a higher than expected prevalence of rapid acetylators. Lymphocyte hypersensitivity to drug metabolites has also been demonstrated in cases of cholestasis induced by halothane (Farrell, NEJM, 1985; 313:1307) and phenytoin (Spielberg, NEJM, 1981; 305:722). Drug metabolites forming adducts with cytochrome-P450 proteins, rather than the parent compound, may initiate the immune-mediated damage described above (Pessayre, JHepatol, 1995; 23(Suppl. 1):16). However, conclusive evidence is, as yet, lacking to establish drug metabolites as a cause of cholestasis in man.

Table 5 Causes of paucity of the intrahepatic bile ducts ('vanishing bile-duct syndromes')
Primary biliary cirrhosis
Primary sclerosing cholangitis
Acquired immunodeficiency syndrome
Sarcoidosis
Autoimmune cholangiopathy
Graft-versus-host disease
Liver allograft rejection
Drugs associated with prolonged cholestasis (see Table 4)
Lymphoma
Histiocytosis X
Behçet's syndrome
Childhood forms (see Table 6)
Idiopathic adult ductopenia

Disorders of intrahepatic bile ducts (Table 5)[52]

Cholangiopathies associated with the neonatal period and childhood are described below under cholestasis in the infant and child. In adults, several cholestatic disorders are associated with progressive damage to the interlobular bile ducts. These diseases, which lead to obliteration of the bile ducts, are known collectively as the 'vanishing bile-duct syndrome', and are sometimes termed 'duct paucity' or 'ductopenia'. Ductopenia is arbitrarily defined as less than 0.5 bile ducts per portal triad, when associated with normal numbers of hepatic arterioles and portal venules. For a definitive number, the biopsy must contain sufficient numbers of portal triads.

The most important causes of chronic cholestasis and bile duct paucity are primary biliary cirrhosis and primary sclerosing cholangitis, which are discussed in Chapters 14.1 and 14.4, respectively. Primary sclerosing cholangitis is usually associated with inflammatory bowel disease. In about 20 per cent of cases only the intrahepatic ducts are involved (Bhatal, Gut, 1969; 10:886; Helzberg, Gastro, 1987; 92:1869). The biliary tree may be normal when examined by cholangiography in other patients with concurrent cholestasis and inflammatory bowel disease, but liver biopsies in these cases may show portal tract oedema, infiltration by chronic inflammatory cells, and in the later stages, fibrosis and obliterative loss of interlobular ducts. This lesion may be part of a spectrum of liver injury in sclerosing cholangitis, but the abnormalities are located in branches that are beyond the resolution of cholangiography; thus the more classic radiological manifestations of primary sclerosing cholangitis in the larger bile ducts are not seen (Wee, AnnIntMed, 1985; 102:581; Ludwig, SemLivDis, 1991; 11: 11). Several cases of sclerosing cholangitis with bile duct paucity have been reported in patients with the acquired immunodeficiency syndrome (Roult, Gut, 1987; 28:1653; Viteri, Gastro, 1987; 92:2014; Forbes, Gut, 1993; 34:116).

Autoimmune cholangiopathy is a term recently applied to a condition which is clinically and histologically indistinguishable from primary biliary cirrhosis but where the serum is negative for antimitochondrial antibody and positive for antinuclear antibody (Michieletti, Gut, 1994; 35:260; Goodman, DigDisSci, 1995; 40: 1232). The condition is probably identical to the overlap syndrome of chronic active hepatitis and primary biliary cirrhosis (Geubel, Gastro, 1976; 71:444; Okuno, DigDigSci, 1987; 32:775). As with

primary biliary cirrhosis, bile duct paucity is common. Some patients show clinical and biochemical improvement with prednisolone (Ben-Ari, Hepatol, 1993; 18:10; Taylor, AmJSurgPath, 1994; 18:91), but in most cases, the disease behaves like primary biliary cirrhosis. Recently, serum antibodies to carbonic anhydrase II, an enzyme present in human bile ducts (Spicer, JHistochemCytochem, 1982; 30:864), were detected in patients with autoimmune cholangiopathy, suggesting that it may be a specific disease entity (Gordon, Gastro, 1995; 108:1802).

Hepatic sarcoidosis may be associated with a severe progressive cholestatic syndrome resembling primary biliary cirrhosis (Rudzki, AmJMed, 1975; 59:373; Murphy, JClinGastro, 1990; 12:555). Apart from cholestasis, the pathological features include periportal inflammation with prominent granulomas, and paucity of the interlobular bile ducts. The destructive bile duct lesion characteristic of primary biliary cirrhosis is occasionally seen (Devaney, AmJSurgPath, 1992; 19:1272). In most cases of hepatic sarcoidosis, granulomatous involvement of other organs, most commonly the lungs, can be demonstrated, and in about 50 per cent of cases the Kveim test is positive. Furthermore, serum IgM level is usually normal and serum is usually, but not always, negative for antimitochondrial antibodies (Fagan, NEJM, 1983; 308:572; Keefe, AmJMed, 1987; 83:977). Sarcoidosis-associated cholestasis may progress to biliary cirrhosis and portal hypertension. Steroids do not appear to be beneficial (Bass, Gut, 1982; 23:417; Pereira-Vima, AmJMed, 1987; 83:144). Ursodeoxycholic acid was effected in one reported case (Becheur, DigDisSci, 1994; 42:789).

Intrahepatic cholestasis is sometimes seen in chronic graft-versus-host disease after allogenic bone marrow transplantation (Chapter 14.5). Liver biopsy shows lymphocytic infiltration of the portal tracts and damage to bile ductular cells (Shulman, Hepatol, 1988; 8:463). In more chronic cases, there is bile duct paucity and the lesion may resemble primary biliary cirrhosis (Knapp, Gastro, 1987; 92:513). Progression to cirrhosis and liver failure can occur (Stechschule, Gastro, 1990; 98:223). A similar clinical and histological picture may be associated with liver allograft rejection (Weisner, Hepatol, 1991; 14:729). Alternative causes of bile duct paucity in a transplanted liver include recurrent primary biliary cirrhosis (Balan, Hepatol, 1993; 18:1392) and primary sclerosing cholangitis (Harrison, Hepatol, 1994; 20:356).

Other causes of cholestasis with bile duct paucity in adults include drugs causing prolonged cholestasis (Table 4), lymphoma, and histiocytosis X (see below) and Behçet's syndrome (Hisoaka, Hepatogast, 1994; 41:267).

Ductopenia in adults is labelled idiopathic when serum is negative for autoantibodies, rectal biopsy and cholangiogram are normal, and sarcoidosis and drug or viral injury can be eliminated (Ludwig, JHepatol, 1988; 7:199–199; Zafrani, Gastro, 1990; 99: 1813; Brugeria, Hepatol, 1992; 15:830). Most of these patients develop progressive cholestasis, often associated with cirrhosis and portal hypertension; however, one reported case was associated with recurring and remitting cholestasis (Faa, JHepatol, 1991; 12:14). In about one-third of cases, family members are affected (Haratake, Gastro, 1985; 89:202). Idopathic adult ductopenia may represent a 'late-onset' variety of non-syndromic bile-duct paucity in childhood (see below), small-duct sclerosing cholangitis, or antimitochondrial antibody-negative primary biliary cirrhosis. Ursodeoxycholic acid has been used with some benefit (Hartmenn, ZGastr, 1993; 31:131).

Cholestasis associated with hepatic infiltration or metabolic disorders

Lymphoma and related disorders[53]

About 10 per cent of patients with Hodgkin's disease develop jaundice, often in the late stages of the disease. Causes include liver infiltration by the lymphoma, tumour compression of the bile duct, and drug hepatotoxicity. Not infrequently, cholestasis is an early clinical feature (Perera, Gastro, 1974; 67:680; Trewby, QJMed, 1979; 189:137; Warner, AmJGastr, 1994; 89:941), sometimes without other features such as fever, lymphadenopathy, and hepatosplenomegaly. The biliary tree is patent by cholangiography. Liver biopsy shows cholestasis but, in most cases, no evidence of neoplastic infiltration. Serial liver biopsies (Hubscher, Hepatol, 1992; 17:70) may show progressive ductopenia and periductal fibrosis. Improvement is seen in only a few cases following successive treatment of the lymphoma (Crosbie, Hepatol, 1997; 26:5). At autopsy, neoplastic infiltration is usually absent or mild. Humoral 'cholestatic factors' have been sought but not identified (Pipken, Gastro, 1979; 77:145).

Patients with non-Hodgkin's lymphoma may also present with jaundice, due to liver infiltration, tumour compression of the biliary tree, or non-obstructive intrahepatic cholestasis (Watterson, Gastro, 1989; 97:1319). Cholestasis may occasionally be a paraneoplastic manifestation of hypernephroma (Utz, MayoClinProc, 1970, 45: 161; Jakobovitz, AustNZJMed, 1981; 11:64) or renal sarcoma (Summerskill, ArchIntMed, 1968; 120:81).

Cholestasis may be a feature of histiocytosis X (Leblanc, Gastro, 1981; 80:134). Extrahepatic manifestations of the disease including skin, bone, and pituitary involvement are usually present. Cholangiography may show lesions resembling those of primary sclerosing cholangitis. Liver biopsies usually show no histiocyte infiltration but sometimes ductopenia and portal fibrosis.

The idiopathic hypereosinophilic syndrome, which involves the liver in about one-third of cases (Harley, AnnIntMed, 1982; 97: 78), may present with cholestatic hepatitis, associated with dense eosinophilic infiltration on liver biopsy and improvement on steroid treatment (Dillon, AmJGastr, 1994; 89:1254). A similar presentation has been reported in a patient with systemic mastocytosis (Safyan, AmJGastr, 1997; 92:1197).

Amyloidosis[54,55]

About one-third of cases of primary amyloidosis have clinical or biochemical evidence of liver involvement (Kyle, MayoClinProc, 1983; 58:665) and most patients have liver involvement at autopsy. The commonest manifestations are hepatomegaly and abnormal liver enzymes (Gertz, AmJMed, 1988; 85:73), which do not correlate with the extent of hepatic amyloid infiltration. About 5 per cent of patients develop cholestatic jaundice, usually in association with hepatomegaly (Peters, Gut, 1994; 35:1232).[54,55] Splenomegaly and ascites are each seen in about 20 per cent of cases. Liver biopsies show changes typical of intrahepatic cholestasis; amyloid deposits are detected by staining with Congo red and examining for green birefringence under polarized microscopy. The diagnosis may be missed if appropriate stains are not performed. The deposits are usually in the periportal regions, but may occasionally be pericentral

(Finkelstein, HumPath, 1981; 12:470). Most patients develop progressive liver failure and mean survival after the onset of jaundice is only 3 months. Recently, cholestatic jaundice has been described in association with a condition related to amyloidosis: light-chain deposition disease (Faa, JHepatol, 1991; 12:75).

Sickle cell disease

Intrahepatic cholestasis may complicate sickle cell disease (Buchanan, JPediat, 1977; 91:21; Johnson, Medicine, 1985; 64:349). It is usually temporary and associated with sickle cell crises but may follow a prolonged course (O'Callaghan, Gut, 1995; 37:144). Liver biopsy shows hepatocyte swelling, sinusoidal dilatation, and Kupffer cell hyperplasia and erythrophagocytosis (Omada, DigDisSci, 1986; 31:247). The cholestasis may be a result of liver hypoxia, caused by sludging of sickle cells in the sinusoids. Exchange transfusion may be of benefit (Shao, AmJGastr, 1995; 90:2048).

Protoporphyria[56]

Hepatic manifestations of protoporphyria are discussed in more detail in Chapter 20.5. Accumulation of porphyrin pigment in the liver may give rise to cholestasis (Bloomer, AmJMed, 1975; 58:869). However, the development of jaundice usually heralds the onset of terminal liver failure. Examination of liver biopsies by polarization microscopy shows brown-black 'Maltese cross' granules, with a characteristic birefringence, in hepatocytes, Kupffer cells, and bile canaliculi (Klatskin, Gastro, 1973; 67:294). These deposits resemble bile thrombi on staining with haematoxylin and eosin. The diagnosis is made by demonstrating increased protoporphyrins in liver, faeces, or red cells. Possible explanations for the cholestasis include obstruction of bile ductules by the precipitated protoporphyrins, and inhibition of plasma membrane enzymes and transporters. Inhibition of Na^+/K^+ATPase has been demonstrated in rat liver (Avner, Gastro, 1983; 85:700).

Cystic fibrosis[57]

The cystic fibrosis transmembrane regulator (**CFTR**) controls apical membrane chloride conductance in many epithelia. Most cases of cystic fibrosis are associated with abnormalities in the CFTR gene. CFTR has recently been demonstrated on the apical membrane of human bile duct epithelial cells (Cohn, Gastro, 1993; 105: 1857). These cells contribute to bile flow by secretion of bicarbonate and water via activation of an apical chloride channel (Alvaro, JCI, 1993; 92:1314; McGill, AmJPhysiol, 1994; 266:G731).

Given this background, cholestasis is surprisingly rare in patients with cystic fibrosis. A case of neonatal cholestasis associated with bile duct paucity has been reported (Furuya, JPediatGastrNutr, 1991; 12:127), but the most common manifestations of the liver disease that complicates about 5 per cent of cases of cystic fibrosis (Scott-Jupp, ArchDisChild, 1991; 66:698; Feigelson, ArchDisChild, 1993: 68:653) are hepatosplenomegaly, mild liver enzyme abnormalities, and portal hypertension. The most common histological abnormality is focal biliary fibrosis sometimes progressing to cirrhosis. Bile duct irregularities are seen on electron microscopy, but cholestasis is not a feature (Linblad, Hepatol, 1992; 16:372).

α_1-Antitrypsin deficiency

Cholestasis is the most common hepatic manifestation of homozygous (ZZ) α_1-antitrypsin deficiency (further discussed in Chapter

20.3) in the neonatal period, and is seen in about 10 per cent of all infants with the ZZ phenotype (Sveger, NEJM, 1976; 294:1316; Pediat, 1978; 62:22). Liver biopsy findings reveal neonatal hepatitis or intrahepatic cholestasis with bile duct paucity (see below). The diagnosis is established by finding typical granules positive for periodic acid–Schiff (**PAS**) staining in hepatocytes on liver biopsy, low serum α_1-antitrypsin levels, and by phenotyping. PAS-positive granules and serum levels of the enzyme are not entirely specific so that phenotyping is required. Fifty per cent of the children die of liver failure, or develop cirrhosis in adolescence, but in 20 per cent the liver disease spontaneously remits (Psacharopoulos, Arch-DisChild, 1983; 58:882).

α_1-Antitrypsin deficiency may also present in adulthood with cirrhosis, portal hypertension, liver failure, and hepatoma (Larsson, ActaMedScand, 1978; 204:345). Cholestasis is seen but is not a prominent feature (Berg, NEJM, 1972; 282:1264; Triger, QJMed, 1976; 49:351). Heterozygous (MZ) α_1-antitrypsin deficiency may also be associated with chronic active hepatitis and cirrhosis in adulthood; some of these patients present with cholestasis (Hodges, NEJM, 1981; 304:557).

Cholestasis may be seen in patients with haemochromatosis (Chapter 20.2) and Wilson's disease (Chapter 20.1), but it is seldom an early feature and usually indicates severe advanced liver disease.

Cholestasis associated with infection[58]

The reported prevalence of cholestasis in patients with septicaemia of non-biliary origin ranges between 1 per cent (Vermillon, ArchIntMed, 1969; 124:611) and 34 per cent (Franson, RevInfDis, 1985; 7:1). The most common associated infections are pneumonia, pyelonephritis, intra-abdominal sepsis, and endocarditis. Causative organisms include *Staphylococcus*, *Pneumococcus*, *Escherichia coli*, *Klebsiella*, *Pseudomonas*, *Haemophilus influenzae*, and Bacteroides (Miller, Gastro, 1976; 71:94; Quale, AmJMed, 1988; 85:615). Cholestasis sometimes accompanies the toxic shock syndrome (Gourley, Gastro, 1981; 81:920) and *Mycoplasma pneumoniae* (Arav-Boyer, JPediatGastrNutr, 1995; 21:459). The infections are usually severe and often associated with renal failure, bone marrow depression, and a high mortality. Mortality is not related to the cholestasis but rather to the severity of the infection and other underlying disease processes (Miller, Gastro, 1976; 71:94).

Cholestasis results in part from the effects of bacterial toxins. Endotoxin causes cholestasis in human volunteers (Blasc, AnnIntMed, 1973; 78:221) and has several effects on rat liver, including a reduction of bile flow, bile acid and organic acid uptake and excretion, reduced $Na^+/K^+ATPase$ activity, and an increase in biliary permeability as measured by horseradish peroxidase excretion (Utilli, Gastro, 1976; 70:248; Utilli, JInfDis, 1977; 136:583; Roelofsen, Gastro, 1994; 107:1075). Bilirubin transport is affected more than bile acid transport. Recent studies indicate that endotoxin administration to rats results in reductions in mRNA and protein for the cMOAT/cMRP/MRP2 canalicular membrane organic anion transporter (Trauner, Gastro, 1997; 113:255). These findings may explain the disproportionate elevation in serum bilirubin (see below).

The effects of endotoxin appear to be mediated by induction of proinflammatory cytokines. Both tumour necrosis factor-α and

interleukin-6 inhibit hepatocyte bile acid uptake and tumour necrosis factor-α inhibits ATP-dependent canalicular bile acid transport; furthermore, the cholestatic effects of endotoxin can be blocked by antibodies to tumour necrosis factor-α (Green, AJP, 1994; 267: G1094; Whiting, Hepatol, 1995; 22:1273; Moseley, AmJPhysiol, 1996; 272:G137). However, about 30 per cent of cases of sepsis-associated cholestasis are associated with organisms that do not produce endotoxins, suggesting that other mechanisms are also operative (Carauna, SGO, 1982; 154:653; Pirovino, Gastro, 1989; 96:1589). Sepsis in rats is associated with decreased hepatocyte intracellular calcium release (Spitzer, AJP, 1987; 253:E130).

In sepsis-associated cholestasis, bilirubin excretion tends to be selectively affected. There is often deep jaundice and a marked (mean ninefold) increase in serum bilirubin, of which 75 to 80 per cent is conjugated. In contrast, pruritus is not a feature (perhaps because patients are so ill) and serum alkaline phosphatase levels are usually less than three times the upper limit of normal. Serum aminotransferases may be normal and are seldom markedly raised. Bromosulphthalein excretion is impaired, but other hepatocellular functions, as measured by galactose elimination capacity, caffeine clearance, and coagulation factor synthesis, are normal or only mildly impaired (Pirovino, Gastro, 1989; 96:1589).

Histological changes are non-specific and include centrilobular cholestasis, a mononuclear portal infiltrate, and mild fatty infiltration. Sometimes there may be changes in the larger intrahepatic ducts (Banks, JClinPath, 1982; 75:1249). Hepatocellular necrosis has been a feature in some series (Carauna, SGO, 1982; 154: 653). Ultrastructural features include dilated canaliculi without microvilli, typical of many intrahepatic cholestatic disorders.

Weil's disease is also associated with conjugated hyperbilirubinaemia and mildly raised liver enzymes, and the diagnosis should be considered in any patient with jaundice, fever, and severe constitutional symptoms. Finally, cholestasis is an occasional feature of several infectious diseases, including toxoplasmosis, brucellosis, malaria, legionnaires' disease, and typhoid fever.[58] Usually the serum aminotransferases are substantially raised, suggesting that the primary pathology is hepatocellular damage.

Cholestasis associated with total parenteral nutrition[59–61]

The prevalence of abnormal liver enzymes in adults receiving total parenteral nutrition is between 25 and 100 per cent, while that of hyperbilirubinaemia between 0 and 46 per cent.[61] These large differences probably reflect the variable presence of other risk factors for liver damage, which include surgery, especially intestinal resection (Stanko, Gastro, 1987; 92:197), inflammatory bowel disease, malignancy, and sepsis. A similar range of prevalence values has been reported in premature infants. However, cholestasis associated with total parenteral nutrition in infants tends to be much more severe, probably because of immaturity of the bile secretory apparatus (Suchy, Gastro, 1981; 80:1037).

Liver biopsies in patients with cholestasis associated with total parenteral nutrition show fat accumulation, especially in the early stages, mild hepatocellular damage and portal inflammation, and variable degrees of cholestasis, especially in infants (Cohen, Arch-PathLabMed, 1981; 105:152).[60] The findings may simulate neonatal hepatitis (Dahms, Gastro, 1981; 81:136), although multinucleated hepatocytes are rare. Ultrastructural findings include fatty infiltration, enlargement of mitochondria and the endoplasmic reticulum, and intrahepatic cholestasis (Dahms, Gastro, 1981; 81:136).

Following prolonged (more than 3 months) total parenteral nutrition, over 50 per cent of infants develop bile duct proliferation and portal fibrosis; about 30 per cent develop cirrhosis, sometimes accompanied by liver failure.[61] The prevalence of fibrosis in adults on prolonged total parenteral nutrition may be lower but about 5 per cent develop severe chronic liver disease (Bowyer, JPEN, 1985; 9:11). There has been one report of a hepatoma (Vileisis, JPaediat, 1982; 100:88) in an infant following prolonged total parenteral nutrition. Cholestasis usually resolves when parenteral feeding is discontinued.

Several factors contribute to the pathogenesis of cholestasis associated with total parenteral nutrition. These include the administration of concentrated solutions of sugar and amino acids.[61] In infants on total parenteral nutrition, the development of hyperbilirubinaemia correlates with the protein content of the feed (Vileisnis, JPaediat, 1980; 96:893). Hyperglycaemia (Marin, Hepatol, 1991; 14:184) and amino acid solutions (Graham, Hepatol, 1984; 4:69) diminish bile flow in rat liver. Amino acids also impair sodium-dependent bile-acid uptake into isolated liver plasma membrane vesicles (Blitzer, AmJPhysiol, 1985; 249:G120; Bucuvalas, PediatRes, 1985; 19:1298). Some of the solutions used in total parenteral nutrition are hypertonic and may decrease bile flow by their osmotic effects.

Another major factor in cholestasis associated with total parenteral nutrition is likely to be absence of oral food intake. First, this decreases the cycling frequency of the bile acid pool and the excretion of biliary bile acid, thereby predisposing to inspissation of bile contents. Second, total parenteral nutrition and lack of oral feeding are associated with intestinal bacterial overgrowth and impaired immunological and barrier function of the intestinal mucosa, leading to increased bacterial translocation and endotoxaemia (Spaeth, Surgery, 1990; 108:240),[61] which also has important cholestatic effects (see cholestasis associated with infection above). Sepsis may often be present is these patients, predisposing to endotoxaemia. Hepatic accumulation of the cholestatic bile acid lithocholic acid may also play a role. Biliary concentrations of lithocholic acid increase in patients with cholestasis associated with total parenteral nutrition (Fouin-Fortnet, Gastro, 1982; 82:93). Furthermore, bowel sterilization with antibiotics, which presumably inhibits formation of lithocholic acid from chenodeoxycholic acid via the bacterial enzyme 7β-dehydroxylase, partially protects against this type of cholestasis (Capron, Lancet, 1983; i:446; Spurr, JPEN, 1989; 13:633).

Approaches to minimizing the incidence and severity of cholestasis related to total parenteral nutrition include avoidance of hyperglycaemia, minimizing excess calories and amino acid content in the infusions, cyclical rather than continuous administration of total parenteral nutrition, and resumption of oral feeding (even in small amounts) as soon as possible. The adverse effects of total parenteral nutrition on the intestinal mucosa may be lessened by adding glutamine to the feed (Souba, JSurgRes, 1990; 48:383). Ursodeoxycholic acid (Lindor, Gastro, 1991; 101:250) has been associated with improvement in liver enzymes in cholestasis related to total parenteral nutrition in children (Beau, JHepatol, 1994; 20:

240) and adults (Kowalski, Gastro, 1994; 106:A615). In a few infants with severe liver disease, where a lack of functioning bowel precludes resumption of oral feeding, combined liver and small bowel transplantation has been performed.

Postoperative cholestasis[62,63]

Cholestasis develops in 10 per cent of patients 1 to 2 weeks after coronary artery bypass surgery and is also seen occasionally following major abdominal surgery. Usually the picture is one of 'pure' intrahepatic cholestasis with normal serum aminotransferases and minimal hepatocellular damage on liver biopsy (LaMont, NEJM, 1973; 288:305). Occasionally there is massive hepatic necrosis (Nunes, ArchSurg, 1970; 100:546). Although the exact mechanisms of cholestasis are obscure, there are probably several contributory factors including: (i) ischaemic liver damage due to hypotension during cardiopulmonary bypass, heart failure, or pulmonary embolism; (ii) extrahepatic obstruction, causes of which include bile duct injury and pancreatitis; and (iii) other factors, including drug reactions, sepsis, and total parenteral nutrition as discussed previously.

Apart from cholestasis, postoperative jaundice also results from excessive haemolysis brought on by blood extravasation, transfusion of stored blood, renal failure, insertion of prosthetic valves, and rarely, transfusion reactions.

Intrahepatic cholestasis of pregnancy[23,24, 64–67]

This disorder is characterized by pruritus with or without jaundice; it usually begins in late pregnancy and disappears at term. It is rare in North America, China, and in most of Europe, occurring between 2 and 20 times in every 10 000 pregnancies. However, in Scandinavia, where the condition was first described in detail (Svanborg, ActaObGyn, 1954; 22:434), it occurs in 1 in 100 pregnancies and in Bolivia and Chile the incidence is high, as much as 1 in 6 in some areas, although it may be declining.[66] The prevalence of the disorder is increased in first-degree relatives (Dalen, AMedScand, 1974; 195:459) and several family clusters of the disease have been reported, with inheritance often occurring as a dominant trait (Reyes, Gut, 1976; 17:709; Holzbach, Gastro, 1983; 85:175). The syndrome is not associated with a specific HLA antigen subtype (Mella, JHepatol, 1996; 24:320).

Several observations support a major role for oestrogens in the pathogenesis of intrahepatic cholestasis of pregnancy. The condition usually presents in the third trimester of pregnancy, when oestrogen levels are highest, and its incidence is increased fivefold in twin pregnancies (Gonzalez, JHepatol, 1989; 9:84). About one-half of patients with a history of intrahepatic cholestasis of pregnancy also develop liver enzyme abnormalities if they take oral contraceptives (Frezza, AmJGastr, 1988; 83:1098). Oestrogens are cholestatic in several animal species and potential mechanisms have been discussed earlier. Excretion of the organic anion bromosulphthalein falls and serum bile acids increase during normal pregnancy (Combes, JCI, 1963; 42:1431) and following oestrogen administration (Mueller, JCI, 1964; 43:1905). The role of progestegens is much less clear; however, recently an association has been reported between intrahepatic cholestasis of pregnancy and oral administration of progesterone.[64]

Sulphation, via the enzyme dihydroepiandrosterone sulpho-transferase, is an important metabolic pathway for oestrogens and is also an important mechanism for inactivating the cholestatic bile acid lithocholic acid. Recently, hepatic sulphation capacity, measured using paracetamol as a probe, was shown to be reduced in pregnancy and following oestrogen administration (Davies, JHepatol, 1994; 21:1127). Such a sulphation defect might result in increased formation of other more cholestatic oestrogen metabolites, such as glucuronides,[22] and might also contribute to lithocholic acid accumulation.

The relative rarity and clinical variability of intrahepatic cholestasis of pregnancy are still unexplained. However, subtle abnormalities in bromosulphthalein retention are found in women with a history of intrahepatic cholestasis of pregnancy (Frezza, ActaObGyn, 1988; 65:577). Bromosulphthalein retention also shows an exaggerated increase following oestrogen administration compared with controls (Kreek, NEJM, 1967; 277:1391). This suggests an increased sensitivity to the cholestatic effects of oestrogens. Similar sensitivities to oestrogens are found in family members of patients, including males (Reyes, Gastro, 1981; 81:226).

Intrahepatic cholestasis of pregnancy tends to recur in successive pregnancies although the course and severity in a given pregnancy are quite unpredictable. It may also appear for the first time in a third or fourth pregnancy, and then usually recurs in subsequent pregnancies. The onset of symptoms is normally in the third trimester but may be as early as the sixth week. Pruritus is the first symptom; jaundice may follow 2 to 3 weeks later but is often absent, when the condition is sometimes termed pruritus gravidarum. Severe abdominal pain and systemic symptoms of chills, arthralgia, and malaise are absent although anorexia and nausea may be present. The liver may be mildly enlarged but splenomegaly is absent.

Serum bilirubin shows a variable rise involving mainly the conjugated fraction. Serum alkaline phosphatase is rarely raised more than threefold, and may be within the normal range for pregnancy. The serum γ-glutamyl transferase level also may be normal and is seldom increased more than twofold, possibly because it is depressed by female sex hormones (Combes, Gastro, 1977; 72: 271). Serum aminotransferases are usually modestly raised but may rarely increase up to 1000 U/l (Wilson, DigDisSci, 1987; 32:665). Serum bile acids are invariably raised, up to 30-fold (Sjovall, CCActa, 1966; 13:207). This rise may precede the rises in liver enzymes and bilirubin, and may be the only biochemical abnormality (Heikkinen, BrJObsGyn, 1981; 88:240). Prothrombin time is prolonged in about 20 per cent of cases and fetal haemorrhage can be induced by bile-acid binding agents. Many patients have fat malabsorption which correlates with the severity of the cholestasis although clinical steatorrhoea is rare (Reyes, Gastro, 1987; 93:584). Liver biopsy is seldom indicated. The histological features are those of 'pure' cholestasis with centrilobular bile staining and a mild periportal mononuclear infiltrate, but minimal cellular damage (Hammerli, Medicine, 1967; 61:367). Ultrastructural changes are also typical of intrahepatic cholestasis (Adlercreutz, AmJMed, 1967; 42:335; Larson-Cohen, ActaMedScand, 1967; 181:257).

Intrahepatic cholestasis of pregnancy must be distinguished from other causes of cholestasis in pregnancy (Section 28).[67] The most important of these is viral hepatitis. Pre-eclampsia and the HELLP syndrome are occasionally associated with jaundice but the other features of these conditions are usually obvious. Fatty liver of pregnancy may present with jaundice in the third trimester, however, patients are usually very ill and have other features of hepatocellular failure. A case of fatty liver coexisting with intrahepatic cholestasis of pregnancy has been described (Vanjah, Gastro, 1991; 100:1123).

The jaundice and pruritus usually resolve within 2 weeks following delivery although, occasionally, resolution can take several months (Olson, Gastro, 1993; 105:267). However, in about one-quarter of cases, there are signs of fetal distress and about 2 per cent of the infants are stillborn (Johnston, AmJObsGyn, 1979; 133:299; Shaw, AmJObsGyn, 1982; 142:621; Fisk, BrJObsGyn, 1988; 95: 1137). [64] Fetal distress may occur without warning, and often manifests as meconium staining during delivery or on diagnostic amniocentesis. Its occurrence is often not predicted by conventional methods of fetal monitoring such as cardiotachography and urinary oestriol estimation, indeed, infants usually have normal development for gestational age (Alsulyman, AmJObsGyn, 1996; 175: 957). The cause is unclear, but examination of placentas from women with intrahepatic cholestasis of pregnancy reveals small infarcts (Costoya, Placenta, 1980; 1:361) and depressed cytochrome P-450-dependent enzyme activities (Pasanen, Placenta, 1997; 18: 37). In addition, fetal serum bile acids are increased (Laatikainen, AmJObsGyn, 1975; 122:852; Shaw, AmJObsGyn, 1982; 142:621) and hyperreactivity of the myometrium to oxytocin has been described (Israel, ActaObsGyn, 1986; 68:581). Finally, women with intrahepatic cholestasis of pregnancy may be malnourished since they can fail to gain weight normally during pregnancy (Reyes, Gastro, 1987; 93:584). The failure to gain weight may be due to fat malabsorption, which correlates with the severity of the cholestasis and inversely with the maternal weight/height index (Reyes, Gastro, 1987; 93:584).

No medical treatment for intrahepatic cholestasis of pregnancy may be necessary if the cholestasis is mild. However, patients should be monitored for signs of fetal distress, and early delivery should be induced if this occurs. In severe cases, some obstetricians advocate diagnostic amniocentesis after 30 weeks and routine induction of delivery as soon as lung maturity, assessed by the lecithin/sphingomyelin ratio, is established (Shaw, AmJObsGyn, 1982; 142: 621; Fisk, BrJObsGyn, 1988; 95:1137). Prothrombin time should be checked and corrected with parenteral vitamin K before delivery.

Several treatments have been tried to relieve maternal symptoms but none are as yet well established. Cholestyramine is sometimes effective in relieving pruritus but has been associated with severe fetal intracranial haemorrhage (Sadler, BrJObsGyn, 1995; 102:169). S-adenosyl methionine reverses oestrogen-induced cholestasis in rats; however, two double-blind trials in intrahepatic cholestasis of pregnancy have provided conflicting evidence regarding a beneficial effect on pruritus and biochemical parameters (Frezza, Gastro, 1990; 99:211; Ribolta, Hepatol, 1991; 13:1084). In open trials, ursodeoxycholic acid has relieved pruritus and lowered serum bile acids and liver enzymes (Palma, Hepatol, 1992; 15:1043; Davies, Gut, 1995; 37:580). Two placebo-controlled trials have now confirmed these findings and one has also suggested that ursodeoxycholic acid may improve fetal prognosis (Isla, Gastro, 1996; 110:1219A; Palma, Hepatol, 1996; 24:373A). In another study, ursodeoxycholic acid was more effective than S-adenosyl methionine in improving pruritus and lowering serum bile acids (Floreani, EurJObsGynReprodBiol, 1996; 67:109). In one study, epomediol was reported to relieve pruritus without affecting serum bile acids or liver enzymes (Gonzalez, JHepatol, 1992; 16:241).

Benign recurrent intrahepatic cholestasis (BRIC)[68–73]

This rare disorder was first reported in 1959[68] and less than 100 cases had been reported by 1989.[69-72] The syndrome is characterized by repeated episodes of unexplained cholestasis occurring over a period of many years and separated by long asymptomatic periods. Ten to fifteen per cent of patients have a relative with the disease and in some families the condition is inherited as a recessive disorder (Goldberg, ArchIntMed, 1967; 120:556; De-Koning, AmJMedGen, 1995; 57:479). Several patients have had episodes of cholestasis during pregnancy. Whether this represents a genuine association with intrahepatic cholestasis of pregnancy or is coincidental remains unclear.[72] In one extended family, including four cases of BRIC, nine family members had intrahepatic cholestasis of pregnancy and two others had cholestasis related to oral contraceptives,[69] suggesting a genetic predispositon to both diseases.

The underlying basis for the disorder is unknown. Hepatic uptake of bile acids[73] and unconjugated bilirubin[30,31] is usually normal during the cholestatic episodes. However, conjugated bilirubin refluxes into serum following injection of radiolabelled unconjugated bilirubin, suggesting an excretory defect. Several abnormalities have been described in patients in between the cholestatic episodes. These include mild defects in indocyanine green and bromosulphthalein excretion,[30,73] consistent with a persisting defect in bile secretion.[30,73] Asymptomatic patients also have a small pool of bile acids with a high turnover rate that contains a relative excess of the hydrophobic (and cholestatic) bile acids deoxycholic and lithocholic acid (Bijleveld, Gastro, 1989; 97:427; Bijleveld, Hepatol, 1989; 9:532). This change in bile composition might result from impaired ileal bile acid uptake with increased colonic dehydroxylation, and might partly explain the propensity to develop cholestasis. Neither bile flow nor hepatocyte uptake of bile acids in an animal model was inhibited by serum from a patient with the disease (Miniuk, Gastro, 1987; 93:1187), suggesting that changes in bile acids result from an intrinsic hepatocyte defect rather than a circulating cholestatic factor.

Recently, Houwn and colleagues (NatureGenet, 1994; 8:380) have performed a genome-wide search for shared chromosomal segments in four distantly related relatives with BRIC, who were assumed to have inherited the disease from a common ancestor several generations back. This was made possible by the availability of high-resolution linkage maps of the human genome. A region on chromosome 18 was identified that contained an extended haplotype which was identical in five of the six chromosomes from these three distantly related individuals. This suggests that BRIC is a recessive disorder which is closely linked to a region on chromosome 18. Further extension of this work has refined the region containing the putative BRIC genetic defect to about 250 kilobases (Houwen, Hepatol, 1997; 26:369A). Using a similar approach, an adjacent segment has been linked to progressive familial intrahepatic cholestasis (Byler's disease, see below) and it is likely that this genetic region codes for a transport protein involved in bile formation

(Wagstaff, Hepatol, 1995; 22:1611; Sela-Herman, BiochemMolMed, 1996; 59:98).

BRIC usually presents in early adulthood, but patients have been identified from 18 months of age to 59 years. Males and females are equally affected. The cholestatic episodes last from 2 to 24 months (usually about 3 months) and may be interspersed with asymptomatic periods of up to 30 years. The episodes are often precipitated by an acute infection, and a seasonal pattern has also been described (Speigal, AmJMed, 1965; 39:682). Symptoms typically begin with malaise, anorexia, and sometimes vomiting, diarrhoea, abdominal pain, and an erythematous maculopapular rash; fever is found in 25 per cent of cases. Jaundice, usually but not always associated with pruritus, follows after 2 to 3 weeks. Occasionally, cough is a prominent feature (Chatila, AmJGastr, 1996; 91:2215). The liver may be enlarged but splenomegaly is not a feature. There may be considerable weight loss.

Laboratory and morphological features are non-specific. Erythrocyte sedimentation rate, serum conjugated bilirubin, and alkaline phosphatase are usually raised. γ-Glutamyl transpeptidase is normal in about 20 per cent of cases;[72] a normal value is unusual in other forms of adult cholestasis apart from progressive familial intrahepatic cholestasis (see below). Serum aminotransferases are often raised, sometimes up to 15-fold. Serum bile acids may be markedly elevated, sometimes before the rise in serum bilirubin and alkaline phosphatase (van Berg Henegouwen, Lancet, 1974; i: 1249).[30] Light microscopic examination of liver biopsies reveals centrilobular cholestasis without hepatic or ductular damage, although there may be a mild portal inflammatory infiltrate (Williams, QJMed, 1964; 33:387).[72] Electron microscopy shows only non-specific features of cholestasis (Biempica, Gastro, 1967; 52:521; Hopwood, Gut, 1972; 13:986). BRIC is essentially a diagnosis of exclusion. Direct cholangiography is often needed to exclude primary sclerosing cholangitis and other extrahepatic bile-duct abnormalities. Until recently, most reported patients had one or more laparotomies before the diagnosis was made.

Treatment is not clearly defined. Steroids (Williams, QJMed, 1964; 33:387), cholestyramine (Spiegal, AmJMed, 1965; 39:682), phenobarbital (Stiehl, NEJM, 1972; 286:858), and ursodeoxycholic acid (Crosignani, Hepatol, 1991; 13:1076; Maggiore, Hepatol, 1992; 16:504) have all been used with unpredictable success.[72] S-Adenosyl methionine has been found to be ineffective in four patients (Everson, Gastro, 1989; 96:1354). The episodes of cholestasis eventually resolve spontaneously. In contrast to other cholestatic syndromes which may present in childhood, growth and development are normal. Although progression to cirrhosis has been reported, most patients have no evidence of chronic liver disease when followed for several decades (Putterman, PostgradMedJ, 1987; 63:295; Nahamuta, Hepatogast, 1994; 41:287).

Cholestasis in the infant and child

For a more detailed discussion of childhood cholestasis see references 74 to 78. Because the bile secretory apparatus does not develop fully until several months after birth (Suchy, Gastro, 1981; 80:1037), infants are particularly prone to develop cholestasis when the liver is exposed to a variety of insults, some peculiar to the neonatal period (Table 6). In about 20 per cent of cases, careful investigation reveals an underlying cause, most commonly in the

Table 6 Causes of intrahepatic cholestasis in infancy [74,75]

Infections	Cytomegalovirus
	Herpes
	Rubella
	Toxoplasmosis
	Syphilis
	Reovirus type III
Metabolic defects	α_1-Antitrypsin deficiency
	Galactosaemia
	Fructose intolerance
	Hypothyroidism
	Hypopituitarism
	Tyrosinaemia
	Bile-acid synthetic defects
	Cystic fibrosis
	Gaucher's disease
	Niemann Pick disease
	Zellweger's syndrome
Chromosomal abnormalities	Down's syndrome
	Turner's syndrome
	Trisomy 17-18
Peroxisomal dysfunction (Zellweger's syndrome)	
Idiopathic	Neonatal hepatitis
	Arteriohepatic dysplasia (Alagille's) (syndromic variant)
	Non-syndromic variant of Alagille's dysplasia
	Progressive familial intrahepatic cholestasis of infancy (Byler's disease) (PFIC)
	Cholestasis with lymphoedema (Aagenes' syndrome)
	North American Indian cholestasis
	Familial chronic intrahepatic cholestasis

form of a viral or bacterial infection such as cytomegalovirus or rubella, or a metabolic defect such as galactosaemia and α_1-antitrypsin deficiency (Danks, ArchDisChild, 1977; 52:360).[75] Recently, a number of enzyme defects in bile acid synthesis have also been described (see below). In the remaining 80 per cent of patients the aetiology is not known. Therefore, classifications of infantile cholestasis have been based on clinical and pathological features that often overlap and are imprecise.

The infantile cholestatic syndromes can be divided into three major pathological groups: extrahepatic biliary atresia, which comprises about two-thirds of the total; neonatal hepatitis; and intrahepatic cholangiopathies with or without hypoplasia of the interlobular bile ducts. These entities probably represent a continuous spectrum, because several aetiological agents (Table 6) can be associated with all three pathological forms, and in a given patient more than one lesion may coexist. For example, some patients with hypoplastic interlobular bile ducts also have a hypoplastic, although patent, extrahepatic biliary bile-duct system and they may initially be misdiagnosed as having extrahepatic biliary atresia (Markowitz, Hepatol, 1983; 3:74). In addition, one lesion may progress to another over time. For example, neonatal hepatitis may progress to paucity of interlobular bile ducts (Dahms, Hepatol, 1982; 2:350). In other children, cholestasis and intrahepatic bile duct paucity may progress or may recur several years after an apparently successful surgical treatment of extrahepatic biliary atresia (Kasai, JPediatSurg, 1975; 10:173; Laurent, Gastro, 1990; 99:1793).

Neonatal hepatitis is more common in males, is associated with premature birth, and infants present before the age of 2 months with cholestatic jaundice and hepatosplenomegaly. An association with reovirus type III has been suggested but not confirmed (Steele, Hepatol, 1993; 21:627). Twenty per cent of patients have the familial condition and have a poorer prognosis than those with the non-familial variety (30 compared with 60 per cent recovery). In contrast, extrahepatic biliary atresia is more common in females, and seldom affects more than one family member. Histologically, neonatal hepatitis is characterized by portal mononuclear inflammation and hepatocyte necrosis of variable degree. Multinucleated giant cells are commonly seen and there may be periportal inflammation. However, in contrast to extrahepatic biliary atresia, bile plugs and bile duct proliferation are rare. The outlook for neonatal hepatitis is good: in over 80 per cent of patients the disease resolves in a few months (Odievre, ArchDisChild, 1981; 156:373).

In most cases of intrahepatic cholestasis of infancy, hepatocellular injury is mild or absent, although there may be periportal inflammation. In some, but not all, cases there is a paucity of bile ducts. All the infective and metabolic causes of childhood cholestasis listed in Table 6 may be associated with histological features of intrahepatic cholestasis with or without a loss of interlobular bile ducts.

Arteriohepatic dysplasia—Alagille's syndrome (also called syndromic intrahepatic bile-duct hypoplasia)[78]

This entity is characterized by chronic intrahepatic cholestasis associated with a loss of the interlobular bile ducts, and a constellation of clinical and radiological anomalies affecting several systems: (i) facies—typically, a prominent forehead, widely-spaced deeply-set eyes, a long nose, and underdeveloped mandible; (ii) eye—posterior embryotoxon on slit-lamp examination; (iii) heart—defects include pulmonary artery hypoplasia, ventricular septal defect, and Fallot's tetralogy; and (iv) skeletal—vertebral body and arch defects and shortening of forearm and hand bones. Usually, not all these abnormalities are present in individual patients. Other features include growth and mental retardation, and hypogonadism. The condition is more common in males and occurs about once in every 70 000 births (Danks, ArchDisChild, 1977; 52:360).

The cause is unknown but the disorder is usually inherited as a dominant trait. Penetrance is high but severity and mode of expression of the disease is variable (LaBreque, Hepatol, 1982; 2:467; Dhorne-Pallet, JMedGenet, 1994; 31:453). Careful screening of 14 families with an affected child revealed abnormalities in at least two organ systems suggestive of Alagille's syndrome in six parents from separate families (Elmslie, JMedGenet, 1995; 32:264). In three cases, the father was affected and in three cases, the mother. Several patients with Alagille's syndrome have been described with a deletion (Schnittger, HumGenet, 1989; 83:239; Anad, JMedGenet, 1990; 27:729; Tielli, AmJMedGen, 1992; 42:35) or balanced translocation (Spinner, AmJHumGen, 1994; 55:238) of a segment on the short arm of chromosome 20. In other patients with a normal karyotype, linkage of the disease to a segment on chromosome 20 has been demonstrated (Hol, HumGenet, 1995; 95:687). Recently the genetic defect has been localized to chromosome 20p12 and shown to be caused by a deletion of JAG-1, encoding a ligand for the notch receptor which mediates cell fate decisions during development (Krantz, NatureGen, 1997; 16:243; Oda, NatureGen, 1997; 16:235).

About 50 per cent of cases present before the age of 3 months. Jaundice tends to be intermittent, although pruritus is usually continuous and can be severe. The liver is always enlarged. Hypercholesterolaemia is marked and often associated with xanthomas. Fat-soluble vitamin deficiency is common. Liver biopsy reveals cholestasis, along with hypoplasia of the interlobular bile ducts that progresses with time (Berman, DigDisSci, 1981; 20:485). In very early cases, there are typical features of neonatal hepatitis (Dahms, Hepatol, 1982; 2:350). Ultrastructural findings include pigment accumulation in the intercellular spaces and in the hepatocytes, especially in vesicles, lysosomes, and in the Golgi regions on the basolateral aspect of the cell. These structures are diminished in the pericanalicular regions, and the 'classic' cholestatic ultrastructural lesions of dilated canaliculi with loss of microvilli are often absent (Valencia-Mayoral, Hepatol, 1984; 4:691), suggesting that there is a secretory defect that lies proximal to the apical canalicular region.

For most patients with extrahepatic manifestations of the syndrome, prognosis is good. Jaundice usually disappears by about 5 years of age and progression to cirrhosis and portal hypertension is seen in only about 10 per cent of cases (Perrault, DigDisSci, 1981; 26:481; Allagille, JHepatol, 1985; 1:561) and over half survive to adulthood. Preliminary evidence suggests that ursodeoxycholic acid lowers liver enzymes and serum cholesterol and improves pruritus in about half of the patients (Krawinkel, JPediatGastrNutr, 1994; 19:4476; Levy, JPediatGastrNutr, 1995; 20:432).[76] In those with progressive liver failure, liver transplantation dramatically improves the outlook (Hoffenberg, JPediat, 1995; 127:220). Hepatocellular carcinoma has been reported in a few patients (Kaufman,

AmJDisChild, 1987; 141:698; Rabiniovitz, JPediatGastrNutr, 1989; 8:26).

Non-syndromic bile duct paucity of intrahepatic bile ducts

These children develop progressive intrahepatic cholestasis in infancy, associated with bile duct paucity. In approximately half of the patients there is an identifiable underlying condition such as cystic fibrosis, α_1-antrypsin deficiency, Down's syndrome, or hypopituitarism (Kahn, Hepatol, 1986; 6:890). Non-syndromic paucity differs in several respects from Allagille's syndrome: (i) the extrahepatic features of Allagille's syndrome are absent; (ii) electron microscopy of liver biopsies shows dilatation of bile canaliculi with loss of microvilli (Kahn, Hepatol, 1986; 6:890), features seen in most forms of cholestasis but often absent in Allagille's syndrome; and (iii) the outlook is poorer—about 50 per cent of these patients develop signs of liver failure by adolescence (Odievre, ArchDisChild, 1981; 56:373; Perrault, DigDisSci, 1981; 26:481). In some cases, however, the condition may resolve spontaneously (Berezin, DigDisSci, 1995; 40:82).

Progressive familial intrahepatic cholestasis (PFIC, Byler's disease)[79,80]

Byler's disease was originally described in seven members of four Amish families descended from one Jacob Byler (Clayton, AmJDisChild, 1969; 117:112). Clinically similar cases have been described in non-Amish patients from many countries and have often been labelled Byler's Syndrome. In about 50 per cent of cases there is an affected relative and PFIC appears to be inherited as an autosomal recessive (Nielsen, ActaPaedScand, 1986; 57:1010). [79] There is accumulating evidence that PFIC is a genetically and phenotypically heterogenous group of disorders.

Initial studies (Carlton, HumMolGen, 1995; 4:1049) on two members of the originally described Amish kindred showed that both members shared extended haplotypes on regions 18q21-q22 on both their chromosomes 18. Recently homozygosity for this haplotype has been demonstrated in affected patients from 11 of 15 Amish familes and 8 of 34 non-Amish families (Bull, Hepatol, 1997; 26:369A) and also, in families with PFIC from Ireland (Bourke, ArchDisChild, 1996; 75:223) and Japan (Tazaya, Hepatol, 997; 26: 384A). Patients with PFIC who are homozygous for this haplotype have been labelled PFIC-1 (Bull, Hepatol, 1997; 26:155). This shared haplotype containing the putative PFIC genetic defect, which has been refined down to 250 kilobases (Bull, Hepatol, 1997; 26:369A) is very close and possibly identical to those regions shared by patients with benign recurrent intrahepatic cholestasis (Houwen, NatureGen, 1994; 8:380), suggesting that both diseases result from defects in either the same gene, or in closely associated genes (van Berge Henegouwen, JHepatol, 1996; 25:395).

The basis for this form of PFIC may be a primary defect of hepatocyte bile-acid excretion. Biliary bile-acid levels are much lower than those found in other infantile cholestatic diseases and the proportion of chenodeoxycholic acid is usually less than 10 per cent of biliary bile acids, although it is the major serum bile acid (Tazawa, JPediatGastrNutr, 1985; 4:32; Jaquemin, EurJPed, 1994; 153:424; Bull, Hepatol, 1997; 26:155)

Affected patients develop pruritus, jaundice, and hepato-splenomegaly after the neonatal period but before 6 months of age. About one-third of patients develop cough or wheeze, usually closely associated with pruritus.[79] Diarrhoea, partially but not completely due to fat malabsorption is a common associated feature. Growth failure and fat-soluble deficiencies are common but mental retardation is uncommon.

Serum alkaline phosphatase and bile acids are usually raised, sometimes markedly so. Unusually for a chronic cholestatic condition, serum cholesterol is only modestly raised and serum γ-glutamyl transferase is typically within the normal range (Maggiore, JPediat, 1987; 111:251).[79] Interestingly, γ-glutamyl transferase in liver tissue is raised to the same degree as in other cholestatic diseases (Chobert; JHepatol, 1989; 8:22). Perhaps the normal level of serum γ-glutamyl transferase is a result of the relative absence of biliary bile acids, which may be important in γ-glutamyl transferase from the bile ductular epithelium.

Liver biopsy findings[80] include intrahepatic cholestasis, which in the early stages may be the only feature (Bull, Hepatol, 1997; 26: 155). In the later stages, hepatocellular ballooning and giant cell transformation are found. Bile duct paucity and fibrosis are seen in over one-half of cases, although portal inflammation is not prominent. Frequently, a characteristic abnormality is found: pericentral hepatic sclerosis.[80] Electron microscopy shows an increased number of microfilaments surrounding the bile canaliculi (De Vos, Gut, 1975; 16:943) which are dilated and lack microvilli. These features are seen in several forms of cholestasis. In addition, however, typical granular structures are seen in bile in the canalicular lumen ('Byler's bile').

Several non-Amish families with PFIC from several parts of the world have been described in whom linkage of the disease to chromosome 18q21-q22 has been excluded (Strautnieks, JMedGen, 1996; 33:833; Anneren, EurJHumGen, 1996; (suppl.1):99; Bull, Hepatol, 1997; 266:155). The disease in these children differed in some respects from that in children with PFIC-1, that is, who are homozygous for the chromosome 18q21-q22 haplotype. Liver biopsies showed more prominent inflammatory changes, a picture resembling neonatal hepatitis (see above). In addition, granular bile was not a feature and biliary chenodeoxycholic acid levels were only modestly depressed. Recently, studies in 19 families with this variant of PFIC, labelled PFIC-2, suggest linkage to a region on chromosome 2, which contains the gene for the sister of P glycoprotein (SPGP) (Thompson, Hepatol, 1997; 26:383A), a promising candidate for the ATP dependent canalicular bile acid transporter (Gerloff, Hepatol, 1997; 26:358A).

Finally, a variant of PFIC has been described, characterized by a high serum γ-glutamyl transferase and more prominent bile ductular proliferation than in PFIC-1 and PFIC-2. Preliminary studies (Deleuze, Hepatol, 1996; 23:904; Jacquemin, Hepatol, 1997; 26:248A), suggest that this variant is associated with a defect in the gene (on chromosome 7) for one of the multidrug resistance (MDR) proteins, MDR-3, a canalicular membrane protein which mediates phospholipid transport into bile. Patients had absence of MDR-3 mRNA and protein in liver and markedly diminished biliary phospholipid levels. A similar cholestatic disease is seen in 'knock-out' mice lacking the equivalent phospholipid transporter. The disease appears to result from bile acid-induced biliary epithelial damage (with consequent release of γ-glutamyl transferase) in the absence of the protective effect of biliary phospholipids.

The course of untreated PFIC is relentlessly progressive. Jaundice may be intermittent in the early stages, but the disease often progresses to cirrhosis and liver failure in adolescence. Partial biliary diversion (Withington, Gastro, 1988; 96:130) may relieve pruritus. Ursodeoxycholic acid improves liver enzymes in about two-thirds of cases and may also improve pruritus, hepatosplenomegaly, and liver fibrosis (Jacquemin, Hepatol, 1997; 25:519). [76] In recent years, several patients have undergone successful liver transplantation (Soubrane, Transpl, 1994; 50:804). [76]

Aagenaes' syndrome

This condition, which may be inherited as an autosomal recessive trait, is characterized by recurrent cholestasis, which usually begins in infancy, and lymphoedema of the lower limbs, which develops later (Aagenaes, ActaPaedScand, 1974; 63:465). Lymphangiograms confirm the presence of severe lymph vessel hypoplasia (Aagenaes, ArchDisChild, 1970; 45:690). Liver biopsies show giant-cell hepatitis, cholestasis, and portal tract fibrosis but no lymph vessel pathology. Progression to cirrhosis is common.

North American Indian cholestasis

This variant (Weber, Gastro, 1981; 81:653), characterized by cholestasis and hepatomegaly in association with facial telangiectasis, was initially described in 14 American Indian children from several families. Progression to cirrhosis and death from liver failure was usual; terminally the jaundice often disappeared. Mental and physical development were normal. Histological features in young children included findings typical of neonatal hepatitis. Later the condition progressed to portal tract fibrosis and cirrhosis. Ultrastructural features included dilated endoplasmic reticulum and canaliculi with loss of microvilli, but the most striking finding was a marked increase in the number of pericanalicular microfilaments, similar to that seen in experimental cholestasis induced by phalloidin (Dubin, Gastro, 1978; 75:450). The primary cause of the condition was therefore thought to be a derangement in microfilament function.

Familial chronic intrahepatic cholestasis

A syndrome characterized by mild cholestasis, hypothyroidism, skin pigmentation, hypertrichosis, facial telangiectasis, and onycholysis has been described in three siblings (Eriksson, Hepatol, 1983; 3: 391). Liver biopsies were normal on light microscopy. The condition is probably due to an undefined inborn error of metabolism.

Zellweger's syndrome

This condition is characterized by progressive cholestasis and hepatomegaly, presenting before 6 months of age and associated with mental retardation, hypotonia, renal cysts, and a characteristic facies. The primary defect lies in the peroxisomes, whose functions include oxidation of fatty acids and side-chain shortening of bile acid precursors (Goldfischer, Science, 1973; 182:62). Therefore, affected patients have increased serum, urine, and biliary levels of bile acid precursors (Hansson, Science, 1979; 203:1107). Liver biopsy findings include cholestasis, bile duct paucity, mild hepatocellular damage, and in the later stages, cirrhosis. The major ultrastructural feature is the virtual absence of peroxisomes. Few patients survive more than a few years.

Defects in bile acid synthesis

A few children with familial intrahepatic cholestasis have had markedly increased serum, urinary, and biliary levels of tri-hydroxycoprostanic acid (Eyssen, BBActa, 1972; 273:212; Hanson, JCI, 1975; 56:577). This accumulation may result from an inherited deficiency of the enzyme which converts trihydroxycoprostanic to varanic acid, a precursor of the most abundant primary bile acid, cholic acid. More recently, deficiencies of 3β-hydroxy-C27-steroid dehydrogenase/isomerase and Δ^4–3-oxosteroid 5β–reductase, two other enzymes of bile acid synthesis, have been demonstrated in several infants with progressive familial intrahepatic cholestasis (Clayton, JCI, 1987; 79:1031; Setchell, JCI 1988; 82:2148; Jacquemin, JPediat, 1994; 125:379). Bile acid replacement with cholic, chenodeoxycholic, or ursodeoxycholic acid resulted in clinical and biochemical improvement (Ichimiya, ArchDisChild, 1990; 65:1121; Daugherty, Hepatol, 1993; 18:1096). It is possible that a relative defect of choleretic bile acids and an accumulation of cholestatic bile-acid precursors are important in the pathogenesis of many cases of progressive familial intrahepatic cholestasis. It is likely that future research will identify further abnormalities of bile acid synthesis in children presently labelled as having idiopathic cholestasis.

Approach to the diagnosis of intrahepatic cholestasis[81]

Investigations should first exclude extrahepatic biliary obstruction and then attempt to establish the cause of the intrahepatic cholestasis. Biliary imaging techniques, including ultrasound, CT scanning, radionucleotide imaging, direct cholangiography, and magnetic resonance cholangiography have obviated the need for diagnostic laparotomy to exclude extrahepatic obstruction. The choice of procedure is determined by the clinical presentation, local expertise, and availability. However, ultrasound examination is usually preferred to exclude dilated intrahepatic ducts because it is specific, low in cost, and non-invasive.

A full history and physical examination with particular attention to the points in Table 7 will correctly distinguish intra- from extrahepatic cholestasis in 80 to 85 per cent of cases (Schenker, AmJDigDis, 1962; 7:449).[79]

Serum bilirubin, serum bile acids, liver biopsy with stains for iron, copper, PAS-positive granules, amyloid, protoporphyrins, liver enzymes, and lipoprotein X add little to diagnostic accuracy. Serum aminotransferase levels in excess of 1000 U/l may occur transiently in acute biliary obstruction due to common duct stones, but usually suggest hepatocellular rather than cholestatic liver injury.

The biliary tree is most accurately delineated by direct cholangiography, usually by the endoscopic retrograde approach. When this method is unsuccessful, cholangiography by the percutaneous approach may be performed. Both techniques have sensitivity and specificity in excess of 95 per cent (Vennes, Gastro, 1983; 84:1615), and usually define accurately the site and nature of the lesion, but they are time consuming, costly, and invasive.

Early studies suggested that ultrasound examination would accurately diagnose the presence of extrahepatic obstruction in 90 per cent of cases by the finding of dilated intrahepatic bile ducts. However, in prospective blinded studies, the accuracy has been lowered to between 60 and 70 per cent (Lapis; AnnIntMed, 1978; 89:613; Matzen, Gastro, 1983; 84:1492; O'Connor, Gastro, 1983; 84:1498). The reasons for the decline in sensitivity include technically inadequate examinations due to bowel gas or to inadequate operator skill, and the failure of the obstructed ducts to dilate when the obstruction is early or intermittent, or when the biliary tree compliance is reduced by sclerosing cholangitis, cirrhosis, or tumour. Therefore, ultrasound may not always be sufficient to exclude large-duct obstruction reliably in clinically equivocal cases and direct cholangiography may be indicated.

The role of other non-invasive imaging techniques in evaluating cholestatic patients is limited. Radionucleotide scanning with HIDA or DISIDA (diisopropyl iminodiacetic acid) is less accurate than ultrasound in distinguishing intra- from extrahepatic cholestasis (Matzen, Gastro, 1983; 84:1492; O'Connor, Gastro, 1983; 84:1498). However, a more refined technique, using a second-generation colloid, may demonstrate abnormalities in some cases of partial obstruction that have mild increases in bilirubin and normal-sized ducts on ultrasound (Lieberman, Gastro, 1986; 90:734). CT scanning is comparable in accuracy to ultrasound in the diagnosis of biliary dilatation (Baron, Radiol, 1982; 145:91; O'Connor, Gastro, 1983; 84:1498), but it is considerably more expensive. However, CT scanning may be used to screen the biliary tree if ultrasound is not technically possible or if pancreatic disease is suspected, since CT provides better images of this organ than does ultrasound. Magnetic resonance cholangiography is a promising biliary imaging technique (Lomanto, AmJSurg, 1997; 174:33), which remains to be compared with direct cholangiography in prospective blinded studies. A suggested investigative approach to the patient with cholestasis is outlined in Table 7.

Eliciting the cause of cholestasis in infancy poses particular problems. Early diagnosis of biliary atresia is vital since the results of surgery are much improved if it is performed before the age of 2 months (Milli-Vergani, Lancet, 1989; i:421; Ohi, JPediatSurg, 1990; 25:442). Ultrasound is much more difficult and less accurate than in adults. Biliary scintigraphy may be useful in distinguishing biliary atresia from neonatal hepatitis (El Tini, ArchDisChild, 1987; 62:180). In equivocal cases, endoscopic retrograde cholangio-pancreatography has been successfully performed (Wilkinson, ArchDisChild, 1991; 66:121). Additional investigations necessary to exclude specific cholestatic disorders in infancy (Table 6) include culture of cerebrospinal fluid, blood, and urine, throat swab, measurement of serum thyroxine and cortisol, sweat chloride, and tests for antibodies to rubella virus, cytomegalovirus, and toxoplasma, as well as α_1-antitrypsin genotyping, examination of urine for reducing sugars and amino acids, and chromosomal analysis.[74, 75]

Management of intrahepatic cholestasis

Treatment of the underlying liver disease

Many liver disorders that cause intrahepatic cholestasis are amenable to treatment, emphasizing the importance of making a correct

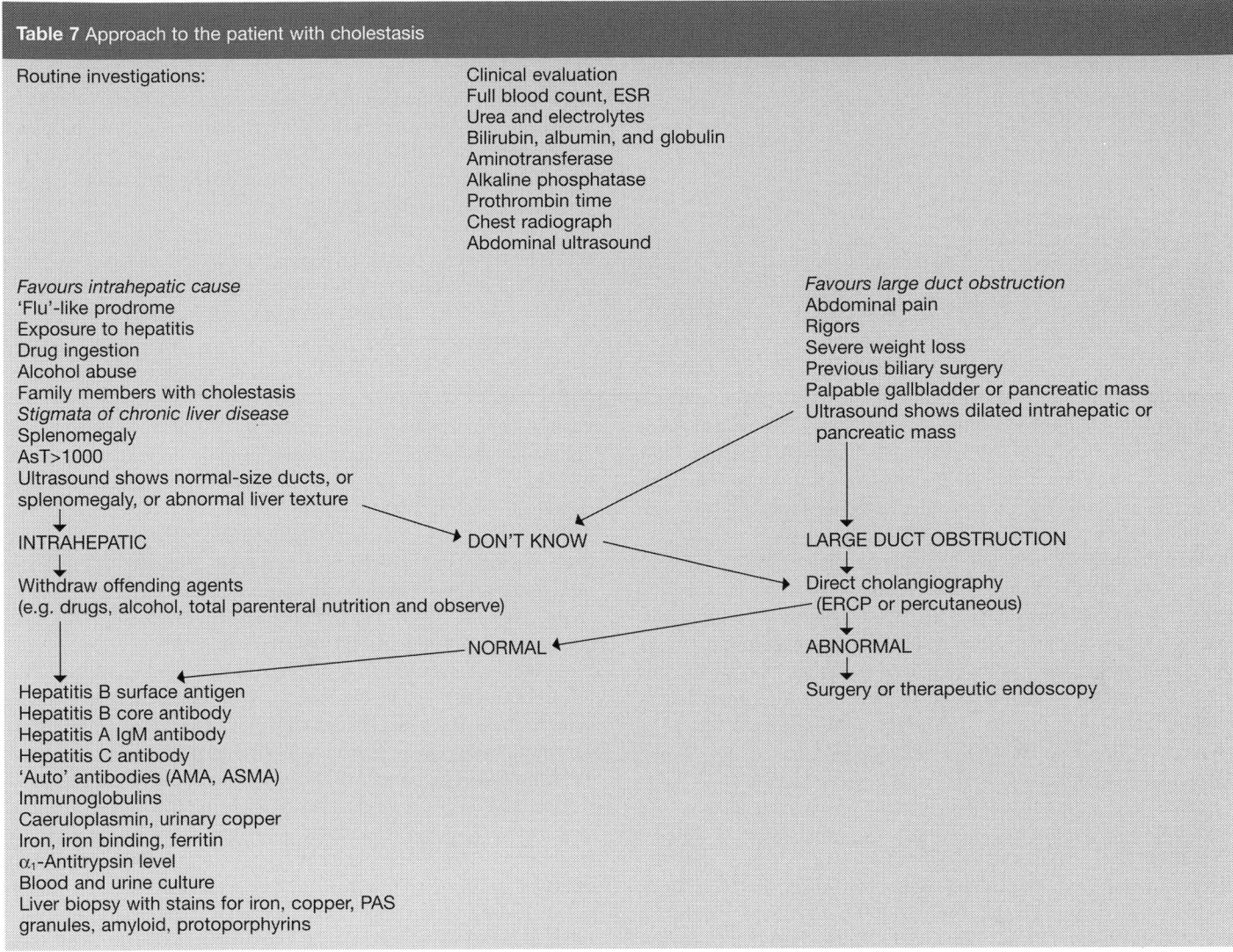

Table 7 Approach to the patient with cholestasis

Routine investigations:

Clinical evaluation
Full blood count, ESR
Urea and electrolytes
Bilirubin, albumin, and globulin
Aminotransferase
Alkaline phosphatase
Prothrombin time
Chest radiograph
Abdominal ultrasound

Favours intrahepatic cause
'Flu'-like prodrome
Exposure to hepatitis
Drug ingestion
Alcohol abuse
Family members with cholestasis
Stigmata of chronic liver disease
Splenomegaly
AsT>1000
Ultrasound shows normal-size ducts, or
splenomegaly, or abnormal liver texture

INTRAHEPATIC

Withdraw offending agents
(e.g. drugs, alcohol, total parenteral nutrition and observe)

Favours large duct obstruction
Abdominal pain
Rigors
Severe weight loss
Previous biliary surgery
Palpable gallbladder or pancreatic mass
Ultrasound shows dilated intrahepatic or
pancreatic mass

DON'T KNOW

LARGE DUCT OBSTRUCTION

Direct cholangiography
(ERCP or percutaneous)

NORMAL

ABNORMAL

Surgery or therapeutic endoscopy

Hepatitis B surface antigen
Hepatitis B core antibody
Hepatitis A IgM antibody
Hepatitis C antibody
'Auto' antibodies (AMA, ASMA)
Immunoglobulins
Caeruloplasmin, urinary copper
Iron, iron binding, ferritin
α_1-Antitrypsin level
Blood and urine culture
Liver biopsy with stains for iron, copper, PAS
granules, amyloid, protoporphyrins

diagnosis. Alcohol, cholestatic drugs, and parenteral nutrition should be withdrawn. Delivery may be induced in women in late pregnancy who have intolerable pruritus. Effective treatments are available for autoimmune hepatitis, Hodgkin's disease, and bacterial infection. Ursodeoxycholic acid may be effective in several types of intrahepatic cholestasis (see below). Finally, liver transplantation is now frequently performed for many chronic progressive cholestatic conditions.

Ursodeoxycholic acid

The endogenous bile acid pool in patients with cholestasis consists mainly of the primary bile acids, cholic and chenodeoxycholic, with relative reductions in pool sizes of the secondary bile acids, deoxycholic and lithocholic. All these bile acids accumulate in the liver in cholestasis. Chenodeoxycholic, deoxycholic, lithocholic, and to a lesser extent cholic acid are hepatotoxic. They cause cholestasis and hepatocellular necrosis when infused *in vivo* and in the isolated perfused liver. They have multiple effects on isolated hepatocytes, some unrelated to the detergent effects of bile acids since they occur at concentrations well below the critical micellar concentrations

(Spivey, JCI, 1993; 92:17). Bile acids at submicellar concentrations insert into cholesterol-rich membranes and form polar compartments with a resulting increase in membrane permeability (Guldutuna, Gastro, 1993; 104:1736). Bile acids cause lipid peroxidation of membranes, which may be mediated by oxygen free radicals (Sokol, Hepatol, 1993; 17:869). At higher concentrations they dissolve cholesterol-rich membranes. Bile acids, again at submicellar concentrations, insert into the inner mitochondrial membrane, with resultant increase in permeability, collapse of the proton gradient, inhibition of oxidative phosphorylation, and ATP depletion (Spivey, JCI, 1993; 92:17; Krakenbuhl, Hepatol, 1994; 19:471; Botla, JPharmExpTher, 1995; 272:930). Finally, bile acids inhibit vesicular transport by inhibiting microtubule-based ATPases (Marks, Gastro, 1995; 108:824).

Ursodeoxycholic acid is present in only trace amounts in normal human bile. Following oral administration, 40 to 50 per cent of ursodeoxycholic acid is absorbed by passive diffusion in the jejunum. Ursodeoxycholic acid is conjugated in the liver, preferentially to taurine but mainly to glycine because taurine stores are limited in humans. The conjugates are excreted into bile and

Table 8 Cholestatic diseases where ursodeoxycholic acid has been used (for details, see text)

Primary biliary cirrhosis
Primary sclerosing cholangitis
Cystic fibrosis
Intrahepatic cholestasis of pregnancy
Benign recurrent intrahepatic cholestasis
Sarcoidosis
Idiopathic adult ductopenia
Drug-induced cholestasis
Cholestasis associated with total parenteral nutrition
Arterio hepatic dysplasia (syndromic and non-syndromic)
Progressive familial intrahepatic cholestasis

constitute 30 to 50 per cent of biliary bile acids during chronic oral administration. The observations that ursodeoxycholic acid induced a greater bile flow than other bile acids (Dumont, Gastro, 1980; 79:82) and was less toxic to hepatocytes than other bile acids (Scholmench, Hepatol, 1984; 4:661) suggested it might be of therapeutic benefit in cholestasis.

Ursodeoxycholic acid has been used in many cholestatic conditions (see Table 8). Its use is usually associated with a fall in serum liver enzymes (alkaline phosphatase, aminotransferases, and γ-glutamyl transferase) and, when elevated, serum bilirubin. Ursodeoxycholic acid also improves biliary excretion of synthetic bile acids, as assessed by scintigraphy, in patients with primary biliary cirrhosis (Jazrawi, Gastro, 1993; 106:134), primary sclerosing cholangitis (Beuers, Hepatol, 1992; 16:707), and cystic fibrosis (Colombo, Hepatol, 1992; 15:677).

However, there remains debate as to whether ursodeoxycholic acid improves symptoms or retards the progression of chronic cholestatic liver diseases. Ursodeoxycholic acid has been most extensively evaluated in primary biliary cirrhosis. In four, large, multicentre trials (Poupon, NEJM, 1991; 324:1548; Heathcote, Hepatol, 1994; 19:1149; Lindor, Gastro, 1994; 106:1284; Coombes, Hepatol, 1995; 22:759), ursodeoxycholic acid at 13 to 15 mg/kg per day effected inconsistent improvements in symptoms (in particular, pruritus and fatigue) and in liver histology. A trend towards a reduction in death or need for liver transplantation was seen, which became significant when the results of three of the trials, involving a total of 550 patients, were combined (Poupon, Gastro, 1997; 113:884) and also following extension of two of the individual trials to 4 years follow-up (Poupon, NEJM, 1994; 330:1342; Lindor, Gastro, 1996; 113:884). However, the beneficial effect of ursodeoxycholic acid on survival appears disappointingly modest.

In two, small, placebo-controlled trials, ursodeoxycholic acid at 13 to 15 mg/kg per day improved serum bilirubin, liver enzymes, and liver histology scores in primary sclerosing cholangitis over a 12-month period (Beuers, Hepatol, 1992; 116:707; Stiehl, JHepatol, 1994; 20:57). However, in a recent multicentre trial, involving 105 patients patients, ursodeoxycholic acid had no effect on survival or transplant requirements, despite improvements in liver enzymes and serum bilirubin (Lindor, Gastro, 1996; 110:A1252).

In cystic fibrosis, ursodeoxycholic acid effects a sustained improvement in liver enzymes, although a higher dose (20 mg/kg per day) seems to be required than in other cholestatic diseases (Colombo, Hepatol, 1992; 16:924; van de Meeberg, ScandJGastro, 1987; 32:369). In a multicentre trial, ursodeoxycholic acid with or without taurine supplementation prevented deterioration of the Schwachman–Kulczycki score, an index of clinical status (Columbo, Hepatol, 1996; 23:1484). Ursodeoxycholic acid may also improve fat malabsorption and nutrition (Cotting, Gut, 1990; 31:918) in cystic fibrosis, however no data are available regarding its effect on progression of liver disease. In two placebo-controlled trials, ursodeoxycholic acid was of benefit in intrahepatic cholestasis of pregnency (Palma, Hepatol, 1996; 24:373A; Isla, Gastro, 1996; 110: 1219A). In other cholestatic conditions, data on ursodeoxycholic acid is largely anecdotal (see relevant sections above). Liver enzymes usually fall and effects on pruritus are variable.

There are several possible mechanisms for the therapeutic effect of ursodeoxycholic acid :

1. Cytoprotection

Coinfusion of ursodeoxycholic acid or its taurine conjugate protects against the cholestasis, biliary protein excretion, and morphological liver damage induced by *in vivo* infusion of chenodeoxycholic acid (Heuman, Gastro, 1991; 100:203), cholic acid (Kitani, AJP, 1985; 248:G407), or lithocholic acid (Scholmerich, JHepatol, 1990; 10: 280). Taurine-conjugated ursodeoxycholic acid also reduces the morphological liver damage associated with extrahepatic obstruction (Krol, Hepatol, 1983; 3:881; Poo, Gastro, 1992; 102:1752), and oestrogens (Utilli, JHepatol, 1990; 11:735).

Coincubation with taurine-conjugated ursodeoxycholic acid (but not unconjugated ursodeoxycholic acid) protects isolated hepatocytes from damage induced by TCDCA, as assessed by intracellular enzyme release (Galle, Hepatol, 1990; 12:486; Heuman, Hepatol, 1991; 14:920). The protective effect is associated with a lowering of intracellular TCDCA levels (Ohiwa, Hepatol, 1993; 17:470) and it may be that ursodeoxycholic acid acts by increasing hepatocellular excretion of other bile acids, perhaps via a calcium–dependent vesicular pathway (see mechanism 2 below). However, others have failed to demonstrate any effect on TCDCA-induced toxicity or intracellular TCDCA levels at the ursodeoxycholic acid concentrations of 0.5 mmol found in serum in cholestasis (Hillaire, Hepatol, 1995; 22:82). It should be remembered, however, that isolated hepatocytes internalize their canalicular membrane to a variable degree; this process might impair bile acid efflux.

Other potential cytoprotective mechanisms include effects on plasma membranes and mitochondria. Taurine-conjugated ursodeoxycholic acid prevents bile-acid induced formation of polar compartments in cholesterol-rich plasma membrames (Guldutuna, Gastro, 1994; 104:1736), and in higher doses prevents membrane dissolution by bile acids (Heuman, Gastro, 1994; 106:1033). Ursodeoxycholic acid prevents the increase in inner mitochondrial membrane permeability and the decline in mitochondrial enzyme activity induced by TCDCA (Krakenbuhl, Hepatol, 1994; 20:1595; Botla, JPharmExpTher, 1995; 272:930). This effect is not seen with taurine-conjugated ursodeoxycholic acid, possibly because it is too polar to insert into the inner mitochondrial membrane.

2. Stimulation of biliary secretion

Ursodeoxycholic acid increases the bile flow in animals more than other bile acids. The most plausible explanation for this hypercholeretic effect is that ursodeoxycholic acid induces biliary bicarbonate secretion via a cholehepatic shunt pathway (Erlinger,

Hepatol, 1990; 11:888). In brief, unconjugated ursodeoxycholic acid is excreted into the bile canaliculus, where, because of its high pK, it becomes protonated. The protonated uncharged ursodeoxycholic acid is then reabsorbed by diffusion into the bile ductular epithelium, and is re-excreted by the hepatocyte. Acceptance of a proton by ursodeoxycholic acid produces a HCO_3^- anion in the bile ductule, which constitutes the osmotic driving force for bile flow. Ursodeoxycholic acid may also directly stimulate bile ductular bicarbonate secretion by activation of an apical membrane chloride channel (Shimo, Gastro, 1995; 109:965). However, a bicarbonate-rich hypercholeresis has not been demonstrated in humans (Knyrim, Hepatol, 1989; 10:134). Furthermore, during ursodeoxycholic acid administration, only small amounts of unconjugated ursodeoxycholic acid are found in bile (Crosignani, Hepatol, 1991; 14:1000). Therefore, the clinical relevance of this hypercholeretic effect is unclear. A more important effect of ursodeoxycholic acid on biliary excretion may be related to the ability of its taurine conjugate to mobilize extracellular calcium, resulting in sustained increases in intracellular calcium cytosolic-membrane translocation of α-PKC, and stimulation of vesicle transport and biliary exocytosis (Beuers, JCI, 1993; 91:2989; Beuers, Gastro, 1996; 110:1553). This effect, observed in rat livers, would serve to reconstitute transporters in the canalicular domain and would explain the stimulation of excretion of synthetic bile acid analogues in primary biliary cirrhosis and primary sclerosing cholangitis (Jazrawi, Gastro, 1994; 106:134).

3. Immunomodulation

The observation that ursodeoxycholic acid lowered serum IgM in patients with primary biliary cirrhosis suggested that it may have immunomodulatory properties. Ursodeoxycholic acid inhibits class I HLA expression on hepatocytes in primary biliary cirrhosis (Calmus, Hepatol, 1990; 11:12) and in primary sclerosing cholangitis (Beuers, Hepatol, 1992; 16:707). However, such expression may be a secondary consequence of cholestasis as it is also seen in experimental biliary obstruction. Ursodeoxycholic acid has been shown to exert inhibitory effects on peripheral blood mononuclear cell proliferation and immunoglobulin production (Yoshikawa, Hepatol, 1992; 16:358). The relevance of these effects to the clinical actions of ursodeoxycholic acid remain unclear, as chenodeoxycholic acid has been shown to have similar immunosuppressive properties (Calmus, Hepatol, 1992; 16:719).

4. Displacement of endogenous bile acids

Probably because of its hydrophilicity and poor detergent properties, ursodeoxycholic acid is less disruptive to liver and other plasma membranes than are other bile acids (Scholmench, Hepatol, 1984; 4:661). Partial replacement of the endogenous bile acid pool by ursodeoxycholic acid should therefore minimize secondary hepatocellular damage from retained endogenous bile acids. In fact, however, enrichment of the bile acid pool with ursodeoxycholic acid is only 30 to 50 per cent in patients with cholestatic liver disease, rather less than the 50 to 60 per cent enrichment attained in patients undergoing gallstone dissolution with ursodeoxycholic acid and much less than the biliary enrichment with chenodeoxycholic acid (80 to 90 per cent) attained during feeding of this bile acid. Furthermore, biliary enrichment with ursodeoxycholic acid during

its administration is mainly at the expense of cholic acid, a relatively hydrophilic and non-toxic bile acid. The cholic acid pool is depleted partly by an inhibitory effect of ursodeoxycholic acid on intestinal absorption of cholic acid (Martheau, Hepatol, 1990; 12:1200; Stiehl, Gastro, 1990; 98:424). In contrast, serum and biliary levels and pool sizes of chenodeoxycholic and deoxycholic acid change little, and the level of lithocholic acid actually increases in patients with cholestasis after administration of ursodeoxycholic acid (Cosignani, Hepatol, 1991; 14:1000; Beuers, Hepatol, 1993; 15:603; Bhatta, AmJGastr, 1993; 88:691). Reasons for the limited biliary enrichment with ursodeoxycholic acid and displacement of the endogenous bile acid pool include: (i) inefficient absorption of orally administered ursodeoxycholic acid of about 50 per cent (Stiehl, Gastro, 1988; 94:1201); (ii) failure of ursodeoxycholic acid (unlike chenodeoxycholic acid) to suppress endogenous bile acid synthesis (Nilsell, Gastro, 1983; 85:1248); and (iii) conversion of administered ursodeoxycholic acid to chenodeoxycholic and lithocholic acid by the intestinal bacterial enzymes 7β-epimerase and 7α-dehydroxylase.

The limited biliary enrichment with ursodeoxycholic acid may be one reason for its limited clinical effects. Indeed, in patients with primary biliary cirrhosis, the return to normal of liver enzymes correlates with the degree of biliary enrichment atttained (Jorgenson, Gut, 1995; 36:935). Potential ways of improving the clinical efficacy of ursodeoxycholic acid currently under evaluation include its administration as a sodium salt, which is better absorbed (Roda, PharmRes, 1994; 11:642), and a 6-fluoro analogue, which attains higher concentrations in bile (Roda, Gastro, 1995; 108:1204). Administration of taurine-conjugated ursodeoxycholic acid is associated with a greater enrichment of the bile acid pool with ursodeoxycholic acid in animals (Rodrigues, Gastro, 1995; 109:564) and in patients with cholestasis (Setchell, Hepatol, 1994; 20:150A), perhaps becauase it has a higher first-pass hepatic extraction than ursodeoxycholic acid (Poupon, BiochemPharm, 1988; 37:209) and is more resistant to 7α-dehydroxylation (Rodrigues, Gastro, 1995; 109:564). Taurine-conjugated ursodeoxycholic acid has a greater hepatoprotective effect on isolated hepatocytes than the unconjugated form, although the opposite is true for isolated mitochondria (see mechanism 1 above). Clinical studies to date in primary biliary cirrhosis suggest similar effects of taurine-conjugated ursodeoxycholic acid and ursodeoxycholic acid on liver enzymes (Crosignani, Hepatol, 1996; 23:111P).

Partial biliary diversion

Children with progressive familial intrahepatic cholestasis may improve dramatically following external biliary drainage via a jejunal conduit (Withington, Gastro, 1988; 95:130). In this series, pruritus disappeared, and serum bile acids and liver enzymes fell to near normal. Furthermore, liver histology improved, consistent with the hypothesis that secondary liver damage is mediated by retained bile acids. Results were less impressive in two children with Alagille's syndrome.

Phenobarbital

Phenobarbital increases bile-acid independent flow, possibly by augmenting hepatic conjugation reactions (Stiehl, EurJClinInv, 1980; 10:307) or by increasing the biliary output of glutathione

(Ballitori, AmJPhysiol, 1989; 256:G22). Phenobarbital administration is associated with variable reductions in serum bilirubin and bile acid levels, and with short-term relief of pruritus in some, although not all, patients with primary biliary cirrhosis, primary sclerosing cholangitis, benign recurrent cholestasis, and infants with a paucity of interlobular bile ducts (Stiehl, NEJM, 1972; 286:858; Bloomer, AmJMed, 1975; 82:310). Clinical benefits are limited by the sedative and dependence-inducing effects of barbiturates, and these agents should not be used as standard therapy.

S-Adenosyl-L-methionine

This agent protects against oestrogen-induced cholestasis in rats (Stramentoli, Gastro, 1981; 80:154), and against the oestrogen-induced defects in plasma membrane Na^+/K^+ATPase activity (Boelsterli, Hepatol, 1983; 3:12) and bile acid transport (Fricker, Hepatol, 1988; 8:1224). Its mechanism of action is unclear but it may stimulate membrane phospholipid synthesis or inactivate toxic oestrogen metabolites.[21] It has been used in intrahepatic cholestasis of pregnancy and in benign recurrent intrahepatic cholestasis with mixed results (see above).

Corticosteroids

Hydrocortisone increases bile-acid independent flow in dogs. Corticosteroids cause a rapid fall in serum bilirubin and relieve pruritus in about 70 per cent of cases of cholestatic viral hepatitis (Summerskill, BMJ, 1958; ii:1499). The mechanism of action is unclear (Williams, Lancet, 1961; ii:392). Corticosteroids are contraindicated in hepatitis B because they may increase the relapse rate, but short-term trials may accelerate recovery in acute drug-induced cholestasis.

Treatment of secondary consequences[47,74, 82]

The steatorrhoea of chronic cholestasis can usually be corrected by a low fat diet (less than 40 g/day), and medium-chain triglyceride supplementation (Cohen, JPediat, 1971; 79:379). In patients who do not respond, the possibilities of pancreatic dysfunction and jejunal villus atrophy should be considered, because pancreatic enzyme replacement or withdrawal of gluten may then be of benefit.

There is some controversy as to whether routine vitamin A supplementation is desirable in patients with chronic cholestasis (Shepherd, BMJ, 1984; 289:1484; Walt, BMJ, 1984; 288:1030). Periodic assessment for night blindness should be performed if cholestasis is severe. In such patients, oral vitamin A (25 000 to 50 000 units/day) will return serum vitamin A levels to normal and may improve vision.

Because serum levels of 1,25-dihydroxyvitamin D are usually normal, and osteomalacia is uncommon, not all patients with cholestasis need vitamin D supplementation. However, patients with long-standing cholestasis who have a poor diet, and get little exposure to sunlight, should receive at least 100 000 units of vitamin D_2 or D_3 intramuscularly every month, or 40 000 units (1 mg) of oral vitamin D_2 or D_3 daily. The dose should be adjusted so as to keep the serum 25-hydroxyvitamin D level in the normal range. An alternative approach is to administer 50 to 100 µg of 25-hydroxyvitamin D daily.

Osteoporosis associated with cholestasis does not respond to vitamin D (Epstein, AmJClinNut, 1982; 36:426).[44,45] However, patients with cholestasis and osteoporosis, even with normal serum levels of vitamin D, tend to have impaired calcium absorption,[44] possibly resulting from fat malabsorption (Kehayoglou, Gut, 1973; 14:653). In these patients, a low fat diet containing at least 1.5 g of calcium per day is recommended. Indeed, dietary supplementation with calcium increases bone density in patients with primary biliary cirrhosis; in the same study, calcitonin was ineffective (Camisasca, Hepatol, 1994; 20:633). Fluoride has also increased bone density in primary biliary cirrhosis (Guanabens, JHepatol, 1992; 15:345); however, use of fluoride in postmenopausal osteoporosis is, despite increases in bone density, not associated with a decreased fracture risk. Recently, etidronate has been shown to be superior to fluoride in preventing bone loss in primary biliary cirrhosis (Guanabens, Gastro, 1997; 113:219). Oestrogen replacement appears to be safe in postmenopausal patients with primary biliary cirrhosis, and does not aggravate the liver disease (Crippin, AmJGastr, 1994; 89:47), but beneficial effects on bone remain to be established. Ursodeoxycholic acid does not influence bone density in primary biliary cirrhosis (Lindor, Hepatol, 1995; 21:389).

In children with cholestasis and established neurological deficits due to vitamin E deficiency, clinical improvement following repletion is modest (Sokol, NEJM, 1985; 313:1580), and routine supplementation after the age of 3 years is recommended. In adults with cholestasis, routine vitamin E (α-tocopherol) replacement is probably not necessary, but patients should be monitored for the development of neurological symptoms and signs. If the cholestasis is moderate, deficiency may be corrected by parenteral vitamin E (200 mg intramuscularly twice monthly) or by large doses of oral vitamin E. In cases of severe cholestasis, these measures are often ineffective (Jeffrey, JHepatol, 1987; 4:307). A water-soluble derivative of vitamin E, 25 units/kg per day linked to polyethylene glycol (D-α-tocopherol–PEG–1000-succinate), has been shown to be effective in returning vitamin E status to normal (Sokol, Gastro, 1987; 93:975) and in effecting some neurological improvement in about 50 per cent and stabilization in most children with chronic cholestasis (Sokol, Gastro, 1993; 104:1727).

When the coagulopathy of vitamin K deficiency is mild, it is seldom a clinical problem and only requires correction by parenteral vitamin K (10 mg) when liver biopsy or surgery is contemplated.

Pruritus is often a distressing symptom in patients with cholestasis and should be treated vigorously to prevent excoriations. The anion-exchange resin cholestyramine is widely used to bind bile acids, although the rationale underlying its use is suspect because of the lack of evidence linking bile acids to pruritus. It is best given 20 to 30 min before meals and particularly in the morning, when most of the bile acid pool is stored in the gallbladder (Javitt, NEJM, 1974; 290:1328). Doses range from 4 to 16 g daily. Other medications must be given at a time when they will not be bound by the resin. Several double-blind trials suggest a benefit from rifampicin at 300 to 600 mg/day over placebo and phenobarbital in cholestatic pruritus (Ghent, Gastro, 1988; 94:488; Bachs, Lancet, 1989; i:574; Cynamon, Gastro, 1990; 98:1913; Podesta, DigDisSci, 1991; 36:216). Other agents not fully evaluated but claimed to be of benefit in treating pruritus, are illustrated in Table 9. Of particular interest are the opiate antagonists naltrexone and nalmefene, in

Table 9 Interventions used in the treatment of pruritus of cholestasis (see ref. 93)
Androgens[34] Cholestyramine (Javitt, NEJM, 1974; 290:1328) Terfenadine (Duncan, BMJ, 1984; 289:22) Rifampicin (Ghent, Gastro, 1988; 94:488) Hydroxyethylrutosides (Hishon, BrJDermatol, 1981; 105:457) Naltrexone (Carson, AmJGastro, 1996; 91:1022) Nalmefene (Thornton, BrMedJ, 1988; 297:1501) Ondansetron (Schworer, Pain, 1995;61:33) Phototherapy (Hanid, Lancet, 1980; ii:530) Plasmapheresis (Lauterberg, Lancet, 1980; ii:1153)

view of the recent evidence implicating endogenous opioids in the pruritus of cholestasis. [35,36]

The hyperlipidaemia of cholestasis seldom requires specific treatment.[37] Phenobarbital (Linarelli, JPediat, 1973; 83:291) and cholestyramine may help, but clofibrate may actually increase serum cholesterol (Schaffner, Gastro, 1969; 57:253). In severe cases complicated by xanthomatous neuropathy, plasmapheresis has been of benefit (Turnberg, Gut, 1972; 13:396). Agents that inhibit cholesterol synthesis have not been adequately assessed and may be toxic in cholestatic conditions.

It should be emphasized that treatment of these secondary consequences may relieve symptoms temporarily, but has only limited effects on the general well being of patients with chronic cholestasis. If effective treatment of the underlying cause is not available and liver function is deteriorating, to the extent that the functional status of the patient is severely impaired, liver transplantation should be considered.

References

1. Popper H. Cholestasis: the future of a past and present riddle. *Hepatology*, 1981; **1**: 187–91.
2. Eppinger H. *Die Leberkrankheiten. Allgemeine und Spezielle Pathologie und Therapie der Leber.* Vienna: Julius Springer, 1937.
3. Watson CJ and Hoffbauer FW. The problem of prolonged hepatitis with particular reference to the cholangiolitic type and to the development of cholangiolitic cirrhosis of the liver. *Annals of Internal Medicine*, 1946; **25**: 195–227.
4. Popper HJ and Szanto PB. Intrahepatic cholestasis (cholangiolitis). *Gastroenterology*, 1956; **31**: 683–700.
5. Sellinger M and Boyer JL. Physiology of bile secretion and cholestasis. In Popper H and Schaffner F, eds. *Progress in liver diseases.* New York: Grune & Stratton, 1990; **9**: 237–59.
6. Oelberg D and Lester R. Cellular mechanisms of cholestasis. *Annual Review of Medicine*, 1986; **37**: 297–317.
7. Reichen J and Simon FR. Cholestasis. In Arias IM, Jakoby WB, Popper H, Schachter D, and Schafritz DA, eds. *The liver. Biology and pathobiology.* New York: Raven Press, 1988: 1105–24.
8. Phillips MJ, Poucell S, and Oda M. Biology of disease mechanisms of cholestasis. *Laboratory Investigation*, 1986; **54**: 593–608.
9. Tuchweber B, Weber A, Roy C, and Yousef IM. Mechanisms of experimentally induced intrahepatic cholestasis. *Seminars in Liver Disease*, 1986; **8**: 161–78.
10. Duffy MC and Boyer JL. Pathophysiology of intrahepatic cholestasis and biliary obstruction. In Ostrow JD, ed. *Bile pigments and jaundice.* New York: Marcel Dekker, 1986: 333–72.
11. Fallon MB, Anderson JM, and Boyer JL. Intrahepatic cholestasis. In Schiff L and Schiff ER, eds. *Diseases of the liver.* 7th edn. Philadelphia: JB Lippincott, 1993: 342–61.
12. Fallon MB, Anderson JM, and Boyer JL. Pathogenesis of cholestasis: past and future trends. *Seminars in Liver Disease*, 1993; **13**: 219–315.
13. Boyer JL. Molecular pathogenesis of cholestasis. In Schmid R, *et al.*, eds. *Molecular biology and clinics.* Dordrecht: Kluwer Academic Publishers, 1996: 87–95.
14. Boyer JL. New concepts of mechanisms of hepatocyte bile formation. *Physiological Reviews*, 1980; **60**: 303–26.
15. Graf J. Canalicular bile salt independent bile formation: concepts and clues from electrolyte transport in rat liver. *American Journal of Physiology*, 1983; **244**: G233–46.
16. Strange RS. Hepatic bile formation. *Physiological Reviews*, 1984; **64**: 1055–102.
17. Coleman R. Biochemistry of bile secretion. *Biochemical Journal*, 1987; **244**: 249–61.
18. Boyer JL, Allen RM, and Oi Cheng Ng. Biochemical separation of Na/K ATPase from 'purified' 'canalicular' enriched plasma membrane fractions from rat liver. *Hepatology*, 1983; **3**: 18–28.
19. Erlinger S. Bile flow. In Arias IM, Boyer JL, Jakoby WB, Fausto N, Schachter D, and Shafritz DA, eds. *The liver. Biology and pathobiology.* New York: Raven Press, 1994: 769–88.
20. Nathanson MH and Boyer JL. Mechanisms and regulation of bile secretion. *Hepatology*, 1991; **14**: 551–66.
21. Schreiber AJ and Simon FR. Estrogen-induced cholestasis; clues to pathogenesis and treatment. *Hepatology*, 1983; **3**: 607–13.
22. Vore M. Estrogen cholestasis. Membranes, metabolites or receptors? *Gastroenterology*, 1987; **93**: 643–9.
23. Kreek MJ. Female sex steroids and cholestasis. *Seminars in Liver Disease*, 1987; **7**: 8–23.
24. Reyes H and Simon FR. Intrahepatic cholestasis: an estrogen-related disease. *Seminars in Liver Disease*, 1993; **13**: 289–301.
25. Schachter D. Fluidity and function of hepatocyte plasma membranes. *Hepatology*, 1984; **4**: 140–51.
26. Anderson JM. Leaky junctions and cholestasis: a tight correlation. *Gastroenterology*, 1996; **110**: 1662–5.
27. Desmet VJ. Cholestasis; extrahepatic obstruction and secondary biliary cirrhosis. In McSween RJ, Anthony PP, and Scheuer PJ, eds. *Pathology of the liver.* Edinburgh: Churchill Livingstone, 1979: 272–305.
28. Popper H. Hepatocellular degeneration and death. In Arias IM, Jacoby WB, Popper H, Schachter D, and Shafritz DA, eds. *The liver. Biology and pathology.* New York; Raven Press, 1988: 1087–103.
29. Scheuer PJ. *Liver biopsy interpretation.* Scheuer PJ, ed. London: Baillière Tindall, 1988; 40–65.
30. Summerfield JA *et al.* Benign recurrent intrahepatic cholestasis: studies of bilirubin kinetics, bile acids and cholangiography. *Gut*, 1980; **21**: 154–60.
31. Bloomer JR, Berk PD, and Howe RB. Hepatic clearance of unconjugated bilirubin in cholestatic liver diseases. *American Journal of Digestive Diseases*, 1974; **14**: 9–14.
32. Murphy GM. Serum bile acids: old and new. In Setchell KDR, Kritchevsky D, and Nair P, eds. *The bile acids; chemistry, physiology and metabolism.* New York: Plenum Press, 1988: IV: 379–404.
33. van Berge Henegouwen GP, Brandt KH, Eyssen H, and Parmentier G. Sulphated and unsulphated bile acids in serum, bile and urine of patients with cholestasis. *Gut*, 1976; **17**: 861–89.
34. Garden JP, Ostrow JD, and Roenigk HH Jr. Pruritus in hepatic cholestasis: pathogenesis and therapy. *Archives of Dermatology*, 1985; **121**: 1415–20.
35. Jones EA and Bergasa NV. The pruritus of cholestasis: from bile acids to opiate antagonists. *Hepatology*, 1990; **11**: 884–7.
36. Bergasa NV and Jones EA. The pruritus of cholestasis: pathogenic and therapeutic implications of opioids. *Gastroenterology*, 1995; **108**: 1582–8.
37. McIntyre N, Harry DS, and Pearson AJG. Progress report: the hypercholesterolaemia of obstructive jaundice. *Gut*, 1975; **16**: 379.
38. Sabesin SM. Cholestatic lipoproteins: their pathogenesis and significance. *Gastroenterology*, 1982; **83**: 704–9.

39. Walshe JM. Copper: its role in the pathogenesis of liver disease. *Seminars in Liver Disease*, 1984; **4**: 252–70.

40. Hay JE. Bone disease in cholestatic liver disease. *Gastroenterology*, 1995; **108**: 276–83.

41. Compston JE. Hepatic osteodystrophy: vitamin D metabolism in patients with liver disease. *Gut*, 1986; **27**: 1073–90.

42. Eastell R *et al*. Rates of vertebral bone loss before and after liver transplantation in women with primary biliary cirrhosis. *Hepatology*, 1991; **14**: 296–300.

43. Hodgson SF *et al*. Bone loss and reduced osteoclast function in primary biliary cirrhosis. *Annals of Internal Medicine*, 1985; **103**: 855–60.

44. Matloff DS *et al*. Osteoporosis in primary biliary cirrhosis: effect of 25-hydroxy vitamin D treatment. *Gastroenterology*, 1982; **83**: 97–102.

45. Herlong HF, Recker RR, and Maddrey WC. Bone disease in primary biliary cirrhosis: historical features and response to 25-hydroxy vitamin D. *Gastroenterology*, 1982; **83**: 103–8.

46. Reed JS, Meredith SC, Nemchausky BA, Rosenberg IH, and Boyer JL. Bone disease in primary biliary cirrhosis: reversal of osteomalacia with 25-hydroxy vitamin D. *Gastroenterology*, 1980; **78**: 512–17.

47. Sokol RJ. Fat-soluble vitamins and their importance in patients with cholestatic liver disease. *Gastroenterology Clinics of North America*, 1994; **23**: 673–705.

48. Zimmerman HJ and Maddrey WC. Toxic and drug induced hepatitis. In Schiff L and Schiff ER, eds. *Diseases of the liver*. Philadelphia: JB Lippincott, 1987: 591–667.

49. Lee WM. Drug-induced hepatotoxicity. *New England Journal of Medicine*, 1995; **233**: 1118–27.

50. Ludwig J and Axelsen R. Drug effects on the liver. An updated tabular compilation of drugs and drug related hepatic diseases. *Digestive Diseases and Sciences*, 1983; **28**: 651–66.

51. Neuberger J. Drug induced jaundice. *Clinics in Gastroenterology*, 1989; **3**: 447–66.

52. Desmet VJ. Cholangiopathies: past, present and future. *Seminars in Liver Disease*, 1987; **7**: 67–76.

53. Birrer MJ and Young RC. Differential diagnosis of jaundice in lymphoma patients. *Seminars in Liver Disease*, 1987; **7**: 269–77.

54. Hoffmann MS, Stein RE, Davidian MM, and Rosenthal WS. Hepatic amyloidosis presenting as severe intrahepatic cholestasis. A case report and review of the literature. *American Journal of Gastroenterology*, 1988; **83**: 783–5.

55. Rubinow A, Koff RS, and Cohen AS. Severe intrahepatic cholestasis in amyloidosis. A report of four cases and a review of the literature. *American Journal of Medicine*, 1978; **64**: 937–46.

56. Bloomer JR. The liver in protoporphyria. *Hepatology*, 1988; **8**: 402–7.

57. Tanner MS and Taylor CJ. Liver disease in cystic fibrosis. *Archives of Diseases of Childhood*, 1996; **72**: 282–4.

58. Zimmerman HJ, Fang M, Utilli R, Seef LB, and Hoofnagle J. Jaundice due to bacterial infection. *Gastroenterology*, 1979; **77**: 362–74.

59. Baker AL and Rosenberg IH. Hepatic complications of total parenteral nutrition. *American Journal of Medicine*, 1987; **82**: 489–97.

60. Withington PB. Cholestasis associated with total parenteral nutrition in infants. *Hepatology*, 1985; **5**: 693–6.

61. Quigley EMM, Marsh MN, Shaffer JL, and Markin RS. Hepatobiliary complications of total parenteral nutrition. *Gastroenterology*, 1993; **104**: 286–301.

62. Moody FG and Thompson DA. Postoperative jaundice. In Schiff L and Schiff ER, eds. *Diseases of the liver*. Philadelphia: JB Lippincott, 1987: 1223–33.

63. Hayes PC and Bouchier IAD. Postoperative jaundice. *Clinics in Gastroenterology*, 1989; **3**: 485–505.

64. Bacq Y, Sapey T, Brechot MC, Fabrice P, Fignon A, and Dubois F. Intrahepatic cholestasis of pregnancy: a French perspective. *Hepatology*, 1997; **26**: 358–64.

65. Reyes H. The enigma of intrahepatic cholestasis of pregnancy: lessons from Chile. *Hepatology*, 1982; **2**: 87–96.

66. Reyes H. The spectrum of liver and gastrointestinal disease seen in cholestasis of pregnancy. *Gastroenterology Clinics of North America*, 1992; **21**: 905–21.

67. Lunzer MR. Jaundice in pregnancy. *Clinics in Gastroenterology*, 1982; **3**: 467–83.

68. Summerskill WHJ and Walshe JM. Benign recurrent intrahepatic 'obstructive' jaundice. *Lancet*, 1959; **ii**: 686–90.

69. de Pagter AGF, van Berge Henegouwen GP, Ten Bokkel Huinink JA, and Brandt KH. Familial benign recurrent intrahepatic cholestasis: interrelationship with intrahepatic cholestasis of pregnancy and from oral contraceptives. *Gastroenterology*, 1976; **71**: 202–7.

70. Schiff L. Idiopathic benign recurrent intrahepatic cholestasis. In Schiff L and Schiff ER, eds. *Diseases of the liver*. Philadelphia: JB Lippincott, 1987: 1473–7.

71. Tygstrup N and Jensen B. Intermittent intrahepatic cholestasis of unknown etiology in five young males from the Faroe Islands. *Acta Medica Scandinavica*, 1969; **185**: 523–30.

72. Brenard N, Geubel AP, and Benhamou JP. Benign recurrent intrahepatic cholestasis. A review of 26 cases. *Journal of Clinical Gastroenterology*, 1989; **11**: 546–51.

73. van Berge Henegouwen GP, Ferguson DR, Hofmann AF, and de Pagter AGF. Familial and non familial benign recurrent cholestasis distinguished by plasma disappearance of indocyanine green but not cholylglycine. *Gut*, 1978; **19**: 345–9.

74. Ballisteri WF. Liver disease in infancy and childhood. In Schiff L and Schiff ER, eds. *Diseases of the Liver*. Philadelphia: JB Lippincott, 1987: 1337–426.

75. Ballesteri WF. Neonatal cholestasis. *Journal of Pediatrics*, 1985; **106**: 171–85.

76. Balistreri WF. Ursodeoxycholic acid in the treatment of paediatric liver disease. In Fromm H and Leuschner U, eds. *Falk Symposium No. 84. Bile acids–cholestasis–gallstones. Advances in basic and clinical bile acid research.* Dordrecht: Kluwer Academic Publishers, 1995: 327–42.

77. Riley CA. Familial intrahepatic cholestatic syndromes. In Suchy FJ, ed. *Liver disease in children*. St Louis: Mosby, 1994: 443–59.

78. Alagille D. Syndromic paucity of interlobular bile ducts (Alagille syndrome or arteriohepatic dysplasia): review of 80 cases. *Journal of Pediatrics*, 1987; **110**: 195–200.

79. Whittington PF, Freese DJ, Alonso EM, Schwarzenberg SJ, and Shaarp HL. Clinical and biochemical findings in progressive familial intrahepatic cholestasis. *Journal of Pediatric Gastroenterology and Nutrition*, 1994; **18**: 134–41.

80. Alonso EM, Snover DC, Montag A, Freese DK, and Whittington PF. Histological pathology of the liver in progressive familial intrahepatic cholestasis. *Journal of Pediatric Gastroenterology and Nutrition*, 1994; **18**: 128–33.

81. Scharschmidt BF, Goldberg HI, and Schmid R. Approach to the patient with cholestatic jaundice. *New England Journal of Medicine*, 1983; **308**: 1515–19.

82. Allagille D. Management of paucity of interlobular bile ducts. *Journal of Hepatology*, 1985; **1**: 561–5.

83. Khandelwal M, Malet PF. Pruritus associated with cholestasis: a review of pathogenesis and management. *Digestive Diseases and Sciences*, 1994; **39**: 1–8.

23.4 Gallstones

R. Hermon Dowling and Neil McIntyre

Introduction

Gallstone disease is common. In industrialized, developed societies the prevalence of gallstones is around 10 per cent, increases progressively with age, and is greater in women than in men (by a factor of at least two). About 25 million Americans, 9 million Germans, and 6 million British, French, and Italian citizens harbour gallbladder stones. In most individuals (66 to 80 per cent), the stones are silent or asymptomatic, and even when complications develop they are seldom fatal. Gallstone disease is therefore not a major cause of death, but because it is so common it is an important cause of morbidity.

Since we wrote this chapter for the first edition there have been appreciable changes in the management of patients with symptomatic gallbladder stones. Laparoscopic cholecystectomy (Chapter 23.6) is now performed worldwide, and although there have been few prospective, randomized controlled trials to compare it with other management options, such as mini-laparotomy (Barkun, Lancet, 1992; 340:116; Majeed, Lancet, 1996; 347:989), 'lap chole' is a well established procedure. Largely as a result of its introduction many of the alternative non-surgical or minimally invasive management options have now been abandoned. Percutaneous cholecystolithotomy, ablation of the gallbladder lumen by 'chemical cholecystectomy', and percutaneous transhepatic insertion of motor-driven rotary 'lithotripts' into the gallbladder to pulverize the stones are no longer used.

The introduction of contact solvents such as methyl t-butyl ether (**MTBE**) and ethyl propionate into the gallbladder, via percutaneous transhepatic catheters or endoscopic retrograde cannulation of the cystic duct, has also been abandoned. Enthusiasm for extracorporeal shock-wave lithotripsy (**ESWL**), to fragment or even pulverize gallbladder stones, has waned. However, in the case of ESWL, the pendulum may have swung too far. We believe that there is still a place for ESWL, albeit a limited one, in a small number of highly selected patients who are unsuitable for, or wish to avoid, laparoscopic or open abdominal surgery. The same is true of oral bile acid treatment. It no longer has novelty value, but remains a viable alternative to elective surgery in some carefully selected symptomatic patients.

This dwindling interest in 'medical' treatments for patients with symptomatic gallbladder stones has been compensated, at least in part, by a greater understanding of gallstone formation. For this reason we have restructured this chapter. New developments in gallstone pathogenesis are described in detail; the discussion of medical/non-surgical treatments, which were covered fully in the first edition, has been greatly reduced.

Open abdominal cholecystectomy was the most commonly performed elective surgical operation. However, since Philipe Mouret from Lyons first performed laparoscopic cholecystectomy in 1987, its use has increased dramatically. In most countries of the developed world, 'lap chole' is not only the most widely practised laparoscopic procedure, it is also the most commonly performed elective surgical operation.

A detailed discussion of the advantages and disadvantages of lap chole over conventional or open abdominal cholecystectomy, is beyond the scope of this chapter (the topic is fully reviewed in Chapter 23.6). However, mortality and morbidity are lower after lap chole than with conventional cholecystectomy. Lap chole causes less postoperative pain and fewer complications than the open approach. Moreover, most patients undergoing lap chole spend less time in hospital and have a shorter period of convalescence. Furthermore, the cosmetic result of lap chole is preferable to that of a subcostal or paramedian incision. For this and other reasons, the concept of 'keyhole surgery' has captured the imagination of the public. However, as noted above, the benefits of the laparoscopic approach, which is undoubtedly popular, have not yet been substantiated by the results of rigorous controlled trials. Critics of lap chole claim that it takes as long, possibly even longer, to perform than conventional surgery. Moreover, whether or not disposable equipment and laser dissection techniques are used, the operating room costs of laparoscopic surgery are at least as great as those incurred with the traditional approach. However, although the basic principles of defining surgical anatomy (cystic duct and cystic artery) are the same with both techniques, the results of many surveys suggest that the prevalence of bile duct injury is greater after laparoscopic cholecystectomy than with the open abdominal approach (Richardson, BrJSurg, 1996; 83:1356).

Classification of gallstone type

In the past, the classification of gallstones was important not only in relation to pathogenesis but also to treatment. Oral bile acid treatment was (and still is) largely confined to patients with cholesterol-rich, potentially dissolvable, gallbladder stones. It is unsuitable for patients with pigment-rich, calcium-containing, non-cholesterol stones. For this reason, much effort was directed into predicting stone composition (and thus the outcome of dissolution treatment). Today, this is seldom relevant; most patients with

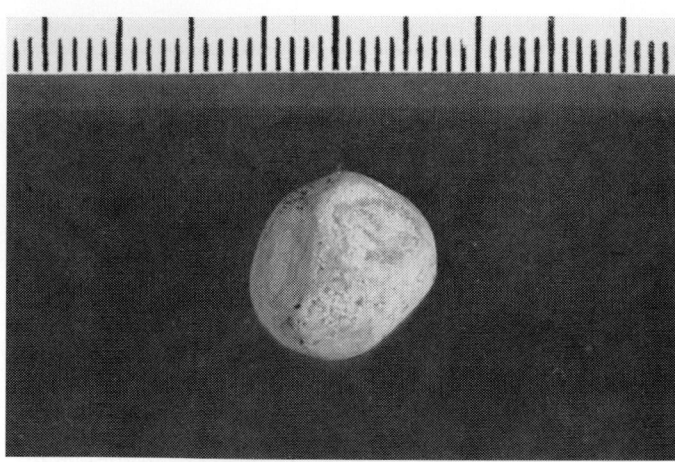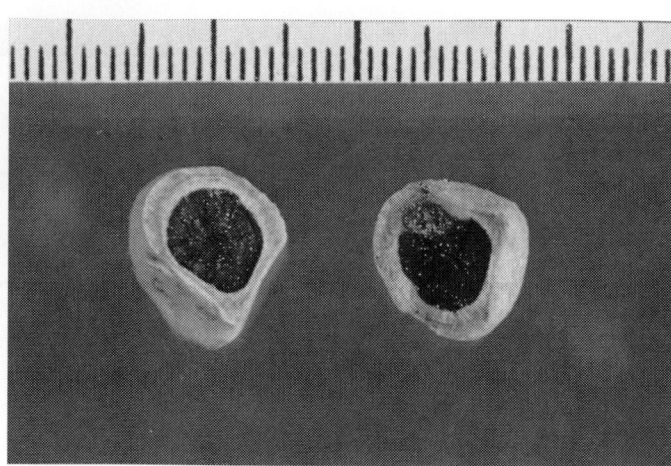

Fig. 1. The appearance of the external surface of gallstones usually provides reliable clues about overall stone composition. Occasionally, however, this can be misleading—as in this example which shows an external appearance suggesting cholesterol and/or calcium-salt gallstones (a), but on examination of the split surface, although the whitish outer rim is indeed mixed in composition (cholesterol, calcium, and a little pigment), the bulk of the stone is made of black polymerized bilirubin (b).

symptomatic gallbladder stones are treated surgically, and the complications of gallbladder stones requiring surgery are just as likely to occur with cholesterol-rich as with calcified non-dissolvable stones. If cholecystectomy is indicated, neither the composition nor the classification of gallstone type is relevant to either surgeon or patient. For this reason, the emphasis nowadays is on the presence or absence of gallbladder stones—which are usually detected by ultrasound. Few patients undergo oral cholecystography, and/or localized CT scanning of the gallbladder, in order to determine stone composition indirectly before a decision is made on treatment/management. However, the pathogenesis of cholesterol-rich stones is fundamentally different from that of stones containing non-cholesterol material. For this reason alone, it remains relevant to consider gallstone structure and composition.

Gallstones used to be subdivided into cholesterol, mixed, and pigment stones—often on the basis of the external appearance of stones retrieved during cholecystectomy or at autopsy. Faceted yellow or yellow/brown stones are usually cholesterol rich (see below); while black, knobbly, and irregular (blackberry or mulberry) stones are usually pigment stones. However, the external appearance of stones is often misleading. Attempts to judge stone composition should also be based on examination of the cut or split surface of the stone (Fig. 1). Most gallstones are then seen to be of mixed composition. Even cholesterol-rich stones usually have a dark or pigmented centre or nucleus, a crystalline interior which often has spoke-like radiations and, depending on the age and size of the stone, a surface layer or rim which may contain calcium salts (Fig. 2). The cut surface may show concentric laminations which, like the rings of a tree trunk, provide clues about the history of the stone and about bile composition at different stages in its evolution.

Gallstones are now classified as cholesterol, black pigment, and brown pigment stones (Soloway, Gastro, 1977; 72:167). Cholesterol stones are the dominant form in industrialized societies. Black pigment stones occur in chronic haemolytic disorders; earthy brown pigment stones are found in association with infection in the biliary tree and occur more commonly in the Orient than in the West.

This classification tells us something about gallstone pathogenesis. It is based not only on the physical properties of stones, but also on studies of their composition using:

(i) chemical analysis;
(ii) scanning electron microscopy of the outer or split surface of the stone;
(iii) X-ray powder diffraction (to study the crystalline content of the stone);
(iv) ixelectron microprobe analysis;
(v) infrared spectroscopy;
(vi) radiology of ultrathin sections, and occasionally;
(vii) staining techniques analogous to those used in histochemistry—for example to show qualitatively the presence of mucus glycoprotein.

Pathogenesis
Bile lipid composition and secretion: supersaturation

More is known about the pathogenesis of cholesterol stones than about that of calcium-containing and 'pure' pigment stones. None the less, many of the principles of lithogenesis are common to all types of stones. Therefore, the mechanisms underlying cholesterol gallstone formation are described in some detail first; the pathogeneses of pigment and calcium stones are discussed only briefly.

The first step in cholesterol gallstone formation is the secretion by the liver of bile supersaturated with cholesterol. Small and his colleagues (Small, Nature, 1966; 211:816; Admirand, JCI, 1968; 47: 1043) were the first to define accurately the physicochemical limits of cholesterol solubility in model and native biles. Cholesterol is virtually insoluble in water and its solubility in bile depends on the detergent properties of bile acids and phospholipids. Thirty years ago, cholesterol was thought to be carried in bile mainly as mixed micelles of bile acids, phospholipids, and cholesterol. Bile became supersaturated with cholesterol because the relative proportions of

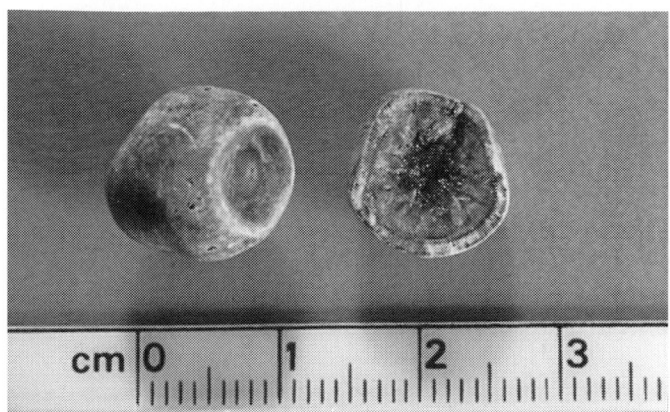

Fig. 2. Example of cholesterol-rich gallstones of mixed composition with a dark, pigment-rich nucleus, spoke-like radiations of cholesterol crystals stained with pigment, and a laminated outer rim containing calcium salts.

cholesterol, bile acids, and phospholipids did not allow cholesterol to be maintained in aqueous solution—in other words there was too much cholesterol, or not enough bile acids and/or phospholipids.

Duodenal marker perfusion studies showed different patterns of 'hypercholesterobilia' in patients with gallstones. Type I hypercholesterobilia is a hypersecretion of cholesterol with normal outputs of the detergent bile acid and phospholipid moeities. In type II there is a deficiency of bile acids and phospholipids. (Bile acid and phospholipid secretion are usually closely linked, so that changes in bile acid secretion tend to be accompanied by corresponding changes in phospholipid output). Type III is a combination of hypersecretion of cholesterol and hyposecretion of bile acids and phospholipids, while type IV is the rare isolated phospholipid deficiency (see below).

Hypersecretion of cholesterol is the most common defect in the genesis of supersaturated bile. It is seen in obese individuals who have an increased incidence of gallstones, and may be the sole bile lipid secretory abnormality in Swedish patients with gallstones (Nilsell, Gastro, 1985; 89:287). In obese subjects, total body cholesterol synthesis is increased as is the hepatic activity of HMG CoA reductase, the rate-limiting enzyme in cholesterogenesis. More important than obesity *per se* is the effect of very rapid weight loss—as a result of dieting, or 'bariatric' surgery (such as gastric stapling) performed to reduce calorie intake. During rapid weight loss, tissue cholesterol is mobilized, taken up by the liver via receptors on the sinusoidal membranes, and secreted into bile. Obese patients losing weight rapidly therefore develop biliary cholesterol hypersecretion and have a high rate of spontaneous gallstone formation (Broomfield, NEJM, 1988; 319:1567; Sugerman, AmJSurg, 1995; 169:91).

Dietary factors also influence biliary cholesterol secretion. These include the total calorie intake and, more controversially, dietary cholesterol. The amounts of refined carbohydrates and dietary fibre may also be important. Indeed, as discussed below, dietary fibre may affect intestinal transit, colonic luminal pH, intestinal bacterial enzymes that metabolize the bile acids, and the formation, solubilization, and absorption of deoxycholic acid.

Lipid-lowering drugs may cause hypercholesterobilia, particularly the fibrates such as clofibrate (see Chapter 2.12). Pregnancy and oestrogen-rich medications can induce biliary cholesterol hypersecretion as can diabetes mellitus, although probably only the insulin-dependent variety. Finally, hyperlipidaemia is associated with biliary cholesterol hypersecretion, but the link is with raised serum triglycerides and not directly with hypercholesterolaemia.

In non-obese individuals who form cholesterol-rich gallbladder stones, the problem seems to be secondary to hyposecretion of bile acids (Reuben, ClinSci, 1985; 69:71) which, in some patients at least, is associated with a small bile acid pool (Vlahcevic, Gastro, 1970; 59:165). This assumes that the small bile acid pool cycles within the enterohepatic circulation at a normal frequency. (In theory, a 50 per cent reduction in pool size could be fully compensated by a twofold increase in enterohepatic cycling frequency since pool size × cycling frequency = secretion rate.) However, this assumption is controversial, mainly for methodological reasons, as pool size and secretion rates are measured by different techniques and the pattern of results for bile lipid secretion varies considerably with the stimulus used during the measurement of so-called steady-state secretion.

The early studies showing that changes in bile acid pool size and in bile lipid secretion are important in the pathogenesis of gallstones remain as valid today as they were two to three decades ago. However, the physicochemical considerations of 30 years ago do not. It is now believed that in dilute hepatic bile, cholesterol is transported not in mixed micelles but in spherical 'packages' of phospholipid and cholesterol, with one or more layers, known as unilamellar and multilamellar vesicles. Video-enhanced, time-lapse photography suggested that cholesterol microcrystals precipitated from these multilamellar vesicles, rather than from micelles (Kibe, Gastro, 1984; 86:1326; Holzbach, Hepatol, 1986; 6:1403). However, this observation may well oversimplify the situation.

The current paradigm of the physicochemical events leading to the nucleation of cholesterol microcrystals is as follows. In small unilamellar vesicles, the molar ratio of cholesterol to phospholipids is low and cholesterol solubility is not in jeopardy. However, as the relative proportion (moles per cent) of cholesterol in bile increases, or the moles per cent of bile acids diminish, the cholesterol:phospholipid ratio in the vesicles increases. This is associated first with aggregation and then with fusion of vesicles to form large multilamellar structures. The stability/instability of these multilamellar vesicles seems to depend on their cholesterol:phospholipid molar ratio. Thus, as the ratio approaches 1:1, the vesicles become unstable and vulnerable to the precipitation of cholesterol microcrystals.

The nature of the relationship between the vesicular cholesterol:phospholipid molar ratio and the stability/instability of multilamellar vesicles is controversial. Most conclusions about this are based on studies of model bile solutions, rather than native human bile, mainly because it is difficult to apply sophisticated physicochemical techniques to complex biological solutions such as bile. Furthermore, there is no non-invasive way of separating vesicles from micelles. The two most commonly used methods of doing so include gel permeation chromatography and density gradient ultracentrifugation. Both methods are subject to artefacts and the two methods yield different results. Thus, when the cholesterol:phospholipid molar ratio predicting vesicular instability is determined by ultracentrification, the result is different from that obtained using elution chromatography. One possible reason for this relates to the type and concentration of bile acids used in the gel permeation technique. In native biles, the total bile acid concentration and individual bile acid compositions vary considerably. Therefore, the somewhat arbitrary choice of 10 mmol taurocholate as the elution buffer may distort the results.

In an attempt to overcome this problem, Donovan and colleagues (JLipRes, 1991; 32:1501) have painstakingly calculated the so-called intermicellar bile acid concentration for individual bile samples. It seems likely that by matching this bile acid concentration and composition, more reliable results will be obtained. Even so, any physical method of separating lipid carriers may distort the subtle relationship between them *in vivo*.

As an alternative approach, several groups have been using proton nuclear magnetic resonance in an attempt to examine the different lipid 'carriers' in native bile. Initial results are encouraging (Groen, JLipRes, 1990; 31:1315; Ellul, FEBS, 1992; 300:30) but further work needs to be done before these complex laboratory techniques can be applied to biological samples.

In addition to the total bile acid and phospholipid molar ratios, recent attention has focused on the impact of qualitative changes in these bile compounds on cholesterol solubility in bile. It now seems that the hydrophobic-hydrophilic balance in individual phospholipids and bile acids may well be important in determining the partitioning of cholesterol between vesicles, micelles, and other putative carriers such as stacked lamellas (Somjen, BBActa, 1990; 1042:28; Cohen, Hepatol, 1993; 18:1522). Thus, the fatty acid composition of biliary phospholipids seems to be important in determining molecular packing within the liposome-like vesicles. The structure of phospholipids is often depicted as a tuning fork, with its prongs corresponding to the two long–chain fatty acids. The first of these, in the sn1 (substitution 1) position, is fully saturated, while the second (sn2) usually contains at least one unsaturated double bond. This leads to rigid angulation of the long-chain fatty acid and the resultant 'knuckle' means that there is less room for packing between adjacent molecules.

Virtually all the phospholipid in bile is present as phosphatidyl choline (lecithin). The dominant phosphatidyl choline molecular species has 16 carbons and no double bonds in the sn1 fatty acid, and 18 carbons with 2 double bonds in the sn2 position (16:0–18: 2). The arachidonic acid-rich phospholipids (16:0–20:4 and 18: 0–20:4) constitute only 10 to 15 and 1 to 1.5 per cent, respectively, of the total biliary phosphatidyl cholines. Despite this, phosphatidyl cholines rich in arachidonic acid seem to be particularly important in influencing cholesterol solubility, the partitioning of cholesterol between different carriers in bile, and gallstone formation. Thus, increased amounts of arachidonic acid-rich phosphatidyl cholines mean that the vesicles can carry less phospholipids than normal, presumably because the bulky, angulated, arachidonic acid-rich phosphatidyl cholines are preferentially shunted from the vesicles into micelles. Cholesterol, however, is left behind in the vesicles with a resultant increase in the cholesterol:phospholipid molar ratio. As indicated above, this in turn favours vesicle aggregation and fusion, the promotion of unstable vesicles, and the formation of cholesterol microcrystals. Similar physicochemical phenomena may occur in bile after feeding fish oils rich in eicosapentaenoic acid. This not only modifies the fatty acid composition of biliary phosphatidyl choline, it also modifies nucleation time, at least as measured (with dubious validity) in duodenal bile (Abel, Gastro, 1997; 263:A1205).

The hydrophobic-hydrophilic balance of bile acids may also be important, in part because of the differing ability of bile acids to solubilize cholesterol (Cohen, AmJPhysiol, 1992; 263:G386). As noted earlier, deoxycholic acid (**DCA**) in particular has been implicated. The specific role of DCA in cholesterol gallstone formation is discussed in detail below.

The genetic control of biliary lipid secretion

Increasing evidence from studies in animals and man suggests that biliary lipid secretion is under genetic control. Carey *et al.* (PNAS, 1995; 92:7729) studied two strains of mice (C57L and SWR) which are susceptible to gallstone formation when fed a lithogenic diet. These animals cannot up- or down-regulate hepatic HMG Co A reductase (the rate-limiting enzyme in cholesterol synthesis) in response to changes in dietary cholesterol intake. Three 'cholesterol gallstone genes' have been mapped in these animals—the so-called *lith 1*, *lith 2*, and *lith 3* genes. They are located on mouse chromosome numbers 2, 10, and 19, respectively, and are associated with a 40, 65, and 90 per cent chance of gallbladder stone formation. Recent studies by the same group (Wang, JLipRes, 1997; 38:1395) suggest that the *lith* genes not only determine biliary cholesterol supersaturation; they also influence mucin gel accumulation, gallbladder site, and gallstone prevalence, especially in male mice of the inbred strains C57L and F-1.

Even stronger evidence in favour of a genetic factor influencing biliary lipid secretion comes from serendipitous observations made in the Netherlands, where an oncology group was studying multiple drug resistance (*mdr*) genes in animals. Smit *et al.* (Cell, 1993; 75: 451) found that the *mdr-2* gene encodes for a protein involved in biliary phospholipid secretion (see also Chapter 2.12). It acts as a 'flippase', transporting phospholipid molecules from the inner to the outer layer of the canalicular membrane. Transgenic knock-out mice lacking the *mdr-2* gene secrete bile acids normally, but their bile contains almost no biliary phospholipids and very little cholesterol. This unique model is interesting as it sheds light on the molecular mechanisms controlling lipid movement across membranes.

Nucleation

The first stage in stone formation is the presence of supersaturated bile, but this alone is insufficient. There must also be an abnormality of nucleation, due to an excess of promoters of crystallization and/or a deficiency of inhibitors. Many other biological fluids, including saliva, urine, and pancreatic secretions, become supersaturated with solutes from time to time during the day. Although stones occasionally form in these fluids, they are rare and occur much less frequently than would be expected on the basis of unstable supersaturation.

Holzbach *et al.* from Cleveland (Holan, Gastro, 1979; 77:611) first emphasized the importance of abnormal nucleation in gallstone formation. Control subjects and those who formed gallstones showed considerable overlap with respect to biliary cholesterol supersaturation, but there was no such overlap in nucleation times—the time taken for microcrystals of cholesterol to appear in isotropic (one-phase) samples of gallbladder bile (Fig. 3). In bile from control subjects the nucleation time was 10 to 14 days or more; in bile from gallstone carriers it was only 1 to 2 days. Since the residence time

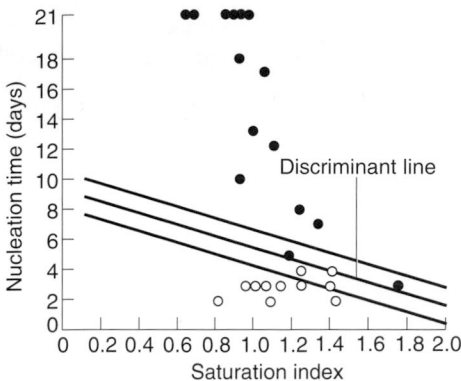

Fig. 3. Nucleation times as a function of saturation index for bile of patients with cholesterol gallstones (○) and controls (●). (Reproduced with permission from Holan, Gastro, 1979; 77:611.)

for bile in the gallbladder is only a matter of hours, nucleation times measured *in vitro* clearly do not relate directly to what happens *in vivo*. They are mainly of comparative value between those with gallstones and those without (controls).

A detailed discussion about the mechanisms controlling nucleation time (more correctly, the cholesterol microcrystal appearance/detection time) is beyond the scope of this chapter, but the situation may be summarized as follows. It is unclear whether the abnormal nucleation found in patients with gallbladder stones is due to an excess of promoters and/or a deficiency of inhibitors of crystallization (Table 1). The most compelling evidence favouring an excess of promoters comes from the work of Strasberg and his colleagues (Gallinger, Hepatol, 1984; 4:177). When samples of gallbladder bile from a patient with gallstones were added to that of healthy control subjects, the long nucleation time of the controls was converted to the rapid nucleation of the gallstone carriers. Indeed, it took only 10 per cent by volume of the bile from a patient with gallstones to convert the slow nucleation time of the healthy subject to an abnormally quick one.

The nature of these promoters and inhibitors of crystallization is unknown but they are likely to be proteins, such as apolipoproteins

Table 1 List of promoters and inhibitors of vesicle aggregation, fusion, and cholesterol microcrystal nucleation
Promoters
Mucin (mucus glycoprotein)
Non-mucin glycoproteins (concanavalin A-bound: aminopeptidases: 130 kDa)
α_1-Acid glycoprotein
Phospholipase C
Immunoglobulins (especially IgM and IgA)
Ionized calcium (vesicle aggregation and fusion)
Deoxycholic acid (? indirect effect)
Arachidonic acid-rich phospholipids (? indirect effect: hydrophobic–hydrophilic balance)
Low density lipoproteins
Transferrin
Fibronectin
Biliary anionic polypeptide fraction
Inhibitors
Apolipoprotein A-I
Apolipoprotein A-II
Helix pomatia-bound protein (120 kDa with 5A/63 kDa subunits)

(Kibe, Science, 1984; 225:514) or mucus glycoprotein (Lee, JCI, 1981; 67:1712; Lee, Science, 1981; 211:1429; LaMont, Hepatol, 1984; 4:51). In turn, the control of biliary mucus glycoprotein synthesis and secretion may be influenced by abnormal bile lipid composition. Thus, when experimental animals are fed a lithogenic diet, the bile becomes supersaturated with cholesterol, and mucus hypersecretion occurs before microcrystals and gallstones appear. It seems, therefore, that the gallbladder mucosa can 'read' changes in the bulk phase of bile within the gallbladder lumen and respond with increased mucus glycoprotein synthesis and release.

These changes may well be mediated by mucosal prostaglandins. In animals, aspirin and other non-steroidal anti-inflammatory drugs (**NSAIDs**) prevent the increase in biliary mucus glycoprotein induced by a lithogenic diet. More importantly, they prevent stone formation. Similar observations have been made in man. In obese individuals losing weight by dieting, high-dose aspirin (1300 mg/day) largely prevented the microcrystal, microstone, and gallstone formation which would otherwise have occurred (Broomfield, NEJM, 1988; 319:1567). Moreover, in the British/Belgian Gallstone Study Group's post-dissolution trial, long-term NSAID ingestion seemed to prevent gallstone recurrence (Hood, Lancet, 1988; ii:1223). Therefore, prevention of the formation of both primary and recurrent gallstones may be achieved by manipulating cholesterol crystal nucleation, rather than by reducing biliary cholesterol saturation. However, the effects of aspirin or NSAIDs on bile composition are controversial. They vary from study to study and from species to species. Moreover, there is scant evidence that chronic aspirin/NSAID ingestion (in patients attending rheumatology clinics) affects the incidence of gallstones. Thus, it is far from clear that gallstone prevention can be achieved safely and economically by the use of these gastro- and entero-toxic drugs. Without further studies this concept must remain speculative.

Stasis: gallbladder motor dysfunction

Before cholesterol gallstones can form, not only must bile become supersaturated with cholesterol and have a nucleation defect, but also there must be sufficient time for the resultant microcrystals of cholesterol to reside within the gallbladder, agglomerate or coalesce, and grow to form macroscopic gallstones. The necessary stasis to permit this sequence of events may be achieved in two ways.

First, the excess mucus may act as a trapping gel to ensnare the crystals and prevent them from being expelled from the gallbladder through the cystic duct. In animal models of gallstone formation, stones invariably originate in the thick viscous layer of surface mucus lining the gallbladder mucosa, rather than 'free' in the gallbladder lumen (Smith, JLipRes, 1987; 28:1088). Whether this applies equally to man is unknown.

Second, gallbladder 'motor dysfunction' has been found in patients with gallstones (see below), mainly impaired gallbladder emptying in response to food or to exogenous cholecystokinin. As gallstone disease is almost invariably associated with histological evidence of chronic cholecystitis, until recently it seemed that the abnormalities in gallbladder motor function seen in patients with gallstones were a secondary phenomenon and not a primary abnormality antedating, and contributing to, gallstone formation. However, there is now strong evidence that the abnormalities in gallbladder motility may be a primary phenomenon (Hay, Sem-LivDis, 1990; 10:159). In animal models of gallstone formation, there is impaired gallbladder emptying as in man. Moreover, like mucus hypersecretion, the changes in gallbladder motility seem to precede stone formation (Doty, Gastro, 1983; 85:168; Pellegrini, Gastro, 1986; 90:143).

Gallbladder motility

A detailed review of the pathophysiology of gallbladder motor dysfunction in gallbladder stone disease is beyond the scope of this chapter but the topic merits further brief discussion. It is naïve to refer to 'gallbladder motor dysfunction' or 'gallbladder hypomotility' without defining further what is meant by these rather loose terms, and considering how the measurements were made. For the most part, abnormal gallbladder motor function of gallstone disease refers to abnormal gallbladder emptying in response to either a test meal or a cholecystokinetic stimulus, such as intravenous cholecystokinin or caerulin, or intraduodenal magnesium sulphate, fat, or amino acids. However, it is worth noting that gallbladder filling and emptying also occur in the interdigestive period when the migrating motor complexes in the intestine, and peptide hormones such as motilin, affect gallbladder motor function.

Methodology
Oral cholecystography

The methods used to study gallbladder emptying are also important since the results vary with the technique used. In the past, oral cholecystography was used to document gallbladder contraction in response to a 'fatty meal' (AFM films). However, although this technique is adequate to document patency or blockage of the cystic duct, a two-dimensional magnified image of the gallbladder (which involves radiation exposure) is unsatisfactory for clinicophysiological studies of three-dimensional gallbladder emptying.

Radionuclide scanning of the gallbladder ('cholescintigraphy')

The use of cholescintigraphy with HIDA (hydroxyimino diacetic acid) (or one of its derivatives) provides dynamic images of: (i) hepatic uptake and biliary excretion of the isotope, (ii) gallbladder uptake, concentration and storage, and (iii) gallbladder emptying. It too is a relatively insensitive technique and, in theory, is also subject to artefacts. Thus, disappearance of the isotope from the area of interest usually signifies contraction/emptying of the gallbladder. But it could also occur if non-isotopic bile displaced HIDA-labelled bile from the gallbladder—even in the absence of volume changes.

Ultrasound

This is probably the most commonly used method of studying 'gallbladder motility'. It depends on measurements of the long and transverse axes of the gallbladder, the volume being calculated using formulas based on the sum of cylinders (Everson, Gastro, 1980; 79: 40) or elipsoids (Dodds, AJR, 1985; 145:1009). It provides a sensitive, well-validated method of estimating gallbladder volume and can even demonstrate minute-by-minute oscillations in volume (Howard, Gut, 1991; 32:1406). However, ultrasound too has its limitations: reductions in volume do correspond accurately to gallbladder emptying, but the method significantly underestimates refilling of the gallbladder, as demonstrated by simultaneous use of

Table 2 Clinical situations where impaired gallbladder emptying is associated with sludge and/or stone formation: indirect evidence that gallbladder motor dysfunction plays a role in the pathogenesis of gallstones

Clinical situation	Citation
Total parenteral nutrition (Sludge from total parenteral nutrition prevented by cholecystokinin)	Messing, Gastro, 1983; 84: 1012
	Roslyn, Gastro, 1986; 91: 313
	Sitzmann, SGO, 1990; 33: 4
High spinal cord injury	Apstein, Gastro, 1987; 92: 966
	Stone, AmJGastro, 1990; 85: 114
Somatostatinoma	Krejs, NEJM, 1979; 301: 285
Chronic octreotide treatment	Stolk, Gut, 1993; 34: 808
	Hussaini, Gut, 1996; 38: 775
Obesity	Palasciano, AmJGastr, 1992; 87:493
Pregnancy	Bolondi, Gut, 1995; 26: 734
Vagotomy ± gastric surgery	Masclee, Gastro, 1990; 98: 1338
? Diabetes mellitus	Shaw, 1993
? Sickle cell disease	Everson, Gastro, 1989; 96: 1307

scintigraphy and ultrasonography (Jazrawi, Gastro, 1995; 109:582).

Parameters measured

Despite differing methods, the consensus of a large number of studies is that gallbladder emptying in response to a variety of cholecystokinetic stimuli, is impaired in carriers of gallbladder stones. However, this does not apply to all individuals with gallstones and several investigators claim that there are 'strong' and 'weak' contractors (reviewed by Duane, Gastro, 1996; 111:823). Indeed, in a small but important prospective study Van der Linden (Tidjschr, Gastro, 1974; 17:121) showed, over a 15-year follow-up period, that the incidence of gallbladder stone development in weak contractors was much greater than that seen in strong contractors. Moreover, studies of gallbladder emptying predict gallstone recurrence in patients treated successfully with ESWL plus oral bile acids (Pauletzki, Gastro, 1996; 111:765). Thus, the results of these studies, when taken together with circumstantial evidence in a number of clinical (Table 2) and animal 'models' of gallbladder stone formation, support the concept that impaired gallbladder emptying is, indeed, a primary event that antedates and contributes to stone formation.

Which component of gallbladder motility is relevant to stone formation?

Depending on the methods used, the following parameters of gallbladder motility can be measured:

(i) the fasting or pre-prandial gallbladder volume;
(ii) the residual or nadir post-prandial gallbladder volume;
(iii) the 'delta' or emptying volume (also known as the ejection volume—the difference between fasting and minimum post-prandial gallbladder volumes);
(iv) the rate of gallbladder emptying (usually expressed in ml/ min);

(v) the speed of gallbladder emptying (expressed as $T_{1/2}$);
(vi) the ejection 'fraction' (the delta volume expressed as a percentage of the fasting gallbladder volume); and
(vii) the percentage of gallbladder emptying.

Given the different methods and the different parameters used, it is not surprising that there is some conflict in the literature about gallbladder emptying in gallstone disease. None the less, the consensus is that both the fasting and the residual post-prandial gallbladder volumes are greater in most patients with cholesterol gallbladder stones than in controls. In some, but not all, studies the speed and extent of gallbladder emptying are also reduced in gallstone carriers.

In theory, once microcrystals of cholesterol have precipitated within the gallbladder, the flushing effect of bile being expelled through the cystic duct (as a result of gallbladder contraction—the speed and extent of gallbladder emptying) could be more important than the effect of stagnation (large residual or post-prandial volume). In practice, however, the incomplete emptying of the gallbladder in response to food seems to be a greater risk factor for stone formation than the vigour of expulsion of bile out of the gallbladder. Furthermore, most investigators find that these observations apply to individuals with cholesterol-rich gallbladder stones, not to those with pigment (non-cholesterol) stones (Behar, Gastro, 1993; 104: 563).

Mechanism for impaired gallbladder emptying in cholesterol gallstone disease

The fact that comparable results are obtained with 'endogenous' or physiological stimuli (such as a test meal) and 'exogenous' stimuli (such as parenteral cholecystokinin), suggests that there is an impaired end-organ (gallbladder) response (Forgacs, Gastro, 1984; 87: 299). Although there are cephalic (probably mediated through the vagus nerve), neural (again mainly autonomic), and hormonal components (principally cholecystokinin but also other regulatory peptides such as motilin, which is particularly important in the interdigestive period), the main mechanism controlling gallbladder emptying is food-stimulated cholecystokinin release from the duodenal and jejunal mucosas. Most investigators find that the profile of meal-stimulated plasma cholecystokinin in response to food is normal in patients with gallbladder stones. This again implies that the defect is in the gallbladder wall. This implication is supported by the results of in vitro studies. When freshly excised strips of full-thickness gallbladder wall (harvested at the time of cholecystectomy) are mounted in an isometric tensiometer, the contractile response to cholecystokinetic agonists (such as cholecystokinin, caerulin, and acetylcholine) is prolonged in patients with gallstones. In fact, the results of dose–response studies suggest that there is up to a 10-fold increase in the amount of agonist required to elicit the same contractile response in strips from patients with gallbladder stones as that seen in strips from control subjects (e.g. transplant donors) (Portincasa, Gut, 1987; 28:A1395). This impaired response does not seem to be due to chronic cholecystitis—at least as judged by histological scoring of a number of indices. However, the microscopic appearance of the muscle in the gallbladder wall varies considerably in patients with gallbladder stones and ranges from myohypertrophy, through myofragmentation and fibrosis, to myoatrophy. Despite this, in a series of patients with cholesterol gallbladder stones, the mean thickness of the muscle layer in the gallbladder wall was twice as great as that in controls. Thus, despite more muscle mass, the contraction of strips in response to agonists such as cholecystokinin was impaired. This suggests that patients with gallstones have 'hypertrophic myopathy' of the gallbladder wall (Portincasa, Gut, 1987; 28:A1395).

A limited number of studies have examined cholecystokinin receptor density either in the gallbladder wall, in cholinergic neurones, or in vesicles prepared from myocyte membranes. Although the results of these studies are inconclusive, it seems that cholecystokinin receptor density/binding is reduced in patients with gallstones.

Relationship between altered bile composition and gallbladder motility

Several lines of evidence suggest that the altered gallbladder motor function, which characterizes gallbladder stone disease, may develop in response to changes in the composition of gallbladder bile. First, in experimental animals fed a lithogenic diet, the gallbladder motor defect is seen when the bile becomes supersaturated with cholesterol before the formation of cholesterol microcrystals or macroscopic stones (Doty, Gastro, 1983; 85:168). Second, in tensiometric studies, when strips of human gallbladder from normal individuals are bathed in abnormal bile from cholesterol gallbladder stone carriers, the contractile response is impaired (Behar, Gastro, 1989; 97:1497). In fact, studies by Behar and colleagues (Gastro, 1995; 108:A442) have shown that the lipid composition (cholesterol:phospholipid molar ratio) of the myocyte membranes is abnormal in animals with supersaturated bile. These observations have been extended to isolated muscle cells where contraction in response to agonists is measured by shortening (Chen, Gastro, 1997; 112:A711). This implies that the gallbladder mucosa absorbs lipids, such as cholesterol, from the gallbladder lumen and, by mechanisms unknown, transports them to the sarcolemmal membrane of the gallbladder myocytes. Alternatively, there could be some sensing mechanism which 'reads' bile composition and responds by affecting gallbladder myocyte membrane composition by mechanisms independent of lipid transport across the gallbladder mucosa. However, it is still not clear how the gallbladder wall 'reads' changes in the composition of bile within the gallbladder lumen. One theory is that gallbladder contraction and the synthesis/secretion of mucus glycoprotein are both influenced by changes in prostaglandin metabolism within the gallbladder wall (Carey, Gastro, 1988; 95:508). Indeed, it has been suggested that the enhanced gallbladder emptying seen in patients with gallstones treated with indomethacin is due to its effect on cyclo-oxygenase (O'Donnell, Lancet, 1992; 339:269).

Intestinal transit (Dowling, CanJGastr, 1997; 11:57)

Although the idea that abnormal intestinal motility might contribute to gallstone formation is not new (Marcus, Gut, 1988; 29:522; Stolk, AmJPhysiol, 1993; 264:G596), it is not widely appreciated. It has been suggested that prolongation of intestinal transit increases bacterial degradation of primary to secondary bile acids in the colon. Bile would then contain a greater proportion of deoxycholate conjugates. This, in turn, would increase biliary cholesterol secretion and saturation thereby enhancing gallstone formation. Reduction of the intestinal transit time would have the opposite effects.

This theory fits with the finding that bile of gallstone carriers contains a higher proportion of deoxycholate than that of control subjects; but the range is large in both groups and there is considerable overlap (Marcus, Gut, 1986; 27:550). However, the total bile acid pool size is often smaller than normal in patients with gallstones (Vlahcevic, Gastro, 1970; 59:165) and it is not known whether it is the relative proportion of deoxycholate or the absolute size of the deoxycholate pool which is more important. The effects of deoxycholic acid feeding are controversial, although apparent differences in response may be explained by differences in experimental design and by the doses of deoxycholic acid used.

Drugs such as lactulose, which accelerate intestinal transit, lower biliary deoxycholate levels and saturation indices (Thornton, BMJ, 1981; 282:1018), while substances which induce constipation have the opposite effect (Marcus, Gut, 1986; 27:550). Shortening of the intestinal transit time could also explain the beneficial effect of a high fibre intake on gallstone formation (Marcus, Gut, 1988; 29: 522).

Octreotide (Dowling, CanJGastr, 1997; 11:57)

Octreotide is a long-acting somatostatin analogue. It is an effective treatment for acromegaly because it inhibits the secretion of growth hormone and insulin-like growth factor-I. Gallstones (mostly cholesterol-rich) are found in 13 to 60 per cent of patients treated with octreotide for 3 to 51 months. Like somatostatin, octreotide inhibits the secretion of many other peptide hormones. It reduces meal-stimulated cholecystokinin release from the small bowel, and this is the principal, but not the only mechanism for the associated impairment of gallbladder contraction. Initially it seemed that this gallbladder hypomotility might promote the gallstone formation seen in patients with acromegaly who are given octreotide (see above).

However, the composition of their gallbladder bile is similar to that found in most patients with cholesterol-rich gallbladder stones (Hussaini, Gastro, 1994; 107:1503). It is supersaturated with cholesterol, and a large proportion of the total biliary cholesterol is found in the vesicular fraction in which there is a high cholesterol: phospholipid molar ratio. Probably as a result, the nucleation of cholesterol microcrystals is more rapid than normal. These changes in bile composition and physical chemistry are associated with a twofold increase in the proportion of deoxycholate conjugates in bile when compared with that seen in stone-free 'controls'. The abnormal bile composition seems to be due to octreotide treatment, rather than to the presence of stones. Thus in paired studies of the same individuals before and during octreotide treatment, the somatostatin analogue doubled the proportion of biliary deoxycholic acid and increased biliary cholesterol saturation—even in the absence of gallstones (Hussaini, Gastro, 1994; 107:1503).

There is strong circumstantial evidence to suggest that these changes are secondary to octreotide-induced changes in intestinal transit. A single injection of octreotide prolongs small bowel transit time in subjects who do not have acromegaly (Fuessl, Digestion, 1987; 36:101; Lembcke, Digestion, 1987; 36:108; Møller, ClinSci, 1988; 75:345; O'Donnell, AlimPharmTher, 1990; 4:177). Transit times in the small and large bowel were found to be prolonged in patients with acromegaly; there was further prolongation of the transit time in the small bowel when they were given a single dose of octreotide, but initially transit through the large bowel seemed relatively unaffected (Hussaini, Gut, 1996; 38:775). However, in patients with acromegaly on long-term therapy with octreotide, paired (before-and-during treatment) studies showed that the drug caused a consistent and significant increase of the large bowel transit time (Veysey, Gut, 1996; 39:S1,A9). Slowing of transit through the large bowel would be expected to increase the proportion of deoxycholate conjugates in bile, as the caecum and colon are thought to be the main site for the conversion of cholic to deoxycholic acid (Morris, ScaJGastr, 1973; 8:425; MacDonald, JLipRes, 1983; 24: 675). The relationship between the octreotide-induced change in intestinal transit and the percentage of deoxycholate in bile has been studied recently and there is a highly significant linear correlation between the large bowel transit time and the percentage of deoxycholate in both the conjugated and unconjugated (newly formed) bile acid fractions in serum and, by implication, in bile (Veysey, ClinSci, 1995; 89:7P).

If prolongation of intestinal transit plays a major role in the development of octreotide-induced gallbladder stones, it is clearly possible that it may also be a factor in conventional gallstone formation. There are studies supporting this hypothesis. When constipation is induced by drugs which reduce intestinal motility, there is an increase in the percentage of deoxycholate, and of cholesterol saturation, in duodenal bile. Conversely, when rapid intestinal transit is induced by the administration of lactulose, senna, or a high fibre diet, there is a fall in the percentage of deoxycholate and in cholesterol saturation (Marcus, Gut, 1986; 27:550; Gut, 1988; 29:522). Furthermore, in a subgroup of women with gallstones, but without obvious risk factors, the mean whole-gut transit time was found to be nearly 20 h longer and their stool output much smaller than in matched control subjects (Heaton, Lancet, 1993; 341:8). In another study, the cholesterol saturation of bile and the percentage of deoxycholate present were linked to changes in both gallbladder and intestinal motility (Shoda, Hepatol, 1995; 21:1291).

Pathogenesis of non-cholesterol stones

As with cholesterol-rich stones (arbitrarily defined, in different studies, as those containing more than 70, 75, or 90 per cent cholesterol by weight on chemical analysis), non-cholesterol stones are usually mixed in composition. They contain polymerized bilirubin (which predominates in black pigment stones), calcium salts, glycoproteins, and undefined amorphous material. In turn, this non-crystalline material may contain epithelial cell debris from the gallbladder mucosa, inflammatory cells, and even bacteria. Indeed bacteria may be seen by scanning electron microscopy of the stone surface or its interior, or may be detected indirectly by the polymerase chain reaction (Lee, Gastro, 1997; 112:A513; Switsuiska, Gastro, 1997; 112:A523). The calcium salts in gallstones are mainly composed of carbonate, bilirubinate, phosphate, and fatty acids. The calcium fatty acid soaps are often loosely described as calcium palmitate, but a variety of long-chain fatty acids may be present. Other calcium salts, such as calcium oxalate, are found rarely in gallstones.

Unconjugated bilirubin is difficult to measure accurately in bile, but it is believed that bilirubin conjugation (which yields mono- and diglucuronides) is incomplete, and that 2 to 5 per cent of the bilirubin secreted into bile is unconjugated. Normally, this is unimportant because, for unknown reasons, both the conjugated (water soluble) and unconjugated (insoluble) forms of bilirubin are associated in bile with micelles, in the so-called 'micellar sink' (Scharschmidt, JCI, 1978; 62:1122). However, in chronic liver disease, and in haemolytic disorders such as sickle cell disease, thalassaemia, and spherocytosis, the capacity of the liver to conjugate bilirubin is exceeded and unconjugated bilirubin escapes into bile where it polymerizes and/or co-precipitates with the calcium cation. In theory, therefore, gallstones associated with chronic haemolysis should consist either of polymerized bilirubin or calcium bilirubinate. In practice they are heterogeneous and contain a miscellany of calcium salts—perhaps because of the phenomenon of 'epitaxy', whereby the presence of one crystalline salt acts as a nidus for the precipitation of others when the spacing of angles or corners on the crystalline lattice corresponds.

In the Far East, 'earthy' brown pigment stones, associated with bacterial and/or parasitic (flukes and worms) infection of the biliary tree, are more common than cholesterol stones. Their formation may also be influenced by stasis in the biliary tree induced by chronic or repeated spasm of the sphincter of Oddi as a result of the widespread use of opium and its derivatives in the Orient.

Maki (AnnSurg, 1996; 164:90)[1] originally proposed that bacterial β-glucuronidase cleaved the mono- and diglucuronides from conjugated bilirubin to yield the unconjugated species, which then coprecipitated with free ionized calcium to form calcium bilirubinate. This explanation may be too simple; the pathogenesis of mixed brown pigment stones is probably complex and multifactorial. However, such a mechanism may modify stone composition in patients with retained common duct stones, and influence it in other types of choledocholithiasis. Thus, cholesterol-rich stones which form in the gallbladder may acquire a laminated outer coat of brown pigment material if they migrate into, and remain in, the common bile duct (Fig. 4). Similarly, stones developing above biliary strictures, or in association with tumours or congenital abnormalities of the bile duct, are likely to be brown pigment stones, as the combination of stasis and infection will contribute to the non-cholesterol concrements. This is important as the friable brown pigment material is insoluble in cholesterol solvents, and stones of this type are not expected to respond to treatment with oral bile acids or contact solvents such as MTBE.

Gallstones containing calcium carbonate

The factors controlling the concentration and secretion of the carbonate ion, and of total, bound, and free ionized calcium, are now well defined. As yet, the same is not true of the other two major 'calcium-sensitive' anions found in gallstones—phosphate and 'palmitate'.

A major stimulus to studies of calcium carbonate secretion and solubility in bile came from two observations made during oral bile acid treatment for gallstone dissolution. First, it was recognized that radio-opaque gallstones do not usually dissolve, although in the American National Cooperative Gallstone Study, gallstones containing a small calcified nidus apparently showed the same dissolution response as those which were completely radiolucent

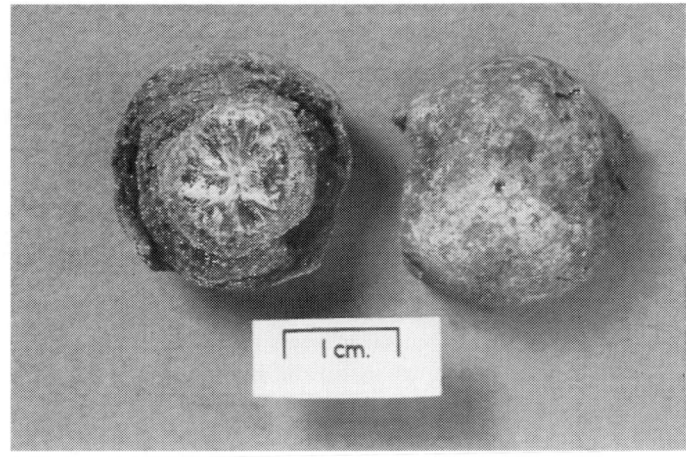

Fig. 4. Example of a brown pigment stone removed from the common bile duct. While the outer layers contain virtually no cholesterol, the inner part of the split stone (left) is made up, almost exclusively, of crystalline cholesterol, suggesting that this cholesterol-rich nucleus began its life in the gallbladder but later acquired a thick amorphous brown pigment coat when it migrated to the biliary tree.

(Schoenfield, AnnIntMed, 1981; 96:257). Second, ursodeoxycholic acid treatment may induce acquired surface gallstone calcification (see later) which then blocks subsequent dissolution. In patients with this complication whose stones were retrieved for analysis at elective cholecystectomy, the surface calcification was invariably due to calcium carbonate.

A further stimulus for research into calcium carbonate stones is that 30 per cent or more of gallstone carriers in Italy (a country representative of other Western industrialized societies) have radio-opaque gallstones.[2,3] Furthermore, it has long been recognized that almost all cholesterol gallstones have a pigment-rich, calcium salt nidus. While this nucleus is usually calcium bilirubinate, it may also contain calcium carbonate. (However, a little pigment goes a long way and, when homogenized, cholesterol stones with a pigment nidus may contain as little as 1 to 2 per cent calcium bilirubinate or carbonate by weight. Moreover, only small amounts of calcium are needed to render a stone radio-opaque. In one study (Rajagopal, Gut, 1988; 29:A1487) the CT attenuation score above which stones were usually CT-dense corresponded with approximately 3 per cent of total calcium by weight.)

In both hepatic and gallbladder bile, the total calcium concentration varies widely (from 1 to 3 mmol in hepatic, and 1 to 10 mmol in gallbladder bile), and is linearly related to bile acid concentration and secretion (Cummings, Gastro, 1984; 87:664; Gleeson, EurJClinIinv, 1995; 25:225). Moreover, attempts to distinguish between patients with radiolucent and radio-opaque gallstones, based on biliary total calcium concentrations, have failed repeatedly; there is a complete overlap in results between patients with gallstones and controls. As most calcium in bile is bound to bile acids, other anions, and mucus glycoprotein, this lack of discrimination based on total calcium is hardly surprising. With the advent of reliable electrodes for measuring free (unbound) ionized calcium (the only species available for interaction with calcium-sensitive anions in the precipitation of calcium salts) it was hoped that there might be some difference between controls and patients with radio-opaque gallstones.

The first step in calcium stone formation is the presence of supersaturated bile in which the (cation $\times$ anion) concentration product exceeds the solubility product, or K'_{SP}, for that salt. In the case of calcium carbonate, the K'_{SP} for $[Ca^{2+}] \times [CO_3^-]$ is approximately 3.8 l/mol, although this has been determined for only one crystalline form of calcium carbonate (calcite), which also exists in other forms such as vaterite, aragonite, and apatite; however, it was determined in an aqueous solution, rather than in bile. In theory, calcium carbonate could precipitate from bile if its K'_{SP} is exceeded either as a result of increased $[Ca^{2+}]$, increased $[CO_3^-]$, or both. When free ionized calcium was measured, using reliable electrodes, its concentration in hepatic bile ranged from 0.7 to 1.1 mmol, while that in gallbladder bile ranged from 0.4 to 1.4 mmol. However, there was complete overlap in the free ionized calcium levels of gallbladder bile in patients with either radiolucent or radio-opaque stones. Indeed, in both groups there was either no (Gleeson, Gastro, 1992; 102:1707), or only a minimal (Knyrim, Hepatol, 1989; 10:134; Schiffman, Gastro, 1990; 99:1452), increase in biliary free ionized calcium concentrations with increasing bile acid concentration.

To date, only a few laboratories have measured free ionized calcium and carbonate ion concentrations in gallbladder bile from control subjects and patients with radiolucent and radio-opaque gallstones (Sutor, JClinPath, 1980; 33:86; Knyrim, Hepatol, 1989; 10:134; Gleeson, Gastro, 1992; 102:1707). These studies show that the mean ion product $[Ca^{2+}] \times [CO_3^-]$ in patients with radio-opaque stones (surface calcification) does indeed exceed the solubility product or K'_{SP} for calcium carbonate (i.e. the calcium carbonate saturation index (**CCSI**) is greater than 1.0, where 1.0 = a saturated solution).

As the free ionized calcium levels in bile from patients with calcified stones were the same as those in patients with radiolucent, presumed cholesterol-rich stones, it follows that the culprit must be the carbonate ion. Carbonate ion concentrations cannot be measured directly in bile but they can be derived from measurements of bile pH, pCO_2, and total CO_2 using the Henderson-Hasselbalch equation. In fact, the main abnormality found in patients with radio-opaque gallstones is a high pH in gallbladder bile. The pH of gallbladder bile is normally about 0.3 of a unit lower than that of hepatic bile. This pH drop was thought to be due to bicarbonate absorption from gallbladder bile, but Moore and his colleagues suggested that it results primarily from hydrogen ion secretion by gallbladder mucosa (Rege, JCI, 1986; 77:21; Schiffman, Gastro, 1990; 99:1452); the CCSI changes dramatically when the pH of gallbladder bile changes by only 0.2 of a pH unit.

Moore postulated, therefore, that hydrogen ion secretion by the gallbladder mucosa is a protective mechanism to ensure the solubility of calcium carbonate in gallbladder bile (the CCSI is always exceeded in the more alkaline hepatic bile but calcium carbonate does not normally precipitate in the ducts because there is no stasis as a result of the continuous flow of bile through the biliary tree). He also suggested that defective mucosal hydrogen ion secretion might be a key factor for calcium carbonate precipitation in the gallbladder. If this hypothesis is true, calcium carbonate precipitation (and the development of calcium carbonate-containing gallstones) might be prevented by reducing the pH of gallbladder bile by only a modest degree, but it is not yet possible to do this.

This complex discussion of calcium carbonate solubility relates only to the formation of supersaturated bile. By analogy with the triple defect in cholesterol gallstone pathogenesis, abnormalities of nucleation and gallbladder motor function might also be present in patients who develop calcified gallstones. To study nucleation time in such individuals, existing methods for detecting crystals in bile would require modification, perhaps by looking for microspheroliths of vaterite, as has been done in duodenal bile (Ros, Gastro, 1986; 91:703). Studies on gallbladder motor function in patients with calcified gallstones have yielded conflicting results. Some investigators found normal gallbladder emptying (Maudgal, BMJ, 1980; 280:141); others found that patients with radio-opaque gallstones have a defect in gallbladder motility similar to that described in association with cholesterol-rich stones (Forgacs, Gastro, 1984; 87:299). However, as noted above, most investigators find that the impaired gallbladder emptying *in vivo*, and the reduced contractile response of strips and myocytes *in vitro*, are confined to patients with cholesterol-rich stones (Bener, Gastro, 1989; 97:1497).

Lessons from epidemiology[4,5]

This section does not attempt to address the question of gallstone epidemiology in detail. Instead, it simply provides a précis of relevant facts and indicates review articles, books, and original source material from which fuller accounts may be obtained.

Methodology

Until 20 years ago, much of our knowledge about gallstone epidemiology came from autopsy studies, findings at laparotomy, and some cholecystographic surveys. All three approaches have serious limitations; of these, post-mortem studies are the most reliable.

Autopsy studies

If carefully performed, autopsies provide information about the presence or absence of stones; their size, shape, and number; their composition (assuming that they were analysed correctly); and their anatomical location—whether they were found in the gallbladder, bile ducts, or elsewhere. They give information about coexisting gallbladder disease and may yield clues about predisposing factors—including age, gender, parity, obesity, and the presence or absence of disorders such as cirrhosis, ileal disease/resection, and congenital or acquired pathology in the biliary tree.

At best, autopsy studies provide information only about prevalence rates—cross-sectional data on the absolute number of individuals, or the percentage of the population studied, who have the disease at one time point. They give no data on the incidence of gallstone disease as a function of time which, arguably, is more valuable information. Moreover, the autopsy rate (the percentage of those dying who undergo autopsy) varies enormously from country to country and seldom, if ever, reaches 100 per cent. All autopsy surveys, therefore, are subject to many types of bias, but particularly the bias of sampling only the elderly: the percentage of individuals dying earlier in adult life is small and this inevitably causes sampling errors. With these caveats, valuable information has emerged from several comparative studies, notably the Prague/Malmo study (Zahor, ScaJGastr, 1974; 9:3) and several others (see Fig. 5).[4,5]

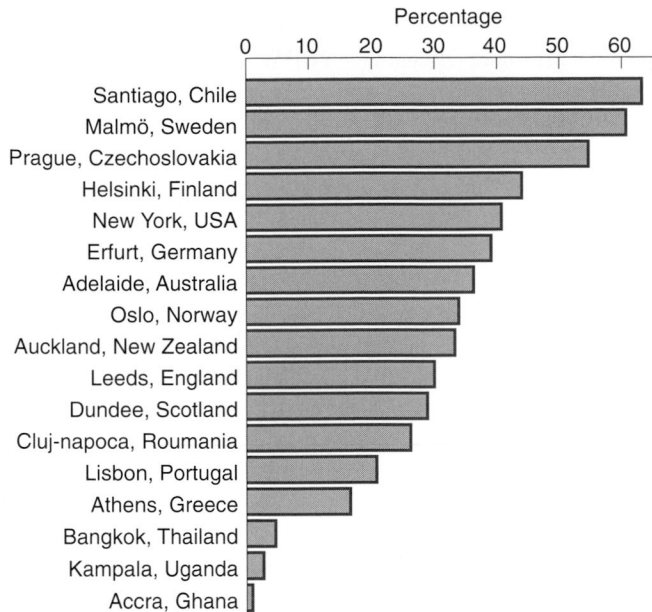

Percentage

Fig. 5. Prevalence of gallstones at autopsy in women aged 70 to 79 years (data taken from reports published since 1951). (Reproduced with permission from Northfield T, Jazrawi R, and Zentler-Munro P, eds. *Bile acids in health and disease.* Dordrecht: Kluwer Academic Publishers, 1990:158.)

Surgery

Cholecystectomy is almost invariably carried out for gallstone disease. Therefore, cholecystectomy rates provide clues about changes in the incidence of advanced gallbladder disease as a function of time. There are many pitfalls in this approach. Surgery is usually performed for complicated gallstone disease; most patients 'earn' their cholecystectomy because of specific, troublesome symptoms. However, we know from large ultrasonographic surveys in Italy and elsewhere that up to 80 per cent of gallstone carriers have either no symptoms or only non-specific symptoms. If it is assumed that no asymptomatic carriers undergo elective surgery, cholecystectomy rates should yield information about the prevalence and incidence of advanced gallstone disease. Clearly this is not the case. Cholecystectomy rates vary considerably from country to country. In Canada in the 1970s, for example, cholecystectomy was carried out five times more commonly per head of population than in the United Kingdom (Lancet, 1973; ii:249; Vayda, NEJM, 1973; 289: 1224).

Cholecystectomy rates are influenced by the number of surgeons in the community, and probably also by the number of radiologists and the radiographic and ultrasound facilities available. Moreover, since the poor, and those living in isolated communities, usually seek medical help only for advanced disease, cholecystectomy rates in different parts of the world may also be related to the affluence of the society.

Cholecystography

Oral cholecystography still provides information about gallstones and the gallbladder which cannot readily be obtained by ultrasonography or other non-invasive methods. Oral cholecystography

was the basis for important surveys of gallstone disease in South Wales (Bainton, NEJM, 1976; 294:1147), the United States (Gracie, NEJM, 1982; 307:798), and one from Israel which compared the prevalence of gallstone disease in Jewish and Arab communities (Gilat, AmJClinNut, 1985; 41:336). However, the irradiation involved in cholecystography, and adverse reactions to iodine-containing contrast media, limit its acceptability for large population surveys. Ultrasonography has replaced oral cholecystography as the investigation of choice for the diagnosis of gallbladder stones.

Ultrasonography

Prevalence studies

In recent years the largest epidemiological studies of gallstone disease have come from Italy: the GREPCO studies from Rome; [2,6] studies from Bologna covering many of the population of Sirmione—a small town on the shores of Lake Garda;[3] and the MICOL study, a multicentre study of over 30 000 individuals from many different centres in Italy (Attili, AmJEpid, 1995; 141:158).

In these surveys ultrasonography, and/or a history of previous cholecystectomy, was the main mode of investigation. Similar but less ambitious studies based on ultrasonography have come from Denmark (Jorgensen, AmJEpid, 1987; 126:912; Gut, 1989;30:528), and from Bristol (Heaton, Gut, 1988; 29:433) and Southampton (Barker, BMJ, 1979; ii:1389) in the United Kingdom. Although there were minor differences in their findings, a broad consensus has emerged which is summarized later.

Incidence studies

To date, most information from ultrasound surveys is cross-sectional in nature. However, having defined a population of gallstone carriers (with and without symptoms) it is possible to follow it for many years to determine the natural history of the untreated disease and the annual incidence of complications. We believe these incidence studies provide the most valuable data obtainable from epidemiological studies of gallstone disease.

Risk factors: surveys of defined populations of gallstone carriers and case–control studies

One of the main functions of epidemiological surveys of gallstone disease is to provide clues about pathogenesis which can then be tested in properly designed, prospective studies. There have been many such surveys in pre-defined populations of individuals with gallstone disease, particularly with regard to: biometric characteristics (age, gender, height, body weight, indices of obesity, number of pregnancies, etc.); dietary factors (intake of calories, carbohydrate, protein, saturated and unsaturated fat, and cholesterol); blood indices (serum lipids, blood glucose and insulin levels, liver function tests, markers of haemolysis, etc.); and social factors such as smoking, alcohol intake, and drug ingestion. The data can be compared with those obtained in control populations, ideally in matched case–control studies such as those reported from Adelaide (Scragg, BMJ, 1984; 288:1113; BMJ, 1984; 289:521) and Oxford (Pixley, BMJ, 1985; 291:11). Again, a broad consensus has emerged from these studies; the following facts emerge from pooling this information with that obtained from the ultrasound studies.

Age

The prevalence of gallstones increases with age. Without other risk factors, they are rare before puberty. Indeed, in most advanced/industrialized societies, gallstones are uncommon before the third decade of life. Thereafter, there is an approximately linear increase in the prevalence of gallstone disease with increasing age, although some studies suggest a plateau around the age of 70 to 80 years.

Gender

In the West, gallstones occur two to three times more often in women than in men. After the age of the menopause, however, the prevalence of gallstones in men tends to catch up with that of women.

The higher frequency of gallstones in women suggests that female sex hormones increase the risk of gallstone formation; indeed, many studies (reviewed by Kern, JLipRes, 1987; 28:828) suggest that both endogenous and exogenous oestrogens (the oral contraceptive pill or hormone replacement therapy) reduce bile flow and adversely affect bile lipid composition. Production of progesterone may also affect the motility of the gallbladder and contribute to bile stasis there in the second half of the menstrual cycle, and particularly during pregnancy (Nilsson, ActaChirScand, 1967; 133:648; Baverman, NEJM, 1980; 302:362; Kern, JCI, 1981; 68: 1228).

There is a complex interplay between potentially confounding risk factors. With advancing age and multiple pregnancies, women tend to become obese; they may also take oral contraceptives containing oestrogens. Therefore, in epidemiological studies, it is necessary to disentangle the confounding influences by performing not only univariate but also multivariate analyses.

Parity

The number of pregnancies is a relative risk factor for gallstones. During pregnancy up to 40 per cent of women show ultrasound evidence of biliary sludge (Maringhini, JHepatol, 1987; 5:218). In most this is reversible; the sludge disappears after delivery; in some women, however, it is not and biliary sludge clearly precedes the development of gallstones (Lee, Gastro, 1988; 94:170). One review[7] suggested that all patients with gallstones develop sludge as the initial step in gallstone formation. Again it is unclear whether this sludge is due solely to gallbladder stasis, resulting from excess circulating progesterone, or whether other mechanisms may be involved.

Body weight

Gallstones are more common in obese people than in the non-obese. In both univariate and multivariate analyses, obesity is one of the most consistent risk factors for gallstone disease. This is due partly to abnormalities in bile lipid secretion and composition (see above, and below). Total body cholesterol synthesis is linearly related to body weight and to the degree of obesity (Miettinen, Circul, 1971; 44:842), and there is a parallel increase of hepatic cholesterol synthesis (Maton, ClinSci, 1982; 62:515) and of biliary cholesterol secretion (Reuben, ClinSci, 1985; 69:71). Whether other pathogenetic mechanisms in gallstone formation are also affected by obesity is not known. Acute weight loss in the obese is also a risk factor for gallstones (Broomfield, NEJM, 1988; 319:1567).

Dietary factors

Since obesity is a risk factor for gallstones, and because calorie intake is usually higher in obese than non-obese individuals, it follows that a high calorie intake may be a risk factor for gallstones.

Carbohydrates may be important. Heaton and his colleagues (Thornton, Gut, 1983; 24:2) showed (in paired, before-and-after studies) that reducing refined carbohydrate intake lowers biliary cholesterol saturation, at least in those with supersaturated bile initially. They also thought dietary fibre important in gallstone pathogenesis; when dietary fibre intake was increased using bran supplements, the biliary cholesterol saturation index in fasting duodenal bile was reduced. However, bran supplements have not consistently lowered biliary cholesterol saturation (Watts, AmJSurg, 1978; 135:321; Huijbregts, EurJClinInv, 1980; 10:487). A high fibre intake shortens intestinal transit, so reducing bacterial degradation of primary to secondary bile acids in the colon; this may explain its beneficial effect on gallstone formation (see below).

The role of dietary fat and its content of saturated and polyunsaturated fatty acids is uncertain. If anything, diets high in polyunsaturated fatty acids, which may be of benefit in lowering serum lipid levels, tend to increase biliary cholesterol saturation (Sturdevant, NEJM, 1973; 288:24). The role of dietary cholesterol as a risk factor for gallstones is also unclear. Cholesterol does not undergo a significant enterohepatic circulation and there is no evidence that dietary cholesterol directly affects biliary cholesterol output and saturation. Nevertheless, two groups showed that low cholesterol diets enhanced the effect of oral chenodeoxycholic and ursodeoxycholic acids in lowering biliary cholesterol saturation (Kupfer, DigDisSci, 1982; 27:1025; Maudgal, BMJ, 1982; ii:851).[8] In theory, high cholesterol diets (and those rich in saturated fatty acids) might increase serum cholesterol levels, but epidemiological evidence implicates hypertriglyceridaemia, not hypercholesterolaemia, as a risk factor for gallstone disease (Ahlberg, DigDisSci, 1979; 24:459).

Genetic and racial factors

Gallstones and supersaturated bile are more common in first-degree relatives of known gallstone carriers than in the general population (Van der Linden, HumHere, 1973; 23:123; Gilat, Gastro, 1983; 84: 242; Negi, Hepatol, 1990; 12:1006).

The prevalence of gallstones varies widely throughout the world (Fig. 5) and, in many cases, genetic factors appear to play a role. The prevalence is highest in native American tribes, not only in the United States and Canada (such as the Pima, Navajo, Chippewa, and Micmac) but also in Central and South America where intermarriage has ensured that almost all of the population have at least some native American genes. The Pima Indians of Arizona have the highest recorded prevalence rate for gallstones (Sampliner, NEJM, 1970; 283:1358). Pima women develop supersaturated bile around the age of puberty; by the age of 25 to 30 years most have borne several children and up to 80 per cent have developed gallstones.

Gallstones are also common in South America, particularly in Chile where their pathogenesis has been well studied. Although native American genes may partly explain the high prevalence in Chile, a high intake of beans (a common component of the Chilean diet) appears to affect biliary cholesterol saturation adversely (Nervi, Gastro, 1989; 96:825; Duane, JLipRes, 1997; 38:1120).

Gallstones are common in developed societies, such as those in Western Europe, North America, and Australasia, where there is a high intake of refined foods and most people have a sedentary lifestyle. In Europe, Sweden has a particularly high prevalence rate. Conversely, gallstones are rare in the rural Japanese population, more common in city dwellers, and more common still when Japanese individuals migrate to live in the United States. Gallstones are seen with approximately the same frequency in North India as in Western countries but are rare in South India (Malhotra, Gut, 1968; 9:290). Gallstones in North India are predominantly cholesterol-rich and similar in composition to stones in the West (Rajagopal, IndJGastro, 1988; 7:9). Gallstones are exceptionally rare in many parts of Africa where the people are physically active, eat a largely vegetarian diet, and have a rapid intestinal transit.

Diseases predisposing to gallstones (Berman, NEJM, 1978; 299:1161)

Hepatic cirrhosis

Gallstones occur two to three times more often in patients with hepatic cirrhosis than in non-cirrhotic controls (Bouchier, Gut, 1969; 10:705; Nicholas, Gastro, 1972; 63:112; Sheen, Hepatol, 1989; 9:538; Grassi, ItalJGastr, 1992; 24:342). However, the prevalence of cholesterol gallstones in patients with chronic liver disease appears to be no different from that in the non-cirrhotic group: the increased frequency is due to non-cholesterol stones. Factors such as hypersplenism, with a shortened red cell survival time, and a reduced activity of hepatic glucuronyl transferase might account for a greater than normal 'spill' of unconjugated bilirubin into bile and the formation of calcium bilirubinate stones (see above). Recent studies from Italy suggest that the duration and severity (Child's class) of cirrhosis are risk factors for cholecystolithiasis, especially in HBsAg-negative patients with a history of alcohol abuse (Benvengre, Digestion, 1997; 58:293).

Ileal disease/resection

Ileal resection interrupts the enterohepatic circulation of bile acids (Playoust, AmJPhysiol, 1965; 208:363) which, in turn, increases biliary cholesterol saturation in animals (Dowling, JCI, 1970; 49:232; 1971; 50:1917) and man (Dowling, Gut, 1972; 13:415). At first sight this seemed to explain the increased prevalence of gallstones in patients with ileal disease or resection. However, in up to 40 per cent of these patients the gallstones are radio-opaque (Heaton, BMJ, 1969; 3:494) and are not the radiolucent, cholesterol-rich stones which would be expected on the basis of bile acid and bile lipid studies.

Haemolysis

As noted above, gallstones are more common in patients with chronic haemolytic disorders such as sickle cell disease, thalassaemia, and spherocytosis than in individuals with normal haematology. In Jamaica, Serjeant et al. (BrJHaemat, 1981; 48:533)

followed a cohort of babies with homozygous sickle cell disease at birth to learn more about the natural history of their disorder. By the age of 10 years up to 40 per cent had developed gallstones, many of which were radio-opaque suggesting that they contained calcium carbonate and not just calcium bilirubinate. (The carbonate ion is small in comparison with bilirubin which is a large anion that 'dilutes' the small calcium cation so that calcium bilirubinate stones may still appear radiolucent. In theory, calcium phosphate could also render gallstones radio-opaque, but this is a comparatively rare calcium salt in gallstones. Usually, therefore, radio-opacity in gallstones signifies the presence of calcium carbonate.)

Vagotomy

Although the evidence that vagotomy predisposes to gallstones is not strong, several studies suggest that truncal vagotomy is a risk factor for cholelithiasis (Sapala, SGO, 1970; 71:196; Tompkins, Surgery, 1972; 71:196; Ihasz, AmJSurg, 1981; 141:48). Others believe that vagotomy is unimportant in gallstone formation (Stempel, Gastro, 1978; 75:608; Shaffer, AnnSurg, 1982; 195:413). The mechanism may result from gallbladder stasis, as gallbladder contraction is under cholinergic as well as hormonal control.

Spinal injury

Apstein (Gastro, 1987; 92:966) clearly showed that high spinal section is associated with a high incidence of gallstones. The mechanism is unknown, but may be due to gallbladder stasis secondary to autonomic (sympathetic) nerve dysfunction in patients with spinal lesions higher than T10.

Drugs

Some of the drugs which increase the risk of developing gallstones have already been discussed. They include:

(i) clofibrate (Persemlides, Gastro, 1974; 66:565);
(ii) oestrogen-rich oral contraceptives and possibly also oestrogen-containing hormone replacement therapy; and
(iii) the somatostatin analogue, octreotide (Wass, BMJ, 1989; 299:1162).

Total parenteral nutrition

This may cause accumulation of sludge and gallstone formation, presumably because it does not stimulate gallbladder contraction like oral ingestion of foods (Lirussi, Gastro, 1989; 96:493).

Presentation of gallstone disease

Gallstones can cause a variety of clinical problems although many patients with gallbladder stones have no symptoms. Stones within the gallbladder may cause 'biliary' pain; they may lead to acute cholecystitis and empyema (Chapter 23.6), or cause cystic duct obstruction. The clinical presentations that may result from gallstones which migrate from the gallbladder, from primary bile duct stones, or from cystic duct stones that cause bile duct obstruction (the Mirizzi syndrome) are considered below under the heading 'Complications of gallstone disease'.

Uncomplicated or 'silent' gallbladder stones

Many patients with cholecystolithiasis have no symptoms due to gallstones. Their stones are usually detected if abdominal radiographic, ultrasound, or CT examinations are carried out for unrelated problems. Right upper quadrant discomfort and indigestion are often attributed to gallbladder stones, but epidemiological studies have shown that 'dyspepsia' and other upper abdominal symptoms, such as post-prandial epigastric discomfort, bloating, heartburn, burping/belching, and fat intolerance, are non-specific. They occur with equal frequency in gallstone carriers and non-gallstone subjects.[2,3] Therefore, a Working Team on this problem considered that patients with gallbladder stones without symptoms, or with the symptoms listed above (often patients with the irritable bowel syndrome), require neither medical nor surgical treatment for gallstones (Schoenfield, GastrInternat, 1989; 2:25).

Symptomatic gallbladder stones

Most investigators agree that 'mild, infrequent but specific gallstone-related symptoms' mean biliary pain, which is defined, clinically and arbitrarily, as a steady epigastric and/or right upper quadrant pain lasting more than 15 to 30 min (Schoenfield, GastrInternat, 1989; 2:25) and unrelated to colonic function (i.e. not relieved by passing stools or flatus) (Podda, GastrInternat, 1989; 2: 107). Even so, in one study, epigastric and/or right upper quadrant pain was of no value in predicting the presence of gallbladder stones (Jorgensen, Hepatol, 1989; 9:856). About 15 per cent (range 10 to 25 per cent) of patients with gallbladder stones have associated choledocholithiasis, and when gallbladder and common bile duct stones coexist we have no reliable way of deciding which of these might be the cause of symptoms. However, unsubstantiated clinical impressions strongly suggest that the natural history of untreated gallbladder stones is more benign than that of bile duct stones (Dowling, Gut, 1983; 24:599).

Cystic duct stones

Gallbladder stones may cause acute, intermittent, or long-term obstruction of the cystic duct; they are usually large, as stones smaller than 2 to 3 mm tend to pass through the duct.[9] The severe pain caused by acute obstruction of the cystic duct cannot be differentiated clinically from that due to acute obstruction of the bile duct (see below). It is presumably due to excessive contraction of the gallbladder trying to expel the stone through the cystic duct. If the pain continues unabated, cholecystectomy should be performed.

Intermittent obstruction of the cystic duct causes episodes of pain, often intense, with spontaneous relief if the stone falls back into the main cavity of the gallbladder. There may be long intervals between the attacks. If ultrasound is performed, a stone may be seen in the neck of the gallbladder during the attack, but shifting to another part of the gallbladder during a pain-free interval.

If a stone impacts in the gallbladder neck or cystic duct in the absence of infection, the gallbladder may enlarge; the contained bile is reabsorbed and the gallbladder fills with mucus. There may be no symptoms, but the organ can become large and easily palpable on abdominal palpation. This may cause confusion if jaundice results from bile duct obstruction due to another stone, as jaundice

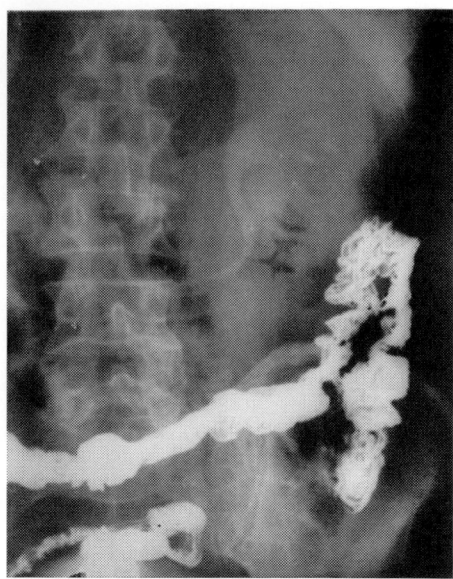

Fig. 6. Gas can be seen in gallstones lying medial to the hepatic flexure of the colon, which is outlined by barium. This is the 'Mercedes Benz' sign, although in this case the appearance is not that of the famous triradiate logo.

associated with a palpable gallbladder is usually attributed to a tumour of the pancreas or ampulla. If the gallbladder is infected, outflow obstruction usually causes an empyema of the gallbladder (see Chapter 23.6).

Investigation of gallbladder stone disease

Detection of gallbladder stones

Ultrasound

Ultrasound examination is the most common and accurate method of detecting gallbladder stones, having a sensitivity of 90 to 95 per cent. It is reasonably accurate for the assessment of stone dimensions, being more precise for top-to-bottom than for side-to-side measurements (the 'bottom' of stones is often impossible to define by ultrasound). Stone number may be difficult to determine by ultrasound if multiple small stones or fragments coalesce. Most investigators believe that ultrasound tells us nothing about stone composition.

Plain radiographs and oral cholecystography (see Chapter 5.5)

Plain abdominal radiographs usually identify only radio-opaque gallstones. Occasionally, however, gas trapped in clefts in gallstones may make them visible on plain radiographs (the so-called 'Mercedes-Benz' sign) (Fig. 6); confusion may arise because there may be marked variation in gallbladder position. Furthermore, calcified costal cartilages, lymph nodes, and blood vessels may be mistaken for radio-opaque stones. Bowel contents may 'mask' the gallbladder.

In approximately 70 per cent of gallstone carriers, the stones are radiolucent; these are usually cholesterol-rich stones which can be dissolved by appropriate therapy. They can be identified by the

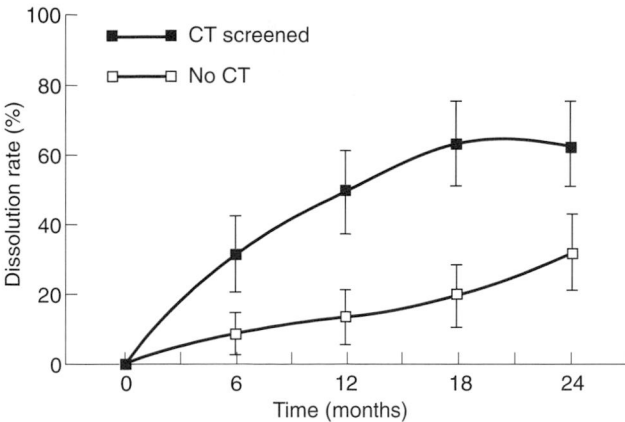

Fig. 7. Actuarial or life table analysis of complete gallstone dissolution rates ($\pm$ SE) in (i) 24 patients screened by CT and (ii) 29 patients with no pretreatment CT (reproduced from Walters, Gut, 1992; 33:375, with permission).

combination of plain abdominal radiography plus oral cholecystography. A plain radiograph of the gallbladder area is mandatory because calcified gallstones may not show up on oral cholecystography as surface calcification of gallstones is masked when the rim abuts on to the adjacent contrast medium. When opacification of the gallbladder is seen on oral cholecystography, it is clear evidence that the cystic duct is patent. Thirty per cent or more of the total population of gallstone carriers have 'non-functioning' or non-opacifying gallbladders by oral cholecystography (Attili, DigDisSci, 1987; 32:349), suggesting the possibility that the cystic duct is blocked; but failure to opacify the gallbladder does not always mean that the cystic duct is blocked.

The results of relatively short (up to 6 years), prospective, longitudinal, epidemiological studies suggest that the natural history of gallbladder stones in patients with a 'non-functioning' gallbladder is benign (Attili, personal communication) and no different from that of stones in patients with a patent cystic duct. Whether it is equally benign in patients with a non-functioning and distended gallbladder (mucocele) is unknown.

The buoyancy of stones in the mixture of bile and contrast material is an important sign. 'Floating' stones, that is, those forming a horizontal layer within the gallbladder when a radiograph of the patient is taken in the erect position, are almost invariably cholesterol-rich and thus dissolvable (Malet, Radiol, 1990; 177:167), while 'sinking' stones are likely to be non-cholesterol in type. Rarely, the trapping of gas within gallstones causes them to float. Since the advent of CT scanning it is clear that air-trapping within gallstones, which causes negative Hounsfield unit values, is more common than originally thought.

Smooth or faceted stones are usually cholesterol-rich, but when gallstones have an irregular contour (the 'mulberry' shape of black pigment stones) one should suspect that they are non-cholesterol in type. Stone contour is often difficult to define on oral cholecystography films.

CT scanning

Localized CT scanning of the gallbladder is much more sensitive than conventional radiography in detecting gallstone calcium. Only 50 per cent of stones which are lucent by CT scanning are also lucent by traditional radiographs; the rest contain enough calcium to render them visible only on CT scans (Rajagopal, JHepatol, 1989; 9:S211; Janowitz, GastrRad, 1990; 15:58). The apparent gallstone density on visual inspection of CT films provides only a rough guide to gallstone opacity, as the appearance depends on the attentuation of the stone, relative to surrounding liver and bile. Furthermore, the apparent attenuation can be modified by altering the 'gain' of the machine.

For several reasons, there is controversy about the usefulness of measuring gallstone attenuation values or CT scores (Hounsfield units, **HU**). First, the gallstone attenuation score is not absolutely constant but varies from patient to patient and from machine to machine. Partial correction for this is possible by using a calcium-containing phantom as a standard every time patients with gallbladder stones are screened. On this basis, we estimate that the maximal overall variation in CT score is no more than $\pm$ 10 HU. However, others claim that it may vary by as much as $\pm$ 50 HU.

Second, we have yet to establish a clinically useful and widely acceptable cut-off point in the maximum HU score measured *in vivo*, which would predict stone composition and dissolvability. Our results suggest that stones with a maximum attenuation value of more than 90 to 100 HU are either non-cholesterol in type (pigment stones) or else contain enough calcium to render complete gallstone dissolution unlikely. Others disagree and think that the cut-off point should be as low as 50 HU or as high as 140 HU. Our recent results suggest that the pretreatment gallstone attenuation score predicts the speed of gallstone dissolution with oral bile acid therapy and that the best results were seen in patients with scores of less than 75 HU (Pereira, DigDisSci, 1997; 42:1175).

Third, in our experience, a maximum score of 100 HU measured *in vivo* corresponds to a mean gallstone composition of only 3 per cent total calcium by weight, when measured *in vitro* on the homogenized stone retrieved at surgery. Indeed, critics of routine CT scanning to select patients with gallstones for dissolution therapy argue that the technique is too sensitive, as it detects tiny amounts of non-cholesterol material (mainly calcium salts) which would not interfere with dissolution.

The CT score, measured *in vivo*, correlates linearly with gallstone composition measured *in vitro* (positively with stone total calcium and calcium carbonate, negatively with stone cholesterol—at least for cholesterol-rich gallstones containing more than 70 per cent cholesterol by weight; Rajagopal, Gut, 1988; 29:A1487; JHepatol, 1989; 9:S211), with gallstone dissolvability *in vitro* (the extent of dissolution being measured in MTBE under arbitrary fixed conditions), and, most importantly, with gallstone dissolvability *in vivo*. Two groups of otherwise comparable patients with similar clinical, gallbladder, and gallstone characteristics were treated with a combination of chenodeoxycholic acid (**CDCA**) plus ursodeoxycholic acid (**UDCA**); the actuarial rate for complete gallstone clearance in patients who had been screened by CT, and had a maximum pretreatment stone CT score of less than 100 HU, was 81 ± 16 per cent at 18 months; it was only 25 ± 10 per cent in those not screened (Walters, Gut, 1989; 30:A1459). Thus, although CT scanning is expensive (even when confined to between five and eight tomographic 'cuts' in the gallbladder area), we believe that routine pretreatment screening of patients with gallstones who are being considered for non-surgical treatment is cost-effective, as it avoids the inappropriate use of expensive oral bile acids, and ESWL plus adjuvant bile acids, in up to 50 per cent of patients who might otherwise be treated ineffectively for periods of up to 2 years (Fig. 7).

Before beginning dissolution therapy the patency of the cystic duct must be established, preferably not more than 1 to 3 months before treatment is started. This is usually done by oral cholecystography (showing gallbladder opacification). If patients are intolerant of cholecystographic contrast media, radionuclide scanning of the gallbladder with HIDA, or one of its derivatives, may be used. Patency of the cystic duct can also be inferred by ultrasound, indirectly but with acceptable accuracy, if there is a significant reduction in gallbladder volume after stimulation of gallbladder contraction by a fatty meal or a cholecystokinetic agent such as cholecystokinin or caerulin.

Management of symptomatic but uncomplicated gallbladder stone disease

Given the wide choice of management options what advice should be given to an individual patient who needs active treatment? The successful management of gallbladder stones depends on the appropriate selection of patients for the different management options, and especially for the various dissolution approaches including oral bile acid treatment. Patients with gallbladder stones causing specific, gallstone-related symptoms of sufficient frequency and/or severity to warrant active treatment can be treated by several different methods (Table 3). Offered the choice, some decide to wait and see what happens; others prefer an elective cholecystectomy in the hope this may lead to permanent resolution of their problems. However, for those who wish to avoid open abdominal or laparoscopic surgery, or who have other diseases which increase the risk of surgery, there are other options.

In theory, the options of simple observation or cholecystectomy apply to stones of any size, number, and composition. However, if the gallbladder is to be left *in situ* (without ablation), most, but not all, (Chiverton, BMJ, 1990; 300:1310) investigators confine these options to patients with a patent cystic duct. This creates a problem because, as mentioned above, 30 per cent or more of the total population of gallstone carriers have 'non-functioning' or non-opacifying gallbladders by oral cholecystography (Attili, DigDisSci, 1987; 32:349). However, the results of relatively short (up to 6 years), prospective, longitudinal, epidemiological studies suggest that, in patients with a 'non-functioning' gallbladder, the natural history of gallbladder stones is benign (Attili, personal communication) and no different from that in gallstone patients with a patent cystic duct.

The treatment options for cholesterol-rich dissolvable gallstones include oral bile acids given alone or with other oral agents, and ESWL alone or with adjuvant oral bile acids. For these treatments the cystic duct must be patent.

Who is suitable for non-surgical treatment of gallbladder stones?

Patients who are symptom free, or who have only vague dyspeptic symptoms, do not require treatment for their gallstones (Schoenfield, GastrInternat, 1989; 2:25). Patients with serious complications (see below) require open abdominal surgery, laparoscopic cholecystectomy, or some form of interventional radiology. Thus, only patients with symptoms which are relatively mild and/or infrequent, but which are definitely related to the presence of the gallstones (see above), are really suitable for non-surgical approaches.

Gallstone dissolution

Pure cholesterol stones (containing 100 per cent cholesterol) should always dissolve completely in unsaturated bile, or with contact solvents such as MTBE or ethyl proprionate. With all types of dissolution therapy the best results are in patients with cholesterol-rich gallbladder stones (those having 70 to 90 per cent cholesterol by weight on chemical analysis; Womack, AnnSurg, 1963; 157:670; Sutor, Gut, 1971; 12:55). Unfortunately, while the composition of stones can be determined accurately following their removal, there is no certain way of determining it *in vivo* (see above).

In the context of selecting patients for dissolution therapy, the major criterion for dissolvability is the lucency of the stones as judged by plain radiography and and oral cholecystography. However, 14 to 20 per cent of lucent stones are non-cholesterol in type (Bell, Gut, 1975; 16:359; Trotman, Gastro, 1975; 68:1563). Indeed, this is a common cause of 'failed' oral bile acid treatment despite adequate therapy with bile acids for 1 year (Gleeson, QJMed, 1990; 279:711).

Gallstone clearance may not depend solely on complete stone dissolution. Cholesterol-rich stones can disintegrate as they dissolve, and even if the resultant particles or debris are not cholesterol-rich (and thus soluble in unsaturated bile or contact solvent) they might pass through the cystic duct, and down the common bile duct, to render the patient free from stones. It is not known how much non-cholesterol material a stone can 'carry' and still be capable of dissolving/disintegrating completely in order to clear the gallbladder. This probably depends on factors such as the density of crystal packing, the distribution/disposition of cholesterol and non-cholesterol material within the stone, and the cohesive properties of 'cement' substances, such as the spongiform mucus glycoprotein skeleton within the stone.

After manual instillation of MTBE through percutaneous, trans-hepatic cholecystic catheters, residual gallstone debris was found in 36 to 65 per cent of patients (Ellul, Gut, 1990; 31:A1214; Leuschner, DigDisSci, 1991; 36:193; 1994; 39:1302).[10] Some of these insoluble non-cholesterol residues (calcium salts, bilirubin granules, mucus glycoprotein, and amorphous debris) seemed to be more common after the use of MTBE than after oral bile acid treatment; why this was so is not known.

Oral bile acid therapy

Oral bile acid treatment is the oldest, most studied, best established, safest, and least-invasive non-surgical method for treating gall-bladder stones; but it is slow, only moderately effective and relatively expensive. The efficacy of oral bile acid therapy in dissolving gallstones depends on the free passage of bile, rendered unsaturated in cholesterol by the treatment, into and out of the gallbladder through the cystic duct.

Chenodeoxycholic acid (CDCA; chenodiol; see Chapter 2.10) was the first bile acid used for treating gallbladder stones (Bell, Lancet, 1972; ii:1213; Danzinger, NEJM, 1972; 286:1).

In 40 to 60 per cent of selected individuals given an appropriate dose of CDCA (15 mg/kg per day; see below) there is complete dissolution of gallbladder stones, as confirmed by two consecutive imaging studies 1 to 3 months apart during continuing therapy (Iser, NEJM, 1975; 293:378). However, CDCA has dose-related side-effects. Diarrhoea occurs in 30 to 60 per cent of patients and there may be a modest increase in plasma cholesterol (10 to 20 mg/dl), usually due to a rise in low-density lipoprotein cholesterol (Albers, Gastro, 1982; 82:638). The serum aminotransferases may increase transiently (up to threefold); liver morphology is usually normal, although minor changes were found on light and electron microscopy in 1 to 3 per cent of patients undergoing liver biopsy (Fisher, Hepatol, 1982; 2:187). These side-effects have limited the popularity and acceptability of CDCA as a monotherapy for gallstones.

Ursodeoxycholic acid (UDCA or ursodiol, the 7β-epimer of CDCA) is largely, but not completely, free of these side-effects (Bachrach, DigDisSci, 1982; 27:737). It rarely causes diarrhoea and does not affect liver function tests. Nor does it cause an increase in plasma cholesterol, perhaps because it does not inhibit primary bile acid synthesis (Carulli, JLipRes, 1980; 21:35; Angelin, JLipRes, 1983; 24:461), although not all investigators agree on this point (Williams, ClinSci, 1980; 58:15P).

UDCA is more potent than CDCA in lowering biliary cholesterol secretion and saturation (von Bergmann, Gastro, 1984; 87:136). A dose of 10 mg UDCA/kg per day is approximately equivalent to 15 mg CDCA/kg per day in its effects on bile lipids and gallstone dissolution; clinical experience suggests that 10 mg/kg per day is the optimal dose of UDCA (Maton, Lancet, 1977; ii:1297; Meredith, Gut, 1982; 23:382).

The combination of UDCA plus CDCA

Many clinicians now use a combination of UDCA and CDCA when oral bile acids are given either alone[11] or together with ESWL (Hood, Lancet, 1988; i:1322).[12] The current consensus, based on many clinical studies, suggests that the combination of UDCA and CDCA is at least as effective as (Stiehl, Gastro, 1980; 79:1192;

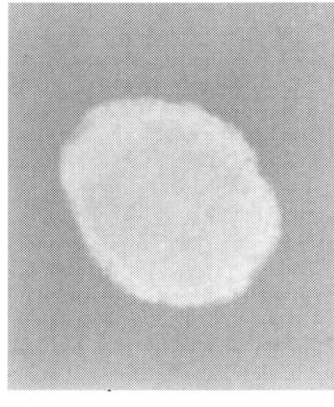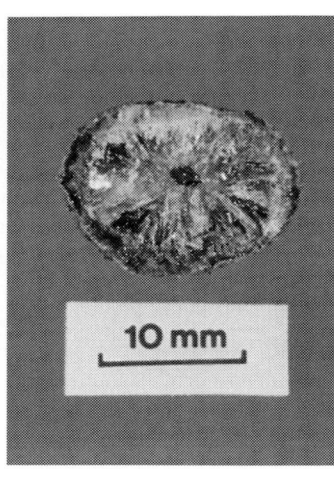

Fig. 8. Split surface of a cholesterol-rich gallstone removed from the gallbladder when the patient came to elective cholecystectomy because of persistent symptoms and failed oral bile acid dissolution therapy. Although the stone had appeared completely radiolucent by plain abdominal radiography and oral cholecystography, and was mainly a cholesterol-rich stone, it was mixed in composition and had a calcium bilirubinate nucleus and a pigment/calcium-rich shell which was apparent on radiography of the stone *in vitro* (b). This cholesterol-poor rim probably explains the failure of the oral dissolution therapy. Such stones often respond to adjuvant oral bile acids after they have been shattered by extracorporeal shock-wave lithotripsy, which 'exposes' the interior of the stone to gallbladder bile rendered unsaturated in cholesterol by oral treatment.

Roehrhasse, DigDisSci, 1986; 31:1032), or possibly better than,[11] monotherapy with either bile acid alone. When given as adjuvant therapy after lithotripsy, however, the Munich group showed that the gallstone clearance rate was no different with UDCA alone than with the combination of UDCA and CDCA (albeit with relatively large UDCA doses).

Because the side-effects of CDCA are dose related, by using one-half of the monotherapeutic dose (7.5 instead of 15 mg/kg per day) the incidence of diarrhoea (Mok, Lancet, 1974; ii:253), abnormal liver function tests (Fisher, Hepatol, 1982; ii:187), and raised serum cholesterol levels (Albers, Gastro, 1982; 82:638) should be reduced. UDCA costs more than CDCA, and by prescribing the two bile acids together, each at one-half of the monotherapeutic dose, the total cost of treatment is less than that of UDCA alone; the toxicity (mainly of CDCA) should be reduced while the dissolution efficacy of the individual bile acids is maintained.

UDCA is reported to cause acquired gallstone surface or rim calcification (Fig. 8) (Bateson, BMJ, 1981; 283:646), and although this is probably a non-specific effect (Frabboni, Hepatol, 1985; 5:1004), occurring as it does spontaneously and during CDCA therapy, it too may be a dose-dependent phenonomen although this has never been established. We believe that the advent of pretreatment CT scanning of the gallbladder may help to eliminate this problem, because it excludes from treatment patients whose gallstones contain small, pre-existing amounts of calcium salts which act as a template for further calcium carbonate precipitation as a result of bile acid-induced, bicarbonate-rich choleresis in ductular epithelial cells (Dumont, Gastro, 1980; 79:82).

Incomplete gallstone dissolution has been reported in patients treated with CDCA (Maton, Medicine, 1982; 61:86), UDCA

(Gleeson, QJMed, 1990; 279:711), and with the combination of the two bile acids (Walters, Gut, 1992; 33:375). At surgery, pigment-rich, non-cholesterol residues were recovered from the gallbladder of some of these patients. Given the limited sensitivity of both oral cholecystography and ultrasonography in detecting individual gallstone particles or remnants measuring less than 2 mm in maximum diameter, it is possible that small residues of this sort are relatively common, even after apparently complete gallstone dissolution/clearance with oral therapy (Shapero, Hepatol, 1982; 2:587; Sommerville, BMJ, 1982; 284:1295; Lanzini, JHepatol, 1986; 3:241). This may occur despite the recommendation that two consecutive normal imaging studies (oral cholecystography, ultrasonography, or both) should be obtained during 1 to 3 months of continued therapy, before stopping treatment.

Other oral agents

Monoterpene mixture

For several years, Bell and his colleagues (Bell, BMJ, 1979; i:24; Ellis, BMJ, 1984; 289:153) studied the preparation 'Rowachol', a mixture of cyclic monoterpenes. In a limited number of patients Rowachol not only dissolved radiolucent gallstones, which were presumed to be cholesterol rich, but also appeared to be effective in some patients with radio-opaque stones. Leuschner et al. (Gut, 1988; 29:428) confirmed this effect of Rowachol in dissolving gallbladder stones and suggested that it also enhanced the efficacy of UDCA when the two treatments were combined. The combination of UDCA and monoterpenes has also been used successfully as adjuvant treatment after ESWL (Darzi, Gut, 1989; 30:A1459).

HMG CoA reductase blockers

When an HMG CoA reductase blocker such as simvastatin, pravastatin, or lovastatin is administered, there is a reduction in biliary cholesterol saturation (Duane, Hepatol, 1988; 8:1147; Hoogerbrugge, Gut, 1990; 31:348) and the effect appears additive to that of oral bile acids. Whether the additional cost of cholesterol synthesis blockers, and the further side-effects which they may produce, will justify the combination of the two treatments for the management of gallbladder stones remains to be seen.

Contact solvent for gallstone dissolution

The aim of contact dissolution was to surround the gallstones with a solvent either for cholesterol (such as MTBE) or for non-cholesterol material (EDTA as a calcium chelator and/or N-acetyl cysteine as a disulphide bond-breaking mucolytic agent). The solvents were introduced directly into the gallbladder through solvent-resistant catheters. This technique, which was fully described in the first edition, has now been abandoned.

Extracorporeal shock-wave lithotripsy

This technique was pioneered in the 1980s at the University of Munich, where it was used by the Department of Surgery (working with the Dornier company) for treating kidney stones (Chaussy, Urol, 1985; 23:59). Paumgattner and his colleagues then applied it to the treatment of gallstones and have now treated over 1000

patients.[12,13] The technique has been used on many thousands of patients with gallstones worldwide.

The original machine used an underwater spark-gap generator; the sudden evaporation of water caused shock waves which were focused on to the target stones with a semi-ellipsoid reflector. The patients had to be submerged in a water bath and were anaesthetized because the treatment was painful. The machine was noisy and the operators wore ear protectors.

Second generation machines operate: (i) on the spark-gap principle; (ii) on the basis of an array of piezoelectric crystals which, when excited, generate shock waves which can be focused because of the arrangement of the crystals; or (iii) by generating shock waves from an electromagnetically activated metal membrane, with focusing of the waves through an acoustic lens. None of the new models require submersion in a water bath.

There are few controlled trials of the efficacy of the different types of machines (Petersen, Gastro, 1988; 94:581; Zuin, JHepatol, 1989; 9:99), but unconfirmed impressions suggest that the spark-gap machines are more powerful, require fewer shocks per treatment and fewer treatments, and fragment stones more effectively and into smaller particles than machines using piezoelectric crystals. However, treatment with spark-gap machines is more painful (60 per cent of patients still requiring some intravenous sedation or analgesia). The piezoelectric and electromagnetic machines are cheaper to install and maintain, and their use is relatively painless, so that anaesthesia and analgesia are rarely required (Albert, SemLivDis, 1990; 10:197).

There are many theoretical questions to be answered about ESWL. There is uncertainty about which component of the shock wave is responsible for stone fragmentation: the entry of the wave through the front surface of the stone, the rebound of the shock wave from the back of the stone, or the negative component of the shock wave producing a cavitation or implosion effect (Coleman, USMedBiol, 1989; 15:213; Lubock, DigDisSci, 1989; 34:999). Furthermore, we are ignorant about the importance of crystal structure and packing, and of planes of cleavage, fissures, crystal orientation, cement substances, and heterogeneous stone composition on the fragmentation responses.

Despite this uncertainty, much is known about the factors governing targeting, fragmentation, and clearance of gallstones after ESWL (plus adjuvant oral bile acid treatment) and about the importance of patient selection in achieving the goal of a symptom-free, stone-free patient without significant side-effects or complications of treatment.

Targeting

In theory, extracorporeal shock waves can be focused on gallstones in all patients. In practice, however, targeting may occasionally be difficult or impossible, particularly in obese patients. In the authors' unit, targeting was unsuccessful in 7 per cent of patients (Ellul, Gut, 1990; 31:A1186), most of whom were markedly overweight. Others have had similar experiences,[14] but in some centres, if targeting of the stones proves difficult or impossible, the results in these patients are ignored rather than included in an 'intention to treat' analysis.

Most lithotripsy machines use either 'in line' or independent ultrasound probes to localize gallstones, but some machines also use fluoroscopic localization of the stones by X-ray, with or without a C-arm, which facilitates patient positioning and optimizes stone localization. In both cases, obesity adversely affects visualization of gallstones; if stones cannot be positioned correctly within the focal zone, one cannot expect fragmentation. The three types of shock-wave generators have different focal volumes. Spark-gap machines have a larger focal volume than piezoceramic devices; electromagnetic machines occupy an intermediate position. The peak pressure zone is not a focal area but an ellipsoid or cigar-shaped focal volume. With piezoelectric devices, the focal zone is 3 to 4 mm in width and 8 to 9 mm long; with spark-gap machines, it is approximately 5 to 8 mm with an active length of 10 to 15 mm.

In theory, these differences in peak pressure volumes have advantages and disadvantages. The pinpoint accuracy of the piezoelectric machines should cause less iatrogenic tissue damage than spark-gap machines, but targeting must be more precise in order to fragment the stones. Because of respiratory and other patient movements, gallbladder stones are not stationary, and the crossed wires of the target oscillate across the surface or subsurface region of the stone 'under attack'. There is an unsubstantiated impression that the less precise focusing of the spark-gap machines results in more effective gallstone fragmentation than that achieved with the other types of lithotriptors (smaller fragments with fewer shocks and/or fewer treatment sessions). However, because the machines generate different peak pressures and shock-wave patterns (duration and height of peak pressure, speed of upstroke and downstroke of the pressure wave, and rebound negative post-shock waves, if any), it is difficult to be certain that the different fragmentation responses seen with the various lithotriptors are due solely to different focal pressure volumes. Furthermore, the influence of operator skill and experience, which also influence the fragmentation response, is difficult to quantify.

Fragmentation

All studies to date show that the speed and efficacy of ESWL plus adjuvant oral bile acids in achieving stone clearance depend on fragment size; the smaller the fragment size, the more rapid the stone clearance. With the optimal voltage setting of the Dornier machine, the Munich group report mean fragment sizes of around 2.5 mm. Ell *et al.* (Gastro, 1990; 99:1439) achieved similar results with a piezoceramic machine, but others have been less successful. As a guiding principle one should aim for a maximum fragment size of 5 mm or less (Podda, GastrInternat, 1989; 2:107), although patients with bigger gallstone fragments (5 to 10 mm in diameter or even larger) may ultimately become free from stones with up to 2 years of adjuvant oral bile acid treatment.

The results of most published studies also show better fragmentation responses with single (solitary) than with multiple stones (Ponchon, Gastro, 1989; 97:457).[12] It is believed that satellite stones absorb or dissipate shock-wave energy so that the efficacy of shock waves directed at the target stone is less. For this reason, some investigators use preliminary oral bile acid treatment for weeks or months before ESWL to dissolve the small satellite stones, thus leaving the large remaining stone (or stones) unimpeded; the benefit of this approach is unproven. Indeed, several investigators claim that the selection criterion of no more than three gallbladder stones (see below) is too restrictive and that the fragmentation response

and subsequent clearance rates are equally good with up to eight gallbladder stones.[14]

There are at least two reasons why there should be more rapid subsequent gallstone clearance in patients with small fragments after ESWL than in those who are left with larger particles. First, after ESWL most patients pass at least some gallstone fragments from the gallbladder through the cystic duct into the intestine and out in the stools; in 21 patients studied for 1 to 3 days after lithotripsy, a total of 555 fragments, measuring up to 8 mm in diameter, were recovered in the stools.[9] Second, the smaller the fragment size the greater the surface area:volume ratio, with more rapid subsequent dissolution in bile rendered unsaturated in cholesterol by oral bile acids. However, the microsurface of the stone fragments is probably very irregular, thus increasing the effective surface area for dissolution; furthermore, fragmentation may well favour disaggregation of the stones into fine particulate matter or biliary sand which, like the small fragments induced immediately after lithotripsy, can migrate out of the gallbladder.

The efficacy of lithotripsy in fragmenting gallstones varies considerably from centre to centre. In the Munich series,[14] and in other large studies from Germany (Ell, DigDisSci, 1989; 34:1006), fragmentation was almost invariable, while in other studies (Ponchon, Gastro, 1989; 97:457; Schoenfeld, Gastro, 1990; 98:A261) ESWL failed to fragment stones adequately in many patients. In the authors' series, fragmentation was achieved in just under 80 per cent of patients; in those with solitary stones the figure was almost 90 per cent, but it was only 55 per cent in those starting with multiple stones (Ellul, Gut, 1990; 31:A1186). Again, obesity seemed important: patients in whom fragmentation was not achieved were, on average, 17 kg heavier than 'fragmenters'. Adipose tissue may attenuate the shock-wave profile, reducing the maximum pressure generated and broadening or flattening the pressure time peak (Ponchon, Gastro, 1989; 97:457).

The need for adjuvant oral bile acid treatment

The Munich group began adjuvant therapy with a mixture of UDCA and CDCA 2 weeks before lithotripsy, and continued for 2 months after disappearance of the gallstones on ultrasound examination in order to dissolve the stone fragments;[12] they reported a 95 to 100 per cent efficacy for single stones and a 67 per cent efficacy for 2 or 3 stones, within 18 months of treatment. The results of a small study from Dublin[14] and of two large studies in the United States have been less encouraging (Schoenfeld, NEJM, 1990; 323:1239; Stern, AmJGastr, 1990; 85:238; Torres, Radiol, 1991; 178:509). In one American study only 8 per cent of patients were stone free at 6 months using ESWL alone, and only 22 per cent were stone free when adjuvant UDCA was also given; in the other, using adjuvant UDCA, 26 per cent were stone free at 6 months. The success rate was higher in patients with solitary stones (48 and 35 per cent).

In the absence of adjuvant bile acid treatment the spontaneous clearance rate of gallstones fragmented by ESWL is unacceptably low in most (Vergunst, AnnSurg, 1989; 210:565) but not all (Fache, Radiol, 1990; 177:719) series. Although many patients pass a small number of gallstone fragments within a few days of ESWL, most of the fragments remain in the gallbladder (an estimated minimum of

85 per cent) and must be dissolved. With lithotripsy of renal stones, most fragments pass out in the urine. This difference between renal and biliary lithotripsy may be explained by the high flow rate of urine through the ureters and the relative stagnation of bile within the gallbladder.

Gallstone clearance

The efficacy of ESWL plus oral bile acids in achieving complete gallstone clearance varies from series to series, but the following generalizations represent a consensus. The best results are in non-obese patients with solitary gallbladder stones, particularly when the maximum stone diameter before ESWL is less than 20 mm. Up to 90 per cent of such patients become stone free after 19 to 24 months of adjuvant bile acid therapy. The response rate with large (2 to 3 cm diameter) stones is around 70 to 80 per cent, while for multiple (two or three) stones it is about 50 to 60 per cent. The results are also better when fragments after ESWL have a maximum diameter size of less than 5 mm.

Side-effects and complications

These have been detailed in many of the articles already quoted; therefore, they will be summarized only briefly here.

Due to the gallstones/fragments

Biliary colic

Since biliary pain is the principle criterion for patient selection, it is not surprising that further attacks of biliary pain may occur until the patient becomes stone free. In different series, some 30 to 40 per cent of patients experience biliary pain at some time after lithotripsy. It is particularly likely during the first 1 to 3 days after ESWL, presumably due to the passage of fragments; thereafter, the incidence is probably no different to that observed before treatment. Whether adjuvant bile acid therapy reduces the frequency of biliary pain is unproven.

Cholestasis/jaundice

The development of abnormal liver function tests and/or clinical features of cholestasis, including frank jaundice, is rare (in the order of 1 to 5 per cent).

Pancreatitis

This is the most serious potential complication of lithotripsy, presumably due to obstruction of the common bile duct by stone fragments (Albert, SemLivDis, 1990; 10:197). It occurs in 1 to 2 per cent of patients, but most attacks are mild and settle spontaneously with conservative treatment.

As a direct result of lithotripsy

Although general or spinal anaesthesia is now seldom necessary, approximately 60 per cent of patients treated with spark-gap machines still require some form of intravenous sedation/analgesia. Patients treated with piezoelectric machines initially required no sedation, anaesthesia, or analgesia. However, this absence of symptoms was 'bought' at the expense of lower efficacy. The patients treated with piezoelectric machines required many more shocks per session (say 2000 to 5000 compared with 500 to 1500) and between 50 and 66 per cent of patients required more than one treatment session. For this reason, several manufacturers have increased the power of the piezoelectric machines with the result that about 30 per cent of patients now experience some discomfort when the machine is used at its maximal setting.

Transient petechiae are visible in the target area on the anterior abdominal wall in about 15 to 20 per cent of patients. They may be more common in thin individuals than in the obese. They usually fade within 24 to 48 h.

Haematuria

Frank haematuria is occasionally seen and is due to transient damage to the kidney; it depends on the positioning of the patient and the type of machine used. It is more common with spark-gap machines, perhaps as a result of the wider focal volume of peak pressure. Microscopic haematuria occurs in 1 to 2 per cent of patients.

Selection criteria

Successful use of ESWL depends on good patient selection. This varies from centre to centre, but most lithotripsy users follow the Munich criteria:

1. *Symptoms.* As for oral bile acid therapy, treatment is confined to patients with specific, gallstone-related symptoms (biliary pain/colic) which are neither too frequent nor too severe: otherwise, surgery is indicated.
2. *Gallbladder 'function'.* Most insist that patency of the cystic duct should be established directly by oral cholecystography (gallbladder opacification) or, less commonly, indirectly by ultrasound. Occasionally, when non-functioning of the gallbladder is associated with ultrasonographic evidence of a stone impacting in the Hartman's pouch/cystic duct area, patients can be treated with ESWL and then patency of the cystic duct returns. To date, experience with this subgroup of patients is anecdotal.
3. *Gallstone characteristics.* The best results are obtained in patients with solitary, radiolucent gallbladder stones measuring less than 20 mm in maximum diameter (see above). Unfortunately, such patients are comparatively rare (at most, 10 per cent of the overall population of gallstone carriers and 2 to 3 per cent of the symptomatic patients; Attili, DigDisSci, 1987; 32:349).

Therefore, most centres treat patients with larger solitary stones (the Munich group arbitrarily limit the maximum diameter to 3 cm), or with two or three stones whose total volume does not exceed that of a single 3-cm stone.

The evidence that the total stone volume is important is wanting. Darzi[14] and others claim successful outcome in patients with up to eight gallbladder stones, while in the authors' unit there is no upper limit to the dimensions of solitary stones. However, we usually confine ESWL to patients with stones which are more than 10 mm in diameter; other groups accept patients for lithotripsy whose stones measure more than 5 mm in diameter. Small stones are sometimes difficult to localize and target with the 'in-line' ultrasound transducer probes; furthermore, patients with stones measuring less than 10 mm in diameter usually respond well to oral bile acid treatment alone. When multiple stones are present it is difficult to assess the results of fragmentation.

With few exceptions (Fache, Radiol, 1990; 177:719),[14] most investigators confine lithotripsy to patients with radiolucent stones (as judged by plain radiography and oral cholangiography), except in research protocols to compare the efficacy of treatment in patients with radio-opaque calcified stones with that in patients with radio-lucent stones. The limited evidence to date suggests that patients with radio-opaque stones can be successfully managed by ESWL, but that the efficacy of treatment is probably only one-half that of completely radiolucent stones.[12] However, the degree of calcification and its distribution within the stone are probably important and one suspects that most successes are with cholesterol-rich stones with a relatively lightly calcified rim, rather than with densely calcified, non-cholesterol stones.

Several groups are currently examining the role of CT scanning, with quantification of stone attenuation values *in vitro* (Barkum, Gastro, 1991; 100:222) and *in vivo*, in assessing the efficacy of lithotripsy. It remains to be seen if routine localized CT scanning of the gallbladder will have the beneficial impact on the efficacy of lithotripsy that it does on the results of oral bile acid therapy alone (Walters, Gut, 1992; 33:375). Unsubstantiated observations suggest that the success rate of lithotripsy plus oral bile acids in clearing the gallbladder of stones with centrally calcified rims is better than that obtained with oral bile acids alone, presumably because the fragmented interior of the stone can be dissolved by unsaturated bile, and with disintegration of the stone there may be spontaneous passage of the fine, non-cholesterol residues.

Exclusion criteria

1. Patients with abnormal bleeding/clotting are normally excluded from ESWL because of the risk of excessive bleeding. Haemo-bilia, and superficial (usually transient) damage to the gallbladder mucosa, is common. When patients were subjected to lithotripsy at various times before elective cholecystectomy, gallbladder mucosal ulceration and bleeding were found at laparotomy 6 and 12 h later, but by 24 to 48 h the mucosa had returned to normal (Stephenson, JPath, 1989; 158:239). Others have studied the effects of ESWL on soft tissue injury in animals and/or in man (Brendel, Lancet, 1983; i:1054; Darzi, Gut, 1990; 31:1110).
2. Pregnancy.
3. The occurrence of cystic, calcified, or vascular abnormalities in the liver or elsewhere in the shock-wave path.
4. The presence of acute complications of gallstone disease, such as acute pancreatitis, cholecystitis, or cholangitis.

ESWL: conclusions/summary

The combination of lithotripsy and adjuvant bile acids results in more rapid and more effective gallstone clearance than is seen with oral bile acid treatment alone. However, the best results are not obtained until 2 years after ESWL. Lithotripsy, therefore, is not dramatically effective and is not a treatment in itself. If the Munich selection criteria are applied, it is suitable for only 20 to 25 per cent of symptomatic patients with gallstones and for less than 5 per cent of the whole population with gallstones (Capocaccia, personal communication). Furthermore, the initial cost of the machines is high as is their maintenance and depreciation. To obtain the best results it seems to be necessary to give adjuvant bile acid therapy,

and this is expensive. For these reasons, many who initially, and enthusiastically, espoused ESWL as a breakthrough, now reject it as a passing fashion. The over-ready acceptance of the technique initially, and the rush to buy lithotripsy machines, was certainly uncritical and excessive. However, the pendulum of opinion may now have swung too far in the other direction, rejecting an important aid to oral bile acids for a selected minority of patients with gallbladder stones. For most patients, laparoscopic cholecystectomy is clearly a more suitable treatment than lithotripsy and the other 'non-surgical' approaches.

The key question: why retain the gallbladder? Is it helpful or harmful to remove a 'functioning' gallbladder?

The question of retaining the gallbladder is controversial. Most patients undergoing cholecystectomy suffer no obvious consequences of losing their gallbladder. Digestion and absorption appear to be unaffected when, after cholecystectomy, the intestine receives a continuous flow of dilute hepatic bile rather than the pulsatile flow of concentrated gallbladder bile which normally occurs in response to meals. However, patients who have previously had a vagotomy and drainage procedure have a high incidence of trouble-some post-vagotomy diarrhoea after cholecystectomy and it is occasionally devastating.

The debate about retention/removal of the gallbladder for gall-stone disease may be summarized as follows:

1. Favouring cholecystectomy is the fact that the gallbladder is seldom histologically normal in patients with cholelithiasis; however, the natural history of this 'histological' chronic cholecystitis is not known.
2. Any technique removing the stones but leaving the gallbladder (oral bile acids, contact solvents, ESWL plus oral treatment, percutaneous cholecystolithotomy, and rotary lithotripsy) has an approximately 50 per cent risk of gallstone recurrence. This is not inevitable and research is now being directed at ways of preventing recurrent stone formation; as yet, none has proven effective and acceptable.
3. There is a theoretical risk of gallbladder cancer in patients with gallbladder stones. More than 95 per cent of gallbladder cancers are associated with cholecystolithiasis. However, gallbladder cancer is rare and in most developed societies the risk of gallbladder cancer arising in patients with gallstone disease is small. Indeed, the risks of death from cholecystectomy are greater than those of dying from gallbladder cancer. In Chile, however, up to 2 to 3 per cent of patients with gallstones ultimately develop gall-bladder cancer; there the case for cholecystectomy is stronger than elsewhere in the developed world. This geographical difference in the incidence of gallbladder cancer may be due to the fact that Chileans have a high carriage rate of mutagenic salmonella (Nervi, personal communication) in their gallbladder bile.
4. In favour of retaining the gallbladder is the philosophy, often strong in the minds of individual patients, that it is pointless, and indeed wrong, to sacrifice a functioning organ unnecessarily.

Although most patients fare well without a gallbladder, cholecystectomy is associated with residual/persisting symptoms in 20 to 30 per cent of patients (Bates, Gut, 1984; 25:A579).

Conceivably, the gallbladder plays other important and useful roles, apart from the storage and concentration of bile. By delivering bile to the intestine to coincide with the arrival of food it could affect upper intestinal homeostasis by neutralizing gastric acid (together with the pancreas), by influencing gut motility, or by modulating the release of gastrointestinal hormones, or it may play a role in immune surveillance. These examples are speculative, but such possibilities should be borne in mind when guiding patients who believe that it is important to retain a functioning gallbladder, even though their ideas may seem misplaced and inappropriate. The whole future of the 'non-surgical' approaches for the management of symptomatic gallbadder stones hinges around this single issue.

Complications of gallstone disease
Mirizzi syndrome

In rare cases a stone impacted in the cystic duct or neck of the gallbladder (or in a cystic duct remnant) causes a localized obstruction of the common hepatic duct, thought to be due to direct pressure and/or secondary inflammatory changes around the duct. This constitutes the 'Mirizzi syndrome' (Mirizzi, JIntChir, 1948; 8: 731), which deserves attention because it may cause diagnostic confusion. A low cystic duct insertion and a close parallel course between the cystic and common hepatic ducts were thought to favour the development of the Mirizzi syndrome (Starling, Surgery, 1980; 88:737), but Cruz et al. pointed out that almost all cystic ducts run parallel to the common hepatic duct in their distal segment (GastrRad, 1983; 8:249). The obstruction of the common hepatic duct may cause right upper quadrant pain, nausea and vomiting, recurrent cholangitis, and jaundice (although partial obstruction can occur without an increase in bilirubin). Prolonged obstruction can cause secondary biliary cirrhosis. Atrophy of the right lobe of the liver resulting from biliary obstruction has also been described with the Mirizzi syndrome (Hadjis, JHepatol, 1987; 4:245).

A fistula may form between the common hepatic duct and the cystic duct or neck of the gallbladder (type II Mirizzi syndrome; Cornud, GastrRad, 1981; 6:265; McSherry, SurgGastr, 1982; 1: 219); the stone itself, lying in the common hepatic duct, may be the cause of the obstruction.

Ultrasound is the most useful initial test. It will show dilated ducts above and normal-sized ducts below the block, and may reveal the stone in the neck of the gallbladder or cystic duct. On cholangiography (percutaneous or endoscopic) the characteristic appearance is of a broad extrinsic impression, 2 to 3 cm long, on the lateral aspect of the common hepatic duct, with dilated ducts above and a normal duct diameter below the narrowing (Fig. 9); the cystic duct and gallbladder do not usually fill with contrast. With an anomalous insertion of the cystic duct the impression may be on the medial side of the common hepatic duct (Koehler, AJR, 1979; 132:1007). It may be possible to see a calcified gallstone close to the narrowing of the bile duct; CT scanning may be particularly useful for identifying the stone (Weiss, DigDisSci, 1986; 31:100). With angiography, there may also be bowing of the hepatic artery (Balthazar, AmJGastr, 1975; 64:144). If fistula formation occurs the

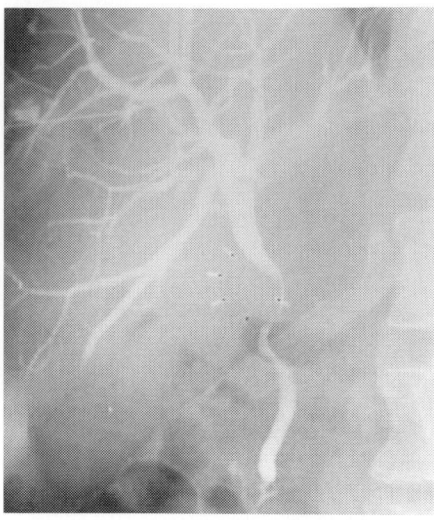

Fig. 9. Percutaneous cholangiography illustrating the Mirizzi syndrome: it shows the characteristic appearance of a broad extrinsic impression on the lateral aspect of the common hepatic duct. Dilated ducts are not obvious in the picture.

stone may be seen in the common hepatic duct on cholangiography, and the fistula itself may be outlined by contrast.

The radiological appearances of the Mirizzi syndrome may be simulated by a tumour of the gallbladder (Musher, AmJGastr, 1976; 66:79) or cystic duct (Walker, AmJGastr, 1982; 77:936; Montefusco, ArchSurg, 1983; 118:1221), by a cholangiocarcinoma, by metastatic disease at the hilum (Glenn, SGO, 1964; 118:93), and by acute cholecystitis (Nolan, BrJRadiol, 1972; 45:821).

Preoperative diagnosis of the Mirizzi syndrome is difficult but important, as intraoperative findings may be similar to those found with carcinoma of the extrahepatic biliary system, which requires a different technical approach (Hayek, AmJMedSci, 1988; 296:74). It is also important to detect a biliobiliary fistula preoperatively as attempts at dissection of the cystic duct or gallbladder neck may damage the common duct.[16] The Mirizzi syndrome has been treated by percutaneous insertion of a self-expandable metallic endoprosthesis (Adam, ClinRadiol, 1993; 48:198). Mirizzi syndrome is considered to be a contraindication to laparoscopic cholecystectomy by some surgeons. However, in one patient in whom the diagnosis was made by endoscopic cholangiography (Meng, BrJSurg, 1995; 82:396), laparoscopic subtotal cholecystectomy and T-tube insertion were performed after laparoscopic ultrasonography was used to clarify the biliary anatomy.

Choledocholithiasis and migratory gallstones

Gallstones usually migrate from the gallbladder via the cystic duct, enter the common bile duct, and then pass into the duodenum through the ampulla. They may also enter the intestine via fistulas between the gallbladder and adjacent parts of the gastrointestinal tract (cholecystogastric, cholecystoduodenal, cholecystojejunal, and cholecystocolic). Stones may pass through connections between two parts of the biliary tract, or rarely from a diseased gallbladder into the cavity of abscesses around that organ.

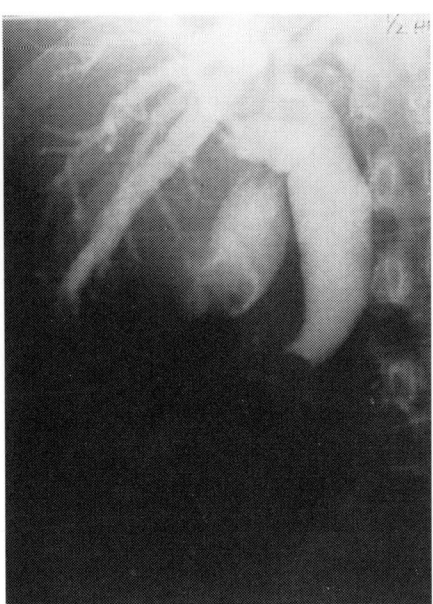

Fig. 10. Stones originating in the gallbladder may be held up for long periods in the common bile duct. In this radiograph there is a stone blocking the common bile duct. Another stone is seen in the gallbladder.

Common duct stones

Stones originating in the gallbladder may be held up for long periods in the common bile duct (Fig. 10); when common duct stones are found following cholecystectomy they must either have been left in the biliary tree (retained stones) or have been formed there *de novo* (primary common duct stones). It seems that stones can exist in the common duct for months or years without symptoms, and without any abnormality in liver function tests; they may be impossible to detect with ultrasound, routine radiography, or CT scanning. Their presence may only become obvious if they obstruct the bile duct and cause pain (which may be intermittent), jaundice, abnormal liver function tests (sometimes without elevation of bilirubin), or cholangitis.

Bile duct pain is usually attributed to distension and increased pressure within the duct and has two phases (see Section 4). The first, due to lesser degrees of increased pressure, is a tolerable fullness and discomfort in the middle and upper abdomen, often associated with nausea. The second pain, usually termed biliary 'colic', is a severe pain, but it is not a true colic as it does not wax and wane and is constant over several (2 to 4) hours. It is usually a central upper abdominal pain, presumably because the biliary tree is embryologically of midline origin, but may be in the right upper quadrant. It usually comes on after the evening meal, often around midnight, and is rarely associated with post-prandial and diurnal indigestion (Spiro, Lancet, 1992; 339:167).

Short episodes of bile duct obstruction may occur when gallbladder stones pass into the intestine, or when a bile duct stone(s) changes its position thus relieving the block; only first phase pain or discomfort may be experienced. There may be a transient alteration in liver function tests. The alkaline phosphatase may rise and there may be an accompanying small increase in serum bilirubin (often with bilirubinuria) and/or aminotransferases; these changes are often mistakenly attributed to viral hepatitis. If the liver function tests return to normal, there may be no further problems, but such cases should probably be investigated by endoscopic cholangiography. If a stone is still present in the bile duct it should be removed, as it may subsequently cause complete biliary obstruction or cholangitis.

Gallstones can also cause prolonged obstruction of the bile duct. This may be associated with severe pain. However, often there is no history of pain, even when the bile duct is completely obstructed and markedly dilated; presumably the intrabile duct pressure and wall tension remain relatively low in these cases. Complete biliary obstruction may occur with a single stone of any size, but in some patients there are multiple stones. Jaundice results and the liver usually enlarges, becoming easily palpable. The gallbladder is rarely palpable when obstructive jaundice is due to gallstones, unless there is also a blocked cystic duct.

In jaundiced patients with bile duct obstruction there will be elevation of the serum bilirubin and bilirubinuria. Serum alkaline phosphatase is usually raised, often to high levels; but in a small proportion of patients, even with complete biliary obstruction, the phosphatase is not increased. There is usually a modest elevation in serum aminotransferases, but in some patients with acute obstruction, particularly those with cholangitis, the aminotransferase levels can be very high (over 1000 U/l). Indeed, biliary obstruction due to gallstones is a relatively common cause of a marked elevation of aminotransferase levels in general clinical practice. This may lead to an erroneous diagnosis of viral hepatitis—a dangerous diagnostic error, particularly when cholangitis is present, as it delays antibiotic therapy and drainage of the bile duct (see below).

Ultrasound is an unreliable method of detecting bile duct stones, even of moderate size, although it does sometimes reveal large stones. Furthermore, a normal ultrasound does not rule out biliary obstruction due to gallstones, even when there is jaundice, as obstruction can occur in the absence of significant dilatation of bile ducts (Greenwald, JAMA, 1978; 240:1983). Oral cholecystography is of no value for detecting the presence of common bile duct stones, and CT scanning has a low sensitivity for this purpose. Endoscopic retrograde cholangiopancreatography (**ERCP**) is both sensitive and specific in this context, and is clearly the investigation of choice in patients when biliary obstruction is suspected, as it also allows the removal of stones.

Routine investigation with ERCP of patients with apparently uncomplicated gallbladder stones is neither practical nor desirable. As ERCP carries a small but definite risk, we need more reliable ways of predicting the presence of common bile duct stones in such patients, and more information on the natural history of these stones.

Management of common duct stones

A number of options are available for the removal of common bile duct stones (Sherman, SemLivDis, 1990; 10:205). Endoscopic sphincterotomy is now the preferred method for the management of most patients with these stones. If the stones are considered too large to be dealt with in this way, surgical removal is the method of choice unless the patient is unfit for surgery; in this case, biliary obstruction can usually be relieved by passing a stent around the stone(s). Contact solvent dissolution and extracorporeal shock-wave lithotripsy have been used to treat bile duct stones. The principles of these methods are described above under the treatment of gallbladder stones, but they are not as easy to apply to bile duct stones and are rarely used. Fragmentation may also be attempted with laser contact lithotripsy, but this technique is in its infancy; at present it is expensive and time-consuming.

Patients in whom common duct stones are left behind at cholecystectomy can have them removed through the tract of the T-tube left in place after surgery. Burhenne (AJR, 1973; 117:388) devised a steerable catheter which, after removal of the T-tube, could be guided via the tract into the bile ducts; this allowed the extraction of stones using a Dormia basket. In skilled hands this is an effective technique which can be performed without sedation or analgesia and which has relatively few complications (Burhenne, AmJSurg, 1976; 131:260).

Endoscopic sphincterotomy

If the need for sphincterotomy is recognized before the initial diagnostic endoscopy, the patient can be prepared for a session involving both procedures; alternatively sphincterotomy can be performed at a later time (and a guide wire or cannula can be left in place on the first occasion to facilitate this). Sphincterotomy involves the cutting, by a hot wire, of the wall of the ampulla, lower bile duct, and duodenum so that an aperture is left which is large enough to permit the passage of the gallstones present in the common bile duct (Fig. 6). The sphincterotome is then removed. The stones can be removed using Dormia basket extraction (which works for stones up to about 15 mm in diameter). Alternatively, a balloon catheter can be introduced and, after inflation of the balloon within the duct to a known diameter of about 8 to 10 mm, it can be pulled through the sphincter to check the size of the channel created. The balloon can then be passed further up the duct and inflated above the level of the stone(s); withdrawal of the catheter then brings the stones down into the duodenum.

It is important initially to check the least diameter of the largest stone present. It is also important to obtain good pictures of the distal intrapancreatic and preampullary common bile duct; if there is narrowing in this region, the passage of stones may be impossible despite adequate sphincterotomy. If the largest stone appears much bigger than the calibre of the distal duct, one can make a sphincterotomy and then check with a balloon whether the narrowed duct can expand, or whether the stone can be made to disintegrate following contact with the balloon catheter. If the stone cannot be removed by this procedure, other methods of stone removal may need to be used, for example a basket which can crush stones, electrohydraulic or laser lithotripsy, or surgical removal. A nasobiliary drain can be introduced and left in position and one can await spontaneous passage of the stone(s), or MTBE can be instilled into the common bile duct (Murray, Gut, 1988; 29:143; Kaye, JHepatol, 1990; 10:337). Alternatively, a stent can be placed across very large stones left in the duct: this may cause the stone(s) to break up; the fragments may pass spontaneously or may be removable at subsequent endoscopy, but often surgical removal is necessary. In very old patients a stent may be an appropriate permanent therapy. If stone extraction fails, it is important to give antibiotics and to drain the bile ducts (by a nasobiliary tube) in order to prevent obstructive cholangitis.

Sphincterotomy may be difficult when the ampulla is in a duodenal diverticulum, when the bile duct is not dilated, or when the ampulla is very small, and the success rate is lower following previous gastric surgery.

We still need to learn more about the natural history of cholecystolithiasis after common bile duct stones have been eliminated endoscopically (Cotton, Surgery, 1982; 91:628; Escourrou, Gut, 1984; 25:598) and, in particular, we need to know whether this history is modified by sphincterotomy.

Cholangitis and septicaemia due to gallstones

This topic is considered in Chapter 23.5.

Pancreatitis

Passage of gallstones through the lower end of the common bile duct is an important cause of acute pancreatitis and is assumed to result from gallstone blockage of the common channel (formed by the junction of the common bile duct and pancreatic duct) which drains into the duodenum via the ampulla.[17] This would allow regurgitation of bile, under pressure, into the pancreatic duct. However, there is often no evidence of an impacted ampullary stone at the time of surgery in patients with gallstone-related acute pancreatitis. The stone may have passed into the gut and it is not surprising that bile duct stones are found more often when surgery is performed early in the course of the illness (Kelly, Surgery, 1982; 92:571; Armstrong, BrJSurg, 1985; 72:551).

Acosta and Ledesma[18] filtered the stools of 36 patients with acute pancreatitis and those of 36 controls with acute biliary disease without evidence of pancreatitis. Within 10 days gallstones were found in the faeces of 34 of the patients with pancreatitis, but in only 3 of the controls. About 70 per cent of them were typical gallbladder stones (small, faceted, and hard); the rest appeared to be of bile duct origin (larger, 'cigar-shaped', and softer). In 24 patients with pancreatitis only one stone was found in the faeces; the others had multiple stones. The stones varied from 1 to 15 mm in their smallest diameter. At surgery, stones were confined to the gallbladder in 20 patients with pancreatitis and were present in the gallbladder and common bile duct in 12. Common bile duct stones were found in 2 of the 4 patients who had had a previous cholecystectomy; in the other 2 patients no stones were found in the biliary tree, but they were found in the faeces. These findings suggest that gallstone pancreatitis is commonly due to transient obstruction of the ampulla by stones migrating into the duodenum from the common bile duct.

It has been suggested that biliary sludge, identified by ultrasonography or by analysis of bile samples (obtained at ERCP, or by duodenal intubation and injection of cholecystokinin), may cause pancreatitis in subjects without gallstones who have no other obvious cause of pancreatitis (Lee, NEJM, 1992; 326:589). Recurrence of pancreatitis was less common when such patients were treated by cholecystectomy or papillotomy.

Anatomical factors may be important in the genesis of acute gallstone pancreatitis. When patients with this condition were compared with controls undergoing cholecystectomy for benign biliary tract disease, the cystic duct was larger, the gallbladder stones were smaller (suggesting easier passage of stones into the common bile duct), the common channel was longer, the angle between the common bile duct and pancreatic duct was greater, and reflux of cholangiographic contrast into the pancreatic duct occurred more commonly (Armstrong, BrJSurg, 1985; 72:551).

The clinical picture of gallstone pancreatitis is like that of other forms of pancreatitis. However, gallstones are a more likely cause in women than in men and in patients over the age of 50 years; furthermore, within the first 48 h of the attack, abnormalities of liver tests (serum bilirubin, aminotransferases, and alkaline phosphatase) and of serum amylase are more pronounced with gallstone pancreatitis. However, these features are of limited diagnostic value in individual cases (McMahon, Lancet, 1979; ii:541; Blamey, AnnSurg, 1983; 198:574; Davidson, BrJSurg, 1988; 75:213). It has been claimed that when the alanine aminotransferase level is greater than or equal to three times the upper limit of normal, the probability that it is gallstone pancreatitis is 95 per cent (Tenner, AmJGastr, 1994; 89:1863).

The likely severity of an attack of pancreatitis can be predicted on the basis of the arterial oxygen saturation, white blood cell count, lactate dehydrogenase, and serum urea (Leese, BrJSurg, 1988; 75: 460). In 'severe' cases of gallstone pancreatitis, urgent ERCP is recommended to detect common duct or ampullary stones, which can be treated by sphincterotomy (Neoptelemos, BrJSurg, 1988; 75: 1035). If cholangitis is also suspected, emergency drainage of the obstructed billiary tree is mandatory.

After recovery from an attack of gallstone pancreatitis, further attacks are common. Cholecystectomy and clearance of stones from the biliary tree should be carried out as soon as the patient is fit enough; this minimizes the frequency of subsequent attacks, although these may still occur due to missed stones or to formation of new bile duct stones (Kelly, Surgery, 1982; 92:571).

Biliary fistulas

Biliary fistulas usually result from long-standing gallstone disease. The most common are those between the gallbladder and intestine, and those connecting two parts of the biliary tract (biliobiliary fistulas). Biliary fistulas that communicate with the skin, the hepatic artery or portal vein, or with structures within the thorax are rare.

Biliary enteric fistulas

The most common type of biliary enteric fistula is cholecystoduodenal, that is, between the gallbladder and the duodenum (about 77 per cent); the next most common is cholecystocolic (about 15 per cent).[19] Less common fistulas are choledochoduodenal, cholecystogastric, cholecystojejunal, and those with multiple communications such as cholecystoduodenocolic, cholecystocholedochoduodenal, and cholecystojejunocolic. Biliary enteric fistulas account for about 1 per cent of surgery for non-malignant biliary tract disease.[19–21]

Biliary fistulas are thought to arise from repeated attacks of biliary tract disease, which cause the gallbladder or common bile duct to become adherent to the serosal surface of nearby viscera. Pressure necrosis, due presumably to the presence of an impacted stone, erodes the wall between two organs and a fistula is formed; [16] the pressure in the obstructed gallbladder or biliary tree then falls. Subsequently, the obstructing stone may migrate across the fistula into the intestine; it may pass out in the stools, but in some cases can cause intestinal obstruction. Biliary enteric fistulas may also result from peptic ulceration, or from pathological processes in the colon or other parts of the gastrointestinal tract (such as diverticular disease, malignancy, or Crohn's disease).

Most patients with biliary enteric fistulas have symptoms like those of chronic cholecystitis or biliary lithiasis. Symptoms of biliary tract disease have usually been present for many years, but sometimes for only a matter of weeks. There may have been long periods of freedom from pain.[19] There may be no change in the nature of the symptoms with development of the fistula, and it is therefore difficult to judge when fistula formation occurs. Most patients with biliary enteric fistulas due to gallstones are women; more than 70 per cent are over 60 years of age and only about 10 per cent are less than 50 years of age, but the average age may be lower in certain populations.[19,21] When biliary enteric fistulas are due to peptic ulcer disease, the average age is lower (around 44 years), there is a marked preponderance of males, and the preceding symptoms are usually typical of the underlying cause.[20] Peptic ulcer is the most common cause of choledochoduodenal fistulas (Constant, AnnSurg, 1968; 167:220). Carcinoma of the gallbladder is quite frequent in patients with biliary enteric fistulas, being found in 14 per cent of the patients of Day and Marks (AmJSurg, 1975; 129:552).

Many fistulas are discovered at surgery for biliary tract symptoms; the surgeon should be alerted to the possibility of a fistula if there are dense adhesions around a small fibrotic gallbladder. A correct preoperative diagnosis is made in 15 to 60 per cent of patients with biliary fistulas, but in some of these cases there is also gallstone ileus. A fistula should be suspected if air is found in the biliary tree on a straight abdominal radiograph (Fig. 11) or during radiological investigations to ascertain the cause of the biliary symptoms. However, air in the biliary tract often goes unrecognized, only to be found on subsequent review of the films. The gallbladder is rarely visualized by oral cholecystography. If air is seen in the biliary tree, or if a fistula is suspected for other reasons, a barium or Gastrografin meal should be performed; contrast may be seen to pass into the gallbladder or bile ducts. If this proves negative, a barium or Gastrografin enema is required (unless the clinical picture makes a colonic fistula more likely in which case the order should be reversed). Patients in whom a fistula is demonstrated radiologically before surgery usually have more severe biliary tract symptoms than those in whom the fistula is found at surgery. In retrospect, a fistula may be suggested by a history of recurrent episodes of jaundice with symptoms of cholangitis; however, these also occur without fistula formation.

The bile in these patients is usually infected and the patients may have obvious signs of infection, often with bacteraemia, at the time of surgery. Patients may also suffer chronically from a biliary 'blind loop' syndrome, particularly if there is a cholecystocolic fistula, when 'bile salt diarrhoea' may be a problem.[16]

Management

The standard approach to management of biliary fistulas in patients without accompanying gallstone ileus is primary repair of the fistula with cholecystectomy. During surgery the whole intestine should be palpated to detect intraluminal gallstones which might subsequently

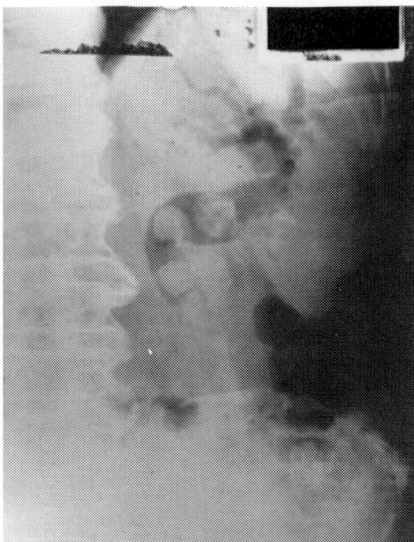

Fig. 11. In this illustration air is seen in the biliary tree on a straight abdominal radiograph. Large stones are also seen in the common bile duct.

obstruct the bowel; operative cholangiography should be performed to detect stones within the biliary tract. If a fistula is suspected preoperatively, the patient should have a full bowel preparation, with antibiotic cover, especially for biliocolic fistulas. If the fistula is found at operation, intravenous antibiotics should be given before it is divided.

In one study, 21 patients with biliary enteric fistulas involving the upper gastointestinal tract were treated conservatively because they had no symptoms related to the biliary tract, they were elderly, or they had other clinical problems; although some died of other causes, those who survived had no symptoms related to the fistula for periods of up to 6 years.[21] However, except in the most extenuating circumstances, conservative therapy is not appropriate for biliocolic fistulas, which should be repaired as soon possible after diagnosis because of the high risk of sepsis.

Gallstone ileus

Gallstone ileus is the term given to mechanical intestinal obstruction caused by a gallstone. Gallstones impact most commonly in the last 50 cm of the terminal ileum (in about 60 per cent of patients with ileus), which is the narrowest part of the small intestine; they obstruct the midileum in 25 per cent of patients and the jejunum in 10 per cent.[19] Less often there is obstruction of the duodenum, although this was the site in 10 per cent of the cases reported by Kasahara *et al.* (AmJSurg, 1980; 140:437), or of the colon or rectum (Anseline, PostgradMedJ, 1981; 57:62; Milsom, DisColRec, 1985; 28:367). Gallstone ileus is almost invariably due to the earlier development of a biliary enteric fistula, most commonly chole-cystoduodenal (although colonic obstruction by a gallstone is usually associated with a cholecystocolonic fistula). Rarely, the condition may occur even after the gallbladder has been removed (Lindsey, ArchSurg, 1975; 110:448) and has been described after the passage of a large stone following endoscopic sphincterotomy (Dunham, Endoscopy, 1981; 13:81). Obstructing gallstones usually measure

more than 2.5 cm in diameter (average 4.5 cm), as smaller stones are usually passed spontaneously in the stools.

When ileus occurs, symptoms of intestinal obstruction are more prominent than those of biliary tract disease.[19] Their exact nature depends on the site of obstruction, bilious vomiting occurring with high obstruction and faeculent vomiting with low obstruction; constipation is relatively common. Several days usually elapse before admission to hospital. Symptoms may be intermittent, suggesting that a stone may cause obstruction at several sites before reaching its final resting place. About one-half of the patients give a prior history suggesting gallbladder disease and in many there is a story of acute biliary tract pain or jaundice; approximately one-quarter have no such history.[19] Although gallstone ileus is a relatively uncommon cause of intestinal obstruction (about 2 to 3 per cent), it is responsible for about 20 per cent of cases of intestinal obstruction in those over 65 years of age, and the average age of patients with gallstone ileus in one series was about 67 years. It is more common in women. Because this condition occurs in older patients, associated diseases such as heart and lung problems and diabetes are common. If perforation of the bowel occurs, the clinical features are those of peritonitis.

The diagnosis may be suspected preoperatively on radiological grounds if, in addition to features of intestinal obstruction such as dilated small bowel loops, there is air in the biliary tree or an obvious change in the position of a gallstone, particularly if it is visible in the intestine. Barium or Gastrografin contrast films may show a biliary enteric fistula, dilatation of the sphincter of Oddi, or a gallstone lodged in the upper small intestine; with high obstruction the gallstone may also be seen by endoscopy. Gallstone ileus should be suspected in all cases of intestinal obstruction in the older age group, especially if there is a history suggesting biliary tract disease. Liver function tests are abnormal in only 20 to 30 per cent of the patients. The accuracy of preoperative diagnosis varies greatly in reported series (from 4 to 88 per cent); it is usually about 40 per cent (van Hillo, Surgery, 1987; 101:273).

Management

In the management of intestinal obstruction due to a gallstone, relief of the obstruction is the first concern, after correction of dehydration and proper preoperative preparation; correction of the biliary fistula is secondary. The stone should be mobilized and removed through an antemesenteric enterotomy, and there should be a thorough search for other stones within the intestinal lumen, as multiple stones are common and may cause recurrent ileus. If there is a perforation at the site of obstruction, or if the bowel wall is not viable, the affected part of the gut should be resected and end-to-end anastomosis performed.

Although some advocate repair of the associated biliary fistula at the first operation (in those considered fit enough for the procedure), most believe that it should be done later.[16] It is necessary to repair the fistula because ileus recurs in a small number of patients (2 to 13 per cent), there is a high incidence of cholangitis, particularly with biliocolic fistulas, and there is an increased risk of carcinoma of the gallbladder.

The average mortality due to gallstone ileus is around 20 per cent, but in some series the mortality has been between 5 and 10 per cent.[16]

Rare biliary fistulas related to gallstones

A bronchobiliary fistula due to gallstone disease is rare. It usually occurs in those who have had many previous upper abdominal operations, usually a cholecystectomy and repeated common duct operations (Boyd, AnnThorSurg, 1977; 24:481). It may also occur as a result of abscesses of the liver or gallbladder, particularly if the gallbladder lies in an anomalous suprahepatic position (Allison, PostgradMedJ, 1987; 63:291).

In one patient, a gallstone eroded through the wall of the left hepatic duct into the portal vein, causing rapid death due to bilaemia (Antebi, AnnSurg, 1973; 177:274).

Spontaneous external biliary fistulas that were once common are now very rare. They result from the formation of adhesions between an inflamed gallbladder and the abdominal wall, with subsequent fistula formation and expulsion of the gallbladder contents, including stones, through the hole in the skin. The external perforation is usually in the right upper quadrant, but may appear at other sites. The condition is almost invariably the result of neglected cholecystitis (Sanowski, AmJGastr, 1978; 70:649).

Haemobilia[22]

Major haemobilia due to any cause is rare, and gallstones account for only about 10 per cent of the cases; most are due to trauma (accidental or iatrogenic). Major haemobilia presents as melaena (90 per cent), haematemesis (60 per cent), biliary pain (70 per cent), and/or jaundice (60 per cent). Haemobilia is rarely considered as a cause of gastrointestinal bleeding unless endoscopy reveals bleeding from the ampulla. On ultrasound examination, clots in the biliary tree give less distinct shadows than stones and the findings are often interpreted as being due to gravel. Cholangiography may reveal filling defects due to clots, which can usually be distinguished from stones. If bleeding continues, the site of haemorrhage can be detected by selective arteriography, or by scintiphotography using labelled red cells or $^{99}Tc^m$-albumin (Miskowiak, ActaChirScand, 1979; 145:125).

Although overt haemobilia due to gallstones is uncommon, small amounts of blood are lost from the gallbladder and common duct in many patients with cholelithiasis; this can only be demonstrated by chemical testing of the stool for blood. Major haemobilia due to stones usually occurs with erosion of the cystic artery, during the formation of a fistula into another organ, or when there is haemorrhagic cholecystitis (Broderick, PostgradMedJ, 1981; 57:396). Major haemobilia may not stop spontaneously, presumably due to the local presence of bile which interferes with coagulation (Sandblom, AnnSurg, 1976; 184:679); fatal haemorrhage can occur.

Most of the blood entering the biliary tree passes into the intestine, but clots do form and it has been claimed that those in the gallbladder rarely may be transformed into stones, which may be either calcified or pigment and cholesterol in nature (Olsen, Surgery, 1982; 92:733; Luzuy, Surgery, 1987; 102:886).

Intrahepatic gallstones

Intrahepatic gallstones are defined as stones found in any of the bile ducts proximal to the junction of the left and right hepatic ducts, even if the junction of the ducts is outside the liver. Stones may also

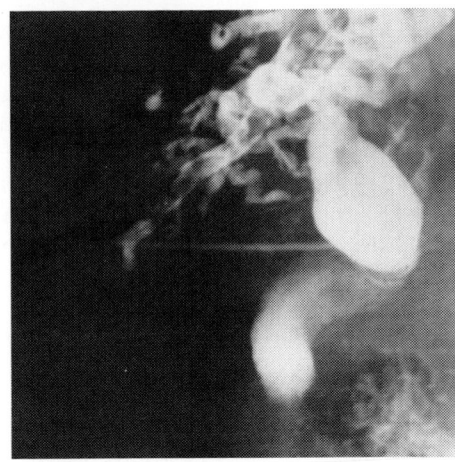

Fig. 12. Percutaneous cholangiography shows intrahepatic gallstones.

be present in the common hepatic duct and/or the common bile duct if they migrated from intrahepatic ducts, or if intrahepatic stone formation was secondary to the presence of stones in the extrahepatic ducts. Intrahepatic stones have been classified on the basis of the location of stones and on the presence or absence of duct stenosis and/or dilatation (Nakayama, WorldJSurg, 1982; 6:802).

Intrahepatic gallstones are common in the Far East where they constitute about 4 to 50 per cent of cases of cholelithiasis, depending on the country.[23] There they are thought to be related to infestation with the parasites *Clonorchis sinensis* and *Ascaris lumbricoides*, which can cause stricture formation and resulting stasis and infection. In Western countries, intrahepatic gallstones tend to be associated with Caroli's syndrome, strictures, tumours, and other ductal abnormalities causing biliary stasis and infection. Bacteria are found in the bile in almost 100 per cent of patients with intrahepatic stones.[24]

Intrahepatic stones are usually dark brown, soft, and friable. The vast majority are calcium bilirubinate stones which result from precipitation of water-insoluble unconjugated bilirubin; this is thought to be released from the bilirubin glucuronides of bile by the action of β-glucuronidase present in biliary bacteria (including *Escherichia coli*, *Clostridium* spp., and *Bacteroides* spp.). Glucaro-1,4-lactone, produced in the liver from glucuronic acid, has a powerful inhibitory effect on β-glucuronidase in bile and may help to limit the production of unconjugated bilirubin. Hepatic formation of glucaro-1,4-lactone seems to be reduced in subjects on a low fat, low protein diet, and this may contribute to intrahepatic stone formation.[1]

Patients with intrahepatic stones experience few symptoms if bile flow is not disturbed and if there is no exacerbation of infection. The most common initial symptom is pain in the right upper quadrant or upper abdomen, followed by jaundice and fever (which may also be presenting features). Lethargy, nausea, and vomiting may also occur, as in other forms of cholelithiasis. If the common bile duct becomes blocked, due either to migration of an intrahepatic stone or to an associated extrahepatic stone, acute obstructive cholangitis is likely to develop; this requires urgent decompression of the obstructed biliary tree, preferably using endoscopic cannulation of the ducts.

In 80 per cent of patients with intrahepatic stones, one or more liver function tests are abnormal. The condition may be detected by ultrasound in about 75 per cent of cases, but when intrahepatic gallstones are suspected the best diagnostic technique is percutaneous cholangiography (Fig. 12), which gives a diagnosis in 97 per cent, compared with 87 per cent with ERCP and 81 per cent by CT scanning.[23] In about 20 per cent of cases the diagnosis is first made at laparotomy; intraoperative cholangiography and ultrasound are then useful for delineating the extent and nature of the disease.

Management of intrahepatic gallstones

The management of intrahepatic gallstones is very difficult and patients should be referred to a specialist hepatobiliary unit. Treatment should be directed primarily at the removal of stones and the relief of biliary obstruction, which may be contributing to the formation of stones. There is, as yet, no satisfactory method for dissolving intrahepatic pigment stones *in vivo*; endoscopic sphincterotomy is not effective and it is extremely difficult to remove these stones by the peroral endoscopic route.

For localized disease, hepatic lobectomy may offer a chance of cure. Success is reported with choledochofiberoscopy, either through a sinus tract established after percutaneous biliary drainage or postoperatively via a T-tube or T-tube tract. Several techniques (such as drills and forceps) can be employed to remove stones or to crush them before removal of the fragments, and cutting instruments can be used to cut narrowed ducts. Laser irradiation via a choledochoscope has been employed to break up the stones.[25] Direct surgical approaches are also used, including lithotomy via an extended choledochotomy with saline washing of the ducts, and scooping or digital evacuation of stones, which is followed by sphincteroplasty or choledochoenterostomy.[26]

It is suggested that patients with intrahepatic stones should be given a high protein, high fat diet in order to enhance the hepatic formation of glucaro-1,4-lactone. One of the most crucial aspects of the management of these patients is the rapid treatment of overt cholangitis (see Chapter 23.5).

References

1. Maki T, Matsushiro T, and Suzuki N. Pathogenesis of the calcium bilirubinate stone. In Okuda K, Nakayama F, and Wong J, eds. *Intrahepatic calculi*. New York: Alan R Liss, Inc., 1984: 81–90.
2. GREPCO (Rome Group for the Epidemiology and Prevention of Cholelithiasis). Prevalence of gallstone disease in an Italian adult female population. *American Journal of Epidemiology*, 1984; **119**: 796–805.
3. Barbara L, *et al.* A population study on the prevalence of gallstone disease. The Sirmione study. *Hepatology*, 1987; **7**: 913–17.
4. Capocaccia L, Ricci G, Angelico F, Angelico M, and Attili AF, eds. *Epidemiology and prevention of gallstone disease*. Lancaster: MTP Press, 1985.
5. Heaton K. Clues from epidemiology. In Northfield T, Jazrawi R, and Zentler-Munro P, eds. *Bile acids in health and disease*. London: Kluwer Academic, 1988: 159–69.
6. GREPCO (Rome Group for the Epidemiology and Prevention of Cholelithiasis). The epidemiology of gallstone disease in Rome, Italy. Part 1: Prevalence data in men; Part 2: Factors associated with the disease. *Hepatology*, 1988; **8**: 904–6; 907–13.
7. Heuman DM, Moore EW, and Vlahcevic ZR. Pathogenesis and dissolution of gallstones. In Zakim D and Boyer TD, eds. *Hepatology: A textbook of liver disease*. Philadelphia: WB Saunders, 1990: 1480–516.
8. Lee DW, *et al.* Effect of dietary cholesterol on biliary lipids in women with and without gallstones. In Paumgartner G, Stiehl A, and Gerok W, eds. *Bile acids and cholesterol in health and disease*. Lancaster: MTP Press, 1983: 237–8.
9. Greiner L, Munks C, Heil W, and Jakobeit C. Gallbladder stone fragments in feces after biliary extracorporeal shock-wave lithotripsy. *Gastroenterology*, 1990; **98**: 1620–4.
10. Thistle JL, *et al.* Dissolution of cholesterol gallbladder stones by methyl *tert*-butyl ether administered by percutaneous transhepatic catheter. *New England Journal of Medicine*, 1989; **320**: 633–9.
11. Podda M, Zuin M, Battezzati PM, Ghezzi C, De Fazio C, and Dioguardi ML. Efficacy and safety of a combination of chenodeoxycholic acid and ursodeoxycholic acid for gallstone dissolution: a comparison with ursodeoxycholic acid alone. *Gastroenterology*, 1989; **96**: 222–9.
12. Sackmann M, *et al.* Shock-wave lithotripsy of gallbladder stones. *New England Journal of Medicine*, 1988; **318**: 393–7.
13. Sauerbruch T, *et al.* Fragmentation of gallstones by extracorporeal shock waves. *New England Journal of Medicine*, 1986; **314**: 818–22.
14. Darzi A, Monson JRT, O'Morain C, Tanner WA, and Keane FBV. Extension of selection criteria for extracorporeal shock wave lithotripsy for gallstones. *British Medical Journal*, 1989; **299**: 302–3.
15. Miller FJ and Rose SC. Percutaneous rotational contact lithotripsy. In *Abstracts of Second International Meeting on Pathochemistry, Pathophysiology and Pathomechanics of the Biliary System*. Bologna, Italy, March 1990: 104.
16. Morrissey KP and McSherry CK. Internal biliary fistula and gallstone ileus. In Blumgart LH, ed. *Surgery of the liver and biliary tract*. Edinburgh: Churchill Livingstone, 1988: 777–89.
17. Imrie CW. Gallstone acute pancreatitis. In Blumgart LH, ed. *Surgery of the liver and biliary tract*. Edinburgh: Churchill Livingstone, 1988: 551–7.
18. Acosta JM and Ledesma CL. Gallstone migration as a cause of acute pancreatitis. *New England Journal of Medicine*, 1974; **290**: 484–7.
19. Glenn F, Reed C, and Grafe WR. Biliary enteric fistula. *Surgery, Gynaecology and Obstetrics*, 1981; **153**: 527–31.
20. Patrassi N, Basoli A, Loriga P, Blandamura V, and Carboni M. Spontaneous internal biliary fistulas. *American Journal of Gastroenterology*, 1975; **64**: 181–6.
21. Zwemer FL, Coffin-Kwart VE, and Conway MJ. Biliary enteric fistulas. *American Journal of Surgery*, 1979; **138**: 301–4.
22. Sandblom P. Haemobilia. In Blumgart LH, ed. *Surgery of the liver and biliary tract*. Edinburgh: Churchill Livingstone, 1988: 1075–89.
23. Nakayama F. Intrahepatic stones. In Blumgart LH, ed. *Surgery of the Liver and Biliary Tract*. Edinburgh: Churchill Livingstone, 1988: 639–45.
24. Tabata M and Nakayama F. Bacteriology of hepatolithiasis. In Okuda K, Nakayama F, and Wong J, eds. *Intrahepatic calculi. Progress in clinical and biological research*, Vol. 152. New York: Allan R Liss, Inc., 1984: 163–74.
25. Kouzo T and Sato H. Endoscopic laser treatment of intrahepatic stones. In Okuda K, Nakayama F, and Wong J, eds. *Intrahepatic calculi. Progress in clinical and biological research*, Vol. 152. New York: Allan R Liss, Inc, 1984: 321–32.
26. Balasegaram M. Surgical treatment of hepatic calculi. In Okuda K, Nakayama F, and Wong J, eds. *Intrahepatic Calculi. Progress in Clinical and Biological Research*, Vol. 152. New York: Allan R Liss, Inc, 1984: 283–301.

23.5 Cholangitis and biliary tract infections

James S. Dooley

Definitions

'Bacterial cholangitis' is a clinical diagnosis based on symptoms and signs of systemic sepsis originating from the biliary tract. Bile, if available, would contain micro-organisms. This finding alone, however, without fever or septicaemia, would not denote cholangitis and is best termed bacterbilia. 'Biliary tract infection' lies in between and should include not only cholangitis but also other infections, for example cytomegalovirus, that damage the biliary system with and without symptoms.

Introduction

Two factors are necessary for the development of cholangitis, as defined clinically: first, the presence of micro-organisms in the bile; second, a rise in biliary pressure. Thus bacteria may be present in the bile, but the patient will remain asymptomatic until there is bile duct or cystic duct obstruction. This causes a rise in pressure within the bile duct or gallbladder, with regurgitation of infected bile into the circulation with resulting systemic features of septicaemia. Although antibiotic therapy is necessary, decompression of the obstructed biliary system is essential for successful treatment.

Epidemiology

Without bile duct or gallbladder pathology, biliary tract infection does not occur. Bile is usually sterile, although micro-organisms have been cultured from the gallbladder, common bile duct, and liver in normal individuals (Edlund, ActaChirScand, 1958; 116: 461). Whether these micro-organisms represent a genuine hepatobiliary flora or contamination at the time of sample collection is not clear (Nielsen, ScaJGastr, 1974; 9:671).

In patients with acute and chronic cholecystitis, gallbladder bile yields bacteria on culture in 30 to 50 per cent of patients (Flemma, AnnSurg, 1967; 166:563). Positive culture is more frequent in acute rather than chronic disease, and when the cystic duct is obstructed.

The incidence of positive culture from common bile–duct bile is greatest (75 to 100 per cent) when obstruction is caused by a calculus or a recurrent benign anastomotic biliary/enteric stricture (Jackaman, BrJSurg, 1980; 67:329). When obstruction is due to carcinoma of the pancreas, positive culture from bile is infrequent (0 to 10 per cent), unless there has been a previous surgical or radiological procedure. Biliary sepsis may occur after a diagnostic endoscopic retrograde cholangiopancreatogram (**ERCP**). Fatal *Pseudomonas* infection has been reported (Allen, Gastro, 1987; 92: 759). Biliary stents are universally associated with colonization of bile with bacteria, and cholangitis occurs frequently after stent blockage.

Micro-organisms

Most infections are caused by aerobic enteric organisms, in particular *Escherichia coli*, *Klebsiella* spp., and *Streptococcus faecalis* (*Enterococcus*) (Leung, GastrEnd, 1994; 40:716). Although previously unusual, *Pseudomonas aeruginosa* is now seen in patients with complicated biliary tract disease who have had multiple invasive procedures, either non-surgical or surgical. Anaerobes, particularly *Bacteroides* spp. and *Clostridium* spp., have been cultured from approximately 40 per cent of infected bile samples (England, JClinMicrobiol, 1977; 6:494). The isolation of anaerobes depends upon early inoculation of the correct culture medium with bile. They are cultured more often from patients who have had multiple biliary operations, or bile duct/bowel anastomoses (Bourgault, ArchIntMed, 1979; 139:1346). Mixed infections with aerobes are the rule.

Blood cultures are positive in about 8 per cent of patients with acute cholecystitis (Kuo, ScaJGastr, 1995; 30:272) and 20 to 30 per cent with cholangitis (Leung, GastrEnd, 1994; 40:716; Sung, JAntimicChemo, 1995; 35:855), and often yield bacteria which match those in bile (Siegman-Igra, ArchSurg, 1988; 123:366; Leung, GastrEnd, 1994; 40:716). This provides useful guidance in the choice of antibiotics before surgery or other biliary intervention.

Clinical features correlating with the presence of bacteria in bile include fever, a raised total count of white cells, neutrophilia, and a raised serum bilirubin concentration (Farinon, EurJSurg, 1993; 159: 531).

Viral, protozoal, and fungal infections of the biliary tract are unusual. Cytomegalovirus, cryptosporidia, and microsporidia are, however, well recognized as playing a role in the picture similar to sclerosing cholangitis seen in AIDS (French, ClinInfDis, 1995; 21: 852) and have been isolated from bile and biopsies from the biliary tract (Cello, AmJMed, 1989; 86:539). Similar opportunistic pathogens are found in AIDS patients with cholecystitis (French, ClinInfDis, 1995; 21:852).

Candida is occasionally detected in bile. Its importance is uncertain although its presence has been associated with a poor prognosis (Marsh, AnnSurg, 1983; 198:42).

Source of infection

Although not proven, the source of biliary micro-organisms is thought to be from the duodenum. The duodenum and jejunum contain only scant Gram-positive organisms under normal circumstances. However, when bile flow is interrupted, the small intestine is colonized by colonic-type organisms (Martini, ClinSci, 1957; 16:35), and these may then ascend into the biliary tree. The higher incidence of infection when gallstones are obstructing the biliary tree has been explained by intermittent biliary obstruction (ball-valve effect) (Scott, Lancet, 1967; ii:790).

An alternative but less convincing source of organisms is from portal venous blood. In animal studies, bacteria delivered to the liver in portal venous blood can be recovered in bile and are viable (Dineen, SGO, 1964; 119:1001). The problem with the portobiliary route as an explanation for biliary infection is that portal venous blood from patients without intestinal disease is usually sterile. Moreover, one would expect the incidence of infection in malignant obstruction to be similar to that due to gallstones, which it is not.

Radiological and endoscopic biliary procedures clearly introduce organisms into the biliary tract. At ERCP, micro-organisms derived from the endoscope or the duodenum may be transferred by the catheter into the bile duct. Diagnostic percutaneous cholangiography should not introduce organisms if done aseptically, but external or internal/external drainage catheters left *in situ* result in colonization of bile, the percentage of patients effected correlating with the duration of drainage. Sealed drainage systems have been designed to reduced this risk (Blenkhaarn, AmJSurg, 1984; 147:318).

Pathogenesis and pathology

As already explained, micro-organisms do not cause problems under normal circumstances in a bile duct in which the pressure is low (8 to 12 cmH$_2$O). An exception is in the immunocompromised individual, where apparently occult cytomegalovirus or cryptosporidia can cause inflammation and fibrosis. However, whether the cholangiographic changes of sclerosing cholangitis seen in these patients are due to infection alone, or to a combination of infection with the impaired bile drainage caused by papillary stenosis, is not known.

For clinical cholangitis to ensue, a high biliary pressure is needed. Experimental data show that regurgitation of bile containing organisms into the circulation occurs when the biliary pressure rises to between 15 and 20 cmH$_2$O (Huang, ArchSurg, 1969; 98:629). Bacteria enter the bloodstream by predominantly intracellular pathways (Raper, Surgery, 1989; 105:352), although lymphatic drainage may be involved. In addition, the phagocytic capacity of the reticuloendothelial cell system is impaired in patients with obstructive jaundice (Drivas, BMJ, 1976; i:1568), so that bacteria are not removed effectively.

Thus bile drainage has to be impaired before clinical features of sepsis appear. The correlation between biliary pressure, biliary micro-organisms and endotoxin, and the clinical picture is speculative, being virtually impossible to study. However, the most severe clinical picture, Reynold's pentad (pain, jaundice, fever, confusion, and hypotension), is usually found in the pathological situation of acute obstructive suppurative cholangitis (Reynolds, AnnSurg, 1959; 150:299)—pus in a completely obstructed high-pressure system. Renal failure also occurs with severe cholangitis and is another indication for urgent bile-duct decompression.

Acute cholecystitis usually occurs when the cystic duct is occluded by a stone. In acute acalculous cholecystitis, when the cystic duct is patent but gallbladder function impaired (see Chapter 23.5), the pathogenetic mechanism is not clear, but is probably multifactorial including increased bile viscosity, mucosal injury due to high bile-acid concentrations or bacterial endotoxin, and ischaemia (Frazee, MayoClinProc, 1989; 64:163).

The pathological end points of biliary tract infection are empyema of the gallbladder with rupture, and pyogenic liver abscess due to untreated biliary sepsis above the bile duct obstruction.

Clinical features and complications

Acute cholecystitis

Patients present with right upper quadrant pain and fever. Tenderness is present over the gallbladder, particularly during inspiration (Murphy's sign). Severe septicaemia is unusual. Imaging is important for diagnosis and ultrasound is the investigation of choice (Health and Policy Committee, American College of Physicians, AnnIntMed, 1988; 109:752). Apart from stones in the gallbladder, signs of acute inflammation include a thickened gallbladder wall (more than 5 mm), a positive sonographic Murphy's sign, pericholecystic fluid, subserosal oedema, intramural gas, or a sloughed mucosal membrane. Technetium-99m IDA scanning (for a non-functioning gallbladder) is a valuable alternative (Krishnamurthy, Hepato, 1989; 9:139). Treatment is usually conservative: nothing by mouth, analgesia, and antibiotics. Early cholecystectomy has become the more favoured policy for acute gallbladder disease.

Empyema of the gallbladder may occur. This may develop silently in the elderly (Thornton, Gut, 1983; 24:1183) so that a high index of suspicion is necessary. Gas gangrene of the gallbladder is a rare complication.

Acute cholangitis

There is a wide spectrum of presentation. Classically there is jaundice, pain, and fever (Charcot's triad) with calculous obstruction, although pain and/or jaundice may be absent. If untreated, Reynold's pentad (Charcot's triad plus confusion and hypotension) may develop. These additional features, together with renal failure, correlate with the pathological finding of acute obstructive suppurative cholangitis. Early decompression of the bile duct is mandatory to prevent further deterioration, including disseminated intravascular coagulopathy and death.

Pyogenic abscess

Cholangitis recognized late, or treated inappropriately, remains the major cause of pyogenic abscess (Yinnon, PostgradMedJ, 1994; 70:436). Other causes include intra-abdominal sepsis with portal pyaemia, penetrating injuries, direct spread from adjacent septic foci (e.g. perinephric abscess), or bacterial infection in an amoebic abscess or cyst.

The presentation of a cholangitis-related abscess is exactly that of acute cholangitis, the presence of the abscess or microabscesses only being discovered on scanning or cholangiography.

Alternatively, patients may present with the classic symptoms and signs of liver abscess (fever, rigors, right upper quadrant pain, enlarged tender liver). Once sepsis is controlled, biliary tract pathology should be ruled out if no other source of infection is obvious.

Congenital intrahepatic biliary dilatation (Caroli's syndrome)

This usually presents in childhood or early adult life with abdominal pain and septicaemia. Jaundice is mild or absent unless there is cholangitis. The liver may have histological features of congenital hepatic fibrosis, part of the spectrum of fibropolycystic disease. Choledochal and renal cysts may be present. Cholangiocarcinoma is a known complication.

Biochemical investigations will show features of cholestasis. Ultrasound and CT scanning will show the dilated segments of the biliary tree, although these may be interpreted as cysts or liver abscesses. Stones within the saccular dilatations alert one to the possibility of Caroli's syndrome. Cholangiography is the diagnostic test.

Recurrent pyogenic cholangitis (oriental cholangiohepatitis)

In this condition, prevalent in Hong Kong and South-East Asia, there are biliary strictures and intra- and extrahepatic brown pigment stones (Ti, BrJSurg, 1985; 72:556). A similar disorder has also been reported in Colombia (Cobo, ArchSurg, 1964; 89:936), Italy (Simi, AmJSurg, 1979; 137:317) and South Africa (Schulman, Radiol, 1987; 162:425). The aetiology is uncertain, but increased portal bacteraemia, nutritional factors, and biliary infestation have been implicated. The condition is characterized by recurrent attacks of fever, rigors, abdominal pain, and jaundice. If a patient from South-East Asia presents with recurrent cholangitis, this diagnosis should be considered.

Biochemical tests will show changes of cholestasis. Ultrasound (Chau, ClinRadiol, 1987; 38:79) and CT scanning (Chan, Radiol, 1989; 170:165) may demonstrate extra- and/or intrahepatic bile-duct dilatation, intraductal stones and air, segmental atrophy, and unilobular involvement.

AIDS-related cholangiopathy

Patients with the acquired immunodeficiency syndrome (**AIDS**) may develop abnormalities of the biliary tree (Cello, AmJMed, 1989; 86:539). They present with one or more of the following: abdominal pain in the right upper quadrant, fever, or raised alkaline phosphatase levels. Ultrasound or CT examination may show duct dilatation. ERCP abnormalities include papillary stenosis (in 60 per cent), diffuse cholangitis (67 per cent), extrahepatic cholangitis

(7 per cent), and intrahepatic cholangitis alone (27 per cent) (Ducreux, AIDS, 1995; 9:875). An AIDS-associated pathogen or malignancy may be identified on ampullary biopsy or bile examination. Recent 1- and 2-year survival rates are reported at 41 and 8 per cent, respectively (Ducreux, AIDS, 1995; 9:875).

Diagnosis and differential diagnosis

In a patient with fever of unknown aetiology, in whom the liver function tests are abnormal, ultrasound scanning is done to search for bile duct dilatation and/or evidence of a common duct stone. If clinical suspicion remains after negative non-invasive imaging, then ERCP clearly is indicated.

When there is good evidence for biliary tract disease and infection, there is an argument for performing ERCP without prior ultrasound or CT scanning as cholangiography is necessary whatever is shown on the non-invasive scan. Stones and primary sclerosing cholangitis may both cause sepsis without duct dilatation.

Differential diagnosis
Acute hepatitis

There may be fever early on, and right upper quadrant pain. However, the liver tests generally show a high level of aminotransferases. Although a high aminotransferase level may occur when there is acute bile-duct obstruction, for example with the passage of a stone, the elevated level usually lasts for only a day or two—in contrast to acute hepatitis when the high level is maintained for longer. Where raised levels of aminotransferase and biliary alkaline phosphatase coexist, as in cholestatic acute hepatitis, ERCP may be necessary to rule out biliary tract disease.

Cholestasis associated with septicaemia

Endotoxin inhibits canalicular organic anion transport (Roelofsen, AmJPhysiol, 1995; 269:G427). Sometimes a rise in alkaline phosphatase and bilirubin is seen associated with Gram-negative septicaemia, presumably due to the same mechanism. Thus abnormal liver function and fever may not indicate a primary hepatic problem. The overall clinical picture should indicate the source of sepsis, but occasionally liver biopsy and/or cholangiography are necessary to establish whether the liver abnormality is primary or secondary.

Drug jaundice

Some drugs may cause a 'pseudocholangitis'—jaundice, fever, and right upper quadrant pain (Keefe, DigDisSci, 1982; 27:701; Nissan, ArchSurg, 1996; 131:670). Again, ultrasound and CT scanning may be helpful in showing normal bile duct calibre. If a drug is suspected, then liver biopsy is indicated. If there is still any diagnostic dilemma, ERCP should be done to rule out biliary tract disease.

Primary sclerosing cholangitis (see Chapter 14.4)

Fever is an unusual presenting feature. More often patients present with malaise, weight loss, itching, and jaundice. There are an increasing number of asymptomatic patients with high alkaline phosphatase levels who are detected during screening at inflammatory bowel disease clinics. The diagnostic test is ERCP.

Necrotic liver tumour

Occasionally, primary liver cell carcinomas undergo necrosis and patients have fever as well as right upper quadrant pain. Liver function tests will show a cholestatic picture. Differentiation between a liver abscess and necrotic tumour may be difficult. Percutaneous needle aspiration, cytology, and/or biopsy may be necessary.

Primary reticuloses (Chapter 24.5)

Lymphoma and Hodgkin's disease may present with fever, often of intermittent Pel–Ebstein type, and evidence of hepatic disease. Other signs such as lymphadenopathy and splenomegaly may support this diagnosis. Imaging may show diffuse enlargement of the liver or focal nodularity, neither being specific. Histological examination of lymph node or liver biopsy should confirm the diagnosis.

Tropical diseases and amoebic abscess

See Section 13.

Investigations and other diagnostic considerations

When there is cholangitis, liver function tests will usually show high levels of alkaline phosphatase and γ-glutamyl transferase. Blood cultures should be taken as the micro-organism(s) responsible may then be identified (Siegman-Igra, ArchSurg, 1988; 12:366). Ultrasonography is indicated and correctly differentiates medical from surgical jaundice in 95 per cent of patients. The remaining 5 per cent have biliary tract disease without bile duct dilatation—for example, when a stone intermittently obstructs the bile duct. Although ultrasound scanning shows common bile-duct stones in only 30 to 50 per cent of patients (Laing, Radiol, 1983; 146:475; Tobin, BMJ, 1986; 293:16), the predictive accuracy of ultrasound for duct stones is greater if, in the absence of visible stones, bile duct dilatation or a technically unsuccessful examination are included as diagnostic criteria (Tobin, BMJ, 1986; 293:6).

Although ERCP is often necessary whatever the result of non-invasive imaging, this does not deny the value of ultrasound and CT scanning for initial screening. Ultrasound is less expensive than CT, does not expose the patient to radiation, but is more operator dependent. Magnetic resonance (MR) cholangiography can demonstrate bile duct stones and strictures but is likely to be reserved for difficult problems, or when a cholangiogram is needed but the patient is unfit for ERCP (Soto, Gastro, 1996; 110:589).

ERCP remains the method of choice to show the biliary system. The success rate is high (95 per cent). Stones may be removed by endoscopic sphincterotomy. If necessary, drainage by nasobiliary tube or endoprosthesis insertion is possible. Although percutaneous transhepatic cholangiography has a similar diagnostic success rate, this route carries greater risks, particularly for therapeutic procedures such as bile drainage.

Intravenous cholangiography provides poor images of the bile duct, and in most institutions has been superseded by ERCP.

Treatment[1]
General considerations

The treatment of cholangitis depends upon the correct choice of antibiotic, together with decompression and drainage of the biliary tree. Prior isolation of the micro-organism responsible is unusual. Thus the antibiotic chosen should be effective for common pathogens, taking into account the sensitivities of micro-organisms in the hospital concerned.

Antibiotics differ in their excretion into bile, their activity against micro-organisms in bile, and their pharmacokinetics in the patient with jaundice; although these are secondary issues, their importance should be appreciated. Thus, although cefotaxime is less well excreted into bile than mezlocillin, the biliary concentrations achieved by both exceed the mean inhibitory concentration of common pathogens to the same degree (approximately 200- to 300-fold) (Dooley, Gut, 1984; 25:988). Ureidopenicillins and cephalosporins are effective in killing biliary bacteria *in vivo* (Helm, Drugs-ExpClinRes, 1981; 7:349). Some antibiotics are ineffective in bile despite secretion. Tetracycline is very well excreted but has a reduced antimicrobial activity in bile (Helm, Infec, 1976; 4:94) and does not eradicate organisms (Helm, DrugsExpClinRes, 1981; 7: 349). This could be due partly to the alkaline pH of bile. In a completely obstructed biliary system, most antibiotics are undetectable in bile (Leung, GastrEnd, 1994; 40:716).[2] Ciprofloxacin is an exception, with biliary concentrations reaching 20 per cent of the serum level (as compared with bile/serum ratios of about four in unobstructed patients) (Leung, GastrEnd, 1994; 40:716). After relief of obstruction, biliary antibiotic concentrations return to the 'unobstructed' range over a few days (Dooley, Liver, 1983; 3:201). For several antibiotics the serum half-life is prolonged (mezlocillin greater than twofold) in patients with obstructive jaundice.

The important issues are the clinical circumstances of sepsis, the spectrum of the antibiotic, the likelihood of resistance, and decompression of the obstructed bile duct. The aim of antibiotic administration is primarily to prevent and treat systemic sepsis rather than to eradicate infection from the biliary system.

Prophylactic antibiotic for biliary procedures

Antibiotics are almost universally used before endoscopic, percutaneous, and surgical procedures on the biliary tract. Trials have established the benefit of prophylactic antibiotics before surgery in reducing postoperative sepsis (septicaemia, wound infection). There are data focusing on antibiotic use before endoscopic procedures (see below) but few for percutaneous cholangiography and bile drainage.

If the whole or part of the biliary system is obstructed, drainage is fundamental to the prevention of subsequent septic complications. Sepsis originating from an obstructed part of the biliary system which is undrained may be suppressed by a systemic antibiotic but is not usually eradicated.

Biliary surgery

The value of antibiotic prophylaxis is well established. A meta-analysis has shown a 9 per cent reduction in risk of wound infection with preoperative antibiotic (Meijer, BrJSurg, 1990; 77:283). A single dose given 1 h before the procedure is as effective as multiple-dose regimens (Strachan, BMJ, 1977; i:1254; Meijers, BrJSurg, 1990; 77:283). Third-generation cephalosporins have no advantage over first- or second-generation types. Cefazolin, cefoxitin, or cefuroxime are used.

ERCP

This is complicated by cholangitis in 1 to 19 per cent of patients, depending on the clinical status of the group studied (Bilbao, Gastro, 1976; 70:314; Huibregtse, Endoscopic Biliary and Pancreatic Drainage; Stuttgart: Thieme Verlag, 1988:121). The cholangitis may be fatal (Bilbao, Gastro, 1976; 70:314; Deviere, Endoscopy, 1990; 22:72).

Scrupulous attention to disinfection of endoscopes is necessary to reduce the risk of introduction of infection into the biliary tract. Death has been reported from introduction of *Pseudomonas aeruginosa* as a result of incomplete disinfection (Allen, Gastro, 1987; 92:759).

Risk factors have been identified which correlate with a higher frequency of bacterbilia and indicate the need for antibiotic prophylaxis. These include a history of cholangitis, raised leucocyte count, previous (diagnostic) ERCP, bile duct dilatation on scanning, fever within 3 days of the procedure, malignant stricture, and hilar stricture (Lai, AmJSurg, 1989; 157:121; Deviere, Endoscopy, 1990; 22:72; Motte, Gastro, 1991; 101:1374; Novello, Gastro, 1992; 103:1367).

For ERCP, the extent of benefit from prophylactic antibiotics is controversial. In the patient with no abnormality found at ERCP, there is general agreement that there is no, or minimal, risk of cholangitis and that antibiotic prophylaxis is not necessary. When bile duct obstruction, due to stone or stricture, is completely relieved at the time of ERCP, the risk of subsequent sepsis is low. Where, however, the bile duct is not drained, or only partially drained, the risk of cholangitis is high (Motte, Gastro, 1991; 101:1374). The explanation for the difference in outcome between studies is almost certainly the inclusion of all of these clinical categories, particularly the last two. Also, studies to date have only investigated the use of antibiotic prophylaxis given before the procedure; none have studied patients given antibiotics after ERCP when it is known whether or not the bile duct has been decompressed.

Bacteraemia alone is not infrequent after ERCP, is abolished by prior antibiotic, and is not necessarily followed by clinical sepsis. Recent trials of antibiotics in the prevention of clinical sepsis have been conflicting. Piperacillin (4 g intravenously) given 30 min before (but not after) ERCP did not significantly reduce cholangitis compared with placebo (4.4 and 6.0 per cent, respectively) (van der Hazel, AnnIntMed, 1996; 125:442). Piperacillin given before as well as after ERCP, until complete drainage was achieved (with one or more ERCP), for a maximum of 7 days, was beneficial with 'clinical failure' (fever or sign of cholangitis or sepsis, during treatment and 48 h after) in only 6 per cent of 34 patients compared with 29 per cent of 34 patients treated with placebo (Deviere, Gastro, 1993; 104:A359). This positive result probably reflects a different patient population as well as antibiotic protocol.

No cholangitis was observed in a group of 50 patients given 2 g of cefotaxime intravenously before ERCP, compared with 8 per cent

(4 of 50 patients) in the placebo group (Niederau, GastrEnd, 1994; 40:533). Prophylaxis with cefotaxime was statistically superior to placebo when the frequency of both bacteraemia and clinical sepsis were combined. With pre- and post-ERCP ciprofloxacin (orally) the low incidence of subsequent cholangitis (1 in 100) was similar to that seen with cefuroxime (intravenous) in a randomized trial (Mehal, EurJGastroHepatol, 1995; 7:641). The ciprofloxacin protocol was less expensive.

In a comparison of pre-ERCP intravenous ticarcillin/clavulinic acid with or without 3 subsequent days of oral amoxycillin/clavulinic acid, the group with post-ERCP antibiotic therapy had a lower rate of 'sepsis' (3 compared with 10 per cent) (Smith, JGastHepatol, 1996; 11:938).

In summary, where biliary tract pathology is expected, the present data support pre-ERCP antibiotic followed by further antibiotic administration for a short period (as yet undetermined) or until bile drainage is complete. If no prophylactic antibiotic is given, but pathology is found at ERCP and drainage is incomplete, then antibiotic should be started. Unless a strict protocol can be established (more difficult when referrals come from many sources) some units will continue to give all patients prophylaxis—and risk the rare but troublesome allergic and other side-effects.

On the basis of current data, there is no one antibiotic regimen that is clearly superior. The antibiotic chosen should cover the likely micro-organisms indicated earlier. Piperacillin, penicillin/clavulinic acid combinations, cephalosporins (e.g. cefuroxime), and fluoroquinolones (e.g. ciprofloxacin) seem effective. Knowledge of the microbiological sensitivities within a hospital is important. In one study imipenem and ciprofloxacin had the highest antimicrobial activities against the micro-organisms isolated (Leung, GastrEnd, 1994; 40:716). However, it should be recognized that adoption of a particular antibiotic policy will change the sensitivities over time (Mohandas, GastrEnd, 1996; 43:175).

Percutaneous cholangiography

Antibiotic prophylaxis is generally used before percutaneous cholangiography, although there are no trial data for this situation. Similarly, prophylaxis is often recommended before T-tube cholangiography. A recent study has questioned this (Chijiiwa, AmJSurg, 1995; 170:356). The volume and speed of injection of contrast are likely to relate to the risk of systemic sepsis; radiologists should be aware of this, and should avoid excess pressure during opacification of the bile duct.

Treatment of acute bacterial cholangitis

Bile duct obstruction, complete or partial, is virtually always present. The exception, ascending sepsis from an intestinal Roux loop through a surgical anastomosis, is very rare and difficult to manage (Matthews, Arch Surg, 1993; 128:269).

Management of acute bacterial cholangitis depends upon appropriate antibiotic treatment followed by biliary decompression, at an interval chosen first according to the severity of sepsis, and second the organization of the ERCP sessions. The patient with acute obstructive suppurative cholangitis (pus under pressure in a completely obstructed bile duct) needs immediate therapy with antibiotics (usually in combination), general supportive measures and resuscitation, and emergency drainage, usually by ERCP. Less severe cholangitis needs urgent antibiotic administration followed by elective ERCP.

At ERCP the ampulla is usually easy to catheterize, although a stone impacted at the lower end of the common bile duct may cause difficulty. If coagulation is normal, the ampulla accessible, and extraction of the stone seems feasible, then sphincterotomy with stone removal should be performed. If the coagulation status precludes sphincterotomy (platelets less than 70×10^9/l; prothrombin greater than 3-s prolongation), if the stone cannot be removed, or if there is a biliary stricture, then a nasobiliary drain should be inserted. Some operators insert an endoprosthesis as an alternative but, in the absence of trial data, a nasobiliary drain through which bile drainage can be demonstrated is preferable.

If ERCP fails or is not possible, then percutaneous transhepatic drainage is done. This is a second choice of treatment because there is likely to be an unavoidable escape of infected bile into the circulation at the time of the procedure.

It should be emphasized that, whichever procedure is done, injection of the biliary tree should be kept to a minimum to avoid increasing the pressure within the system.

Surgery can be used to relieve biliary obstruction, but in the presence of severe sepsis the morbidity and mortality are higher than those reported with non-surgical approaches.

A randomized study in patients with acute cholangitis showed that emergency endoscopic bile drainage is significantly safer (mortality 10 per cent, morbidity 34 per cent) than surgical drainage (mortality 33 per cent, morbidity 66 per cent) (Lai, NEJM, 1992; 326:1582).

In acute cholangitis, studies have not shown one antibiotic regimen to be superior to all others. The spectrum should cover *E. coli* and *Klebsiella* spp. The usual satisfactory response to cephalosporins argues against the necessity to use an antibiotic that is effective against *Streptococcus faecalis* (*Enterococcus*). *Pseudomonas* spp. are an unusual primary isolate, often occurring after previous biliary intervention (e.g. stenting). Anaerobes (*Bacteroides* and *Clostridium* spp.) may be present, and metronidazole should be added in severe cholangitis.

In the patient with acute cholangitis of mild to moderate severity (no hypotension, confusion, or renal dysfunction), a single antibiotic is usually used. The choice of appropriate agents is wide, including ampicillin, amoxycillin, mezlocillin, piperacillin, second-generation cephalosporins, and ciprofloxacin. Because of the concern over renal toxicity (Desai, AmJMed, 1988; 85:47; Gerecht, ArchIntMed, 1989; 149:1279) aminoglycosides are usually held in reserve for more severe cholangitis. If cover for anaerobes is thought necessary, metronidazole may be added.

Piperacillin is as effective as the combination of ampicillin with tobramycin (Thompson, SGO, 1990; 171:275; Muller, SGO, 1987; 165:285). Second-generation cephalosporins have not been fully evaluated for acute cholangitis. Data on cefoperazone (third generation), which has activity against *Pseudomonas* spp., compared with ampicillin plus tobramycin is conflicting (Muller, SGO, 1987; 165:285; Bergeron, AntimicrobAgentsChemother, 1988; 32:1231). In a randomized study, ciprofloxacin was as effective for acute cholangitis as the combination of ceftazidime, ampicillin, and metronidazole (all give intravenously) (Sung, JAntimicChemo, 1995; 35: 855). In all patients, blood cultures are essential before an antibiotic is given, as are bile cultures at the time of biliary decompression, to

redirect therapy if resolution of sepsis is slower than expected. Incomplete biliary decompression should be considered as an alternative explanation.

In the patient with the clinical features of acute obstructive suppurative cholangitis (jaundice, fever, pain, confusion, hypotension), a more aggressive approach is appropriate. An aminoglycoside may be added together with metronidazole to the basic Gram-negative cover. Emergency biliary decompression is mandatory.

Recurrent bacterial cholangitis where better bile drainage cannot be achieved

This occurs in the unusual patient with partial biliary obstruction, often a recurrent anastomotic stricture which cannot be improved upon by surgical operation or non-surgical techniques (e.g. balloon dilatation). Recurrent cholangitis of a mild degree can be troublesome. If better drainage cannot be achieved, then the patient, usually ambulant at home, should be given a course of oral antibiotics. There are no comparative data to guide the choice, which lies between ampicillin/amoxycillin (with or without a β-lactamase inhibitor), cephalosporin, cotrimoxazole, and ciprofloxacin. A single antibiotic or rotating antibiotics may be successful (van den Hazel, EurJClinMicrob, 1994; 13:662). Since no treatment will sterilize the bile, rotating antibiotics is theoretically more appropriate.

Pyogenic abscess (see Chapter 13.1.1)

If there is underlying biliary pathology, treatment is as for cholangitis—antibiotic therapy and drainage of the biliary system with removal of the stone(s) if present. Antibiotic therapy should, however, be continued for longer than for cholangitis alone, oral treatment being used for approximately 4 weeks after initial parenteral administration. Patients presenting primarily with symptoms and signs of liver abscess, in whom scanning (ultrasound or CT) shows a liver abscess, should be treated with percutaneous aspiration or drainage under scanning control, and antibiotics (Stenson, ArchIntMed, 1983; 143:126). In the absence of another obvious cause, cholangiography should be done to rule out any underlying biliary tract pathology.

Recurrent pyogenic cholangitis

Recurrent pyogenic cholangitis requires intensive treatment with antibiotics and, if this measure alone fails, early drainage of the biliary system is necessary (Choi, BrJSurg, 1989; 76:213). Interventional radiological techniques are valuable (Kalan, AJR, 1985; 145:809), as well as endoscopic sphincterotomy. Surgical drainage operations and local resection may be necessary (Kashi, AnnRCSurg, 1989; 71:387).

Caroli's syndrome

Recurrent cholangitis may be extremely resistant to antibiotics (Summerfield, JHepatol, 1986; 2:141). If stones are shown in the common duct then endoscopic sphincterotomy may allow their retrieval. Despite patency of the common duct, however, recurrent sepsis may still occur because of stones and obstruction within the dilatations of the intrahepatic biliary system. Surgical resection of an affected area may be possible (Nagasue, AnnSurg, 1984; 200: 718).

Primary sclerosing cholangitis

In the case of diffuse disease, antibiotics alone are all that is available. If there is a dominant common-duct or hilar stricture, it should be treated either by non-surgical balloon dilatation (Lee, Hepatol, 1995; 21:661), endoprosthesis insertion, or by surgical operation, although the last should be avoided in patients who are likely to require transplantation. For recurrent cholangitis in the ambulant patient with primary sclerosing cholangitis without a remediable stricture, oral antibiotics should be prescribed along the lines discussed under 'antibiotic choice' above. In severe cholangitis, admission to hospital and administration of parenteral antibiotics will be necessary.

Benign biliary strictures

Recurrent cholangitis usually denotes a partial stricture requiring therapy. Non-surgical stenting and balloon dilatation have a similar outcome with a symptom-free interval of approximately 1 year (Gillams, Gut, 1989; 30:A1458). If sufficient biliary system remains accessible, then surgery in a specialist unit should be considered.

For low-grade recurrent cholangitis in ambulant patients, oral antibiotics usually abort or shorten the attack. There is unlikely to be culture-proven identification of the micro-organism responsible. Cotrimoxazole, ampicillin, cephalosporins, and ciprofloxacin are useful antibiotics.

Sepsis above a hilar cholangiocarcinoma

Sepsis above a hilar cholangiocarcinoma *de novo* is unusual, and usually follows a diagnostic ERCP or intervention by the endoscopic or percutaneous route. If surgery is contemplated, it should be done after sepsis is controlled. If an endoprosthesis is in place, it should be replaced. Where individual intrahepatic duct segments are obstructed, the outcome is poor since drainage of all segments is not possible, and antibiotic therapy will only temporize. Long-term antibiotics are usually necessary.

Prognosis of acute cholangitis: predictive factors

The prognosis of acute obstructive cholangitis is poor unless the treatment is correct and prompt. In the wider clinical spectrum of cholangitis, attempts have been made to analyse risk factors for mortality so as to judge which patients should have antibiotics and elective therapy, and which need aggressive treatment and rigorous monitoring.

One such study using multivariate analysis identified acute renal failure, cholangitis associated with liver abscesses or cirrhosis, cholangitis secondary to a high malignant biliary stricture, percutaneous transhepatic cholangiography, female gender, and age as factors predicting mortality (Gigot, AnnSurg, 1989; 209:435). The clinical value of a scoring system based on such an analysis needs to be confirmed in a prospective study but should provide a guide to plan management.

References

1. van den Hazel S, Speelman P, Tytgat GNJ, Dankert J, and van Leeuwen DJ. Role of antibiotics in the treatment and prevention of acute and recurrent cholangitis. *Clinics in Infectious Diseases*, 1994; **19**: 279–86.
2. van Delden OM and van Leeuwen DJ. The relevance of biliary secretion and other features of antibiotics in biliary tract disease. In Tytgat GNJ and Huibregtse K, eds. *Bile and bile duct abnormalities*. Stuttgart: Thieme Verlag, 1989: 15–20.

The gallbladder and laparoscopic cholecystectomy

K. E. F. Hobbs

'The diseased gall bladder is one of the most frequent specimens submitted to the surgical pathology laboratory'.[1] Disease of the gallbladder has long been recognized and successful cholecystectomy was first performed in 1882 by Carl Langenbuch, Professor of Surgery in Berlin. It is now one of the commonest operations in general surgery and young surgeons in training are introduced to the techniques of cholecystectomy early in their careers.

Since 1989 the operation is increasingly being carried out laparoscopically, and with greater frequency than ever before. This is probably due more to the aesthetically pleasing high technology and television techniques used than to a greater need. Both the conventional and laparoscopic techniques are usually straight-forward and uncomplicated and so many unnecessary, and sometimes inappropriate, cholecystectomies are done. Unfortunately, when the surgeon is caught unawares by an unusual anatomical or pathological anomaly, or by lack of appropriate experience with the new technologies, the results for the patient may be disastrous.

In this chapter the pathology of non-malignant gallbladder disease will be reviewed together with the current approach to the problems produced.

Development

The embryology and normal anatomy of the gallbladder is reviewed in Section 1 but it is essential for surgeons and diagnosticians, especially interventional radiologists, to appreciate the anatomical anomalies which may produce diagnostic and therapeutic problems. The organ may be totally absent, be divided by a septum in a single organ, or exist as two (Fig. 1) or three separate gallbladders. It may be ectopic, intrahepatic, left sided, transverse, or retrodisplaced. It may be suspended on a mesentry—the so-called 'floating' gallbladder. The commonest variation of all is the presence of a 'Phrygian cap' (Fig. 2), which may have a similar aetiology to the congenital septum.

The cystic duct may be absent (Fig. 3(a)) or very long, and can join the rest of the biliary tract in a variety of ways (Fig. 3(b)). Usually it joins the common hepatic duct in the free edge of the lesser omentum or hepatoduodenal ligament to form the common bile duct. This junction may take place far distally, close to the choledochoduodenal junction, or more proximally, even occasionally joining with the right or left hepatic ducts. Accessory

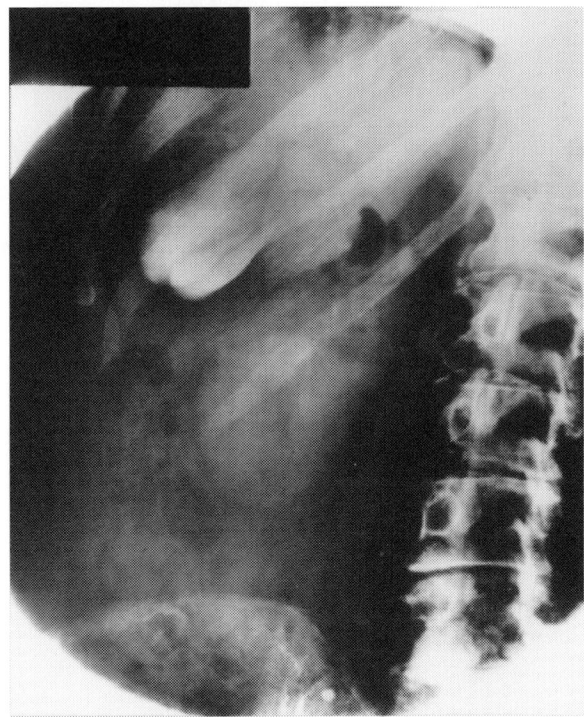

Fig. 1. Oral cholecystogram showing a double gallbladder (by courtesy of Dr R. Dick).

ducts occasionally enter the gallbladder from the right lobe of the liver.

The junction of the cystic and common hepatic ducts and the origin and course of the cystic artery can be related in different ways (Fig. 4). The artery itself is variable and can arise from any branch of the hepatic arterial supply, can be single or double, and can pass in front of or behind the biliary duct system. Sometimes the right hepatic artery is, deceptively, closely related to the gallbladder and appears to the operating surgeon to be the cystic artery. This can result in the inadvertent ligation of the vessel, although this does not produce serious problems.

It is important that these variations in normal anatomy are appreciated by the operating surgeon, to avoid any potentially catastrophic damage to the biliary system, and by the interventional radiologist when placing a catheter for hepatic embolization or

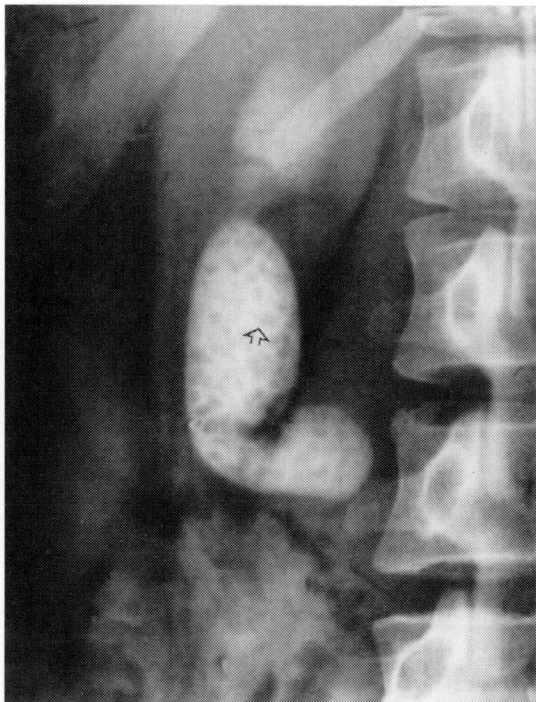

Fig. 2. Oral cholecystogram showing gallstones in a gallbladder with a 'Phrygian cap' (by courtesy of Dr R. Dick).

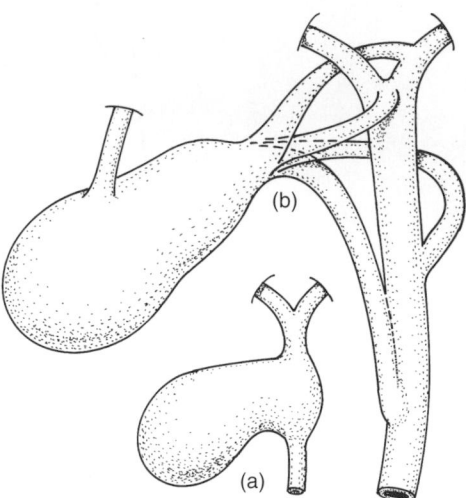

Fig. 3. (a) A drawing of the gallbladder with an absent cystic duct. (b) A composite drawing showing common variations of the anatomy of the cystic duct.

infusion chemotherapy, if infarction of the gallbladder or chemical cholecystitis is to be prevented (Rabinovitch, AnnSurg, 1958; 148: 161; Pietrafitta, JSurgOncol, 1986; 31:287; Korn, Surgery, 1988; 103:496).

The variations in anatomical structure may contribute to pathological problems. The 'floating' gallbladder, in which the organ is suspended by a mesentery, may undergo torsion (Gross, ArchSurg, 1936; 32:131) that can mimic acute cholecystitis. This was first recognized in 1898 (Wendel, AnnSurg, 1898; 27:199). A septate

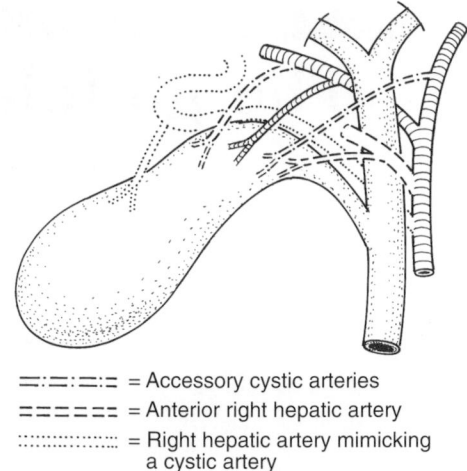

=:=:=:= = Accessory cystic arteries
====== = Anterior right hepatic artery
::::::::::::::: = Right hepatic artery mimicking a cystic artery

Fig. 4. A composite drawing showing common variations of the anatomy of the cystic artery (or arteries).

gallbladder and gallbladders with strictures or 'hourglass' deformities are not uncommon in surgical specimens or at autopsy (Deutch, PostgradMedJ, 1986; 62:453) and the presence of a septum can mimic a stone on cholecystography (Bova, AJR, 1983; 140:287). Total agenesis, although rare, has been reported and is associated with a high incidence of duct stones and biliary tract carcinoma (Bennion, ArchSurg, 1988; 123:257).

Pathology of gallbladder disease

Stones in the gallbladder are one of the most common diseases in the Western world with a prevalence of about 20 per cent in the adult population, women having a higher prevalence than men. They are associated with both acute and chronic inflammatory and obstructive processes and may be risk factors in the development of gallbladder cancer. However, the gallbladder may become inflamed in the absence of gallstones, and other pathological processes can also cause clinical problems.

Mechanisms of inflammation

The causes of acute inflammation of the gallbladder are probably multifactorial and are summarized in Fig. 5. Biliary stasis and changes in bile salt concentration have been observed, in animals, to be associated with changes in prostaglandin concentrations in the tissues. Prostaglandin E (the 'inflammatory' prostaglandin) is raised, and prostaglandin F (the 'anti-inflammatory' prostaglandin) is reduced in inflamed gallbladders (Kaminski, Hepatogast, 1987; 34: 70). These changes are associated with inflammation and resultant mucosal trauma. Mucosal trauma can also be produced by the presence of stones, or by ischaemia, and may release phospholipases that change bile lecithins into lysolecithins which in turn can increase the mucosal damage. As a result, inflammation and ischaemia are self-perpetuating and can lead to gangrene and perforation of the wall.

There is an increased risk of gallbladder disease in patients taking oestrogens, and in obesity. Both can contribute to the inflammatory processes. Oestrogens (Petitti, Gastro, 1988; 94:91) may increase the lithogenicity of bile, while obese patients (Petitti, AmJPrevMed,

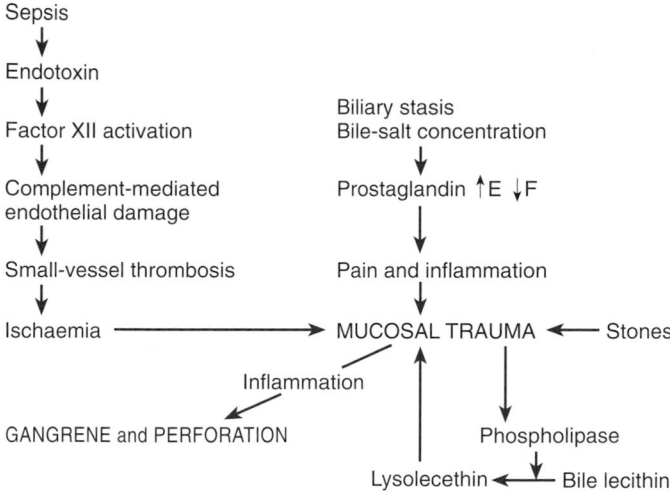

Fig. 5. Diagram to illustrate the interrelation between various factors which predispose to gallbladder inflammation.

1988; 4:327) have reduced gallbladder contractility. Furthermore, in an attempt to lose weight they often take a low-calorie, low-fat diet which may favour bile stasis and further increase the likelihood of stone formation (Marzio, DigDisSci, 1988; 33:4).

Biliary sludge, which is a 'gelation of gallbladder mucin with entrapment of "particulate matter" nucleated from bile', may be implicated in the formation of gallbladder stones (Carey, Gastro, 1988; 95:508) even though it can sometimes resolve spontaneously.

Acute calculous cholecystitis

This is probably the commonest type of acute cholecystitis. The development, presentation, and management of gallstones is reviewed elsewhere (Chapter 23.4). Patients with gallbladder stones are always at risk of developing acute inflammation and it is estimated that about 1 per cent of such patients develop this complication each year (Editorial, Lancet, 1990; 335:21).

Acute acalculous cholecystitis or 'necrotizing cholecystitis'

There are reports that between 6 and 17 per cent of all cases of acute cholecystitis develop in the absence of gallstones, and some evidence that this is increasing in frequency.[2] The diagnosis is often missed and is therefore associated with a high mortality, of up to 90 per cent in some series.

Fifty per cent of patients have no identifiable predisposing cause, while many are seen in intensive therapy units. The condition may follow recent surgery, multiple injuries, burns, recent childbirth, severe sepsis, or drug overdose. The reason for these associations is unknown but may be related to the increased production of bile pigment following multiple blood transfusions, an increase in bile viscosity as a result of dehydration, or an increase in bile stasis associated with parenteral nutrition,[3] assisted ventilation, and opiate therapy (Glenn, AnnSurg, 1979; 189:458).

Acalculous cholecystitis can occur in children in association with congenital duct narrowing, local inflammation, and pressure on the duct by nodes. It may occur in patients with systemic lupus erythematosus (Swanepoel, BMJ, 1983; 285:251) and has been seen in patients with AIDS associated with cryptosporidium and cytomegalovirus infection.[4] In these patients, biliary disease progresses after cholecystectomy and the prognosis is very poor.

A particularly virulent form known as emphysematous acalculous cholecystitis is rare; it results from infection with gas-forming organisms (Ruby, JAMA, 1983; 249:248). Bubbles may be seen rising from the fundus of the gallbladder on ultrasound, giving rise to the so-called 'champagne sign' (Nemcek, AJR, 1988; 150: 575). This has been reported after hepatic artery embolization in the treatment of hepatic tumours (Nakamura, CardvascIntRadiol, 1986; 9:152).

Chronic cholecystitis

This can occur with or without gallstones[2] and is the commonest pathological problem in patients with gallbladder disease. Histologically there is pronounced fibrosis and muscular hypertrophy of the wall. The mucosa is flat and atrophic, Rokitansky–Aschoff sinuses (epithelially lined diverticula) extend from the mucosa into the adventitia. There may be an infiltrate of a few inflammatory cells, lymphoid follicles, and granulomatous foreign-body giant cell reactions. Vessels often show endarteritis obliterans; dystrophic calcification may occur and the mucosa may demonstrate cholesterosis (the strawberry gallbladder).[5]

Less common causes of cholecystitis include salmonella and staphylococcal infections, and leptospirosis in children. Xanthogranulomatous cholecystitis is associated with chronic infection, usually in the presence of gallstones and with many histiocytes in the wall (Howard, AmSurg; 1991, 57:821). This condition is difficult to distinguish from carcinoma of the gallbladder macroscopically, and perioperative frozen section histology is indicated. The gallbladder should be removed totally, or in part if total removal is considered to be unsafe. The organ may also be affected in polyarteritis nodosa, Crohn's disease, and sclerosing cholangitis.[6]

Gallbladder disease in diabetes mellitus

Gallbladder stones and cholecystitis are probably more common in patients with diabetes mellitus, and there are many reports in the older literature suggesting that these patients are at greater risk of death during an attack of acute cholecystitis than non-diabetic patients. Early elective surgery has therefore been advocated (Ransohoff, AnnIntMed, 1987; 106:829; Reiss, DigSurg, 1987; 4:37). However this assumed ominous association is perhaps no longer valid as the management of these very sick patients has improved greatly in recent years, and the question of timing of surgery and the management of asymptomatic gallstones in diabetic patients must be reconsidered. Elective surgery is still strongly advised for symptomatic patients (Reiss, DigSurg, 1987; 4:37).

Gallbladder polyps and adenomas

Benign tumours are rare. Sometimes called 'hyperplastic cholecystoses' (Aguirre, AmJRoentRadTherNuclMed, 1969; 107:1), they can be classified as epithelial (adenomas), supporting tissue tumours (haemangiomas, lipomas, leiomyomas, and granular cell tumours), and benign pseudotumours, which include hyperplasia

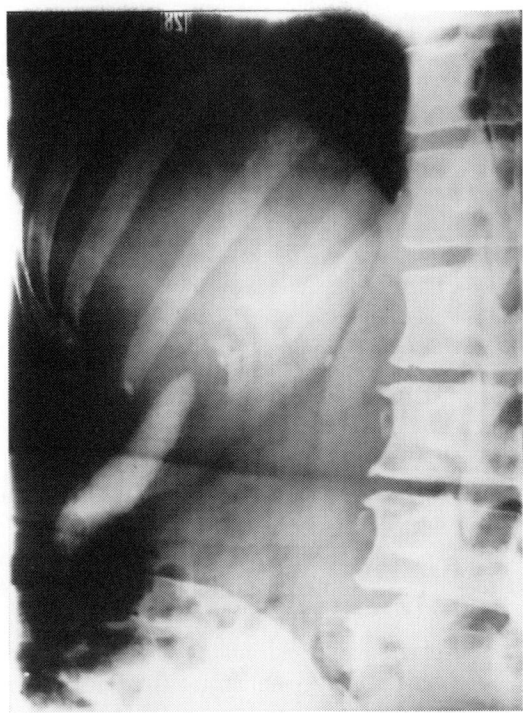

Fig. 6. Cholecystogram showing adenomyomatosis of the gallbladder wall: the diverticula in the wall are filled with contrast (by courtesy of Dr R. Dick).

(adenomatous and adenomyomatous), heterotopia (mucosa of gastric intestinal pancreatic and liver origin), polyps (inflammatory and cholesterol), and miscellaneous lesions (fibroxanthogranulomatous inflammation and parasitic infection) (Christensen, ArchPathol, 1970; 90:423). Although these are usually benign, malignant change may occur especially in larger ones (Kozuka, Cancer, 1984; 54: 2277; Mogilner, JPediatSurg, 1991; 26:223).

Adenomyomatosis of the gallbladder has a pathology that in many ways resembles that of diverticulosis of the colon and is due to hyperplasia of the tissues of the gallbladder wall with outpouching of the mucosa (Berk, Radiol, 1983; 146:593). It may give rise to symptoms which are suggestive of gallbladder disease. The characteristic finding on investigation is that diverticula within the thick wall of the gallbladder fill with contrast on cholecystography (Fig. 6). The condition is cured by cholecystectomy (Meguid, AmJSurg, 1984; 147:260).

In cholesterolosis, triglycerides and cholesterol esters are incorporated in macrophages in the gallbladder wall.[6] If these project into the lumen they produce the macroscopic change known as a 'strawberry gallbladder'. The condition does not respond to bile-acid therapy nor is it associated with cholesterol gallstones, supersaturation of the bile with cholesterol, hyperlipidaemia, obesity, or atherosclerosis (Berk, Radiol, 1983; 146:593).

Torsion, gangrene, and infarction

Torsion and gangrene are rare problems which present as an acute emergency (Schlinkert, MayoClinProc, 1984; 59:490) and they were mentioned earlier. Torsion may occur in gallbladders with a long mesentery and infarction may follow. On occasions infarction follows intra-arterial injection of embolic material, cytoxic drugs, or surgical ligation of the hepatic artery used in an attempt to treat liver tumours.

Trauma

Trauma to the gallbladder is rare because the organ is protected by the liver, kidney, and costal arch. It may occasionally be subjected to laceration following stabbing or abdominal blunt trauma; injury is commoner in males than females and the age of the patients is relatively young. The injury can be classifed as contusion, avulsion, or laceration (perforation). One-half of patients present with clinical signs or associated injuries which require laparotomy, the other half have a delayed diagnosis. Often at the time of laparotomy the biliary trauma is missed. Intraoperative recognition of biliary tract damage needs a high index of suspicion (Parks, BrJSurg, 1995; 82:1303). On occasions the gallbladder may suffer iatrogenic damage, being punctured inadvertently during attempts at liver biopsy.

Presentation of gallbladder disease
Acute

Patients with acute gallbladder disease present with symptoms and signs of an 'acute abdomen'. There is rapid onset of severe upper abdominal pain; it is usually in the midline initially, but may radiate to the right upper quadrant, shoulder tip, or right scapular region, because of shared sensory innervations. The skin over the shoulder tip and the central diaphragmatic peritoneum are both supplied by the fourth and fifth cervical nerves. Sensory stimuli arising as a result of inflammation of the latter (travelling up the phrenic nerve) are interpreted by the brain as arising from the former. The peritoneum over the more lateral parts of the right hemidiaphragm and the skin of the posterior chest wall also share a common sensory innervation, which explains pain referral to the shoulder blade area when the subphrenic peritoneum is irritated. The severe pain is associated with general gastrointestinal disturbances of nausea, vomiting, and anorexia. The patient has difficulty in finding a comfortable resting position and the pain may be exacerbated by deep breathing.

Clinically there are physical signs of right-sided peritoneal irritation with varying degrees of tenderness, guarding, and guarding on inspiration (Murphy's sign). The patient may be pyrexial and, especially in those cases of acalculous disease seen in the intensive care unit, may be very toxic. There may be mild jaundice if the inflammatory process extends to the common bile duct and impairs bile flow[7] (Edlind, ActaChirScand, 1983; 149:597; Fox, SGO, 1984; 159:13).

Chronic

The symptoms and signs of chronic cholecystitis can be vague and non-specific. Typically they include right upper quadrant abdominal pain or discomfort, often following a heavy meal. This pain may be referred through into the back in the region of the shoulder blade. Other less specific symptoms include feelings of bloating, distension, and excessive flatulence. Sometimes they consist of non-specific 'indigestion'. Often symptoms are present for many years and it is not unusual for patients to recognize, after a curative cholecystectomy, that they had been suffering for a considerable period of time without realizing they had organic disease.

Clinical signs are usually absent, although occasionally there may be some tenderness in the right upper quadrant, and a palpable gallbladder may be found if the cystic duct has become blocked by a stone and the gallbladder is full of mucus (a mucocele).

Investigation of gallbladder disease

All patients with suspected gallbladder disease should have some standard blood tests carried out to give a baseline, and to exclude other occult disease, especially chronic liver disease. In addition to haemoglobin and blood cell analyses these should include clotting studies, and liver function tests measuring bilirubin, alkaline phosphatase, aspartate and alanine transferases, and serum albumin. Patients presenting with symptoms and signs suggestive of acute cholecystitis should also have the serum amylase measured to exclude acute pancreatitis, which must be part of the differential diagnosis.

Normal results from these tests do not exclude gallbladder disease. Conversely, an inflamed gallbladder alone, in the absence of stones in the hepatic or common bile duct, may cause the alkaline phosphatase, bilirubin, serum amylase, and the white cell count to be raised.[7] In acute acalculous cholecystitis about 50 per cent of patients show a rise in bilirubin and 70 per cent a rise in the white cell count (Fox, SGO, 1984; 159:13).

All patients should have any abnormalities of blood clotting corrected before interventional investigations are undertaken. Clotting may be impaired if there is biliary tract obstruction as lack of bile may reduce absorption of fat-soluble vitamin K and so interfere with prothrombin synthesis. Furthermore, gallbladder disease may sometimes complicate occult chronic liver disease with impaired clotting.

Straight abdominal radiography

Straight radiography of the abdomen is usually not helpful in the management of patients with gallbladder disease as only 10 per cent of gallstones are radio-opaque (Fig. 7) and other pathological processes will not be seen. It may demonstrate pneumobilia if there is a communication between the biliary tract and the gut, following a previous surgical procedure or a spontaneous cholecystenteral fistula produced by a gallstone eroding through the wall of the gallbladder into the gut (Fig. 8).

Cholecystography

Until the advent of ultrasound examinations this was the standard method for investigating the gallbladder. However, it is notoriously inaccurate and is rarely used these days as the sole diagnostic test since false positive and false negative results are common. A gallbladder septum can mimic a stone (Bova, AJR, 1983; 140: 287) and, conversely, in histologically confirmed chronic acalculous disease, the preoperative cholecystogram may be normal.[7] At the Royal Free Hospital in London the number of oral cholecystograms requested has fallen from 512 in 1975 to 9 in 1995 (data supplied by Dr R. Dick, Department of Diagnostic Radiology). The most common indications for this investigation now are to assess gallbladder function when litholytic or lithotriptic treatments are being

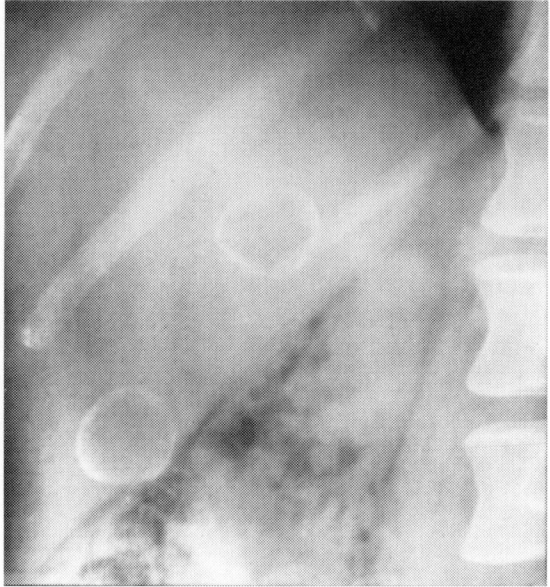

Fig. 7. Radio-opaque gallstones shown on a straight abdominal radiograph (by courtesy of Dr R. Dick).

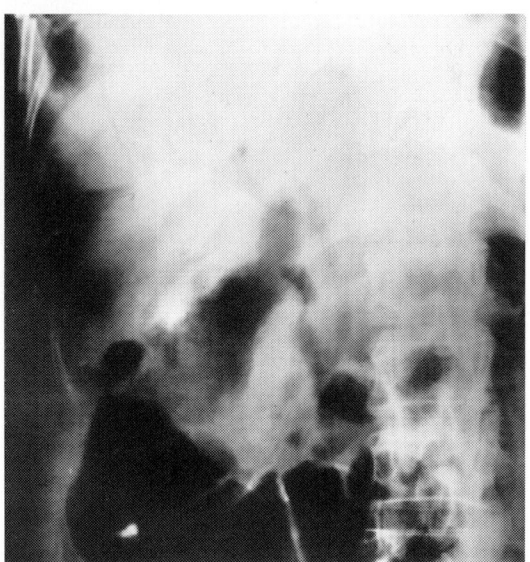

Fig. 8. Pneumobilia shown on a straight abdominal radiograph of a patient who has a choledocho-enteral anastomosis (by courtesy of Dr R. Dick).

considered or following an equivocal ultrasound scan. In this situation the findings on cholecystography may complement those of the ultrasound and lead to a definitive diagnosis.

Intravenous cholangiography

This investigation, too, is rarely used routinely in these days of radionuclide and ultrasound scans although, with the advent of laparoscopic cholecystectomy, it is being explored as a positive alternative to perioperative cholangiography or preoperative endoscopic retrograde cholangiopancreatography (**ERCP**) for demonstrating the biliary tree and the presence or absence of biliary tract stones. It seems to offer a cost-effective modality for biliary

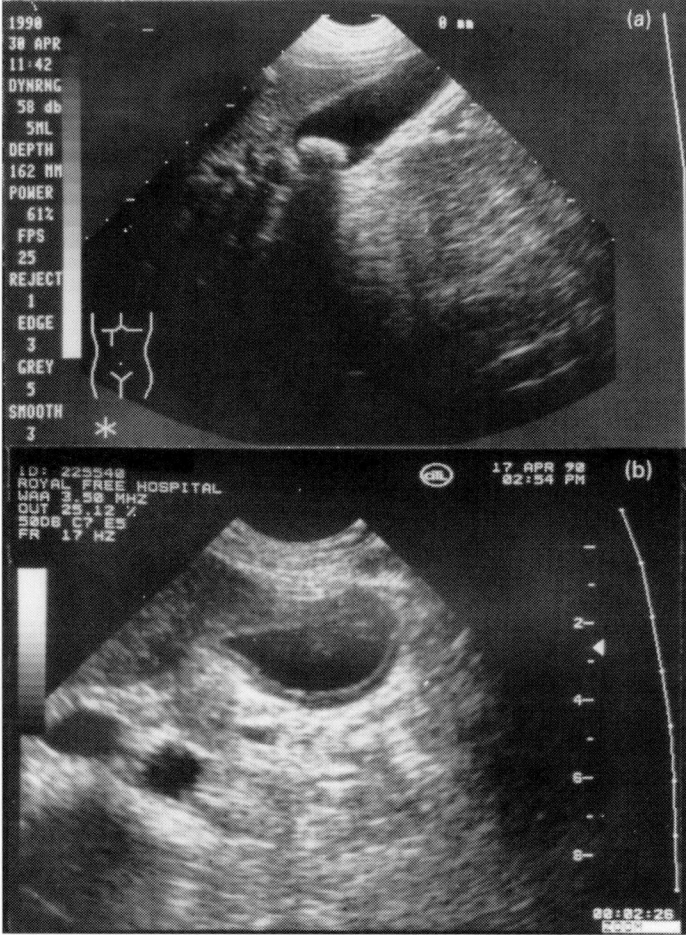

Fig. 9. (a) Ultrasound showing stones in a gallbladder. (b) Ultrasound scan showing the 'halo' of subserosal oedema (by courtesy of Dr L. Berger).

tract imaging (Bloom, BrJSurg, 1996; 83:755), but is associated with mild to moderate adverse reactions and is not as accurate as ultrasonography combined with biochemical liver function tests for this purpose (Thompson, BrJSurg, 1996, 83:724). When biliary tree imaging is indicated, it is best carried out by direct injection of radio-opaque contrast using either the percutaneous transhepatic or endoscopic retrograde techniques.

Ultrasound scan

This is perhaps the investigation of choice in patients with suspected gallbladder disease. However, it is operator dependent and it is therefore essential that the investigation is carried out at least under the supervision of an experienced ultrasonographer. It can demonstrate luminal stones (Fig. 9(a)), distension, thickening of the wall, gas in the wall in the rare condition of emphysematous acute cholecystitis (see above), the halo sign of subserosal oedema (Fig. 9(b)), and it may be possible in an acutely inflamed gallbladder to elicit an 'ultrasound Murphy's sign', where marked tenderness is elicited by pressure with the probe over the inflamed organ.

Non-visualization of the gallbladder on ultrasound usually indicates a gallbladder abnormality. This may happen in the presence of congenital abnormalities, when the organ is contracted, when there is extraneous shadowing due to gas surrounding or within the gallbladder or its wall, or when the bile is thick and isoechogenic with the liver (Hammond, JClinUltrasound, 1988; 16:77).

Ultrasound has been used to monitor the changes in gallbladder contraction after the administration of a fatty meal as a test of function. This may be valuable in diagnosing acalculous gallbladder disease (Hederstrom, ActaRadiol, 1988; 29:207) in the absence of any other signs of disease of the organ.[8]

Endoluminal ultrasound at the time of upper gastrointestinal endoscopy is a new technique which is reported by its enthusiastic supporters to be a valuable diagnostic aid in the investigation of biliary tract pathology (Prat, Lancet, 1996; 347:75).

Computed tomography (CT) and magnetic resonance imaging (MRI)

Although gallstones may be shown using either of these methods, they are probably less valuable in diagnosis of patients with gallstone disease than ultrasound. However, the full potential of MRI in the investigation of biliary tract disease, and especially gallbladder stones, is yet to be explored.[9]

Radioisotope techniques

Investigations using technetium radioisotopes (hepatobiliary iminodiacetic acid (HIDA), di-isopropyl iminodiacetic acid (DISIDA), and *p*-di-isopropyl iminodiacetic acid (PIPIDA)) are of value in the evaluation of patients with acutely inflamed gallbladders, when they can demonstrate a patent biliary tract associated with non-filling of the gallbladder (see Chapter 6.6). This technique has a sensitivity in excess of 90 per cent in acute disease (Swayne, Radiol, 1986; 160: 33). It may be further improved by adding intravenous low-dose morphine sulphate. This appears to lower the incidence of non-visualization of the gallbladder, probably due to constriction of the sphincter of Oddi (Vasquez, NuclMedComm, 1989; 9:217). Even in the few patients with an inflamed gallbladder who do demonstrate HIDA filling of the organ, there is usually a visible abnormality, associated with an extrabiliary leak (Warshauer, AJR, 1987; 149:505), peritoneal spillage, or increased pericholecystic 'activity' (Swayne, Radiol, 1986; 160:33). HIDA, DISIDA, AND PIPIDA have now all been superseded by a third-generation radioisotope Mebrofenin (trimethyl bromohepatobiliary iminodiacetic acid). This is now the only one licensed by the European Union.

Cholecystokinin provocation testing

This is used in an attempt to identify if pain thought to be of biliary origin can be induced by an injection of cholecystokinin, a related octapeptide sincalide, or a structurally similar decapeptide ceruletide, all of which stimulate gallbladder contraction. Some claim a fatty meal is equally effective. More objective studies of gallbladder function after stimulation include radiological and scintigraphic techniques. Studies of correlation between the results of these tests and cure of symptoms by cholecystectomy are inconclusive and it must be concluded that routine use of cholecystokinin tests for selection of patients with suspected biliary pain for cholecystectomy is of unproven value.[2]

Summary

Disease of the gallbladder, especially chronic acalculous disease, may sometimes be very difficult to diagnose accurately. It may therefore be necessary to employ various investigative procedures. In one study sonography, oral cholecystography, and biliary scintigraphy reviewed together produced a diagnostic accuracy of 88 per cent (Raptopoulos, AJR, 1986; 147:721). It is likely that over the next few years mini-endoscopy of the gallbladder and cystic duct or intraluminal ultrasound, techniques only recently available, will be employed and may aid diagnosis in difficult cases (Foerster, Endoscopy; 1988, 20:316).

Differential diagnosis

Acute cholecystitis

Acute cholecystitis presents with symptoms and signs of an acute abdomen and, although a careful history and clinical examination may suggest the diagnosis, other serious pathological processes can mimic it and must be considered in the differential diagnosis. These include acute problems arising above the diaphragm (from the heart, lungs, or pleura) or within the abdomen as a result of acute pancreatitis, perforated peptic ulcer, or acute appendicitis. Since each may be life threatening, an early and accurate diagnosis must be made, even by laparoscopy where this is available, or by laparotomy following resuscitation and exclusion of cardiorespiratory problems if doubt still exists.

There has been a noticeable increase in the age of patients with this condition as well as an increasing rate of associated diabetes mellitus and acalculous cholecystitis.[10]

Chronic cholecystitis

Since the symptoms can be so vague and variable, a differential diagnosis in these patients must include the possibility of disease of practically all abdominal and thoracic organs, as well as problems arising from the spine. Many patients are subjected to every radiological and endoscopic procedure available in an attempt to exclude disease of other organs before their chronic cholecystitis is eventually diagnosed.

Conversely, many patients have their gallbladder removed in the mistaken belief that it is responsible for symptoms arising from disease elsewhere. Cases when symptoms recur after the inappropriate operation are labelled, equally inappropriately, 'post-cholecystectomy syndrome'.

Complications of gallbladder disease

Acute inflammation of the gallbladder may predispose to local pericystic abscess formation or, if the cystic duct is obstructed, the pus may collect within the organ producing an empyema; very occasionally the organ can become gangrenous and rupture. These are life-threatening conditions that require urgent drainage. Unfortunately, especially in elderly patients and despite the presence of pus, symptoms may be minimal and the patient afebrile. Because the diagnosis is not made early, this can result in a high mortality of 25 per cent (Thornton, Gut, 1983; 24:1183).

A stone contained within the gallbladder may ulcerate through the wall into an adjacent loop of bowel. If it is large enough it can cause mechanical obstruction of the gut giving rise to 'gallstone ileus' (see Chapter 23.4). Although this is a well reported condition beloved of authors of surgical textbooks, it only accounts for between 1 and 4 per cent of all cases of intestinal obstruction (Hillo, Surgery, 1987; 101:273).

Carcinoma of the gallbladder may arise in a chronically diseased organ and is discussed fully in Chapter 22.2.2. Benign tumours or adenomas of the gallbladder may become malignant and it is usually recommended that they should be treated by surgical excision, especially when they exceed 1 cm in diameter (Koga, ArchSurg, 1988; 123:26).

Treatment

Asymptomatic gallbladder stones (see also Chapter 23.4)

Consideration of the correct management of patients who have gallbladder stones diagnosed during the course of investigations for other unrelated problems frequently leads to heated discussion at medical meetings. Asymptomatic gallstones are very common because the prevalence of stones in the population is reported as being at least 17 per cent (Godrey, Gut, 1984; 25:1029) and modern diagnostic techniques reveal asymptomatic stones in patients who are being investigated for other clinical problems. Most stones are symptomless in both sexes and the risk of developing symptoms is only of the order of 1 per cent per year (Editorial, Lancet, 1990; 335:21). This is less than the risk of elective surgery.[11] In one series only 10 per cent of asymptomatic patients followed for a median of 46 months developed symptoms of biliary calculi and only 7 per cent of these required surgery (McSherry, AnnSurg, 1985; 202:59).

Conversely, one group has expressed caution about adopting this conservative approach. They argue that by reducing the number of elective operations associated with a low morbidity, more patients will require emergency surgery with its associated higher morbidity and so suffer a disadvantage (Diettrich, ArchSurg, 1988; 123:810). However, this theoretical concern is not substantiated, because urgent surgery carried out by a skilled team carries no higher a risk than elective surgery (Pickleman, ArchSurg, 1986; 121:930).

In some countries, such as Saudi Arabia, it is suggested that the silent gallstone may not be innocent and there is a report of a 21 per cent incidence of problems developing during a 38-month study period in one group of women patients (Jaddou, AnnSaudiMed, 1996; 16:123).

Cholelithiasis in patients with diabetes mellitus

Patients with diabetes mellitus have been said to present a special problem. Traditionally, prophylactic cholecystectomy has been recommended because of reports of increased mortality resulting from acute cholecystitis in these patients. However, in a recent study of the data, it appears this traditional teaching is based on studies carried out before 1980 and the authors believe that the recommendation that prophylactic cholecystectomy is necessary for diabetics with silent gallstones should be reconsidered (Ransohoff, AnnIntMed, 1987; 106:829).

Gallstones in the elderly

Much discussion has surrounded the management of elderly patients with stones in the common bile duct which have been removed endoscopically. If they remain asymptomatic should they have their gallbladders removed? Certainly cholecystectomy appears to be safe in older patients who have no significant associated illness and a laparoscopic approach may be even safer (Watkins, Geriat, 1993; 48:48). Although it is difficult to give unqualified advice, one report suggests that if the cystic duct remains patent there is no need for elective surgery, but if it is occluded on ERCP then the gallbladder should be removed to avoid a possible high complication and associated mortality rate (Worthley, BrJSurg, 1988; 75:796). However, more studies are needed to explore this still unresolved problem.

Gallstones in children

There is some evidence that these are being recognized more frequently in childhood as a result of haematological disorders, total parenteral nutrition, ileal problems, or prolonged fasting. In the absence of biliary obstruction, conservative management may result in spontaneous dissolution of the stones. Otherwise they should be managed as in adults by open or laparoscopic cholecystectomy and removal of any duct stones (Rescorla, SemPediatSurg, 1992; 1:98).

Conservative measures

The traditional conservative treatment of patients with chronic cholecystitis has been a low-fat diet. This was based on the theory that cholecystokinin release will be less (if the diet is low in fat), causing less stimulation of the diseased gallbladder. However, gallbladder contraction is equally stimulated by a high- or a low-fat diet and both of these situations result in only marginally less contraction than that produced by a cholecystokinin infusion (Mogadam, AmJGastr, 1984; 79:745). Despite a low-fat diet, many patients continue to have recurrent symptoms, but they prefer to tolerate them rather than entertain the possibility of surgery. As they may develop an attack of acute cholecystitis at any time, they should be warned of this and advised to have an elective procedure.

Acute cholecystitis

The time-honoured treatment of patients presenting with an attack of acute cholecystitis has been initially conservative, with gastro-intestinal rest, intravenous fluids, and antibiotics, in anticipation that the acute inflammatory process will settle; it usually does. They are then allowed to leave hospital to return after an interval of about 6 weeks for an elective cholecystectomy. This was believed to be safer than an urgent operation. This traditional approach has now been questioned as a result of several prospective studies which have demonstrated quite clearly that the morbidity and mortality of an operation during the acute phase of the disease is no greater than if it is delayed for 6 weeks (McArthur, BrJSurg, 1975; 62:850; Jarvinen, AnnSurg, 1979; 191:501; Norrby, BrJSurg, 1983; 70:163). Furthermore, it is clear that these patients always run the risk of developing a further acute attack of cholecystitis or some other complication of gallstone disease, such as jaundice or pancreatitis, during the 6-week waiting period. Their return to work is delayed by the same 6 weeks. For these reasons few clinicians now advise

their patients to delay the operation once the diagnosis has been confirmed in patients classified as having a low operative risk. The treatment of choice is early and definitive surgery. This is both medically and economically beneficial. High-risk patients should have percutaneous gallbladder drainage directed by ultrasound, at least as an initial procedure (Avrahami, IntSurg, 1995; 80:111), both surgery and drainage being carried out with prophylactic antibiotic cover.[10,12]

Cholecystectomy

Details of the classic operation of open cholecystectomy through a subcostal Kocher's incision are well described in surgical texts and will not be discussed here, except to draw attention to the value and safety of a 'fundus first' or 'retrograde' approach to the removal of the diseased organ. This differs from the traditional approach which involves dissection and ligation of the cystic duct and artery at their origin adjacent to the common hepatic duct. The fundus first technique is especially important when the anatomy is obscured by the local disease processes. Under these conditions it reduces, significantly, the possibility of damage to the main hepatic duct by inadvertent ligation.[13]

The results of cholecystectomy, both elective and acute, in patients of all ages have greatly improved recently (Pickleman, ArchSurg, 1986; 121:930). It is thus necessary to exercise caution when comparing the results of new approaches to gallbladder stones with the reported results of surgery carried out some time ago. Elective biliary surgery in experienced hands is relatively safe even in the elderly (Houghton, BrJSurg, 1985; 72:220). The current death rate following cholecystectomy alone varies from 0.1 to 2.5 per cent in patients over 70 years old. Deaths are mainly due to cardiovascular problems. Complication rates, mainly due to biliary, pulmonary, and wound problems, are 3.6 per cent and these rise to 17 per cent following concomitant exploration of the bile ducts. Thus although gallbladder surgery is safe, mortality and morbidity increases with age and exploration of the bile ducts (Girard, CanJSurg, 1993; 36:75).[12]

What has contributed to the recent improvement in surgical morbidity and mortality? Probably the main factor is the appreciation that a diseased gallbladder is likely to contain infected bile and so prophylactic antibiotic therapy is indicated. The risk factors for biliary sepsis include age (over 60 years), obstructive jaundice, a history of cholangitis or previous biliary surgery, stones in the common bile duct, and a clinical history lasting more than 3 years. The infecting organisms are of gut origin and include *Escherichia coli*, *Klebsiella* spp., *Pseudomonas* spp., *Proteus* spp., *Streptococcus faecalis*, *Bacteriodes fragilis*, *Clostridium* spp., and *Staphylococcus aureus* (Aloj, DigSurg, 1988; 5:185). Postoperative infection from these organisms can be significantly reduced by the prophylactic use of a single perioperative dose of a cephalosporin antibiotic. In the absence of obvious infection its value is not improved by continuing therapy after surgery.

The septic complications of biliary tract surgery have been reduced so significantly that it is now mandatory to treat all patients having cholecystectomy with appropriate antibiotics (Kellum, Arch-Surg, 1987; 122:918).

In common with all surgical procedures there is a very real risk of patients developing venous thrombosis and pulmonary embolism following cholecystectomy. This is especially so in women taking the contraceptive pill. Women being offered elective surgery should therefore be advised to discontinue the contraceptive pill for 3 months prior to surgery, and all patients should receive prophylactic treatment designed to reduce the incidence of venous thrombotic problems.

The question of cholecystectomy in patients with concurrent liver disease frequently causes concern for fear of excessive haemorrhage and delay in healing. Many studies have been undertaken to find out if wound healing is delayed in jaundiced patients, but the results of such studies are confusing. Wound healing is certainly delayed by concurrent jaundice in experimental rats (Arnaud, AmJSurg, 1981; 141:593), but in humans any impaired healing is probably related to the patient's general clinical condition and not the raised bilirubin levels (Greaney, BrJSurg, 1979; 66:478; Armstrong, BrJSurg, 1984; 71:267).

Cholecystectomy in patients with cirrhosis demands that care is comparable with that given to cirrhotic patients having major surgery for portal hypertension. The morbidity and mortality can then be acceptably low, although still higher than in normal patients. Sepsis and bleeding, which are common complications in these sick patients, need aggressive treatment (Kogut, ArchSurg, 1985; 120: 1310; Sirinek, ArchSurg, 1987; 122:271). It was at one time argued that cirrhosis was a contraindication to major abdominal surgery. However, experience has shown that this is not so in skilled hands, but it should not be undertaken lightly for fear of encountering uncontrollable haemorrhage.

Mini-cholecystectomy

A fairly recent change in technique involves using a short, 5-cm subcostal incision—a so-called mini-cholecystectomy. It is claimed that recovery is faster and hospital stay shorter than following the classic operation (O'Dwyer, BrJSurg, 1990; 77:1189).

Laparoscopic cholecystectomy

The introduction of laparoscopic techniques for carrying out surgical procedures has had a revolutionary effect on the practice of surgery within the last decade. Gynaecologists had used the technique for some years previously for intraperitoneal inspection of the pelvic viscera and associated minor surgical procedures; but it has been used extensively since the development of fibre-optic laparoscopes and miniature colour television cameras. It is an aesthetically very pleasing technique which can display magnified, albeit two dimensional, colour pictures of the intraperitoneal organs on a series of television screens around the operating table, the operating room, the hospital and, sometimes, the city or even across continents. Video recordings can be made and used as teaching material, in medicolegal situations, or even given to the patient to take home to entertain friends and family in place of holiday pictures. As a result of this development the incidence of cholecystectomy, sometimes for very dubious reasons, has increased greatly and enhanced surgical bank accounts worldwide.

The first publications on laparoscopic cholecystectomy appeared as recently as 1989 and 1990 from France and the United States (Dubois, PressMed, 1989; 18:980; Perissat, SurgEndosc; 1990, 4:1;

Reddick, AmJSurg, 1990; 160:485). Initially the reports promised faster surgery, minimal scars, very short hospital stay, minimal postoperative discomfort, and early return to normal activities. Unfortunately, not all these expectations have been realized and some even question if it offers any major advance at all. Some serious complications have been encountered. These occur mainly when the procedure is carried out by surgeons without adequate training and experience. As a result, a more conservative, critical approach to the procedure is now developing and, hopefully, it is being carried out more appropriately by surgeons with proper training (Cuschieri, AmJSurg, 1991; 161:385; Perissat, WorldJSurg, 1992; 16:1074). I believe there is no doubt that laparoscopic cholecystectomy really does represent a major advance in surgery of the biliary tract.

The operation is carried out under general anaesthesia after the stomach has been emptied through a nasogastric tube and the bladder through a urethral catheter. The peritoneal cavity is inflated with carbon dioxide to a pressure of between 12 and 15 mmHg by means of a small cannula inserted through the umbilicus. This is replaced with a 1-cm trocar through which is passed a laparoscope with an attached miniature television camera. All subsequent procedures are displayed on television screens. The whole peritoneal cavity is first examined.

Three additional cannulas are introduced: one of 1 cm in diameter to the right of the linear alba in the epigastrium and two 0.5-cm instruments, one in the right hypochondrium and one a little lower in the midclavicular line. By appropriate manipulation of the laparoscope a clear picture of the gallbladder and its adjacent structures is obtained (Plate 1(a)), and holding, cutting, and ligating instruments are introduced through the three additional ports. The peritoneum covering the cystic duct and artery and the neck of the gallbladder is removed and they are mobilized from surrounding tissues (Plate 1(b)) before application of clips and subsequent division. The gallbladder is dissected from its bed, haemostasis being obtained using electrocautery, and it is removed through one of the 1-cm stab incisions, sometimes after mechanically crushing the contained stones.

If excessive fibrosis and inflammation, or the presence of portal hypertension, make total removal of the gallbladder hazardous, subtotal cholecystectomy can be safely carried out in an attempt to avoid conversion to an open procedure (Crosthewaite, JRCollSurgEdinb, 1995; 40:20). The gallbladder fossa in the liver is flushed with saline, haemostasis is checked, the pneumoperitoneum is released, and the incision is closed with absorbable subcuticular sutures.

Some surgeons routinely carry out perioperative percutaneous cholangiography. A cannula is introduced through a separate needle puncture in an appropriate part of the anterior abdominal wall and the tip of the cannula is guided into the cystic duct before it is clipped and divided. Radio-opaque contrast in injected. This demonstrates the choledochal anatomy and the presence or absence of ductal stones. There is a great deal of, often heated, discussion between advocates of the procedure as a routine step and those who consider it an unnecessary waste of time—reminiscent of the earlier similar discussions in relation to the value of operative cholangiography during open surgery. There is similar lack of agreement between clinicians in relation to the value of routine or selective preoperative ERCP for the same purpose (Welbourn, Gut, 1995; 37:576; Tanaka, WorldJSurg, 1996; 20:267).

When hepatic duct stones are identified before or during cholecystectomy they can be removed either preoperatively by ERCP, at the time of surgery by formal surgical removal (a procedure to be undertaken only by the very skilled laparoscopic surgeon), or after surgery by ERCP. Each approach has its advocates but there is no study which can give absolute advice, rather the decision should be governed by local expertise.

Recovery from the operation is usually rapid. Most patients take a cup of tea soon after recovery from anaesthesia and suffer only minimal discomfort, requiring only one injection of analgesic medication followed by mild oral analgesics. Many are fit for discharge from the clinic a few hours after the procedure and most return to work within 1 or 2 weeks.

Any variation from this recovery pattern should draw the surgeon's attention to the possibility of a complication: a bile leak or, even more serious, biliary tract damage. Such a patient needs careful observation and early investigation if recovery continues to be unsatisfactory. Early measurement of biochemical liver function tests, coupled with an ultrasound examination of the abdomen and an ERCP, will identify any problem. If a problem is identified the patient should be further managed in a centre with specialist hepatobiliary expertise.

The incidence of general postoperative complications, such as chest and wound infections, seems to be lower than following open surgery, but the incidence of inadvertent biliary tract damage is higher. In one survey of American institutions (which reported their complications) a mean rate of bile duct injury was reported as being 0.6 per cent (Deziel, AmJSurg, 1993; 165:9), while a European survey reported an incidence of 4 in 1203 operations (Cuschieri, AmJSurg, 1991; 161:385).

It is quite clear from the reported experience that, if a serious technical problem is encountered during laparoscopic cholecystectomy, the operation should be converted immediately to the conventional open procedure.

It is difficult to obtain exact data to support the view that the operation offers a significantly better outcome than the open operation since the few comparative studies which truly compare the laparoscopic with an open mini-incision cholecystectomy have been carried out in major specialist centres where the incidence of complications is, in any case, low. It is an impression gained from increased referral rates of biliary tract complications that the incidence of biliary damage is higher than following the open operation. Review of recent literature[14] suggests the following:

1. Symptomatic outcome and recovery in 3 to 6 months following cholecystectomy irrespective of the surgical approach.
2. General complication rates are similar following all operations, but postoperative pulmonary function is better following laparoscopic cholecystectomy and postoperative pain is less.
3. Biliary tract complications may be more frequent following the laparoscopic approach.
4. Postoperative hospital stay and time to return to work seem to be less following laparoscopic or mini-cholecystectomy when compared with conventional open cholecystectomy.

5. The training and experience of the operating surgeon dictate the likelihood of complications.

However, patient satisfaction following the now almost standard laparoscopic approach to cholecystectomy is good mainly because they are left with fewer and almost invisible abdominal scars.

'We must not forget that the optimal method of management of gall bladder disease will not rest on rigid unthinking devotion to any one technique but on judicious selection of the most appropriate method or combination of methods for the individual circumstances' (Paterson-Brown, BrJSurg, 1991; 78:132).

Operative cholecystostomy

It is argued that in patients who are very acutely ill, cholecystostomy is a preferable procedure to cholecystectomy. However, recent studies suggest that although it may appear to be a safe procedure in the acute situation (Winkler, BrJSurg, 1989; 76:693), its advantage over a more radical one is doubtful. In patients with diabetes or elderly patients with gangrenous or necrotic gallbladders it may offer a poor chance of rapid recovery and reduction of the septic process (Burdiles, Hepatogast, 1989; 36:136; Reiss, DigDis, 1993; 11:55). Probably, operative cholecystectomy is no more dangerous and may even be more effective than cholecystostomy (Gutman, DigDis, 1988; 5:189). In some situations where total cholecystectomy is judged to be unduly hazardous, a partial resection may be safe and effective (Ibrarullah, HPBSurgery; 1993, 7:61).

Percutaneous cholecystostomy

The percutaneous transhepatic approach to cholecystostomy is being explored as this avoids a major formal surgical procedure.[15] This should be a transhepatic approach because in 70 per cent of cases the gallbladder fundus lies conveniently behind the liver margin and in 13 per cent the right hemicolon lies between the fundus of the gallbladder and the skin, making an approach from below unacceptably hazardous. Percutaneous cholecystostomy has been used to treat patients with hydrops and empyema, gallbladder stones, and biliary obstruction due to malignant disease.

The technique is to use a 22-gauge removable hub or Chiba needle for initial access. A Seldinger wire or trocar is then passed and various sizes of pigtail catheters are inserted, finally passing a 12-F single or double lumen catheter. This approach to the gallbladder with ultrasound guidance is reported anecdotally to be life saving in some patients with empyema and subsequent cholecystectomy may be unnecessary (Eggermont, ArchSurg, 1985; 120:1354; Hawkins, SemIntRadiol, 1985; 2:97; Vogelzan, Radiol, 1988; 168:29). Early reports of the technique inevitably come from enthusiastic and experienced workers, so the results must be interpreted with caution. No prospective studies have yet been undertaken to investigate if this approach is preferable to, or safer than, a formal surgical operation which, even in very sick patients, now carries an acceptably low complication rate in experienced hands. Furthermore, no comparative studies have been made between this technique and laparoscopic cholecystectomy, but it will be only a temporary acute treatment and further definitive measures will have to be considered when the patient's condition improves.[16]

Other techniques for managing gallbladder stones

Other percutaneous measures being carried out by interventional radiologists include attempts to flush out stones broken by ultrasound lithotripsy or to dissolve them with substances such as methyl terbutyl ether (**MTBE**) (Chapter 23.1). Although MTBE does not appear to produce significant damage to the gallbladder mucosa and it does cause large stones to break allowing the pieces to be flushed out, there may be resultant changes in hepatic enzyme levels. The technique has promise in the management of gallbladder stones, but it is too early to say whether there will be any long-term advantages over other treatment modalities (Heaton, CurrOpinGastro, 1985; 1:696).

Dissolution of gallbladder stones using bile salts is discussed in Chapter 23.4.

Although the potential of ultrasound lithotripsy is being explored in the treatment of patients with biliary tract stones, the technique is even more experimental in relation to the treatment of gallbladder stones. To reduce gallbladder stones to 2 mm in diameter for their safe passage through the biliary system, either multiple shocks or adjuvant bile-salt therapy is needed (Bird, JHepatol, 1989; 9:99). The results of *in vivo* controlled clinical studies are awaited.

Post-cholecystectomy syndrome

This is a vague diagnosis applied to symptoms experienced by patients after cholecystectomy. Twenty-five per cent or more of patients will complain of pain, dyspepsia, and other symptoms which they relate to the operation weeks to years afterwards.[17] Frequently, they are similar to those experienced before the operation. In many cases this is due to the fact that the operation was carried out for the wrong reason and the pathology causing the symptoms is extrabiliary, such as reflux oesophagitis, gastritis, *Helicobacter pylori* infection, peptic ulcer, or functional bowel disorders. In only a very small proportion of cases, perhaps as low as 2 to 5 per cent, is the problem genuine. This group truly suffers biliary dyskinesia or true post-cholecystectomy syndrome. It is either related to gallstones being left unobserved in the biliary tract, to the iatrogenic induction of a choledochoduodenal fistula, or to a functional motility disturbance with organic disease. In cases where the symptoms are genuine, multiple costly investigations are needed. The most frequent finding in biliary dyskinesia is an abnormally high tone in the sphincter of Oddi, although this is very difficult to elicit. An alternative technique recently described to investigate sphincter of Oddi dysfunction induced by prostigmine morphine provocation involves quantitative hepatobiliary scintigraphy (Madacsy, EurJNucMed, 1995; 22:227).

Retained biliary stones are treated endoscopically but, apart from this situation, true post-cholecystectomy syndrome is an exclusion diagnosis which is treated medically by diet and spasmolytics, such as sublingual nitroglycerine, or occasionally surgically by closing any choledochoduodenal fistula or carrying out a sphincterotomy of the sphincter of Oddi. However, interventional procedures should only be employed when all conservative measures have failed, accepting that often the results are unsatisfactory.[17]

References

1. Frierson HF Jr. The gross anatomy and histology of the gall bladder, extrahepatic bile ducts, Vaterian system and minor papilla. *American Journal of Surgical Pathology*, 1989; **13**: 146–62.
2. Kang JY and Williamson RC. Cholecystitis without gall stones. *HPB Surgery*, 1990; **2**: 83–103.
3. Power R, Mrdeza MA, and Block GE. Association of cholecystitis and parenteral nutrition. *Nutrition*, 1970; **6**: 125–30.
4. Hinnant K and Rotterdam H. Acalculus cholecystitis in the aquired immunodeficiency syndrome. *Progress in AIDS Pathology*, 1990; **2**: 151–62.
5. Johnson CD *et al.* Calculus disease and cholecystitis. In Millward Sadler GH, Wright R, and Arthur MJP, eds. *Wright's liver and biliary disease*, 3rd edn. London: Saunders, 1992: 1457–88.
6. Williamson RCN. Acalculus disease of the gallbladder. *Gut*, 1988; **29**: 860–72.
7. Lee AW, Proudfoot WH, and Griffen WO. Acalculous cholecystitis. *Surgery, Gynecology and Obstetrics*, 1984; **159**: 33–5.
8. Kane RA. The biliary system. (Review.) *Clinics in Diagnostic Ultrasound*, 1988; **23**: 75–137.
9. Brink, JA and Borrello JA. MR imaging of the biliary sytem. *MRI Clinics of North America*, 1995; **3**: 143–60.
10. Reiss R and Deutsch AA. State of the art in the diagnosis and management of acute cholecystitis. (Review.) *Digestive Diseases*, 1993; **11**: 55–64.
11. Den Besten L. Asymptomatic gallstones. In Blumgart LRH, ed. *Surgery of the liver and biliary tract*. London: Churchill Livingstone, 1988.
12. Govma DJ and Obertop H. Acute calculus cholecystitis. What is new in diagnosis and therapy? *HPB Surgery*, 1992; **6**: 69–78.
13. Espiner HJ. Emergency cholecystectomy: towards guaranteed safety. In Wilson DH and Marsden AK, eds. *Care of the acutely ill and injured*. London: Wiley, 1982: 385–7.
14. Downs SH, Black NA, Devlin HB, Royston CMS, and Russell RCG. Systemic review of the effectiveness and safety of laparoscopic cholecystectomy. *Annals of the Royal College of Surgeons of England*, 1996; **78(3)** Pt II: 241–323.
15. van Sonnenberg E *et al.* Diagnostic and therapeutic percutaneous gall bladder procedures. *Radiology*, 1986; **160**: 23–6.
16. Vrahami R *et al.* The role of percutaneous transhepatic cholecystostomy in the management of acute cholecystitis in high risk patients. *International Surgery*, 1995; **80**: 111–14.
17. Lasson A, Fork F-T, and Ekberg O. Decision making in post-cholecystectomy pain and biliary dyskinesia. *Digestive Diseases*, 1989; **7**: 288–300.

24

The liver in diseases of other systems

24.1 The liver in cardiovascular and pulmonary disease

Neil McIntyre and Peter Collins

The liver in cardiovascular disease

Hepatic abnormalities occur as a result of a variety of cardiovascular diseases. A palpable liver and/or abnormal liver function tests are often found in patients with conditions such as myocardial infarction, hypotension, shock, heart failure, and constrictive pericarditis. In some cases the hepatic involvement is such that the overall clinical picture may erroneously be attributed to liver disease *per se*. The liver is also involved in many generalized cardiovascular conditions, such as polyarteritis nodosa and hereditary haemorrhagic telangiectasia, and may be affected by some of the drugs used to treat cardiovascular diseases (Table 1). Jaundice is a frequent transient complication of cardiac surgery.

Heart failure and the liver

The aetiology of congestive heart failure is changing. Rheumatic heart disease is no longer the most common cause, as it was in the mid-1950s, and has been replaced by congestive heart failure due to coronary artery disease and hypertension. With advances in therapy, many more patients survive long periods with severe congestive

Table 1 Cardiac/circulatory drugs causing liver disease[1,2]

Liver condition	Drug
Acute hepatitis	Acebutolol, aprindine, benzarone, captopril, diltiazem, enalapril, hydralazine, labetalol, linisopril, methyldopa, metoprolol, nifedipine, quinidine, verapamil
Chronic hepatitis/cirrhosis	Benzarone, labetalol, methyldopa
Cholestasis, cholestatic hepatitis	Atenolol, captopril, disopyramide, enalapril, hydralazine, methyldopa, prajmaline, procainamide, propafenone, warfarin
Granulomatous hepatitis	Diltiazem, hydralazine, perhexilene, procainamide, quinidine, quinine
Phospholipidosis	Amiodarone
Non-alcoholic steathepatitis	Amiodarone, perhexiline

heart failure; the liver may suffer because of hepatic congestion and a decreased poor blood supply.

Symptoms

Most patients with heart failure have no symptoms due to hepatic congestion.[3] However, right upper quadrant pain may occur with acute heart failure, or with exacerbations of chronic heart failure. Nausea and vomiting can also result from severe heart failure, but it is not known whether they are due to hepatic or intestinal congestion.[4] Heart failure is a rare, but reported cause of hepatic encephalopathy and coma[5,6] (Kaymakcalan, AmJMed, 1978; 65: 384; Kisloff, DigDisSci, 1976; 21:895), and hepatic congestion can also cause severe hypoglycaemia which may induce stupor (Mellinkoff, NEJM, 1952; 247:745; Benzing, Circul, 1969; 40:209). Fulminant hepatic failure may result from previously unrecognized cardiomyopathy and treatment of the heart condition may improve the liver failure (Wiesen, DigDis, 1995; 13:199). In patients with hepatic failure due to cardiomyopathy, symptoms suggesting cardiac failure may be absent; echocardiography or catheterization may be needed to make the correct diagnosis, which may be suggested by the presence of hepatic congestion on liver biopsy (Hoffman, JClinGastro, 1990; 12:306). Clinical features simulating acute hepatitis have also been described in patients with left-sided heart failure (Cohen, Gastro, 1978; 74:583; Parisi, ItalJGastr, 1990; 22: 133).

Signs

Hepatomegaly occurs in 95 to 99 per cent of patients with moderate to severe heart failure.[3] The liver is palpable in many patients (often more than 5 cm below the right costal margin) and is usually tender, firm, and smooth.[7] Palpable splenomegaly occurs in about 20 per cent of patients with heart failure without cardiac cirrhosis, and in about 80 per cent of those with cardiac cirrhosis.[8]

Ascites occurs in approximately a quarter of patients with liver involvement secondary to cardiac failure;[3,7,8] in about one-third of these the ascitic fluid protein content is over 30 g/l (Pillay, SAMedJ, 1963; 37:379). Peripheral oedema is, of course, more common, occurring in 75 per cent of patients with acute or chronic congestive heart failure, and pleural effusion is present in 20 to 25 per cent,[3] but both are usually the direct result of the heart failure rather than hepatic congestion.

Liver function tests in heart failure

In the following paragraphs we discuss the effect of heart failure on the results of individual liver function tests. In a recent study of 552 patients with chronic heart failure, followed for up to 13 years, abnormal liver tests (bilirubin, aspartate aminotransferase, γ-glutamyl transpeptidase, and alkaline phosphatase) were related to mortality, as was the plasma urate. Of all variables, aspartate aminotransferase accounted for the greatest variance, followed by serum bilirubin (Batin, EurHeartJ, 1995; 16:1613).

Serum aminotransferases

Serum aminotransferases, glutamate dehydrogenase, and lactate dehydrogenase are all elevated in congestive heart failure[7,9] (Bang, ActaMedScand, 1959; 164:385; Betro, AmJClinPath, 1973; 60:679). Aspartate and alanine aminotransferases rise in up to a third of patients, and show similar increases; an increased lactate dehydrogenase is found in 20 to 60 per cent of patients.

In a series of 175 patients with acute and chronic heart failure,[7] aspartate aminotransferase was elevated in 49 per cent of those with acute heart failure, but in only 5 per cent of those with chronic heart failure; 80 per cent of the high levels were between 40 and 80 U/l. Alanine aminotransferase results paralleled, but were less marked than, those of aspartate aminotransferase. Very high values of aspartate aminotransferase (1000–10 000 U/l) can occur with an acute onset of severe heart failure, especially if it is associated with hypotension or shock[11] (Killip, Circul, 1960; 21:646; Ross, AmJGastr, 1981; 76:511), and they correlate well with the degree of centrilobular hepatic necrosis.

Increased venous congestion and decreased hepatic perfusion both contribute to the elevation of aminotransferases, although centrilobular hypoxia and/or necrosis are probably the major factors.

The increases in aspartate and alanine aminotransferases and lactate dehydrogenase correlate with increases in systemic venous pressure, pulmonary capillary wedge pressure and cardiac index, but the correlation coefficients are low, suggesting that other factors must also be involved[9] (West, AmJMedSci, 1961; 241:350).

Very high enzyme levels in congestive heart failure are often misinterpreted as evidence of viral or drug-induced hepatitis (Logan, AnnIntMed, 1962; 56:784). The following clinical features suggest that circulatory failure is the cause of liver cell necrosis:[10]

(1) the presence of chronic heart failure;
(2) a recent episode of acute circulatory failure;
(3) hepatomegaly (which is unusual in severe viral hepatitis); and
(4) the early appearance of renal insufficiency—this tends to be a late development in severe viral hepatitis.

Myocardial infarction is a common occurrence in patients with congestive heart failure of ischaemic aetiology, and modest elevations of aspartate aminotransferase (<200 U/l) may result from the resulting myocardial necrosis. Assay of other enzymes helps to identify a myocardial infarct. The aspartate aminotransferase–alanine aminotransferase ratio is high with infarction, and an increase in serum creatine phosphokinase (**CPK**), which is mainly of muscle origin, also suggests that an increased aspartate aminotransferase is cardiac rather than hepatic in origin. The CPK–MB fraction is highly specific for the heart.

Serum bilirubin

Jaundice is found in less than 20 per cent of patients with liver damage due to congestive heart failure, and depends on the severity of the heart failure, as evidenced by right atrial pressure, pulmonary wedge pressure, and cardiac index.[3,8,9] However, the serum bilirubin is elevated in 20 to 80 per cent of patients with congestive heart failure; it rarely exceeds 85 μmol/l and is usually less than 50 μmol/l.[7,9,11] Unconjugated bilirubin is usually higher than conjugated bilirubin[9] (Zieve, JLabClinMed, 1951; 38:446; Levine, AmJMed, 1964; 36:541). The elevated serum bilirubin falls quickly with resolution of heart failure, usually becoming normal within 3 to 7 days.[4]

When obvious jaundice is found with heart failure, pulmonary infarction should be suspected (Rich, BullJHopkHosp, 1926; 38:75). Biliary disease, and other complications such as sepsis, haemolysis, or drugs, should also be considered. Severe hyperbilirubinaemia has, however, been reported in a small number of patients with congestive heart failure alone[5,6] (Kaymakcalan, AmJMed, 1978; 65:384).

The mechanism(s) underlying the rise in bilirubin in heart failure is poorly understood. A high unconjugated bilirubin suggests poor hepatic uptake or conjugation of bilirubin. Obstruction of bile canaliculi by distended veins and sinusoids in the congested liver does not appear to be an important cause of the rise in bilirubin.[12] There is only a weak correlation between the bilirubin elevation and the increased central venous and pulmonary wedge pressures, and the decrease in cardiac index.[4,11] In one report, three patients with congestive heart failure had bilirubin levels over 300 μmol/l; these high serum bilirubins seemed to correlate with histological evidence of extensive hepatic necrosis.[11] Very high bilirubin levels are usually accompanied by abnormalities of other liver function tests, such as the serum aspartate aminotransferase, prothrombin time, and bromsulphthalein retention[11] (Killip, Circul, 1960; 21:646; Logan, AnnIntMed, 1962; 56:784), which also suggests that liver damage is the cause for the rise in bilirubin.

Patients with advanced mitral valve disease may show an impairment in the elimination of conjugated bilirubin, due probably to a reduced liver blood flow (Bohmer, EurHeartJ, 1994; 15:10).

Serum alkaline phosphatase

Serum alkaline phosphatase rises by about 10 to 20 per cent in patients with congestive heart failure[9,11] (Felder, Circul, 1950; 2:256); much higher levels are uncommon (West, AmJMedSci, 1961; 241:350). There appears to be no correlation between the rise in alkaline phosphatase and the increases of aspartate aminotransferase or bilirubin in patients with hepatic damage due to heart failure.[9] At higher levels the alkaline phosphatase appears related to the degree of hepatomegaly and elevation of the jugular venous pressure.[7]

Intrahepatic biliary obstruction due to a high intrahepatic pressure may play a role in the alkaline phosphatase rise associated with congestive heart failure,[7] as the highest values were found in patients with enormously distended livers. Hepatocellular dysfunction and changes in cell membrane permeability may also affect the levels. Elevated levels of alkaline phosphatase usually return to normal about 1 week after improvement in cardiac status.

Prothrombin time

Prolonged prothrombin times are found in 80 to 90 per cent of patients with acute and chronic heart failure.[3,4,7] Decreased hepatic synthesis of vitamin K-dependent clotting factors may be responsible, as the prothrombin time is not altered by vitamin K administration. Return of the prothrombin time to normal usually takes 2 to 3 weeks following the successful treatment of the heart failure. Caution should therefore be exercised when treating patients in heart failure with warfarin and dicumarol derivatives (Kliesch, JAMA, 1960; 172:223).

Serum proteins

Serum albumin is low in about 30 to 50 per cent of patients with congestive heart failure, and the incidence, and degree of change, appears to be similar in acute and chronic failure.[7] The changes were not marked; in 75 per cent of those with reduced albumin the values were between 25 and 29 g/l (normal range 30–45 g/l). The lowest values were in patients with high right-sided pressures due to rheumatic heart disease or cor pulmonale. Values less than 15 g/l are rarely found.

The serum albumin level does not correlate with the degree of histological damage to the liver[7] (Felder, Circul, 1950; 2:286). Lower values appear to correlate with the extent of ascites and oedema. Causes of the low albumin probably include decreased hepatic synthesis, leakage from a congested intestine, and poor nutrition. With treatment of the heart failure, the serum albumin tends to rise over a period of one or more months.

Mild hyperglobulinaemia occurred in about 50 per cent of patients with heart failure, being more common in acute (60 per cent) than chronic failure (37 per cent); in 75 per cent of these the serum globulins were only slightly elevated—to between 35 and 41 g/l (normal range 20–35 g/l). Again, the highest levels were found in patients with very high right-sided pressures. Resolution was uncommon following treatment of the congestive failure.[7]

Bromsulphthalein retention

The bromsulphthalein retention test is abnormal in 78 to 100 per cent of patients with congestive heart failure, and seems to correlate well with the elevation of central venous pressure[11,12] (Evans, AmJMed, 1952; 13:704; West, AmJMedSci, 1961; 241:350). This test is rarely used nowadays but the results found in early studies remain of interest.

The influence of systemic haemodynamics on liver function abnormalities in chronic heart failure

Systemic haemodynamics and biochemical profiles were analysed in 133 patients with chronic heart failure.[9] Patients with a normal or moderately impaired cardiac index had normal liver function, whereas those with marked impairment of the cardiac index (<1.5 l/min/m²) had deranged liver tests. There was a correlation with the reduction in cardiac index and the height of the right atrial and pulmonary wedge pressures. Reduced forward flow and passive backward congestion both appeared to be contributory factors, but non-haemodynamic factors were also thought to be important.

There is a correlation between the diameter of the portal vein and the right atrial pressure in patients with heart disease, and it has even been suggested that right atrial pressure might be assessed by measurement of the portal vein diameter using regression analysis (Strohm, IntMed, 1981; 8:138).

Passive hepatic congestion can cause a mottled hepatic enhancement on computed tomography (CT) scanning. This could represent a potential pitfall in the use of dynamic bolus-enhanced CT scanning for the detection of focal hepatic masses (Moulton, AJR, 1988; 151:939).

The pathogenesis of liver dysfunction in congestive heart failure

Congestive heart failure causes a number of pathophysiological effects which, alone or in combination, result in liver cell damage. The main factors are thought to be:

(1) decreased hepatic blood flow;
(2) increased hepatic venous pressure with subsequent oedema of the perisinusoidal area and atrophy of hepatocytes; and
(3) decreased arterial oxygen saturation which could result in hepatocellular hypoxia.

The single most important factor in both acute and chronic heart failure appears to be hypoxia of the liver cells, resulting in centrilobular necrosis[13] (Cohen, Gastro, 1978; 74:583).

Hepatic blood flow

If hepatic arterial blood flow falls, due to a decreased cardiac output, hypoxia of the liver can result[14,15] (Greenway, PhysiolRev, 1971; 51:23; Acero, GastroHepato, 1984; 7:334). The liver has a dual blood supply, receiving about 17 to 34 per cent of its blood flow from the hepatic artery, and 66 to 83 per cent via the low-pressure portal vein, in which the oxygen saturation is relatively high (Bradley, JCI, 1945; 24:890; Bradley, Gastro, 1963; 44:403). Thus much of its oxygen supply comes from the portal vein.

If patients cannot increase their cardiac output, there is a fall in splanchnic blood flow with exercise, and a reduced hepatic blood flow; the oxygen requirement of the liver does not change, and oxygen extraction increases.[14,15] Hepatic venous oxygen saturation may therefore fall sharply on exercise in patients with congestive heart failure; the reduction is roughly proportional to the impairment of cardiac function (Bishop, JCI, 1955; 34:1114). If the oxygen supply to the liver is inadequate, centrilobular damage may result; the central zone (zone 3) is particularly sensitive to hypoxia (Rapaport, RevPhysiolBiochemPharmacol, 1976; 76:129).

Increased venous pressure

An increased venous pressure probably contributes to the hepatic dysfunction of congestive heart failure. Splanchnic blood volume increases in moderate and severe congestive heart failure;[15] much of the extra blood is contained within the hepatic and portal venous systems. The splanchnic blood volume correlates with the degree of portal hypertension, which in turn is related to the systemic venous pressure; bromsulphthalein retention also correlates with systemic venous pressure[11] (Evans, AmJMed, 1952; 13:704).

Whether right-sided heart failure *per se* can cause centrilobular necrosis is debatable; in 26 patients with varying degrees of cor pulmonale there was no correlation between serum enzyme activities and the clinical signs of right heart failure (Refsum, ClinSci, 1963; 25:369). In another study, only 3 of 11 patients who appeared to have congestion alone had abnormal aminotransferase levels and all were less than five times normal; however, when moderate or marked centrilobular necrosis is present, serum aminotransferases tend to be more than five times normal (Bynum, DigDisSci, 1979; 24:134).

The liver has a relatively non-compliant capsule; compression of the liver, leading to an increase in hepatic resistance, may contribute to decreased hepatic blood flow when there is passive congestion. However, hepatic parenchymal resistance has not been shown to rise significantly under these circumstances.[15,16] Furthermore, in an experimental model of raised hepatic venous pressure in the cat, hepatic oedema did not occur (Lautt, CircRes, 1977; 41:787). In human livers an increased venous pressure caused electron microscopic changes in hepatocytes, but only centrilobular cell atrophy occurred, and other factors appeared to be necessary in order to produce centrilobular hepatic cell necrosis (Safran, AmJPathol, 1967; 50:447).

Arterial hypoxia

Arterial hypoxia does not appear to be an important cause of liver damage in congestive heart failure, as it is relatively uncommon in this condition (Evans, AmJMed, 1952; 13:704). In patients with hepatic impairment secondary to severe heart failure the arterial oxygen saturation was about 89 per cent,[12] and centrilobular necrosis on biopsy correlated poorly with arterial hypoxia in patients with heart failure.[11] Liver tests were normal in patients with hypoxia due to lung disease without heart failure (Shorey, AmJPhysiol, 1969; 216:1441; Whelan, AusAnnMed, 1969; 18:243), and the hepatic storage and excretory transfer maximum of bromsulphthalein were also normal. Experimental studies of arterial hypoxia in animals have also failed to show significant hepatic dysfunction (Shorey, AmJPhysiol, 1969; 216:1441).

Pathology of the liver in congestive heart failure

Macroscopic features

The liver in congestive heart failure is enlarged and purple in colour with rounded edges. At autopsy a cut section usually shows the 'nutmeg' appearance associated with venous distension[11,17]— regular deep-brown centrilobular zones alternating with yellow or pale-tan periportal zones. When cardiac sclerosis is present, the capsular surface is pitted and granular; on the cut surface poorly circumscribed areas of parenchymal granularity or nodularity emerge from periportal zones, the nodules being less than 1 to 2 mm in diameter. This picture differs from true cirrhosis because of the very small size of the nodules, their non-uniform distribution, poor circumscription, and their origin from periportal regions.

In one patient with severe congestive heart failure there was a large collateral vein between the right and middle hepatic veins, a feature that occurs in the Budd–Chiari syndrome (Middleton, JUS, 1994; 13:479).

Microscopic features

Heart failure may cause the histological changes of chronic passive congestion and centrilobular necrosis, but hepatic morphology can be normal. Of 75 patients with heart failure, 47 had a normal needle liver biopsy or evidence only of passive congestion.[3]

With mild congestion due to an elevated venous pressure, centrilobular hepatocytes become compressed and atrophic, and the adjacent sinusoids are engorged with blood. If there has not been severe or chronic congestion, little else is seen.[11] With increasing congestion more marked hepatocellular compression with atrophy is seen, with an extension further from the central veins. Increased brown pigment in the centrilobular liver cells is a constant finding.[11]

With prolonged heart failure and severe hepatic congestion centrilobular necrosis increases, and fibrosis develops with bridging between central veins.[17] In an autopsy series of 1000 cases, the severity of chronic passive congestion correlated with cardiac weight and chamber enlargement; centrilobular necrosis correlated best with profound hypotension, renal failure, and with acute tubular necrosis and adrenal cortical-medullary junction necrosis, two lesions associated with shock. In these patients there was a good correlation between chronic passive congestion and centrilobular necrosis.[13] However, centrilobular necrosis can occur in severe heart failure without hypotension or shock[5,6] (Kisloff, DigDis, 1976; 21:895; Kaymakcalan, AmJMed, 1978; 65:384), suggesting that it is a low cardiac output, causing decreased blood flow and parenchymal hypoxia, which is the main prerequisite for centrilobular necrosis (Ross, AmJGastr, 1981; 76:511); shock is an extreme example of a low output state.

Centrilobular necrosis in heart failure may be associated with an inflammatory reaction consisting of polymorphonuclear leucocytes, or lymphocytes and plasma cells, and this picture may depend on the duration of ischaemia.[17]

Cardiac sclerosis consists of fibrosis of the central veins and of the centrilobular region, with or without bridging to other central veins or portal tracts. In one study cardiac sclerosis was the most common form of hepatic fibrosis, occurring in 48 per cent of cases.[17]

Regenerative hyperplasia may be seen in periportal zones, the parenchyma showing a variable increase in the number of hepatocytes within liver-cell plates. In most cases with plate-thickening alone, 'twinning' of liver cells occurs, with three to five liver cells forming the plates. Affected cells are often enlarged, with a pale cytoplasm and enlarged and pleomorphic nuclei. Nodular regenerative hyperplasia has been found in a small number of cases.

Cardiac cirrhosis appears to be relatively uncommon, and can be considered as a progression from cardiac sclerosis. Central–central and central–portal fibrosis, and fibrous scars adjacent to a parenchyma showing early nodularity, are the main histological findings. The incidence varies with the population studied and the histological definition of cirrhosis. In one study of 790 patients dying of heart disease, 35 (4.4 per cent) were considered to have cardiac cirrhosis at postmortem (Koletsky, AmJMedSci, 1944; 207: 421). In another study only 1.7 per cent of 407 patients were thought to have cirrhosis (Garvin, AmJMedSci, 1943; 205:515). If fibrosis alone is considered a criterion of cirrhosis, then this occurs in about 10 per cent of adults dying of heart disease (Kotin, AmJPathol,

1951; 27:561). In a recent study Wanless *et al.* (Hepatol, 1995; 21: 1232) found evidence of thrombosis in small and medium-sized hepatic veins in patients with congestive heart failure, and suggested that congestive cirrhosis is a response to intrahepatic thrombosis, which may begin in sinusoids, propagates occasionally to hepatic veins, and causes secondary local portal vein thrombosis, ischaemia, parenchymal extinction, and fibrosis.

Shock liver

Shock liver is a severe hepatic derangement following a hypotensive or ischaemic insult[10,16] (Kantrowitz, NEJM, 1967; 276:591; Nunes, ArchSurg, 1970; 100:546; Bergens, ActaMedScand, 1978; 204:417). It occurs with haemorrhage, coronary thrombosis, sepsis (including ascending cholangitis and peritonitis), postoperative hypotension, and pulmonary embolism[16] (Das, JAMA, 1974; 230:1558; Bloth, ActaMedScand, 1976; 200:281). It is also well documented in congestive heart failure[5,6] (Kisloff, DigDis, 1976; 21:895; Kaymakcalan, AmJMed, 1978; 65:384). Liver injury resulting from hypotension is frequently associated with dysfunction of other organs (Tilney, AnnSurg, 1973; 178:117). Ischaemic hepatitis can also occur in cirrhotic patients after variceal bleeding (Henrion, JClinGastro, 1993; 16:35; Kamiyama, JClinGastro, 1996; 22:126).

The clinical picture varies from an isolated finding of very high aminotransferase levels after an episode of hypotension, to fulminant hepatic failure after acute circulatory failure, often in the setting of established chronic heart failure.[10] Jaundice, marked elevation of hepatic enzymes, and hepatic encephalopathy can all occur (Killip, Circul, 1960; 21:646). It is the duration rather than the cause of the shock that is important in the development of the syndrome. Shock of less than 24 h duration rarely causes central liver cell necrosis, although brief periods of hypotension may cause a marked increase in aminotransferases. Shock of more than 24 h does so invariably.[16] The clinical outcome depends entirely on the severity of the underlying heart disease.

Laboratory data

There is a rapid elevation of serum aminotransferases, with peak levels of 8 to 100 times the upper reference limit within 24 h (Loosli, SchMedWoch, 1981; 111:499). They fall rapidly if there is an improvement in the cardiovascular state, being less than twice normal within about 6 days. Lactate dehydrogenase is usually higher than in patients with viral hepatitis, and is almost entirely hepatic in origin. Serum bilirubin increases in most patients but rarely to more than four times normal. Alkaline phosphatase may increase up to twice normal; the prothrombin time is not usually increased by more than two seconds. Serum albumin and proteins are unaffected (Gibson, AustNZJMed, 1984; 14:822; Bergens, ActaMedScand, 1978; 204:417).

Pathological findings

In a series of 200 routine unselected autopsy cases there was evidence of central liver cell necrosis in 34, and in 32 of these there was a clear association with shock.[16] In another study, on patients with fulminant hepatic failure, due to transient circulatory failure in the presence of chronic heart disease, there was marked

congestion of central veins with sinusoidal distension, and necrosis was invariably centrilobular. Local haemorrhage, with extravasation of red cells and rupture of the sinusoids, was common. Eosinophilic staining of involved areas contrasted sharply with basophilic staining of normal liver cells. Polymorphonuclear leucocytic infiltration was often present, to a varying degree, but in some cases there was no inflammatory infiltration. Architectural disruption was a constant finding but varied in amount from case to case.[10]

Some have suggested that diffuse hepatic calcification, visible on radiographs, may be a consequence of ischaemic hepatic injury (Shibuya, Gastro, 1985; 89:196; Nguyen, AMJRadiol, 1986; 147: 596; Munoz, Hepatol, 1988; 8:476).

Pathophysiology of shock liver

The main mechanism proposed for the development of centrilobular necrosis is a severe decrease in cardiac output, the resulting hepatic hypoxia causing damage to the hepatocytes (Cohen, Gastro, 1978; 74:583; Bynum, DigDisSci, 1979; 24:129).[10,13] In a porcine model of cardiogenic shock liver, blood flow through the hepatic artery and portal vein was reduced to about a third. There was a marked increase in hepatic and preportal splanchnic vascular resistance, indicating that cardiogenic shock induced a striking vasospasm in the hepatic vascular bed; this appears to be due largely to an exquisite responsiveness of splanchnic vascular smooth muscle to endogenously released angiotensin II (Bulkley, AmJSurg, 1986; 151:87).

Hypoxia *per se* does not produce centrilobular necrosis, and in experimental shock, hepatic necrosis is not prevented by hyperbaric oxygen (Ratliff, AmJPath, 1967; 51:341). Splanchnic ischaemia may result in absorption of endotoxin from the intestinal lumen, causing portal endotoxaemia. In a rat model intraportal infusion of endotoxin resulted in a rise in serum aminotransferases and caused focal coagulative hepatocellular necrosis. However, when portal endotoxaemia was superimposed on poor hepatic perfusion there was massive hepatic necrosis and excessive elevation of serum aminotransferases (Shibayama, PatholResPract, 1987; 182:817).

Acute myocardial infarction

Many patients with acute myocardial infarction have abnormal liver function tests, even in the absence of congestive cardiac failure or significant hypotension (that is, systolic pressure <100 mmHg) (Das, JAMA, 1974; 230:1558), but there is usually no clinical evidence of hepatic involvement.

The serum total bilirubin is elevated in 50 per cent of patients, mainly due to an increase in unconjugated bilirubin (Cowan, PostgradMedJ, 1981; 57:9). Bromsulphthalein retention is increased (Das, JAMA, 1974; 230:1558). Aspartate aminotransferase levels rise with the myocardial necrosis, but alanine aminotransferase and lactate dehydrogenase levels are not consistently raised. Abnormalities are greater on the first and third days postinfarction than on the fifth.

The cause of these changes is uncertain. Cardiac output falls significantly in the first few days after an uncomplicated myocardial infarction (Murphy, AmJCard, 1963; 11:587). When myocardial ischaemia was induced in cats, by ligation of the left anterior descending coronary artery, total liver blood flow fell by 60 per cent

Table 2 Causes of constrictive pericarditis

Idiopathic
Infections
  Bacterial
  Tuberculosis
  Fungal—histoplasmosis
  Syphilitic
  Parasitic disease
    Amoebiasis
    Echinococcal disease
  Viral
Neoplastic disease
  Primary mesothelioma
  Secondary neoplasm: lung, breast, Hodgkin's disease and
    lymphoma
Post-traumatic
  Cardiac surgery
  Right ventricular myocardial infarction
  Dressler's syndrome
Connective tissue disease
  Rheumatoid arthritis
  Systemic lupus erythematosus
Radiation therapy
Uraemia
Mulibrey nanism
Secundum atrial septal defect (association)

at 5 h, supporting the idea that liver ischaemia plays a role in the changes seen in man (Galvin, Experientia, 1979; 35:1602). However, hepatic clearance of unconjugated bilirubin is relatively independent of blood flow, and some of the extra serum bilirubin may come from myoglobin released from necrotic myocardium. A reduced caloric intake during the first few days after infarction might also increase the serum bilirubin (Cowan, PostgradMedJ, 1981; 57:13).

Hypoxic hepatitis (an aminotransferase of at least 20 times the upper limit of normal with no other identifiable cause) occurred in 2.6 per cent of 766 patients admitted to a coronary care unit, and in 22 per cent of those with a low cardiac output (Henrion, JHepatol, 1994; 21:696). These patients had a higher central venous pressure and a lower hepatic blood flow.

Constrictive pericarditis and confusion with cirrhosis

Diffuse thickening of the pericardium causes pericardial constriction with restriction of ventricular filling. It is often due to tuberculosis, but has been described in a number of other conditions (Table 2). (One triumph of the late Hans Popper was to identify syphilis as the cause of constrictive pericarditis from the appearance of granulomas seen in the liver biopsy!)

The symptoms of constrictive pericarditis are initially relatively mild, and the patient may complain of little other than fatigue, slight breathlessness on effort, fullness of the abdomen, and slight dependent oedema. The condition is often confused with cirrhosis because it causes hepatomegaly and often splenomegaly, and in the later stages there may be jaundice and marked ascites. In one case acute hepatic failure occurred and hepatic coma was a presenting feature (Arora, AmJGastr, 1993; 88:430). The Budd–Chiari syndrome (Chapter 21.3), due to obstruction of hepatic venous outflow, also causes hepatomegaly, splenomegaly, and ascites formation, and may be closely mimicked by constrictive pericarditis (Solano,

AmJMed, 1986; 80:113). Constrictive pericarditis can be distinguished from cirrhosis and the Budd–Chiari syndrome because there are characteristic features in the jugular venous wave form and on cardiac auscultation, but these features are often missed.

Constrictive pericarditis may also be confused with malignant disease, myocardial disease (when the differentiation may be very difficult), with other causes of obstruction to right ventricular inflow, and with right ventricular infarction.

The pulse is usually of small volume and may diminish during inspiration. Atrial fibrillation occurs in about a third of cases. The blood pressure is usually low. The jugular venous pressure is high and may rise paradoxically during inspiration. The most striking feature in the jugular wave form is a prominent 'y' descent during early diastole, which may be accompanied by an 'x' descent early in systole when the atrium relaxes. The apical impulse is usually difficult to feel. The heart sounds are usually quiet, but there may be a loud, early third sound, or 'pericardial knock', over the right ventricle.

Chest radiography may show a large heart due to pericardial thickening, and pericardial calcification may also be seen. Echocardiography and CT scanning are useful diagnostic procedures for revealing thickened pericardium and pericardial calcification, and cardiac catheterization allows the distinction to be made between constrictive pericarditis and cirrhosis and the Budd–Chiari syndrome, although it may not allow it to be differentiated from some of the cardiac conditions that can cause confusion. When constrictive pericarditis is present, pericardial stripping leads to reversal of the clinical findings.

Hepatic pulsations in constrictive pericarditis

The liver is usually considered non-pulsatile in constrictive pericarditis. However, clinically evident pulsation of the liver has been reported, and confirmed by recording of external hepatic and jugular venous pulsations using piezoelectric sound wave transducers (Manga, BrHeartJ, 1984; 52:465; Coralli, AmJCard, 1986; 58:370). For this to occur, free communication must be present between the right atrium and inferior vena cava; this may occasionally be lost in constrictive pericarditis if there is narrowing at the junction between the right atrium and the inferior vena cava. Pulsation may also be lost in the presence of centrilobular fibrosis or cirrhosis (Dunn, AmJMedSci, 1973; 265:174).

Clinically, the pulsations are detected as a movement of the liver away from the palpating hand, corresponding to a prominent 'x' or 'y' descent of the jugular venous pulse; movement of the liver toward the palpating hand occurs when blood refluxes into the inferior vena cava and hepatic veins during the rapid increase of right atrial pressure which occurs after the 'y' descent (culminating in the 'a' wave).

Tricuspid incompetence

Functional tricuspid incompetence is commonly the result of severe right heart failure; the dilated right ventricle causes general dilatation of the valve ring and also pulls down the chordae which are attached to the edge of the valve (Loffenbach, BrHeartJ, 1957; 19:395). Organic tricuspid incompetence results from disease of the valve, and is usually due to rheumatic valvulitis; congenital tricuspid incompetence is rare (Barritt, BrHeartJ, 1956; 18:133).

With tricuspid incompetence the right ventricular pressure is transmitted into the larger veins. A 'cv' wave is seen in the neck; the liver enlarges, often quite markedly, and can be felt to pulsate. The systolic pulsation of the liver in tricuspid incompetence must be differentiated from that transmitted from the abdominal aorta. If two fingers are placed some distance apart on the surface of the enlarged liver, they separate with each pulse in tricuspid incompetence ('expansile pulsation'). The distinction is also easy if there are ventricular extrasystoles; these cause ventricular contraction with regurgitation of blood across the tricuspid valve, but without ejection of much blood into the aorta (thus explaining the absence of a second heart sound and the lack of a pulse wave in peripheral arteries). If one hand is held over the liver, and the other over a peripheral artery, then, with tricuspid incompetence, pulsation will be felt over the liver with each ventricular extrasystole (and a systolic wave will be observed in the jugular pulse), but no pulse will be felt in the peripheral artery. This 'coupled hepatic pulse' is found in patients with tricuspid incompetence and either ventricular extrasystoles or ventricular bigeminy; in the latter, two hepatic pulsations are found for each aortic pulsation (Terry, AmHeartJ, 1959; 57:158).

In a hepatic pulse tracing, tricuspid incompetence is characterized by a marked systolic wave and plateau, and by giant systolic waves in the jugular pulse tracing. In tricuspid incompetence associated with Bjork–Shiley prostheses, liver pulse tracings were found to have a higher sensitivity and specificity for detecting the incompetence than jugular venous pulse tracings, because the latter were found to show carotid pulse artefacts (Scheck-Krejca, EurHeartJ, 1986; 7:973). Pulsed Doppler hepatic vein blood flow patterns have been used to evaluate the degree of tricuspid regurgitation; they correlated well with right atrial and right ventricular diastolic pressure estimations measured during right heart catheterization (Pennestri, AmJCard, 1984; 54:363; Sakai, AmHeartJ, 1984; 108:516), and may therefore be helpful as a non-invasive method of evaluating tricuspid regurgitation.

In the presence of cardiac cirrhosis or significant centrilobular fibrosis the hepatic systolic pulsation of tricuspid incompetence may be lost (Calleja, AmJMed, 1961; 30:302; Dunn, AmJMedSci, 1973; 265:174).

Other forms of hepatic pulsation associated with heart disease

The normal liver pulse consists of 'a' and 'v' waves; the 'a' wave due to atrial contraction is followed in ventricular systole by a 'systolic collapse', due to a decrease in liver volume when the hepatic veins empty into the inferior vena cava early in ventricular contraction when the atrium relaxes. The 'v' wave then occurs in systole, when there is obstruction to the flow of blood from the atrium to the ventricle, and the hepatic volume increases again. These waves correspond to the 'a' and 'v' waves in the jugular pulse.

Hepatic pulsations occur in heart diseases other than tricuspid incompetence and constrictive pericarditis (Table 3), and can be confirmed by liver and jugular venous recordings. A pulsating liver was reported many years ago with tricuspid stenosis (Turnbull, Heart, 1911; 3:243), which causes an 'a-wave' liver pulse due to vigorous atrial contraction. Palpable presystolic hepatic pulsation

Table 3 Pulsations of the liver

Condition	Pulsation
Tricuspid stenosis	Giant a wave
Tricuspid incompetence and stenosis	Giant a wave, s (systolic) wave
Cor pulmonale	a wave
Atrial septal defect	a wave
Myocarditis	a wave
Ebstein's anomaly	a wave
Constrictive pericarditis	a = v, y>x
Budd–Chiari syndrome	a = v, y rapid

due to an 'a-wave' liver pulse may also be found in other conditions in which there is systolic, diastolic, or systolic and diastolic overloading of the right atrium; these are listed in Table 4 (George, ClinCard, 1988; 11:349).

Congenital heart disease and its association with liver disease

In a recent study, 65 infants and children with haemodynamic abnormalities were investigated to assess the effect of heart disease on hepatic function (Mace, AmJDisChild, 1985; 139:60). Fifty-four had various types of congenital heart disease; eight had cardiomyopathy, pulmonary hypertension, or shock secondary to other causes; two were normal; and one suffered from cardiomyopathy 9 years after successful repair of Fallot's tetralogy. Abnormalities of liver function were noted in most or all of the patients showing a haemodynamic abnormality, and the degree of change in the liver tests was related to the cardiac status. When patients' haemodynamic status improved with treatment, the results of liver function tests returned towards normal; worsening of the cardiac status was associated with deterioration in liver function.

Table 4 Causes of atrial hepatic pulsation

1. Systolic overloading of the right atrium
   Obstruction to right atrial outflow
     (a) Tricuspid atresia
     (b) Rhythm disturbances—complete AV block
   Obstruction to right ventricular outflow
     (a) Pulmonary artery atresia
     (b) Valvular or infundibular pulmonary stenosis (or both)
     (c) Pulmonary hypertension
   Restriction of right ventricular filling
     (a) Pericardial effusion, constrictive pericarditis
     (b) Ebstein's anomaly
2. Diastolic overloading of the right atrium
   Left to right shunt at atrial level
   Atrial septal defect
   Patent foramen ovale
   Lutembacher syndrome
   Rupture of sinus of Valsalva into right atrium
   Anomalous pulmonary veins
3. Combination of 1 and 2
   Congestive heart failure
   Primary myocardial disease with congestive heart failure
   Myocarditis

Tumours of the heart affecting the liver

Cardiac myxoma

Of 11 patients with cardiac myxoma, most showed increased levels of bilirubin, alkaline phosphatase, and lactate dehydrogenase, and total protein and albumin levels were reduced in all of them. There were also abnormalities of alpha- and gammaglobulins. These changes were attributed not to heart failure or malnutrition, but to the immune response thought to be operating in patients with cardiac myxoma (Kluge, SGO, 1972; 134:288).

Right atrial tumours causing the Budd–Chiari syndrome

In one patient a right atrial myxoma caused the Budd–Chiari syndrome because the tumour prolapsed from the right atrium into the inferior vena cava; successful removal of the tumour resulted in rapid improvement of the clinical condition (Cujec, AnnThorSurg, 1987; 44:658). There are other reports of the Budd–Chiari syndrome caused by malignant right atrial tumours, but in these the malignant process was uniformly fatal (Watts, BrHeartJ, 1947; 9:175; Feingold, ArchIntMed, 1971; 127:292). One was a primary myosarcoma of the right atrium. Thrombus caused by the tumour involved the entire length of the inferior vena cava, causing acute vena caval obstruction, and it extended into the iliac and femoral veins. Both hepatic veins contained thrombus. There was no evidence of malignancy elsewhere (Theodossi, JPath, 1979; 128:159).

Hepatic infarction

Hepatic infarction was an uncommon condition until the more widespread use of liver transplantation. Previously the most commonly reported causes were polyarteritis nodosa (Pass, AmJPathol, 1969; 11:503) and septic emboli (Mowrey, AnnIntMed, 1954; 40: 1145). Other causes include acute bacterial endocarditis (Henrich, Gastro, 1976; 68:1602), neoplasm of the liver and gallbladder (Carroll, JClinPath, 1963; 16:133), atherosclerosis (Seeley, HumPath, 1972; 3:265), and cholesterol emboli (Castleman, NEJM, 1973; 289:1360). Even rarer associations are with haemorrhagic necrotizing enteropathy (Ishii, JAmGeratSoc, 1975; 23:512), systemic scleroderma (MacMahon, SGO, 1972; 134:10), diabetic ketoacidosis (Ng, Gastro, 1977; 73:804), and ulcerative colitis (Hirsh, Gastro, 1980; 78:571).

Hepatic infarction is rare because the liver has a dual blood supply from the hepatic artery and the portal vein, and because it has an extensive arterial collateral circulation (Michels, JAMA, 1960; 172:125).

The clinical features of infarction include abdominal pain, in either the epigastrium or right upper quadrant, which may be associated with nausea, vomiting, jaundice, and fever. There are no pathognomonic laboratory tests.

In the past the condition was rarely diagnosed in life (Chen, ArchPathLabMed, 1976; 100:32). At autopsy infarcts are usually sharply demarcated, extending in a wedge shape to the periphery of the liver. Microscopically there is parenchymal necrosis in the centrilobular zone with survival of the portal tracts, hepatic veins, and intralobular stroma (Parker, JPath, 1955; 70:521).

Nowadays the most useful investigation is probably computed tomography (**CT**) or magnetic resonance imaging; in five patients with hepatic infarction, contrast-enhanced CT scans showed well-defined hepatic infarcts (Adler, AJR, 1984; 142:315). CT examination in 18 cases of proven hepatic infarction (15 post-transplant, two following laparoscopic cholecystectomy, and one after trauma) revealed 55 lesions, 53 of which which could be classified into three shapes—wedge shaped (18), which tended to be peripheral; rounded or oval (26), which were central or peripheral; and irregularly shaped, low-attenuation lesions running parallel to bile ducts (9) (Holbert, AJR, 1996; 166:815).

Polyarteritis nodosa

Polyarteritis nodosa may affect the hepatic vessels. Postmortem studies reveal involvement of the liver in 42 to 71 per cent of cases (Harris, ArchIntMed, 1939; 63:1163; Mowrey, AnnIntMed, 1954; 40:1145). Twenty-one per cent had hepatomegaly and 12 per cent were jaundiced; in only a small number (6 per cent) were other liver function tests abnormal.

There is usually a swinging fever and polymorphonuclear leucocytosis. The hepatic arteries, arterioles, and portal vein radicles may show infiltration with neutrophils, lymphocytes, eosinophils, and plasma cells, and there may be fibrinoid necrosis of the media, fibrosis with scarring, and sometimes calcification of the periportal tissues (Mowrey, AnnIntMed, 1954; 40:1145). Rupture of intra- and extrahepatic arterial aneurysms may occur (Dzwonczyk, AnnSurg, 1959; 115:479).

In 230 patients with polyarteritis nodosa, hepatic infarction occurred in 15 per cent (Mowrey, AnnInnMed, 1956; 40:1145), and in a study of 54 patients with hepatic infarction 42 per cent were due to the disease (Pass, AmJPathol, 1969; 11:503). Massive infarction has been described in association with polyarteritis nodosa (Wooling, Gastro, 1951; 17:479; Haratake, ActaPathJpn, 1988; 38: 89); for this to occur, simultaneous occlusion of both the hepatic arterial and portal venous systems would be needed, because of the complex and collateral blood supply of the liver. This was found in two of the four patients described by Wooling et al. (Gastro, 1951; 17:479).

Liver involvement in giant cell arteritis

Giant cell arteritis is characterized by granulomatous inflammation of medium- and large-sized arteries. It may affect many organs, including brain, heart, kidneys, and liver. Abnormal liver tests are common and liver biopsy may show non-caseating granulomas (McCormack, DigDis, 1978; 23:725). There is usually an elevation of alkaline phosphatase and aspartate aminotransferase, and increased retention of bromsulphthalein with normal bilirubin (Wadman, ActaMedScand, 1972; 192:327). In one study normal liver tissue was found on light microscopy, but mitochondrial abnormalities and a disorganized endoplasmic reticulum were found by electron microscopy, with cellular debris in liver sinusoids (Terwindt, ActaMedScand, 1966; 179:307).

Hereditary haemorrhagic telangiectasia

Hereditary haemorrhagic telangiectasia (Rendu–Osler–Weber disease) is an inborn error of vascular structure, with dominant inheritance and an incidence of about 1 to 2 : 100 000 in Europe. Nearly all patients have visible telangiectases on the lips, face, tongue, and/or fingertips, and similar lesions are present on the mucous membranes of the nose and gastrointestinal tract. They usually develop in the second and third decades and increase in number with age. Patients may also have pulmonary arteriovenous malformations which may allow paradoxical emboli to occur; therapeutic embolization should be considered for these lesions.

The clinical picture is usually one of frequent epistaxes, of bleeding after dental extractions or cuts, heavy menstrual bleeding, or iron deficiency due to occult gastrointestinal bleeding. Severe gastrointestinal bleeding may also occur. Not all patients with hereditary telangiectasia have a pronounced bleeding tendency. Cardiac failure may be a feature, especially in the older age group, and is probably due to the accompanying high cardiac output. There is usually a strong family history.

The liver is commonly involved in this condition and at autopsy most patients exhibit hepatic pathology (Daly, AmJMed, 1976; 60: 723). About 50 per cent develop right upper quadrant pain. The liver is often enlarged, and the spleen is enlarged in 50 per cent of cases. There is often a bruit over the liver, and sometimes a thrill (Bernard, Gastro, 1993; 105:482). Liver function is reasonably well preserved, with only slight rises in alkaline phosphatase and bilirubin levels, noted in several papers as a 'cholestatic' picture. Some patients have portal hypertension, but few develop portal systemic encephalopathy. Bleeding from oesophageal varices has been treated successfully by hepatic arterial ligation (Zentler-Munro, Gut, 1989; 30:1293).

The vascular derangement in the liver includes telangiectasia, arteriovenous fistulas, connective tissue formation with fibrosis, and atypical cirrhosis (Martini, Gut, 1978; 19:531). Three types of liver involvement have been proposed (Martini, Gastroenterologia, 1955; 83:157):

1. Telangiectasia in the liver with fibrosis and/or cirrhosis.
2. Cirrhosis and no telangiectases.
3. Telangiectases in the liver without fibrosis or cirrhosis.

Hepatic involvement has usually been confirmed by examination of biopsy or autopsy specimens or by angiography, but recently hepatic vascular malformations (almost all at a late stage of hepatic vascular derangement) have been identified using sonography, CT scanning, or magnetic resonance imaging (Bernard, Gastro, 1993; 105:482; Buscarini, AJR, 1994; 163:1105). Although real-time colour Doppler and pulsed Doppler sonography did not show intrahepatic arteriovenous shunts, they revealed dilatation, tortuosity, and increased flow in the hepatic artery, and the occasional presence of arterioportal shunts, portovenous shunts, and multiple shunts between hepatic veins (Naganuma, AJR, 1995; 165:1421).

In one female aged 33 years a liver transplant was performed for a high-output cardiac failure together with liver failure, due to biliary necrosis with refractory biliary sepsis (Bauer, JHepatol, 1995; 22:586). Biliary pathology was also found in a 65-year-old woman with hereditary haemorrhagic telangiectasia and a high cardiac output; intrahepatic gallstones caused ascending cholangitis and secondary biliary cirrhosis (Mendoza, EurJGastroHepatol, 1995; 7: 999). Intrahepatic stones have been attributed to narrowing of bile ducts due to the hepatic fibrosis which is found (Ball, ArchPathLabMed, 1990; 114:423). Nodular hyperplasia of the liver has also been described in this condition (Wanless, ArchPathLabMed, 1986; 110:331)

Thoracoabdominal aneurysm

Marked congestive hepatomegaly has been reported in association with a large thoracoabdominal aortic aneurysm (Sigal, Gastro, 1984; 87:1367); it was due to partial venous obstruction at the confluence of the hepatic veins and inferior vena cava. This is a very rare complication of unruptured aortic aneursyms, but rupture of an abdominal aortic aneurysm may cause obstruction of the inferior vena cava (Snider, Surgery, 1974; 75:613; Gertner, Surgery, 1978; 83:605).

Jaundice has been reported after surgery for a ruptured abdominal aortic aneurysm (Tilney, AnnSurg, 1973; 178:117). It is usually mild, and probably due to liver dysfunction resulting from hypovolaemic shock combined with an increased bilirubin load due to massive blood transfusion. Severe jaundice is relatively rare but has been reported, the bilirubin exceeding 400 µmol/l (Hermreck, AmJSurg, 1977; 134:745). Obstructive jaundice, due to extrahepatic obstruction of the common bile duct, occurs rarely due to expansion of an abdominal aortic aneurysm (van Someren, GastrEnd, 1993; 39:85), or to its rupture (Dickinson, TransPathSoc, 1981;42:77; Lieberman, DigDisSci, 1983; 28:88).

Fistula formation between the abdominal aorta and the inferior vena cava is very rare, but in one patient it caused a dramatic clinical picture with marked congestive hepatomegaly, a very high jugular venous pressure, and hepatic encephalopathy (Collier, EurJGastroHepatol, 1991; 3:649).

Cardiac surgery

Despite improvements in pre- and perioperative surgical and anaesthetic techniques, jaundice still occurs following cardiopulmonary bypass surgery. Early retrospective studies suggested many possible causes for this syndrome, including the age of the patient and bypass time (Robinson, Thorax, 1967; 22:232), preoperative heart failure and sepsis (Lockey, Thorax, 1967; 22: 165), hypoxia (Kantrowitz, NEJM, 1967; 276:591), blood transfusion (Geller, ArchIntMed, 1950; 86:908), hypothermia (Kingsley, Thorax, 1966; 21:91), and shock (Sanderson, AnnSurg, 1967; 165: 217).

In a later study 'post-pump' jaundice developed in 20 per cent of 248 consecutive patients undergoing cardiopulmonary bypass operations (Collins, Lancet, 1983; ii:1119). The prognosis was poor; 25 per cent of jaundiced patients died in the postoperative period but only 1 per cent of the non-jaundiced patients. Jaundice was associated with multiple valve replacement, high transfusion requirements, and long bypass time, but also occurred after uncomplicated operations. It did not appear associated with hypotension, hypoxia, hypothermia, or heart failure. It was suggested that jaundice may be due in part to a defective hepatic excretion of bilirubin. There was no evidence to support post-pump haemolysis; 75 per cent of the bilirubin was conjugated. Septicaemia did not appear to be a factor. No histological evidence of 'shock liver' was found in those patients who came to postmortem.

In another study, aspartate and alanine aminotransferase levels increased significantly during the 2 weeks following cardiac bypass; more than 25 per cent of patients had a high alkaline phosphatase level after 2 weeks. The raised aspartate aminotransferase may have resulted from skeletal muscle damage, haemolysis, myocardial damage, and/or liver damage. The serum bilirubin was up in about 25 per cent of patients. Lactate dehydrogenase isoenzyme analysis suggested myocardial or erythrocyte damage in all of the 14 patients in whom this was performed (Olsson, ScaJThorCardiovascSurg, 1984; 18:217), and liver or skeletal muscle damage in 10. An increased activity of lactate dehydrogenase isoenzyme 5 on the first postoperative day was thought to suggest liver damage.

The cause of liver damage was not clear, but there was usually no evidence of general hypoperfusion. The incidence of postoperative non-A non-B hepatitis was 9 per cent. Therefore although haemodilution, hypothermia, and cardioplegia have improved, signs of transient liver damage still occur. This did not appear to increase morbidity in this study. The high incidence of hepatitis continues to be a cause for concern with this type of surgery.

Acute liver failure following cardiac surgery in children

Acute liver failure is a rare complication of low cardiac output in children after cardiac operations. In one report, 11 of 1979 children undergoing cardiac surgery developed this condition; six of them died from myocardial failure (Jenkins, JThoracCardiovascSurg, 1982; 84:865). Six had had modified Fontan procedures for tricuspid atresia, and four of these died. The greatest risk of hepatic failure occurred in children with a low cardiac output for more than 24 h, and all the patients had very high right atrial pressures. Seven patients developed hepatic disease during the first or second postoperative day; in the remaining four it was not detected until 6 to 9 days. Viral hepatitis seemed an unlikely cause, none received halothane and there was no clinical or bacteriological evidence of septicaemia.

The clinical picture was that of acute hepatocellular failure, with marked elevation of the aspartate aminotransferase level. Alkaline phosphatase levels were normal but there was marked prolongation of the prothrombin time. All the patients developed acute renal failure. Hypoglycaemia occurred in seven patients and was profound in two; it could only be detected by routine testing of blood glucose, as all patients were lethargic or comatose for other reasons. Restoration of hepatic perfusion pressure caused a rapid decline of aspartate aminotransferase levels, suggesting a low cardiac output as the primary aetiological factor.

In a group of 15 patients following a modified Fontan operation for single ventricle, or for tricuspid or mitral atresia, most had abnormal liver function. In three of them hepatic venous oxygen saturation was monitored and showed a marked decrease to below 20 per cent, with subsequent hepatic dysfunction. It was suggested that low cardiac output and hepatic hypoperfusion may be more important than a high central venous pressure in causing hepatic dysfunction in these cases (Matsuda, JThoracCardiovascSurg, 1988; 96:219). Takano *et al.* (JThoracCardiovascSurg, 1994; 108:700) considered that a hepatic venous oxygen saturation value below 25 per cent during the first 24 h after a Fontan operation predicts the occurrence and severity of acute liver dysfunction. They suggested monitoring of the hepatic venous oxygen saturation during this period.

Abnormalities of liver function tests were found in 40 of 66 patients who underwent a Fontan procedure in the previous 1 to 14 years (Cromme-Dijkhuis, JThoracCardiovascSurg, 1993; 106:

1126). Earlier reports described hepatic cirrhosis developing after modified 'Fontan' operations (right atrial–right ventricular conduits) for tricuspid atresia (Stanton, Circul, 1981; 2:140; Lemmer, JThoracCardiovascSurg, 1983; 86:757). The histological findings were of fibrous septa bridging central veins. Necrosis and subsequent fibrosis spread to incorporate some portal tracts in the later stages. Increased hepatic venous pressure and decreased hepatic blood flow are thought to be the main cause of the damage.

Hepatitis B transmission

Five patients operated upon by a cardiac surgeon incubating hepatitis B were infected with hepatitis B virus (Haerem, ActaMedScand, 1981; 21:389). Patients infected during open-heart surgery and cardiopulmonary bypass run a particular risk of becoming HBsAg carriers.

Over 4 to 5 years, 67 of 243 patients undergoing cardiac transplantation subsequently became HBsAg positive. The HBsAg subtype in 63 of them was ay, suggesting a common source of infection. The infection appeared to be transmitted at the time of endomyocardial biopsy, performed on the same day and in the same room after biopsy of HBsAg-positive patients (Drescher, JHospInf, 1994; 26:81).

Herpes simplex hepatitis following coronary artery bypass surgery

Herpes simplex hepatitis has been reported in one patient undergoing coronary artery bypass surgery (Williams, AmHeartJ, 1985; 110:679). Steroids were started 5 days postoperatively for postcardiotomy syndrome, and at 8 days liver enzymes were markedly deranged. On day 10 disseminated intravascular coagulation developed and death occurred following laparotomy for massive upper gastrointestinal tract bleeding. Postmortem examination revealed necrosis of the liver; herpes simplex virus was seen in some hepatocytes on microscopic examination, and it was cultured from the liver and spleen.

Prosthetic valve-induced haemolysis causing gallstones

There were early reports of a significant increase of pigment gallstones in patients in whom prosthetic heart valves were inserted (Merendino, AnnSurg, 1973; 177:694). Thirty-one per cent of males had gallstones at 3 years following valve implant. These patients often developed an acquired chronic haemolytic state, but most had evidence of only mild haemolysis.

Budd–Chiari syndrome due to pacemaker-induced thrombosis

Lu *et al.* (JGastHepatol, 1995; 10:355) reported the development of the Budd–Chiari syndrome in a 34-year-old female several years after the insertion of a permanent pacemaker. Echocardiography and superior and inferior cavography revealed thrombus extending from the superior vena cava, through the right atrium, and into the inferior vena cava. Clinical symptoms improved after removal of the pacemaker and thoracotomy and thrombectomy.

Hepatic trauma

Hepatic trauma has been described following cardiopulmonary bypass (Eugene, JCardiovascSurg, 1986; 27:100). The hepatic damage may have been associated with the insertion of thoracic tubes following median sternotomy, or possibly by laceration by the falciform ligament secondary to traction on the chest wall.

Rupture of the liver secondary to external cardiac massage

Laceration of the liver was found in about 3 per cent of postmortems performed following external cardiac massage (Baringer, NEMJ, 1961; 265:62; Silberberg, SGO, 1964; 119:6; Paaske, DanMedBull, 1968; 15:225; Jeresaty, ArchIntMed, 1969; 124:588); most of these patients had undergone vigorous massage. Children appear more susceptible to this liver injury due, perhaps, to their small size and high-lying diaphragm (Thaler, NEJM, 1962; 267:500).

Traumatic laceration presents with clinical signs of intra-abdominal haemorrhage and shock, and signs of haemoperitoneum with peritonism. Surgical repair is the only effective management. The mortality associated with surgery is, as one would expect, very high, being over 40 per cent (Dumoulin, AnnMedIntern, 1981; 132:26).

The liver in pulmonary disease

Hepatic abnormalities are less common with primary pulmonary disease than with cardiovascular disease. Clinical evidence of liver disease and abnormal liver function tests are noted occasionally in pulmonary disorders, and a number of diseases affect both the liver and lungs; for example, cystic fibrosis (Chapter 20.4), sarcoidosis (Chapter 14.2), and histiocytosis X.

Altered liver function with chronic respiratory disease

Early studies suggested that aminotransferases and lactate dehydrogenase may increase in chronic pulmonary disease, but only when the arterial oxygen content is very low (Refsum, ClinSci, 1963; 25:369). Subsequently, aspartate aminotransferase and alanine aminotransferase, total bilirubin, alkaline phosphatase, and γ-glutamyl transferase were all found to be significantly higher in patients with chronic respiratory insufficiency than in controls (Bayego, RevClinEsp, 1982;166:137); all patients with these abnormalities had a Po_2 below 60 mmHg. Having assessed the relative importance of arterial oxygen saturation, arterial carbon dioxide, and right ventricular pressure, the authors concluded that hypoxia was the sole factor contributing to the abnormal liver function tests.

Acute hypoxia impairs bromsulphthalein clearance in patients (Kaufman, NEJM, 1950; 242:90; Leevy, JAMA, 1961; 178:151), guinea-pigs, and mice (Shorey, AmJPhysiol, 1969; 216:1441), affecting transport between liver cells and bile canuliculi. Animal studies suggest that severe hypoxia is necessary before hepatic excretory function is affected; the addition of 5 per cent CO_2 reduced the adverse effect of hypoxia on hepatic excretion of bromsulphthalein, at least partly, by increasing Po_2. Severe hypoxia also inhibited the hepatic transport of fluorescein in anaesthetized rats (Hanzon, ActaPhysiolScand, 1952; 101:268; Reese, BrJExpPath, 1960; 41:527); the mechanism is unclear but may be related to increased permeability of damaged hepatocytes (Bayego, RevClin Esp, 1982; 166:135).

Whelan et al. (AustAnnMed, 1969; 216:243) found no impairment of hepatic function, despite hypoxia ranging from 44 to 83 mmHg Po_2, in patients with chronic bronchitis (with or without emphysema); they suggested that a degree of heart failure is necessary to produce abnormalities of liver function tests. Heart failure may play a part in causing centrilobular liver cell necrosis. In a study of 35 patients with respiratory failure, 35 patients with congestive cardiac failure, and 47 patients with both types of failure, neither simple passive liver congestion nor isolated hypoxaemia appeared adequate to account for abnormalities of liver function, except for an increase of alkaline phosphatase. The coexistence of both factors was thought to be necessary (Xarau, RevClinEsp, 1979; 155:97).

Severe asthma

Elevation of aspartate and alanine aminotransferases has been reported in severe asthma (Colldahl, ActaMedScand, 1960; 166:399), more often during status asthmaticus than during recovery, and the increase in enzymes may be related to the severity of the attack (El-Shaboury, BMJ, 1964; i:1220).

Obstructive sleep apnoea and ischaemic hepatitis

An obese patient developed massive centrilobular hepatic necosis, severe coagulopathy, encephalopathy, and acute renal failure. This acute liver disease was attributed to liver cell hypoxia resulting from severe arterial hypoxaemia due to obstructive sleep apnoea; this was demonstrated by measurement of nocturnal blood oxygen saturation, the results of a polysomnographic study, and normal baseline pulmonary function tests (Mathurin, Gastro, 1995; 109:1682).

Pneumonia

It has been recognized for many years that the liver may be affected in patients with pneumococcal pneumonia. Jaundice has been reported in 3 to 26 per cent of cases, even after the advent of antibiotic therapy (Curphey, AmJMedSci, 1938; 196:348; Zimmerman, JLabClinMed, 1950; 35:556; Radford, MedJAust, 1967; 2:678; Douglas, AustNZJMed, 1974; 4:346). It usually appears between the third and sixth day of the illness, and tends to be associated with consolidation of the right lower lobe. The liver may or may not be enlarged, but hepatic tenderness is common, and the spleen is occasionally palpable. Fever tends to last longer in jaundiced patients but the presence of jaundice does not appear to be associated with a worse prognosis. In some cases liver tests suggest a hepatocellular disturbance (Zimmerman, JLabClinMed, 1950; 35:556; Radford, MedJAust, 1967; 2:678); the serum bilirubin is usually around 70 μmol/l and may reach 350, but there is only a modest elevation in those with raised aminotransferases and some show a slight increase in alkaline phosphatase. Others have noted a cholestatic picture (Fahrlender, Gastro, 1964; 47:590; Theron, JPath, 1972; 106:113).

The rise in bilirubin has been attributed to a non-specific response to infection; the mechanism is unknown, but hypoxia, fever, and direct toxicity have been implicated (Zimmerman, Gastro, 1979; 77:362). In many series there was a striking male predominance in the incidence of jaundice. In one study most had glucose 6-phosphate dehydrogenase deficiency (Tugwell, Lancet, 1973; i:968), a sex-linked trait with full expression in males and in female homozygotes. This suggests that an acute haemolysis may contribute to the jaundice (although bilirubinuria is also present), which explains why jaundice associated with lobar pneumonia is so common in Africans (Gelfand, SAMedJ, 1942; 16:432) and Afro-Americans (Turner, SouthMedJ, 1943; 36:603), in whom there is a high prevalence of glucose 6-phosphate dehydrogenase deficiency.

Few histological abnormalities are seen on liver biopsy (Clain, CentrAfrMedJ, 1964; 10:217). Abnormal bromsulphthalein retention has been documented (Zimmerman, JLabClinMed, 1950; 35:556); however, fever alone can affect this test (Blaschke, AnnIntMed, 1973; 78:221). Microsomal function is impaired in some patients, as indicated by a decrease in antipyrine metabolism (Sonne, ClinPharmTher, 1985; 37:701), therefore caution should be exercised when patients with pneumonia are treated with drugs metabolized by the liver.

Legionnaire's disease (Chapter 13.1.1)

Liver function tests are often abnormal in legionnaire's disease. There are increases in aspartate aminotransferase and alkaline phosphatase in about 50 per cent of reported cases (Kirby, AnnIntMed, 1978; 89:297; Kirby, Medicine, 1980; 59:188). Elevations of bilirubin are less common, occurring in about 20 per cent of patients. The increase in aminotransferases was thought to be relatively specific for legionnaire's disease, but it is seen in many other pneumonias, including psittacosis and mycoplasma pneumonia (Yu, AmJMed, 1982; 73:357). Cytomegalovirus pneumonia can also cause an elevation of aminotransferases and alkaline phosphatase (Oill, AmJMed, 1977; 62:413).

Jaundice, when it does occur, appears to be associated with severe illness. It is rarely a presenting feature of the disease but this has been reported (Verneau, GastrClinBiol, 1987; 11:254).

Biopsy findings include a chronic portal infiltrate, a sinusoidal polymorphonuclear neutrophil infiltrate, Kupffer cell hyperplasia, and centrilobular congestion (Weisenburger, ArchPathLabMed, 1981; 105:130; Winn, HumPath, 1981; 12:401). A rare histological finding, mitochondrial margination, has been reported in liver cells in a case of legionnaire's disease (Verneau, GastrClinBiol, 1987; 11: 254).

Liver involvement in carcinoma of the lung

Liver involvement is found unexpectedly in 28 to 37 per cent of patients with small cell lung cancer (Matthews, CancChemoRep, 1973; 4:63; Ihde, AmRevRespDis, 1981; 123:500); the liver is a frequent site of recurrence. Peritoneoscopy with biopsy appears the most sensitive method of detecting liver secondaries, as it detects cases missed on blind biopsy; radionuclide and CT scanning are the most accurate non-invasive procedures (Mulshine, JClinOncol, 1984; 2:733). Extrahepatic biliary obstruction is reported rarely, although one study described 12 patients with small cell lung cancer presenting with jaundice; five had pancreatic metastases causing

extrahepatic bile duct obstruction, and they responded to chemotherapy with resolution of jaundice; seven had diffuse hepatic metastases without extrahepatic obstruction, and they remained icteric despite treatment (Johnson, AnnIntMed, 1985; 102:487).

Intravascular bronchiolo-alveolar tumours rarely spread to extrapulmonary sites. However, there are at least two reports of metastatic spread to the liver (Dial, Cancer, 1983; 51:452; Gledhill, JClinPath, 1984; 37:279).

Sarcoidosis, tuberculosis, histoplasmosis, and cystic fibrosis

See Chapter 14.2 (sarcoidosis), Chapter 13.1.1 (tuberculosis), Chapter 13.2 (histoplasmosis), and Chapter 20.4 (cystic fibrosis).

Histiocytosis X

Histiocytosis X is a term used to describe a group of clinical disorders (Letterer–Siwe disease, Hand–Schuller–Christian disease, and eosinophilic granuloma) in which there is proliferation of histiocytes, which include macrophages of the monuclear phagocytic system and cells of the dendritic cell family; both are accessory cells in the immune response, presenting antigen or mitogen to T lymphocytes. The Langerhans cell, the dendritic cell of the dermis, is considered to be the key cell in the active lesions of histiocytosis X (Favara, HumPath, 1983; 14:663).

This uncommon condition occurs worldwide. The aetiology and pathogenesis are unknown. The disease spectrum is very wide, ranging from involvement of one bone in eosinophilic granuloma, to a disseminated disease involving skin, lymph nodes, lung, liver, thymus, spleen, and bone marrow. Patients often have skin lesions, otitis media, lytic bone lesions, diabetes insipidus, and lymphadenopathy. Lung lesions are common, with destruction of alveoli and infiltration of the airways, resulting in focal cystic changes and airways obstruction; lung disease may be complicated by infections and problems related to aspiration. Extensive pulmonary fibrosis is a late fatal complication of this disease.

Liver involvement occurs in about 40 to 60 per cent of those with disseminated disease. Usually there is only hepatomegaly, without other overt hepatic manifestations, but some patients become jaundiced and may show marked abnormalities of liver function tests. Jaundice has been considered an ominous sign (Lahey, JPediat, 1962; 60:664). The clinical picture may be of prolonged cholestasis with a cholangiographic picture identical to that of primary sclerosing cholangitis (Leblanc, Gastro, 1981; 80:134; Thompson, Gut, 1984; 25:526). Hepatic fibrosis, biliary cirrhosis, and portal hypertension may develop (Grosfeld, AmJSurg, 1976; 131:108) with splenomegaly and bleeding from oesophageal varices; the spleen may also be directly involved by the disease. The biliary cirrhosis may result either from lesions in the biliary tract (Heitner, SAMedJ, 1978; 53:768) or from histiocytic infiltration of the parenchyma (Parker, AmJClinPath, 1963; 40: 624). In one patient there was an association with erythropoietic protoporphyria, which may have been exacerbated by the liver disease (Graham-Brown, JRSM, 1984; 77:238).

The liver is a useful organ to biopsy for diagnostic purposes even when there are no features suggesting hepatic disease (Jurco, HumPath, 1983; 14:1059). Light microscopy may show granulomas containing histiocytic cells; if they are absent, electron microscopy may show the Langerhans cells which have distinct cytoplasmic granules (Birbeck granules); sinusoidal and portal histiocytes may be hypertrophied. There may be periportal ductular proliferation, cholestasis, and even bile lakes.[18]

Effect of drugs used in pulmonary disease on liver function

Inhaled disodium chromoglycate has been reported as causing an illness like primary biliary cirrhosis in one patient (Rosenberg, ArchIntMed, 1978; 138:989). There was marked eosinophilia and cutaneous vasculitis with an elevation of aspartate and alanine aminotransferases, alkaline phosphatase, and serum IgG and IgM, and positive tests for antimitochondrial antibody and rheumatoid factor, suggesting an immunological mechanism. The tests, including the positive antimitochondrial antibody, returned to normal after stopping the drug. Liver biopsy showed portal areas expanded by eosinophils, lymphocytes, and plasma cells, and the presence of granulomas.

One report suggested that theophylline might have caused elevations of aspartate aminotransferase in children on long-term treatment with this drug for asthma; these changes occurred when they became ill during an epidemic of influenza, and their blood levels were in the toxic range. The drug had been well tolerated previously (Schuller, ImmunolAllergPract, 1981; 111:27).

References

1. Strickler BHCh. *Drug-induced hepatic injury*, (2nd edn). Amsterdam: Elsevier, 1992.
2. Farrell GC. *Drug-induced liver disease*. Edinburgh: Churchill Livingstone, 1994.
3. White TJ, Leevy CM, Brusca AM, and Gnassi AM. The liver in congestive heart failure. *American Heart Journal*, 1955; 49: 250–7.
4. Dunn GD, Hayes P, Breen KJ, and Schenker S. The liver in congestive heart failure: a review. *American Journal of Medical Sciences*, 1973; 265: 174–89.
5. Moussavian SN, Dincsoy HP, Goodman S, Helm RA, and Bozian RC. Severe hyperbilirubinemia and coma in chronic congestive heart failure. *Digestive Diseases and Sciences*, 1982; 27: 175–9.
6. Gadeholt H and Haugen J. Centrilobular hepatic necrosis in cardiac failure: one case with severe acute jaundice. *Acta Medica Scandinavica*, 1964; 176: 525–7.
7. Richman SM, Delman AJ, and Grob D. Alterations in indices of liver function in congestive heart failure with particular reference to serum enzymes. *American Journal of Medicine*, 1961; 30: 211–25.
8. Garvin CF. Cardiac cirrhosis. *American Journal of Medical Sciences*, 1943; 205: 515–18.
9. Kubo SH, Walter BA, John DHA, Clark M, and Cody RJ. Liver function abnormalities in chronic heart failure: influence of systemic hemodynamics. *Archives of Internal Medicine*, 1987; 147: 1227–9.
10. Nouel O, Henrion J, Bernuau J, Degott C, Rueff B, and Benhamou JP. Fulminant hepatic failure due to transient circulatory failure in patients with chronic heart disease. *Digestive Diseases and Sciences*, 1980; 25: 49–52.
11. Sherlock S. The liver in heart failure: relation of anatomical, functional and circulatory changes. *British Heart Journal*, 1957; 13: 273–93.
12. Losowsky MS, Ikram H, Snow HM, Hargreave FE, and Nixon FE. Liver function in advanced heart disease. *British Heart Journal*, 1965; 27: 578–84.
13. Arcidi JM, Moore GW, and Hutchins GM. Hepatic morphology in cardiac dysfunction: a clinicopathologic study of 100 subjects at autopsy. *American Journal of Pathology*, 1981; 104: 160–5.
14. Myers JD and Hickman JB. An estimation of the hepatic blood flow and splanchnic oxygen consumption in heart failure. *Journal of Clinical Investigation*, 1948; 27: 620–7.
15. Rapaport E, Weisbart MH, and Levine M. The splanchnic blood volume in congestive heart failure. *Circulation*, 1958; 18: 581–7.
16. Ellenberg M and Osserman KE. The role of shock in the production of central liver cell necrosis. *American Journal of Medicine*, 1951; 11: 170–8.
17. Lefkowich JH and Mendez L. Morphological features of hepatic injury in cardiac disease and shock. *Journal of Hepatology*, 1986; 2: 313–27.
18. Ishak KG and Sharp HL. Developmental abnormality and liver disease in childhood. In MacSween RNM, Anthony PP, and Scheuer PJ, eds. *Pathology of the liver*. 2nd edn. Edinburgh: Churchill Livingstone, 1987: 66–98.

24.2 The effect of gastrointestinal diseases on the liver and biliary tract

R. W. Chapman and Peter W. Angus

The hepatobiliary system and the alimentary tract are closely linked, not only anatomically but also physiologically and biochemically. It is not surprising, therefore, that the liver is especially vulnerable to the development of complications of many different gastrointestinal diseases. This chapter will attempt to classify and elucidate the effect of various gastrointestinal diseases on the hepatobiliary system.

Hepatobiliary complications of inflammatory bowel diseases

The first association between colonic ulceration and liver disease was made in 1874 by Thomas; he described a young man who died of a 'much enlarged, fatty liver in the presence of ulceration of the colon'.[1] The association was confirmed by Lister in 1899, who reported a patient with ulcerative colitis and secondary diffuse hepatitis.[2] Since then the close relationship between inflammatory bowel disease and various hepatobiliary disorders has become well established. These disorders are listed in Table 1.

In the last decade, a different concept of hepatobiliary disorder in inflammatory bowel disease has emerged. It is now apparent that the major hepatobiliary diseases seen in association with both ulcerative colitis and Crohn's disease, namely pericholangitis, primary sclerosing cholangitis, cholangiocarcinoma, and most cases of chronic active hepatitis, represent different aspects of the same spectrum of hepatobiliary disease.

Prevalence of liver disease

The prevalence of liver disease in patients with ulcerative colitis and Crohn's disease has varied widely in different series. The discrepancy between the series may be largely due to differences in the number of patients included with severe, active, or extensive inflammatory bowel disease, and also in the methods used to identify liver involvement.

Abnormal liver function tests are found in over half of patients with inflammatory bowel disease requiring surgery and are due to a number of factors such as malnutrition, sepsis, and blood transfusions with the subsequent risk of viral infection. However, significant liver disease is much less common. The true prevalence of hepatobiliary abnormality is difficult to determine as it would involve obtaining liver histology and cholangiography on an unselected group of patients with inflammatory bowel disease. Most series, therefore, have relied upon detecting persistent abnormalities

Table 1 Hepatobiliary diseases associated with inflammatory bowel disease		
	Ulcerative colitis	**Crohn's disease**
Primary sclerosing cholangitis	+	+
Small-duct primary sclerosing cholangitis (pericholangitis)	+	+
Chronic active hepatitis	(+)	−
Cirrhosis	+	+
Cholangiocarcinoma	+	(+)
Hepatocellular carcinoma	(+)	−
Fatty liver	+	+
Granulomas	(+)	+
Amyloidosis	(+)	+
Gallstones	−	+*
Hepatic abscess	−	+
Drug reactions	+	+
Primary biliary cirrhosis	(+)	−

+ =Definite association; (+)=possible association; − =no association.
* Crohn's disease involving the terminal ileum.

on serum biochemical testing before proceeding to hepatic biopsy or endoscopic retrograde cholangiography.

In an early study from Oxford (Perret, QJMed, 1971; 40:211), 5 to 6 per cent of 300 unselected adult patients with ulcerative colitis had significant histological abnormalities on hepatic histology compared with 10 per cent of 100 unselected patients with Crohn's disease; none of these patients underwent cholangiography. A group of 336 Norwegian patients with ulcerative colitis and persistently abnormal liver function tests were investigated using cholangiography by Schrumpf et al.[3] More than 14 per cent of patients had some form of hepatobiliary disease and 5 per cent of all patients had primary sclerosing cholangitis, although most were asymptomatic. Similar results were obtained in 1500 Swedish patients with ulcerative colitis (Olsson, Gastro, 1991; 100:1319). In this thorough study, endoscopic cholangiography was obtained in 65 of 72 patients with elevated values of serum alkaline phosphatase. Primary sclerosing cholangitis was diagnosed in 3.7 per cent of the ulcerative colitis group. The prevalence was 5.5 per cent in patients with extensive colitis and only 0.5 per cent in patients with distal disease. These figures may be an underestimate, as a study from the Mayo Clinic has shown that standard liver function tests may be normal despite the presence of primary sclerosing cholangitis on cholangiography (Balasubramanian, Gastro, 1989; 95:1385).

The prevalence of hepatobiliary abnormalities with normal liver function tests has been investigated in a study from Sweden (Broome, Gut, 1990; 31:468). Liver biopsies were assessed from 74 patients with ulcerative colitis and normal liver function tests. Fifty per cent had a completely normal liver biopsy. The biopsies of three patients with total colitis displayed concentric periductular fibrosis and the rest showed minimal portal inflammation or fatty infiltration. The patients were then followed for a mean of 18 years. None of the three patients with concentric fibrosis developed abnormal liver function tests; cholangiography was not performed. Two other patients developed chronic liver disease; cirrhosis in one and autoimmune chronic hepatitis and cholangiocarcinoma in the other.

In summary, approximately 5 per cent of adult patients with inflammatory bowel disease will have significant hepatobiliary disease. Although the number of patients with hepatobiliary abnormality is approximately the same for ulcerative colitis and Crohn's disease, severe significant liver disease is more commonly seen in patients with ulcerative colitis and when it occurs in Crohn's disease it is usually associated with extensive colonic involvement.

The relationship of primary sclerosing cholangitis with inflammatory bowel disease

Primary sclerosing cholangitis is a chronic cholestatic liver disease characterized by an obliterative inflammatory fibrosis which usually involves the whole biliary tree.[4,5] A full description of the aetiology, clinicopathological features, and management of primary sclerosing cholangitis is provided (see Chapter 14.4). In this section the close relationship between primary sclerosing cholangitis and inflammatory bowel disease, particularly ulcerative colitis, will be discussed.

Approximately 70 per cent of Caucasian patients with primary sclerosing cholangitis have coexisting ulcerative colitis (Table 2) and primary sclerosing cholangitis is the most common form of chronic liver disease found in ulcerative colitis. Some believe that all patients with primary sclerosing cholangitis will develop inflammatory bowel disease. Three studies from different parts of the world have reviewed the clinical features of patients with ulcerative colitis and primary sclerosing cholangitis.[3-5] The findings from all three studies have been remarkably consistent. Paradoxically, the colitis is usually total but symptomatically mild, often with no rectal bleeding, and is frequently characterized by prolonged remissions. Interestingly, in patients with ulcerative colitis and primary sclerosing cholangitis there is a male predominance, with a male–female ratio of 2:1, which contrasts with the slight female predominance of primary sclerosing cholangitis in isolation (Rabinovitz, Hepatol, 1991; 11:7)

Cigarette smoking has been recognized as a protective factor against the development of ulcerative colitis. Two recent studies suggested that cigarette smoking may also protect against the development of primary sclerosing cholangitis. This protective effect was more marked in patients with primary sclerosing cholangitis than ulcerative colitis and was seen in patients with and without inflammatory bowel disease (Loftus, Gastro, 1996; 110:1496; Van Erpeciun, Gastro, 1996; 110:503). The mechanism of protection in both disorders remains unknown.

Although the symptoms of ulcerative colitis usually develop before those of sclerosing cholangitis, the onset of primary sclerosing cholangitis may precede the symptoms of colitis by up to 4 years. Although large-scale studies have not been performed, there is some evidence that the prevalence of liver abnormality may be higher in children than adults. Abnormal liver function tests were detected in 60 per cent of 34 children with ulcerative colitis; abnormalities were most commonly seen in total colitis. Cholangiography was only performed in two patients, one of whom had sclerosing cholangitis (Nemeth, Liver, 1990; 10:239). The outcome of the hepatobiliary disease is completely unrelated to the activity, severity, or clinical course of the colitis. This is borne out by the fact that colectomy makes no difference to the clinical progression or to the mortality of patients with primary sclerosing cholangitis. Indeed, liver disease may develop some years after a total colectomy has been performed (Cangemi, Gastro, 1989; 96:790). Patients with combined ulcerative colitis and primary sclerosing cholangitis may have a worse prognosis from liver disease than patients with primary sclerosing cholangitis alone (Wiesner, Hepatol, 1989; 10:430).

The increased frequency of bile-duct cancer, including carcinoma of the gallbladder, in patients with ulcerative colitis is well established (Ritchie, QJMed, 1974; 43:263). It is also clear that carcinoma of the bile duct may develop in patients with longstanding primary sclerosing cholangitis and ulcerative colitis. There is accumulating evidence that patients with both primary sclerosing cholangitis and ulcerative colitis have an increased neoplastic potential to develop colonic and bile-duct cancer compared with those with ulcerative colitis alone. In a retrospective case–control study, 40 patients with both primary sclerosing cholangitis and ulcerative colitis were each matched to 2 control patients of the same age with extensive colitis of a comparable duration but without primary sclerosing cholangitis. The cumulative risk of developing colorectal dysplasia or carcinoma in the group with primary sclerosing cholangitis was 9, 31, and 50 per cent after 10, 20, and 25 years of disease duration compared with 2, 5, and 10 per cent, respectively, in the group with ulcerative colitis alone. Cholangiocarcinoma

Table 2 Prevalence of inflammatory bowel disease in patients with primary sclerosing cholangitis

Institution (year published)	Number of patients	Percentage with inflammatory bowel disease
Royal Free Hospital (1980)	29	72
Mayo Clinic (1980)	50	70
Yale (1987)	53	62
King's College Hospital (children) (1987)	13	77
Oslo (1989)	60	98

complicating primary sclerosing cholangitis was detected in 17 per cent of patients (Broome, Hepatol, 1995; 22:1404). Furthermore, cholangiocarcinoma developed significantly more often in patients with colonic dysplasia or carcinoma, thus suggesting that these patients may constitute a high-risk subgroup requiring increased colonic and biliary surveillance. However, further prospective studies are needed to confirm these findings.

Orthotopic liver transplantation is the only effective treatment for primary sclerosing cholangitis, and the presence of inflammatory bowel disease does not affect the outcome but is associated with a higher rate of severe acute graft rejection (Miki, BrJSurg, 1995; 82: 114). Colon cancer represents the most common cause of death after liver transplantation and increased colonic surveillance is required (Narumi, Hepatol, 1995; 22:451). Patients with ulcerative colitis treated by colectomy with an ileal reservoir (pouch) are sometimes affected by a non-specific inflammation of the pouch (pouchitis). This complication is more common in patients who have primary sclerosing cholangitis (Penna, Gut, 1996; 38:234), although there is no good explanation for this association.

There are fewer reports of primary sclerosing cholangitis associated with Crohn's disease, and the prevalence of bile-duct carcinoma is not increased in Crohn's disease. The explanation for these apparent differences in prevalence between the two diseases is unclear but may be related to the less frequent occurrence of total colonic involvement in patients with Crohn's disease.

Small-duct primary sclerosing cholangitis—'pericholangitis'

Pericholangitis is a histological diagnostic term that has been used to describe inflammatory reactions in the portal zones of the liver which are characterized by periductular inflammation and fibrosis. For many years, the term 'pericholangitis' has been synonymous with involvement of the liver in inflammatory bowel disease (Mistilis, AnnIntMed, 1965; 63:1). Some patients with pericholangitis have been shown to progress to cirrhosis of the liver and cholangiocarcinoma (Boden, Lancet, 1959; ii:245). However, it has become clear that most patients with histological pericholangitis and persistently abnormal liver function tests will have cholangiographic appearances diagnostic of primary sclerosing cholangitis at endoscopic retrograde cholangiography (Blackstone, DigDisSci, 1978; 23:579; Shepherd, QJMed, 1983; 52:503). A minority of patients with ulcerative colitis will have persistently abnormal liver function tests, together with histological appearances such as concentric fibrosis, but have normal bile ducts at cholangiography. The term 'small-duct primary sclerosing cholangitis' has been proposed to

replace the term 'pericholangitis' in this group of patients as the evidence suggests that these conditions are all part of the same disease spectrum. Wee and Ludwig have described two patients who progressed from small-duct primary sclerosing cholangitis to develop extrahepatic biliary involvement diagnostic of sclerosing cholangitis.[6] It is clear that patients with small-duct sclerosing cholangitis are just as likely to develop cholangiocarcinoma as patients with large-duct disease.

A number of other portal tract lesions such as chronic periportal inflammation and/or increased cellularity of portal tracts have also been described as 'pericholangitis' in patients with ulcerative colitis.

In view of the confusing use of the term pericholangitis, which has been applied to a heterogeneous mixture of hepatobiliary disorders by different authors, it has been proposed that the term and concept of pericholangitis should be abandoned (Desmet, JPath, 1987; 151:247).[6]

Chronic active hepatitis

Chronic active hepatitis has been reported to occur in association with ulcerative colitis (Olsson, ScaJGastr, 1975; 10:331). However, piecemeal necrosis on liver histology can accompany the classic bile-duct changes of primary sclerosing cholangitis on cholangiography[4] and it seems likely that most patients with chronic active hepatitis and inflammatory bowel disease will have either large- or small-duct primary sclerosing cholangitis. The diagnosis of chronic active hepatitis should not be made in patients with inflammatory bowel disease unless cholangiography is normal. The diagnostic difficulties are compounded by the presence of circulating serum autoantibodies such as antinuclear antibodies, smooth muscle antibodies, antineutrophil cytoplasmic antibodies, and elevated serum immunoglobulins in some patients with primary sclerosing cholangitis.[4] Moreover, both autoimmune chronic active hepatitis and primary sclerosing cholangitis are associated with an increased prevalence of the tissue antigens HLA B8 and HLA DR3 (Donaldson, Hepatol, 1991; 13:189; Manage, Hepatol, 1993; 18:1334), and overlap syndromes exist (Gahike, JHepatol, 1996; 24:699). It is unclear from current evidence whether the prevalence of chronic active hepatitis without underlying sclerosing cholangitis is increased in patients with inflammatory bowel disease.

Cirrhosis

The incidence of cirrhosis associated with inflammatory bowel disease has varied in different series between 1 and 5 per cent (Tumen, AnnIntMed, 1947; 26:542; Holdsworth, QJMed, 1965; 34: 211; Lupinetti, AmJSurg, 1980; 139:113; Schrumpf, ScaJGastr,

1980; 15:689). Most patients are classified as having biliary cirrhosis and, since patients with sclerosing cholangitis can present with portal hypertension and established cirrhosis with no preceding symptoms, it seems likely that most of these patients will have underlying endstage primary sclerosing cholangitis. However, not all patients with cirrhosis and inflammatory bowel disease will have primary sclerosing cholangitis, and it is possible that some cases may be due to chronic hepatitis C infection (Broome, Gut, 1994; 35:84) associated with previous blood transfusions. Patients with cirrhosis may present with the typical symptoms of liver failure including jaundice, ascites, and variceal haemorrhage. Although the variceal bleeding usually occurs from veins in the oesophagus, patients with concomitant inflammatory bowel disease who have undergone total proctocolectomy may bleed from peristomal varices some 6 to 13 years after formation of the ileostomy stoma (Wiesner, Gastro, 1986; 90:316).

Cholangiocarcinoma

The first case of biliary tract cancer and ulcerative colitis was reported by Parker and Kendall in 1954 (Parker, BMJ, 1954; ii: 1030). Since that time, the association between cholangiocarcinoma and ulcerative colitis has been well established. A recent large study from the Cleveland Clinic has reported a prevalence rate of 0.5 per cent (Mir-Madjlessi, DigDisSci, 1987; 32:145). The relative risk of developing bile-duct cancer in ulcerative colitis has recently been estimated as between 20 and 30 times that of a normal population.

Bile-duct cancer develops in patients with long-standing total colitis. Colectomy does not protect against the development of the tumour, which can occur some 20 years after the removal of the colon. Early studies did not report any evidence of associated hepatobiliary diseases (Ritchie, QJMed, 1974; 43:268), but more recent studies have shown that most patients have either large- or small-duct primary sclerosing cholangitis which can precede the development of carcinoma by many years (Converse, AmJSurg, 1975; 121:39; Mir-Madjlissi, DigDisSci, 1987; 32:145).[4] Five of twelve patients who died from primary sclerosing cholangitis, and who came to autopsy at the Mayo clinic, had cholangiocarcinoma (Wee, HumPath, 1985; 16:719). In two patients the tumour was multifocal in origin. The reason why some patients with primary sclerosing cholangitis go on to develop biliary cancers is unknown and no risk factors have been identified. Although bile-duct carcinoma has been reported in association with Crohn's disease, it occurs much more rarely (Berman, DigDisSci, 1980; 25:795; Choi, DigDisSci, 1994; 39:667).

The clinical presentation of bile-duct cancer is that of progressive cholestatic jaundice. Cholangiography usually reveals a narrow bile-duct stricture, although differentiation from primary sclerosing cholangitis can be difficult. The tumour usually pursues a progressive course and prognosis is very poor, with a median survival of 5 months (Rosen, AnnSurg, 1991; 213:21). Liver transplantation for isolated cholangiocarcinoma occurring in primary sclerosing cholangitis has been disappointing, with rapid recurrence of tumour (Stieber, IntSurg, 1989; 74:1).

Hepatocellular carcinoma

Two recent case reports have described the development of fibrolamellar hepatocellular cancer in male patients with ulcerative colitis

and primary sclerosing cholangitis. Neither patient was cirrhotic (Klompmaker, BMJ, 1988; 296:1445; Snook, Gut, 1989; 30:243). In the single patient who received a transplant the tumour recurred in the donor liver (Klompmaker, BMJ, 1988; 296:1445).

Fatty change

Fatty liver or steatosis is said to be the most common type of hepatobiliary lesion found in patients who have inflammatory bowel disease. It has been recorded as occurring in 45 per cent of patients with ulcerative colitis who undergo colectomy (Eade, AnnIntMed, 1970; 72:457) and in 40 per cent of patients with Crohn's disease who undergo similar surgery (Eade, AnnIntMed, 1970; 74:518). The presence of fatty liver is related to the general state of health of these patients and the severity of the underlying colitis rather than any other specific factor. This is reflected by the fact that, in an unselected series, fatty liver was found in only 6.3 and 4 per cent of patients with ulcerative colitis and Crohn's disease, respectively (Perret, QJMed, 1971; 40:187). Moreover, the incidence of fatty change in patients with ulcerative colitis at autopsy is similar to that of other debilitated patients (Palmer, AmJMed, 1964; 36:856). The pathogenesis of fatty liver in inflammatory bowel disease is unknown. It is probably multifactorial, secondary to causes such as poor nutrition, drugs, bacterial and chemical toxins, and unsuspected alcohol abuse. The steatosis is usually of the macrovesicular type and all types of distribution, including diffuse, periportal, and centrilobular, have been described in patients with inflammatory bowel disease.

There are no symptoms associated with fatty liver, although on abdominal examination, hepatomegaly may be detected. Treatment of the underlying bowel disorder and improvement in the general health of the patient will normally result in a resolution of the fatty change. There is no evidence that the lesion progresses to chronic liver disease. In view of improvements in the management of inflammatory bowel disease, the incidence of fatty change has probably fallen.

Gallstones

Patients with Crohn's disease of the small bowel have an increased incidence of gallstones. The reported incidence in patients with Crohn's ileitis, ileal resection, or intestinal bypass ranges from 13 to 34 per cent (Cohen, Gastro, 1971; 60:243; Baker, AmJDigDis, 1974; 19:109; Marks, AmJDigDis, 1977; 22:1097; Hangaas, Hepatogast, 1990; 37:83). However, the incidence of gallstones in patients with ulcerative colitis and those with Crohn's disease confined to the colon is about 5 per cent and does not differ from that of the general population. Total colectomy with ileoanal anastamosis does not predispose to the formation of cholesterol gallstones (Galatola, EurJClinInv, 1995; 25:534). The increased rate of formation of gallstones in patients with inflammation or absence of the terminal ileum is due to a reduction in bile-salt absorption, leading to depletion of the bile-salt pool (see Chapter 23.4). As a result, the concentration of biliary bile salts falls and there is a relative increase in the concentration of biliary cholesterol. Thus, bile may become supersaturated with cholesterol, which in turn increases cholesterol precipitation in the gallbladder and predisposes to the formation of cholesterol gallstones. There may be additional factors predisposing to gallstones in these patients as in one series an unusually high percentage of calcified stones was found (57 per cent) and solitary cholesterol stones were only present in a minority (Heaton, BMJ, 1969; 3:494).

Amyloidosis

Hepatic amyloidosis is a rare complication occurring in less than 1 per cent of patients with inflammatory bowel disease; it is much more commonly associated with Crohn's disease than ulcerative colitis. The development of amyloid can occur in association with Crohn's disease involving either the small or large bowel.

The amyloid deposition in the liver is found in the media of portal blood vessels and in the sinusoidal wall, and eventually leads to atrophy and disappearance of hepatocytes. In addition to inflammatory bowel disease, most patients who develop amyloidosis have either extraintestinal foci of suppuration or arthropathy. Although regression of amyloidosis has been reported after colectomy (Fausa, ScaJGastr, 1977; 12:657), in most patients the prognosis is poor.

Granulomas

Granulomas are occasionally seen in the liver biopsy specimens of some patients with Crohn's disease, some of whom may show a moderate elevation of serum alkaline phosphatase (Meyer, Gastro, 1967; 53:301; Eade, AnnIntMed, 1970; 74:518; Eade, ScaJGastr, 1971; 6:199). The granulomas can be present in portal tracts as well as in the parenchyma. The presence of hepatic granulomas in patients with Crohn's disease often reflects granulomas in the bowel. There have been a few isolated reports of hepatic granulomas occurring in association with ulcerative colitis but the relationship remains unproven.

Liver abscess

Intra-abdominal abscess is a frequent complication of Crohn's disease. However, the development of hepatic abscess in association with inflammatory bowel disease is very uncommon. The abscesses are often multiple and are associated with a high mortality (Greenstein, QJMed, 1955; 56:505). Streptococci, especially *Streptococcus milleri*, are the most frequent organisms isolated from the abscesses (Mir-Medjlessi, Gastro, 1986; 91:987).

Primary biliary cirrhosis

Five patients have been described recently with concomitant ulcerative colitis and primary biliary cirrhosis. It remains unclear whether these cases represent a true association or have occurred by chance (Kato, JClinGastro, 1985; 7:425; Bush, Gastro, 1987; 92:2009).

The effect of malabsorption syndromes on the hepatobiliary system

There are a large number of hepatobiliary abnormalities that may occur in patients with various malabsorptive disorders (Table 3). The hepatobiliary abnormalities are subdivided into those which are closely associated with the primary disease process and those in

Table 3 Malabsorptive disorders associated with hepatobiliary disease

Coeliac disease
Crohn's disease
Tropical sprue
Whipple's disease
Chronic pancreatitis
Cystic fibrosis
Jejunoileal bypass
Short bowel syndrome

which the liver dysfunction is due to the secondary nutritional consequences of malabsorption rather than the primary gut disease itself. This section will concentrate mainly on those liver abnormalities associated with primary gut disease. The effects of malnutrition on the liver are described in Chapter 29.2.

Coeliac disease and the liver

Unlike inflammatory bowel disease, the relationship between coeliac disease and liver disease has not been extensively studied. Consequently, the incidence and exact nature of chronic liver disorders that occur in association with coeliac disease are unclear. In a Swedish study, Hagander et al. (Lancet 1977; ii:270) examined the case records of 74 consecutive adult patients with coeliac disease.

Abnormalities of liver function tests were found in 39 per cent of the 74 patients and histological evidence of liver injury in 16 per cent. Liver biopsies were obtained in 13 patients; 7 of those were found to have cirrhosis and/or chronic active hepatitis and 5 were described as having 'reactive hepatitis'. Three of the patients with cirrhosis subsequently died of the effects of chronic liver disease.[7] In 19 of the 29 patients with elevated serum enzymes, several of the levels were measured before and after the institution of a gluten-free diet. A significant reduction was observed in many patients after gluten withdrawal.

In another Scandinavian study from Lindberg et al. (Lancet, 1978; i:390), elevated aminotransferase levels were noted not only in children with coeliac disease, but also in children with allergies to cow's milk and other proteins. It was suggested that the development of hepatic dysfunction in this context was related to the severity of the mucosal lesion rather than the specific disease entity. In a study of 132 patients with coeliac disease, 47 per cent had elevated liver function tests. Liver biopsies were performed in 37 patients and findings were normal in 5; non-specific changes were described in 25 patients and chronic active hepatitis was demonstrated in 5 patients (Jacobsen, ScaJGastr, 1990; 25:656). It is unclear from published data whether the incidence of chronic active hepatitis is truly increased in patients with coeliac disease, although both disorders are associated with the HLA B8, DR3 phenotype.

The reported association between coeliac disease and primary biliary cirrhosis also remains unproven. Less than 20 patients have been described with both disorders, usually in isolated case reports (Logan, Lancet, 1978; ii:230) and the association may be spurious. Recently, three patients were reported with coexisting coeliac disease and primary sclerosing cholangitis; two of the patients were suffering from ulcerative colitis (Hay, AnnIntMed, 1988; 109:713).

Gallbladder contractility is sluggish in untreated coeliac disease (Low-Beer, NEJM, 1975; 292:961; Maton, Gastro, 1985; 88:391), probably as a result of impaired release of cholecystokinin from the diseased small intestine (Maton, Gastro, 1985; 88:391). However, there is no evidence to suggest an increased incidence of gallstones in coeliac disease.

Tropical sprue and hepatic dysfunction

Very few studies of liver function have been reported in patients with tropical sprue. In one study, liver function tests and liver biopsies were performed in eight patients with mild to severe tropical sprue (Floch, AmJDigDis, 1963; 8:344). Only minimal abnormalities in liver function were noted and no significant changes were found on hepatic histology.

Whipple's disease and the liver

The liver is involved in most patients with Whipple's disease (Haubrich, Gastro, 1960; 39:454). The characteristic macrophages positive for periodic acid–Schiff staining are usually seen on liver biopsy, and are most frequently observed in the Kupffer cells (Upton, AmJClinPath, 1952; 22:755).

Cystic fibrosis (see also Chapter 20.4)

Approximately 7 to 10 per cent of patients with cystic fibrosis develop a biliary cirrhosis, often preceded by cholestasis and fatty liver (Feigelson, ArchDisChild 1993; 68:653). There is an increased prevalence among male patients bearing the haplotype B7, DR15, DQ6 (Duthie, JHepatol, 1995; 23:532). A prior history of meconium ileus is also associated with liver disease in later life (Colombo, JPaediat, 1994; 124:393). Strictures of the distal common bile duct are common (Gaskin, NEJM, 1988; 318:340), but these stenoses probably do not contribute to the development of significant liver disease. In a cholangiographic study of 104 adult patients with cystic fibrosis, those with significant liver disease had biliary changes confined to the intrahepatic biliary tree (O'Brien, Gut, 1992; 33: 387).

Although it is unpredictable, cirrhosis may develop between 4 and 15 years of age and some patients suffer from bleeding oesophageal varices secondary to portal hypertension (Psacharopoulos, Lancet, 1981; ii:78).

Treatment with high-dose ursodeoxycholic acid (18 to 22 mg/kg per day) has been shown to improve liver function tests, but has no effect on nutritional status in malnourished patients (Merli, JPaediatGastrNutr, 1994; 19:198). Longer-term studies are needed to assess the effects of ursodeoxycholic acid on the prognosis of the liver disease.

Hepatobiliary disease after surgical bypass operations for obesity

A number of surgical procedures have been tried for the treatment of morbid obesity. From the mid-1950s to the mid-1970s the jejunoileal bypass operation was widely performed. In this procedure the proximal jejunum is anastomosed to the terminal 10 cm of distal ileum. The subsequent profound malabsorption produces significant weight loss in the majority of patients. However, in view of serious hepatic side-effects, the operation has largely been abandoned and replaced by gastric procedures which have few or no serious liver complications.

The cause of hepatic damage following jejunoileal bypass is unknown. A number of possible mechanisms have been advanced including: (i) bacterial overgrowth of the isolated intestinal segment leading to production of hepatotoxins, (ii) malnutrition caused by the malabsorption, and (iii) miscellaneous causes such as concurrent viral infections or toxicity due to anaesthetic agents. There is no convincing evidence in favour of any of these theories.

The majority of patients undergoing jejunoileal bypass will develop mild elevations of serum transaminases, although the enzymes usually return to normal after stabilization of body weight. However, approximately 5 per cent of patients who have undergone jejunoileal bypass will develop significant liver injury (Buchwald, AmJSurg, 1974; 127:48). The symptoms of liver dysfunction are non-specific and include malaise, anorexia, nausea, and vomiting.

There is often a disparity between serum biochemical tests and the severity of hepatic injury judged histologically (Solhang, ScaJGastr, 1976; 11:793), although patients with severe liver damage usually have hypoalbuminaemia, coagulopathy, and elevated aminotransferase and bilirubin levels. The presence of an elevated serum bilirubin at 3 months following a bypass procedure is associated with a poor prognosis; indeed, a level of 50 mmol/1 or more carries a mortality rate of 50 to 75 per cent (Weissman, AmJSurg, 1977; 134:253).

Most obese patients will have a fatty liver before surgery, although there is no correlation between the amount of fat present in the liver biopsy and the degree of obesity. The severity of fatty liver is increased by jejunoileal bypass surgery. Some patients develop more severe liver injury with evidence of periductular fibrosis, portal inflammation, and bile-duct proliferation. Occasionally, a histological picture similar to alcoholic hepatitis may develop, with infiltration of neutrophil polymorphs, Mallory body formation, and hepatic necrosis. The presence of pericentral fibrosis often precedes the development of cirrhosis (Marubbio, SurgClinNAm, 1979; 59: 1079). These various types of hepatic injury are sometimes seen in obese patients who have not undergone bypass surgery, particularly in the presence of diabetes mellitus (see Chapter 24.8) and in patients who have undergone massive small-bowel resection with short bowel syndrome (Peura, Gastro, 1980; 79:128).

Significant liver damage usually occurs within 3 to 12 months after intestinal bypass (Spin, AmJSurg, 1975; 130:88). Initial treatment is usually carried out by means of hyperalimentation (Heimburger, AmJSurg, 1975; 129:229), but reanastomosis may be required if no improvement is seen. The response of the hepatic damage to reanastomosis is unclear (Geiss, ArchSurg, 1976; III: 1362).

References

1. Thomas CH. Ulceration of the colon with a much enlarged fatty liver. *Transactions of the Pathology Society of Philadelphia*, 1873; **4**: 87–8.
2. Lister JD. A specimen of diffuse ulcerative colitis with secondary diffuse hepatitis. *Transactions of the Pathological Society of London*, 1899; **50**: 130–5.

3. Schrumpf E, Fausa O, Kolmannskog F, Elgjo K, Ritland S, and Gjome E. Sclerosing cholangitis in ulcerative colitis. A follow-up study. *Scandinavian Journal of Gastroenterology*, 1982; **17**: 33–9.

4. Chapman RW, *et al.* Primary sclerosing cholangitis—a review of its clinical features, cholangiography and hepatic histology. *Gut*, 1980; **21**: 870–7.

5. Wiesner RH and LaRusso NF. Clinicopathologic features of the syndrome of primary sclerosing cholangitis. *Gastroenterology*, 1980; **79**: 200–6.

6. Wee A and Ludwig J. Pericholangitis in chronic ulcerative colitis: primary sclerosing cholangitis of the small ducts? *Annals of Internal Medicine*, 1985; **102**: 581–7.

7. Ludwig J. Small-duct primary sclerosing cholangitis. *Seminars in Liver Disease*, 1991; **11**: 11–17.

24.3 The effect of skin diseases on the liver

J. Hughes and M. Rustin

Introduction

The skin is a complex structure which has multiple functions other than that of acting as a physical barrier. It is responsible for thermoregulation, prevents loss of essential body fluids, protects the body against toxic environmental chemicals and ultraviolet radiation, and manufactures a proportion of the body's vitamin D supplies. The skin also plays a vital role in the immune system, and is an important organ of sensation.

There are many conditions involving both skin and liver. This chapter examines the effect of cutaneous disease on the liver, briefly reviews the features of those disorders in which both the skin and liver are involved, and describes the hepatotoxic effects of therapies used in skin disease.

Toxic epidermal necrolysis

Toxic epidermal necrolysis is an uncommon disorder characterized by local and widespread blistering and erosion of the skin and mucous membranes, resembling partial thickness burns (Plate 1).[1] Microscopically there is full-thickness subepidermal blistering and necrosis, and a sparse or absent dermal infiltrate. It is most commonly seen as an idiopathic reaction to a host of drugs, especially sulphonamides, anticonvulsants, and non-steroidal anti-inflammatory drugs (Table 1), although it may be seen after viral infections and immunization (Schopf, ArchDermatol, 1991; 127:839). Sepsis and hypovolaemia are the most serious complications and attention to fluid balance, temperature control, and prevention of secondary infection is imperative. Intensive care nursing is usually necessary. There is no specific therapy and treatment with high-dose

Table 1 Drugs causing toxic epidermal necrolysis

Sulphonamides, especially Septrin
Carbamazepine
Barbiturates
Non-steroidal anti-inflammatory drugs (especially phenylbutazone derivatives)
Allopurinol
Aspirin
Antibiotics, e.g. penicillin, erythromycin
Paracetamol
Chlormezanone

corticosteroids is of no proven benefit. There are a handful of recent reports showing a favourable response to cyclosporin (Zaki, BrJDermatol, 1995; 133:337). The mortality of this condition varies according to the age of the patient and whether there are any coexisting diseases, but remains on average at about 25 per cent (Revuz, ArchDermatol, 1987; 123:1160). The liver may be congested and the aminotransferases may be raised as part of the widespread systemic upset associated with this condition.[1]

Other conditions associated with extensive skin loss

Widespread areas of skin loss may also occur in other conditions such as pemphigus vulgaris, staphylococcal scalded skin syndrome, and severe forms of epidermolysis bullosa. These cause major systemic upset as seen in toxic epidermal necrolysis. Thermal burns, depending on their severity, also cause similar problems. Elevation of liver enzymes, and in extreme cases liver failure, may occur in the acute stage of hypovolaemic shock that follows extensive full-thickness burns.

Erythroderma is a less life-threatening condition but one that compromises cutaneous function. It is a descriptive term for inflammation involving 90 per cent or more of the body surface and may be caused by eczema, psoriasis, drugs, cutaneous lymphomas, Sézary syndrome, and leukaemias. Increased cutaneous blood flow may lead to hypothermia and high-output cardiac failure. Excess fluid loss and secondary sepsis are common sequelae. Hypoalbuminaemia may occur as a result of a general increase in metabolic rate and a decrease in albumin synthesis (Worm, BrJDermatol, 1981; 104:389). The liver enzymes are generally normal and, where liver biopsies have been performed, liver architecture is usually unaffected.

Psoriasis

Psoriasis is a common inflammatory skin condition which affects 2 per cent of the population in the United Kingdom.[2] It is characterized by the formation of erythematous plaques with an adherent silver scale on extensor surfaces, particularly the elbows, knees, and hands, and on the base of the spine and the scalp. The nails are frequently involved. Hyperproliferation of the epidermis is the hallmark of the disorder with an approximately 10-fold increase in cell turnover at affected sites together with a neutrophilic and CD8 lymphocytic dermal inflammatory cell infiltrate.

The cause of psoriasis is not known. There is a strong genetic component and 30 per cent of patients with psoriasis have an affected first-degree relative (Barker, Lancet, 1991; 338:227). In susceptible people emotional stress, physical trauma, streptococcal infection, and certain drugs such as lithium, chloroquine, and β-blockers may trigger or exacerbate the condition.[2] Smoking may also be a risk factor, especially in patients with palmo-plantar psoriasis (Williams, BMJ, 1994; 308:428).

Excessive alcohol may exacerbate psoriasis (Poikolainen, BMJ, 1990; 300:780). One study showed alcohol misuse in patients with psoriasis to be as high as 38 per cent (Higgins, AlcAlc, 1992: 27: 595). The effect of stress needs to be considered. Psoriasis may be precipitated by stress and the disease is associated with anxiety and poor self-esteem. (Ramsay, BrJDermatol, 1988; 118:195). Increased alcohol consumption is a recognized response to stress and therefore debate has occurred as to whether alcohol misuse is a cause or consequence of psoriasis. However, there is evidence that alcohol does provoke psoriasis, and that abstinence is associated with re-mission (Vincenti, JRArmyMedCorps, 1987; 133:77).

Rarely, psoriasis may become extensive and unstable and erythrodermic psoriasis may result. There may be excessive water loss, inability to maintain the core temperature, increased risk of infection, and hypoproteinaemia. If sheets of erythema and sterile pustules form, this is known as acute generalized pustular psoriasis and may be provoked by steroid withdrawal. The patient is toxic and needs intensive nursing and immunosuppressive treatment, usually methotrexate, acitretin, or cyclosporin A. A raised level of bilirubin or hypoalbuminaemia may occur in either of these two serious forms of the condition, as a result of oligaemia, sepsis, and general toxicity (Warren, BMJ, 1974; ii:406).

Lichen planus

Lichen planus is a self-limiting papular eruption that is character-ized by intensely pruritic violaceous papules (Plate 2).[3,4] Oral involvement is characterized by lace-like patterning and ulceration and may be found in up to 65 per cent of patients (Strauss, OralSurg, 1989; 68:406). Genital involvement occurs in 25 per cent of men with the disorder[4] and in an unknown percentage in women, and the nails are involved in up to 16 per cent of patients (Scott, ArchDermatol, 1979; 115:1197). Histology is identical whether the disease is idiopathic or due to a a drug eruption. There is a dense band-like lymphocytic infiltrate at the dermoepidermal junction with basal cell degeneration and hypergranulosus.

A cutaneous eruption similar to lichen planus may occur after ingestion of drugs or contact with certain chemicals (Halevy, JAm-AcadDermatol, 1993; 29:249). The list of drugs that can induce lichenoid drug reactions include gold, penicillamine, antimalarials, β-blockers, and thiazide diuretics.

The aetiology of lichen planus is unknown but it has been postulated that T lymphocytes initiate the basal layer abnormalities (De Panfilis, JCutPath, 1983; 10:52). Grafting of involved skin on to 'nude' or immunoincompetent mice brings about a resolution of the histopathological changes seen in lichen planus (Gilhar, BrJDermatol, 1989; 120:541). A tentative genetic predisposition has been suggested by familial cases of lichen planus and a significant association with both HLA A3 (Lowe, BrJDermatol, 1976: 95:169) and HLA DR1 (Powell, BrJDermatol, 1986; 114:473).

There appears to be an association between lichen planus and liver disease. Raised levels of liver enzymes have been found in 7 to 52 per cent of patients (Korkij, JAmAcadDermatol, 1984; 11:609; Monk, JAmAcadDermatol, 1985; 12:122) and a link between erosive oral lichen planus and cirrhosis has been reported (Ayala, JAm-AcadDermatol, 1986; 14:139).

Primary biliary cirrhosis has been described in association with lichen planus. It was initially described in patients with primary biliary cirrhosis receiving treatment with penicillamine, which is known to cause a lichenoid drug reaction (Seehafer, ArchDermatol, 1981; 117:140). However, lichen planus was subsequently reported in patients with primary biliary cirrhosis unrelated to therapy (Graham-Brown, Lancet, 1981; ii:1046), although this association was recognized to occur rarely, with one large study identifying 7 out of 268 patients with primary biliary cirrhosis (2.6 per cent) having lichen planus (Powell, JAmAcadDermatol, 1983; 9:540).

An association between lichen planus and hepatitis C has also been reported (see Chapter 25.6).

Sarcoidosis

Sarcoidosis of the liver is discussed fully in Chapter 14.2. The commonest cutaneous manifestation of sarcoidosis is erythema no-dosum occurring in 25 to 30 per cent of cases (Saboor, BrJHospMed, 1992; 48:293). This is characterized by bilateral tender red nodules on the extensor surfaces of the lower legs. The coexistence of erythema nodosum and bilateral hilar lymphadenopathy is as-sociated with a good prognosis. Sarcoidosis in the skin presents as orange-brown granulomatous papules or nodules which may co-alesce into plaques and there may be infiltration of scars (Plate 3). Lupus pernio is a bluish-red shiny eruption which occurs most frequently on the nose, cheeks, and ears. However, there are a large number of other manifestations of cutaneous sarcoidosis and these include hypopigmentation, ulceration, palmo-plantar and ungual types, vasculitis, and an annular eruption.[5]

Skin tumours that metastasize to the liver

The commonest skin cancer, basal cell carcinoma, virtually never metastasizes although rare cases have been reported (Farmer, Can-cer, 1980; 46:748). Squamous cell carcinomas metastasize slowly to local draining lymph nodes, although spread via the bloodstream is uncommon. The occurrence of metastases in this tumour is unpredictable.

Advanced cutaneous malignant melanoma commonly meta-stasizes (Plate 4). The incidence of this tumour is increasing in the United Kingdom. Scotland has the highest occurrence with an incidence rate per year of 7.9 per 100 000 men and 10.4 per 100 000 women (Mackie, Lancet, 1992; 339:971). Exposure to ultraviolet light and sunburn, especially when intermittent, is thought to be the most important environmental factor in the pathogenesis of melanoma (Koh, NEJM, 1991; 325:171).

The prognosis of malignant melanoma is determined by the vertical depth or Breslow thickness of the tumour. The 5-year survival is inversely proportional to tumour thickness and those patients who have a Breslow thickness of 1 mm or less have a 5-year survival of approximately 90 per cent. If the tumour is in a vertical growth phase then prognosis is less good, which explains why occasionally patients with thin lesions develop metastases (Clark, JNCI, 1989; 89:1893). Patients who have a melanoma with a Breslow thickness of 1 to 3 mm have a 5-year survival of approximately 70 per cent and those with a thickness of 3 to 3.5 mm or greater have a 5-year survival of around 40 per cent. Deep tumours tend to metastasize early to local lymph nodes or more widely to the liver, lungs, bone, and brain.

Primary sarcomas of the skin are rare but also have metastatic potential. Another rare cutaneous malignancy, the Merkel cell tumour, which is derived from neuroendocrine cells, has a high incidence of secondary spread. Metastases, including hepatic secondaries, are rare in the classic form of Kaposi's sarcoma but relatively common in the endemic and HIV-related forms of the disease. A number of tumours such as breast and colon may metastatize both to the liver and to the skin.

Dermatomyositis

Dermatomyositis is an acquired inflammatory myopathy which is associated with a characteristic rash (Bohan, NEJM, 1975; 292:244). A violaceous or heliotrope eruption occurs on the face, especially the periorbital area, associated with oedema. A shiny, erythematous rash may be found elsewhere, particularly on the dorsal aspects of joints and overlying the knuckles, a finding known as Gottron's sign (Plate 5). Dilated nail-fold capillaries and ragged cuticles are common.

Approximately one-quarter of all adult patients with dermatomyositis have an underlying malignancy (Callen, ArchDermatol, 1980; 116:295) and this figure increases with age. Hence, although there are no specific liver changes associated with this disorder, there may be hepatic metastases in the patients with malignancy-associated dermatomyositis. Both aspartate and alanine aminotransferase levels may be elevated, but the enzymes are derived from damaged muscle fibres and not from the liver.

Dermatitis herpetiformis

The relationship between dermatits herpetiformis and coeliac disease was first described in the 1960s and is now well established (Marks, Lancet, 1966; ii:1280). Approximately 1 per cent of patients with coeliac disease have pruritic vesiculo-bullous lesions, which characteristically involve the elbows, buttocks, knees, shoulders, and scalp in young people.[6] The diagnosis is confirmed by immunofluorescent studies on uninvolved skin showing the presence of granular deposits of IgA in the papillary or upper dermis (Fry, BrJDermatol, 1974; 90:137). The majority of patients with dermatitis herpetiformis have some features of a gluten-sensitive enteropathy with villous atrophy, crypt hyperplasia, and cellular infiltration of the lamina propria of the small intestine (Brow, Gastro, 1971; 60:355).

In one series, abnormal liver function tests were found in 17 per cent of patients with dermatitis herpetiformis (Wojnarowska, ActaDermVen, 1981; 61:165). In half of these, a raised bilirubin level may have been attributable to dapsone treatment. In most patients, abnormal liver function tests improve after gluten withdrawal. Dermatitis herpetiformis responds rapidly to treatment with dapsone and in patients who cannot tolerate dapsone, sulphapyridine or sulphamethoxypyridazine are alternative treatments. Withdrawal of dietary gluten is advised. Long-term therapy is necessary.

Mastocytosis

Mastocytosis describes a spectrum of clinical disorders that are characterized by the proliferation of mast cells in one or more organ systems, most commonly the skin.[7] The clinical manifestations result from the release of inflammatory mediators derived from mast cells (Metcalfe, JInvDermatol, 1991; 96:2S). It may occur in all races and the sex incidence is equal. There are four types of cutaneous mastocytosis, the most common being urticaria pigmentosa (Soter, JInvDermatol, 1991; 96:32S). The other forms are solitary mastocytoma, diffuse cutaneous mastocytosis, and telangiectasia macularis eruptiva perstans. In urticaria pigmentosa, multiple reddish-brown macules, papules, or rarely nodules are present on the skin. Lesions may urticate spontaneously or after pressure (Darier's sign) and may be associated with pruritus, flushing, dermographism, and petechiae, especially when there is extensive involvement.

Solitary mastocytomas are uncommon and account for less than 5 per cent of patients with cutaneous mastocytosis. They are isolated brown nodules which usually present in the postnatal period. Rubbing may induce blister formation. Diffuse erythrodermic cutaneous mastocytosis occurs most often in infants and presents with doughy, yellowish infiltration of the skin and tense blisters. Owing to the large mast cell load in this form of the disease, systemic manifestations are common and may include flushing, diarrhoea, headache, abdominal pain, hypotension, and, very rarely, shock (Stein, PediatrDermatol, 1986; 3:365). The term telangiectasia macularis eruptiva perstans is descriptive of the individual lesions and pruritus is usually absent.

Hepatic involvement is frequently found in patients with mastocytosis, and hepatomegaly was present in 40 per cent of adults with the disorder in one series of 58 patients (Travis, Medicine, 1988; 67:345). In the same series of 58 patients, 30 per cent had a raised level of serum alkaline phosphatase. In a second recent series of 41 patients with mast cell disease, 24 per cent had hepatomegaly and 54 per cent had elevated levels of serum alkaline phosphatase, aminotransferases, or γ-glutamyl transferase (Mican, Hepatol, 1995; 22:1163). Analysis of liver biopsies performed on 25 patients from this series showed that systemic mastocytosis is commonly associated with hepatic mast cell hyperplasia, fibrosis, and, less commonly, nodular regenerative hyperplasia, portal venopathy, and/or veno-occlusive disease. Other studies have noted similar findings, with hepatic mast cell infiltration as a frequent finding (Yam, AmJMed, 1986; 80:819; Horny, Cancer, 1989; 63:532). Severe liver disease with ascites is rare in mastocytosis and has a poor prognosis (Mican, Hepatol, 1995; 22:1163).

Kawasaki disease

Kawasaki disease is an acute vasculitis which is characterized by fever, an erythematous psoriasiform-like rash on the body, swelling and redness of the hands and feet followed by desquamation of the fingertips, mucosal inflammation (the 'strawberry red tongue'), and cervical lymphadenopathy (Plate 6). Associated cardiac involvement with the development of myocarditis, pericarditis, and coronary artery aneurysms is not uncommon and must be excluded (Gersony, JAMA, 1991; 265:2699). The aetiology of Kawasaki disease is not known, but a superantigen toxin has been implicated following isolation of toxin-producing staphylococcal or streptococcal strains from patients with the disorder (Leung, Lancet, 1993; 342:1385; Curtis, Lancet, 1994; 343:299). A recent report suggested that active or recent parvovirus B19 infection may also be implicated (Nigro, Lancet, 1994; 343:1260), but other series have failed to confirm this finding (Yoto and Cohen, Lancet, 1994; 344:58).

Treatment with early high-dose intravenous immunoglobulin and aspirin has improved the prognosis of this disease with regard to its cardiac complications (Newburger, NEJM, 1986; 315:341).

Ten to fifteen per cent of children with Kawasaki disease develop upper abdominal pain during their illness (Melish, HospPract, 1982; 17:99). In one series, hepatomegaly was noted in 14.5 per cent and a non-specific increase in serum aminotransferases was found in 31 per cent of cases (Burns, JPediat, 1991; 118:680). There is also a known association with hydrops of the gallbladder, although its pathogenesis remains unclear (Magilavy, Pediat, 1978; 61:699; Mofenson, NYStateJMed, 1980; 80:249). A recent report described three patients with Kawasaki disease and liver involvement who had histological evidence of intrahepatic cholangitis and necrosis of the intrahepatic bile duct epithelium (Bader-Meunier, JPediat, 1992; 120:750). Intrahepatic cholangitis in a child who had persistent hepatomegaly has been reported previously (Edwards, JPediat-GastrNutr, 1985; 4:140). Vasculitis, portal inflammation, fatty degeneration, and severe hepatic congestion have all been reported at autopsy and could contribute towards hepatic dysfunction (Ohshio, PediatPath, 1985; 4;257).

Neurofibromatosis

The neurofibromatoses include two separate genetic disorders, neurofibromatosis type 1 and 2, in which affected persons have tumours involving neural tissue and cutaneous and other pathological features.

Neurofibromatosis type 1

Neurofibromatosis type1 or von Recklinghausen's disease is the most common neurocutaneous disorder, occurring in 1 in 2500 to 7800 persons.[8] It is inherited in an autosomal dominant mode with a high rate of spontaneous mutations and a wide spectrum of clinical findings. The gene for this disease has been localized to chromosome 17q11.2.(Schmidt, AmJMedGen, 1987; 28:771). It is a large gene which may explain why the frequency of new mutations is as high as 50 per cent (Riccardi, CurrProbPediat, 1992; 22:66). Cutaneous features of this disorder include café-au-lait spots which may be present at birth or develop during infancy, axillary freckling which is pathognomonic of neurofibromatosis, and cutaneous neurofibromas which are soft flesh-coloured papules and nodules. Other types of neurofibromas include subcutaneous neurofibromas involving nerves, nodular plexiform neurofibromas in the subcutis involving dorsal nerve roots, and diffuse plexiform neurofibromas which may involve all layers of skin and penetrate deeply into muscle, bone, and viscera. There are occasional reports of plexiform neurofibromas involving the liver, which may be extensive, as in the case of a 15-year-old girl where infiltration had occurred into the porta hepatis and intrahepatic portal branches of the liver leading to hepatomegaly and right upper quadrant tenderness (Kakitsubata, PaediatrRadiol, 1994; 24:66). Extrahepatic biliary obstruction leading to obstructive jaundice has also been reported (Meyer, Ann-IntMed, 1982; 97:722).

Neurofibromatosis type 2

Neurofibromatosis type 2 is an autosomal dominant condition which occurs less frequently than type 1. The disorder occurs in 1 in 30 000 to 50 000 persons and is characterized by the development of bilateral acoustic neuromas (Evans, JMedGenet, 1992; 29:841). Skin manifestations are not as common as in type 1 disease and liver involvement is extremely rare.

Tuberous sclerosis

Tuberous sclerosis is an autosomal dominant disease with multisystem hamartomas and a wide range of clinical variability and severity.[8] Two gene linkages (9q34 and 16p13) have been found with equal frequency in approximately 90 per cent of patients with tuberous sclerosis and further research is in process (Kwiatkowski, ArchDermatol, 1994; 130:348). The skin lesions may clinch the diagnosis as they are usually distinctive. They include hypo-pigmented patches or 'ash-leaf macules', most easily seen under Wood's modified ultraviolet light, and four types of cutaneous hamartomas pathognomic of the disease. These are facial angiofibromas, the forehead plaque, shagreen patches, and periungual fibromas (Osborne, ArchDisChild, 1988; 63:1423).

Hepatic hamartomas are more common in females with the disorder and are usually asymptomatic (Jozwiak, ArchDisChild, 1992; 67:1363). They are usually benign malformations known as angiomyolipomas which involve smooth muscle, fat, and blood vessels, but occasionally portal fibrosis may also be found.

Drugs used in the treatment of skin disease and their effects on the liver

The effects of drugs on the liver are covered fully in Section 17. There are a number of agents used widely in the treatment of skin disease that are known to cause hepatic side-effects.

Retinoids

Synthetic retinoids have had an established role in the treatment of psoriasis, disorders of keratinization such as Darier's disease, severe types of ichthyosis, pityriasis rubra pilaris, and acne.[9] Three retinoids have been marketed for use: etretinate, which has now been replaced by acitretin, used primarily in psoriasis, and iso-tretinoin used in severe acne (owing to its sebosuppressive effects). All three are teratogenic; pregnancy is contraindicated for 2 years following the administration of acitretin and etretinate and for 1 month after isotretinoin. The main side-effects are dryness of the skin and mucous membranes causing cheilitis and conjunctivitis and reversible alopecia. Increases in serum cholesterol and tri-glycerides may occur in up to 20 per cent of patients on 3 months of treatment with acitretin or etretinate (Kragballe, ActaDermVen, 1989; 69:35). If these changes do not respond to dietary measures or dosage reduction then retinoid treatment should be stopped, especially in patients at high risk for cardiac disease.

A transitory rise in serum aminotransferases has been noted in up to 20 per cent of patients treated with retinoids although the significance of this is uncertain. Acute hepatitis progressing to chronic liver disease is rare but recognized (Van Ditzhuijsen, J Hepatol, 1990; 11:185). Liver biopsies carried out in a series of patients on long-term etretinate showed no consistent abnormalities (Roenigk, BrJDermatol, 1985; 112:77). It is recommended that serum liver function tests are measured at the beginning of therapy with acitretin or isotretinoin and intermittently thereafter, if persistently abnormal the dose should be reduced or treatment stopped.[9]

Methotrexate

Methotrexate is an effective treatment for severe psoriasis which is unresponsive to topical treatments. It is a derivative of folic acid which inhibits DNA synthesis and cell division by competitive inhibition of the enzyme dihydrofolate reductase. In use from the 1950s onwards (Gubner, AmJMedSci, 1951; 221:17), the standard dose is from 10 to 25 mg given orally once a week and adjusted according to the response of the patient. The drug is a known teratogen and affects both spermatogenesis and oogenesis, which may result in decreased fertility.

Liver damage is one of the most important unwanted side-effects of methotrexate.[10] This may range from mild hepatitis to fibrosis, cirrhosis, and rarely, fulminant hepatic failure. Approximately 15 per cent of patients will develop mild fibrosis and less than 1 per cent moderate fibrosis or cirrhosis. Histological changes secondary to methotrexate commence with increased collagen in the space of Disse progressing to fibrosis and eventually micronodular cirrhosis. Fatty infiltration is not uncommon although hepatocellular damage is not usually a feature.

Patients taking methotrexate who are at increased risk of developing liver damage include those with a high cumulative dosage, alcohol consumption in excess of 10 units per week, diabetics, obese patients, and the elderly (Whiting-O'Keefe, AmJMed, 1991; 90:711). Patients with rheumatoid arthritis who are treated with methotrexate are significantly less susceptible to liver damage than those with psoriasis. This difference has been attributed to lower doses used in rheumatoid arthritis and less associated alcohol consumption and obesity.

Monitoring of patients on methotrexate is of vital importance and if patients are selected beforehand and reviewed regularly then methotrexate has been shown to be a relatively safe therapy (Van Dooren-Greebe, BrJDermatol, 1994; 130:204). Conventional serum tests of liver function are relatively insensitive and non-specific, and may not accurately reflect the degree of liver injury. Other methods to look at progression of liver damage such as ultrasound and MRI have generally proved unsatisfactory. Liver histology is still the most accurate way of assessing methotrexate toxicity but debate exists as to when and how often liver biopsy should be performed. Recommendations[11,12] suggest that, unless a short course of treatment is envisaged, liver biopsy should be carried out after every cumulative dose of 1.5 g or if liver function tests become persistently abnormal. It should also be carried out in those patients at risk of developing methotrexate liver damage, or with a pre-existing liver disorder. However, percutaneous liver biopsy has attendant risks and each individual case must be carefully considered.

Azathioprine

Azathioprine is a 6-mercaptopurine derivative and immuno-suppressive agent frequently used in dermatological practice, often in combination with systemic steroids as a steroid sparing agent. Skin diseases for which azathioprine is an established treatment include the bullous disorders pemphigus and pemphigoid, eczema (particularly of the photosensitive type), actinic reticuloid, systemic lupus erythematosus, and dermatomyositis (Anstey, JRSM, 1995; 88:155). Cholestasis and elevation of liver enzymes are only occasionally seen during therapy and are usually reversible on withdrawal of the drug. Very rarely, azathioprine induces a hypersensitivity reaction which may include cholestatic jaundice, portal fibrosis, hepatocellular necrosis, fever, and shock (Saway, AmJMed 1988; 84:960).

Cyclosporin

This immunosuppressant is now well established as one of the systemic treatments of choice for severe psoriasis. It is also used regularly in a wide variety of cutaneous disorders including atopic eczema, pyoderma gangrenosum, Behçet's disease, epidermolysis bullosa acquisita, lichen planus, pemphigus, and bullous pemphigoid. The standard dose of cyclosporin for these skin conditions is between 3 and 5 mg/kg per day, given in two divided doses; it is usually well tolerated. Monitoring of renal function and blood pressure is mandatory because long-term use of this drug in transplant recipients has been found to cause an irreversible reduction in the glomerular filtration rate associated with characteristic renal histopathological changes (Mihatsch, SemDiagPath, 1988; 5:104). Cyclosporin is metabolized predominantly by the hepatic cytochrome P450 enzyme system with only 6 per cent excreted unaltered in the urine. Caution is therefore necessary when cyclosporin is given to patients with pre-existing liver disease as the risk of further damage is potentiated and increased blood levels may be expected (Wadhwa, TherDrugMonit, 1987; 9:399).

A rise in serum bilirubin, alkaline phosphatase, and amino-transferases may be seen.[13] Hyperbilirubinaemia is the most common alteration in liver function noted and occurs in up to 50 per cent of patients taking this drug. These changes are usually asymptomatic and return to normal on dosage reduction. Their significance is unclear.

Ketoconazole

This broad-spectrum azole antifungal drug is now rarely prescribed because of its association with serious cholestatic, hepatocellular, and mixed cholestatic–hepatocellular patterns of injury. The incidence of liver damage in patients taking the drug is in the region of 1 in 70 000, a lower figure than first reported (Lewis, Gastro, 1985; 86:503). The patients most at risk are those over 50 years (especially women), those with pre-existing liver disease, alcoholics, and those who have previously received potentially hepatotoxic drugs. Shorter courses (less than 14 days) of the drug have reduced the incidence of hepatic side-effects but, as the newer azoles have a lower affinity for cytochrome P450, they are usually preferred as first-line therapy (Stricker, JHepatol 1986; 3:399).

Itraconazole

Itraconazole is a broad-spectrum triazole antimycotic with a low reported incidence of hepatic injury. The recommended dose for adults is between 100 and 200 mg and the length of treatment varies according to the type and severity of the infection. It is now the preferred treatment for superficial and deep mycoses, including those caused by *Actinomycetes* and *Candida* species and in pityriasis versicolor. There is increased usage of this drug in HIV disease. In one short series, six patients developed liver damage on a prolonged course of itraconazole, but three of the six were already receiving drugs that could potentially cause liver damage (Lavrijsen, Lancet, 1992; 340:251).

Terbinafine

The recently developed antifungal drug terbinafine is a fungicidal allylamine. It is prescribed at a dose of 250 mg per day in adults and 125 mg per day in children and the treatment course may vary from 1 week for superficial infections to 6 months for advanced onychmycosis involving the toenails. Terbinafine has effective fungicidal activity against nail and skin infections caused by dermatophyte fungi.

Asymptomatic transient increases in liver enzymes occur in 0.5 per cent of those on the drug. There have been rare reports of a mixed cholestatic–hepatocellular type of hepatitis occurring as an idiosyncratic reaction (van't Wout, JHepatol, 1994; 21:115). There may be a loss of taste which is reversible on stopping treatment.

Griseofulvin

This previously widely-used antifungal drug is still effective, especially in the treatment of tinea corporis, but the newer and faster-acting agents are now generally preferred. The dose is 1 g daily in adults and 10 mg/kg per day in children. Length of treatment is variable and depends on the clinical response. Hepatic side-effects are rare but reports include intrahepatic cholestasis (Chiprut, Gastro, 1976; 70:1141), the exacerbation of acute intermittent porphyria (Redecker, JAMA, 1964; 188:466), and drug-induced lupus erythematosus.

Chinese herbal treatment

Traditional Chinese herbal therapy is becoming an increasingly popular treatment for eczema and a wide range of different disorders. A double-blind study using a quality controlled product, Zemaphyte, has shown great benefit in patients with recalcitrant atopic eczema (Sheehan, Lancet, 1992; 340:13). When treatment is prescribed by a Chinese herbal therapist, a patient is given an individualized prescription which may contain from 10 to 25 different ingredients from a choice of hundreds of plants, fungi, animal material, or minerals. The usual mode of administration is to boil the mixture and to take the decoction daily as a form of herbal 'tea'. The benefit gained from this treatment is considerable but its use is

unregulated. In a recent series (Perharic, VetHumTox, 1995; 6:562), symptomatic liver damage was reported in nine patients taking Chinese herbal therapy and in all but one case, which had a fatal outcome, the liver function tests returned to normal between 1 and 6 months after stopping the treatment. The mechanism of toxicity was unclear and thought to be idiosyncratic. No dose-related effect was seen. In another report, two patients developed an acute hepatitic illness whilst on Chinese herbal therapy which settled after discontinuing treatment. In one of the patients there was a clear recurrence of symptoms and biochemical evidence of liver damage soon after resuming Chinese herbs (Kane, Gut, 1995; 36:146).

Spironolactone

The aldosterone antagonist diuretic spironolactone is used in the treatment of hirsutism and in hyperandrogenetic conditions such as polycystic ovary syndrome as a consequence of its weak anti-androgenetic properties (Shaw, JAmAcadDermatol, 1991; 24:236). Hepatic toxicity is extremely rare and there are only two reported cases (Renkes, JAMA, 1995; 273:376). Spironolactone has been shown to cause tumours, including liver tumours, in rats when used at doses 25 to 100 times higher than those used in humans (Brest, ClinTher, 1986; 8:586). No reported cases of spironolactone-related tumours in humans have been reported.

Cyproterone acetate

Women suffering from acne or hirsutism, often secondary to the polycystic ovary syndrome, may be treated with the antiandrogen cyproterone acetate in combination with ethinyloestradiol. The oral contraceptive preparation Dianette contains a small dose of cyproterone acetate (2 mg daily) and 35 µg of ethinyleostradiol; it is not recommended solely for contraception, but should be used in women who have androgen-dependent skin conditions. Cyproterone acetate is contraindicated in patients with pre-existing liver disease. There have been occasional reports of hepatic dysfunction, most commonly cholestatic jaundice, although fatal fulminant hepatitis has occurred (Parys, BrJUrol, 1991; 67:312). These reports were in patients who had advanced prostatic carcinoma and were on high-dose cyproterone acetate (100 mg three times daily) given for periods of up to 2 years. However, recent reports point towards a rare link between prolonged use of high-dose cyproterone acetate and the development of hepatocellular carcinoma. In one case report a 75-year-old man with carcinoma of the prostate developed hepatocellular carcinoma after 18 months of treatment with cyproterone acetate at a dose of 100 mg three times daily (Ohri, BrJUrol, 1991; 67:213). Three further cases of liver cancer were reported in patients who had been treated with cyproterone acetate for sexual precocity at doses varying between 100 and 300 mg daily for periods of 9 to14 years (Watanabe, Lancet, 1994; 344:1567). In a recent isolated report a healthy female with no other risk factors developed hepatocellular carcinoma after 14 years of taking Dianette (Rudiger, Lancet, 1995; 345:452).

Psoralens

Psoralens are photosensitizers which cross-link with DNA in the presence of ultraviolet light. This reaction is utilized when psoralens are given in combination with long-wavelength ultraviolet A light

(**PUVA**) for conditions such as psoriasis, cutaneous T-cell lymphoma, and vitiligo.[14] PUVA has been rarely associated with hepatitis (Bjellerup, JAmAcadDermatol, 1981; 4:481) and is known to induce liver microsomal enzymes (Bickers, JInvDermatol, 1982; 79:201).

Antituberculous therapy

Cutaneous tuberculosis generally accounts for only a small proportion of cases of extrapulmonary tuberculosis. However, with the emergence of HIV disease over the last 10 years, the skin manifestations of the opportunist *Mycobacterium avium-intracellulare* have become a relatively common finding in patients with this disorder.

Lupus vulgaris, which causes a progressive plaque with characteristic 'apple-jelly' appearance, is one of the more familiar forms. Atypical mycobacterial infections presenting as indolent nodules or pustules with sporotrichoid spread are not uncommon and most cases are caused by *M. marinum* with domestic fish tanks as the source of infection.

Hepatic reactions caused by antituberculous therapy are dealt with fully in Section 17. Severe hepatotoxic reactions necessitating a change in therapy occur in fewer than 5 per cent of patients receiving triple therapy with isoniazid, rifampicin, and pyrazinamide (O'Brien, JAMA, 1991; 265:3323). Adverse effects on the liver are more likely to occur in older patients, those with underlying liver disease, and in alcoholics. Isoniazid is usually the cause of any hepatic damage.

Danazol

Danazol is a synthetic anabolic steroid with androgenic effects. In dermatology, it is used in the treatment of the rare familial and autoimmune condition C1-esterase inhibitor deficiency which causes life-threatening angio-oedema and urticaria. It may cause modest increases in serum aminotransferases and, very rarely, cholestatic jaundice (Qaseem, PostgradMedJ, 1992; 68:984). There are also isolated and extremely rare cases of danazol-induced hepatocellular adenomas, usually occurring after prolonged treatment (Khan, ArchPathLabMed, 1991; 115:1054). Danazol can induce aminolaevulinic acid (ALA) synthetase activity and hence may precipitate porphyria.

Stanozolol

Stanozolol is similar in structure to danazol and is used in chronic venous disease, Raynaud's disease, hereditary angio-oedema, urticaria, cryofibrinogenaemia, and for the vascular manifestations of Behçet's disease because of its fibrinolytic effect. Like danazol, slight elevation of liver enzymes may be seen and porphyria precipitated (Helfman, JAmAcadDermatol, 1995; 33:254). Very rarely stanozolol may induce hepatic tumours and peliosis hepatitis with prolonged treatment (Soe, Liver, 1992; 12:73).

Lupus-like syndromes and hepatitis secondary to drugs

A large number of drugs such as sulphasalazine, hydralazine, and methyldopa are known to cause an acute lupus-like disease, although only approximately 5 per cent of cases of systemic lupus erythematosus are drug induced.[7] Abnormal laboratory findings such as antinuclear, ribonucleoprotein, and single-stranded DNA antibodies are common, but antibodies against double-stranded DNA are hardly ever present (Schoen, AmJMed, 1981; 71:5). Rarely, an acute hepatitis may be seen as part of the more usual syndrome of fever, arthralgia, myalgia, and pleuropericarditis.

References

1. Roujeau J-C et al. Toxic epidermal necrolysis. *Archives of Dermatology*, 1990; **126**: 37–42.
2. Barker JNWN. The pathophysiology of psoriasis. *Lancet*, 1991; **338**: 227–30.
3. Boyd AS and Nelder KH. Lichen planus. *Journal of the American Academy of Dermatology*, 1991; **25**: 593–619.
4. Arndt KA. Lichen planus. In Fitzpatrick TB et al., eds. *Dermatology in general medicine*. 3rd edn. New York: McGraw-Hill, 1987: 967–73.
5. Savin JA. Sarcoidosis. In Champion RH, Burton JL, and Ebling FJG, eds. *Textbook of dermatology*. 5th edn. Oxford: Blackwell Scientific Publications, 1992: 2383–406.
6. Fry L. Dermatitis herpetiformis. *Baillière's Clinical Gastroenterology*, 1995; **9**: 371–93.
7. Longley J, Duffy TP, and Kohn S. The mast cell and mast cell disease. *Journal of the American Academy of Dermatology*, 1995; **32**: 545–61.
8. Zvulunov A and Esterly N. Neurocutaneous syndromes associated with pigmentary skin lesions. *Journal of the American Academy of Dermatology*, 1995; **32**: 915–35.
9. Retinoids: present and future. *Journal of the American Academy of Dermatology*, 1992; **27**(2): S1–46.
10. Neuberger J. Methotrexate and liver disorders. *Prescribers Journal*, 1995; **35**: 158–63.
11. Workshop of the Research Unit of the Royal College of Physicians of London: Department of Dermatology, University of Glasgow; British Association of Dermatologists. Guidelines for management of patients with psoriasis. *British Medical Journal*, 1991; **303**: 829–35.
12. Roenigk, et al. Methotrexate in psoriasis: revised guidelines. *Journal of the American Academy of Dermatology*, 1988; **19**: 145–56.
13. Fradin M, Ellis C, and Voorhees J. Management of patients and side-effects during cyclosporine therapy for cutaneous disorders. *Journal of the American Academy of Dermatology*, 1990; **23**: 1265–75.
14. British Photodermatology Group guidelines for PUVA. *British Journal of Dermatology*, 1994; **130**: 246–55.

24.4 The liver in urogenital diseases

Juan Rodés and Vicente Arroyo

This chapter includes hepatic disturbances observed in some urogenital diseases, such as hypernephroma and prostatic carcinoma, as well as those associated with haemodialysis and renal transplantation. Renal cyst diseases and the liver are discussed in Chapter 11.2.

The nephrogenic hepatic dysfunction syndrome

This syndrome was first described by Stauffer in 1961 (Stauffer, Gastro, 1961; 40:694) in five patients with hypernephroma without hepatic metastases. These patients had abnormal standard liver function tests and hepatomegaly which completely disappeared upon removal of the tumour. This syndrome has also been observed in patients with renal sarcoma (Farrow, Cancer, 1968; 22:556) and xanthogranulomatous pyelonephritis (Vermillion, AnnSurg, 1970; 171:130). Strict confirmation of this syndrome requires the following criteria: (1) return to normal of liver function tests after nephrectomy and (2) absence of hepatic metastases at autopsy.[1]

The incidence of this syndrome is unknown. The clinical picture is characterized by the presence of hepatomegaly, fever, weight loss, anaemia, high alkaline phosphatase, prolonged prothrombin time, and impaired excretion of sulphobromophthalein (Table 1). In some patients thombocytosis may be observed, probably as a paraneoplastic manifestation. No relationship has been found between

the development of this syndrome and the histological characteristics of the renal cancer.

Liver biopsy shows only minimal changes, including steatosis, spotty necrosis, moderate lymphocyte infiltration in the portal tracts, and haemosiderosis. There is no relationship between the hepatic morphological lesions and the degree of alteration in liver function tests. A patient with progressive hepatic failure has been reported in whom the liver biopsy showed minimal changes (Summerskill, ArchIntMed, 1967; 120:81). Hepatic granulomas have also been described in a patient with hypernephroma. This lesion has been considered to be a paraneoplastic manifestation as it disappears after nephrectomy (Chagnac, AmJGastr, 1985; 89:989). Cholestatic jaundice has been reported in two patients with carcinoma of the kidney (Jakobovits, AustNZJMed, 1981; 11:64). More recently, a case of renal cell carcinoma associated with extensive peliosis hepatis has also been reported (Otani, ActaPathJpn, 1992; 42:68).

The pathogenesis of nephrogenic hepatic dysfunction is unknown. It has been suggested that it may be due to the presence of undetected micrometastases in the liver, with disappearance after nephrectomy, as reported for lung metastases (Gilbert, BrJUrol, 1975; 47:259). This, however, is unlikely since liver metastases were not detected at necropsy in some cases. An alternative hypothesis is that this syndrome is due to a 'hepatotoxic hormone' produced by the tumour itself. Unfortunately, no clinical or experimental study has confirmed this hypothesis (Hanask, InvestUrol, 1971; 8:399).

Recognition of this syndrome is clinically important for two reasons: (1) renal cancer should be considered in the diagnosis of any patient with fever, hepatomegaly, abnormal standard liver function tests, and normal or only minimally altered hepatic histology, and (2) patients with kidney tumours and abnormal standard liver function tests do not necessarily have hepatic metastases.[1]

Recently, eight cases of renal cell carcinoma producing α-fetoprotein have been reported (Minamoto, JSurgOncol, 1994; 55:215). The serum α-fetoprotein levels in these patients ranged from 152 to 234 700 ng/ml. Histologically, these tumours consist of clear-cell carcinoma with several morphological variants. Clinically, most cases show extensive metastases and the prognosis is very poor compared to that of conventional renal cell carcinoma.

Haemodialysis and the liver

Patients treated with haemodialysis frequently present abnormal standard liver function tests. Approximately 30 per cent of haemodialysis patients show mild elevation of transaminases (Parfrey,

Table 1 Clinical and laboratory features of 30 patients with well-documented nephrogenic hepatic dysfunction syndrome	
	Percentage of patients
Clinical features	
fever	71
weight loss	66
abdominal mass	47
hepatomegaly	47
splenomegaly	36
Haematological and biochemical data	
impaired BSP excretion	100
increased alkaline phosphatase	94
thrombocytosis	68
prolonged prothrombin time	66

BSP, sulphobromophthalein.

ProcEDTA, 1982; 19:153). Hepatitis B, D, C, and G viruses are the main cause of liver disease in such patients. Other aetiological factors include drugs, iron overload from repeated blood transfusions, cytomegalovirus, Epstein–Barr virus, bacterial infections, or foreign bodies. Finally, some liver and renal diseases have a common aetiogy such as amyloidosis, diabetes, or vasculitis.

Hepatitis B

With the extensive use of haemodialysis in the 1960s it became apparent that viral hepatitis was a major problem associated with this therapy (Friedman, Lancet, 1966; ii:675, Eastwood, Ann-IntMed, 1968; 69:58). In 1972 it was found that patients submitted to chronic haemodialysis were at great risk of acquiring hepatitis B virus infection (Marmin, BrMedBull, 1972; 28:169). Subsequently, several studies confirmed the high incidence of hepatitis B virus infection in haemodialysis units; at least one serological hepatitis B virus marker was positive in about 40 per cent of the patients, and chronic HBs antigenaemia was found in 10 to 15 per cent (Gahl, Nephron, 1974; 24:58; Ware, Hepatol, 1983; 3:315). The prevalence of serological markers in patients dialysed at home is lower (5–6 per cent), suggesting that transmission of hepatitis B virus from other patients or hospital personnel may be important in the spread of hepatitis B virus infection in haemodialysis units. Most HBsAg carriers are discovered before entering the haemodialysis programme. However, between 5 and 10 per cent of the patients become HBsAg positive after starting haemodialysis in spite of preventive measures (Hawe, BMJ, 1971; 1:540). Many sources, including transfusions (Jones, Lancet, 1967; ii:675), needles (Syndman, AmJEpid, 1976; 104:563), and dialysis machinery (Patisson, Lancet, 1973; i:172), have been implicated in the spread of hepatitis B virus infection. Between 40 and 60 per cent of HBsAg-positive patients with chronic renal failure present HBeAg and DNA polymerase activity in the serum and can therefore transmit the infection to other patients, relatives, and staff members in the dialysis unit (Werner, AnnIntMed, 1978; 89:310). It is important to point out that the incidence of hepatitis B virus infection among patients and staff members in haemodialysis units has declined dramatically with the introduction of infection control strategies. In fact, in the latest annual survey in the United States, reported by Alter et al. (ASAIOTrans, 1991; 37:97), the annual incidence of hepatitis B virus infection among patients had fallen to only 0.1 per cent in 1989 with a prevalence of 1.4 per cent; the annual incidence among staff members had declined to 0.1 per cent with a prevalence of 0.3 per cent.

The illness resulting from hepatitis B virus infection in the dialysis patient is usually asymptomatic (shown only by elevated transaminases and appearance of HBsAg in the blood), while relatives or staff members display a more severe course (London, NEJM, 1969; 281:571). In fact, in a multicentre study (27 countries) carried out in Europe (Jacobs, ProcEDTA, 1977; 14:4) 16 of the 778 staff members of dialysis units who contracted hepatitis died as a consequence of acute hepatic failure. This different outcome between dialysed patients and staff members may be due to immunodeficiency occurring in renal patients compared with the normal immune response of the healthy counterparts. Dialysis patients who develop acute hepatitis B virus infection have about a 60 per cent chance of becoming chronic HBsAg carriers (London,

KidneyInt, 1977; 12:51). Male patients are more prone than female patients to becoming chronic carriers after hepatitis B virus infection. Interestingly, only 5 per cent of dialysis-related cases of acute hepatitis B subsequently develop persistent elevation of aminotransferases due to chronic hepatitis (Nilsen, NEJM, 1971; 285:1157). A study using monoclonal hepatitis B surface antibody suggested that the prevalence of HBsAg in haemodialysis patients may be higher (Fujita, Gastro, 1986; 91:1357). It has been shown that active viral replication in these patients promotes histological progression (Harnett, AmJKidneyDis, 1988; 11:210). The high risk of chronicity as well as progression of liver disease in haemodialysis patients has been attributed to depressed cell-mediated immunity (Lee, AmJNephrol, 1991; 11:98).

Liver disease in chronic HBsAg carriers receiving haemodialysis is characteristically asymptomatic. The serum aminotransferases are slightly increased. Initially, the histology of the liver is also mild with moderate inflammatory infiltration and liver cell necrosis. However, the course of the disease may be progressive, leading to more severe forms such as chronic hepatitis and cirrhosis. This explains the high incidence of hepatitis B virus advanced chronic liver disease found in patients treated for many years with haemodialysis (Degott, Liver, 1983; 3:377; Franceschini, RenFail, 1994; 16:491).

Serum transaminases are the most commonly used screening test for detecting liver disease in haemodialysis patients. However, minor and/or transient abnormalities of serum transaminases in these patients should be interpreted with caution since they may be elevated as a consequence of extrahepatic lesions (skeletal muscle injury or cardiac lesions). Initial screening with HBsAg, anti-HBs, and hepatitis B virus DNA is recommended for everyone on entering the haemodialysis unit, in order to define potential hepatitis B virus carriers as well as those subjects vulnerable to hepatitis B virus infection.

Prevention of hepatitis B virus infection in haemodialysis includes segregation of HBsAg positive from HBsAg negative patients, the use of a dedicated dialysis machine for HBsAg positive patients (dialyser membranes are permeable to hepatitis B virus), and regular serological screening for HBsAg and anti-HBs, in addition to routine cleaning and disinfection procedures.[2]

To avoid the spread of hepatitis B virus among dialysis patients and staff members, vaccination against hepatitis B is recommended. However, it has been demonstrated that haemodialysis patients have a lower anti-HBs response than healthy persons, probably in relation to their poor immunological responsiveness. The percentage of these patients showing antibody response to hepatitis B vaccine has been reported to be 50 to 60 per cent.[3–6] Bruguera et al. found that a higher dose (40 μg rather than 20 μg) and a schedule of four injections gave a better anti-HBs response than a regimen using three injections (AmJNephrol, 1990; 8:547). However, a controlled trial showed that the incidence of hepatitis B virus infection in haemodialysis patients who received the vaccine was similar to that in the placebo group, indicating poor protective efficacy of the hepatitis B virus vaccine in such patients.[5] This may be due to the fact that anti-HBs levels induced by vaccination may decline by the time of infection and therefore the patients are no longer protected against hepatitis B virus infection. Despite its limitations, hepatitis B virus vaccination is useful in the haemodialysis population. It has been suggested that vaccination of patients before the

Table 2 Prevalence (%) of anti-hepatitis C virus antibodies in haemodialysed patients according to geographical area

	Prevalence (%)
United States	13–16
South America	
Brazil	35–68
Venezuela	39
Far East	
Japan	29
Hong Kong	22
Europe	
Italy	43
Spain	35–54
France	23–39
Bulgaria	60
Poland	48
South Africa	23

Data taken from ref. 7.

development of advanced chronic renal disease will further increase the effectiveness of the vaccine against hepatitis B virus infection.[2]

Finally, it is important to note that interferon has demonstrated similar efficacy in these patients and in those without chronic renal disease (Perillo, NEJM, 1990; 323:301).

Hepatitis D

Hepatitis D virus infection is not a major problem in haemodyalisis. Several reports have indicated the absence of hepatitis D virus infection in hepatitis B virus-infected haemodialysed patients.[2] However, hepatitis D virus infection should be considered in these patients when there is a rapidly deteriorating liver disease.

Hepatitis C

Hepatitis C virus infection is very common among haemodialysed patients. The prevalence of anti-hepatitis C virus ranges from 13 to 68 per cent according to geographical area (Table 2).[7] However, it is important to take into account that these results were obtained by using the first-generation test, a less specific technique than the second-generation test (RIBA) or detection of hepatitis C virus RNA by the polymerase chain reaction (**PCR**). A recent report highlights the limitations of the second-generation serological test for hepatitis C virus infection in haemodialysed patients since there was a high false-negative rate for detection of hepatitis C virus infection by serology alone (Bukh, JInfDis, 1993; 168:1343). Therefore, to detect the presence of viraemia the determination of hepatitis C virus RNA is recommended in haemodialysed patients (Chan, Hepatol, 1993; 17:5). Hepatitis C virus infection is less common in patients on continuous peritoneal dialysis. The prevalence of hepatitis C virus infection in this group of patients ranges from 0 to 17 per cent. The reasons for these differences have not yet been fully evaluated.[8]

The clinical features of acute hepatitis C virus infection among haemodialysis patients are similar to those of acute hepatitis B virus infection. In most patients the illness is either asymptomatic or associated with mild symptoms. Furthermore, in a recent study conducted in chronic hepatitis C virus infection by Pol *et al.*

(KidneyInt, 1993; 44:1097), only 31 per cent of the patients with hepatitis C virus RNA in the blood had abnormal liver tests. However, the clinical consequences of hepatitis C virus infection in haemodialysis patients are more severe than was initially considered. In three studies, liver biopsy demonstrated that the incidence of chronic hepatitis, cirrhosis, and even hepatocellular carcinoma is relatively high. Therefore, liver biopsy is the most accurate way to assess severity of liver injury in these patients (Caramelo, AmJKidneyDis, 1993; 22:282; Gilli, Nephron, 1993; 61:293; Rao, AmJMed, 1993; 94:241).

It is a matter of debate whether haemodialysis is a risk factor for transmission or whether the high prevalence of hepatitis C virus infection reflects acquisition from other exposure. In this sense, it is important to consider that the incidence of hepatitis C virus infection in chronic renal failure patients not yet requiring haemodialysis is about 20 per cent (Fabrizi, NephrolDialTranspl, 1994; 9: 1615); there is also a close relationship between the duration of haemodialysis and the increased prevalence of hepatitis C virus infection (Chauvean, KidneyInt 1993; 43:5149; Knudsen, KidneyInt, 1993; 4:1353; Niu, AmJKidneyDis, 1993; 22:568; Oguchi, ClinNephrol, 1993; 38:36), indicating that haemodialysis *per se* is a risk factor for hepatitis C virus transmission. Although most episodes of hepatitis C virus infection in dialysis units have been thought to be related to blood transfusion, there may be other modes of transmission. Nowadays the frequency of blood transfusion has been reduced because of the introduction of erythropoietin. In addition, the screening of blood products in the past several years for hepatitis C virus has also diminished the risk of hepatitis C virus infection through blood transfusion. At present, the prevalence of hepatitis C virus infection in haemodialysis units has been reduced from 43 to 21 per cent (Simon, KidneyInt, 1994; 46:504). However, an outbreak of acute hepatitis C was described among patients undergoing haemodialysis on dialysis machines without completely disposable circuits. The introduction of disposable circuits stopped the spread of hepatitis C virus within the unit, suggesting that the outbreak of hepatitis was due to the dialysis system, again providing evidence for transmission of hepatitis C virus by haemodialysis (Chiaramonte, Nephron, 1992; 61:287). Using hepatitis C virus genotyping, it has been found that 50 per cent of haemodialysis patients not receiving blood transfusions had the same strain of hepatitis C virus (Badalamenti, JAmSocNephrol, 1993; 4:332A), further suggesting that hepatitis C virus infection may be spread through haemodialysis techniques. However, reuse of dialysers has not been associated with hepatitis C virus transmission (Lion, AmJKidneyDis, 1993; 21:288). These discrepancies suggest that, at present, it is not clear whether these patients should be segregated. From the results reported, it seems logical that hepatitis C virus infection among haemodialysis patients may be spread through haemodialysis techniques. However, at present there is no clear policy to prevent the spread of hepatitis C virus infection among haemodialysis patients. This should be defined in the near future according to the results obtained in prospective longitudinal studies through determination of hepatitis C virus RNA in these patients.

Nowadays, there is limited information regarding the treatment of hepatitis C virus-infected haemodialysis patients. Data obtained by Koenig (JAmSocNephrol, 1993; 4:301) suggests that interferon showed a positive response in 20 per cent of the patients. However, more extensive and prolonged clinical trials are necessary to know the real efficacy of interferon in the treatment of haemodialysis-infected patients.[9]

The risk to staff and family members of contracting hepatitis C from haemodialysed patients is not well known. However, in two studies (Mitsui, Hepatol, 1992; 16:1109; Forseter, AmJInfec-Control, 1993; 21:5), the risk to staff of acquiring hepatitis C after needle-stick accidents was over 10 per cent. The risk to sexual partners and family members is much lower (Chan, Gastro, 1993; 104:862).

Hepatitis G

The hepatitis G virus is a recently identified RNA virus. In a recent publication (Masuco, NEJM, 1996; 334:1485) it was reported that 16 out of 519 haemodialysis patients (3.1 per cent) presented hepatitis G virus RNA in the blood as compared with 0.9 per cent of healthy blood donors. None of these 16 patients showed evidence of active liver disease, although seven were also infected with hepatitis C virus. The transmission was probably through blood transfusion. It is possible that the incidence of hepatitis G virus infection among haemodialysed patients varies according to the geographical area investigated. Its prevalence in haemodialysis patients has also been investigated in our unit (Forns, Nephrol-DialTranspl, 1997; 12:956) and we have found that hepatitis G virus RNA was present in 26 per cent of haemodialysed patients and in 4.6 per cent of blood donors. In addition, 52 per cent of the patients infected with hepatitis G virus were co-infected with other hepatitis viruses (hepatitis B virus or hepatitis C virus). Liver test abnormalities were more frequent in patients infected by hepatitis C virus or hepatitis B virus (71 per cent) than in patients infected by hepatitis G virus alone (16 per cent), suggesting that hepatitis G virus infection is not a frequent cause of chronic liver disease in these patients. Although 80 per cent of hepatitis G virus-infected patients had received blood products, the transfusion rate was not different from other patients. Time on haemodialysis was significantly shorter in patients infected by hepatitis G virus alone compared to patients infected by hepatitis C virus or hepatitis B virus, indicating that blood transfusion could be one of the main factors implicated in hepatitis G virus transmission in patients on haemodialysis. To know the clinical importance of hepatitis G virus infection in haemodialysed patients further clinical data are required.

Other hepatic lesions

Other hepatic lesions which occasionally affect haemodialysis patients include spontaneous liver haematoma, haemorrhagic cholecystitis, diffuse hepatic calcification, hepatic infarction, liver deposition of silicone, haemosiderosis, and haemochromatosis.

Spontaneous haemorrhagic complications of haemodialysis are diverse and have occasionally been observed in the liver and in the gallbladder. Although hepatic haematoma has been reported in a few patients, an incidence of 1.5 per cent has been published among haemodialysis patients with manifestations of spontaneous bleeding (Borra, AnnIntMed, 1980; 93:574). The clinical picture of hepatic haematoma is characterized by upper quadrant pain, tenderness on palpation of the liver, fever, a decrease in haematocrit, and an increase in alkaline phosphatase levels. Radio-isotope scanning, ultrasonography or CT scan provide supportive evidence of this

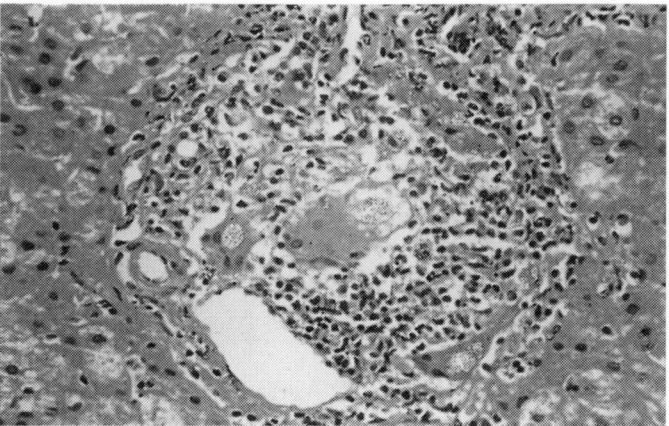

Fig. 1. Silicone deposit in the liver. Granules of a brilliant material are seen within several multinucleated cells in a portal tract. This material was refractile, but not refringent under polarized light (H and E × 180).

complication. Management is dependent on the extent and location of liver injury. Central haematomas can simply be evacuated, whereas haematomas causing subcapsular tear and bleeding may require partial hepatectomy. Haemorrhagic cholecystitis (McFadden, AmJGastr, 1987; 82:1081) is usually associated with right-side abdominal pain, fever, nausea, vomiting, and leucocytosis. Radionuclide scanning is useful for confirming this diagnosis. The treatment is cholecystectomy.

Only one haemodialysis patient has been reported with microscopic diffuse hepatic calcification (Sugiura, AmJGastr, 1987; 82:786). The calcifications were found in the intracellular and extracellular space, and were round or rod-shaped and single or multiple in distribution. Calcium was deposited as calcium phosphate.

Recently, hepatic infarction was reported as developing on a patient with systemic lupus erythematosus and chronic renal failure treated with haemodialysis (Kaplan, AmJKidneyDis, 1995; 26:785). This complication is very uncommon as haemodialysis patients have a decreased tendency for vascular thrombosis. However, this may not be true in the presence of circulating antiphospholipid antibodies as occurs in patients with systemic lupus erythematosus.

Particles of silicone have been observed in the livers of patients treated with haemodialysis (Leong, Lancet, 1981; i:889; Leong, NEJM, 1982; 306:135). The hepatic lesion is characterized by the presence of granulomas associated with varying degrees of inflammation and fibrosis (Fig. 1). The incidence of this lesion in haemodialysis patients is about 50 per cent. Silicone tubing is the source of particulate contamination in haemodialysis. Although most blood lines are made of polyvinyl chloride, silicone is still widely employed in the pump-blood segment because of its non-occluding properties. The spillage or fragmentation and release of plastic particles into the blood may occur anywhere in the blood-tubing set; however, the blood-pump segment is most susceptible because of the mechanical stress imposed by the action of the pump (Laohapand, ProcEDTA, 1982; 19:143). Most of these patients are asymptomatic, although in some patients fever and malaise may occur. It has been suggested that hepatic silicone deposition could be a cause of chronic hepatic dysfunction in haemodialysis patients (Parfrey, ProcEDTA, 1982; 19:153).

Renal transplant and the liver

Hepatic dysfunction, recognized by increased levels of transaminases, is frequently seen in renal transplant patients. In the 1970s the reported incidence varied from 7 to 67 per cent (Arnoff, CanMedAssJ, 1973; 108:43; Ireland, ArchIntMed, 1973; 123:29; Barnes, SGO, 1975; 141:171; Mores, AnnSurg, 1978; 188:783; Allison, QJMed, 1992; 83:355). In most patients chronic liver disease is due to hepatitis virus infection, particularly hepatitis B virus and hepatitis C virus.[2,10] Other hepatic lesions have been described due to renal transplantation *per se* or as a consequence of immunosuppression therapy; for example, peliosis hepatis (Degott, Gut, 1978; 19:748), idiopathic portal hypertension (Nataf, Gut, 1978; 20:235), hepatic veno-occlusive disease (Marubbio, Gastro, 1975; 69:739), nodular regenerative hyperplasia (Bradfeldt, DigDisSci, 1981; 26:271), and cholestasis (Bruguera, Nephrol, 1984; 4: 227).

Hepatitis B

Renal transplantation and associated therapeutic immunosuppression affects the outcome of infected hepatitis B virus patients (Cohen, AnnIntMed, 1976; 84:275; Parfrey, KidneyInt, 1985; 28: 959; Parfrey, Transpl, 1985; 39:610). Prospective studies using sequential liver biopsy have demonstrated that hepatitis B virus infection in renal transplant recipients usually leads to a severe form of chronic liver disease. Pol *et al.* (Lancet, 1990; 335:878) showed histological worsening of the liver during the post-transplant period in 80 per cent of hepatitis B virus-infected patients. Such patients may develop chronic hepatitis, cirrhosis, and even hepatocellular carcinoma (Parfrey, Transpl, 1984; 37:461). It was found that hepatitis B virus renal transplant patients had a lower post-transplant survival than patients not infected with hepatitis B virus (Pirson, NEJM, 1979; 296:194), although others have reported different results (Rivolta, TransplProc, 1987; 19:2153; Huang, Transpl, 1990; 49:540; Pol, Lancet, 1990; 335:878), indicating that the survival of renal transplanted patients with hepatitis B virus infection was similar to that of patients negative for hepatitis B virus. Recently, Hiesse *et al.* (ClinTranspl, 1992; 46:461) reported on a large series of patients: the 10-year post-transplant survival of hepatitis B virus-positive renal transplanted patients was, in fact, significantly lower than that found in the hepatitis B virus-negative patients, confirming previous results reported by Pirson and co-workers (NEJM, 1979; 296:194). These results are in contrast with the survival rate observed in hepatitis B virus-infected patients submitted to haemodialysis, in whom the outcome was similar to that observed in haemodialysed patients without hepatitis B virus infection. Therefore, at present, chronic renal hepatitis B virus patients with active viral replication (hepatitis B virus DNA positive) should be treated with haemodialysis rather than renal transplantation (Harnett, AmJKidneyDis, 1988; 12:210; Friedlander, AmJNephrol, 1989; 3:204). The poor results of renal transplantation among hepatitis B virus patients may be explained by increased viral replication with reappearance of, or an increase in the serum of, hepatitis B virus DNA, HBsAg and HBeAg, following apparent clearance of previous hepatitis B virus infection (Nagington, Lancet, 1977; ii:558; Dusheiko, Hepatol, 1983; 3:330; Rao, Transpl, 1991; 51:331). These effects are probably secondary to immunosuppressive therapy which may increase hepatitis B virus replication by the activation of the glucocorticoid-responsive element, contained in the hepatitis B virus genome, that may increase the transcription of hepatitis B virus genes (Degos, Gastro, 1988; 94: 151). In a preliminary study it has been found that the outcome of those renal transplant patients infected by hepatitis B virus treated with cyclosporin was better than in those treated with azathioprine (Sandrini, NephrolDialTranspl, 1990; 5:525), suggesting that cyclosporin should be used as immunosuppressive therapy in these patients. However, more extensive controlled clinical trials are required to confirm this result. On the other hand, attempts to reduce the dose of prednisone after renal transplantation are probably appropriate and beneficial.[2]

The effect of hepatitis B virus infection on graft survival is controversial. Some authors have suggested that graft survival is shortened (London, NEJM, 1977; 296:241). However, other researchers have been unable to detect any effect of hepatitis B virus infection on graft survival (Chatarjee, NEJM, 1974; 291:62). Nevertheless, it is possible that the reported differences may have reflected the unrecognized presence of HBsAg-negative/hepatitis B virus DNA-positive renal transplant recipients in whom graft survival is superior to that of truly hepatitis B virus-negative patients (Degos, Gastro, 1988; 94:151; Dienstag, Gastro, 1988; 94:235).

At present, it is not clear whether interferon produces a significant HBeAg and HBsAg seroconversion; long-term follow-up studies are not yet available.[10]

As a consequence of the effective control of hepatitis B virus infection in haemodialysis units, the number of hepatitis B virus-positive patients undergoing evaluation for renal transplantation has declined in the past 10 years. Nowadays, renal transplantation should only be considered in patients with mild liver disease without hepatitis B virus replication. In those patients with advanced liver disease without viral replication simultaneous kidney–liver transplantation may be indicated.[10]

Hepatitis D

Hepatitis D virus infection is an infrequent clinical condition in renal transplant recipients. Kharsa *et al.* (Transpl, 1987; 44:221) reported three cases of fulminant hepatitis among 300 renal transplant recipients. In two of these three cases, direct staining of liver tissue identified hepatitis D virus, indicating that this virus should be considered as a cause of fulminant hepatitis in renal transplant recipients.

Hepatitis C

The prevalence of hepatitis C virus infection in renal transplant patients is very high, ranging from 11 to 49 per cent. It is important to indicate that this prevalence has been confirmed in two studies using hepatitis C virus RNA (Table 3).

The source of transmission of hepatitis C virus comes from infection acquired during haemodialysis and from blood transfusion.[9] Another possible source of hepatitis C virus infection is solid organ transplantation. Studies conducted so far have given highly discordant results. In a retrospective study, Roth *et al.* (AnnIntMed, 1992; 57:490) found this kind of hepatitis C virus transmission to be uncommon. In contrast, Pereira *et al.* (NEJM, 1992; 327:910) reported that nearly all the recipient organs from anti-hepatitis C virus-positive donors became infected with the

Table 3 Hepatitis C virus infection in renal allograft recipients

Author	EIA-I	EIA-III	HCV RNA
Roth USA (AnnIntMed, 1992; 117:470)	179/596 (30)	—	—
Ponz, Spain (KidneyInt, 1991; 40:748)	32/67 (48)	—	—
Baur, Germany (AnnHemat, 1991; 62:68)	27/272 (10)	—	—
Klauser, Austria (TransplProc, 1992; 24:286)	43/324 (13)	—	—
Huang, China (Transpl, 1992; 53:763)	59/120 (49)	—	—
Morales, Spain (TransplProc, 1992; 24:78)	66/200 (33)	—	—
Pol, France (JHepatol, 1992; 15:202)	20/127 (24)	—	—
Stempel, USA (Transpl, 1993; 55:273)	76/176 (11)	—	—
Chan, Hong Kong (Gastro, 1993; 104:862)	—	19/185 (10)	18/19 (95)
Roth, USA (KidneyInt, 1994; 45:238)	—	109/641 (17)	39/53 (74)

EIA-I, EIA-III: The numbers of hepatitis C virus-positive patients to the total numbers of patients tested are given; HCV RNA: the numbers of hepatitis C virus RNA-positive patients to EIA-positive patients are stated. Percentages are given in parentheses.
Data taken from ref. 9.

virus. In renal transplant recipients, Vincenti *et al.* (Transpl, 1994; 57:826) did not find hepatitis C virus infection in recipients of kidneys from anti-hepatitis C virus- and hepatitis C virus RNA-positive donors, whereas Tesi *et al.* (Transpl, 1994; 57:826) reported that 56 per cent of the recipients of kidneys from hepatitis C virus infected donors became hepatitis C virus RNA-positive after transplantation. These results clearly indicate that although hepatitis C virus infection may be acquired by organ tranplantation, the risk varies widely from one centre to another. It is very difficult to explain this variation in hepatitis C virus transmission. Possibilities worth exploring include differences in diagnostic techniques for hepatitis C virus detection and in the numerous steps of the transplantation procedure.[11] Recently, it has been shown that washing the donated kidney by a modified pulsatile perfusion preservation procedure can eliminate up to 99 per cent of the viral burden (Zucker, Transpl, 1994; 57:832). Although these results are encouraging, further studies are needed to confirm these findings.

In the past the determination of transaminases was considered the best surrogate marker to detect liver disease among renal transplant patients; however, it has been shown that this is not the best procedure, since 33 to 52 per cent of anti-hepatitis C virus-positive patients have normal transaminases (Ponz, KidneyInt, 1991; 40:748; Roth, Transpl, 1991; 51:396). In addition, progression to cirrhosis has been demonstrated in serial liver biopsy specimens from renal transplant recipients infected with hepatitis C virus (Rao, AmJMed, 1993; 94:241). Therefore, since these patients may progress to cirrhosis, liver biopsy is essential to detect those patients at high risk of developing this lesion.

The outcome of renal transplant recipients infected with hepatitis C virus was thought to be identical to that of non-infected patients. However, it has been found that hepatitis C virus-infected renal transplant recipients have a lower long-term survival from 5 years after transplantation. Consequently, although the natural history for hepatitis C virus infection in transplant recipients is unknown, it should not be considered a benign entity. Further prospective long-term follow-up is needed because chronic hepatitis C may be an asymptomatic and indolent process until symptoms of endstage liver disease develop, even hepatocellular carcinoma (Arita, TransplProc, 1992; 24:1538), 10 to 25 years after the original infection (Bruguera, JClinGastro, 1990; 12:298).

Various percentages of co-infection with hepatitis B virus and hepatitis C virus may be observed, depending on the geographical area of the studies. Huang *et al.* (Transpl, 1992; 53:763) from Hong Kong found that about 50 per cent of their patients were hepatitis B virus and hepatitis C virus positive. Among 120 patients studied, 21 per cent of the dually infected patients were found to have cirrhosis, compared with none in the hepatitis C virus-positive and hepatitis B virus-negative group. These authors concluded that the co-infection by hepatitis B virus and hepatitis C virus leads to severe forms of liver disease in renal transplant recipients.

At present, hepatitis C virus infection is not considered an absolute contraindication for renal transplantation. However, before considering renal transplantation, hepatitis C virus-infected patients should be tested for hepatitis C virus RNA and submitted to liver biopsy in order to detect advanced liver disease at an early stage. Patients with mild or moderate chronic hepatitis should be considered for renal transplantation while patients with more advanced liver disease should remain on haemodialysis, or should be considered for kidney–liver transplantation.[8]

No available data regarding the efficacy and tolerance of interferon in the management of hepatitis C virus infection have yet been reported in kidney recipients. It has been suggested that interferon may increase the risk of acute rejection; however, this issue is still under discussion.[7] Nevertheless, nowadays it is not known whether interferon is useful in the treatment of these patients. In a preliminary report Koenig, (KidneyInt, 1994; 44: 1507) found that interferon was as effective in non-uraemic patients, although more side-effects were detected.

Hepatitis G

Up to now there are no available data regarding the prevalence and clinical importance of hepatitis G virus infection among renal transplant recipients.

Other hepatic lesions

One hepatic lesion which is undoubtedly related to renal transplantation is peliosis hepatis, as it is not observed in haemodialysed patients or in liver biopsies performed on the day of transplantation. This lesion consists of sinusoidal dilatation and blood-filled spaces, without endothelial lining, located predominantly in centrilobular areas. The development of this lesion has been related to immuno-suppresion therapy, particularly azathioprine (Izumi, JHepatol, 1994; 20:129). The estimated prevalence of peliosis hepatis in renal transplant patients is 2 to 4 per cent (Degott, Gut, 1978; 19: 748), and it is more frequent in males than females. The clinical manifestations of peliosis hepatis in renal transplant patients are variable. In some cases it is clinically latent, whereas in others it may produce hepatomegaly, portal hypertension, oesophageal varices, and ascites. Renal graft rejection is relatively common in patients with peliosis hepatis. The prognosis of this lesion depends on the degree of portal hypertension. In some renal transplant recipients it has been shown that peliosis hepatis causes severe fibrosing liver lesions. The course of vascular hepatic disease is not modified by azathioprine withdrawal (Cavalcanti, Transpl, 1994; 58:315).The mechanism of peliosis hepatis in renal transplanted patients is not known, although it may be related to a blockage of liver blood flow at the junctions of the sinusoid and centrilobular veins (Paradina, Histopath, 1976; 1:225).

Idiopathic portal hypertension causing ascites, oesophageal varices, and gastrointestinal bleeding has been described in renal transplant patients treated with azathioprine. In all these cases perisinusoidal fibrosis was demonstrated by electron microscopy. This lesion may be the cause of portal hypertension, through a partial obstruction of hepatic sinusoids (Yoshimura, SurgToday, 1994; 24:1111). A fatal case of partial obstruction due to nodular regenerative hyperplasia of the liver was reported following renal transplantation (Bradfett, DigDisSci, 1981; 26:271). More recently it has been reported that nodular regeneration is also associated with the administration of azathioprine (Mion, Gut, 1991; 32:715).

Approximately 5 per cent of renal transplant patients develop acute cholestasis secondary to azathioprine therapy, which resolves slowly after drug withdrawal (Bruguera, Nephrol, 1984; 4:227). Fatal hepatic veno-occlusive disease has also been reported in a renal transplant patient receiving azathioprine (Marubbio, Gastro, 1975; 69:739).

Prostatic carcinoma and the liver

In addition, to hepatic metastases (see Chapter 22.3.1), which are uncommon, patients with prostatic carcinoma may present obstructive jaundice due to infiltration of the subhepatic tissues around the common bile duct (Ben-Ishay, IsrlJMedSci, 1975; 11: 838; Chen, AnnIntMed, 1990; 112:881) or as a consequence of a lesion resembling sclerosing cholangitis (Taylor, JClinGastro, 1993; 16:143). This biliary obstruction may improve or disappear with orchidectomy and with the administration of stilboestrol.

Patients with prostatic carcinoma may be treated with diethyl-stilboestrol. Although this drug has been used for more that 50 years, its metabolism and toxicity are still not completely understood. It is considered that diethylstilboestrol is excreted, almost exclusively in the bile, as a glucuronide with very weak oestrogenic activity (Smith, ActaEnd, 1974; 185(suppl.):149). Therefore, the liver excretes di-ethylstilboestrol and probably has a relatively low parenchymal level of biologically active oestrogen.

In about 30 to 50 per cent of treated patients with prostatic cancer diethylstilboestrol may produce a slight increase of transaminases within 2 weeks of starting treatment (Kontturi, BMJ 1969; 4:204).

With continued treatment, values usually return to normal. This study also showed that 20 per cent of patients presented a moderate increase of serum bilirubin which returned to basal values 1 month later. In addition to these findings Ishibe (JUrol, 1975;113:829) found that those patients with a poor response to treatment with synthetic female sex hormone showed an increase of alkaline phos-phatase during follow-up. In these cases the diagnosis of hepatic metastases was not discarded. These two reports show that during treatment with oestrogen great individual variations occur in liver function tests of patients with prostatic cancer. Since several of these patients may have liver function test alterations before treatment with oestrogen, the dosage of diethylstilboestrol should be adjusted according to liver function. In addition, patients with a history of chronic liver disease are known to be more sensitive to the toxic effects of synthetic hormones and the risk of worsening of liver disease is very high (Konturi, ScaJUrolNephrol, 1972; 6:289).

In humans diethylstilboestrol can induce several malignancies (vaginal and cervical adenomas, clear-cell adenocarcinoma, renal cell carcinoma, endometrial carcinoma, and papillomatosis of the male breast). In the liver, tumour-like lesions reported with diethylstilboestrol therapy are peliosis hepatis, focal nodular hyperplasia (Moesner, ActaMedScand, 1977; 85:119, Puppala, PostgradMed, 1979; 65:227), angiosarcoma (Hoch-Laegth, JAMA, 1978; 240:1510; Ham, DigDisSci, 1980; 25:879), and hepatocellular carcinoma (Brooks, JUrol, 1982; 128:1044). Interestingly, in all the cases of hepatic malignancy associated with diethylstilboestrol the drug had been taken over a long period of time (3–5 years).

In the 1970s cyproterone acetate was introduced in the treatment of prostatic carcinoma. This drug, a synthetic 21-carbon steroid with marked progestational activity, effectively inhibits testosterone-induced growth of the prostate and seminal vesicles in the rat. The mechanism responsible for its antiandrogenic action is suppression of plasma testosterone levels by inhibiting the C21–19 desmolase enzymatic activity in the testes and at the target cell by competitively inhibiting the binding of dehydrotestosterone to cytoplasmic and nuclear binding proteins (Smith, JUrol, 1973; 110:106). Cy-proterone acetate has been used in man, not only to treat prostatic cancer, but also in the treatment of hypersexuality and sexual deviation, and in women for the treatment of severe acne and hirsutism. More recently it has been used at higher doses in combination with growth hormone for treating growth-hormone deficiency children with short stature at puberty. Initially, it was considered that this drug was not hepatotoxic. However, it has been shown that about 15 to 20 per cent of patients may develop a transient and slight increase of transaminases after 6 weeks or even several months of therapy (Crombie, BrJUrol, 1987; 59:44; Roila, AnnOncol, 1993; 4:701). However, liver function in these patients became normal 4 to 9 weeks after treatment. None the less, in other patients hepatitis was very severe (Meijers, EurJCanClinOnc, 1986; 22:112; Lévesque, Lancet, 1989; i:215; Blake, Gut. 1990; 31:556; Parys, BrJUrol, 1991; 67:312; Drakos, EurJCan, 1992; 28A:1931; Dourakis, JHepatol, 1994; 20:350). The mechanism responsible for this hepatotoxicity is under discussion. However, in a recent publication it has been suggested that this drug may induce the synthesis of transforming growth factor β-1 in rat hepatocytes together with an enhanced sensitivity to undergo apoptosis, that, in turn, would induce hepatic necrosis (Oberhammer, Hepatol, 1996;

23:329). As a consequence of these reports, most researchers recommend that hepatic function should be assessed 2 and 4 weeks after initiating therapy and every 2 months thereafter (Roila, Ann-Oncol, 1993; 4:701).

Recently, there have been reports that patients receiving cyproterone acetate have developed hepatocellular carcinoma (Ohri, BrJUrol, 1991; 67:213; Roila, AnnOncol, 1993; 4:701; Kattan, AmJClinOncCanClinTrials, 1994; 17:390; Watanake, Lancet, 1994; 344:1567; Rudiger, Lancet, 1995; 345:452). All were treated with high doses of cyproterone acetate. These tumours were observed in prostate carcinoma patients, during puberty in women with Turner's syndrome, and in a woman receiving cyproterone acetate in combination with an oral contraceptive for more than 10 years. The mechanism by which cyproterone acetate intake may cause hepatocellular carcinoma is, at present, not well understood. However, experimental studies have shown that cyproterone acetate induces DNA adduct formation and DNA repair activities in rat hepatocytes (Topinka, Carcinogenesis, 1993; 14:423; Martelli, Carcinogenesis, 1995; 16:1265). In addition, these DNA adducts may accumulate in liver cells (Werner, Carcinogenesis, 1995; 16:2369), facilitating the development of hepatocellular carcinoma.

Bladder cancer and the liver

Patients with superficial bladder cancer are usually treated with intravesical bacillus Calmette–Guérin (**BCG**). BCG is commonly given in three clinical settings: (1) prophylaxis in tumour-free patients, (2) treatment of residual tumour in patients with papillary transitional cell carcinoma other than carcinoma *in situ*, and (3) treatment of patients with carcinoma *in situ*. Long-term studies of BCG therapy have reported favourable responses in 50 to 89 per cent of patients and it is considered that this treatment probably exerts its antitumoral effect through immune mechanisms or as a consequence of an inflammatory reaction induced by the intravesical instillation of BCG.[12] Complications of this therapy include local side-effects such as haematuria, cystitis, granulomatous prostatitis, bladder contractures, and renal abscess. These local side-effects occur either as an inflammatory reaction to BCG, or infection secondary to contact with BCG-contaminated urine (Lamm, JUrol, 1992: 147:596). Systemic side-effects such as granulomatous hepatitis, pneumonitis, azotaemia, and pancytopenia have also been described (Lamm, UrolClinNAm, 1992; 19:565). The systemic side-effects are believed to be the result of either a hypersensitivity

reaction to BCG, or clinical illness caused by BCG mycobacteria (Lage, JUrol, 1986; 135:916). Granulomatous hepatitis and/or pneumonitis occur in 0.7 per cent of treated cases. Patients present after multiple intravesical BCG instillations with high fever, severe illness, and abnormal liver function tests (Marans, JUrol, 1987; 137:111). Liver biopsies show intrahepatic granulomas without mycobacteria in most patients. Recently a patient with mycobacteraemia and granulomatous hepatitis occurring after the initial intravesical instillation of BCG has been reported (Proctor, AmJ-Gastr, 1993; 88:1112). Treatment of systemic BCG infection in acutely ill patients with isoniazid, rifampicin, and ethambutol is recommended (Lamm, JUrol, 1992; 147:597). Granulomatous hepatitis should be considered as an important side-effect of intravesical instillation of BCG for bladder cancer, and its presence should be taken into account in any patient with persistent fever and abnormal liver function tests after BCG instillation.

References

1. Strickland RC, and Schenker S. The nephrogenic hepatic dysfunction syndrome: a review. *Digestive Disease*, 1977; **22**: 49–55.
2. Martin P, and Friedman LS. Chronic viral hepatitis and the management of chronic renal failure. *Kidney International*, 1995; **47**: 1231–41.
3. Crosnier J, *et al.* Randomized placebo controlled trial of hepatitis B surface antigen vaccine in French haemodialysis units II. Haemodialysis patients. *Lancet*, 1981; i: 797–800.
4. Köhler H, *et al.* Active hepatitis B vaccination of dialysis patients and medical staff. *Kidney International*, 1984; **25**: 124–8.
5. Stevens CE, *et al.* Hepatitis vaccine in patients receiving hemodialysis. Immunogenecity and efficacy. *New England Journal of Medicine*, 1984; **311**: 496–501.
6. Bruguera M, *et al.* Immunogenicity of a recombinant hepatitis B vaccine in haemodialysis patients. *Postgraduate Medical Journal*, 1987; **63** (suppl): 155–8.
7. Pol S. Hepatitis C virus infection in haemodialysed patients and kidney allograft recipients. *Advances in Nephrology*, 1995; **24**: 315–30.
8. Davis CL, *et al.* Hepatitis C virus in renal diseases. *Current Opinion in Nephrology and Hypertension*, 1994; **3**: 164–73.
9. Roth D. Hepatitis C virus: The nephrologist's view. *American Journal of Kidney Diseases*, 1995; **25**: 3–15.
10. Goffin E, Pirson Y, and van Ypersele de Strihou. Implications of chronic hepatitis B or hepatitis C for renal transplant candidates. *Nephrology, Dialysis, Transplantation*, 1995; **10** (suppl. 6): 88–92.
11. Sánchez-Tapias JM and Rodés J. Dilemmas of organ transplantation from anti-HCV- positive donors. *Lancet*, 1995; **345**: 469–70.
12. Catalona WJ. Urothelial tumors of the urinary tract. In Walsh PC, Ratik AB, Stamey TA, and Vaughan DE, eds. *Campbell's urology*. Philadelphia: Saunders, 1992: 1094–158.

24.5 The effect of haematological and lymphatic diseases on the liver

Miguel Bruguera

Liver abnormalities are frequently seen in patients with haematological diseases. The changes are due either to liver involvement by the haematological disorder, to the measures employed for its treatment, or to a concurrent and independent disease. Occasionally, clinical evidence of liver disease is the first manifestation of a primary haematological condition. This chapter summarizes the hepatic abnormalities found in the different haematological diseases. Hepatic complications related to bone marrow transplantation are described in Chapter 14.5.

Hodgkin's disease

Frequency

Hepatic involvement in Hodgkin's disease is regarded as evidence of stage IV disease. Thus, it has a wide variation depending on the duration of the disease.[1] The prevalence ranges from 5 to 14 per cent in liver biopsies obtained at the time of diagnosis of Hodgkin's disease, increases to 30 per cent during the course of disease, and becomes as high as 60 per cent in autopsy series.

Liver infiltration is more common in the aggressive histological subtypes of Hodgkin's disease—the lymphocyte-depleted and the mixed cellularity varieties. The lymphocyte-predominant type has the lowest incidence.[2] Splenic involvement correlates closely with the risk of hepatic involvement. When multiple nodules are found in the spleen, the likelihood of hepatic infiltration is high (Colby, Cancer, 1982; 49:1848). There is a single instance reported of liver infiltration in the absence of splenic Hodgkin's disease (Falk, Cancer, 1979; 43:1146).

Histology

Hepatic infiltration in Hodgkin's disease occurs multifocally in the portal tracts. Sometimes, large infiltrates coalesce forming large tumour nodules. The diagnosis of liver involvement requires the finding of Reed–Sternberg cells, admixed with lymphocytes, eosinophils, plasma cells, and atypical histiocytes. The finding of atypical histiocytes, even without Reed–Sternberg cells, is highly suggestive of hepatic involvement by Hodgkin's disease (Fig. 1).[2]

Non-caseating epithelioid granulomas, either in the hepatic lobules or in the portal tracts, may be seen in 10 per cent of liver biopsies (Kadin, NEJM, 1974; 27:1277). They often occur in patients without involvement of the liver by Hodgkin's disease.[3]

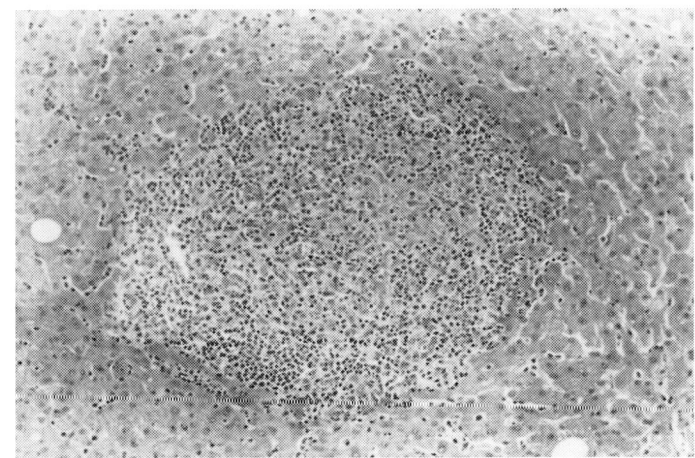

Fig. 1. Hodgkin's disease. Nodular infiltrate in the parenchyma composed of atypical histiocytes, eosinophils, and lymphocytes (HE × 60).

Non-specific inflammatory infiltrates of portal tracts are seen in a high proportion of cases (Leslie, HumPath, 1984;15:808). They should not be mistaken for liver involvement by Hodgkin's disease. Sinusoidal dilatation is present in many patients with systemic (B) symptoms (Bruguera, Liver, 1987; 7:76) and reverses when disease activity is abolished with chemotherapy. Peliosis hepatis has been documented in one patient (Bhaskar, AmJGastr, 1990; 85:628).

Clinical features

Patients with liver involvement often remain asymptomatic. An enlarged liver is a common finding, but does not necessarily indicate hepatic infiltration.

Jaundice is rare as an initial manifestation but relatively frequent in late stages,[4] resulting from extensive liver infiltration by tumour (Levitan, AmJMed, 1961; 30:99) or extrahepatic biliary obstruction produced by hilar adenopathies (Perera, Gastro, 1974; 56:680). A few patients exhibit a syndrome of idiopathic intrahepatic cholestasis, for which none of the known causes of jaundice can be implicated (Piken, Gastro, 1979; 77:145; Lieberman, JClinGastro, 1986; 8:304). A paraneoplastic hormonal effect unrelated to the bulk of tumour has been suggested as a cause for jaundice. Cholestasis may remit with chemotherapy. In a few patients presenting with jaundice associated with fever and severe hepatic failure (acute cholestasis of Hodgkin's disease) liver biopsy demonstrates tumoural infiltration in the liver with loss of bile ducts in portal tracts (Trewby, QJMed, 1979; 48:137; Lefkowitch, ArchPathLabMed, 1985; 109:424; Hubscher, Hepatol, 1993; 17:70; Cervantes, AnnHemat, 1996; 72:357). The development of Hodgkin's disease several years after the diagnosis of primary sclerosing cholangitis has been reported (Man, Hepatol, 1993; 18:1127).

Liver function tests are of little value in diagnosing liver involvement. Increased serum alkaline phosphatase activity is found in many patients with hepatic infiltration, but may also be associated with non-specific histological changes, such as granulomas or sinusoidal dilatation.[3] An isolated elevation of serum alkaline phosphatase activity may represent a minor form of the syndrome of idiopathic cholestasis of Hodgkin's disease (Carreras, MedicinaClin, 1987; 89:43).

Non-Hodgkin's lymphomas
Frequency

Liver involvement in non-Hodgkin's lymphoma is more common than in Hodgkin's disease. Liver biopsies obtained at diagnosis of lymphoma show hepatic infiltration in about 15 per cent of the cases. Around 100 cases have been reported in which the liver was the only tissue affected by the lymphoma (Strayer, Gastro, 1980; 78:1571; Osborne, Cancer, 1985; 56:2902; DeMent, AmJClinPath, 1987; 88:255; Anthony, JClinPath, 1990; 43:1007; Scoazec, Hepatol, 1991; 13:870; Oshawa, DigDisSci, 1992; 37:1105). Primary lymphomas of the liver account for 0.4 per cent of all extranodal lymphomas. Criteria for diagnosis of primary lymphoma are: (i) absence of lymphadenopathy or splenomegaly, (ii) normal abdominal and thoracic computed tomographic scans, and (iii) normal bone marrow and blood counts (Caccamo, ArchPathLabMed, 1986; 110:553).

Histology

Hepatic infiltration is more common in low-grade lymphocytic (small cell) lymphomas than in high-grade (large cell, histiocytic) lymphomas,[2] but primary lymphomas of the liver more frequently belong to the large cell type. The hepatic infiltration consists of a well-circumscribed nodular infiltration of portal tracts by packed malignant cells, which may infiltrate the sinusoids when the disease evolves to a leukaemic phase. Large tumour nodules effacing the hepatic architecture may be observed.[5,6]

Immunohistochemistry may help to characterize the lymphoid infiltrates present in liver biopsies (Verdi, Hepatol, 1986; 6:6; Voight, GastrClinBiol, 1989; 13:343). The demonstration of monoclonality supports the diagnosis of lymphoma.

Epithelioid granulomas are found in up to 10 per cent of liver biopsies from patients with non-Hodgkin's lymphoma (Braylan, Cancer, 1977; 39:1146); they do not indicate that the liver is affected by the lymphoma.

Clinical features

Hepatic infiltration with non-Hodgkin's lymphoma is usually silent. Mild to moderate elevations of serum alkaline phosphatase may be present. Jaundice is uncommon and, when it occurs, is more likely to be due to extrahepatic obstruction at the liver hilum than to hepatic infiltration.[7] Exceptionally, jaundice with liver failure is the first clinical manifestation of lymphoma. The diagnosis should be suspected if there is liver enlargement and lactic acidosis. Neither feature is seen when acute liver failure is due to viral or toxic agents. Diagnosis must be confirmed histologically before starting chemotherapy; liver transplantation should be avoided (Saló, AmJGastr, 1993; 88:774; Zafrani, Hepatol, 1993; 3:428; Gargot, EurJGastroHepatol, 1994; 6:843; Woolf, DigDisSci, 1994; 6:1351). Untreated patients follow a rapid course to death. Liver tissue examination reveals massive tumoural infiltration of sinusoids, and replacement of hepatic cords by malignant cells. Lymphomas presenting as severe hepatic failure are of various histological types, such as Burkitt-type and small or large cell lymphoma. Cases previously reported as malignant histiocytosis would probably now be classified as large cell lymphomas (Colby, Gastro, 1982; 82:339). Healthy carriers of hepatitis B virus with non-Hodgkin's lymphoma have experienced severe reactivation of hepatitis B followed by liver failure and death after withdrawal of chemotherapy (Pariente, DigDisSci, 1988; 33:1185; Pinto, Cancer, 1990; 65:878).

Primary lymphoma usually affects middle-aged people and presents with abdominal pain and B symptoms (fever, weight loss, and night sweats), but without ascites or jaundice. There is a consistent increase in serum alkaline phosphatase activity and a less constant increase in serum aminotransferases. Ultrasound and CT scans are not specific, and may be confused with hepatocellular carcinoma or metastases. The lesions are hypo- or hyperechoic on sonography, and of low density in CT scans. Diagnosis of lymphoma can only be achieved by liver biopsy.

One primary lymphoma of the extrahepatic bile duct has been documented (Nguyen, Cancer, 1982; 50:2218).

Peripheral T-cell lymphoma

Some patients with non-cutaneous, peripheral T-cell lymphoma have presented with hepatosplenomegaly but without lymphadenopathy (Gaulard, Hepatol, 1986; 6:864; Falini, Blood, 1990; 75:434; Farcet, Blood, 1990; 75:2213; Gaulard, AmJPath, 1990; 137:617). The white blood count was normal and liver function tests only slightly modified. One patient presented with jaundice mimicking acute hepatitis (King, JClinGastro, 1994; 19:234).

Diagnosis is based on the histology of the liver, which is characterized by sinusoidal infiltration by atypical lymphoid cells. Immunotyping shows that tumour cells express the γ/δ cell receptor, suggesting that their origin is the small population of normal cells expressing the γ/δ receptor. In the spleen, infiltration by these cells is diffuse and predominates in the sinuses.

Chronic lymphoid leukaemia

Patients with chronic lymphoid leukaemia often have mild to moderate liver enlargement. Functional impairment of the liver is a late manifestation.[8] Extensive lymphocytic infiltration is seen in portal tracts, sometimes associated with periportal fibrosis that may lead to portal hypertension (Schwartz, HumPath, 1981; 12:432). Nodular regenerative hyperplasia of the liver has been reported (Rozman, MedicinaClin, 1988; 92:26).

Hairy cell leukaemia

Hairy cell leukaemia is a lymphoproliferative disorder characterized by the proliferation of mononuclear cells which harbour atypical hair-like cytoplasmic projections, in peripheral blood, bone marrow, spleen, liver, and lymph nodes. The liver is always infiltrated by leukaemic cells which invade both portal tracts and sinusoids.[9] They may be identified by the halo-like clear cytoplasm around rounded or indented nuclei, and by the demonstration of a tartrate-resistant acid phosphatase activity (Grouls, PatholResPract, 1984; 178:332). The finding of intra-acinar cavities lined by leukaemic cells and filled by red cells is very characteristic of hairy cell leukaemia.[10]

Liver enlargement is found in less than 40 per cent of patients, and serum biochemical abnormalities are rarely seen.[9]

Monoclonal gammopathies

In multiple myeloma, hepatomegaly is found in 15 to 40 per cent of cases. It is usually mild to moderate and sometimes accompanied by splenomegaly; other manifestations of liver involvement are uncommon (Thomas, ArchIntMed, 1973; 132:195; Perez-Soler, AmJHemat, 1985; 20:25). Jaundice is rarely seen. Two histological patterns of hepatic infiltration can be observed: (i) diffuse sinusoidal and portal tract infiltration and (ii) large nodules simulating metastatic carcinoma. Amyloid deposition is exceedingly uncommon. There is one report of primary extramedullary plasmocytoma of the liver, which presented as a painful liver with a single nodule in segment VII; it was successfully treated by surgical resection, (Weichold, AmJSurgPath, 1995; 19:1197).

Various liver lesions have been described in patients with Waldenstrom's macroglobulinaemia: infiltration of malignant cells into portal tracts giving rise to portal hypertension (Brooks, BMJ, 1976; i: 689), massive blastic infiltration revealed by hepatic failure (Beau, GastrClinBiol, 1984; 8:57), amyloidosis, light-chain deposits (Rodrigo-Saez, RevEspEnfermAparDig, 1987; 71:55), peliosis hepatis (Voinchet, Gastro, 1988; 95:482), and nodular regenerative hyperplasia (Wanless, AmJMed, 1981; 70:1203).

Acute leukaemia

Hepatic involvement in acute leukaemia is usually mild and silent at the time the disease is diagnosed. Infiltration by leukaemic cells is localized in portal tracts in acute lymphoblastic leukaemia, and in portal tracts and sinusoids in acute myeloblastic leukaemia. A slight elevation of serum alkaline phosphatase activity and a mild to moderate liver enlargement may be noted.

Post-transfusion chronic viral hepatitis, drug-induced hepatotoxicity, or bacterial and fungal infections affecting the liver may occur in patients with leukaemia. Exceptionally, massive infiltration of the liver by leukaemic cells has presented as fulminant liver failure (Zafrani, Hepatol, 1983; 3:428).

Focal hepatic candidiasis is being recognized with increasing frequency in patients with acute leukaemia (Haron, AmJMed, 1987; 83:7; Thaler, AnnIntMed, 1988; 108:88). Clinically, it presents as a well-tolerated and prolonged fever, unresponsive to broad-spectrum antibiotics, when the neutropenia following chemotherapy is returning to normal. There is hepatomegaly, abdominal pain, and minimal liver impairment, other than a raised serum alkaline phosphatase activity. The finding of 'bull's eye' lesions on ultrasound examination is characteristic (Eiff, Blut, 1990; 60:242). At laparoscopy, white nodules, 0.5 to 2 cm in diameter, displaying a nipple-like prominence can be seen on the liver surface (Bladé, AnnHemat, 1992; 64:240). Liver biopsy, guided by ultrasound or peritoneoscopy, reveals yeasts and pseudohyphae of *Candida* spp. within a granulomatous reaction. Prolonged treatment with amphotericin B is required, often in association with other antifungal drugs. Patients with hepatic candidiasis have been treated with cytosine arabinoside, which often induces extensive lesions in the mucosa of the gastrointestinal tract, favouring local invasion by *Candida* spp.

Chronic myeloproliferative disorders
Myeloid metaplasia

Liver involvement in primary myelofibrosis, also termed agnogenic myeloid metaplasia, is common and due to any of following mechanisms, individually or in combination: extramedullary haematopoiesis, increased hepatic blood flow, haemosiderosis secondary to either blood transfusions or to ineffective erythropoiesis, and post-transfusion chronic viral hepatitis.

Histology

Hepatic extramedullary haematopoiesis is found in 90 to 100 per cent of patients with myeloid metaplasia.[11] Because of this high frequency, its demonstration is often used to confirm the diagnosis of primary myelofibrosis. However, care should be taken when patients with agnogenic myeloid metaplasia are submitted to liver biopsy because of the risk of bleeding related to platelet dysfunction. A transjugular approach (Lebrec, JHepatol, 1996; 25(Suppl 1):20) or a 'plugged' percutaneous liver biopsy (Sawyerr, JHepatol, 1993; 17:81) should be considered.

In the early stages, extramedullary haematopoiesis is confined to the sinusoids, whereas portal tract involvement is a feature of more advanced disease.[12] The three haemopoietic cell lines are usually represented, but the most commonly observed are megakaryocytes, which are often dysplastic (Fig. 2). Sinusoidal dilatation is found in one-half of the cases, and it is probably related to the obstruction of blood flow by sinusoidal foci of haematopoietic cells. An increase of the reticulin network is present in 30 to 40 per cent of cases. It has been attributed to some factor released by dysplastic megakaryocytes which induces transformation of Ito cells in fibroblasts (Roux, Gastro, 1987; 92:1067). Haemosiderin deposition in hepatocytes and Kupffer cells is always present.

Clinical features

Liver enlargement is found in nearly all patients. The size of the liver correlates with the stage of the disease, and increases following splenectomy (Towell, AmJMed, 1987; 82:371). Such an increase is usually gradual over several years, but is rapidly progressive in some patients. In some of the latter, fatal hepatic failure of obscure origin has been reported after the splenectomy (Perez Villa, MedicinaClin, 1988; 91:108; Lopez Guillermo, ActaHaem, 1991; 85:1847). Palpable splenomegaly is also a common finding; its absence makes the diagnosis of agnogenic myeloid metaplasia unlikely.

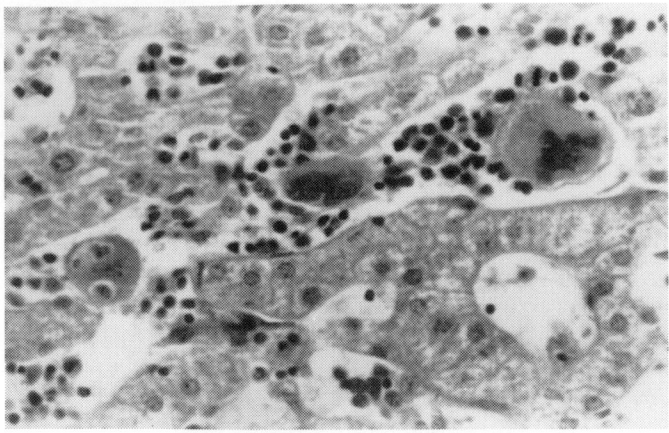

Fig. 2. Marked sinusoidal infiltration by haemopoietic cells in idiopathic myelofibrosis. Note the presence of bizarre megakaryocytes (HE × 375).

Ascites and oesophageal varices develop in about 7 per cent of patients. Portal hypertension is caused by an increased intrahepatic vascular resistance related to sinusoidal fibrosis, and to infiltration by haemopoietic cells (Dubois, Hepatol, 1993; 17:246). Nodular regenerative hyperplasia related to an obstruction of intrahepatic portal vein branches is another well recognized cause of portal hypertension (Wanless, Hepatol, 1990; 12:1166).

Abnormal liver function tests can be detected in 40 to 60 per cent of patients.[12] High serum alkaline phosphatase activity is the most common abnormality and seems to reflect the severity of sinusoidal dilatation rather than the grade of hepatic myeloid metaplasia.

Polycythaemia vera

Liver involvement is uncommon in polycythaemia vera. Patients in whom the disorder evolves into myelofibrosis develop myeloid metaplasia. Other patients may present with an acute or chronic Budd–Chiari syndrome. Polycythaemia vera is found in over 40 per cent of patients with Budd–Chiari syndrome, although this proportion may be even higher since a latent myeloproliferative disorder is demonstrated in many patients with idiopathic Budd–Chiari syndrome by *in vitro* erythroid colony formation in the absence of erythropoietin.[13]

Chronic myeloid leukaemia

At presentation 50 per cent of patients display mild to moderate hepatomegaly, without altered liver function tests (Cervantes, Blood, 1982; 60:1298). In blastic phases of the disease, liver enlargement increases due to the sinusoidal infiltration by immature cells. Serum alkaline phosphatase activity also increases.

A single patient has been reported in whom the initial manifestation of blast crisis was acute hepatic failure due to massive infiltration of the liver by leukaemic cells (Ondreyco, Cancer, 1981; 48:957).

Myelodysplasias

Myelodysplasias are a group of chronic haematological disorders characterized by variable degrees of cytopenia in the presence of quantitatively normal or rich bone marrow, dyshaemopoietic features, and frequent evolution to acute leukaemia. Hepatic involvement can occur through two mechanisms. In patients with sideroblastic anaemia or refractory anaemia, the liver often shows iron deposition due both to frequent transfusions and to increased iron absorption as a result of decreased iron utilization by bone marrow. Infiltrative hepatomegaly is observed in patients with refractory anaemia with excess of blasts or with chronic myelomonocytic leukaemia.

Haemolytic anaemias

Sickle-cell disease

Sickle-cell disease is an inherited disorder of haemoglobin producing chronic haemolytic anaemia with recurrent acute haemolytic crisis. The liver is commonly involved as a result of viral hepatitis transmitted by blood transfusion, iron overload, jaundice due to biliary tract obstruction by gallstones, cardiac dysfunction due to secondary haemochromatosis, or to a clinical disorder unique in sickle-cell disease, termed 'hepatic crisis'.[14] The latter presents with upper right abdominal quadrant pain, fever, jaundice, leucocytosis, and a variable elevation of hepatic serum enzymes, mimicking acute cholecystitis. With general supportive care, clinical improvement is seen within several days, but occasionally the disease follows a fulminant course to death. Some young patients exhibit extreme hyperbilirubinaemia, not associated with pain or fever. Jaundice resolves over several weeks without permanent sequelae.

Histologically, the liver consistently shows intrasinusoidal obliteration by sickled red blood cells and Kupffer cell erythrophagocytosis, which may result in impairment of intrahepatic blood flow. Other histological changes that may be detected are iron deposition, which is often massive, chronic hepatitis, and cirrhosis.[15]

Cholelithiasis is frequently observed in patients with sickle-cell disease (40 to 80 per cent). Gallstones are related to haemolysis and may cause cholecystitis and bile duct obstruction.

Thalassaemia

In patients with thalassaemia, major chronic liver disease is due to haemochromatosis related to ineffective erythropoiesis and/or posttransfusion viral hepatitis B or C (Pastore, VoxSang, 1983; 44:14). Massive iron deposition is found in the liver and other organs. Heart failure due to haemochromatosis is the main cause of death in these patients (Barry, BMJ, 1974; 2:16). It has been suggested that repeated blood transfusions protect against the development of serious hepatic disease.

Paroxysmal nocturnal haemoglobinuria

Paroxysmal nocturnal haemoglobinuria is a chronic haemolytic anaemia related to an acquired defect in the membrane of red cells that renders them especially sensitive to the lytic action of complement when blood pH falls. Besides haemolysis, the disease is associated with a high tendency to develop venous thrombosis.

Budd–Chiari syndrome and portal vein thrombosis are consequences of the disease (Grossman, AmJSurg, 1974; 127:733; Leibowitz, BrJHaemat, 1981; 48:1). Up to 10 per cent of cases of Budd–Chiari syndrome may be related to paroxysmal nocturnal haemoglobinuria (Sobrino, MedicinaClin, 1987; 88:773).

One patient with paroxysmal nocturnal haemoglobinuria presented with abdominal pain and anicteric cholestasis. Endoscopic retrograde cholangiopancreatography showed a radiological pattern of sclerosing cholangitis, which was interpreted as ischaemic cholangiopathy (Huong, Gastro, 1995; 109:1338).

Other haematological diseases
Haemophilia

Chronic viral hepatitis is common in haemophiliac patients. Up to 90 per cent of the patients have serological markers of past or ongoing hepatitis B virus infection; 50 to 70 per cent are anti-HCV positive, and 25 per cent of hepatitis B carriers have hepatitis δ-virus superinfection (Rizzetto, JInfDis, 1982; 145:18; Brettler, Blood, 1990; 76:254; Rumi, AnnIntMed, 1990; 129:379). Nearly 70 per cent of the patients have altered liver function tests; in most, chronic active hepatitis or cirrhosis related to chronic viral infection is found on liver biopsy (Hay, Lancet, 1985; i:1495). The risk of hepatitis is higher in patients treated on a regular basis than in those treated according to need, and higher in those who started treatment at an earlier age (Colombo, ScaJHaematol, 1984; 33:341).

Needle liver biopsy is a hazardous procedure in these patients, even under the cover of clotting-factor concentrates, and should be avoided (Aledort, Blood, 1995; 66:67); however, it has been carried out without problems by some authors (Mannucci, JClinPath, 1978; 31:779; Preston, Lancet, 1978; ii:592).

Exclusion of blood donors infected by hepatitis B and C virus, as well as the introduction of effective viral inactivation procedures such as pasteurization of factor VIII concentrates, has reduced the risk of hepatitis (Mannucci, AnnIntMed, 1990; 113:27; Schwartz, NEJM, 1990; 323:1800).

Aplastic anaemia (see Chapter 25.3)

Aplastic anaemia is a rare complication of viral hepatitis. In up to 10 per cent of patients, development of aplastic anaemia follows a recent episode of hepatitis, which is rarely due to hepatitis B virus (Casciato, ArchIntMed, 1978; 138:1557) or to hepatitis C virus (Gruber, AnnHemat, 1993; 66:157), but is more often due to a still unidentified non-A, non-B, non-C virus (Pol, AnnIntMed, 1990; 113:435; Hibbs, JAMA, 1992; 267:2051). The role of parvovirus B19 is being investigated, particularly in those patients who have developed aplastic anaemia following liver transplantation (Langnas, Hepatol, 1995; 22:1661). A direct injury of stem cells has been postulated for the pathogenesis of this complication. Bone marrow transplantation yields similar efficacy in patients with hepatitis-related aplastic anaemia and in those with anaemia of unknown aetiology.

Anabolic steroids given for long periods of time as treatment for aplastic anaemia can induce peliosis hepatis (Bagheri, AnnIntMed, 1974; 81:610) and hepatocellular adenoma (Hernandez Nieto, Cancer, 1977; 40:1761).

Mastocytosis

Subclinical hepatic involvement is frequent in systemic mastocytosis. Hepatosplenomegaly is common and due to infiltration by mast cells. Identification of mast cells in paraffin-embedded sections stained with haematoxylin and eosin is difficult, but they may be recognized in sections stained with Giemsa or toluidine blue. Tissue eosinophilia is often seen (Yam, AmJClinPath, 1980; 73:48). Portal hypertension attributed to mast cell infiltration and sinusoidal fibrosis has occasionally been reported (Ghandur-Mnaymneh, ArchPathLabMed, 1985; 109:76; Narayan, PostgradMed J, 1989; 65:394). Mast cell infiltration of the bile duct walls may cause a cholangiopathy radiographically similar to primary sclerosing cholangitis (Baron, Gastro, 1995; 109:1677).

Essential mixed cryoglobulinaemia

Essential mixed cryoglobulinaemia is a condition clinically characterized by purpura, arthralgias, and glomerulonephritis, associated with circulating mixed (IgM–IgG) cryoprecipitable globulins. Earlier reports suggested an association of this syndrome with hepatitis B virus infection (McIntosh, QJMed, 1976; 45:23; Levo, NEJM, 1977; 296:1501), but this could not be confirmed in other studies (Popp, AnnIntMed, 1990; 92:379).

Stronger support for an association between essential mixed cryoglobulinaemia and hepatitis C virus infection has been gained from recent studies (Ferri, ArthRheum, 1991; 34:1606; Agnello, NEJM, 1992; 327:1490; Misiani, AnnIntMed, 1992; 117:573; Marcellin, Gastro, 1993; 104:272; Lunel, Gastro, 1994; 106:1291), based on the high prevalence of anti-HCV and HCV RNA in the serum cryoprecipitates of patients with essential mixed cryoglobulinaemia. Cryoglobulinaemia is found in about one-third of patients with chronic hepatitis C, but the proportion of patients with clinical expression of essential mixed cryoglobulinaemia is much lower (Patlowski, Hepatol, 1994; 19:841). The mechanisms by which hepatitis C virus infection allows cryoprecipitable immune complexes to deposit in vascular tissue causing tissue injury remain to be determined. Interferon transiently improves the biochemical and clinical manifestations of essential mixed cryoglobulinaemia in parallel to its effect on virological markers of hepatitis C virus (Misiani, NEJM, 1994; 330:751).

References

1. Givler RL, Brunk SF, Hass CA, and Guleserian HP. Problems of interpretation of liver biopsy in Hodgkin's disease. *Cancer*, 1971; **28**: 1335–42.
2. Jaffe ES. Malignant lymphomas: pathology of hepatic involvement. *Seminars in Liver Disease*, 1987; **7**: 257–68.
3. Belliveau RE, Wiernik PH, and Abt AB. Liver enzymes and pathology in Hodgkin's disease. *Cancer*, 1974; **34**: 300–5.
4. Birrer MJ and Young RC. Differential diagnosis of jaundice in lymphoma patients. *Seminars in Liver Disease*, 1987; **7**: 269–77.
5. Lotz MJ, Thomas LB, and Johnson BC. Pathological staging of 100 consecutive patients with non-Hodgkin's lymphomas. *Cancer*, 1976; **37**: 266–70.
6. Kim H, Dorfman RF, and Rosenberg SA. Pathology of malignant lymphomas of the liver: application in staging. *Progress in Liver Diseases*, 1976; **5**: 683–94.

7. Boddie AW, Eisenberg BL, Mullins JD, and Schlichtemeier AL. The diagnosis and treatment of obstructive jaundice secondary to malignant lymphoma: a problem in multidisciplinary management. *Journal of Surgical Oncology*, 1980; **14**: 111–23.

8. Sweet DL, Golomb HM, and Ultmann JE. The clinical features of chronic lymphocytic leukaemia. *Clinics in Haematology*, 1987; **6**: 185–202.

9. Yam LT, Janckila AJ, and Chan CM. Hepatic involvement in hairy cell leukaemia. *Cancer*, 1983; **51**: 1487–504.

10. Roquet ML, Zafrani ES, and Farcet JP. Histopathological lesions of the liver in hairy cell leukemia: a report of 14 cases. *Hepatology*, 1985; **5**: 496–500.

11. Ligumski M, Polliack A, and Benbassat J. Nature and incidence of liver involvement in agnogenic myeloid metaplasia. *Scandinavian Journal of Haematology*, 1978; **21**: 81–93.

12. Pereira A, Bruguera M, Cervantes F, and Rozman C. Liver involvement at diagnosis or primary myelofibrosis: a clinicopathological study of twenty-two cases. *European Journal of Haematology*, 1988; **40**: 355–61.

13. Valla D, *et al*. Primary myeloproliferative disorders and hepatic vein thrombosis. A prospective study of erythroid colony formation *in vitro* in 20 patients with Budd–Chiari syndrome. *Annals of Internal Medicine*, 1985; **103**: 329–34.

14. Omata M, Johnson CS, Tong MS, and Tatter D. Pathogical spectrum of liver diseases of sickle cell disease. *Digestive Diseases and Sciences*, 1986; **31**: 247–56.

15. Bauer TMN, Moore GW, and Hutchins GFM. The liver in sickle cell disease. A clinicopathologic study of 70 patients. *American Journal of Medicine*, 1980; **69**: 833–7.

24.6 The effect of endocrine diseases on liver function

Pierre M. Bouloux and Yolanta T. Kruszynska

Introduction

Liver dysfunction is associated with many disorders of the endocrine system. The propensity of several of these to be gradual in onset, and to present with subtle, non-specific symptoms such as lethargy, weight loss, nausea and depression, may, when associated with perturbed 'liver function tests', prompt a hepatological referral. A number of inappropriate and potentially harmful investigations may be performed, before the correct underlying endocrine diagnosis is established. Obesity and diabetes mellitus are commonly associated with abnormal liver function tests. Severe 'thyroid liver disease' once formed an important part of hepatological practice[1] but with the advent of effective treatment for thyrotoxicosis, severe liver disease due to thyroid dysfunction is now seldom seen, though abnormalities of liver function tests are often found. Adrenal insufficiency, though rare, may also increase serum aminotransferase levels, while hepatomegaly may be found in patients with acromegaly.

Liver dysfunction may be a consequence of treatment. Octreotide, a somatostatin analogue used in the treatment of acromegaly and other endocrine tumours, is associated with a high risk of cholelithiasis. Rarely, sulphonylureas, antithyroid drugs, and ketoconazole used in the treatment of Cushing's syndrome may be associated with severe liver dysfunction, while the C17-alkylated androgenic steroids and synthetic oestrogens may cause cholestasis.

Certain liver tumours may have an endocrine basis. The oral contraceptive pill and anabolic steroids may be associated with the development of hepatic adenomas and hepatocellular carcinoma, respectively. Endocrine cancers often metastasize to the liver, and deposits from thyroid, adrenal, and gonadal cancers are not infrequently associated with liver dysfunction. Paraganglionomas (extra-adrenal phaeochromocytomas) may occasionally occur at the hilum of the liver and present with features of biliary obstruction.

Some diseases affect both the endocrine system and the liver. Examples include the autoimmune deficiency syndrome, syphilis, sarcoidosis, haemochromatosis, histiocytosis X, idiopathic fibrotic syndromes, and some lymphomas. Rarely, hydatid disease occurs both in the liver and the pituitary–hypothalamic region.

Obesity

Abnormalities of liver function tests, particularly minor elevations of serum alanine aminotransferase and γ-glutamyl transpeptidase are commonly found in obese subjects. Serum alkaline phosphatase and aspartate aminotransferase are raised less often. Abnormalities are particularly common in morbidly obese subjects but are also frequent in subjects with less severe degrees of obesity. Abnormal liver function tests are more likely to be found in those with a predominantly central (visceral) distribution of body fat, which can be assessed anthropometrically by the waist–hip ratio or by computed tomography (**CT**) scan. This distribution of body fat is also associated with an increased prevalence of hyperlipidaemia, glucose intolerance, hypertension, and atherosclerosis. The underlying liver pathology in the absence of other causes of liver disease is fatty liver of varying severity. The liver may be enlarged. The fatty infiltration is usually diffuse but occasionally may be non-uniform. Ultrasound examination reveals increased echogenicity when fatty change involves more than 30 per cent of hepatocytes (Celle, DigDisSci, 1988; 33:467), and a reduced attenuation value is found on CT scanning (Nomura, Radiol, 1987; 162:845). Hepatic triglyceride content measured by ^{13}C-nuclear magnetic resonance correlates well with the percentage of fat assessed by morphometric analysis of liver biopsies ($r = 0.9$) (Petersen, Hepatol, 1996; 24: 114).

Liver histology shows varying degrees of fatty infiltration, ranging from simple steatosis without inflammation to steatosis accompanied by an inflammatory cell infiltrate and necrosis of liver cells ('steatonecrosis') (see Chapter 2.12) and, in more severe cases, fibrosis and cirrhosis. In some cases the appearances may be indistinguishable from alcoholic steatohepatitis, including the presence of Mallory hyaline (Ludwig, MayoClinProc, 1980; 55:434). Lipogranulomas and glycogen in hepatocyte nuclei may also be found.[2–4] Steatosis is present in virtually all patients with morbid obesity; steatohepatitis is less common, being found in 20 to 30 per cent.[2,6] Cirrhosis for which no other cause is evident is found in 2 to 3 per cent[2,6] (Andersen, IntJObes, 1984; 8:97). An elevated serum aspartate aminotransferase may be associated with more severe histological abnormalities,[2] but in most studies there is little relationship between histological findings and serum biochemical abnormalities; fibrosis and even cirrhosis may be present with normal serum aspartate aminotransferase, alanine aminotransferase, and γ-glutamyl transpeptidase levels[2,4] (Galambos, Gastro, 1978; 74:1191).

A more central distribution of body fat is predictive of fatty liver, even in morbidly obese subjects (Kral, Metabolism, 1993; 42:548;

Goto, IntJObes, 1995; 19:841). Visceral (intra-abdominal) adipocytes are more sensitive to lipolytic stimuli than adipocytes in subcutaneous fat depots. High lipolytic rates in intra-abdominal adipocytes increase the delivery of non-esterified fatty acids to the liver via the portal vein. Hepatic uptake of non-esterified fatty acids is proportional to their concentration in portal venous blood. Some fatty acids taken up by the liver will be oxidized and a proportion used for ketogenesis. However, in the presence of normal or increased basal and postprandial insulin levels, the greater proportion of fatty acids taken up in excess of energy requirements will be re-esterified to triglyceride. If very low density lipoprotein (VLDL) synthesis and secretion fail to keep pace with the increased rate of triglyceride production, triglyceride accumulates in hepatocytes. Excessive dietary fat (reaching the liver as chylomicron remnants) and fructose, which enhances fatty acid esterification (see Chapter 2.11), will also promote hepatic triglyceride deposition. The increased triglyceride in the liver may result in increased lipid peroxidation, generation of cytotoxic intermediates, and recruitment of inflammatory cells. Increased non-esterified fatty acid supply to the liver may also reduce hepatic insulin sensitivity, in part by impairing insulin's action on hepatic glucose production after meals (see Chapter 2.11).

Weight loss induced by a low-calorie diet containing an adequate amount of protein is associated with improvement or return to normal of serum alanine aminotransferase, aspartate aminotransferase, γ-glutamyl transpeptidase, and alkaline phosphatase levels[3] (Eriksson, ActaMedScand, 1986; 220:83; Palmer, Gastro, 1990; 99:1408), reduction in liver size and liver fat content as determined by CT scanning (Nomura, Radiol, 1987; 162:845), and a marked reduction or reversal of fatty change on follow-up liver biopsy[3] (Eriksson, ActaMedScand, 1986; 220:83). However, rapid weight reduction (more than 1.6 kg/week), inadequate protein intake, and starvation may be associated with an initial increase in inflammatory changes, and pericellular and portal fibrosis[3] (Rozenthal, AmJDigDis, 1967; 12:198; Drenick, NEJM, 1970; 282:829; Capron, DigDisSci, 1982; 27:265; Powell, Hepatol, 1990; 11:74).

Fatty liver without evidence of inflammation or fibrosis in moderately obese subjects shows little progression with time, and from the purely hepatological viewpoint is a very benign condition.[5] The development of fatty liver hepatitis ('steatonecrosis') may be associated with increasing fibrosis and eventually cirrhosis[4] (Powell, Hepatol, 1990; 11:74). However, in the absence of additional factors, such as jejunoileal bypass or diabetes (see below), this would appear to be an extremely slow and relatively rare event given the low prevalence (2–3 per cent) of non-alcohol-related cirrhosis in morbidly obese patients[2, 6] (Andersen, IntJObes, 1984; 8:97). It is unclear whether the duration of obesity is important in determining which patients will eventually develop fibrosis and cirrhosis. About 10 per cent of obese children have hepatic steatosis with elevated serum aminotransferases (Vajro, JPediat, 1994; 125:239), and even at this early stage liver biopsy may reveal fibrosis (Kinugasa, JPediatGastrNutr, 1984; 3:408; Shaffer, SemLivDis, 1992; 12:429).

Diabetes mellitus

Liver function tests

Abnormal liver function tests may be found in 10 to 20 per cent of patients with diabetes. Mild increases in serum alkaline phosphatase and γ-glutamyl transpeptidase are the most frequent abnormalities, but alanine aminotransferase and, less commonly, aspartate aminotransferase may also be increased. The prevalence varies in different populations (Table 1). Abnormal liver function tests are more often found in patients with non-insulin-dependent (type II) diabetes mellitus than in patients with insulin-dependent (type I) diabetes. When the disease first presents, the serum albumin concentration may be low. Orrell *et al.* (DiabetResClinPrac, 1990; 10:51) found no relationship between abnormalities of liver function tests and blood glucose control, or duration of diabetes. In approximately half of their patients serum alanine aminotransferase levels returned to normal when repeated 6 months later. The biochemical changes correlate poorly with the hepatic histology, which may show increased glycogen deposition, fatty liver, cirrhosis, or biliary tract disease.

Many patients with type II diabetes are obese with a 'visceral pattern' of distribution of body fat; obesity and fatty liver (see above) rather than hyperglycaemia can account for a large proportion of abnormal test results. Weight reduction may result in both an improvement of glucose tolerance and return to normal of the liver function tests (Eriksson, ActaMedScand, 1986; 220:83). Apart from fatty liver, other factors may also contribute to the high prevalence of abnormal liver function tests in Type II diabetes. In some populations, diabetic patients have a higher incidence of infection with viruses causing chronic liver disease, due to repeated hospital exposure and contamination of instruments used for blood sampling (Douvin, NEJM, 1990; 322:57; Polish, NEJM, 1992; 326:721). The risk is highest in countries with high prevalence rates of hepatitis B and C. In a study from Beirut, hepatitis B virus antibody positivity was found in 51 per cent of diabetic patients compared to 25 per cent in healthy control subjects (Khuri, DiabetCare, 1985; 8:250). Although, type I diabetic patients may have an impaired immune response to vaccination with hepatitis B surface antigen (Pozzilli, Diabetolog, 1987; 30:817), there is no evidence for defective clearance of hepatitis B virus in diabetic patients (Kew, JClinMicrobiol, 1976; 4:467; Khuri, DiabetCare, 1985; 8:250). Gray *et al.* (DiabetMed, 1995; 12:244) studied the prevalence of hepatitis C virus antibody positivity in 200 type II diabetic patients (100 white Caucasian, 50 Afro-Caribbean, and 50 Asian patients) enrolled in a UK multicentre study of diabetic control. Patients were selected on the basis of their serum alanine aminotransferase: half of the patients having an increased alanine aminotransferase at entry and 3 years later, the other half having a persistently normal alanine aminotransferase. The prevalence of hepatitis C virus antibody positivity was significantly increased in the patients with an elevated serum alanine aminotransferase (Afro-Caribbean 28 per cent versus 4 per cent, white Caucasians 12 per cent versus 0 per cent, both $p < 0.05$; Asian, 8 per cent versus 0 per cent, not significant). An increased prevalence of viral hepatitis in type II diabetic patients in Japan could explain their threefold increased risk of death from cirrhosis (6.4 per cent of deaths) and from hepatocellular carcinoma (7.8 per cent of deaths) (Sasaki, DiabetResClinPrac, 1989; 7:33).

Diabetes may occasionally be due to high rates of alcohol consumption even in the absence of significant pancreatic damage or cirrhosis. Many of these patients will have abnormal liver function tests and fatty liver on biopsy. In some, the diabetes disappears rapidly with abstention from alcohol (Phillips, JAMA, 1971; 217:1513); the diabetes is probably due to alcohol-induced insulin

	Patients (n)	Percentage of test results above reference range					Comment
		AST	ALT	γGT	ALP	Bilirubin	
Foster (1980)[a]	60	3.3	10	16.7	18.3	10	34 = insulin treated 26 = non-insulin treated
Salmela (1984)[b]	57 IDDM	3.5	5.3	10.5	5.3	21.1	'IDDM' may include some insulin-treated NIDDM
	118 NIDDM	5.1	22.9	23.7	5.1	10.2	
Orrell (1990)[c]	411	6.4	8.3	15.2	nd	nd	50% insulin treated

Table 1 Prevalence of abnormal liver function tests in patients with diabetes mellitus

AST, aspartate aminotransferase; ALP, alkaline phosphatase; ALT, alanine aminotransferase; γGT, γ-glutamyl transpeptidase; IDDM, insulin-dependent diabetes mellitus; NIDDM, non-insulin-dependent diabetes mellitus; nd, not determined.
[a] Foster, PostgradMedJ, 1980; 56: 767.
[b] Salmela, DiabetCare, 1984; 7: 248.
[c] Orrell, DiabetResClinPrac, 1990; 10: 51.

resistance (Avogaro, DiabetMetabRev, 1993; 9:129) and/or fatty liver. In the long term a high alcohol intake is associated with central obesity, fatty liver, and insulin resistance, and these factors could account for the increased risk of type II diabetes in alcoholics without cirrhosis (Lindegard, BMJ, 1985; 2:1529; Holbrook, AmJEpid, 1990; 132:902; Balkau, Diabetolog, 1992; 35:39).

Thus, in certain populations an increased prevalence of undiagnosed liver disease or excessive alcohol consumption could contribute to the higher frequency of abnormal liver function tests in diabetic patients. In some of these the diabetes may, in part, be a consequence of the liver disease (see Chapters 2.11 and 24.2). Haemachromatosis and excessive alcohol consumption may also cause diabetes by their effects on pancreatic insulin secretion.

Increased serum aminotransferase levels may be found during ketoacidosis (Knight, Diabetes, 1974; 23:126). Sometimes this is due to accompanying pathology such as myocardial infarction and cardiac failure. However, often no additional explanation is found. Very high aminotransferase levels found in ketoacidotic patients in some earlier studies (Cryer, Diabetes, 1969; 18:781) may have been due to interference in the assay by elevated acetoacetate levels (Chen, Diabetes, 1970; 19:730). Hepatic infarction complicating diabetic ketoacidosis has been reported (Ng, Gastro, 1977; 73:804). Very high aspartate aminotransferase and alanine aminotransferase levels may also be found following hypoglycaemic coma, particularly when this is prolonged (Soler, BMJ, 1985; 291:1541). Since there is no accompanying rise in serum creatine phosphokinase levels, the liver would appear to be the source of the elevated transaminases. In most type I diabetic patients stabilized on insulin, liver function tests are normal, although elevated transaminase levels are occasionally found in patients with very labile blood glucose control in the absence of ketoacidosis or hypoglycaemia (Olsson, JClinGastro, 1989; 11:541; Lenaerts, JClinGastro, 1990; 12:93).

Hepatomegaly and increased liver glycogen content

Hepatomegaly may be found in patients with poorly controlled diabetes and during and following episodes of ketoacidosis (Goodman, AnnIntMed, 1953; 39:1077; Bronstein, NEJM, 1959; 261: 1314). There may be associated abdominal pain and the liver may be tender on palpation. In type I diabetes, hepatomegaly is largely due to increased hepatic glycogen. The liver size returns to normal with glycaemic control, although there may be an initial further enlargement as the administered insulin augments hepatic glycogen synthesis and prevents its degradation. In type II diabetes, steatosis is the main cause of hepatomegaly, though glycogen content is also increased. Liver size is usually unaffected by diabetic control in type II diabetes mellitus but it may decrease with weight loss and a reduction in liver fat content (see above).

Early studies found increased hepatic glycogen in up to 75 per cent of patients with diabetes[7] (Wasatjerna, ActaMedScand, 1972; 191:225). The prevalence is likely to be less now with improvements in diabetic control. While overinsulinization can lead to increased hepatic glycogen content, more often hyperglycaemia secondary to inadequate insulin availability accounts for the increased glycogen in both type I and type II diabetes mellitus. Hyperglycaemia inhibits the degradation of liver glycogen (see Chapter 2.11); insulinopenic diabetic rats have markedly increased hepatic glycogen stores in the fasted state which are reduced by control of their diabetes with insulin (Friedman, JBC, 1963; 238:2899). The perivenous hepatocytes contain more glycogen than the periportal cells. The glycogen is present both in the cytoplasm and the nuclei of hepatocytes, causing a characteristic vacuolization of liver cell nuclei (Nagore, JPath, 1988; 156:155). Nuclear glycogen is not specific for diabetes. It may be found in patients with Wilson's disease, chronic active hepatitis, biliary tract disease, sepsis, and cirrhosis. It may also be found in subjects with fatty liver associated with obesity in the absence of diabetes or glucose intolerance.

In children with very poorly controlled diabetes, gross hepatomegaly due to the excessive glycogen deposition may be associated with failure of growth, truncal obesity, delayed puberty, and hyperlipidaemia ('Mauriac syndrome') (Mauriac, PressMed, 1946; 54: 826; Lestradet, SemHopPar, 1964; 40:1030; Najjar, ClinPediat, 1974; 13:723). The syndrome was more often seen with once-daily short-acting insulin injection regimens which would induce alternate cycles of over- and under-insulinization. To prevent ketoacidosis in type I diabetes with a once daily injection of short-acting insulin, the dose has to be very large to last 24 h. This in turn may lead to overeating during the day, increased hepatic glycogen deposition, and obesity. Periods of hyperglycaemia inhibit the breakdown of hepatic glycogen (see Chapter 2.11). In some children the syndrome is primarily due to overinsulinization. This results in hypoglycaemic episodes which stimulate the release of counter-regulatory hormones, leading to rebound hyperglycaemia and insulin resistance, and an inappropriate further increase in the insulin dose (Rosenbloom, AmJDisChild, 1977; 131:881); the periods of hypoglycaemia often went unrecognized before the advent of home blood glucose monitoring. Increased release of glucocorticoids as part of the stress response during periods of hypoglycaemia or ketosis may contribute to the Cushingoid appearance of some children with the Mauriac syndrome. With the development of central obesity, increased hepatic delivery of fatty acids to the liver augments hepatic glycogen deposition and also leads to steatosis. Growth failure does not appear to be due to a disturbance of the growth hormone–insulin-like growth factor-1 axis in these children (Mauras, Metabolism, 1991; 40:1106). Improved glycaemic control achieved by more appropriate insulin delivery (often entailing a reduction in the total insulin dose) and dietary measures leads to regression of hepatomegaly, improved growth and sexual development. With home blood glucose monitoring, better education, and more appropriate insulin regimens, the Mauriac syndrome is rarely seen nowadays.

Fatty liver and cirrhosis in diabetes mellitus

Fatty liver is common in patients with type II diabetes mellitus but infrequent in patients with type I diabetes except during periods of very poor control (see above). Most series which give figures for the frequency of fatty liver in diabetes are biased, since usually only those diabetic patients with some abnormality of liver size or function will undergo biopsy. Wasatjerna et al. (ActaMedScand, 1972; 191:225) found hepatic steatosis in two-thirds of 100 unselected patients with type II diabetes mellitus. Using ultrasonography Foster et al. (PostgradMedJ, 1980; 56:767) found that 23 per cent of 60 unselected diabetic patients (34 on insulin, 26 on oral hypoglycaemic agents) had an abnormally 'bright' liver ultrasound echo pattern consistent with a fatty liver. Since ultrasound will only detect moderate to severe degrees of steatosis (involving more than 30 per cent of hepatocytes) this is probably an underestimate of the prevalence of steatosis in diabetes.

Cirrhosis appears to be more common in patients with diabetes than in the general population[2,7] (Sasaki, DiabResClinPrac, 1989; 7:33; Balkau, JClinEpid, 1991; 44:465). Autopsy studies have suggested that the prevalence of cirrhosis in diabetic patients is about twice as high as in the normal population.[7] Clearly, this association may in part be explained by diabetes complicating cirrhosis (Chapter 25.2), since it is difficult to be certain of the time of onset and duration of either cirrhosis or diabetes mellitus. In some populations, alcohol-related deaths, including cirrhosis, are more common in diabetic patients (Balkau, Diabetolog, 1992; 35:39) so that undiagnosed alcoholic cirrhosis could contribute to the increased frequency of cirrhosis in diabetes. However, the most likely explanation is the high prevalence in obese type II diabetic patients of fatty liver and severe steatohepatitis which may progress to cirrhosis.

Fatty liver in patients with type II diabetes mellitus is due primarily to their associated obesity. More than 80 per cent of patients with type II diabetes mellitus are obese, with a predominantly central (visceral) distribution of body fat. Hepatic fat content measured by CT correlates with the degree of central adiposity in patients with type II diabetes mellitus (Banerji, IntJObes, 1995; 19:846), as it does in obese subjects with normal glucose tolerance (Goto, IntJObes, 1995; 19:841). An important

issue is whether diabetes increases the risk of fatty liver, steatohepatitis, and cirrhosis over and above that which can be attributed to the accompanying obesity. Adipose tissue lipolytic rates are higher in obese patients with type II diabetes mellitus compared with equally obese non-diabetic subjects, both basally and after meals, due to a combination of insulin resistance and impaired insulin secretion. Thus, given the key role of increased hepatic non-esterified fatty acid delivery in the pathogenesis of fatty liver in obese patients (see above), one would predict that diabetes would increase the risk of fatty liver.

Several studies suggest that while the prevalence of fatty liver may be no higher in diabetic patients than in non-diabetic patients matched for a similar degree of obesity, the frequency of more severe histological findings, steatohepatitis, fibrosis, and cirrhosis may be increased.[2, 6] Silverman et al.[2] studied hepatic histology in morbidly obese subjects scheduled for gastric bypass. They found steatohepatitis in 48 per cent and cirrhosis in 9.7 per cent of 31 obese subjects with type II diabetes mellitus, compared to 32.6 per cent and 2.2 per cent, respectively, in 46 similarly obese subjects with normal glucose tolerance. Similar results were obtained in an autopsy study of 349 patients with varying degrees of obesity; diabetes was associated with a 2.6-fold increase in the prevalence of steatohepatitis; the prevalence of fibrosis increased with increasing obesity in diabetic patients but not in those without diabetes[6] (Fig. 1). In various series of non-alcoholic steatohepatitis, obesity is found in about 90 per cent and diabetes in 25 to 40 per cent[4] (Ludwig, MayoClinProc, 1980; 55:434; Powell, Hepatol, 1990; 11: 74).

These studies are consistent with the idea that type II diabetes may promote the development of more severe hepatic lesions (steatohepatitis, fibrosis, and eventually cirrhosis) in patients predisposed to fatty liver by virtue of their visceral obesity. The term 'diabetic hepatitis' (Nagore, JPath, 1988; 156:155) is best avoided as the changes are not specific to diabetes and in many patients may precede the development of diabetes (Batman, Histopath, 1985; 9: 237; Eriksson, ActaMedScand, 1986; 220:83). This in turn suggests an alternative, albeit less likely, explanation for the association of diabetes with these more severe manifestations of fatty liver, namely that diabetes is a consequence of the more severe hepatic changes that might be expected to increase hepatic and peripheral tissue insulin resistance (see Chapter 2.11). Cytokines such as tumour necrosis factor-α released from inflammatory cells have been shown to interfere with insulin receptor signalling (Hotamisligil, Science, 1996; 271:665), while collagenization of the hepatic sinusoids (Falchuk, Gastro, 1980; 78:535) may impair access of insulin to hepatocytes; in some patients (those unable to compensate by secreting more insulin) hepatic glucose production and plasma glucose levels may rise. Retrospective studies do not allow us to distinguish between these alternative explanations for the association of diabetes and severe manifestations of fatty liver in obese patients.

Hepatic subcapsular steatosis may be found in type I diabetic patients on continuous ambulatory peritoneal dialysis treated with intraperitoneal insulin (Wanless, ModPathol, 1989; 2:69; Grove, VirchArchA, 1991; 419:69; JClinPath, 1994; 47:274). This is likely to be due to the local high concentrations of insulin and possibly glucose contained in the dialysis fluid which will promote esterification of non-esterified fatty acids and triglyceride synthesis in the subcapsular hepatocytes.

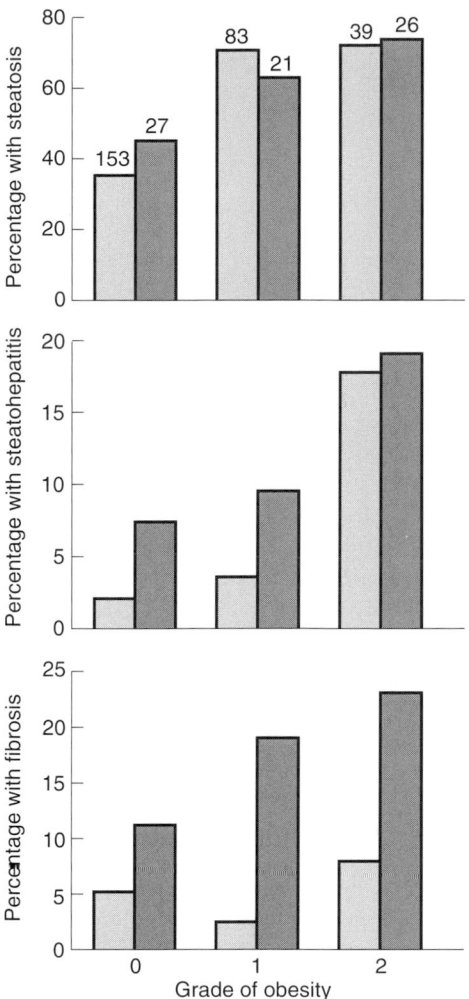

Fig. 1. Prevalence of steatosis, steatohepatitis, and fibrosis in 349 autopsy cases with varying severity of obesity: grade 0 (<10 per cent above ideal body weight); grade 1, (10–39 per cent above ideal body weight or abdominal fat pad 1–3 cm thick, or described as moderately obese); grade 2 (at least 40 per cent above ideal weight or fat pad >3 cm thick, or described as massively or grossly obese). ▪, 275 non-diabetic subjects, ▪, 74 type II diabetic subjects. Numbers over the bars are the number of patients in each group. There was no difference in the prevalence of steatosis in the diabetic and non-diabetic patients, but there was an increased prevalence of steatohepatitis and fibrosis in the diabetic patients ($p < 0.05$ and $p < 0.001$, respectively). (Redrawn from ref. [6] with permission.)

Management of diabetic patients with abnormal liver function tests

It is important to exclude haemochromatosis, alcohol-related liver disease, viral hepatitis, or other coincidental primary liver disease. However, most diabetic patients with abnormal liver function tests will be found to have a fatty liver. Since steatohepatitis can, albeit infrequently, progress to cirrhosis, and since these more severe manifestations of fatty liver may be increased in frequency in patients with type II diabetes mellitus, careful evaluation of diabetic patients with abnormal liver function tests and/or hepatomegaly is indicated. Weight loss combined with good diabetic control should

prevent progression. However, as already noted, histological changes do not correlate with abnormal liver function tests (Galambos, Gastro, 1978: 74:1191) and, indeed, the conventional liver function tests may remain within the reference range until the degree of fatty change is extreme (Nakamura, TohokuJExpMed, 1980; 132:473). Imaging studies of all type II diabetic patients with moderate or severe obesity is impractical and there is a need for simple ways of identifying those patients at risk.

Gallstones

Obesity and hypertriglyceridaemia are important risk factors for cholesterol-rich gallstone formation. Since obesity and hypertriglyceridaemia are common in patients with type II diabetes mellitus, it is not surprising that studies that have not controlled for these variables have found a two to threefold higher prevalence of gallstones in type II diabetic patients than in the general population (Stone, Gastro, 1988; 95:170; Mitsukawa, AmJGastr, 1990; 85:981). Whether diabetes *per se* increases the risk of gallstone formation is unclear. Studies that have controlled for obesity have failed to demonstrate an increase in gallstone formation in diabetic patients (Ikard, SGO, 1990; 171:528).

Factors that are thought to predispose to gallstone formation in diabetic patients include decreased gallbladder contractility and altered bile composition. Diminished gallbladder contractility and an increase in the residual volume after gallbladder contraction have been found in diabetic patients (Braverman, AmJGastr, 1986; 81: 960; Stone, Gastro, 1988; 95:170). Stone et al. (Gastro, 1988; 95: 170) found that these defects were independent of the level of diabetic control, obesity, or the presence of peripheral neuropathy, but others have shown that hyperglycaemia can inhibit gallbladder contraction (DeBoer, Hepatol, 1993; 17:1022). Autonomic neuropathy might explain diminished gallbladder contractility in a minority of patients as a similar abnormality is seen following bilateral vagotomy. There is little evidence that bile composition differs between diabetic and control subjects matched for degree of obesity. Haber et al. (Gut, 1979; 20:518) compared the bile from 27 patients with type II diabetes mellitus and a non-diabetic group matched for degree of obesity and found no significant difference between the cholesterol saturation, molar percentages of bile acids, phospholipid, and cholesterol in the two groups. Normal bile composition was also found in patients with type I diabetes (Meinders, DigDisSci, 1981; 26:402). However, treatment may affect the lithogenicity of bile in patients with diabetes. Insulin treatment of Pima Indians which significantly improved diabetic control was associated with a reduction in bile acid pool size and a 58 per cent increase in the cholesterol saturation index. Furthermore, diabetic patients are often advised to increase their dietary intake of poly-unsaturated fatty acids and this may also increase biliary cholesterol saturation (Sturdevant, NEJM, 1973; 288:24).

Diabetic patients with cholecystitis have higher operative morbidity and mortality rates following both emergency and elective biliary tract surgery (Sandler, Gastro, 1986; 91:157; Ransohoff, AnnIntMed, 1987; 106:829). Complications such as perforation and emphysematous cholecystitis were reported in up to 25 per cent of patients. Infection with multiple organisms is very common in the postoperative period. The main risk appears to be in diabetic patients who have concomitant renal, cardiac, and peripheral vascular disease. Such patients therefore require close monitoring perioperatively, with careful microbiological examination, including bile culture during surgery and from the T-tube postoperatively. Cholecystectomy was previously recommended for asymptomatic diabetic patients with gallstones, a practice which has been questioned (Pellegrini, Gastro, 1986; 91:245; Friedman, AnnIntMed, 1988; 109:913).

Effects of oral hypoglycaemic agents on the liver

The sulphonylureas may rarely cause an intrahepatic cholestasis accompanied by a mild to moderate inflammatory infiltrate and necrosis of liver cells predominant in the portal zones. This usually occurs within the first few weeks of treatment. This was more common with the first-generation sulphonylureas, occurring in 0.5 to 1 per cent of patients treated with chlorpropamide and about 0.3 per cent of those treated with tolbutamide; it may be seen rarely in patients treated with glibenclamide and newer agents (Gregory, ArchPathol, 1967; 84:506; Van Thiel, Gastro, 1974; 67:506; Wongpaitoon, PostgradMedJ, 1981; 57:244; Schneider, AmJGastr, 1984; 79:721; Del-Val, JHepatol, 1991; 13:375). The serum bilirubin, alkaline phosphatase, and γ-glutamyl transpeptidase levels may be very high with little increase in aminotransferases, consistent with cholestasis. There is often an accompanying eosinophilia and fever. Complete resolution can be expected on stopping the drug, although this may be slow. It may be possible to treat patients who develop cholestasis during chlorpropamide or tolbutamide therapy with one of the newer agents (glibenclamide, glipizide, etc.) without cross-reactivity (Rumboldt, ActaDiabLat, 1984; 21:387). In some patients, the extent of hepatocellular necrosis is more pronounced, with a marked increase in serum aminotransferase levels. Such a hepatitic reaction has been reported with glibenclamide (Goodman, AnnIntMed, 1987; 106:837) as well as older agents such as chlorpropamide, tolbutamide, and acetohexamide, and may occasionally be fatal (Schneider, AmJGastr, 1984; 79:721).

Mild and transient elevations of serum aminotransferases were reported in a few patients shortly after starting treatment with glibenclamide (Martin, MedJAust, 1969;2:433; O'Sullivan, BMJ, 1970; 2:572) but it is difficult to know whether these were due to the drug or the diabetes/obesity (see above). The biguanides are not associated with hepatotoxicity.

The liver in thyroid disease

Abnormal 'liver function tests' are commonly found in patients with primary thyroid disease. Liver damage may be secondary to the effects of thyroid hormone excess or deficiency or to the effects of antithyroid drugs on liver function. Elevated serum aspartate aminotransferase and alanine aminotransferase levels in patients with thyroid disease are not necessarily indicative of hepatic injury; in patients with hypothyroidism skeletal muscle is the main source of these enzymes. Similarly, in patients with thyroid crisis, rhabdomyolysis may lead to a massive release of myoglobin and increased serum bilirubin levels as a result of the increased conversion of haem to bilirubin.

Abnormalities of liver function in patients with autoimmune thyroid disease may also be due to coexisting primary liver disease due to an increased prevalence of autoimmune chronic active hepatitis and primary biliary cirrhosis. This association and the effects of liver disease on plasma thyroid hormone levels and transport are discussed in Chapter 25.2.

Thyrotoxicosis

Hepatic dysfunction in association with hyperthyroidism has long been recognized. In perhaps the earliest description of thyrotoxicosis, Karl Basedow described a patient with an enlarged liver and episodes of jaundice. Early studies (Weller, AnnIntMed, 1933; 7:687) of patients dying of untreated thyrotoxicosis described a spectrum of pathological changes ranging from marked hepatic inflammation, fatty liver with focal necrosis through atrophy to cirrhosis in 10 to 40 per cent of cases. This cirrhosis was often considered specific for hyperthyroidism (cirrhosis Basedowiana–Haban) (for early references see ref.[1]). Some of these histological changes may have been due to associated congestive cardiac failure, infection, or malnutrition associated with the catabolic state. With early diagnosis and effective treatment, severe liver disease in association with hyperthyroidism is rare nowadays.

Hepatic histology of patients presenting with thyrotoxicosis may be normal or suggest mild non-specific liver injury. On light microscopy, vacuolization of hepatocytes, balloon degeneration, nuclear glycogen, and mild portal infiltration of mononuclear cells may be found; electron microscopy may reveal hyperplasia of the smooth endoplasmic reticulum, a paucity of cytoplasmic glycogen, and increased numbers and size of mitochondria, which contain more crystae (Klion, AmJMed, 1971;50:317). A predominantly centrilobular cholestasis may be found in thyrotoxic patients with elevated alkaline phosphatase and γ-glutamyl transpeptidase levels (Sola, Liver, 1991; 11:193). In severe hyperthyroidism associated with congestive cardiac failure, centrizonal necrosis and perivenular fibrosis may be found (Myers, JCI, 1950; 29:1060). Rarely, this lesion may be found in patients presenting with cholestasis and jaundice in the absence of congestive cardiac failure (Yao, AmJMed, 1989; 86:619). In these patients it may be secondary to relative hypoxia of the perivenous region because hyperthyroidism increases hepatic oxygen consumption but either has no effect on hepatic blood flow (Myers, JCI, 1950; 29:1069) or increases it to a lesser extent than oxygen consumption (Wahren, JCI, 1981; 67:1056); increased oxygen demands are therefore met by increased oxygen extraction, accentuating the low oxygen tension in the centrilobular zones.

The reported incidence of abnormal 'liver function tests' in patients with untreated thyrotoxicosis varies from 15 to 76 per cent[8-10] (Thompson, MilitMed, 1978; 143:548). The most common finding is an increased serum alkaline phosphatase. The elevation can originate from liver, bone, or both; more often it reflects thyroid hormone enhancement of bone turnover (Tibi, ClinChem, 1989; 35:1427). Huang et al.[8] found that 76 per cent of thyrotoxic patients had at least one biochemical abnormality. Serum aspartate aminotransferase, alanine aminotransferase, alkaline phosphatase, γ-glutamyl transpeptidase, and bilirubin were elevated in 27 per cent, 37 per cent, 64 per cent, 17 per cent, and 5 per cent, respectively. Of 34 patients with an elevated serum alanine aminotransferase, 62 per cent showed a gradual return of the enzyme to normal during propylthiouracil therapy as serum thyroxine (T4) and triiodothyronine (**T3**) declined, but 38 per cent showed a transient asymptomatic further elevation of serum alanine aminotransferase levels. Overt hepatitis occurred in one patient. Changes in serum total alkaline phosphatase paralleled those of γ-glutamyl transpeptidase, despite a significant increase in the bone isoenzyme. This suggests that bone healing is occurring during the early phase of treatment. Serum levels of the liver-specific glutathione-*S*-transferase, a very sensitive indicator of hepatocellular damage, are also increased in hyperthyroidism (Beckett, BMJ, 1985; 291: 427; Tibi, ClinChem, 1989; 35:1427).

Abnormal bromosulphthalein retention occurs in 8 per cent of hyperthyroid patients, and the antipyrine half-life is significantly shortened[10] (Eichelbaum, NEJM, 1974; 290:1040). Cholic acid synthesis and pool size are decreased in hyperthyroidism but chenodeoxycholic acid kinetics are unchanged (Pauletzki, Hepatol, 1989; 9:852). This results in a reduced ratio of cholic acid to chenodeoxycholic acid in bile and serum but unchanged total serum bile acid levels (Kosuge, ClinSci, 1987; 73:425; Pauletzki, Hepatol, 1989; 9:852).

Jaundice is uncommon. It occurs in long-standing severe thyrotoxicosis associated with congestive cardiac failure, and in thyroid storm (see below), or in association with autoimmune liver disease. Thyroxine decreases hepatic bilirubin UDP-glucuronyltransferase activity (Steenbergen, Hepatol, 1989; 9:314) and hyperthyroidism may induce a mild unconjugated hyperbilirubinaemia in subjects with Gilbert's syndrome (Greenburger, AmJMed, 1964; 36:840). Rarely, jaundice due to intrahepatic cholestasis may develop in the absence of congestive cardiac failure or thyroid storm (Jansen, NethJMed, 1982; 25:318; Yao, AmJMed, 1989; 86:619).

The development of thyrotoxicosis in patients with established cirrhosis may lead to a marked deterioration in liver function tests. Thompson *et al.* (Gastro, 1994; 106:1342) reported a patient with primary biliary cirrhosis who had a fivefold increase in serum aminotransferases with jaundice as a result of the development of Graves disease and proximal muscle weakness. Clinical examination, radiological and cardiovascular investigations excluded heart failure and biliary obstruction. With treatment of her hyperthyroidism, serum aminotransferases declined to their previous stable level, and the bilirubin decreased over 6 weeks from 244 to 16 μmol/l.

In summary, mild elevations of serum alkaline phosphatase and aminotransferases may occur in untreated thyrotoxicosis but resolve with effective therapy[8-10] (Thompson, MilitMed, 1978; 143: 548; Beckett, BMJ, 1985; 291:427). Part of the rise in alkaline phosphatase and aminotransferases may sometimes be of bone or muscle origin, respectively (Cooper, AnnIntMed, 1979; 90:164; Tibi, ClinChem, 1989; 35:1427). Transient asymptomatic elevation of transaminase levels occurs in one-third of patients treated with propylthiouracil (see below).

Effects of thyroid hormone on liver metabolism

Thyroxine increases hepatic gluconeogenesis, glycogenolysis, and hepatic glucose production in the basal state (Sandler, JClinEndoc, 1983; 56:479). Increased muscle protein catabolism and adipose tissue lipolysis provide the amino acid and glycerol substrates for the enhanced glucose production (see Chapter 2.11). Increased gluconeogenesis from amino acids implies a greater amino nitrogen load that must be eliminated. This is achieved by increased basal rates of urea synthesis, though the enhancement of urea synthesis in response to an amino acid load in patients with untreated hyperthyroidism is normal (Marchesini, Metabolism, 1994; 43: 1023). Gluconeogenesis and urea synthesis are energy-requiring processes, but they probably account for only a small part of the enhanced hepatic oxygen consumption induced by excess thyroid hormone. Much of the enhanced hepatic oxygen consumption may be due to the stimulation of a mitochondrial proton leak; the dissipation of the proton gradient across the mitochondrial membrane will mean impaired adenosine triphosphate (**ATP**) regeneration, increased heat production, and an increased rate of respiratory chain electron transport to maintain ATP levels (Harper, CanJPhysPharm, 1994; 72:899). The relative hypoxia of perivenous hepatocytes (see above) may lead to increased glycolytic rates to maintain ATP levels; the marked increase in the amount of flavin adenine dinucleotide (**FAD**)-linked glycerol-3-phosphate dehydrogenase in hyperthyroidism (Muller, PNAS, 1994; 91:10581) would increase the efficiency with which reducing equivalents generated during glycolysis are transported from the cytosol to the mitochondria.

In thyrotoxicosis, serum concentrations of proteins secreted by the liver, such as albumin and thyroxine-binding globulin, are normal. However, sex hormone binding globulin is increased. Cholesterol synthesis and clearance are also increased in thyrotoxicosis; the effect on clearance predominates so that cholesterol levels tend to be low.

Thyroid storm and the liver

The clinical spectrum of thyrotoxicosis ranges in severity from asymptomatic biochemical abnormalities to a severe metabolic crisis associated with a high mortality rate. The main clinical features of thyroid storm are fever, mental status aberration, and evidence of multisystem involvement. Body temperature is usually above 38.5 °C. The resting pulse rate may exceed 140 beats/min, with a high propensity for atrial dysrrhythmias; cardiac failure may supervene. Cerebral dysfunction is manifest as severe agitation, delerium, or frank psychosis, progressing in some instances to stupor and coma. Gastrointestinal and hepatic involvement may dominate the presentation in thyroid storm, with nausea, vomiting, frank diarrhoea, and marked hepatic dysfunction manifested by jaundice. Indeed, unexplained jaundice in a severely thyrotoxic patient, in conjunction with fever and marked tachycardia (more than 140 beats/min), has a strong predictive value for the appearance of storm. Known precipitants of thyroid storm are listed in Table 2. It should be noted that atypical presentations of storm may occur, particularly in patients with 'apathetic thyrotoxicosis'. Such patients lack the florid manifestations of thyrotoxicosis and may not have a goitre or exophthalmos. They have a tendency to lapse into semistupor and death with none of the usual signs of thyrotoxicosis. Thyroid crisis has more rarely presented with abdominal pain and fever, coma, status epilepticus, non-embolic cerebral infarction, and acute renal failure associated with rhabdomyolysis. Rhabdomyolysis is associated with a marked increase in serum aspartate aminotransferase, alanine aminotransferase, and creatine kinase levels, and contributes to the rise in serum bilirubin levels as a result of the degradation of haem from released myoglobin.

Table 2 Precipitants of thyroid crisis

Conditions causing a rapid rise in thyroid hormone levels
  Thyroid surgery
  Withdrawal of antithyroid drug therapy
  Vigorous thyroid palpation
  Iodinated contrast dyes
Conditions associated with acute or subacute non-thyroidal illness
  Non-thyroidal surgery
  Infection
  Cerebrovascular accident
  Pulmonary thromboembolism
  Parturition
  Diabetic ketoacidosis
  Emotional stress
  Trauma

The pathophysiology of thyroid storm does not differ fundamentally from that of thyrotoxicosis in general. The development of thyroid storm may be due in part to a sudden rise in the free T4 and T3 levels, possibly associated with a transient depression of the thyroxine–binding globulin level. This may be particularly relevant in the context of sepsis or other intercurrent illness. Other mechanisms may also be operative. These include:

(1) an increase in catecholamine secretion in stress situations (thyrotoxic patients are very sensitive to catecholamine levels and normally have reduced plasma adrenaline and noradrenaline levels);

(2) decreased clearance of thyroid hormone during systemic illness; and

(3) enhanced generation of the metabolically active T3 congener, triiodoacetic acid.

Effects of antithyroid drugs on the liver

Increased serum levels of aspartate aminotransferase and alanine aminotransferase occur in about 30 per cent of patients treated with propylthiouracil (Liauw, AnnIntMed, 1993; 118:424). The rise in aminotransferases appears to be dose related, so that aspartate aminotransferase and alanine aminotransferase levels are highest during the first few weeks of treatment, falling rapidly with reduction of the dose of propylthiouracil. In most patients serum aminotransferases return to normal despite continued propylthiouracil treatment. Bilirubin levels remain normal unless hepatitis develops. This occurs very rarely but may be severe (Levy, ClinPediat, 1993; 32:25). It is unrelated to the dose of propylthiouracil used and can develop at any time, but usually occurs within the first 2 to 3 months of treatment. Liver histology shows varying degrees of hepatocellular necrosis, which can be massive. Rarely, the clinical and histological picture is one of an autoimmune chronic active hepatitis (Levy, ClinPediat, 1993; 32:25).

Abnormalities of liver function are much less common with carbimazole and methimazole. These agents may induce cholestasis, which is probably an idiosyncratic reaction to the drugs (Blom, ArchIntMed, 1985; 145:1513; Arab, JClinEndoc, 1995; 80:1083). An elevation of the bilirubin, alkaline phosphatase, and γ-glutamyl transpeptidase levels are the predominant abnormalities, but there may also be a mild rise in serum aminotransferase levels. Liver dysfunction presents within 2 to 3 weeks of initiation of treatment.

The predominant finding on liver biopsy is intrahepatic cholestasis. Cholestasis may progress despite discontinuation of treatment and may take several months to resolve (Arab, JClinEndoc, 1995; 80: 1083).

Hypothyroidism

Serum aspartate aminotransferase and alanine aminotransferase levels are often increased in patients with untreated hypothyroidism (Doran, JRSM, 1978; 71:189; Klein, ArchIntMed, 1984; 144:123). The increase is usually less than three times the upper limit of normal but in occasional patients may be quite marked. The accompanying rise in serum creatine phosphokinase and aldolase levels suggests that skeletal muscle is the source of the increase in serum aminotransferases. Both increased release and diminished clearance contribute to their increased plasma levels. Elevated aspartate aminotransferase and alanine aminotransferase levels were found in 84 per cent and 60 per cent, respectively, of patients with untreated hypothyroidism (Doran, JRSM, 1978; 71:189). Ninety-six per cent of these patients had an elevated creatine phosphokinase up to six times the upper limit of normal; much higher creatine phosphokinase levels may occasionally be found. Serum alkaline phosphatase, γ-glutamyl transpeptidase, and bilirubin levels are usually normal and the serum transaminase levels are restored to normal rapidly after initiation of thyroid hormone replacement. Liver histology is usually normal in patients with untreated hypothyroidism and elevated aminotransferases. However, one study found central congestive hepatic fibrosis without myxoedematous infiltration in patients with myxoedematous ascites who had no evidence of cardiac failure; it was suggested that this may be a specific hypothyroid hepatic lesion (Baker, AnnIntMed, 1972; 77: 927).

Myxoedema ascites has a high protein concentration (Clancy, MedJAust, 1979; 2:415; Klein, ArchIntMed, 1984; 144:123). It is often intractable and associated with pleural and pericardial effusions. The ascites and other effusions resolve with thyroid hormone replacement.

Thyroid status affects bile acid synthesis and bilirubin excretion; the antipyrine half-life is prolonged (Eichelbaum, NEJM, 1974; 290:1040). A single case of cholestasis and jaundice associated with hypothyroidism in an adult has been reported (Ariza, JAMA, 1984; 252:2392). In experimental hypothyroidism, bile flow is diminished due to a decrease in both bile-salt independent canalicular flow and diminished bile salt output (Steenbergen, Hepatol, 1989; 9:314). This reduction in bile flow may in part be due to an increase in membrane cholesterol–phospholipid ratio and diminished membrane fluidity, which may affect a number of canalicular membrane transporters and enzymes, including the Na^+,K^+-ATPase. Certain key enzymes in cholesterol and bile-acid synthesis (HMG-CoA reductase and cholesterol-7-α-hydroxylase) are reduced,[11] and the fraction of bile acids conjugated with glycine is increased, possibly due to decreased availability of dietary taurine for conjugation. The activity of bilirubin UDP-glucuronyltransferase is increased and the biliary excretion of bilirubin diminished (Steenbergen, Hepatol, 1989; 9:314).

A persistent unconjugated hyperbilirubinaemia in the newborn may suggest the diagnosis of congenital hypothyroidism. The mechanism is unclear. It may be due to delayed maturation of bilirubin

UDP-glucuronyltransferase activity; in one infant with congenital hypothyroidism there was no measureable hepatic activity of this enzyme prior to initiation of thyroid hormone replacement (Labrune, JPediatGastrNutr, 1992; 14:79). The hypercholesterolaemia, gallbladder hypotonia (Losada, JClinEndocr, 1957; 17:133), and decreased bile flow in hypothyroidism suggests an increased predisposition to gallstones, but this association has yet to be established.

Liver function test abnormalities in patients with thyroid dysfunction that do not resolve quickly with thyroid hormone treatment in hypothyroid patients or with antithyroid drugs in those with thyrotoxicosis should raise the possibility of associated primary liver disease. Propylthiouracil may also be a cause of persistently elevated transaminase levels, in which case levels should fall with reduction of the dose of the drug. Overtreatment of patients with hypothyroidism may result in mild elevations of serum aminotransferases and plasma glutathione S-transferase (Beckett, BMJ, 1985; 291:427; Gow, JClinEndocr, 1987; 64:364).

Addison's disease

Mild elevations of serum aspartate aminotransferase and alanine aminotransferase may be found in patients with Addison's disease. Olsson et al. (AmJGastr, 1990; 85:435) reported four patients with Addison's disease who had elevated aspartate aminotransferase and alanine aminotransferase levels at presentation; in all four, serum transaminase levels were restored to normal within 1 week of corticosteroid replacement therapy. Three patients with elevated alanine aminotransferase (and to a lesser extent aspartate aminotransferase) levels in the months preceding diagnosis of Addison's disease were reported by Boulton et al. (Gastro, 1995; 109:1324); in all cases transaminase levels reverted to normal after starting glucocorticoid therapy. No other cause of elevated transaminase levels was identified in these patients.

The reason for the elevated transaminase levels in some patients with Addison's disease is unclear. Increased hepatic release of alanine aminotransferase and aspartate aminotransferase is suggested by reports of a mild lymphocytic infiltrate on liver biopsy (Nerup, DanMedBull, 1974; 21:201; Olsson, AmJGastr, 1990; 85:435). However, elevated transaminase levels in Addison's disease may also be found in the presence of normal hepatic histology (Boulton, Gastro, 1995; 109:1324).

An increased serum alanine aminotransferase is often regarded as being a relatively specific indicator of hepatic damage (see Chapter 5.1). However, myopathic disorders can also cause significant elevations of serum alanine aminotransferase; the aspartate aminotransferase and alanine aminotransferase levels in these patients often increase by the same order of magnitude (Thomson, BMJ, 1960; 2:1276; Helfgott, AmJMed, 1993; 95:447; Morse, JPaediat, 1993; 122:254). Thus, theoretically, skeletal muscle could be the source of increased transaminase levels in patients with Addison's disease; diminished clearance of the enzymes in hypovolaemic patients might also be a factor. The slightly delayed bromosulphthalein elimination reported in Addison's disease (Rowntree, MayoClinProc, 1931; 207) could also be due to hypovolaemia and diminished liver blood flow.[12]

Acromegaly

The liver and spleen may be enlarged in active acromegaly. Autopsy studies suggested that hepatosplenomegaly was common in acromegalic patients (Gordon, CanMedAssJ, 1962; 87:1106; Sorber, ArchIntMed, 1974; 134:415). However, more recent studies, employing ultrasound or computed tomography, suggest that hepatosplenomegaly is uncommon (Ezzat, DigDis, 1992; 10:173; Avagnina, Metabolism, 1996; 45:109). In patients with clinically significant hepatomegaly and/or splenomegaly, other causes should be excluded before invoking excess growth hormone as the cause (Sorber, ArchIntMed, 1974; 134:415; Ezzat, DigDis, 1992; 10:173).

Standard liver function tests are normal in acromegaly. Occasional patients with very active disease may have a slightly elevated serum alkaline phosphatase of bone origin due to increased bone turnover. In patients with an increase in liver size, the hepatic extraction of indocyanine green and oxygen is increased (Preisig, JCI, 1966; 45:1379). Galactose elimination capacity is increased in acromegaly even in patients without significant hepatomegaly (Avagnina, Metabolism, 1996; 45:109). It falls to normal with restoration of normal growth hormone and insulin-like growth factor-1 levels by hypophysectomy or octreotide treatment. Since splanchnic and liver blood flow are unchanged in acromegaly, the enhanced galactose elimination capacity may be due to increased expression of galactokinase rather than an increase in the number of functional liver cells or enhanced hepatic perfusion. Growth hormone and insulin-like growth factor-1 increase the transcription of a number of genes in the liver, and effects of growth hormone and insulin-like growth factor-1 excess on liver enzymes could also explain the increased excretory capacity for bromosulphthalein in acromegaly.

Trans-sphenoidal hypophysectomy is currently the treatment of choice for microadenomas causing acromegaly. With incomplete excision, radiotherapy may be indicated. Because the optimal effect of irradiation on growth hormone levels may be delayed for several years, it is customary to reduce growth hormone levels medically in the interim, either with a dopamine agonist such as bromocriptine, or with the somatostatin analogue octreotide. Octreotide is used in doses of 100 to 500 µg thrice daily subcutaneously. Prolonged treatment with octreotide predisposes to biliary sludging, gallstone formation, and cholecystitis. Gallbladder contraction and bile excretion are both impaired in patients treated with octreotide (Van Liessum, JClinEndoc, 1989; 69:557; Zhu, DigDisSci, 1994; 39:284). These effects may be due to direct effects of somatostatin on the gallbladder and biliary tree which contain somatostatin receptors, and to inhibition of secretion of a number of hormones that regulate bile secretion, including cholecystokinin, secretin, motilin, vasoactive intestinal peptide, and gastrin (Marteau, Digestion, 1989; 42:16).

Since gallbladder contractility is restored by 8 h after the last subcutaneous injection of octreotide, it has been suggested that the risk of cholelithiasis may be reduced if patients on long-term octreotide treatment take one of their daily meals about 8 h after their last injection (Hopman, DigDisSci, 1992; 37:1685). This meal should contain sufficient protein and fat to ensure an adequate release of cholecystokinin and effective gallbladder contraction.

Cushing's syndrome

Fatty liver may occur in patients with Cushing's syndrome. It may be diffuse (Benamouzig, GastrClinBiol, 1991; 15:865) or localized

(Christian, ArchIntMed, 1983; 143:1605), and may in part be related to the high prevalence of truncal obesity and insulin resistance in patients with Cushing's syndrome. The development of severe fatty liver may be associated with an elevation of serum alanine aminotransferase and γ-glutamyl transpeptidase levels. Elevated serum γ-glutamyl transpeptidase levels may be found in about 50 per cent of patients with Cushing's syndrome, but serum alanine aminotransferase and aspartate aminotransferase levels are usually normal (Sato, EndocrinolJpn, 1984; 31:705). An autopsy study suggested that moderate to severe fatty liver may be found in about 50 per cent of patients with Cushing's syndrome (Soffer, AmJMed, 1961; 30:129) but others have suggested a lower prevalence (Sato, EndocrinolJpn, 1984; 31:705). Fatty liver may also develop after prolonged high-dose corticosteroid therapy (Itoh, Acta-HepatoGastroenterol, 1977; 24:415); the hepatic fat content may decrease rapidly following steroid withdrawal (Steinberg, Gastro, 1952; 21:304). Increased liver glycogen may also be found. This is common in patients with hepatic steatosis but may occur in the absence of excess hepatic triglyceride. It may be a consequence of hyperglycaemia in patients with associated diabetes or it could be due to the stimulation of glycogen synthesis by glucocorticoids. Fatal fat embolism involving the lungs and systemic organs has been reported in association with severe fatty liver in Cushing's syndrome (Moran, ArchPathol, 1962; 73:300; Jones, NEJM, 1965; 273:1453). This complication may be more likely to occur after abrupt cessation of steroid therapy.

Ketoconazole used in the treatment of Cushing's syndrome may rarely cause severe liver dysfunction (Lake-Bakaar, BMJ, 1987; 294:419). The clinical picture may suggest a predominantly hepatocellular injury with very high serum aminotransferases and modest increase in the alkaline phosphatase or a mixed hepatocellular/cholestatic injury with more marked increase in serum alkaline phosphatase levels. Massive liver cell necrosis and liver failure may occur. Severe liver injury with jaundice occurs after at least 10 days of treatment, thus the risk of serious hepatotoxicity is greater with more prolonged treatment than with short courses. An elevation of serum transaminase levels and alkaline phosphatase may be seen within a few days of starting treatment (McCance, ClinEndoc, 1987; 27:593). In many patients the enzyme abnormalities may be transient but it is important to monitor these closely as they could signal early hepatotoxicity. Most patients recover when the drug is stopped, liver function tests returning to normal within about 3 months. Liver function tests should be performed at baseline, after 10 days, and then twice a month during ketoconazole treatment (Lake-Bakaar, BMJ, 1987; 294:419).

Sex steroids and the liver

Anabolic androgenic steroids

The C17 alkylated androgenic steroids are hepatotoxic and can produce acute cholestatic jaundice. The alkyl group at position C17 appears to be essential for cholestasis, although isolated cases of cholestasis and jaundice have been reported with esterified testosterone (Yoshida, JClinGastro, 1994; 18:268) which lacks a C17-alkyl group. A mild degree of hepatic dysfunction is seen in the majority of patients on high doses of androgens, while relatively few develop cholestasis and jaundice.[14] Jaundice usually develops

after 2 to 5 months or more of treatment. Anorexia, nausea, and occasionally vomiting may precede the development of jaundice and there may be significant weight loss. Pruritus is variable; it may be severe or absent.[14] Renal failure may also occur (Gurakar, JOklStateMedAssoc, 1994; 87:399). Liver function tests reveal an elevated serum bilirubin and mild elevation of serum aspartate aminotransferase and alanine aminotransferase levels. The serum alkaline phosphatase is normal or mildly elevated in most patients; fewer than 5 per cent have an alkaline phosphatase more than three times the upper normal limit.[14] The prognosis in patients developing cholestatic jaundice is generally good, although it may initially progress after stopping the drug and may be very slow to resolve. There are rare reports of progression to cirrhosis.[14]

Peliosis hepatis (sinusoidal distension and blood-filled spaces in the liver) is particularly associated with the use of anabolic steroids.[13,14] Peliosis hepatis is more likely to occur in patients treated with anabolic steroids (Haupt, AmJSportsMed, 1984; 12:469; Lowdell, BMJ, 1985; 291:637) than in athletes, in whom this complication is extremely rare but can occur (Cabasso, MedSciSportsExer, 1994; 26:2). It may be asymptomatic or result in hepatomegaly, tenderness in the right hypochondrium, liver failure, or intraperitoneal haemorrhage. It can appear at any time during treatment with anabolic steroids and does not seem to be related to the dose used.[13] Liver biopsy is diagnostic; ultrasound, CT scan, or angiography may all be helpful in diagnosis.[14] Regression of peliosis hepatis may occur after discontinuation of anabolic steroid treatment.[13] Anabolic steroids may be associated with the development of hepatic adenomas, hepatocellular carcinoma, cholangiocarcinoma, hepatic angiosarcoma, and focal nodular hyperplasia.[13,14]

Mild elevations of serum aspartate aminotransferase, alanine aminotransferase, and alkaline phosphatase levels may be found in athletes using anabolic steroids (Alen, BrJSportsMed, 1985; 19:15; O'Connor, MilitMed, 1990; 155:72); serum creatine phosphokinase is also elevated (Boone, IntJSportsMed, 1990; 11:293) and thus skeletal muscle may contribute to the increased serum transaminase levels (Strauss, PhysSportsMed, 1983; 11:87).

Oral contraceptive pill

Synthetic oestrogens, particularly those with a C17-ethinyl group may cause an acute cholestasis.[15,16] Cholestasis in patients on the oral contraceptive pill occurs with increased frequency in those with a family history of cholestasis of pregnancy, suggesting a genetic susceptibility.[15] The cholestasis is of canalicular type, most pronounced in the central area, and not associated with evidence of portal inflammation or parenchymal injury. It usually occurs within the first 2 months of treatment and tends to be insidious in onset with pruritus and mild jaundice, pale stools, and dark urine. Synthetic oestrogens decrease bile flow, biliary secretion of bile acids, and decrease the activity of the liver membrane Na^+,K^+-ATPase, possibly by reducing membrane lipid fluidity.[15,16] However, the exact mechanism of oestrogen-induced cholestasis remains unclear.

Liver function returns rapidly to normal on stopping the oral contraceptive pill. Failure of liver tests to return to normal should suggest an underlying hepatobiliary disorder that has been unmasked by the use of the oral contraceptive pill. In such patients there may be more marked derangement of liver function tests during the cholestatic phase.

In patients with an underlying tendency to thromboembolism, the oral contraceptive pill may precipitate hepatic venous occlusion and a Budd–Chiari syndrome (Lewis, DigDisSci, 1983; 28:673; Chapter 21.3). In a case-control study, the relative risk of hepatic vein thrombosis in oral contraceptive users was 2.37, comparable to that for stroke, myocardial infarction, and venous thromboembolism (Valla, Gastro, 1986; 90:807).

The occurrence of hepatic adenomas in oral contraceptive pill users was described a few years after their introduction (Baum, Lancet, 1973; 2:926). Most of the adenomas were found in women who had taken oral contraceptive steroids for several years. Focal nodular hyperplasia is also associated with use of the oral contraceptive pill. The tumours are generally painless and the patient asymptomatic. Ten per cent of lesions are pedunculated. They may increase in size during pregnancy. They are often very vascular and may occasionally rupture, causing catastrophic haemoperitoneum. Most lesions regress spontaneously with discontinuation of treatment (Edmondson, AnnIntMed, 1977; 86:180). Very rarely they may become malignant, although the association between hepatocellular carcinoma and oral contraceptive use is disputed (Goodman, Hepatol, 1982; 2:440; Forman, BMJ, 1986; 292:1357).

Cyproterone acetate

This antiandrogen used in the treatment of hirsutism, precocious puberty, and prostatic carcinoma may cause severe liver damage (Levesque, Lancet, 1989; 8640:215; Blake, Gut, 1990; 31:556; Hirsch, IsrJMedSci, 1994; 30:238). The drug is very lipophilic and stored in fat. Excretion is via bile (70 per cent) and urine (30 per cent). By 1995, 91 cases of cyproterone acetate-induced hepatotoxicity (32 fatal), occurring in men treated for prostatic cancer, had been reported to the Committee on Safety of Medicines (UK). The hepatic reactions included cholestasis, hepatitis, and fulminant liver failure. Hepatotoxicity typically occurred in men receiving the highest doses of cyproterone acetate (300 mg/day) for several months. Hepatocellular carcinoma has also been reported in prostate cancer patients treated with cyproterone acetate (Kattan, AmJClinOncCanTrials, 1994; 17:390) and in women who had been treated with a high dose of the drug at puberty (Watanabe, Lancet, 1994; 344:1567).

Histiocytosis X (Langerhans' cell histiocytosis)

Hepatosplenomegaly is common in the disseminated forms of this condition (Letterer–Siwe syndrome and Hand–Schuller–Christian disease), which also frequently causes diabetes insipidus and more rarely panhypopituitarism. Children are usually affected in the first years of life but it may present in adults (Novice, Cancer, 1989; 63: 166). Hepatomegaly is associated with infiltration of the portal areas with Langerhan cell histiocytes. In patients with rapidly progressive disseminated disease, hepatic involvement may result in ascites and oedema due to hypoalbuminaemia, coagulopathy, and jaundice, and is associated with a very poor prognosis. In some patients the disease follows a more protracted course and may either go into spontaneous remission or be cured by combinations of corticosteroids and chemotherapy. Hepatosplenomegaly is also common in these patients (Leblanc, Gastro, 1981; 80:134), who rarely may go on to develop intrahepatic cholestasis and jaundice and/or cirrhosis with portal hypertension and bleeding from oesophageal varices (Grosfeld, AmJSurg, 1976; 131:108). These sequelae may be seen even if the disease is cured; the portal tract areas initially infiltrated by histiocytes are involved in a progressive fibrotic reaction which may lead to the disappearance of intrahepatic bile ducts. Cholangiographic appearances may resemble those found in sclerosing cholangitis but are more localized and do not usually involve the extrahepatic bile ducts (Leblanc, Gastro, 1981; 80:134). Rarely, histiocytic infiltration of the gallbladder may occur. Splenomegaly may be due to infiltration of the spleen with histiocytes or secondary to portal hypertension.

References

1. Lichtman SS. The liver in hyperthyroidism. In *Diseases of the liver, gallbladder and bile ducts*. London: Henry Kimpton, 1953: 924–39.
2. Silverman, JF, O'Brien KF, Long S, *et al*. Liver pathology in morbidly obese patients with and without diabetes. *American Journal of Gastroenterology*, 1990; 85: 1349–55.
3. Andersen T, Gluud C, Franzmann M-B, and Christoffersen P. Hepatic effects of dietary weight loss in morbidly obese subjects. *Journal of Hepatology*, 1991; 12: 224–9.
4. Bacon BR, Farahvash MJ, Janney CG, and Neuschwander-Tetri BA. Nonalcoholic steatohepatitis: an expanded clinical entity. *Gastroenterology*, 1994; 107: 1103–9.
5. Tell MR, James OFW, Burt AD, Bennett MK, and Day CP. The natural history of nonalcoholic fatty liver: a follow-up study. *Hepatology*, 1995; 22: 1714–19.
6. Wanless IR and Lentz JS. Fatty liver hepatitis (steatohepatitis) and obesity: an autopsy study with analysis of risk factors. *Hepatology*, 1990; 12: 1106–10.
7. Creutzfeldt W, Frerichs H, and Sickinger K. Liver disease in diabetes mellitus. *Progress in Liver Disease*, 1970; 13: 371–407.
8. Huang MJ and Liaw YF. Clinical association between thyroid and liver diseases. *Journal of Gastroenterology and Hepatology*, 1995; 10: 344–50.
9. Fong TL, McHutchison JG, and Reynolds TB. Hyperthyroidism and hepatic dysfunction. A case series analysis. *Journal of Clinical Gastroenterology*, 1992; 14: 240–4.
10. Ashkar FS, Miller R, Smoak WM, and Gilson AJ. Liver disease in hyperthyroidism. *Southern Medical Journal*, 1971; 64: 462–5.
11. Mayer D. Hormones and 7-α-hydroxylation of cholesterol. In Matern S, Hackenschmidt J, Back P, and Gerok W, eds. *Advances in bile research*. Stuttgart: Schattauer Verlag, 1975: 61–7.
12. McIntyre N, Mulligan R, and Carson E. BSP Tm and S: a critical re-evaluation. In Paumgartner G and Preisig R, eds. *The liver: quantitative aspects of structure and function*. Karger: Basel, 1973: 417–27.
13. Soe KL, Soe M, and Gluud C. Liver pathology associated with the use of anabolic–androgenic steroids. *Liver*, 1992; 12: 73–9.
14. Ishak KG and Zimmerman HJ. Hepatotoxic effects of the anabolic/androgenic steroids. *Seminars in Liver Disease*, 1987; 7: 230–6.
15. Reyes H and Simon FR. Intrahepatic cholestasis of pregnancy: an estrogen-related disease. *Seminars in Liver Disease*, 1993; 13: 289–301.
16. Reichen J and Simon FR. Cholestasis. In Arias IM, Boyer JL, Fausto N, Jakoby WB, Schachter DA, and Shafritz DA, eds. *The liver: biology and pathobiology*, (3rd edn). New York: Raven Press, 1994: 1291–326.

24.7 Musculoskeletal diseases and the liver

J. van den Bogaerde and H. L. C. Beynon

Introduction

Rheumatologists treat connective tissue diseases and other conditions with an autoimmune aetiology. Although the pathogenesis of rheumatological diseases is poorly understood, diseases as diverse as rheumatoid arthritis and systemic vasculitis respond to immunosuppressive regimens. A better understanding of their immunogenetics and pathogenesis might lead to more rational and successful treatment regimens.

Connective tissue diseases may cause abnormalities of liver function tests as well as a variety of histological changes. The severity of the underlying connective tissue disease influences the course of the liver disease, and immunosuppressive treatment can affect liver enzymes. Generally, the symptoms of the connective tissue disease dominate the clinical presentation, and liver involvement rarely causes diagnostic or therapeutic problems. Frequently, however, deranged liver function tests, in conjunction with evidence of other organ involvement, may pose major diagnostic and therapeutic challenges to the practising clinician.

This chapter will discuss connective tissue diseases and the liver, and briefly consider hepatic effects of drugs such as methotrexate and non-steroidal anti-inflammatory drugs (**NSAIDs**), which are often used to treat patients with these diseases. As patients with a wide range of connective tissue diseases are treated with NSAIDs, this will be the first topic of discussion.

Drugs used in musculoskeletal diseases (see also Section 17)
NSAID-associated hepatotoxicity

Liver damage due to NSAIDs is well recognized and has been extensively reviewed (Fry, GastrClinNAm, 1995; 24:875). Although the absolute risk of NSAID-induced liver disease is low (9/100 000), NSAID use appeared to double the risk of liver disease in current users (Garcia Rodriguez, ArchIntMed, 1994; 154:311). Aspirin is the most widely used NSAID and may result in a mild elevation of aminotransferase enzymes (Lewis, ClinPharmTher, 1984; 3:128). Aspirin-related hepatotoxicity is dose dependent (Tolman, Gastro, 1978; 74:205), and is usually found in patients taking large doses over a long time (Kanda, AmJHospPharm, 1978; 35:33). Aspirin use rarely results in jaundice, but hepatic failure and death have been described (Zimmerman, ArchIntMed, 1981; 141:333).

Reports of NSAID-induced hepatotoxicity are usually derived from case reports and phase III trials (Fry, GastrClinNAm, 1995; 24:875). Sulindac has been shown to be more harmful than other NSAIDs (Garcia Rodriguez, BMJ, 1992; 305:865; Garcia Rodriguez, ArchIntMed, 1994; 154:311). Seventy-five per cent of patients with sulindac-induced liver damage were female, cholestatic damage was found in 50 per cent, often with a striking eosinophilia, and 25 per cent had biochemical evidence of hepatitis (Tarazi, Gastro, 1993; 104:569).

Diclofenac has been associated with a threefold elevation in aminotransferases in 2 per cent of users (Helfgott, JAMA, 1990; 264:2660). Another study of 180 patients with diclofenac-associated hepatotoxicity reported jaundice in 75 per cent, with a mortality rate of 3.8 per cent (Banks, Hepatol, 1995; 22:820). As with most of the other NSAIDs, liver damage is caused by an idiosyncratic mechanism (Helfgott, 1990; Fry, GastrClinNAm, 1995; 24;875). Isolated reports have appeared implicating most NSAIDs in liver disease; one drug, fenzlozic acid, was withdrawn as a result of hepatic damage (Hart, AnnRheumDis, 1970; 29:684).

Before initiating long-term NSAID use, aminotransferase levels should be measured; if they are elevated, an underlying cause should be sought (Fry, GastrClinNAm, 1995; 24:875). During NSAID therapy, monitoring of aminotransferase levels should be undertaken, and if aminotransferase levels double, the drug should be withdrawn (Fry, 1995). Since toxicity is idiosyncratic, the same NSAID drug should never be reintroduced, and a different class should be given under strict supervision. It is essential to warn the patient that over-the-counter preparations could contain the offending NSAID.

Paracetamol

In the United States in 1987, 60 000 cases of paracetamol overdose were reported (Smilkstein, NEJM, 1988; 319:1557), making this the most common cause of acute drug-induced liver failure in developed countries. Intake of more than 15 g is found in 80 per cent of patients with serious cases of toxicity (Zimmerman, ArchIntMed, 1981; 141:333). Lower doses are dangerous in alcoholics, malnourished patients, or those using drugs such as isoniazid, phenytoin, and omeprazole, which affect the P-450 enzyme system (Lauterburg, Gut, 1988; 29:1153; Burk, ResCommChemPathPharm, 1990; 69:115; Diaz, Gastro, 1990; 99:737). Greater awareness of paracetamol toxicity, and early treatment with *N*-acetylcysteine, has resulted in lower mortality.

Methotrexate therapy and the liver

Methotrexate is an immunosuppressive agent widely used in the management of patients with connective tissue diseases. It blocks lymphocyte proliferation by inhibiting dihydrofolate reductase. Methotrexate is often used in the management of psoriasis (10 to 25 mg/week) and rheumatoid arthritis (7.5 to 15 mg/week, as a single or divided dose). Recognized hepatic side-effects include mild fibrosis in 15 per cent of patients, and moderate fibrosis or cirrhosis in less than 1 per cent of patients (Neuberger, PrescribersJ, 1995; 35:158). Patients with psoriasis are more prone to fibrosis than those with rheumatoid arthritis, which may reflect the higher cumulative dose used. Methotrexate therapy at doses of 15 mg/week is reported to result in a 17 to 60 per cent drop-out in the first year, with gastrointestinal, pulmonary, and infectious complications exceeding hepatic complications (Schnabel, RheumInt, 1996; 15:195). The drug is excreted by the kidney, so risk of toxicity is increased in the elderly patient with renal impairment, and is theoretically increased in patients with mild renal impairment who take NSAIDs.

Guidelines for patients with psoriasis and rheumatoid arthritis who use methotrexate (Workshop, BMJ, 1991; 303:829; Kremer, ArthRheum, 1994; 37:316; Neuberger, PrescribersJ, 1995; 35:158) emphasize the importance of regular liver function tests, the assessment of pre-existing liver disease, particularly when daily alcohol use exceeds 15 g/day, and the documentation of preceding hepatitis B and C infection. Although patients with psoriasis may require a liver biopsy after a cumulative dose of 1.5 g of methotrexate, patients with rheumatoid arthritis should only undergo a biopsy if monthly aminotransferases are consistently elevated or if serum albumin decreases. The issue of biopsy in patients on long-term methotrexate therapy is not resolved, and the attitudes of informed patients and physicians differ (Ferraz, ClinExpRheumatol, 1994; 126:6215). The mortality following liver biopsy is between 0.12 and 0.33 per cent (Gilmore, Gut, 1995; 36:437). Recent reports have found that 5 or 10 yearly liver biopsies for patients with rheumatoid arthritis are not cost-effective (Bergquist, ArthRheum, 1995; 38:326).

Connective tissue diseases
Systemic lupus erythematosus

Systemic lupus erythematosus is a group of multisystem inflammatory diseases, characterized by a wide range of autoantibodies directed against both intra- and extracellular antigens.[1] Anti-dsDNA antibodies are characteristic of systemic lupus erythematosus. Other antibodies, such as antiendothelial IgG antibodies, have been described in 74 per cent of patients with this disease (Rosenbaum, ClinExpImmun, 1988; 72:450). It is often held up as the paradigm of a disease mediated by the deposition of immune complexes.

The revised American College of Rheumatology criteria are widely used in clinical practice, since they encompass the heterogeneous manifestations of the disease (Tan, ArthRheum, 1982; 25:1271). The presence of four or more of the criteria, not necessarily at the same time, is sufficient to make the diagnosis of systemic

Table 1 Hepatic complications and associations in systemic lupus erythematosus (SLE)	
Enzyme elevation	From SLE NSAIDs and aspirin Antiphospholipid syndrome with thrombi
Hepatitis	Granulomatous Chronic active Cholestatic Viral Alcoholic
Steatosis	From SLE Steroid use
Nodular regenerative hyperplasia	With and without antiphospholipid syndrome
Rare associations	Budd–Chiari syndrome (antiphospholipid syndrome) Primary biliary cirrhosis Sclerosing cholangitis

lupus erythematosus. The criteria for the diagnosis of the disease are: malar (butterfly) rash; discoid rash; photosensitivity; oral ulcers; non-erosive arthritis; serositis (pleuritis or pericarditis); renal involvement, with proteinuria or cellular casts; haematological involvement (haemolytic anaemia or leucopenia); central nervous system involvement, with psychosis or epilepsy; immunological disorder (lupus erythematosus test, anti-DNA, or anti-Sm); and positive antinuclear antibody.

The prevalence of systemic lupus erythematosus in the United Kingdom is 1 in 3000, with a female to male ratio of approximately 10:1.[2] The aetiology of this disease is unknown, although it probably represents a combination of genetic and environmental factors (Walport, ClinRheumDis, 1982; 8:3; Kahaleh, ClinExpRheumatol, 1992; 10(Suppl. 7):51).[2] Immune complexes may constitute the major proinflammatory stimulus of systemic lupus erythematosus. Circulating immune complexes are produced by autonomous, polyclonal B-cell activation and persist as a result of failure of the monocyte phagocytic system to clear them.[1] The trigger for the formation of immune complexes is the breakdown of tolerance to autoantigens, possibly as a result of microbial and viral antigenic mimicry, or an abnormality of idiotypic networks.[2]

Liver involvement is frequently reported in patients with systemic lupus erythematosus (see Table 1).

Liver enzyme elevations, usually aminotransferases, occur in 23 to 50 per cent of patients with systemic lupus erythematosus (Miller, QJMed, 1984; 53:401; van Hoek, NethJMed, 1996; 48:244). In clinical practice, haemolysis as a result of this disease may cause an increase in unconjugated bilirubin, and myositis may result in an elevation of serum alanine and aspartate aminotransferases. Alkaline phosphatase is usually not elevated in patients with lupus. Abnormal enzyme values may be related to microthrombi in the livers of patients with antiphospholipid syndrome (Inam, PostgradMedJ, 1991; 67:385). Hepatomegaly has been reported in up to 55 per cent of patients (Cairns, JClinPath, 1996; 49:183; van Hoek, 1996).[3] Fatty change is the most common histological finding (Runyon, AmJMed, 1980; 69:187). Steroid use has been implicated in patients with steatosis, but this condition has been found in patients with lupus who were not using steroids (Atsumu, Lupus, 1995; 43:

2258). Centrilobular necrosis and progressive fibrosis have also been described (Runyon, 1980).

Liver granulomas have been described in patients with lupus (Estes, Medicine, 1971; 50:85; Runyon, AmJMed, 1980; 69:187). Liver vasculitis is very rare but has been reported (Dubois, JAMA, 1964; 190:104), as have hepatic rupture, hepatic infarction, giant cell hepatitis, inflammation of portal tracts, and hepatic amyloidosis (Dohen, JGastro, 1994; 29:3628; Atsumi, Lupus, 1995; 4:225; Garcia Tobaruela, Lupus, 1995; 41:757; van Hoek, NethJMed, 1996; 48:244). In a retrospective analysis, liver disease, not related to any other disease, was described in 43 of 238 patients, and histological examination in 33 of these demonstrated abnormalities which included chronic active hepatitis and cirrhosis; an unusual cholestasis with canalicular casts was seen in 3 of the 4 patients with cirrhosis (Runyon, AmJMed, 1980; 69:187).

Systemic lupus erythematosus has developed in patients with primary biliary cirrhosis (Miller, QJMed, 1984; 53:401; Nachbar, Dermatology, 1994; 188(4):313), and Budd–Chiari syndrome has been described in patients with systemic lupus erythematosus and lupus coagulant (Asherson, JRheum, 1989; 16:219). Sclerosing cholangitis is also rarely associated with systemic lupus erythematosus (Alberti Flor, AmJGastr, 1984; 79:889).

NSAIDs are commonly used in patients with systemic lupus erythematosus and sometimes cause liver damage. Immunosuppressive therapy may result in infections, both systemic and hepatic, and there is also an increased risk of malignancy, which may involve the liver. The incidence of non-Hodgkin's lymphoma is fourfold higher in patients with lupus than in the general population (Abu Shakra, ArthRheum, 1996; 39:1050). It is noteworthy that this study demonstrated that patients with lupus were at lower risk of malignancy than patients with rheumatoid arthritis or systemic sclerosis.

The antiphospholipid antibody syndrome

The antiphospholipid antibody syndrome is characterized by a range of autoantibodies which bind to negatively charged phospholipids (phosphatidylserine and phosphatidylcholine). This syndrome presents clinically with recurrent thromboembolic disease or multiple miscarriages.

Antiphospholipid antibodies occur alone (the primary syndrome) or in combination with other connective tissue diseases or drugs (the secondary syndrome). These antibodies are paticularly common in systemic lupus erythematosus (30 to 50 per cent) and Sjögren's syndrome (Asherson, JRheum, 1986; 13:416; Bowles, RheumDisClinNAm, 1990; 16:471). They may also be found in diverse conditions such as scleroderma, Behçet's disease, psoriatic arthritis, and dermatomyositis. Drugs such as phenytoin, hydralazine, chlorpromazine, and quinidine are responsible for approximately one-tenth of patients with antiphospholipid antibodies.

In clinical practice there are three commonly performed tests which detect antibody against negatively charged phospholipid. These are the lupus anticoagulant test, the cardiolipin antibody test, and the false-positive VDRL test. Although thrombotic complications dominate the clinical presentation, the partial thromboplastin time is characteristically increased. Less than 10 per cent of patients with the primary or secondary antiphospholipid antibody syndromes develop thrombotic complications, probably because of low titres or varying antibody specificities. One group of antiphospholipid antibodies binds to β_2-glycoprotein I, and the presence of these antibodies may predict a worse clinical outcome, particularly in pregnant patients (Harris, Lancet, 1990; 336:1505; Katano, HumRepro, 1996; 11:509; Tsutsumi, ArthRheum, 1996; 39:1466).

Thrombotic complications represent the main clinical manifestation of the antiphospolipid antibody syndrome, and large and small venous or arterial thromboses, usually without inflammation (Bowles, RheumDisClinNAm, 1990; 16:471; Gastineau, AmJHemat, 1995; 19:265), have been reported. Hepatic manifestations include the Budd–Chiari syndrome (Mackworth Young, JHepatol, 1986; 3:83; Van Steenbergen, JHepatol, 1986; 3:87; Asherson, JRheum, 1989; 16:219) and chronic active hepatitis (Saeki, Hepatogast, 1993; 40:499). Inferior vena cava obstruction (Terabayasji, Gastro, 1986; 91:219) and sclerosing cholangitis (Kirby, AmJMed, 1986; 81:1077) have been reported in patients with antiphospholipid antibodies. In a single patient, hepatic microthrombosis, renal thrombosis, and Addison's disease were documented (Inam, PostgradMedJ, 1991; 67:385).

Other manifestations of the antiphospholipid antibody syndrome include: (i) pulmonary thromboembolic disease; (ii) recurrent fetal loss; (iii) cerebral thrombosis, dementia, and epilepsy; (iv) livedo reticularis, digital gangrene, and skin ulcers; (v) heart valve vegetations and valvular insufficiency (Chartash, AmJMed, 1989; 86:407; Beynon, BrHeartJ, 1992; 67:281); and (vi) thrombocytopenia and haemolytic anaemia.

Rheumatoid arthritis

Rheumatoid arthritis is the commonest inflammatory disease of synovial joints, with a prevalence of approximately 1 per cent in the United Kingdom. It is a true multisystem disease, but joint involvement is usually the predominant feature.[4] Although the aetiology is unknown, there is an association with DR3 and DR4 HLA antigens (Bowles, RheumDisClinNAm, 1990; 16:471). It is widely believed that an infectious organism, in a genetically predisposed individual, results in abnormal cytokine and T-cell regulation (Mu, ArthRheum, 1996; 39:931). Inflammation of synovial tissue leads to pannus formation with eventual cartilage and joint destruction. Perivascular T- and B-cell infiltration, as well as immune complex deposition, has been demonstrated in synovial tissue, skin, and rheumatoid nodules (Vollertsen, RheumDisClinNAm, 1990; 16:445), suggesting a vasculitic aetiology in this disease.

Rheumatoid arthritis is a clinical diagnosis, but the revised American Rheumatism Association criteria of 1987 are widely used to establish the diagnosis (Arnett, ArthRheum, 1988; 31:315). The presence of four or more of the following criteria are sufficient to make the diagnosis: (i) morning stiffness (lasting longer than 1 h, for more than 6 weeks); (ii) arthritis of three or more areas (objective swelling for more than 6 weeks); (iii) arthritis of the hand joints; (iv) symmetrical arthritis; (v) rheumatoid nodules; (vi) serum rheumatoid factor (the laboratory method must diagnose this factor in less than 5 per cent of control subjects); and (vii) radiographic changes (anteroposterior wrist and hand radiographs).

Hepatic involvement is a recognized extra-articular complication of rheumatoid arthritis. Biochemical evidence of hepatic dysfunction is often seen in patients with rheumatoid arthritis, and as many as one-half of patients with rheumatoid arthritis have raised alkaline phosphatase levels (Cockel, AnnRheumDis, 1971; 30:166; Webb, AnnRheumDis, 1975; 34:70; Mills, AnnRheumDis, 1982; 41:295). In one series of 98 patients with rheumatoid arthritis, 45 had elevated alkaline phosphatase, 23 elevated γ-glutamyl transferase, and 12 had elevation of both enzymes (Spooner, JClinPath, 1982; 35:638). Isoenzyme analysis showed that in those with elevation of both, alkaline phosphatase derived from the bone in approximately half. One patient in this series had concomitant primary biliary cirrhosis, but overt liver disease was not seen in the rest, despite the enzyme abnormalities. Some authors have proposed that alkaline phosphatase and γ-glutamyl transferase elevations in patients with rheumatoid arthritis correlate with levels of acute-phase proteins and the erythrocyte sedimentation rate (Lowe, AnnRheumDis, 1978; 37:428).

Enzyme elevations in patients with rheumatoid arthritis are not associated with consistent histological changes in the liver. Liver biopsies were performed on 117 unselected patients with rheumatoid arthritis, many of whom had normal liver function tests (Rau, AnnRheumDis, 1975; 34:198). Abnormal hepatic histology was found in 65 per cent, with steatosis present in 22 per cent. Up to 3 per cent of patients with rheumatoid arthritis have hepatic fibrosis before initiation of methotrexate therapy. Patients may have mild inflammatory changes, mainly involving portal tracts, with occasional fat-containing hepatocytes, and scattered foci of liver cell necrosis. Hepatic rupture and intrahepatic haemorrhage have been described in a patient with rheumatoid arthritis (Hocking, ArchIntMed, 1981; 141:792).

Synovial fluid of patients with rheumatoid arthritis was shown to produce interleukins 1 and 6 in sufficient quantities to induce serum amyloid A production by hepatic cells (McNiff, Cytokine, 1995; 7:209). Rheumatoid arthritis is a well-recognized cause of secondary amyloidosis (Pai, ScaJRheum, 1993; 225:2489; al Janadi, ClinImmunPath, 1994; 711:337), in which liver involvement is well described.

Juvenile rheumatoid arthritis

Juvenile rheumatoid arthritis has been documented in children as young as 3 years, although patients are generally older than 10 years. Females are more commonly affected than males. Systemic onset of juvenile chronic rheumatoid arthritis is called Still's disease and is characterized by fever, hepatosplenomegaly, polyserositis, coagulopathy, lymphadenopathy, and rash. This subset of patients with juvenile rheumatoid arthritis may be associated with liver enlargement and aminotransferase elevation (Schaller, JPediat, 1971; 79:139). In patients with hepatic involvement, periportal mononuclear cell infiltration, Kupffer cell hyperplasia, and steatosis are seen. The hepatomegaly and liver cell dysfunction regress during remission of the systemic disease. Focal hepatic lesions have also been seen in patients with juvenile rheumatoid arthritis (Agarwal, JRheum, 1994; 213:5801), as well as a macrophage-activation syndrome associated with hepatosplenomegaly and bone marrow infiltration (Stephan, ClinExpRheumatol, 1993; 114:4516). Adult-onset Still's disease may also be associated with hepatomegaly and abnormal aminotransferase elevation (Larson, Medicine, 1984; 63: 82).

Treatment of young patients with NSAIDs may also cause liver dysfunction, although children may be more resistant to aspirin-induced hepatotoxicity than adults (Fry, GastrClinNAm, 1995; 24: 875). The use of methotrexate in children with juvenile rheumatoid arthritis, at doses of 10 to 15 mg/week, has been shown to be at least as safe as in adults and may become the treatment of choice in children with this disease (Giannini, DrugSafety, 1993; 95:32539).

Felty's syndrome

Felty's syndrome is characterized by the triad of rheumatoid arthritis, leucopenia, and splenomegaly. Severe joint disease and extra-articular features may be seen (Sienknecht, AnnRheumDis, 1977; 36:500). An association between Felty's syndrome, nodular regenerative hyperplasia, and portal hypertension has been described (Blendis, AnnRheumDis, 1978; 37:183). Nodular regenerative hyperplasia is a diffuse hepatic regenerative process and differs from cirrhosis by not having fibrous septa (Dachman, AJR, 1987; 148: 717). Conditions such as partial nodular transformation, focal nodular hyperplasia, and hepatocellular adenomatosis (usually seen in young women taking oral contraceptives) must be differentiated from nodular regenerative hyperplasia (Sherlock, AmJMed, 1966; 40:195; Evans, BrJSurg, 1980; 67:175). In one study, 12 of 18 patients with Felty's syndrome had abnormal liver findings, 5 with nodular regenerative hyperplasia and 7 with portal fibrosis or abnormal lobular architecture (Thorne, AmJMed, 1982; 73:35). One-third of the 12 had portal hypertension, which caused bleeding in a significant number. Only 7 of the 12 with abnormal histology had abnormal biochemistry, suggesting that in patients with Felty's syndrome, portal hypertension and oesophageal varices should be excluded even if liver function tests are normal.

Mixed connective tissue disease

Mixed connective tissue disease is characterized by the overlap of the clinical features of systemic lupus erythematosus, progressive systemic sclerosis, Sjögren's syndrome, and polymyositis. High levels of antibody to RNP (ribonucleoprotein of extractable nuclear antigen) are invariably found. Raynaud's phenomenon, dactylitis (sausage fingers), and pulmonary hypertension are frequently found. Renal disease is not usually prominent, and if present is responsive to steroid therapy.

Hepatomegaly has been described, but serious liver disturbance is rare. Of 61 patients with mixed connective tissue disease, only 4 had evidence of liver disease (Marshall, ArchIntMed, 1983; 143: 1817). Chronic active hepatitis and cirrhosis was documented in one patient, steatosis in another, and the remaining two patients had liver congestion secondary to pulmonary hypertension. The presence of autoimmune hepatitis in patients with mixed connective tissue disease should be suspected if anti-smooth muscle antibodies are found, and occasional associations with Budd–Chiari syndrome, thyroiditis, or Sjögren's syndrome have been documented (Maeda, DigDisSci, 1988; 33:1487; Wada, JpnJMed, 1991; 30:278; Tomsic, AnnRheumDis, 1992; 51:544).

Sjögren's syndrome

Sjögren's syndrome is a chronic autoimmune disease of unknown aetiology, which is characterized by lymphocytic infiltration and destruction of epithelial exocrine glands.[1] The Epstein–Barr virus as well as human retroviruses have been implicated in the pathogenesis of Sjögrens syndrome (Fox, JImmunol, 1986; 137:3162; Miyasaka, ScaJRheum, 1986; 61(Suppl.):123). Primary Sjögren's syndrome has an incidence of 1 in 2500 and is more commonly seen in women over 50 years of age. Objective demonstration of dry eyes (Schirmer's test), dry mouth (parotid flow rate), and lymphocytic salivary gland infiltrate are required to make the diagnosis in addition to abnormal autoantibodies. Both antinuclear and rheumatoid factor (IgM anti-IgG) antibodies may be present in titres exceeding 1/320. The most specific antibodies are anti-SS A (Ro) and anti-SS B (La), but these are also seen in systemic lupus erythematosus. Secondary Sjögren's syndrome is more common than the primary syndrome and is found in association with rheumatoid arthritis (20 per cent) and systemic lupus erythematosus (30 per cent), as well as progressive systemic sclerosis.

The following are clinical features of Sjögren's syndrome: (i) xerostomia, keratoconjuctivitis sicca, salivary gland enlargement; (ii) bronchitis, interstitial lung fibrosis, lymphocytic interstitial pneumonitis (Ferreiro, AmJMed, 1987; 82:1227), mucus inspissation, infection, pleuropericarditis, nasal and upper airway dryness in 50 per cent; (iii) arthritis, Raynaud's phenomenon; (iv) lymphadenopathy, splenomegaly; (v) renal tubular acidosis, interstitial nephritis, glomerulonephritis; and (vi) hepatitis, (vii) myositis, (viii) neuropathy, (ix) B-cell lymphoma.

Hepatomegaly has been documented in 25 per cent of patients, and alkaline phosphatase levels may also be elevated in 25 per cent of patients with Sjögren's syndrome; antimitochondrial antibody is found in approximately 10 per cent of patients (Whaley, QJMed, 1973; 42:513; Webb, AnnRheumDis, 1975; 34:70), and lymphocytic infiltration of the liver may be seen. Sjögren's syndrome is common in patients with chronic liver disease and may accompany chronic active hepatitis (35 per cent) or cryptogenic cirrhosis (24 per cent) (Golding, AmJMed, 1973; 55:772).

Acute cholecystitis has been described in conjunction with Sjögren's syndrome, but the association is probably coincidental. A patient with primary biliary cirrhosis, CREST, and Sjögren's syndrome has been described (Ito, IntMed, 1995; 34:451). Sjögren's syndrome may be found in patients with sclerosing cholangitis, mixed connective tissue disease, or primary biliary cirrhosis (Montefusco, AmJSurg, 1984; 147:822; Rutan, Gastro, 1986; 90:206; Wada, JpnJMed, 1991; 30:278; Skopouli, BrJRheum, 1994; 33:745).

Primary Sjögren's syndrome may be associated with vasculitis, particularly of the central nervous system (Fox, JImmunol, 1986; 137:3162), but hepatic involvement has been documented. Secondary Sjögren's syndrome is associated with all the vasculitic and pulmonary complications of the primary connective tissue disease.

Corticosteroids should only be used in patients with primary Sjögren's syndrome in the face of visceral organ involvement and vasculitis. Local therapy should be used for mouth dryness and keratoconjuctivitis sicca.

Systemic sclerosis

Systemic sclerosis is a mulitsystem connective tissue disease of unknown origin, which is commoner in women than in men (Tamaki, ArchDermRes, 1991; 283:366). It is characterized pathologically by the overproduction of connective tissue and collagen.

Patients may present with widespread vascular damage and microvascular obliteration.

Clinically, there is a disease spectrum ranging from limited systemic sclerosis with skin thickening of the face, arms below the elbow, and legs below the knee, to diffuse systemic sclerosis with widespread skin thickening. The rare syndrome of systemic sclerosis without scleroderma is characterized by typical internal organ involvement without the skin thickening. Anticentromere antibodies are found in up to 70 per cent of patients with limited systemic sclerosis, and antitopoisomerase antibodies in as many as 40 per cent of patients with diffuse systemic sclerosis (Tamaki, ArchDermRes, 1991; 283:366; Isenberg, BMJ, 1995; 310:795). Although the aetiology is unknown and the pathogenesis remains uncertain, there is evidence that vascular and endothelial cell activation play an important role in fibroblast activation (Denton, BrJRheum, 1995; 34:1048).

The association between systemic sclerosis, both limited and diffuse, and primary biliary cirrhosis has been well documented (Murray Lyon, BMJ, 1970; i:258; Reynolds, AmJMed, 1971; 50:302; O'Brien, Gastro, 1972; 62:118). Only 3 to 4 per cent of patients with systemic sclerosis also have primary biliary cirrhosis, and systemic sclerosis usually precedes the latter. The presence of antimitochondrial antibodies in patients with systemic sclerosis should alert the clinician to the possibility of primary biliary cirrhosis. Antimitochondrial antibodies may be found in approximately one-third of patients with systemic sclerosis. Hepatic fibrosis may also occur in patients with systemic sclerosis (Gruschwitz, Hautarzt, 1994; 4511:78791).

Eosinophilic fasciitis

Eosinophilic fasciitis is an uncommon disease, which may be confused with scleroderma. Symmetrical swelling and induration of the distal parts of the limbs occurs; the hands, feet, and trunk are involved less frequently, and eosinophilia is found in 90 per cent of cases. Antinuclear antibodies and thyroiditis are sometimes associated, and rare patients with granulomatous or a reactive hepatitis have been described (Jacobs, ArchIntMed, 1985; 145:162; Loeliger, ClinRheum, 1991; 10:440; Siberry, ArchDermatol, 1994; 130:884).

Dermatomyositis/polymyositis

Liver involvement is rarely found in patients with poly/dermatomyositis. Muscle involvement may result in enzyme elevations, which can mistakenly be attributed to the liver. Chronic active hepatitis, biliary cirrhosis, peliosis hepatitis, and Wilson's disease have been described in these patients (Buonanno, PoliclinicoSezMed, 1969; 76:117; Lorcerie, RevMedInt, 1990; 11:25; el Alaoui Faris, RevNeurol, 1994; 150:391). Primary or metastatic liver disease may result in dermatomyositis (Allan, Gastro, 1972; 62:1227; Leaute, NEJM, 1995; 333:1083).

Vasculitides and liver disease

Wegener's granulomatosis, microscopic polyangiitis, polyarteritis nodosa, and Churg–Strauss syndrome

Systemic vasculitis may be defined as an inflammatory disorder of the blood vessels, which usually results in necrosis of the vessel wall with subsequent vascular occlusion. There are a group of diseases such as Wegener's granulomatosis and polyarteritis nodosa in which vasculitis appears to represent the primary pathology. There can be no definitive classification of vasculitis as long as the aetiology and pathogenesis of the condition remain unknown in most cases. Even when vasculitis has been associated with a specific infection such as hepatitis B virus, the clinical features and pathology may be diverse, ranging from polyarteritis nodosa to localized vasculitic lesions affecting the skin and kidneys.

Wegener's granulomatosis and microscopic polyarteritis form part of the spectrum of primary systemic vasculitides. Both principally affect small blood vessels and lead to focal necrotizing glomerulonephritis. The pathological changes are similar in both conditions, with a leucocytoclastic vasculitis and fibrinoid necrosis of small muscular arteries, although the presence of granulomas is a feature of Wegener's granulomatosis and not microscopic polyarteritis. The clinical syndromes are also similar, and both may present with pulmonary–renal syndromes although destructive lesions of the upper and lower respiratory tracts are specifically found in Wegener's granulomatosis (Fauci, AnnIntMed, 1983; 98:76).

The utilization of antineutrophil cytoplasmic antibodies (ANCA) has contributed to the serological diagnosis of Wegener's granulomatosis and microscopic polyarteritis. Two main types of ANCA have been identified: antiproteinase 3 and antimyeloperoxidase, which correspond to cANCA and pANCA, respectively. Surprisingly, patients with cANCA do not have pANCA, and vice versa (Niles, AnnRevMed, 1996; 47:303). Although exceptions to the rule occur, cANCA are more typical of Wegener's granulomatosis, and pANCA or cANCA may be found in microscopic polyarteritis (Niles, 1996; Penas, BrJDermatol, 1996; 134:542).

Churg–Strauss syndrome is a systemic necrotizing granulomatous vasculitis, predominantly affecting medium-sized vessels, and is diagnosed in individuals with asthma, eosinophilia of more than 1500/mm^3, and vasculitis of two or more extrapulmonary sites (Lanham, Medicine, 1984; 63:65). Pulmonary infiltrates are characteristic, and although nasal polyps may occur, nasal cartilage involvement, sinusitis, and otitis are rare (Chumbley, MayoClinProc, 1977; 52:477). Although rare, ANCA antibodies have been documented in a patient with Churg–Strauss syndrome (Nakagawa, NipponKyobuShikkanGakkaiZasshi, 1995; 33:543).

Polyarteritis nodosa is a systemic, non-granulomatous vasculitis, affecting medium-sized and small arteries. Clinically, it may be difficult to distinguish from microscopic polyarteritis, and in the past these two diseases were considered together. Hepatitis B virus infection is found in 10 to 20 per cent of patients. Liver involvement is common; cirrhosis, acute and chronic hepatitis, hepatic infarction, and hepatic arteriole involvement have been documented (Duffy, Medicine, 1976; 55:19; Cowan, PostgradMedJ, 1977; 53:89). Rupture of intra- or extrahepatic arterial aneurysms may occur. Hepatomegaly may be seen in 20 per cent of patients, but bilirubin and liver enzyme elevations are documented in approximately 10 per cent. Acute cholecystitis may be the presenting manifestation of polyarteritis nodosa (LiVolsi, Gastro, 1973; 65:115). Patients with hepatitis B-associated polyarteritis nodosa may deteriorate during treatment with immunosuppressive agents such as steroids and cyclophosphamide. In these patients, initial brief steroid therapy may be used to control the serious complications of polyarteritis

nodosa, followed by plasma exchange and antiviral therapy (interferon or vidarabine) (Guillevin, CurrOpinRheum, 1997; 9:31).

Vasculitides may involve a variety of organs, and abnormal liver function tests have been described in all types of primary vasculitic syndromes (Camilleri, QJMed, 1983; 52:141; Gambari, ScaJRheum, 1989; 18:171; Yoshimoto, NipponKyobuShikkanGakkaiZasshi, 1989; 27:1545).

In general, combination therapy with prednisolone and cyclophosphamide, or prednisolone and methotrexate, is used to induce remission in the primary systemic vasculitides. Azathioprine is widely used as a steroid-sparing agent for maintenance therapy.

Behçet's disease

Behçet's disease is a systemic vasculitis, which occurs predominantly in young men. The aetiology of this disease is unknown. The diagnosis is confirmed by the presence of recurrent oral ulceration with two out of the following four other criteria: recurrent genital ulceration, typical eye lesions (uveitis or iridocyclitis), typical skin lesions (erythema nodosum, skin ulcers), or a positive pathergy test. Other systems such as the lungs, gastrointestinal tract, joints, and veins may be involved.

A necrotizing vasculitis involving arteries, arterioles, and veins is found (O'Duffy, RheumDisClinNAm, 1990; 15:423). Thrombosis is initiated by inflammation of veins, and Behçet's disease may be a more important cause of venous occlusion than systemic lupus erythematosus (O'Duffy, 1990). Vena caval obstruction as well as Budd–Chiari syndrome have been documented (Kansu, QJMed, 1972; 41:151).

Polymyalgia rheumatica and giant cell arteritis

Polymyalgia rheumatica is relatively common with a reported prevalence of 500 per 100 000 in the population over 50 years old (Chuang, AnnIntMed, 1982; 97:672). The disease has the following characteristics (Cohen, RheumDisClinNAm, 1990; 16:325): (i) patients are usually more than 50 years old; (ii) pain or stiffness of shoulder, hip, or neck; (iii) erythrocyte sedimentation rate of more than 40 mm/h; (iv) rapid response to relatively low-steroid dose (15 mg/day); and (v) exclusion of other connective tissue or primary muscle diseases.

Giant cell arteritis is a vasculitic disease, predominantly affecting branches of the carotid artery, in particular the temporal artery. Peripheral arteries may be involved in 10 per cent of patients (Klein, AnnIntMed, 1975; 83:806). The prevalence is 223 per 100 000 in patients older than 50 years (Machado, ArthRheum, 1988; 31:745). Headache, temporal artery tenderness of tortuosity, and jaw claudication are common and specific findings. Constitutional symptoms are present in one-half of patients, and optical and neurological symptoms are present in one-third (Hunder, RheumDisClinNAm, 1990; 16:399; Machado, 1988).

Polymyalgia rheumatica and giant cell arteritis are often associated (Bruckle, ZRheumatol, 1989; 48:1). Patients with giant cell arteritis have polymyalgic symptoms in approximately 50 per cent of cases. The prevalence of giant cell arteritis in patients with polymyalgia rheumatica is lower, and probably occurs in 15 per cent of unselected patients (Chuang, AnnIntMed, 1982; 97:672).

The incidence of liver abnormalities in patients with polymyalgia rheumatica or giant cell arteritis is 40 to 60 per cent (Wadman, ActaMedScand, 1972; 192:377). Alkaline phosphatase or aminotransferase levels may be elevated in approximately 50 per cent of patients (Hall, Lancet, 1972; ii:48). Enzyme levels may return to normal when the disease is treated with steroids. Liver biopsy is usually non-specific, but steatosis, hepatic granulomas, and portal tract inflammation have been seen (Long, Lancet, 1974; i:77). Cholestasic liver disease has been documented in patients with giant cell arteritis (Ilan, ClinRheum, 1993; 12:219; Achar, PostgradMedJ, 1995; 71:59). Arteritis of hepatic arterioles and arterioli, and granulomatous hepatitis have been documented in patients with giant cell arteritis (de Bayser, Gastro, 1993; 105:272). The correlation between abnormal liver histology and biochemical tests is poor.

References

1. Beynon HL, Athanassiou P, and Davies KA. Role of the endothelium in systemic lupus erythematosus and Sjögren's syndrome. In Savage COS and Pearson JD, eds. *Immunological aspects of the vascular endothelium*. Cambridge: Cambridge University Press, 1995: 124–52.
2. Walport MJ. Systemic lupus erythematosus. In Lachman PJ, Peters DK, Rosen FS, and Walport MJ, eds. *Clinical aspects of immunology*, 5th edn. Boston: Blackwell Scientific Publishers, 1993: 1161–204.
3. Rothfield NF. Systemic lupus erythematosus. Katz WA, ed. *Rheumatic Diseases: diagnosis and management*. Philadelphia: JB Lippincott Co, 1977: 765.
4. Wolheim FA. Rheumatoid arthritis, the clinical picture. In Maddison PJ, Isenberg DA, Woo P, and Glass DN, eds. *Oxford textbook of rheumatology*. Oxford: Oxford Medical Publications, 1993: 639–66.

25

The effect of liver disease on other systems

25.1 The effect of liver disease on the cardiovascular system, lungs, and pulmonary vasculature

Peter Collins, Jean-Pierre Benhamou, and Neil McIntyre

Cardiovascular system

Liver disease can have profound effects on the cardiovascular system. Cirrhotics tend to have a high cardiac output, unduly large in relation to oxygen consumption, and a low peripheral resistance; this hyperkinetic state may also occur with obstructive jaundice. Most cirrhotics also have an increased plasma volume, even when there is no obvious fluid retention. Left ventricular function may be impaired, particularly in patients with ascites.

The hyperkinetic syndrome in cirrhosis (see also Section 9)

Cirrhosis, of varying aetiologies, is associated with a hyperdynamic circulatory state[1,2] (Siegel, ArchSurg, 1974; 108:282; Groszmann, Hepatol, 1994; 20:1359), and there is often clear clinical evidence of increased peripheral blood flow. The hyperdynamic state is more obvious with recumbency, suggesting translocation of excessive blood volume from the peripheral to the central circulation (Bernardi, JHepatol, 1995; 22:1205).

The hyperdynamic circulatory state is more pronounced the greater the degree of hepatic decompensation; as liver function and clinical status improve the cardiac output falls. Multivariate analysis revealed that changes in cardiac output and systemic vascular resistance were significantly and independently correlated with changes in serum albumin and bilirubin, plasma prothrombin and gastrointestinal bleeding (Valla, GastrClinBiol, 1984; 8:321). No relationship was found between the hyperkinetic syndrome and the hepatic venous pressure or the presence of ascites. Valla *et al.* concluded that liver failure is partly responsible for the hyperkinetic state of cirrhosis, but that portal hypertension *per se* might also play a role (Lebrec, Hepatol, 1983; 3:550). The magnitude of the haemodynamic changes in the hyperkinetic state also correlates with the severity of cirrhosis as assessed by a modified Pugh's classification (Braillon, Gut, 1986; 27:1204; Meng, JGastHepatol, 1994; 9:148).

Studies on the coronary (Zobl, Circul, 1962; 26:808), cerebral (Posner, JCI, 1960; 39:1246), and renal (Lancestremere, JCI, 1962; 41:1922) circulations in cirrhotic patients suggested that blood flow through these regional beds was either normal or decreased. Middle cerebral artery flow velocity was decreased in patients in Child's groups B and C who had no clinical evidence of encephalopathy (Dillon, EurJGastroHepatol, 1995; 7:1087).

When blood flow to the hand and forearm was measured by venous occlusion plethysmography, and forearm muscle blood flow by arteriovenous differences and forearm muscle temperature,[2] cirrhotic patients with high cardiac indices were found to have an increased blood flow to the hand and forearm. It was suggested that flow to both skin and skeletal muscle was increased, but direct measurement of forearm skeletal muscle blood flow (by clearance of xenon-133) revealed no difference between cirrhotics and controls (Lunzer, Gut, 1973; 14:354). Peripheral vasodilatation may therefore be entirely cutaneous in origin. Fernandez-Seara *et al.* (Gastro, 1989; 97:1304) reported an increased blood flow to the legs in cirrhotics. Others found a higher than normal peripheral blood flow and deep body temperature, and a lower vascular resistance, in the forearm of cirrhotics, but these differences were not found in the calves (Okumura, ScaJGastr, 1990; 25:883). This regional difference in blood flow in cirrhotics may be due partly to impaired sympathetic activity, and might be linked to the distribution of spider naevi and the presence of palmar erythema.

Although they have a high peripheral flow, cirrhotics show a reduced flow of portal blood through the liver,[3] as scarring and distortion of the liver increase hepatic vascular resistance, causing a rise in portal venous pressure. This does not necessarily imply a low total splanchnic portal venous flow, as portal blood can also return to the heart via the collaterals which develop in portal hypertension. Indeed, the splanchnic circulation is the major site of peripheral arteriolar dilatation in studies on animals with portal hypertension (Cohn, AmJMed, 1972; 53:704; Groszmann, AmJMed, 1972; 53:715; Kotelanski, Gastro, 1972; 63:102; Vorobioff, Gastro, 1984; 87:1120), mesenteric flow increasing with chronic portal hypertension (Blanchet, EurJClinInv, 1982; 12:327; Vorobioff, AmJPhysiol, 1983; 244:G52). Furthermore, studies in man suggest that a hyperdynamic splanchnic circulation is a major factor determining the development and severity of portal hypertension (Sabba, Hepatol, 1991; 13:714; Groszmann, Hepatol, 1994; 20: 1359).

Pathophysiology of the hyperkinetic state in cirrhosis

The cause(s) of the haemodynamic changes of cirrhosis is far from clear. Many have studied sympathetic activity, and the role of noradrenaline and other vasoactive substances of endogenous origin. Sympathetic nervous system activity is increased in cirrhosis (Ring-Larsen, Hepatol, 1982; 2:304) as evidenced by an increased plasma noradrenaline. However, patients without ascites showed normal plasma noradrenaline levels (Henriksen, Gut, 1984; 25:1034); unfortunately most of the work in this field has been done on patients with ascites as well as a hyperdynamic syndrome.

Plasma levels of renin and angiotensin also increase in cirrhotics with ascites but the peripheral vascular response to these substances, and to noradrenaline, seems to be impaired in cirrhotics. In alcoholic cirrhotics the peripheral vascular response to infused noradrenaline was impaired compared with that of normal controls (Lunzer, Lancet, 1975; ii:382). With head-up tilting the arterial pressure was lower in cirrhotics than in controls, despite higher plasma noradrenaline and renin activity (Bernardi, Digestion, 1982; 25:124); similar results were obtained by this group with exercise (Bernardi, JHepatol, 1991; 12:207).

Resistance to the pressor effect of angiotensin II has also been observed in cirrhosis (Laragh, JCI, 1963; 42:1179), and in dogs following bile duct ligation (Finberg, ClinSci, 1981; 61:535). From studies on rats with carbon tetrachloride-induced cirrhosis it was concluded that the decreased pressor response to angiotensin II resulted from a postreceptor defect in angiotensin action (Murray, CircRes, 1985; 57:424).

The impairment of cardiovascular reactivity to sympathetic drive, and to renin and angiotensin, is clearly one factor that might help to explain the hyperdynamic circulation of cirrhotics.

Many other endogenous compounds have been incriminated as causes of the hyperdynamic circulation (Abelmann, Hepatol, 1994; 20:1356), including prostacyclins (Sitzmann, AnnSurg, 1989; 209:322), vasoactive intestinal polypeptide (Hunt, ArchIntMed, 1970; 139:994) and glucagon (Benoit, AmJPhysiol, 1984; 247:G486; Yonekawa, NipponGekaGakkaiZass, 1986; 87:781), false neurotransmitters (Mespoli, ArchSurg, 1981; 116:1129), and substance P (Hortnagl, Lancet, 1984; i:480).

Recently major emphasis has been placed on the role of the vascular-endothelium-derived vasodilator, nitric oxide (NO). In 1991 Vallance and Moncada (Lancet, 1991; 337:776) suggested that increased synthesis and release of NO, induced directly by endotoxin or indirectly by cytokines, could explain peripheral vasodilatation in cirrhosis. Subsequently Vallance and his colleagues (Calver, ClinSci, 1994; 86:303) found that the response to local inhibition of NO synthesis in the forearm arterial bed was no different in cirrhotics and controls; they concluded that increased production of NO by the induction of NO synthase was unlikely to account fully for the vasodilatation seen in mild to moderate alcoholic cirrhotics. However, it was found that the infusion of L-NMMA, an inhibitor of NO synthase, caused a greater reduction in forearm blood flow and a bigger increase in vascular resistance in decompensated than in compensated cirrhotics (Campillo, Hepatol, 1995; 22:1423). An increased NO content of expired air in Child–Pugh class C cirrhotics showed a significant negative correlation with pulmonary vascular resistance but not with systemic vascular resistance (Sogni, JHepatol, 1995; 23:471). The NO hypothesis has been reviewed by Bomzon and Blendis (Hepatol, 1994; 20:1343) and by Sogni et al. (JHepatol, 1995; 23:218). It was felt that the NO hypothesis cannot at present explain all of the features of the hyperdynamic circulation of patients with cirrhosis.

Cardiovascular function in obstructive jaundice

Some patients with obstructive jaundice have a hyperkinetic circulation similar to that found in cirrhotic patients (Saito, NipponGekaGakkaiZass, 1981; 82:483); dogs with experimental obstructive jaundice had a tendency to hypotension, a diminished peripheral resistance, and an increased cardiac output (Shasha, ClinSci, 1976; 50:533). The mechanisms are unclear. There appears to be a blunted response to vasoactive agents, such as intravenous angiotensin II and noradrenaline, in conscious, bile duct ligated dogs (Finberg, ClinSci 1981; 61:535; Bonzon, Hepatol, 1984; 4:1093). There is also, from 4 weeks after obstruction, a blunted renal response to volume expansion with saline and an associated reduction in renal blood flow. Jaundice may therefore induce a state in which the cardiovascular system cannot respond appropriately, probably due to an impairment of the contractile response of cardiac and vascular smooth muscle to sympathetic stimulation (Bonzon, IsrJMedSci, 1986; 22:81).

Plasma volume in cirrhosis of the liver (see Section 9)

The plasma volume tends to be elevated in cirrhosis (Bateman, JCI, 1949; 28:539; Dykes, QJMed, 1961; 30:297) even if there is no obvious fluid retention as oedema or ascites. It has been argued that, in patients with ascites, renal sodium retention is a response to hypovolaemia resulting from leakage of plasma into the ascitic fluid (Gabuzda, JCI, 1954; 33:780; Sherlock, Gut, 1963; 4:95). However, the plasma volume, measured with [^{131}I]albumin and ^{51}Cr-labelled erythrocytes, was elevated in all groups of cirrhotics, including patients with ascites, functional renal failure, and portacaval anastomoses (Lieberman, JCI, 1967; 46:1297). The increased plasma volume may be due partly to splanchnic venous congestion, as it correlates with the wedged hepatic venous pressure, but the plasma volume remained high after portacaval shunting (Lieberman, JCI, 1967; 46:1297) and normal values for plasma volume have been found in portal hypertension due to an extrahepatic obstruction.[1]

Cirrhotic cardiomyopathy[4]

Clinical signs of heart failure are uncommon in cirrhotics without another cause of heart disease, perhaps because their marked peripheral vasodilatation reduces ventricular afterload.[4] However, some of the 14 cirrhotics described by Murray et al.[1] showed radiological evidence of ventricular enlargement, and/or ECG evidence of left venticular enlargement; two had a severe cardiomyopathy and one died of heart failure. Furthermore, some cases of overt heart failure have now been described in cirrhotics after liver transplantation, transjugular intrahepatic portosystemic stent shunt (**TIPSS**) and surgical portacaval shunting.[4] It has been known for some time that alcoholic cirrhotics may show a blunted ventricular response to physiological or pharmacological stress. This also appears to be true for non-alcoholic cirrhotics.

Gould *et al.* (JCI, 1969; 48:860) found that while left ventricular diastolic pressure and pulmonary artery pressure increased with exercise in alcoholic cirrhotics, the mean stroke index showed little change; it decreased in some patients—a highly abnormal response under the circumstances. In a later study on physical work capacity there were no significant differences between biopsy-proven alcoholic cirrhotics (abstinent at the time) and controls, in terms of systolic time intervals, echocardiographic indices, and resting left ventricular ejection fraction (Kelbaek, AmJCard, 1984; 54:852). However, on exercise, ventricular wall compliance was reduced and left ventricular ejection fraction was lower in the cirrhotics, suggesting a latent left ventricular impairment that manifests itself with physical exertion.

The ratio pre-ejection period : left ventricular ejection time increases in patients with cardiomyopathy; it was found to be higher than normal in cirrhotics (Bernardi, Hepatol, 1991; 12:207), and impairment of cardiovascular function correlated with the severity of the cirrhosis. Recently, exercise capacity was found to be reduced in cirrhotics; with exercise the peak heart rate was lower than in controls and the left ventricular ejection fraction did not increase, an increase in stroke volume being accompanied by an increase in end-diastolic volume (Grose, JHepatol, 1995; 22:326). At maximal exercise, cardiac output was subnormal in cirrhotics, as it increased by only 97 per cent while there was an increase of 300 per cent in healthy subjects: most of the patients showed autonomic reflex abnormalities.

The situation is more complicated in cirrhotics with ascites. After paracentesis their cardiac output may increase (Knauer, NEJM, 1967; 276:491) or stay the same (Kowalski, JCI, 1953; 32: 1025). If there is gross ascites and a high intra-abdominal pressure, paracentesis increases cardiac output, stroke volume, ventricular stroke work (right and left), and the mean rate of systolic ejection (Guazzi, AmJMed, 1975; 59:165); the fall in intra-abdominal and right atrial pressures correlates with the amount of fluid removed, and there is a direct relationship between the normalization of right atrial pressure and improvement of cardiac function. Paracentesis caused a fall in right atrial pressure in another study (Panos, Hepatol, 1990; 4:662); there was an initial increase in cardiac output without change in pulmonary capillary wedge pressure. From 3 to 12 h the cardiac output and wedge pressure fell, indicating a need for therapeutic plasma expansion. Ascites also appeared to cause compression of the right atrium; the ratio of right atrial size to left atrial size (measured by two-dimensional echocardiography) was significantly lower in patients with ascites, the ratio increasing following paracentesis.

The mechanism by which cardiac output increases after paracentesis is unclear. A mechanical effect seems plausible. Tense ascites increases intra-abdominal pressure, causing diaphragmatic elevation and less diaphragmatic descent on inspiration; both factors raise intrapleural pressure and so reduce effective cardiac filling pressure. Removal of ascites would augment filling of the cardiac chambers, increase venous return, and, by Starling's mechanism, increase stroke volume.

Ascites with cirrhosis may also be associated with pericardial effusion. Of 27 patients studied by echocardiography, 63 per cent had a pericardial effusion, 27 per cent showed impaired left ventricular function, while in 30 per cent there was abnormal systolic motion of the mitral valve and/or septum which became normal with resolution of the ascites (Shah, ArchIntMed, 1988; 148:585).

When angiotensin was infused in alcoholic cirrhotics in order to bring their low peripheral resistance back to the normal range, the cardiac output did not change despite a marked increase in the pulmonary wedge pressure; this failure of the cardiac output to rise with an increase in the left ventricular filling pressure was clearly an abnormal response (Limas, Circul, 1974: 49:755).

Both the inotropic (contractile force) and chronotropic (heart rate) responses of the heart to β-adrenergic agonists are impaired in patients with cirrhosis. In one study, cirrhotics showed only a non-significant increase in stroke volume with infusion of dobutamine (Mikulic, ClinPharmTher, 1983; 34:56). Another group found that the dose of isoproterenol required to increase the heart rate by 25 beats/min was three times higher in cirrhotics than in controls (Ramond, BrJClinPharm, 1986; 21:191). These results are analogous to the impaired peripheral vascular responses of cirrhotics to an increase in sympathetic drive or the infusion of noradrenaline (see above). There have been similar findings in animal studies (Lee, Hepatol, 1990; 12:481).[4]

The above points strongly suggest that the heart is abnormal in many patients with cirrhosis—that there is a 'cirrhotic cardiomyopathy'. As early as 1949, histological abnormalities were found in the hearts of cirrhotics at autopsy (Spatt, AnnIntMed, 1949; 31: 479), and were confirmed in later studies (Hall, AmJPathol, 1953; 29:993; Loyke, AmJMedSci, 1955; 230:627; Lunseth, ArchIntMed, 1958; 102:405). But most of the patients were alcoholic cirrhotics and the histological changes might have been due to alcohol rather than cirrhosis *per se*; this has been a problem in the interpretation of abnormalities of cardiac function during life. Studies in chronic alcoholics showed prolonged systolic time intervals but some were still drinking and the results may have been due to the acute effects of alcohol (Spodick, NEJM, 1972; 287:677; Levi, BrHeartJ, 1977; 39:35; Askanas, AmHeartJ, 1980; 99:9). Alcohol itself affects ventricular function and left atrial size, as shown by echocardiography (Kino, BrHeartJ, 1968; 37:149; Matthews, AmJCard, 1981; 47:520); after prolonged abstinence no deterioration of cardiac function was found in one study (Reeves, AmHeartJ, 1978; 95:578).

Ma and Lee[4] suggested that the mechanisms that cause 'cirrhotic cardiomyopathy' are quite different from those underlying alcoholic heart muscle disease; the latter may be due to impairment of contractile protein synthesis or the production of protein–acetaldehyde adducts in cardiac muscle cells (Preedy, AlcAlc, 1994; 29:141; Harcombe, ClinSci, 1995; 88:263). They pointed out[4] that cardiac β-adrenergic receptors and their postreceptor signal transduction pathway play a key role in modulating myocardial contractile function. Brodde *et al.* (Science, 1986; 231:1584) removed atrial tissue at open heart surgery and found that both cardiac contractility and the β-adrenergic receptor density in the atria correlated positively with β-adrenergic receptor density in circulating lymphocytes from the same patients; they suggested that lymphocytes may be a surrogate for studying receptor density in other tissues of interest. Soon afterwards it was found that β-adrenergic receptor density was reduced in lymphocytes from decompensated cirrhotics (Gerbes, Lancet, 1986; i:1584).

Unfortunately, because of the difficulty in obtaining heart muscle from living humans, most of the studies in this area have been done on animals. In rats with biliary cirrhosis, cardiomyocyte plasma membrane β-adrenoceptor density was reduced without change in receptor binding affinity (Ma, AmJPhysiol, 1994; 267:G87); this may also be true in the carbon tetrachloride-induced rat model of cirrhosis (Zavecz, FASEBJ, 1994; 8:870A). β-Adrenoceptor function may also be desensitized *in vivo* (Lee, Hepatol, 1990; 20:481), due in part to sustained high levels of blood noradrenaline in decompensated cirrhotics[4]; other factors are probably involved in cirrhotic cardiomyopathy as cAMP production is not only impaired at the receptor level, but also at the G-protein and adenyl cyclase levels (Ma, Gastro, 1996; 110:1191).

The β-adrenoreceptors and G-proteins are surrounded by the plasma membrane; changes in its physico-chemical properties would almost certainly affect the functioning of these membrane proteins (see Chapter 2.12). Myocardial plasma membrane fluidity has been shown to affect β-adrenoceptor function in rat heart. The less fluid plasma membrane from the hearts of cirrhotic rats showed a 40 per cent decrease in isoproterenol-stimulated cAMP production; incubation with a fatty acid analogue, which restored fluidity to normal values, also brought isoproterenol-stimulated cAMP production back to values seen in control membranes (Ma, AmJPhysiol, 1994; 267:G87).

The concept of a 'cirrhotic cardiomyopathy' is a relatively new one. It deserves further study.

The heart in Wilson's disease

The heart disease of haemochromatosis is well documented (see Chapter 20.2). Little attention has been paid to the heart in Wilson's disease. Scheinberg and Sternlieb[8] found the heart to be hypertrophied in five out of nine patients with Wilson's disease; on histological examination interstitial fibrosis and varying degrees of sclerosis of intramyocardial small vessels were found in all nine patients; interstitial or perivascular myocarditis was found in seven. One patient died, 'almost certainly because of a cardiac arrhythmia', but this was thought to be unrelated to his Wilson's disease. There seemed to be no evidence that the pathological changes in the heart were proportional to the cardiac concentrations of copper. However, in a study of 53 patients with Wilson's disease 18 had ECG abnormalities—including left ventricular or biventricular hypertrophy, early repolarization, ST depression and T-wave inversion, premature atrial or ventricular contractions, atrial fibrillation, sinoatrial block, and Mobitz type I atrioventricular block (Kuan, Chest, 1987; 91:579). One of these patients died of repeated ventricular fibrillation, another of dilated cardiomyopathy.

Systemic hypertension and ischaemic heart disease in cirrhosis

It is widely believed that systemic hypertension is less common in cirrhotics than in a control population. In an autopsy study of 782 cirrhotic patients, previously recorded blood pressures were lower than in controls (Hall, AmJPathol, 1953; 29:993). However, in another autopsy study 8 per cent of patients dying with cirrhosis had hypertensive heart disease (Lunseth, ArchIntMed, 1958; 102:405). The increased prevalence of hypertension in the general population of chronic alcoholics is well known (Klatsky, NEJM, 1977; 296:1194), but little account has been taken of the presence or absence of liver disease.

In a retrospective study (Heikal, EurJGastroHepatol, 1993; 5:463) of 153 cirrhotics 20 (13 per cent) had arterial hypertension (diastolic pressure >95 mmHg, and/or systolic pressure >160 mmHg on three separate but consecutive occasions). In the group as a whole the mean systolic and diastolic pressures, analysed by gender and age, did not differ significantly from those in a reference population of over 7400 adults. Mean pressures were significantly higher in those with Pugh's A grade than with grades B and C. Systemic hypertension preceded a diagnosis of cirrhosis in 15 of the 20 patients, and was equally common in alcoholic and non-alcoholic liver disease. Complications of hypertension were rare; one patient had hypertensive retinopathy, another ischaemic heart disease. The severity of the hypertension appeared to decrease with follow-up; antihypertensive drug requirements were reduced in nine patients, and four were able to stop treatment.

It is generally believed that patients with cirrhosis are less likely to develop coronary atherosclerosis. Up to the age of 55 years moderate to severe coronary atherosclerosis was only about 50 per cent as common in cirrhotics as in non-cirrhotic patients, but after 65 years the differences were much more marked (Hall, AmJPathol, 1953; 29:993). However, of 108 patients dying with cirrhosis, 48 per cent had serious heart disease, 24 per cent moderate or severe arteriosclerotic heart disease, 8 per cent hypertensive heart disease, and smaller numbers had valvular, congenital, or infective heart diseases (Lunseth, ArchIntMed, 1958; 102:405). Although not a direct comparative study, it was suggested that serious heart disease, including ischaemic heart disease, may be less common in patients with cirrhosis than in the rest of the population.

Ahrens (BullNYAcadMed, 1950; 26:151) found aortic atheroma in hyperlipidaemic patients with primary biliary cirrhosis, but paradoxically its extent seemed inversely related to plasma lipid levels. Four patients with marked cutaneous xanthomatosis had minimal atheroma; three patients without xanthomas had arterial lesions which were disproportionately severe in relation to the patients' age and gender. Many believe ischaemic heart disease to be uncommon in primary biliary cirrhosis, but Schaffner (Gastro, 1969; 57:253) quoted three series in which it was present in some patients; in his own series of over 50 patients, four had had a myocardial infarct and two had severe angina.

In a more recent study the incidence of atherosclerotic death was a little higher in patients with primary biliary cirrhosis than would have been expected in American Caucasians generally, but this difference was not statistically significant and it was concluded that the hyperlipidaemia of primary biliary cirrhosis does not increase the risk of atherosclerosis (Crippin, Hepatol, 1992; 15:858). Unfortunately, because a broad, densely staining beta band and a high total serum cholesterol and triglyceride may be found in primary biliary cirrhosis (and other types of obstructive jaundice), a diagnosis of type IIa or type III hyperlipoproteinaemia is sometimes made and inappropriate dietary or other advice is then given on this basis. Dietary measures do not reduce the hypercholesterolaemia of obstructive jaundice (see also Chapter 2.12). This subject deserves further study.

Gallbladder disease and myocardial infarction

There are conflicting reports on the relationship between gallbladder disease and ischaemic heart disease. One study showed no association (Paul, Circul, 1963; 28:20), another an increased relative risk for women (Petitti, JAMA, 1979; 242: 1150). Two studies suggested a small reduction in the risk of myocardial infarction following cholecystectomy (Bortnichak, AmJEpid, 1985; 121:19; Strom, AmJEpid, 1986; 124:420) but the evidence was inconclusive.

Bacterial endocarditis in cirrhosis

Because bacteraemia is relatively common in patients with cirrhosis, one might expect an increased incidence of bacterial endocarditis. Snyder et al. (Gastro, 1977; 73:1107) found bacterial endocarditis at autopsy in 1.8 per cent of 557 cirrhotics and 0.9 per cent of 3658 non-cirrhotic patients ($p < 0.06$), and during life in 0.34 per cent of 3806 cirrhotics and in 0.1 per cent of 37 345 non-cirrhotic patients admitted to hospital ($p < 0.001$). However, a later report of 2352 autopsies revealed no significant relationship between cirrhosis and bacterial endocarditis (Denton, DigDisSci, 1981; 26:935); indeed it was argued that cirrhotics may be protected from bacterial endocarditis by their impaired coagulation, as a sterile thrombus of platelets and fibrin seems to be important for bacterial aggregation (Weinstein, NEJM, 1974; 291:832).

A more recent paper reported 10 cases of bacterial endocarditis in cirrhotics (McCashland, AmJGastr, 1994; 89:924). In eight the responsible organism was *Staphylococcus aureus*. In six the mitral valve was affected, in two the aortic valve, and in the other two both valves were involved. Eight of the 10 patients died. Of 92 patients with endocarditis and/or bacteraemia due to *Streptococcus bovis* 51 per cent had colonic pathology and 56 per cent documented liver disease or dysfunction (Zarkin, AnnSurg, 1990; 211:786).

Fatal right-sided endocarditis was reported in two patients following peritoneovenous shunting for ascites (Valla, ArchIntMed, 1983; 143:1801). In both there was a staphylococcal septicaemia but one suffered recurrent endocarditis due to *Corynebacterium xerosis*. No clinical manifestation of tricuspid valve dysfunction was noted in either patient. The right-sided endocarditis was recognized only at autopsy, and was thought to be due to contamination of the venous line. Right-sided endocarditis may also be seen in drug addicts with liver disease as a result of intravenous injections (Roberts, AmJMed, 1972; 53:7).

Pyogenic pericarditis as a complication of benign bile duct stricture

Acute pyogenic pericarditis resulted from the perforation of a left lobe liver abscess into the pericardium (Colovic, DigSurg, 1987; 4: 45). The abscess was due to cholangitis from a stricture at the site of a choledochojejunostomy. Initial treatment of the pericarditis (with repeated evacuations, pericardectomy and drainage) was unsuccessful, but the condition resolved with biliary reconstruction and drainage of the hepatic abscess.

Right atrial spread of hepatocellular carcinoma

Hepatocellular carcinoma may extend into the portal and hepatic veins in the form of a tumour thrombus. Such a thrombus may rarely extend into the right atrium and subsequently the right ventricle and, as a result, can cause impairment of cardac function or provide a source of pulmonary emboli. The diagnosis is not usually made during life, but if a right atrial lesion is suspected the diagnosis may be supported or confirmed by echocardiography, CT scanning, and/or angiography (Baba, IntJCardiol, 1995; 47:281), or with the addition of [^{67}Ga]citrate scintigraphy which may demonstrate a hot area above the diaphragm (Noguchi, AnnNuclMed, 1995; 9:39).

The ECG in liver disease

It was suggested many years ago that sinus bradycardia may occur with obstructive jaundice[5] (Song, SAMedJ, 1983; 64:548). Postulated mechanisms include depression of sinus node function by bile acids,[6] or direct damage to myocardial fibres,[7] but these proposals came from studies of animal hearts bathed in bile acids. In patients with moderate to severe cholestasis no correlation was found between total serum bile acid concentration and sinus rate, P-R interval, or corrected QT interval (Song, SAMedJ, 1983; 64:548).

Obstructive jaundice has been associated with cardiac arrest in asystole; the patient, with bile duct malignancy, subsequently had prolonged episodes of sinus arrest with intervening sinus bradycardia and atrial escape, and junctional and ventricular arrhythmias. The arrhythmias disappeared, and the markedly prolonged sinus node recovery time returned to normal after relief of the jaundice by bile duct drainage. The sinus node dysfunction recurred when jaundice returned (Bashour, AnnIntMed, 1985; 103:384).

Several groups have found evidence of autonomic dysfunction in patients with chronic liver disease (Kempler, Lancet, 1989; ii: 1332; Thuluvath, QJMed, 1989; 72:737; MacGilchrist, AmJGastr, 1990; 85:288). This has been documented in terms of decreased variability of the R-R interval (Dillon, AmJGastr, 1994; 89:1544; Isobe, JGastHepatol, 1994; 9:232) and prolongation of the QT interval, and both appear to be related to the severity of the liver disease. Kempler et al. (Lancet, 1992; 340:318; ZGastr, 1993; 31:96 (Suppl. 21)) noted a relationship, in alcoholic and non-alcoholic patients, between the severity of autonomic damage and prolongation of the QT interval corrected for heart rate (QTc). A prolonged QT interval appears to increase the risk of sudden death in a variety of clinical conditions, and this also appears to be the case in patients with alcoholic liver disease (Day, Lancet, 1993; 341: 1423). Recently it was found that the maximum QT interval in any lead, corrected for heart rate (QTcmax), showed significant improvement after liver transplantation in patients with endstage liver disease (Mohamed, Hepatol, 1996; 23:1128); other indices of parasympathetic and sympathetic function also improved.

Three patients with cirrhosis, treated with ornipressin for variceal bleeding, developed bradycardia which ceased after the drug was discontinued; one of them also developed ventricular tachycardia of the 'torsades de pointes' type (Kupferschmidt, SchRundMedPrax, 1996; 85:340). 'Torades de pointes' with prolongation of the QT interval also occurred in a patient with cirrhosis and a hepatocellular carcinoma after 10 days of treatment with terfenadine; the ECG abnormalities disappeared after withdrawal of the drug (Kamisako, IntMed, 1995; 34:92). In another cirrhotic patient terfenadine was associated with prolongation of the QT interval and the secondary appearance of sustained ventricular ectopic beats (Venturini, RecProgressMed, 1992; 83:21).

In 22 children with acute hepatocellular failure there were prolonged P-R and QTc intervals, and premature excitation and ST-T wave changes; myocarditis was blamed for the cardiac disturbances (Sumdaravalli, IndPaediat, 1977; 14:631).

In one woman with fulminant hepatic failure the ECG showed dramatic ST-segment elevation, suggesting diffuse myocardial injury, but subsequent studies (including autopsy) did not reveal a cause for this change (Rosenbloom, Chest, 1991; 100:870). In a man with fulminant hepatic failure due to hepatitis B infection there were ECG changes suggesting myocardial infarction, but this was not confirmed at autopsy; it was suggested that the ECG changes resulted from a high level of plasma catecholamine (Hayashi, JpnJMed, 1988; 27:1988).

Cardiac involvement in viral hepatitis

Features suggesting cardiac involvement, such as palpitations, dyspnoea and chest pain, hypotension and sinus bradycardia, were reported many years ago in patients with viral hepatitis (Dehn, AmHeartJ, 1946; 31:183; Adler,Cardiologia,1947; 11:111). Cardiac complications,including prolonged hypotension, progressive cardiomegaly, pulmonary oedema, arrhythmias (atrial fibrillation, ventricular ectopics), other ECG abnormalities (P-wave, T-wave, and S-T segment changes, and an abnormal axis), and even sudden death were described more recently in acute viral hepatitis (Gordon, JMedVirol, 1989; 28:219); the hepatitis in such cases was usually fulminant (Bell, JAMA, 1971; 218:387). At autopsy subendothelial and epicardial petechiae were commonly found, and haemorrhage into the intraventricular septum has been described (Lucke, AmJPathol, 1944; 20:471).

The heart disease may be due to a myocarditis, possibly due to a direct effect of the virus or to an immune-mediated mechanism (Miller, AnnIntMed, 1973; 79:276; Ursell, HumPath, 1984; 15: 481). Inflammatory infiltration with lymphocytes has been observed (Wood, ArchPathol, 1946; 41:345; Saphir, AmJMedSci, 1956; 231: 168). One case of fulminant hepatic failure and severe myocarditis was reported in association with Coxsackie B virus infection (Read, PostgradMedJ, 1985; 61:749).

Pericarditis with effusion has been described in patients who have recovered from acute hepatitis B (Miller, AnnIntMed, 1973; 79:76; Adler, Pediat, 1978; 61:716).

Cardiac complications were reported in four of 643 patients treated with interferon for chronic hepatitis C: two had a second-degree atrioventricular block, one a severe sinus bradycardia; the other patient had a myocarditis (Kouno, JpnJClinMed, 1994; 52: 1914). Two case reports suggested that interferon may induce coronary vasospasm, causing chest pain/angina and ECG changes of myocardial ischaemia (Tanaka, Angiol, 1995; 46:1139; Yamazaki, RespirCircul, 1993; 41:805); it was was also considered to be the cause of left ventricular dysfunction when interferon was given to treat a recurrence of hepatitis C following a liver transplant (Mateo, DigDisSci, 1996; 41:1500). Cardiotoxicity due to interferon was

also described in patients treated with the drug for solid and lymphoid tumours (Sonnenblick, Chest, 1991; 99:557).

Hepatitis B causing vasculitis/polyarteritis nodosa

Vasculitis associated with hepatitis B may present as a transient serum sickness type illness, with polyarthritis and an urticarial or exanthematous skin rash (Alpert, NEJM, 1971; 285:185), or with the clinical presentation of polyarteritis nodosa (Gocke, JExpMed, 1971; 134:330), a well-recognized complication of acute and chronic hepatitis B infection (Sestoft, ScaJGastr, 1971; 6:495; Martini, CanMedAssJ, 1972; 106:508). The polyarteritis nodosa appears associated with circulating surface antigen (HBsAg) or antibody (anti-HBs) and with hepatitis B Ag–Ab complexes (Gocke, Lancet, 1970; ii:1149; Trepo, JClinPath, 1974; 27:863). It may affect the arteries to the gut and, rarely, causes mesenteric vascular occlusion with infarction and perforation of the intestine (Anuras, AmJSurg, 1980; 140:692).

In areas endemic for hepatitis B, vasculitis is more prevalent. Over 4 years six cases of hepatitis B virus-associated vasculitis were reported in Eskimo residents of south-western Alaska (MacMahon, JAMA, 1980; 244:2180): four had cardiac involvement with congestive failure; two had evidence of pericarditis. Features of liver disease were mild and overshadowed by involvement of other organs. In some, vasculitis followed a recent infection, demonstrating that long-term carriage is not a prerequisite for the development of vasculitis.

Guillevin *et al.* (Medicine, 1995; 74:238) studied 41 patients with hepatitis B virus-associated polyarteritis nodosa, describing it as an acute disease, occurring shortly after infection, and with the characteristics of classical polyarteritis nodosa. It is not an antineutrophil anticytoplasmic antibody (**ANCA**)-mediated vasculitis. Most patients were first given corticosteroids; all were included in a trial of an antiviral agent (35 vidarabine, six α-interferon) plus plasma exchange; mean duration of follow-up was 70 months. A half seroconverted to anti-HBeAb; a quarter also seroconverted to anti-HBsAb. Thirty-three patients were alive at the end of follow-up and recovered from polyarteritis nodosa, and 19 were also thought to have been cured of the HBV infection. Of the eight deaths, three were thought to be directly attributable to the polyarteritis.

Congenital heart disease and liver disease
Congenital hepatic fibrosis

Congenital hepatic fibrosis is a rare recessive disease that presents in children with hepatomegaly, portal hypertension, oesophageal varices, and normal liver function. It is found occasionally in association with congenital heart disease, including congenitally corrected 'l-transposition', patent foramen ovale, subpulmonary stenosis (mild), and ventricular septal defect (Lieberman, Medicine, 1971; 50:277; Maveh, Gut, 1980; 21:799).

Alagille syndrome associated with congenital heart disease

The Alagille or arteriohepatic dysplasia syndrome (Section 26) comprises unusual facies, congenital heart disease, vertebral anomalies, and intrahepatic biliary atresia (Watson, ArchDisChild, 1973; 48:459; Alagille, JPediatr, 1975; 86:63). The most common heart lesion is pulmonary stenosis; other associated malformations are atrial septal defect, tetralogy of Fallot (Greenwood, Pediat, 1976; 58:243), and coarctation of the aorta. Pulmonary atresia, overriding aorta and ventricular septal defect (pseudo truncus arteriosus) were reported in a patient with arteriohepatic dysplasia who had both extra- and intrahepatic biliary atresia (Kocoshis, JPediat, 1981; 99: 436).

Lungs and pulmonary vasculature

Pulmonary dysfunction is a well-recognized complication of chronic liver disease. Intrapulmonary and portal–pulmonary shunting, increased closing volume and ventilation–perfusion mismatching, pulmonary hypertension and failure of hypoxic pulmonary vasoconstriction all occur in cirrhosis. There may be significant oxygen desaturation in cirrhotics, particularly those with oesophageal varices. Primary biliary cirrhosis is associated with diffuse interstitial and obstructive airways disease. Pleural effusions occur commonly in cirrhotic patients, with and without ascites.

The chest radiograph in liver disease

When diseases involve the liver and the lungs (e.g. cystic fibrosis, α1-antitrypsin deficiency, sarcoidosis, tumour metastases, histiocytosis X, hydatid disease, etc.) characteristic changes may be seen on the chest radiograph.

Dilatation of the azygous vein and lateral displacement of the left paravertebral line secondary to hemiazygous vein enlargement were found in chest radiographs taken during supine expiratory tomography in patients with portal hypertension (Doyle, ClinRadiol, 1961; 12:114). Of 304 patients with suspected portal hypertension, none exhibited azygous vein enlargement when erect inspiratory chest radiographs were performed (Moult, Gut, 1975; 16:57). However, mediastinal 'pseudotumours' have been reported due to aneurysmal dilatation of the azygous vein, hemiazygous vein, or oesophageal varices, and they may be confused with malignant neoplasms (Moult, Gut, 1975; 16:57; Dunn, JAMA, 1982; 247: 1873).

Hepatic tumours or abscesses may show elevation of the diaphragm, particularly on the right side. Lung secondaries may be seen in patients with either primary or secondary malignant disease of the liver. With ascites there is usually marked elevation of both sides of the diaphragm with upward displacement of the heart; pleural effusion, usually right sided, is commonly associated with ascites (see below). In a study on 10 patients with the hepatopulmonary syndrome (see below) the chest radiograph showed medium-sized (1.5–3.0 mm) nodular or reticulonodular opacities (McAdams, AJR, 1996; 166:1379). The opacities, which were always in the lung bases, were bilateral in nine and unilateral in one. CT scans showed basilar dilatation of lung vessels with a larger than normal number of visible branches.

Pulmonary function changes in cirrhosis of the liver

Several indices of lung function are affected in cirrhosis. Restrictive and obstructive lung abnormalities have been found in cirrhotics

with ascites; vital capacity, maximum voluntary ventilation, functional residual capacity, total lung capacity, residual volume/total lung capacity ratio, and forced expiratory volume were all reduced in cirrhotics when compared with controls. Unfortunately, details of smoking habits were omitted from this study.[9]

Vital capacity, functional residual capacity, and expiratory reserve volume have been found to be significantly decreased in cirrhotics without ascites, without significant change in FEV_1.[10] These changes were attributed to mechanical compression of lung tissue by interstitial oedema, which causes early airway closure in expiration. Closing volumes were found to be increased in cirrhotic patients inhaling ^{133}Xe, which suggests gas trapping in the lung (Ruff, JCI, 1971; 50:2403).

With ascites, and the associated diaphragmatic elevation and decreased intrathoracic volume, lung tissue is compressed; this may cause alveolar collapse and atelectasis. Restrictive and obstructive abnormalities of lung function are found in cirrhotics with ascites; in one study vital capacity, maximum voluntary ventilation, functional residual capacity, total lung capacity, residual volume/total lung capacity ratio, and forced expiratory volume were all reduced when compared with controls, but details of smoking habits were not presented.[9] In 12 patients paracentesis (a mean of 7.4 litres) increased forced vital capacity, forced expiratory volume at 1 s, total lung capacity, functional residual capacity, inspiratory capacity, expiratory reserve volume, diffusing capacity, and alveolar volume. However, Kco (diffusing capacity corrected by alveolar volume) decreased significantly (Chao, JHepatol, 1994; 20:101). It was thought that an increase in lung volumes and ventilation to the lower lungs with unfavourable ventilation–perfusion matching might explain the discrepancy between changes in diffusing capacity and Kco after large-volume paracentesis.

The presence or absence of ascites might explain the decrease in FEV_1 seen in some studies,[9] and the absence of change in FEV_1 in other studies.[10]

Functional residual capacity was measured by helium gas dilution, using a water-sealed spirometer, in children with α1-antitrypsin deficiency, biliary atresia, neonatal hepatitis, and congenital hepatic fibrosis, and in healthy children of similar ages; children with severe liver disease were not significantly smaller than healthy children, but they had a reduced functional residual capacity (Greenough, ArchDisChild, 1988; 63:850). The reduced lung volume may have resulted from compression due to hepatosplenomegaly and ascites.

The 'hepatopulmonary syndrome'; the effect of cirrhosis on arterial oxygen saturation and gas exchange

Mild hypoxaemia is common in cirrhotics, occurring in approximately a third; severe hypoxia is uncommon in the absence of associated cardiopulmonary disease.[11] Desaturation is seen most commonly in patients with oesophageal varices. Hypoxaemia may also occur, though far less commonly, in patients with non-cirrhotic portal hypertension (Pettei, JPediatGastrNutr, 1995; 20:343).

The term 'hepatopulmonary syndrome' was coined by Kennedy and Knudson in 1977 (Chest, 1977; 72:305). It is defined as the combination of liver disease, an increased alveolar–arterial gradient while breathing room air, and evidence of intrapulmonary vascular dilatations.

The more severely hypoxic cirrhotic patients may exhibit dyspnoea, cyanosis, clubbing, spider naevi, hypocapnia, orthodeoxia (arterial deoxygenation, accentuated by the upright position with improvement during recumbency), and platypnoea (dyspnoea in the upright position which improves during recumbency).[10] Orthodeoxia and platypnoea are related to the gravitational effect of posture on lung blood flow: standing increases the blood flow to dilated pulmonary vessels at the lung bases; these are poorly ventilated and so there is a further fall in Pao_2.

There are several possible causes of the hepatopulmonary syndrome (mild and severe) which may coexist. Changes in the affinity of haemoglobin for oxygen (due to an increased intra-erythrocyte concentration of 2,3-diphosphoglycerate), ascites, and portopulmonary shunting appear relatively unimportant as causes of severe hypoxia.[11]

Early measurements of pulmonary diffusing capacity in patients with cirrhosis revealed either normal or slightly reduced values (Heinemann, AmJMed, 1960; 28:239; Heinemann, Circul, 1960; 22:154), except in patients with primary biliary cirrhosis (see below). In a more recent study, on patients being evaluated for liver transplantation, single-breath diffusing capacity for carbon monoxide (DLco) was the most commonly affected test of lung function (Hourani, AmJMed, 1991; 90:693), but it does not appear that a defect in pulmonary diffusing capacity plays a significant role in the arterial oxygen desaturation seen in patients with cirrhosis.

Use of the term 'hepatopulmonary syndrome' implies the presence of intrapulmonary vascular dilatations. Gross pulmonary arteriovenous fistulas are not a feature of cirrhosis. Tiny star-like pulmonary arteriovenous fistulae, like cutaneous spider naevi, are found (Berthelot, NEJM, 1966; 74:291), and act as small arteriovenous shunts. When macroaggregated albumin particles, labelled with technetium-99m, were administered to cirrhotics in the sitting position, up to 70 per cent of the injected particles traversed the pulmonary vasculature, but only 6 per cent or less passed through the lungs in normal controls (Robin, TrAAP, 1975; 88:202). This work has been confirmed by others (Wolfe, AmJMed, 1977; 63: 746).

Intrapulmonary vascular dilatations or arteriovenous shunting can also be demonstrated by contrast-enhanced echocardiography and pulmonary arteriography.[11] Contrast-enhanced echocardiography involves the intravenous injection either of indocyanine green or of agitated saline, which provides a stream of bubbles 60 to 90 μm in diameter. Usually only the right heart chambers are opacified by these procedures. When there are intrapulmonary or intracardiac shunts, indocyanine green or microbubbles opacify the left heart chambers, and the two types of shunt can be distinguished on the basis of the timing of the opacification. Several studies using contrast-enhanced echocardiography have confirmed the presence of intrapulmonary shunts in patients with cirrhosis (Hind, Gut, 1981; 22:1042; Krowka, Chest, 1990; 97: 1165), and this technique is probably the most useful screening test for intrapulmonary vasodilatation (Abrams, Gastro, 1995; 109: 1283). Pulmonary angiography is a more invasive technique, and its role is not yet clearly established, although it is valuable for ruling out pulmonary hypertension.

To explain why supplemental oxygen improves oxygenation more than would be expected from true 'anatomic' shunts, a new mechanism, 'diffusion-perfusion impairment' or 'alveolar–capillary oxygen disequilibrium', has been proposed, linked to the presence of intrapulmonary vascular dilatations: 'because the capillary is dilated and has an expanded diameter, oxygen molecules from adjacent alveoli cannot diffuse to oxygenate hemoglobin in erythrocytes at the centre stream of venous blood. At the same time, supplemental oxygen provides enough driving pressure to partially overcome this relative diffusion defect.'[11] This problem would be exacerbated by the increased cardiac output, which reduces the transit time through the lung vasculature and the amount of time for oxygen diffusion.

Defect in pulmonary hypoxic vasoconstriction

The combination of arterial hypoxaemia and low pulmonary vascular resistance in cirrhotics is largely unexplained. There may be a defective pulmonary vasoconstrictor response to hypoxia in some cirrhotics; this would result in perfusion/ventilation mismatch, which would contribute to arterial hypoxia. Right and left heart catheterization was performed in patients with severe alcoholic cirrhosis, and in controls with systolic murmurs, hyperkinetic heart syndrome, and intracardiac left to right shunts; in the cirrhotics breathing of a hypoxic mixture (10 per cent oxygen in nitrogen) for 10–15 min failed to increase pulmonary vascular resistance, which rose in all control patients (Daoud, JCI, 1972; 51:1076).

When patients with biopsy-proven cirrhosis breathed either 11 per cent O_2 or 100 per cent O_2, a mild to moderate ventilation–perfusion mismatch was found. Clear differences were shown in liver tests, systemic and pulmonary haemodynamics, and in gas exchange in response to hypoxia and hyperoxia, between cirrhotic patients with and without cutaneous spider naevi. Hypoxic vasoconstriction was not fully abolished, and diffusion equilibrium for oxygen was reached in cirrhosis. Cirrhotic patients with a greater degree of hepatocellular failure exhibit an inadequate pulmonary vascular tone, which leads to ventilation-perfusion inequality and subsequent hypoxia (Rodriguez-Roisin, AnnRevRespDis, 1987; 135:1085).

The idea that ventilation-perfusion mismatch contributes to the arterial hypoxia is supported by other studies. In one of these, 11 cirrhotics with moderate to severe hypoxaemia (Pao_2 < 78 mmHg in air) underwent pulmonary angiography, contrast echocardiography, and measurement of arterial blood gases; none had ascites, one a pleural effusion. The response to almitrine bismesilate (which improves ventilation-perfusion mismatch in hypoxaemia associated with obstructive pulmonary disease) was compatible with a diffuse abnormality of the pulmonary vascular bed at the precapillary or capillary level (Krowka, MayoClinProc, 1987; 62:164). No significant correlation was found between the degree of hypoxaemia and either serum total bilirubin or aspartate aminotransferase. However, hepatic dysfunction always preceded hypoxaemia.

One reason for studying the underlying mechanism of the hepatopulmonary syndrome is the hope that a treatment might be found for the hypoxia. Attempts at medical therapy have proved disappointing,[11] although Song et al. (Pediat, 1996; 97:917) claimed some improvement of the clinical features of the hepatopulmonary syndrome in three children treated with long-term aspirin. Clearly we need to identify the biochemical mediator(s) of the low pulmonary vascular tone. The damaged liver may fail to produce, or may detoxify, a substance with an effect on the pulmonary vasculature. It is still unclear whether the severity of the pulmonary abnormalities is related to the degree of liver failure, although some data support this hypothesis (Ericksson, JHepatol, 1988; 7:529).

Hypoxia was considered a contra-indication to liver transplantation. However, there are now reports showing improvement of oxygenation and reduction of shunting following transplantation in some patients. In one, macroaggregated technetium-labelled lung scans were normal after transplantation, with no significant uptake over kidneys or brain, and there was an improvement in arterial Po_2 values on breathing 100 per cent oxygen (Stoller, Hepatol, 1990; 11:1954). Erickson and her colleagues (Hepatol, 1990; 12:1350) described six patients whose severe ventilation-perfusion mismatch and shunting improved after transplantation. In one patient transplantation for autoimmune hepatitis did not lead to improvement of platypnoea and orthodeoxia. Pulmonary angiography showed large pulmonary arteriovenous shunts which were treated successfully with coil embolotherapy (Poterucha, Hepatol, 1995; 21: 96).

There is still concern about a high surgical mortality in severely hypoxic patients, whether the recipient can be safely oxygenated during anaesthesia, and whether all intrapulmonary vascular dilatations are reversible after transplantation (Krowka, Hepatol, 1990; 11:138). Orthotopic liver transplantation was performed in nine children with cirrhosis-related hypoxaemia (Hobeika, Transpl, 1994; 57:224). The five patients with a Pao_2 greater than 60 mmHg lost their hypoxaemia after surgery and the intrapulmonary shunts closed; the four patients with a Pao_2 below 60 mmHg all died. In one patient with hepatopulmonary syndrome there was less dyspnoea, and an improvement in arterial oxygenation and calculated shunt fraction, after a transjugular portosystemic shunt was performed; liver transplantation was subsequently performed without difficulty (Riegler, Gastro, 1995; 109:978).

Pulmonary function in primary biliary cirrhosis

In 25 patients with primary biliary cirrhosis, lung volumes and diffusing capacity for carbon monoxide (DLco) were measured. Eighteen had clear evidence of liver disease (i.e. they were 'symptomatic', with jaundice, pruritus, xanthomata, hyperpigmentation, and/or hepatosplenomegaly); the others were asymptomatic.[12] Nine (36 per cent) had decreased diffusing capacity, which was not present in any of the controls. Abnormal lung function tests were found almost exclusively in symptomatic patients. Smoking did not seem to be responsible for the abnormalities. Decreased diffusing capacity has been found by others, and is usually attributed to the presence of associated diseases such as fibrosing alveolitis and Sjögren's syndrome (Golding, AmJMed, 1973; 55:772; Rodriques-Roisin, Thorax, 1981; 36:208). In a recent study, alveolar diffusing capacity was reduced in 24 of 61 patients (39 per cent) with primary biliary cirrhosis (Costa, Liver, 1995; 15:196). It appeared unrelated to smoking, the stage of the liver disease, or the presence of Sjögren's syndrome. There was a correlation with complete or incomplete

CREST syndrome and with the presence of anticentromere antibodies.

Both obstructive (Clarke, AnnRheumDis, 1978; 37:42) and/ or restrictive (Rodriques-Roisin, Thorax, 1981; 36:208) types of pulmonary disease have been found with primary biliary cirrhosis, and again were attributed to associated autoimmune conditions such as progressive systemic sclerosis or Sjögren's syndrome, rather than to the primary biliary cirrhosis. In a large study,[12] 12 per cent of the patients were found to have bronchial asthma. However, in a more recent paper describing three patients with primary biliary cirrhosis and asthma, the prevalence of asthma in 266 cases of primary biliary cirrhosis was only about 2.2 per cent (Terasaki, JGast, 1995; 30:667).

The lung function abnormalities in primary biliary cirrhosis are similar to those found in sarcoidosis, another granulomatous disease. Widespread granulomas have been found in the lungs of some patients with primary biliary cirrhosis, which may account for the decreased diffusing capacity. Airways obstruction can occur due to the presence of granulomas in and around bronchi, bronchioles, and capillaries (Stanley, NEJM, 1972; 287:1282). Primary biliary cirrhosis can be differentiated from sarcoid liver disease by the finding of serum mitochondrial antibodies and a negative Kveim test (Olsson, Chest, 1979; 75:663).

Spiteri et al. (Gut, 1990; 31:208) studied the cell population obtained by bronchoalveolar lavage in 10 patients with primary biliary cirrhosis, but without pulmonary symptoms, and with normal lung function and a normal chest radiograph. They examined the lymphoid and non-lymphoid cells using immunocytochemical methods. Six of the 10 appeared to have a subclinical alveolitis. In these patients the lymphocyte count in the lavage was elevated, the CD4/CD8 ratio was increased, and some of the T cells showed markers of activation; there was an increase in dendritic cells in the non-lymphoid cell population. These changes are also seen in sarcoidosis. The authors suggested that there is a granuloma-producing mechanism in the lung similar to that occurring in the liver.

The granulomatous pattern found in the lungs of some patients with primary biliary cirrhosis may be associated with a type 3 response, which suggests an association between primary biliary cirrhosis and interstitial lung disease. A patient with long-standing primary biliary cirrhosis had a severe illness due to a lymphoid interstitial pneumonia which was confirmed by open-lung biopsy; the initial pulmonary infiltrate consisted of unilateral nodules mimicking neoplastic disease, but it progressed to involve both lungs in a diffuse interstitial process. It cleared spontaneously but recurred on two subsequent occasions (Weissman, AmJMedSci, 1983; 285: 21).

Pulmonary hypertension

Pulmonary hypertension is more prevalent in patients with chronic liver disease and portal hypertension than in normal people (McDonnell, AnnRevRespDis, 1983; 127:437). The association was first reported in 1952 (Mantz, ArchPathol, 1952; 52:91). Of 507 patients with portal hypertension, but without known pulmonary hypertension, 10 (2 per cent) had primary pulmonary hypertension (Hadengue, Gastro, 1991; 100:520); in a series of mainly alcoholic cirrhotic patients there was a reported incidence of 0.25 per cent.

Pulmonary hypertension may develop fairly rapidly in patients with portal hypertension, but does not appear to be related to the Child–Pugh score.

Pulmonary hypertension complicates portal hypertension from many causes, for example cirrhosis (Lebrec, AmRevRespDis, 1979; 120:849), chronic hepatitis (Cryer, AmJMed, 1977; 63:604), extrahepatic portal hypertension (Cohen, Hepatol, 1983; 4:588), and non-cirrhotic portal hypertension, but the prevalence seems even higher after surgical shunting for portal hypertension. Transjugular intrahepatic portosystemic shunting (**TIPS**) may also cause an increase in pulmonary artery pressure (van der Linden, Hepatol, 1996; 23:982), as the major haemodynamic change after TIPS placement appears to be an increase in pulmonary vascular resistance.

Patients with pulmonary hypertension show some typical clinical features (Hadengue, Gastro, 1991; 100:520). Most complain of dyspnoea on exertion, 20 to 30 per cent of exertional syncope, and a smaller number complain of precordial chest pain and occasional haemoptysis. Most have a loud pulmonary second sound and/or a pulmonary systolic murmur; pulmonary incompetence may result, and heart failure (sometimes with tricuspid incompetence) is relatively common. Patients may die from causes related to pulmonary hypertension, usually in association with a relatively low cardiac output.

Two main morphological types of pulmonary hypertension have been described: 'thromboembolic' (Naeye, Circul, 1960; 22:376) and 'plexogenic' (Segel, BrHeartJ, 1968; 30:575; Lebrec, AmRevRespDis, 1979; 120:849).

With thromboembolic pulmonary hypertension, which appears to be a less severe form, thrombus, or inflammatory reaction to thrombus, is found in small muscular pulmonary arteries and arterioles. Organization of the thrombotic material may cause fibrous mural pads, occlusive non-vascular or vascular fibrous tissue, and fibrous septa. This form might be expected if portacaval shunting allowed multiple emboli to reach the lung from thrombi in portal, splenic, and superior mesenteric veins. Since this mechanism was first suggested (Mantz, AMAArchPath, 1951; 52:91) others have confirmed the association of microemboli with cirrhosis. Of six cases of pulmonary hypertension associated with portal vein thrombosis, five had postmortem evidence of recurrent emboli (Naeye, Circul, 1960; 22:376). In two cases of pulmonary hypertension following portacaval shunts there was postmortem evidence of recurrent pulmonary microemboli but no source of thrombus was found (Senior, Circul, 1968; 37:88). In two other patients with a portacaval shunt pulmonary hypertension was considered to be 'primary' (Levine, JPediat, 1973; 83:964; Bernthal, JClinGastro, 1983; 5:353;).

The lesions of plexogenic pulmonary hypertension are distal to the branch points of muscular pulmonary arteries, and characterized by vascular dilatation, medial thinning, and luminal obstruction by loose connective tissue with interspersed vascular channels and occasional fibrin deposits (Morrison, AmJMed, 1980; 69:513). This plexogenic arteriopathy appears to be associated with more severe forms of portal hypertension. The underlying mechanism is unknown, but this type of pulmonary hypertension is associated with pulmonary vasoconstriction (Lebrec, AmRevRespDis, 1979; 120: 849). It has been suggested that a vasoconstrictive agent originating in the splanchnic bed might be destroyed in the liver in normal subjects; portal-systemic shunting would allow it direct access to the pulmonary vasculature. In animal models certain prostaglandins cause pulmonary and portal vein vasoconstriction (Kitamunra, JpnJPhysiol, 1976; 26:687). Other substances which may cause pulmonary vasoconstriction are serotonin and adenine nucleotides, which may be derived from aggregating platelets (Levine, JPediat, 1973; 83:964).

Plexogenic pulmonary hypertension has been found in patients with macronodular cirrhosis and evidence of associated autoimmune disease, for example positive antinuclear antibody, positive latex agglutination for a rheumatoid factor, antimitochondrial antibody, and hypergammaglobinaemia (Morrison, AmJMed, 1980; 69:513). This suggests that both the lung and liver abnormalities might be autoimmune in nature. Plexiform lung lesions have also been described in association with chronic active hepatitis (Cohen, AmJMed, 1965; 39:127; Cryer, AmJMed, 1977; 63:604). Alcoholic cirrhosis with portal and plexiform pH has been described in the presence of microangiopathic haemolytic anaemia (Pare, AmJMed, 1983; 74:1093); the severe plexiform dilatation of the pulmonary microvasculature was considered to be the site of intravascular fragmentation of red cells, thus causing the haemolytic anaemia.

Plexiform pulmonary hypertension was found at autopsy in a 16-year-old girl who had had a portacaval shunt performed at 12 years of age for her Von Gierke's disease (type I glycogen storage disease). She had a sudden death. At autopsy there were well-demarcated hepatic nodules, but no cirrhosis, and changes in the lungs of plexiform pulmonary hypertension with hypertrophy of the small and medium-sized arteries plus plexiform lesions (Pizzo, Pediat, 1980; 65:341).

There is at present no effective treatment for pulmonary hypertension associated with liver disease. The prognosis is poor, although there are some long-term survivors, and the condition is considered a contra-indication to liver transplantation.

The pulmonary effects of variceal sclerotherapy

The adult respiratory distress syndrome has been associated with sodium morrhuate sclerotherapy (Monroe, Gastro, 1983; 85:693). Radiographic studies have shown that sclerotherapy material rapidly enters the systemic circulation (Barsoum, BrJSurg, 1978; 65:588). This sclerosant contains several fatty acids, including oleic and linoleic acid, which are toxic to the lung (Ashburgh, JSurgRes, 1968; 8:417). Respiratory distress, with bilateral alveolar/interstitial infiltrates and pulmonary oedema on chest radiography, occurred within 8 to 36 h of sclerotherapy in 2 of 30 patients (Cahill, JTrauma, 1974; 14:73). When sodium morrhuate was injected mixed with $^{99}Tc^m$-labelled albumin microspheres in 11 patients with hepatic cirrhosis, most of the label remained in the region of the oesophagus, the remainder presumably reaching the pulmonary circulation; there were no changes in DLco 1 h after sclerotherapy (Connors, AnnIntMed, 1986; 105:539). The authors suggested that the amount of sclerosant reaching the lungs would have little deleterious effect on the pulmonary vasculature. However, in another study, computed tomography (**CT**) scanning of the chest 48 h following endoscopic sclerotherapy with ethanolamine oleate suggested that the sclerosing agent had passed into the pulmonary vessels; subsegmental atelectasis, dilatations of peripheral vessels, and/or high density collections and small nodular or irregular lesions were observed, probably representing embolic and/or interstitial pneumonitis (Ikezoe, ActaRadiol, 1987; 28:415).

In studies on an acute sheep model, intravenous injection of sodium morrhuate caused marked but transient pulmonary hypertension; pulmonary oedema was not evident. These deleterious pulmonary effects may have been due to the activation of the complement and kinin systems rather than direct vascular injury (Musso, AnnIntMed, 1987; 106:640).

Oesophagobronchial fistulas have been reported as a rare complication of endoscopic sclerotherapy (Carr-Locke, Gut, 1982; 23: 1005; Wilborn, JClinGastro, 1988; 10:81). The first case reported was fatal; the other patient responded to medical therapy consisting of enteral feeding, H2 antagonists and antibiotics; the fistula closed spontaneously.

Pleural effusions are also a rare complication of endoscopic sclerotherapy (Hughes, GastrEnd, 1982; 28:62). Acute respiratory insufficiency occurred after endoscopy for bleeding oesophageal varices, due to diaphragmatic restriction caused by air left in the stomach after the procedure (Crawford, BMJ, 1984; 288:1639).

Hepatic hydrothorax

This term is used to describe a large pleural effusion in the presence of cirrhosis, but in the absence of primary pulmonary or cardiac disease (Morrow, AnnIntMed, 1958; 49:193). An incidence as high as about 5 to 6 per cent has been reported in cirrhotics with clinically detectable ascites (Johnston, AnnIntMed, 1964; 61:385; Lieberman, AnnIntMed, 1966; 64:341). About 67 per cent of the effusions are right-sided, 17 per cent left-sided, and 17 per cent bilateral. They may be massive and/or recurrent (Emerson, Lancet, 1955; i:487; Esteve, JClinNutrGastro, 1986; 1:139).

Pleural effusions in cirrhosis have been attributed to one or to a combination of the following factors; hypoalbuminaemia, azygous hypertension, lymphatic obstruction, or the presence of diaphragmatic holes which allow communication between the peritoneal and pleural cavities.

Small holes have been detected in the diaphragm by several methods. Intraperitoneally injected blue dye has been shown to traverse a small diaphragmatic hole at autopsy in an ascitic patient (Emerson, Lancet, 1955; i:487). Radio-isotopes injected into the peritoneal cavity *in vivo* have been shown to pass into the pleural space in patients with a hydrothorax (Vargas-Tank, ScaJGastr, 1984; 19:294). Holes have been demonstrated on the superior surface of the diaphragm at postmortem in patients with ascites and hydrothorax (Lutherman, ArchIntMed, 1970; 125:114).

Although these effusions are usually associated with ascites, right-sided hepatic hydrothorax can occur in the absence of clinically detectable ascites (Singer, Gastro, 1977; 73:575; Frazer, MedJAust, 1983; 2:520; Llaneza, DigDisSci, 1985; 30:88; Rubinstein, Gastro, 1985; 88:188;). Ascitic fluid secreted from the liver surface may enter the thoracic cavity directly as a result of the negative intrathoracic pressure; however, in one patient without clinical ascites transdiaphragmatic flow into the right pleural effusion was demonstrated by scintigraphy after intraperitoneal injection of [^{99}Tc^m]tin colloid (Schroder, NukMed, 1991; 3:104).

A prospective study of 22 patients with chronic liver disease and ascites and left-sided pleural effusions revealed that four (18 per

cent) of them were due to tuberculosis. Therefore, all left-sided pleural effusions in cirrhotics with ascites should be fully investigated (Mirouze, DigDisSci, 1981; 26:984).

Hepatic hydrothorax usually responds to diuretics, but when there is a large effusion, repeated thoracocentesis may be necessary. Some patients may require pleural obliteration with tetracycline or another agent (Falchuk, Gastro, 1977; 72:319). In a series of 22 patients with tension hydrothorax, due to small one-way valves in the diaphragm (Crawford, ArchIntMed, 1982; 142:194), 18 were treated successfully by chest tube insertion and creation of a LeVeen peritoneovenous shunt; after emptying the abdomen of its fluid load, a sclerosing agent (nitrogen mustard or tetracycline) was injected into the pleural cavity to ensure closure of the defects (LeVeen, AmJSurg, 1984; 148:210). More recently TIPSS has been used successfully to treat many patients with hepatic hydrothorax. In two patients, thoracotomy allowed the identification of the diaphragmatic defects, and their repair by chemical and traumatic pleurodesis, followed by postoperative peritoneal and pleural drainage (Rubinstein, Gastro, 1985; 88:188).

Pleural effusion has also been noted during the prodrome or in the early icteric phase of acute viral hepatitis (Gross, Gastro, 1971; 60:898; Katsilabros, Gastro, 1972; 63:718), particularly in hepatitis B infection (Owen, NEJM, 1974; 291:963; Cocchi, JPediatr, 1976; 89:329; Tabor, Gastro, 1977; 73:1157).

Hepatobronchial fistulas complicating liver abscess

Pleuropulmonary fistulas are the most common complication of right-sided liver abscess (Ochsner, AmJSurg, 1938; 40:292; Diffenbauch, ArchSurg, 1960; 81:934). Direct perforation seems the most likely cause; however, an abscess can occur without apparent pleural involvement and it is possible that lymphatic channels through the bare area of the diaphragm may explain this anomaly. In one report diagnostic percutaneous cholangiography demonstrated transfer of contrast medium into the bronchi, probably via lymphatics between the mid portion of the right liver and the right lower lung (Okuda, Gastro, 1973; 65:124); the usual drainage route would be toward the porta hepatis.

Pulmonary complications of amoebic liver abscess (Chapter 13.3.1)

Amoebic liver abscess is the most common complication of intestinal amoebiasis, occuring in about 8 per cent of patients (Ralls, Radiol, 1979; 132:125). Abscesses frequently occur on the right side of the liver (80 per cent), and about 25 per cent are multiple (DeBakey, SGO, 1951; 92:209). Pleuropulmonary involvement occurs in about 7 per cent of patients (Adams, Medicine, 1977; 56:315), causing hepatobronchial fistula (47 per cent), pleural effusions and empyema (29 per cent), lung abscess (14 per cent), and consolidation (10 per cent). Elevation of the right hemidiaphragm is a non-specific finding, occurring in about 50 per cent of patients with amoebic liver abscess without direct pulmonary involvement.

The need for early diagnosis and treatment of hepatic involvement of amoebic infection has been emphasized (Fulton, AustRadiol, 1982; 26:60). Grey scale ultrasound now provides a non-invasive tool for the early diagnosis of liver and lung involvement.

Treatment of the basal pneumonia and/or cavitation with metronidazole and postural drainage is successful in the majority of patients. Empyema is usually treated with intermittent aspiration and metronidazole. If aspiration is ineffective, then surgery is indicated.

Pulmonary complications of hepatic echinococcosis (Chapter 13.4.2)

Alveolar echinococcosis of the liver behaves as a malignant tumour of the intrahepatic biliary system, whereas hydatid cyst echinococcosis behaves as a benign hepatic tumour. The major presenting symptoms of alveolar echinococcosis are obstructive jaundice and/or an irregular, enlarged liver mimicking hepatic carcinoma (Miguet, ArchFrMalAppDig, 1976; 65:9). Lung metastases are observed in hepatic alveolar echinococcosis in about 10 per cent of patients (Levrak, AnnGastroHep, 1973; 9:37). These metastases are usually clinically silent and occur from 3 to 20 years after the discovery of the primary hepatic lesions. Hepatic alveolar echinococcosis has been reported with metastasis to the right atrium (Etlevent, JCardiovascSurg, 1986; 27:671); secondary pulmonary lesions in this case produced the presenting symptoms, while the hepatic disease was silent. The right atrial metastasis was presumably due to migration of the disease from the hepatic veins.

Pulmonary emboli associated with liver disease

Pulmonary embolism may occur from thrombus in the hepatic veins in patients with the Budd–Chiari syndrome, in patients with hepatic venous thrombosis associated with hepatocellular carcinoma (see earlier), or in patients who have an underlying thrombotic disorder, such as protein C or protein S deficiency.

Fatal pulmonary thromboembolic disease has been found in association with portal vein thrombosis in a woman who had been taking oral contraceptives (Capron, JClinGastro, 1981; 3:295). The pulmonary vascular disease may have been independent of the portal thrombosis, but some authors have suggested that pulmonary embolism may result directly from portal vein thrombosis (Mantz, ArchPathol, 1951; 52:91; Owen, NEJM, 1953; 249:919; Naeye, Circul, 1969; 22:376).

In a patient with the Budd–Chiari syndrome due to thrombosis of the inferior vena cava and hepatic veins, faecal pulmonary embolization was found to be the cause of death at autopsy (Smith, NEJM, 1978; 298:1069). Ileal diverticulitis had caused an ileovenous fistula, and the extensive collateral circulation which had developed as a result of the Budd–Chiari syndrome permitted direct pulmonary embolization of faecal material from the diverticulum.

The embolism of bile to the lungs is a very rare finding. All reported cases had marked obstructive jaundice of long duration, usually associated with some kind of hepatic trauma, often iatrogenic. It is described after percutaneous liver biopsy (Brown, AnnIntMed, 1952; 36:1529), percutaneous cholangiography (Koehler, Anesthesiol, 1978; 49:210), and severe hepatic trauma due to gunshot injury (Doyle, ArchPathLabMed, 1968; 85:559). Bile emboli were found at postmortem in a patient with sclerosing adenocarcinoma of the common hepatic duct on whom several invasive procedures had been carried out (Balogh, ArchPathLabMed, 1984; 108:814). It has been suggested that little or no microscopic reaction occurs in vessel walls in the lung unless the pulmonary bile emboli are infected. For biliary embolism to occur, it seems likely that a bile duct must have communicated with a hepatic vein, and that there must have been a higher pressure in the biliary system than in the hepatic veins.

Fatal air embolism occurred 4 months after the placement of a LeVeen peritoneovenous shunt for the treatment of intractable ascites. It resulted from perforation of the caecum during cauterization of a mucosal vascular malformation via a flexible colonoscope (Hirst, AmJGastr, 1981; 76:453). Gastrointestinal perforation from any cause is therefore an indication for immediate closure of the shunt.

References

1. Murray JF, Dawson AM, and Sherlock S. Circulatory changes in chronic liver diseases. *American Journal of Medicine*, 1958; **24**: 358–67.
2. Kontos HA, Shapiro W, Mauck HP, and Patterson JL. General and regional circulatory alterations in cirrhosis of the liver. *American Journal of Medicine*, 1964; **37**: 526–35.
3. Bradley SE, Inglefinger FJ, and Bradley GP. Hepatic circulation in cirrhosis of the liver. *Circulation*, 1952; **5**: 419–29.
4. Ma Z and Lee SS. Cirrhotic cardiomyopathy: getting to the heart of the matter. *Hepatology*, 1996; **24**: 451–9.
5. Wood P. *Diseases of the heart and circulation*, 3rd edn. London: Eyre and Spottiswoode, 1968: 232.
6. Schamroth L. *Introduction to electrocardiography*, 7th edn. Oxford: Blackwell, 1980: 27.
7. Sobotka H. *Physiological chemistry of the bile*. Baltimore: Williams and Wilkins, 1937: 133.
8. Scheinberg IH and Sternlieb I. *Wilson's disease*. Philadelphia: WB Saunders, 1984: 110.
9. Yao EH, Kong B, Hsue G, Zhou A, and Wang H. Pulmonary function changes in cirrhosis of the liver. *American Journal of Gastroenterology*, 1987; **81**: 352–4.
10. Fujiwara K. Pulmonary function in patients with cirrhosis of the liver. *Japanese Journal of Chest Diseases*, 1982; **41**: 422–9.
11. Lange PA and Stolle JK. The hepatopulmonary syndrome. *Annals of Internal Medicine*, 1995; **122**: 521–9.
12. Uddenfeldt P, Bjerle P, Danielsson A, Nystrom L, and Stjernberg N. Lung function abnormalities in patients with primary biliary cirrhosis. *Acta Medica Scandinavica*, 1988; **223**: 549–55.

25.2 The effect of liver disease on the endocrine system

Yolanta T. Kruszynska and Pierre M. Bouloux

Introduction

The liver is involved in the metabolism of many steroid and peptide hormones. It synthesizes plasma hormone binding proteins whose levels influence plasma hormone levels and their tissue distribution. It is a major target tissue for many hormones, and it produces hormones (for example, insulin-like growth factor-I (**IGF-I**)) that influence the synthesis and secretion of hormones by other endocrine glands. It is therefore not surprising that the metabolic disturbance of liver disease may cause abnormalities of neuro-endocrine function and circulating hormone levels. Moreover, some liver disorders, particularly those with an autoimmune basis, may be associated with endocrine disorders (for example, autoimmune thyroid disease).

Abnormalities of circulating hormone levels may be due to impaired hepatic metabolism of a hormone, to a compensatory increase in hormone production because of tissue resistance to its action, to abnormalities of plasma hormone binding proteins, or to effects of liver disease or its treatment on hormone secretion. The hepatologist needs to be aware of the effect of liver disease on the endocrine system and plasma hormone levels to enable him or her to interpret the results of endocrine tests correctly. In addition, it is important to recognize that certain endocrine presentations, such as hypogonadism or glucose intolerance, may be due to liver disease and may be the presenting complaint.

Glucose intolerance and diabetes in liver disease

The liver plays a key role in glucose and insulin metabolism. In the postabsorptive and fasted states it releases glucose (derived from glycogen or gluconeogenesis) into the circulation for use by other tissues. After meals it switches from net glucose production to net glucose uptake, and stores glucose (taken up from plasma or synthesized by gluconeogenesis) as glycogen. It thus helps to limit the rise in plasma glucose levels after carbohydrate ingestion while ensuring a supply of glucose to extrahepatic tissues in the postabsorptive and fasted states. The liver is also the major site of insulin metabolism; about 60 per cent of the insulin secreted into the portal vein is removed by the liver on first pass (Blackard, Diabetes, 1970; 19:302). It is thus not surprising that abnormalities of glucose and insulin metabolism are found in patients with liver

disease. The role of the liver in carbohydrate and insulin metabolism is discussed in detail in Chapter 2.11.

Prevalence of impaired glucose tolerance and diabetes in liver disease

Most patients with cirrhosis show impaired glucose tolerance despite normal fasting blood glucose levels, and there is a higher prevalence of overt diabetes mellitus in cirrhotics than in the general population. Glucose intolerance is also common in patients with acute viral hepatitis (Record, ClinSci, 1973; 45:677; Chupin, Diabetes, 1978; 27:661), fatty liver (Rehfeld, Gastro, 1973; 64:445), autoimmune chronic active hepatitis (Alberti, ClinSci, 1972; 42:591), and toxic liver damage (Record, ClinSci, 1975; 49:473). Increased blood glucose levels are also seen after meals in patients with liver disease (Marchesini, Hepatol, 1981; 1:294; Stewart, EurJClinInv, 1983; 13:397; Kruszynska, ClinSci, 1992; 83:597).

The prevalence of impaired glucose tolerance in cirrhosis depends on the diagnostic criteria used and the type of patients studied. Using WHO criteria,[1] impaired oral glucose tolerance is found in 60 to 80 per cent of patients with cirrhosis[2] (Fig. 1). Intravenous glucose tolerance is traditionally assessed by measuring the rate at which the blood glucose falls after an intravenous bolus of glucose. The results are expressed as the slope of the logarithm of blood glucose concentration against time (K_G). Most studies have shown a lower K_G value in cirrhotic patients than in matched controls[3-5] (Greco, Diabetolog, 1979; 17:23; Magnusson, ScaJ-Gastr, 1987; 22:301), even when patients with fasting hyperglycaemia are excluded[3,4] (Greco, Diabetolog, 1979; 17:23). In cirrhotics with normal fasting glucose levels a good correlation was found between K_G (intravenous glucose tolerance) and oral glucose tolerance[3]. A direct correlation was also found in the 145 cirrhotic patients studied by Conn *et al.*,[2] although the inclusion of patients with overt diabetes mellitus might have strengthened the relationship in their study. Like diabetic patients without liver disease (Brunzell, JClinEndoc, 1976; 42:222), cirrhotic patients with fasting hyperglycaemia (whole blood glucose > 6.7 mmol/l) have a K_G value of less than 1.0 per cent per min (Fig. 2).[2,3]

The prevalence of diabetes in cirrhotics is two to four times higher than that seen in the general population,[6] a relationship not explained by the high prevalence of diabetes mellitus in haemochromatosis as this is an uncommon cause of cirrhosis. Bloodworth

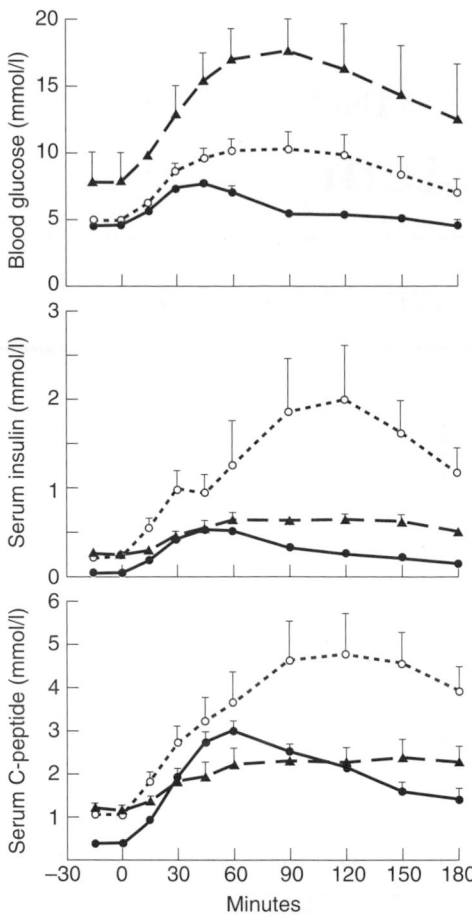

Fig. 1. Blood glucose, serum insulin, and C-peptide levels after an overnight fast and after ingestion of 75 g glucose at $t = 0$ min in seven non-diabetic cirrhotic patients (○), eight diabetic cirrhotic patients (▲), and eight normal control subjects (●). Mean ± SEM. (Reproduced from Kruszynska *et al.*, Metabolism, 1995; 44:254, with permission.)

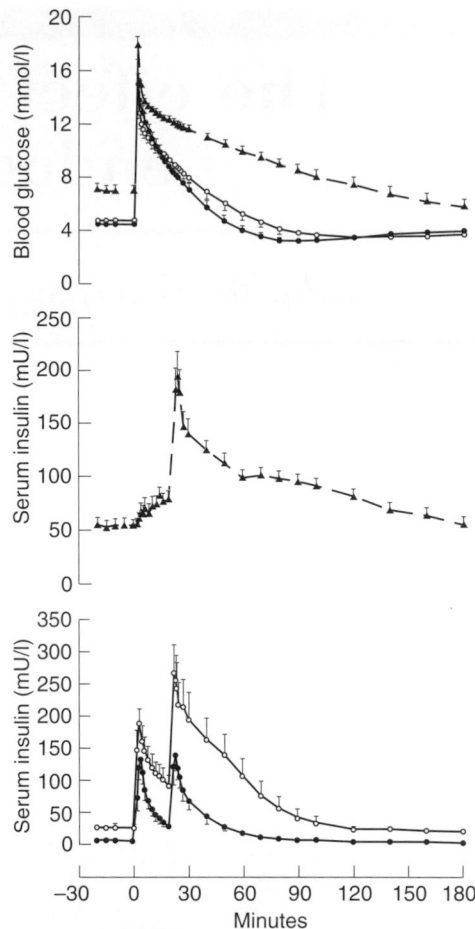

Fig. 2. Blood glucose and serum insulin levels after intravenous glucose (0.3 g/kg) at $t = 0$ min and intravenous tolbutamide (300 mg) at $t = 20$ min in 12 non-diabetic cirrhotic patients (fasting blood glucose < 6.7 mmol/l) (○), eight diabetic cirrhotic patients (▲), and 10 normal control subjects (●). Mean ± SEM. (Reproduced from ref. 3, with permission.)

(ArchIntMed, 1961; 108:95) analysed 27 050 consecutive autopsies performed between 1937 and 1960 and found diabetes in 5.6 per cent of cirrhotics compared with 3.0 per cent in the general population; for the autopsies performed between 1955 and 1960 the corresponding figures were 12 per cent and 5.5 per cent. These figures are in accord with the results of numerous clinical studies reviewed by Creutzfeldt *et al.*[6] In populations with a high prevalence and incidence of type II diabetes, the frequency of diabetes in cirrhosis may be as high as 40 per cent (Kingston, Gastro, 1984; 87:688). It is not clear whether diabetes is associated with cirrhosis of a particular aetiology (other than haemochromatosis). In many early studies alcoholic, biliary, and autoimmune cirrhosis were all included as 'nutritional cirrhosis'. Most studies have been retrospective and inevitably suffer from selection bias. Information on alcohol consumption, use of diabetogenic medications, the presence of a family history of diabetes, and on the criteria used for the diagnosis of diabetes is either lacking or inadequate. Some studies have suggested a stronger association between diabetes and alcoholic cirrhosis (Frankel, ArchIntMed, 1950; 86:376; Bloodworth, ArchIntMed, 1961; 108:95). However, Blanco *et al.*[7] found the prevalence of glucose intolerance to be similar in alcohol-abusing

and non-abusing cirrhotics. In a study of 401 cirrhotic patients the main risk factors for glucose intolerance were severity of liver disease, a family history of diabetes, and age.[7] Muller *et al.* (EurJClinChemClinBioch, 1994; 32:749) found no increase in the prevalence of diabetes in cirrhotics with a first-degree type II diabetic relative. Their 'diabetic' cirrhotics, however, had normal fasting blood glucose concentrations and the number of cirrhotics with a known diabetic relative was small. In patients with cirrhosis due to haemochromatosis, diabetes is more common in those who have a first-degree relative with diabetes (Dymock, AmJMed, 1972; 52:203).

Overview of glucose metabolism and mechanisms of hyperglycaemia (see Chapter 2.11)

In the postabsorptive and fasted states, the liver releases glucose for use by other tissues. At rest this rate is approximately 2 mg/kg/min and is matched by a similar rate of tissue glucose uptake; insulin levels are low, and 75 to 85 per cent of this basal glucose uptake is insulin-independent. Brain accounts for most of this and skeletal muscle for only 15 to 20 per cent.

Because insulin plays only a small role in promoting tissue glucose uptake in the fasted state, an impairment of insulin-mediated glucose uptake by muscle has little effect on fasting glucose levels. Fasting hyperglycaemia is primarily due to hepatic over-production of glucose (Ferrannini, DiabetMetabRev, 1989; 5:711). Most cirrhotics have normal basal glucose production rates and fasting glucose levels despite marked insulin resistance.[8,9] Diabetic cirrhotics with fasting hyperglycaemia have increased basal hepatic glucose production[10] which is due largely to their marked impairment of insulin secretion (see below); hepatic insulin resistance and hyperglucagonaemia may also contribute to the increased hepatic glucose production in diabetic cirrhotics.

Insulin stimulates glucose uptake by skeletal muscle, heart muscle, and adipocytes. It also enhances hepatic glucose uptake by its effects on certain liver enzymes. In other tissues, glucose uptake is not influenced by insulin. After meals or glucose ingestion, the rise in insulin levels suppresses glucose output by the liver and markedly stimulates glucose uptake by muscle; the accompanying rise in glucose levels enhances glucose uptake (by mass action) by insulin-dependent and non-insulin-dependent tissues (other than brain). Hyperglycaemia also helps to suppress hepatic glucose output. Skeletal muscle takes up about 50 to 60 per cent of an oral glucose load; the liver accounts for 20 to 35 per cent.

Most cirrhotics are resistant to the effects of insulin on glucose metabolism. Glucose disposal during a hyperinsulinaemic glucose clamp (see Chapter 2.11) is about 50 per cent lower in cirrhotics than in normal subjects[3,9–12] (Proietto, ClinEndoc, 1984; 21: 677). This is mainly due to diminished muscle glucose uptake and storage as glycogen (Kruszynska, Hepatol, 1988; 118:337; Selberg, JCI 1993; 91:1897). Skeletal muscle insulin insensitivity is the main cause of glucose intolerance in non-diabetic cirrhotics, although portosystemic shunting also plays a role by causing a small increase in the amount of glucose entering the systemic circulation, particularly during the first 30 min after glucose ingestion; inhibition of hepatic glucose output is normal. These factors are discussed in Chapter 2.11 (also see Chapter 2.11 Fig. 6). Insulin secretory abnormalities also contribute to glucose intolerance in non-diabetic cirrhotics. In diabetic cirrhotics there are striking abnormalities of insulin secretion and the ability of glucose *per se* to promote tissue glucose uptake and inhibit hepatic glucose output ('glucose effectiveness') is impaired.[3] In diabetic cirrhotics not only is there a further impairment of muscle glucose uptake but also less inhibition of hepatic glucose output, resulting in an even greater glucose load entering the systemic circulation and hence marked hyperglycaemia (Fig. 1).

The total amount of glucose taken up by muscle after a glucose load may be similar to that of normal subjects (Leatherdale, ClinSci, 1980; 59:191) because later during the glucose tolerance test the higher plasma glucose levels and much higher insulin levels compensate for the insulin resistance (Fig. 1).

Insulin secretion and clearance in liver disease

Fasting and postprandial plasma insulin levels are raised in nearly all patients with cirrhosis, including those with diabetes.[3–5,8–12]

In cirrhotics hepatic extraction of insulin falls[12,13] (Kruszynska, ClinSci, 1992; 83:597). In hyperinsulinaemic cirrhotics with portal hypertension arterial serum insulin levels exceeded those in the hepatic vein.[13] This suggests that extrahepatic shunting allows a large amount of secreted insulin to escape initial hepatic removal. The observation that the insulin clearance defect is more marked for secreted insulin[12] (Kruszynska, ClinSci, 1992; 83:597) or insulin infused into the portal vein (Nygren, Metabolism, 1985; 34: 48) than for insulin infused into the systemic circulation also suggests that reduced first-pass hepatic uptake of insulin due to portosystemic shunting is important.

Studies using serum C-peptide levels and the C-peptide : insulin molar ratio (during steady state) as indices of pancreatic insulin secretion and hepatic insulin extraction, respectively (Polonsky, Diabetes, 1986; 35:379)(see Chapter 2.11) have indicated that both hypersecretion and decreased clearance contribute to the fasting and postprandial hyperinsulinaemia of cirrhosis[12] (Proietto, ClinEndoc, 1984; 21:657; Kruszynska, ClinSci, 1992; 83:597); decreased clearance is quantitatively more important. Measurements of C-peptide (the clearance of which is normal in cirrhosis[12]) and insulin secretion rates have drawn attention to the importance of insulin secretory defects in the glucose intolerance of cirrhosis as well as in the aetiology of overt diabetes.

Insulin secretion in non-diabetic cirrhotics (see Chapter 2.11)

Non-diabetic cirrhotics have increased insulin responses to glucose, and to secretagogues such as arginine and sulphonylureas. The insulin hypersecretion appears to be due to an increase in the maximal secretory capacity (Kruszynska, Hepatol, 1995; 22:238A) and is thus similar to the islet adaptation found in normoglycaemic insulin-resistant obese subjects (Beard, JClinEndoc, 1987; 65:59). Cirrhotics with high insulin secretion rates to intravenous glucose have better oral and intravenous glucose tolerance than cirrhotics with 'normal' secretion rates.[3,12]

For normal glucose tolerance, both the total amount of insulin secreted and the timing are important (Bruce, Diabetes, 1988; 37: 736; Mitrakou, NEJM, 1992; 326:22). Insulin secretion is normally much higher after oral than intravenous glucose (McIntyre, JClinEndoc, 1965; 25:1317; Shapiro, Diabetes, 1987; 36:1365). This 'incretin' effect of oral glucose is due in part to release of glucose-dependent insulinotropic peptide and glucagon-like peptide-1 [7–36 amide] from the gut during glucose absorption (Kreymann, Lancet, 1987; ii:1300; Creutzfeldt, DiabetMetabRev, 1992; 8:149; Nauck, JClinEndoc, 1993; 76:912). These gut hormones may also be important for augmenting the early insulin response to oral glucose (i.e. before a marked increase in plasma glucose levels)[14] (Nauck, Diabetolog, 1986; 29:46). Cirrhotics show less enhancement of insulin secretion with oral glucose relative to the intravenous route, and by contrast with normal subjects show a good correlation between insulin secretion rates after oral and intravenous glucose.[12] Many have a blunted early C-peptide response to oral glucose[11,12,14] (Johnston, Lancet, 1977; i:10) which may contribute to their glucose intolerance (see Chapter 2.11).

The reduced 'incretin effect' and blunted early C-peptide response is not due to reduced secretion of glucose-dependent insulinotropic peptide and glucagon-like peptide-1 [7–36 amide];

fasting levels of both are higher in cirrhotics than controls, and both rise to higher levels after oral glucose[14] (McDonald, Metabolism, 1979; 28:300). It is possible that some cirrhotics are resistant to the action of these gut hormones. A parasympathetic autonomic neuropathy which is common in cirrhosis (Thuluvath, QJMed, 1989; 72:737) could also explain the blunted early insulin response to oral glucose; insulin secretion is delayed and glucose tolerance impaired after truncal vagotomy (Humphrey, BMJ, 1975; 2:112).

Most studies have contained many alcoholic cirrhotics. Chronic alcohol abuse may result in a reversible impairment of insulin secretion (Sereny, Metabolism, 1978; 27:1041); it may also be associated with significant hyperinsulinaemia in the absence of cirrhosis or impaired glucose tolerance (Nyboe Andersen, Metabolism, 1983; 32:1029). However, the insulin secretory abnormalities are not confined to alcoholic cirrhotics (Megyesi, Lancet, 1967; ii:1051; Iwasaki, JClinEndoc, 1978; 47:774). Furthermore, they may be found in patients who have abstained from alcohol for many months or years. The possibility that the abnormality is secondary to malnutrition (Pezarossa, Metabolism, 1986; 35:984) or potassium depletion (Podolsky, NEJM, 1973; 288:644) should also be considered, as correction of these abnormalities may improve glucose tolerance (see also Chapter 2.11).

Insulin secretion in diabetic cirrhotics

Diabetic cirrhotics (i.e. with fasting hyperglycaemia) have a marked impairment of insulin secretion to oral and intravenous glucose[3] (Kruszynska, Metabolism, 1995; 44:254) (Figs 1 and 2). More of their serum immunoreactive insulin is due to proinsulin and its derivative des–31,32-proinsulin, which may account for up to 15 per cent of measured 'insulin' (Kruszynska, Metabolism, 1995; 44:254). Insulin secretion in response to a sustained intravenous glucose stimulus is normally biphasic, a rapid rise in insulin within 1 to 3 min of a rise in glucose level (first phase), followed by a return to baseline by 6 to 10 min, and then a gradual increase (second phase). Once the fasting blood glucose rises above 6.7 mmol/l, cirrhotics lose their first–phase insulin response to an intravenous glucose stimulus,[3] they may have a prompt insulin response to other secretagogues such as intravenous tolbutamide or arginine, although this is lower than in non–diabetic cirrhotics[3] (Fig. 2). More marked fasting hyperglycaemia is associated with loss of the insulin response to intravenous tolbutamide as well. Measurement of insulin and C-peptide during sequential hyperglycaemic clamps at 12, 19, and 28 mmol/l glucose, and in response to a maximally stimulating dose of arginine at each of these glucose levels, suggested a marked decrease in maximal insulin secretory capacity (Kruszynska, Hepatol, 1995; 22:238A). Cirrhotics with little insulin response to non-glucose secretagogues require insulin for control of their diabetes, whereas those with a good insulin response to tolbutamide can usually be well controlled on sulphonylureas.

The genesis of diabetes mellitus in cirrhosis

Insulin resistance is not sufficient for the development of overt diabetes in cirrhosis. A defect of insulin secretion is also required. This is very similar to findings in type II diabetes. In some patients this defect of insulin secretion (see above) may arise from alcoholic damage to the pancreas, in which case diabetes may develop in the absence of significant liver disease or peripheral tissue insulin resistance. However, alcoholic pancreatic damage probably accounts for only a small proportion of cirrhotic patients who develop diabetes because most of these patients have hyperglucagonaemia, fasting and in response to arginine (see below); alcoholic pancreatic damage characteristically causes impaired glucagon secretion (Sjoberg, DiabetCare, 1989; 12:715; Larsen, ActaEnd, 1991; 124:510). Insulin deficiency may also be due to autoimmune destruction of islet β-cells (type I diabetes) or to pancreatic islet iron deposition and islet β-cell loss in patients with haemochromatosis (Rahier, Diabetolog, 1987; 30:5). Most patients with cirrhosis who develop diabetes probably have a genetic predisposition to type II diabetes. The higher prevalence of diabetes in cirrhotics with a family history of diabetes supports this view.[7] The abnormalities of insulin secretion found in diabetic cirrhotic patients are very similar to those found in patients with type II diabetes mellitus.

Prospective studies of normoglycaemic first-degree relatives of type II diabetic patients, and studies in some populations at high risk for type II diabetes, have shown that insulin resistance and hyperinsulinaemia in non-diabetic subjects are predictive of subsequent diabetes (Taylor, Diabetes, 1994; 43:735; Lillioja, NEJM, 1993; 329:1988). It is thought that insulin resistance induces a compensatory increase in insulin secretion and hyperinsulinaemia to maintain normal glucose metabolism but that diabetes eventually develops when insulin secretion becomes impaired. It is not clear whether normal islets can fail after prolonged insulin resistance or whether a coexistent islet defect is necessary. The finding of subtle abnormalities of insulin secretion in non-diabetic relatives of type II diabetic patients supports the latter hypothesis (Taylor, Diabetes, 1994; 43:735; Polonsky, Diabetes, 1995; 44:705). It would seem that as in type II diabetes, insulin insensitivity in patients with cirrhosis eventually leads to islet β-cell failure in those with a genetic predisposition to diabetes. Other factors, such as the effects of alcohol or cytokine production on pancreatic islet function, may also be important.

Management of diabetes in patients with liver disease

There have been no controlled studies of the short- and long-term benefits of different treatment regimes for patients with cirrhosis who also have diabetes, and there is a need for studies in this area. Patients with hyperglycaemia of sufficient severity to cause symptoms clearly require control of their diabetes. Diabetic cirrhotics with a good long-term prognosis are at risk of long-term microvascular and macrovascular complications of diabetes. There are no good data on the prevalence of these complications in cirrhotics with overt diabetes. In a study of 72 patients with diabetes and haemochromatosis aged 20 to 70 years (mean 48 years), 12 (14 per cent) had a history of ischaemic heart disease compared to two of 43 patients with haemochromatosis without diabetes (4.7 per cent) (Dymock, AmJMed, 1972; 52:203). Diabetic retinopathy is common in diabetic haemochromatotic patients (Griffiths, Diabetes, 1971; 20:766), and nephropathy and neuropathy also occur. Diabetic complications are also frequent in patients who have autoimmune liver disease and insulin-dependent diabetes. Retinopathy, neuropathy, nephropathy, and macrovascular disease (ischaemic heart disease/strokes) are seen in diabetic patients who develop cirrhosis, but these complications appear to be uncommon in cirrhotics who develop diabetes. It may be that the natural history of cirrhosis is such that there may be insufficient time for the development of these complications. Kingston *et al.* (Gastro, 1984; 87:688), in a study of 49 diabetic cirrhotics (mainly due to hepatitis B), found neuropathy in 37 per cent and background retinopathy in 18 per cent. An angiographic study found a 27 per cent prevalence of moderate or severe coronary artery disease in 37 patients over the age of 50 with endstage liver disease undergoing liver transplantation; diabetes was the most important risk factor (Carey, Transpl, 1995; 59:859). The incidence of renal dysfunction after liver transplantation may be greater in diabetic patients (Trail, Surgery, 1993; 114:650). Thus, with more patients being considered for liver transplantation more attention needs to be given to the prevention of these long-term complications of diabetes.

Diabetic patients undergoing liver transplantation have an increased risk of bacterial and fungal infections (Wahlstrom, Transpl-Proc, 1991; 23:1565; Trail, Surgery, 1993; 114:650). Good diabetic control should diminish this risk. In patients with severe liver disease who are not candidates for liver transplantation, the risk of long-term diabetic micro- and macrovascular complications is not a primary consideration. However, there are good reasons for attempting to achieve good glycaemic control. First, diabetes will be associated with enhanced mobilization of adipose tissue fatty acids, and increased muscle protein catabolism, as well as impaired tissue glucose utilization and hyperglycaemia. Thus decreased effective tissue insulinization might play a major role in the asthenia and tissue wasting that are prominent features in many patients with chronic liver disease. Secondly, poorly controlled diabetes will predispose to infection, particularly fungal infection.

Many cirrhotics have a normal fasting blood glucose level but a 2 h blood glucose after oral glucose consistent with a diagnosis of diabetes according to WHO criteria.[1] Serum insulin levels in these patients are often very high, due to a combination of delayed hypersecretion and decreased clearance. Symptomatic reactive hypoglycaemia 3 to 4 h after an oral glucose load is common in this group. At present there is no evidence that these patients will benefit from attempts to lower their postprandial blood glucose levels, although those with reactive hypoglycaemia will respond to dietary measures.

Patients with postprandial hyperglycaemia and only minor increases of fasting blood glucose concentration should be treated initially by a trial of diet. Since decreased tissue sensitivity to insulin and impaired insulin secretion are associated with diets in which the carbohydrate content is restricted to below 40 per cent of energy, it is recommended that the carbohydrate intake should be between 45 and 55 per cent of energy as tolerated. This should be in the form of complexed carbohydrates with low glycaemic indices and rich in soluble fibre. Foods such as pulses, oats, barley, and pasta are recommended. Small quantities of sucrose (less than 30 g/day) may be permitted as part of a mixed meal, but should be avoided in the form of rapidly absorbed drinks. Such a high carbohydrate/low glycaemic index diet, rich in soluble fibre, has been shown to lower the glucose and insulin responses to meals in cirrhotic patients (Jenkins, AmJGastr, 1987; 82:223; Jenkins, AmJGastr, 1989; 84:732). The diet should be low in saturated fat (less than 10 per cent of total energy), and with a polyunsaturated/saturated fatty acid ratio of 1.0 or more. The intake of total fat should be about 30 to 35 per cent of total energy. In countries where the intake of olive oil is traditionally high, a higher intake of fat is permissible, providing this is in the form of mono- and polyunsaturated fatty acids. These recommendations with respect to the lipid composition of the diet, as well as being associated with decreased cholesterol and triglyceride levels in diabetic patients, may also improve glycaemic control, perhaps by increasing the sensitivity to insulin.

In the event of dietary failure (persistent postprandial blood glucose elevation with levels of 6.0 mmol/l or greater before the next meal) consideration should be given to additional measures. The two options available are treatment with an oral hypoglycaemic agent or with insulin. Since about 55 to 60 per cent of the digestible carbohydrates in modern Western diets are in the form of polysaccharides (starch), inhibitors of small intestinal α-glucosidases, such as acarbose, may be tried to delay carbohydrate absorption. These agents have no effect on fasting blood glucose levels but cause a dose-dependent reduction in postprandial blood glucose and insulin levels. Side-effects including flatulence, diarrhoea, and abdominal pain are dose-dependent but tend to diminish with time. Treatment should be started with small doses (25 mg with each of the three main meals). Acarbose has little effect on the blood glucose response to ingestion of monosaccharides and disaccharides, and it is important therefore that patients adhere to the dietary guidelines discussed above (i.e. intake of complexed carbohydrate) if acarbose is to be effective.

Biguanides (metformin) should be avoided in patients with liver disease, particularly those who are at risk of acute complications (bleeding, renal impairment, sepsis) because of the risk of lactic acidosis. Sulphonylureas are generally well tolerated but should be used cautiously especially in alcoholic patients and in patients with inadequate and erratic food intake. Hypoglycaemia is the most important adverse effect. As most sulphonylureas are metabolized by the liver their plasma half-life may be considerably prolonged, thus increasing the risk of hypoglycaemia. Although glibenclamide has a plasma half-life of only 2 to 3 h, it is an important cause of prolonged hypoglycaemia (2–3 days) with a risk similar to that of chlorpropamide (Ferner, BMJ, 1988; 296:949). Fatal cases have been reported with doses as low as 2.5 mg/day. The reasons for the prolonged hypoglycaemic effect of glibenclamide are unclear, but it may be due to an uncharacterized active metabolite or accumulation of the drug in pancreatic islets. The very slow intestinal absorption of the drug will also result in prolonged exposure. Glibenclamide is thus best avoided in patients with liver disease.

Tolbutamide and glipizide, which are both short acting, rapidly absorbed, and have a low risk of hypoglycaemia when used in standard doses, are probably the sulphonylureas of choice in patients with liver disease. Tolbutamide has a short duration of action (6–10 h), but may aggravate the tendency to water retention; glipizide or gliclazide (both longer acting) are alternatives that are usually well tolerated.

The decision to start insulin, when sulphonylureas are ineffective or poorly tolerated, will depend on the therapeutic targets set for any particular patient. Good self-monitoring of blood glucose concentration is of paramount importance. As fasting blood glucose concentrations are often only modestly raised, these patients may be best managed by a regime of multiple injections of a short-acting insulin 30 to 45 min before each main meal; an intermediate-acting insulin may then be introduced before the evening meal or at bedtime in accordance with the blood glucose response. Patients with liver disease appear to be more prone to fasting and nocturnal hypoglycaemia in association with intermediate-acting insulins. However, this is poorly documented in formal clinical studies. Also unclear is the extent to which hormonal and physiological counterregulatory mechanisms are disturbed in patients with liver disease and whether the glucose threshold for development of neuroglycopenic symptoms is affected by coexistent liver disease. Studies addressing these issues would help in the clinical management of these patients.

Glucagon

Fasting plasma glucagon levels are increased two- to sixfold in cirrhotic patients and they show a greater rise in glucagon levels after intravenous arginine (Marco, NEJM, 1973; 28:1107; Kruszynska, Hepatol, 1995; 22:441A) and in response to a protein meal (Marchesini, Gastro, 1983; 85:283). Extremely high plasma glucagon levels may be found in patients with fulminant hepatic failure (Vilstrup, EurJClinInv, 1986; 16:193). Unlike insulin, glucagon is cleared mainly by the kidney (Sherwin, JCI, 1976; 57:722; Bastl, AmJPhysiol, 1977; 233:F67; Jaspan, Diabetes, 1977; 26:887); the portal:peripheral glucagon concentration ratio is much lower than for insulin (Blackard, Diabetes, 1974; 23:199) and it has been estimated that first-pass hepatic glucagon extraction is only about 15 to 25 per cent (Sherwin, Gastro, 1978; 74:1224; Jaspan, AmJPhysiol, 1981; 240:E233). Thus, while diminished glucagon clearance might contribute to the higher fasting plasma glucagon levels in cirrhotics, it cannot (given the low first-pass hepatic extraction of glucagon) explain the greater rise in glucagon levels that is seen within 5 min of an intravenous arginine bolus. In keeping with the lower hepatic extraction ratio for glucagon than for insulin, Sherwin et al. (Gastro, 1978; 74:1224) showed that the metabolic clearance rate of infused glucagon was normal in cirrhotics with and without portacaval shunts, and they concluded that the hyperglucagonaemia of cirrhosis was due to increased glucagon secretion. However, plasma glucagon levels were higher in their patients with surgical portocaval shunts or large varices on endoscopy than in patients without evidence of portal systemic shunting, who had normal glucagon levels. An increase in glucagon levels in cirrhotics after portacaval anastomosis was also reported by Dudley et al. (Gut, 1979; 20:817). These observations led to the idea that portosystemic shunting in cirrhosis is the major factor that leads to increased pancreatic glucagon secretion and hyperglucagonaemia. Studies in rats would support this view: hyperglucagonaemia due to increased glucagon secretion develops after portal vein ligation (Sikuler, AmJPhysiol, 1987; 253: G110) or portacaval anastomosis (Kravetz, AmJPhysiol, 1987; 252: G257) in the absence of cirrhosis. However, normal glucagon levels were found in non-cirrhotic patients with portal vein block and extensive collaterals or surgical portosystemic shunts (Smith-Laing, Diabetolog, 1980; 19:103), and some consider hepatocellular function to be the major determinant of increased plasma glucagon levels (Smith-Laing, Diabetolog, 1980; 19:103; Kabadi, AmJGastr, 1984; 79:715; Lewis, JLabClinMed, 1991; 117:67).

Plasma glucagon levels in normal subjects are suppressed after glucose ingestion or during an intravenous glucose infusion. Both hyperglycaemia and hyperinsulinaemia mediate this suppression. The acute glucagon response to intravenous arginine is also progressively attenuated as plasma glucose (and hence insulin) levels are raised. In cirrhotic patients this regulation of basal and stimulated glucagon levels by glucose and insulin is disturbed. In response to oral glucose ingestion, or a moderate increase in plasma glucose levels achieved by intravenous glucose administration, the fall in plasma glucagon levels is often less than in controls despite higher insulin and glucose levels (Dudley, Gut, 1979; 20:817; Greco, Diabetolog, 1979; 17:23; McDonald, Metabolism, 1979; 28:300; Kruszynska, Hepatol, 1995; 22:441A).

Failure to achieve complete suppression of plasma glucagon levels by hyperglycaemia in many of the earlier studies may have been due in part to an increased contribution of enteroglucagon (molecular weight of approximately 9000 Da) to plasma immunoreactive glucagon in cirrhosis (Dudley, Gut, 1979; 20:817). Enteroglucagon cross-reacts in many glucagon assays and does not undergo acute changes in response to changes in blood glucose concentration or when glucagon secretion is stimulated by amino acids. However, even when a specific antiglucagon antibody is used, impaired suppression of glucagon levels by hyperglycaemia is found (Kruszynska, Hepatol, 1995; 22:441A). Complete suppression of fasting glucagon levels can be achieved at very high glucose levels (c. 28 mmol/l); however, while there is a progressive decrease in the acute glucagon response to arginine with increasing glucose concentrations, the acute response to intravenous arginine remains higher than in normal subjects even when measured at a blood glucose concentration of 28 mmol/l (Kruszynska, Hepatol, 1995; 22:441A).

Fasting and stimulated glucagon levels may be much higher in diabetic cirrhotic patients than in matched non-diabetic cirrhotics (McDonald, Metabolism, 1979; 28:300; Kruszynska, Hepatol, 1995; 22:441A). Suppression of basal plasma glucagon levels, and the acute glucagon response to intravenous arginine by hyperglycaemia is markedly impaired in diabetic cirrhotics (Kruszynska, Hepatol, 1995; 22:441A). Impaired insulin secretion and chronic hyperglycaemia could explain the more marked abnormalities of glucagon secretion in the diabetic cirrhotics by comparison with cirrhotics without diabetes, as similar abnormalities are found in those with type II diabetes mellitus, in whom they are improved by insulin therapy (Muller, NEJM, 1970; 283:109; Raskin, AmJMed, 1978; 64:988).

The mechanism for increased glucagon secretion in cirrhosis is unclear. Glucagon secretion is increased in non-diabetic cirrhotics despite increased circulating levels of insulin,[2-5,8-14] somatostatin (Verrillo, Metabolism, 1986; 35:130), and glucagon-like peptide-1 [7-36 amide][14] which, together with glucose, are the main inhibitors of islet α-cell glucagon secretion. However, gastric inhibitory polypeptide levels are increased in cirrhosis[14] (McDonald, Metabolism, 1979; 28:300), and in cirrhosis the glucagon-secreting α-cells may be more sensitive to the stimulatory effects of gastric inhibitory polypeptide (Dupre, JClinEndoc, 1991; 72:125). The enhanced glucagon secretion has also been attributed to increased ammonia levels in cirrhosis. Marchesini et al. (DigDis, 1982; 27:406) reported increased plasma glucagon levels in cirrhotics after intravenous administration of ammonium salts, but no such increase was found by others (Doffoel, GastrClinBiol, 1981; 5: 1087). Although fasting glucagon levels correlate with plasma ammonia levels, Kabadi and colleagues suggested that the increased glucagon levels may in part explain the elevated plasma ammonia levels rather than vice versa (Gastro, 1985; 88:750). Another theory put forward to explain glucagon hypersecretion in cirrhosis or liver failure is deficiency of a factor produced by the liver that normally inhibits glucagon secretion by islet α-cells (Kabadi, DiabetRes, 1993; 23:41). Secretion of this factor is believed to increase with increasing liver glycogen content (Kabadi, DiabetRes, 1993; 23:41). However, the further enhancement of glucagon secretion in cirrhosis by the presence of diabetes does not support this hypothesis because diabetic patients (normal or cirrhotic) characteristically have increased liver glycogen content, particularly when poorly controlled (see Chapter 24.6).

The significance of the abnormalities of glucagon secretion for hepatic glucose and amino acid metabolism in cirrhosis is unclear. Cirrhotic patients appear relatively resistant to the effects of glucagon: the rise in plasma cyclic AMP and glucose (Feruglio, ClinSci, 1966; 30:43; Francavilla, Gastro, 1978; 75:1026; Keller, JClinEndoc, 1982; 54:961; Petrides, Metabolism, 1994; 43:85) and hepatic glucose output in response to intravenous glucagon are impaired (see Chapter 2.11). Furthermore, in cirrhosis there is impaired stimulation of gluconeogenesis (Sherwin, Gastro, 1978; 74:1224) and urea synthesis (Fabbri, Hepatol, 1993; 18:28) by glucagon, and resistance to its haemodynamic effects (Pak, JHepatol, 1994; 20:825). While low hepatic glycogen stores may account for a smaller output of glucose from the liver in response to an intravenous bolus or infusion of glucagon, chronically elevated glucagon levels may also impair the acute response through downregulation of glucagon receptors (Bhathena, JCI, 1978; 61:1488; Soman, Nature, 1978; 272: 829; Authier, Endocrinol, 1992; 131:447) and postreceptor signalling mechanisms (Honge, MolEndocrin, 1990; 4:481). Increased basal glucagon levels may be necessary for maintenance of normal fasting glucose levels in cirrhosis (Chapter 2.11) but do not appear to play a role in glucose intolerance. This may not be true in overtly diabetic cirrhotics in whom increased glucagon secretion and lack of suppression by hyperglycaemia may contribute to their impaired suppression of hepatic glucose production and hyperglycaemia (Del Prato, JCI, 1987; 79:547; Petrides, Hepatol, 1994; 19:616). These issues are discussed in Chapter 2.11. The role of glucagon in the splanchnic hyperaemia and portal hypertension of cirrhosis is discussed in Chapter 7.2.

Growth hormone
Normal physiology

Growth hormone is a polypeptide of 191 amino acids in humans (molecular weight 21 500). About 5 to 15 per cent of circulating growth hormone is due to a biologically less-active 176 amino acid isoform. Secretion of growth hormone from the anterior pituitary is under the influence of hypothalamic regulatory peptides (Fig. 3). Growth hormone releasing hormone increases growth hormone synthesis and release; somatostatin inhibits growth hormone release. A number of other peptides synthesized and released from the hypothalamus may also stimulate growth hormone secretion, independently of growth hormone releasing hormone, by interacting with specific receptors on the pituitary somatotrophs, but their physiological role is at present unclear. Insulin-like growth factors which mediate many of the growth effects of growth hormone inhibit both the hypothalamic release of growth hormone releasing hormone and the pituitary response to this peptide, thus providing a feedback control of growth hormone secretion. In this respect

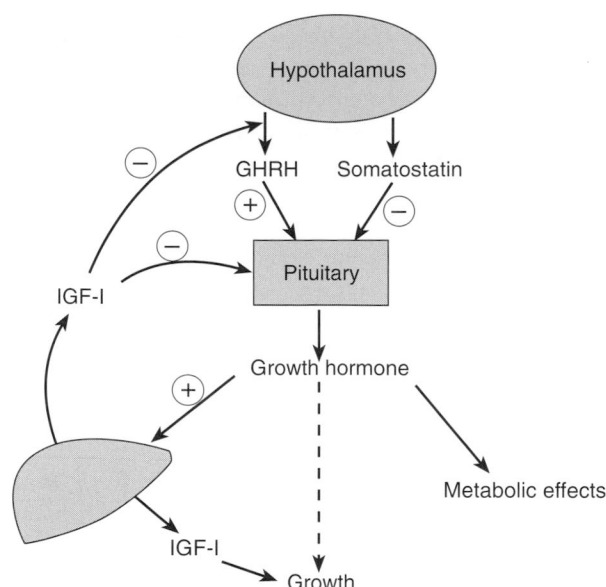

Fig. 3. Growth hormone (GH) secretion is regulated by hypothalamic hormones: somatostatin inhibits and growth hormone releasing hormone (GHRH) stimulates GH secretion. The growth effects of GH are mostly indirect and mediated via insulin-like growth factor-I (IGF-I). The liver is the main source of circulating IGF-I. IGF-I inhibits GH secretion by inhibiting the release of GHRH and the pituitary response to this peptide. GH secretion is enhanced by stress, exercise, hypoglycaemia, and certain amino acids, and inhibited by increased levels of fatty acids, ketone bodies, and glucose. Increased GH levels in liver disease may partly be due to impaired IGF-I production. GH has direct metabolic effects. Many of these are 'anti-insulin'. The high GH levels in cirrhosis may contribute to insulin resistance.

insulin-like growth factor-I is considerably more potent than insulin-like growth factor-II. Growth hormone itself stimulates somatostatin release from the hypothalamus and increases local pituitary production of insulin-like growth factor-I, thus providing possible short-loop autocrine or paracrine feedback control of its own secretion. Many neuropeptides, neurotransmitters, peripheral hormones, and metabolites modulate growth hormone secretion. It is stimulated by stress, fasting, exercise, hypoglycaemia, and certain amino acids, especially arginine. A rapid fall in plasma levels also stimulates growth hormone release. Conversely, growth hormone secretion is suppressed in normal individuals by a glucose load, and by elevated plasma non-esterified fatty acid levels. Thyroid hormones play an important role in the regulation of growth hormone synthesis and secretion; growth hormone responses to hypoglycaemia, sleep, and arginine are impaired in patients with hypothyroidism. High levels of corticosteroids also impair growth hormone secretion, possibly by increasing hypothalamic release of somatostatin.

Growth hormone secretion is pulsatile with a periodicity of 3 to 4 h. Between pulses, serum growth hormone falls with a half-life of approximately 15 to 20 min to very low levels (<0.5 mU/l (<0.25 μg/l)). Physiological modulation of growth hormone secretion is achieved by variation in the amplitude rather than the frequency of pulses, although both amplitude and frequency increase at puberty and decline after the age of 40 years. Pulses are higher during the first part of the night during deep sleep, so that about two-thirds of growth hormone secretion occurs during the 12-hour overnight period. The liver, and to a lesser extent the kidney, are the main sites of growth hormone clearance, although there is some uncertainty as to their relative contributions. Hepatic growth hormone clearance is receptor mediated; about 10 to 20 per cent of the growth hormone delivered to the liver is removed during a single trans-hepatic passage. Estimates of the contribution of the liver to total growth hormone clearance vary between 50 and 95 per cent (Bratusch-Marrain, EurJClinInv, 1979; 9:257; Taylor, JClinEndoc, 1972; 34:395).

Growth hormone in serum associates with a specific high-affinity binding protein, which is identical to the extracellular domain of the growth hormone receptor, from which it is derived (in man) by proteolytic cleavage (Baumann, Nutrition, 1993; 9:546). Since the liver is the tissue with the highest abundance of growth hormone receptors, the liver is also the major source of growth hormone binding protein, and plasma growth hormone binding protein levels reflect hepatic growth hormone receptor status. In contrast to the marked variations in growth hormone concentrations due to pulsatile secretion, growth hormone binding protein levels are relatively constant (Snow, JClinEndoc, 1990; 70:417; Ho, ClinEndoc, 1993; 38:143). Normally, serum growth hormone binding protein concentrations are similar to basal growth hormone levels and some 30 to 50 per cent of circulating growth hormone is bound. The molecular size of the growth hormone–growth hormone binding protein complex (80–85 kDa) prevents glomerular filtration and limits the extravascular distribution of growth hormone. In addition, growth hormone binding protein competes with cellular receptors for growth hormone binding (Mannor, JClinEndoc, 1991; 73:30; Amit, Metabolism, 1992; 41:732). Thus, growth hormone binding protein serves to delay growth hormone clearance and dampen the marked oscillations in plasma growth hormone levels (Baumann, JClinEndoc, 1987; 64:657). There is effective transfer of growth hormone from growth hormone binding protein to hepatic growth hormone receptors because the affinity of growth hormone binding protein for growth hormone is much lower than that of the growth hormone receptor (Baumann, Nutrition, 1993; 9:546); high growth hormone binding protein levels actually enhance the hepatic effects of growth hormone *in vivo* (for example, insulin-like growth factor-I production and hence growth) by prolonging plasma growth hormone half-life (Mannor, JClinEndoc, 1991; 73:30; Veldhuis, JCI, 1993; 91:629). The effect of growth hormone binding protein levels on growth hormone actions in peripheral tissues that have few growth hormone receptors (Martini, Endocrinol, 1995; 136:1355) is unclear.

Many of the growth promoting effects of growth hormone are mediated by insulin-like growth factor-I and -II, although it also has direct effects on cartilage and bone. Its anabolic actions on protein, amino acid, and nitrogen metabolism (Chapter 2.13) are both direct and via insulin-like growth factor-I. By contrast, the 'insulin-antagonistic' metabolic effects, which serve to shift fuel utilization away from glucose towards fat, are due to direct effects of growth hormone on skeletal muscle, adipose tissue, and hepatic metabolism. The role of growth hormone in the insulin resistance and glucose intolerance of patients with liver disease is discussed in Chapter 2.11.

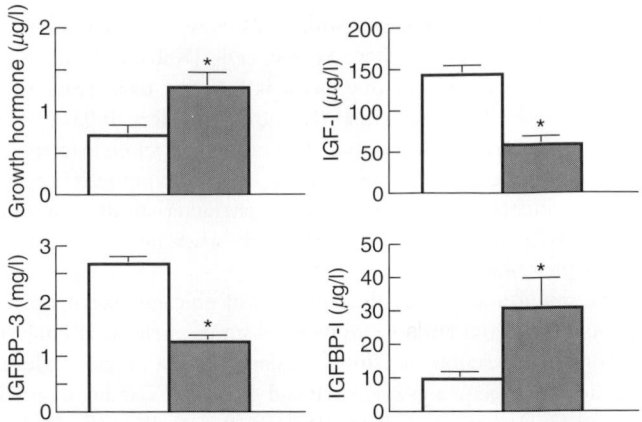

Fig. 4. Fasting arterial plasma growth hormone, insulin-like growth factor-I (IGF-I), and insulin-like growth factor binding proteins-1 and -3 (IGFBP-1 and -3) in 22 cirrhotic patients ■ (19 alcoholic, three post-hepatitic; Child's grading: A = 6, B = 10, C = 6), and 27 normal subjects □ matched for age and sex. Mean ± SEM. *, $p < 0.001$ versus controls. (Data from ref. 15 with permission.)

Disturbances of growth hormone in liver disease

Basal and mean daily growth hormone levels are increased in cirrhosis[15–17] (Samaan, ArchIntMed, 1969; 124:149; Caufriez, JEndocrInv, 1991; 14:317) (Fig. 4). Increased growth hormone levels may also be found in patients with acute viral hepatitis (Hernandez, JLabClinMed, 1969; 73:25; Record, ClinSciMolMed, 1975; 49:473), chronic active hepatitis (Becker, Lancet, 1969; ii: 1035), and in patients with schistosomal hepatic fibrosis and marked portal hypertension (Assaad, Metabolism, 1990; 39:349). The diurnal pattern of serum growth hormone is markedly disturbed in patients with cirrhosis, due primarily to an increased frequency of growth hormone pulses;[17] pulse amplitude may also be increased in some patients[17] (Stewart, EurJClinInv, 1983; 13:397; Kruszynska, unpublished observations). Daytime secretion in cirrhotics accounts for a larger proportion of total daily growth hormone secretion.

Many patients with cirrhosis have a paradoxical increase in serum growth hormone levels in response to an oral glucose load (Samaan, ArchIntMed, 1969; 124:149; Shankar, HormMetRes, 1988; 20:579); stimulation of growth hormone secretion may also be seen in response to an intravenous bolus of thyrotrophin releasing hormone (Zanoboni, JClinEndoc, 1977; 45:576; Salerno, HormMetRes, 1982; 14:482; Assaad, Metabolism, 1990; 39:349) which does not normally elicit a rise in growth hormone levels. These responses of serum growth hormone to oral glucose and thyrotrophin releasing hormone are similar to those found in many patients with acromegaly, and in patients with poorly controlled diabetes (Vierhapper, HormMetRes, 1983; 15:4). Samaan *et al.* (ArchIntMed, 1969; 124:149) suggested that a paradoxical rise in growth hormone after glucose ingestion was more likely in cirrhotic patients with impaired glucose tolerance than in those with normal glucose tolerance. However, in the study of Conn and Daughaday (JLabClinMed, 1970; 76:678) a paradoxical growth hormone response to oral glucose was no more likely in the cirrhotics with overt diabetes than in those with normal or impaired glucose tolerance, though the number of patients studied was small. The growth hormone response to arginine and insulin-induced hypoglycaemia in cirrhotics may be exaggerated (Muggeo, ArchIntMed, 1979; 139:1157), normal (Shankar, HormMetRes, 1988; 20:579), or reduced.[18] Caution is required in the interpretation of the two studies reporting a normal or subnormal growth hormone response to insulin-induced hypoglycaemia[18] (Shankar, HormMetRes, 1988; 20:579) because an equivalent hypoglycaemic stimulus was not achieved due to insulin resistance in the cirrhotics. The increase in growth hormone levels after glucose ingestion may contribute to the markedly disturbed daytime growth hormone levels (Stewart, EurJClinInv, 1983; 13:397). In chronic alcoholic patients without significant liver disease, the growth hormone response to insulin-induced hypoglycaemia may be impaired (Chalmers, BMJ, 1978; I: 748) returning to normal with abstinence.

The aetiology of the increased basal growth hormone levels and abnormal growth hormone responses to glucose and other stimuli in cirrhosis is unclear. In general, higher serum growth hormone levels are found in patients with liver disease who have established cirrhosis (Becker, Lancet, 1969; ii:1035; Hernandez, JLabClinMed, 1969; 73:25). Cuneo et al.[17] found higher mean daily growth hormone secretion rates in cirrhotics with poor liver function as assessed by Child–Pugh score but in most other studies growth hormone levels did not correlate with severity of liver disease[16] (Baruch, JClinEndoc, 1991; 73:777; Caufriez, JEndocrInv, 1991; 14: 317).

Impaired hepatic production and low circulating insulin-like growth factor-I levels[15-17,19] (Wu, JLabClinMed, 1988; 112: 589) (Fig. 4), resulting in impaired feedback inhibition of growth hormone secretion, are probably the most important factors in the increased growth hormone secretion in cirrhosis. In men with marked feminization associated with portosystemic shunting, oestrogens may contribute to the abnormal growth hormone secretory patterns, since in women growth hormone pulses are more frequent and their basal growth hormone levels higher (Bertherat, EurJEndocr, 1995; 132:12; Ho, HormRes, 1996; 45:67).

Hepatic growth hormone resistance

Low hepatic insulin-like growth factor-I production despite increased circulating growth hormone levels implies hepatic resistance to growth hormone in patients with liver disease[15-17] (Bucuvalas, JPediat, 1990; 117:397; Buzzelli, AmJGastr, 1993; 88:1744). There is little evidence that decreased hepatocyte mass *per se* plays a role in the impaired insulin-like growth factor-I production. As discussed below, many factors, particularly nutritional state and insulin, affect the hepatic insulin-like growth factor-I response to growth hormone. Protein–calorie malnutrition and insulin deficiency induce hepatic resistance to growth hormone by reducing the number of hepatic growth hormone receptors and by postreceptor mechanisms (Maes, Endocrinol, 1986; 118:377; Straus, MolEndocrin, 1990; 4:91; Thissen, EndocrRev, 1994; 15:80). Malnutrition is common in patients with chronic liver disease and could contribute to the hepatic resistance to growth hormone. Although systemic insulin levels are high in patients with cirrhosis, portosystemic shunting and sinusoidal capillarization may result in relative hepatic hypoinsulinaemia. Since portal insulin delivery seems

to be important for a normal insulin-like growth factor-I response to growth hormone (Russell-Jones, JMolEndocr, 1992; 9:257), hepatic hypoinsulinaemia could contribute to hepatic growth hormone resistance. Plasma growth hormone binding protein levels, which reflect hepatic growth hormone receptor status, are a major determinant of the response to a given dose of growth hormone (Martha, JClinEndoc, 1992; 75:1464). Growth hormone binding protein levels are reduced in cirrhosis[17] (Baruch, JClinEndoc, 1991; 73:777; Hattori, Metabolism, 1992; 41:377) and reduced growth hormone receptor expression has been found in cirrhotic liver (Chang, Hepatol, 1990; 11:123). Thus, hepatic resistance to the effects of growth hormone in terms of insulin-like growth factor-I production may partly be due to fewer growth hormone receptors.

Abnormalities of growth hormone action may contribute to the stunted growth seen in young patients with chronic liver disease. Children with Alagille syndrome (chronic cholestasis associated with a paucity of interlobular bile ducts, characteristic facies, skeletal and cardiac abnormalities (Alagille, JPediat, 1987; 110:195; Chapter 23.3) frequently show growth retardation in the absence of malnutrition. There is evidence that resistance to growth hormone may contribute to their growth disturbance. Children with Alagille syndrome have high serum growth hormone and growth hormone binding protein levels but their insulin-like growth factor-I levels are very low, and similar to those found in growth hormone deficient children. Unlike growth hormone deficient children, serum insulin-like growth factor-I levels do not increase when growth-retarded children with Alagille syndrome are treated with recombinant human growth hormone (Bucuvalas, JClinEndoc, 1993; 76:1477). This impairment in the insulin-like growth factor-I response to growth hormone is similar to that seen in cirrhosis but is found when liver synthetic function is good and in the absence of portal hypertension.

Growth hormone clearance in cirrhosis

Although the liver plays an important role in growth hormone metabolism, evidence for delayed growth hormone clearance in cirrhosis is inconclusive. Owens et al. (EurJClinInv, 1973; 3:284) found a lower growth hormone metabolic clearance rate in a very heterogeneous group of patients with liver disease, half of whom had ascites which might well have influenced the calculation of kinetic parameters. Others have reported normal total and hepatic growth hormone clearance in cirrhotics with advanced liver disease[15] (Taylor, JClinEndoc, 1972; 34:395). The fractional hepatic extraction of growth hormone may be enhanced when growth hormone levels increase, for example in response to an infusion of arginine or with exercise (Bratusch-Marrain, EurJClinInv, 1979; 9: 257). This increase in hepatic growth hormone uptake is not explained by changes in hepatic plasma flow. The most likely explanation is an increase in the proportion of free growth hormone with increasing plasma levels because of partial saturation of growth hormone binding protein at growth hormone levels above 20 mU/l (10 µg/l) (Baumann, Nutrition, 1993; 9:546; Veldhuis, JCI, 1993; 91:629). This would favour binding and clearance by hepatocyte growth hormone receptors; it would also enhance renal growth hormone clearance. In view of the lower growth hormone binding protein levels in patients with cirrhosis (Baruch, JClinEndoc, 1991; 73:777; Hattori, Metabolism, 1992; 41:377), one would predict saturation of growth hormone binding proteins at growth hormone levels found in many fasting cirrhotics; an increase in the free growth hormone fraction could explain the normal growth hormone clearance found in cirrhosis[15] (Taylor, JClinEndoc, 1972; 34:395).

Insulin-like growth factors and their binding proteins

Normal physiology

Insulin-like growth factor-I and -II are polypeptides (c. 7.5 kDa) similar in structure to proinsulin, with which they share about 50 per cent homology. Insulin-like growth factor-I, and to a lesser extent insulin-like growth factor-II, mediate many of the somatotrophic effects of growth hormone and play an important role in bone metabolism (Chapter 25.10). Insulin-like growth factor-I increases lean body mass through its effects on protein and amino acid metabolism (Chapter 2.13.1). Both peptides have insulin-like effects on glucose metabolism in muscle and liver. Circulating levels of insulin-like growth factor-I and, to a much lesser extent, insulin-like growth factor-II are increased by growth hormone. Most tissues express insulin-like growth factor-I and -II but hepatocytes show the highest expression of their mRNAs and the liver is the main source of circulating insulin-like growth factors. Growth hormone stimulates the transcription of the gene in hepatocytes and the release of insulin-like growth factor-I into the circulation, which in turn inhibits growth hormone release from the pituitary by modulating hypothalamic factors that increase somatostatin release (Berelowitz, Science, 1981; 212:1279) and by inhibiting the pituitary somatotroph response to growth hormone releasing hormone (Morita, Endocrinol, 1987; 121:2000). The liver thus plays a central role in an important endocrine feedback loop.

Regulation of hepatic insulin-like growth factor-I production

Nutritional state and many hormones affect the hepatic insulin-like growth factor-I response to growth hormone. Insulin is a prerequisite for growth hormone stimulated insulin-like growth factor-I synthesis (Maiter, Endocrinol, 1989; 124:2604; Bini-Schnetzler, AmJPhysiol, 1991; 260:E846). Underinsulinized diabetic patients have low serum insulin-like growth factor-I levels (despite high growth hormone levels) that are increased by intensive insulin treatment (Amiel, Diabetes, 1984; 33:1175); their splanchnic output of insulin-like growth factor-I and plasma insulin-like growth factor-I levels increase within hours during intravenous insulin administration (Brismar, JClinEndoc, 1994; 79:872). Insulin deficiency impairs the hepatic insulin-like growth factor-I response to growth hormone by decreasing hepatic growth hormone receptor number (Baxter, BBResComm, 1978; 84:350; Roupas, MolCellEndocrinol, 1989; 61:1) and by a post-growth hormone receptor mechanism. Insulin may also regulate insulin-like growth factor-I production independently of growth hormone (Phillips, Diabetes, 1990; 40:1525). Thyroid hormone (Wolf, Endocrinol, 1989; 125:2905) and glucocorticoids (Miell, JEndocr, 1993; 136:525) also enhance the insulin-like growth factor-I response to growth hormone, while somatostatin (Serri, Endocrinol, 1992; 130:1816) and oestrogens (Murphy, Endocrinol, 1988; 122:352) are inhibitory.

Hepatic insulin-like growth factor-I production is profoundly influenced by nutritional factors. Caloric restriction, protein deficiency alone, or protein–calorie malnutrition all result in a state of hepatic growth hormone resistance with respect to insulin-like growth factor-I synthesis and secretion (Isley, JCI, 1983; 71:175; Thissen, EndocrRev, 1994; 15:80–101; Weller, AmJPhysiol, 1994; 266:E776; Oster, JCI, 1995; 95:2258). In addition, the quality of protein administered (in terms of essential amino acid content) can affect the insulin-like growth factor-I response to refeeding of fasted individuals (Clemmons, Metabolism, 1985; 34:391).

Plasma transport of the insulin-like growth factors

Plasma levels of insulin-like growth factor-I and -II show little variation over a 24-hour period, despite marked fluctuations in growth hormone levels. This constancy is in part due to their association with specific binding proteins (**IGFBPs**) so that less than 1 per cent of circulating insulin-like growth factor is in the free form. Six distinct highly homologous IGFBPs have been cloned (Jones, EndocrRev, 1995; 16:3; Thissen, EndocrRev, 1994; 15:80). The liver is the main site of synthesis of IGFBPs 1–4 but they are also synthesized by many tissues. About 75 per cent of circulating insulin-like growth factor-I and -II is found in a 150 kDa complex, the rest in complexes less than 50 kDa. IGFBP-3 is the insulin-like growth factor binding component of the 150 kDa complex. It has a very high affinity for the insulin-like growth factors, and once associated with insulin-like growth factor it also binds an acid-labile subunit to form a stable ternary complex. The serum half-life of insulin-like growth factor in this 150 kDa ternary complex is 12 to 16 h (Baxter, PNAS, 1989; 86:6898). Unable to cross the capillary endothelial barrier, this 150 kDa complex serves as the body's main storage of insulin-like growth factors. IGFBP-1 and IGFBP-2 are the binding proteins in the smaller 50 kDa complexes. IGFBP-1 binds insulin-like growth factor-I and -II with equal affinity, while IGFBP-2 preferentially binds insulin-like growth factor-II. IGFBP-1 and IGFBP-2 seem to have little effect in slowing the exit of insulin-like growth factors from the circulation and the insulin-like growth factors in this pool disappear from the circulation with a half-life of 20 to 30 min (Baxter, PNAS, 1989; 86:6898; Lewitt, JEndocr, 1993; 136:253).

The IGFBPs play an important role in regulating tissue delivery of the insulin-like growth factors. They can either potentiate or inhibit insulin-like growth factor action by influencing insulin-like growth factor interaction with tissue receptors (Zapf, EurJEndocr, 1995; 132:645). The importance of the IGFBPs becomes apparent when one considers the insulin-like metabolic effects of the insulin-like growth factors. Insulin-like growth factor-I and -II bind with high (approximately equal) affinity to the insulin-like growth factor-I receptor, which is structurally very similar to the insulin receptor with which it seems to share many of the intracellular signalling pathways. Both insulin-like growth factors can also bind with low affinity to the insulin receptor. At physiological concentrations, the growth and insulin-like metabolic effects are mediated via the insulin-like growth factor-I receptor; at high free concentrations they can also signal via the insulin receptor (De Meyts, HormRes, 1994; 42:152; Froesch, Diabetolog, 1985; 28:485). Since their potency on glucose metabolism in skeletal muscle is 5 to 10 per cent that of insulin (Poggi, Endocrinol, 1979; 105:723; Zapf, JCI, 1986;

77:1768; Guler, NEJM, 1987; 317:137), and the plasma concentration of insulin-like growth factors is about 100 nM (1000 times that of insulin) (Baxter, HormRes, 1994; 42:140), it is evident that the hypoglycaemic potential of the circulating insulin-like growth factors is huge. Due to sequestration of the insulin-like growth factors in the 150 kDa ternary complex comprising the insulin-like growth factor, IGFBP-3 and the acid-labile subunit, most of this hypoglycaemic activity is not expressed.

Regulation of insulin-like growth factor binding proteins (IGFBPs)

The IGFBPs are under complex hormonal and nutrient control, providing a further level at which the tissue delivery of insulin-like growth factors is regulated. IGFBP-1 undergoes acute variations in plasma levels, decreasing after meals or glucose ingestion and rising during fasting. The liver is the main site of IGFBP-1 production and insulin is the main regulator, inducing a rapid inhibition of IGFBP-1 gene transcription (Suwanickul, JBC, 1993; 258:17063); plasma IGFBP-1 levels are inversely correlated with estimated portal venous insulin concentrations (Yki-Jarvinen, JClinEndoc, 1995; 80:3227) and splanchnic output and plasma levels fall rapidly when insulin is infused intravenously (Brismar, JClinEndoc, 1994; 79:872). Glucagon (Hilding, JClinEndoc, 1993; 77:1142) and somatostatin (Ezzat, JClinEndoc, 1992; 75:1459) stimulate IGFBP-1 production. The resulting fall in IGFBP-1 levels after meals may increase free insulin-like growth factor-I in the interstitium of peripheral target tissues, thereby promoting glucose and amino acid uptake and inhibiting protein breakdown. IGFBP-3 and IGFBP-2 do not undergo acute changes in plasma levels in response to metabolic events but are regulated by growth hormone and insulin-like growth factor-I. Growth hormone, acting via insulin-like growth factor-I increases the synthesis and secretion of IGFBP-3 from hepatic non-parenchymal cells (Villafuerte, Endocrinol, 1994; 134:2044). Malnutrition, chronic protein restriction, and growth hormone deficiency decrease IGFBP-3 levels (Thissen, EndocrRev, 1994; 15:80–101; Oster, JCI, 1995; 95:2258). IGFBP-2 levels rise within 24 h of fasting.[20] IGFBP-2 levels are increased in growth hormone deficiency and malnutrition (Counts, JClinEndoc, 1992; 75:762; Thissen, EndocrRev, 1994; 15:80–101).

Insulin-like growth factors and their binding proteins in liver disease

Serum insulin-like growth factor-I and -II levels are reduced in patients with cirrhosis[19] (Buzzelli, AmJGastr, 1993; 88:1744) (Fig. 4) and in a variety of other liver diseases[16] (Wu, JLabClinMed, 1988; 112:589). Low serum insulin-like growth factor-I levels are thought to be a major cause of the increased growth hormone levels in cirrhosis through impaired feedback inhibition of growth hormone secretion. Circulating levels of IGFBPs are also disturbed in liver disease, with a reduction in IGFBP-3 and an increase in IGFBP-1 and IGFBP-2[16,20] (Fig. 4). Less of the circulating insulin-like growth factor is found in the large 150 kDa complex and more in the rapidly turning over smaller complexes. There is no evidence that the binding of insulin-like growth factor-I to IGFBP3 is impaired (Moller, JClinEndoc, 1995; 80:1148) due to proteolytic cleavage of IGFBP-3, as has beeen found in poorly

controlled type I diabetic patients (Bereket, JClinEndoc, 1995; 80: 2282) and in other severely ill or malnourished patients (Giudice, JClinEndoc, 1995; 80:2279). Low serum insulin-like growth factor-I levels in liver disease are mainly due to impaired hepatic insulin-like growth factor-I synthesis. However, a redistribution of insulin-like growth factors to smaller molecular weight short-lived complexes, may also enhance their clearance and contribute to the low plasma levels.

It is generally assumed that decreased hepatocellular function is the main cause of low plasma insulin-like growth factor-I levels in patients with chronic liver disease. However, this does not explain the increased hepatic production of IGFBP-1 in cirrhosis.[15,16] Furthermore, Donaghy and colleagues[16] found no difference in insulin-like growth factor-I levels between cirrhotics in Child–Pugh groups A, B, or C, and while IGFBP-1 levels were higher in the group B than group A cirrhotics, there was no further increase in the Child–Pugh group C cirrhotics with very poor liver function. In a large group of patients with alcoholic liver disease, serum insulin-like growth factor-I levels showed a stronger correlation with a composite protein–calorie malnutrition score than with liver function (Mendenhall, AlcAlc, 1989; 24:319) suggesting that malnutrition may also be an important determinant of the low insulin-like growth factor-I levels. In patients without liver disease, insulin-like growth factor-I levels provide a sensitive index of acute changes in nutritional state (Clemmons, AmJClinNutr, 1985; 41: 191); insulin-like growth factor-I levels correlate better with nitrogen balance than do such hepatic markers as retinol binding protein and thyroxine binding prealbumin (Underwood, HormRes, 1986; 24:166; Minuto, JPEN, 1989; 13:392). Low insulin-like growth factor-I and IGFBP-3 levels accompanied by high IGFBP-1 levels are found in anorexia nervosa and other malnourished patients who have an acquired growth hormone resistant state (Counts, JClinEndoc, 1992; 75:762; Oster, JCI, 1995; 95:2258; Ross, EurJEndocr, 1995; 132:655). Malnutrition may be an important determinant of the hepatic growth hormone resistance and abnormal insulin-like growth factor-I, IGFBP-1, and IGFBP-3 levels in chronic liver disease. It could also underlie the prognostic value of insulin-like growth factor-I and IGFBP-3 for survival in alcoholic cirrhosis (Moller, Hepatol, 1996; 23:1073) as nutritional state is an important prognostic factor in patients with cirrhosis (Muller, Hepatol, 1992; 15:782). In addition to protein–calorie malnutrition, deficiencies of specific nutrients, such as zinc, that may occur in some cirrhotic patients (see Chapter 29.2) may also result in hepatic growth hormone resistance and impaired insulin-like growth factor-I production (McNall, JNutr, 1995; 125:874).

As discussed earlier, insulin plays a key role in the regulation of plasma insulin-like growth factor-I and IGFBP-1 levels; through its effects on insulin-like growth factor-I it also influences IGFBP-3 levels. Low insulin-like growth factor-I and IGFBP-3 levels, and increased IGFBP-1 levels, are also found in type I diabetes (Holly, DiabetMed, 1990; 7:618; Bereket, JClinEndoc, 1995; 80:1312). Studies in animals (Russell-Jones, JMolEndocr, 1992; 9:257) and humans (Yki-Jarvinen, JClinEndoc, 1995; 80:3227) have suggested that the portal route of insulin delivery is important for normal regulation of insulin-like growth factor-I and IGFBP-1 production. In type I diabetic patients on subcutaneous insulin injections, loss of the normal portal-peripheral insulin concentration gradient may contribute to the abnormalities of the insulin–like growth factor-I–growth hormone axis. In cirrhosis, portosystemic shunting and sinusoidal capillarization may similarly result in hepatic under-insulinization despite high systemic insulin levels, and may contribute to the low insulin–like growth factor-I and IGFBP-3, and increased IGFBP-1 levels. Plasma glucagon levels are increased in cirrhosis. However, since the liver is resistant to glucagon in cirrhosis it is unlikely that glucagon is the cause of the increased hepatic synthesis of IGFBP-1[15] (Hilding, JClinEndoc, 1993; 77: 1142); however, the low insulin–like growth factor-I levels could contribute to increased glucagon secretion in cirrhosis (Kerr, JCI, 1993; 91:141).

Many cells besides hepatocytes produce insulin–like growth factor-I and IGFBPs. It is unclear whether local tissue production of insulin–like growth factor-I and the IGFBPs is disturbed in liver disease and to what extent individual tissues rely on locally produced versus circulating insulin–like growth factor-I. The observation that administration of a blocking antibody to insulin–like growth factor-I results in a transient rise in protein turnover (Koea, JEndocr, 1992; 135:279) suggests that at least part of the effect on protein metabolism is mediated by circulating insulin–like growth factor-I. In view of the frequency of malnutrition in cirrhosis (Lautz, ClinInvest, 1992; 70:478) and its impact on the outcome of transplantation (Pikul, Transpl, 1994; 57:469), insulin–like growth factor-I may have a place in the nutritional management of patients with liver disease (see Chapter 2.13.1). In children with endstage liver disease, plasma insulin–like growth factor-I levels are restored to normal after liver transplantation but IGFBP-1, IGFBP-2, and IGFBP-3 levels are higher than in normal control subjects during the first year.[20] These abnormalities correlated with nutritional indices such as triceps skin-fold thickness and mid-upper arm circumference. The increased levels of these binding proteins may limit tissue insulin–like growth factor-I availability and thus provide a basis for growth failure after successful liver transplantation in some children.[20]

Insulin-like growth factors and extrapancreatic tumour hypoglycaemia

Hepatocellular carcinoma is one of the more common extrapancreatic tumours known to be associated with hypoglycaemia. While hypoglycaemia may develop as a late manifestation in patients with liver failure (Chapter 2.11), in patients with hepatocellular carcinoma it may present relatively early, at a time when the tumour is slow-growing and well differentiated. Hypoglycaemia presenting early in the course of hepatocellular carcinoma (in the absence of liver failure) is common in South-East Asia (McFazdean, AmJMed, 1969; 47:220) but rare in Western countries. The hypoglycaemia in these patients may be severe and difficult to control; as in patients with other extrapancreatic tumours, hypoglycaemia is due to both an impairment of hepatic glucose production and increased glucose utilization, particularly by skeletal muscle (Benn, ClinEndoc, 1990; 32:769; Moller, Diabetolog, 1991; 34:17; Wing, Metabolism, 1991; 40:508; Eastman, JCI, 1992; 89:1958). Serum non-esterified fatty acids and growth hormone levels are low during hypoglycaemia, suggesting an impaired counter-regulatory response. All these metabolic abnormalities are found in the presence of very low, often unmeasureable, serum insulin levels.

Megyesi and colleagues, over 20 years ago, reported increased plasma levels of 'non-suppressible insulin like activity' in some patients with extrapancreatic tumour hypoglycaemia (Megyesi, JClinEndoc, 1974; 38:931). Insulin-like growth factor-I and -II were isolated in 1976 (Rinderknecht, PNAS, 1976; 73:2365) and shown to account for the 'non-suppressible insulin-like activity' in plasma. Several groups subsequently reported modest increases of serum insulin-like growth factor-II levels (but low insulin-like growth factor-I) in some but not all patients with tumour-related hypoglycaemia (Daughaday, JClinEndoc, 1981; 53:289; Ron, JClinEndoc, 1989; 68:701); in other series insulin-like growth factor-II levels were either normal or just above the normal reference range, while insulin-like growth factor-I levels were again low or normal.[21,22] Normal serum insulin-like growth factor-II levels were often found despite evidence of increased insulin-like growth factor-II mRNA and insulin-like growth factor-II protein levels in tumours associated with hypoglycaemia.[21] (Daughaday, NEJM, 1988; 319: 1434; Lowe, JClinEndoc, 1989; 69:1153). As discussed earlier, patients with cirrhosis characteristically have low serum insulin-like growth factor-I and insulin-like growth factor-II levels. Not surprisingly therefore, in cirrhotic hepatocellular carcinoma patients with hypoglycaemia, serum insulin-like growth factor-I and -II levels have been consistently low, and although insulin-like growth factor-II levels tended to be higher in hypoglycaemic than in normoglycaemic cirrhotic hepatocellular carcinoma patients, the differences were not significant (Wu, JLabClinMed, 1988; 112:589; Wing, Metabolism, 1991; 40:508). The role of the insulin-like growth factors in hypoglycaemia complicating hepatocellular carcinoma and other non-islet-cell tumours thus remained unclear until recently.

There is now good evidence that tumours associated with hypoglycaemia produce increased amounts of insulin-like growth factor-II precursor forms ('**big IGF-II**') with molecular weights in the range 10 to 17 kDa compared to 7.5 kDa for mature insulin-like growth factor-II, due to abnormal processing of pro- insulin-like growth factor-II which contains an 89 amino acid C-terminal extension[21–24] (Daughaday, NEJM, 1988; 319:1434). A variable C-terminal extension, and abnormal glycosylation, result in marked heterogeneity of 'big IGF-II' in sera of patients with tumour hypoglycaemia.[24] Shapiro et al.[21] found that 'big IGF-II' accounted for 48 to 72 per cent of total serum insulin-like growth factor-II in six patients with hepatocellular carcinoma with hypoglycaemia, but for only 6 to 40 per cent in five normoglycaemic patients with hepatocellular carcinoma. Interestingly, increased serum levels of big IGF-II have also been found in chronic hepatitis B carriers without evidence of tumour.[23] At the receptor level some 'big IGF-II' species may be more potent than mature insulin-like growth factor-II;[21] however, the main mechanism by which unregulated tumour production of 'big IGF-II' induces hypoglycaemia is by increasing tissue insulin-like growth factor bioavailability.

As discussed earlier, insulin-like growth factor-I and -II circulate in plasma bound in a large 150 kDa ternary complex and smaller 50 kDa complexes. Formation of the 150 kDa complex is important for sequestration of insulin-like growth factors in the circulation. Although 'big IGF-II' and mature insulin-like growth factor-II bind equally well to IGFBP-3, in patients with hypoglycaemia due to excessive 'big IGF-II' production the association of IGFBP-3 and its bound insulin-like growth factor with the acid-labile subunit to form the stable 150 kDa ternary complex is impaired[22,24] (Baxter, JClinEndoc, 1995; 80:2700). The result is that most plasma insulin-like growth factor in these hypoglycaemic patients is found in complexes of less than 50 kDa, which can readily leave the circulation to interact with tissue insulin-like growth factor-I and insulin receptors. Increased action of insulin-like growth factor-II at the level of the hypothalamus/pituitary leads to inhibition of growth hormone secretion; this inhibits normal insulin-like growth factor-I and -II production and aggravates the situation by decreasing plasma levels of IGFBP-3 and the acid-labile subunit. The low growth hormone levels may also account for the markedly increased IGFBP-2 levels found in patients with hypoglycaemia due to 'big IGF-II' producing tumours (Zapf, JCI, 1990; 86:952; Blum, GrowthRegul, 1993; 3:100; Baxter, JClinEndoc, 1995; 80: 2700); high IGFBP-2 levels may further promote the redistribution of insulin-like growth factor-II to lower molecular weight complexes. The increased tissue bioavailability of insulin-like growth factors may account for the occasional association of non-islet cell tumour hypoglycaemia with acromegaloid skin changes (Trivedi, ClinEndoc, 1995; 42:433).

Management

Large amounts of intravenous glucose may be required. Studies on small numbers of patients with tumour-associated hypoglycaemia have shown that growth hormone may be useful in the management of these patients pending definitive treatment or in patients with inoperable tumours (Wing, Metabolism, 1991; 40:508; Teale, AnnClinBioch, 1992; 29:314; Hunter, ClinEndoc, 1994; 41:397; Agus, JPediat, 1995; 127:403). Prednisolone (Anderson, SAMedJ, 1967; 41:505; Foger, JIntMed, 1994; 236:692) and glucagon (Samaan, AnnIntMed, 1990; 113:404) have also been used, with some success, to reduce glucose requirements in patients with tumour-associated hypoglycaemia. Growth hormone is important for counter-regulation of hypoglycaemia. It is also important for the synthesis of the protein components (IGFBP3 and the acid-labile subunit) of the circulating 150 kDa insulin-like growth factor complex that serves to restrict access of the insulin-like growth factors to tissues and thereby limit their hypoglycaemic potential. Suppression of growth hormone secretion by insulin-like growth factor-II may thus contribute to the hypoglycaemic effect of increased tissue insulin-like growth factor-II delivery. Prednisolone may inhibit tumour 'big IGF-II' production; it increases levels of the acid-labile subunit and decreases IGFBP-2 levels and thereby increases the proportion of plasma insulin-like growth factor-II in the 150 kDa complex, as well as opposing the actions of insulin (and by implication those of the insulin-like growth factors) on hepatic glucose production and peripheral tissue glucose utilization. Alleviation of hypoglycaemia is consistently associated with a restoration of the 150 kDa insulin-like growth factor ternary complex, regardless of whether total or 'big' insulin-like growth factor-II levels fall. Since prednisolone and growth hormone may increase the proportion of insulin-like growth factor-II in the 150 kDa complex by different mechanisms, their combined effects may be additive (Baxter, JClinEndoc, 1995; 80:2700).

Hypoglycaemia complicating hepatocellular carcinoma in cirrhotic patients may be particularly difficult to manage because of resistance to the actions of growth hormone and glucagon that is characteristic of patients with cirrhosis. One would predict markedly impaired responses of insulin-like growth factor-I, IGFBP-3, and the acid-labile subunit to growth hormone, and a subnormal glycaemic response to glucagon. Thus, in patients with hypoglycaemia due to hepatocellular carcinoma complicating cirrhosis, prednisolone may be tried first in an attempt to lower glucose requirements, though large doses may be needed. Targeted chemotherapy may also be effective, although there may be an initial worsening of hypoglycaemia (Hunter, ClinEndoc, 1994; 41:397).

Thyroid hormones
Normal physiology

Thyroid hormones are essential for normal growth and development and play a key role in the regulation of energy metabolism, thermogenesis, and neuromuscular activity. Although thyroxine (T_4) is quantitatively the main hormone secreted by the thyroid, thyroid hormone action is mediated by the binding of 3,3',5-tri-iodothyronine (T_3) to specific nuclear receptors (Fig. 5) which in turn control the transcription of thyroid-regulated genes (Brent, AnnRevPhysiol, 1991; 53:17). Thyroxine has a much lower affinity for the nuclear T_3 receptors than T_3, and should be regarded as a pro-hormone that requires conversion to T_3 by 5' monodeiodination of the outer ring (Fig. 6). T_3 bound to nuclear receptors may come either from the circulation or local tissue 5' deiodination of T_4. The relative importance of these two sources varies between tissues; skeletal muscle, liver, and kidney rely mainly on circulating T_3, whereas more than 60 per cent of brain and pituitary T_3 is produced locally. Tissue thyroid status thus depends not only on normal secretion of thyroxine but also on normal thyroid hormone metabolism and delivery of T_3 to nuclear T_3 receptors, and on T_3 receptor function.

In normal subjects the thyroid secretes about 110 nmol (86 µg) of T_4 and 5 nmol of T_3 (3 µg) each day. The deiodination of the outer ring of T_4 in extrathyroidal tissues results in the delivery of a further 40 nmol of T_3 into the circulation. About 45 nmol of secreted T_4 undergoes deiodination of the inner tyrosyl ring in extrahepatic tissues to produce the biologically inactive 3,3',5'-tri-iodothyronine (reverse T_3) (Fig. 6); the remaining 20 to 25 nmol of T_4 undergoes oxidative deamination or glucuronidation, sulphation, and excretion in bile. A large proportion of unmetabolized T_4 excreted in bile is reabsorbed in the intestine and delivered back to the liver. The liver plays an important role in the transport, storage, and metabolism of thyroid hormones, and is a major target tissue for their action. In man 10 to 30 per cent of the total extrathyroidal pool of T_4 is in the liver (Oppenheimer, JCI, 1967; 46:762). It is the main site of extrathyroidal conversion of T_4 to the biologically active T_3 for release into the circulation and delivery to other tissues. It is also the main site of removal of reverse T_3 and of thyroid hormone degradation and excretion. The liver synthesizes thyroxine-binding globulin, thyroxine-binding prealbumin, and albumin, which bind most of the circulating T_4 and T_3 and thereby influence their total plasma concentrations.

Thyroxine in plasma is almost completely (>99.95 per cent), and T_3 only slightly less (>99.5 per cent), bound to thyroxine-binding globulin, thyroxine-binding prealbumin, and albumin. The total

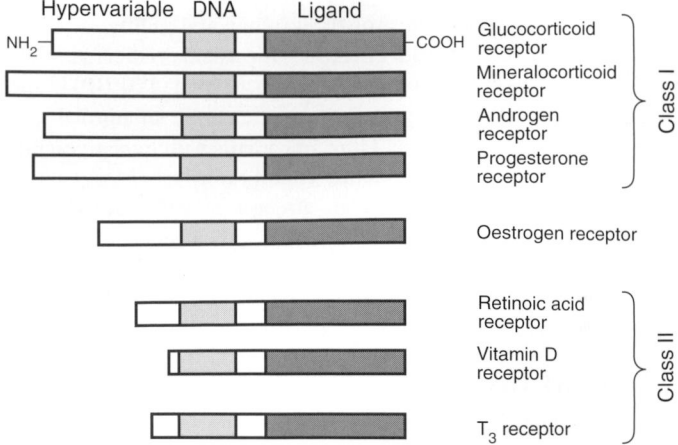

Fig. 5. Superfamily of steroid-thyroid hormone receptors. All contain highly homologous central DNA binding domains, a less well-conserved C-terminal ligand binding domain, and an N-terminal hypervariable transactivation domain that enhances the transcriptional regulatory activities of the receptor. Near the C terminus is a highly conserved region important for receptor dimerization. Class I receptors and the oestrogen receptor form homodimers. These homodimers with bound ligand bind to palindromic hormone response elements (HREs) in the DNA that contain hexamers separated by three base pairs. Class II receptors bind to direct repeat elements with hexamers separated by 0–5 bases. They may bind as homodimers with or without bound hormone, but can also form heterodimers with other class II receptors (e.g. T_3 and retinoic acid receptor heterodimers). Whereas class II receptors are located in the nucleus in the absence of ligand, class I receptors are cytosolic, and move to the nucleus following hormone binding.

concentration of T_4 and T_3 in plasma largely reflects the concentrations and binding affinities of these three proteins. Although thyroxine-binding globulin is the least abundant of these, it has the highest binding affinity and is quantitatively the most important; 70 to 80 per cent of circulating T_3 and T_4 are bound to thyroxine-binding globulin, 15 to 20 per cent to thyroxine-binding prealbumin, and 5 to 10 per cent to albumin (Table 1). The affinities for T_3 are lower than for T_4 so that plasma concentrations of T_3 are much lower than those of T_4; the molar ratio of T_4 to T_3 in plasma is 50 to 100 : 1, even though delivery of T_4 into the circulation is only two to three times that of T_3. The thyroid binding proteins, by providing a large, rapidly exchangeable pool of circulating T_4, help to ensure that the flux of T_4 across cell membranes exceeds the rate of cellular removal of T_4 and thus promote the equilibration of cytosolic and plasma free T_4 so that the intracellular thyroid hormone concentrations, that determine biological activity, are proportional to the free hormone concentrations. The free hormone concentration within the thyrotrophin and thyroid stimulating hormone secreting cells of the hypothalamus and anterior pituitary, respectively, is a major determininat of thyrotrophin and thyroid stimulating hormone secretion, and hence thyroid hormone production rate.

Hepatic uptake of thyroid hormones

Studies employing [^{131}I]T_4 have shown that the liver takes up about 5 to 10 per cent of T_4 during a single passage (Mendel, AmJPhysiol, 1988; 255:E110). This is much higher than can be accounted for by the amount of free T_4 delivered to the liver, and a large proportion of T_4 bound to albumin is also available for hepatic uptake during its passage through the hepatic sinusoids. Because there is also a high rate of T_4 efflux from hepatocytes into sinusoidal plasma

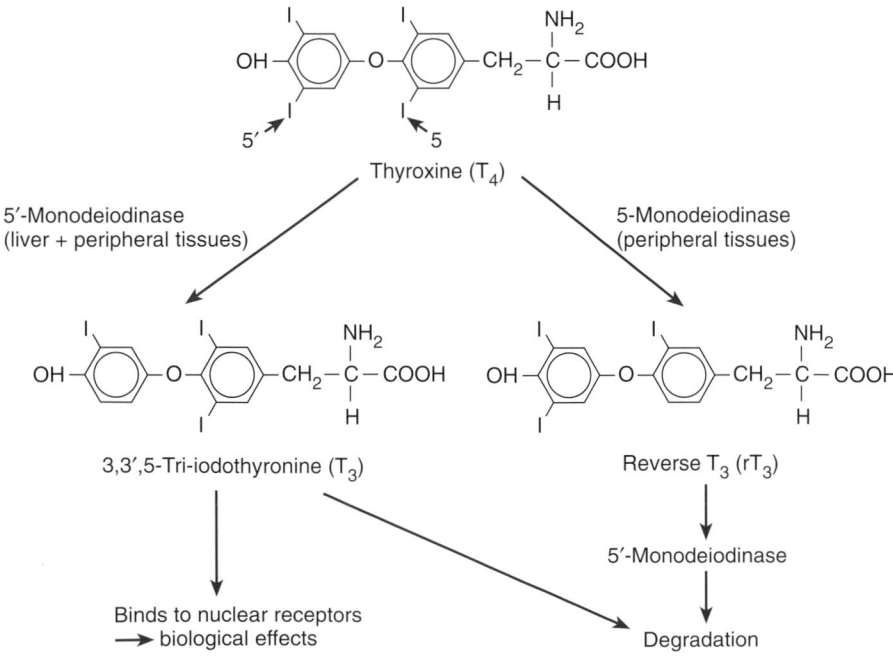

Fig. 6. Thyroid hormone metabolism. T_4 and reverse T_3 (rT_3) share the same hepatic uptake mechansism. In addition 5′ deioidination of T_4 and rT_3 is performed by the same type 1 5′ monodeiodinase. The impaired conversion of T_4 to T_3 and impaired hepatic clearance of rT_3 in liver disease may be due to decreased hepatic uptake and/or decreased activity of the hepatic 5′ monodeiodinase.

Table 1 Thyroid hormone binding proteins in serum				
	Serum concentration (mg/dl)	Affinity constant (per mole)		Serum half-life (days)	T_4-binding capacity (μg/dl)
		T_4	T_3		
Thyroxine-binding globulin (TBG)	1.5	1×10^{10}	5×10^8	5	20[a]
Thyroxine-binding prealbumin (TBPA)	25	7×10^7	2×10^7	2	200
Albumin	4000	7×10^5	1×10^5	15	2000

From ref. 30.
[a] Normally only about one-third of TBG in plasma contains T_4.

(Cavalieri, JCI, 1966; 45:939; Mendel, AmJPhysiol, 1988; 255: E110;) net hepatic uptake of T_4 is low. This is evident if one considers that the metabolic clearance rate of T_4 in man is only about 0.9 ml/min, with the liver accounting for some 35 per cent of this; assuming an hepatic plasma flow of 650 ml/min one can estimate that net hepatic T_4 uptake is less than 0.05 per cent of that presented to the liver. Influx of thyroid hormones is energy dependent and the hepatocyte intracellular concentration of the free hormone has been found to be somewhat higher than in plasma (Mooradian, Endocrinol, 1985; 117:2449; Oppenheimer, JCI, 1985; 75:147). An active stereospecific transport mechanism has been suggested; T_4 and reverse T_3 may share the same uptake mechanism, while that for T_3 appears to be different (De Jong, AmJPhysiol, 1994; 266:E44). Efflux of thyroid hormones appears to be passive and determined by the concentration gradient of the free hormone. Some authors have suggested that hepatocyte uptake of T_3 is by passive diffusion rather than by an active transport process (Weisiger, AmJPhysiol, 1992; 262:G1104).

Thyroid hormones in liver disease

Most patients with liver disease are clinically euthyroid. In general they have normal free T_4 and free T_3 levels, and a normal or slightly elevated thyroid stimulating hormone level.[25-28] However, total circulating thyroid hormone levels may be markedly abnormal and may complicate the biochemical diagnosis of thyroid disease. There are many factors that account for the abnormalities of plasma thyroid hormone levels, including alterations in the plasma levels of thyroid binding proteins, altered binding of T_3 and T_4 to their carrier proteins, diminished hepatic conversion of T_4 to T_3, and impaired hepatic clearance of reverse T_3.[29] Thyroxine-binding prealbumin levels are reduced in cirrhotics in parallel with the fall in serum albumin levels; levels fall within days in acute liver disease (Skrede, ScaJCLI, 1975; 35:399). Thyroxine-binding globulin levels may be increased or decreased, depending on the aetiology and stage of liver disease. The abnormalities in plasma thyroid hormone levels vary between acute and chronic liver disease, and are influenced by the aetiology and severity of liver disease, the presence of intercurrent illness, and dietary intake. Table 2 summarizes the alterations in thyroid function tests that may be found in euthyroid patients with liver disease. Estimation of free T_4 and T_3 concentrations or their respective free indices, together with measurement of thyroid stimulating hormone is essential for accurate interpretation of thyroid function tests in patients with liver disease.

Acute and chronic viral hepatitis

Plasma T_4 levels rise during the course of acute viral hepatitis, returning to normal with recovery (Gardner, AnnIntMed, 1982; 96: 450; Ross, AmJMed, 1983; 74:564; Hegedus, Metabolism, 1986; 35: 495). Plasma free T_4 levels may be normal or increased. This increase in total T_4 levels is primarily due to increased plasma levels of thyroxine-binding globulin, which in some studies have been found to correlate with the rise in plasma aspartate aminotransferase levels (Gardner, AnnIntMed, 1982; 96:450). In addition there is impaired hepatic conversion of T_4 to T_3. Total T_3 levels are very variable but free T_3 levels may be markedly reduced. Biologically inactive reverse T_3 levels are increased; this is probably due to impaired hepatic clearance of reverse T_3 with an unaltered production rate, as is found in a variety of 'sick' patients without liver disease (Kaptein, JCI, 1982; 69:526) and in patients with cirrhosis.[29] (Nomura, JCI, 1975; 56:643). Serum thyroid stimulating hormone levels are usually normal, but the need for increased T_4 production may be associated with the development of a goitre during the course of acute viral hepatitis; Hegedus (Metabolism, 1986; 35:495) found a 50 per cent increase in thyroid gland volume on ultrasound in 23 patients with acute viral hepatitis, which returned to normal 3 to 6 months after recovery.

In patients with chronic viral hepatitis (chronic active or chronic persistent hepatitis on biopsy), without evidence of decompensation, total T_4 and thyroxine-binding globulin levels are often increased but free T_4, thyroid stimulating hormone, T_3, and reverse T_3 levels are usually normal (Borzio, Gut 1983; 24:631; Itoh, AmJGastr, 1986; 81:444; Orbach, AmJPhysiol, 1989; 86:39). By contrast, in fulminant hepatitis plasma total T_4 and T_3 levels are very low, in association with a marked impairment of thyroxine-binding globulin (and thyroxine-binding prealbumin) synthesis; reverse T_3 levels are increased. An increase in the reverse T_3/T_4 ratio and the T_4/T_3 ratio was associated with a particularly poor prognosis (Kano, GastrJap, 1987; 22:344).

Cirrhosis

Serum total T_4 levels are usually normal but may be slightly increased or decreased in some patients in association with increased or decreased synthesis of thyroxine-binding globulin (Table 2).[25, 26] The daily production rate of T_4 in patients with alcoholic cirrhosis is normal[29] or mildly reduced (Chopra, JCI, 1976; 58: 32). Studies employing radiolabelled T_4 showed a reduced rate of

Table 2 Alterations of serum thyroid function tests in liver disease and in the 'low T_3' syndrome

	Total T_4	Free T_4	Total T_3	Free T_3	Total reverse T_3	TSH	TBG	TBPA
Liver disease								
Acute hepatitis	↑	↑	↓	↓	↑	↑	↑	↓
Cirrhosis	↓	↑	↓	↓	↑	↑→	↓	↓
PBC and CAH	↑	→	↑	↓	→	↑	↑	→
HCC	↑	→	↑	→	↑	↑→	↑	↓
Low T_3 syndrome	→	↑→	↓	↓	↑	→	→	↓→

CAH, chronic active hepatitis; HCC, hepatocellular carcinoma; PBC, primary biliary cirrhosis; TBG, thyroxine-binding globulin; TBPA, thyroxine-binding prealbumin; TSH, thyroid stimulating hormone.

hepatic T_4 uptake and a diminished hepatic thyroid hormone pool size in cirrhosis (Cavalieri, JCI, 1966; 45:939). The most consistent findings are decreased serum total and free T_3 levels[25,26] (reflecting diminished hepatic conversion of T_4 to T_3), and an increased reverse T_3 level due to its impaired hepatic removal.[29] Serum thyroid stimulating hormone levels are either normal or mildly elevated. The thyroid stimulating hormone response to thyrotrophin releasing hormone may be normal (Chopra, JClinEndoc, 1974; 39:501) or subnormal (Van Thiel, JEndocrInv, 1986; 9:479). Green et al. (ClinEndoc, 1977; 7:453), in a study of 23 cirrhotics of varying aetiology, found that many patients had a delayed thyroid stimulating hormone response to thyrotrophin releasing hormone, suggestive of hypothalamic–pituitary dysfunction. Agner and colleagues (ActaMedScand, 1986; 220:57) found that the subnormal thyroid stimulating hormone response to thyrotrophin releasing hormone in alcoholic cirrhotics was corrected by pretreatment with a dopamine-receptor blocking agent such as metoclopramide, implying that it may be due to increased dopaminergic inhibition of thyroid stimulating hormone release by the pituitary.

The abnormalities of plasma T_3 and reverse T_3 in patients with alcoholic cirrhosis correlate with the severity of liver damage. Decompensated cirrhotic patients may have very low total and free T_3 levels (Becker, ActaMedScand, 1988; 224:367; Guven, EurJMed, 1993; 2:83). Their total T_4 levels may also be low in association with marked reductions in thyroxine-binding globulin and thyroxine-binding prealbumin levels. Since T_3 and reverse T_3 (rT_3) bind to the same plasma binding proteins, the plasma reverse T_3/T_3 ratio provides a parameter that is largely independent of binding protein levels, and reflects the impairment of hepatic uptake and conversion of T_4 to T_3, and the impaired hepatic removal of reverse T_3.[29] The reverse T_3/T_3 ratio was found to correlate well with liver function as measured by the aminopyrine breath test (Hepner, AnnIntMed, 1979; 139:1117). In a large heterogeneous group of patients with endstage liver disease, Van Thiel and colleagues (Hepatol, 1985; 5:862) found that those with a high rT_3/T_3 ratio were more likely to die while awaiting liver transplantation.

The plasma thyroid hormone profile in patients with cirrhosis resembles the low T_3 syndrome (Table 2) found in many 'sick' patients and in normal subjects during caloric deprivation.[30] It may be regarded as an adaptive hypothyroid state that is important for preserving total body protein stores during fasting and illness (Gardner, NEJM, 1979; 300:579; Kaptein, JClin Endoc, 1985; 22:1). Thus while the low T_3 state in cirrhosis may reflect diminished

hepatocellular function, it may also be due to diminished caloric intake and the same factors that determine the low T_3 levels in other sick patients. The low T_3 and increased reverse T_3 levels in cirrhosis may be due to a diminished capacity of the hepatic microsomal 5'-deiodinase (type 1) since the conversion of T_4 to T_3, and the metabolism of reverse T_3, are both mediated by this enzyme. But it could also be due to impaired hepatic uptake of T_4 and reverse T_3 as is seen in the low T_3 syndrome associated with fasting and various non-thyroidal illnesses (Van der Heyden, AmJPhysiol, 1986; 251: E156). Lim et al.[31] showed that serum from jaundiced patients inhibited the uptake of T_4 and reverse T_3 by isolated rat hepatocytes, and that bilirubin and non-esterified fatty acids in conjunction with a low serum albumin concentration could account for this inhibitory effect. Bilirubin and non-esterified fatty acids added to normal serum had additive effects on hepatocyte T_4 uptake which correlated with the bilirubin/albumin and non-esterified fatty acid/albumin molar ratios. Comparable non-esterified fatty acid/albumin and bilirubin/albumin molar ratios might be expected in many decompensated cirrhotic patients.

Autoimmune liver disease

There is an increased prevalence of autoimmune thyroid disease in patients with autoimmune chronic active hepatitis (Thompson, AmJDigDis, 1973; 18:111) or primary biliary cirrhosis (Crowe, Gastro, 1980; 78:1437; Culp, MayoClinProc, 1982; 57:365). Primary sclerosing cholangitis may be associated with Riedel's thyroiditis (Bartholomew, NEJM, 1963; 269:8). Hypothyroidism develops in 10 to 25 per cent of patients with primary biliary cirrhosis (Sherlock, NEJM, 1973; 289:674; Crowe, Gastro, 1980; 78:1437; Culp, Mayo-ClinProc, 1982; 57:365; Elta, DigDisSci, 1983; 28:971); it may predate the diagnosis of liver disease or occur during its course. Thyrotoxicosis is rare in association with primary biliary cirrhosis but common in patients with autoimmune chronic active hepatitis. In both primary biliary cirrhosis and chronic active hepatitis, plasma total T_4 levels are often increased due to increased plasma thyroxine-binding globulin levels.[25,27,28]. Plasma total and free T_3 levels are often low due to impaired conversion of T_4 to T_3,[25,27] although Shussler and colleagues[28] found elevated total T_3 levels in chronic active hepatitis. Plasma free T_4 levels are normal. Serum thyroid stimulating hormone levels and thyroidal radio-iodine uptake tend to be low, and the thyroid stimulating hormone response to thyrotrophin releasing hormone may be subnormal, particularly in patients with active liver disease.[27] Because total T_4 levels are often increased in primary biliary cirrhosis and patients with chronic active hepatitis, the diagnosis of hypothyroidism may be missed unless a free T_4 and thyroid stimulating hormone level are measured. Autoimmune thyroid disease in these patients is associated with high titres of thyroid autoantibodies (thyroid microsomal and/or thyroglobulin) and patients with primary biliary cirrhosis will often have dimished lacrimation, suggestive of sicca syndrome.

Hepatocellular carcinoma

Elevated serum total T_4 levels due to increased thyroxine-binding globulin levels may be found in up to 40 per cent of patients with hepatocellular carcinoma (Nelson, ArchIntMed, 1979; 139:1063; Gershengorn, JClinEndoc, 1982; 42:907; Kalk, Hepatol, 1982; 2:72; Alexopoulos, BrJCanc, 1988; 57:313). Free T_4 and T_3 levels are generally normal and the patients are clinically euthyroid. The increase in serum thyroxine-binding globulin levels is thought to be due to increased thyroxine-binding globulin production rather than impaired clearance, since elevated thyroxine-binding globulin levels have been found in the tumour tissue and also in areas of the liver free of tumour in these patients, many of whom had an active cirrhosis due to hepatitis B (Hutchinson, Hepatol, 1991; 14:116). The circulating thyroxine-binding globulin in patients with hepatocellular carcinoma often has a lower affinity for T_4 which may, in part, be due to alterations in its glycosylation state (Reilly, JClinEndoc, 1983; 57:15; Du, ClinSci, 1990; 78:551).

Drugs

Many therapeutic agents commonly used in patients with liver disease interfere with thyroid hormone metabolism and distribution. Frusemide (in large doses) may increase plasma free T_4 levels by displacing T_4 from thyroxine-binding globulin; serum total T_4 and T_3 levels are reduced. Phenytoin may decrease plasma total and free T_4 concentrations into the hypothyroid range in up to 30 per cent of normal subjects; an erroneous diagnosis of hypothyroidism is avoided by measuring plasma thyroid stimulating hormone levels, which are unaffected by phenytoin. Dopamine or glucocorticoid administration can suppress thyroid stimulating hormone secretion and lower plasma T_4 and T_3 levels, while sulphonylureas in high dosage may inhibit normal thyroid gland function. Propranolol inhibits the hepatic conversion of T_4 to T_3. Normal subjects receiving more than 200 mg propranolol often have mild elevation of free T_4 and a corresponding reduction in T_3. Lipid-soluble radiographic iodine-containing contrast media inhibit the peripheral conversion of T_4 to T_3, and displace T_4 from hepatic (and possibly renal) storage sites, resulting in increased plasma T_4 and low T_3 levels together with an increase in plasma reverse T_3. The conversion of T_4 to T_3 within pituitary thyroid stimulating hormone secreting cells is also inhibited, resulting in an increased secretion of thyroid stimulating hormone. These hormonal changes are maximal after 4 to 7 days and persist for up to 3 to 4 weeks. These hormonal changes do not occur after administration of water-soluble contrast agents.

Thyroid dysfunction (hypo- or hyperthyroidism) may develop in 3 to 10 per cent of patients treated with α-interferon for chronic viral hepatitis. Hypothyroidism is more common but may be preceded by transient thyrotoxicosis. The risk of thyroid dysfunction increases with duration of treatment but bears little relationship to the dose of interferon used. It is unusual for thyroid disease to present in patients treated with α-interferon for less than 8 weeks. This might explain why thyroid dysfunction is seen more commonly with interferon treatment of chronic hepatitis C than chronic hepatitis B, for which treatment regimens have generally been shorter. α-Interferon-induced thyroid dysfunction is thought to have an autoimmune basis. In the majority of patients there is a thyroiditis; some patients present with features typical of Graves' disease or Hashimoto's. Thyroid autoantibodies are induced in 30 to 50 per cent of those treated but there is a poor correlation with clinical thyroid dysfunction (Mayet, Hepatol, 1989; 10:24). Some authors have reported that thyroid dysfunction during interferon treatment is more likely to develop in patients with pre-existing thyroid autoantibodies, particularly thyroid microsomal antibodies (Watanabe, AmJGastr, 1994; 89:399; Wada, AmJGastr, 1995; 90:1366) but this was not found in other studies[32] (Lisker-Melman, Gastro, 1992; 102:2155). It has been suggested that interferon may induce the expression of MHC class II antigens on thyrocytes with consequent activation of cytotoxic T cells directed against thyroid cells.

Thyroid function and thyroid autoantibodies should be checked prior to initiation of α-interferon treatment, and serum thyroid stimulating hormone and free T_4 should be monitored during treatment. It should be noted that thyroid autoantibodies and clinical thyroid dysfunction may appear in the months following treatment. The development of thyroid dysfunction during interferon treatment may be associated with a rise in serum transaminases (Chapter 24.6) (Berris, DigDisSci, 1991; 36:1657). In many patients thyroid function may return to normal following interferon withdrawal.[32] In view of this potential for recovery, radical therapy such as thyroidectomy or ^{131}I ablation should not be considered as first-line treatment in thyrotoxic patients. Thyroid autoantibodies eventually disappear following withdrawal of α-interferon (Mayet, Hepatol, 1989; 10:24; Lisker-Melman, Gastro, 1992; 102:2155).

Parathyroid hormone and osteocalcin (see also Chapter 25.10)

Parathyroid hormone

Parathyroid hormone (**PTH**) is an 84-amino-acid peptide (molecular weight 9300). PTH synthesis and secretion are under feedback control by the plasma (free) calcium ion concentration. Mild hypomagnesemia also stimulates PTH secretion but magnesium is much less potent than calcium. Synthesis of PTH is inhibited by high levels of α1,25-dihydroxyvitamin D_3. Biological activity of PTH resides in the N-terminal amino acids 1 to 34. PTH, together with vitamin D (see Chapter 25.10), acts on bone, kidney, and gut to regulate calcium homeostasis and maintain extracellular calcium ion levels (Fig. 7). PTH acts on the kidney to stimulate calcium reabsorption, and on bone to increase bone resorption. Normally, bone resorption and bone formation are tightly coupled. The kidney filters about 5 to 7 g of calcium each day. Most but not all of this is reabsorbed, and there are additional obligatory losses in sweat and from the gut. PTH acts indirectly to enhance the intestinal absorption of dietary calcium by increasing the renal conversion of

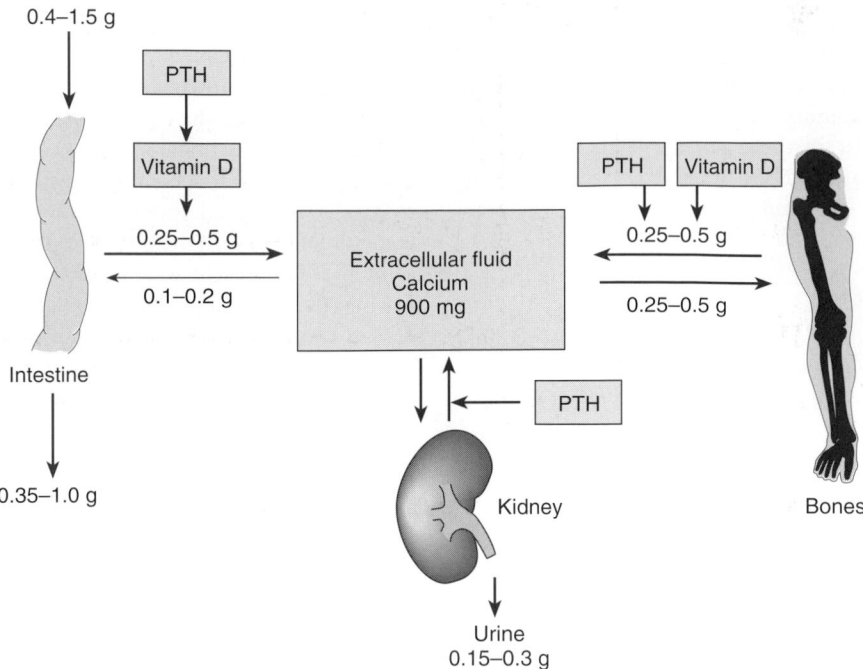

Fig. 7. Sites of action of PTH to maintain extracellular calcium. Figures represent approximate quantities of elemental calcium transferred per 24 h. Approximately 900–1500 g calcium is stored in bone.

25-hydroxyvitamin D_3 to the active hormone, $\alpha1,25$-di-hydroxyvitamin D_3 and thereby offset these obligatory losses. In the presence of inadequate dietary calcium intake or vitamin D deficiency/disturbed metabolism (see Chapter 25.10), the over-riding effects of PTH to maintain extracellular calcium ion concentration will lead to negative calcium balance (especially from bone).

Because about 90 per cent of the protein-bound calcium (c. 35 per cent of total) is associated with albumin, total plasma calcium concentration may be low in patients with liver disease and hypoalbuminaemia. Ionized calcium levels are usually normal but may be low, especially in patients abusing alcohol. Low ionized calcium levels are also found in patients with fulminant hepatic failure. Most patients with chronic liver disease are in negative calcium balance, and osteoporosis is very common in all forms of chronic liver disease. Osteomalacia is rare even in patients with cholestatic disease (Stellon, Bone, 1986; 7:181; Chapter 25.10). The aetiology of bone disease is complex. Poor nutrition and malabsorption are important; malabsorption of calcium and phosphate are common in both cholestatic and hepatocellular liver disease (Kehayoglou, Lancet, 1968; I:715; Whelton, Gut, 1971; 12: 978; Bengoa, Hepatol, 1984; 4:261; Mitchison, Gastro, 1988; 94: 463). The coupling between bone resorption and bone formation is also disturbed.

Relevant factors may include decreased physical activity, effects of alcohol, hypogonadism, diminished hepatic insulin-like growth factor-I production, and the effects of glucocorticoid treatment in patients with autoimmune liver disease or after liver transplantation. These are discussed in Chapter 25.10. PTH has also been implicated in the increased prevalence of osteoporosis in alcoholic patients. Alcohol ingestion can acutely inhibit the secretion of PTH, resulting in reduced ionized calcium levels, hypercalciuria, and increased urinary magnesium excretion (Laitinen, NEJM, 1991; 324:721). PTH levels may subsequently increase to supranormal levels with restoration of serum calcium levels. It has been suggested that recurrent cycles of hypoparathyroidism and hyperparathyroidism could contribute to the development of alcohol-related bone disease (Laitinen, NEJM, 1991; 324:721; Lalor, QJMed, 1986; 59:497). Severe hypomagnesemia, which may occasionally be found in chronic alcoholic patients, can also produce a state of functional hypoparathyroidism and hypocalcaemia.

Circulating PTH includes the intact, biologically active hormone (PTH 1–84) and a family of closely related fragments that include the midportion of PTH and C terminus of PTH and are biologically inactive in calcium homeostasis. Intact PTH has a very short circulating half-life (2–3 min). The liver and kidney are the main sites of clearance, the liver accounting for about 70 per cent of the total (Martin, JCI, 1977; 60:808; Canterbury, JCI, 1975; 55:1245; Segre, JCI, 1981; 67:438). C-terminal fragments are released back into the circulation. Their circulating half-life is longer (20–30 min) than that of intact PTH. The main C-terminal fragments disappear from the circulation after hepatectomy (Segre, JCI, 1981; 67:438). The kidney is the main site of clearance of C-terminal fragments and they accumulate after nephrectomy and in patients with chronic renal failure. Although low levels of amino-terminal fragments may be detected in the liver and kidney, they are not released back into the plasma, and under most circumstances intact PTH(1–84) is the only biologically active form in plasma. The presence of circulating biologically inactive fragments of PTH has complicated the measurement of PTH in plasma. Most 'mid-region' PTH assays predominantly recognize C-terminal fragments. While 'mid-region'

PTH assays are reliable for the diagnosis of primary hyperparathyroidism, serum PTH levels obtained using these 'mid-region' assays in patients with altered PTH metabolism (renal failure and liver disease) may be difficult to interpret.

Some patients with hepatic osteomalacia may develop secondary hyperparathyroidism with increased serum PTH levels and other evidence of increased PTH activity (increased urinary cyclic AMP excretion, decreased tubular phosphate reabsorption, bone histological changes of osteitis fibrosa) (Compston, DigDis, 1980; 25:29; Davies, DigDisSci, 1983; 28:145). Increased serum PTH levels (using a 'mid-region' PTH assay) were also found in patients with primary biliary cirrhosis despite normal or slightly elevated serum calcium and 25-hydroxyvitamin D_3 levels (Fonseca, JClinEndoc, 1987; 64:873). These authors suggested that mild vitamin D deficiency and secondary hyperparathyroidism may be early features. However, because of abnormal handling of PTH in liver disease, caution is needed in the interpretation of serum PTH levels. Kirch *et al.* (JClinEndoc, 1990; 71:1561) in a large group of cirrhotic patients of differing aetiologies (70 per cent alcoholic), found increased PTH levels using a 'mid-region' assay but normal levels of the biologically active intact PTH(1–84). Levels of biologically inactive PTH C-terminal fragments were inversely related to serum albumin and prothrombin times but did not correlate with levels of intact PTH(1–84). Increased levels of C-terminal PTH fragments in liver disease have also been reported by others (Rittinghaus, ActaEnd, 1986; 111:62).

Osteocalcin

Osteocalcin (bone Gla-protein) is a 49-amino-acid non-collagenous peptide, synthesized and secreted by bone osteoblasts. The serum concentration is believed to reflect the rate of bone formation and osteoblast activity. The peptide is activated by vitamin K-dependent carboxylation. Decreased serum osteocalcin levels with a relative decrease in the active carboxylated form were found in patients with primary biliary cirrhosis (Fonseca, JClinEndoc, 1987; 64:873). Decreased osteocalcin levels have also been found in patients with alcoholic liver disease, cholestatic liver disease, haemochromatosis, and chronic active hepatitis; the lowest levels were found in the patients with the poorest liver function (Diamond, Gastro; 1989; 96:213). Low osteocalcin levels are consistent with the findings from histological studies of bone showing that decreased bone formation is the main cause of bone disease in cholestatic and hepatocellular liver disease (Chapter 25.10).

Adrenal hormones
Normal physiology

The adrenal cortex secretes glucocorticoids (including cortisol, cortisone, and 11-deoxycorticosterone), mineralocorticoids (mainly aldosterone), and androgens. Mineralocorticoid metabolism is discussed elsewhere. Cortisol synthesis and secretion from the adrenal gland is stimulated by ACTH. Cortisol production is influenced by the diurnal rhythm of ACTH secretion, stress, and negative feedback by cortisol. Plasma ACTH and cortisol levels peak between 07.00 and 08.00 h, assuming a normal sleep time from midnight to 07.30 h (Van Cauter, HormRes, 1990; 34:45). Levels then fall, interrupted by occasional secretory peaks, to reach their nadir around midnight, rising again 2 to 4 h after the onset of sleep. This rhythm persists despite considerable peturbation of the system, including sleep deprivation. Stress is the most important stimulus to ACTH and cortisol release; it induces the release of corticotrophin releasing hormone from hypothalamic neurones into the hypophyseal portal system to stimulate pituitary ACTH release. The observation that the ACTH and cortisol response to insulin-induced hypoglycaemia is generally greater than that elicited by a maximally stimulating dose of corticotrophin releasing hormone, suggests that in addition to corticotrophin releasing hormone there are other releasing factors. Antidiuretic hormone and catecholamines (but not circulating adrenaline or noradrenaline) potentiate corticotrophin releasing hormone-induced ACTH release. Serotonin may also increase ACTH release while opioids are inhibitory. An increase in plasma cortisol decreases ACTH release and pro-opiomelanocortin synthesis by inhibiting hypothalamic corticotrophin releasing hormone synthesis and by decreasing the responsiveness of the pituitary to corticotrophin releasing hormone.

Plasma transport of glucocorticoids

About 80 to 85 per cent of plasma cortisol is bound with high affinity to cortisol-binding globulin, and about 10 to 15 per cent with much lower affinity to albumin. However, with increasing cortisol concentrations, cortisol-binding globulin becomes saturated (above *c*. 690 nmol/l [25 µg/l]) and a larger proportion is then associated with albumin. Since the rate of dissociation from albumin is more rapid than from cortisol-binding globulin, albumin-bound cortisol is more readily available to tissues. Only the free hormone is physiologically active. However, in the various tissues, the binding of cortisol from the free pool to intracellular receptors, steroid-metabolizing enzymes, and other proteins, shifts the equilibrium towards dissociation of plasma protein–cortisol complexes, and the dissociated hormone can then be taken up. In the liver, which has a relatively long sinusoidal transit time, some cortisol-binding globulin-bound cortisol may be taken up (after its dissociation) in addition to the free and albumin-bound hormone. The physiological mechanisms that control the plasma cortisol level respond to the free rather than total cortisol levels. Thus, with variations in cortisol-binding globulin levels, the free cortisol concentration is maintained within the normal range even though total cortisol levels change.

Cortisol-binding globulin also binds corticosterone and prednisolone with high affinity but binding of prednisone, cortisone, dexamethasone, and methylprednisolone is negligible. Cortisol-binding globulin has a structure similar to that of several members of the serine protease superfamily that includes α1-proteinase inhibitor, α1-chymotrypsin, and thyroxine binding globulin (Hammond, EndocrRev, 1990; 11:65). The cortisol-binding globulin–cortisol complex is cleaved by neutrophil-derived elastase at sites of inflammation. Thus, in addition to serving as a reservoir of cortisol, and slowing its clearance, cortisol-binding globulin may target the delivery of glucocorticoids to sites of infection and inflammation (Hammond, JClinEndoc, 1990; 71:34).

Cortisol metabolism

In the liver the enzyme 11β-hydroxysteroid dehydrogenase plays a key role in the metabolism of cortisol; it converts cortisol to inactive cortisone. The reverse reaction is catalysed by 11-oxo-steroid reductase, and administered cortisone is largely converted to active cortisol in the liver. The liver is the main site of cortisol degradation. Hepatic conjugation of the cortisol and cortisone metabolites with sulphate and glucuronide enhances their water solubility and renal clearance. Normally, roughly equivalent amounts of the conjugated metabolites of cortisol and cortisone are excreted in the urine. Only about 1 per cent of the cortisol produced daily is excreted unchanged in the urine. The plasma concentration of cortisol is about 1000 times that of aldosterone in man; conversion of cortisol to cortisone in the kidney collecting tubules by 11-β-hydroxysteroid dehydrogenase is important for preventing cortisol from binding to the mineralocorticoid receptor and causing a state of mineralocorticoid excess (Funder, Science, 1988; 242:583).

Cortisol in liver disease

Plasma cortisol concentration in the morning after an overnight fast is usually normal in patients with cirrhosis[18,33] (Johnston, HormMetRes, 1982; 14:34). Cirrhotic patients with poor liver function may have low cortisol-binding globulin[34] (Doe, JClinEndoc, 1964; 24:1029) and albumin levels. This may result in low morning total cortisol levels, but the biologically active free cortisol levels are usually normal;[18] they may even be somewhat higher than in matched normal subjects though still within the normal range.[34] There may be a loss or blunting of the diurnal cortisol rhythm, particularly in decompensated cirrhotics and those with alcoholic liver disease[34] (Tucci, Gastro, 1966; 50:637; McCann, JClinEndoc, 1975; 40:1038) with a tendency to higher total and free cortisol levels in the evening than in matched normal subjects. A blunting of the diurnal cortisol rhythm may also be found in alcoholic patients without significant liver disease (Kirkman, Metabolism, 1988; 37:390; Wand, JClinEndoc, 1991; 72:1290). It tends to return to normal with abstinence (Risher-Flowers, AdvAlcSubstAb, 1988; 7:37; Iranmanesh, JAndrol, 1989; 10:54).

Patients with autoimmune chronic active hepatitis may have features suggestive of Cushing's syndrome, including abdominal striae, facial mooning, acne, bruising and hirsuties, prior to treatment with corticosteroids. There is a paucity of data on cortisol metabolism in these patients. Plasma cortisol levels may be elevated but this is due to increased cortisol-binding globulin levels. Elevated cortisol-binding globulin levels are also found in patients with non-autoimmune chronic active hepatitis (Orbach, AmJMed, 1989; 86: 39). Plasma free cortisol and urinary 24-hour free cortisol excretion were normal in the patient studied by Orbach et al. (AmJMed, 1989; 86:39), and were normally suppressed by dexamethasone (0.5 mg 6 hourly for 2 days). However, due to delayed cortisol clearance in patients with raised cortisol-binding globulin levels there may be impaired suppression of the morning plasma cortisol levels with an overnight dexamethasone (1 mg) suppression test.

In keeping with the importance of the liver for cortisol metabolism, clearance of cortisol is reduced in cirrhosis (Peterson, JCI, 1960; 39:320; Zumoff, JCI, 1967; 46:1735; McCann, JClinEndoc, 1975; 40:1038; Kawai, JClinEndoc, 1985; 60:848). The clearance of synthetic glucocorticoids, prednisolone, and dexamethasone is also impaired (Kawai, JClinEndoc, 1985; 60:848). Renner et al. (Gastro, 1986; 90:819) found that in decompensated alcoholic cirrhotic patients prednisolone clearance correlated directly with galactose

elimination capacity, and that with declining liver function a larger proportion of plasma prednisolone was non-protein bound. The urinary cortisol metabolite profile is abnormal in cirrhosis. There is an increase in the ratio of cortisol metabolites (tetrahydrocortisol and its isomer 5α-tetrahydrocortisol) to tetrahydrocortisone, irrespective of the aetiology of liver disease, implying a deficiency of 11β-hydroxysteroid dehydrogenase[33] (Zumoff, JCI, 1967; 46: 1735). Other abnormalities include a reduction in the tetrahydrocortisol/5α-tetrahydrocortisol ratio (due to either deficiency of 5α-reductase or stimulation of 5β-reductase activity) and an increased proportion of unconjugated cortisol metabolites.[33]

However, the reduction in cortisol metabolism does not result in increased plasma cortisol levels because of the negative feedback effect on ACTH secretion. Patients with non-alcoholic liver disease and most alcoholic cirrhotic patients have an appropriate reduction in 24 h cortisol production rate[33,34] (McCann, JClinEndoc, 1975; 40:1038). In non-abstinent patients with alcoholic liver disease 24 h cortisol production rates are very variable; some patients show an appropriate reduction but others may have 24 h cortisol production rates within or above the normal range, despite a marked impairment of cortisol metabolism, resulting in increased plasma cortisol levels and urinary free cortisol excretion.[33] Although, their cortisol level at around 09.00 hours may be within the normal range, it tends to be higher than in patients with non-alcoholic liver disease[33] (Smals, JRoyCollPhys, 1977; 12:36). It has been suggested that this impairment of cortisol feedback at the hypothalamic pituitary level in some alcoholic patients may explain the development of pseudo-Cushing's syndrome.[33]

Pseudo-Cushing's syndrome

Alcohol-induced 'pseudo-Cushing's' is an uncommon syndrome occurring in chronic alcoholic patients. Most patients have abnormal liver function tests (Smals, JRoyCollPhys, 1977; 12:36; Kirkman, Metabolism, 1988; 37:390). In addition to the clinical features suggestive of Cushing's syndrome, such as muscle wasting, thin skin, bruising, abdominal striae, central obesity, moon face (due to parotid enlargement), hypertension, and glucose intolerance, biochemical findings may be identical to those found in pituitary-dependent Cushing's syndrome (Rees, Lancet, 1977; i:726; Kapcala, AmJMed, 1987; 82:849; Kirkman, Metabolism, 1988; 37:390; Groote Veldman, EndocrRev, 1996; 17:262). Plasma ACTH and free cortisol levels are increased, there is a loss of the normal diurnal cortisol rhythm and impaired suppression of plasma cortisol and ACTH levels with dexamethasone. Urinary excretion of free cortisol and its metabolites is increased, and there is impaired suppression of urinary free cortisol and 17-hydroxycorticosteroids during a 'low dose' dexamethasone (0.5 mg 6 hourly for 2 days) suppression test (Kapcala, AmJMed, 1987; 82:849). With 'high dose' dexamethasone (2.0 mg 6 hourly for 2 days) suppression of urinary free cortisol excretion is comparable to that in Cushing's disease. The abnormalities of cortisol metabolism resolve within days to weeks of cessation of alcohol consumption (Rees, Lancet, 1977; i:726; Smals, JRoyCollPhys, 1977; 12:36; Lamberts, JAMA, 1979; 242:1640; Kapcala, AmJMed, 1987; 82:849) but may cause diagnostic confusion. A corticotrophin-releasing hormone test performed after administration of dexamethasone (2 mg/day for 2 days) may help in the differentiation of pseudo-Cushing's from true Cushing's: in all subjects with true Cushing's syndrome a serum cortisol level above 38 nmol/l (14 μg/l) was found 15 min after the injection of corticotrophin-releasing hormone (Yanovski, JAMA, 1993; 269: 2232).

The observation that plasma cortisol levels and 24-hour cortisol production rates tend to be higher in patients with alcoholic cirrhosis than in patients with non-alcoholic chronic liver disease[33] has led to the suggestion that in some alcoholic patients there is a failure to downregulate ACTH secretion in response to increased plasma free cortisol levels arising from the impaired hepatic metabolism of cortisol. It would appear that ethanol is capable of inducing resistance to the suppressive effects of glucocorticoids on ACTH secretion (Kirkman, Metabolism, 1988; 37:390).

Cortisol response to insulin-induced hypoglycaemia in cirrhosis

Decreased plasma ACTH and cortisol responses to insulin-induced hypoglycaemia have been found in patients with endstage non-alcoholic liver disease[18] as well as in some alcoholic patients without significant liver disease (Marks, ProcRoySocMed, 1977; 70: 338; Chalmers, BMJ, 1978; 1:745). In alcoholics without significant liver disease the cortisol response to ACTH is normal (Berman, JClinEndoc, 1990; 71:712) but in endstage liver disease this may also be impaired, implying both a defect at the hypothalamic–pituitary level and an impaired response of the adrenal glands.[18] McDonald et al. found that the impairment of the plasma cortisol response to insulin-induced hypoglycaemia and to ACTH was most marked in patients with the poorest liver function as assessed by Child–Pugh score.[18] Studies in bile-duct ligated cholestatic rats also suggested an impaired ACTH/corticosterone response to stress (Swain, JCI, 1993; 91:1903). The significance of these findings in terms of recovery from hypoglycaemia and adequacy of the adrenal response to stress situations such as sepsis and gastrointestinal bleeding is unclear. The possibility of an inadequate cortisol response to stress should be borne in mind when dealing with the critically ill hypotensive patient.

Sex hormones
Normal physiology

Testosterone, the major circulating androgen in men, is synthesized and secreted by the testicular Leydig cells. Normal daily production rate is 4 to 8 mg. The testes also secrete 5α-dihydrotestosterone (50–100 μg/day), a more potent metabolite of testosterone. However, most of the circulating 5α-dihydrotestosterone is derived from reduction of the A ring of testosterone in peripheral tissues. Only a small proportion of the 5α-dihydrotestosterone produced in peripheral tissues is released into the circulation, and plasma levels do not correlate with peripheral formation (Toscano, JCI, 1987; 79: 1653). Normal plasma testosterone levels in men range from 3 to 12 μg/l (10–42 nmol/l), with a mean value of 6 to 7 μg/l (20–24 nmol/l); plasma levels of 5α-dihydrotestosterone are about one-tenth those of testosterone. Less potent androgens include androstenedione, secreted by the testes and the adrenals, and dehydroepiandrosterone and its sulphate, which are mainly of adrenal origin. These weaker androgens probably require conversion to

testosterone for androgenic activity, although less than 10 per cent of plasma testosterone in men is derived from this source.

A small fraction of plasma testosterone (<1 per cent) is converted to oestradiol, the main biologically active oestrogen. Androstenedione is the main source of the less potent oestrone (Fig. 8). Skin, fat, and muscle are the main sites of conversion, which is mediated by a cytochrome P-450-dependent aromatase. Only a fraction of the peripherally produced oestrogen enters the circulation. Peripheral conversion accounts for about 70 per cent of the oestradiol released into the circulation in men; direct testicular secretion accounts for only 20 per cent. Brain, including the hypothalamus, is also an active site of conversion of testosterone to oestradiol which is involved in the regulation of gonadotrophin secretion. Normal oestradiol and oestrone levels in men are below 50 ng/l (184 pmol/l) and 60 ng/l (222 pmol/l) respectively.

In women, production of oestradiol varies during the menstrual cycle (250–500 μg/24 h), plasma levels are lower in the early follicular phase (60–100 ng/l (0.22–0.37 nmol/l)) than during the luteal phase (200–700 ng/l (0.73–2.57 nmol/l)). Oestrone is produced mainly by peripheral conversion of androstenedione. In premenopausal women the ovaries and adrenals each contribute about 50 per cent of total daily androstenedione production (3 mg/day); after the menopause ovarian production declines markedly and the adrenals are the main source. In normal lean premenopausal women about 1 to 1.5 per cent of androstenedione is converted to oestrone; after the menopause this increases to 2 to 3 per cent so that total oestrone production (40 μg/day) remains unchanged. Plasma testosterone levels in women (c. 0.35 μg/l (1.21 nmol/l)) are about 5 per cent those found in men. Nearly half of this comes from the ovaries. The remainder is derived from conversion of androstenedione (c. one-third), and to a lesser extent dehydroepiandrosterone, of adrenal origin to testosterone in fat, muscle, and possibly liver.

Testosterone production is stimulated by luteinizing hormone (**LH**), which regulates the enzymatic steps leading to production of testosterone from its precursor pregnenolone. LH secretion in turn is inhibited by testosterone in a negative feedback fashion, at both the hypothalamic and pituitary levels (Fingelstein, JClinEndoc, 1991; 73:609). Spermatogenesis is primarily controlled by follicle stimulating hormone (**FSH**), which acts on Sertoli cells to modulate the production of a variety of protein factors that regulate and coordinate sperm development; the hormone inhibin produced by Sertoli cells exerts negative feedback control of FSH secretion. LH acts indirectly by stimulating testosterone secretion; high local concentrations of testosterone (50–100 μg/100 g) are necessary for normal spermatogenesis. Sertoli cell secretion of androgen-binding protein (which has the same amino acid sequence as sex hormone binding globulin but differs in its carbohydrate content) into the lumen of the seminiferous tubules helps to ensure these high local concentrations of testosterone. Androgen deficiency due to primary testicular disease is associated with elevated plasma LH levels. If spermatogenesis is decreased, plasma FSH levels are also raised. In hypothalamic–pituitary disease, plasma gonadotrophin levels are low.

The liver is the main site of degradation of androgens and oestrogens. Testosterone is degraded to water-soluble 17-ketosteroids such as androsterone and etiocholanolone. Oestrogens are metabolized largely by hydroxylation and oxidation reactions. The

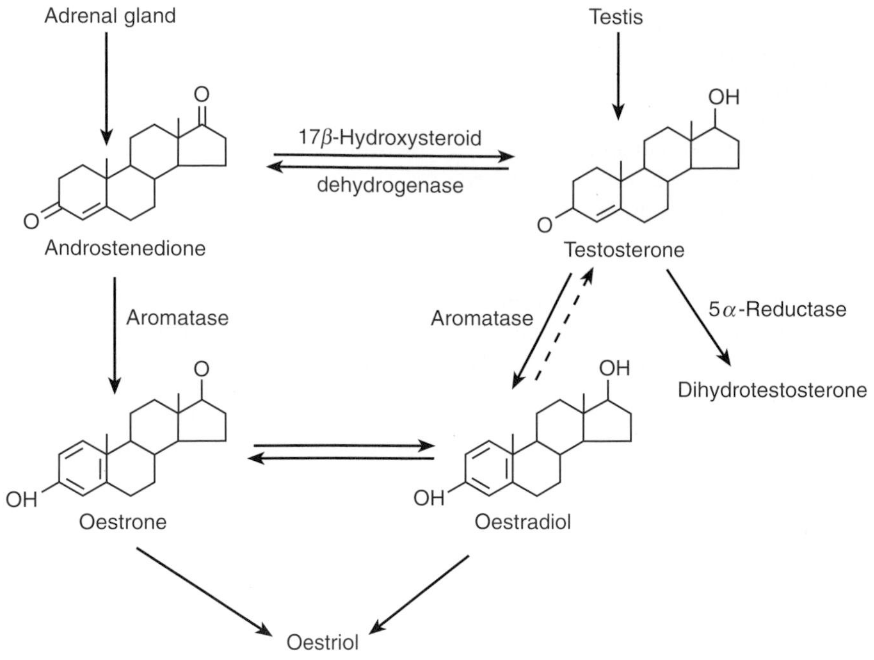

Fig. 8. Peripheral pathway for conversion of androgens to oestrogens. In males most blood oestradiol originates from testosterone. In liver disease activity of the cytochrome P-450-dependent aromatase is increased, resulting in increased oestrone and oestriol formation. In men with cirrhosis as much as 15 per cent of circulating testosterone may be derived from androstenedione compared to 1 per cent in normal men.

17-ketosteroids and oestrogen metabolites are then conjugated with sulphate or glucuronide and excreted in the urine. The bulk (c. 70 per cent) of the urinary 17-ketosteroids are derived from the adrenal cortex and not from the metabolism of testosterone.

Sex steroid transport in blood

Circulating testosterone and 5α-dihydrotestosterone are mainly bound to sex hormone binding globulin (high-affinity, low-capacity binding) and albumin (low-affinity, high-capacity binding) with only 1 to 4 per cent in the free form. Sex hormone binding globulin is a glycoprotein synthesized by the liver (Petra, JSteroid-BiochMolBiol, 1991; 40:735). In addition to testosterone, it binds oestradiol with a much lower affinity. Androstenedione, de-hydroepiandrosterone, and oestrone, which lack the 17β-hydroxy group, do not bind to sex hormone binding globulin (Dunn, JClin-Endoc, 1981; 53:58). Binding of androgens to sex hormone binding globulin slows their plasma clearance. Thus, the metabolic clearance rate of testosterone (0.6 1/min in men and 0.3 1/min in women) is lower than that of androstenedione and dehydroepiandrosterone which circulate free or bound to albumin, and have high hepatic extraction ratios and clearance rates (c. 1.0 1/min) that resemble splanchnic plasma flow. Unbound testosterone and oestradiol have generally been considered to be the biologically active fraction. However, because of the low-affinity binding to albumin, the albumin-bound fraction of these hormones is readily available for tissue extraction; the sum of free plus albumin-bound testosterone provides a good estimate of bioactive androgen.

Hepatic sex hormone binding globulin production is increased by oestrogens and decreased by administration of androgen (Selby, AnnClinBioch, 1990; 27:532). Insulin and insulin-like growth factor-I may, however, be the major regulators (Yki-Jarvinen, JClin-Endoc, 1995; 80:3227; Plymate, Metabolism, 1990; 39:967).

Thyroid hormone also stimulates sex hormone binding globulin synthesis, and levels are low in hypothyroidism (Selby, AnnClin-Bioch, 1990; 27:532). Sex hormone binding globulin levels have a major influence on plasma free testosterone levels. An increase in sex hormone binding globulin in response to oestrogen lowers the free testosterone level; conversely a rise in testosterone lowers sex hormone binding globulin levels and increases the unbound testosterone fraction. Changes in sex hormone binding globulin levels have much less effect on measured oestrogen levels because the affinity of sex hormone binding globulin for oestradiol is much lower than for testosterone, and in men circulating oestradiol levels are an order of magnitude below the K_a of sex hormone binding globulin for oestradiol.

In some androgen-responsive target tissues testosterone is converted by steroid 5α-reductase to 5α-dihydrotestosterone, which is the main cellular mediator of androgen action. In other tissues testosterone itself is active. Thus, testosterone itself mediates the anabolic actions on muscle (Mooradian, EndocrRev, 1987; 8:1) and stimulates the female pattern of axillary and pubic hair growth in both sexes (Randall, ClinEndoc, 1994; 40:439) but 5α-dihydrotestosterone is essential for the development of external male genitalia and the development of the full male pattern of facial and body hair growth and androgenic alopecia. The intracellular androgen receptor (Chang, Science, 1988; 240:324; Faber, JBC, 1991; 266:10743; Jenster, MolEndocrin, 1991; 5:1396) can bind testosterone or 5α-dihydrotestosterone, but its affinity for 5α-di-hydrotestosterone is higher. Binding of androgen to the receptor causes the receptor to be released from an inactive complex of proteins. The active receptor with its bound ligand then binds to specific chromosomal DNA sequences ('androgen response element') to regulate gene expression (Fig. 5). Specificity of the response probably depends on formation of a complex with a number of transcriptional factors as well as binding to the androgen response element (Adler, PNAS, 1992; 89:11660). In blood stem cells there is a specific 5β-dihydrotestosterone receptor, and enhancement of red cell production in response to erythropoietin by testosterone requires its conversion to 5β-dihydrotestosterone (Gardner, CurrTopHaematol, 1983; 4:123; Ammus, AdvIntMed, 1989; 34:191).

Sexual dysfunction in men with liver disease

Cirrhosis is associated with hypogonadism and signs of feminization. Hypogonadism is associated with testicular atrophy, impotence, and loss of libido. Signs of feminization include loss of body hair, a female distribution of body hair, a redistribution of body fat, and gynaecomastia (Kew, Hepatol, 1988; 8:429). Vascular spider naevi and palmar erythema are also regarded by many as signs of feminization, as they occur with increased frequency during normal pregnancy, and may be found in men with prostatic carcinoma treated with high doses of oestrogens. Benign prostatic hypertrophy occurs less frequently in cirrhosis (Stumpf, ArchIntMed, 1953; 91: 304; Frea, UrolRes, 1987; 15:311). Most published figures (see below) concerning the prevalence of these complications are based on studies of selected patients in hospital, and of patients with long-standing disease. The abnormalities are more commonly found in patients with de-compensated liver disease, and in patients with alcoholic cirrhosis in whom they tend to be more pronounced than in men with cirrhosis due to other causes.[35,36] In patients with well-compensated, non-alcoholic liver disease gynaecomastia and sexual dysfunction are uncommon. In haemachromatosis, however, gonadal failure may precede the development of cirrhosis (see later).

Hypogonadism and associated hormonal changes

Hyogonadism has been reported in as many as 70 to 80 per cent of men with cirrhosis;[36–40] clinical and histological evidence of testicular atrophy is found in over 50 per cent of patients[35] (Bennett, AmJClinPath, 1950; 20:814; Van Thiel, Gastro, 1974; 67: 1188). The gonadal atrophy in alcoholic cirrhotic men reflects a reduction in mass of the seminiferous tubules which account for 90 to 95 per cent of the testicular volume, and there are gross abnormalities of seminal fluid composition (Van Thiel, Hepatol, 1981; 1:39). Leydig cell failure is manifest by a marked reduction in testosterone production (Gordon, JClinEndoc, 1975; 40:1018), and as much as 15 per cent of circulating testosterone in cirrhotic men may be derived from the peripheral conversion of androstenedione produced by the adrenals, compared to 1 per cent in normal men. Total plasma testosterone levels are often decreased in cirrhotic patients,[35,36,38–41] falling with increasing severity of liver disease as assessed by Child–Pugh score[39,41] (Kley, Gastro, 1979; 76: 235; Gluud, Metabolism, 1987; 36:373; Becker, ActaMedScand, 1988; 224:367). Testosterone responses to small doses of human chorionic gonadotrophin, which has predominant LH activity, are diminished.[35]

While liver disease *per se* is associated with hypogonadism,[36, 39–41] most studies have been conducted in alcoholic cirrhotic men, many of whom will have continued to consume alcohol up to the time of investigation. Alcohol itself affects gonadal and hypothalamic–pituitary function (Chapter 15.3). Ethanol inhibits testosterone production by blocking 17α-reductase and 17,20-desmolase activities which are key enzymes in the biosynthetic

pathway. Excessive alcohol intake in normal volunteers inhibits testosterone production, resulting in decreased testosterone levels with a secondary rise in LH; after 1 to 2 weeks of heavy alcohol intake, testosterone levels remain low and LH levels also become subnormal (Gordon, ClinExpRes, 1978; 2:259). Ethanol also inhibits spermatogenesis; it may compete with retinol for an alcohol dehydrogenase enzyme in the testes which is important for converting retinol to retinal (the aldehyde form of vitamin A) that is essential for normal spermatogenesis (Van Thiel, Science, 1974; 196:941). Alcohol abuse, even in the absence of liver disease, causes hypogonadism and a variety of sexual disorders (Van Thiel, Gastro, 1974; 67:1188). Testosterone levels tend to be lower in alcoholic than in non-alcoholic cirrhotic men matched for severity of liver disease,[36,42] consistent with a direct toxic effect of alcohol on the testes. Thus, in alcoholic cirrhosis the effects of alcohol and cirrhosis may be additive, and alcohol is undoubtedly a factor in the high prevalence rates of hypogonadism found in alcoholic cirrhotics;[37, 43] sexual function may improve with abstinence[37] (Van Thiel, Gastro, 1983; 84:677). Van Thiel has suggested a much lower prevalence of gonadal dysfunction in men with well-compensated non-alcoholic liver cirrhosis (Hepatol, 1981; 1:39). In endstage liver disease, some[40] but not all studies[42] have suggested that the prevalence of hypogonadism may be equally high in alcoholic and non-alcoholic cirrhotic patients. In patients with endstage liver disease the relative importance of liver disease *per se* and such factors as nutritional state, weight loss, and intercurrent illness, all of which can produce a transient secondary hypogonadism and biochemical androgen deficiency (Semple, QJMed, 1987; 64:601; Handelsman, EndMetClinNAm, 1994; 23:839), is unclear.

Sex hormone binding globulin levels are increased in men with cirrhosis[39] (Johnson, ClinSci, 1984; 66:369; Gluud, Metabolism, 1987; 36:373; Guechot, Gastro, 1987; 92:203; Becker, ActaMedScand, 1988; 224:367). Possible explanations for increased hepatic production of sex hormone binding globulin in liver disease are the low levels of insulin-like growth factor-I and possibly hepatic underinsulinization due to portosystemic shunting and capillarization of hepatic sinusoids. Abnormal glycosylation of sex hormone binding globulin (Terasaki, JClinEndoc, 1988; 67:639) could prolong its circulating half-life. Because of the increased sex hormone binding globulin levels in cirrhotic men, free testosterone levels are decreased more consistently than total testosterone levels. In patients with very poor liver function and encephalopathy, hepatic synthesis of sex hormone binding globulin may be impaired resulting in very low total testosterone levels (DeBesi, ActaEnd, 1989; 120:271).

There is no correlation between impotence and the low plasma testosterone levels in patients with liver disease and treatment with testosterone has generally been ineffective.[37] Other hormonal changes associated with cirrhosis include increased plasma levels of androstenedione, decreased dehydroepiandrosterone and dehydroepiandrosterone sulphate, and increased levels of oestrone (Table 3). Plasma oestradiol concentrations are usually normal in well-compensated disease,[35,36] but may increase with increasing severity of liver disease, particularly in alcoholic cirrhotics (Chopra, AnnIntMed, 1973; 79:198; Guechot, Gastro, 1987; 92:203). The increase in oestradiol levels is due to increased peripheral conversion of testosterone to oestradiol, and not to a reduction in oestradiol metabolism; this is normal or even increased[35] (Olivo, Steroids,

Table 3 Sex steroid hormone changes in cirrhosis

Hormone	Men	Premenopausal women	Postmenopausal women	References Men	References Women
Testerone	↓	→↓	→	1–10	19–21
5α-Dihydrotestosterone	↓	→	↓	8	20, 22, 23
DHEA	↓	↓	↓	1, 11	
DHEA-sulphate	↓	↓	↓	1, 9, 11	20–22
Androstenedione	↑	→↑	→↑↓	1, 9, 10	20–23
Oestrone	↑	↑	↑	2, 10, 12	19–23
Oestradiol	→↑	↓	→	1, 5, 7, 10, 12	19, 21
Oestriol	↑	↑	↑	12	19
Progesterone	↑	↓	↓	13	19
Luteinizing hormone	↑→↓	→↓	→↓	2–5, 7, 9	20, 24
FSH	↑→↓	→↓	→↓	2–5, 7	20, 24
Prolactin	→↑	→↑	→↑	4, 7, 14, 15	20, 24
SHBG	↑	→↑	↑→	3, 16–18	21–24

DHEA, dehydroepiandrosterone; FSH, follicle stimulating hormone; SHBG, sex hormone binding globulin.

References:
1. Bannister, QJ Med, 1987; 63: 305–13.
2. Wang, JHepatol, 1993; 18: 101–5.
3. Handelsman, ClinEndoc, 1995; 43: 331–7.
4. Wang, Hepatogast, 1991; 38: 531–4.
5. Baker, QJMed, 1976; 45: 145–78.
6. Zifroni, Hepatol, 1991; 14: 479–82.
7. Van Thiel, Hepatol, 1981; 39: 39–46.
8. Chopra, AnnIntMed, 1973; 79: 198–203.
9. Bannister, BMJ, 1986; 293: 1191–3.
10. Kley, Gastro, 1979; 76: 235–41.
11. Bahnsen, EurJClinInv, 1981; 11: 473–9.
12. Green, Gut, 1976; 17: 426–30.
13. Farthing, Gut, 1982; 23: 276–9.
14. Morgan, Gut, 1978; 19: 170–4.
15. Van Thiel, JEndocInv, 1986; 9: 479–86.
16. Gluud, Metabolism, 1987; 36: 373–8.
17. Becker, ActaMedScand, 1988; 224: 367–73.
18. Johnson, ClinSci, 1984; 66: 369–76.
19. Valimaki, JClinEndoc, 1984; 59: 133–8.
20. Becker, JHepatol, 1991; 13: 25–32.
21. Bannister, ClinEndoc, 1985; 23: 335–40.
22. Becker, DanMedBull, 1993; 40: 447–59.
23. Becker, Hepatol, 1991; 13: 865–9.
24. Bell, EurJEndoc, 1995; 132: 444–9.

1975; 26:47). Conversion of androstenedione to oestrone is increased in cirrhosis (Gordon, JClinEndoc, 1975; 40:1018; Van Thiel, Metabolism, 1979; 28:536). Adipose tissue is an important site of aromatization of androstenedione to oestrone. This conversion may be enhanced by increased delivery of androstenedione to adipose tissue as a result of decreased hepatic clearance of androstenedione in patients with significant portosystemic shunting (Van Thiel, Gastro, 1980; 78:81). Guechot et al. (Gastro, 1987; 92:203) found a strong correlation between the hepatic extraction ratios of androstenedione and indocyanine green in patients with alcoholic cirrhosis. However, Wang and colleagues found no correlation between changes in sex hormone levels and the severity of portal hypertension in patients with cirrhosis due to hepatitis B virus infection.[38]

Increased conversion of androstenedione to oestrone and of testosterone to oestradiol in cirrhosis could also be due to altered hepatic steroid metabolism. The hepatic expression of certain forms of cytochrome P-450 concerned with metabolism of sex steroids shows marked gender differences. Portal vein ligation of male rats resulted in a marked reduction of male-specific cytochrome P-450 isoforms, responsible for 16α- and 6β-hydroxylation of androstenedione, associated with a corresponding decrease in metabolism of androstenedione via these pathways; the conversion of androstenedione to oestradiol increased seven- to 15-fold (Farrell, JCI, 1988; 81:221). The sexually dimorphic pattern of hepatic steroid-metabolizing enzymes is in part determined by the pattern of hypothalamic–pituitary hormone release. Growth hormone is known to be important (Kobliakov, EurJBioch, 1991; 195:585); feminization of hepatic steroid metabolism occurs in rats treated with growth hormone (Mode, Endocrinol, 1981; 108:2103).

Whether the elevated growth hormone levels in many patients with cirrhosis influence hepatic sex steroid metabolism is unknown.

Plasma LH and FSH levels are usually normal or increased in patients with well-compensated cirrhosis[38,40] (Van Thiel, Hepatol, 1981; 1:39; DeBesi, ActaEnd, 1989; 120:271) but are often decreased in patients with endstage liver disease (Pugh's grades B and C).[38–41] Reduced gonadotrophin production may be a key to the development of overt hypogonadism. Bannister et al. (BMJ, 1986; 293:1191), in a small group of alcoholic cirrhotic men, found a decreased amplitude and frequency of LH pulses, despite normal basal LH levels, in those with overt hypogonadism and testicular atrophy, but normal LH pulsatility and raised basal LH levels in those with subclinical primary testicular failure. Primary testicular failure is normally associated with elevated LH levels. Thus, normal or low plasma LH concentrations in the presence of low free testosterone levels suggest a hypothalamic–pituitary defect. The response of LH and FSH to gonadotrophin releasing hormone is variable.[35,39,40] Peak responses are usually normal or increased but the incremental responses are often diminished in those with elevated basal LH and FSH levels[40] (Van Thiel, Hepatol, 1981; 1:39); the peak LH and FSH response may be delayed in patients with endstage liver disease, irrespective of aetiology.[39] Decreased plasma testosterone and LH concentrations with preserved pituitary gonadotrophin responses to gonadotrophin releasing hormone strongly suggest that diminished LH production in 'sick' cirrhotics and those with overt hypogonadism is due to a hypothalamic defect. Decreased LH and FSH responses to clomiphene, particularly in alcoholic cirrhotic patients (Van Thiel, Hepatol, 1981; 1:39) is in keeping with a hypothalamic defect. Hypothalamic dysfunction would explain the diminished pulsatile LH secretion (Bannister, BMJ, 1986; 293:1191), as this depends on episodic release of gonadotrophin releasing hormone from hypothalamic neurones into the pituitary portal blood.

Testicular endocrine dysfunction is improved by successful liver transplantation in alcoholic and non-alcoholic cirrhotic patients.[39, 42,44] Sexual function may also improve in some patients.[42] Handelsman *et al.*[39] reported a progressive improvement but not normalization, in sex hormone levels at 6 and 12 months after successful liver transplanation for endstage non-alcoholic liver disease. At 12 months plasma total and free testosterone levels had increased to 71 and 66 per cent of normal, sex hormone binding globulin levels had decreased to normal and (despite the increase in testosterone levels), basal LH and FSH levels increased to levels that were approximately twice those found in normal men. Plasma oestrone and androstenedione levels also fall after transplantation.[44] Whether the residual abnormalities reflect an irreversible component or are due to the effects of treatment with glucocorticoids, cyclosporin, or other drugs is unclear.

Feminization

Clinical features of feminization, including gynaecomastia, loss of body hair, and a redistribution of body fat occur in 20 to 50 per cent of patients with cirrhosis. Gynaecomastia is usually bilateral but may be unilateral. Vascular spider naevi and palmar erythema are often regarded as signs of feminization but their appearance in women with alcoholic hepatitis or cirrhosis who have evidence of oestrogen deficiency casts some doubt on the role of oestrogens in their pathogenesis. The plasma levels of a number of proteins whose synthesis is enhanced by oestrogens, including sex hormone binding globulin, prolactin, growth hormone, and thyroxine binding globulin are increased in these patients. By contrast with hypogonadism, feminization usually occurs only in the presence of cirrhosis, although gynaecomastia can appear in acute alcoholic hepatitis and may be found in young men with chronic active hepatitits without cirrhosis. Feminization may be more common in alcoholic cirrhosis than in other forms of liver disease[35] (Summerskill, NEJM, 1960; 262:1) but not all studies have found this (Powell, MedJAust, 1971; 1:941; Mowat, Gut, 1976; 17:345). It often occurs as a side-effect of spironolactone treatment (see below).

The biochemical basis for feminization remains unclear. Serum oestradiol levels are normal in most cirrhotic men with gynaecomastia and other feminizing features. Some studies have suggested a relationship with plasma oestrone levels (Green, Gut, 1976; 17:426) which are frequently raised in cirrhotic patients. However, because the feminizing potency of oestrone (and of oestriol which is also raised) is much less than that of oestradiol the importance of increased plasma oestrone and oestriol levels remain unclear. Other metabolites of oestradiol such as 16-hydroxyoestrone are increased in cirrhosis and may be biologically active. It has been suggested that the relative concentrations of free testosterone and oestradiol levels may be more important than oestradiol levels *per se*. Because of the increased sex hormone binding globulin levels in cirrhosis, and the greater affinity of sex hormone binding globulin for testosterone than for oestradiol, the free testosterone : free oestradiol ratio may be markedly decreased in patients with cirrhosis, falling with increasing severity of liver disease (Kley, Gastro, 1979; 76:

235). The presence of abnormal isoforms of sex hormone binding globulin in cirrhosis may result in increased tissue availability of oestradiol (Terasaki, JClinEndoc, 1988; 67:639). Increased local oestrogen synthesis in the breast may occur from androgens (notably androstenedione) that have escaped hepatic metabolism as a result of portosystemic shunting.

Altered end-organ sensitivity to sex steroids could also be a factor leading to feminization. Increased hepatic expression of oestrogen receptors has been suggested as a potential mechanism leading to feminization of hepatic metabolism. Alcohol increases hepatic oestrogen receptor content (Eagon, ArchBiochemBiophys, 1981; 211:48). However, findings in patients with cirrhosis have been conflicting. Increased hepatic oestrogen receptor concentrations in alcoholic cirrhotics, particularly those with superimposed alcoholic hepatitis, were found by Villa *et al.* (Hepatol, 1988; 8:1610), while others found decreased levels (Becker, ScaJGastr, 1992; 27:355; Becker, DanMedBull, 1993; 40:447). Hepatic oestrogen receptor concentrations are normal in patients with non-alcoholic liver disease (Villa, Hepatol, 1988; 8:1610; Becker, DanMedBull, 1993; 40: 447). Low hepatic androgen receptor levels were found in a small group of patients with cirrhosis of varying aetiology (Bannister, Liver, 1988; 8:28). The oestrogen/androgen receptor status of other target organs in men with hypogonadism/ feminization is unknown.

Drugs

Spironolactone is a common cause of gynaecomastia and impotence in patients with and without liver disease. Spironolactone and its metabolites act partly by reducing testosterone synthesis by inhibiting the cytochrome P-450-dependent 17-hydroxylase complex, and partly by binding competitively to tissue androgen receptors. Spironolactone treatment is associated with a fall in serum testosterone levels and a rise in oestradiol levels (Rose, AnnIntMed, 1977; 87:398). Except for the unchanged sex hormone binding globulin levels, these hormonal changes are similar to those found in cirrhotic patients not treated with spironolactone. Thus, spironolactone may contribute to hypogonadism and feminization in some patients. Indeed, spironolactone has been used successfully in dosages of 100 to 200 mg daily for the treatment of idiopathic hirsutism (Jeffcoate, ClinEndoc, 1993; 39:143). Potassium canrenoate, which is metabolized to canrenone (a metabolite of spironolactone), may be as good as spironolactone in the management of ascites, but has less anti-androgenic activity and may be less likely to cause gynaecomastia (Andriulli, Digestion, 1989; 44:155). Many other drugs commonly used in patients with liver disease may contribute to hypogonadism, including cimetidine (androgen receptor antagonist) (Van Thiel, ScaJGastr, 1987; 136:24), propranolol, thiazide diuretics, glucocorticoids, sulphasalazine (Toovey, Gut, 1981; 22:445), and drugs that stimulate prolactin secretion.

Ovarian dysfunction in women

Ovarian endocrine failure in alcoholic cirrhotic women is manifested by loss of libido, irregular menses, loss of secondary sexual characteristics such as breast and pelvic fat, and ovulatory failure (Van Thiel, ClinEndMetab, 1979; 8:499). A paucity of developing follicles, and few or no corpora lutea, was found at autopsy in women aged 20 to 40 dying of alcoholic cirrhosis (Jung, ArchPathol, 1972; 94:265). Menopause often occurs at an earlier age in cirrhotic and non-cirrhotic female alcoholic patients.[45] The pathways for steroid synthesis in the testes and ovaries are similar and it is likely that hypogonadism in alcoholic cirrhotic patients is in part due to direct toxic effects of alcohol on ovarian function. However, as in men, liver disease *per se* is important. Valimaki *et al.* (ActaObGyn, 1995; 74:462) found no difference in ovarian size or follicular development by ultrasonography in alcoholic women without significant liver disease admitted for detoxification, compared to a matched control group. Amenorrhoea and oligomenorrhoea are common in women with endstage non-alcoholic liver disease. Amenorrhoea tends to be more common in patients with cirrhosis and hepatocellular failure than in patients with predominantly biliary disease and cholestasis. Indeed, patients with primary biliary cirrhosis have a high frequency of menorrhagia (Cundy, Gut, 1990; 31:337) and age at menopause appears similar to that of control subjects (Becker, Hepatol, 1991; 13:865). Amenorrhoea is also usual in patients presenting with autoimmune chronic active hepatitis (with or without cirrhosis) but regular menses resume when the liver disease is controlled by corticosteroids, and then they have little trouble conceiving, although there may be a higher fetal wastage (Steven, QJMed, 1979; 48:519). Recovery of menstruation and fertility can be expected in the vast majority of premenopausal women with amenorrhoea associated with endstage liver disease after successful liver transplantation (Cundy, Gut, 1990; 31:337). The need for oestrogen replacement therapy should be considered in those failing to menstruate within 1 year of transplantation.

Hormone levels (Table 3)

Sex hormone changes in women with chronic liver disease have been less well characterized than in men. Premenopausal alcoholic cirrhotic women with secondary amenorrhoea are oestrogen deficient. Their urinary total oestrogen excretion is subnormal and similar to that found in normal postmenopausal women; oestriol makes a bigger contribution to their total oestrogen excretion compared to normal premenopausal women.[46] Plasma oestradiol and progesterone levels are reduced, while plasma oestrone levels are increased.[46] (Van Thiel, ClinEndMetab, 1979; 8:499). Plasma testosterone and androstenedione levels are usually normal.

Postmenopausal women with either alcoholic or non-alcoholic cirrhosis have increased oestradiol and oestrone levels by comparison with normal postmenopausal women. Their testosterone levels are generally normal and most studies have found low androstenedione, dehydroepiandrosterone and dehydroepiandrosterone sulphate levels[45,47,48] (Jasonni, Steroids, 1983; 41:569), though increased androstenedione levels have also been found (Carlstrom, ActaEnd, 1986; 111:75; Eriksson, JSterBioch, 1989; 32:427; Becker, Hepatol, 1991; 13:865). Grun *et al.* (KlinWschr, 1987; 65:411) found that androstenedione levels increased in decompensated cirrhotic patients. As in cirrhotic men, sex hormone binding globulin levels are often increased in alcoholic and non-alcoholic cirrhotic women[46] (Becker, Hepatol, 1991; 13:865), and may rise with abstinence in alcoholic cirrhotic patients.[50] Plasma prolactin levels are generally normal in both pre- and postmenopausal women with chronic liver disease (see below).

Hypothalamic pituitary dysfunction

Despite the low plasma oestradiol levels, LH and FSH levels are not increased in cirrhotic women; inappropriately low LH and FSH levels are found in amenorrhoeic cirrhotic women (pre- or postmenopausal) irrespective of the aetiology of liver disease (Bell, EurJEndocr, 1995; 32:444). In response to intravenous gonadotrophin releasing hormone they have a normal increase in LH and FSH levels, suggesting that the defect is at the level of the hypothalamus rather than the pituitary[46] (Bell, EurJEndocr, 1995; 32:444). In sick patients the abnormalities of gonadotrophin and sex hormone levels may be due in part to the effects of systemic illness (Woolf, JClinEndoc, 1985; 60:444; Dong, ClinEndoc, 1992; 36:399) or malnutrition (Handelsman, JAndrol, 1985; 6:144; Handelsman, EndMetClinNAm, 1994; 23:839). However, liver disease *per se*, and possibly portosystemic shunting (Farrell, Gastro, 1986; 90:299), are likely to be important since the abnormalities of plasma gonadotrophin levels may be found in cirrhotic patients in the absence of weight loss or malnutrition.

Prolactin

Increased secretion of prolactin is an important cause of hypogonadism and impotence in men, and of amenorrhoea in women. Prolactin is under inhibitory hypothalamic dopaminergic regulation. Prolactin inhibits hypothalamic gonadotrophin releasing hormone release and directly inhibits ovarian progesterone and oestradiol secretion. Thus, hyperprolactinaemia inhibits sex steroid synthesis in both sexes. In men, prolactin inhibits testosterone production and also decreases the activity of 5α-reductase in peripheral tissues (Magrini, ActaEnd, 1977; 212:143), resulting in impaired conversion of testosterone to the more potent androgen, 5α-dihydrotestosterone. Prolactin levels are normal in most patients with liver disease[45,46,50] although there is a very wide range, with about 8 per cent of male and 17 per cent of female patients having prolactin levels above the reference range.[51] Prolactin levels are unrelated to the aetiology of liver disease[40,49,50] (Van Thiel, Hepatol, 1981; 1:39). In some[49] but not all[50] studies, hyperprolactinaemia was more commonly found in patients with established cirrhosis than in patients with non-cirrhotic liver disease, and in cirrhotic men prolactin levels correlated with the severity of liver disease as assessed by Pugh's grading.[40] Prolactin responses to intravenous thyrotrophin releasing hormone have been found to be normal[46] (Green, Gut, 1977; 18:843) or increased (Panerai, JClinEndoc, 1977; 45:134). Basal and stimulated prolactin levels may be higher in cirrhotics with encephalopathy than those without encephalopathy (Van Thiel, JEndocrInv, 1986; 9:479).

The mechanism of hyperprolactinaemia in liver disease is unclear. Since prolactin secretion is stimulated by an increase in circulating oestrogen levels, the increased plasma oestrone levels in cirrhotic men (particularly those in Pugh's grades B and C) might be expected to play a role. However, prolactin levels do not correlate with plasma oestrogen levels (Van Thiel, Metabolism, 1978; 27:1778). Brain delivery of oestradiol may be enhanced in cirrhosis despite a reduction in the free plus albumin-bound fraction of oestradiol (Sakiyama, JClinEndoc, 1982; 54:1140). The presence of abnormal isoforms of sex hormone binding globulin in cirrhosis may result in increased availability of sex hormone binding globulin-bound oestradiol (Terasaki, JClinEndoc, 1988; 67:639).

The clinical manifestations of hypogonadism or the presence of gynaecomastia do not correlate with plasma prolactin levels[50] (Farthing, Gut, 1982; 23:276). Thus, hyperprolactinaemia cannot be invoked to explain the high prevalence of either hypogonadism or feminization in patients with liver disease.

Endocrine dysfunction in haemochromatosis

Endocrine dysfunction is common in patients with haemochromatosis.[51-55]

Diabetes

The reported prevalence of diabetes in haemochromatosis is very variable. The differences partly reflect varying definitions of diabetes as well as the severity of haemochromatosis. Many patients previously classified as having diabetes (Stocks, QJMed, 1973; 168: 733) would now be regarded as having impaired glucose tolerance.[1] Earlier diagnosis of patients with haemochromatosis may also account for a lower prevalence of diabetes in recent studies compared with earlier reports (Niederau, Gastro, 1996; 110:1107). Niederau et al.[51] in a study of 163 patients with haemochromatosis diagnosed between 1959 and 1983 found diabetes at presentation in 6 per cent of 45 precirrhotic patients but in 71 per cent of 112 patients with cirrhosis. Adams et al. (AmJMed, 1991; 90:445) found that 23 per cent of haemochromatotic patients had diabetes at the time of presentation.

The aetiology of diabetes in haemochromatosis is multifactorial. Most patients with haemochromatosis are insulin resistant. This may be due to effects of cirrhosis (see above) or to iron overload; insulin resistance is an early finding in patients with transfusional iron overload (Merkel, NEJM, 1988; 318:809). Patients with overt diabetes have impaired insulin secretion. This is probably due to the heavy iron deposition in the islet β-cells and the exocrine pancreas. The morphology of the islets tends to be well preserved and quite different from that in either type I or type II diabetes mellitus (Rahier, Diabetolog, 1987; 30:5). Diabetes appears to be more common in haemochromatotic patients with a first-degree relative with diabetes (Dymock, AmJMed, 1972; 52:203; Saudek, ClinEndMetab, 1992; 6:807), suggesting that a genetic predisposition to diabetes may be important in some patients.

The presence of diabetes in haemochromatotic patients is associated with a worse prognosis[51,53] (Niederau, Gastro, 1996; 110:1107). Patients are at risk of long-term microvascular (retinopathy, neuropathy, nephropathy) and macrovascular complications of diabetes. Good diabetic control is important to decrease the risk of these and to slow their progression (DCCT, NEJM, 1993; 329:977; DCCT, Diabetes, 1995; 44:968). Diabetic haemochromatotic patients are more likely to require insulin for control of their diabetes if they have cirrhosis: in the study of Niederau et al.[51] 62 per cent of those with cirrhosis were on insulin at presentation, compared to 40 per cent of those without cirrhosis. Depletion of body iron stores does not eliminate the need for insulin, but insulin requirements may fall; diabetic control may also

be improved in about half of the patients treated with sulphonylureas or diet. Some patients on oral hypoglycaemic agents may be able to stop these, though diabetes may progress with longer-term follow-up as it does in patients with non-insulin-dependent diabetes mellitus. Over a 2-year follow-up period, about 10 per cent of those with normal or impaired glucose tolerance at presentation show a deterioration of glucose tolerance despite iron depletion. The principles of management are similar to those outlined earlier. Some insulin-treated patients may have diabetes that is difficult to control. Defective glucose counter-regulation has been suggested. Some patients may have deficient growth hormone responses.[55] However, iron deposits are not found in the glucagon secreting islet α-cells (Rahier, Diabetolog, 1987; 30:5) and plasma glucagon levels are usually increased (Nelson, JClinEndoc, 1979; 48:412).

Hypogonadism and gynaecomastia

Decreased gonadal function is an early and common manifestation in men with haemochromatosis.[51-55] It may antedate the presence of liver disease and often goes unrecognized as a manifestation of haemochromatosis[52,54] (Adams, AmJMed, 1991; 90:445). Hypogonadism is less common in women, presumably owing to the protective effects of iron loss from menstruation. In men the clinical picture includes impotence, decreased libido, testicular atrophy, loss of body hair, and decreased frequency of shaving. These manifestations do not correlate with the severity of liver disease. Gynaecomastia is uncommon in the early stages but may be present in cirrhotic patients with portal hypertension, and may develop during testosterone replacement therapy (see below). In most patients hypogonadism is due to gonadotrophin deficiency (Walton, QJMed, 1983; 205:99). Plasma LH, FSH, and testosterone levels are low, and the LH response to gonadotrophin releasing hormone is impaired. There may be a normal increase in plasma testosterone levels in response to human chorionic gonadotrophin. Plasma oestrogens are usually normal. Sex hormone binding globulin levels may be normal or increased (Walton, QJMed, 1983; 205:99). Haemochromatotic patients with established cirrhosis have higher sex hormone binding globulin levels so that their free testosterone levels may be very low.[54,55] Although primary testicular involvement may also be present (presumably secondary to cirrhosis), the pituitary defect predominates. Rarely, patients may present with primary testicular failure, in which case low testosterone and high LH levels may be found.

The impaired gonadotrophin production appears to be due to iron deposition in the pituitary gonadotrophs (Bergeron, AmJPathol, 1978; 93:295). Pituitary iron deposition can be demonstrated by MRI scan (Balducci, JEndocrInv, 1990; 13:1). By contrast, little iron is found in the testes; when present it is in the vessel walls rather than in the germinal epithelium (Mowat, Gut, 1976; 17: 345). Impotence is more common, and more severe, in diabetic haemochromatotics than those without diabetes.[54] This may be due to associated diabetic autonomic neuropathy or vascular disease. Testicular biopsy in hypogonadal patients shows atrophy of the germinal epithelium with fewer or absent Leydig cells. The testicular changes are not necessarily irreversible.

In most patients hypogonadism is not influenced by depletion of body iron stores by venesection.[51,53-55] However, in the occasional patient, venesection may lead to an increase in plasma gonadotrophin and testosterone levels with loss of hypogonadal symptoms (Cundy, ClinEndoc, 1993; 38:617; Gama, PostgradMedJ, 1995; 71:297; Kelly, AnnIntMed, 1984; 101:629). Recovery of spermatogenesis in a patient with documented azoospermia has also been reported (Siemons, JClinEndoc, 1987; 65:585). Age may be an important determinant of the potential for recovery; all the reports of recovery of sexual function with iron depletion have been in patients under 45 years at presentation.

Management

In the absence of diabetes, symptomatic improvement and normal sexual function can be expected with androgen replacement therapy that increases plasma testosterone levels into the normal range (Matsumoto, EndMetClinNAm, 1994; 23:857). In addition to maintenance of normal secondary sexual characteristics and lean body mass, testosterone replacement may be important for normal erythropoiesis. Normal erythropoiesis is important to allow an adequate frequency of venesection and de-ironing (O'Hare, AnnIntMed, 1985; 102:871). Testosterone therapy may also be beneficial in relation to osteoporosis that is common in haemochromatotic patients. Gynaecomastia occasionally develops during treatment as a result of aromatization of testosterone to oestradiol in peripheral tissues. Because of testosterone's sodium retaining properties, fluid retention may develop during treatment but is usually only a problem in cirrhotic patients with poor liver function. In view of the potential for recovery of gonadal function following successful depletion of body iron stores, it is suggested that in younger men testosterone therapy should be interrupted at intervals to assess gonadotrophin and testosterone production (Siemons, JClinEndoc, 1987; 65:585). A course of gonadotrophin treatment may be considered in men with hypogonadotrophic hypogonadism who desire fertility (Selvais, PostgradMedJ, 1993; 69:241).

Thyroid dysfunction

Thyroid dysfunction occurs with increased frequency (8–20 per cent)[51] (Edwards, ClinHaematol, 1982; 11:411; Edwards, ArchIntMed, 1983; 143:1890). Hypothyroidism is much more common than hyperthyroidism. Thyroid stimulating hormone levels are raised, and the thyroid stimulating hormone response to thyrotrophin releasing hormone is normal,[55] suggesting primary hypothyroidism. The thyroid gland is fibrotic and loaded with iron (McDonald, ArchIntMed, 1960; 105:686). Iron deposition is probably the main cause of damage since an increased prevalence of hypothyroidism is also found in patients with thalassaemia and iron overload (Maggiolini, Endocrinol, 1995; 3:91). However, high titres of thyroid autoantibodies may be found in haemachromatosis (Edwards, ArchIntMed, 1983; 143:1890); perhaps the exposure of cellular antigens secondary to iron toxicity leads to further autoimmune thyroid damage. Occasional patients may develop hypothyroidism secondary to impaired pituitary thyroid stimulating hormone release (Thomas, ClinEndoc, 1984; 21:271).

Adrenal hormones

Basal plasma cortisol and ACTH levels, and their responses to insulin-induced hypoglycaemia, are usually normal in patients with haemochromatosis.[55] Thomas (ClinEndoc, 1984; 21:271) reported a patient with postural hypotension due to primary aldosterone deficiency. The patient had iron deposits in the zona glomerulosa of the adrenal cortex with sparing of the other zones. Such a pattern of iron deposition appears to be common in haemochromatosis (Bergeron, AmJPathol, 1978; 93:295). However, Walsh *et al.* (ClinEndoc, 1994; 41:439) in a cross-sectional study of 19 haemochromatotics found normal cortisol responses to ACTH and insulin-induced hypoglycaemia, and normal regulation of plasma aldosterone levels. It would seem that adrenocortical dysfunction is rare.

Prolactin and growth hormone

Basal prolactin levels tend to be low in hypogonadal haemochromatotic patients and they have a subnormal prolactin response to intravenous thyrotrophin releasing hormone[55] (Walton, QJMed, 1983; 205:99). Similarly, basal growth hormone levels are usually normal but the growth hormone response to insulin-induced hypoglycaemia may be impaired.[55]

Osteoporosis

The prevalence of osteoporosis is increased in haemochromatosis. Diamond *et al.* (AnnIntMed, 1989; 110:435) found osteoporosis in 10 of 22 men aged 35 to 62 years. Both cortical and trabecular bone density were decreased. The abnormalities were more marked in the haemochromatotic men with hypogonadism. However, osteoporosis and fractures may be found in the absence of hypogonadism (Eyres, Bone, 1992; 13:431). It is likely that many factors contribute to the osteopenia in these patients. In addition to androgen deficiency, iron interference with osteoid mineralization (deVernejoul, JClinEndoc, 1982; 54:276; deVernejoul, AmJPathol, 1984; 116:377), lower 25-hydroxyvitamin D levels (Chow, Gastro, 1985; 88:865; Diamond, AnnIntMed, 1989; 110:435), poorly controlled diabetes (McNair, ActaEnd, 1979; 90:463), and impaired insulin-like growth factor-I production in those with cirrhosis or poorly controlled diabetes may all play a role.

Endocrine manifestations of liver tumours

Primary hepatic tumours may rarely be associated with metabolic and endocrine abnormalities resulting from tumour production and release of hormones (or their precursors), hormone-releasing factors, or other substances that influence circulating levels of active hormone produced in other tissues. Hypoglycaemia due to tumour production of insulin-like growth factor-II precursors ('big' IGF-2) was discussed earlier.

Erythrocytosis

Hepatocellular carcinoma is one of the more common tumours to produce erythrocytosis (Schonfield, NEJM, 1961; 265:231; Jacobson, SAMedJ, 1978; 53:658), which is found in up to 10 per cent of patients in areas with a high incidence of hepatocellular carcinoma (McFadzean, Blood, 1958; 13:427; Kew, Cancer, 1986; 58:2485; Teniola, TropGeogMed, 1994; 46:20). There is an increase in the haemoglobin and packed cell volume but these may be masked by the expanded plasma volume in many cirrhotic patients, necessitating determination of red cell mass for diagnosis. Erythrocytosis may increase the risk of hepatic and portal venous thrombosis that is fairly common in these patients (Chapter 22.2.1). The increase in red cell mass is probably due to overproduction of erythropoietin by the tumour (Kan, Blood, 1961; 18:592; Nakao, AmJMedSci, 1966; 251:161; Lehman, AmJMed, 1969; 35:439). Raised plasma erythropoetin levels are more commonly found than erythrocytosis (Kew, Cancer, 1986; 58:2485). This may be explained by the expanded plasma volume in cirrhosis, bleeding episodes, concomitant iron deficiency, or hypogonadism (see above), but it could also be due to a lower biological activity of erythropoietin of tumour origin. Erythropoietin production by hepatocellular carcinoma tissue has been demonstrated by immunohistochemical staining and by demonstration of a high level of expression of its mRNA (Sakisaka, Hepatol, 1993; 18:1357; Muta, IntMed, 1994; 33:427). Successful resection of the tumour leads to a fall in erythropoietin levels and reduction in red cell mass (Muta, IntMed, 1994; 33:427; Funakoshi, BBResComm, 1993; 195:717).

Hypercalcaemia

Hypercalcaemia is found in about 10 per cent of patients with primary liver tumours (Ihde, AmJMed, 1974; 56:83; Oldenburg, ArchSurg, 1982; 117:1363; Van Leeuwen, ScaJGastr, 1991; 188(Suppl):108). While it may be associated with osteolytic metastases, in most patients it occurs in the absence of metastatic bone deposits and appears to be due to production of humoral factors by the tumour. Hypercalcaemia is more commonly associated with cholangiocarcinoma than with hepatocellular carcinoma (Oldenburg, ArchSurg, 1982; 117:1363) and may be particularly common with the sclerosing variant of cholangiocarcinoma (Omata, Gastro, 1979; 77:31A). In four hypercalcaemic hepatocellular carcinoma patients without bony metastases Panesar et al. (ClinEndoc, 1991; 35:527) found low serum phosphate levels, decreased tubular reabsorption of phosphate, increased hydroxyproline–creatinine ratios, and increased excretion of nephrogenous cyclic AMP, consistent with increased activity of a PTH-like hormone in bone and kidney; however, serum PTH levels were suppressed. Unlike patients with hyperparathyroidism, there is a tendency to hypochloraemic alkalosis (Oldenburg, Arch Surg, 1982; 117:1363).

Parathyroid hormone related peptide (**PTHrP**) which has a high degree of homology at the N-terminus (first 13 amino acids) with PTH, has been identified as the main mediator of humoral hypercalcaemia in non-haematological malignancies (Burtis, NEJM, 1990; 322:1106; Kao, MayoClinProc, 1990; 65:1399); this is probably also true of hypercalcaemia associated with primary liver tumours. Knill-Jones et al. (NEJM, 1970; 282:704) demonstrated an arterio-hepatic venous gradient for immunoreactive PTH in a patient with cholangiocarcinoma and hypercalcaemia. Cholangiocarcinoma but not hepatocellular carcinoma has been shown to express PTHrP even in the absence of hypercalcaemia; mixed types of primary liver tumour contained PTHrP only in areas of cholangiocellular differentiation (Roskans, Histopath, 1993; 23:519). This could explain the higher incidence of hypercalcaemia in association with cholangiocarcinoma than with hepatocellular carcinoma, although probably only a small percentage of tumours that produce PTHrP will secrete enough biologically active material to cause hypercalcaemia

(Dunne, JPath, 1993; 171:215). Other factors may also play a role in some patients; Ikeda et al. (Cancer, 1988; 61:1813) reported a patient with hypercalcaemia who was found to have a tenfold increase in prostaglandin E levels in the tumour compared with adjacent normal liver. The significance of this finding is unclear in view of the very high rate of prostaglandin metabolism by the liver and lungs so that circulating levels are unlikely to increase to levels necessary for stimulation of bone resorption (Caro, AmJMed, 1979; 66:337). Prostaglandin production by tumour cells is probably only important in inducing osteolysis in the region surrounding metastases in bone. Successful tumour resection (Oldenburg, ArchSurg, 1982; 117:1363), liver transplantation (Knill-Jones, NEJM, 1970; 282:704), or tumour embolization (Roche, Radiol, 1979; 133:315) may restore the serum calcium to normal.

Isosexual precocity and gonadotrophin secretion

Hepatoblastoma and hepatocellular carcinoma in young boys may rarely be associated with sexual precocity. This is due to human chorionic gonadotrophin (**hCG**) production with stimulation of testicular testosterone production (Braunstein, AnnIntMed, 1973; 78:857; McArthur, AmJMed, 1973; 54:390; Reeve, InvestCellPath, 1980; 3:151; Nakagawara, Cancer, 1985; 56:1636). The syndrome occurs only in males because whereas either hCG or LH can stimulate testicular steroid synthesis, initiation of ovarian steroid synthesis requires FSH as well. In adult men gynaecomastia may develop as a result of tumour production of hCG, or the conversion of dehydroepiandrosterone to oestrone and oestradiol by the tumour (Kew, NEJM, 1977; 296:1084; Kirschner, CancerRes, 1981; 41:1447). In women, amenorrhoea with breast enlargement and galactorrhoea has been reported (Reeve, InvestCellPath, 1980; 3:151); menstruation returned following tumour resection. Production of either hCG or prolactin by the hepatocellular carcinoma may have been responsible.

Other tumour-associated endocrine syndromes

hCG has the same α-subunit as thyroid stimulating hormone and can act via the thyroid stimulating hormone receptor to stimulate growth of thyroid cells. In early pregnancy high hCG levels cause a rise in thyroid hormones. Hyperthyroidism may rarely be associated with hepatocellular carcinoma secreting very large amounts of hCG (Reeve, InvestCellPath, 1980; 3:151; Fradkin, NEJM, 1989; 320:640). Carcinoid syndrome is usually due to hepatic metastases but it may very rarely be due to a primary biliary or liver tumour (Primack, Cancer, 1971; 27:1182). Cox et al. (VirchArchA, 1975; 366:15) described a young girl with severe hypertension due to renin production by a benign hepatoma which resolved following tumour resection.

References

1. WHO Study Group. *Diabetes mellitus*. Technical Report Series 727. Geneva: WHO, 1985; 80–2.
2. Conn HO, Schreiber W, and Elkington SG. Cirrhosis and diabetes. II. Association of impaired glucose tolerance with portal-systemic shunting in Laennec's cirrhosis. *Digestive Diseases*, 1971; **16**: 227–39.

3. Kruszynska YT, Harry DS, Bergman RN, and McIntyre N. Insulin sensitivity, insulin secretion and glucose effectiveness in diabetic and non-diabetic cirrhotic patients. *Diabetologia*, 1993; **36**: 121–8.

4. Marchesini G, Pacini G, Bianchi G, Patrono D, and Cobelli C. Glucose disposal, B-cell secretion, and hepatic insulin extraction in cirrhosis; a minimal model assessment. *Gastroenterology*, 1990; **99**: 1715–22.

5. Letiexhe MR, *et al*. Insulin secretion, clearance, and action on glucose metabolism in cirrhotic patients. *Journal of Clinical Endocrinology and Metabolism*, 1993; **77**: 1263–8.

6. Creutzfeldt W, Frerichs H, and Sickinger K. Liver diseases and diabetes mellitus. In Popper H, and Schaffner F, eds. *Progress in liver disease*, Vol. 3. New York: Grune and Stratton, 1970: 371–407.

7. Blanco DCV, Gentile S, Marmo R, Carbone L, and Coltorti M. Alterations of glucose metabolism in chronic liver disease. *Diabetes Research and Clinical Practice*, 1990; **8**: 29–36.

8. Kruszynska YT, Meyer-Alber A, Darakhshan F, Home PD, and McIntyre N. Metabolic handling of orally administered glucose in cirrhosis. *Journal of Clinical Investigation*, 1993; **91**: 1057–66.

9. Petrides AS, Groop LC, Riely CA, and DeFronzo RA. Effect of physiologic hyperinsulinaemia on glucose and lipid metabolism in cirrhosis. *Journal of Clinical Investigation*, 1991; **88**: 561–70.

10. Petrides A, Vogt C, Schulze-Berge D, Matthews D, and Strohmeyer G. Pathogenesis of glucose intolerance and diabetes mellitus in cirrhosis. *Hepatology*, 1994; **19**: 616–27.

11. Taylor R, Heine RJ, Collins J, James OFW, and Alberti KGMM. Insulin action in cirrhosis. *Hepatology*, 1985; **5**: 64–71.

12. Kruszynska YT, Home PD, and McIntyre N. The relationship between insulin sensitivity, insulin secretion and glucose tolerance in cirrhosis. *Hepatology*, 1991; **14**: 103–11.

13. Bosch J, *et al*. Role of spontaneous portal-systemic shunting in hyperinsulinism of cirrhosis. *American Journal of Physiology*, 1984; **247**: G206-G212.

14. Kruszynska YT, Ghatei MA, Bloom SR, and McIntyre N. Insulin secretion and plasma levels of glucose-dependent insulinotropic peptide and glucagon-like peptide 1 [7–36 amide] after oral glucose in cirrhosis. *Hepatology*, 1995; **21**: 933–41.

15. Moller S, Juul A, Becker U, Flyvberg A, Skakkebaek NE, and Henriksen JH. Concentrations, release, and disposal of insulin-like growth factor (IGF)-binding proteins (IGFBP), IGF-I, and growth hormone in different vascular beds in patients with cirrhosis. *Journal of Clinical Endocrinology and Metabolism*, 1995; **80**: 1148–57.

16. Donaghy A, Ross R, Gimson A, Hughes SC, Holly J, and Williams R. Growth hormone, insulin-like growth factor-I, and insulin-like growth factor binding proteins 1 and 3 in chronic liver disease. *Hepatology*, 1995; **21**: 680–8.

17. Cuneo RC, *et al*. Altered endogenous growth hormone secretory kinetics and diurnal GH-binding protein profiles in adults with chronic liver disease. *Clinical Endocrinology*, 1995; **43**: 265–75.

18. McDonald JA, Handelsman DJ, Dilworth P, Conway AJ, and McCaughan GW. Hypothalamic–pituitary adrenal function in end-stage non-alcoholic liver disease. *Journal of Gastroenterology and Hepatology*, 1993; **8**: 247–53.

19. Shmueli E, Stewart M, Alberti KGMM, and Record CO. Growth hormone, insulin-like growth factor-I and insulin resistance in cirrhosis. *Hepatology*, 1994; **19**: 322–8.

20. Holt RIG, Jones JS, Stone NM, Baker AJ, and Miell JP. Sequential changes in insulin-like growth factor I (IGF-I) and IGF-binding proteins in children with end-stage liver disease before and after successful orthotopic liver transplantation. *Journal of Clinical Endocrinology and Metabolism*, 1996; **81**: 160–8.

21. Shapiro ET, Bell GI, Polonsky KS, Rubenstein AH, Kew MC, and Tager HS. Tumour hypoglycaemia : relationship to high molecular weight insulin-like growth factor II. *Journal of Clinical Investigation*, 1990; **85**: 1672–9.

22. Zapf J, Futo E, Peter M, and Froesch ER. Can 'big' insulin-like growth factor II in serum of tumor patients account for the development of extrapancreatic tumor hypoglycaemia. *Journal of Clinical Investigation*, 1992; **90**: 2574–84.

23. Daughaday WH, Wu J-C, Lee S-D, and Kapadia M. Abnormal processing of pro-IGF-II in patients with hepatoma and in some patients with hepatitis B virus antibody-positive asymptomatic individuals. *Journal of Laboratory Clinical Medicine*, 1990; **115**: 555–62.

24. Daughaday WH, Trivedi B, and Baxter RC. Serum 'big insulin-like growth factor II' from patients with tumor hypoglycaemia lacks normal E-domain O-linked glycosylation, a possible determinant of normal propeptide processing. *Proceedings of the National Academy of Sciences, USA*, 1993; **90**: 5823–7.

25. Liewendahl K, Helenius T, Tanner P, and Salaspuro M. Serum free thyroid hormone concentrations and indices in alcoholic liver cirrhosis, primary biliary cirrhosis and chronic active hepatitis. *Acta Endocrinologica Supplementum*, 1983; **251**: 21–6.

26. L'age M, Meinhold H, Wenzel KW, and Schleusener H. Relations between serum levels of TSH, TBG, T_4, T_3, rT_3 and various histologically classified chronic liver diseases. *Journal of Endocrinological Investigation*, 1980; **4**: 379.

27. Sheridan P, Chapman C, and Losowsky MS. Interpretation of laboratory tests of thyroid function in chronic active hepatitis. *Clinica Chimica Acta*, 1978; **86**: 73–80.

28. Shussler GC, Schaffner F, and Korn F. Increased serum thyroid hormone binding and decreased free hormone in chronic active liver disease. *New England Journal of Medicine*, 1978; **299**: 510–15.

29. Faber J, Francis Thomsen H, Lumholtz IB, Kirkegaard C, Siersbaek-Nielsen K, and Friis T. Kinetic studies of thyroxine, 3,5,3′-triiodothyronine, 3,3′5′-triiodothyronine, 3′5′-diiodothyronine, 3,3′-diiodothyronine, and 3′-monoiodothyronine in patients with liver cirrhosis. *Journal of Clinical Endocrinology and Metabolism*, 1981; **53**: 978–84.

30. Utiger RD. The thyroid: physiology, thyrotoxicosis, hypothyroidism, and the painful thyroid. In Felig P, Baxter JD, and Frohman LA, eds. *Endocrinology and metabolism*, (3rd edn). New York: McGraw-Hill, 1995: 435–519.

31. Lim C-F, *et al*. Inhibition of thyroxine transport into cultured rat hepatocytes by serum of nonuremic critically ill patients: effects of bilirubin and nonesterified fatty acids. *Journal of Clinical Endocrinology and Metabolism*, 1993; **76**: 1165–72.

32. Baudin E, *et al*. Reversibility of thyroid dysfunction induced by recombinant alpha interferon in chronic hepatitis C. *Clinical Endocrinology*, 1993; **39**: 657–61.

33. Stewart PM, Burra P, Shackleton CHL, Sheppard MC, and Elias E. 11β-Hydroxysteroid dehydrogenase deficiency and glucocorticoid status in patients with alcoholic and non-alcoholic liver disease. *Journal of Clinical Endocrinology and Metabolism*, 1993; **76**: 748–51.

34. Rosman PM, Farag A, Benn R, Tito J, Mishik A, and Wallace EZ. Modulation of pituitary-adrenocortical function: decreased secretory episodes and blunted circadian rhythmicity in patients with alcoholic liver disease. *Journal of Clinical Endocrinology and Metabolism*, 1982; **55**: 709–17.

35. Baker HWG, *et al*. A study of the endocrine manifestations of hepatic cirrhosis. *Quarterly Journal of Medicine*, 1976; **45**: 145–78.

36. Bannister P, Oakes J, Sheridan P, and Losowsky MS. Sex hormone changes in chronic liver disease: a matched study of alcoholic versus non-alcoholic liver disease. *Quarterly Journal of Medicine*, 1987; **63**: 305–13.

37. Gluud C, *et al*. No effect of oral testosterone treatment on sexual dysfunction in alcoholic cirrhotic men. *Gastroenterology*, 1988; **95**: 1582–7.

38. Wang YJ, *et al*. Changes of sex hormone levels in patients with hepatitis B virus-related postnecrotic cirrhosis: relationship to severity of portal hypertension. *Journal of Hepatology*, 1993; **18**: 101–5.

39. Handelsman DJ, Strasser S, McDonald JA, Conway AJ, and McCaughan GW. Hypothalamic–pituitary–testicular function in end-stage non-alcoholic liver disease before and after liver transplantation. *Clinical Endocrinology*, 1995; **43**: 331–7.

40. Wang YJ, Wu JC, Lee SD, Tsai YT, and Lo KJ. Gonadal dysfunction and changes in sex hormones in postnecrotic cirrhotic men: a matched study with alcoholic cirrhotic men. *Hepato-Gastroenterology*, 1991; **38**: 531–4.

41. Zifroni A, Schiavi RC, and Schaffner F. Sexual function and testosterone levels in men with nonalcoholic liver disease. *Hepatology*, 1991; **14**: 479–82.

42. van Thiel DH, Kumar S, Gavaler JS, Tarter RE. Effect of liver transplantation on the hypothalamic–pituitary gonadal axis of chronic alcoholic men with advanced liver disease. *Alcoholism: Clinical and Experimental Research*, 1990; **14**: 478–81.

43. Gavaler JS, and van Thiel DH. Gonadal dysfunction and inadequate sexual performance in alcoholic cirrhotic men. *Gastroenterology*, 1988; **95**: 1680–4.

44. Guechot J, *et al*. Effect of liver transplantation on sex-hormone disorders in male patients with alcohol-induced and post-viral hepatitis advanced liver disease. *Journal of Hepatology*, 1994; **20**: 426–30.

45. Becker U, *et al*. Menopausal age and sex hormones in postmenopausal women with alcoholic and non-alcoholic liver disease. *Journal of Hepatology*, 1991; **13**: 25–32.

46. Valimaki M, Pelkonen R, Salaspuro M, Harkonen M, Hirvonen E, and Ylikahri R. Sex hormones in amenorrheic women with alcoholic liver disease. *Journal of Clinical Endocrinology and Metabolism*, 1984; **59**: 133–8.

47. Becker U. The influence of ethanol and liver disease on sex hormones and hepatic oestrogen receptors in women. *Danish Medical Bulletin*, 1993; **40**: 447–59.

48. Bannister P, Sheridan P, and Losowsky MS. Plasma concentrations of sex hormones in postmenopausal women in non-alcoholic cirrhosis. *Clinical Endocrinology*, 1985; **23**: 335–40.

49. Bell H, Raknerud N, Falch JA, and Haug E. Inappropriately low levels of gonadotrophins in amenorrheic women with alcoholic and non-alcoholic cirrhosis. *European Journal of Endocrinology*, 1995; **132**: 444–9.

50. Morgan MY, Jakobovits AW, Gore MBR, Wills MR, and Sherlock S. Serum prolactin in liver disease and its relationship to gynaecomastia. *Gut*, 1978; **19**: 170–4.

51. Niederau C, Fischer R, Sonnenberg A, Stremmel W, Trampisch HJ, and Strohmeyer G. Survival and causes of death in cirrhotic and in non-cirrhotic patients with primary haemochromatosis. *New England Journal of Medicine*, 1985; **313**: 1256–62.

52. Milman N. Hereditary haemochromatosis in Denmark 1950–1985. *Danish Medical Bulletin*, 1991; **38**: 385–93.

53. Niederau C, Stremmel W, and Strohmeyer GW. Clinical spectrum and management of haemochromatosis. *Baillère's Clinics in Haematology*, 1994; **7**: 881–901.

54. Cundy T, Bomford A, Butler J, Wheeler M, and Williams R. Hypogonadism and sexual dysfunction in haemochromatosis: the effects of cirrhosis and diabetes. *Journal of Clinical Endocrinology and Metabolism*, 1989; **69**: 110–16.

55. Lufkin EG, Baldus WP, Bergstralh EJ, and Kao PC. Influence of phlebotomy treatment on abnormal hypothalamic–pituitary function in genetic haemochromatosis. *Mayo Clinic Proceedings*, 1987; **62**: 473–9.

25.3 Haematological abnormalities in liver disease

Atul B. Mehta and Neil McIntyre

Liver disease produces a diverse range of haematological effects (Table 1). Those which primarily concern red cells, white cells, and platelet number and function are considered here. Liver disease has important effects on haemostasis which are considered in Chapter 25.4. Hypersplenism is covered in Section 10.

The liver has an important role as a haematopoietic organ in fetal life. Although the yolk sac is the first haemopoietic organ in the fetus, erythropoiesis is detectable in fetal liver as early as 6 weeks (Knoll, ActaHaem, 1949; 2:369). It is virtually confined to the marrow at birth, and under normal physiological circumstances the

Table 1 Combination of haematological abnormalities with abnormal liver function tests

Abnormality	Haematological indices	Primary liver disease	Disease in other systems
Red cells			
Anaemia	Increased MCV (macrocytic)	Many liver diseases	Alcoholism
			Vitamin B_{12}/folate deficiency
			Haemolysis (reticulocytes up)
	Low MCV/MCHC (microcytic)	With iron deficiency	Thalassaemia
	Normochromic, normocytic	With dilutional anaemia	Anaemia of chronic disease
	High reticulocyte count	With hypersplenism	Haemolysis
	Low reticulocyte count	With marrow aplasia (viral hepatitis)	Paroxysmal nocturnal haemoglobinuria ($\pm$ Budd–Chiari syndrome)
Normal haemoglobin	Increased MCV	Mild liver disease	Alcoholism
	Low MCV	With iron deficiency	Thalassaemia trait
Erythrocytosis		Hepatocellular carcinoma	
		Viral hepatitis (rare)	
White cells			
	Increased	With infection, neoplasia inflammation	Myeloproliferative disorder
			Leukaemia, lymphoma, drugs
	Neutrophils increased	With bacterial infection or steroid therapy	
	Lymphocytes increased	Viral infections	
	Eosinophils increased	Parasitic infection	Connective tissue disorders
		Drug hepatitis	
		Chronic active hepatitis (rare), sarcoidosis	
	Monocytes increased		Tuberculosis, leukaemia
	Basophils/mast cells increased		Myeloproliferative disease
			Mastocytosis
	Decreased	With infection, marrow aplasia, or hypersplenism	Infections (typhoid, SBE, tuberculosis, septicaemia), leukaemia
	Lymphocytes decreased	Liver disease	Viral infections
Platelets	Increased	And haemorrhage, neoplasia, infection, inflammation	Myeloproliferative disorder
	Decreased	With hypersplenism, viral hepatitis	Leukaemia/lymphoma
			Connective tissue disorders
			Paroxysmal nocturnal haemoglobinuria

liver has no haemopoietic role later in life. Transient erythropoiesis occurs within the grafted organ after liver transplantation (Schlitt, Hepatol, 1995; 21:689) and transmission of leucocytes (especially lymphocytes) from within the donor organ to the recipient leads to coexistence of autologous and allogeneic leucocytes, i.e. chimerism (Schlitt, Transplant Mediz, 1996; 8:9).

Extramedullary haemopoiesis is found in adult liver in certain pathological states, for example myelofibrosis, and massive compensatory hepatic myeloid metaplasia can occur after splenectomy for myelofibrosis (Towell, AmJMed, 1987; 82:371). Fetal liver infusion has been used to repopulate the adult bone marrow in patients with aplastic anaemia (Bhargawa, Thymus, 1987; 10:103). Granulocyte precursors and megakaryocytes are also present in fetal liver, but production of these cells does not become significant until haematopoiesis is established in the marrow (Hesseldahl, ActaAnat, 1971; 78:274).

Cultures of slices of fetal liver sustain erythropoiesis, whereas cell suspensions from the same liver do not (Fontebuoni, PSEBM, 1978; 158:201); this suggests an important facilitatory role for the fetal liver microenvironment. Exogenous erythropoietin stimulates erythropoiesis in these cultures. Studies of the fetal erythropoietin response to haemorrhage suggest that the liver itself, but not kidney, is an important source of erythropoietin in the fetus (Zanjani, JLabClinMed, 1977; 89:640).

In adults, the kidney is the main source of erythropoietin and the liver the site of its clearance. However, liver can produce erythropoietin in uraemic (especially anephric) subjects, in response to hypoxia or haemolysis, or when hepatocytes are regenerating (Fisher, IsrJMedSci, 1971; 7:991; Fried Blood, 1972; 40:671; Simon, BMJ, 1980; 280:892).

Serum erythropoietin levels are frequently raised in patients with hepatocellular carcinoma (Kew, Cancer, 1986; 58:2485; and see below under 'Erythrocytosis'). Liver is an important source of thrombopoietin, the primary regulator of platelet production within bone marrow.[1] It also plays an important role in the metabolism of iron, vitamin B_{12}, and folate, and in the clearance of inflammatory cytokines (e.g. tumour necrosis factor, interleukin-1) (see below and ref.[2]). Thus although liver disease in adults is not a direct cause of defective haemopoiesis, the liver has an important role in facilitating bone marrow function and there is a suboptimal marrow response to anaemia and thrombocytopenia in patients with liver disease.

Anaemia in liver disease

Anaemia occurs in up to 75 per cent of patients with chronic liver disease.[3-5] It is characteristically of moderate severity, and is either normochromic normocytic or moderately macrocytic. Several mechanisms may be involved, and it is exacerbated by complications of chronic liver disease, for example haemorrhage or haemolysis. The anaemia of uncomplicated chronic liver disease results from a combination of haemodilution, shortened red cell survival, and a reduced bone marrow response to anaemia.

Cirrhotic patients with chronic anaemia have significantly reduced erythropoietin levels when compared with patients with chronic anaemia due to iron deficiency (Siciliano, Hepatol, 1995; 22:1132). However, cirrhosis without anaemia is not associated with low erythropoietin levels, and erythropoietin therapy does not lead to a sustained improvement in haemoglobin (Pirisi, JHepatol, 1994;

21:376). Thus a relative reduction in erythropoietin levels is unlikely to be the sole mechanism explaining an inadequate bone marrow response to anaemia. Chronic inflammation can lead to relative unresponsiveness of erythroid progenitors to erythropoietin.[2] Furthermore, increased serum levels of inflammatory cytokines (e.g. tumour necrosis factor, interleukin-1) occur in cirrhosis (Tilg, IntJClinLabRes, 1993; 23:179) and may also suppress the bone marrow.

Patients with cirrhosis have a low oxygen-haemoglobin affinity, which increases tissue oxygen availability and leads to better tolerance of anaemia (Astrup, ScaJCLI, 1973; 31:311). Chronic liver disease often results in splenomegaly and hypersplenism, which may be associated with pooling of red cells, excessive red cell destruction, and haemodilution. An elevated plasma volume occurs in chronic liver disease; while this is partly due to the hypersplenism and to fluid retention with portal venous congestion, other endocrine changes may play a role (see Chapters 8.1 and 25.1). Sheehy and Berman[4] showed that this expansion of plasma volume is an important contributory factor to the anaemia of chronic liver disease, and while portocaval shunt procedures may reduce the increased plasma volume, it does not usually return to normal (Lieberman, JCI, 1967; 46:1297). Leucopenia and thrombocytopenia are additional manifestations of hypersplenism (see Section 10) but their degree is not necessarily related to splenic size, suggesting that other mechanisms (for example reduction in serum thrombopoietin) are frequently important.

Liver disease and haematinic metabolism

Iron metabolism

A low or normal serum iron concentration with a low or normal total iron binding capacity is frequently found in uncomplicated cirrhosis, and is compatible with the 'anaemia of chronic disorder' which is commonly seen in inflammatory and neoplastic disorders ([2]; Bentley, ClinHaem, 1982; 11:465). However, most reported series do not clearly define their population of patients with 'uncomplicated' cirrhosis. Bleeding from oesophagitis, peptic ulceration, or oesophageal varices, compounded by the haemostatic defects of chronic liver disease, occurs in up to 70 per cent of patients with liver disease[3-5] and causes iron deficiency. Many reported series have included patients with alcohol-induced liver disease, and alcohol has a suppressant action on haemopoiesis (Section 15; Sullivan, JCI, 1964; 43:2048; Straus, SemHemat, 1973; 10:183) and may increase iron absorption from the gastrointestinal tract (Charlton, BMJ, 1964; 2:1427). Patients with idiopathic haemochromatosis are considered as a separate group (see Chapter 20.2).

The study of iron kinetics in patients with cirrhosis has yielded discrepant results in different series[4] (Bovin, NouvRevFrHemat, 1961; 1:3; Conrad, Gastro, 1962; 43:385). If one excludes patients with obvious iron deficiency, a major haemolytic process, alcoholism (Conrad, SemHemat, 1980; 17:149), or idiopathic haemochromatosis, one can conclude that plasma iron turnover, red cell iron utilization, and erythrocyte iron turnover are normal or reduced in patients with cirrhosis[3] (Chapman, Gastro, 1983; 84:143).

These data confirm that the bone marrow response to anaemia is inadequate, as occurs in the anaemia of chronic disease.

Accurate assessment of iron stores is important in patients with chronic liver disease, but conventional laboratory investigations can be misleading. An important practical point is that hepatic inflammation and necrosis tend to increase serum ferritin (Prieto, Gastro, 1975; 68:528) so that a raised value does not necessarily indicate iron overload, and a normal value does not exclude iron deficiency. The rise in red cell mean corpuscular volume (**MCV**) which accompanies chronic liver disease and alcohol ingestion can also mask iron deficiency, which normally lowers the MCV. Serum iron levels are subject to widespread physiological variation in normal individuals; mean serum iron levels are higher in the morning than the afternoon, may fall during menstruation, and rise in women taking the contraceptive pill (Cavill, ClinHaem, 1982; 11:259).

Serum iron is bound to a beta globulin (transferrin, which is synthesized in the liver) and total iron binding capacity largely depends on the transferrin concentration. Thus, a high total iron binding capacity generally indicates iron deficiency (though 'false' elevations of total iron binding capacity do sometimes occur, for example in pregnancy) . Many acute and chronic diseases (for example infection, rheumatoid arthritis) lower the total iron binding capacity; it then fails to reflect iron stores in these patients (Bentley, JClinPath, 1974; 27:786). The total iron binding capacity is often lowered in patients with liver disease due to reduced hepatic synthesis of transferrin. The degree of saturation of transferrin by iron can yield additional information.

A low saturation generally indicates iron deficiency (but it may be falsely low in pregnancy and chronic diseases). Increased saturation is usually considered an early indicator of iron overload, and on this basis is a useful screening test for hereditary haemochromatosis (Edwards, ClinHaem, 1982; 11:411). However, in other forms of liver disease, iron studies sometimes give a false picture of iron overload. Patients with active liver disease tend to have increased serum iron and serum ferritin, probably reflecting release of iron and ferritin from damaged liver cells (Bacon, SemLivDis, 1984; 4:181); transferrin levels may fall due to reduced hepatic synthesis, and transferrin saturation may therefore rise. This pattern is common in viral hepatitis (particularly hepatitis C virus; Arber, DigDisSci, 1994; 39:2656), reflecting hepatocellular damage. Biopsy measurement of liver iron content may be required to distinguish such 'spurious' iron overload from true iron overload. The serum transferrin receptor level should not be affected by liver disease or inflammation, and may be a more reliable laboratory index of iron defiency in patients with liver disease (Ferguson, JLabClinMed, 1992; 19:385).

Vitamin B_{12} and folic acid metabolism

The liver is an important storage organ for both vitamin B12 and folic acid,[6] and chronic liver disease may be associated with several clinically significant disorders of their metabolism.

The liver stores 5 to 10 mg of vitamin B_{12}, representing 50 to 90 per cent of body stores.[7] Intrinsic factor is required for the absorption of B_{12} from the diet, and there is a significant enterohepatic recirculation of B_{12}.[6,7] Lack of intrinsic factor (for example in pernicious anaemia, or following gastrectomy or acute gastritis) causes a significant disturbance of this recycling mechanism and leads to depletion of liver stores (Grasbeck, PSEBM, 1958; 97:780). Pernicious anaemia has been reported in association with primary biliary cirrhosis, presumably as an associated autoimmune disease (Arikan, WienMedWoch, 1994; 17:426). Alcohol can inhibit B_{12} absorption (Lindenbaum, AnnNYAcadSci, 1975; 252:228). Alcoholic liver disease, in common with most other liver diseases causing hepatic necrosis, is associated with a reduction of liver B_{12} content accompanied by an increase in serum B_{12} concentration (Jones, JLabClinMed, 1957; 49:422; Baker, AmJClinNut, 1964; 14:1). Elevated serum B12 binding capacity is occasionally seen in cirrhosis, but more specifically with hepatocellular carcinoma (Burger, JCI, 1975; 56:1262; Mexo, ScaJCLI, 1975; 35: 683), reflecting either tumour production or modification of the binding protein, transcobalamin I; a particular association has been reported with the fibrolamellar variant of hepatocellular carcinoma (Paradinas, BMJ, 1982; 285:840).

Liver stores of folic acid are sufficient for only 4 to 5 months (Herbert, TRAAP, 1962; 75:307). Alcohol-induced liver disease and poor nutrition often result in disordered folate metabolism (Chapter 29.2; Weir, BiochemPharm, 1985; 34:1; Lindenbaum, SemLivDis, 1987; 7:169). Alcoholism is associated with impaired folate absorption from the intestine as well as decreased hepatic stores.[6-8] Hepatic necrosis, as in viral hepatitis, may lead to release of stored folates from the damaged liver, and to increased urinary folate excretion (Retief, BMJ, 1969; 2:150).

Red cell disorders and haemolytic syndromes in liver disease

As many of the features of haemolytic anaemia (raised bilirubin concentration, reduced or absent haptoglobins, and shortened red cell survival) are found in uncomplicated chronic liver disease, their significance in the absence of anaemia may be difficult to evaluate. Jandl[9,10] found red cell life-span reduced by about 50 per cent in cirrhotics, with the spleen as a major site of red cell destruction. The reticulocytosis so frequently seen in chronic liver disease (Jarold, JCI, 1949; 28:286) reflects the attempt of bone marrow to compensate for this shortened survival, but production is often inadequate and anaemia results.

The causes of the haemolytic anaemia may be broadly categorized into extracorpuscular and intracorpuscular, although there is a substantial interplay between these factors. There are two major extracorpuscular causes, hypersplenism and lipid abnormalities; the latter induce alterations in the red cell membrane. The spleen plays a central role in 'conditioning' the red cell, whereby the spleen progressively erodes the membrane of red cells entrapped within its specialized circulation, causing spherocytosis and haemolysis (Cooper, SemHemat, 1980; 17:103). Some red cell shape abnormalities induced by lipid changes (for example target cell formation) may partially correct the process of splenic conditioning and serve to reduce the haemolytic rate.

Abnormalities of red cell shape[11] (Hall, AmJMed, 1960; 28:541; Table 2)

Macrocytosis

Macrocytosis is found in approximately two-thirds of patients with chronic liver disease (Werre, BrJHaemat, 1970; 19:223) and in up

Table 2 Abnormal red cell morphology in association with abnormal liver function tests

Abnormality	Primary liver disorders	Disease in other systems
Macrocytes	Many types of liver disease	Megaloblastic anaemia
		Hypothyroidism, cytotoxic drugs
Target cells	Many types of liver disease	Thalassaemia
		Other haemoglobinopathies
		Hyposplenism, e.g. SLE, coeliac disease
Spherocytes	Zieve's syndrome	Hereditary spherocytosis
		Autoimmune haemolytic anaemia
		Burns
Echinocytes	Severe chronic liver disease	Haemolytic anaemia
Acanthocytes	Very severe disease (especially alcoholic)	Abetalipoproteinaemia
	(Spur-cell anaemia)	Anorexia nervosa/malnutrition
		McLeod phenotype
Burr cells	Hepatorenal syndrome	Renal failure
Fragmented cells (schistocytes)		Thrombotic thrombocytopenic purpura
		Microangiopathic haemolytic anaemia
		DIC, HELLP syndrome
		Some haemoglobinopathies
Stomatocytes	Alcoholic cirrhosis	Alcoholism
Tear-drop poikilocytes		Haemolytic anaemias
		Primary and secondary myelofibrosis
Nucleated red cells	Acute fatty liver of pregnancy	Many causes
Punctate basophilia		Infections, e.g. malaria
		Heavy metal poisoning
		Haemolytic/dyserythropoietic anaemia
Rouleaux		Myeloma/macroglobulinaemia/lymphoma
Autoagglutination		Autoimmune haemolytic anaemia
Sickle cells		Sickle-cell disease

to 90 per cent of alcoholics (Wu, Lancet, 1974; i:829; Morgan, ClinLabHaemat, 1981; 3:35). Bingham, in his classic papers (Blood, 1959; 14:694; Blood, 1960; 15:244), described three types of macrocytosis in liver disease. 'Thin' macrocytosis is the most common and involves an increase in red cell diameter with little or no increase in mean cell volume; it has no clear association with anaemia,[11] is not usually associated with megaloblastic erythropoiesis, and resolves with improvement in liver function. 'Target' macrocytosis is a condition wherein 10 per cent or more of thin macrocytes have formed target cells. True or 'thick' macrocytosis is associated with a more marked increase in MCV, is less common, and frequently associated with megaloblastic erythropoiesis; Bingham reported it only in patients with moderately advanced chronic liver disease.

The precise mechanisms responsible for the macrocytosis of liver disease are unclear, but an increase in red cell membrane cholesterol and phospholipid content (Cooper, SemHemat, 1980; 17:103) is likely to be important. Other mechanisms include the reticulocytosis associated with haemolysis and/or bleeding, and disturbances of vitamin B_{12} and folic acid metabolism. Bingham concluded from cross-transfusion studies that there was an intrinsic abnormality in bone marrow erythropoiesis, and it is likely that alcoholics and patients with chronic liver disease do indeed have disturbed erythropoiesis which is macronormoblastic.

Target cells

In routine blood films target cells are seen in most patients with significant liver disease, as their red cell membrane contains more cholesterol, or more cholesterol and phospholipid, than that of normal cells. Surface area expands without corresponding change in volume and so the cells become 'bowl' or 'saucer' shaped.

Although this shape is obvious in wet films and on scanning electron microscopy, drying prior to staining distorts the cells (Fig. 1) and in conventional blood films they appear as 'target' cells (Barrett, JPathBact, 1938; 46:603). As target cells are also seen in familial lecithin-cholesterol acyltransferase deficiency,[12] their presence in liver disease may result from low lecithin-cholesterol acyltransferase activity and the transfer of lipid to red cells from cholesterol-rich lipoprotein particles. As volume should not increase with expansion of the membrane, target cell formation is unlikely to be the reason for the macrocytosis (with a high MCV) often seen in chronic liver disease. Target cells are also seen in thalassaemia and this condition should be suspected in the presence of a low MCV. Because the surface area : volume ratio increases in liver disease, red cells tend to show increased resistance to osmotic lysis.

Echinocytes, burr cells

In conventional blood films red cells from cirrhotics often appear normal, except for the presence of target cells. However, in wet films or on scanning electron microscopy, many patients have spiculated red cells or 'echinocytes' (Fig. 2) in the blood (Grahn, AmJMed, 1968; 45:78). Sometimes, when the numbers are very large and the cells have many spicules, spiky red cells are seen in conventional blood films. The presence of echinocytes appears to be related to changes in high-density lipoproteins (**HDLs**); purified HDLs from blood containing echinocytes transform normal red cells into echinocytes within seconds, and there is a close correlation between the echinocyte count and the ability of a patient's HDL to transform normal red cells.[13] The cells rapidly revert to normal on incubation with albumin or normal HDL. HDL-induced echinocytosis is not accompanied by enrichment with cholesterol or

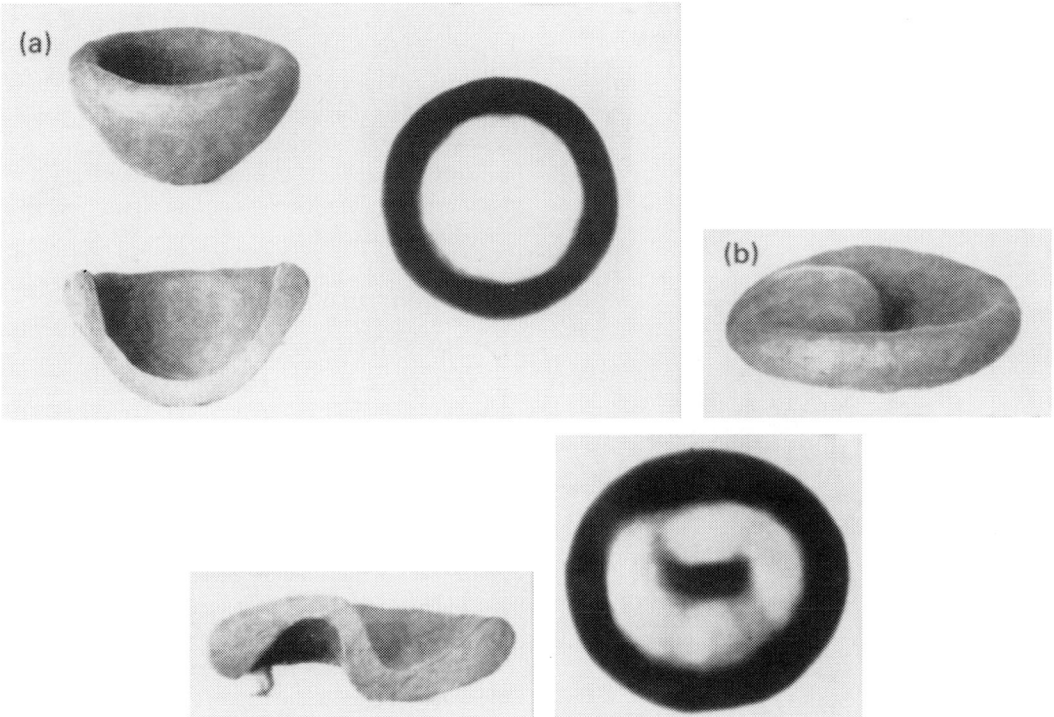

Fig. 1. Models explaining the appearance of (a) target cells in wet films and (b) target cells in conventional blood films (from Barrett, JPatholBacteriol, 1938; 46:603).

phospholipid, a suggested mechanism for echinocytogenesis in liver disease (Cooper, SemHemat, 1970; 7:296), although *in vivo*, as one would expect, red cells in liver disease do tend to have a high cholesterol : phospholipid ratio. Echinocytosis appears to be due to reversible, saturable binding of abnormal HDL by the red cell surface. The pathophysiological significance of these red cell shape changes is unknown, and there is no clear relationship between the echinocyte count and the haemoglobin level.

Acanthocytes

Red cells of bizarre shape (Fig. 3), structurally identical to the acanthocytes of abetalipoproteinaemia, are seen occasionally in the blood of cirrhotics, in association with an overt and often severe haemolytic anaemia; this syndrome is called 'spur-cell' anaemia (Smith, NEJM, 1964; 271:396; Silber, NEJM, 1966; 275:639). The term 'spur-cell' anaemia should only be used when acanthocytes are present; their shape is quite different from that of echinocytes[11] (Beecher, Blood, 1972; 40:333), but the distinction is not always made (Powell, AustNZJMed, 1975; 5:101). The cirrhosis is usually, but not invariably, alcoholic in origin. The liver disease tends to be severe with jaundice, ascites, encephalopathy, and/or gastro-intestinal haemorrhage, preceding or following the development of haemolysis; although patients may survive many months with acanthocytosis, the prognosis of the underlying liver disease is poor. Acanthocytes have also been seen in severe liver disease in neonates or children with haemolytic anaemia (Marie, ArchFrancPediat, 1967; 24:585; Tchernia, ArchFrancPediat, 1968; 25:729; Balistreri, Pediat, 1981; 67:461).

Only a small proportion of the red cells in these patients are acanthocytes; most of the remaining cells are typical echinocytes.

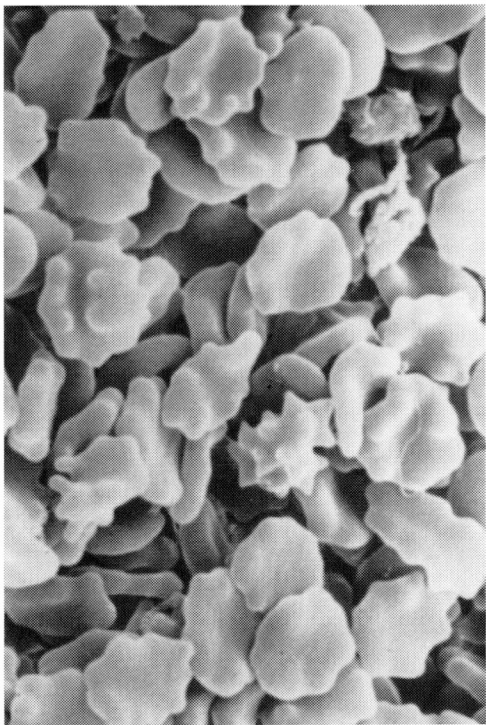

Fig. 2. The appearance of echinocytes on scanning electron microscopy.

Echinocytes, but not acanthocytes, have been produced *in vitro* by incubating normal red cells in sera from patients with spur-cell anaemia. It was suggested that the shape change is caused by marked

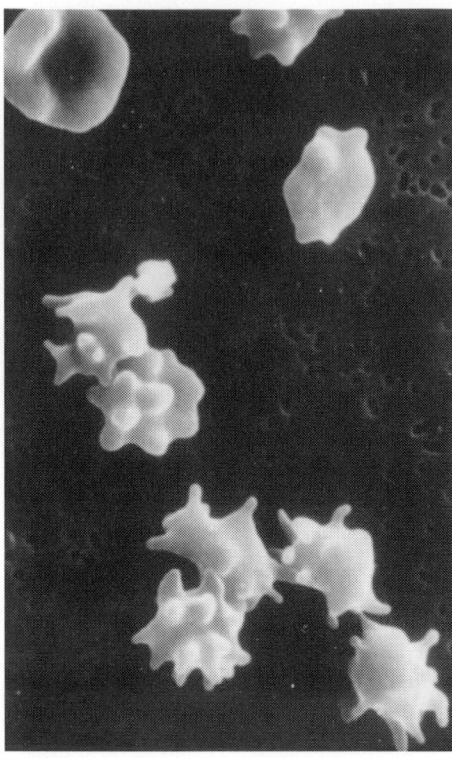

Fig. 3. The appearance of acanthocytes on scanning electron microscopy.

elevation of the membrane cholesterol–phospholipid ratio (Cooper, SemHemat, 1970; 7:296); however, the cholesterol : phospholipid ratio is just as high in familial lecithin-cholesterol acyltransferase deficiency in which target cells are seen, but acanthocytes and echinocytes are absent.[12] It was suggested, on the basis of a single case in which splenectomy was performed, that acanthocytes may be produced *in vivo* by splenic modification of echinocytes (Cooper, NEJM, 1974; 290:1279); however, splenectomy itself has been reported to cause acanthocytosis (Beecher, Blood, 1972; 40:333). The underlying mecnanism responsible for the formation of acanthocytes remains unclear; nor is it known why they are so uncommon (as compared to echinocytes) in the peripheral blood of patients with cirrhosis.

It has been assumed that haemolytic anaemia is caused because the abnormal shape of acanthocytes causes them to be trapped in the spleen (Douglass, AnnIntMed, 1968; 68:390). However, haemolytic anaemia is not a feature of the acanthocytosis of abeta-lipoproteinaemia.

There is no known treatment for the acanthocytosis associated with liver disease. In at least two cases in which splenectomy was performed the patients died. It was claimed that infusion of polyunsaturated phosphatidylcholine caused regression of spur-cell anaemia, but in this study the abnormal cells, seen in many patients, were probably echinocytes and not acanthocytes (Salvioli, Gut, 1978; 19:844). Olivieri *et al.* (BrJHaemat, 1988; 70:483) found an increased intrinsic membrane proteolytic activity in red cells from a patient with acanthocytes, and a similar increase in normal red cells incubated in the patient's plasma (which presumably caused echinocyte formation). This activity normalized *in vivo* following

plasma exchange; the authors did not record the effect on erythrocyte structure and the patient died. Sato *et al.* (ActaHepatolJpn, 1994; 35:689) suggested that spur-cell anaemia induces disseminated intravascular coagulation; treatment of a patient with spur-cell anaemia aimed at controlling endotoxaemia (polymyxin B and kanamycin sulphate) seemed to improve the endotoxaemia and the haemorrhagic tendency resulting from the disseminated intravascular coagulation.

Extracorpuscular abnormalities
Zieve's syndrome

In 1958 Zieve (AnnIntMed, 1958; 48:471) described a group of patients with alcoholic liver disease who showed evidence of mild, short-lived haemolytic anaemia associated with jaundice and hypertriglyceridaemia. He suggested that this was a distinct syndrome, the hyperlipoproteinaemia causing the haemolysis, but others reject this idea (Blaas, AmJMed, 1966; 40:283); Wisloff and Boman argued that Zieve's 'syndrome' represents the association of some common and independent phenomena in alcoholic subjects (ActaMedScand, 1979; 205:237).

Hepatic histology in these cases usually reveals a fatty liver, but there may be associated fibrosis, alcoholic hepatitis, or cirrhosis. Veyrac *et al.* suggested that the fatty change can mask acute alcoholic hepatitis which may be revealed by a repeat biopsy (NouvPresseMed, 1982; 11:2003). The hyperlipidaemia is usually a marked hypertriglyceridaemia with hypercholesterolaemia, a type V pattern on electrophoresis with increased chylomicrons and very low density lipoproteins. The hyperlipidaemia and the haemolysis usually respond rapidly to the withdrawal of alcohol.

In early studies during the acute phase, increased plasma lipids were found to be associated with increased red cell cholesterol and phospholipid (particularly lecithin), but there was no clear relationship between plasma and red cell lipid levels, which fell during remission, though not necessarily to normal. These changes were associated with a reduction in red cell osmotic fragility (Westerman, JLabClinMed, 1968; 72:665). During the acute phase the half-life of both autologous and transfused red cells was reduced, but incubation of red cells with acute-phase plasma did not increase their lipid levels *in vitro*, nor did they undergo premature destruction *in vivo*. As haemolysis occurred only for a short period during the acute phase, it was suggested that an unidentified extracorpuscular factor, present at that time, was the cause of the haemolysis (Balcerzak, AmJMedSci, 1968; 255:277).

Goebel *et al.* (EurJClinInv, 1975; 5:83) proposed an abnormality of red cell pyruvate kinase activity during the acute phase of Zieve's syndrome. Subsequently they reported that red cells in the acute phase contained less vitamin E, relative to their content of polyunsaturated fatty acids, and were particularly sensitive to lysis induced by hydrogen peroxide; they suggested that the combination of the low vitamin E and altered membrane lipid composition caused increased oxidation of glutathione, thus causing a pyruvate kinase instability which triggered haemolytic anaemia (Goebel, BrJHaemat, 1977; 35:573).

The status of Zieve's syndrome remains uncertain, as jaundice, mild haemolysis, and marked hyperlipidaemia may all occur independently in alcoholics. Cases are still described (Ng, ChinJGastro, 1991; 8:24), but unfortunately the full-blown syndrome is, in our experience, extremely rare and therefore difficult to study in detail.

Wilson's disease

In 1934 Sjovall and Wallgren (ActaPsychNeurol, 1934; 9:435) described a patient who, aged 10 years, suffered two episodes of haemolysis; 3 years later Wilson's disease was diagnosed. Subsequently, similar cases were described (Brinton, ProcRoySocMed, 1947; 40:556; Cartwright, JCI, 1954; 33:1487; Gruter, DeutschZfNervenh, 1959; 179:401; Scheinberg, Gastro, 1959; 37: 550; Walshe, ArchDisChild, 1962; 37:253). In 1965 Carr *et al.* (ProcRoySocMed, 1965; 58:614) diagnosed Wilson's disease at the time of haemolysis in a 10-year-old girl whose elder sister died, age 7 years, with jaundice and haemolytic anaemia; cirrhosis had been found at autopsy.

In 1967 McIntyre *et al.* (NEJM, 1967; 276:439) reported three cases. In two boys, aged 12 and 9 years, the diagnosis of Wilson's was made during the haemolytic episode; the third patient, aged 21, was a known case of Wilson's disease whose penicillamine dosage had been reduced to only 0.9 g/week 4 years earlier. In all three cases ascites appeared soon after haemolysis. The serum bilirubin rose, but there was either no increase in aspartate aminotransferase or only a moderate rise. During haemolysis urinary copper levels were very high, serum copper was raised, and in the one case in which red cell copper was measured it was several times higher than normal.

Subsequently the association of haemolysis with Wilson's disease has been more widely recognized (Deiss, AnnIntMed, 1970; 73: 413; Hamlyn, BMJ, 1977; 2:660; Forman, AmJHemat, 1980:9:269; Degenhardtm, DMedWoch, 1994; 119:1421).

There are several important clinical points. The episodes of haemolysis, which may be very severe, are brief. They are usually mistaken for an attack of acute viral hepatitis even though they are often associated with ascites; indeed, early appearance of ascites in a young person with liver disease should suggest the possibility of Wilson's disease. In some patients with haemolysis the course is that of fulminant hepatic failure (Adler, AmJDisChild, 1977; 131: 870; Roche-Sicot, AnnIntMed, 1977; 86:301). Haemoglobinuria and renal failure may occur. Despite jaundice, with a high conjugated bilirubin, bilirubin may be absent from the urine; the reason for this is not clear. This absence of bilirubinuria may suggest haemolysis, but it may also deflect attention from the coexisting liver disease, as there may be little or no change in aminotransferase levels or alkaline phosphatase (see Chapter 5.1). Conversely, when deep jaundice is present this may hinder the recognition of underlying haemolysis, though this is usually evident from the haemoglobin level and reticulocyte count.

Although haemolysis is characteristically an early presentation of Wilson's disease, cirrhosis is already present. The quickest method of making the diagnosis of Wilson's at the time of haemolysis is to ask an ophthalmologist to look for Kayser–Fleischer rings (see Section 4), although these are not always present. When severe acute haemolysis occurs in children or young people, Wilson's disease should be considered, particularly if there are features of liver disease; the only other likely diagnosis is acute viral hepatitis occurring in patients with glucose 6-phosphate dehydrogenase deficiency. The serum caeruloplasmin may be normal (Degenhardt, DMedWoch, 1994; 119:1421).

The mortality following haemolysis is high, either early from fulminant hepatic failure or during the next few months as a result of decompensated liver disease. However, many patients recover and if the diagnosis is not made they may have no further manifestations of Wilson's disease for many years. There is no known treatment for the haemolysis; neither haemodialysis nor peritoneal dialysis appear particularly effective, although they remove copper from the blood. In severe and fulminant cases liver transplantation should be considered. Penicillamine therapy should be started in those who recover and should be continued in adequate dosage for life, as haemolysis can recur years later if the dose is inadequate or if penicillamine is stopped (see Chapter 20.1). Haemolysis has been described in a patient receiving zinc sulphate as treatment for Wilson's disease (Shimon, IsrJMedSci, 1993; 10:646). Siblings should be screened for the disease.

The haemolyic episodes in Wilson's disease are analogous to the naturally occurring 'enzootic jaundice' of sheep in which large amounts of copper accumulate in liver until, for unknown reasons, a large amount is suddenly released into the bloodstream, causing severe haemolysis, jaundice, and often death from renal impairment associated with haemoglobinuria (Todd, BrVetJ, 1963; 119:161; Todd, VetRec, 1965; 77:498). The mechanism for the sudden release of copper from the liver is not known. The haemolysis appears to be due to a direct toxic effect of copper on erythrocytes.

Other extracorpuscular abnormalities

Approximately 10 to 30 per cent of subjects undergoing transjugular intrahepatic portosystemic shunts (**TIPSS**) develop intravascular haemolysis due to traumatic red cell damage (Conn, Hepatol, 1996; 23:177; Sanyal, Hepatol, 1996; 23:32) and it may be clinically significant. It tends to settle spontaneously within about 2 weeks, and thereafter there is an increase in the haemoglobin and platelet count and a reduction in spleen size (Jalan, EurJGastroHepatol, 1996; 8:381).

Widespread endothelial injury can lead to platelet activation and to consumption thrombocytopenia, renal failure, microangiopathic haemolytic anaemia, and neurological manifestations. This constellation of abnormalities (haemolytic uraemic syndrome or thrombotic thrombocytic purpura) has been reported in association with hepatitis A (Furgiuele, TexasMed, 1981; 77:55; Cronin, IrMedJ, 1983; 76:357). Disseminated intravascular coagulation (see Chapter 25.4) can also lead to haemolytic anaemia.

An autoimmune haemolytic anaemia with a positive direct antiglobulin test may occur in association with autoimmune liver disease. It has been most frequently reported in association with chronic active hepatitis (Pengelly, PostgradMedJ, 1971; 47:683; Lightwood, VoxSang, 1973; 24:331; Portell, RevClinEsp, 1982; 164: 101; Girino, ClinRheum, 1986; 5:92) but may also occur in primary biliary cirrhosis (Orlin, Gastro, 1980; 78:576). Coombs-positive haemolytic anaemia is also found in children with giant cell hepatitis; the hepatitis is thought to be autoimmune in nature but it is unusual to find the autoantibodies usually associated with autoimmune hepatitis; however, smooth muscle antibodies were found in one such case (Weinstein, JPediatGastrNutr, 1993; 17:313). One patient with cirrhosis suffered from autoimmune haemolytic anaemia, interstitial lung disease, and autoimmune hypothyroidism; she appeared to have antibodies to hepatitis C virus with a second-generation

RIBA test, but was negative for serum hepatitis C virus RNA (Sousa, EurJGastroHepatol, 1994; 6:1067).

Intracorpuscular defects in liver disease

Apart from abnormalities of membrane lipids, intrinsic disturbances of the red cell are uncommon in patients with uncomplicated chronic liver disease. However, the metabolic simplicity of the mature red cell, and its inability to perform protein synthesis and thereby renew its complement of enzymes, renders it uniquely susceptible to injuries to its enzymatic machinery. Thus, instability of the glycolytic enzyme pyruvate kinase (Goebel, BrJHaemat, 1977; 35:573) may occur with alcohol-induced red cell and liver damage, and play a role in exacerbating the haemolysis. Haemolytic anaemia is more frequent in children with glucose 6-phosphatase dehydrogenase deficiency who develop viral hepatitis than in normal children[14] (Kattamis, JPediat, 1970; 77:422) and reduction of hepatocyte glucose 6-phosphatase dehydrogenase levels in glucose 6-phosphatase dehydrogenase deficient individuals may exacerbate and prolong the hyperbilirubinaemia seen with haemolytic episodes (Oluboyede, JLabClinMed, 1979; 93:783).

Sideroblastic anaemia is due to a defect in haem synthesis. It leads to deficient iron utilization, may therefore cause iron overload, and should be considered in the differential diagnosis of haemochromatosis. It is reported in alcoholic liver disease (Chapter 15.4; Kushner, AdvIntMed, 1977; 22:229).

Vitamin E deficiency may exacerbate haemolysis in chronic cholestatic liver disease, particularly in children (Fernandez-Zamorano, JMed, 1988; 19:317).

Erythrocytosis

In contrast to anaemia, erythrocytosis has been reported in 3 to 12 per cent of patients with hepatocellular carcinoma (Jacobsen, SAMedJ, 1978; 53:658); as many as 23 per cent may have raised serum erythropoietin concentrations by radio-immunoassay (Kew, Cancer, 1986; 58:2485). Paraneoplastic production of erythropoietin is the main mechanism, but local hypoxia of the tumour may also result in increased hepatic release of erythropoietin (Pirisi, Hepatol, 1995; 22:148).

There is evidence that the erythropoietin-like activity elaborated by cultured hepatic tumour cells is structurally different from normal human erythropoietin (Okabe, Cancer, 1985; 55:1918), and may therefore be functionally different. Transient erythrocytosis has been reported early in the course of infectious hepatitis (Bank, MedChirDig, 1974; 3:321).

Viral hepatitis and bone marrow aplasia

A transient, mild depression of haemoglobin, white cell, and platelet counts occurs commonly with acute viral hepatitis, as with other viral infections, and is occasionally quite persistent (Havens, AmJMed Sci, 1946; 212;129; Kivel, AmJDigDis, 1961; 6:1017; Firkin, BMJ, 1978; ii:1534; Vande-Stouwe, Gastro, 1983; 85:186).

An association of viral hepatitis with aplastic anaemia emerges from epidemiological surveys. Viral hepatitis appears to be an aetiological factor in up to 13 per cent of patients with aplastic

anaemia;[15] it seems particularly important in the Far East where hepatitis is more prevalent (Alter, ClinHaem, 1978; 7:431; Young, BrJHaemat, 1986; 62:1). Marrow aplasia is, however, a rare complication of viral hepatitis, first reported in 1955 (Lorenz, Wein-MedWoch, 1955; 105:19). Community-based surveys are lacking, but of 5500 children in hospital, seen over 20 years in Thessaloniki (Greece), only four (0.07 per cent) developed aplasia (Pikis, ScaJInfectDis, 1988; 20:109); a similar incidence was found in other studies (Ajlouni, BrJHaemat, 1974; 27:345; Losowsky, ClinGastroent, 1980; 9:3). All four children died, and this high mortality rate has been confirmed[15] (Camitta, NEJM, 1982: 306:645 and 712). Although the aplasia is usually complete and affects all three cell lineages in the marrow, incomplete aplasias, such as pure red cell aplasia (Iacopino, Haematol(Pavia), 1986; 71:217; Ide, AmJGastr, 1994; 89:257) and agranulocytosis (Nishimoto, ActaPathJap, 1987; 37:155), have been reported with acute hepatitis A and B and with post-transfusion non-A non-B hepatitis.

Sporadic cases of aplastic anaemia have been reported following hepatitis A (Smith, AmJHemat, 1978; 5:247; Domenech, Acta-Haem, 1986; 76:227) and hepatitis B (Nakamura, TohokuJExpMed, 1975; 116:101; Casciato, ArchIntMed, 1978; 138:1557; Kindmark, ActaMedScand, 1984; 215:89; McSweeney, AmJMed, 1988; 85: 255), but most appear to be a consequence of infection with non-A non-B infection[15-17] (Perillo, JAMA, 1981; 245:494; Bannister, BMJ, 1983; 286:1314; Cargnel, AmJGastr, 1983; 78:245; Sandberg, ScaJInfectDis, 1984; 16:403). Most patients with hepatitis-associated aplastic anaemia do not have antibodies to hepatitis C (Pol, AnnIntMed, 1990; 113:435; Hibbs, JAMA, 1992; 267:2051). However, most patients have not been tested for hepatitis C virus RNA, which makes it difficult to rule hepatitis C infection out completely. Hepatitis C virus RNA was demonstrated in serum and peripheral blood cells (but not in bone marrow stem cells) in one patient with hepatitis C virus-associated aplastic anaemia (Peters, DigDisSci, 1995; 40:763). In a study of 10 patients with hepatitis-associated aplastic anaemia, Brown et al. (NEJM, 1997; 336:1059) found no association with any of the known hepatitis viruses.

Marrow failure usually follows 1 to 3 months after the onset of hepatitis, but longer periods have been reported. Males are considered more likely to develop aplasia after hepatitis than females (Hagler, Medicine, 1975; 54:139), and it is primarily a disorder of younger persons with a median age in one series of 18 years (Ajlouni, BrJHaemat, 1974; 27:345). The hepatitis is usually mild and aplasia characteristically occurs as the hepatitis begins to improve (Foon, AnnIntMed, 1984; 100:657).

The pathogenesis of hepatitis virus-induced aplastic anaemia remains poorly understood; there are several excellent reviews[18-20] (Peters, DigDisSci, 1995; 40:763). One possibility is that the virus is directly cytotoxic to haemopoietic progenitor cells as well as to hepatocytes. Hepatitis B virus has been studied in this regard, studies being facilitated both by the extensive characterization of the molecular structure of the virus and of the immunological consequences of infection (see Section 12). Hepatitis B virus DNA has been detected in peripheral blood myeloid cells (Hoar, Blood, 1985; 66:1251) and bone marrow (Romet-Lemonne, Lancet, 1983; ii:732; Yoffe, JInfDis, 1986; 153:471) of patients with hepatitis, and the virus has been shown to inhibit both haemopoietic and lymphoid colony growth in vitro (Zeldis, JCI, 1986; 78:411). If the virus were truly cytopathic for haemopoietic cells, however, one would expect a higher incidence of aplastic anaemia after hepatitis B.

In one series (Tsakis, NEJM, 1988; 319:393) the incidence of aplastic anaemia was 28 per cent (9 of 32) in patients undergoing liver transplantation for acute sporadic non-A non-B hepatitis. None had previous evidence of haematological dysfunction, there were no other apparent causes for the marrow aplasia, and aplastic anaemia was not seen in any other patients (over 1400) undergoing liver transplantation for other indications (in some of whom transfusion-related hepatitis C must have occurred). In one study of children undergoing transplantation for fulminant hepatic failure the incidence of aplastic anaemia was 33 per cent, with a mortality of 42 per cent (Cattral, Hepatol, 1994; 20:813), but this high incidence was not found at another liver transplant centre (Forbes, NEJM, 1989; 320:122). It is possible that successful liver transplantation simply permits a high expression of aplastic anaemia, not usually evident because fulminant non-A non-B hepatitis *per se* has a mortality rate close to 90 per cent (O'Grady, Gastro, 1988; 94: 1186).

Indirect mechanisms of haemopoietic suppression may operate with hepatitis. Hepatic failure may prevent hepatic metabolism of a marrow toxin, thus enhancing the myelotoxic effect of certain drugs or toxins[20] (Watananukul, ArchIntMed, 1977; 137:898). However, aplastic anaemia complicates mild as well as fulminant viral hepatitis, and presents typically when the hepatitis is resolving.

A further possibility is that the bone marrow damage (and possibly much of the liver damage) is immunologically mediated. Several immunological abnormalities have been reported among patients with hepatitis-associated aplastic anaemia. Foon *et al.* (AnnIntMed, 1984; 100:657) studied 16 young male patients and found a reduction in total circulating T lymphocyte levels, reduced T-cell mitogen responses, and decreased B lymphocyte and serum immunoglobulin levels. The reductions in humoral immunity are the opposite of those typically seen in acute or chronic hepatitis (Dienstag, Gastro, 1983; 83:439); in another study there was actually a polyclonal plasma cell proliferation in a patient with hepatitis-associated aplastic anaemia (Nishimoto, ActaPathJpn, 1987; 37: 155). Hermann *et al.* (JImmunol, 1986; 136:1629) established an interleukin-2-dependent T-cell line, from a patient with hepatitis-associated aplastic anaemia, which had an activated suppressor cell phenotype, produced γ-interferon in a dysregulated fashion, and inhibited haemopoietic colony growth *in vitro*. Kojima *et al.* found a significantly lower peripheral blood helper : suppressor T lymphocyte ratio in five children with hepatitis-associated aplastic anaemia than in 16 children with idiopathic aplasia (BrJHaemat, 1989; 71: 147); four of the five also had a striking increase in activated suppressor T lymphocytes, which may mediate haemopoietic suppression (Mehta, BrJHaemat, 1989; 72:287). Brown *et al.* (NEJM, 1997; 336:1059) have also reported a consistent increase in peripheral blood activated CD8 + T lymphocytes.

Treatment of hepatitis-associated aplasia

Hepatitis-associated aplastic anaemia is transient in some patients and recovers spontaneously (Havens, AmJMedSci, 1946; 212:219; Kivel, AmJDigDis, 1961; 6:1017; Firkin, BMJ, 1978; 2:1534) so that supportive therapy with antibiotics and blood products is appropriate initially. There are a few reports of successful response

to immunosuppressive therapy with either antithymocyte globulin (Champlin, NEJM, 1983; 308:113) or high-dose methyl-prednisolone (Ozsoylu, ScaJHaematol, 1984; 33:309). Four patients with pure red cell aplasia appear to have been treated successfully with prednisolone or transfusion (Ide, AmJGastr, 1994; 89:257). Such therapy is usually of only limited value in severe aplastic anaemia and the prognosis for haemopoietic recovery is poor, but improving (Cattral, Hepatol, 1994; 20:813). Allogeneic bone marrow transplantation is probably the treatment of choice for severely affected patients with a histocompatible donor; a number of studies have reported a successful outcome (Camitta, Blood, 1974; 43:473; Royal Marsden, BMJ, 1974; i:363; Witherspoon, AmJHemat, 1984; 17:269; Kojimas, ActaHaem, 1988; 79:7; Brown, NEJM, 1997; 336: 1059).

White cell changes in liver disease

Leucocyte abnormalities in liver disease may be due to the underlying disease or its therapy, and range from neutrophilia to neutropenia and lymphopenia.[8] Leucocytosis occurs in response to infection, haemorrhage, haemolysis, and malignancy. In patients with cirrhosis and systemic inflammatory response syndrome leucocyte activation is evident from measurement of leucocyte adhesion molecule expression, and there is elevation of serum interleukin-6 (Rosenbloom, JAMA, 1995; 274:58). Specific changes in different diseases are dealt with elsewhere in the appropriate chapters. Alterations in lymphocyte function which are of potential pathogenetic significance are also covered under the specific diseases.

Eosinophilia

Eosinophilia is frequently seen in association with parasitic diseases, but can occur in other situations. Croffy *et al.* (DigDisSci, 1988; 33: 233) reported four young males with steroid-responsive chronic hepatitis; all presented with unexplained hypereosinophilia and relapse of the hepatitis was heralded by an increase in the eosinophil count. Eosinophilia has also been reported in association with hepatic vein thrombosis (Walker, ArchIntMed, 1987; 147:2220), hepatocellular carcinoma (Salame, GastroentBelg, 1988; 51:141), drug allergy, and graft rejection.

More recently, transient eosinophilia (either absolute (>500 × 10^9/litre) or relative (>6 per cent of white blood cells)) was noted in 9 of 23 patients with primary biliary cirrhosis (Wirth, SchMedWoch, 1993; 123:2278); the highest number of eosinophils noted was 1385 × 10^9/litre (19 per cent of white blood cells). The eosinophilia seemed to be an indicator of an early disease state with florid bile duct lesions. Eosinophils are also found in the portal tracts in primary biliary cirrhosis (Terasaki, Hepatol, 1993; 17:206), and it has been suggested that eosinophils and the cationic protein released from them may contribute to cellular damage. Serum eosinophilic cationic protein was high in patients with primary biliary cirrhosis, when compared to levels in healthy subjects and patients with cirrhosis or chronic viral hepatitis; there was no difference in the level between symptomatic and asymptomatic patients with primary biliary cirrhosis (Miyaguchi, IntHepatolComm, 1994; 2:285).

Because ursodeoxycholic acid appeared to lower the eosinophil count, Wirth *et al.* (SchMedWoch, 1994; 124:810) thought that this might contribute to its beneficial effect. Yamazaki *et al.* (AmJGastr,

1996; 91:516) also found higher relative and absolute eosinophilia with primary biliary cirrhosis; they noted that it was higher in patients with early histological changes, correlated with the basophil count and serum IgA levels, and that it was markedly reduced by treatment with ursodeoxycholic acid. Ursodeoxycholic acid treatment also leads to improvement in the imbalance of lymphocyte subsets in primary biliary cirrhosis (Ikeda, JGastHepatol, 1996; 11: 366).

Leucopenia

A mild leucopenia is frequently encountered in patients with chronic liver disease, and reflects either hypersplenism or a toxic effect on the bone marrow (e.g. of infection, alcohol, or toxic metabolites from the gastrointestinal tract which have not been neutralized by the liver). In addition to causing leucopenia, alcohol has well-recognized toxic effects on neutrophils and also on lymphocyte function, which cause defects in both cellular and humoral immunity (Girard, Hemat/OncolClinNAm, 1987; 1:321; and Chapter 15.4). Reduced clearance of IgG-coated autologous red cells has been demonstrated in alcoholic cirrhosis (Gomez, NEJM, 1994; 331:1122) and suggests defective macrophage Fc-receptor function with functional hyposplenism. Many of the reported studies on white cell numbers and function in liver disease include substantial numbers of patients with alcoholic cirrhosis, and it is difficult to distinguish between the general effects of liver disease and complications of alcohol abuse.

Increased susceptibility to infection is well recognized in chronic liver disease, and this is likely to be due to a combination of mechanisms. Specific areas of haematological interest are disturbances of neutrophil function, lymphocyte function, and of complement activation.

Neutrophil function

Casassus et al. (AnnMedIntern, 1985; 136:213) found normal bone marrow granulocyte colony growth in cirrhotics; the leucocyte response to hydrocortisone stimulation was reduced, suggesting a disturbance in the late maturation compartment of granulocyte differentiation. Although the chemotactic response of neutrophils from cirrhotics is normal when tested in normal serum, chemotaxis may be inhibited in the presence of the patient's serum (Demeo, NEJM, 1972; 286:735; Maderazo, JLabClinMed, 1975; 85:621; Van Epps, AmJMed, 1975; 58:200). Demeo et al. suggested that this was due to low levels of alternative pathway complement components; low levels of these components have been reported in chronic liver disease. Inhibition of chemotaxis by ascitic fluid from cirrhotics is even greater than by serum, and proportional to the local concentration of C3 (Horing, JGastHepatol, 1995; 10:186). Hypocomplementaemia also occurs in hepatitis C viraemia (Itch, AmJGastr, 1994; 89:2019). High levels of IgA, often found in patients with alcoholic and cryptogenic cirrhosis (Campbell, ClinExpImmun, 1981; 45:81), may form aggregates or complexes and thus inhibit chemotaxis (Kemp, ClinExpImmun, 1980; 40:388). Similar defects of neutrophil motility have been observed in children with chronic liver disease (Maggiore, AmJDisChild, 1983; 137:768).

The degree of the functional defects found *in vitro* appears to parallel the severity of the liver disease[21] (Wyke, Gut, 1980; 21: 643), supporting the notion that the defects are secondary to impaired hepatic synthesis of complement components and opsonins. One study, in chronic active hepatitis, reported an inverse correlation between complement concentrations and the biochemical severity of the liver disease.[21] It is of interest that defects of serum opsonization are uncommon with primary biliary cirrhosis, and complement deficiency is also uncommon in this disease; indeed, complement activation and hypercatabolism, perhaps related to elevated IgM levels, are characteristic of this condition (Potter, JLabClinMed, 1976; 88:427; Lingren, JLabClinMed, 1985; 105:432).

Immunoglobulin-producing cells and liver disease

Hyperglobulinaemia is a well-recognized feature of cirrhosis (Feizi, Gut, 1968; 9:193; Jensen, ArchIntMed, 1982; 142:2318). It has been suggested that this polyclonal hypergammaglobulinaemia is initiated by immunization with enteric organisms normally filtered by the liver (Triger, Lancet, 1973; i:1494; Stobo, DigDisSci, 1979; 24:737). However, cirrhosis may be associated with a state of generalized immunological hyperactivity, perhaps as a result of a defect of immune regulation. Berger et al. (DigDisSci, 1979; 24:741) found that peripheral blood mononuclear cells from cirrhotics with hypergammaglobulinaemia had a normal proportion of B cells, but that IgG and IgA synthesis was markedly increased in these cells.

A high frequency of hepatitis B surface antigen and antibody in serum has been reported from patients with essential mixed cryoglobulinaemia, and it has been suggested that hepatitis B virus is involved in the pathogenesis of this syndrome (Realdi, ZImmunitat, 1974; 147:114; Levo, NEJM, 1977; 296:1501); other reports did not confirm this association (Popp, AnnIntMed, 1980; 92:379; Zarski, GastrClinBiol, 1984; 8:845). Type II mixed cryoglobulinaemia frequently occurs with hepatitis C virus infection (Misiani, AnnIntMed, 1992; 117:537), and circulating immune complexes and hypocomplementaemia were found some years ago in patients with non-A non-B hepatitis (Dienstag, Lancet, 1979; i:1265).

Benign monoclonal gammopathy has been reported in association with primary biliary cirrhosis and other types of cirrhosis (Parlier, NouvPresseMed, 1982; 11:3841; Hendrick, QJMed, 1986; 231:681); the absence of distinctive clinical, biochemical, and immunological features suggests that the association may be fortuitous.

In spite of the hypergammaglobulinaemia, the erythrocyte sedimentation rate is not raised by inflammation, infection, or neoplasia to the extent that one would expect in patients without chronic liver disease; this is largely due to the lower fibrinogen levels found in cirrhosis, and to the lower kininogen levels (Lujkan, ActaHepatoGastroenterol, 1975; 22:89).

Liver disease and platelets

Defects of platelet number and function are well documented in patients with chronic liver disease, contributing significantly to their haemostatic abnormalities. Alcoholic liver disease is associated with additional abnormalities which are probably a consequence of the toxic effect of alcohol on platelet production and function (Mikhailides, BMJ, 1986; 293:715; Girard, Hemat/OncolClinNAm, 1987; 1:321; Hillbom, BMJ, 1987; 295:581; and Chapter 15.4).

Several studies have examined platelet kinetics in patients with chronic liver disease. Similar results are seen whether the platelets are labelled with 111In (Toghill, Gut, 1983; 24:49; Schmidt, ScaJHaematol, 1985; 34:39; Noguchi, Hepatol, 1995; 22:1682) or 51Cr (Kummer, SchMedWoch, 1971; 101:1816; Toghill, JClinPath, 1977; 30:367; Stein, JLabClinMed, 1982; 99:217; Schmidt, ScaJHaematol, 1983; 30:465). These studies demonstrate diverse mechanisms for the thrombocytopenia of liver disease, including a shortened platelet mean lifetime (i.e. accelerated platelet destruction), platelet pooling in an enlarged spleen, and inability of the bone marrow to compensate adequately for thrombocytopenia even though platelet production increases. Liver disease may also reduce thrombopoietin production.[1] There is no clear relationship between abnormalities of platelet kinetics and the severity of the liver disease; very low counts often accompany portal hypertension and splenomegaly in patients with relatively normal liver function tests.

There is growing evidence of impaired platelet function in chronic liver disease (Thomas, NEJM, 1967; 276:1344; Thomas, AnnNYAcadSci, 1972; 201:243, and see below), and of impairment of aggregation by intrinsic platelet defects and circulating inhibitors of aggregation. Qualitative platelet abnormalities, assessed by template bleeding times and platelet aggregation studies, may correlate with the severity of both acute and chronic liver disease (Rubin, QJMed, 1977; 46:339; Rubin, DigDisSci, 1979; 24:197). The causes of the functional abnormalities are probably similar to the underlying causes of the thrombocytopenia, and include platelet activation (Luzzatto, ActaHaem, 1987; 77:101), perhaps by adhesion to incompletely endothelialized sinusoids (Stein, JLabClinMed, 1982; 99:217); enzymatic alteration of the platelet membrane (Greenberg, Blood, 1979; 53:916); and metabolic factors associated with the cirrhotic process or its causes (Kummer, SchMedWoch, 1971; 101: 1816; Schmidt, ScaJHaematol, 1985; 34:39).

Normal platelets enriched with cholesterol show increased aggregability by ADP and adrenaline (Kramer, JBC, 1982; 257:6844). Platelets in liver disease tend to be cholesterol-rich but their aggregability is diminished, probably because the arachidonic acid content of platelet phospholipids is reduced (Owen, JLipRes, 1981; 22:423); this may reduce production of proaggregatory thromboxane A2 (Laffi, Gastro, 1986; 90:274; Laffi, Hepatol, 1988; 8:1620). Further work is needed to establish the haemostatic significance of these findings in liver disease.

Cross-incubation studies suggested the possibility of a circulating inhibitor of platelet aggregation in chronic liver disease (Ballard, ArchIntMed, 1976; 136:316). Fibrin degradation products are known inhibitors but they may only be important in very severe liver disease (Rubin, DigDisSci, 1979; 24:197). High-density lipoproteins (HDL) isolated from patients with cirrhosis inhibited ADP-induced platelet aggregation, and this effect of cirrhotic HDL seemed to be related to its high apolipoprotein E content (Desai, Lancet, 1989; i:613); there appeared to be no relationship to the aetiology of the cirrhosis or the severity of the disease. Apolipoprotein E-enriched HDL1 from normal plasma also impairs reactivity of platelets to several agonists, apparently by binding to saturable sites on the cell surface (Desai, JLipRes, 1989; 30:831). Recently, studies from the same laboratory presented evidence suggesting that apolipoprotein E exerts its antiplatelet effect by enhancing endogenous nitric oxide (NO) synthesis; it markedly elevated platelet NO synthase activity and intraplatelet levels of cGMP, while NO synthesis inhibitors restricted its inhibitory action (Riddell, JBC, 1997; 272:89). It was also reported recently that the basal cytosolic calcium content in platelets from cirrhotic patients was lower than that of controls (Forrest, JHepatol, 1996; 25:312). Incubation of normal platelets in fresh plasma from patients with cirrhosis caused a fall in their cytosolic calcium; this did not occur if the plasma or serum had been frozen. There was an increase in cytosolic calcium when platelets from cirrhotics were incubated in control plasma.

Platelets from patients with cirrhosis also exhibit a defect in the von Willebrand factor-binding domain (Jaschonek, ZGastr, 1993; 31:8). The resulting defect in primary haemostasis, that is, the vWF-mediated attachment of platelets to exposed subendothelium, might contribute to the increased risk of haemorrhagic complications in cirrhotics.

A raised level of platelet-associated immunoglobulin is found in some patients with chronic liver disease (Landolfi, ScaJHaematol, 1980; 25:417; Barrison, BrJHaemat, 1981; 48:347), suggesting that antibody-mediated platelet destruction may contribute to shortened platelet survival. Bassendine et al. (Gut, 1985; 26:1074) found high levels of platelet-associated immunoglobulin in 40 per cent of 62 patients with primary biliary cirrhosis; a similar incidence of autoimmune platelet destruction occurs in alcoholic cirrhosis (Harrison, BrJHaemat, 1981; 48:347) and chronic active hepatitis (Landolfi, ScaJHaematol, 1980; 25:417).

Recently, Pereira et al. (AmJHaemat, 1995; 50:173) demonstrated a high prevalence (>60 per cent) of platelet-associated immunoglobulin in a group of 36 patients with chronic liver disease of diverse aetiology. They went on to show that the platelet-associated immunoglobulin reacted specifically against the platelet glycoproteins IIb/IIIa (4 of the 36), Ib/IX complexes (12 of 36), or against both (7 of 36). These are often the autoantigens in classical idiopathic autoimmune thrombocytopenia (**AITP**), and platelet autoantibodies in AITP have similar specificity (He, Blood, 1994; 83:1031). These data suggest that an immune mechanism may induce or aggravate thrombocytopenia in chronic liver disease as it does in AITP. The level of platelet-associated immunoglobulin does not usually correlate with the platelet count (nor did the level of specific autoantibodies in the Pereira study). It is therefore likely that other factors (e.g. serum thrombopoietin level, splenic size, and reticuloendothelial cell function) influence the degree of thrombocytopenia.

Acute immune thrombocytopenia has been reported in association with hepatitis A (Kleinman, Hepatogast, 1982; 29:144; Ibarra, Blut, 1986; 52:371), hepatitis B (Lever, BMJ, 1987; 295: 1519), and primary hepatic lymphoma (Aghai, Cancer, 1987; 60: 2308). Selinger et al. (AnnIntMed, 1987; 107:686) and Chalmers et al. (ScotMedJ, 1987; 32:152) have also reported immune thrombocytopenia in patients with primary biliary cirrhosis.

Chronic hepatitis C infection appears to be particularly associated with immune thrombocytopenia (Nagamine, JHepatol, 1996; 24:135): thrombocytopenia was found in 41 per cent, and a raised platelet-associated immunoglobulin in 88 per cent of 368 patients with chronic hepatitis C; a significantly smaller rise in platelet-associated immunoglobulin occurred in 47 per cent of 53 patients with chronic hepatitis B. In another study 10 per cent of 139 patients with 'autoimmune thrombocytopenia' had antibodies

Table 3 Causes of thrombocytopenia in patients with liver disease

Deficient platelet production*
  Bone marrow hypoplasia, e.g. following viral hepatitis
  Exposure to toxins/physical agents, e.g. organic chemical
    exposure
  Marrow infiltration, e.g. metastatic carcinoma
  Ineffective thrombopoiesis, e.g. folate deficiency, alcohol
  Reduced thrombopoietin, e.g. chronic liver disease of diverse
    aetiology
Accelerated platelet destruction
  Autoimmune
    e.g. chronic liver disease of diverse aetiology,* especially
    primary biliary cirrhosis, hepatitis C virus
    acute viral hepatitis**
    drug induced (e.g. rifampicin)
  Other immunological mechanisms*
    e.g. graft-versus-host disease, post-transfusion, immune
    complex-mediated, drug-induced, allergic states,
    anaphylaxis, AIDS, etc.
  Non-immune processes
    disseminated intravascular coagulation**
    microangiopathic processes,* e.g. thrombotic
    thrombocytopenic purpura, haemolytic–uraemic syndrome
    giant haemangioma*
  Other
    e.g. some infections, massive transfusion**
Pooling*
  e.g. Hypersplenism, post-liver transplantation

* Coagulation tests typically normal or minimally deranged.
** Coagulation tests typically markedly deranged.

to hepatitis C virus, suggesting that hepatitis C virus infection might have triggered autoimmune thrombocytopenia in a proportion of these patients (Pawlotsky, JHepatol, 1995; 23:635).

Treatment of thrombocytopenia

An accurate diagnosis is essential in planning appropriate treatment (Table 3). A coagulation profile should be performed (see Chapters 2.14.3 and 25.4). Markedly abnormal coagulation in association with abnormal liver function tests and profound thrombocytopenia ($<20 \times 10^9$/l) suggests an acute illness (e.g. disseminated intravascular coagulation) with multiple organ failure and accelerated utilization of platelets and coagulation factors, or prominent hepatocellular injury associated with AITP (e.g. acute viral hepatitis). Normal or near-normal coagulation, however, with liver disease and thrombocytopenia suggests stable chronic liver disease or a microangiopathic process. A bone marrow aspirate will usually be required to assess bone marrow platelet production, and a trephine biopsy may be necessary to exclude marrow infiltration. Other tests that are useful in clinical assessment include a template bleeding time, platelet function tests, thromboelastography, further tests of coagulation and fibrinolysis (Chapters 2.14.3 and 25.4), and measurement of antiplatelet antibodies.

Treatment should, whenever possible, be directed at the cause. However, the choice and timing of treatment will be influenced by whether the patient is bleeding or at risk of serious spontaneous bleeding, and whether surgery or an invasive procedure is planned.

Some patients with chronic liver disease exhibited an increase in the platelet count lasting several weeks following the administration of recombinant erythropoietin; non-responders had a significantly lower baseline platelet count and showed less of an improvement in their haematocrit (Pirisi, JHepatol, 1994; 21:376).

Treatment of the bleeding patient

Stable patients who are not bleeding do not generally require therapy. The risk of bleeding is higher, at a given level of the platelet count, in patients who have infection or coexistent abnormalities of coagulation, and efforts should be made to correct these (Chapter 25.4). Other factors that increase susceptibility to haemorrhage are abnormal platelet function (due for example to drugs, liver disease itself, or renal failure) and deficient bone marrow platelet production. Furthermore, when there is an associated increase in the platelet lifespan and reduced platelet turnover, platelets are older and do not function as well. By contrast, patients with accelerated platelet destruction and increased turnover have young platelets and are less likely to bleed, particularly if they have normal coagulation. Platelet transfusion therapy is of very little benefit in the presence of accelerated platelet destruction, particularly when immune mediated; such therapy may actually cause thrombosis in situations where there is microangiopathy, for example thrombotic thrombocytopenic purpura or haemolytic–uraemic syndrome (Harkness, JAMA, 1981; 246:1931).

Patients who are actively bleeding need blood component support, coagulation factor therapy, and treatment aimed at elevating the platelet count. Platelet transfusions are indicated if there is deficient platelet production, and one should try to maintain a platelet count above 50×10^9/litre. Intravenous desmopressin (0.3 μg/kg) may be useful for patients in whom qualitative platelet dysfunction is suspected (Manucci, Blood, 1988; 72:1449). If an autoimmune mechanism of accelerated platelet destruction is suspected, a trial of specific therapy may be indicated. Intravenous immunoglobulin is particularly valuable in this setting as it acts rapidly, is usually effective, is not immunosuppressive, and a response is unlikely in the absence of immune destruction. Other therapies for AITP include prednisolone, immunosuppressive therapy, and splenectomy (George, NEJM, 1994; 331:1207).

Splenectomy is of established value in the treatment of uncomplicated immune thrombocytopenia (Rosse, ClinHaemm, 1983; 12:267). A favourable outcome has also been reported in those thrombocytopenic patients with chronic liver disease in whom there was good evidence for autoimmune platelet destruction (Skootsky, ArchIntMed, 1986; 146:555); however, the role of splenectomy in most thrombocytopenic patients with chronic liver disease and hypersplenism is controversial (El-Khishen, SGO, 1985; 160:233; and Section 10).

Noguchi et al. (Hepatol, 1995; 22:1682) used partial splenic–arterial embolization in 22 cirrhotics with thrombocytopenia; their platelet-associated immunoglobulin G was higher than in controls. The mean splenic infarction ratio was 55 per cent. As expected, the platelet count rose and platelet survival time increased; perhaps surprisingly the platelet-associated immunoglobulin G level showed an inverse relationship with the platelet count.

Alvarez and his colleagues (AmJGastr, 1996; 91:134) described 11 patients with cirrhosis who had a significant improvement in their thrombocytopenia after a transjugular intrahepatic portosystemic shunt (TIPSS). However, in another study (Sanyal, Hepatol, 1996;

23:32) there was no significant change in white cell or platelet counts in 60 patients undergoing TIPSS for variceal bleeding or ascites, and TIPSS was not recommended as a method of improving the platelet count.

Treatment before surgery or other invasive procedures

Elective surgery and associated blood component therapy for patients with chronic liver disease should be carefully planned in advance. Those who have recently undergone surgery, or for whom an elective invasive procedure is planned, should receive therapy aimed at correcting coagulation and maintaining a platelet count greater than 50×10^9/litre (Rintel, Hemat/OncolClinNAm, 1994; 8:1131). A lower count (e.g. 30×10^9/litre) may be permissible, if thrombocytopenia is due to accelerated platelet destruction and/or a less invasive procedure is planned. However, a higher count (e.g. 100×10^9/litre) may be required if there is persisting abnormal coagulation, deficient platelet production, or if surgery is planned on critical sites such as the eyes or brain (Lundberg, JAMA, 1994; 271:777).

High platelet counts

Most patients with chronic liver disease have a low platelet count, especially those with splenomegaly. A normal or raised count may occur as a response to infection, inflammation, neoplasia, bleeding, and iron deficiency; these are the most common causes of secondary thrombocytosis and all occur frequently in chronic liver disease. In the context of a patient with chronic liver disease, however, these conditions should be suspected even if the platelet count is normal (e.g. $>300 \times 10^9$/litre). Primary thrombocythaemia, occurring as part of a myeloproliferative disorder, may present as liver disease in the form of hepatic or portal venous thrombosis.

Nickerson *et al.* (Cancer, 1980; 45:315) reported raised platelet counts in two children with hepatoblastoma; tumour extract from one patient contained elevated levels of thrombocytopoietin. The authors speculated that liver tumours may elaborate thrombopoietin in a manner analogous to erythropoietin production (see above).

Acute haematological and hepatic problems in pregnancy

The syndrome of haemolysis, elevated liver enzymes, and low platelets (**HELLP**; Weinstein, AmJObsGyn, 1982; 142:159; Weinstein, ObsGyn, 1985; 66:657) occurs in as many as 10 per cent of pregnancies associated with eclampsia (Sibai, AmJObsGyn, 1986; 155:501). It has also been reported in normotensive pregnancies (Aarnoudse, BrJObsGyn, 1986; 93:145). Both maternal and fetal outcome are poor in pregnancies associated with pre-eclampsia and HELLP (Lopez-Llera, AmJObsGyn, 1976; 124:681). The pathogenesis is uncertain but probably involves several pathological processes, including microangiopathic haemolytic anaemia disseminated intravascular coagulation and thrombotic thrombocytopenic purpura.[22] The presence of haemolysis in HELLP syndrome is strongly suggested by the presence of red cell fragments and burr cells in the peripheral smear.

Burroughs *et al.* (QJMed, 1982; 31:481) emphasized the importance of the peripheral blood smear in the diagnosis of acute fatty liver of pregnancy. They found that the presence of nucleated red cells, basophilic stippling, and large platelets distinguished fatty liver of pregnancy from eclampsia.

Haematological aspects of liver transplantation[23]

Increasing numbers of transplants are being performed worldwide (see Chapter 30.5). An important consequence has been the need to supply these patients with blood component support. The average consumption in our unit is declining and is currently 6 to 8 units each of red cell concentrate, platelet concentrate, and fresh frozen plasma (Smith, TransfusMed, 1993; 3:97). This usage is comparable to that reported from other centres (Farrar, Transfusion, 1988; 28: 474; Ramsey, Hemat/OncolClinNAm, 1994; 6:117). Improvements in surgical technique, management of coagulopathies, and case selection, and the use of the serine protease inhibitor aprotinin have all contributed to this trend. The figures for average consumption conceal the fact that the occasional patient requires massive transfusion support. Similar problems arise when treating gastrointestinal haemorrhage in patients with liver disease; they require careful management following established guidelines (BSH Guidelines, ClinLabHaemat, 1988; 10:265).

Red cell antibodies and immune haemolysis have been found during the first or second week following transplantation (Petz, TransfusMedRev, 1987; 1:85). Donor lymphocytes within the transplanted organ are thought to be the source of such antibodies, which are directed against antigens on recipient red cells. The relevant antibodies are usually anti-A or anti-B made by group O donor lymphocytes; they appear in 38 per cent of ABO unmatched liver transplants (Ramsey, Transfusion, 1987; 27:552). Although haemolysis is usually mild and short-lived (Yang, TransplProc, 1988; 20: 295), significant haemolysis followed by renal failure has been reported (Dzik, Transfusion, 1987; 27:550). Immune haemolysis in these heavily transfused patients can also be due to delayed transfusion reactions (Reisner, Transfusion, 1987; 27:526). A further risk to all recipients of blood products is non-A non-B hepatitis (Seeff, CurrOpinGastro, 1989; 5:378).

Thrombocytopenia is frequently present in the early postoperative phase following liver transplantation (Plevak, TransplProc, 1988; 20:630; and personal observations). Dilution following massive transfusions, immune destruction, suboptimal bone marrow compensation, and accelerated consumption are all contributory factors. There is good experimental evidence for increased fibrinolytic activity, platelet activation, and sequestration of activated platelets in the graft (Porte, JHepatol, 1994; 21:592). Thrombopoietin levels are low in cirrhotic patients before transplantation and rise after the procedure, presumably due to production by the transplanted organ (Martin, AnnIntMed, 1997; 127: 285).

References

1. Kaushansky K. Thrombopoietin: the primary regulator of platelet production. *Blood*, 1995; **86**: 419–31.

2. Means RT and Krantz S. Progress in understanding the pathogenesis of the anaemia of chronic disease. *Blood*, 1992; **80**: 1639–47.

3. Kimber C, Deller DJ, Ibbotson RH, and Lander H. The mechanism of anaemia in chronic liver disease. *Quarterly Journal of Medicine*, 1965; **34**: 33–64.

4. Sheehy TW and Berman A. The anaemia of cirrhosis. *Journal of Laboratory and Clinical Medicine*, 1960; **56**: 72–82.

5. Phillips DL and Keeffe EB. Hematologic manifestations of gastrointestinal disease. *Hematology/Oncology Clinics of North America*, 1987; **1**: 207–28.

6. Chanarin I. *The megaloblastic anaemias*, (2nd edn). Oxford: Blackwell, 1979.

7. Hillman RS. Hematopoietic agents: growth factors, minerals and vitamins. In Harriman JG, Linbird LE, Molinoff TB, Ruddon RW, and Gillman AG, eds. *The pharmacologic basis of therapeutics*, (9th edn). New York: Macmillan, 1996: 1323–37.

8. Berman L, Axelrod AR, and Horan TN. The blood and bone marrow in patients with cirrhosis of the liver. *Blood*, 1949; **4**: 511–33.

9. Jandl JH. The anemia of liver disease: observations on its mechanism. *Journal of Clinical Investigation*, 1955; **34**: 390–403.

10. Jandl JH, Greenberg MS, and Yonemoto RH. Clinical determination of the sites of red cell sequestration in hemolytic anaemias. *Journal of Clinical Investigation*, 1956; **35**: 842–67.

11. Bessis M, Weed RI, and Le Blond PF (eds). *Red cell shape: physiology, pathology, ultrastructure*. New York: Springer-Verlag, 1973.

12. Glomset JA, Assmann G, Gjone E and Norum KR. Lecithin: cholesterol acyltransferase deficiency and fish eye disease. In Scriver CR, Beaud AL, Sly WS, and Valle D, eds. *The metabolic bases of inherited diseases*, (7th edn). New York: McGraw Hill, 1995: Ch. 60, 1933–51.

13. Owen JS *et al.* Erythrocyte echinocytosis in liver disease. Role of abnormal plasma high density lipoproteins. *Journal of Clinical Investigation*, 1985; **76**: 2275–85.

14. Luzzatto L and Mehta AB. Glucose-6-phosphatase dehydrogenase deficiency. In Scriver CR, Beaud AL, Sly WS, and Valle D, eds. *The metabolic bases of inherited diseases*, (7th edn). New York: McGraw Hill, 1995: Ch 111, 3367–98.

15. Zeldis JB, Dienstag JL, and Gale RP. Aplastic anaemia and non-A non-B hepatitis. *American Journal of Medicine*, 1983; **74**: 64–8.

16. Camitta BM, Storb R, and Thomas ED. Aplastic anemia. *New England Journal of Medicine*, 1982; **306**: 645–52, 712–18.

17. Kurtzman G and Young N. Viruses and bone marrow failure. *Clinical Haematology*, 1989; **2**: 51–68.

18. Baranski B and Young N. Haematologic consequences of viral infection. *Hematology/Oncology Clinics of North America*, 1987; **1**: 167–81.

19. Young N and Mortimer P. Viruses and bone marrow failure. *Blood*, 1984; **63**: 729–37.

20. Young NS. Drugs and chemicals as agents of bone marrow failure. In Gale RP and Testa N, eds. *Bone marrow damage*. New York: Marcel Decker, 1988: 131–57.

21. Wyke RJ, Rajkowic IA, and Williams R. Impaired opsonization by serum from patients with chronic liver disease. *Clinical and Experimental Immunology*, 1983; **51**: 91–8.

22. Letsky EA (ed.) Haematological disorders in pregnancy. *Clinics in Haematology*, 1985; **14**: 3.

23. Petz LD. Hematologic aspects of liver disease. *Current Opinions in Gastroenterology*, 1989; **5**: 372–7.

25.4 Haemostasis in liver disease

Marie-Helene Denninger

Introduction

As described in Chapter 2.14.3, the liver plays a major role in regulating haemostasis, synthesizing most of the clotting factors and coagulation inhibitors, as well as some proteins of the fibrinolytic system, and clearing from the circulating blood the activated enzymes of the clotting and of the fibrinolytic systems. Thus, haemostatic abnormalities are prone to occur in patients with liver disease. These abnormalities include clotting protein deficiencies due to impaired synthesis; synthesis of abnormal clotting proteins; quantitative and qualitative platelet defects; enhanced fibrinolytic activity due to impaired clearance of fibrinolytic activators; and disseminated intravascular coagulation. The abnormalities tend to be similar, whatever the type of liver damage (viral or toxic hepatitis, toxic or metabolic cirrhosis), except with cholestasis or when there is a particular clinical setting, such as infection or pregnancy; thus they depend mainly on the degree of hepatocellular insufficiency.[1]

Impaired synthesis of clotting factors
Decreased clotting factor levels
Factors II, VII, IX, and X

In hepatocellular insufficiency, factor VII is usually the first to be decreased, probably due to its short half-life (Table 1 Chapter 2.14.3)[1], followed by factors II and X. Factor IX is usually the last to be affected. Thus, the most often affected clotting factors, especially at an early stage of liver disease, are factors II, VII, IX, and X. Moreover, these clotting factors may be decreased before any other evidence of liver damage.[1,2] The decreased level of these vitamin K-dependent proteins, associated with normal levels of the other clotting factors, may suggest vitamin K deficiency, and in mild or moderate hepatocellular insufficiency the differential diagnosis from moderate vitamin K deficiency is somewhat difficult to establish. However, if these defects are unresponsive to parenteral administration of vitamin K, it can be assumed that the hepatic synthesis of clotting factors is impaired, since in hepatocellular insufficiency the administration of vitamin K is ineffective in correcting the levels of these factors to normal. Nevertheless, an acquired vitamin K-dependent carboxylation deficiency has been described in parenchymal liver disease,[3] based on specific immunoassay for abnormal des-γ-carboxyprothrombin induced by vitamin K antagonists or absence (**PIVKA II**) (Chapter 2.14.3). Under normal conditions, hepatic carboxylation occurs efficiently, and thus abnormal prothrombin is undetectable in normal plasma.

Conversely, abnormal prothrombin is the predominant component of the prothrombin species in patients on oral anticoagulant treatment. Undercarboxylated prothrombin has, however, been found in plasma of patients with different types of liver diseases such as cirrhosis or hepatitis, although at a considerably lower level than that found in patients with vitamin K deficiency or with oral anticoagulant therapy.[3] Undercarboxylated prothrombin is present in the plasma of more than 90 per cent of patients with liver disease, and the level of this abnormal prothrombin is not modified by treatment with vitamin K. Thus, in liver disease, moderate impairment of vitamin K-dependent carboxylation is superimposed on protein synthesis deficiency. This mechanism is unclear and could be related to premature release of prothrombin precursor by diseased liver, as well as to deficiency of the vitamin K-dependent carboxylase. In any case, this impaired vitamin K-dependent carboxylation does not modify the circulating level of native prothrombin.

Vitamin K deficiency

In adults dietary vitamin K deficiency is rare. It nevertheless occurs in chronically ill patients with little oral intake, and in critically ill patients in intensive care units, without oral intake of or supplementation with exogenous vitamin K, or in patients treated with antibiotics. Vitamin K deficiency more often complicates diseases associated with biliary obstruction, since bile salts are necessary for vitamin K absorption (Chapter 2.14.3) (Hawkins, JExpMed, 1936; 63:795). Thus vitamin K-dependent protein deficiencies affecting clotting factors II, VII, IX, and X, as well as coagulation inhibitors protein C and S, are observed in obstructive jaundice, cholangitis, and biliary cirrhosis.[4] The defects are usually moderate except when there is a total mechanical obstruction of bile ducts by tumours, such as pancreatic head carcinoma. In this latter case, the levels of factors II, VII, IX, and X can be decreased to less than 10 per cent of normal (<10 U/dl) while factor V and fibrinogen levels, both acute-phase reactants, are elevated.[5]

Factor V

Factor V is synthesized in the liver in the absence of vitamin K. Thus, a decreased level of factor V associated with decreased levels of factors II, VII, IX, and X is an indicator of hepatocellular insufficiency which can then be distinguished from simple vitamin K deficiency (Table 1). Nevertheless, factor V is less sensitive than vitamin K-dependent factors to liver damage.[2] Thus, decrease in factor V usually occurs later, with deterioration of hepatocyte

Table 1 Haemostatic evaluation in patients with different conditions in liver disease

	Normal range	Vitamin K deficiency/ common bile duct obstruction	Hepatocellular insufficiency /alcoholic cirrhosis	Fulminant hepatitis	Acute liver failure + DIC (Reye's syndrome)	Acute Budd–Chiari syndrome	Liver transplantation		
							Pre-anhepatic period	Anhepatic period	Reperfusion period
Ivy bleeding time (min)	≤10	8	13	7					
Platelet count (×10^9/l)	150–400	250	110	300	129	75	213	150	128
APTT (s)	36–37	50	65	90	89	99	53	65	61
Ratio	≤1.2	1.4	1.8	2.5	2.5	2.8	1.5	1.8	1.7
PT (%)	75–110	30	40	<10	10	22	45	40	32
Factor II (%)	75–110	25	35	<10	34	16	54	42	53
Factor VII+X (%)	75–110	15	32	<10	10	16	45	38	34
Factor V (%)	75–110	85	45	25	<10	19	46	37	21
Fibrinogen (g/l)	2–4	2.3	2	2.5	0.40	0.90	3.10	2.90	2.10
ELT	>3 h	>3 h	1 h 30	>3 h	2 h		>3 h	20 min	>3 h
Protamine sulphate gelation test	Negative	Negative	Negative	Negative	Positive on diluted plasma 1:8	Positive on diluted plasma 1:2	Negative	Negative	Positive on diluted plasma 1:2
t-PA antigen (ng/ml)	1–12						22	82	48
PAI-1 activity (UI/ml)	0–5						11.8	0	>50

PT, Prothrombin time; APTT, activated partial thromboplastin time; ELT, euglobulin lysis time; PAI, plasminogen activator inhibitor; t-PA, tissue type plasminogen activator.

function, and a marked factor V decrease is more likely to be observed in severe liver disease.[4]

Fibrinogen

As for factor V, the synthesis of fibrinogen is sustained in mild or moderate liver disease. Thus, hypofibrinogenaemia is less frequent than defects in other clotting proteins and does not occur until there is severe liver damage.[4]

Factors XI, XII, prekallikrein, high molecular weight kininogen

Factors XI, XII, and high molecular weight kininogen (**HMWK**) are usually moderately decreased (Saito, Blood, 1976; 48:941). They are not sensitive indicators of the degree of hepatocellular insufficiency[6] and, moreover are not routinely measured. By contrast, prekallikrein decreases early in liver disease (Wong, Ann-IntMed, 1972; 77:205), as do factors II, VII, and X, and it is mainly affected by liver damage.

Factor XIII, fibrin stabilizing factor

Factor XIII level is frequently decreased in liver disease, and the degree of the defect is function of the degree of hepatocellular insufficiency.[5]

Decreased coagulation inhibitor levels
Antithrombin III

Antithrombin III (**AT III**) level is decreased in hepatocellular insufficiency. The decrease is not usually severe[6] and parallels that

of factor V. The AT III decrease is somewhat correlated with prolongation of the prothrombin time.[2] In cirrhotic patients metabolic studies of AT III have shown that the low levels of AT III were associated with a decreased absolute catabolic rate, indicating decreased synthesis (Chan, ClinSci, 1981; 60:681). This synthesis is only affected by general damage to the liver. By contrast, in patients with primary or secondary liver carcinoma, AT III synthesis is not significantly affected[2] (Rubin, ThrombRes, 1980; 18:353) as hepatocyte function is usually preserved in large areas of the liver. Antithrombin III levels are moderately low in patients with primary liver carcinoma and metabolic studies have shown a normal absolute catabolic rate, suggesting normal AT III production with increased catabolism. When ascites is present in cirrhotic patients the metabolism of AT III is modified since ascites represents an extravascular compartment where AT III accumulates (Chan, ClinSci, 1981; 60:681).

Protein C, protein S

Protein C deficiency parallels the deficiency of other vitamin K-dependent factors II, VII, and X. However, the level of protein S remains significantly greater, probably due to extrahepatic synthesis of protein S, as it is not synthesized only in the liver like protein C and factors II, VII, and X, but also by endothelial cells (Chapter 2.14.3).

Although it is not an acute phase reactant, α_2-macroglobulin rises in liver disease, as does α_1-antitrypsin.[2] No C_1-inhibitor decrease has been observed.

Although levels of natural occurring inhibitors of blood clotting are decreased in hepatocellular insufficiency, clinical evidence of thromboembolism is rarely noted.This is probably due to the balance maintained between these inhibitors and the procoagulant factors II, VII, IX, and X, the levels of which are equally depressed.[6] By contrast, the occurrence of thromboembolic manifestations in a patient with hepatocellular insufficiency must lead to suspicion of a disequilibrium between pro- and anticoagulant physiological mechanisms, and thus a more pronounced defect in one of the coagulation inhibitors. However, when the level of AT III, protein C or protein S is found to be lower than expected as compared with clotting factor levels, only a familial enquiry would allow confirmation of a hereditary defect.

Increased clotting factor levels

High plasma levels of factors II, VII, IX, X, XI and XII (that is, above 150 per cent of normal (>150 U/dl)) have been described in patients with biliary tract disease, such as primary biliary cirrhosis, cholestatic drug reaction, and common bile duct obstruction.[7,8] This increase, associated with an increase of many other plasma proteins, is thought to be due to a non-specific increase in the synthesis of liver-produced proteins with cholestasis[8] and is not related to changes in serum bilirubin or alkaline phosphatases.[7] A moderate increase in factors II, VII, XI, and XII has been observed in patients with chronic active hepatitis.[8] Increased levels of factor VII have been observed in mild liver disorders characterized by considerable inflammation[9,10] (Paramo, SemThrombHaemost, 1993; 19:184) as well as in congenital biliary atresia.[4] Factor V is an acute phase reactant and increased levels occur in obstructive jaundice, cholangitis, biliary cirrhosis, congenital biliary atresia, and primary or secondary liver carcinoma.[4] Elevated fibrinogen levels are also observed in these latter conditions as fibrinogen is an acute phase reactant. Increase in fibrinogen can also be observed in mild hepatitis[2,4] and in cirrhosis. Thus, in cirrhosis, depending on the stage of the disease and the extent of liver damage, the fibrinogen level may be elevated, normal, or low. Elevated levels of factor V and fibrinogen may only reflect the non-specific increase observed in inflammatory states.

Factor VIII

By contrast with the other clotting factors, factor VIII level is usually elevated in acute and chronic liver disease, whatever the aetiology[11] (Meili, ThrombDiathHaemorrh, 1970; 24:61; Van Outryve, ScaJHaematol, 1973; 11:148); this is true for cirrhosis, hepatitis, and primary or secondary liver carcinoma.[4] The degree of increase in factor VIII level can be significantly greater than the mild increases observed during pregnancy or in a number of disease states[12] and may attain more than 1000 per cent of normal (1000 U/dl) in advanced hepatic cirrhosis or acute hepatitis. Factor VIII, von Willebrand factor antigen, and von Willebrand factor activity are increased[12] (Maisonneuve, JClinPath, 1977; 30:221) as a function of hepatocellular insufficiency.[11] The multimeric pattern of von Willebrand factor has been found to be normal in chronic liver diseases.[11,12] Increased factor VIII level might reflect extrahepatic synthesis associated with decreased catabolism by the diseased liver.[2]

Abnormal protein synthesis
Fibrinogen

Functional abnormalities of the fibrinogen molecule are known as dysfibrinogenaemias. They are characterized by impairment of fibrinoformation, as evidenced by the association of a normal fibrinogen level measured immunochemically, with a low to undetectable fibrinogen level measured by a functional test. Most frequently dysfibrinogenaemias are constitutional and discovered by chance, since they rarely cause haemorrhagic manifestations (Galanakis, ClinLabMed, 1984; 4:395). Indeed, some of them have been associated with thromboembolic manifestations. Acquired dysfibrinogenaemias are most often associated with liver disease, and have been observed in patients with primary hepatocellular carcinoma and severe cirrhosis[13] (Von Felten, NEJM, 1969; 280:405). By contrast with constitutional dysfibrinogenaemia, the functional defect is not due to any molecular or structural defect of the polypeptide chains of the patient's fibrinogen but to delayed polymerization of the fibrin monomer[13] (Lane, BrJHaemat, 1977; 35:301). This defective polymerization results from an abnormal glycosylation of the fibrinogen molecule (Soria, Coagulation, 1970; 3:37), due to a postranslational defect in fibrinogen synthesis, causing an increase in the sialic acid content of the molecule (Palascak, JCI, 1977; 60:89). Increased levels of sialyl transferase have been demonstrated in liver patients with dysfibrinogenaemia;[14] this also causes hypersialation of other proteins. Removal of excess sialic acid restores fibrinogen function. Fetal fibrinogen has also been shown to be hypersialated as compared to normal adult fibrinogen (Galanakis, AnnNYAcadSci, 1983; 408:640). The similarities between fetal fibrinogen and hepatocellular carcinoma-associated dysfibrinogen led to the suggestion that there is a regenerative mechanism going on in the hepatocytes in hepatocellular carcinoma. In patients with acquired dysfibrinogenaemia, the clinical and laboratory findings are similar to those in patients with constitutional dysfibrinogenaemia; there may be considerable impairment of fibrinoformation, resulting in a very prolonged thrombin time. Such gross abnormalities appear predominantly in advanced cirrhosis or hepatocellular carcinoma and are associated with a poor prognosis. However, milder forms of abnormal fibrin polymerization are relatively frequent in liver disease and have been observed most frequently in cirrhosis, chronic hepatitis, and acute liver failure, but not in obstructive jaundice[15]; they seem to be associated with more severely impaired liver function than in similarly affected patients without this clotting defect (Green, Gut, 1977; 18:909). Discrete or moderate prolongation of thrombin time, related at least in part to this functional defect, is frequently encountered in liver diseases.[1] These mild abnormalities are usually associated with fibrinogen levels still in the normal range, although measured by functional assay.

Circulating fibrinogen derivatives resulting from fibrinogen degradation (Mosesson, JBC, 1972; 247:5210) due to enhanced plasma fibrinolytic activity may be present in the plasma of patients with liver disease. They also exhibit abnormal polymerization due to the proteolytic loss of functional sites and are thus less or more clottable according to their degree of degradation.

Prothrombin

The abnormal type of prothrombin described above (des-γ-carboxyprothrombin, **DCP**, PIVKA II) has been reported to be significantly increased in the plasma of 90 per cent of patients with primary hepatocellular carcinoma[16,17,18] (Soulier, Gastro, 1986; 91:1258). Des-γ-carboxyprothrombin is also detectable in the plasma of patients with secondary carcinoma of the liver, although at significantly lower levels[16] than in patients with chronic active hepatitis or cirrhosis (see above). In hepatocellular carcinoma the abnormal vitamin K-dependent carboxylation affects not only prothrombin but all vitamin K-dependent blood coagulation proteins[17] (Lefrère, ThrombHaem, 1987; 58:1092). It is not the result of a deficiency in plasma vitamin K[17] (Furukawa, Cancer, 1992; 69:31) although pharmacological doses of vitamin K can transiently suppress DCP in some tumours.[16,18] Plasma DCP can be used as a marker for the diagnosis and screening of hepatocellular carcinoma, as long as vitamin K deficiency has been eliminated. However, plasma DCP does not correlate with serum α-fetoprotein levels[16,18] and its specificity seems to be superior to that of α-fetoprotein.[18,19] However, used together, DCP and α-fetoprotein assays increase the accuracy of biological diagnosis of hepatocellular carcinoma, identifying up to 85 per cent of the patients[16,18] (Denninger, JHepatol, 1991; 12:261).

There is some evidence that the DCP found in the circulation originates from tumour cells (Ono, AmJGastr, 1990; 85:1149). Successful tumour resection results in correction of DCP level, and non-surgical treatment results in a marked reduction of DCP level which increases with recurrence of the disease[16,18,19] (Fujiyama, DigDisSci, 1991; 36:1787; Kusano, CancChemoPharm, 1992; 31: S146). Plasma DCP levels greater than 0.1 AU/ml (100 ng/ml), measured by immunoassay, strongly suggest the presence or recurrence of hepatocellular carcinoma.[18] Elevated levels of plasma DCP are not found in patients with solitary tumours smaller than 2 cm in size, but are found in multiple tumours and have been found to correlate with tumour size in patients with medium- to large-sized hepatocellular carcinoma.[19] The mechanism responsible for the production of DCP by malignant hepatocytes has not yet been elucidated. However, the abnormal γ-carboxylation process associated with human hepatocellular carcinoma does not seem to be due predominantly to the defective gene expression of the carboxylase in human malignant hepatocytes but rather to the vitamin K content of the tumours, which has been found to be lower than that of non-tumourous liver. The vitamin K content of DCP-secreting tumours has been found to be significantly lower than that of non-secreting tumours. It is not known if this is due to a decreased uptake of vitamin K by the malignant cells or to an increased turnover (Huisse, Cancer, 1994; 74:1533).

Modifications of coagulation factor levels not usually observed in hepatocellular insufficiency have been found in hepatocellular carcinoma. A factor V level higher than expected from the reduced prothrombin time has been suggested as a diagnostic marker of hepatocellular carcinoma (Lefrère, ThrombHaem, 1988; 60:468). Likewise, the finding of a discordance between the plasma levels of vitamin K-dependent clotting factors with a particularly low level of factor II as compared to factors VII and X has been suggested as a way of improving the biological diagnosis of hepatocellular carcinoma, when used with α-fetoprotein and DCP assays. This particular decrease in factor II level has not been found to be related to a qualitative abnormality nor to be correlated in any way to the presence of DCP (Denninger, JHepatol, 1991; 12:261).

Plasma urokinase-type plasminogen activator antigen (**u-PA**) has also been characterized as a tumour-associated antigen, and the combination of urokinase-type plasminogen activator and α-fetoprotein has been shown to increase the accuracy of detection of primary liver cancer in chronic liver diseases (Huber, CancerRes, 1992; 52:1717).

Unusual coagulation disorders
Acquired isolated clotting factor deficiencies

Occurrence of acquired deficiency of a single clotting factor is rare and must therefore be distinguished carefully from quantitative or qualitative hereditary deficiency, as well as from the result of the inhibitory activity of a specific antibody. Nevertheless, isolated clotting factor deficiencies have been reported in a small number of cases and may be related to abnormality of liver synthesis. Thus, isolated factor II deficiency causing a bleeding diathesis unresponsive to vitamin K therapy has been described in a patient receiving multi-drug therapy. The abnormality resolved spontaneously (Karpatkin, ThrombDiathHaemorrh, 1962; 8:221).

Several cases of acquired isolated factor X deficiency unresponsive to vitamin K have been described[20] (Baver, Pediat, 1969; 44:1007). In one case the defect caused severe bleeding, and was attributed to the toxic effect of the fungicide methylbromide[20]. As in the case of acquired factor II deficiency the patients recovered spontaneously. In one case, isolated factor X deficiency was associated with malignancy of the liver (Bolandrina, GazIntMedChir, 1964; 69:63). The association of acquired isolated factor X deficiency with amyloïdosis is well known, although not frequently observed (Korsan-Bengsten., ThrombDiathHaemorrh, 1962; 7:558; Pechet, AnnIntMed, 1964; 61:315; Furie, NEJM, 1977; 297:81; Krause, AmJClinPath, 1977; 67:170; Greipp, NEJM, 1979; 301:1050). In these patients the deficiency is attributed to enhanced clearance of circulating factor X, due to the 'capture' of factor X by amyloid fibrils (Furie, NEJM, 1981; 304:827; Camoriano, NEJM, 1987; 316:1133). Acquired factor X deficiencies have also been reported in patients with respiratory tract infections and the use of erythromycin has been incriminated (Hosker, PostgradMedJ, 1983; 59:514).

Isolated factor VII deficiencies have been described in a significant number of cases of Gilbert, Rotor (Seligsohn, Lancet, 1970; 1:1398), and Dubin–Johnson syndrome (Seligsohn, QJMed, 1970; 39:569). Some patients with the Dubin–Johnson syndrome had moderate but significant decreases of factor VII level below 42 per cent of normal (42 U/dl) and the deficiency was not corrected by vitamin K. More than 30 per cent of relatives had factor VII levels below 42 per cent of normal (42 U/dl) (Seligsohn, QJMed, 1970; 39:569). No relationship has been evidenced between the congenital hyperbilirubinaemia and the factor VII defect.

Acquired, isolated factor VII deficiency, not responsive to vitamin K, has also been described in patients with homocystinuria resulting from cystathionine synthase deficiency. Factor VII level was about 20 per cent of normal (20 U/dl). This deficiency was found to be related to homocysteine accumulation and was corrected by a low-methionine diet (Munnich, JPediat, 1983; 102:730). Although no liver disease was demonstrated in this case, it is included here to aid differential diagnosis.

Congenital deficiency of factor II, VII, IX, and X (Borgschulte syndrome)

A patient with severe haemorrhagic diathesis and constitutional deficiency of factors II, VII, IX, and X observed over a period of 3 years has been described. The defect was only partially correctable by vitamin K. Although the mechanism of this deficiency remained obscure, and the patient had no demonstrable liver disease, defective utilization of vitamin K at the hepatic level was suggested (McMillan, NEJM, 1966; 274:1313).

Fibrinolysis

The frequency of enhanced fibrinolysis in cirrhosis was first described in 1914 (Goodpasture, BullJHopkHosp, 1914; 25:330) and since then has been well recognized (DeNicola, ThrombDiathHaemorrh, 1958; 2:290; Fletcher, JCI, 1964; 43:681; Tytgat, ActaHaem, 1968; 46:265). The enhanced circulating fibrinolytic activity in liver disease is explained by the decreased hepatic synthesis of the inhibitors α_2-antiplasmin (**α2AP**) and plasminogen activator inhibitor (**PAI-1**), as well as by the decreased hepatic clearance of tissue type plasminogen activator (**t-PA**) (Chapter 2.14.3). Nevertheless, abnormalities of the fibrinolytic system vary somewhat according to the stage and to the type of the liver disease. Thus, an increased PAI-1 level may occur as an early marker of liver damage and is found in mild and severe cirrhosis.[21] An increase of PAI-1 has also been described in patients with infectious hepatitis or malignant disease of the liver, whereas the t-PA level remained normal;[22] this may be related to the fact that PAI-1 is an acute phase reactant. However, a decrease of PAI-1 occurs with progressive impairment in liver function[23] and the importance of the liver in the synthesis of PAI-1 is suggested by the positive correlation between the PAI-1 and albumin levels.[23]

α_2-Antiplasmin level is decreased in both mild and severe cirrhosis and correlates with liver synthetic function (Aoki, CCActa, 1978; 84:99). Moreover, in cirrhosis, the binding of α_2AP to fibrin is reduced, causing an increased susceptibility of fibrin clots to lysis.[21] Decreases in PAI-1 and α_2AP thus favour increase of circulating fibrinolytic activity.[21]

Marked elevation of t-PA level is observed in liver cirrhosis in association with abnormal liver function tests[22] and is a marker of severe liver disease. By contrast, in patients with infectious hepatitis or malignant disease of the liver, the level of t-PA is usually normal and enhanced fibrinolytic activity is less frequent.[4] Elevated levels of t-PA are often found in cirrhotics and particularly in alcoholic cirrhotics[24]; more than 40 years ago a decreased euglobulin lysis time due to enhanced fibrinolytic activity was found more often in such patients than in patients with acute liver failure (Ratnoff, BullJHopkHosp, 1949; 84:29). Patients with alcoholic cirrhosis are more prone than normal subjects to develop increased systemic fibrinolytic activity after stimulation such as physical exercise, stress, or administration of vasoactive substances such as nicotinic acid or adrenaline (Weiner, AmJMedSci, 1963; 246:294; Das, BrJHaemat, 1969; 17:431). In these patients, the stress and vascular

stimulation induced by surgical procedures may again cause an increased fibrinolytic state. In most of them, the increase in t-PA is counterbalanced by the elevated levels of PAI-1, but when the PAI-1 level decreases due to the progression of liver damage, there is a shift in balance and the euglobulin lysis time shortens as an inverse function of the fibrinolytic activity[24] (Hersch, Blood, 1987; 69: 1315). The t-PA increase is correlated with bilirubin[23] and γ-glutamyltransferase levels[22] and with the severity of the disease. Thus, a significantly greater increase of t-PA has been demonstrated in patients with liver cirrhosis of Child C type as compared to patients with Child A or Child B, whereas PAI-1 plasma levels were significantly decreased in Child C patients.[23,25] It is important to identify patients prone to hyperfibrinolysis because enhanced fibrinolysis represents a haemorrhagic risk factor and predisposes to soft-tissue haemorrhage after trauma as well as intracranial bleeding[22] (Francis, Haemostasis, 1984; 14:460). Patients with cirrhosis and hyperfibrinolysis are also at greater risk of gastrointestinal bleeding.[25] In patients with alcoholic cirrhosis fibrinolytic activity parallels alcohol consumption; alcohol seems to have a specific role in the enhancement of fibrinolysis, independently of liver damage (Meade, BMJ, 1979; i:153; Laug, JAMA, 1983; 250: 772; Lee, Fibrinolysis, 1995; 8:49).

Plasminogen level is also decreased in hepatocellular insufficiency and, as in the case of α_2-antiplasmin, the decrease correlates with the degree of liver damage.

Elevated levels of fibrinogen/fibrin degradation products are a common finding in moderate to severe liver disease[2]; their genesis is controversial,[2] although probably related at least in part to enhanced fibrinolytic activity. Fibrinogen/fibrin degradation products are cleared in part by the reticuloendothelial system (Chapter 2.14.3), and therefore severe hepatocellular insufficiency causes an increase in their level. Fibrinogen/fibrin degradation products act as pseudosubstrates for thrombin, interfering with the incorporation of fibrin monomers in the polymerization process. Thus, elevated circulating levels of fibrinogen/fibrin degradation products exert a global anticoagulant activity due to antithrombin activity and inhibition of fibrinogen polymerization (Marder, JBC, 1969; 244: 2111). The presence in circulating blood of high titres of fibrinogen/fibrin degradation products thus impairs the already poor clotting function of patients with liver disease. A schematic depiction of the regulation of fibrinolytic activity by the liver is represented in Figs 1 and 2.

Disseminated intravascular coagulation

Disseminated intravascular coagulation is the consequence of non-compensated formation of thrombin and leads to the formation of platelet thrombi and fibrin within the circulation. Disseminated intravascular coagulation is thus associated with activation and consumption of circulating platelets, and consumption of factors V, VIII, VII, II, and XIII, proteins C and S, AT III, plasminogen, and α_2 plasmin inhibitor (**α2PI**).[4,26] The circulating levels of these factors decrease as a function of their rate of utilization and degradation.[26] Platelet dysfunction is often observed as a result of earlier activation.[26] Severe disseminated intravascular coagulation is most often due to the massive contact of tissue factor with

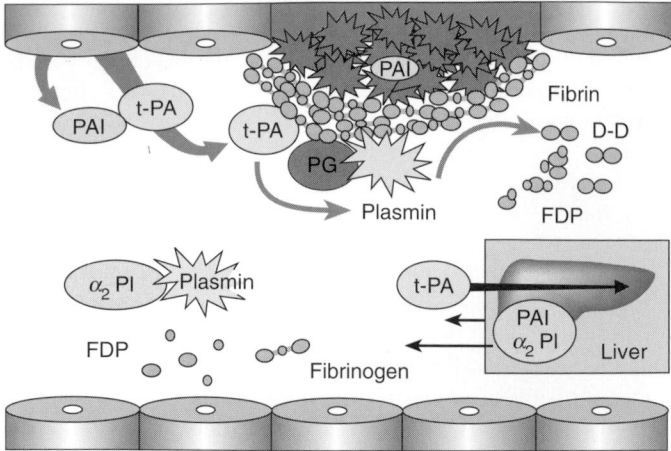

Fig. 1. Schematic respresentation of the role of the liver in regulation of the fibrinolytic system. Tissue type plasminogen activator (t-PA) produced by endothelial cells binds to fibrin as well as circulating plasminogen (PG). In this ternary complex t-PA activity is greatly enhanced and transforms PG to plasmin, which proteolytically degrades fibrin to fibrin degradation products (FDP) among which are D-dimers (D–D). Thus fibrinolysis is restricted to fibrin formed at the site of the lesion. Natural inhibitors of t–PA and plasmin are, respectively, plasminogen activator inhibitor (PAI) produced by endothelial cells, by the liver, and present in platelets (PT), and α_2 plasmin inhibitor (α_2PI) produced by the liver. α_2PI essentially inhibits circulating plasmin. The role of the liver is to clear the fibrinolysis activator t-PA from the circulating blood and to synthesize fibrinolysis inhibitors PAI and α_2PI, thus limiting circulating fibrinolytic activity.

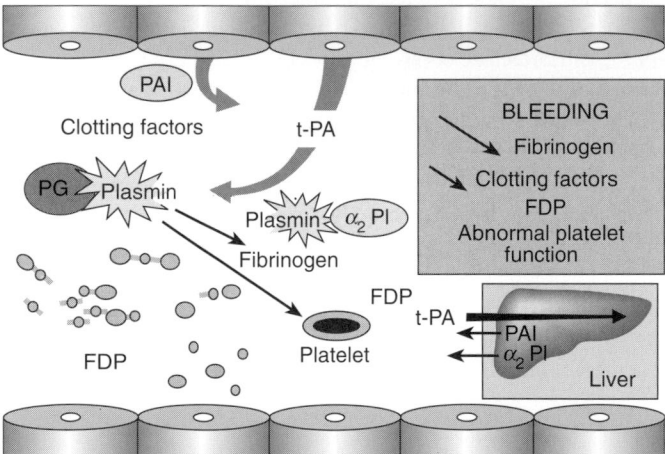

Fig. 2. Schematic representation of hyperfibrinolytic state in liver disease. When tissue type plasminogen activator (t-PA) is insufficiently cleared by diseased liver and/or produced in excess, the inhibitory capacities of plasminogen activator inhibitor (PAI) and of α_2 plasmin inhibitor (α_2PI) are overwhelmed, especially if their liver synthesis is decreased. Thus t-PA transforms circulating PG into massive amounts of plasmin that proteolytically degrades circulating fibrinogen and clotting factors, impairs platelet function, and produces fibrinogen degradation products (FDP) with anticoagulant activity, thus favouring bleeding.

circulating blood. In this case, it is generally possible to circumvent haemorrhage, but most damage is due to the extensive occurrence of microvascular thrombi which impair blood flow and cause ischaemic

organ necrosis, thus leading to irreversible morbidity and mortality.[26] However, low to moderate disseminated intravascular coagulation is found in association with many pathological states.[26]

Intravascular coagulation enhances the activation of the fibrinolytic system; and moderate to extensive fibrinolysis occurs as a secondary event, acting as a defence mechanism.[26] However, systemic fibrinolysis may contribute to clotting impairment by proteolysis of clotting factors, production of fibrin and fibrinogen degradation products, and impairment of platelet function.[26, 27] With a few exceptions, the biological diagnosis of disseminated intravascular coagulation is not easy to make, especially in liver disease, because similar biological signs are observed in both occurrences,[4,26,28] even though they result from two different mechanisms— consumption and degradation in disseminated intravascular coagulation, and impaired production or clearance in liver disease. Thus, in liver disease, the concept of disseminated intravascular coagulation and its contribution to the clotting abnormalities has long been controversial. Support for the idea of disseminated intravascular coagulation in liver disease came from the observation of accelerated catabolism[28] or shortened half-lives of prothrombin, plasminogen, and fibrinogen.[29] The release of tissue 'thromboplastin like' material by necrotic liver had been claimed to be the trigger producing coagulation activation and disseminated intravascular coagulation in severe liver failure,[28, 29] disseminated intravascular coagulation in turn being responsible for further hepatic necrosis (Rake, Lancet, 1971; ii:1215) and thus contributing to hepatic failure. However, the strongest support for disseminated intravascular coagulation came from radiofibrinogen studies that indicated a shortened half-life of radiofibrinogen in liver disease with its possible correction by heparin[29] (Tytgat, JCI, 1971; 50:1690; Coleman, AnnIntMed, 1975; 83:79). However, increased fibrinogen turnover is not pathognomonic of disseminated intravascular coagulation and can be produced by primary fibrinolysis[4] as well as by several other mechanisms (Straub, SemThrombHaemost, 1977; 4:29). Moreover, the observed heparin reversal effect has not been confirmed[30] (Stein, JLabClinMed, 1982; 99:217).

In patients with disseminated intravascular coagulation without liver disease, the more reliable biological findings are elevated levels of the coagulation activation markers D-dimer and fibrinopeptide A, a depressed level of AT III, thrombocytopenia, and a positive protamine sulphate test or ethanol gelation test indicative of the presence of fibrin monomer.[26] Unfortunately, depressed AT III level and thrombocytopenia are common findings in liver disease in the absence of disseminated intravascular coagulation and therefore they cannot be used for the diagnosis of disseminated intravascular coagulation in this context. It is, nevertheless, well–recognized that the decreased ability of damaged liver to clear activated clotting factors from the circulating blood favours activation of coagulation; excessive amounts of thrombin have been found to be generated in liver disease (Takahashi, AmJHemat, 1989; 32:30). Thus, considerable interest has been devoted to the measurement of coagulation activation markers in liver disease, with the hope that this would provide clear evidence of disseminated intravascular coagulation. Therefore, fibrinopeptide A, a peptide selectively cleaved from fibrinogen by thrombin; thrombin–antithrombin III complexes (**TAT**) formed by the rapid binding of thrombin to its inhibitor; and the cross-linked fibrin degradation products, D-dimers, have all been examined in liver disease. However, although these markers constitute direct or indirect indicators of thrombin formation, they are not specific for disseminated intravascular coagulation.

Increased fibrinopeptide A levels have been found in patients with cirrhosis and chronic hepatitis (Coccheri, BrJHaemat, 1982; 52: 503; Violi, Haematol(Pavia), 1984; 69:655; Marongiu, ThrombRes, 1985; 37:287). However, moderate increases of fibrinopeptide A occur in other clinical conditions in the absence of disseminated intravascular coagulation, and in a recent study it has been demonstrated that the (slight) increase observed in patients with cirrhosis was significantly lower than that measured in patients with disseminated intravascular coagulation, and was not consistent with the amount of thrombin needed to cause disseminated intravascular coagulation. Moreover, in this study, coagulation abnormalities, especially hypofibrinogenaemia and thrombocytopenia, could not be related to plasma fibrinopeptide A levels in these patients, strongly indicating that disseminated intravascular coagulation was not the main cause of the coagulation defects; significant disseminated intravascular coagulation could be excluded in more than 80 per cent of the studied cirrhotic patients.

Elevated levels of TAT have been reported in chronic active hepatitis, decompensated liver cirrhosis, endstage liver disease, and fulminant liver failure (Langley, EurJClinInv, 1990; 20:627; Kemkes-Matthes, ThrombRes, 1991; 64:253; Pernambuco, Hepatol, 1993; 18:1350) and related to disseminated intravascular coagulation. However, even if TAT is sensitive and specific for detecting thrombin generation, this is not always associated with disseminated intravascular coagulation, and elevated TAT levels are not pathognomonic of disseminated intravascular coagulation (Takahashi, AmJHemat, 1991; 36:76).

Whereas fibrinogen/fibrin degradation products are only indicative of plasmin activity[26] and may be either fibrinogen (see above) or fibrin plasmic derivatives (Mosesson, JBC, 1972; 247: 5210), the cross-linked fibrin plasmic derivatives, D-dimers, are fibrin specific. D-dimers are thus direct indicators of the fibrinolytic process and indirect indicators of thrombin activity. However, increased D-dimer levels do not necessarily indicate that generalized intravascular fibrin formation has occurred, and may simply be the consequence of clinically irrelevant forms of fibrin deposition which may even be extravascular. They can also be due to disseminated intravascular coagulation triggered independently by occult concomitant disorders, such as neoplasia (hepatocellular carcinoma) or thromboembolism (portal vein thrombosis) (Yudelman, Blood, 1978; 51:1189; Mombelli, Blood, 1982; 60:381). Elevated levels of D-dimer may also be a reflection of impaired clearance. In liver disease, the finding of increased coagulation activation markers (indicative of thrombin activity) does not indicate, even in the presence of high levels as in acute liver failure (Pernambuco, Hepatol, 1993; 18:1350):

(1) that disseminated intravascular coagulation is necessarily present;

(2) whether, if present, disseminated intravascular coagulation is responsible for such significant haemostatic abnormalities that they are clinically relevant; or

(3) that coagulation disorders induced by disseminated intravascular coagulation overwhelm those produced by the defective liver.

Consumption coagulopathy is a rare complication in liver disorders[30,31] (Mombelli, ThrombHaem, 1987; 58:758; Tanaka, TohokuJExpMed, 1987; 153:179) and disseminated intravascular coagulation is neither a basic nor a frequent abnormality in cirrhosis.[31] A low incidence of disseminated intravascular coagulation has been found at autopsy (Oka, ThrombHaem, 1979; 42: 564). The coagulopathy of disseminated intravascular coagulation is, if present, a minor determinant of the haemostatic defect. However, it is also widely recognized that liver disease, and especially advanced liver failure, constitutes a considerable risk for disseminated intravascular coagulation occurrence[31] in the presence of complicating disorders such as infections and shock,[1,31] and of other predisposing conditions such as pregnancy; and in these cases superimposed disseminated intravascular coagulation must be suspected. For this reason the administration of clotting factor concentrates which enhance the risk of precipitating disseminated intravascular coagulation must be avoided in liver disease. By contrast, administration of AT III concentrates may be beneficial or even life-saving in some cases (Langley, JHepatol, 1988; 7:S144). In severe hepatic failure the challenge is to distinguish worsening of hepatic function from superimposed disseminated intravascular coagulation due to complicating events. Attributing haemostatic failure to disseminated intravascular coagulation might lead to underestimation of the degree of liver failure, while the failure to identify it as disseminated intravascular coagulation might lead to the overestimation of the degree of liver failure.

Quantitative and qualitative platelet defects

Liver disease may affect platelet number or function, thus impairing primary haemostasis.[2]

Quantitative platelet defects

Common causes of thrombocytopenia in acute and chronic liver disease include increased splenic sequestration, impaired production by the bone marrow (Cohen, NEJM, 1961; 264:1294), folic acid deficiency, increased destruction due to immune mechanisms or disseminated intravascular coagulation[32] (Pitney, SemHemat, 1971; 8:65), and sepsis.

In normal subjects, 30 per cent of the platelet pool is sequestered in the spleen (Aster, JCI, 1966; 45:645) and these platelets are unavailable for immediate haemostasis.[2] In cirrhotics with portal hypertension, up to 90 per cent of platelets may be sequestered in the spleen (Harker, JCI, 1969; 48:963; Kutti, ScaJHaematol, 1972; 9:351), when it is massively enlarged. These entrapped platelets are destroyed by reticuloendothelial cells.[33] There is a negative correlation between the platelet count and splenic volume, and a positive correlation between the platelet count and platelet survival time.[32] In cirrhotics, increased platelet destruction by the spleen may also be mediated by immune mechanisms, and there is a negative correlation between the platelet count and platelet-associated IgG.[32] The suggested mechanism is that in liver cirrhosis, non-specific IgG adhere to the platelet surface with the formation of platelet-associated IgG. This non-specific binding of IgG could be related to a platelet membrane abnormality[1] similar to the erythrocyte membrane abnormality observed in liver cirrhosis (Harada, JKurumeMedAssoc. 1984; 47:1031), and which could be responsible for neoantigenicity of the platelet membrane surface.[32] However, in a number of cases, thrombocytopenia cannot be explained by increased splenic sequestration. Thrombocytopenia persists in about half of the cirrhotic patients submitted to portal-systemic shunting procedures, even though portal pressure decreased as well as the size of the spleen[34] (Soper, AmJSurg, 1982; 144:700). The platelet count improved in these patients when the portal perfusion of the liver was maintained.[33] When liver damage or chronic hepatocellular insufficiency is induced in experimental animals, thrombocytopenia occurs rapidly but improves with reversal of liver damage.[33] Thus, it has been suggested that thrombocytopenia might be due to the impaired synthesis of a 'thrombopoiesis stimulating factor' produced by the liver.[33] Since then, a cytokine, thrombopoietin (**TPO**), has been identified, which plays a major role in regulating megakaryocyte and platelet production. Thrombopoietin mRNA is expressed in the liver, as well as in kidney, spleen, and bone marrow (Vignon, Oncogene, 1993; 8: 2607; De Sauvage, Nature, 1994; 369:533; Lok, Nature, 1994; 369: 565). Moreover a study of plasma TPO levels in patients with thrombocytopenia, including patients with hepatitis or cirrhosis, has shown an inverse relationship between these levels and the platelet count (Nichol, Blood, 1995; 86:1474). The correction of central thrombocytopenia by hepatic transplantation in a cirrhotic patient with hepatocellular carcinoma could be related to such a regulating mechanism (Bettan, AnnIntMed, 1987; 106:170).

Qualitative platelet defects

Prolonged bleeding times and abnormal platelet aggregation are well documented and were reported many years ago in severe liver disease associated with bleeding manifestations[4,35] (Mandel, NEJM, 1961; 265:56; Thomas, NEJM, 1967; 276:1344). Impairment of platelet aggregation correlates with the degree of hepatocellular insufficiency, but not with the platelet count nor with the aetiology of liver disease. Patient platelet volumes have been shown to be smaller than normal. Thus, a deficiency of larger haemostatically active platelets could explain the functional defect (Rubin, DigDisSci, 1979; 24:197).

Specific effects of alcoholism

In alcoholism platelet disorders are not only due to the liver disease resulting from chronic drinking, but also result from active ingestion of ethanol. The first reported platelet disorder related to alcoholism was thrombocytopenia (King, NEJM, 1929; 200:482; Morlock, ArchIntMed, 1943; 72:69). This was generally attributed to splenic sequestration or folic acid deficiency (McPherson, Lancet, 1953; i: 1120; Herbert, AnnIntMed, 1963; 58:977). Nevertheless, splenomegaly is not common,[36] especially in patients without cirrhosis, and thrombocytopenia in alcoholic patients does not depend on low folate levels (Cowan, JLabClinMed, 1973; 81:64). There is a direct toxic effect of alcohol on blood platelets[37] (Sullivan, JCI, 1964; 43: 2048) and the deleterious effects of alcohol on platelet production, survival, function, and structure (Sahud, NEJM, 1972; 286:355;

Cowan, ThrombDiathHaemorrh, 1975; 33:310) have been demonstrated. The mechanism of the impairment of thrombopoiesis by alcohol is unknown[36], but could involve a direct toxic effect on bone marrow (Sullivan, JCI, 1964; 43:2048) which affects utilization or cellular metabolism of folate.[36] The decreased platelet lifespan is not due to increased splenic sequestration but depends on sustained high plasma alcohol levels.[36] Thrombocytopenia, defined as a platelet count less than $100 \times 10^9/l$, is uncommon in patients who are not severely ill from their chronic alcoholism, but it occurs in about 25 per cent of severely affected alcoholic patients (Cowan, AnnIntMed, 1971; 74:37). Even so, there is no relation between the severity of the liver disease and the occurrence or severity of thrombocytopenia.[36] Alcohol-related thrombocytopenia is corrected by cessation of ethanol ingestion[37] (Ryback, ArchIntMed, 1970; 125:475; Cowan, AnnIntMed, 1971; 74:37). The recovery occurs spontaneously[36] and rebound thrombocytosis has been observed[38] (Haselager, Lancet, 1977; i:774).

The haemostatic capacity of platelets may be considerably impaired in alcoholic patients as, in addition to thrombocytopenia, multiple platelet functional defects can occur. They include defective platelet aggregation, decreased release of thromboxane A_2, which enhances platelet aggregation, and increased vascular release of a potent platelet anti-aggregant and vasodilator, prostacyclin (**PGI2**)[38] (Landolfi, Blood, 1984; 64:679). Like thrombocytopenia, functional abnormalities may correct after abstinence and there is a link between platelet abnormalities and the amount of ethanol ingested.[38] However, in the absence of splenomegaly and thrombocytopenia, no relationship has been demonstrated between platelet function and histological or functional liver tests (Stein, JLabClinMed, 1982; 99:217; Mikhailidis, BMJ, 1986; 293: 715; Mikhailidis, BMJ, 1987; 295:1062). Bleeding time correlates significantly with impairment of platelet aggregation, thromboxane A_2 release, platelet count, and estimated ethanol consumption, and reverts to normal with abstinence. Thus, in alcoholic patients, there is great variability in the results of platelet aggregation tests and the measurement of bleeding time, which may be normal or abnormal depending on the time of sampling and whether the patient is abstinent or not.

Acute liver failure

In acute liver failure due to fulminant or subfulminant hepatitis, haemostatic abnormalities are severe and involve all the clotting and fibrinolytic proteins synthesized by the liver. The fall in the levels of clotting factors, inhibitors, prekallikrein, plasminogen, and α_2AP is usually greater than that seen in other liver diseases.[24,39] Even so, the degree of deficiency varies among the different proteins and with the degree of liver damage.

The levels of vitamin K-dependent proteins are extremely low, with the exception of protein S. In our experience the levels of factors II, VII, IX, and X, and of protein C are less than 20 per cent of normal (20 U/dl) in 90 per cent of patients at the most critical stage of the disease, while the protein S level is lower than 20 per cent of normal (20 U/dl) in only 27 per cent of patients. This is probably due to extrahepatic synthesis of protein S by endothelial cells (see above). Factor V level is usually less affected than the level of factors II, VII, IX, and X except with toxic hepatitis. By contrast with protein S, this cannot be explained by megakaryocyte synthesis of factor V, since platelet factor V cannot be effective unless platelets are activated. Factor V is less than 30 per cent of normal (30 U/dl) at the most critical stage of the disease in more than 80 per cent of patients, and less than 20 per cent of normal (20 U/dl) in 60 per cent of patients. Similar figures have been found for AT III. Plasminogen deficiency parallels that of factors II, VII, IX, and X. However, at the early stages of the disease, fibrinogen is normal and thus contrasts with the very low levels of other clotting proteins. The fibrinogen level then gradually decreases to less than 1 g/l with the progression of liver damage. In our experience, fibrinogen was less than 0.80 g/l in over 40 per cent of patients, and in more than 50 per cent of the patients who did not recover; it was less than 0.80 g/l in only 30 per cent of patients who recovered. A plasma fibrinogen level less than 1 g/l was previously considered to indicate severe and massive damage of hepatocytes and to indicate a poor prognosis[2] (Clark, ScaJGastr, 1973; Suppl. 19:63; Herold, HelvMedActa, 1973; 37:5; Dymock, BrJHaemat, 1975; 29:385.

As indicated in earlier reports the factor VIII level is usually very high, being above 1000 per cent of normal (1000 U/dl) in fulminant viral hepatitis (Straub, SchMedWoch, 1966; 96:1199).[39, 40] The factor VIII increase is less marked in toxic fulminant hepatic failure—in a series of patients with fulminant hepatic failure, most of whom had paracetamol poisoning, all three components of factor VIII complex were increased (Langley, ThrombHaem, 1985; 54:693). This is not always observed in *Amanita phalloides* poisoning (Menache, ProbRéan, 1968; 499; Aledort, ProgLivDis, 1976; 22:350).[40] The factor XIII level is low but is usually more than 20 per cent of normal (20 U/dl).[39] The fall in α_2AP level depends on the degree of liver damage (Pernambuco, Hepatol, 1993; 18:1350).[2,24]

The platelet count is usually normal on admission,[39] contrasting, as the fibrinogen level, with the severe deficiencies of clotting factors; and platelet function, as evaluated by bleeding time measurement, is normal in the absence of associated factors such as drugs or renal insufficiency. Nevertheless, platelets of patients with fulminant hepatic failure function abnormally, exhibiting many structural abnormalities and showing a poor response to aggregating agents (Rubin, QJMed, 1977; 46:339). Increased platelet adhesion to glass beads has been reported (Langley, ActaHaem, 1982; 67:124) but it was not found to correlate with an increase of any member of the factor VIII complex (Langley, ThrombHaem, 1985; 54:693). Severe thrombocytopenia with a platelet count less than 50×10^9/l may occur within 4 to 5 days after patient admission.[39] The low platelet count has been related to defective production due to defective hepatic synthesis of a stimulating factor (see above) or to a viral effect (Kelly, Gut, 1986; 27:339). Megakaryocyte number is normal or elevated,[39] suggesting peripheral destruction in at least some cases. Thrombocytopenia is now rarely observed since hepatic transplantation is generally performed rapidly in critically ill patients. Increased fibrinolytic activity, evidenced by a shortened euglobulin lysis time, has only been observed in fatal cases in our experience. Given so, there are gross abnormalities of the fibrinolytic system in fulminant hepatic failure and the limited clinical evidence of fibrinolysis has been reported to be due to sustained fibrinolytic inhibitory activity (Pernambuco, Hepatol, 1993; 18:1350). As stated above, acute liver failure strongly predisposes to disseminated intravascular coagulation, and high levels of TAT as well as D-dimer have been found in patients with fulminant hepatic failure

(Pernambuco, Hepatol, 1993; 18:1350). In our experience overt disseminated intravascular coagulation has been observed only exceptionally in this context. The unusual finding of a factor V level inferior to the levels of factors II, VII, and X seen in *Amanita phalloides* poisoning, or the occurrence of a positive protamine sulphate test (Takahashi, AmJHemat, 1989; 32:30) should lead to the suspicion of superimposed disseminated intravascular coagulation.

Some patients with severe disseminated intravascular coagulation and a grossly prolonged prothrombin time, but without liver disease, are sometimes referred inappropriately to a liver disease intensive care unit because of a suspicion of fulminant hepatic failure.

Prognostic factors

In acute liver failure, the need to identify patients whose chances of survival would be enhanced by early orthotopic liver transplantation has led to the search for useful prognostic factors (Munoz, Gastro, 1991; 100:1480; Otte, JHepatol, 1991; 12:386). To assess outcome in these patients many variables have been studied (Christensen, Gastro, 1984; 19:90) and coagulation data have been retained as prognostic indicators (Tygstrup, SemLivDis, 1986; 2:129). Thus, different indices of coagulation which may give an accurate prediction of terminal failure have been investigated.

The prothrombin time, available in most laboratories, has long been used to assess the severity of fulminant hepatic failure (O'Grady, Gastro, 1989; 97:439; Harrison, BMJ, 1990; 301:964). However, the prothrombin time suffers from marked reagent-dependent and inter-laboratory variations, which preclude comparisons between different institutes and the establishment of universal guidelines. It was recommended that prothrombin time should be expressed as the international normalized ratio (**INR**) (Munoz, Gastro, 1991; 100:1480; O'Grady, Gastro, 1991; 10:1480). However, the INR system of prothrombin time standardization which was tailored for monitoring oral anticoagulant therapy (Poller, SemThrombHaemost, 1986; 12:13) is not valid for hepatocellular insufficiency (see below). Moreover, prothrombin time does not seem to differentiate survivors from non-survivors (Cordova, AmJClinPath, 1986; 85:579).

Independent clotting factors have also been investigated and factor VII and prekallikrein had been indicated as sensitive indexes of liver damage (Dymock, BrJHaemat, 1975; 29:385; Gazzard, Gut, 1976; 17:489; Orlando, Haemostasis, 1982; 11:73; Cordova, AmJClinPath, 1986; 85:579). The half-life of factor VII is short and increase in factor VII level was thought to be the earliest sign of recovery. However, correction of factor VII has never been observed before that of factor V in patients with fulminant hepatic failure who recovered.

In our experience at Hôpital Beaujon the prognosis has been found to be favourable when the levels of factors II, VII, X, protein C, and plasminogen are maintained above 20 per cent of normal (20 U/dl) and the level of AT III above 30 per cent of normal (30 U/dl). By contrast, levels of AT III and especially of factor V below 10 per cent of normal (10 U/dl) have been found to indicate a very poor prognosis. In earlier reports, univariate analysis of prognostic factors in patients with fulminant hepatitis of various causes had already shown a significant relationship between survival and factor V level (Alagille, RevIntHep, 1954; 4:1; Rueff, AnnMedIntern, 1971; 122:373). This has been confirmed in a multivariate analysis where the most significant differences between survivors and non-survivors of fulminant hepatic failure were age and factor V level. In this study, the factor V level was found to be the most sensitive independent coagulation prognostic indicator in patients with fulminant hepatitis B infection (Bernuau, Hepatol, 1986; 6: 648) if the inter- and intra-assay variability and the conditions of the factor V level measurement were satisfactory. Freeze–thawing of the plasma samples leads to underestimation of factor V level, and the level of factor V differs according to the species of the reagent used for the assay (Denninger, Hepatol, 1992; 16:Abstr. 931).

Criteria for emergency liver transplantation have been proposed. According to the London criteria, liver transplantation is indicated in fulminant hepatic failure, if:

1. In the case of paracetamol overdose, arterial blood pH is below 7.3 or if prothrombin time is above 100 s and is associated with a serum creatinine level above 300 μmol/l, and with grade III or IV encephalopathy.
2. In cases without paracetamol overdose, three of the following indices are found: age between 10 and 40 years, non-A, non-B or drug-induced hepatitis, jaundice-encephalopathy lasting more than 7 days, prothrombin time above 50 s, and serum bilirubin above 300 μmol/l (O'Grady, Gastro, 1989; 97:439).

According to the Clichy criteria, liver transplantation is indicated in fulminant hepatic failure, except for paracetamol-induced fulminant hepatic failure, when confusion or coma is associated with a factor V level below 20 per cent of normal (<20 U/dl) and age below 30 years, or a factor V level below 30 per cent of normal (< 30 U/dl) and age greater than 30 years (Bernuau, Hepatol, 1991; 14:49A), the factor V level being measured using a rabbit thromboplastin reagent. These Clichy criteria are used by several groups (Devictor, Hepatol, 1992; 16: 1156; Belghiti, BrJSurg, 1995; 82:986; Bismuth, AnnSurg, 1995; 222:109; Durand, Hepatol, 1995; 21:929; Van Hoek, Hepatol, 1995; 23:109). In a study of 81 patients with fulminant liver failure, a French group concluded that both Clichy and London criteria for emergency liver transplantation had insufficient positive and negative predictive values (Pauwels, JHepatol, 1993; 17:124). However, because this study was retrospective (Bernuau, Hepatol, 1993; 19:486; O'Grady, Hepatol, 1993; 19:485) and did not provide critical therapeutic features (Bernuau, Hepatol, 1993; 19:486), its conclusions are likely to be invalid.

Recently factor VIII : V ratios have been used as a predictor of outcome in paracetamol-induced fulminant hepatic failure, and predictive accuracy has been found to be 95 per cent for the conjunction of a factor VIII : V ratio greater than 30, with an admission coma grade of III or IV (Pereira, Gut, 1992; 33: 98; Bradberry, Lancet, 1995; 346:646). Elevated factor VIII : V ratios are consistent with the low factor V level due to impaired synthesis and the high factor VIII level observed in fulminant hepatic failure. Nevertheless, it should be emphasized that the limit value given for the factor VIII : V ratio may vary according to the aetiology of the fulminant hepatic failure, as different degrees of factor VIII increase have been observed in viral and toxic fulminant hepatic failure.

Haemostatic changes in liver surgery
Orthotopic liver transplantation

In orthotopic liver transplantation, increased blood loss constitutes a significant contributory factor to postoperative morbidity, including surgical, immunological, and infectious complications, as well as single or multiorgan failure. Blood loss also correlates significantly with postoperative mortality (Starzl, NEJM, 1984; 311:1658; Kirby, BrJSurg, 1987; 74:3).[41,42] Thirty years ago the first liver transplanted patient died of haemorrhage due to haemostatic impairment (Starzl, SGO, 1963; 117:659) and until recently bleeding complications have been the most frequent cause of death (Bismuth, AnnIntMed, 1987; 107:337).[43,44] Thus, the most difficult problem during and after liver transplantation has been the prevention of bleeding (Starzl, Hepatol, 1982; 2:614; Butler, Transfusion, 1985; 25:120; Neuhaus, ThrombHaem, 1993; 19:183).[43] Blood clotting abnormalities are a major contributing factor to high blood loss (Haagsma, Liver, 1985; 5:123), and a better understanding of haemostatic impairment during the different stages of orthotopic liver transplantation has led to the use of more specific therapy and thus to diminished transfusion requirement.[41,43]

In the pre-anhepatic period, there are usually no major changes in clotting and fibrinolytic indices (Kang, AnesthAnalg, 1985; 64: 888; Owen, MayoClinProc, 1987; 62:761), which reflect the patient's preoperative status, or are the result of transfusion of fresh frozen plasma.[45] Signs of hypercoagulability were described occasionally in earlier reports, mainly in patients with liver tumour (Howland, ArchSurg, 1974; 108:605).

Significant changes in blood clotting occur during the anhepatic period: increased fibrinolytic activity, as shown by shortened clot lysis time[46] (Blecher, ArchSurg, 1968; 96:331; Pechet, JLabClinMed, 1968; 73:91; Groth, ArchSurg, 1969; 98:31) or thromboelastography (Kang, AnesthAnalg, 1985; 64:888), and without signs of disseminated intravascular coagulation, has been reported in a number of studies.[45,47] This primary hyperfibrinolysis is due to a massive increase in circulating t-PA that reaches a peak at the end of the anhepatic period[42,48] (Palareti, Fibrinolysis, 1988; 2: 61; Porte, TransplProc, 1989; 21:3542) and which has been described in association with high intraoperative blood loss. This t-PA increase is explained by the combination of increased intravascular release[42] and lack of hepatic clearance due to the absence of liver (Böhmig, ThrombDiathHaemorrh, 1969; 21:332; Homatas, ActaHepatoSplenol, 1969; 2:14; Dinbar, Surgery, 1970; 68:269; Bakker, Hepatol, 1992; 16:404), as previously demonstrated by liver exclusion in experimental animals (Alican, ArchSurg, 1970; 101: 590; Dinbar, Surgery, 1970; 68:269; Korninger, ThrombHaem, 1981; 46:658). Fibrin and fibrinogen degradation products are elevated as the result of primary fibrinolysis (Bakker, Hepatol, 1992; 16:404; Groenland, SemThrombHaemost, 1993; 19:213) and there is a decrease in PAI-1[42,48,49] as well as in α_2AP.[42] There are a few changes in factors II, V, VII, IX, XI, and XII, suggesting a steady-state balance between the loss of the clotting factors and the administration of fresh frozen plasma,[45] although a more pronounced decrease of fibrinogen and factor VIII has been observed.[45]

We have found an increase in t-PA level associated with a very shortened euglobulin lysis time, a total lack of PAI-1 activity, and a moderate fibrinogen and α_2AP decrease. The protamine sulphate gelation test has not been found to be positive at this stage of orthotopic liver transplantation (Table 1).

The therapeutic use of aprotinin, a fibrinolysis inhibitor, has reduced blood loss in orthotopic liver transplantation and this, together with meticulous coagulation monitoring which allows maintenance of sufficient levels of clotting factors, has caused t-PA-induced systemic fibrinolysis to become of minor importance in orthotopic liver transplantation (Welte, SemThrombHaemost, 1993; 19:297). It has recently been suggested that the lytic state observed during liver transplantation could be due in part to the presence of trypsin-like activity associated with decreased levels of protease inhibitors, especially α_1-antitrypsin, and to a lesser extent to the participation of urokinase plasminogen activator (u-PA) (Legnani, Transpl, 1993; 56:568).

At the reperfusion period, disseminated intravascular coagulation has been observed, starting with perfusion of the graft liver and paralleling the bleeding tendency[50] (Harper, Transpl, 1989; 48:603) and associated with a decrease of factors II, V, VII, VIII, IX, X, fibrinogen, AT III, and platelet counts[46] (Flute, BMJ, 1969; 3:20; Groth, ArchSurg, 1969; 98:31; Böhmig, SemThrombHaemost, 1977; 4:57). In disseminated intravascular coagulation, increased thrombin production induces platelet activation and may impair platelet function, so that platelet dysfunction may be involved in the pathophysiology of post-reperfusion bleeding (Himmelreich, BloodCoagFibrinol, 1991; 2:51). The decrease in platelet aggregability found after revascularization of the graft liver[50] is probably multifactorial and due not only to thrombin but also to mediators released from leucocytes (Riess, Transpl, 1992; 52:482). Moreover, the University of Wisconsin solution (Belzer UW-CSS solution) used for cold storage of the liver has also been shown to inhibit collagen- and ADP-induced platelet aggregability. During reperfusion, small amounts of UW solution enter the circulation[50], and may contribute to the observed platelet defect. We have experienced a massive post-reperfusion bleeding in which the essential haemostatic abnormality was a grossly prolonged Ivy bleeding time associated with moderate thrombocytopenia, but which stopped readily with platelet transfusion. The particular platelet count drop observed after graft reperfusion cannot be attributed exclusively to disseminated intravascular coagulation[43] and platelet sequestration in the grafted liver has also been seen.[51]

At this stage, the severity of coagulation abnormalities seems to be due primarily to the quality of the donor liver[46] (Böhmig, SemThrombHaemost, 1977; 4:57) and the degree of ischaemic damage to the graft[52] (Mieny, Gastro, 1968; 55:179; Pechet, JLabClinMed, 1968; 73:91). Endothelial injury may occur during ischaemic liver preservation (Otto, Transpl, 1986; 42:122) and cause coagulation after graft reperfusion (Böhmig, SemThrombHaemost, 1977; 4:57; Suzumura, TransplProc, 1988; 20: 622 (Suppl. 1)). Improvement in preservation techniques seems to have reduced the signs of disseminated intravascular coagulation previously observed, and in later reports only minor coagulation abnormalities suggesting disseminated intravascular coagulation were observed[45,53] (Kang, AnesthAnalg, 1985; 64:888; Bellani, TransplProc, 1987; 19:71 (Suppl. 3)). In our experience, discrete or moderate signs of disseminated intravascular coagulation are most often observed with the reperfusion of the graft liver. The most frequent signs, in decreasing order of frequency, are a moderate decrease in factor V

level (not observed during the hyperfibrinolytic state of the anhepatic period), a discrete to moderate decrease in fibrinogen level, both already described,[45] and a positive protamine sulphate gelation test. In some patients, clearcut signs of disseminated intravascular coagulation occurred at this time, including a decrease in platelet count and factor V and fibrinogen levels, and a positive protamine sulphate gelation test. When measured, the PAI-1 level was greatly increased (Virji, TransplProc, 1989; 21:3540), as was α_2AP, but to a lesser extent. A moderate increase in D-dimer and TAT has been observed, as described earlier (Bakker, ThrombHaem, 1993; 69:25), as well as a decrease in t-PA level[42] (Palareti, Fibrinolysis, 1988; 2:61). However an 'explosive' and very transient increase of t-PA, not described in earlier reports, has been found to occur immediately after graft reperfusion[49] (Porte, TransplProc, 1989; 21:3542; Virji, TransplProc, 1989; 21:3540), followed by a gradual decrease. It was suggested that this peak would be missed if no blood sample was taken within 10 min after reperfusion.[49] We have never observed this fibrinolytic peak, probably because our blood samples are generally taken later, after the beginning of reperfusion; we have found fibrinolytic activity, measured by euglobulin lysis time, always to be normal at this stage.

A recent study has suggested that both platelet disorders and increased fibrinolytic activity were largely responsible for the haemostatic defect observed after graft reperfusion.[52]

The fall in the platelet count observed during and after orthotopic liver transplantation[51] (Hutchison, ArchSurg, 1968; 97: 27) may persist for several days postoperatively[51] (Hutchison, ArchSurg, 1968; 97:27; Owen, MayoClinProc, 1987; 62:761) and has been attributed to platelet sequestration in the graft liver. This sequestration seems to be due to the accumulation of platelets in the sinusoids, and to phagocytosis by Kupffer cells. Platelet counts lower than 50×10^9/litre are usually observed postoperatively and are then a major cause of bleeding complications, especially when they are associated with major functional impairment due to renal insufficiency.

Thrombotic manifestations

Arterial thrombosis remains a life-threatening complication requiring urgent retransplantation (Tygstrup, SemLivDis, 1986; 2: 129) and portal vein and hepatic artery thrombosis are major causes of mortality in children.[54] During the postoperative period of orthotopic liver transplantation a hypercoagulable state has been described due to diminished inhibition of coagulation and fibrinolytic activity; this may contribute to the thrombotic complications (Velasco, Transpl, 1992; 53:1256). Thrombotic complications cannot be prevented by infusion of AT III concentrates and/or unfractionated heparin.

Auxiliary liver transplantation

In auxiliary liver transplantation a liver graft is transplanted without removal of the diseased host liver. Thus, the anhepatic phase is avoided and there is no increase in t-PA (Bakker, Hepatol, 1992; 16: 404) nor in fibrinogen/fibrin degradation product levels (Groenland, SemThrombHaemost, 1993; 19:213) and PAI level remains high (Knot, Fibrinolysis, 1988; 2:111). Then, during auxiliary liver transplantation, no major haemostatic change occurs.[43] However, changes in haemostasis similar to those observed after graft re-perfusion in orthotopic liver transplantation, with increased TAT levels (Reuvers, AnnSurg, 1986; 204:552; Porte, Fibrinolysis, 1988; 2:67 (Suppl. 3)), are observed with reperfusion of the auxiliary graft (Bakker, ThrombHaem, 1993; 69:25; Groenland, SemThromb-Haemost, 1993; 19:213).

Hereditary coagulation deficiencies and liver transplantation

Haemophilia A has been cured by orthotopic liver transplantation performed for endstage liver disease (Gibas, Gastro, 1988; 95:192); factor VIII coagulant activity increased within 6 to 18 h of successful liver transplantation (Bontempo, Blood, 1987; 69:1721). Factor IX deficiency of haemophilia B was immediately corrected by ortho-topic liver transplantation (Merion, Surgery, 1988; 104:929).

A lifelong familial bleeding diathesis due to excess of t-PA has also been cured by orthotopic liver transplantation. Although the specific defect leading to excess t-PA in the patient and relatives was not known, correction by orthotopic liver transplantation sug-gested that abnormal hepatic regulation of fibrinolysis was involved in this familial haemorrhagic disease (Humphries, AmJClinPath, 1994; 102:816).

In a 20-month-old child with homozygous protein C deficiency and the dramatic thrombotic manifestations associated with this condition, orthotopic liver transplantation was successfully per-formed as primary therapy (Casella, Lancet, 1988; ii:435).

Conversely, a severe factor XI deficiency (2 per cent of normal, 2 u/dl) has been acquired by liver transplantation (Clarkson, Ann-IntMed, 1991; 115:877). This led to the suggestion that, if possible, routinely used preoperative coagulation tests should be performed in the donor before transplantation.

Liver resection

Postoperative decreases in clotting factors have been observed due to loss of hepatic parenchyma and post-hepatectomy liver failure (Ro, ScaJGastr, 1973; 8:71; Conard, NouvPresseMed, 1976; 5:2519; Nagino, Surgery, 1995; 117:581). Some reports have described post-hepatectomy disseminated intravascular coagulation (Takeda, ThrombRes, 1990; 57:289; Tsuzuki, Surgery, 1990; 107:172). How-ever, in a recent study of 100 patients without cirrhosis who underwent resection of two or more segments of the liver for biliary tract carcinoma, disseminated intravascular coagulation occurred in only 2 per cent. In an earlier report, a transitory increase in fibrinolytic activity and a positive ethanol gelation test were reported in a few patients (Conard, NouvPresseMed, 1976; 5:2519). How-ever, in a more recent study (Bakker, Hepatol, 1992; 16:404) plasma degradation products of fibrin and fibrinogen and t-PA levels re-mained low after partial hepatic resections.

Peritoneovenous shunt

Ascitic fluid of cirrhotic patients is known to contain procoagulants and fibrinolytic activators[55,56] (Pettinson, BrJObsGyn, 1981; 88:160; Patrassi, EurJClinInv, 1985; 15:161), with significantly higher levels of plasmin–antiplasmin complexes and t-PA than those found in plasma (Patrassi, EurJClinInv, 1985; 15:161). Disseminated intra-vascular coagulation has been observed following peritoneovenous

shunting, especially by the Le Veen technique[56] (Lerner, JAMA, 1978; 240:2064; Harmon, AnnIntMed, 1979; 90:774; Salem, Gut, 1983; 24:412), while plasma hyperfibrinolysis has been observed in plasma after reinfusion of concentrated ascites. Although this is in apparent contrast, it may be assumed that, depending on both the route and technique of ascites reinfusion, the balance may be shifted towards activation of coagulation or fibrinolysis.[55]

Liver diseases associated with pregnancy

Late pregnancy is associated with a physiological hypercoagulable state due to an increase in procoagulant factors associated with decreased inhibitory and fibrinolytic activity (Stirling, Thromb-Haem, 1984; 52:176; Wright, BrJHaemat, 1988; 69:253). In normal pregnancy, there is a progressive increase in clotting factor levels, such as factors II, VII, X, V, and fibrinogen (Stirling, ThrombHaem, 1984; 52:176), and von Willebrand factor can reach 500 per cent (500 U/dl) at the third trimester.[57] There is a gradual decrease in protein S, which reaches its lowest level at the end of pregnancy, and an increase in the level of PAI-2, a plasminogen activator inhibitor similar to PAI-1, but produced exclusively by the placenta. A progressive increase in D-dimer and TAT complex levels is also found in normal pregnancy.[57] Thus, especially in the third trimester, pregnancy predisposes to disseminated intravascular co-agulation or thrombosis in the presence of associated risk factors.

HELLP syndrome

HELLP syndrome (haemolysis, elevated liver enzymes, low platelet count syndrome) occurs in 5 to 10 per cent of women with preg-nancy-induced hypertension and is characterized by haemolysis, elevated liver enzymes, and thrombocytopenia with a platelet count less than $100 \times 10^9/l$ (Sibai, AmJObsGyn, 1986; 155:501). It does not seem to be a unique disorder, but rather a variant of pre-eclampsia.[58] In this syndrome, the occurrence of disseminated intravascular coagulation is controversial since routine coagulation tests have rarely shown abnormalities indicative of this condition (Beller, AustNZJObsGyn, 1985; 25:83; Weinstein, ObsGyn, 1985; 66:657; Burrows, ObsGyn, 1987; 70:334). The use of more sensitive methods suggested coagulation activation in this syndrome (Greer, AmJObsGyn, 1985; 152:113; Weenink, ClinObstetGynecol, 1985; 28:37; Weiner, ObsGyn, 1988; 72:847). A more recent report showed that compensated disseminated intravascular coagulation was found in women with HELLP syndrome but not in women with preg-nancy-induced hypertension without HELLP syndrome.[59] Mean values of platelet count, AT III and protein C were significantly lower in the patients with HELLP, whereas TAT complexes and fibrin/fibrinogen degradation products were significantly higher. There was no significant difference in prothrombin time, activated partial prothrombin time, or positivity of the ethanol gelation test in the presence or absence of HELLP syndrome.[59]

On routine tests, the most prominent abnormality observed in HELLP is a low platelet count.[58] Thrombocytopenia may be severe with platelet counts less than $50 \times 10^9/l$. The continuous mild activation of coagulation may result in intravascular fibrin deposition, leading to organ dysfunction.[59] Such fibrin deposits have in fact been observed in the liver, kidney, and placenta of these patients[60] (Aarnoudse, BrJObsGyn, 1986; 93:145; Hill, JPath, 1989; 156:291). As suggested, the pathogenesis of this syndrome is local triggering of platelet aggregation in damaged placental vessels with subsequent production of small amounts of thrombin. Incomplete neutralization of thrombin by naturally occurring anticoagulants at the damaged endothelial cell surface might then cause mild disseminated intravascular coagulation, thus explaining the observed haemostatic abnormalities (Weenink, ClinObstetGynecol, 1985; 28:37). Major haemorrhage rarely occurs in patients with HELLP syndrome, but minor bleeding is common, as well as postoperative oozing after Caesarean section (Sibai, AmJObsGyn, 1986; 155:501). In the absence of bleeding, platelet transfusion has only been recommended when platelet counts are less than $20 \times 10^9/l$ or less than $50 \times 10^9/l$ before Caesarean section.[58] Therapeutic intervention against the observed coagulation activation has not been demonstrated to influence the course of the HELLP syndrome[59] and thus heparin therapy is uneffective.

Fatty liver of pregnancy

Fatty liver of pregnancy is rare and occurs in the second half of pregnancy, most often in the third trimester. Until 10 years ago, the illness was considered fulminant in nature, resulting in acute hepatic failure, bleeding diathesis, and coma. Since then, early diagnosis and delivery, and meticulous control of coagulation, have led to considerable improvement[61] (Bernuau, Gut, 1983; 24:340). Pregnancy and liver disease both predispose to disseminated intravascular coagulation (see above) and the combination of these two conditions causes mild to severe disseminated intravascular coagulation in most cases of fatty liver of pregnancy (Laursen, ActaObGyn, 1983; 62:403). Haemostatic abnormalities observed in fatty liver of pregnancy thus link those observed in hepatocellular insufficiency with those induced by disseminated intravascular coagulation and vary from mild or moderate to very severe deficiencies, depending on the degree of hepatocellular damage and on the stage of the disease. These abnormalities include prolongation of activated partial prothrombin time and prothrombin time, diminution of platelet count,[62] reduction of factor II, VII, and X levels, and a more pronounced or marked decrease of factor V, fibrinogen, and AT III levels; AT III levels may be undetectable in some cases.[62] The protamine sulphate gelation test is usually positive[62] and elevated fibrin/fibrinogen degradation products have been found.[62] An elevated D-dimer level is not useful diagnostically in this situation as D-dimer levels are increased in normal late pregnancy.[57] In our experience, this marked decrease of factor V level and AT III, as compared to factors II, VII, and X levels, and the pronounced fibrinogen decrease and positive protamine sulphate gelation test, which are not observed in hepatocellular insufficiency, are indicative of superimposed disseminated intravascular coagulation.

In fatty liver of pregnancy, the seriousness of disseminated intravascular coagulation has been thought to be responsible for fatal complications such as gastrointestinal bleeding (Holzbach, ObsGyn, 1974; 43:740; Cano, JAMA, 1975; 231:159), renal failure[61] (Laursen, ActaObGyn, 1983; 62:403) and postpartum bleeding (Hatfield, DigDis, 1972; 17:167; Liebman, AnnIntMed, 1983; 98:330). Heparin therapy has never been proven to be efficacious in this condition and may even aggravate bleeding.[61] The therapeutic effect of heparin requires AT III, and in severe acquired deficiency of AT III the effect of heparin may

be diminished. It was previously found that severe AT III depression in fatty liver of pregnancy could be a major cause of persistent intravascular clotting, and that replacement of AT III favourably improves the prognosis. Antithrombin III concentrates are now available for replacement therapy and have been used successfully in fatty liver of pregnancy[63] (McGehee, Blood, 1985; 66:282a (Suppl. 1)).

Most cases of jaundice during pregnancy are due to viral hepatitis, bile duct obstruction, or obstetric cholestasis. The haemostatic abnormalities observed are those usually found in viral hepatitis and bile duct obstruction, but with partial compensation due to the elevated levels of factors II, VII, X, V, and fibrinogen observed in normal pregnancy, especially in the third trimester. In obstetric cholestasis there is no coagulopathy and prothrombin time is normal.[62]

Budd–Chiari syndrome and portal vein thrombosis

Budd–Chiari syndrome is a rare condition characterized by hepatic venous outflow obstruction often due to thrombosis and is responsible for structural and functional abnormalities of the liver. The clinical manifestation may be either acute, with severe hepatocellular dysfunction, or chronic, with relatively preserved hepatocellular function (Dilawari, Medicine, 1994; 73:21; Frank, MayoClinProc, 1994; 69:877). In coagulation studies performed in 45 consecutive patients with chronic Budd–Chiari syndrome we found mean values of 59 per cent (59 U/dl) and 55 per cent (55 U/dl) for factor II and factor V, respectively, and significantly higher values of 64 per cent (64 U/dl) for protein C and 77 per cent (77 U/dl) for protein S and AT III.[64] In the acute presentation with fulminant hepatic failure, levels of clotting factors II, VII, X, and V may be less than 20 per cent (20 U/dl), and the fibrinogen level less than 1 g/l with a positive sulphate gelation test (Table 1). In patients with portal vein thrombosis, abnormalities of routine coagulation tests may be absent, or mild to moderate when they are those observed in moderate hepatocellular insufficiency. In only a few patients have we found associated moderate decreases of factor V and protein S, suggesting compensated mild disseminated intravascular coagulation as already described (Robson, Hepatol, 1993; 18:853). A myeloproliferative disorder is considered a major cause of hepatic as well as portal vein thrombosis (Valla, AnnIntMed, 1985; 103:329; Valla, Gastro, 1988; 94:1063; Pagliuca, QJMed, 1990; 76:981). Haemostatic abnormalities which constitute thrombosis risk factors have been reported only occasionally; of these the most common is the presence of acquired lupus anticoagulant, antiphospholipid antibodies, or anticardiolipin antibodies (Pomeroy, Gastro, 1984; 86:158; Terabayashi, Gastro, 1986; 91:219; Steenbergen, JHepatol, 1986; 3:87; Asherson, JRheum, 1989; 16:219; Stinson, AmJHemat, 1990; 35:281; Ouwendijk, Gut, 1994; 35: 1004).

In Budd–Chiari syndrome, inherited deficiencies of protein C[64] (Bourlière, Gut, 1990; 31:949), AT III (Ludwig, MayoClinProc, 1990; 65:51), and protein S[64] have been reported, as well as the occurrence of factor V Leiden (Denninger, Lancet, 1995; 345:525). Inherited deficiencies of protein C (Valla, Gut, 1988; 29: 856), protein S (Sas, ThrombHaem, 1985; 54:724), and AT III (Valla, Gastro, 1988; 94:1063) have also been reported in portal vein thrombosis. Because of overall clotting factor deficiencies caused by associated liver failure, measurement of physiological coagulation inhibitor levels are not usually informative, nor is the activated protein C resistance test indicative of the presence of factor V Leiden (see below). Inherited defects can only be established by family studies,[64] and inherited coagulation deficiencies have probably been underestimated in those conditions.[64] Anticardiolipin antibodies can be detected and the presence of factor V Leiden can easily be demonstrated by DNA analysis, even in the case of hepatocellular insufficiency. In hepatic and portal vein thrombosis, as stated before (Dilawari, Medicine, 1994; 73:21) important aetiological factors are related to hypercoagulability of blood, and we must look for an association of different thrombosis risk factors, including coagulation abnormalities.

Evaluation of haemostasis in liver diseases

In liver disease haemostatic testing is used either to estimate the degree of hepatocellular function, or to assess coagulation and fibrinolytic abnormalities (in patients with bleeding, before invasive procedures and surgery, or after replacement or corrective therapy). Less frequently, tests are done to look for the aetiology of thrombotic manifestations in patients with Budd–Chiari syndrome or portal thrombosis. This section deals with the coagulation tests routinely used in clinical practice, especially in patients with liver diseases. More information can be obtained from exhaustive reviews[65] (Hassouna, Hemat/OncolClinNAm, 1993; 7:1161). In liver diseases the most frequently used tests for haemostasis evaluation are: platelet count, bleeding time, prothrombin time, activated partial prothrombin time, individual clotting factor assays, euglobulin clot lysis time, protamine sulphate gelation test and D-dimer assay.

Platelet count

Normal platelet count is 150 to 400 $\times$ 10^9/l. Adequate haemostasis is assured even with a platelet count as low as 50 $\times$ 10^9/l as long as the platelets are functional. Thrombocytosis, with platelet counts above 500 $\times$ 10^9/l, predisposes to thrombosis, but is rarely observed in liver diseases in the absence of a pronounced inflammatory state or myeloproliferative disease. The finding of a low platelet count must necessarily lead to examination of the blood smear to estimate platelet number and to look for platelet aggregates that, if present, cause underestimation of the platelet count. Those platelet aggregates may occur artefactually when **EDTA** (ethylenediaminetetraacetic acid) is used as an anticoagulant in the sampling tube. To avoid this artefact, the platelet count may be performed on a prediluted blood sample, obtained by direct finger puncture using a simple disposable device consisting of a calibrated micropipette linked to a reservoir containing haemolysing solution (Unopet, Becton-Dickinson, Cowley, Oxford, UK). When there is persistence of an unexpected and unexplained thrombocytopenia, platelet-associated antibodies may be looked for.

Bleeding time

The bleeding time is the time that elapses between the moment when a small standard cut is made and the moment when the bleeding stops. The method of Duke (Duke, JAMA, 1910; 55:1185), performed on the ear lobe, is no longer used because of its lack of sensitivity. Bleeding time is generally measured by a modified Ivy method (Ivy, JLabClinMed, 1941; 26:1812; Mielke, ThrombHaem, 1984; 52:210), using a disposable template device designed to standardize the cut (Simplate, General diagnostics, Division of the Warner-Lambert Company, Morris Plain, NJ, USA; Surgicut, Ortho Diagnostic Systems, Carpinteria CA, USA). The device is held on the forearm while maintaining a constant back pressure of 40 mmHg with a pressure cuff on the upper arm. For reliable results, the bleeding time should be measured with meticulous attention to the recommendations given by the template device manufacturer. This test is simple to perform and is painless.

Bleeding time is obviously dependent on platelet count and function. The most common choice of upper limit is between 9 and 10 min[66] (Poller, ClinLabHaemat, 1984; 6:369); a bleeding time greater than 15 min in the absence of severe thrombocytopenia is quite abnormal and indicates severe impairment of platelet function of acquired or genetic origin. The most frequent acquired causes of prolonged bleeding time are drugs, renal insufficiency, and liver disease, and the most frequent genetic cause is von Willebrand disease. Many drugs, and not only antiplatelet drugs, may have the capacity to prolong the bleeding time in a given patient, and patients must be questioned carefully about the use of drugs. Bleeding time is also affected by the haematocrit and may be prolonged with a haematocrit less than 30 per cent (Eberst, AmJMed, 1994; 96:168). Thus, when thrombocytopenia is associated with impaired renal function and a low haematocrit, a common occurrence in liver transplant patients in the postoperative period, severe impairment of primary haemostasis may occur, and constitutes a major cause of haemorrhage. A prolonged bleeding time is common in patients with cirrhosis (see above), even when platelet counts are considered to be safe for invasive procedures (Blake, BMJ, 1990; 301:12), i.e. above 100 $\times$ 10^9/l, and an independent correlation of serum bilirubin concentration with bleeding time has been reported. Bleeding time should therefore be measured before invasive procedures such as percutaneous liver biopsy, arteriography, or surgical procedures (Blake, BMJ, 1990; 301:12) in patients with poor hepatic function. Although there is no proven link between prolonged bleeding time and haemorrhagic risk in patients with chronic liver disease, the finding of a prolonged bleeding time should make one cautious in deciding about or performing invasive procedures.[66] In the case of a prolonged bleeding time, a transjugular liver biopsy could be performed instead of a percutaneous liver biopsy. However, a normal bleeding time does not preclude haemorrhagic manifestations. If a patient has been treated recently with an antiplatelet drug, it would be sensible to delay percutaneous liver biopsy or another invasive procedure such as arteriography until 7 to 10 days after cessation of treatment, even if the bleeding time is found to be normal.

Prothrombin time

Prothrombin time is the clotting time of a citrated platelet-poor plasma sample to which thromboplastin has been added. Thromboplastin is made up from tissue factor, phospholipid, and calcium ions (Quick, JBC, 1935; 109:73). Prothrombin time studies the extrinsic pathway of factor X activation, thrombin formation, and fibrinoformation. Prothrombin time is thus sensitive to decreases in plasma levels of factors II, VII, X, V, and to a lesser extent of fibrinogen. The most frequent causes of prolonged prothrombin time are oral anticoagulant therapy and hepatocellular insufficiency. Prothrombin time is sensitive to the presence of abnormal fibrinogens, but rarely detects lupus anticoagulants. It is expressed in seconds as compared to a normal control, or as the ratio of the patient prothrombin time to the control prothrombin time, or as a percentage of normal. The reagents used are of animal or human origin, and the results depend on the sensitivity, and thus on the origin, of the thromboplastin used.[67] In patients on oral anticoagulant therapy, a standardized mode of expression of prothrombin time, the international normalized ratio (INR), that overcomes the variable sensitivities of the different thromboplastin reagents, has been recommended[67] in order to allow comparison of prothrombin time from different laboratories and thus to improve treatment monitoring. The INR is the ratio of the patient prothrombin time to the control prothrombin time elevated to the power of the international sensitivity index (**ISI**) of the thromboplastin used. The ISI characterizes a given thromboplastin compared to the corresponding reference thromboplastin. The INR corresponds thus to the prothrombin time ratio that would be obtained with the reference thromboplastin, and thus to a standardized prothrombin time result whatever the reagent used. However, this mode of expression of prothrombin time, especially designed for monitoring oral anticoagulant treatment, must be restricted exclusively to this situation. It is prohibited for other purposes, especially for use in patients with liver impairment where it has been shown to be an invalid method as different reagents do not give the same INR for the same sample (Kovacs, ThrombHaem, 1994; 71:678). This is probably because the ISI of commercial thromboplastins is established using platelet-poor plasma of patients on oral anticoagulants. In these patients, the prolongation of prothrombin time is due not only to the decrease of vitamin K-dependent factors II, VII, IX, and X, but also to the presence of high levels of PIVKA that interfere to a varying extent with the normal clotting factors in the prothrombin time test (Duckert, SchRundMed (Praxis), 1977; 66:293) according to the different sensitivities of the used thromboplastins. By contrast, patients with liver impairment do not exhibit high plasma PIVKA levels, and may show a decrease of factor V level which is not observed in orally anticoagulated patients. In orally anticoagulated patients and in patients with liver impairment, the prolongation of prothrombin time has a different basis; therefore the use of a single system of standardization is inappropriate.

Reagents used to perform prothrombin time generally contain a heparin inhibitor. Thus prothrombin time is insensitive to the presence of heparin, at least in the therapeutic range. However, if a large amount of heparin is present in the sample, the inhibitory capacity of the reagent will be overwhelmed and prothrombin time will be very prolonged and uninterpretable. Prothrombin time, like thrombin time, assesses the process of fibrinoformation and both tests are highly sensitive to fibrinoformation impairment. Thus in the presence of high levels of fibrinogen/fibrin degradation products (**FDP**), of dysfibrinogenaemia, or of any antithrombin, prothrombin time may be prolonged, as in the case of hyperfibrinogenaemia. Individual clotting factor levels may then be found to be normal, since the assays are performed on a dilution of plasma that produces a decrease of the inhibitory effect.

Activated partial thromboplastin time

Activated partial thromboplastin time is the clotting time of citrated platelet-poor plasma to which is added phospholipids, an activator (silica, kaolin, or ellagic acid), that may vary according to the manufacturer, and calcium ions. It is expressed in seconds as compared to the result with a control platelet-poor plasma, or better as the ratio of the sample to the control activated partial thromboplastin time. This test studies the contact phase, the intrinsic pathway of factor X activation, thrombin formation, and fibrinoformation. It is thus sensitive to decreases of plasma levels of factors XII, XI, VIII, IX, X, V, II, and of fibrinogen, but insensitive to factor VII deficiency. The specificity and sensitivity vary with the origin of the reagent (D'Angelo, AmJClinPath, 1990; 94:297) and each laboratory must define its normal range. This test is sensitive to the presence of heparin and is widely used to monitor heparin therapy. Heparin sensitivity varies greatly from one reagent to another and each laboratory has to define its therapeutic range. Activated partial thromboplastin time is also sensitive to lupus anticoagulants, but is less sensitive than prothrombin time to fibrinoformation impairment. In liver diseases activated partial thromboplastin time may be found to be moderately to highly prolonged, according to the degree of liver failure. In the case of moderate deficiencies of factors II, IX, X, and V, associated with a high level of factor VIII, the activated partial thromboplastin time may be normal.

Thrombin time/thrombin clotting time

Thrombin time is the clotting time of citrated platelet-poor plasma to which is added exogenous thrombin of human or animal origin. This test studies fibrinoformation, is sensitive to the fibrinogen level, and may thus be prolonged when this level is low or high (Carr, SouthMedJ, 1986; 79:563). Thrombin time is sensitive to the presence of abnormal fibrinogen, and to the presence of antithrombin inhibitors of any type. It is thus prolonged in the presence of heparin, fibrin or fibrinogen degradation products, monoclonal immunoglobulins, and antithrombin-specific antibodies. Prolongation of thrombin time is responsible for prolongation of prothrombin time, and to a lesser extent of activated partial thromboplastin time. In the case of a very prolonged prothrombin time and activated partial thromboplastin time, thrombin time must be measured together with the reptilase time. Reptilase is a snake enzyme which transforms fibrinogen to fibrin but is insensitive to heparin. Prolongation of thrombin time with a normal reptilase time indicates the presence of heparin in the sample, and then prolongation of prothrombin time and activated partial thromboplastin time must not be interpreted as evidence of haemostatic abnormalities. If both thrombin time and reptilase time are prolonged, this indicates impairment of fibrinoformation.

Fibrinogen

Testing of fibrinogen is now widely performed by a functional, chronometric method based on the measurement of thrombin time. A high concentration of exogenous thrombin is added to diluted platelet-poor plasma and the amount of clottable fibrinogen is derived from the measured clotting time (Clauss, ActaHaem, 1957; 17:237). When the thrombin time is prolonged due to the presence of fibrinogen/fibrin degradation products, other thrombin inhibitors, or abnormal fibrinogen, the fibrinogen measurement by this functional test will be an underestimate. Dysfibrinogenaemias are characterized by functional abnormalities of the fibrinogen molecule, leading to impaired fibrinoformation, and thus to erroneously low levels of fibrinogen as measured by functional tests. In this case measurement of fibrinogen level by another non-functional method such as heat precipitation or immunological testing will give a higher result.

Prothrombin time, activated partial thromboplastin time, and thrombin time are used as screening tools, that constitute the basis of specialized clot-based coagulation assays. When the results of prothrombin time and activated partial thromboplastin time are outside the normal range, further investigation is required. For instance, in the presence of prolonged prothrombin time and activated partial thromboplastin time, provided the thrombin time, and thus fibrinoformation, is normal, the expected abnormality is probably related to factor II, VII, X, and V, or fibrinogen, and the activities of these different factors can be measured separately. Clotting factors VII and X are generally assayed simultaneously in a first step, for practical and economical purposes. The normal range for clotting factor II, VII, X, and V is 75 to 110 per cent (75–110 U/dl). In the case of isolated prolonged activated partial thromboplastin time, with normal prothrombin time and thrombin time, the abnormality is probably related to clotting factors VIII, IX, XI, or XII, only studied by activated partial thromboplastin time, or to the presence of a circulating anticoagulant. The distinction between deficiency of clotting factor and inhibitor is easily made by mixing the study sample with a normal platelet-poor plasma. The normal range for clotting factors VIII, IX, and XI is 60 to 150 per cent (60–150 U/dl). The normal range for factor XII has not been defined since even a pronounced decrease of this factor does not cause clinical manifestations. The only haemostatic abnormality able to prolong prothrombin time without changes in other coagulation tests is factor VII deficiency.

Fibrinolytic activity

Whole blood clot lysis time is the time taken for lysis to occur in a clot of whole blood incubated at 37 °C. This test is insensitive and able to detect only severe hyperfibrinolysis. In the plasma clot lysis time, platelet-poor plasma is clotted and the lysis time measured. This test is only slightly more sensitive than the previous one. These two methods are affected by the plasma t-PA, plasminogen, and fibrinogen levels, but also by the level of inhibitors. Isoelectric precipitation of the plasmatic euglobulins containing plasminogen, fibrinogen, and t-PA leaves most inhibitors in solution. Thus, study of the lysis time of the clot formed with the euglobulin precipitate dissolved in buffer and recalcified, allows assessment of t-PA activity in a system mostly devoid of fibrinolytic inhibitors (Von Kaulla, ProgChemFibrinThromb, 1975; 1:131; Kluft, ProgChemFibrin-Thromb, 1976; 2:57). The response is much more quickly obtained than with the above-described tests, since in acute hyperfibrinolysis the euglobulin lysis time is less than 30 min, and is about 1 h in the case of moderately elevated fibrinolytic activity (normal is above

3 h). This inexpensive and relatively rapid test is thus most useful clinically. Moreover, a hyperfibrinolytic state can be demonstrated by this single test.

Fibrinogen/fibrin degradation products

Fibrinogen/fibrin degradation products (FDP) can be detected by latex agglutination tests, in which latex particles coated with antifibrinogen antibodies agglutinate when fibrinogen or FDP are present (Merskey, PSEBM, 1969; 131:871). The tests must be performed on serum to avoid fibrinogen interference, and a blood sample different from that used to study haemostasis must be obtained. Elevated FDP levels are, however, only indirect indicators of increased fibrinolytic activity that can be assessed directly by euglobulin lysis time. They are not useful for differentiating disseminated intravascular coagulation from increased fibrinolysis as they originate from both fibrin and fibrinogen. They can also be overestimated in the case of incomplete clotting (i.e where non-clotted fibrinogen is left in serum), which may occur in advanced liver disease or in the case of dysfibrinogenaemia. Thus, FDP measurement may advantageously be replaced by euglobulin lysis time assessment plus a D-dimer assay.

Fibrin monomers

Fibrin monomers can be determined with the ethanol (Breen, AnnIntMed, 1968; 69:1197) or protamine sulphate (Gurewich, AnnIntMed, 1971; 75:895; Niewiarowski, JLabClinMed, 1971; 77:665) gelation or paracoagulation tests. These tests utilize the ability of ethanol or protamine sulphate to induce end-to-end aggregation of circulating soluble fibrin monomers produced by thrombin, and thus the formation of a pseudo-clot or of a gel. Positive results are observed in disseminated intravascular coagulation, and the protamine sulphate test has been described as the most sensitive and clinically applicable test for detecting circulating soluble fibrin.[26] This latter test is performed on serial plasma dilutions until no more paracoagulation can be evidenced. Thus, the higher the plasma dilution at which the test is still found positive, the higher the fibrin monomer level. This simple, rapid, non-expensive, and informative test must nevertheless not be used alone but in association with other coagulation tests. It must also be remembered that, in the case of blood dilution, i.e. after transfusion, this test may become negative.

Coagulation activation markers

Fibrinopeptide A is an activation peptide released from fibrinogen by the specific proteolytic action of thrombin (Chapter 2.14.3). Thus its release indicates that thrombin has formed in blood, and identifies an hypercoagulable or a prothrombotic state. Other markers of thrombin formation, such as prothrombin activation peptide $F1+2$ and thrombin–antithrombin complex (TAT), have been identified, and specific antibodies directed against these markers have been prepared (Nossel, JCI, 1974; 54:43; Lau, JBC, 1979; 254:8751; Pelzer, ThrombHaem, 1988; 59:101; Pelzer, ThrombHaem, 1991; 65:153). Enzyme linked immunosorbent assays (**ELISA**) for these markers are commercially available. Elevated levels of fibrinopeptide A and other coagulation activation markers are found in a number of pathological conditions (Boisclair, BloodRev, 1990; 4:25) and these markers increase during pregnancy.[57]

Thus they are not pathognomonic of disseminated intravascular coagulation. Artefactual increases of fibrinopeptide A are frequent, and so the routine use of fibrinopeptide A testing is limited.

Likewise, D-dimer, the specific degradation product of cross-linked fibrin can be measured using various commercially available ELISA or latex agglutination tests (Kroneman, BloodCoagFibrinol, 1990; 1:91). Both methods are useful for biological diagnosis of disseminated intravascular coagulation,[26] but the ELISA method is the only one that can be used for diagnostic exclusion of deep venous thrombosis and pulmonary embolism (Bounameaux, ThrombHaem, 1994; 71:1) because of the lack of specificity of the latex method. There is an increase in D-dimer level with age, during pregnancy, and in conditions associated with an inflammatory state, and thus, increased D-dimer levels are frequently found in liver diseases. It must also be emphasized that D-dimer is directly indicative of fibrinolytic activity, and that in conditions in which extravascular or haemostatic fibrin deposits may have formed, e.g. neoplasia or in the postoperative period, elevated D-dimer levels are likely to be demonstrated by a method as sensitive as the ELISA test.

Coagulation inhibitors

None of the above-mentioned coagulation screening tests identifies a decrease of AT III, protein C, or protein S levels, or resistance to activated protein C (Chapter 2.14.3). Such defects can only be suspected on the basis of an individual or familial clinical history. When screening for deficiencies of inhibitors, it is best to use a functional assay first, so that both quantitative and qualitative defects are detected. Functional assays can be performed using clotting or chromogenic methods. However, chromogenic methods only study the catalytic activity of the enzyme and not its full inhibitory capacity. Measurement of protein S activity is delicate and immunological assay of both total and free active protein S are required. As in the case of isolated clotting factor deficiency, if the activity of an inhibitor is found to be decreased, an immunological assay must be performed to distinguish a quantitative from a qualitative deficiency (Pabinger, ThrombHaem, 1992; 68:470; Kottke-Marchant, Hemat/Oncol-ClinNAm, 1994; 8:809).

The activated protein C-resistance test consists of two activated partial prothrombin times, one in the presence and one in the absence of a fixed amount of activated protein C, and is a simple and reliable method to detect a poor anticoagulant response to activated protein C, associated in most cases with the presence of the mutated factor V, factor V Leiden, responsible for thrombophilia (De Ronde, ThrombHaem, 1994; 72:880; Le, Blood, 1995; 85:1704) (Chapter 2.14.3). Nevertheless, this test is not reliable with liver and haemostatic impairment, and it is then better to look for the presence of factor V Leiden by direct DNA analysis (Beauchamp, Lancet, 1994; 344:694). Likewise, AT III, protein C, and protein S are synthesized by the liver and in the case of liver impairment, with decreased synthesis of clotting factors, the results of the inhibitor assays are not informative, as is the case with vitamin K deficiency or treatment with vitamin K antagonists, as protein C and protein S are vitamin K-dependent proteins (Chapter 2.14.3).

Haemostatic evaluation in liver transplantation

In liver transplantation haemostasis tests should be performed at intervals of 0.5 to 2 h, depending on the stage of the surgical procedure.[43] In our institute the tests listed below are performed preoperatively, at least once in the pre-anhepatic and anhepatic periods, and at the reperfusion period. They are then repeated more or less frequently according to the degree of the observed abnormalities. The tests performed are: platelet count, activated partial prothrombin time, prothrombin time, measurement of factors II, VII + X, V, and fibrinogen levels, measurement of euglobulin lysis time, and protamine sulphate gelation test. Thromboelastography consists of the graphic monitoring of the different stages of the coagulation process and can be performed on plasma as well as on total blood; it has been used to monitor haemostatic changes during liver transplantation (Owen, Mayo-ClinProc, 1987; 62:761; Porte, Fibrinolysis, 1988; 2:67 (Suppl. 3)). Nevertheless, this method, which studies the global coagulation process, does not allow differentiation of disseminated intravascular coagulation from a hyperfibrinolytic state or other abnormalities responsible for impaired coagulation.[1]

Haemostatic evaluation before percutaneous liver biopsy

Although it has been established that percutaneous liver biopsy is easy and safe when performed by experienced physicians,[68,69] the procedure is not trivial and the decision to perform liver biopsy must be based on assessment of the risks and benefits.[69] Of the complications occurring after percutaneous liver biopsy, haemorrhage is the most frequent (Ali, NZMedJ, 1978; 88:237; Knauer, Gastro, 1978; 74:101; Perrault, Gastro, 1978; 74:103; Wright, SouthMedJ, 1991; 84:889; Janes, AnnIntMed, 1993; 118:96), and bleeding into the abdomen or chest is the principal major complication of liver biopsies performed in transplant recipients.[68] Although earlier reports did not show a correlation between bleeding and clotting indices, haemostatic evaluation was then limited and biopsies were not done in patients with severe clotting disorders (Ewe, DigDisSci, 1981; 26:388). Differences in haemorrhagic complications may thus be related to differences in haemostatic requirements. Most centres require prothrombin time above 40 to 60 per cent of normal, or no more prolonged than 3 to 6 s as compared to normal, as well as platelet counts above 60 to $100 \times 10^9/l$[70-73] (McGill, Gastro, 1990; 99:1396). A few investigators require normal bleeding time.[66,69] Thus, as stated before, haemostasis must be evaluated before percutaneous liver biopsy in patients with poor liver function and especially in the cirrhotic patient. In our institute, haemostatic requirements before blind percutaneous liver biopsy are as follows: bleeding time 10 min or less; activated partial prothrombin time ratio 2 or less; factors II, VII + X, and V levels greater than 40 per cent; fibrinogen 1 g/l or higher; euglobulin lysis time 3 h or more; and platelet count greater than $50 \times 10^9/l$. In the case of isolated abnormal activated partial prothrombin time, even mildly prolonged, the procedure is delayed and factor VIII, IX, or XI deficiency as well as the presence of inhibitor are looked for. If those requirements are not met, a transjugular liver biopsy is performed instead of percutaneous liver biopsy. Liver biopsy with plugging of the needle track is an alternative to transjugular liver biopsy, especially when focal lesions have to be examined. Nevertheless, the haemorrhagic risk is not negligible and this technique may even be associated with an increased risk of haemorrhage (Sawyerr, JHepatol, 1993; 17:81). The efficiency, accuracy and safety of ultrasound-guided liver biopsy with plugging of the needle track has been assessed in patients at high risk for haemorrhage and prospectively classified in different groups on the basis of coagulation parameters (Zins, Radiol, 1992; 184:841). Serious bleeding complications were encountered in some patients with major coagulation disorders, that is bleeding time greater than 15 min, activated partial prothrombin time ratio above 2, clotting factor II, VII + X, and V levels less than 35 per cent, euglobulin lysis time less than 2 h, and platelet counts below $50 \times 10^9/l$. No serious complication occurred in the 32 patients with moderately severe coagulation defects (i.e. bleeding time ranging from 12 to 15 min, activated partial prothrombin time ratio between 1.5 and 2, clotting factor II, VII + X, and V levels from 35 to 50 per cent, euglobulin lysis time from 2 to 2.5 h, and platelet counts from 50 to $80 \times 10^9/l$. Likewise, in an earlier report of a series of 100 plugged liver biopsies in patients with similar clotting abnormalities, no major bleeding was observed (Tobin, DigDisSci, 1989; 34:13).

It must be noted that massive intraperitoneal bleeding after capsular perforation has been reported in all cases of death following transjugular liver biopsy. Serious thought must therefore be given before deciding to perform transjugular liver biopsy in a patient with hereditary haemorrhagic disease such as haemophilia or von Willebrand disease; one must balance the risk of haemorrhage if no replacement therapy is undertaken, with risk of viral infection if replacement therapy is given, and with the benefit to be gained by inspection of the liver biopsy.

Comments

It must be remembered that the quality of laboratory data depends largely on the quality of the sample. The following recommendations must be followed carefully. Blood samples must be obtained directly into the sampling tube to avoid platelet and coagulation activation and, if possible, after a frank venepuncture to avoid the contact of blood with tissue factor. The ratio between the volume of blood sample and the volume of anticoagulant present in the sampling tube must be carefully respected (usually 9 volumes of blood : 1 volume of trisodium citrate 0.13 M) since this ratio is designed to allow reliable results. Sampling tubes must be used strictly as indicated by the manufacturer. As soon as the blood has been taken, the sampling tubes must be immediately, but gently tilted so as to allow mixing of blood with the anticoagulant. The sample, kept at room temperature, never in melting ice or in a fridge, must be sent rapidly to the laboratory, at least within 2 h.

In most instances close communication between the pathologist and the clinician—making the pathologist aware of the patient's condition, and the clinician being well-informed about the specificity and sensitivity of the laboratory tools used in coagulation testing—will improve the quality of patient's diagnosis and treatment.

Examples of routine haemostatic evaluation in patients with variable conditions in liver disease are given in Table 1.

Management of haemostatic abnormalities in liver disease

In liver disease, even in the presence of multiple and sometimes severe haemostatic abnormalities, haemorrhages rarely occur in the absence of trauma, lesions, or invasive procedures, and thus systematic correction of clotting defects is not necessary. Gastrointestinal bleeding is most often due to ruptured oesophageal varices and not correlated with clotting abnormalities. In the latter, treatment consists essentially of the control of bleeding by mechanical devices, and in transfusion to control the blood pressure. In acute or fulminant hepatitis, bleeding is rare but monitoring of clotting factor levels, especially of factor V level, is essential for prognosis. In this particular situation, there is no indication for infusion of fresh frozen plasma; it is not useful and artificially changes an essential prognostic criterion, i.e. the factor V level. Similarly, infusion of clotting factor concentrates and prothrombin complex concentrates is unnecessary and, moreover, contra-indicated in liver disease, as these substances contain activated clotting factors[74] (Blatt, AnnIntMed, 1972; 81:766) that are not cleared by the diseased liver and thus are responsible for disseminated intravascular coagulation occurrence[74] (Menaché, BrJHaemat, 1975; Suppl. 31:247; Marassi, ThrombHaem, 1978; 39:248; Anderson, MedJAust, 1990; 153:352). Nevertheless, in the case of lesions, trauma, haemorrhage, or before surgery or invasive procedures, replacement therapy may be necessary. In these occurrences viroinactivated or securized fresh frozen plasma may be used to maintain clotting factor levels at least equal to or above 30 per cent of normal (30 U/dl), and a fibrinogen level equal to or above 1 g/l. Fresh frozen plasma is effective for correcting most of the clotting defects associated with liver disease (Spector, NEJM, 1966; 275:1032), since it contains coagulation factors, coagulation inhibitors, and fibrinolytic inhibitors. Moreover, fresh frozen plasma does not contain activated clotting factors and does not cause disseminated intravascular coagulation.[74] Replacement therapy is not necessary when clotting factor levels are above 40 per cent of normal (40 U/dl). Vitamin K administration is only useful in cholestasis causing low levels of vitamin K-dependent factors. When thrombocytopenia is present, platelet counts are generally only moderately low and platelet infusions are not usually useful.

By contrast, in the case of prolonged bleeding time, desmopressin (deaminodearginovasopressin, Minirin®, Ferring) may be used for tentative correction (Burroughs, BMJ, 1985; 291:1377; Mannucci, Blood, 1986; 67:1140) in the absence of contra-indication and especially of thrombotic risk[75] (Mannucci, AnnRevMed, 1990; 41:55; Hartmann, Lancet, 1995; 345:1302). Desmopressin is infused intravenously, 0.3 µg/kg body weight, in 50 to 100 ml of normal saline, over 20 min. In the case of haemorrhage, or before surgery, an excessive increase in fibrinolytic activity may be corrected by antifibrinolytic drugs. Aprotinin (Trasylol, Bayer AG, Leverkusen, Germany) is a single-chain polypeptide of 6512 kDa derived from bovine lungs (Verstraete, Drugs, 1985; 29:236). It is a potent naturally occurring serine protease inhibitor. By inhibiting trypsin, kallikrein, and plasmin, aprotinin affects fibrinolytic, coagulation, and complement systems. Aprotinin is a potent antifibrinolytic drug when given intravenously as a bolus of 250 000 to 500 000 KIU (kallikrein inhibitory units), i.e. 125 to 250 UphE (European Pharmacopoeia Units). The half-life of aprotinin is short, less than 2 h, and the administration of additional 125 000 KIU is often necessary 1 to 2 h later. Lysine analogues such as ε-aminocaproic acid, 0.1 g/kg body weight, or tranexamic acid, 10 mg/kg body weight, may also be used, but are contra-indicated in the case of disseminated intravascular coagulation or renal insufficiency since they increase the occurrence of thrombotic complications (Naeye, Blood, 1962; 19:694; Gralnick, AmJClinPath, 1971; 56:151).

Aprotinin has a low toxicity and large doses are well tolerated (Soilleux, AnesthAnalg, 1995; 80:349), thus it is currently used to reduce blood loss in liver transplantation[76] and appears to be more efficacious than the previously used ε-aminocaproic acid (Scudamore, AmJSurg, 1995; 169:546). However, in this setting, large doses (i.e. initial bolus of 2 million KIU, followed by an infusion of 0.5 million KIU/h) do not appear to offer additional benefit as compared to low doses (i.e. an initial bolus of 0.5 million KIU followed by an infusion of 150 000 KIU/h) (Soilleux, AnesthAnalg, 1995; 80:349). Although a higher risk of thrombosis due to high-dose aprotinin was not observed in early reports[76] a fatal thrombotic event was described recently (Baubillier, Transpl, 1994; 57:1664).

Because aprotinin is of bovine origin, anaphylactoid reactions may occur. Such reactions are rare (Freeman, CurrMedResOpin, 1983; 8:559; Wuthrich, Lancet, 1992; 340:173; Dewachter, Anaesth, 1993; 48:1110); even so, one should be aware of possible previous aprotinin exposure before treatment. Antihistamine receptor drugs can then be administrated before aprotinin.

In the case of disseminated intravascular coagulation, the efficacy of heparin therapy is disputed and uncertain, since it depends on the AT III level. Moreover, heparin therapy favours haemorrhagic manifestations. By contrast, administration of AT III concentrates may be beneficial,[63] especially in the case of acute fatty liver of pregnancy (McGehee, Blood, 1985; 66:282a (Suppl. 1)). Antithrombin III concentrates should be administered so that a plasma level of 120 per cent (120 U/dl) is reached and maintained above 80 per cent (80 U/dl) during treatment (Menache, Hemat/Oncol-ClinNAm, 1992; 6:1115). In liver transplantation, systematic administration of AT III concentrates has not been demonstrated to have any effect on blood loss nor on the occurrence of postoperative thrombotic complications (Coccheri, SemThrombHaemost, 1993; 19:268). In disseminated intravascular coagulation, treatment of haemorrhagic manifestations involves the maintenance of coagulation factor levels to at least 30 per cent of normal (30 U/dl) and fibrinogen to at least 1 g/l by the use of fresh frozen plasma; transfuse platelets if the platelet count is less than $50 \times 10^9/l$, or if the bleeding time is above 15 min. If there is excessive fibrinolytic activity, as measured by euglobulin lysis time, aprotinin may be used, but lysine analogues are contra-indicated (see above).

In Budd–Chiari syndrome and portal vein thrombosis, anticoagulant therapy, although it does not modify the existing thrombus, prevents thrombosis extension and may be expected to stop the course of the disease. Anticoagulant therapy is initiated with heparin (Hartmann, JohnsHopkMedJ, 1980; 146:247). In the case of poor haemostatic function with low clotting factor levels, unfractionated standard heparin may be replaced by fractionated low molecular weight heparin.[77] Standard heparin therapy is monitored by activated partial prothrombin time, or by heparinaemia when activated partial prothrombin time is prolonged before treatment. Low molecular weight heparin therapy is monitored by

heparinaemia. In both cases heparinaemia may be assessed by the plasma antifactor Xa activity.[77] The therapeutic range for standard heparin curative therapy is 0.3 to 0.6 UI anti-Xa/ml and for low molecular weight heparin (LMWH) curative therapy it is 0.5 to 1 UI anti-Xa/ml. A dreadful complication of heparin therapy is heparin-induced immune thrombocytopenia. Thus, as soon as possible, when coagulation factor levels are equal to or above 40 per cent of normal (40 U/dl), the anticoagulant treatment should be switched from heparin to vitamin K antagonists and long-term oral anticoagulant treatment must be maintained (Ouwendijk, Gut, 1994; 35:1004). It must be remembered that the INR mode of expression of prothrombin time cannot be used in the presence of liver disease (see above). Then, assessment of the decrease of the vitamin K-dependent factors II and VII + X levels as compared with factor V level, may be used for treatment monitoring.

Thrombolytic therapy has been used successfully on occasion, especially when given early for a recent thrombosis[78] (i.e. before the thrombus has organized). The thrombolytic agents used are: urokinase, streptokinase, or recombinant tissue-type plasminogen activator (r-tPA). In Budd–Chiari syndrome, the local infusion of urokinase, 4000 U/min for 4 h, associated with heparin, 5000 U as a bolus and then 1000 U/h, resulted in dissolution of half the thrombus. Angioplasty was then performed and urokinase continued at a rate of 10 000 U/h overnight for a total dose of 1.08 million U. Additional lysis occurred and the remaining thrombus was extracted with a balloon catheter into the vena cava.[78] Streptokinase therapy has also been used in hepatic vein thrombosis. A bolus of 250 000 U was been administered intravenously, followed by 150 000 U/h with heparin therapy (Sholar, AnnIntMed, 1985; 103:539). Similarly r-tPA has been used in portal[79] and hepatic[80] vein thrombosis. A bolus of 20 mg r-tPA was given locally[79] or infused intravenously,[80] followed by 40 mg over 30 min[80] or by low molecular weight heparin (LMWH) therapy.[79] Application of the thrombolytic agent directly to the clot through a catheter seems most likely to be effective.[78] Otherwise, the infused agent can be directed away from the clot. Moreover, direct application minimizes haemorrhagic risk due to the lower dose administered as compared with systemic administration.[78]

References

1. Mammen EF. Coagulation abnormalities in liver disease. Perplexing thrombotic and hemorrhagic disorders. *Hematology/Oncology Clinics of North America*, 1992; **6**: 1247–57.
2. Colman RW and Rubin RN. Blood coagulation. In Arias IM, Jakoby WB, Popper H, Schachter D, and Shafritz DA, eds. *Liver biology and pathobiology*, 2nd edn. New York: Raven Press, 1988: 1033–42.
3. Blanchard RA, Furie BC, Jorgensen M, Kruger SF, and Furie B. Acquired vitamin K-dependent carboxylation deficiency in liver disease. *New England Journal of Medicine*, 1981; **305**: 242–8.
4. Roberts HR and Cederbaum AI. The liver and blood coagulation: physiology and pathology. *Gastroenterology*, 1972; **63**: 297–320.
5. Walls WB and Losowsky MS. The hemostatic defect of liver disease. *Gastroenterology*, 1971; **60**: 108–19.
6. Deutsch E. Blood coagulation changes in liver disease. *Progress in Liver Diseases*, 1965; **2**: 69–83.
7. Arnman R, Iwarson S, and Olsson R. The clinical significance of increased plasma levels of liver-synthesized coagulation factors in liver disease. *Scandinavian Journal of Gastroenterology*, 1977; **12**: 387–9.

8. Cederblad G, Korsan-Bengtsen K, and Olsson R. Observations of increased levels of blood coagulation factors and other plasma proteins in cholestatic liver disease. *Scandinavian Journal of Gastroenterology*, 1976; **11**: 391–6.

9. Brozovic M. Acquired disorders of coagulation. In Bloom AL and Thomas AT, eds. *Haemostasis and thrombosis*. Edinburgh: Churchill Livingstone, 1987: 519–34.

10. Fiore L, Levine J, and Deykin D. Alterations of haemostasis in patients with liver disease. In Zakim D and Boyer TD, eds. *Hepatology: a textbook of liver disease*. Philadelphia: WB Saunders, 1990: 546–71.

11. Hofeler H and Klingemann HG. Fibronectin and factor VIII–related antigen in liver disease. *Journal of Clinical Chemistry and Clinical Biochemistry*, 1984; **22**: 15–19.

12. Green AJ and Ratnoff OD. Elevated antihemophilic factor (AHF, factor VIII) procoagulant activity and AHF-like antigen in alcoholic cirrhosis of the liver. *Journal of Laboratory and Clinical Medicine*, 1974; **83**: 189–97.

13. Gralnick HR, Givelbar H, and Abrams E. Dysfibrinogenemia associated with hepatoma. *New England Journal of Medicine*, 1978; **299**: 221–6.

14. Francis JL and Armstrong DJ. Sialic acid and sialotransferase in the pathogenesis of acquired dysfibrinogenemia. In Haverkate F, Henschen A, Nieuwenhuizen W, Straub PW, eds. *Fibrinogen–structure, functional aspects, metabolism*. Berlin: Walter, 1983.

15. Green FG, Thomson JM, Dymock IW, and Poller L. Abnormal fibrin polymerization in liver disease. *British Journal of Haematology*, 1976; **34**: 427–39.

16. Liebman HA *et al*. Des-γ-carboxy (abnormal) prothrombin as a serum marker of primary hepatocellular carcinoma. *New England Journal of Medicine*, 1984; **310**: 1427–31.

17. Yoshikawa Y, Sakata Y, Toda G, and Oka H. The acquired vitamin K-dependent γ-carboxylation deficiency in hepatocellular carcinoma involves not only prothrombin, but also protein C. *Hepatology*, 1988; **8**: 524–30.

18. Weitz IC and Liebman HA. Des-γ-carboxy (abnormal) prothrombin and hepatocellular carcinoma: a critical review. *Hepatology*, 1993; **18**: 990–7.

19. Kasahara A, *et al*. Clinical evaluation of plasma des-γ-carboxy prothrombin as a marker protein of hepatocellular carcinoma in patients with tumors of various sizes. *Digestive Diseases and Sciences*, 1993; **38**: 2170–6.

20. Graham JB, Barrow EM, and Wynne TR. Stuart clotting defect III: an acquired case with complete recovery. In Brinkhous KM, ed. *Hemophilia and other hemorrhagic states*. Chapel Hill: University of North Carolina Press, 1959: 158–66.

21. Leebeek FWG, Kluft C, Knot EAR, De Maat MPM, and Wilson JHP. A shift in balance between profibrinolytic and antifibrinolytic factors causes enhanced fibrinolysis in cirrhosis. *Gastroenterology*, 1991; **101**: 1382–90.

22. Tran-Thang C, Fasel-Felley J, Pralong G, Hofstetter JR, Bachmann F, and Kuithof EKO. Plasminogen activators and plasminogen activator inhibitors in liver deficiencies caused by chronic alcoholism or infectious hepatitis. *Thrombosis and Haemostasis*, 1989; **62**: 651–3.

23. Huber K, Kirchheimer JC, Korninger C, and Binder BR. Hepatic synthesis and clearance of components of the fibrinolytic system in healthy volunteers and in patients with different stages of liver cirrhosis. *Thrombosis Research*, 1991; **62**: 491–500.

24. Boks AL, Brommer EJP, Schalm SW, and Van Vliet HHDM. Hemostasis and fibrinolysis in severe liver failure and their relation to hemorrhage. *Hepatology*, 1986; **6**: 79–86.

25. Ferro D, *et al*. Prevalence of hyperfibrinolysis in patients with liver cirrhosis. *Fibrinolysis*, 1993, 7: 59–62.

26. Bick RL. Disseminated intravascular coagulation. In Perplexing thrombotic and hemorrhagic disorders. *Hematology/Oncology Clinics of North America*, 1992; **6**: 1259–85.

27. Bachmann F. Disseminated intravascular coagulation. *Diseases of the mouth*. Chicago: Year Book Medical Publishers, 1969: 1–44.

28. Rake MO, Flute PT, Pannell G, and Williams R. Intravascular coagulation in acute hepatic necrosis. *Lancet*, 1970; 534–7.

29. Verstraete M, Vermylen J, and Collen D. Intravascular coagulation in liver disease. *Annual Review of Medicine*, 1974; **25**: 447–55.

30. Mombelli G, Fiori G, Monotti R, Haeberli A, and Straub PW. Fibrinopeptide A in liver cirrhosis: evidence against a major contribution of disseminated intravascular coagulation to coagulopathy of chronic liver disease. *Journal of Laboratory and Clinical Medicine*, 1993; **121**: 83–90.

31. Carr JM. Disseminated intravascular coagulation in cirrhosis. *Hepatology*, 1989; **10**: 103–10.

32. Aoki Y, Hirai K, and Tanikawa K. Mechanism of thrombocytopenia in liver cirrhosis: kinetics of indium-111 tropolone labelled platelets. *European Journal of Nuclear Medicine*, 1993; **20**: 123–9.

33. Aseni P, Frangi M, Beati C, Vertemati M, and Romani F. Is thrombocytopenia in liver failure dependent on an inadequate synthesis of thrombopoietic stimulating factor by the liver? *Medical Hypothesis*, 1988; **26**: 217–19.

34. Galambos JT. Evaluation and therapy of portal hypertension. In Smith LH, ed. *Cirrhosis*. Philadelphia: WB Saunders, 1979: 286.

35. Ratnoff OD. Disordered hemostasis in hepatic disease. In Schiff L, ed. *Diseases of the liver*. Philadelphia: Lippincott, 1969: 147–64.

36. Cowan DH. Effect of alcoholism on hemostasis. *Seminars in Hematology*, 1980; **17**: 137–47.

37. Lindenbaum J and Hargrove RI. Thrombocytopenia in alcoholics. *Annals of Internal Medicine*, 1968; **68**: 526–32.

38. Mikhailidis DP, Barradas MA, and Jeremy JY. The effect of ethanol on platelet function and vascular prostanoids. *Alcohol*, 1990; **7**: 171–80.

39. Guillin MC, Menache D, Barge J, Fueff B, and Fauvert R. Les troubles de l'hémostase au cours des hépatites virales graves: étude clinique, anatomique et biologique. *Annales de Medicine Interne*, 1971; **122**: 605–12.

40. Meili EO, Frick PG, and Straub PW. Coagulation changes during massive hepatic necrosis due to *Amanita phalloides* poisoning. *Helvetica Medica Acta*, 1970; **35**: 304–13.

41. Bontempo FA, *et al*. The relation of preoperative coagulation findings to diagnosis, blood usage, and survival in adult liver transplantation. *Transplantation*, 1985; **39**: 532–6.

42. Dzik WH, Arkin CF, Jenkins RL, and Stump DC. Fibrinolysis during liver transplantation in humans. Role of tissue-type plasminogen activator. *Blood*, 1988; **71**: 1090–5.

43. Porte RJ, Knot EAR, and Bontempo FA. Hemostasis in liver transplantation. *Gastroenterology*, 1989; **97**: 488–501.

44. National Institutes of Health consensus development conference statement: liver transplantation. *Hepatology*, 1984; **4**: 1078–108.

45. Lewis JH, *et al*. Liver transplantation. Intraoperative changes coagulation factors in 100 first transplants. *Hepatology*, 1989; **9**: 710–14.

46. Von Kaulla KN, Kayne H, Von Kaulla E, Marchioro TL, and Starzl TE. Changes in blood coagulation before and after hepatectomy or transplantation in dogs and man. *Archives of Surgery*, 1966; **92**: 71–9.

47. Groth, CG. Changes in coagulation. In Starzl TE, Putman CW, eds. *Experience in hepatic transplantation*. Philadelphia: Saunders, 1969: 159–75.

48. Arnoux D, Boutiere B, Houvenaeghel M, Rousset-Rouviere A, Le Treut P, and Sampol J. Intraoperative evolution of coagulation parameters and t-PA/PAI balance in orthotopic liver transplantation. *Thrombosis Research*, 1989; **55**: 319–28.

49. Porte RJ, Bontempo FA, Knot EAR, Lewis JH, Kang YG, and Starzl T. Systemic effects of tissue plasminogen activator associated fibrinolysis and its relation to thrombin generation in orthotopic liver transplantation. *Transplantation*, 1989; **47**: 978–84.

50. Himmelreich G, Hundt K, Isenberg C, Bechstein WO, Neuhaus P, and Riess H. Thrombocytopenia and platelet dysfunction in orthotopic liver transplantation. *Seminars in Thrombosis and Haemostasis*, 1993; **19**: 209–12.

51. Plevak DJ, *et al*. Thrombocytopenia after liver transplantation. *Transplantation Proceedings*, 1988, **20** (Suppl. 1): 630–3.

52. Porte RJ, *et al*. Role of the donor liver in the origin of platelet disorders and hyperfibrinolysis in liver transplantation. *Journal of Hepatology*, 1994; **21**: 592–600.

53. Lewis JH, Bontempo FA, Kang YG, Spero JA, Ragni MV, and Starzl TE. Intraoperative coagulation changes in liver transplantation. In Winter PM, Kang YG, eds. *Hepatic transplantation*. New York: Praeger, 1986: 142–50.

54. Busuttil RW, Brenis JJ, and Hiatt JR. Pediatric liver transplantation. In Maddrey WC, ed. *Transplantation of the liver*. New York: Elsevier Science, 1988: 309–30.

55. Wilde JT, Cooper P, Kennedy HJ, Triger DR, and Preston FE. Coagulation disturbances following ascites recirculation. *Journal of Hepatology*, 1990; **10**: 217–22.

56. Schwartz ML, Swaim WR, and Vogel SB. Coagulopathy following peritoneovenous shunting. *Surgery*, 1979, **85**: 671–6.

57. Cadroy Y *et al*. Evaluation of six markers of haemostatic system in normal pregnancy and pregnancy complicated by hypertension or pre-eclampsia. *British Journal of Obstetrics and Gynaecology*, 1993; **100**: 416–20.

58. McCrae KR, Samuels P, and Schreiber AD. Pregnancy-associated thrombocytopenia: pathogenesis and management. *Blood*, 1992; **80**: 2697–714.

59. De Boer K, Buller HR, Ten Cate JW, and Treffers PE. Coagulation studies in the syndrome of haemolysis, elevated liver enzymes and low platelets. *British Journal of Obstetrics and Gynaecology*, 1991; **98**: 42–7.

60. Wallenburg HCS. Changes in the coagulation system and platelets in pregnancy-induced hypertension and preeclampsia. In Sharp F, Symonds EM, eds. *Hypertension and pregnancy*. Ithaca, NY: Perinatology Press, 1987: 227–44.

61. Bernuau J, Levardon M, and Huisse MG. La stéatose hépatique aiguë gravidique: une maladie aisément curable. *Gastroenterologie Clinique et Biologique*, 1987; **11**: 128–32.

62. Pockros PJ, Peters RL, and Reynolds TB. Idiopathic fatty liver of pregnancy: findings in ten cases. *Medicine*, 1984; **63**: 1–10.

63. Schwarz R. Clinical studies using antithrombin III in patients with acquired antithrombin III deficiency. *Seminars in Hematology*, 1994; **31**: 52–9.

64. Hadengue A, Denninger MH, Shouval D, Erlinger S, and Benhamou JP. Budd–Chiari Syndrome due to hepatic vein thrombosis: underestimated protein C and protein S deficiencies. *Hepatology*, 1992; **16**: Abstr. 819.

65. Bowie EJ and Owen CA. Clinical and laboratory diagnosis of hemorrhagic disorders. In Ratnoff OD and Forbes CD, eds. *Disorders of haemostasis*. Philadelphia: WB Saunders, 1991:48–74.

66. Burroughs AK and Blake J. Bleeding time in patients with hepatic cirrhosis. *British Medical Journal*, 1990; **301**: 494–5.

67. Hirsh J and Poller L. The International Normalized Ratio. *Archives of Internal Medicine*, 1994; **154**: 282–8.

68. Van Thiel DH, Gavaler JS, Wright H, and Tzakis A. Liver biopsy. Its safety and complications as seen at a liver transplant center. *Transplantation*, 1993; **55**: 1087–90.

69. Garcia-Tsao G and Boyer JL. Outpatient liver biopsy: how safe is it? *Annals of Internal Medicine*, 1993, **118**: 150–3.

70. Edmondson HA and Schiff L. Needle biopsy of the liver. In Schiff L, ed. *Diseases of the liver*. 4th edn. Philadelphia: JB Lippincott, 1975:247–63.

71. Menghini G and Ghergo GF. Needle biopsy of the liver. In Bockus HL, ed. *Gastroenterology*. Philadelphia: WB Saunders, 1976; III:88–112.

72. Isselbacher K and La Mont JT. Diagnostic procedures in liver disease. In Harrison TR, ed. *Principles of internal medicine*. New York: McGraw Hill, 1977:1580–4.

73. Sherlock S. Needle biopsy of the liver. In Sherlock S, ed. *Diseases of the liver and biliary system*. 7th edn. London: Blackwell Scientific, 1985: 28–37.

74. Cederbaum AI, Blatt PM, and Roberts HR. Intravascular coagulation with use of human prothrombin complex concentrates. *Annals of Internal Medicine*, 1976, **84**: 683–7.

75. Lusher JM. Myocardial infarction and stroke: is the risk increased by desmopressin? In Mariani G, ed. *Desmopressin in bleeding disorders*. New York: Plenum Press, 1993:347–53.

76. Bechstein WO, *et al*. Aprotinin in orthotopic liver transplantation. *Seminars in Thrombosis and Hemostasis*, 1993; **19**: 262–7.

77. Hull RD and Pineo GF. Treatment of venous thromboembolism with low molecular weight heparins. *Hematology/Oncology Clinics of North America*, 1992; **6**: 1095–103.

78. Frank JW, Kamath PS, and Stanson AW. Budd–Chiari syndrome: early intervention with angioplasty and thrombolytic therapy. *Mayo Clinic Proceedings*, 1994; **69**: 877–81.

79. Bizollon T, Bissuel F, Detry L, and Trepo C. Fibrinolytic therapy for portal vein thrombosis. *Lancet*, 1991; **337**: 1416.

80. Assouline D, *et al*. Successful systemic thrombolysis of hepatic vein thrombosis in a patient with promyelocytic leukemia treated with all-trans retinoic acid. *American Journal of Hematology*, 1995, **48**: 291–2.

25.5 Effect of liver disease on the gastrointestinal tract

R. W. Chapman and Peter W. Angus

Disorders involving every part of the gastrointestinal tract have been described in patients with acute and chronic liver disease. While lesions such as oesophageal varices can be clearly linked to the direct pathophysiological effects of liver disease, in many cases the reasons for the association between liver disease and the gut are less clear. This chapter describes the gastrointestinal syndromes that can occur in patients with liver diseases, listed according to the major organ or area involved.

Mouth

Examination of the lips and mouth may reveal a number of abnormalities in patients with liver disease. Inspection of the mucous membranes may detect jaundice, anaemia, or dehydration; palatal petechiae indicate thrombocytopenia or septicaemia; while the presence of foetor hepaticus suggests hepatic encephalopathy.

Oral xanthomas occasionally develop as a complication of hypercholesterolaemia in patients with chronic cholestatic liver disease. The lesions are flat, plaque-like, and irregular; they may be found under the tongue, on the buccal mucosa, or in areas of angular cheilitis.[1] Oral lichen planus has been described in a number of patients with primary biliary cirrhosis (Graham-Brown, BrJDermatol, 1982; 106:699), but it is unclear whether this is a chance association. Several patients with primary biliary cirrhosis have developed lichen planus-like lesions in the mouth as part of a hypersensitivity reaction to penicillamine (Seehafer, ArchDermatol, 1981; 117:140). Telangiectasias in and around the mouth may give a clue to the presence of hepatic angiomas in patients with Osler–Weber–Rendu syndrome (hereditary telangiectasia) and are also occasionally seen in patients with primary biliary cirrhosis and the **CREST** (Calcinosis, Raynaud's, (o)Esophagitis, Sclerodactyly, Telangiectasia) syndrome.

The majority of patients with primary biliary cirrhosis (approximately 75 per cent) develop keratoconjunctivitis sicca or Sjögren's syndrome (Alarcon-Segovia, AnnIntMed, 1973; 79:31; Crewe, Gastro, 1980; 78:1437). Xerostomia usually occurs late in the disease. Apart from dryness of the mouth, patients may develop cheilosis, buccal ulceration, fissuring of the tongue, and enlargement of the parotid salivary glands. Biopsy of the salivary glands reveals lymphocyte infiltration, ductal hyperplasia, and acinar destruction.[1] As in the liver, the disease is probably initiated by immunological damage to duct endothelium.

Oesophagus

Although varices are the most important oesophageal complication of cirrhosis, a number of other oesophageal disorders may occur in patients with cirrhosis (the pathophysiology and management of varices are discussed in Section 7).

The frequency and pathological importance of gastro-oesophageal reflux in cirrhosis are controversial. In patients with massive ascites, one might expect raised intra-abdominal pressure to predispose to reflux of gastric contents into the oesophagus. Early studies suggested that reflux was common in cirrhotics, particularly in the presence of ascites (Simpson, Gastro, 1968; 55:17; Nebel, DigDisSci, 1977; 22:1101). A number of subsequent investigations failed to find either evidence of impaired function of the lower oesophageal sphincter or increased reflux in cirrhotics, whether or not ascites was present (Van Thiel, Gastro, 1977; 72:842).[2] Most of these results were based on measurements of the pressure at the lower oesophageal sphincter or short-term recording of oesophageal pH, both of which have relatively poor specificity and sensitivity for detecting acid reflux. During 3 h of postprandial monitoring of oesophageal pH, episodes of acid reflux were considerably more common in non-drinking alcoholic cirrhotics than controls; episodes of reflux were more prolonged in cirrhotics than in non-cirrhotics with known reflux; in contrast to previous studies, no link was found between gastro-oesophageal reflux and the presence of ascites.[3]

Since alcohol itself causes relaxation of the lower oesophageal sphincter and impairs oesophageal acid clearance (Kaufman, Gut, 1978; 19:336), oesophageal reflux is likely to be more severe when alcoholic cirrhotic patients are actively drinking. Importantly, whether or not acid reflux is increased in cirrhotic patients, it does not appear to contribute to variceal haemorrhage, since the frequency of variceal bleeding does not appear to be influenced by the presence or severity of acid reflux.[2,3] Oesophageal reflux appears to play an important part in the pathogenesis of persistent oesophageal ulceration following injection sclerotherapy of oesophageal ulcers. These ulcers are resistant to treatment with H_2-antagonists but respond to omeprazole.[4]

Approximately 4 per cent of patients with primary biliary cirrhosis have evidence of scleroderma.[5] Usually this takes the form of the CREST syndrome and most of these patients have positive anticentromere antibodies.[4] Oesophageal involvement with scleroderma results in atrophy of the muscle coats, dilatation of the lumen, and loss of tone in the lower sphincter. The principal symptoms are of lower oesophageal dysphagia and acid reflux, which may be complicated by peptic structure. Telangiectasias of the oesophagus have been described in patients with primary biliary cirrhosis with the CREST syndrome, and these lesions may occasionally be a source of bleeding (Reynolds, AmJMed, 1971; 50:302).

Endoscopic injection sclerotherapy for oesophageal varices in patients with cirrhosis may produce a number of local oesophageal complications (Ayres, AnnIntMed, 1983; 98:900; Jeffe, BrJSurg, 1984; 71:85). Ulceration is common and may be complicated by bleeding. Strictures may develop in the lower third of the oesophagus but are usually amenable to simple dilatation. Perforation after flexible endoscopic sclerotherapy usually results from full-thickness necrosis of the oesophageal wall by sclerosant. Fortunately this complication is rare and, if recognized early, usually settles with conservative management (Shemesh, ArchSurg, 1986; 121: 243).

Endoscopic ligation of oesophageal varices appears to be associated with a lower risk of local oesophageal complications than variceal sclerosis. Bleeding from ulcers at the site of banding has been described, but severe oesophageal ulceration and stricturing appear to be much less common.[6] There may be temporary dysphagia after the procedures, presumably due to partial occlusion of the oesophageal lumen by the banded varix. Until recently, endoscopic variceal ligation required the use of an overtube to facilitate multiple passages of the endoscope for the placement of each ligation band. The overtube has been associated with injuries to the upper oesophagus and hypopharynx including laceration, bleeding, dissection, and perforation.[7]

Stomach and duodenum
Portal hypertensive gastropathy

After variceal haemorrhage the gastric mucosa is the most common source of upper gastrointestinal bleeding in patients with cirrhosis and portal hypertension.[8–10] In the past, gastric mucosal bleeding in patients with liver disease was attributed to a range of lesions including 'haemorrhagic gastritis', 'diffuse gastric erosions', 'gastric red spots' or 'gastric petechiae'.[8–12] It is now recognized that mucosal lesions such as these are very common in cirrhosis, and are features of a distinct entity now known as portal hypertensive gastropathy.[12–14]

The changes of portal hypertensive gastropathy are most marked in the mucosa of the fundus and body of the stomach. The endoscopic appearances include a pattern of fine, erythematous speckling or 'scarlatina' type rash, reddening and streaks, and a fine, white, reticular mosaic pattern separating red, oedematous mucosa with an appearance 'like snake skin'.[12–15] Severe gastropathy is characterized by the presence discrete gastric red spots ('cherry red spots') and areas of diffuse, haemorrhagic mucosal change ('haemorrhagic gastritis').[12,15] In large endoscopic studies of asymptomatic cirrhotic patients, more than 50 per cent have had features of portal hypertensive gastropathy, the most frequent finding being the characteristic mosaic pattern or snake skin-like appearance in the proximal stomach.[15,16]

There is no clear relation between the severity of portal hypertensive gastropathy and the size of oesophageal varices, the degree of hepatic dysfunction, or the level of portal hypertension.[12,15] Although gastropathy occurs in patients with extrahepatic portal venous thrombosis, the changes are found less frequently than in those with cirrhosis. Portal hypertensive gastropathy is more common in patients who have undergone variceal sclerotherapy.[12,16]

The pathophysiology of this condition is incompletely understood. The term 'gastritis' was commonly used to describe the appearance of the gastric mucosa in cirrhosis, but biopsies do not usually show inflammatory-cell infiltration.[12,17] The characteristic histological findings are suggestive of vascular congestion, with dilation and tortuosity of submucosal veins and ectasia of mucosal capillaries and venules.[12] Because the vascular changes in portal hypertensive gastropathy are largely submucosal, deep mucosal biopsies may be needed to demonstrate the characteristic changes. Increased total gastric blood flow has been demonstrated in experimental portal hypertension and in patients with portal hypertensive gastropathy.[13,18] The mucosal changes appear to result from a combination of increased total gastric blood flow, changes in blood-flow distribution, and stasis as a result of the increase in portal vascular resistance and portal venous congestion. These vascular changes are associated with a range of functional mucosal defects that predispose the portal hypertensive gastric mucosa to injury from agents such aspirin, bile acids, and alcohol.[13] Once the mucosa is breached the increase in total gastric blood flow may contribute to the risk of significant bleeding. No significant association has been found with *Helicobacter pylori* infection.[19]

The reported frequency with which portal hypertensive gastropathy has apparently caused acute upper gastrointestinal bleeding in cirrhotic patients ranges between 10 and 50 per cent; this wide range may largely be explained by variation in the timing of endoscopy and in the aetiology and severity of the liver disease in different studies.[8–10] Acute gastric bleeding normally occurs in those with severe gastropathy. Bleeding from the portal hypertensive gastric mucosa responds poorly to treatment with H_2-blockers, antacids or sucralfate.[16] Propranolol reportedly arrested active bleeding, reduced the risk of rebleeding from gastric mucosal lesions in cirrhotic patients, and improved the endoscopic grading of portal hypertensive gastropathy.[20] Portacaval shunting appears to reduce the risk of bleeding greatly and is an effective treatment for acute haemorrhage from portal hypertensive gastropathy,[21] but the procedure is associated with considerable operative risks and long-term side-effects. Although no large studies are available, several case reports have demonstrated the efficiency of the transjugular intrahepatic portosystemic stent shunt (TIPSS) in such cases.

A number of studies describe a pattern of mucosal vascular abnormality in patients with portal hypertension in which the predominant feature is vascular ectasia affecting the antral mucosa.[15–22] The characteristic appearance is of prominent, friable, longitudinal red stripes on the antral mucosal radiating out from the pylorus giving a 'watermelon stripe' appearance, or a picture of fused, flat, red mucosal lesions. The terms gastric antral vascular ectasia (**GAVE**) or 'watermelon stomach' have been used to describe this lesion. While the classical appearance of portal hypertensive gastropathy is seen in patients with portal hypertension, GAVE also occurs in patients without liver disease or portal hypertension.[23] Whether, in cirrhotic patients, this endoscopic pattern of mucosal abnormality represents an entity that is distinct from severe portal hypertensive gastropathy is unclear.[15,22] Bleeding from antral lesions is common and is difficult to control with pharmacological therapy or portal decompression.

Acute gastric erosions

Upper gastrointestinal bleeding is also a significant problem in patients with acute liver failure. These patients commonly develop acute erosions of the oesophagus, stomach, or duodenum; the presence of abnormal clotting contributes to the risk of bleeding. Severe upper-gastrointestinal bleeding from erosions was reportedly the cause of death in almost one-fifth of these patients (Bailey, Gut, 1976; 17:389). To prevent this potentially devastating complication, H_2-antagonists should be given routinely to reduce gastric acidity (McDougall, Lancet, 1977; i: 617). Non-steroidal anti-inflammatory drugs must be avoided.

Peptic ulcer

The prevalence of peptic ulcer appears to be increased in cirrhosis: in large series, ulcers were reported in between 10 and 16 per cent of patients with cirrhosis.[24–27] Although the prevalence of peptic ulcer is considerably lower than this in the general community, [22–28] epidemiological studies of peptic ulcer in cirrhotics have generally not included an adequate control group. Thus factors such as age, sex distribution, smoking habits, and frequency of upper gastrointestinal investigation of the cirrhotic population, rather than liver disease itself, may in part explain an apparently higher risk of peptic ulceration than in the community as a whole. As in the general population, duodenal ulcers are more common than gastric ulcers,[26] but there is some evidence that the normal male predominance in duodenal ulcer is lost.[25] Although peptic ulcers appear to be common in patients with cirrhosis, they are often asymptomatic and are identified as the cause of only about 6 to 16 per cent of acute upper-gastrointestinal haemorrhage. [9,26, 27]

There is some evidence that the frequency of peptic ulcer varies among different forms of liver disease. In a study of 510 patients awaiting liver transplantation, duodenal ulceration was found in 12.2 per cent of alcoholics compared to 4.2 per cent of non-alcoholics; the prevalence of gastric ulcers was also higher in the alcoholic group.[29, 30] While in one early series, peptic ulcers were found in more than 30 per cent of patients with primary biliary cirrhosis, a much lower incidence was reported in a more recent series.[26] This may reflect reduced use of analgesic and anti-inflammatory drugs in these patients. Patients treated with corticosteroids for hepatitis B-negative chronic active hepatitis appear to be at low risk of developing peptic ulceration.[26]

Although in animal experiments, basal and maximal stimulated outputs of gastric acid are markedly increased following the construction of a portocaval shunt, in man there is little evidence of a similar affect on acid secretion.[31] Early reports that portocaval anastomosis increased the risk of peptic ulceration in cirrhotic patients were not substantiated by a large, prospective, controlled study, which showed that ulcers occurred no more frequently in shunted patients than controls with equally advanced liver disease.[24] Moreover, this study demonstrated that portocaval shunting did not exacerbate pre-existing ulcer.

If cirrhosis does predispose to peptic ulceration, the mechanism is unclear. It has been suggested that there may be impaired hepatic clearance of gastrin or other compounds that stimulate the acid secretion. Although there is little evidence that gastric acid secretion in the cirrhotic population as a whole is increased compared with controls,[31] cirrhotics with duodenal ulcers have higher gastric acid secretion than those without ulcers. While there is increasing evidence that in portal hypertension the abnormal mucosal circulation may predispose the gastric mucosa to injury, there are no data at present to indicate that portal hypertensive vasculopathy contributes to the development of chronic peptic ulcer. *Helicobacter pylori* infection is central to the pathogenesis of peptic ulceration. It is unclear whether the increased rate of peptic ulceration in cirrhotics can be explained by higher rates of *Helicobacter* colonization.[19] Nor is it clear whether eradication of *Helicobacter* returns the risk of peptic ulceration in cirrhotics to that in the general population.

Pancreas

Excess alcohol causes injury in both the liver and pancreas; it is not surprising, therefore, that evidence of pancreatic damage is commonly found in patients with alcoholic liver disease. In a recent review of 1022 patients who developed alcoholic liver disease, pancreatitis was found in 28 per cent at autopsy.[32] Other autopsy studies have found an equal or even greater prevalence of pancreatic disease in alcoholic cirrhotics (Sobel, Gastro, 1963; 45:341; Morin, Gastro, 1969; 56:727), while studies of pancreatic function in largely alcoholic cirrhotic populations have reported abnormalities in 40 per cent or more of patients (Van Goidsenmoven, AmJDigDis, 1963; 8: 160; Zieve, AmJDigDis, 1967; 12:303). The most common pathological finding in these patients is chronic fibrotic pancreatitis; of these approximately one-third have calcific change. Acute pancreatic damage is found less commonly and may represent an early stage in the development of chronic disease (Van Thiel, Gastro, 1981; 81: 594).[32] The presence of pancreatic damage does not seem to be related to the severity of alcoholic liver disease.[32] Indeed, why some alcoholic patients develop severe pancreatitis but have little or no liver disease, while others with advanced alcoholic liver disease have little evidence of pancreatic damage, is unknown.

Signs of pancreatic damage are also commonly found in patients with primary biliary cirrhosis. Abnormal pancreatograms are found in more than 40 per cent of these patients and many have elevated serum pancreatic isoamylase or immunoreactive trypsin (Fonseca, JClinPath, 1986; 39:638).[32] Immunoreactive trypsin and the flow rates of duodenal juice in response to secretin–pancreozymin stimulation are significantly reduced. Since these abnormalities of pancreatic structure and function were closely linked to the presence of Sjögren's syndrome, it was suggested that, in primary biliary cirrhosis, pancreatic hyposecretion is a component of the sicca or dry gland complex.[33] Other studies provide evidence that cholestasis itself may inhibit exocrine pancreatic secretion in these patients.[34, 35] Overt exocrine pancreatic failure, severe enough to produce steatorrhoea, appears to be very uncommon.[34,35]

Endoscopic pancreatography is abnormal in approximately 10 to 50 per cent of those with primary sclerosing cholangitis.[33] The changes seen on pancreatography vary from isolated strictures of the main pancreatic duct to classical chronic pancreatitis. However, these changes are seldom associated with clinically significant impairment of pancreatic function (Palmer, Gut, 1984; 25:424).[33]

Serum pancreatic amylase isoenzymes and pancreatic lipase are elevated in 34 per cent of patients with fulminant hepatic failure.[36] Although the presence of encephalopathy makes it difficult to confirm the diagnosis of pancreatitis clinically in these patients, approximately one-third are found to have acute pancreatic damage at autopsy.[37] While in other clinical conditions acute pancreatitis carries a significant mortality, at present there is no evidence that the finding of 'biochemical pancreatitis' worsens the prognosis of patients with acute liver failure.[36]

The pathogenesis of pancreatitis in fulminant hepatic failure is not understood. The acute pancreatitis that occasionally occurs in those with acute viral hepatitis has been attributed to either direct or immune-mediated cytopathic effects of the virus (Morante, PostgradMedJ, 1986; 62:407).[34,37] Although such effects may be important in those with viral hepatitis, it does not explain the occurrence of pancreatitis in hepatic failure caused by paracetamol overdose or halothane toxicity.[36]

Small-bowel function/malabsorption

Fat malabsorption is common in patients with chronic liver disease. Approximately 50 per cent of adults and more than 90 per cent of children with various types of cirrhosis have increased faecal fat excretion (Burke, BMJ, 1966; 2:1050; Marin, Gastro, 1969; 56:727; Weber, Pediat, 1972; 50:73).[38,39] Although, in most of these patients, steatorrhoea is mild (less than 15 g/day), in about 10 per cent there is severe steatorrhoea with faecal fat excretion exceeding 25 to 30 g daily (Mavin, Gastro, 1969; 56:727).[39]

A number of factors may be responsible for fat malabsorption in patients with liver disease. Bile-acid uptake, synthesis, and secretion are all impaired in patients with significant parenchymal liver damage or cholestasis.[40] As a result, in some patients, intra-duodenal bile-acid concentrations may fall to levels that are insufficient to achieve adequate solubilization and micellar incorporation of dietary lipid, cholesterol, and fat-soluble vitamins. This mechanism appears to be largely responsible for steatorrhoea in patients with non-alcoholic cirrhosis and chronic cholestatic liver disease.[34,35] Indeed, in these patients, fat malabsorption is usually restricted to those with subnormal duodenal bile-acid concentrations and impaired micellar lipid incorporation.[39] Although pancreatic exocrine secretion may be reduced in patients with primary biliary cirrhosis, this seems to be of far less importance in the pathogenesis of fat malabsorption than failure of bile-acid secretion, since even in patients with severe steatorrhoea the pancreatic output of lipase is not sufficiently reduced to limit intestinal lipolysis.[34,35]

There is little evidence that liver disease itself significantly affects the absorptive capacity of the small-bowel mucosa. A number of investigations have failed to detect any consistent abnormalities of small-bowel structure or function in non-alcoholic patients with portal hypertension and malabsorption (Astaldi, AmJDigDis, 1963; 5:603; Losowsky, Gastro, 1968; 56:589; Mavin, Gastro, 1969; 56:727). Furthermore, in cirrhotic patients, portocaval anastomosis produces no substantial change in intestinal absorption of fat or protein (Fisher, AnnSurg, 1968; 187:41). In contrast, the venous and lymphatic obstruction that occurs in Budd–Chiari syndrome

may cause structural abnormalities of the small-bowel mucosa and protein-losing enteropathy (Tsuchiya, Gastro, 1978; 75:114).

A number of studies report an association between coeliac disease and primary biliary cirrhosis (Logan, Lancet, 1978; i: 230; Olsson, ScaJGastr, 1982; 17:625). Dermatitis herpetiformis and intestinal villous atrophy have also been described in patients with primary biliary cirrhosis (Gabrielsen, Dermatologica, 1985; 170:31; Walton, ClinExpDerm, 1987; 12:46). It seems unlikely that this association is due to a direct effect of the liver disease on the small bowel, nor is it likely that coeliac disease causes primary biliary cirrhosis. Malabsorption and villous atrophy respond to gluten restriction in the normal way, but there is no improvement in the liver disease (Olsson, ScaJGastr, 1982; 17:625). Coeliac disease has now also been reported in three patients with primary sclerosing cholangitis; whether this is more than a chance association is as yet unclear (Hay, AnnIntMed, 1988; 109:713).

In non-alcoholic cirrhotics and patients with cholestatic liver disease, malabsorption is usually limited to fat and fat-soluble vitamins. However, in patients with alcoholic liver disease there may be a mixed malabsorption syndrome, in part related to the effects of chronic alcohol abuse on the gut and in part due to the underlying liver disease. In actively drinking chronic alcoholics, jejunal perfusion experiments have demonstrated marked malabsorption of sodium and water, and a similar effect was reproduced in normal volunteers following chronic infusion of the jejunum with alcohol (Krasner, Gut, 1976; 17:245; Mekhjian, Gastro, 1977; 72: 1280). Alcohol has also been shown to deplete brush-border enzymes (lactose, sucrose, and alkaline phosphatase) and appears directly to inhibit absorption of glucose, amino acids, and vitamin B_{12} (Van Thiel, Gastro, 1981; 81:594). Poor diet, malnutrition, and deficiencies of substances such as folate and magnesium may also contribute to the impairment of intestinal absorptive function in alcoholics (Van Thiel, Gastro, 1981; 81:594).[38]

Whatever the cause, much of the diarrhoea and malabsorption resolves with alcohol withdrawal and adequate nutrition, but in those with established alcoholic cirrhosis, steatorrhoea often persists long after alcohol consumption has ceased. This may, in part, be due to continuing deficiency of intestinal bile acids. However, in alcoholic cirrhotics, chronic pancreatic disease is common (Sobel, Gastro, 1963; 45:341)[32] and in many of these patients chronic severe steatorrhoea may be primarily pancreatic in origin; improvement normally follows pancreatic enzyme replacement therapy (Mavin, Gastro, 1969; 56:727).

Patients with liver disease may develop deficiencies of fat-soluble vitamins as a result of poor micellar solubilization and absorption of these compounds; those with inadequate diets, and jaundiced patients with chronic cholestatic disease, appear to be particularly at risk. Hepatic vitamin A stores are large and vitamin A deficiency is usually only seen in patients with long-standing liver disease. Vitamin A deficiency is mainly described in patients with primary biliary cirrhosis, the lowest levels being found in the most severely cholestatic. Impaired dark adaptation is the major clinical finding, while true night blindness is relatively uncommon (Herlong, Hepatol, 1981; 1:348; Walt, BMJ, 1984; 288:1030).

Low serum vitamin E is also mainly found in patients with chronic cholestasis.[40] Vitamin E-deficient children with chronic liver disease develop a typical neurological syndrome that responds to parenteral vitamin E (Rosenblum, NEJM, 1981; 304:503). However, even in patients with primary biliary cirrhosis who have severe vitamin E deficiency, clinically apparent neurological problems are uncommon.[41] A sensorimotor neuropathy has been noted in some of these patients, but this responds poorly to vitamin E replacement.[41]

Vitamin K stores in the body are small and readily depleted by poor diet and impaired absorption. Vitamin K deficiency may be largely responsible for abnormal clotting in patients with cholestasis and is readily correctable with parenteral vitamin K. In patients with established parenchymal liver disease, there may be only a partial response to vitamin K replacement, since hepatic synthesis of clotting factors is also likely to be impaired.

Vitamin D is obtained from the diet, but can also be synthesized by ultraviolet irradiation of the skin. Vitamin D deficiency may develop in patients with chronic cholestatic or parenchymal liver disease, but it seems likely that this is entirely due to impaired intestinal absorption. Poor exposure to sunlight, inadequate diet, excess urinary loss of vitamin D metabolites, and interruption of the enterohepatic circulation of 2-hydroxyvitamin D may be further factors.[42,45] 25-Hydroxylation of vitamin D does not appear to be significantly reduced in patients with chronic liver disease. Poor intestinal absorption of both calcium and vitamin D has been demonstrated in patients with chronic cholestasis. Malabsorption of calcium may be partly due to vitamin D deficiency, but precipitation of calcium by excess luminal fat may also be important.[42]

Although early studies suggested a high prevalence of osteomalacia in patients with cirrhosis, recent reports, using more rigorous diagnostic criteria, indicate that its prevalence is relatively low.[42,43] Jaundiced patients with chronic cholestasis appear to be most at risk. Osteomalacia is prevented in these patients by vitamin D prophylaxis and the disease responds well to both oral and parenteral vitamin D (Reed, Gastro, 1980; 78:512). It is now evident that osteoporosis is the major cause of bone problems in patients with chronic liver disease (Herlong, Gastro, 1982; 83: 103).[42,43] The pathogenesis of osteoporosis in these patients is unclear. It seems that it is not simply due to vitamin D deficiency and calcium malabsorption. Osteoporosis is not prevented by vitamin D prophylaxis, and at present there are no clearly established guidelines for treatment or prophylaxis.

Colon

A range of changes are described in the colonic mucosa in cirrhotic patients, including mucosal oedema, erythematous telangiectatic macular lesions, spider naevi-like or angiodysplastic lesions, and non-specific colitis. The changes may be patchy or diffuse, and, at colonoscopy, can be found in between 30 and 50 per cent of patients with portal hypertension. The term 'portal hypertensive colopathy' has been used to describe these mucosal lesions.[15,44] On histological examination, the findings are similar to those of portal hypertensive gastropathy, with the major features being dilated mucosal capillaries, a thickened basement membrane, and oedema without mucosal inflammation.[15] The importance of the portal hypertensive colonic mucosa as a source of overt gastrointestinal bleeding or anaemia is unclear.

In large colonoscopic series, rectal varices are described in between 40 and 80 per cent of patients with portal hypertension.[15,

44] The wide variation in the frequency of reporting these lesions may reflect problems in differentiating varices from haemorrhoids. Haemorrhoids do not appear to be more common in patients with portal hypertension and, in contrast to rectal varices, are rarely a source of major gastrointestinal haemorrhage. The key to differentiating rectal varices from haemorrhoids is the finding of large, feeding, collateral veins that commence well above the anal verge.[44] Lower-gastrointestinal bleeding has been reported in 1 to 4 per cent of patients with rectal varices. A number of approaches can be used to control bleeding from rectal varices, including local sclerotherapy or banding, and portal decompression by surgery or TIPSS.

References

1. Shaffner F and Bach N. Gastointestinal syndromes in primary biliary cirrhosis. *Seminars in Liver Disease*, 1988; **8**: 263–71.
2. Eckardt VF and Grace ND. Gastro-oesophageal reflux and bleeding oesophageal varices. *Gastroenterology*, 1979; **76**: 39–42.
3. Arsene D, *et al.* Gastro-oesophageal reflux and alcoholic cirrhosis. *Journal of Hepatology*, 1987; **4**: 250–8.
4. Gimson A, Polson R. Westby D, and Williams R. Omeprazole in the management of intractable oesophageal ulceration following injection sclerotherapy. *Gastroenterology*, 1990; **99**: 1829–31.
5. Powell FC, Schroeter AL, and Dickson ER. Primary biliary cirrhosis and the CREST syndrome: a report of 22 cases. *Quarterly Journal of Medicine*, 1987; **62**: 75–82.
6. Laine L and Cook D. Endoscopic ligation compared with sclerotherapy for treatment of oesophageal variceal bleeding. *Annals of Internal Medicine*, 1995; **123**: 280–7.
7. Holderman WH, Etzkorn KD, Patel SA, and Watkins JL. Endoscopic findings and overtube related complications associated with oesophageal variceal ligation. *Journal of Clinical Gastroenterology*, 1995; **21**: 91–4.
8. Thomas E, Rosenthal WD, Rymer W, and Katz D. Upper gastrointestinal haemorrhage in patients with alcoholic liver disease and oesophageal varices. *American Journal of Gastroenterology*, 1977; **72**: 623–9.
9. Mitchell CJ and Jewell DP. The diagnosis of the site of upper gastrointestinal haemorrhage in patients with portal hypertension. *Endoscopy*, 1977; **9**: 131–5.
10. Mitchell KJ, MacDougall BRD, Silk DBA, and Williams R. A prospective reappraisal of emergency endoscopy in patients with portal hypertension. *Scandinavian Journal of Gastroenterology*, 1982; **17**: 965–8.
11. Rector WG and Reynolds TB. Risk factors for haemorrhage from oesophageal varices and acute gastric erosions. *Clinics in Gastroenterology*, 1985; **14**: 139–53.
12. McCormick TT, *et al.* Gastric lesions in portal hypertension; inflammatory gastritis or congestive gastropathy. *Gut*, 1985; **26**: 1226–32.
13. Sarfeh IJ and Tarnawski A. Gastric mucosal vasculopathy in portal hypertension. *Gastroenterology*, 1987; **93**: 1129–31.
14. Baxter J. Dobbs B. Portal hypertensive gastropathy. *Journal of Gastroenterology and Hepatology*, 1988; **3**: 635–44.
15. Viggiano TR and Gostout CJ. Portal hypertensive intestinal vasculopathy: a review of the clinical, endoscopic and histological features. *American Journal of Gastroenterology*, 1992; **87**: 944–54.
16. Papazian A, *et al.* Portal hypertensive gastric mucosa: an endoscopic study. *Gut*, 1986; **27**: 1199–203.
17. Brown RS, *et al.* Gastritis and cirrhosis—no association. *Journal of Clinical Pathology*, 1981; **134**: 744–8.
18. Ohta M, *et al.* Portal and gastric mucosal haemodynamics in cirrhotic patients with portal hypertensive gastropathy. *Hepatology*, 1994; **20**: 1432–6.
19. Fraser AG, Pounder RE, and Burrough AK. Gastric secretion and peptic ulceration in cirrhosis. *Journal of Hepatology*, 1993; **19**: 171–82.
20. Hosking SW, Kennedy HJ, Seddon I, and Triger DR. The role of propranolol in congestive gastropathy of portal hypertension. *Hepatology*, 1987; **7**: 437–41.

21. Orloff MJ, Orloff MS, Orloff SL, and Haynes KS. Treatment of bleeding from portal hypertensive gastropathy by portacaval shunt. *Hepatology*, 1995; **21**: 1011–17.

22. Payen JL, *et al*. Severe portal hypertensive gastropathy and antral vascular ectasis are distinct entities in patients with cirrhosis. *Gastroenterology*, 1995; **108**: 138–44.

23. Jabbari M, *et al*. Gastric antral vascular ectasia; the watermelon stomach. *Gastroenterology*, 1984; **87**: 1165–70.

24. Phillips MM, Ramsby GR, and Conn HO. Portocaval anastomosis and peptic ulcer: a non-association. *Gastroenterology*, 1975; **68**: 121–31.

25. Tabaqchali S and Dawson AM. Peptic ulcer and gastric secretion in patients with liver disease. *Gut*, 1964; **5**: 417–21.

26. Kirk AP, Dooley JS, and Hunt RH. Peptic ulceration in patients with chronic liver disease. *Digestive Diseases and Sciences*, 1980; **25**: 756–60.

27. Fraser AG, Pounder RE, and Burrough AK. Gastric secretion and peptic ulceration in cirrhosis. *Journal of Hepatology*, 1993; **19**: 171–82.

28. Langman MJS and Cook AR. Gastric and duodenal ulcer and their associated diseases. *Lancet*, 1976; **i**: 680–3.

29. Rabinovitz M, *et al*. Combined upper and lower gastrointestinal endoscopy: a prospective study in alcoholic and non-alcoholic cirrhosis. *Alcoholism: Clinical and Experimental Research*, 1989, **13**: 790–4.

30. Rabinovitz M, *et al*. Prevalence of duodenal ulcer in cirrhotic males referred for liver transplantation. Does aetiology of cirrhosis make a difference? *Digestive Diseases and Sciences*, 1990; **35**: 321–6.

31. Lenz HJ, *et al*. Increased sensitivity of gastric acid secretion to gastric in cirrhotics with porto-caval shunt. *Journal of Clinical Investigation*, 1987; **79**: 1120–4.

32. Renner IG, Savage WT, Stace NH, Pantoja JL, Schultheis WM, and Peters RL. Pancreatitis associated with alcoholic liver disease. A review of 1022 autopsy cases. *Digestive Diseases and Sciences*, 1984; **29**: 593–9.

33. Epstein O, Chapman RWG, Lake-Bakaar C, Foo AY, Rosalki SB, and Sherlock S. The pancreas in primary biliary cirrhosis and primary sclerosing cholangitis. *Gastroenterology*, 1982; **83**: 1177–82.

34. Lanspa SJ, Chan ATH, Bell JS, Go VLW, Dickson RR, and Dimagno EP. Pathogenesis of steatorrhoea in primary biliary cirrhosis. *Hepatology*, 1985; **5**: 837–42.

35. Ros E, Garcia-Puges A, Reixach M, Cuso E, and Rodes J. Fat digestion and exocrine pancreatic function in primary biliary cirrhosis. *Gastroenterology*, 1984; **87**: 180–7.

36. Ede R, Moore KP, Marshall WJ, and Williams R. Frequency of pancreatitis in fulminant hepatic failure using isoenzyme markers. *Gut*, 1988; **29**: 778–81.

37. Ham JM and Fitzpatrick P. Acute pancreatitis in patients with acute hepatic failure. *Digestive Diseases and Sciences*, 1973; **18**:1079–83.

38. Linscheer WG. Malabsorption in cirrhosis. *American Journal of Clinical Nutrition*, 1970; **23**: 488–92.

39. Badley BWD, Murphy GMS, Bouchier IAD, and Sherlock S. Diminished micellar phase lipid in patients with chronic non-alcoholic liver disease and steatorrhoea. *Gastroenterology*, 1970; **58**: 781–9.

40. Heaton KW. Bile salts. In Wright R, Millward-Sadler GR, Alberti KGMM, and Karran S, eds. *Liver and biliary disease*. London: Baillière Tindall, 1985: 283–4.

41. Jeffrey GP, *et al*. Vitamin E deficiency and its clinical significance in adults with primary biliary cirrhosis and other forms of chronic liver disease. *Journal of Hepatology*, 1987; **4**: 307–17.

42. Compston JE. Hepatic osteodystrophy: vitamin D metabolism in patients with liver disease. *Gut*, 1995; **27**: 1073–90.

43. Diamond TH, Stiel D, Lunzer M, McDowell D, Ecckstein RP, and Posen S. Hepatic osteodystrophy. Static and dynamic bone histomorphometry and serum Gla-protein in 80 patients with chronic liver disease. *Gastroenterology*, 1989; **96**: 213–21.

44. Ganguly S, Sarin S, Bhatia V, and Lahoti D. The prevalence and spectrum of colonic lesions in patients with cirrhotic and non cirrhotic portal hypertension. *Hepatology*, 1995; **21**: 1226–31.

25.6 The effect of liver disease on the skin

J. Hughes and M. Rustin

Introduction

The cutaneous features of chronic liver disease are well known and include jaundice, palmar erythema, and spider naevi (see also Section 4). Jaundice is detected first in the sclerae and then affects the skin in a more widespread fashion. Occasionally, jaundice needs to be distinguished from carotenaemia, lycopenaemia (orange staining of the palms and soles secondary to drinking large amounts of tomato juice), or mepacrine or busulphan ingestion.

Palmar erythema starts on the hypothenar eminence in a speckled pattern and, if the associated liver disease progresses, it spreads to the finger pulps and becomes more confluent. Erythema may also be observed on the plantar aspects of the feet. The erythema has a pulsatile nature and blanches on pressure (Sarkany, ClinExpDerm, 1988; 13:152).

Patients who have multiple and disfiguring spider naevi can now be treated effectively with the tunable pulsed dye laser (Hruza, ArchDermatol, 1993; 129:1026). 'Paper-money skin' is the term used to describe fine thread-like capillaries which may be seen in association with spider naevi on the upper chest and back.

Leuchonychia or white nails may occur in up to 80 per cent of patients with chronic liver disease (Terry, Lancet, 1954; ii:248). This finding may be preceded by the formation of multiple transverse white bands across the nails (Jenson, ActDermVen, 1981; 63:261).

Pruritus (see also Section 4)

The pathogenesis of the pruritus of cholestasis is still unknown and therapy has been mainly empirical.[1] Pruritus is one of the most common and distressing symptoms associated with liver disease. It is a subjective phenomenon which may vary from patient to patient and occasionally be so severe that sleep is disturbed or it may lead to suicidal ideation. Intractable pruritus has been an indication for liver transplantation (Maddrey, Hepatol, 1988; 8:948). Skin changes are usually secondary to scratching, with widespread excoriations and, occasionally, with lichenification (thickening of the skin), nodular prurigo, or secondary infection arising from peturbation of the skin barrier.

The most commonly used drug for the pruritus of cholestasis is the anion exchange resin cholestyramine, with colestipol as an alternative. These resins work by binding to bile acids in the intestine, leading to increased excretion. Cholestyramine has been thought to enhance the faecal excretion of an unknown pruritogen secreted in bile

(Garbutt, JCI, 1972; 51:2781). Most patients respond to treatment initially, but often the beneficial effects are transient. Bloating, constipation, or diarrhoea are relatively common side-effects and may limit the use of these drugs.

Antihistamines are occasionally used and, although there is no evidence to suggest that histamine acts as a mediator in this form of pruritus, they may be helpful, possibly because of their sedative effect (Duncan, BMJ, 1984; ii:1289).

The hepatic enzyme-inducing antibiotic rifampicin has been used in the management of pruritus with good effect (Cynamon, Gastro, 1990; 98:1013). The mode of action by which rifampicin relieves itching is not known although, interestingly, it has been shown to increase the serum concentration of bile acids (Galeazzi, DigDisSci, 1980; 25:108).

The bile acid ursodeoxycholic acid has been reported to ameliorate pruritus in some patients with primary biliary cirrhosis (Poupon, NEJM, 1991; 324:1548). Methotrexate, also being evaluated in the treatment of primary biliary cirrhosis, has been found to be helpful if used for longer than 6 months (Bergasa, Hepatol, 1992; 16:516). Propofol, an anaesthetic agent used as a hypnotic, has also been reported to relieve itching (Borgeat, Gastro, 1993; 104:244).

Other uncontrolled trials of useful antipruritic treatments include metronidazole, phototherapy, carbamazepine, lignocaine, and androgens.[1]

Recently, evidence has emerged to suggest that the pruritus of cholestasis may not be associated with increased concentrations of bile acids but be mediated via a central effect, similar to that of opiates.[1] Studies using the opiate antagonists naloxone (Bergasa, Gastro, 1992; 102:544) and nalmefene (Thornton, BMJ, 1988; 297: 1501) in the treatment of cholestasis-induced pruritus have shown promising results. Naloxone is only available in parenteral form and is therefore unsuitable for long-term treatment. Nalmefene and naltrexone are administered orally and may be a useful therapeutic option once they have been fully evaluated.

Congenital diseases affecting the liver and the skin

Argininosuccinic aciduria

This rare autosomal recessive disease is caused by a deficiency of the enzyme argininosuccinase, leading to increased levels of arginosuccinic acid in the blood, urine, and cerebrospinal fluid. It is characterized by mental retardation, ataxia, seizures, hepatomegaly, and liver enzyme abnormalities (Brenton, JMentalDeficRes, 1974; 18:1). The hair of affected patients tends to be dry and brittle and trichorhexis nodosa may be noted on light or electron microscopy.

Ataxia telangiectasia

Ataxia telangectasia is an autosomal recessive disorder in which telangiectases of the skin, and other cutaneous features, are associated with progressive cerebellar ataxia and recurrent respiratory infections. There are abnormalities of humoral and cellular immunity, with thymic abnormalities and deficiencies of IgA, IgG, and IgE, and an increase in IgM (Peterson, ImmunolToday, 1989; 10:313). The abnormal gene locus is on chromosome 11q22–23.

Atrophy and dryness of the skin may be found in conjunction with the telangiectases and the hair may be prematurely grey. Pigmentary disorders and eczema are occasionally present (Cohen, JAmAcadDermatol, 1984; 10:431).

There is an increase in neoplastic disorders in patients and their families (Swift, NEJM, 1987; 316:1289). Lymphomas and leukaemias are the most common tumours but others have been reported, including hepatoma (Weinstein, ArchPathLabMed, 1985; 109:1000).

Alagille's syndrome (see also Section 26)

Alagille's syndrome, also known as arteriohepatic dysplasia, is a congenital anomaly comprising hepatic, ocular, facial, skeletal, and cardiac abnormalities. It is usually inherited as an autosomal dominant trait and the underlying genetic abnormality is proposed to be located on chromosome 20p (Hol, HumGenet, 1995; 95:687). There is a wide variation in expression of the disease. Abnormalities found in affected children may include cholestastic jaundice, with a decreased number of interlobular bile ducts; characteristic facies which include micrognathia, a prominent chin, and flattening of the nasal bone; pulmonary artery stenosis; and butterfly-like vertebrae (Weston, JAmAcadDermatol, 1987; 16:117). Pruritus, multiple xanthomas, and hyperlipidaemia may be present secondary to the chronic liver disease which leads to cirrhosis (Gottrand, Atheroscl, 1995; 115:233). The only definitive treatment available is liver transplantation (Cardona, Transpl, 1995; 60:339).

Anderson Fabry disease

This rare X-linked disorder is caused by a deficiency of α-galactosidase A, which results in the deposition of glycolipid in the skin and viscera. The first symptoms occurring between the ages of 5 and 15 years are lance-like excrutiating pains, vasomotor disturbances, and the appearance shortly after puberty of multiple dark red or black telangiectatic and occasionally scaly papules known as angiokeratomas. These are distributed in a variable fashion over the thighs, hips, buttocks, scrotum, and the periumbilical area. Angiokeratomas may be absent or less widespread in female carriers.

Cardiac abnormalities include conduction defects and coronary artery disease. The locus of the gene responsible for Anderson Fabry disease is in the middle of the long arm of the X chromosome. The condition may be diagnosed by blood enzyme analysis and the prognosis is poor, with death in the fourth or fifth decade from ischaemic heart disease, stroke, or renal failure.

Histiocytoses

Langerhans cell histiocytosis is the term that is now used to encompass the following four diseases—eosinophilic granuloma, Letterer–Siwe disease, histiocytosis X, and Hand–Schüller–Christian disease; they show overlapping features and are thought to represent part of a clinical spectrum. Langerhans cell histiocytosis is a rare disorder and there has been a debate as to whether there is a reactive or, less likely, a malignant accumulation of Langerhans cells in various tissues (Chu, Lancet, 1987; i:208). This disease usually affects children but can occasionally occur in adults. Cutaneous findings include a seborrhoeic dermatitis-like scalp eruption with greasy yellow-brown scales, which may also involve the trunk, groin, and perianal area. Flexural lesions may erode and ulcerate. In adults, a granuloma annulare-like appearance has been reported (Lichtenwald, ArchDermatol, 1991; 127:1545).

Treatment is usually with PUVA (psoralen with long-wavelength ultraviolet light) or monochemotherapy.

Gaucher's disease

Gaucher's disease (see Chapter 20.7) is a rare inborn error of metabolism, inherited in an autosomal recessive mode, causing an accumulation of complex lipid substances in macrophages within the liver, spleen, and bones (Balicki, Medicine, 1995; 74:305).

In the adult or type 1 form of Gaucher's disease, diffuse pigmentation secondary to haemosiderosis or deposition of melanin is usually noted. Easy tanning is characteristic and there may be multiple pigmented macules (Goldblatt, BrJDermatol, 1984; 111: 331). If marked liver involvement is a feature, then telangiectasia may be present.

Type II childhood Gaucher's is a more devastating form of the disorder and may present with severe ichthyosis. At birth, this form of skin involvement leads to the appearance known as 'collodion baby' where the infant is covered in a lamellar, hyperkeratotic membrane, of which Gaucher's may be a rare underlying cause (Lipson, ArchDisChild, 1991; 66:667). Treatment of this condition is with enzyme replacement.

Eruptive neonatal angiomatosis

Infants affected by this rare disorder develop multiple, dome-shaped, cutaneous haemangiomata at birth or during the first few weeks of life. Visceral and, in particular, hepatic involvement is common and the subsequent arteriovenous shunting may lead to high-output cardiac failure (Keller, Cutis, 1979; 23:295). Hepatic artery ligation or selective embolization may be necessary to improve cardiac function (Johnson, Pediat, 1984; 73:546). Complications such as biliary obstruction and the Kasabach–Merritt syndrome, in which a secondary consumptive coagulopathy develops, have been reported (Wishnik, JPaediat, 1978; 92:960).

Infections

Viral hepatitis

Hepatitis B

Most dermatological manifestations of hepatitis B infection are thought to be associated with immune complex formation (Gupta, JImmunol, 1984; 132:1223).

Hepatitis B is known to cause a serum sickness syndrome in 20 to 30 per cent of initial cases, usually 1 to 6 weeks before the onset of clinical hepatitis. Urticaria and angio-oedema are the commonest cutaneous manifestations, although petechiae, palpable purpura, and erythema multiforme-like lesions may occur, confirming an underlying vasculitic process (Popp, ArchIntMed, 1981; 141:623). Rarely, maculopapular and lichenoid eruptions and erythema nodosum have been associated with acute hepatitis B infection (Maggiore, JAmAcadDermatol, 1983; 9:602). Systemic manifestations include fever, arthralgia or arthritis, and headache.

Hepatitis B infection is one of the causes of Gianotti–Crosti syndrome, which is a papular eruption occurring in children in response to a viral trigger (Spear, ArchDermatol, 1984; 120: 891)(Plate 1). Dull red papules occur on the thighs and buttocks, then on the arms and finally the face. There is often an asymmetrical distribution. The skin lesions fade over a period of 2 to 8 weeks with mild desquamation. Generalized lymphadenopathy may be present and mild constitutional symptoms such as fever and lassitude often accompany the rash (Taieb, BrJDermatol, 1986; 115: 49). Treatment is symptomatic.

Hepatitis C

Hepatitis C virus (**HCV**) is associated with a number of dermatological disorders and, when patients present with these conditions, evidence of HCV infection must be sought as antiviral therapy may be of benefit.[2]

There have been numerous reports of essential mixed cryoglobulinaemia (type II or III) occuring in association with HCV, although no link has been found with type I cryoglobulinaemia (Agnello, NEJM, 1992; 327:1490). HCV RNA has been detected in more than 90 per cent of sera or cryoprecipitates from patients with essential mixed cryoglobulinaemia and is now considered as the main causative agent of this disorder (Lunel, Gastro, 1994; 106: 1291). The cutaneous manifestations of mixed cryoglobulinaemia are varied and include mild purpuric vasculitis, urticaria, ulcerative lesions with or without necrosis, Raynaud's phenomenon, and Sjögren's syndrome (Plate 2).[2]

Polyarteritis nodosa most commonly occurs in association with hepatitis B, but a few recent series have reported the prevalence of HCV to be as high as 5 to 20 per cent in patients with polyarteritis nodosa, suggesting that HCV rarely may be the cause of polyarteritis nodosa (Carson, JRheum, 1993; 20:304).

HCV infection has also been linked to the occurrence of porphyria cutanea tarda, and in a number of series of Southern European patients the prevalence of HCV markers has been as high as 76 to 95 per cent in patients with this condition (Herrero, Lancet, 1993; 341:788). Cases of porphyria cutanea tarda occurring in patients with HCV have been reported in the United States (Koester, JAmAcad Dermatol, 1994; 31:1054) and at lower prevalences elsewhere, for example in Ireland (Murphy, Lancet, 1993;

341:1534) and the Netherlands (Siersema, Liver, 1992; 12:56). All these prevalence rates are significantly higher than in the general population. The most likely hypothesis is that HCV-related liver disease can trigger porphyria cutanea tarda in genetically predisposed patients.

Recent data have suggested that lichen planus (see also Chapter 24.3) may be associated with HCV-related liver disease. There have been reports that the prevalence of HCV in patients with lichen planus ranges from 4 to 38 per cent (Cribier, JAmAcadDermatol, 1994; 31:1070), but it is not known whether these figures reflect the overall prevalence of HCV infection in the general population and this association remains to be proven. Similarly, a possible link between HCV and Sjögren's syndrome has been raised, although there is currently no direct evidence to substantiate this claim (Aceti, Lancet, 1992; 339:1425).

Human immunodeficiency virus

HIV infection commonly affects the liver and the skin and may present in numerous ways. Specific skin conditions are more common in HIV disease; seborrhoiec dermatitis is present in over 70 per cent of patients with the condition. Kaposi's sarcoma is a vascular tumour and an AIDS-defining diagnosis. Human herpes hominid virus 8 is thought to have an aetiological role in this malignancy. Infections and inflammatory and neoplastic disorders of the skin are all more common in HIV disease[3] and there are some shared features with the specific skin disorders found in patients who are immunosuppressed, for example after liver transplantation.

Bacterial (see also Chapter 13.1.1)

Severe systemic bacterial infections with septicaemia may lead to liver enzyme abnormalities and, in extreme cases, liver failure. If disseminated intravascular coagulation is a sequel to infection it may cause a rapid onset of extensive and symmetrical purpura of the extremities. Lesser changes include petechiae, purpuric papules, haemorrhagic bullae, and acral cyanosis. Meningococcaemia is estimated to cause a rash in between 40 and 90 per cent of cases. Early petechial skin lesions are caused by organisms in the capillary endothelium which together with disseminated intravascular coagulation may cause necrosis of the vessel wall or thrombosis (Bannister, JMedMicrobiol, 1988; 26:161). The earliest skin lesions may be pinpoint pink macules occurring in a widespread fashion including the palms and soles. This eruption is usually followed by purpura. Rarely, morbilliform or urticarial eruptions may arise in the early stages of infection (Baxter, Lancet, 1988; i:1166).

Syphilis

Hepatitis may occur as an uncommon complication of secondary syphilis. The skin manifestations of this stage of the disease are well known and include a widespread, symmetrical erythematous or copper-coloured maculopapular rash which characteristically affects the palms and soles. However, syphilis is the 'great imitator' in the skin as well as in other systems; the lesions may be psoriasiform or pustular, or may be so subtle that they pass unnoticed. In flexural areas the papules enlarge to form moist grey-white or pink discs known as condylomata lata, which harbour large numbers of organisms and are highly infectious. 'Snail-track ulcers' or superficial mucosal erosions form in one-third of patients with secondary syphilis and are also highly infectious. They may be found on the lips, tongue, oral mucosa, external genitalia, vagina, or rectum. Patchy 'moth-eaten' alopecia may occur as may telogen effluvium (WHO, Treponemal infections, Technical Report Series No 674, Geneva, 1982).

Lyme disease

Lyme disease is a multisystem inflammatory disease caused by *Borrelia burgdorferi*.[4] The characteristic skin eruption of early Lyme disease is known as erythema chronicum migrans (Berger, RevInfDis, 1989; 11:1475). It begins as a centrifugally expanding, erythematous macular lesion with a central papule that follows the bite of an *Ixodes* tick infected with the spirochaete *B. burgdorferi*. Over the following few weeks, central clearing of the skin lesion may occur. Treatment with appropriate antibiotics such as doxycycline or amoxycillin is important to prevent secondary neurological or cardiac sequelae.

Patients with Lyme disease have been noted to have liver function abnormalities in the absence of a clinical hepatitis. In one study, 20 out of 73 patients (27 per cent) with untreated early Lyme disease had abnormal liver enzymes with an increase in γ-glutamyl transferase as the most common finding (Kazakoff, ArchFamMed, 1993; 2:409). In another small group of 16 patients with late Lyme disease, 3 were found to have abnormal levels of serum aminotransferases, but no comment was made as to whether these results could have been linked to treatment (Melski, ArchDermatol, 1993; 129:709). Histological studies have noted the presence of lymphoplasmocellular infiltrates in the liver and spleen, but their clinical significance is uncertain (Duray, RheumDisClinNAm, 1989; 15:691).

Autoimmune conditions
Primary biliary cirrhosis

Primary biliary cirrhosis is well known to be associated with xanthelasma and hyperpigmentation of the skin, although these changes are less commonly seen now the disorder is diagnosed at an earlier stage, often via routine blood testing.[5] Pruritus is a common presenting complaint in approximately 50 per cent of cases (Christensen, Gastro, 1980; 78:236).

There is a strong association with other autoimmune conditions such as scleroderma and Sjögren's syndrome. Limited cutaneous sclerosis (CREST syndrome—calcinosis, Raynaud's phenomenon (o)esophageal hypomotility, sclerodactyly, and telangiectasia) occurs in approximately 16 per cent of patients with primary biliary cirrhosis and diffuse cutaneous sclerosis in 9 per cent (Culp, MayoClinProc, 1982; 57:365) (Plate 3).

Lupus

Systemic lupus erythematosus is a multisystem disease which may affect the liver and the skin.[6] Cutaneous features can be classified as chronic, subacute, and acute. The chronic manifestations occur in 15 to 20 per cent of patients with the disease[3] and include discoid lupus erythematosus, most often seen on the face, ears, and scalp; lupus panniculitis; and mucosal and chilblain lupus. Subacute lupus erythematosus, classically associated with Ro antibodies,

affects the upper trunk and has two variants, the papulosquamous and annular-polycyclic forms.

Acute cutaneous lupus erythematosus (estimated to occur in 30 to 50 per cent of patients with the systemic disease) includes localized and widespread indurated erythema and bullous lupus erythematosus.

A recent study of 73 patients with systemic lupus erythematosus found that the commonest cutaneous manifestations were photosensitiviy (63 per cent), butterfly rash (51 per cent), urticaria (44 per cent), non-scarring alopecia (40 per cent), chronic discoid lupus erythematosus (25 per cent), and chilblain lupus (20.5 per cent) (Yell, BrJDermatol, 1996; 135:355).

Wegener's granulomatosis

Wegener's granulomatosis is a rare multisystem disease characterized by a necrotizing granulomatous vasculitis. The upper respiratory tract and kidneys are the most commonly involved sites (Fauci, AnnIntMed, 1983; 98:76).

Although rare, gastrointestinal involvement has been reported and, in one case, sclerosing cholangitis was an atypical manifestation of Wegener's granulomatosis (Leavitt, CurrOpinRheum, 1992; 4:16).

Skin involvement may either cause vasculitis or pyoderma gangrenosum-like lesions, which may occur anywhere but are highly suggestive of Wegener's granulomatosis if they have a periorificial distribution (Jorizzo, JInvDermatol, 1993; 100:106S).

Antineutrophil cytoplasmic antibodies with a characteristic cytoplasmic staining occur in more than 90 per cent of patients with extensive Wegener's granulomatosis (Kallenberg, AmJMed, 1992; 93:675). Cyclophosphamide is the mainstay of treatment and rare cases of hepatotoxicity secondary to this drug have been reported (Snyder, MayoClinProc, 1993; 68:1203).

Polyarteritis nodosa (see also Chapter 24.1)

Hepatitis B has been linked to the occurrence of polyarteritis nodosa and 10 to 50 per cent of patients who develop this condition carry hepatitis B surface antigen (Baker, Gastro, 1972; 62;105), although this association may have been overstated. Systemic polyarteritis nodosa is a multisystem necrotizing vasculitis involving both small and medium-sized vessels. Cutaneous lesions occur in 20 to 50 per cent of patients, with palpable purpura being the most common (Thomas, ClinExpDerm, 1983; 8:47). Other skin features of polyarteritis nodosa include large 'punched out' ulcers, digital gangrene, or livedo reticularis, occasionally seen with ulcerating nodules.

Graft-versus-host disease

Graft-versus-host disease (**GVHD**) affecting the liver is covered fully in Chapter 14.7. Acute graft-versus-host disease occurs 1 to 8 weeks after transplantation and starts as a purplish-red maculopapular eruption on the palms and soles, spreading to the face, limbs, and trunk (Harper, BMJ, 1987; 295:401). Desquamation of the skin usually follows and, in severe forms, toxic epidermal necrolysis may ensue. Bullous, ulcerated, and follicular forms of graft-versus-host disease have all been described (Lycka, ArchDermatol, 1988; 124:1442). Skin biopsy is a non-invasive and sensitive diagnostic test.

Chronic graft-versus-host disease may be localized or generalized and usually occurs 3 to 4 months after transplantation following the acute form. The localized form appears as indurated hyper-pigmented areas which eventually soften and atrophy. The chronic form is a lichenoid eruption with a variable finding of lichen planus-like changes in the buccal mucosa (Barrett, ArchDermatol, 1984; 120:1461).

In the late chronic phase, sclerodermatous changes occur and these may be complicated by ulceration, subcutaneous calcification, hyperpigmentation, alopecia, dystrophic nail changes, and eye changes.

Neoplastic conditions
Hepatocellular carcinoma

Cutaneous conditions seen in hepatocellular carcinoma are non-specific and include paraneoplastic syndromes such as acanthosis nigricans, dermatomyositis, erythema gyratum repens, and para-neoplastic acrokeratosis or Bazex's syndrome. In the latter syndrome, erythema and scaling develop in acral sites, and nail dystrophy and hyperkeratotic plaques may mimic psoriasis. Pityriasis rotunda is an ichthyotic skin condition with widespread annular scale which is more commonly seen in patients of African or Asian origin and is particularly linked to an underlying hepatocellular carcinoma (Leibowitz, ArchDermatol, 1983; 119:607).

Carcinoid syndrome (see also Chapter 22.3.2)

Carcinoid syndrome is a result of secretory factors released by a carcinoid tumour, the primary usually being located in the gut with secondary liver metastases. Skin signs of carcinoid syndrome such as flushing do not generally occur until liver metastases have developed. Paroxysms of flushing tend to involve the face, neck, and upper part of the trunk and are usually spontaneous, although exertion and alcohol may trigger an attack. The flushing may vary in colour from pink-orange to bright red and from purplish-blue to a blanching white. In time, persistent erythema develops on the face and neck and poikiloderma and telangiectasiae may also be present. Treatment of the hepatic metastases by excision or embolization usually causes regression of the erythema and telangiectases.

The flushing is thought to be a result of kinin, prostaglandin, histamine, and substance P release in combination with serotonin secretion. Long-acting somatostatin analogues such as octreotide given subcutaneously may provide relief from the flushing (Oates, NEJM, 1986; 315:702).

Occasionally, a pellagra-like dermatitis may occur on light-exposed skin in patients with the carcinoid syndrome (Castiello, ArchDermatol, 1972; 105:574). This may present with hyper-keratosis, scaling, and a grey-black hyperpigmentation of the skin which is most marked on the legs, forearms, and trunk. Treatment with niacin will cause resolution of these lesions. The rationale for this vitamin deficiency is that its precursor tryptophan is diverted into producing increased amounts of serotonin.

Occasionally, carcinoid tumours metastasize to the skin where they cause firm, tender nodules. Rarely, carcinoid syndrome is

associated with the development of scleroderma, although a common pathogenesis is not known (Durward, PostgradMedJ, 1995; 71:299).

Effects of immunosuppression
Liver transplantation

Skin infections, infestations, malignancies, and other dermatoses are seen more frequently in patients who have received organ transplants than in the normal population.[7] The effects of carcinogens such as ultraviolet radiation may be potentiated by immunosuppressive drugs leading to an increased incidence of both premalignant skin lesions and squamous cell carcinoma (Gupta, ArchDermatol, 1986; 122:1288). Overall, a threefold increase in malignancies is found in recipients of organ transplants compared with age-matched control groups (Penn, SGO, 1986; 162:603). These include lymphoma, Kaposi's sarcoma, anogenital cancer, and both melanoma and non-melanoma skin cancer (Hertzler, AmJMedSci, 1995; 309:278).

Preventative measures with sun avoidance are important in recipients of liver transplants, and a prompt biopsy should be taken of any suspicious skin lesion. In view of the increased risk of infection, unexplained skin lesions should also be stained and cultured to look for bacterial, viral, fungal, and typical or atypical mycobacterial infections (Leyden, ArchDermatol, 1985; 121:855).

Alcohol and alcoholic liver disease

Characteristic stigmas of alcoholic liver disease including spider naevi, palmar erythema, and leuchonychia are widely recognized, but also commonly occur in chronic liver disease due to other causes. However, vascular lesions such as spider naevi and palmar erythema are more common in patients with alcoholic cirrhosis than in patients with viral or cryptogenic cirrhosis (Strauss, ArqGastro-SaoPaulo, 1990; 27:46). A prospective study showed that numbers and size of spider naevi in patients with alcoholic liver disease correlated well with both presence and frequency of bleeding from oesophageal varices (Foutch, AmJGastr, 1988; 83:723). Patients with spider naevi greater than 15 mm in diameter had an 80 per cent risk of variceal bleeding.

Flushing and plethoric facies are linked to alcohol misuse. In susceptible individuals, there may be fine telangiectasia and persistent facial erythema, often without spider naevi or palmar erythema. The underlying mechanism is thought to be chronic vasodilatation and loss of vasoregulatory control mechanisms.

Alcohol may also exacerbate but not cause rosacea. In particular, it can trigger the flushing and vasomotor instability associated with the condition.

The relationship of alcohol with psoriasis has been covered in Chapter 24.3.

Cutaneous infections such as cellulitis are more common in patients who abuse alcohol and are due to a combination of factors including immune dysfunction, trauma, and poor nutrition and hygiene (Adams, MedClinNAm,1984; 68:179). In one survey of patients attending an alcohol misuse clinic, the incidence of chronic fungal skin infections (tinea pedis, onychomycosis, and pityriasis versicolor) was 33 per cent as opposed to an incidence of 5 to 10 per cent of these conditions in the general population (Higgins, AlcAlc, 1992; 27(Suppl):95).

Nutritional deficiencies in patients with alcoholic liver disease that are severe enough to cause cutaneous manifestations are rare in the United Kingdom. Pellagra caused by niacin deficiency presents with an erythematous and photosensitve scaly dermatitis on the face and arms, characteristically in association with diarrhoea and dementia. The skin changes eventually form a dusky, brown-red coloration, similar to resolving severe sunburn.

Scurvy is secondary to vitamin C deficiency, and follicular keratosis with corkscrew hairs are the earliest cutaneous changes. Later, perifollicular haemorrhages, stomatitis, bleeding gums, epistaxes, and ecchymoses occur (Leung, AnnEmergMed, 1981; 10: 652).

Recently, a link between discoid eczema and alcohol misuse has emerged, with affected patients having no history of atopic eczema.

Drugs and chemicals affecting the liver and skin

Porphyria

Of the hepatic porphyrias, the skin is affected in porphyria cutanea tarda, variegate porphyria, hepatoerythropoietic porphyria, and hereditary coproporphyria (see Chapter 20.5).

Porphyria cutanea tarda

This is caused by a reduced activity of the uroporphyrinogen decarboxylase in the haem biosynthetic pathway and can have a hereditary or acquired aetiology. Patients present with blistering on light-exposed areas, usually the dorsal aspect of the hands and the face, with milia formation and atrophic scarring (Grossman, AmJMed, 1979; 67:277) (Plate 4). Hyperpigmentation is a common feature but mottled hypopigmentation may also occur. Skin fragility and hypertrichosis, initially facial and more prominent in women, may also be noted. Sclerodermatous-like plaques, often located on the upper chest, are a rare association.

The sporadic or acquired type makes up the majority of cases and uroporphyrinogen decarboxylase activity is reduced by approximately 50 per cent in the liver. In susceptible people additional factors are necessary to precipitate porphyria cutanea tarda, and these include iron therapy, oestrogen use such as the oral contraceptive pill or hormone replacement therapy, alcohol abuse, or exposure to polyhalogenated cyclic hydrocarbons.

Familial porphyria cutanea tarda is extremely rare and is inherited in an autosomal dominant fashion. In this type, uroporphyrinogen decarboxylase is deficient in non-hepatic tissues as well as the liver. The diagnosis is made by the finding of increased uroporphyrin in the plasma or urine.

Treatment includes the identification and avoidance of, or abstinence from, precipitating factors, sun avoidance and the wearing of sunscreens, and venesection or low-dose chloroquine therapy (Ashton, BrJDermatol, 1981; 111:609).

Variegate porphyria

This rare autosomal disorder is caused by a deficiency of the enzyme protoporphyrinogen oxidase. The majority of patients with the variegate porphyria trait are asymptomatic, but of those who are symptomatic, 50 per cent have skin disease alone and 70 per cent have cutaneous involvement (Eales, IntJBiochem, 1980; 12:837). The neurovisceral features of variegate porphyria are confusional states, abdominal pain, or peripheral neuropathy. All the features are precipitated by drugs, pregnancy, or reduced carbohydrate intake.

The diagnosis is made by the finding of increased faecal excretion of protoporphyrin and coproporphyrin. Treatment of acute attacks is by haematin infusion to reduce the excretion of porphyrins, and carbohydrate loading to reduce the production of porphyrins and their precursors. Supportive care is also important. The skin lesions can be prevented by sunscreens and sun avoidance.

Variegate porphyria presents in a similar fashion to porphyria cutanea tarda, with blister formation on the sun-exposed areas such as the face, neck, and the dorsum of the hands. The skin is fragile and may blister after trauma. Healing leads to milia and the formation of tissue paper scars. Hypertrichosis also occurs, mainly confined to the cheeks with hyper- or hypopigmentary changes. Diffuse thickening of the hands and fingers may rarely be seen, similar to the changes found in scleroderma.

Hereditary coproporphyria

Hereditary coproporphyria is a rare autosomal dominant disorder of porphyrin metabolism caused by a partial deficiency (approximately 50 per cent) of the enzyme coproporphyrinogen oxidase. The gene locus for this enzyme has been found on chromosome 9 (Grandchamp, HumGenet, 1983; 64:180). There is marked elevation of faecal coproporphyrin, even between acute attacks.

The acute attacks are similar but less severe than in variegate porphyria and cutaneous photosensitivity is only seen in 30 per cent of cases (Brodie, QJMed, 1977; 46:229). The disease is more often symptomatic in females and may be triggered by menstruation, pregnancy, and the contraceptive pill. The treatment is the same as in variegate porphyria.

Hepatoerythropoietic porphyria

This extremely rare disorder is due to a homozygous deficiency of uroporphyrinogen decarboxylase activity. Severe photosensitivity occurs in the first year of life and total sun avoidance is imperative. Blistering occurs with marked scarring, hyperpigmentation, and sclerodermatous skin changes (Czarnecki, ArchDermatol, 1980; 116:307).

α_1-Antitrypsin deficiency

Deficiency of the protease inhibitor α_1-antitrypsin (see Chapter 20.3) may rarely be associated with the cutaneous findings of panniculitis, vasculitis, urticaria, and angio-oedema (Rubinstein, AnnIntMed, 1977; 86:742). Nodular panniculitis is the most frequent association and α_1-antitrypsin deficiency accounts for up to 14 per cent of cases (Smith, JAmAcadDermatol, 1989; 21:1192). It presents with tender, single or multiple subcutaneous nodules, usually on the lower legs although a more generalized form may occur. The nodules may liquefy or ulcerate and heal with scarring. The age of onset may be from infancy to old age. Treatment is difficult although dapsone and infusions of α_1-proteinase inhibitor concentrate have been used to good effect (Smith, ArchDermatol, 1987; 123:1655).

Haemochromatosis

This disorder of iron deposition is discussed in Chapter 20.2. The characteristic skin change is a grey-brown or 'bronze' pigmentation, particularly on the face, flexural creases, and sun-exposed areas. This is secondary to excessive melanin formation.

Vinyl chloride

Industrial workers exposed to polyvinyl chloride who are HLA DR5, B8, or DR3 positive are at risk of developing a scleroderma-like disorder with associated Raynaud's phenomenon (Black, Lancet, 1983; i:53). Although rare, angiosarcoma of the liver (2 per cent of all primary tumours of the liver) has been linked to exposure with polyvinyl chloride (Creech, JOccMed, 1974; 16:150). The risk of a person who works with polyvinyl chloride developing angiosarcoma of the liver is 10 to 15 times that of the general population (Tamburro, SemLivDis, 1984; 4:158).

Phenytoin

The anticonvulsant phenytoin may rarely cause a hypersensitivity syndrome consisting of rash, fever, tender generalized lymphadenopathy, hepatosplenomegaly, arthralgia, leucocytosis with eosinophilia, and an associated hepatitis (Stanley, ArchDermatol, 1978; 14:1350). The rash is usually an erythroderma with periorbital and facial oedema and pinhead-like sterile pustules on the face and scalp, resolving with marked desquamation known as toxic pustuloderma (Chopra, BrJDermatol, 1996; 134:1109).

The hepatic damage is variable and submassive necrosis and lobular, cholestatic, and granulomatous hepatitis have all been reported (Mullick, AmJClinPath, 1980; 74:442).

Nephritis, pneumonitis, and other haematological abnormalities have also been reported in the phenytoin hypersensitivity syndrome (Rosenthal, Cancer, 1982; 49:2305) and it may be severe enough to cause pseudolymphoma (Harris, BrJDermatol, 1992; 127:403).

Studies of the rearrangements of T-cell receptor genes are useful to look for clonal expansion and to differentiate the condition from true lymphoma.

Wilson's disease and penicillamine treatment

Patients with Wilson's disease who have been treated with high-dose D-penicillamine as a copper-chelating agent may develop elastosis perforans serpiginosa as a rare complication (Sahn, JAmAcadDermatol, 1989; 20:279). This condition causes pseudoxanthoma elasticum-type changes with 'plucked-chicken skin' developing on the neck and axilla, and erythematous, keratotic, annular, or serpiginous lesions also occurring on the neck, axilla, antecubital fossa, and penis (Plate 5). These lesions may occasionally ulcerate or form cribriform scarring. Electron microscopy of the affected skin shows a characteristic bramble bush-like appearance of the coarse elastic fibres of the skin with extreme variation in thickness of the collagen fibres (Hashimoto, JAmAcadDermatol, 1981; 4:300).

References

1. Bergasa NV and Jones EA. The pruritus of cholestasis. *Seminars in Liver Disease*, 1993; **13**: 319–27.
2. Pawlotsky JM, Dhumeaux D, and Bagot M. Hepatitis C virus in dermatology: a review *Archives of Dermatology*, 1995; **131**: 1185–93.
3. Goodman DS, *et al*. Prevalence of cutaneous disease in patients with acquired immunodeficiency syndrome (AIDS) or AIDS-related complex. *Journal of the American Academy of Dermatology*, 1987; **17**: 210–20.
4. Symposium on Lyme disease. *American Journal of Medicine*, 1995; **98** (Suppl. 4A).
5. Kaplan MM. Primary biliary cirrhosis. *New England Journal of Medicine*, 1987; **316**: 521–8.
6. Gilliam JN and Sontheimer RD. Distinctive cutaneous subsets in the spectrum of lupus erythematosus. *Journal of the American Academy of Dermatology*, 1981; **4**: 471–5.
7. Abel EA Cutaneous manifestations of immunosuppression in organ transplant recipients. *Journal of the American Academy of Dermatology*, 1989; **21**: 167–79.

25.7 Effect of liver disease on the urogenital tract

Juan Rodés and Vicente Arroyo

It is well known that both acute and chronic liver disease (hepatic cirrhosis, acute and chronic Budd–Chiari syndrome, hepatocellular carcinoma, alcoholic hepatitis, and fulminant hepatic failure) in addition to renal sodium and water retention may induce hepatorenal syndrome. This association is discussed in other sections of the book. This chapter reviews other renal disturbances associated with hepatic disease: (i) acute renal failure in obstructive jaundice; (ii) glomerular abnormalities in hepatic cirrhosis, viral infection with hepatitis B and hepatitis C; and (iii) renal tubular acidosis in chronic liver disease. In addition, the influence of hepatic cirrhosis on the prostate is also discussed.

Acute renal failure in obstructive jaundice

The natural route for the excretion of bile is the biliary tract. When this route is blocked, the kidney becomes the main excretory organ for the biliary products. Therefore, the jaundiced patient is critically dependent on the kidney for survival. Unfortunately, kidney function may deteriorate during obstructive jaundice.

For many decades (Clairmont, MittGrenzgebMedChir, 1910; 22:159) it has been recognized that surgery in patients with obstructive jaundice is associated with a high risk of acute renal failure which contributes to postoperative mortality (Dawson, BMJ, 1964; i:810; Dawson, BrJSurg, 1965; 52:663).[1,2] Initial studies reported an incidence of renal failure from 7 to 20 per cent. The postoperative mortality rate for these patients ranged from zero to 27 per cent, with renal failure as a major contributing cause in 30 to 40 per cent of cases. Nowadays, however, the rate of postoperative renal failure among patients with obstructive jaundice is lower, probably due to better treatment with appropriate preoperative rehydration aimed at maintaining urine flow at the time of surgery (Parks, BrJSurg, 1994; 81:437).[2] Renal failure may occur in association with any disease causing obstruction of the biliary tract, including calculi, tumour, and chronic pancreatitis. Although impairment in renal function usually occurs immediately after surgery, it may also develop preoperatively.[1] Acute renal failure (acute tubular necrosis) in these patients is characterized by a severely reduced endogenous creatinine clearance, high levels of blood urea nitrogen and serum creatinine, a urinary sodium concentration greater than 10 mEq/day, and urine-to-plasma osmolality ratio lower than unity.

Patients with jaundice who develop acute tubular necrosis are severely ill and most have cholangitis, sepsis, and arterial hypotension.

Microscopical examination of the kidney shows either mild degenerative changes and dilatation of the distal tubules with bile casts, or frank tubular cell necrosis with bile casts, inflammatory infiltration, oedema, and with glomerular and peritubular fibrin deposition.[1] The mechanism of renal failure in these patients remains poorly understood. However, several factors have been implicated in its development, such as endotoxaemia (Bailey, BrJSurg, 1976; 63:774), hyperbilirubinaemia (Armstrong, BrJSurg, 1984; 71:234), increased serum levels of bile salts (Aoyagi, JLabClinMed, 1968; 71:686; Green, JAmSocNephrol, 1995; 5:1853), renovascular fibrin deposition (Wardle, BMJ, 1970; iv:472), alterations in systemic and renal haemodynamics,[3] and fluid depletion (Sitges-Serra, BrJSurg, 1992; 79:553). It is possible that the mechanism responsible for acute renal failure in obstructive jaundice is multifactorial. It is considered that gut-derived endotoxin may be the initial cause of renal dysfunction in these patients, since systemic endotoxaemia is demonstrated in about 50 per cent of patients in the postoperative period whilst renal failure is very uncommon in the absence of endotoxaemia (Bailey, BrJSurg, 1976; 63:774; Wilkinson, BMJ, 1976; ii:1415). The crucial role of endotoxaemia has received further support because the oral administration of bile salts not only prevents endotoxaemia but also the development of renal failure in patients with obstructive jaundice (Cahill, BrJSurg, 1983; 70:590; Pain, BrJSurg, 1991; 78:467). The effects of endotoxin are probably mediated through the action of various cytokines, as these substances are able to alter renal haemodynamics in addition to their direct toxic action on the kidneys. In fact, cytokines may produce renal haemodynamic disturbances by inducing arterial hypotension with concomitant release of renal vasoconstrictors (Tracey, SGO, 1987; 164:425; Van der Poll, BrJIntensCare, 1992; 2:99), and by distributing intrarenal blood flow away from the renal cortex (Yarger, JClinInvest, 1976; 57:408). The renal toxic action of the cytokines may be due to their procoagulant activity, with induction of disseminated intravascular coagulation that may explain the deposition of fibrin in the renal tubules and in the glomeruli. Moreover, cytokines may also produce intrarenal sequestration of neutrophils, which in turn leads to a neutrophil-mediated release of cytotoxins (Cotran, KidneyInt, 1989; 35:969; Dinarello, AdvImmunol, 1989; 44:153).

In addition to endotoxaemia there are other factors that may play an important role in the development of acute tubular necrosis in these patients. One of the mechanisms recently investigated is the appearance of extracellular fluid depletion that has been detected in experimental studies and in patients with obstructive jaundice. Valverde *et al.* (AnnSurg, 1992; 219:73) showed a marked increase in atrial natriuretic peptide (**ANP**) in the plasma of rabbits submitted to ligation of the common bile duct. In the same study it was demonstrated that these high levels of ANP were associated with an increase of plasma aldosterone, renin, and antidiuretic hormone, suggesting that these hormones were produced in response to the reduced extracellular volume and that the raised levels of ANP may explain the reduced vascular reactivity in response to hypovolaemia (Green, JAmSocNephrol, 1995; 5:1853). This predisposition to arterial hypotension may explain the pathological changes of focal tubular necrosis that are often found in the kidneys when renal failure develops in association with obstructive jaundice (Green, Surgery, 1986; 100:14). At present the cause of this hypovolaemia is poorly understood, although it seems plausible that it may result from preoperative fluid depletion. In fact, it has been shown in experimental studies that ligation of the common bile duct is followed by a 15 per cent fall in the plasma volume (Gillet, JSurgRes, 1971; 11:447; Martínez-Ródenas, BrJSurg, 1989; 76:461). These changes were associated in this experimental model with hypodipsia, hypophagia, and an impaired capacity to concentrate urine, suggesting that these factors are the cause of this volume depletion. These findings have been confirmed in human studies (Sitges-Serra, BrJSurg, 1992; 79:553). Finally, it has been demonstrated that the administration of indomethacin, which inhibits the renal synthesis of prostaglandins, may induce the development of acute renal failure in patients with jaundice (Kramer, ClinSci, 1995; 88:39), suggesting that prostaglandins, as vasodilator substances, may also play an important role in the maintenance of renal plasma flow in these patients (Uemura, ScaJGastr, 1989; 24:705).

As indicated, preoperative rehydration is essential to prevent the development of renal failure in these patients. In addition, the administration of non-steroidal anti-inflammatory drugs and aminoglycosides should be avoided as these drugs may precipitate the development of renal failure. The administration of mannitol was considered the best treatment to prevent the development of renal failure in obstructive jaundice (Dawson, BMJ, 1965; i:82). However, in a more recent, prospective, controlled clinical trial (Gubern, Surgery, 1988; 103:39), not only was it shown that perioperative mannitol administration was ineffective, but also that it produced renal functional deterioration in the treated group compared with the control group. Therefore mannitol is of doubtful value in the treatment of these patients. Antiendotoxin therapy, using bile salts or lactulose, has shown conflicting results and at present it is not fully accepted that use of these drugs may prevent renal failure in patients with jaundice.[2] Biliary drainage has been used to reduce the problems associated with obstructive jaundice as it may improve the clinical condition by reversing endotoxaemia. However, it is not yet clear whether this procedure is of benefit.[2] Haemodialysis is required in patients with obstructive jaundice and oliguric acute renal failure.

Glomerular abnormalities

The association between liver disease and histological glomerular abnormalities has been widely recognized during the last 25 years.

The glomerular alterations observed in cirrhosis of the liver and hepatitis B and C infection are discussed in this chapter. Other diseases causing hepatic and glomerular lesions, such as schistosomiasis, malaria, infectious mononucleosis, legionnaires' disease, obstructive jaundice, biliary atresia, amyloidosis, autoimmune chronic hepatitis, primary biliary cirrhosis, haemochromatosis, α_1-antitrypsin deficiency, nodular regenerative hyperplasia, sickle-cell disease, collagen disease, toxaemia, and acute fatty liver of pregnancy, are discussed in other chapters.

Cirrhosis of the liver

In autopsy studies the frequency of histological glomerular abnormalities in cirrhosis varies from 11.7 to 100 per cent. In 1133 patients with cirrhosis reported from 1863 to 1984, an abnormality was detected in about 53 per cent.[3] The figure is very high in biopsy studies, where glomerular alteration was present in 98.6 per cent of the 140 cases reported in the literature between 1965 and 1987.[3] The higher incidence of changes observed in biopsy studies was related to the fact that patients who underwent biopsy were selected on the basis of clinical and laboratory evidence of renal disturbances at the time of the procedure, whereas the autopsy studies were performed in consecutive cases. However, in a recent prospective study in unselected patients with non-alcoholic cirrhosis in whom renal biopsy was performed at the time of liver transplantation, glomerular abnormalities were observed in all the cases, although most had only minor changes. These data also suggest that glomerular histological alterations are secondary to the hepatic dysfunction and independent of the aetiology of cirrhosis.[4]

The most frequent glomerular changes observed in patients with cirrhosis are periglomerular fibrosis and hyaline thickening of the basement membrane, hypercellularity of both endothelial and epithelial cells, and a mild to marked thickening of the mesangium by a fibrillar material positive for periodic acid–Schiff staining. Endothelial cells are swollen and vacuolated and stain positively for lipids. In some cases there is obliteration of the glomerular lumen. This lesion has been termed 'hepatic glomerulosclerosis' (Bloodworth, LabInvest, 1959; 8:962) (Fig. 1). Ultrastructural examination reveals the presence of electron-dense osmophilic deposits in the capillary wall and mesangium, thickening of the basement membrane, an increased amount of mesangial matrix, fusion and focal destruction of foot processes, and oedema of the cytoplasm of podocytes (Sakaguchi, LabInvest, 1965; 14:533; Fisher, AmJPath, 1968; 52:869; and Callard, AmJPathol, 1975; 80:329).

Immunofluorescence studies have drawn attention to the relationship of these glomerular changes and the presence of subendothelial and mesangial deposits of IgA, IgG, IgM, and complement (Callard, AmJPathol, 1975; 80:329; Nochy, ClinNephrol, 1976; 6:422).[3,4] Several patterns of glomerular lesions have been recognized in hepatic cirrhosis including IgG and IgM mesangial deposition, glomerulosclerosis devoid of immunoglobulin, proliferative glomerulonephritis, classic membranous or membranoproliferative lesions, and rapidly progressive glomerulonephritis.[4] However, they can be classified into two types according to the presence or absence of cellular proliferation (Berger, AdvNephrol, 1978; 7:3). In the type without proliferation, which is the most common type of glomerular lesion observed in patients with cirrhosis, the deposits are mainly mesangial, and IgA is the

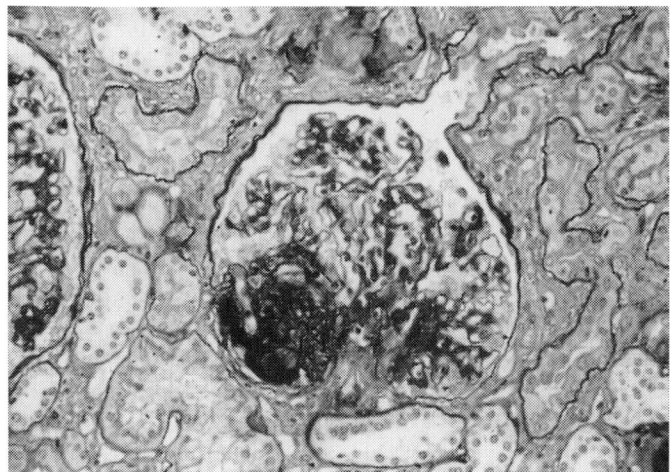

Fig. 1. Light microscopy of glomerular alterations seen in hepatic cirrhosis. The nodules in the tuft are sparsely cellular and uniformly stained: nodular glomerulosclerosis (periodic acid–Schiff, ×336).

predominant immunoglobulin detected in the deposits, although IgG and/or IgM are also present. Clq is found in about one-third of the cases. These patients are asymptomatic. The glomerular lesion associated with proliferative changes is uncommon. The incidence of this lesion among the population with cirrhosis has been estimated to be around 1.7 per cent (Nakamoto, VirchArchA, 1981; 392:45). In this type of lesion IgA deposits are intramembranous. Mallory body (alcoholic hyaline) antigen has also been found within immune complexes and in the glomeruli with cirrhosis-associated IgA nephropathy (Burns, JClinPath, 1983; 36: 751). These patients present overt proteinuria (which may be in the nephrotic range), haematuria, and occasionally rapidly progressive glomerulonephritis. A syndrome simulating Henoch–Schönlein purpura has also been described in these patients (Aggarwal, AmJ KidneyDis, 1992: 20:400). The deposit of immunoglobulins is as prominent in patients with proliferative changes as in those without proliferation.

The pathogenesis of glomerular abnormalities in patients with cirrhosis is unknown, but probably involves immune complex deposition.[5] Recently, it has been shown that there is a close relationship between chronic infection with hepatitis C virus and type II mixed cryoglobulinaemia. Antihepatitis C viral antibody, hepatitis C viral core antigens, and hepatitis C-RNA can be found in cryoglobulins and in the renal deposits of patients with hepatitis C virus infection associated with mixed (IgG–IgM) cryoglobulinaemia. On the other hand, it has been estimated that 50 to 75 per cent of patients with 'essential' mixed IgG–IgM cryoglobulinaemia have underlying chronic hepatitis C virus infection (see later).[6] These findings suggest that in patients with concurrent cirrhosis and hepatitis C virus infection the development of glomerular lesions may be explained by the above-mentioned mechanism.

In addition to cryoglobulinaemia, hypocomplementaemia is also frequent in patients with cirrhosis (Druet, ClinExpImmun, 1973; 15:483; Kourulsky, AmJMed, 1973; 55:783). Hypocomplementaemia could be due to the activation of complement and/or reduced hepatic production. However, a more frequent finding is the elevation of serum IgA (Bene, AmJClinPath, 1988;

89:767). In normal subjects, IgA is present in the circulation as monomeric units, mainly of the IgA1 subclass, and is synthesized by plasma cells chiefly in the bone marrow and spleen. IgA is transported into bile by endocytic transfer mediated by a secretory component across intrahepatic and extrahepatic biliary epithelium (Nagura, JImmunol, 1981; 126:587). At mucosal sites, IgA is synthesized and secreted actively as A1 or A2 dimers, polymerized by J chain, and transported by binding to the secretory component. The bowel is the main site of IgA production in response to antigenic challenge (Woodroffe, ContribNephrol, 1984; 40:51). Most dimeric IgA produced by the bowel is secreted into the intestinal lumen; however, a small proportion of this IgA passes to the portal circulation and reaches the liver (Lemaître-Coelho, EurJImmun, 1977; 7:588). Serum dimeric IgA in patients with cirrhosis is increased sevenfold compared with controls; the monomeric form is increased 2.5-fold (André, Lancet, 1977; i:97). The mechanism of the increased circulating plasma levels of monomeric and dimeric IgA in patients with cirrhosis may be reduced catabolism and/or increased synthesis (Delacroix, JCI, 1983; 71:358). Defective elimination of IgA-containing immune complexes has been demonstrated. An IgA–IgG aggregate utilized to stimulate IgA immune complexes is cleared slowly by the liver in patients with cirrhosis compared with normal subjects. Although splenic clearance is disproportionately increased, this increment fails to return the overall clearance rate to normal. Clearance time via specific asialoglycoprotein receptors is also prolonged in patients with cirrhosis, suggesting defective processing of IgA or IgA immune complexes (Roccatello, LabInvest, 1993; 69:714). Therefore, IgA deposition in the liver of patients with cirrhosis may reflect abnormalities in both the synthesis and the clearance of IgA and its associated immune complexes. Furthermore, the deposition of IgA in the kidney could be the cause of the glomerular lesion in these patients (Sancho, ContribNephrol, 1984; 40:93).

In some patients with advanced cirrhosis, deposition of a lipid material in the glomerular basement membrane, mesangium, and endothelial regions, has been found, similar to that previously described in patients with lecithin–cholesterol acyltransferase deficiency (Hovig, LabInvest, 1978;38:540). The role of this abnormality in the development of glomerulosclerotic lesions of patients with cirrhosis remains to be elucidated (Grone, LabInvest, 1989; 60:443).

Hepatitis B virus infection

Chronic hepatitis B virus (**HBV**) infection is also associated with several types of glomerular diseases, such as membranous nephropathy, mesangiocapillary glomerulonephritis, crescentic glomerulonephritis, polyarteritis nodosa, and systemic necrotizing vasculitis. Serum sickness-like syndrome may be observed in patients with acute HBV infection.

Serum sickness-like syndrome appears in 10 to 25 per cent of patients infected with HBV. The symptoms include fever, arthralgias, arthritis, skin rash, and in a few patients proteinuria that may be associated with haematuria. The outcome of this syndrome is benign and spontaneous resolution is the rule (Onion, AnnIntMed, 1971; 75:29; Duffy, Medicine, 1976; 55:19).

The first study suggesting that HBV may lead to the development of membranous nephropathy was described in 1969

(Feizi, Lancet, 1969; ii:873), and in 1971 the hepatitis surface antigen (**HBsAg**) was identified in the glomerular capillary wall together with IgG and C3 (Combes, Lancet, 1971; ii:234). Later, the three hepatitis B antigens (HBsAg, HBeAg, and HBcAg) were found in the subepithelial immune complexes of patients with this HBV-associated nephropathy (Takekoshi, NEJM, 1979; 300:814; Johnson, KidneyInt, 1990; 37:663). This syndrome is four times more frequent in males than in females.[3] Although it has been reported in adults it is more frequent in children, particularly in Asia (Levy, KidneyInt, 1991; 40 (Suppl. 35):S24; Lin, KidneyInt, 1991; 40(Suppl 35):S-46). These patients usually show microscopic haematuria, granular casts, proteinuria, and hypoalbinaemia; most present an overt nephrotic syndrome without renal insufficiency. The complement level is normal but in some cases cryo-globulinaemia may be detected (Levo, NEJM, 1977; 296:1501). Spontaneous resolution of this membranous nephropathy is common in patients with seroconversion of HBeAg to anti-HBeAg (65 per cent within the first year and 85 per cent within the second year of seroconversion) (Hsu, ClinNephrol, 1983; 20:121). However, a few patients develop renal failure requiring haemodialysis (Klein-knecht, JPediat, 1979; 95:946; Montoliu, AmJNephrol, 1985; 5:372). The administration of corticosteroids is not advisable in these patients because they may worsen the HBV infection. Antiviral therapy with interferon has proved to be effective in the treatment of HBV-associated glomerulopathy (Lisker-Melman, AnnIntMed, 1989; 11:479).

In these patients other histological patterns have been reported, such as mesangiocapillary glomerulonephritis, mesangial pro-liferative glomerulonephritis, and crescentic glomerulonephritis (Johnson, KidneyInt, 1990; 37:663; Lai, ModPathol, 1992; 5:262). Subepithelial electron-dense deposits are observed on electron microscopy.[3] Immunofluoresence studies show IgG, IgA, and IgM together with C1q and C4 along the glomerular basement membrane and mesangial areas (Iida, Nephron, 1990; 54:18).

Polyarteritis nodosa associated with HBV infection (see also Chapter 12.1.2.3) is more common in Western countries than in Asia. These patients present similar clinical manifestations to those patients with idiopathic polyarteritis nodosa, such as fever, cu-taneous leucocytoclastic vasculitis, livedo reticularis, neuropathy, myalgias, otitis, orchitis, arthritis, and pulmonary manifestations. Symptomatic acute hepatitis in the preceding 6 months is common and a moderate increase of transaminases may be detected in about half of the cases at presentation of polyarteritis nodosa. Antineutrophil cytoplasmic antibodies are positive in around 10 per cent of the cases. Liver biopsy reveals moderate or severe chronic hepatitis. Aneurysms are more frequent in the coeliac and renal territories. The renal manifestations include haematuria, pro-teinuria, and azotaemia.[6] Although spontaneous remission has been reported, it is very uncommon (Trepo, JClinPath, 1974; 27:863). The administration of steroids and cyclophosphamide has been shown to be useful in the treatment of these patients. However, it should be taken into account that this therapy may increase viral replication. Furthermore, these reports were based on uncontrolled clinical trials (Frohnert, AmJMed, 1967; 43:8; Oriente, ClinRheum, 1986; 5:193). Combination therapy, with steroids directed at the immune-mediated vasculitis and vidarabine or interferon as antiviral therapy, has been used in these patients with promising results; viral replication was no longer present in about 50 per cent of the

patients at the end of follow-up (Guillevin, JRheum, 1993; 20:289).

Hepatitis C virus infection

During the last few years evidence has been presented indicating a close relationship between type II mixed essential cryoglobulinaemia and chronic hepatitis C virus (**HCV**) infection. Most patients with type II mixed essential cryoglobulinaemia have antibodies to HCV, HCV-RNA in the serum, and chronic liver disease (chronic hepatitis or cirrhosis) (Misiani, AnnIntMed, 1992; 117:573), and approxi-mately 50 per cent of patients with chronic HCV infection have cryoglobulins. However, almost all patients with glomerulonephritis and cryoglobulinaemia have chronic HCV infection (Pasquariello, AmJNephrol, 1993; 13:300). Renal histology consists of a mem-branoproliferative glomerulonephritis with mesangial proliferation, lobulation of the glomeruli, thickening of the glomerular capillary wall as a consequence of the presence of subendothelial deposits, and intraglomerular thrombi. Clinical manifestations included arterial hypertension, oedema, and hepatomegaly. Moderate increases of aminotransferases are observed in about 75 per cent of cases. Rheumatoid factor and hypocomplementaemia were detected in all the patients and mixed IgG–IgM cryoglobulins in two-thirds of them. Haematuria, proteinuria (being in the nephrotic range in more than 50 per cent of the patients), and decreased glomerular filtration rate were also observed in all the patients (Johnson, NEJM, 1993; 328:464). The administration of steroids is contraindicated as they enhance the replication of HCV.[6] Interferon has been used in these patients and the results obtained indicate that this drug may be of benefit. In those patients in whom interferon was able to eliminate HCV-RNA, an improvement in renal function was also observed (Misiani, NEJM, 1994; 330:756). However, at present, the real efficacy of interferon in the treatment of these patients remains unknown. Therefore, controlled clinical trials and risk–benefit ana-lyses are required to determine the optimal dose and duration of therapy for patients with HCV-associated glomerulonephritis with mixed IgG–IgM cryoglobulinaemia.[6]

Renal tubular acidosis

Renal tubular acidosis is defined as the inability of the renal tubule to acidify the urine in the presence of a normal glomerular filtration rate (Morris, NEJM, 1969; 281:145). Renal tubular acidosis has been classified into two major types, distal and proximal (Rodriguez-Soriano, AnnRevMed, 1969; 20:363). In type I (distal), or classic renal tubular acidosis, the distal tubule is unable to maintain the steep lumen–peritubular hydrogen-ion gradient. The distal disease can, in turn, be subdivided into hypokalaemic, hyperkalaemic, and incomplete forms. In the hypokalaemic form, urine pH does not fall inappropriately, and acidosis is a consequencce of decreased acid excretion. This form of distal renal tubular acidosis can be inherited, drug induced, or associated with various systemic conditions. Im-paired distal tubular acidification with hyperkalaemia can be associated with mineralocorticoid deficiency, urinary tract ob-struction, and administration of distal diuretics (amiloride). In the incomplete distal form, acidosis is absent, although urinary pH remains inappropriately high following acid loading.[7] Type II (proximal) renal tubular acidosis is due to abnormal proximal tubular function resulting in an impaired reabsorption of bicarbonate. In this form more than 15 per cent of the filtered bicarbonate load is not reabsorbed and it is excreted in the urine.

Renal tubular acidosis may occur in various liver diseases.[8] Type I has been observed in patients with autoimmune chronic hepatitis (Read, Gut, 1963; 4:378; Garcia-Puig, ClinNephrol, 1980; 13:287), primary biliary cirrhosis (Parés, Gastro, 1981; 80:681), and alcoholic cirrhosis (Paré, ArchIntMed, 1984; 144:941; Cecchin, NEJM, 1993; 329:1927). Both types have been recognized in Wilson's disease (Leu, JFormosanMedAss, 1977; 76:829). Finally, an isolated acidifying defect of the proximal tubule has been reported in paediatric patients receiving liver transplants and treatment with FK506 (O'Gorman, ClinTranspl, 1995; 9:312). Nevertheless, renal tubular acidosis is more common in primary biliary cirrhosis, Wilson's disease, and alcoholic liver cirrhosis (30 to 57 per cent of cases).

The clinical manifestations of patients with distal renal tubular acidosis and chronic liver disease are similar to those of patients with renal tubular acidosis but without hepatic lesions. Most patients, however, present an incomplete distal form. Hence, the finding of hypokalaemia, hyperchloraemia, acidaemia, osteomalacia, or nephrolithiasis is very infrequent.[7] In primary biliary cirrhosis a decrease of plasma levels of uric acid has been reported in relation to distal renal tubular acidosis (Izumi, Hepatol, 1983; 3:719). Patients with the proximal disease may, in addition, have other clinical manifestations, such as glycosuria, aminoaciduria, and high levels of β_2-microglobulin in the urine. Whether renal tubular acidosis increases the risk of hepatic encephalopathy is controversial. Theoretically, acidosis or hypokalaemia associated with the disease facilitate renal ammoniogenesis. The increased urinary pH may divert some of this ammonia into the renal venous blood (Shear, NEJM, 1969; 280:1). This hypothesis, however, has not been confirmed by other researchers (Paré, ArchIntMed, 1984; 144:941).

The pathogenesis of renal tubular acidosis associated with chronic liver disease is not clearly understood, although several mechanisms have been considered. It has been suggested that in patients with autoimmune chronic hepatitis, renal tubular acidosis is the consequence of a cell-mediated immune response to Tamm–Horsfall glycoprotein, a protein produced in the kidney and present in the cells of the ascending limb of the loop of Henle and the distal tubule (Tsantoulas, BMJ, 1974; iv:491). On the other hand, in Wilson's disease, as well as in primary biliary cirrhosis, copper-induced tubular lesions appear to play an important pathogenetic role. Significantly higher plasma and urinary copper levels have been observed in patients with primary biliary cirrhosis and renal tubular acidosis, as well as a correlation between these parameters and the minimal urinary pH after an ammonium chloride load (Parés, Gastro, 1981; 80:681). Treatment with D-penicillamine may reverse this abnormality (Walshe, Lancet, 1968; i:775; Leu, AmJMedSci, 1970; 260:381), probably by decreasing the copper content in the kidney. The development of cytological alterations in the epithelium of the renal tubules, when a copper–albumin complex is given to mice (Vogel, AmJPath, 1960; 36:669), makes it seem likely that copper itself may be the major cause of renal tubular acidosis in such patients. Bile acids may be another primary cause in the development of renal tubular acidosis in chronic liver disease as they are elevated in these patients and may be toxic to cell membranes. Magnesium deficiency may also produce the distal

disease in patients with cirrhosis. The administration of this element reverses this abnormality (Cohen, Magnesium, 1986; 5:39). Decreased delivery of sodium to the distal nephron appears to play a central pathogenetic role in renal tubular acidosis in patients with alcoholic cirrhosis; intense activity of sodium reabsorption has been observed in patients with this disease (Perez, PSEBM, 1977; 154: 562). The administration of diuretics, sodium sulphate, or sodium phosphate, which increase distal sodium delivery, may produce a lowering of urine pH. On the other hand, there is a close relationship between distal sodium delivery and reabsorption and the urinary excretion of hydrogen ions (Kurtzmann, KidneyInt, 1983; 24:807). Nevertheless, whether reduced delivery of sodium is the cause of an abnormal acidification in alcoholic cirrhosis or an epiphenomenon that unmasks another underlying defect remains to be elucidated.

The prostate and alcoholic hepatic cirrhosis

Testicular atrophy, decreased testicular production, prostatic atrophy, and gynaecomastia are frequent signs of endocrine dysfunction in male patients with alcoholic cirrhosis (Van Thiel, JLabClinMed, 1983; 101:21). Several studies have shown that the incidence of benign prostatic hypertrophy is lower among patients with alcoholic cirrhosis than in the general population (Stumpf, ArchIntMed, 1953; 91:304; Robson, JUrol, 1964; 92:307; Frea, UrolRes, 1987; 15:311; Morrison, AmJEpid, 1992; 135:974). Chronologically, benign prostatic hypertrophy appears later in the patient with alcoholic cirrhosis than in the normal population. Stromal hyperplasia is the most common histological finding in patients with concurrent cirrhosis and benign prostatic hypertrophy, whereas in the general population both stromal and epithelial hyperplasia are present equally. This is interesting because oestrogens induce stromal hyperplasia whereas androgens produce epithelial hyperplasia (Gavaler, AlcoholClinExpRes, 1987; 11:349). Thus, the different histological pattern of prostatic hypertrophy in patients with cirrhosis could be related to the high ratio of oestrogen to testosterone present in the plasma of these patients.

Interestingly enough, although the prevalence of prostatic carcinoma is not significantly different in patients with cirrhosis compared with normal subjects, no patient with advanced liver disease developed prostatic cancer. However, in those patients with cirrhosis with clinical hyperoestrogenism (manifested by at least two of the following criteria: gynaecomastia, palmar erythema, spider angiomas, testicular atrophy, or female hair distribution) the incidence of prostatic carcinoma was not reduced from that in the non-hyperoestrogenic group (Robson, Geriat, 1966; 21:150). These results are surprising since the response of prostatic carcinoma to oestrogens has been well recognized for many years and a lower incidence of prostatic carcinoma in the hyperoestrogenic group would be predicted. This interesting clinical aspect requires further research.

References

1. Bomzon A, Jacob G, and Better O. Jaundice and the kidney. In Epstein M, ed. *The kidney in liver disease*. 4th edn. Philadelphia: Hanley and Belfus, 1996: 423–46.

2. Fogarty BJ, *et al*. Renal dysfunction in obstructive jaundice. *British Journal of Surgery*, 1995; **82**: 878–84.

3. Eknoyan G. Glomerular abnormalities in liver disease. In Epstein M, ed. *The kidney in liver disease*, 4th edn. Philadelphia: Hanley and Belfus, 1996: 123–50.

4. Newell GC. Cirrhotic glomerulonephritis: incidence, morphology, clinical features and pathogenesis. *American Journal of Kidney Diseases*, 1987; **9**:183–90.

5. Kawaguchi K and Koike M. Glomerular lesions associated with liver cirrhosis. An immunochemical and clinicopathological analysis. *Human Pathology*, 1986; **17**: 1137–43.

6. Adler SG, Cohen AR, and Glassock RJ. Secondary glomerular diseases. In Brenner BM, ed. *The kidney*, 5th edn. Philadelphia: WB Saunders, 1996: 1498–596.

7. Oster JR and Perez GO. Derangements of acid–base homeostasis in liver disease. In Epstein M, ed. *The kidney in liver disease*, 4th edn. Philadelphia: Hanley and Belfus, 1996: 109–22.

8. Rodés J, Parés A, Rimola A, and Bruguera M. Renal tubular function in chronic cholestasis. In Gentillini P, Popper H, Sherlock S, and Teodori U, eds. *Problems in intrahepatic cholestasis*. Basel: S Karger, 1979: 132–6.

25.8 The nervous system in liver disease

Johannes Bircher and Hermann Menger

Since the discovery of portal–systemic encephalopathy interest in the relationship between the nervous system and the liver has remained high. Two excellent reviews in the 1960s summarized various neurological manifestations in patients with advanced chronic liver disease. In the meantime abnormalities of the liver have been detected in many neurological diseases, but only a few have been thoroughly investigated using modern methods.

This chapter focuses on aspects which are not covered in other sections of the book. An overview of the more important conditions with references is given in Table 1, and details are added in the text. Rare associations are summarized in Table 2.

Inborn errors of metabolism

In infants and children, different metabolic disorders of the liver may result in more or less irreversible brain damage, due for example to hyperbilirubinaemia (Hansen, ActaPaedScand, 1986; 75:513), hyperammonaemia, or hypoglycaemia.[3] A case of citrullinaemia was reported in association with isolated ACTH deficiency, rapidly developing coma (Ishii, Rinsho-Shin, 1992; 32: 853). Some congenital malformations of the central nervous system may also be associated with metabolic defects of the liver, e.g. multiple cerebellar heterotopias in ornithine carbamoyl transferase deficiency (Harding, EurJPed, 1984; 141:215).

Transient neonatal hyperammonaemia

Patients with congenital hyperammonaemias have a positive family history (76 per cent), onset in the first week of life (67 per cent), and neurological manifestations (Mufti, JPMA, 1993; 43:232). Elevation of plasma ammonia concentrations in these newborns is unexplained. In a few children it may lead to lethargy, apnoea, seizures, and coma and therefore justifies vigorous treatment. Prospective treatment of urea cycle disorders to avoid neonatal hyperammonaemic coma was described (Maestri, JPediat, 1991; 119: 923). Peritoneal dialysis and exchange transfusions have been used as main therapeutic measures, but they have not as yet been evaluated critically (Giacoia, AmJPerinat, 1986; 3:249).

Reye's syndrome

Reye's syndrome (Reye, Lancet, 1963; 2:749) characteristically presents with severe hyperemesis, and irritability followed by lethargy and coma. The syndrome occurs mostly in children (until 1994 there were only 28 cases of adult onset reported in the literature) (Rangel Guerra, RevInvestClin, 1994; 46:417) and usually follows 3 to 5 days after an influenza-like illness or varicella. A history of prior treatment with aspirin can be elicited in 95 per cent of patients. It is estimated, however, that less than 0.1 per cent of children receiving aspirin for a viral illness subsequently suffer from Reye's syndrome.

In the mildest form no change in consciousness occurs, and patients remain only irritable or lethargic (grade 1 and 2 encephalopathy). Plasma aspartate aminotransferase (**AST**) and alanine aminotransferase (**ALT**) are 3 to 30 times normal, but serum bilirubin is not elevated. In more severe forms of the disease an agitated delirium (grade 3) may progress to frank coma and decerebrate or decorticate posturing, hyperventilation (grade 4), flaccid paralysis, and respiratory failure (grade 5). The rate of progression may be quite variable, i.e. a few hours to a few days. In survivors, recovery of consciousness may occur within 24 to 96 hours, but longer-lasting brain damage has also been observed. Liver biopsy typically shows microvesicular steatosis with little necrosis or inflammatory changes. On electron microscopy mitochondria are swollen and pleomorphic, the matrix is greatly expanded and the matrix substance thickened and coarsely granular or flocculent (Partin, NEJM, 1971; 285:1339). Similar changes of the mitochondria were also observed in the brain of a patient (Partin, JNeuropathExpNeurol, 1975; 34:425) and it is now believed that Reye's syndrome is a generalized mitochondrial disease (Brown, JInherMetDis, 1991; 14:436; van Coster, Neurology, 1991; 41: 1815).

Biochemical changes include mild to severe hyperammonaemia, depending on the severity of the syndrome. Presumably the intramitochondrial part of the urea cycle is disturbed. In line with abnormal function of mitochondria, β-oxidation and glyconeogenesis are reduced. Increased glycolysis to cover energy demands leads to glycogen depletion and may be followed by hypoglycaemia (Osterloh, MedToxAdvDrugExp, 1989; 4:272).

The diagnosis should be suspected in any child or adolescent who develops vomiting 2 to 5 days after an influenza-like illness or after varicella, and early vigorous treatment should be instituted. In mild cases admission to hospital and generous energy supply by intravenous glucose (10–20 per cent) and fluid replacement is essential. When encephalopathy develops, transfer to an intensive care unit is needed, intracranial pressures should be monitored, and a programme to prevent excessive increases in intracranial pressures

Table 1 The liver in different neurological diseases

Condition of liver	Neurological manifestations	References
Congenital disorders of urea cycle enzymes (irrespective of specific enzymatic disorder)	Multiple cerebellar heterotopias	Batshaw, NEJM, 1980; 302:482
	Delayed myelination	Clancy, ElectroencephalogrClinNeurophys, 1991; 78:222
	Cerebral atrophy, microcephaly	Clayton, JInherMetDis, 1991; 14:478
	Mental retardation	Dolma, ClinNeuropathol, 1988; 7:10
Inborn errors of bile acid metabolism	Seizures, EEG abnormalities	Ebels, ArchDisChild, 1972; 47:47
	Coma	Finkelstein, JPediat, 1990; 117:897
	Pyramidal signs	Harding, EurJPed, 1984; 141:215
	Spastic paraparesis	Kendall, JNeurolNeurosurgPsych, 1983; 46:28
	Spastic quadriplegia	Lemay, JPediat, 1992; 121:725
	Distal muscle atrophy	Msall, NEJM, 1984; 310:1500
	Decreased vibration sense	Shigeto, Rinsho-Shin, 1992; 32:729
	Bucco-facio-lingual dyspraxia	Shiro, Rinsho-Shin, 1992; 32:752
	Episodes of drowsiness	Verma, ElectroencephalogrClinNeurophys, 1984; 57:105
Transient neonatal hyperammonaemia	Lethargy, seizures, coma	Giacoia GP, AmJPerinat, 1986; 3:249
	Mental retardation	Yoshimo, Neuropediatrics, 1991; 22:198
	Spastic quadriplegia	
	Epilepsy	
Reye's syndrome with microvesicular fatty change	Prodromal illness (generally influenza or varicella)	Bove, Gastro, 1975; 69:685
		Brown, JInherMedDis, 1991; 14:436
		Chi, ActaPaedJpn, 1990; 32:426
	Nausea, vomiting	Heubi, Hepatol, 1987; 7:155
	Lethargy possibly progressing to coma and death	Hukin, PediatrNeurol, 1993; 9:134
		Osterloh, MedToxAdvDrugExp, 1989; 4:272
	Gradual recovery after 1–4 days of coma	Partin, NEJM, 1971; 285:1339
		Partin, JNeuropathExpNeurol, 1975; 34:425
	Raised intracranial pressure	Pranzatelli, ClinNeuropharmacol, 1987; 10:96
		Reye, Lancet, 1963; 2:749
		Taly, IndJMedSci, 1990; 44:237
		van Coster, Neurology, 1991; 41:1815
		Schubert, ProgLivDis, 1972; 4:489
Acute necrotizing encephalopathy of childhood	Coma, convulsions, vomiting, hyperpyrexia	Mizuguchi, JNeurolNeurosurgPsych, 1995; 58:555
Alper's disease with microvesicular fatty change, liver cell loss, bridging fibrosis, etc.	Progressive neuronal degeneration of childhood	Blackwood, ArchDisChild, 1963; 38:193
		Egger, JClinPediat, 1987; 26:167
	Developmental delay	Frydman, AmJMedGen, 1993; 43:31
	Intractable epilepsy and brain atrophy	Harding, Brain, 1986; 109:181
		Harding, JChildNeurol, 1990; 5:273
	Visual and sensory symptoms	Harding, JNeurolNeurosyrgPsych, 1995; 58:320
	Severe microcephaly	Huttenlocher, ArchNeurol, 1976; 33:186
	Fetal akinesia	Jellinger, ActaNeuropath, 1970; 16:125
		Werfing, ActaPaedScand, 1967; 56:295
Wilson's disease (see Chapter 19.1)	Presentation with tremor or disturbed gait	Dobyns, MayoClinProc, 1979; 54:35
		Kendall, Neuroradiol, 1981; 22:1
	Intellectual deterioration	Lingam, Neuropediatrics, 1987; 18:11
	Ataxia, clumsiness, choreoathetosis	Lossner, PsychiatrNeurolMedPsycholLeipz, 1990; 42:585
		Saito T, EurJPed, 1987; 146:261
	Dysarthria	Walshe JM, ArchDisChild, 1962; 37:253
	Multiple reversible cerebral lesions (MRI)	See also ref. 4
Acute intermittent porphyria (see Chapter 19.5)	Acute stages	Christensen, UgeskrLaeger, 1991; 153:2237
	Neuropsychological impairment	Doss, ActaMedAustr, 1990; 17:94
	Emotional disturbances	Duhalde, RevMedChile, 1990; 118:1129
	Acute peripheral neuropathy	King, Neurology, 1991; 41:1300
	Autonomic neuropathy (e.g. hypertension)	Ranz, Hepatol, 1993; 18:1404
		Mustajoki, BMJ, 1975; 2:310
	Latent stage	Tishler, AmJPsychiat, 1985; 142:1430
	Slowed ulnar nerve conduction velocity	See also ref. 3
	Progressive weakness	
	Central pontine myelinolysis	
Sarcoidosis (detectable by liver biopsy) (see Chapter 13.2)	Parenchymatous disease of CNS; seizures	Delaney, AnnIntMed, 1977; 87:336
		Herring, JNeurolSci, 1969; 9:405
	Aseptic meningitis	Man, CanJNeurSci, 1983; 10:50
	Cranial neuropathies	Mende, FortschrNeurolPsychiatr, 1990; 58:7
	Hydrocephalus	Silverstein, ArchNeurol, 1965; 12:1
	Myopathy	Stern, ArchNeurol, 1985; 42:909
	Diabetes insipidus	
	Hemiparesis	
	Organic psychosis	

Table 1 continued

Condition of liver	Neurological manifestations	References
Vitamin B$_1$ deficiency associated with alcohol-related liver disease	Acute Wernicke's encephalopathy	Wood, MetabBrainDis, 1995; 10:57
Vitamin E deficiency due to cholestasis resulting from for example: Infantile obstructive cholangiopathy Cystic fibrosis Primary biliary cirrhosis Primary sclerosing cholangitis	Reversible changes of visual evoked potentials Hypo- to areflexia Ophthalmoplegia, other disorders of eye movements Peripheral neuropathy with axonal dystrophy and patchy demyelination Proximal muscle weakness, ataxia Decreased proprioception Psychomotor dysfunction	Alvarez, JPediat, 1985; 107:422 Arria, AmJClinNut, 1990; 52:383 Elias, Lancet, 1981; 2:1319 Guggenheim, JPediat, 1982; 100:51 Knight, Gastro, 1986; 91:209 Messenheimer, AnnNeurol, 1984; 15:499 Rosenblum, NEJM, 1981; 304:503 Sokol, JPediat, 1983; 103:197 Sokol, NEJM, 1984; 310:1209 Sokol, JPediat, 1987; 111:830 Sokol, AdvPediat, 1990; 37:119 Sokol, Gastro, 1993; 104:1727 Werlin, AnnNeurol, 1983; 13:291
Vitamin K deficiency due to cholestasis	Cerebral haemorrhage	Sutor, KlinPadiatr, 1995; 207:89
Viral hepatitis Acute hepatitis A, B, or other	1. Guillain–Barré syndrome	Dunk, BrJVenerDis, 1982; 58:269 Huet, CanMedAssJ, 1980; 122:1157 Murthy, JAssocPhysInd, 1994; 42:27 Niermeijer, BMJ, 1975; 4:732 Ono, IntMed, 1994; 33:799 Ninet, NouvPresseMed, 1983; 12:103 Penner, Gastro, 1982; 82:576 Schuchardt, DMedWoch, 1984; 109:1160 Walle, Hepatogast, 1981; 28:305
	2. Mononeuritis 3. Polyarteritis nodosa 4. Seventh cranial nerve palsy 5. Encephalitis	Pelletier, Digestion, 1985; 32:53 Lehmann, Therapiewoche, 1983; 33:6849 Gupta, JAssocPhysInd, 1992; 40:419 Davis, ActaNeurolScand, 1993; 87:67
Hepatitis B vaccination	Spontaneous reports of Guillain–Barré syndrome and other neurological events Central nervous system demyelination	Shaw, AmJEpid, 1988; 127:337 Herroelen, Lancet, 1991; 338:1174
Recovery after fulminant hepatic failure	Permanent cortical or generalized brain atrophy	O'Brien, Gut, 1987; 28:93 Toda, AmJGastr, 1983; 78:446
Anticonvulsant-induced liver changes (see Epilepsy, Section 17)		See ref. 5
Cirrhosis Alcoholic With chronic viral (usually with marked portal–systemic shunting)	1. Cerebral atrophy with neuropsychological abnormalities, hepatic 'dementia' in the aged	Bernthal, Hepatol, 1987; 7:107 Mendez, JAmGeriatSoc, 1989; 37:259 Read, QJMed, 1967; 36:135 Tarter, Gastro, 1984; 86:1421 Victor, Medicine, 1965; 44:345 Zeneroli, JHepatol, 1987; 4:283
	2. Paraplegia due to demyelination of corticospinal fibres (not responsive to treatment of portal–systemic encephalopathy)	Bechar, JNeurolSci, 1970; 11:101 Bourgeois, Neurology, 1992; 42:983 Jeske, Nervenarzt, 1991; 62:130 Lebovics, ArchIntMed, 1985; 145:1921 Mendoza, EurNeurol, 1994; 34:209 Mumford, PostgradMedJ, 1990; 66:218 Misumi, JpnJMed, 1988; 27:333 Pant, Neurology, 1968; 18:134 Rab, BrJClinPract, 1985; 39:244 Read, QJMed, 1967; 36:135 Scobie, ArchIntMed, 1964; 113:805 Sobukawa, IntMed, 1994; 33:718
	3. Cerebellar and basal ganglia disorder, choreoathetoid movements (not responsive to treatment of portal–systemic encephalopathy)	Read, QJMed, 1967; 36:135 Toghill, JNeurolNeurosurgPsych, 1967; 30:358 Victor, Medicine, 1965; 44:345 Yokota, JNeurol, 1988; 235:487
	4. Pontine spongy degeneration of white matter	Thornberry, ArchPathLabMed, 1984; 108:564

Table 1 continued

Condition of liver	Neurological manifestations	References
	5. Subclinical peripheral neuropathy, reduced nerve conduction velocities	Chari, JNeurolSci, 1977; 31:93 Dayan, Lancet, 1967; 2:133 Fierro, ElectroencephalogrClinNeurophys, 1988; 70:442 Knill-Jones, JNeurolNurosurgPsych, 1972; 35:22 Seneviratne, JNeurolneurosurgPsych, 1970; 33:609
	6. Encephalomyelopathy with spastic triparesis	Bourgeois, ActaNeurolBelg, 1992; 92:41
	7. Autonomic neuropathy	Gonzalez-Reimers, DrugAlcDep, 1991; 27:219 Kempler, GastrJ, 1990; 50:187 Khosla, JAssocPhysInd, 1991; 39:924
Sclerotherapy of oesophageal varices	Irreversible paraplegia	Seidman, Hepatol, 1984; 4:950

Table 2 Rare associations of central nervous system and liver disease

Clinical conditions	References
Alagille syndrome with intracranial haemorrhage	Hoffenberg, JPediat, 1995; 127:220
Ataxia telangiectasia with hepatocellular carcinoma	Weinstein, ArchPathLabMed, 1985; 109:1000
Creutzfeldt–Jakob disease and liver dysfunction	Tanaka, Neurology, 1992; 42:1249 Lanska, Neurology, 1993; 43:236
Olivopontocerebellar degeneration and liver cirrhosis	Agamanolis, Neurology, 1986; 36:674 Kawahara, BrainDev, 1988; 10:312
von Recklinghausen's disease with obstructive jaundice	Meyer, AnnIntMed, 1982; 97:722
von Recklinghausen's disease with hepatic Schwannoma and angiosarcoma	Lederman, Gastro, 1987; 92:234
Primary biliary cirrhosis, Sjögren's syndrome, and recurrent transverse myelitis	Rutan, Gastro, 1986; 90:206
Subarachnoid haemorrhage with polycystic kidneys and liver disease	Kuroiwa, NoShinkeiGeka, 1992; 20:905
Liver metastasis from intracranial meningioma	Jenkinson, PostgradMedJ, 1987; 63:199
Niemann–Pick disease type C with cholestatic liver disease and ataxia, nystagmus, supranuclear ophthalmoplegia, spastic tetraparesis, choreoathetosis, seizures, dementia	Kelly, JPediat, 1993; 123:242
Peripheral neuropathy and fatal alcoholic hepatitis-like disease due to amiodarone	Lim, BMJ, 1984; 288:1638
Peripheral neuropathy and alcoholic hepatitis-like liver lesions due to perhexiline	Pessayre, Gastro, 1979; 76:170
Zellweger syndrome with cirrhosis and hypo- to arreflexia, seizures, psychomotor retardation	Setchell, Hepatol, 1992; 15:198

instituted. Hyperthermia should be prevented and sedatives must be avoided.

Acute necrotizing encephalopathy of childhood

The hallmark of this encephalopathy, proposed to be a novel entity, is multiple necrotic brain lesions showing a symmetrical distribution. This was noted in previously healthy children after respiratory tract infections, with presenting symptoms of coma, convulsions, vomiting, hyperpyrexia, and hepatomegaly. Based on the characteristic combination of clinical and pathological findings, acute necrotizing encephalopathy of childhood should be distinguished from previously known encephalopathies, including Reye's syndrome (Mizuguchi, JNeurolNeurosurgPsych, 1995; 58: 555).

Alper's disease

An unknown metabolic defect with recessive inheritance is postulated in Alper's disease, the progressive neuronal degeneration of childhood. Typically it manifests itself at the age of 1 to 15 months by developmental delay and failure to thrive, followed by intractable epilepsy, with progressive brain atrophy on computed tomography, particularly in occipital areas. Liver involvement may not be conspicuous clinically but, depending on the stage of the disease, liver biopsy reveals a microvesicular fatty change, ongoing liver cell necrosis, diffuse bile-duct proliferation, together with heavy liver cell loss, collapse of plates, and bridging fibrosis.

Organic brain syndromes

In patients with organic brain syndromes, whether or not associated with affective disorders, acute intermittent porphyria and subclinical portal–systemic encephalopathy should be suspected. Both may occur intermittently and diagnosis may be difficult, if personality disorders or old age (Mendez, JAmGeriatSoc, 1989; 37:259) appear to be predominant clinically. The conditions are covered in Section 9 and Chapter 20.5.

Sarcoidosis

Sarcoidosis of the central nervous system may present with protean manifestations including focal or multifocal parenchymal disease of the CNS, meningeal inflammation and scarring, hydrocephalus, cranial or peripheral neuropathy, and myopathies. Since the neurological manifestations are non-specific, tissue diagnosis should be sought elsewhere. If no lymph node appears suitable, liver biopsy is indicated. It must be realized, however, that liver involvement may be patchy. A negative biopsy does therefore not exclude sarcoidosis. Furthermore, the finding of granulomas in the liver is not specific for sarcoidosis, since many other conditions may also lead to granulomatous changes (see Chapter 14.2).

Chronic cholestasis and vitamin E deficiency

Since bile acids are essential for the absorption of fat-soluble vitamins, cholestasis may lead to deficiencies of vitamins A, D, E, and K. Vitamin E deficiency has been associated with a progressive ataxic neurological syndrome in children with infantile obstructive cholangiopathy. Early signs are hypotonia and areflexia. In addition, the advanced clinical picture includes truncal ataxia, dysmetria, decreased vibratory sensation, decreased proprioception, gait disturbance, and ophthalmoplegia (Rosenblum, NEJM, 1981; 304: 503). Although the clinical manifestations tend to be more prominent as the children grow older, particularly after 5 years (Guggenheim, JPediat, 1983; 102:577), muscle wasting, areflexia, ptosis, and ataxia have been observed at 2 years of age and earlier (Sokol, JPediat, 1983; 103:197; Chaine, AnnMedIntern, 1988; 139: 198).

In adults, reversible delay in visual evoked potentials (P100 peak latency) has been observed in a patient with cystic fibrosis and cirrhosis (Messenheimer, AnnNeurol, 1984; 15:499). Other manifestations include ophthalmoplegia, peripheral neuropathy with axonal dystrophia, patchy demyelination, ataxia, proximal muscle weakness, and psychomotor dysfunction. Early diagnosis of the condition is important, because advanced lesions may be only partially reversible. Presumably neurological manifestations due to vitamin E deficiency may result from any of the cholestatic conditions, irrespective of their aetiology.

Serum vitamin E levels tend to be below 4 mg/ml, the lower limit of the normal range. In some cases, however, they are normal. Since vitamin E is carried with lipoproteins, serum vitamin E levels should be expressed per total lipids. In deficiency states levels will then consistently be below 0.6 to 0.8 mg/g, the lower limit of the normal range (Sokol, NEJM, 1984; 310:1209). Oral replacement therapy may be unsatisfactory because of poor bioavailability (Sokol, JPediat, 1983; 103:197). Intramuscular vitamin E substitution by repeated injections of, for example, α-tocopherylacetate may be an emotional burden for small children. α-Tocopheryl polyethylene glycol 1000 succinate in a final oral dose of 20 IU/kg/day has been reported to raise vitamin E levels in cholestasis and to improve neurological manifestations (Sokol, JPediat, 1987; 111:830; Sokol, AdvPediat, 1990; 37:119; Sokol, Gastro, 1993; 104:1727).

Neuropathies associated with viral hepatitis

Several cases of Guillain–Barré syndrome have been reported (Murthy, JAssocPhysInd, 1994; 42:27), mostly related to acute hepatitis B, but also in one case without evidence for hepatitis B, but with anti-A IgM by radioimmunoassay (Dunk, BrJVenerDis, 1982; 58:269), in another case without serological markers for hepatitis A and B (Ninet, NouvPresseMed, 1983; 12:103), and following fulminant viral hepatitis A (Ono, IntMed, 1994; 33:799). Neurological manifestations occurred either 7 days before onset of jaundice simultaneously with clinical signs of acute hepatitis, 1 to 2 weeks after onset of jaundice, or up to 5 weeks after an apparently uneventful recovery from acute hepatitis. In the last case, immune complexes were found in the serum and C3 was reduced during the phase of polyradiculitis, when the liver disease was in remission (Penner, Gastro, 1982; 82:576). Neurological recovery occurred in all patients within weeks to months. The only fatal case is of doubtful origin (Schuchardt, DMedWoch, 1984; 109:1160).

Rare instances of mononeuritis, associated with acute hepatitis A or B, involved the facial, trigeminal, auditory, and several peripheral nerves. The temporal relationship to the onset of jaundice varied from -40 to + 21 days. Clinical presentation of neuritis was generally sudden and recovery slow, the latter requiring 1 month to more than 2 years (Pelletier, Digestion, 1985; 32:53). Seventh cranial nerve palsy was reported in a case of viral hepatitis B (Gupta, JAssocPhysInd, 1992; 40:419).

Periarteriitis nodosa is a systemic disease. It involves primarily renal vessels, thereby leading to hypertension, proteinuria, haematuria, and renal failure. However, peripheral neuropathy (mononeuritis multiplex), amyotrophy, and myalgia are also frequent, and evidence for past or ongoing hepatitis B is found in about one-third of cases. Thus, the simultaneous manifestation of disease in several parts of the nervous system is the consequence of multiple vascular lesions rather than a specific association. Nevertheless, a case presenting as mononeuritis multiplex should, among other investigations, lead to a search for hepatitis B.

A reversible encephalitis developed in a 7-year-old girl 5 days after onset of a hepatitis A (Davis, ActaNeurolScand, 1993; 87:67).

A postmarketing surveillance for neurological adverse events after hepatitis B vaccination revealed 10 cases of Bell's palsy, nine of Guillain–Barré syndrome, five each of convulsions, lumbar radiculopathy, and optic neuritis, four of transverse myelitis, and three of brachial plexus neuropathy. The study involved a plasma-derived hepatitis B vaccine given to 850 000 persons. In view of limitations of the spontaneous reporting used in this study, the causal relationship between vaccination and neurological adverse events has remained questionable (Shaw, AmJEpid, 1988; 127:337). Central nervous system demyelination after immunization with recombinant hepatitis B vaccine was discussed in one case (Herroelen, Lancet, 1991; 338:1174).

Sequelae after fulminant hepatic failure

Although most survivors of fulminant hepatic failure recover full function of the central nervous system, exceptions have been noted. In these cases hepatic failure was due to paracetamol intoxication, hepatitis B, or non-A, non-B hepatitis, respectively. The lesions involved unilateral cranial nerve palsies, infarction of the right middle cerebral artery area (O'Brien, Gut, 1987; 28:93), and diffuse brain atrophy (Toda, AmJGastr, 1983; 78:446). The role of cerebral oedema for the development of irreversible lesions requires further clarification.

Neuropsychiatric conditions associated with portal–systemic encephalopathy

Although portal–systemic encephalopathy is generally thought to be a functional disorder of the brain (see Section 9) several organic lesions have been described (Table 1). Cerebral atrophy has been documented by computed tomography and correlated with neuropsychological findings (Bernthal, Hepatol, 1987; 7:107). Irreversible paraplegia due to myelopathy with loss of fibres of the corticospinal motor system has been described in several patients with long-standing portal–systemic shunting. Other neurological findings include cerebellar and basal ganglia disease with varying movement disorders, including choreoathetoid movements. Reduced nerve conduction velocities found in patients with cirrhosis are not generally associated with clinical signs of peripheral neuropathy.

Guanabens (GastroHepato, 1983; 6:119) found that 1 per cent of cirrhotics suffered from cerebrovascular accidents. In 80 per cent they were due to cerebral haemorrhages related to prolonged prothrombin times.

Neurological complication of sclerotherapy

In one patient, sclerotherapy of oesophageal varices has been followed by irreversible paraplegia due to occlusion of a spinal artery and consecutive ischaemic infarction of the spinal cord (Seidman, Hepatol, 1984; 4:950).

Neurological deficits associated with liver transplantation

Encephalopathies and neuropathies have been observed after liver transplantation, yet their relation to the procedure cannot be judged adequately, unless the relevant neurological investigations have been carried out preoperatively and reveal postoperative changes (Höckerstedt, JHepatol, 1992; 16:31). Postoperative neurological findings occurred in 76 cases, i.e. 23 per cent of the adult and 8 per cent of the paediatric patients (Menegaux, Transpl, 1994; 58:447; Patchell, Ann Neurol, 1994; 36:688). The most frequent diagnosis was encephalopathy (59 per cent), revealed by changes in mental status: agitation or obtundation, coma, catatonia, severe depression,

and insomnia occurred in decreasing order of frequency. Other common neurological complications were seizures of various causes (12 per cent), brachial plexus or peripheral nerve injuries (20 per cent), strokes (7 per cent), and central nervous system infections (7 per cent). The latter were due to *Staphylococcus aureus*, *Streptococcus*, and *Toxoplasma gondii*. Apparently, neuropathies due to femoral–axillary venous bypasses, catheterization injuries, nerve compression, and surgical retraction occur during the transplant procedure (Moreno, ActaNeurolScand, 1993; 87:25). Tremor and mental changes followed by seizures were the most frequent complications related to cyclosporin or FK506. Imipenem and desferrioxamine were responsible for one case of confusion and coma, respectively. Post-transplant mortality was higher in patients with neurological findings (14 per cent in adults and 50 per cent in children) than in patients without them (5 per cent and 7 per cent, respectively). In another series the most frequently encountered central nervous system lesions were cerebrovascular complications (infarcts, haemorrhages, anoxic–ischaemic encephalopathies, approximately 40 per cent), CNS infections (c. 15 per cent), and central pontine myelinolysis (c. 11 per cent) (Singh, Medicine, 1994; 73:110). One patient with a very complicated postoperative course lapsed into coma 12 h after liver transplantation and never regained consciousness until death 38 days after surgery (Soffer, ActaNeuropath, 1995; 90:107). He had postoperative impairment of liver function and submassive liver necrosis at autopsy.

Anticonvulsant-induced liver disease

Phenytoin, carbamazepine, and phenobarbital are strong inducers of the microsomal drug metabolizing enzyme system. Clinical correlates are occasional slight increases of serum aminotransferases and more marked increases of γ-glutamyltransferase. Liver biopsy generally shows hepatocytes with abundant, faintly eosinophilic, homogeneous or finely granular cytoplasm due to hypertrophy of endoplasmic reticulum. Uni- or paucicellular necrosis may be seen in some cases. These changes are considered to be adaptive and have no pathological significance (Jacobsen, ActaMedScand, 1976; 199:345). Replacement of carbamazepine with oxcarbazepine returned the function of the hepatic cytochrome P-450 enzyme system to normal (Isojarvi, Epilepsia, 1994; 35:1217). Valproate, ethosuximide, diazepam, and clonazepam have no enzyme-inducing properties.

Acute liver damage due to phenytoin and carbamazepine, although uncommon, has been well described. It may be hepatocellular, cholestatic, or granulomatous, and is frequently associated with signs of hypersensitivity (De Vriese, Medicine, 1995; 74:144). Similar lesions have also been described with phenobarbital. The acute liver lesion induced by valproate strongly resembles Reye's syndrome, except for the preceding viral illness which is lacking. Vigabatrin, lamotrigine, and gabapentin are well tolerated new antiepileptic drugs. Only the risk–benefit ratio of felbamate has recently been compromised by fatal liver disease in a number of patients (see Section 16 and refs [5-7]).

References

1. Read AE, Sherlock S, Laidlaw J, and Walker JG. The neuro-psychiatric syndromes associated with chronic liver disease and an extensive portal–

systemic collateral circulation. *Quarterly Journal of Medicine*, 1967; **36**: 135–50.

2. Victor M, Adams RD, and Cole M. The acquired (non-Wilsonian) type of chronic hepatocerebral degeneration. *Medicine*, 1965; **44**: 345–96.

3. Stanbury JB, Wyngaarden JB, Fredrickson DS, Goldstein JL, and Brown MS, eds. *The metabolic basis of inherited disease*. New York: McGraw-Hill, 1983.

4. Scheinberg H and Sternlieb I. *Wilson's disease. Major problems in internal medicine*. Philadelphia: WB Saunders, 1984: 23.

5. Stricker BHC. Drug-induced hepatic injury. In: Dukes MNG, ed. *Drug-induced disorders*, 2nd edn, Vol. 5. Amsterdam: Elsevier Science Publishers, 1992.

6. Schmidt D and Krämer G. The new anticonvulsant drugs. Implications for avoidance of adverse effects. *Drug Safety*, 1994; **11**: 422–31.

7. Smith MC and Bleck TP. Convulsive disorders: toxicity of anticonvulsants. *Clinics in Neuropharmacology*, 1991; **14**: 97–115.

25.9 Musculoskeletal problems in liver disease

J. van den Bogaerde and H. L. C. Beynon

Introduction

Diseases which primarily involve the liver may present with musculoskeletal manifestations (Golding, AmJMed, 1973; 55:772). Recently, hepatitis C virus has emerged as an important aetiological factor in many rheumatic diseases. Certain metabolic diseases, in particular haemochromatosis and Wilson's disease, involve the liver and joints. Other diseases, such as inflammatory bowel disease and sarcoidosis, result in pathology of both liver and musculoskeletal systems.

The following definitions are relevant:

Arthritis: swelling and inflammation of synovial tissue, with deformity, redness, and loss of function.
Polyarthritis: arthritis of more than four joints at the same time.
Oligoarthritis: arthritis of two to four joints at the same time.
Enthesopathy: inflammation of tendon or ligament insertions to bone (entheses).
Arthralgia: pain in a joint(s); swelling is not observed, but loss of function may be present.

Viral hepatitis
Acute viral infections

A transient polyarthralgia/arthritis may be seen in the prodromal phase of acute viral hepatitis. Although arthralgias are more common, frank arthritis is also well recognized, more commonly in adults than in children (Duffy, Medicine, 1976; 55:19; Bamber, Gut, 1983; 24:561). The distribution of joint involvement is usually symmetrical, with small joints of the hands and feet most frequently involved, followed by shoulders, knees, and elbows. Urticarial or maculopapular rashes, usually of the legs, may accompany the joint symptoms. Joint symptoms usually precede jaundice, but in 5 per cent of patients, joint symptoms and jaundice develop simultaneously.

Patients with hepatitis A infection develop arthralgia in approximately 10 per cent of cases, but arthritis has not been reported (Bamber, Gut, 1983; 24:561). In contrast, patients with hepatitis B may present with a symmetrical polyarthritis which resembles rheumatoid arthritis. Arthritis has even been documented following hepatitis B vaccination (Schnitzer, CurrOpinRheum, 1996; 8:341). The pathogenesis of arthritis in patients with hepatitis B infection has not been elucidated, but immune complexes may play a role (Onion, AnnIntMed, 1971; 75:29; Duffy, Medicine, 1976; 55:19; Collins, ClinImmunPath, 1983; 26:137). During the prodromal phase of hepatitis B, surface antigen (HBsAg) is present in excess, while antibody levels are low. This promotes immune complex formation, and serum complement levels fall as the resulting immune complexes are opsonized. Diagnostic confusion with acute rheumatoid arthritis is possible, since swelling is symmetrical, morning stiffness is prominent, and subcutaneous nodules may be found (Duffy, 1976). In contrast to rheumatoid arthritis, joint fluid is not inflammatory, with white cell counts of less than 1000 cells/mm^3 in the joint fluid. Plain radiographs show no joint abnormalities, and symptoms tend to settle spontaneously after approximately 20 days.

Epstein–Barr virus (**EBV**) infection may cause acute arthralgia. Up to 50 per cent of patients with EBV infection have abnormal liver function tests, and about 5 per cent have hepatomegaly. Arthralgia and myalgia are common complaints, which may persist in some patients. Parvovirus B19 may present with hepatitis and arthralgia, and has been aetiologically linked to rheumatoid arthritis (Schnitzer, CurrOpinRheum, 1996; 8:341).

The joint symptoms related to acute viral hepatitis usually settle in 6 weeks, but chronic arthritis may follow parvovirus and hepatitis B virus infection (Siegel, AmFamilyPhysician, 1996; 54:2009).

Chronic viral infections
Hepatitis C

A great deal of interest has been generated recently by data showing that hepatitis C virus (**HCV**) is associated with mixed cryoglobulinaemia syndrome, as well as porphyria cutanea tarda and membranoproliferative glomerulonephritis (Agnello, NEJM, 1992; 327:1490; Johnson, NEJM, 1993; 328:465; Gumber, AnnIntMed, 1995; 123:615; Wener, JRheum, 1996; 23:953).

Cryoglobulins are immunoglobulins which precipitate in the cold. Type I cryoglobulinaemia consists of a monoclonal cryoglobulin (such as in multiple myeloma). Type II cryoglobulinaemia has monoclonal and polyclonal cryoglobulins, while type III consists only of polyclonal cryoglobulins (Brouet, AmJMed, 1974; 57:775). IgM anti-IgG antibodies (rheumatoid factor) are often found in mixed (types II and III) cryoglobulinaemias. The mixed cryoglobulinaemias are associated with chronic bacterial, viral, or protozoal infections; lymphoproliferative disorders; connective tissue diseases such as systemic lupus erythematosus; and liver diseases (Gorevic, AmJMed, 1980; 69:287; Invernizzi, ActaHaem, 1983; 70:73). When measuring cryoglobulins, blood should be kept at 37°C until the serum has separated, and the serum is then stored at 4°C for 5 days. A serum level of more than 0.05 g/l on two occasions is sufficient to make the diagnosis of cryoglobulinaemia (Wong, ClinExpImmun, 1996; 104:25).

Historically, no underlying cause was identified in 30 to 55 per cent of patients presenting with mixed cryoglobulinaemia, and these patients were classified as having 'essential' mixed cryoglobulinaemia. Hepatitis C antibody was first demonstrated in patients with type II 'essential' cryoglobulinaemia in 1990 (Pascual, JInfDis, 1990; 162:569), and subsequent studies have confirmed HCV serological positivity in up to 90 per cent of these patients (Durand, Lancet, 1991; 337:449; Ferri, ClinExpRheum, 1991; 9: 621; Ferri, Infec, 1991; 19:417; Agnello, NEJM, 1992; 327:140). One-third of HCV-infected patients have circulating cryoglobulins (Clifford, Hepatol, 1995; 21:613). While type III cryoglobulins may be more prevalent in unselected patients with HCV infection, type II cryoglobulins are found in higher concentration, and are more likely to lead to complications (Wong, ClinExpImmun, 1996; 104: 25). The presence of HCV RNA in the cryoprecipitates argues strongly that the HCV is of pathological significance (Wong, 1996). There is no association between HCV genotypes and cryoglobulinaemia (Wener, JRheum, 1996; 23:953). The DR2 class II MHC molecule appears to confer some protection against HCV-associated cryoglobulinaemia (Congia, Hepatol, 1996; 24:1338).

Immunoglobulin complex deposition with a decrease in complement levels is found in patients with mixed cryoglobulinaemia syndrome, resulting in polyarthritis, arthralgia, leucocytoclastic or necrotizing vasculitis, glomerulonephritis, and peripheral neuropathy (Apartis, JNeurolNeurosurgPsych, 1996; 60:661). Cerebral infarction has also been described in these patients (Petty, Mayo-ClinProc, 1996; 71:671). It has been suggested that the incomplete manifestations of the mixed cryoglobulinaemia syndrome in HCV-infected patients could explain the chronic fatigue, sicca syndrome, peripheral neuropathy, lung involvement, polyarthritis, and lichen planus which have all been reported in patients with HCV infection.

An association between lymphoproliferative diseases and HCV infection has also been described (Ferri, JAMA, 1994; 272:355). HCV infection is associated with salivary gland inflammation in 49 per cent of asymptomatic patients (Pawlotsky, Hepatol, 1994; 19:841), and has also been reported in antibody negative (anti-Ro or La) cases of sicca syndrome (Pawlotsky, 1994).

Although some tantalizing data have been presented implicating HCV in diseases such as polyarteritis nodosa, polymyositis, systemic lupus erythematosus, rheumatoid arthritis, and thyroiditis (Cupps, ProbIntMed, 1981; 21:1; Hirohata, IntMed, 1992; 31:493), the consensus is that these are probably chance associations (Wener, JRheum, 1996; 23:953). Since the mixed cryoglobulinaemia syndrome due to HCV infection causes 75 per cent rheumatoid factor seropositivity (Pawlotsky, Hepatol, 1994; 19:841; Clifford, Hepatol, 1995; 21:613) and a chronic deforming polyarthritis, differentiation between this syndrome and conditions such as rheumatoid arthritis may be difficult. It would however seem prudent to include an HCV serological test in patients with chronic arthritis, particularly if hepatotoxic drugs such as methotrexate are being considered.

Once the diagnosis of HCV infection and mixed cryoglobulinaemia syndrome has been made, treatment options include chloroquine, low-dose steroids, or interferon-α (Misiani, NEJM, 1994; 330:751). Interferon-α may increase symptoms of fatigue and myalgias in these patients, but may be useful in treating HCV infection as well as mixed cryoglobulinaemia syndrome (Misiani, NEJM, 1993; 328:1121; Misiani, 1994). Complications such as thrombocytopenia may accompany interferon therapy (Kimura, ActaMedScand, 1994; 85:329). Joint disease may be treated with short-term steroid therapy, but long-term immunosuppression is not recommended (Gane, Gastro, 1996; 110:167; Wener, JRheum, 1996; 23:953) due to the danger of increasing viral replication and worsening hepatitis.

Autoimmune hepatitis (see Chapter 14.3)

Autoimmune hepatitis is a disease of unknown aetiology; 80 per cent of patients are female. Chronic hepatitis is characteristic, but up to one-third of patients present with an acute hepatitis. Immune-mediated inflammation of hepatocytes occurs, and the autoimmune haplotype (HLA A1/B8/DR8) and the C4A null allele are over-expressed in these patients (Vergani, AnnItalMedInt, 1996; 11:119). Non- organ-specific autoantibodies are typically detected in patients with autoimmune hepatitis. Anti-smooth muscle and antinuclear antibodies are characteristic of adult patients with autoimmune hepatitis, while anti-liver/kidney microsomal type 1 (**LKM 1**) antibodies are reported in younger patients. Anti-LKM 1 antibodies may also be found in patients with hepatitis C infection, but the antigen specificity differs from patients with autoimmune hepatitis (Vergani, 1996). Anti-LKM 3 antibodies have also been documented in autoimmune hepatitis and hepatitis D patients (Strassburg, Gastro, 1996; 111:1576). Anticentromere and antineutrophil cytoplasmic antibodies (pANCA) have been documented in patients with autoimmune hepatitis (Onozuka, RinshoByori, 1996; 44:877; Seibold, EurJGastroHepatol, 1996; 8:1095).

Ten to fifty per cent of patients with autoimmune hepatitis present with arthralgia at some stage during the course of the disease. Large joint involvement is usual, but symptoms may be confined to the small joints of the hands. Arthritis is less common, but confusion with rheumatoid arthritis may occur since joint erosions have occasionally been reported, and rheumatoid factor is frequently detected (Barnardo, Gut, 1973; 14:800). Lymphocyte infiltration of joints may also be similar to rheumatoid arthritis. Rash, pleurisy, ulcerative colitis, and serositis have all been described. Autoimmune hepatitis responds to long-term immunosuppression, and joint symptoms should be managed symptomatically.

Primary biliary cirrhosis (Chapter 14.1)

Primary biliary cirrhosis is an uncommon autoimmune disease of unknown aetiology, characterized by the destruction of small bile ducts. Patients usually present with jaundice and pruritus in the fourth to the seventh decades, and up to 90 per cent of patients are female. High titres of antimitochondrial antibody (**AMA**) are typical, and serum IgM level is usually raised. AMA is usually found in less than 1 per cent of the general population (Turchany, AmJGastr, 1997; 92:124), and although patients with primary biliary cirrhosis without AMA have been described, it has been suggested these these patients may have a disease which is distinct from primary biliary cirrhosis (Sanschez Pobre, JClinGastro, 1996; 23;191). Patients with primary biliary cirrhosis have an increased incidence of other autoimmune diseases such as thyroiditis, scleroderma, Sjögren's syndrome, and rheumatoid arthritis.

Primary biliary cirrhosis may be associated with rheumatoid arthritis, Sjögren's syndrome, diffuse and limited scleroderma, polymyalgia rheumatica, systemic lupus erythematosus, thyroiditis, Raynaud's syndrome, haemolytic anaemia, uveitis, and polymyositis/dermatomyositis (Clarke, AnnRheumDis, 1978; 37:42; Miller, ArchPathLabMed, 1979; 103:505; Schaffner, PostgradMed, 1979; 65:97; Culp, MayoClinProc, 1982; 57:365; Hall, AnnIntMed, 1984; 100:388; Rutan, Gastro, 1986; 90:206; Milosevic, JClinGastro, 1990; 12:332). Immune complexes are sometimes found (Gupta, AmJMed, 1982; 73:192), but are probably of minor importance in the pathogenesis of the disease. Immune complex tests may be falsely positive due to reactive IgM molecules which are associated with this disease.

The most common joint involvement in patients with primary biliary cirrhosis is an erosive, non-deforming synovitis involving the hands and ankles (Clarke, AnnRheumDis, 1978; 37:42; Schaffner, PostgradMed, 1979; 65:97). Proximal and distal interphalangeal joints are often involved. An association between cutaneous xanthomas and cortical bone erosions has been noted, suggesting that cholesterol deposition might have contributed to bone erosions. Subperiosteal bone resorption and osteopenia may be visible on radiography (Clarke, 1978). A study has shown periostitis in 35 per cent of patients with primary biliary cirrhosis (Epstein, Gut, 1981; 22:203).

Metabolic and genetic liver diseases

Haemochromatosis (Chapter 20.2)

An MHCV-like gene which is mutated in genetic haemochromatosis has been identified in patients (Feder, NatureGen, 1996; 13:399). Arthritis develops in 50 per cent of patients with homozygous haemochromatosis, and may be the presenting symptom (Dymock, AnnRheumDis, 1970; 29:469; Rosner, AmJMed, 1981; 70:870). The second and third metacarpophalangeal and proximal interphalangeal joints are usually involved (Rosner, 1981; Adamson, Radiol, 1983; 147:377), and wrist and knee joints are less commonly affected. Haemochromatosis is an important differential diagnosis in patients with symmetrical polyarthritis involving the metacarpophalangeal joints and should be excluded when considering the diagnosis of rheumatoid arthritis.

Calcium pyrophosphate deposition is one of the major and frequent manifestations of joint disease of haemochromatosis and increases with time. In one study, crystal deposition was seen in 7 of 18 patients at the first examination, and 13 of 18 patients 10 years later (Hamilton, QJMed, 1981; 50:321). In 12 of the 13 patients with calcium pyrophosphate deposition, two or more joints were involved, and involvement became more pronounced with age. Calcium pyrophosphate deposition is found in patients with genetic haemochromatosis, and also those with iron overload due to blood transfusions, so iron molecules may play a role in crystal deposition (Dymock, AnnRheumDis, 1970; 29:469). Venesection does not reduce crystal deposition (Hamilton, 1981). Arthritis can be worsened by crystal deposition, causing recurrent attacks of pseudogout (Atkins, QJMed, 1970; 39:71).

Radiologically, joint space narrowing and bone cysts are seen, articular cartilage is destroyed, and calcification in the triangular ligament of the wrist and the menisci and cartilages of the knee is a characteristic feature (Adamson, Radiol, 1983; 147:377). Joint space narrowing of the fourth and fifth metacarpophalangeals is more pronounced in haemochromatosis than in primary chondrocalcinosis, and hook-like osteophytes on the radial aspect of the metacarpal heads are typical.

Wilson's disease (Chapter 20.1)

Joint and bone problems are common complications of this disease (Golding, AnnRheumDis, 1977; 36:99; Menerey, JRheum, 1988; 15:331). Osteopenia is the most common rheumatological complication and is seen in 25 to 50 per cent of patients, probably due to proximal renal tubular acidosis (Mindelzun, Radiol, 1970; 94: 127). Arthropathy is also commonly seen, and has been reported in up to 50 per cent of adults. Premature osteoarthritis, periarticular subchondral cysts, osteochondritis dessicans, and chondromalacia patellae may all be found. The longer the duration of disease, the more severe the arthritis becomes. Synovial fluid is usually clear and viscous, with less than 1000 mononuclear cells/mm^3. Multiple calcified loose bodies at the wrist with marked osteophyte formation are well described. Prominent calcified entheses may be seen, and chondrocalcinosis of the large joints such as the hips, spine, and knees are also a feature of this disease (Golding, 1977).

Copper has been found in articular cartilage, suggesting a role for oxygen-derived free radicals in joint disease (Menerey, JRheum, 1988; 15:331). Penicillamine-induced arthropathy may complicate therapy in patients with Wilson's disease (Walshe, ProcRSocMed, 1977; 70(Suppl. 3):4).

Miscellaneous joint disease in patients with liver abnormalities

Inflammatory bowel disease

Inflammatory bowel disease is associated with a wide range of extraintestinal manifestations, including peripheral arthritis in 20 per cent, ankylosing spondylitis in 3 to 5 per cent, sclerosing cholangitis, uveitis, and dermatological complications (Greenstein, Medicine, 1976; 55:401; Baillie, Geriat, 1985; 40:53; Harmatz, MedClinNAm, 1994; 78:1387). Extraintestinal manifestations may be caused by cross-reactivity to bacterial antigens (Levine, GastrClinNAm, 1995; 24:633). Peripheral arthritis, skin disease, and uveitis are symptoms which resolve during medically induced remission of disease or after surgery (Greenstein, 1976). The frequency of axial arthritis is increased in HLA B27-positive patients (Levine, 1995). Axial joint involvement is typically independent of inflammatory bowel disease activity. Although bowel involvement is usually obvious, some patients may have arthritis in the absence of bowel symptoms, and may present years later with overt bowel disease (Levine, 1995).

Periostitis

Periostitis has been reported in all types of chronic liver disease, and in one series was reported in up to 29 per cent of patients with chronic liver disease (Epstein, Gut, 1981; 22:203). Bilateral involvement of the distal ends of the tibia and fibula is the commonest pattern seen, but distal radius and ulna may also be affected. Patients complain of pain and tenderness over the distal ends of the long bones, and radiology confirms the diagnosis as it shows periosteal proliferation.

Hypertrophic osteoarthropathy

Hypertrophic osteoarthropathy is characterized by clubbing of fingers and toes, and periosteal proliferation of long bones. Synovitis, producing arthritis or arthralgia, is associated with hypertrophic osteoarthropathy but is not required to make the diagnosis (Martinez-Lavin, JRheum, 1993; 20:1386; Martinez-Lavin, CurrOpinRheum, 1997; 9:83). The association between cirrhosis and hypertrophic osteoarthropathy been known for more than a hundred years, and has been called hypertrophic hepatic osteoarthropathy (Epstein, Gut, 1981; 22:203). Hypertrophic osteoarthropathy may be generalized or localized, and has been described in patients with lung disease (cystic fibrosis, chronic lung infections, lung cancer), cardiac disease (cyanotic heart lesions, infective endocarditis), intestinal diseases (inflammatory bowel disease, laxative abuse), mediastinal tumours, primary hyperthyroidism, and the POEMS syndrome of polyneuropathy, organomegaly, endocrinopathy, M protein, and skin changes (Martinez-Lavin, 1997). Hypertrophic osteoarthropathy has been reported in hepatic diseases such as primary biliary cirrhosis, alcoholic cirrhosis, sclerosing cholangitis, biliary atresia, and bile duct and hepatic carcinoma (Reginato, ArthRheum, 1980; 23:1391; Rothberg, PediatrRadiol, 1983; 13:44; Varju, ClinExpRheumatol, 1986; 4:375; Huaux, AnnRheumDis, 1987; 46:342); it has been reported in alcoholics without cirrhosis.

The pathogenesis of this condition is not known, but may be related to shunting of blood through the lungs, which occurs in conditions such as cirrhosis and cyanotic heart disease. Megakaryocytes are usually filtered from the blood by the lung microvasculature, but if they enter the systemic circulation as a result of shunting, they concentrate at the distal ends of bones and activate endothelial cells and platelets (Varju, ClinExpRheumatol, 1986; 4:375).

Sarcoidosis (Chapter 14.2)

Sarcoidosis is a multisystem disorder of unknown aetiology, characterized by the presence of non-caseating granulomas in various tissues (Chesnutt, West JMed, 1995; 162:519). The overall prevalence is in the order of 1/5000 in the normal population (DeRemee, MayoClinProc, 1995; 70:177), and the clinical features depend on the severity of the disease in the affected organs. The pathogenesis of sarcoidosis probably involves abnormal interactions between external antigens, T cells, intercellular adhesion molecules, and cytokine networks (Petterson, CurrOpinRheum, 1997; 1:62).

The commonest organs involved include the lungs, eyes, skin, nervous system, musculoskeletal system, kidneys, endocrine organs, liver, and the heart. Liver involvement is usually subclinical, but liver function tests are often abnormal (DeRemee, MayoClinProc, 1995; 70:177). Intrahepatic cholestasis, portal hypertension, and Budd–Chiari syndrome have all been described.[1] Liver biopsy demonstrates non-caseating granulomas in up to 80 per cent of patients, and is often used as a diagnostic test in patients with sarcoidosis. The most common rheumatological manifestation of sarcoidosis is an acute sarcoid arthritis as part of Loffgren's syndrome (DeRemee, 1995), but a chronic arthritis resembling rheumatoid arthritis has been described, as well as spinal involvement which may look like ankylosing spondylitis. Bone involvement in sarcoidosis may occur in up to 33 per cent of cases, patients may be asymptomatic or complain of tenderness and stiffness of adjacent joints. Radiologically, punched-out cysts involving the cortex and the medulla of the phalanges are typical.[2] Acute and chronic granulomatous myopathy or a palpable nodular myopathy may complicate systemic sarcoidosis (Matsuo, SkeletalRadiol, 1995; 24:535; Petterson, CurrOpinRheum, 1997; 1:62).

References

1. Sherlock S. The liver in sarcoidosis. In Geraint James D, ed. *Sarcoidosis and other granulomatous disorders*. New York: Marcel Dekker, 1994: 375–85.
2. Rizzato G and Montemurro L. The locomotor system in sarcoidosis. In Geraint James D, ed. *Sarcoidosis and other granulomatous disorders*. New York: Marcel Dekker, 1994: 349–68.

The effect of liver disease on bone

Juliet Compston

Liver disease may affect the bones in several ways. First, generalized disturbances of bone remodelling and mineralization can cause metabolic bone disease. Secondly, localized skeletal lesions may occur; these are most commonly neoplastic, but may occasionally be infective. Thirdly, periosteal new bone formation sometimes occurs in chronic liver disease.

Metabolic bone disease

Two major forms of metabolic bone disease occur in association with liver disease, osteoporosis and rickets or osteomalacia.

Osteoporosis

Definition

Osteoporosis is characterized by low bone mass and disruption of bone architecture, resulting in reduced bone strength and increased risk of fragility fracture, particularly in the spine, hip, and radius. The increased risk of osteoporosis associated with chronic liver disease should be considered in the context of its high prevalence in the general population; in the United Kingdom approximately 250 000 fractures due to osteoporosis occur annually, with an estimated cost to the health services of £750 million. The incidence of fragility fractures rises with age, and women are more commonly affected than men. The estimated remaining lifetime risk of any fragility fracture in a 50-year-old Caucasian woman is around 40 per cent; in men of this age, the figure approaches 13 per cent.

Clinical manifestations

The morbidity and mortality resulting from osteoporosis are solely attributable to fracture. Hip fractures occur mainly in very elderly people and have a mortality at 6 months of around 20 per cent, whereas the incidence of Colles' fractures of the distal radius starts to increase around the time of the menopause and reaches a peak at about 65 years of age. Vertebral fractures may be asymptomatic and only one-third or so come to medical attention. Nevertheless, the morbidity of these fractures, although poorly characterized, is likely to be considerable, with spinal deformity, pain, and disability. A minority of patients present with acute and severe back pain at the level of the affected vertebra, which often radiates around to the front of the chest or abdomen. The natural history of the pain is extremely variable, but some patients continue to suffer severe pain for many years.

Vertebral fractures are the most commonly reported manifestation of osteoporosis in patients with chronic liver disease. This may reflect predominantly axial, trabecular bone loss or may be a consequence of the shortened lifespan of these patients, many of whom die before the ninth and tenth decades of life when hip fractures are most common

Diagnosis

The problems that have arisen in the past over the diagnosis of osteoporosis relate to its heterogeneous skeletal distribution and the lack of definite clinical or radiological changes until bone loss is advanced, often with fracture. The development of non-invasive techniques that enable accurate and precise measurements of bone mass at clinically relevant sites has revolutionized the diagnosis of osteoporosis and has provided a means by which fracture risk may be predicted.

A number of techniques are available for assessment of bone mineral density (Table 1).[1] The method of choice is dual-energy X-ray absorptiometry because of its low radiation dose, good precision, and application to both axial and appendicular skeleton. This and most of the other methods generate a bone mineral density expressed in g/cm^2 and hence represent an areal rather than a true volume density (Compston, Bone, 1995; 16:5). Spinal measurements are performed in the lumbar spine, usually L1–L4; the presence of vertebral deformity artefactually increases bone mineral density, as may scoliosis, extraskeletal calcification, and osteophytes. Dual-energy X-ray absorptiometry has now largely superseded the technique of dual-photon absorptiometry, which was based on similar principles but employed a radioactive source.

The rationale for the use of bone densitometry in clinical practice is based on the demonstration, in prospective studies, of a relation between bone mass and fracture risk. For every decrease of 1 SD in bone density, fracture risk increases two- to three-fold; the strength of this association compares favourably with that between blood pressure and stroke or serum lipid profile and coronary heart disease. Since the gradient of fracture risk across bone density is continuous, there is no cut-off point below which fracture will always occur and above which it will not. None the less, for diagnostic purposes, thresholds have been proposed that are based on T scores, SD scores derived from values in healthy premenopausal women (WHO Study Group, WHO TechRepSer 843, 1994; Compston, BMJ, 1995; 310:1507). The proposed diagnostic classification is as follows:

Table 1 Measurement of bone mineral density			
Method	**Site**	**Accuracy (%)**	**Precision (%)**
Dual-energy X-ray absorptiometry	Spine	5–10	1
	Femur	5–10	2–3
	Whole body	1–2	1
Single X-ray absorptiometry	Radius	2–5	1–2
Single-photon absorptiometry	Radius	2–5	1–2
Quantitative computed tomography	Spine	5–10	2–4
	Radius	5–10	2–4
Broad band ultrasonic attenuation	Os calcis	Uncertain	2–4

- osteopenia: T score between −1 and −2.5;
- osteoporosis: T score below −2.5;
- established osteoporosis: T score below −2.5 with one or more fragility fractures.

Studies of the prevalence of osteoporosis associated with chronic liver disease predate this classification and have generally employed a criterion of a bone mineral density of 2 SD or more below the mean age- and sex-matched reference value (Z score below −2). The World Health Organization densitometric criteria apply to measurements of bone mineral density at the spine or hip or, less commonly, the radius and are based on studies in women. Appropriate criteria in men have not been established.

Radiology

Radiological osteopenia is a relatively insensitive index of low bone mass. However, radiology plays an important part in the diagnosis of vertebral deformities (Fig. 1). In recent years, quantitative approaches to the assessment of vertebral deformity have been developed that take into account differences in vertebral shape between and within normal individuals. These are based on changes in the ratio of anterior, middle, and posterior vertebral heights, a reduction of 3 SD or more generally being regarded as significant (Eastell, JBoneMinRes, 1991; 6:207).

Prevalence in liver disease

Osteoporosis has been described in association with a large variety of liver diseases including primary biliary cirrhosis, chronic active hepatitis, sclerosing cholangitis, alcoholic liver disease, cryptogenic cirrhosis, idiopathic haemochromatosis, glycogen storage disease, and primary benign hepatoma.[2] Most studies have concerned patients with chronic cholestatic liver disease, although there are reports in patients with chronic active hepatitis and alcoholic liver disease. Because trabecular and cortical osteoporosis often exist independently of one another, their prevalence has to be defined

separately. The implications of bone loss in these two types of bone also differ: vertebral fractures are mainly a consequence of trabecular bone loss, whereas both cortical and trabecular bone loss are important in fractures of the radius and femur.

Trabecular osteoporosis

Clinical descriptions of spinal osteoporosis in patients with chronic liver disease date back to the early part of the twentieth century (Seidel, MunchMedWoch, 1910; 57:2033). Estimates of its prevalence were generally based either on radiological changes or histomorphometric assessment of trabecular bone volume in the iliac crest. Such studies, carried out mainly in selected groups of patients with chronic cholestatic liver disease, reported a wide variation in the percentage of patients with osteoporosis, from as low as 9 per cent up to 60 per cent (Ahrens, Medicine, 1950; 29: 299; Atkinson, QJMed, 1955; 99:299; Long, Gut, 1978; 19:85; Compston, DigDisSci, 1980; 25:28; Herlong, Gastro, 1982; 83:103; Cuthbert, Hepatol, 1984; 4:1; Stellon, Bone, 1986; 7:181). These reported variations clearly reflect a variety of factors, including patient selection and diagnostic criteria. Data obtained using newer and more appropriate techniques are now emerging, but most studies so far have included only small numbers of selected patients (Table 2). Using either quantitative computed tomography or dual-photon absorptiometry, two studies on chronic alcohol abusers, of 8 and 17 patients, respectively, have shown an increased prevalence of osteoporosis (defined as a vertebral bone mineral density more than 2 SD below the normal mean) (Bikle, AnnIntMed, 1985; 103: 42; Feitelberg, Metabolism, 1987; 36:322); some increase in the prevalence of spinal osteoporosis was also reported in a selected group of 15 premenopausal women with primary biliary cirrhosis (Hodgson, AnnIntMed, 1985; 103:855).

In a larger and unselected study of 64 patients with chronic liver disease, 9 per cent were found to have a spinal bone mineral density more than 2 SD below the age-matched mean reference value: most of these had corticosteroid-treated chronic active hepatitis and, furthermore, the mean spinal bone mineral density in corticosteroid-treated patients was lower than in those not treated with corticosteroids (Rose, EurJGastroHepatol, 1991; 3:63). However, in a prospective study of 16 women treated with corticosteroids for chronic active hepatitis, increased rates of bone loss were observed at a predominantly cortical site in the radius (Clements, EurJ-GastroHepatol, 1993; 5:543).

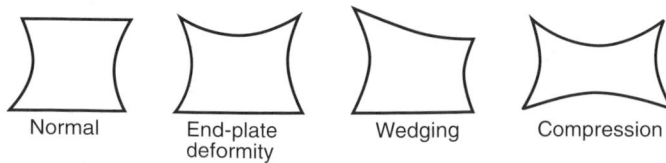

Normal   End-plate   Wedging   Compression
                deformity

Fig. 1. Changes in vertebral shape associated with osteoporosis.

Table 2 Prevalence studies of spinal trabecular osteoporosis in chronic liver disease

Authors	Year	No. studied	Liver disease	Selection of patients	Method used	No. abnormal	Percentage abnormal
Bikle *et al.*	1985	8	Alcoholic liver disease	Yes	Quantitative CT	5	62.5
Hodgson *et al.*	1985	13	Primary biliary cirrhosis	Yes	Dual-photon absorptiometry	2	15.4
Feitelberg *et al.*	1987	17	Alcoholic liver disease	Yes	Dual-photon absorptiometry	2	11.8
Diamond *et al.*	1990	115	Mixed	No	Quantitative CT	18	16
Bonkovsky *et al.*	1990	133	Mixed	No	Dual-photon absorptiometry	33	26
Rose *et al.*	1991	64	Mixed	No	Quantitative CT	6	9.4

Osteoporosis is defined as a bone mineral density more than 2 SD below the normal mean value.

More recently, two large studies of patients with chronic liver disease have been reported. One reported a prevalence of spinal osteoporosis of 16 per cent in a large unselected group of patients (Diamond, 1990, Gut; 31:82); a higher prevalence of 26 per cent was found in a study of 133 unselected patients (Bonkovsky, Hepatol, 1990; 12:273). Finally, in a study of bone disease in patients with primary sclerosing cholangitis (Hay, Hepatol, 1991; 14:257), spinal bone mineral density was significantly reduced in those with advanced disease but normal in newly diagnosed patients. In 50 per cent of the advanced group, spinal bone mineral density was below an arbitrary fracture threshold (0.98 g/cm^2).

Cortical osteoporosis

The first quantitative demonstration of cortical osteoporosis in chronic liver disease (Paterson, ScaJGastr, 1967; 2:293) employed metacarpal morphometry. Subsequent studies, using either this technique or single-photon absorptiometry, confirmed this finding in chronic cholestatic liver disease (Wagonfeld, Lancet, 1976; ii: 391; Herlong, Gastro, 1982; 83:103; Matloff, Gastro, 1982; 83:97; Kato, ClinRadiol, 1982; 33:313; Stellon, QJMed, 1985; 57:783), chronic active hepatitis (Stellon, Gastro, 1985; 89:1078), and alcoholic liver disease (Nilsson, ClinOrthopRelRes, 1973; 90:229; Mobarhan, Hepatol, 1984; 4:266) (Table 3). There is some evidence that the prevalence of cortical osteoporosis may be higher than that of trabecular osteoporosis; thus in one study (Kato, ClinRadiol, 1982; 33:313) around 20 per cent of women with primary biliary cirrhosis were found to have cortical thinning whilst in another (Rose, EurJGastroHepatol, 1991; 3:63) a prevalence of 16 per cent was found in 64 patients with chronic liver disease. Finally, in two large studies of patients with mixed chronic liver disease, reported prevalence rates of osteoporosis were 23 per cent at the distal radius site (Diamond, Gut, 1990; 31:83) and between 13 and 39 per cent at the proximal femur (Bonkovsky, Hepatol, 1990; 12:273).

As would be expected, studies of patients in the early stages of liver disease have shown little evidence of significant metabolic bone disease. Thus bone density in the proximal femur was normal at the time of presentation of primary biliary cirrhosis in all of 25 patients, although bone mineral content in the forearm was reduced in three of these (Mitchison, Gastro, 1988; 94:463).

Fracture prevalence in liver disease

There have been no studies of the incidence of fractures in patients with chronic liver disease. In a selected group of 15 women with primary biliary cirrhosis, a prevalence rate of 13 per cent was found for vertebral fractures (Hodgson, AnnIntMed, 1985; 103:855), and in 31 patients with alcoholic liver disease a prevalence rate of 32 per cent for peripheral fractures (Wilkinson, BrJAddic, 1985; 80:65). In a study of 115 unselected patients with chronic liver disease, the prevalence rates for both spinal and peripheral fractures were twice those found in an age- and sex- matched control group, hypogonadal and cirrhotic patients being at greater risk (Diamond, Gut, 1990; 31:82).

Pathophysiology of bone loss in chronic liver disease

Bone remodelling occurs at discrete sites located on the trabecular bone surface, a quantum of bone being resorbed by osteoclasts and subsequently replaced by osteoblasts (Fig. 2).[3]

Under normal circumstances, the amount of bone formed within each remodelling unit is similar to that resorbed, so that there is no net change in the amount of bone. If, however, the amount of bone formed is less relative to the amount initially resorbed, there will be net bone loss. This is one of the basic mechanisms of bone loss at the cellular level in osteoporosis, and may theoretically be due to an increase in the amount of bone resorbed, a decrease in that formed, or a combination of the two. Once bone formation within the unit has ceased, bone loss is irreversible. The other mechanism of bone loss at this level is an increase in the number of remodelling units activated along the trabecular bone surface, which leads to potentially reversible bone loss (Fig. 3). These two mechanisms may operate separately or simultaneously and their contribution to bone loss can to some extent be assessed by standard histomorphometric techniques.

Present evidence on the cellular pathophysiology of bone loss associated with chronic liver disease is conflicting, but most data indicate that decreased bone formation contributes to bone loss (Fig. 4). The mean wall thickness, a measure of the amount of bone formed within individual remodelling units, is reduced in primary biliary cirrhosis (Stellon, Hepatol, 1987; 7:137), chronic active

Table 3 Prevalence studies of osteoporosis—peripheral measurements

Authors	Year	No. studied	Liver disease	Selection of patients	Method used	No. abnormal	Percentage abnormal
Paterson and Losowsky	1967	38	Mixed	Yes	Metacarpal morphometry	3	8.3
Epstein et al.	1981	83, 61	Primary biliary cirrhosis, parenchymal liver disease	No, No	Metacarpal morphometry, metacarpal morphometry	17, 14	20.0, 22.5
Matloff et al.	1982	10	Primary biliary cirrhosis	Yes	Single-photon absorptiometry	6	60
Mobarhan et al.	1984	56	Alcoholic liver disease	Yes	Single-photon absorptiometry (d)	18*	32
Cuthbert et al.	1984	11	Primary biliary cirrhosis	Yes	Single-photon absorptiometry (d)	1	9.1
Stellon et al.	1985	36	Chronic active hepatitis	No	Metacarpal morphometry, single-photon absorptiometry (d), single-photon absorptiometry (m)	3, 5, 4	8.3, 13.9, 11.1
Bikle et al.	1985	8	Alcoholic liver disease	Yes	Metacarpal morphometry, single-photon absorptiometry (m)	2, 2	25, 25
Hodgson et al.	1985	15	Primary biliary cirrhosis	Yes	Single-photon absorptiometry (d)	2	13.3
Stellon et al.	1986	36	Primary biliary cirrhosis	No	Single-photon absorptiometry (d), single-photon metacarpal morphometry	4, 2, 3	11.1, 5.6, 8.3
Mitchison et al.	1988	25	Primary biliary cirrhosis	No	Single-photon absorptiometry (d)	3	12
Diamond et al.	1990	115	Mixed	No	Single-photon absorptiometry (d)	26	23
Bonkovsky et al.	1990	133	Mixed	No	Dual-photon absorptiometry: femoral neck Ward's triangle greater trochanter	33 17 51 33	26 23 39 25
Rose et al.	1991	64	Mixed	No	Single-photon absorptiometry (m)	10	15.6

(d) Distal radius (trabecular and cortical bone); (m) mid-radius (mainly cortical bone).
* More than 1.5 SD below the normal mean value.
Except where otherwise indicated, osteoporosis is defined as a bone mineral content more than 2 SD below the normal mean value.

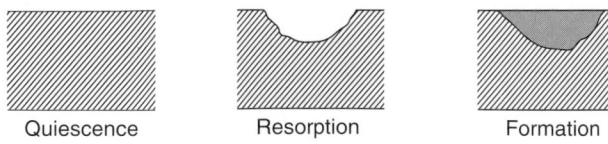

Quiescence   Resorption   Formation

Fig. 2. Schematic representation of the sequence of events within a bone remodelling unit. The sequence of events is always that resorption precedes formation.

hepatitis (Stellon, Gut, 1988; 29:378), and alcoholic liver disease (Mobarhan, Hepatol, 1984; 4:266); reduced rates of bone formation at both tissue and cellular levels were demonstrated in these and other studies (Herlong, Gastro, 1982; 83:103; Cuthbert, Hepatol,

1984; 4:1; Quanabens, AmJGastr 1990; 85:1356) when comparison is made with most control data (Frost, Bone Histomorphometry, Second International Workshop, 1977; 445; Melsen, CalcifTissRes, 1978; 26:99; Vedi, Bone, 1983; 5:69). Further evidence in support of reduced osteoblastic function is provided by measurements of osteoid seam width and its determinants. The mean osteoid seam width depends on three factors, the rate of matrix synthesis, the rate of its maturation, and finally, the mineral apposition rate. In primary biliary cirrhosis, most studies have reported a reduced (Matloff, Gastro, 1982; 2:97; Stellon, Bone, 1986; 7:181) or normal (Hodgson, AnnIntMed, 1985; 103:855) mean osteoid seam width, which, in conjunction with the demonstrated prolonged maturation period and normal or low mineral apposition rate, indicates a

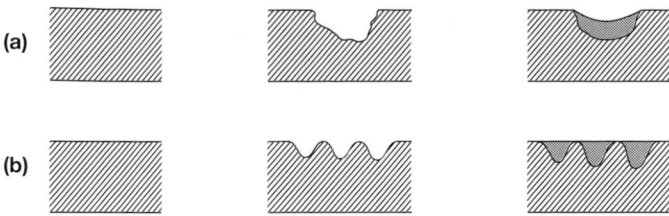

Fig. 3. Mechanisms of bone loss at the level of the remodelling unit. In (a) the amount of bone formed within the unit is less than that resorbed, leading to irreversible bone loss. This may result from an increase in the amount resorbed, a decrease in the amount formed, or a combination to the two. In (b) the number of remodelling units along the trabecular bone surface is increased, leading to potentially reversible bone loss at the end of the resorption phase of remodelling.

reduced rate of matrix synthesis. Similarly, in chronic active hepatitis a normal mean osteoid seam width has been reported together with a prolonged maturation rate and reduced mineral apposition rate (Stellon, Gut, 1988; 29:378). In both primary biliary cirrhosis and chronic active hepatitis an increased bone-formation period, $sigma_f$, has been demonstrated (Stellon, Hepatol, 1987; 7:137, Stellon, Gut, 1988; 29:378), indicating impaired function of osteoblasts rather than a reduction in their lifespan.

Most studies in alcoholic liver disease also indicate that osteoblast dysfunction plays an important part in bone loss (Crilling, CalcifTissInt, 1988; 43:269; Diamond, AmJMed, 1989; 86:282), although in one study the rate of matrix synthesis was normal (Morbahan, Hepatol, 1984; 4:266). There is some evidence that ethanol has direct effects on osteoblast function: indices of bone matrix formation and mineralization were significantly lower in current drinkers than abstainers, as assessed both by bone histomorphometry and concentrations of serum osteocalcin, a marker of bone formation (Diamond, AmJMed, 1989; 86:282). In a study of 50 alcoholic males (Crilly, CalcifTissInt, 1988; 43:269), there was histomorphometric evidence of a greater reduction in osteoblast function in drinkers than abstainers, with prolongation of the bone-formation period in the drinkers. Low serum osteocalcin has been consistently reported in alcoholics with and without liver disease (Pietschmann, BoneMin, 1990; 8:103; Lindholm, JClinEndoc, 1991; 73:118; Pepersack, JBoneMinRes 1992; 7:383; Peris, JBoneMinRes

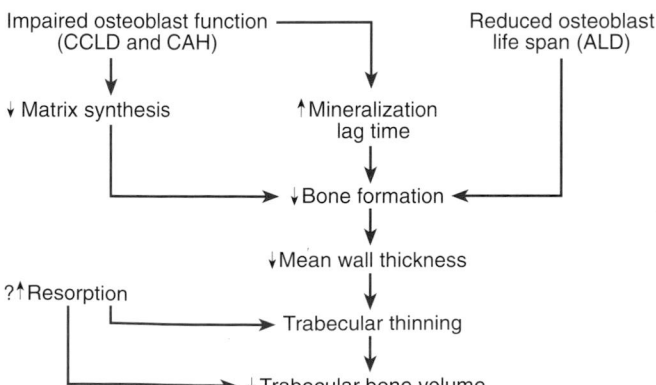

Fig. 4. Proposed pathophysiology of trabecular bone loss in chronic liver disease. CCLD, chronic cholestatic liver disease; CAH, chronic active hepatitis; ALD, alcoholic liver disease.

1994; 9:1607; Laitenen, BoneMin, 1994; 24:171); the rapid increase in serum osteocalcin following ethanol withdrawal provides further evidence that ethanol has a direct toxic effect on osteoblasts and is consistent with densitometric data which indicate that bone loss associated with alcoholism is reversible (Lindholm, JClinEndoc, 1991; 73:118; Peris, JBoneMinRes, 1994; 9:1607).

Thus several studies in primary biliary cirrhosis, and one in chronic active hepatitis, have provided convincing evidence that bone formation is reduced, both in amount and rate. However, one study (Shih, CalcifTissInt, 1987; 41:187) has shown increased mean wall thickness and bone formation rates in primary biliary cirrhosis; inspection of the data reveals very low rates of bone formation in the small number of controls studied, values in most patients being lower than those reported in large control series (Melsen, CalcifTissRes, 1978; 26:99; Vedi, Bone, 1983; 5:69). Problems with the control data may also account for the apparent increase in mean wall thickness found in the patient group, since the controls had lower values than a group of patients with primary osteoporosis who were also included in the study.

Whether bone resorption is increased in patients with chronic liver disease is controversial. Depth of resorption cavities is difficult and time-consuming to measure and no data are yet available in such patients. However, the surface extent of resorption cavities along the trabecular bone surface, which may provide information about the activation frequency of bone remodelling units, has been assessed in several studies. These have mostly shown a normal or reduced surface extent of resorption, consistent with low-turnover disease, in patients with primary biliary cirrhosis (Hodgson, Ann IntMed, 1985; 103:855; Shih, CalcifTissInt, 1987; 41:187), chronic active hepatitis (Stellon, Gut, 1988; 29:378), and alcoholic liver disease (Mobarhan, Hepatol, 1984; 4:266; Bikle, AnnIntMed, 1985; 103:42). However, three studies have reported an increased surface extent of resorption cavities in patients with primary biliary cirrhosis (Cuthbert, Hepatol, 1984; 4:1; Stellon, Hepatol, 1987; 7:137; Mitchison, Gastro, 1988; 94:463); this does not necessarily indicate an increased resorption rate but might reflect impaired bone formation at sites of previous resorption, a view supported by the observation, in two of these studies, that osteoclasts were sparse. In addition, the identification of resorption cavities is subjective and sometimes difficult. Most studies have failed to show any biochemical evidence of increased resorption, for example raised serum parathyroid hormone or increased urinary hydroxyproline or calcium excretion, although there is a report (Fonseca JClinEndoc, 1987; 64:873) that serum parathyroid hormone was frequently elevated in vitamin D-replete patients with primary biliary cirrhosis. Finally, the observation that resorption surfaces and serum parathyroid hormone fell after 6 months of vitamin D therapy (Cuthbert, Hepatol, 1984; 4:1) would suggest the presence of secondary hyperparathyroidism and increased resorption.

In a study of 80 patients with chronic liver disease, significant reductions in bone turnover were found in patients with alcoholic and cholestatic liver disease and with haemochromatosis, although bone formation rates in those with chronic active hepatitis were normal; in addition, a significant positive correlation was observed between bone formation rate and serum osteocalcin (Diamond, Gut, 1989; 96:213). Wall width and erosion depth were not assessed in this study. The results of a more recent study (Hodgson, Bone,

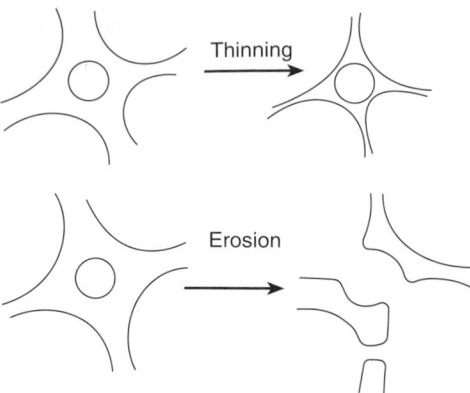

Fig. 5. Structural mechanisms of trabecular bone loss at the microanatomical level.

1993; 14:819) of bone remodelling and turnover in 12 pre-menopausal women with primary biliary cirrhosis confirmed the reduction in wall width reported earlier and also showed, for the first time, that erosion depth was normal. In contrast to most previous studies, however, bone turnover was increased and positively related to severity of cholestasis.

In summary, there is evidence from a number of studies that low bone turnover and remodelling imbalance, due to reduced bone formation, play an important part in the development of osteoporosis in patients with chronic liver disorders. Nevertheless, in a minority of studies, increased bone turnover has been demonstrated; the apparent disparity between these and other reports may be explained by factors such as the severity and aetiology of the underlying liver disease, patient selection, and drug therapy. In addition, it is possible that sequential or intermittent changes in bone turnover may occur, as has been postulated in postmenopausal osteoporosis.

Effects of liver disease on bone

At the microanatomical level, trabecular bone loss may be associated either with trabecular thinning, in which case bone architecture is relatively well preserved, or with erosion and removal of trabeculae, leading to a much greater loss of connectedness of the bone structural pattern (Fig. 5). These changes are largely determined by the accompanying changes in bone remodelling; low-turnover disease predisposes to trabecular thinning while an increased rate of activation of bone remodelling units, with or without an increase in resorption depth (high-turnover disease), will lead to increased trabecular penetration and greater loss of connectedness. The only two studies in which structural changes have been assessed, one in primary biliary cirrhosis (Stellon, Hepatol, 1987; 7:137) and the other in chronic active hepatitis (Stellon, Gut, 1988; 29:378), have shown significant trabecular thinning with little loss of connectedness in patients when compared to age- and sex-matched controls; this provides further evidence in favour of low-turnover bone disease.

Pathogenesis of osteoporosis associated with chronic liver disease

The pathogenesis of osteoporosis associated with liver disease is multifactorial. Steroid therapy may be an important factor in the development of osteoporosis in some patients (Hahn, ArchIntMed, 1978; 138:882; Eastell, JIntMed 1995; 237:439). In a randomized, controlled study of 36 patients with primary biliary cirrhosis, prednisolone therapy at an initial dose of 30 mg daily reducing to a maintenance dose of 10 mg daily was associated with approximately twice the rate of bone loss in the proximal femur when compared to the control group (Mitchison, Hepatol, 1989; 10:420). However, smaller doses of corticosteroids in women with chronic active hepatitis (mean daily dose of prednisolone 5.5 mg) were not associated with increased spinal bone loss in another study (Clements, EurJGastroHepatol, 1993; 5:543). Secondary hyperparathyroidism resulting from calcium malabsorption and/or vitamin D deficiency will also predispose to bone loss, particularly in cortical bone (Parfitt, AmJClinNut, 1982; 36:1014). Hypogonadism is an important pathogenetic factor both in men (Green, Gut, 1977; 18:843; Diamond, AnnIntMed, 1989; 110:430; Diamond, Gut, 1990; 31:82) and in women (Bannister, ClinEndoc, 1985; 23:335; Cundy, Gut, 1991; 32:202). In alcoholic liver disease, factors such as malnutrition and heavy tobacco consumption may further increase bone loss, and trauma plays an important part in the increased fracture risk that has been demonstrated in these patients; in addition, alcohol may have a direct toxic effect on osteoblasts (De Vernejoul, ClinOrthopRelRes, 1983; 179:107).

Finally, there is some evidence that hyperbilirubinaemia may impair the proliferative capacity of osteoblasts (Janes, JCI, 1995; 95: 2581).

Treatment of osteoporosis associated with chronic liver disease

Although there have been rapid advances in recent years in the treatment of postmenopausal osteoporosis, very few studies have addressed the problems of treating osteoporosis in patients with chronic liver disease. Hormone replacement therapy, which prevents menopausal bone loss and reduces fracture risk in normal women, has not been evaluated in patients with chronic liver disease. Oestrogen therapy is widely believed to be contraindicated in such patients, although there is little evidence to support this contention. Transdermal preparations, which avoid the hepatic first-pass effect and produce more physiological circulating concentrations of oestrogens, have similar bone-sparing effects to oral therapy and may be preferable in patients with chronic liver disease.

There have been no randomized, controlled studies of hormone replacement therapy in patients with chronic liver disease. In a retrospective study of 203 women with primary biliary cirrhosis, (Crippen, AmJGastr, 1994; 89:47), 16 postmenopausal women receiving hormone replacement therapy showed a significant increase in spinal bone mineral density after 1 year, compared with effects in 91 untreated women. Definitive conclusions cannot be drawn from these data because of the study design and further, prospective studies are required.

Although there is controversy over the role of calcium supplementation in the prevention or reduction of bone loss, the general consensus is that a daily calcium intake of around 1 g should be advised in premenopausal women, the figure in peri- and postmenopausal women being of the order of 1.5 g (Heaney, ClinObstetGynecol, 1987; 50:833). This can be achieved by dietary means or by the use of calcium supplements. In one study in which the effects of calcium supplementation were examined in women with primary biliary cirrhosis, metacarpal bone loss was prevented by either calcium gluconate or hydroxyapatite (Ossopan) (Epstein, AmJClinNut, 1982; 36:426). Reduction in bone loss by Ossopan has also been reported in patients with corticosteroid-treated, chronic active hepatitis (Stellon, PostgradMedJ, 1985; 61:791).

Reports of the effects of vitamin D on bone mass, measured either as iliac crest trabecular bone volume or bone mineral content in the radius, have produced conflicting results (Wagonfeld, Lancet, 1976; ii: 391; Herlong, Gastro, 1982; 83:103; Matloff, Gastro, 1982; 83:97; Cuthbert, Hepatol, 1984; 4:1), but the treatment period was too short in all these studies for long-term effects on bone mass to be determined accurately and the effects on spinal trabecular bone mineral content were not studied.

In a study of 203 women with primary biliary cirrhosis (Crippin, AmJGastro, 1994; 89:47), beneficial effects of calcium and vitamin D supplementation on lumbar spine bone mineral density could not be demonstrated.

A number of other agents have been evaluated in postmenopausal osteoporosis; these include bisphosphonates, calcitonin, anabolic steroids, and sodium fluoride. A significant reduction in spinal bone loss in patients with chronic liver disease treated for 1 year with vitamin D, calcium and calcitonin has been reported (Floreani, JHepatol, 1991; 12:217); however, the study was non-randomized and patients were selected for treatment on the basis of low bone density.

In view of the high prevalence of osteopenia and osteoporosis in patients with chronic liver disease, bone densitometry should be routinely performed at diagnosis and repeated every 1 to 2 years if initially normal. If low bone density is documented, hormone replacement therapy should be considered in all peri- and post-menopausal women. In premenopausal women with secondary amenorrhoea, oestrogen therapy should also be prescribed. In men with osteoporosis, hypogonadism should be corrected and bis-phosphonate therapy may be considered, although at present there are no reported trials of any treatment in male osteoporosis, re-gardless of liver function. In all treated patients, bone density should be monitored at 1- to 2-year intervals. Risk factors should be modified whenever possible. Corticosteroid therapy should be lim-ited to a minimum and the dose constantly reviewed, smoking and excessive alcohol consumption discouraged, regular physical exercise advocated, and a good nutritional state maintained where possible. In view of the high prevalence of vitamin D deficiency in patients with chronic liver disease and the potential role of secondary hyperparathyroidism in hepatic osteoporosis, supplementation should be routinely prescribed; daily oral doses of between 400 and 4000 IU result in normal serum 25-hydroxyvitamin D con-centrations in most cases (Davies, DigDisSci, 1983; 28:145) and are not associated with hypercalcaemia. Finally, calcium supplements should be advised in patients with dietary intakes below 1 g daily.

Post-transplantation bone disease

Since the first report of bone disease after liver transplantation (Weaver, AmJGastro, 1983; 78:102), osteoporosis has emerged as a common and serious complication of this procedure. In a study of 36 consecutive adults undergoing orthotopic liver transplantation (Haagsma, JHepatol, 1988; 6:94), the development of vertebral

fractures was reported in 38 per cent within the first postoperative year, the majority of these occurring between 3 and 6 months. Subsequent studies have confirmed this high fracture incidence, with rates for all fractures varying between 17 and 65 per cent (Eastell, Hepatol, 1991; 14:296; McDonald, Hepatol, 1991; 14:613; Porayko, TransplProc, 1991; 23:1462; Navasa, BrJRheum, 1994; 33: 52; Meys, AmJMed, 1994; 97:445). In the largest prospective study to date (Porayko, TransplProc, 1991; 23:1462), fracture incidence was studied in 146 patients surviving transplantation for over 6 months. Fracture rate was highest in patients with primary biliary cirrhosis (43 per cent) and primary sclerosing cholangitis (31 per cent); another complication of transplantation, namely avascular necrosis, was reported in 8 per cent of patients. Fracture incidence is also high in children who have undergone liver transplantation (Hill, PediatrRadiol, 1995; 25:S112).

Measurement of bone density following liver transplantation has revealed rapid bone loss in the first 3 to 6 months post-transplantation. The rate of spinal bone loss during the first 3 months post-transplant was 15 per cent/year, with a subsequent increase of the next 9 months of 6 per cent/year (Eastell, Hepatol, 1991; 14:296). Other studies have also reported high rates of bone loss in the spine (MacDonald, Hepatol, 1991; 14:613; Meys, AmJMed, 1994; 97:445; Abdelhadi, ScaJGastr, 1995; 30:1210) and in the radius and femur (Abdelhadi, ScaJGastr, 1995; 30:1210). Although there does appear to be some reduction in the rate of bone loss after 6 months or so, it is uncertain whether preoperative bone mass is eventually regained and the rapid loss occurring in the first few months after transplantation may result in irreversible disruption of bone architecture.

The pathogenesis of bone loss after transplantation is poorly understood. The high doses of corticosteroids used for immuno-suppression are likely to play an important part and other immuno-suppressive agents, such as cyclosporin A, may also have adverse skeletal effects. Many patients have low bone mass preoperatively and are thus at greater risk of sustaining fractures postoperatively. Other pathogenetic factors may include sex-hormone deficiency and immobilization. In a recent study, large but transient increases in plasma parathyroid hormone concentrations were reported during the first month after transplantation (Compston, JHepatol,1996; 25: 715), raising the possibility that post-transplantation bone loss is largely parathyroid hormone-mediated, perhaps as a result of large doses of corticosteroids. Histomorphometric studies indicate that most of the changes responsible for bone loss occur within the first few months (MacDonald, Hepatol, 1991; 14:613), with an increase both in bone turnover and resorption depth. These data suggest that treatment is most likely to be effective if given in the peri-operative period and that antiresorptive agents such as bis-phosphonates may be effective. This is an important area for future research, since the sequelae of bone loss result in permanent pain and disability in a significant proportion of patients.

Rickets and osteomalacia
Definition

Rickets and osteomalacia are conditions characterized by defective mineralization of bone, which may lead to softening of the bones and skeletal deformity. One of the earliest clinical descriptions of rickets, the term applied to the childhood form of the disease, is attributed to a British physician, Daniel Whistler, in 1645. Osteomalacia, the adult equivalent of rickets, was described 100 years later by Thomas Cadwalader, a physician from Philadelphia. The cause of rickets and osteomalacia remained unknown until the early part of this century, when it became established that the majority of cases were due to vitamin D deficiency.

Clinical features

Because in childhood bone growth is actively proceeding, the clinical manifestations of rickets differ from those of osteomalacia. Rickets commonly leads to difficulty in walking, short stature, and characteristic skeletal deformities, including frontal bossing, craniotabes (abnormal softening of the skull bones, which can often be indented), visible widening of the epiphyses at the wrist and ankle, bowing of the legs, prominence of the costochrondral junctions, pigeon chest, and spinal kyphosis.

In adults, skeletal deformities are much less common and the clinical symptoms and signs are frequently ill defined and non-specific. Bone pain is the most common symptom, but this varies considerably in its quality, localization, and other characteristics, and is often misdiagnosed. Moreover, a few patients with histologically severe osteomalacia have no bone pain, whereas others with much milder disease may have apparently severe pain. Many patients can point to the bones as the source of their pain and there may be tenderness on palpation or pressure over certain sites, particularly the ribs, pelvis, and tibiae, although this feature is also variable. Proximal muscle weakness occurs in some cases, leading to the characteristic waddling gait, difficulty in rising from the sitting position, in walking up and down stairs, and in lifting heavy objects from a height. Its severity varies widely and appears to be related more to the cause than to the severity of osteomalacia; patients with privational vitamin D deficiency and osteomalacia are often particularly affected. Skeletal deformities such as protrusio acetabuli, coxa vara, and spinal kyphosis occur occasionally, and pathological fractures are a late manifestation of the disease. From the foregoing discussion it is clear that, except in advanced cases, it is often difficult to make a clinical diagnosis of osteomalacia and it is therefore important to have a high index of suspicion in patients who are at risk.

Diagnosis

The classical biochemical changes that occur in vitamin D deficiency are hypocalcaemia, hypophosphataemia (provided renal function is normal), and a raised plasma alkaline phosphatase. Measurement of these indices provides a useful screening test in patients with suspected osteomalacia but they are not uniformly reliable and symptomatic; histologically proven osteomalacia has been reported in the absence of any biochemical abnormality (Chalmers, JBoneJt-Surg, 1967; 49(B): 403; Compston, Lancet, 1978; ii: 1). A raised plasma alkaline phosphatase is the most common biochemical abnormality in osteomalacia (Peach, JClinPath, 1982; 35:625), but assessment of its significance in patients with chronic liver disease is difficult unless the isoenzymes are measured separately.

Specific radiological changes occur relatively early in rickets and are generally best seen at the wrists. The lower ends of the radius and ulna become widened, indistinct and cupped, producing the so-called 'frothing champagne glass' appearance. The distance between the calcified end of the shaft and the epiphysis is increased, and the presence of subperiosteal osteoid may produce a double contour along the longitudinal axis of the shaft. In contrast, characteristic radiological changes occur at a much later stage in osteomalacia and, even in advanced disease, are by no means invariable. There may be reduced radiodensity of bone, coarsening of the trabecular pattern, and loss of corticomedullary differentiation in the phalanges. More specific changes include Looser's zones or pseudofractures, which, if bilateral and symmetrical, are virtually pathognomonic of osteomalacia. Pathological fractures and, finally, phalangeal subperiosteal resorption due to secondary hyperparathyroidism may also occur.

Because of the lack of specific clinical, biochemical, and radiological changes in many cases of osteomalacia, histological examination of bone provides the only accurate method of diagnosis. Unlike osteoporosis, osteomalacia is a generalized skeletal disease and thus a biopsy taken from a single site is representative. Histologically, osteomalacia is characterized by defective mineralization that leads to accumulation of osteoid (unmineralized bone); this appearance, however, is not specific and may occur in a variety of other bone disorders. Quantitative assessment of mineralization, which is essential for accurate documentation of osteomalacia, requires the use of double tetracycline labelling, in which two, time-spaced doses of a tetracycline are given to the patient before biopsy.[4] Tetracyclines are taken up at the mineralization fronts in bone and can be visualized by fluorescence microscopy; this allows measurement of both the linear extent and rate of mineralization, from which many dynamic indices related to bone formation can be calculated. The diagnostic histomorphometric criteria of osteomalacia are first an increase in the mean osteoid seam width, and second a prolongation of the mineralization lag time, calculated from the mean osteoid seam width and the bone formation rate at tissue level.[5] Failure to use these strict criteria rigorously has led to inaccurate estimates of the prevalence of osteomalacia associated with chronic liver disease, and accounts for much of the enormous variation reported in earlier studies (Table 4). In the absence of tetracycline labelling, mineralization fronts can be demonstrated by stains such as toluidine blue, and the surface extent of those fronts can be used to assess the linear extent of mineralization; however, mineralization rates and lag time cannot be derived.

Prevalence of osteomalacia

The reported prevalence of osteomalacia in chronic liver disease varies widely, from zero to nearly 70 per cent (Table 4). More recent studies, which have employed strict histomorphometric criteria, have shown that hepatic osteomalacia is rare and virtually restricted to parts of the world, such as the United Kingdom, where ultraviolet irradiation is low and fortification of foods with vitamin D is uncommon. Although much of the reported variation in prevalence can be accounted for by the use of incorrect histological criteria, other contributing factors include the selection of patients for study and variations in the severity of liver disease in those studied. The first clinical case reports of osteomalacia in patients with chronic liver disease date back to the 1930s and 1940s (Gerstenberger, MonatsschrKinderheilkd, 1933; 56:217; Mayor, BeitrPath, 1942; 106:408; Fraser, JPediat, 1943; 23:410). Following the development

Table 4 Reported prevalence of histological osteomalacia

Authors	Year	Country	No. studies	Liver disease	Selection of patients	Assessment of mineralization	Number with osteomalacia	Percentage with osteomalacia
Atkinson et al.	1956	UK	25	Mixed	Yes	No	9	36
Paterson and Losowsky	1967	UK	11	Mixed	Yes	No	0	0
Kehayoglou et al.	1968	UK	12	Primary biliary cirrhosis	Yes	No	1	8.3
Compston et al.	1977	UK	11	Primary biliary cirrhosis	Yes	Yes	4	36.4
Long et al.	1978	UK	32	Mixed	Yes	No	22	68.8
Compston et al.	1980	UK	32	Chronic cholestatic liver disease	No	Yes	4	12.5
Herlong et al.	1982	USA	15	Primary biliary cirrhosis	Yes	Yes*	0	0
Matloff et al.	1982	USA	10	Primary biliary cirrhosis	Yes	Yes*	0	0
Dibble et al.	1982	UK	29	Mixed	Yes	Yes	9	31.0
Recker et al.	1983	USA	27	Primary biliary cirrhosis	No	Yes*	0	0
Cuthbert et al.	1984	USA	11	Primary biliary cirrhosis	No	Yes*	)	0
Morbarhan et al.	1984	USA	9	Alcoholic liver disease	Yes	Yes*	0	0
Lalor et al.†	1986	UK	22	Alcoholic liver disease	No	Yes	5	22.7
Stellon et al.	1986	UK	36	Chronic cholestatic liver disease	No	Yes*	0	0
Stellon et al.	1988	UK	34	Chronic active hepatitis	No	Yes*	0	0
Mitchison et al.	1988	UK	33	Primary biliary cirrhosis	No	Yes*	1	3

* Double tetracycline labelling given prior to biopsy.
† Quarterly Journal of Medicine 1986.

of techniques for preparing undecalcified bone sections and for staining mineralization fronts in bone, prevalence studies based on histological criteria became possible. The demonstration of increased osteoid amount in a proportion of patients with chronic liver disease (Atkinson, QJMed, 1956; 99:299) was followed, some years later, by more definite evidence of impaired mineralization in biopsies from 4 of 11 selected patients with primary biliary cirrhosis (Compston, Lancet, 1977; i: 721). Subsequently, evidence was claimed for osteomalacia in 22 of 32 patients with chronic liver disease, 50 per cent of whom were receiving high-dose parenteral vitamin D prophylactically (Long, Gut, 1978; 19:85); however, mineralization was not assessed in this study, and in many of those classified as abnormal, osteoid amount was well within the normal range of most published control data. Another study in a similar patient population, using stricter histological criteria, reported evidence of osteomalacia in only 4 of 32 unselected patients with primary biliary cirrhosis (Compston, DigDisSci, 1980; 25:28). Subsequent unselected studies from Europe and the United States have

confirmed a low prevalence of osteomalacia in chronic liver disease. Indeed, only one properly documented case has been described from the United States (Reed, Gastro, 1980; 78:512), other recent American studies reporting zero prevalence (Herlong, Gastro, 1982; 83:103; Matloff, Gastro, 1982; 83:97; Recker. In Frame B, Potts ST, eds. *Clinical Disorders of Bone Mineral Metabolism*. Amsterdam: Excerpta Medica, 1983:227; Cuthbert, Hepatol, 1984; 4:1). Although there is no doubt that osteomalacia is seen in a small percentage of patients with chronic liver disease in the United Kingdom, most recent studies indicate that the prevalence is falling, possibly reflecting the trend towards earlier diagnosis of liver disease and the resulting change in its clinical spectrum. Thus no osteomalacia was reported in 36 unselected British patients with primary biliary cirrhosis (Stellon, Bone, 1986; 7:181), and only one possible case of osteomalacia found in 33 patients investigated for bone disease at the time of diagnosis of primary biliary cirrhosis (Mitchison, Gastro, 1988; 94:463). Fewer data are available in patients with other forms of chronic liver disease; although osteomalacia has been described both in chronic active hepatitis and alcoholic liver disease, it appears to be rare and no evidence of it was found in a study of 36 patients with chronic active hepatitis (Stellon, Gastro, 1985; 89:1078).

Rickets in infants and children with liver disease

Rickets is a relatively common complication of hepatobiliary disease in infants and young children; in one study (Kobayashi, Arch DisChild, 1974; 49:641), radiological evidence of rickets was reported in 59 per cent of 21 infants with neonatal hepatitis and in two of four with intrahepatic cholestasis. As in adults, vitamin D deficiency has a major pathogenetic role, although its cause differs slightly. Thus malabsorption of dietary vitamin D appears to be the main cause of vitamin D deficiency in patients with cholestatic disease (dietary intake being the main source of the vitamin in infants), while in neonatal hepatitis, impaired hepatic production of 25-hydroxyvitamin D may be a contributory factor (Kobayashi, ArchDisChild, 1979; 54:367; Kooh, JPediat, 1979; 94:879). Treatment with parenteral vitamin D (Kobayashi, ArchDisChild, 1974; 49:641; Kooh, JPediat, 1979; 94:870), oral 25-hydroxyvitamin D_3 (Daum, JPediat, 1976; 88:1041), and parenteral 1,25-dihydroxyvitamin D_3 (Heubi, JPediat, 1979; 94:977) have all been shown to be effective in the healing of rickets associated with cholestatic disease, whereas high doses of oral vitamin D may be ineffective (Kooh, JPediat, 1979; 94:870). Since neither oral 25-hydroxyvitamin D_3 nor parenteral 1,25-dihydroxyvitamin D_3 are widely available, either intravenous vitamin D, 3000 IU/day, or intramuscular vitamin D, 30 000 IU/week, are recommended (Kooh, JPediat, 1979; 94:870; Kobayashi, ArchDisChild, 1979; 54:367). In mild or moderate neonatal hepatitis, however, oral administration of 2000 to 5000 IU vitamin D/day may be effective (Yu, MedJAust, 1971; 1:790).

In a study of radial bone mineral content and vitamin D status in 56 infants and children with chronic cholestatic liver disease (Argao, Pediat, 1993; 91:1151), bone mineral content was reduced at all ages, most values being between 2 and 4 SD below the mean reference value; although 29 per cent had low serum 25-hydroxyvitamin D, no correlations were found between bone mineral content and vitamin D status. The low bone-mineral content demonstrated in these patients may therefore partly reflect delayed growth and malnutrition, although values remained low even after correction for weight–age and height–age.

Pathogenesis of osteomalacia associated with chronic liver disease (Fig. 6)

Vitamin D deficiency

Vitamin D deficiency is the major factor responsible for the development of osteomalacia in chronic liver disease (Fig. 6). Its cause has been the subject of many investigations, most of which have centred around various aspects of vitamin D metabolism. These are considered in more detail below.

Vitamin D metabolism[6] (Fig. 7)

Vitamin D may be obtained from endogenous and exogenous sources. Endogenous synthesis occurs in the skin where 7-dehydrocholesterol is converted, in the presence of ultraviolet

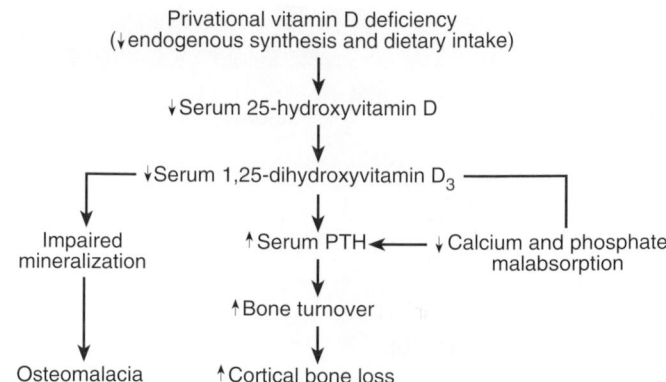

Fig. 6. Pathogenesis of osteomalacia and secondary hyperparathyroidism in chronic liver disease.

irradiation, to vitamin D_3 (cholecalciferol) (Kobayashi, JNutr SciVitaminol, 1973; 19:123). Vitamin D may also be obtained from the diet; however, studies in the United Kingdom and the United States have demonstrated that, under normal circumstances, endogenous synthesis provides quantitatively the most important source of the vitamin, dietary intake being relatively unimportant except in infants and the house-bound and very elderly (Haddad, Nature, 1973; 244:515; Preece, QJMed, 1975; 44:575). Vitamin D undergoes 25-hydroxylation, almost exclusively in the liver, to form 25-hydroxyvitamin D, the major circulating form of the vitamin (Ponchon, JCI, 1969; 48:2032); at the concentrations normally found circulating in plasma, this metabolite has no biological activity. The serum concentration of 25-hydroxyvitamin D does, however, provide a reasonable assessment of vitamin D status in an individual. The major active metabolite of vitamin D, 1,25-dihydroxyvitamin D_3, is formed from 25-hydroxyvitamin D, mainly in the kidney (Fraser, Nature, 1970; 228:764).

Vitamin D metabolism in chronic liver disease[6] (Fig. 8)

A number of studies have demonstrated low serum 25-hydroxyvitamin D in a high proportion of patients with chronic liver disease,

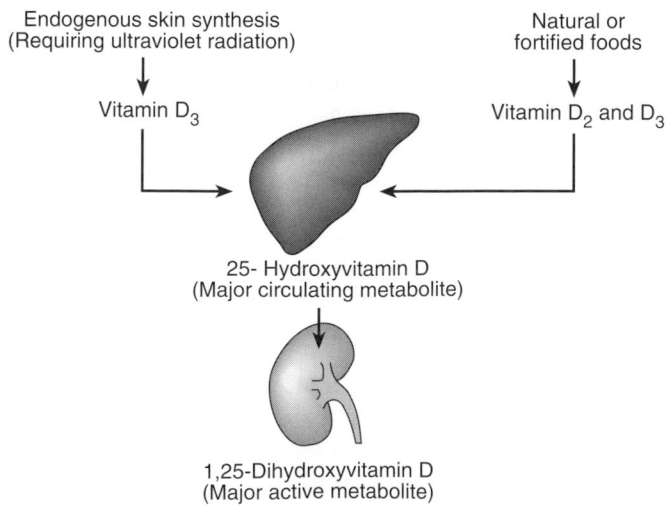

Fig. 7. Outline of the major steps in vitamin D metabolism.

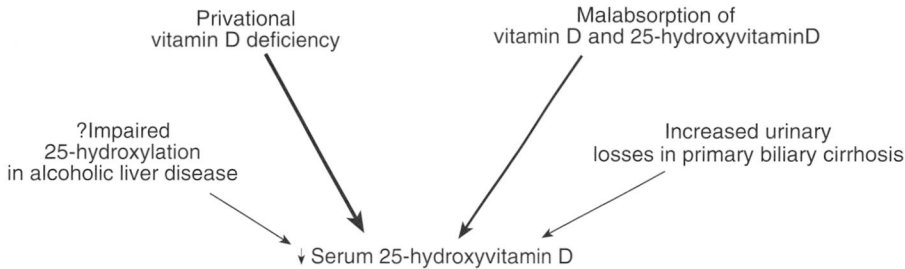

Fig. 8. Pathogenesis of vitamin D deficiency in chronic liver disease.

indicating that vitamin D deficiency is common in these individuals (Ajdukiewicz, Digestion, 1974; 10:332; Long, Lancet, 1976; ii: 650; Compston, Lancet, 1977; i:721; Dibble, QJMed, 1982; 51:89; Bengoa, Hepatol, 1984; 4:261). Although one report suggested that hepatic production of 25-hydroxyvitamin D was impaired in chronic cholestatic liver disease (Wagonfeld, Lancet, 1976; ii:391), most subsequent studies have shown no significant impairment of 25-hydroxylation (Skinner, Lancet, 1977; i:720; Krawitt, Lancet, 1977; ii:1246; Long, CCActa, 1978; 85:311; Jung, Gut, 1979; 20:840). In alcoholic liver disease, the data are more conflicting, evidence for (Hepner, DigDisSci, 1976; 21:527; Jung, Gut, 1978; 19:290; Mawer, ClinSci, 1985; 69:561) and against (Lund, ActaMedScand, 1977; 202:221; Posner, Gastro, 1978; 74:866) impairment of 25-hydroxylation being reported.

Malabsorption of vitamin D and 25-hydroxyvitamin D has been demonstrated in a number of studies (Thompson, JCI, 1966; 45:94; Compston, Lancet, 1977; i:721; Krawitt, Lancet, 1977; ii:1246; Stamp, Lancet, 1974; ii:121). Treatment with cholestyramine may further decrease absorption of the vitamin (Thompson, Gut, 1969; 10:717). In alcoholic liver disease, two studies have found evidence of vitamin D malabsorption (Lund, ActaMedScand, 1977; 202: 221; Meyer, JMolMed, 1978; 3:29), whilst normal absorption was reported in another (Barragry, Gut, 1979; 20:559).

Other factors that may contribute to vitamin D deficiency in chronic liver disease include increased urinary excretion of vitamin D metabolites in patients with cholestasis (Krawitt, Lancet, 1977; ii:246), and reduced exposure to ultraviolet irradiation and/or low dietary vitamin D intake (Jung, Gut, 1979; 20:840). Although serum concentrations of the specific protein that binds vitamin D and 25-hydroxyvitamin D are low in chronic liver disease (Haddad, JCI, 1976; 58:1217), this reduction is functionally unimportant because of the very low saturation of the binding protein. Finally, there is evidence that endogenous synthesis of vitamin D is unimpaired in the presence of jaundice (Jung, Gut, 1970; 29:840; Long, ClinSci, 1980; 59:293).

In summary, although malabsorption of vitamin D and 25-hydroxyvitamin D has been demonstrated in patients with chronic liver disease, this cannot fully account for vitamin D deficiency in patients with normal exposure to ultraviolet irradiation, and increased urinary excretion of metabolites is unlikely to be quantitatively significant in most cases. Moreover, hepatic production of 25-hydroxyvitamin D appears to be adequate even in the presence of severe liver disease, and formation of the active metabolite, 1,25-dihydroxyvitamin D3, is normal, as would be expected (Mawer, ClinSci, 1971; 40:39; Kaplan, Gastro, 1981; 81:681). Thus it seems likely that privational factors, that is, reduced exposure to ultraviolet

irradiation and low dietary intake, are mainly responsible for vitamin D deficiency associated with chronic liver disease (Fig. 8). This would be consistent with the extreme rarity of hepatic osteomalacia in the United States, where the availability of ultraviolet irradiation is greater than in the United Kingdom, and the observation that small doses of oral vitamin D are usually effective in healing osteomalacia in patients with chronic liver disease (Davies, Dig-DisSci, 1983; 28:145).

Calcium and phosphate malabsorption

Malabsorption of calcium and phosphate has been reported in both cholestatic and parenchymatous liver disease (Kehayoglou, Lancet, 1968; i:715; Whelton, Gut, 1971; 12:978; Long, CCActa, 1978; 87: 353; Bengoa, Hepatol, 1984; 4:261). The improvement in malabsorption reported after administration of parenteral vitamin D or oral 25-hydroxyvitamin D3 (Bengoa, Hepatol, 1984; 4:261) or oral 1,25-dihydroxyvitamin D3 (Farrington, Gut, 1979; 20:616) indicates that malabsorption is, at least partly, due to vitamin D deficiency. Precipitation of calcium salts by unabsorbed fats within the intestinal lumen may also contribute to calcium malabsorption.

Prevention and treatment of hepatic osteomalacia

The high prevalence of vitamin D deficiency associated with chronic liver disease demonstrated in many studies suggests that vitamin D supplementation should be routine in these patients.

Established hepatic osteomalacia is responsive to either oral or parenteral vitamin D preparations, including high doses of parenteral vitamin D or 50 μg daily of oral 25-hydroxyvitamin D3 (Compston, Gut, 1979; 20:133), parenteral 1,25-dihydroxyvitamin D3, 15 μg/month (Long, BMJ, 1978; 1:75), or oral 1-α-hydroxyvitamin D3, 2 μg/day (Compston, BMJ, 1979; 2:309). However, in keeping with the evidence that hepatic osteomalacia is due mainly to privational vitamin D deficiency, small doses of oral vitamin D have also been shown to be effective; on economic and safety grounds, this is the preferred treatment. The dose recommended is between 400 and 4000 IU daily, depending on the degree of vitamin D malabsorption present (Davies, DigDisSci, 1983; 28:145). Response to treatment is best assessed by bone biopsy after a period of approximately 18 months.

Secondary hyperparathyroidism associated with hepatic osteomalacia

Secondary hyperparathyroidism occurs in patients with hepatic osteomalacia and presumably results from vitamin D and/or calcium deficiency. Thus a raised serum immunoreactive parathyroid hormone has been reported in some patients with osteomalacia, together with decreased tubular phosphate reabsorption, increased urinary cAMP excretion, and histological evidence of osteitis fibrosa (Compston, DigDisSci, 1980; 25:28, Dibble, ClinEndoc, 1981; 15: 373; Davies, DigDisSci, 1983; 28:145). Histologically, hyperparathyroidism leads to increased bone turnover and accelerated cortical bone loss, which may increase the risk of osteoporosis in later years. It is therefore important to ensure that treatment of hepatic osteomalacia is continued until mineralization has returned to normal, and the changes of secondary hyperparathyroidism have resolved completely.

Skeletal metastases from hepatoma

Skeletal metastases from hepatoma are relatively rare, occurring in 7 to 16 per cent of cases (Okazaki, Cancer, 1985; 55:1991; Kuhlman, Radiol, 1986; 160:175). The sites most commonly affected are the ribs, spine, femur, pelvis, and humerus; the metastases are osteolytic, vascular, and may be expansile with associated soft-tissue masses (Golimbu, Radiol, 1985; 154:617; Kuhlman, Radiol, 1986; 160:175). The skeletal lesions are associated with bone pain and may progress to pathological fracture; these symptoms usually appear before any clinical manifestation due to the liver disease itself. The metastases can be demonstrated by a variety of techniques, including plain radiography, CT scanning, and nuclear scintography using Tc-methylene diphosphonate, gallium, or [^{131}I]antiferritin immunoglobulin. The prognosis of patients with skeletal metastases is surprisingly good, median survival in one study being 14.9 months, with a maximum survival of 4.5 years (Kuhlman, Radiol, 1986; 160:175).

Periostitis associated with chronic liver disease

Periostitis has been reported in all types of chronic liver disease and commonly occurs in the absence of finger clubbing. The distal end of the tibia and fibula are most commonly affected, usually in a symmetrical fashion, and in some cases the distal radius and ulna are also affected. In a prospective study of 74 patients with primary biliary cirrhosis and 54 with other forms of chronic liver disease, periostitis was found in 35 per cent of the patients with primary biliary cirrhosis, in 29 per cent of those with chronic active hepatitis, and in 23 per cent of the other patients (Epstein, Gut, 1981; 22: 203). The main symptom is pain over the affected area, and bone tenderness is a common clinical sign. The diagnosis is established by plain radiography of the affected area.

References

1. Riggs BL and Wahner HAW. Bone densitometry and clinical decision making in osteoporosis. *Annals of Internal Medicine*, 1988; **108**: 292.
2. Compston JE. Hepatic osteodystrophy: vitamin D metabolism in patients with liver disease. *Gut*, 1986; **27**: 1073–90.
3. Parfitt AM. The cellular basis of bone remodelling. The quantum concept re-examined in light of recent advances in cell biology of bone. *Calcified Tissue International*, 1984; **36**: 537–45.
4. Frost HM. Tetracycline-based analysis of bone remodelling. *Calcified Tissue Research*, 1969; **3**: 211–37.
5. Parfitt AM. The physiologic and clinical significance of bone morphometric data. In Recker R, ed. *Bone histomorphometry. Techniques and interpretations.* Boca Raton, CA: CRC Press, 1983; 143–223.
6. Haussler MR and McCain TA. Basic and clinical concepts related to vitamin D metabolism and action. *New England Journal of Medicine*, 1977; **297**: 974–83: 1041–50.

25.11 Infections in liver disease

Antoni Rimola and Miquel Navasa

Patients with severe liver disease frequently develop bacterial infections. However, in contrast to other complications which commonly occur in these patients, such as gastrointestinal bleeding, ascites, hepatic encephalopathy, bile secretion impairment, or coagulopathy, little attention has been paid to infections complicating the course of patients with acute and chronic liver failure. Since most studies dealing with this subject have been done in cirrhotic patients, this chapter mainly reviews the incidence, predisposing factors, clinical and laboratory features, diagnosis, treatment, and prophylaxis of bacterial infections in cirrhosis. Nevertheless, the important aspects of infectious complications in patients with acute liver failure are also discussed.

Bacterial infections in cirrhosis

The incidence of bacterial infections in cirrhotic patients admitted to hospital is very high. In several studies, 30 to 50 per cent of cirrhotics presented with bacterial infections at admission, or developed this type of complication during hospitalization.[1-4] Most bacterial infections in cirrhotic patients are hospital-acquired. Fifteen to 35 per cent of cirrhotics admitted to hospital develop nosocomial infections;[1-4] these figures contrast sharply with the hospital–acquired infection rate in the general hospital population (5–7 per cent)[5] (Horan, MMWR, 1986; 35(1SS):17; EPIME Working Group, JHospInf, 1992; 20:1; Dinkel, JHospInf, 1994; 28: 297).

Urinary tract infections, peritonitis, respiratory infections, and bacteraemia are the most frequent infections reported in cirrhotics. Table 1 shows the overall incidence of infection and the incidence of different types of infection found in several studies, including large series of cirrhotic patients.

Factors predisposing to infection in cirrhosis

The high incidence of infections in cirrhosis may be explained by the existence in most of these patients of several abnormalities in the defence mechanisms against infection, e.g. depression of the reticuloendothelial system and granulocyte function, and impairment of non-specific humoral and cell-mediated immunity systems. Alterations in the enteric flora and the intestinal barrier may also play a role in the pathogenesis of bacterial infections in cirrhosis. Finally, invasive procedures frequently performed in cirrhotics increase the risk of infection in these patients. Because of the highly frequent infectious complications and the multiple derangements in the defence mechanisms, cirrhosis might be considered as a form of acquired immunodeficiency (Runyon, JHepatol, 1993; 18:271).

Iatrogenic factors

In addition to procedures well known to predispose to infection, such as intravenous or urethral catheters, cirrhotic patients are frequently subjected to other diagnostic or therapeutic manoeuvres which may alter the natural defence barriers and which therefore increase the risk of bacterial infection.

Patients who require oesophageal tamponade with a Sengstaken–Blakemore or Linton–Nachlas tube for the treatment of variceal haemorrhage are especially prone to develop aspiration pneumonia. This complication occurs in approximately 10 per cent of patients treated with oesophageal tamponade, although an incidence of 25 per cent may be reached in cirrhotics with profound hepatic encephalopathy (Johansen, ScaJGastr 1973; 8:81; Novis, Gut, 1976; 17:258; Teres, Gastro, 1978; 75:566; Chojkier, DigDisSci, 1980; 25: 267; Hunt, DigDisSci 1982; 27:413; Panes, GastroHepato, 1985; 8: 13). Therefore, prophylactic tracheal intubation of cirrhotic patients with gastrointestinal haemorrhage and profound hepatic encephalopathy is advisable to reduce the risk of aspiration pneumonia. Endoscopic sclerotherapy for bleeding oesophageal varices, particularly emergency sclerotherapy, is associated with bacteraemia, with an incidence ranging from 5 to 30 per cent (Rolando, JHepatol, 1993; 18:290; Selby, GastrEnd, 1994; 40:680). Nevertheless, although sclerotherapy has been implicated in the development of serious infective complications, such as purulent meningitis (Toyoda, IntMed, 1994; 33:706) and bacterial peritonitis (Bac, AmJGastr, 1994; 89:659), bacteraemia is usually a transient phenomenon and routine prophylaxis with antibiotics is not recommended.

Table 1 Incidence of bacterial infection in cirrhosis			
	Percentage		
	Range	**Average**	**Reference no.**
Patients with infection	33–47	40	1–4
Patients with:			
urinary tract infection	12–29	18	1–4, 6
peritonitis[a]	7–23	15	7–14
respiratory infection	6–10	8	1–4
bacteraemia	4–9	6	7, 15–17
other infections	3–6	5	1–4

[a] Percentage in relation to patients with ascites.

The placement of a transjugular intrahepatic portosystemic stent for the treatment of bleeding oesophageal varices is not associated with the development of significant bacterial infections.

Unselected cirrhotic patients undergoing surgical procedures, especially abdominal surgery in non-bleeding patients, are prone to develop bacterial infections during the postoperative period; the incidence of such complications ranges between 10 and 30 per cent (O'Hara, AnnSurg, 1975; 181:85; Aranha, AmJSurg, 1982; 143:55; Doberneck, AmJSurg 1983; 146:306; Garrison, AnnSurg, 1984; 199:648; Bloch, ArchSurg, 1985; 120:669). However, the risk of infection following surgical operations for the treatment of portal hypertension is very low in carefully selected patients (Cello, AmJSur, 1981; 141:257; Harley, Gastro, 1986; 91:802).

Cirrhotic patients with a peritoneovenous shunt (LeVeen shunt) frequently develop infectious complications, particularly spontaneous bacteraemia and peritonitis. In several series, the incidence of bacterial infections after the insertion of a LeVeen shunt for the treatment of ascites was approximately 20 per cent (Greig, AmJSurg, 1980; 139:125; Bernhoft, ArchSurg, 1982; 117:631; Kravetz, GastroHepato, 1982; 5:347; Rubinstein, Gut, 1985; 26: 1070; Smadja, AnnSurg, 1985; 201:488). Nevertheless, this incidence can be drastically reduced by using appropriate antibiotic prophylaxis (Ginès, NEJM, 1991; 325:829).

Other invasive procedures often performed in cirrhotic patients, such as diagnostic or therapeutic paracentesis and endoscopy, are associated with a very low risk of clinically relevant infection (Liebowitz, NYStateJMed 1962; 62:2223; O'Connor, Endoscopy, 1983; 15:21; Shorvon, Gut, 1983; 24:1078; Runyon, ArchIntMed, 1986; 146:2259; Botoman, GastrEnd, 1986; 32:342; Menghof, Liver, 1988; 8:167).

Changes in the intestinal flora and in the intestinal barrier

Whereas aerobic (facultative) Gram-negative bacilli are present in low numbers in the small bowel of normal subjects (Simon, Gastro, 1984; 86:174), the concentration of these micro-organisms is significantly increased in the jejunal flora of many cirrhotic patients.[18-20] This abnormal small bowel colonization in cirrhosis may increase the possibility of aerobic Gram-negative bacteria invading the bloodstream and causing infections of enteric origin in these patients.

In addition, recent experimental studies have reported an increased passage of bacteria from the intestinal lumen to extra-intestinal sites, including regional mesenteric lymph nodes (a phenomenon known as bacterial translocation) and the systemic circulation (Sorell, Gastro, 1993; 104:1722; Llovet, Gut, 1994; 35: 1648; Runyon, JHepatol, 1994; 21:792; Garcia-Tsao, Gastro, 1995; 108:1835). One possible cause for bacterial translocation in cirrhosis is the aforementioned small bowel bacterial overgrowth. Another possibility is a disruption of the intestinal mucosal barrier. This possibility is supported by the finding that the caecal submucosa of rats with experimentally induced cirrhosis and ascites becomes markedly oedematous and inflamed, probably as a consequence of portal hypertension (Garcia-Tsao, Gastro, 1995; 108:1835). Furthermore, haemorrhagic shock in portal hypertensive rats is associated with an increased bacterial translocation to mesenteric lymph nodes (Sorell, Gastro, 1993; 104:1722), suggesting that

hypovolaemia secondary to haemorrhage, a frequent event in cirrhotic patients, may increase the alteration in the intestinal barrier and, secondarily, increase the possibility of bacterial infection of enteric origin. Finally, other conditions capable of altering the host immune defence mechanisms, such as glucocorticoid administration, immunosuppression, or protein depletion, may also account for increased bacterial translocation in cirrhosis. Cirrhotic rats with ascites develop bacteraemia more frequently after intratracheal instillation of *Streptococcus pneumoniae* than cirrhotic animals without ascites (Mellencamp, JInfDis, 1991; 163:102), thus suggesting the existence of a general impairment in body barriers (including the intestinal mucosal barrier) in advanced cirrhosis.

However, it is difficult to extrapolate the results of experimental studies to humans as experiments are conducted under controlled circumstances, which can influence the pathogenicity of the flora, and animal models may have a different natural resistance to bacterial infection than human beings. It is important to remark that very few studies have been performed in humans, and their significance is not clear. Although an increased incidence of bacterial translocation has been reported in several groups of patients, such as subjects with inflammatory bowel disease, intestinal obstruction, and abdominal trauma (Reed, CircShock, 1994; 41:1; Sedman, Gastro, 1994; 107:643), there are no data on the prevalence of bacterial translocation in patients with cirrhosis.

Depression of reticuloendothelial system activity

Although the reticuloendothelial system (also called the mononuclear phagocytic system) is widely distributed throughout the body, approximately 90 per cent of this defence system is in the liver, Kupffer cells and endothelial sinusoidal cells being the major components.[21-25] The special intravascular location of the hepatic reticuloendothelial system is thus considered as the main defence mechanism against bacteraemia and other infections acquired by a haematogenous route, such as spontaneous bacterial peritonitis (Beeson, JExpMed, 1945; 81:9; Rogers, BacteriolRev, 1960; 24:50).

The phagocytic activity of the reticuloendothelial system can be assessed either by its uptake of radioactive isotope-labelled particles (e.g. hepatosplenic scintigraphy) or by measuring the plasma disappearance rate of particles which, once injected into the circulation, can only be eliminated from the bloodstream by the action of reticuloendothelial system cells. Using these techniques, several groups have demonstrated that many cirrhotic patients show marked depression of reticuloendothelial system function, particularly of the hepatic reticuloendothelial system fraction (Mundschenk, JNuclMed, 1971; 12:711; Cooksley, BrJHaemat, 1973; 25:147; Habibian, SouthMedJ, 1975; 68:5; DeNardo, JNuclMed 1976; 17: 449; Horisawa, Gastro, 1976: 71:210; Huet, Gastro, 1980; 78:76; Lahnborg, ScaJGastr, 1981; 16:481; Winkler, ClinPhysiol, 1984; 4: 135). In one investigation,[26] a series of cirrhotic patients was divided into two groups, according to whether their reticuloendothelial system phagocytic activity was normal or depressed, and were then observed over a long period. It was found that only patients with depression of the reticuloendothelial system developed bacteraemia and/or spontaneous bacterial peritonitis (with a probability of 35 per cent at 1 year of follow-up), whereas these infections did not occur in patients with normal function of the reticuloendothelial system. The incidence of other types of

Table 2 Mechanisms of the depression of the reticuloendothelial system in cirrhosis
Intrahepatic shunting
Intrinsic defects in reticuloendothelial cells
Reduced serum opsonic activity

Circumstances worsening the reticuloendothelial function:
    alcohol intake
    malnutrition
    hypovolaemia, shock
    surgery
    corticosteroid therapy

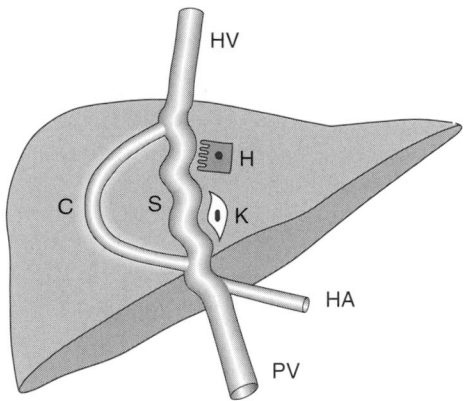

Fig. 1. Intrahepatic shunting in cirrhosis. In normal subjects, virtually all the blood reaching the liver via the hepatic artery (HA) and portal vein (PV) circulates through the sinusoids (S), thus being purified by contacting hepatocytes (H) and reticuloendothelial system cells (mainly Kupffer cells, K). In cirrhotic patients an important proportion of hepatic blood flow circulates through intrahepatic shunts (possibly neoformed capillaries, (C), thus escaping from the action of reticuloendothelial cells located in the sinusoids and reaching the hepatic veins (HV) and the general circulation whithout being adequately 'filtered' by the liver. In this case, the dysfunction of the hepatic reticuloendothelial system in cirrhosis is due to abnormalities in the hepatic microcirculation rather than an intrinsic alteration of reticuloendothelial cells.

infection was similar in both groups of patients. More recently, the maximum removal capacity of the reticuloendothelial system, as an estimation of its functional reserve, has been evaluated in cirrhotic patients by administering increasing amounts of albumin millimicrospheres.[27] In this study, the maximum removal capacity of the reticuloendothelial system significantly correlated with serum albumin, prothrombin index, Pugh score, aminopyrine breath test, galactose elimination capacity and plasma indocyanine green clearance. Impaired maximum removal capacity was associated with increased risk of spontaneous bacterial peritonitis and poorer prognosis during follow-up. All these results strongly suggest that the risk of acquiring bacteraemia and spontaneous bacterial peritonitis in cirrhosis is directly related to the degree of dysfunction of the reticuloendothelial system in these patients.

The pathogenesis of the depression of phagocytic activity of the reticuloendothelial system in cirrhosis is not clear. However, several mechanisms have been proposed (Table 2). Most studies suggest that this alteration could be due to the intrahepatic shunting of blood, which then escapes the phagocytic action of the reticuloendothelial system cells located in the liver sinusoids.[26] According to this theory, a significant amount of hepatic blood flow would circulate through anatomical or functional intrahepatic shunts which, therefore, would not be available for blood–tissue exchange (Fig. 1) (Groszmann, Gastro, 1977; 73:201; Huet, JCI, 1982; 70: 1234; Hoefs, JLabClinMed, 1984; 103:446). On the other hand, some authors have found that in cirrhosis there is a reduction in the phagocytic capacity of monocytes, which are considered as Kupffer cell precursors (Hassner, BMJ, 1981; 282:1262; Holdstock, JClinPath, 1982; 35:972; Olmos, GastroHepato, 1985; 8:334). Furthermore, an impaired function of macrophage Fcγ receptors has also been described in alcoholic cirrhosis (Gomez, NEJM, 1994; 331:1122). All these studies suggest an intrinsic defect in reticuloendothelial system cells in these patients. Finally, serum opsonic activity is markedly reduced in most cirrhotic patients, probably as a consequence of a decreased serum concentration of complement and fibronectin, substances that normally stimulate the phagocytosis of micro-organisms by enhancing their adhesiveness to the reticuloendothelial cell surface (Fig. 2) (Fox, Gut, 1971; 12: 574; Finlayson, Gastro, 1972; 63:653; Potter, Gut, 1973; 14:451; Simberkoff, JLabClinMed, 1978; 91:831; Matsuda, CCActa, 1982; 118:91; Akalin, QJMed, 1985; 56:431; Naveau, Hepatol, 1985; 5: 819). In addition, cirrhotic patients frequently suffer from other conditions (shown in Table 2), such as alcoholism, malnutrition, or acute hypovolaemia, or undergo surgical procedures which may exacerbate their pre-existent dysfunction of the reticuloendothelial system (Saba, Surgery, 1969; 65:802; Altura, PSEBM, 1972; 139: 935; Holper, Surgery, 1974; 76:423; Kaplan, AmJPhysiol, 1976; 230:7; Carr, CanJPhysPharm, 1978; 56:299; Saba, AmJMed, 1980; 68:577; Galante, JReticulSoc, 1982; 32:179; Soper, JSurgRes, 1984; 37:431; McGregor, JAMA, 1986; 256:1474).

Abnormalities of humoral immunity

Cirrhotic patients show a normal or enhanced specific humoral immunity; many studies report a high titre of antibodies against several micro-organisms, particularly bacteria of enteric origin, and even against dietary products (Bjorneboe, Lancet, 1972; 1:58; Triger, Lancet, 1972; 1:60; Prytz, ScaJGastr, 1973; 8:433; Simjee, Gut, 1975; 16:871; Turunen, Gut, 1981; 22:849; Bercoff, GastrClinBiol, 1984; 8:503; Teare, AlcAlc, 1993; 28:11).

By contrast non-specific humoral immunity is depressed in cirrhosis. Serum bactericidal and opsonic activities and serum levels of complement and fibronectin have been found to be reduced in most cirrhotic patients.[28–30] Furthermore, the non-specific antimicrobial capacity of ascitic fluid in cirrhosis varies greatly from patient to patient, and this variability may be involved in the pathogenesis of spontaneous bacterial peritonitis.[31–33] Runyon reported a highly significant inverse correlation between the opsonic activity of ascitic fluid and the risk of developing peritonitis in patients admitted to hospital with ascites (most being cirrhotics).[34] In this study, 15 per cent of patients with a reduced opsonic activity developed spontaneous bacterial peritonitis during hospital stay, whereas this complication did not occur in any patient with increased opsonic activity in ascitic fluid.

Opsonic activity of ascitic fluid in cirrhosis is directly correlated with the concentration of defence substances, such as immunoglobulins, complement, and fibronectin, and with the concentration

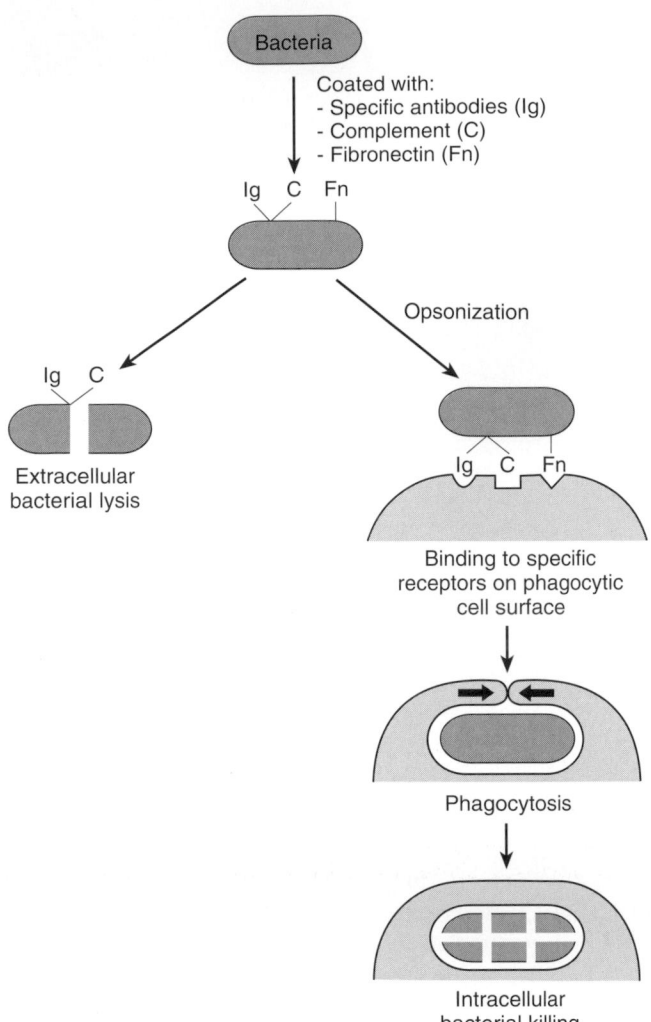

Fig. 2. Mechanisms of bacterial killing. Bacteria can be lysed extracellularly by the action of complement (C), alone or in combination with specific antibodies (immunoglobulins, Ig). Intracellular bacterial killing involves humoral-specific (Ig) and non-specific (complement, C, and fibronectin, Fn) opsonization, followed by the binding of opsonized bacteria to the surface of phagocytic cells (mainly reticuloendothelial cells, other macrophages, and granulocytes), and the engulfment and intracellular digestion of bacteria.

of total protein in ascites.[32,33] Interestingly, the concentration of total protein in ascitic fluid, a very easy measurement in clinical practice, correlates very well with the risk of spontaneous bacterial peritonitis in cirrhosis with ascites. Runyon demonstrated that patients with protein concentration in ascitic fluid below 10 g/l developed peritonitis during hospital stay with a significantly higher frequency than those with a greater protein content in ascites (15 per cent versus 2 per cent, respectively).[35] Subsequently, other authors showed that a low ascitic fluid protein concentration (lower than 10 g/l) and high serum bilirubin levels (greater than 2.5 mg/dl (43 μmol/l)) were independently associated with an increased probability of the first episode of spontaneous bacterial peritonitis during long-term follow-up in cirrhotics with ascites.[36, 37] Finally, in another study cirrhotic patients who had recovered from their first episode of spontaneous bacterial peritonitis, and in

whom the ascitic fluid protein content was lower than 10 g/l, had a greater probability of recurrent episodes of peritonitis than those whose protein concentration in ascitic fluid was higher than 10 g/l (77 versus 33 per cent, respectively, after 1 year).[38] Although other authors have chosen an ascitic protein concentration of less than 15 g/l for selecting patients with a particularly increased probability for spontaneous bacterial peritonitis,[39,40] from the results of the investigations described above it seems clear that a protein concentration in ascitic fluid of 10 g/l is an adequate cut-off value for establishing the risk of peritonitis in cirrhotic patients with ascites.

The reason for the variation in the antimicrobial properties, the concentration of defence substances, and the total protein content in ascitic fluid in cirrhotic patients is unknown, although several authors have suggested that all these indices could be related (a) to the serum levels of the defence proteins involved in antibacterial mechanisms of ascitic fluid; (b) to the degree of portal hypertension and hepatic insufficiency, and (c) to the volume of water diluting ascitic fluid solutes (Hoefs, Hepatol, 1981; 1:249; Hoefs, JLab-ClinMed, 1983; 102:260). This last possibility is supported by the finding that diuretic-induced reduction of water in ascitic fluid increases the total protein concentration and the antibacterial power of ascites (Runyon, Hepatol, 1986; 6:396) and by the common observation in clinical practice that spontaneous bacterial peritonitis occurs predominantly in cirrhotics with large-volume ascites.

Alterations in cell-mediated immunity

Many *in vitro* and *in vivo* studies have demonstrated that most cirrhotic patients show a depression in cell-mediated immunity. Both the proliferation and activation of T lymphocytes incubated with several immunostimulant substances, and the response to the intradermal injection of common antigens (delayed hypersensitivity) are markedly reduced in many decompensated cirrhotic patients.[41-44] Although the precise mechanism of the immunoincompetence in cirrhosis is unclear, a close relationship between impairment of cell-mediated immunity and malnutrition exists in these patients.[41-44] In addition, a large number of lymphoid alterations have been described in alcoholic patients, including peripheral blood lymphopenia, reduced *in vitro* response of circulating peripheral blood mononuclear cells to both phytohaemagglutinin and concanavalin A, and reduced *in vitro* interleukin-2 production, as well as impaired natural killer and/or lymphokine-activated killer cell activity (Berstein, Lancet, 1974; ii: 488; Thestrup-Pedersen, ClinExpImmun, 1976; 24:1; Charpentier, ClinExpImmun, 1984; 58:107; Yoshioka, ClinExpImmun, 1984; 56:668; Mutchnick, AlcoholClinExpRes, 1988; 12:155). Although alcohol induces a specific but transient impairment of T-lymphocyte activation, which is reversed after ethanol withdrawal (Spinozzi, Gastro, 1993; 105:1490), most of the immune alterations observed in alcoholic subjects may be related to the underlying liver disease and associated malnutrition rather than to the alcohol intake itself, because when selected alcoholic patients without relevant hepatic failure and/or malnutrition are studied, there is no evidence of lymphopenia or depressed *in vitro* proliferative response to mitogens (Drew, ClinExpImmun, 1984; 57:459; Spinozzi, JAMA, 1987; 257: 316).

In spite of the many studies investigating cell-mediated immunity disorders in cirrhosis, there have been no investigations assessing the role of these alterations in the pathogenesis of infection in cirrhotic patients. Moreover, the types of infection usually observed in immunocompromised patients without liver disease are very different from those presented by cirrhotic patients. Subjects suffering from acquired immunodeficiency syndrome, or patients treated with immunosuppressive drugs after organ transplantation, frequently develop infections caused by herpes group viruses, opportunistic bacteria, fungi, and protozoa,[45] all very unusual causes of infection in cirrhotic patients.

Neutrophil leucocyte dysfunction

A high proportion of cirrhotic patients show altered neutrophil leucocyte function at different levels. The most frequent disturbance is a marked reduction of chemotaxis, probably caused by the presence of substances in the serum which are capable of inhibiting granulocyte migration (DeMeo, NEJM, 1972; 286:735; Maderazo, JLabClinMed, 1975; 85:621; Feliu, EJClinInv, 1977; 7:571; Altin, Gut, 1983; 24:746; Rajkovik, Hepatol, 1986; 6:252). The nature of these chemotactic inhibitory substances has not yet been determined. Furthermore, the phagocytic and bacterial killing capacity of neutrophils has been found to be reduced in many cirrhotic patients (Feliu, EJClinInv, 1977; 7:571; Rajkovik, Hepatol, 1986; 6:252).

The role of leucocyte dysfunction as a factor favouring infection in cirrhosis is unclear. No differences in granulocyte function were found between infected and non-infected cirrhotics in two studies in which this issue has been examined.[46,47] Furthermore, the types of infection frequently developed by patients with congenital or acquired neutrophil function abnormalities (mainly chronic granulomatous diseases and recurrent staphylococcal and fungal infections) (Gallin, AnnIntMed, 1980; 90:520; Tauber, AmJMed, 1981; 70:1237), are very different from the infections developed by cirrhotic patients. Nevertheless, although leucocyte dysfunction does not seem to play a major role in the susceptibility of cirrhotic patients to bacterial infections, some factors capable of altering leucocyte function, such as alcoholism, malnutrition, and diabetes (Brayton, NEJM, 1970; 282:123; McGregor, JInfDis, 1978; 138:747; Gallin, RevInfDis, 1981; 3:1196; Horwitz, RevInfDis, 1982; 4:104), which are frequently associated with cirrhosis, could increase the degree of leucocyte impairment in these patients, and therefore be involved in the pathogenesis of bacterial complications in cirrhosis.

Bacteraemia and spontaneous bacterial peritonitis

Bacteraemia is the presence of bacteria in the bloodstream. In this chapter, the term 'bacteraemia' also includes the more classical term of 'septicaemia'. As in non-cirrhotic patients, bacteraemia in cirrhotics can be secondary to localized infections or can occur without any apparent source of infection, the latter being called spontaneous, primary, or idiopathic bacteraemia.

Spontaneous bacterial peritonitis is the infection of a previously sterile ascitic fluid, with no apparent intra-abdominal source of infection. Although spontaneous bacterial peritonitis can theoretically appear in any patient with ascites (Horina, Nephron 1993; 65:633), this type of infection is presented almost exclusively in cirrhotics with ascites.

Bacteraemia, particularly the spontaneous type, and spontaneous bacterial peritonitis usually occur in cirrhotic patients with advanced liver disease. Since the pathogenesis of bacteraemia and spontaneous bacterial peritonitis is similar, both infectious complications are discussed together.

Pathogenesis

Approximately 50 per cent of the episodes of bacteraemia presented by cirrhotic patients are secondary to localized infections, particularly of the urinary tract, and respiratory and soft-tissue infections.[1,4,7,15,17,48,49] It is possible that secondary bacteraemia in cirrhosis could be favoured by disturbances in the defence mechanisms normally acting against localized infections, such as neutrophil dysfunction and the reduction of humoral defence factors present in most of these patients (see above). The other 50 per cent of bacteraemic episodes are spontaneous. Since spontaneous bacteraemia is caused predominantly by enteric organisms[1,4,7,15,48,49] (Whipple, AnnIntMed, 1950; 33:462; Caroli, SemHopPar, 1958; 34:472; Tisdale, Gastro, 1961; 40:141; Martin, ArchIntMed, 1962; 109:555), the most accepted pathogenic mechanisms for this type of infection are the following:

(1) the depression of the hepatic reticuloendothelial system, which represents a failure of the liver in 'filtering' these bacteria, thereby allowing the passage of micro-organisms from the bowel lumen to the systemic circulation via the portal vein[26,50] (Caroli, SemHopPar, 1958; 34:472);

(2) as discussed above, the relative increase of aerobic Gram-negative bacilli in the jejunal flora in cirrhosis and the possible alteration in the intestinal barrier caused by circumstances decreasing mucosal blood flow (e.g. acute hypovolaemia or splanchnic vasoconstrictor drugs)[18-20] (Sorell, Gastro, 1993; 104:1722); and

(3) as also shown above, bacterial translocation, or the process by which enteric bacteria can cross the mucosa and infect the mesenteric lymph nodes, and reach the bloodstream through the intestinal lymphatic circulation (Sorell, Gastro, 1993; 104:1722; Llovet, Gut, 1994; 35:1648; Runyon, JHepatol, 1994; 21:792; Garcia-Tsao, Gastro, 1995; 108:1835; Runyon, Hepatol, 1995; 21:1719).

To explain the mechanism of spontaneous bacteraemia caused by non-enteric bacteria, it can reasonably be assumed that these micro-organisms enter the circulation from the skin or the upper respiratory tract, this pathogenesis being favoured in many cases by therapeutic or diagnostic procedures which rupture the natural mucocutaneous barriers. Whatever the source of the bacteria reaching the bloodstream, a bacteraemic event could be more prolonged and, therefore, could more readily become clinically significant in cirrhotic patients than in non-cirrhotic subjects, because of the marked depression of the reticuloendothelial system in the former (Fig. 3). This assumption is supported by experimental data demonstrating that cirrhotic rats had more prolonged bacteraemia than normal animals after intravenous injection of *Escherichia coli* (Rutenburg, PSEBM, 1959; 101:279).

According to the most accepted hypothesis on the pathogenesis of spontaneous bacterial peritonitis, the mechanism by which cirrhotic patients with ascites develop this type of infection is the

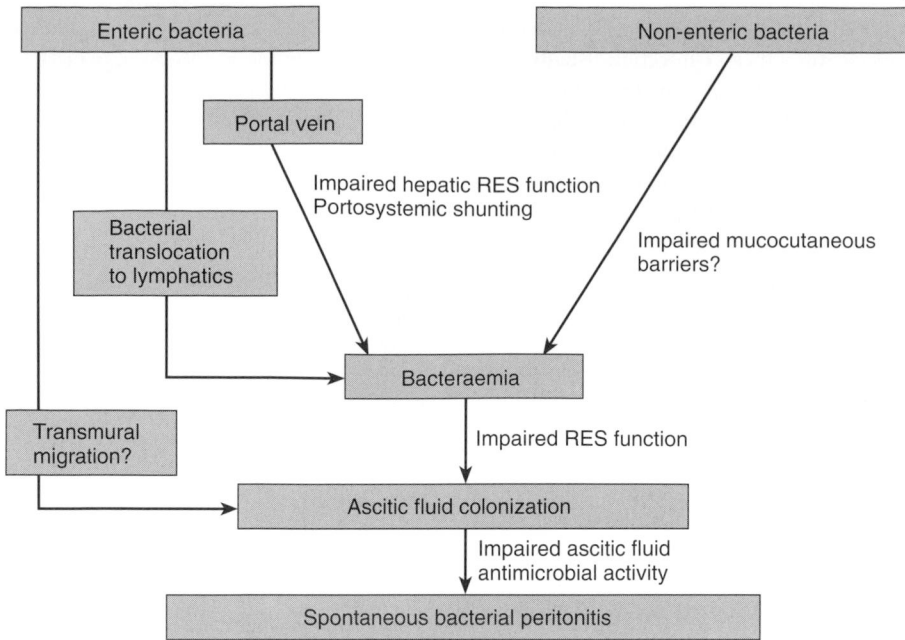

Fig. 3. The currently most accepted theory on the pathogenesis of bacteraemia and spontaneous bacterial peritonitis in cirrhosis. RES: reticuloendothelial system.

colonization of the ascitic fluid from an episode of bacteraemia.[51] Although the passage of micro-organisms from the bloodstream to the ascites has never been documented, it can be assumed that bacteria present in the circulation easily reach the ascites because of the constant fluid exchange between these two compartments. Once micro-organisms have colonized the ascites, the development of peritonitis would depend on the defensive capacity of ascitic fluid. Patients with a decreased antimicrobial activity of ascitic fluid would develop spontaneous bacterial peritonitis (Fig. 3). The passage of enteric organisms from the bowel lumen to the peritoneal cavity through the intestinal wall, another theoretical mechanism for development of spontaneous bacterial peritonitis, has never been demonstrated clinically or experimentally. Finally, the transfallopian route has been reported as an exceptional and anecdotal pathogenic mechanism of spontaneous bacterial peritonitis in occasional cases (Stassen, Gastro, 1985; 88:804; Brinson, JClinGastro, 1986; 8:82).

Clinical and laboratory data

The clinical manifestations of secondary bacteraemia often overlap the symptoms and signs of the localized infection causing it. In these cases, however, a marked worsening of liver and renal function is frequently observed. The clinical picture of spontaneous bacteraemia varies from one patient to another. Fever is the most prominent sign in this type of infection and is the only clinical manifestation in approximately 50 per cent of the patients.[48] In the remaining cases, fever is associated with clinical signs of impaired liver function and severe sepsis, such as hepatic encephalopathy, renal failure, gastrointestinal haemorrhage (particularly due to erosive gastritis), and septic shock.[16,48,49] The development of septic shock in a cirrhotic patient with bacteraemia is especially ominous, since most patients with this complication die within a few hours or days in spite of adequate treatment. Although most cirrhotic patients with bacteraemia show leucocytosis and

neutrophilia, a decreased white blood cell count is not infrequent.[49,50] In cases with severe sepsis, metabolic acidosis, hypoxaemia, and hypoglycaemia are common (Nouel, ArchIntMed, 1981; 141:1477).

The clinical picture of spontaneous bacterial peritonitis has been described in detail in several excellent articles.[11,14,51-54] Abdominal pain and fever are the most frequent signs presented by cirrhotics with spontaneous bacterial peritonitis. Most patients complain of diffuse abdominal pain and often have rebound tenderness. However, it is important to point out that in some cases abdominal pain is localized or absent, particularly in the early stages of the infection or in patients with hepatic encephalopathy, which may result in misdiagnosis. Fever, although present in most cases, is not usually a prominent feature. Other clinical features frequently observed in patients with spontaneous bacterial peritonitis are hepatic encephalopathy, gastrointestinal motility disturbances (vomiting, diarrhoea, or ileus), oliguria, and septic shock. As in bacteraemic patients, the development of septic shock in subjects with spontaneous bacterial peritonitis has a very poor prognostic significance. The frequency of presentation of these signs depends mainly on when spontaneous bacterial peritonitis is diagnosed; the clinical picture in patients with early diagnosis is usually less expressive; approximately 10 per cent of cirrhotic patients with spontaneous bacterial peritonitis have no new symptoms when the infection is diagnosed.[14]

The most outstanding laboratory finding in patients with spontaneous bacterial peritonitis is an increase in the ascitic fluid leucocyte count, due exclusively to a marked rise in the number of polymorphonuclear leucocytes. The average value of the polymorphonuclear cell count in ascitic fluid in cirrhotics with spontaneous bacterial peritonitis reported in recent studies[54,55] is approximately 7000 per millilitre. Nevertheless, although most patients with spontaneous bacterial peritonitis show an increased ascitic fluid polymorphonuclear count, the minimum poly-morphonuclear count which allows discrimination between infected ascites and non-infected ascites in cirrhosis has been debated for years. There is now general agreement that 250 polymorphonuclear leucocytes per millilitre of ascitic fluid can be reasonably used as this cut-off point and, therefore, is useful for establishing the diagnosis of spontaneous bacterial peritonitis and, more importantly, for making the decision to start antibiotic therapy, since this figure has a good sensitivity, specificity, and diagnostic accuracy in cirrhotics with ascites.[14,56] Several authors have reported a decrease in pH and an increase in lactate concentration in ascitic fluid from patients with spontaneous bacterial peritonitis. The pH of ascitic fluid is lower than 7.35 and the arterial blood–ascitic fluid pH gradient higher than 0.10 in most cases of spontaneous bacterial peritonitis. Similarly, many patients with spontaneous bacterial peritonitis shows a lactate concentration in ascitic fluid greater than 25 mg/dl (2.8 mmol/l) and an ascitic fluid–arterial lactate gradient greater than 20 mg/dl (2.2 mmol/l)[12,56] (Brook, DigDisSci, 1981; 26:1089; Gitlin, Hepatol, 1982; 2:408; Garcia-Tsao, Hepatol, 1985; 5:91; Sceama-Clergue, Gut, 1985; 26:332; Yang, Hepatol, 1985; 5:85; Pinzello, Hepatol, 1986; 6:244; Stassen, Gastro, 1986; 90:1247). However, since the incidence and magnitude of the changes in ascitic fluid pH and lactate concentration vary greatly in patients with spontaneous bacterial peritonitis studied by different authors, these alterations are difficult to interpret, thus limiting their diagnostic value (Reynolds, Gastro, 1986; 70:455; Runyon, Hepatol, 1991; 13:929).

Microbiological data

The micro-organisms isolated in secondary bacteraemia obviously depend on the type of localized infection causing the episode. Gram-negative bacilli are the most common organisms responsible for bacteraemia secondary to abdominal and urinary tract infections, and Gram-positive cocci are usually isolated in bacteraemia resulting from respiratory, soft tissue, and intravenous catheter-related infections.

Most cases of spontaneous bacteraemia and spontaneous bacterial peritonitis in cirrhosis are caused by bacteria normally present in the intestinal flora (Table 3). Individually, *E. coli* is the most common organism isolated from patients with these types of infection. However, ascitic fluid cultures are negative in a high proportion of patients with a clinical and laboratory picture of spontaneous bacterial peritonitis; this condition, the so-called 'culture-negative neutrocytic ascites', is currently considered as a variant of spontaneous bacterial peritonitis.[57,58] This is due mainly to the fact that the number of bacteria in ascitic fluid in patients with spontaneous bacterial peritonitis is usually very small (the concentration of organisms is lower than 1 organism/ml in most patients).[59] To increase the probability of isolating causative organisms in this infection it is recommended that media normally used for blood culture (aerobic and anaerobic bottles) are inoculated at the bedside with a large volume of ascitic fluid (10 ml or more).[59] Nevertheless, approximately 30 to 50 per cent of the patients with spontaneous bacterial peritonitis reported in recent large series had negative cultures despite use of the most accurate microbiological methods.[54,55,60,61]

Positive ascitic fluid cultures are obtained in approximately 5 per cent of cirrhotic patients with ascites without clinical or biological

Table 3 Micro-organisms isolated in spontaneous bacteraemia and peritonitis of cirrhotic patients[a]

	Spontaneous bacteraemia (85 episodes)	Spontaneous bacterial peritonitis (190 episodes)
Gram-negative bacilli	50 (57)	152 (77)
Staphylococci	17 (19)	2 (1)
Streptococcus pneumoniae	9 (10)	19 (9)
Other streptococci	6 (7)	17 (8)
Enterococcus faecalis	0	4 (2)
Anaerobic organisms	5 (6)	1 (1)
Other	1 (1)	3 (2)

[a] More than one organism was isolated in some episodes. Percentages in parentheses.

signs of spontaneous bacterial peritonitis when ascitic fluid is routinely cultured. The significance of this condition, usually called 'asymptomatic bacterascites', is unclear, although it may represent the stage of bacterial colonization of ascitic fluid shown in Fig. 4. Some cases of asymptomatic bacterascites progress to authentic spontaneous bacterial peritonitis, while others may resolve spontaneously (Kline, Gastro, 1976; 70:408; Forné, GastroHepato, 1986; 9:351; Chu, DigDisSci, 1995; 40:561).

The same bacteria are isolated from ascitic fluid and blood cultures in 30 to 40 per cent of patients with spontaneous bacterial peritonitis.[53,60] In other patients, blood cultures are positive but ascitic fluid culture is negative; in these cases, as in non-cirrhotic patients with haematogenous infections, it is reasonable to accept that the bacteria isolated from blood cultures are the causative organisms of spontaneous bacterial peritonitis.

Diagnosis

The existence of a bacteraemia or spontaneous bacterial peritonitis should always be suspected when a cirrhotic patient develops fever,

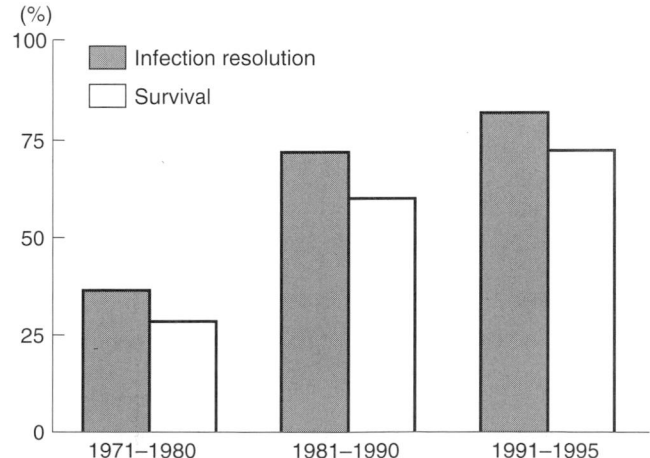

Fig. 4. Rates of infection resolution and hospital survival in different series of cirrhotic patients with spontaneous bacterial peritonitis treated in the Liver Unit from Barcelona over the past decades.

hepatic encephalopathy without a clear precipitating factor, acute renal function impairment without any apparent cause, or shock unrelated to a hypovolaemic event. When there is abdominal pain in a cirrhotic patient with ascites there must always be a high index of suspicion of spontaneous bacterial peritonitis. Therefore, whenever these signs appear, blood samples for cultures and total and differential white blood cell count, and ascitic fluid samples (if ascites is present) for cultures and cell count should be taken immediately and processed. Since spontaneous bacterial peritonitis is present at the time of admission in a relatively high proportion of cirrhotic patients referred to hospital for ascites, the tests of ascitic fluid should be performed on admission. Urine culture and sediment and chest radiography (in patients with hepatic encephalopathy) should also be performed, since most urinary tract infections occur without signs suggesting urinary tract involvement (see later), and pneumonia can be clinically unapparent in patients with profound encephalopathy.

Bacteraemia can only be diagnosed on the basis of isolation of the responsible organisms in blood cultures. The diagnosis of spontaneous bacterial peritonitis is usually easily established from the clinical and laboratory data described above. The most important criterion required for the diagnosis of spontaneous bacterial peritonitis in a cirrhotic patient with ascites is the existence of an ascitic fluid polymorphonuclear count greater than $250/mm^3$, in the absence of clinical, laboratory, and radiological data suggesting secondary peritonitis. Since most cases of spontaneous bacterial peritonitis are culture-negative, the isolation of causative organisms is not essential for diagnosis.[54,55,57,58,60,61]

Almost all episodes of peritonitis in cirrhotic patients with ascites are spontaneous. Therefore, infection of the ascitic fluid in these patients should always be considered as spontaneous bacterial peritonitis unless there are clinical or laboratory features indicating the possibility of a secondary peritonitis. The probability of secondary peritonitis is increased when a patient shows one of the following features:

(1) persistent and selectively localized abdominal pain;
(2) total protein concentration greater than 10 g/l, glucose less than 50 mg/dl (2.8 mmol/l), or lactic dehydrogenase greater than the upper limit of normal for serum; and
(3) the isolation of more than one type of micro-organism from the ascitic fluid culture, particularly when cultures grow anaerobic bacteria.[53,62]

Based on these criteria, together with the response of the ascitic fluid cell count to appropriate antibiotic therapy, an algorithm useful for differentiating spontaneous from secondary bacterial peritonitis has been proposed.[63]

Treatment

Until the 1980s, the development of a serious bacterial infection in patients with advanced liver disease usually had ominous prognostic significance. This is no longer the case. Figure 4 illustrates the change in the prognosis of severely infected cirrhotic patients; it shows the progressive increase in the rate of resolution of infection, and in survival, in different series of cirrhotics with spontaneous bacterial peritonitis treated in our Liver Unit (Barcelona) over the past two decades. Although improved general management of

patients with advanced liver failure may have played a role in the improvement of the prognosis of cirrhotics with severe bacterial infections, other important reasons could be earlier diagnosis of infectious complications and, therefore, earlier commencement of antimicrobial therapy, and better selection of antibiotics to be used in these patients[64] (Arroyo, Infec, 1994; 22(Suppl. 3):S1). The importance of early diagnosis and the symptoms and signs on which the suspicion of severe infection must be established have been stressed earlier.

Since bacteraemia and spontaneous bacterial peritonitis are severe infections, antimicrobial therapy must be started immediately they are suspected and, thus, before identification of the causative organisms and knowledge of their in vitro sensitivity. Until the 1980s, combinations of aminoglycosides and ampicillin or first- or second-generation cephalosporins were the antibiotic regimes habitually used in these patients. However, these regimes were associated with a relatively low efficacy and a high risk of nephrotoxicity.[65,66] In 1984, a prospective, randomized trial comparing the efficacy and safety of tobramycin combined with ampicillin versus cefotaxime in cirrhotic patients with severe infections (mostly spontaneous bacterial peritonitis) demonstrated the superiority of cefotaxime administration in terms of a higher rate of resolution of infection, a lower incidence of side-effects, and greater survival.[67] Since then, cefotaxime has been considered as one of the first-choice antibiotics for initial empiric therapy in severely infected cirrhotics (Rimola, DiagMicrobInfDis, 1995; 22:141). Based on the results of several studies reassessing the usefulness of cefotaxime in patients with spontaneous bacterial peritonitis, the high efficacy and safety of this antimicrobial agent has remained almost unmodified up to the present in these patients regardless of its wide use and the progressive reduction in its dosage.[54,55,60,67-69] The usefulness of other antibiotics has also been investigated in patients with spontaneous bacterial peritonitis: e.g. several second- and third-generation cephalosporins (ceftriaxone, ceftizoxime, and cefonicid), aztreonam, amoxicillin–clavulanic acid and different quinolones. All of them, with the exception of aztreonam, have shown adequate therapeutic efficacy and safety, although regimes including penicillin derivatives are associated with a relatively high incidence of super-infections.[70-75] Interestingly, in a recent study it was reported that oral administration of ofloxacin (a quinolone which is very effective against organisms commonly causing peritonitis in cirrhosis, with high bioavailability and adequate distribution to ascitic fluid after oral administration) is as effective as intravenous cefotaxime in uncomplicated spontaneous bacterial peritonitis.[76] Table 4 summarizes the results obtained in studies investigating the efficacy and safety of different antibiotic regimes used as empirical antimicrobial therapy in cirrhotic patients with spontaneous bacterial peritonitis.

In spite of the high rate of resolution of infection obtained with current antibiotic regimes, the mortality rate in patients with severe bacterial infection still remains relatively high. As shown in Table 4, approximately 20 to 40 per cent of patients with spontaneous bacterial peritonitis died while in hospital. Prognostic factors in patients with this type of infection have recently been investigated in several studies;[54,61,69] the most important clinical features adversely influencing the prognosis are nosocomial acquisition of the infection, advanced degree of severity of the underlying liver disease, and the existence of complications related to the peritonitis,

Table 4 Results obtained with different antibiotic regimens in the treatment of cirrhotic patients with spontaneous bacterial peritonitis

	Reference	No. of patients	Infection resolution (%)	Nephrotoxicity (%)	Superinfection (%)	Hospital survival (%)
Tobramycin + ampicillin	67	38	56	7	16	61
Cefotaxime:						
2 g/4 h	67	37	85	0	0	73
2 g/6 h	54	213	77	0	0	62
2 g/6 h	55	66	77	0	1	69
2 g/8 h						
5-day therapy	60	43	93	0	0	67
10-day therapy	60	47	91	0	0	58
2 g/12 h	55	70	79	0	1	79
Other cephalosporins:						
ceftriaxone	71, 72	48	94	0	0	63
ceftizoxime	73	25	88	0	0	84
cefonicid	72	30	94	0	0	70
Aztreonam	68	28[a]	71	0	14	57
Amoxicillin–clavulanic acid	74	27	85	0	7	63
Oral pefloxacin + other antibiotics	75	15	87	0	7	60
Oral ofloxacin	76	64[b]	84	0	1	81

[a] The study only included spontaneous bacterial peritonitis caused by Gram-negative organisms.
[b] The study only included non-complicated spontaneous bacterial peritonitis, that is, without septic shock, profound hepatic encephalopathy, gastrointestinal haemorrhage, ileus, or severe renal failure.

such as shock, ileus, or renal dysfunction. Furthermore, patients with spontaneous bacterial peritonitis with a markedly increased inflammatory response to the ascitic fluid infection (estimated by high circulating and ascitic fluid levels of tumour necrosis factor-α and interleukin-6, two cytokines involved in the initial steps of inflammation) showed a greater hospital mortality rate and a higher incidence of renal failure during the infectious episode than those with lower levels of these cytokines (Propst, EurJClinInv, 1993; 23: 832; Navasa, JHepatol, 1994; 21(Suppl. 1):S48). These results raise the possibility of modulating the inflammatory response as a coadjuvant therapy in severely infected cirrhotic patients.

Another important feature concerning the outcome of patients with spontaneous bacterial peritonitis is their poor mid- and long-term prognosis. The cumulative survival of patients recovering from the first episode of spontaneous bacterial peritonitis has been estimated as low as 38 per cent at 1 year and 16 per cent at 3 years of follow-up.[38] Therefore, since the current survival probability in cirrhotic patients undergoing liver transplantation is much better than these figures, this therapeutic procedure should be considered in these patients following resolution of the first episode of this infection.

Prophylaxis

Several groups of cirrhotic patients have been identified as being at particular risk of acquiring bacterial infections. The most important of these groups are patients with marked derangements in their defence mechanisms, patients with circumstances (particularly gastrointestinal bleeding) contributing to the impairment of these mechanisms, patients with previous episodes of severe infections, and patients who undergo invasive procedures.[26,35–38,50,77,78] Table 5 summarizes the groups of patients with an especially increased risk of infection. It is, therefore, logical that most studies

investigating the possibility of prevention of infection in cirrhosis have involved the cirrhotic populations mentioned above.

Since bacterial infections in cirrhosis are predominantly caused by bacteria of enteric origin, most of these studies have been done to assess the efficacy of intestinal decontamination in these patients. The pioneer study consisted of a prospective, randomized, controlled trial on the prophylactic effect of 6-hourly administration of oral non-absorbable antibiotics (gentamicin, neomycin, colistin, vancomycin, and nystatin, in different combinations) in a large series of cirrhotic patients with gastrointestinal haemorrhage.[77] Patients prophylactically treated with oral non-absorbable antibiotics showed a lower incidence of infection than those who did not receive these drugs (16 per cent versus 35 per cent, respectively), this difference being particularly apparent when only infections caused by enteric organisms were considered (4 per cent versus 21 per cent, respectively). Infections caused by non-enteric bacteria were observed with a similar frequency in both groups of patients. These results indicate that intestinal decontamination is useful in preventing infection in cirrhotic patients with gastrointestinal bleeding.

However, the high frequency of administration and cost of the antibiotic regimes described above led to the investigation of other antimicrobial agents for the prevention of infection in cirrhotic patients. In this setting, norfloxacin has been investigated in several controlled studies. It is a quinolone antibiotic, poorly absorbed when orally administered, but very effective *in vitro* against enterobacteria and capable of producing selective intestinal decontamination (that is, the elimination of aerobic Gram-negative bacilli from the faecal flora without changes in other micro-organisms) in cirrhotic patients after a few doses (Gines, GastroHepato, 1990; 13:325). In one of these studies, the oral administration of 400 mg/12 h of norfloxacin was very useful in reducing

Table 5 Cirrhotic populations with increased risk of infection

	Reference	Infection	Risk
Cirrhotic patients with:			
impaired reticuloendothelial function	26	Bacteraemia and/or spontaneous bacterial peritonitis	35% at 1 year
decreased total protein content in ascitic fluid (<10 g/l)	35, 36, 37	Spontaneous bacterial peritonitis	15% in-hospital; 20–40% at 1 year
increased serum bilirubin levels (>2.5 mg/dl)	37	Spontaneous bacterial peritonitis	40% at 1 year
gastrointestinal haemorrhage	77, 78	Bacteraemia, spontaneous bacterial peritonitis, and other infections	35% in-hospital
previous episodes of spontaneous bacterial peritonitis	38	Spontaneous bacterial peritonitis	69% at 1 year

the incidence of infection in cirrhotic patients with gastrointestinal haemorrhage.[78] In this investigation, bacterial infectious complications occurred in 10 per cent of the patients receiving norfloxacin and in 37 per cent of the patients from the control group. This difference was due to a reduced incidence of infections caused by enteric bacteria in the treated group. In another study, a markedly low incidence of in-hospital spontaneous bacterial peritonitis was reported in patients with ascitic cirrhosis with low ascitic fluid protein content when prophylactically treated with 400 mg/day of norfloxacin during the whole period of hospitalization (0 per cent in the treated group versus 22 per cent in the control group).[39] Finally, in a multicentre, double-blind, placebo-controlled trial, long-term administration of 400 mg/day of norfloxacin was very effective in reducing the probability of spontaneous bacterial peritonitis recurrence in patients who had recovered from an episode of this type of infection (20 per cent in the treated group versus 68 per cent in the placebo group at 1 year).[79] The one-year probability of recurrence of spontaneous bacterial peritonitis caused by Gram-negative bacilli was only 3 per cent in the treated group, whereas it was 60 per cent in the placebo group. Interestingly, in this study norfloxacin administration caused selective intestinal decontamination throughout the study period (mean follow-up period of 6 months, with a range of 1–19 months) without overgrowth of resistant, potentially pathogenic bacteria or increased faecal concentration of *Candida* spp.

More recently, the effectiveness of antibiotics other than norfloxacin has also been investigated. In two studies, cirrhotic patients with ascites receiving long-term oral administration of ciprofloxacin (750 mg once a week)[40] or trimethoprim–sulphamethoxazole (one double-strength tablet five times a week),[80] respectively, showed a reduced incidence of spontaneous bacterial peritonitis as compared to patients not receiving prophylaxis. In these investigations, the incidence of the infection was approximately 3 per cent in treated patients and 25 per cent in control patients. In another controlled study, systemic antibiotic therapy consisting of 10-day administration of ofloxacin (400 mg/day, first intravenously, then orally) plus intravenous amoxicillin–clavulanic acid before each endoscopic examination was also effective in preventing bacterial infection in cirrhotic patients with gastrointestinal haemorrhage (20 per cent in the treated group versus 66 per cent in the control group).[81]

Urinary tract infections

Urinary tract infections are the most frequent infectious complication in cirrhosis (Table 1). As in the non-cirrhotic population, cirrhotic patients with indwelling urethral catheters are highly predisposed to develop urinary tract infections. The incidence is markedly higher in female than in male cirrhotics.[1,6,82] Among female patients, some authors have reported an higher susceptibility to urinary tract infection in patients with primary biliary cirrhosis than in patients with other types of chronic liver disease,[83] although this finding has not been observed by other investigators.[82,84] A direct correlation between the physical presence of tense ascites and the development of urinary tract infection has been reported (Bercoff, Lancet, 1985; i:987; Bellaïche, GastrClinBiol, 1994; 18:96). Bercoff *et al.* suggested that this finding was related to incomplete bladder emptying observed in most of their patients, particularly in those with alcoholic cirrhosis (Bercoff, Lancet, 1985; i:987).

Many urinary tract infections in cirrhosis are oligo- or asymptomatic. In symptomatic cases, fever is the most common clinical manifestation. A significant increase in the number of leucocytes in fresh urine sediment is only observed in about 60 per cent of cirrhotic patients with urinary tract infection. Therefore, bacteriuria alone is found in a high proportion of urinary tract infections in cirrhotics.[6,83,85] However, the potential role of these infections in causing bacteraemia should not be underestimated.[1]

Most urinary tract infections in cirrhotic patients are caused by Gram-negative bacilli.[1,6,83,85] Therefore, although urine cultures for identification and *in vitro* sensitivity testing of causative organisms are always recommended, cases requiring immediate therapy should be given co-trimoxazole, quinolones (norfloxacin, ciprofloxacin, or ofloxacin), or amoxicillin–clavulanic acid, since these agents are very active against Gram-negative bacteria and reach high concentrations in urine. Recurrence of the infection after adequate therapy is not uncommon and it has been reported to be particularly frequent in patients with primary biliary cirrhosis.[85]

Pneumonia

Community-acquired pneumonia is a frequent complication in subjects with active alcoholism (Adams, MedClinNAm, 1984; 68: 179). Alcohol intake depresses leucocyte and reticuloendothelial cell function, impairs cell-mediated immunity, and profoundly alters the local defence mechanisms of the respiratory tract (Laurenzi, AmRevRespDis, 1966; 93:134; Krumpe, MedClinNAm, 1984; 68: 201). *Streptococcus pneumoniae* is the causative organism in most lower respiratory tract infections in alcoholics. However, a significant number of cases of pneumonia in these patients are caused by other pathogens normally present in the oropharyngeal area, especially anaerobic bacteria or *Haemophilus influenzae*, or by Gram-negative bacilli, particularly *Klebsiella pneumoniae*. All these organisms should be considered when selecting empiric therapy for lower respiratory tract infection in alcoholic subjects. In contrast to alcoholic subjects, non-alcoholic cirrhotics do not seem to be especially predisposed to develop community-acquired pneumonia. In the authors' experience, characteristics of community-acquired pulmonary infections in patients with cirrhosis of non-alcoholic origin do not differ from those seen in the general population (Levy, Chest, 1988; 92:43). Nevertheless, a decrease in pulmonary defence mechanisms against *Streptococcus pneumoniae* has recently been reported in rats with experimentally induced cirrhosis (Mellencamp, JInfDis, 1991; 163:102).

Hospital-acquired pneumonia is predominantly caused by Gram-negative bacilli and staphylococci[45] (Bradcher, MedClinNAm, 1983; 67:1233; Craven, EurJClinInfDis, 1989; 8:1). These organisms may reach the lungs through inhaled air, bronchial aspiration of pharyngeal secretions (frequently colonized by Gram-negative bacilli in hospitalized patients), or via the haematogenous route. Some procedures or clinical conditions, such as tracheal intubation, oesophageal tamponade, or hepatic encephalopathy, clearly represent predisposing factors for pneumonia in cirrhotic patients. Although the identification of the responsible organisms in hospital-acquired pneumonia is important for the selection of antibiotic treatment, organisms causing pneumonia cannot be isolated in many patients, even with a very aggressive diagnostic approach. In such cases, the empiric administration of third-generation cephalosporins should be considered as the first choice of antibiotic because of their wide spectrum of antibacterial activity and low risk of adverse effects, although in cases with a reasonably high probability of pneumonia caused by *Pseudomonas* spp. (i.e. pneumonia developed in patients admitted to intensive care units and under mechanical ventilation) a combination of antimicrobial agents effective against this type of organism should be administered. As in community-acquired pneumonia, there is no specific information about hospital-acquired pneumonia in cirrhotic patients. In the authors' experience there are no significant differences between cirrhotics and non-cirrhotic patients with severe underlying diseases in relation to the clinical and laboratory characteristics and the final outcome of this type of infection.

Tuberculosis

Alcoholic subjects are classically considered as prone to develop pulmonary tuberculosis (Adams, MedClinNAm, 1984; 68:179; Feingold, SouthMedJ, 1976; 69:1336). The response to antituberculous drugs is poorer and the relapse rate higher among alcoholics than in non-alcoholic patients (Hudolin, AnnNYAcadSci, 1975; 252:353). Since the relationship between the existence of cirrhosis and the risk of acquiring pulmonary tuberculosis has not been investigated, it is not known whether alcoholics are predisposed

to this type of infection because of the alcoholism itself, their social circumstances, or because of underlying hepatic disease.

Another classical association is that between alcoholism and peritoneal tuberculosis (Burack, AmJMed, 1960; 28:510). However, this association has not been found by all workers investigating large series of patients with this type of infection (Borhanmanesh, AnnIntMed, 1972; 76:567; Dineen, AnnSurg, 1976; 184:717). Since peritoneal tuberculosis can be observed in non-alcoholic cirrhotic patients, the development of this infection in cirrhotic patients could be related to the hepatic disease rather than alcoholism. The most common clinical picture of peritoneal tuberculosis in cirrhotic patients consists of low-grade fever and ascites with a high protein content and increased lymphocyte count (Palmer, Gut, 1985; 26: 1296; Scully, NEJM, 1986; 315:952; Cellier, EurJGastroHepatol, 1994; 6:831). Tuberculous infection should be suspected when left-sided pleural effusion develops in alcoholic patients with ascites. It is not always possible to isolate *Mycobacterium tuberculosis* from ascitic fluid cultures, and the response to the intradermal injection of tuberculin is frequently negative in cirrhotic patients. In most cases, therefore, the diagnosis of this infection must be established on the basis of the findings at laparoscopy and by peritoneal biopsy (Rodriguez de Lope, Endoscopy, 1982; 14:178; Cellier, EurJGastroHepatol, 1994; 6:831). At laparoscopy, the peritoneum usually appears hyperaemic with multiple white nodules on its surface. Typical tuberculous granulomata (central necrosis with Langhans giant cells) are frequently observed in the biopsies taken from these nodules. Special stains are also useful to identify mycobacteria in the granulomata. Martinez-Vazquez *et al.* (Gut, 1986; 27:1049) reported that most patients with peritoneal tuberculosis show an increased concentration of adenosine deaminase in ascitic fluid. Response to antituberculous drugs in cirrhotic patients with peritoneal tuberculosis is usually good (Dutt, AnnIntMed, 1986; 104:7).

Other infections

Soft-tissue infections, particularly lymphangitis of the lower extremities and abdominal wall, are relatively frequent in cirrhotic patients with ankle oedema or ascites.[1,4,86] These infections are commonly related to deficient hygienic standards and unapparent skin injuries. However, since lymphangitis usually does not resolve until the underlying oedema or ascites disappears, local factors related to increased interstitial water content or to raised cutaneous and subcutaneous tissue distension may play a role in the pathogenesis of this infective complication. Lymphangitis is commonly caused by Gram-positive cocci. Therefore antimicrobial therapy in cirrhotics with lymphangitis should cover these organisms. Nevertheless, as several cases of lower extremity cellulitis caused by Gram-negative bacilli have been reported recently,[86] needle aspiration of the lesions to identify the causative organisms seems advisory. In some cases of cellulitis due to Gram-negative organisms a haematogenous route of infection has been suggested.[86]

In a classical investigation including all admissions and necropsy studies performed over 20 years in a general hospital Snyder *et al.* reported that cirrhotic patients showed a greater incidence of bacterial endocarditis than non-cirrhotic patients (0.34 versus 0.10 per cent of admissions, and 1.8 versus 0.9 per cent of postmortem studies, respectively).[87] The authors explained this finding on the basis of the high risk of cirrhotics developing bacteraemia, with the consequent possibility of colonizing the endocardium. However, these results have been questioned by other investigators who were not able to confirm an increased incidence of endocarditis in cirrhotic patients.[88] Endocarditis complicating the course of cirrhosis frequently arises on a previously normal endocardium[87] and predominantly involves the mitral valve.[89] Although Gram-positive cocci are the most common causative organisms, particularly *Staphylococcus aureus*,[89] some cases are caused by enterobacteria.[87] Prognosis of endocarditis in cirrhotic patients is usually ominous.[89]

Cirrhotic patients with hydrothorax, a quite common condition in cirrhotics with ascites, can develop spontaneous bacterial empyema, that is, the infection of a pre-existing hydrothorax without any concomitant pneumonia.[1,90,91] Although spontaneous bacterial empyema is rarely observed, its interest derives from the fact that this infective complication has only been described in cirrhotic patients. Almost half of the cirrhotic patients with spontaneous bacterial empyema also have spontaneous bacterial peritonitis.[91] Diagnosis of empyema is based on laboratory findings in pleural fluid similar to those in ascitic fluid of spontaneous bacterial peritonitis, mainly an increased polymorphonuclear cell count. The most frequent causative organisms are Gram-negative bacilli, particularly *E. coli*.[91] The pathogenesis of spontaneous bacterial empyema is also thought to be the same as that of spontaneous bacterial peritonitis, i.e. the colonization of a previously sterile hydrothorax from a bacteraemia,[90] although in cases coexisting with spontaneous bacterial peritonitis passage of infected ascites from the abdominal cavity through the diaphragm has been suggested.[91] Recommended therapy consists of the administration of parenteral antibiotics without the need for pleural drainage.[91]

Bacterial infections in acute liver failure

Patients with acute liver failure, particularly those with fulminant hepatitis, are at great risk of acquiring severe infections. Although an incidence of infection of 20 to 40 per cent was reported in early studies,[92-94] the incidence of infection in patients with fulminant hepatic failure has been found to be very much greater in more recent investigations, ranging from 50 to 80 per cent.[95-97] The most frequent infections in these patients are bacteraemia, particularly of the spontaneous type, followed by urinary tract infections and respiratory infections. The predominant organisms isolated are staphylococci, streptococci, and Gram-negative bacilli, [95-98] although fungi (especially *Candida* spp.) can be isolated in 40 per cent of patients with fulminant hepatic failure.[96,99] Most fungal infections are clinically silent and coexist with bacterial infection. Serial microbiological analysis, white blood cell count, and chest radiological examination seem to be the best methods for early detection of bacterial and fungal complications in these patients.

Prophylactic administration of antibiotics effective against the most frequently isolated bacteria and fungi is recommended in patients with acute liver failure. In a retrospective study, selective intestinal decontamination with poorly absorbable oral antibiotics was useful in reducing the risk of infection from enterobacteria in patients with acute liver failure.[97] In a prospective, controlled trial, prophylaxis with systemic antimicrobial agents (intravenous cefuroxime) with or without enteral decontamination (oral administration of colistin + tobramycin + amphotericin B), was effective in reducing the infection rates of patients with fulminant liver failure, although there was not any significant effect on survival.[100] However, it should be noted that a reduction in infection is an important consideration in patients with fulminant liver failure in whom active sepsis may be considered as a contra-indication for liver transplantation, which is the only therapeutic option in many cases (Caraceni, Lancet, 1995; 345:163).

The pathogenesis of infectious complications in patients with acute liver failure is multifactorial. These patients frequently undergo invasive procedures, such as intravenous and urethral catheterization, tracheal intubation, and mechanical ventilation, which are potential vehicles of infection. Physical immobility in comatose patients is another predisposing factor to infection, particularly lower respiratory tract infection. On the other hand, serum complement concentration is markedly decreased in most patients with acute liver failure[95] (Fox, Gut, 1971; 12:574; Kosmidis, ClinExpImmun, 1972; 11:31; Thompson, ClinExpImmun, 1973; 14: 335; Wyke, Gut, 1980; 21:643; Wyke, ClinExpImmun, 1982; 50: 442). The reduction of serum complement in these patients is associated with defective serum opsonization of bacteria and yeasts and with several granulocyte function abnormalities, mainly a reduced neutrophil chemotaxis and adherence capacity[29,95] (Altin, Gut, 1983; 24:746). In addition, Kupffer cell dysfunction, deficient fibronectin production, and impairment of cell-mediated immunity have been also reported in patients with acute liver failure (Imawari, DigDisSci, 1985; 30:1028; Muto, Lancet, 1988; 1:72). Finally, it has been shown recently that bacterial translocation occurs in experimental acute liver injury (Kasravi, Hepatol, 1996; 23:97).

References

1. Rimola A, Bory F, Planas R, Xaubet A, Bruguera M, and Rodés J. Infecciones bacterianas agudas en la cirrosis hepática. *Gastroenterología y Hepatología*, 1981; **4**: 453–8.
2. Andreu M, *et al.* Fiebre en el enfermo con cirrosis hepática: Estudio prospectivo durante 6 meses. *Medicina Clínica* (Barcelona), 1985; **84**: 433–6.
3. Clemente-Ricote G, *et al.* Infecciones bacterianas en la cirrosis hepática. *Gastroenterología y Hepatología*, 1986; **9**: 285–90.
4. Caly WR, and Strauss E. A prospective study of bacterial infections in patients with cirrhosis. *Journal of Hepatology*, 1993; **18**: 353–8.
5. Bennett HJV, and Brachman PS, eds. *Hospital infections*, 3rd edn. Boston: Little Brown and Co., 1992.
6. Gómez J, Vilardell F, Casals L, and Prats G. Infecciones urinarias del cirrótico. *Revista Española de Enfermedades del Aparato Digestivo*, 1979; **56**: 321–6.
7. Clumeck N, Estenne M, Canhoff R, Reding P, and Cornil A. Septicémie et péritonite 'spontanée' chez le cirrhotique. *Nouvelle Presse Medicale*, 1979; **8**: 2655–8.
8. LeCarrer M, Poupon RY, Petit J, Ballet F, and Darnis F. Les infections du liquide d'ascite chez le cirrhotique: Etude clinique et biologique de 36 épisodes observés au cours d'une année. *Gastroenterologie Clinique et Biologique*, 1980; **4**: 640–5.
9. Lévy VG, Theis C, Denis C, and Denis J. Critères cytologiques de l'infection de l'ascite au cours des cirrhoses. *Gastroenterologie Clinique et Biologique*, 1982; **6**: 736–9.
10. Kammerer J, Dupeyron C, Vuillemin N, Leluan G, and Fouet P. Apport des examens cytologiques et bactériologiques du liquide d'ascite cirrhotique

au diagnostic de péritonite bactérienne. A propos de 610 rélèvements chez 156 malades. *Medicine et Chirurgie Digestive*, 1982; **11**: 243–51.

11. Pinzello G, Simonetti RG, Craxi A, DiPiazza S, Spano C, and Pagliaro L. Spontaneous bacterial peritonitis: A prospective investigation in predominantly nonalcolic cirrhotic patients. *Hepatology*, 1983; **3**: 545–9.

12. Attali P, Turner K, Pelletier G, Ink O, and Etienne JP. pH of ascitic fluid: diagnostic and prognostic value in cirrhotic and noncirrhotic patients. *Gastroenterology*, 1986; **90**: 1255–60.

13. Almdal TP and Skinhoj P. Spontaneous bacterial peritonitis in cirrhosis. Incidence, diagnosis and prognosis. *Scandinavian Journal of Gastroenterology*, 1987; **22**: 295–300.

14. García-Tsao G. Spontaneous bacterial peritonitis. *Gastroenterology Clinics of North America*, 1992; **21**: 257–75.

15. Graudal N, Milman N, Kikegaard E, Korner B, and Thomsem AC. Bacteremia in cirrhosis of the liver. *Liver*, 1986; **6**: 297–301.

16. Almdal T, Skinhoj P, and Friis H. Bacteremia in patients suffering from cirrhosis. *Infection*, 1986; **14**: 68–70.

17. Kuo C-H, Changchien C-S, Yang C-Y, Sheen I-S, and Liaw Y-F. Bacteremia in patients with cirrhosis of the liver. *Liver*, 1991; **11**: 334–9.

18. Martini GA, Phear EA, Ruebner E, and Sherlock S. The bacterial content of the small intestine in normal and cirrhotic subjects: relation to methionine toxicity. *Clinical Science*, 1956; **16**: 35–51.

19. Lal D, Gorbach SL, and Levitan R. Intestinal microflora in patients with alcoholic cirrhosis: urea-splitting bacteria and neomycin resistance. *Gastroenterology*, 1972; **62**: 275–9.

20. Casafont-Morencos F, DeLasHeras-Castaño G, Martin-Ramos L, López-Arias MJ, Ledesma F, and Pons-Romero F. Small bowel bacterial overgrowth in patients with alcoholic cirrhosis. *Digestive Disease and Science*, 1995; **40**: 1252–6.

21. Bjorneboe M, and Prytz H. The mononuclear phagocytic functions of the liver. In Ferguson A, and McSween RNM, eds. *Immunological aspects of the liver and gastrointestinal tract*. Lancaster: MTP Press, 1976: 251–89.

22. Biozzi C and Stiffel C. The physiopathology of the reticuloendothelial cells of the liver and spleen. In Popper H, and Schaffner F, eds. *Progress in liver diseases, II*. New York: Grune and Stratton, 1965: 166–91.

23. Bradfield JWB. Reticulo-endothelial blockade: a reassessment. In Wise E, and Knook DL, eds. *Kupffer cells and other liver sinusoidal cells*. Amsterdam: Elsevier/North Holland Biomedical Press, 1977: 365–72.

24. Jones EA and Summerfield JA. Kupffer cells. In Arias IM, Jakoby WB, Popper H, Schacter D, and Shafritz DA, eds. *The liver: biology and pathobiology*, 2nd edn. New York: Raven Press, 1988: 683–704.

25. Saba TM. Physiology and physiopathology of the reticuloendothelial system. *Archives of Medicine*, 1970; **126**: 1031–52.

26. Rimola A, Soto R, Bory F, Arroyo V, Piera C, and Rodés J. Reticuloendothelial system phagocytic activity in cirrhosis and its relation to bacterial infections and prognosis. *Hepatology*, 1984; **4**: 53–8.

27. Bolognesi M, *et al*. Clinical significance of the evaluation of hepatic reticuloendothelial removal capacity in patients with cirrhosis. *Hepatology*, 1994; **19**: 628–34.

28. Fierer J and Finley F. Deficient serum bactericidal activity against *Escherichia coli* in patients with cirrhosis of the liver. *Journal of Clinical Investigation*, 1979; **63**: 912–21.

29. Rajkovik IA and Williams R. Mechanisms of abnormalities in host defences against bacterial infection in liver diseases. *Clinical Science*, 1985; **68**: 247–53.

30. Rolando N and Wyke RJ. Infections. *Gut*, 1991; (Suppl.): S25–S28.

31. Akalin G, Laleli Y, and Telatar H. Bactericidal and opsonic activity of ascitic fluid from cirrhotic and non-cirrhotic patients. *Journal of Infectious Diseases*, 1983; **147**: 1011–17.

32. Runyon BA, Morrissey RL, and Hoefs JC. Opsonic activity of human ascitic fluid. A potentially important protective mechanism against spontaneous bacterial peritonitis. *Hepatology*, 1985; **5**: 634–7.

33. Runyon BA. Opsonic activity of human ascitic fluid. *Hepatology*, 1986; **6**: 546.

34. Runyon BA. Patients with deficient ascitic fluid opsonic activity are predisposed to spontaneous bacterial peritonitis. *Hepatology*, 1988; **8**: 632–5.

35. Runyon BA. Low-protein-concentration ascitic fluid is predisposed to spontaneous bacterial peritonitis. *Gastroenterology*, 1986; **91**: 1343–6.

36. Llach J, *et al*. Incidence and predictive factors of first episode of spontaneous bacterial peritonitis in cirrhosis with ascites: relevance of ascitic fluid protein concentration. *Hepatology*, 1992; **16**: 724–7.

37. Andreu M, *et al*. Risk factors for spontaneous bacterial peritonitis in cirrhotic patients with ascites. *Gastroenterology*, 1993; **104**: 1133–8.

38. Tító L, Rimola A, Ginès P, Llach J, Arroyo V, and Rodés J. Recurrence of spontaneous bacterial peritonitis in cirrhosis: frequency and predictive factors. *Hepatology*, 1988; **8**: 27–31.

39. Soriano G, *et al*. Selective intestinal decontamination prevents spontaneous bacterial peritonitis. *Gastroenterology*, 1991; **100**: 477–81.

40. Rolanchon A, *et al*. Ciprofloxacin and long-term prevention of spontaneous bacterial peritonitis: results of a prospective controlled trial. *Hepatology*, 1995; **22**: 1171–4.

41. Hsu CCS and Leevy CM. Inhibition of PHA-stimulated lymphocyte transformation by plasma from patients with advanced cirrhosis. *Clinical and Experimental Immunology*, 1971; **8**: 749–57.

42. O'Keefe SJ, El-Zayadi AR, Carrhaher TE, Davis M, and Williams R. Malnutrition and immunoincompetence in patients with liver disease. *Lancet*, 1980; **ii**: 615–17.

43. Franco D, *et al*. Nutrition and immunity after peritoneovenous drainage of intractable ascites in cirrhotic patients. *American Journal of Surgery*, 1983; **146**: 652–7.

44. Nouri-Aria KT, Alexander GJM, Portmann BC, Hegarty JE, Eddleston ALWF, and Williams R. T and B cell function in alcoholic liver disease. *Journal of Hepatology*, 1986; **2**: 195–207.

45. Mandell G, Bennett JE, and Dolin R, eds. *Mandell, Douglas and Bennett's Principles and practice of infectious diseases*, 4th edn. New York: Churchill Livingstone, 1995.

46. Yousif-Kadaru AGM, Rajkovic IA, Wyke RJ, and Williams R. Defects in serum attractant activity in different types of chronic liver disease. *Gut*, 1984; **25**: 79–84.

47. Garcia-Gonzalez M, Boixeda D, Herrero D, and Burgaleta C. Effect of granulocyte–macrophage colony-stimulating factor on leukocyte function in cirrhosis. *Gastroenterology*, 1993; **105**: 527–31.

48. Javaloyas M, Ariza J, and Gudiol F. La bacteriemia en el paciente con cirrosis hepática. Análisis etiopatogénico y pronóstico de 92 casos. *Medicina Clínica* (Barcelona), 1984; **82**: 612–16.

49. Barnes PF, Arevalo C, Chan LS, Wong SF, and Reynolds TB. A prospective evaluation of bacteremic patients with chronic liver disease. *Hepatology*, 1988; **8**: 1099–103.

50. Rimola A, Arroyo V, and Rodés J. Infective complications in acute and chronic liver failure: Basis and control. In Williams R, ed. *Critical care medicine. Liver failure*. London: Churchill Livingstone, 1986; 93–111.

51. Hoefs JC and Runyon BA. Spontaneous bacterial peritonitis. *Disease-a-month*, 1985; **31**: 1–48.

52. Correia JP and Conn HO. Spontaneous bacterial peritonitis: Endemic or epidemic?. *Medical Clinics of North America*, 1975; **59**: 963–81.

53. Hoefs JC, Canawati HN, Sapico FL, Hopkins RR, Weiner J, and Montgomerie JZ. Spontaneous bacterial peritonitis. *Hepatology*, 1982; **2**: 399–407.

54. Toledo C, *et al*. Spontaneous bacterial peritonitis in cirrhosis: predicitve factors of infection resolution and survival in patients treated with cefotaxime. *Hepatology*, 1993; **17**: 251–7.

55. Rimola A, *et al*. Two different dosages of cefotaxime in the treatment of spontaneous bacterial peritonitis in cirrhosis: results of a prospective, randomized, multicenter study. *Hepatology*, 1995; **21**: 674–9.

56. Albillos A, *et al*. Ascitic fluid polymorphonuclear cell count and serum to ascites albumin gradient in the diagnosis of bacterial peritonitis. *Gastroenterology*, 1990; **98**: 134–40.

57. Runyon BA and Hoefs JC. Culture-negative neutrocytic ascites: a variant of spontaneous bacterial peritonitis. *Hepatology*, 1984; **4**: 1209–11.

58. Terg R, *et al*. Analysis of clinical course and prognosis of culture-positive spontaneous bacterial peritonitis and neutrocytic ascites. Evidence of the same disease. *Digestive Disease and Science*, 1992; **37**: 1499–504.

59. Runyon BA, Canawati HN, and Akriviadis EA. Optimization of ascitic fluid culture technique. *Gastroenterology*, 1988; **95**: 1351–5.

60. Runyon BA, McHutchison JG, Antillon MR, Akriviadis EA, and Montano AA. Short-course versus long-course antibiotic treatment of spontaneous bacterial peritonitis. A randomized controlled study of 100 patients. *Gastroenterology*, 1991; **100**: 1737–42.

61. Llovet JM, *et al.* Short-term prognosis of cirrhotics with spontaneous bacterial peritonitis: multivariate study. *American Journal of Gastroenterology*, 1993; **88**: 388–92.

62. Runyon BA and Hoefs JC. Ascitic fluid analysis in the differentiation of spontaneous bacterial peritonitis from gastrointestinal tract perforation into ascitic fluid. *Hepatology*, 1984; **4**: 447–50.

63. Akriviadis EA and Runyon BA. Utility of an algorithm in differentiating spontaneous from secondary bacterial peritonitis. *Gastroenterology*, 1990; **98**: 127–33.

64. Navasa, M. Treatment of spontaneous bacterial peritonitis and other severe bacterial injections in the setting of cirrhosis. In Arroyo V, Bosch J, and Rodes J, eds. *Treatments in hepatology*. Barcelona: Masson, S.A., 1995: 109.

65. Cabrera J, *et al.* Aminoglycoside nephrotoxicity in cirrhosis. Value of urinary beta2-microglobulin to discriminate functional renal failure from acute tubular damage. *Gastroenterology*, 1982; **82**: 97–105.

66. Moore RD, Smith CR, and Lietman PS. Increased risk of renal dysfunction due to interaction of liver disease and aminoglycosides. *American Journal of Medicine*, 1986; **80**: 1093–7.

67. Felisart J, *et al.* Cefotaxime is more effective than is ampicillin–tobramycin in cirrhotics with severe infections. *Hepatology*, 1985; **5**: 457–62.

68. Ariza J, *et al.* Aztreonam vs. cefotaxime in the treatment of Gram-negative spontaneous bacterial peritonitis in cirrhotic patients. *Hepatology*, 1991; **14**: 91–8.

69. Follo A, *et al.* Renal impairment after spontaneous bacterial peritonitis in cirrhosis: incidence, clinical course, predictive factors and prognosis. *Hepatology*, 1994; **20**: 1495–501.

70. Ariza J, *et al.* Evaluation of aztreonam in the treatment of spontaneous bacterial peritonitis in patients with cirrhosis. *Hepatology*, 1986; **6**: 906–10.

71. Mercader J, Gomez J, Ruiz J, Garre MC, and Valdes M. Use of ceftriaxone in the treatment of bacterial infections in cirrhotic patients. *Chemotherapy*, 1989; **35** (Suppl. 2): 23–6.

72. Gómez-Jiménez J, *et al.* Randomized trial comparing ceftriaxone with cefonicid for treatment of spontaneous bacterial peritonitis in cirrhotic patients. *Antimicrobial Agents and Chemotherapy*, 1993; **37**: 1587–92.

73. Rimola A, *et al.* Efficacy of ceftizoxime in the treatment of severe bacterial infections in patients with cirrhosis. *Drug Investigation*, 1992; **4**(Suppl. 1): 35–7.

74. Grange JD, *et al.* Amoxicillin–clavulanic acid therapy of spontaneous bacterial peritonitis: a prospective study of twenty-seven cases in cirrhotic patients. *Hepatology*, 1990; **11**: 360–4.

75. Silvain C, Breux JP, Grollier G, Rouffineau J, Bezq-Giraudon B, and Beauchant M. Les septicémies et les infections du liquide d'ascite du cirrhotique peuvent-elles être traitées exclusivement par voie orale? *Gastroenterologie Clinique et Biologique*, 1989; **13**: 335–9.

76. Navasa M, *et al.* Randomized, comparative study of oral ofloxacin versus intravenous cefotaxime in spontaneous bacterial peritonitis. *Gastroenterology*, 1996; **111**: 1011–17.

77. Rimola A, *et al.* Oral, nonabsorbable antibiotics prevent infection in cirrhosis with gastrointestinal hemorrhage. *Hepatology*, 1985; **5**: 463–7.

78. Soriano G, *et al.* Norfloxacin prevents bacterial infection in cirrhotics with gastrointestinal hemorrhage. *Gastroenterology*, 1992; **103**: 1267–72.

79. Gines P, *et al.* Norfloxacin prevents spontaneous bacterial peritonitis recurrence in cirrhosis: results of a double-blind, placebo-controlled trial. *Hepatology*, 1990; **12**: 716–24.

80. Singh N, Gayoswski T, Yu VL, and Wagener MM. Trimethoprim–sulfamethoxazole for the prevention of spontaneous bacterial peritonitis in cirrhosis: a randomized trial. *Annals of Internal Medicine*, 1995; **122**: 595–8.

81. Blaise M, Pateron D, Trinchet J-C, Levacher S, Beaugrand M, and Pourriat J-L. Systemic antibiotic therapy prevents bacterial infection in cirrhotic patients with gastrointestinal hemorrhage. *Hepatology*, 1994; **20**: 34–8.

82. Rabinovitz M, Prieto M, Gavaler JS, and Van Thiel DH. Bacteriuria in patients with cirrhosis. *Journal of Hepatology*, 1992; **16**: 73–6.

83. Burroughs AK, Rosenstein IJ, Epstein O, Hamilton-Miller JMT, Brumfit W, and Sherlock S. Bacteriuria and primary biliary cirrhosis. *Gut*, 1984; **25**: 133–7.

84. Floreani A, Bassendine MF, Mitchison H, Freeman R, and James OFW. No specific association between primary biliary cirrhosis and bacteriuria. *Journal of Hepatology*, 1989; **8**: 201–7.

85. Butler P, Hamilton-Miller JMT, McIntyre N, and Burroughs AK. Natural history of bacteriuria in women with primary biliary cirrhosis and the effect of antimicrobial therapy in symptomatic and asymptomatic groups. *Gut*, 1995; **36**: 931–4.

86. Corredoira JM, *et al.* Gram-negative bacillary cellulitis in patients with hepatic cirrhosis. *European Journal of Clinical Microbiology and Infectious Diseases*, 1994; **13**: 19–24.

87. Snyder N, Atterbury CE, Correia JP, and Conn HO. Increased concurrence of cirrhosis and bacterial endocarditis. A clinical and postmortem study. *Gastroenterology*, 1977; **73**: 1107–13.

88. Hernandez-Denton J, Rubio C, Velazquez J, and Ramirez G. Bacterial endocarditis in cirrhosis. *Digestive Disease and Science*, 1981; **26**: 935–7.

89. McCashland TM, Sorell MF, and Zetterman RK. Bacterial endocarditis in patients with chronic liver disease. *American Journal of Gastroenterology*, 1994; **6**: 924–7.

90. Flaum MA. Spontaneous bacterial empyema in cirrhosis. *Gastroenterology*, 1976; **70**: 416–17.

91. Xiol X, *et al.* Spontaneous bacterial empyema in cirrhotic patients: a prospective study. *Hepatology*, 1996; **23**: 719–23.

92. Mummery RV, Bradley JM, and Jeffries DJ. Microbiological monitoring of patients with hepatic failure with particular reference to extracorporal porcine liver perfusion. *Lancet*, 1971; **ii**: 60–4.

93. Bailey RJ, Woolf IL, Cullens H, and Williams R. Metabolic inhibition of polymorphonuclear leucocytes in fulminant hepatic failure. *Lancet*, 1976; **i**: 1162–3.

94. Nusinovici V, Crubille C, Opolon P, Ptouboul JP, Darnis F, and Caroli J. Hepatites fulminantes avec coma. Revue de 137 cases. I. Complications. *Gastroenterologie Clinique et Biologique* 1977; **1**: 861–73.

95. Larcher VF, Wyke RJ, Mowat AL, and Williams R. Bacterial and fungal infection in children with fulminant hepatic failure: possible role of opsonization and complement deficiency. *Gut*, 1982; **23**: 1037–43.

96. Rolando N, Alexander GJM, Harvey F, Brahm J, Philpott-Howard J, and Williams R. Microbial infection: a common, covert complication of fulminant hepatic failure, denoting a poor prognosis. *Hepatology*, 1987; **7**: 1065.

97. Salmeron JM, *et al.* Selective intestinal decontamination in the prevention of bacterial infection in patients with acute liver failure. *Journal of Hepatology*, 1992; **14**: 280–5.

98. Wyke RJ, Gimson AES, Canalese J, and Williams R. Bacteraemia in patients with fulminant hepatic failure. *Liver*, 1982; **2**: 42–5.

99. Rolando N, *et al.* Fungal infection: a common, unrecognised complication of acute liver failure. *Journal of Hepatology*, 1991; **12**: 1–9.

100. Rolando N, *et al.* Prospective controlled trial of selective parenteral and enteral antimicrobial regimen in fulminant hepatic failure. *Hepatology*, 1993; **17**: 196–201.

26

Paediatric liver disease

26 Paediatric liver disease*

O. Bernard and M. Hadchouel

As many causes of liver diseases in children are discussed in other parts of this book, this chapter will deal mostly with the practical approach to children with liver disease, emphasizing diagnosis, treatment, and discussing a few entities not dealt with in detail elsewhere.

Cholestasis in children

Cholestatic diseases, presenting most often in the neonatal period, account for most admissions to hospital in units specializing in the care of children with liver diseases, and for 80 per cent of cases going on to liver transplantation.

Neonatal cholestasis

Aetiology

The neonate is especially prone to cholestasis after any kind of liver injury. Cholestasis may result from one or more factors, including immaturity of biliary excretory function, intra- or extrahepatic bile-duct injuries, metabolic abnormalities of hepatocytes, and external factors such as bacterial or viral infections or total parenteral nutrition.

The main causes of neonatal cholestasis are indicated in Table 1. It is worth noting that diseases of the extrahepatic bile ducts only account for a very small proportion of neonatal cholestasis, and, therefore, an ultrasonographic search for dilatation of the bile ducts yields limited results in this age group. Among these conditions, lithiasis of the common bile duct (Debray, JPediat, 1993; 122:385) is the least rare; it is due to pigment stones and presents either with cholestatic jaundice, sepsis, or intermittently acholic stools. Diagnosis relies on ultrasonography showing dilated bile ducts and sometimes the calculi themselves. In a fair number of cases, spontaneous resolution occurs. When jaundice persists or when signs of sepsis are present, an interventional radiological procedure will allow washing and drainage of the bile duct. Surgery is thus indicated only when interventional radiology fails. Spontaneous perforation of the bile ducts (Chardot, EurJPaediatSurg, 1996; 6: 341) usually takes place at the junction between the cystic and the common bile duct, and may be ischaemic in origin. It presents with acute biliary peritonitis or a localized biliary collection or bile-duct stenosis. Surgical treatment, extremely urgent in case of acute biliary peritonitis, is necessary in all cases.

* Much of the text describing tyrosinaemia, galactosaemia, and fructosaemia in this Section has been taken from Professor A.P. Mowat's work in the first edition: we have provided material to update it.

Diseases involving both extra- and intrahepatic bile ducts are a major part of the causes of neonatal cholestasis. Biliary atresia is described in Chapter 11.1. Sclerosing cholangitis with neonatal onset is a disease that may be of genetic origin (Amédée-Manesme, JPediat, 1987; 111:225; Baker JPediatGastrNutr, 1993; 17:317). Neonates present with cholestatic jaundice, sometimes mimicking biliary atresia, which resolves spontaneously after a few months. The disease then evolves towards biliary cirrhosis, portal hypertension, and liver failure within 5 to 10 years, and eventually requires liver transplantation (Debray, JPediat, 1994; 124:49).

Intrahepatic cholestasis

There are numerous causes of intrahepatic cholestasis in the newborn.

Infections

In neonates with antenatal infections caused by cytomegalovirus, toxoplasmosis, syphilis or rubella, cholestatic hepatitis is usually part of a multisystem disorder, including thrombocytopenia, haemolytic anaemia, and involvement of the central nervous system. Hepatitis resolves spontaneously within a few months without sequelæ except in a few cases of cytomegalovirus infection where portal hypertension develops (Ghishan, Hepatol, 1984; 4:684). Both perinatal sepsis and postnatal infection of the urinary tract by *Escherichia coli* may be associated with hepatitis and cholestatic jaundice. Liver lesions are thought to be due to the combination of the immaturity of bile secretion with the action of bacterial toxins on hepatocytes and intrahepatic bile ducts. Under appropriate antibiotic treatment, cholestasis resolves within a few days. Persisting cholestasis after the infection is cured requires investigation for another associated cause of cholestasis. As far as infections are concerned, it is worth noting (i) that perinatal viral hepatitis due to herpes simplex, echo-, adeno- or herpes hominis-6 virus does not result in cholestasis, but rather an acute hepatitis, sometimes with liver-cell failure, and (ii) that perinatal contamination with hepatitis B or C virus does not cause neonatal cholestasis.

Paucity of the interlobular bile ducts

Paucity of the interlobular bile ducts is characterized by a lack of visible interlobular ducts in more than 50 per cent of portal tracts provided there are more than 10 complete portal tracts on the biopsy sample.[1] The syndromatic type (Alagille syndrome) is described in Chapters 11.1 and 23.3. Non-syndromatic paucity of

Table 1 Main causes of neonatal cholestasis

Disorders of extrahepatic bile ducts only (5%)
Cholelithiasis
Perforation of the bile ducts
Congenital dilatation of the bile ducts (choledocal cyst)
Congenital stenosis

Disorders of extra and intrahepatic bile ducts (47%)
Biliary atresia
Sclerosing cholangitis

Disorders intrahepatic in origin (47%)
Infections (neonatal hepatitis):
   Antenatal (cytomegalovirus, toxoplasmosis, rubella, syphilis)
   Perinatal (neonatal sepsis)
   Postnatal (*E. coli* urinary-tract infection)
Paucities of interlobular bile ducts:
   Syndromatic (Alagille syndrome)
   Non-syndromatic
Genetic diseases with recessive autosomal inheritance:
   α_1-antitrypsin deficiency
   Progressive familial intrahepatic cholestasis (Byler disease)
   Cystic fibrosis
   Niemann–Pick disease type C
   Gaucher disease
   Respiratory-chain disorders*
   Peroxysomal disorders
   Defect in primary bile-acid synthesis
Benign neonatal cholestasis
Others:
   Liver angiomas
   Adrenal insufficiency
   Pituitary deficiency
   Post-haemolytic
   Parenteral nutrition-associated

Numbers in parentheses indicate the percentage of each group of causes in the experience of the Pediatric Hepatology Service of Bicêtre Hospital.
* Genetic transmission not always autosomal-recessive.

interlobular bile ducts is not a genuine entity but rather a peculiar histopathological picture that calls for a further search for an associated condition such as α_1-antitrypsin deficiency, sclerosing cholangitis, peroxisomal disorders, or extreme prematurity.

Genetic disorders

Several genetic disorders associated with neonatal cholestasis are described in Chapters 20.3 and 23.3. The two main genetic deficiencies of enzymes of primary bile-acid synthesis known so far, 3β-hydroxy-C_{27}-steroid dehydrogenase/isomerase and Δ^4–3-oxosteroid 5β-reductase, were initially described in children with neonatal cholestasis (Clayton, JCI 1987; 79:1031; Setchell, JCI, 1988; 82:2148). Diagnosis relies on analysis of the patient's urine with fast atom-bombardment mass spectrometry, which shows the abnormal metabolites. Treatment uses cholic and/or cheno-deoxycholic acid. Children with 3β-hydroxy-C_{27}-steroid dehydrogenase/isomerase deficiency may present with cholestasis later on during infancy or childhood; their disease is characterized by lack of pruritus, normal serum γ-glutamyl-transferase activity and total serum bile-acid concentration, spontaneous evolution towards cirrhosis and liver-cell failure, and remarkable efficacy of treatment with ursodeoxycholic acid and cholic acid.[2] Δ^4–3-oxosteroid 5β-reductase deficiency has also been described in association with severe neonatal liver failure (Shneider, JPediat, 1994; 124:234).

Progressive familial intrahepatic cholestasis of childhood was first described in the Byler family and usually bears the name Byler's disease.[3] It is characterized clinically by chronic, sometimes relapsing, cholestasis, often presenting in the neonatal period. There is early pruritus, low or normal serum cholesterol, raised serum bile acids, morphologically normal extra- and intrahepatic bile ducts on cholangiography, presence of interlobular bile ducts in portal tracts, although they are sometimes small and may be difficult to see, and lobular fibrosis of various extent. Spontaneous evolution is always lethal, with progression of fibrosis and liver failure. It is actually a heterogeneous group with at least two separate entities, as follows.

(1) The first type of progressive familial intrahepatic cholestasis is characterized by persistently normal serum γ-glutamyl trans-peptidase activity and by an earlier onset, often during the neonatal period (Maggiore, JPediat, 1987; 111:251; Maggiore, JPediat-GastrNutr, 1991; 12:21; Whitington, JPediatGastrNutr, 1994; 18:124). It leads to death with liver failure within a few years, rarely after adolescence, and with little or no endoscopic signs of portal hypertension. This disease may be due to a defect in bile-acid secretion into bile (Tazawa, JPediatGastrNutr, 1985; 4:32; Jacquemin, EurJPed, 1994; 153:424). In the original Byler family, the disease may be genetically linked to a locus on chromosome 18 that is also associated with benign recurrent intrahepatic cholestasis (Carlton, HumMolGenet, 1995; 4:1049). Forty per cent of patients benefit from ursodeoxycholic therapy (Jacquemin, Hepatol, 1997;

25:519). Some children improve considerably after surgical partial external biliary diversion (Whitington, Gastro, 1988; 95:130). In other patients both treatments fail and liver transplantation is necessary (Soubrane, Transpl, 1990; 95:130). In a subgroup of patients, cholestasis is associated with renal tubular defect, refractory diarrhoea, and/or arthrogryposis (De Rocco, EurJPed, 1995; 154:835).

(2) The second type of progressive familial intrahepatic cholestasis is characterized by raised serum γ-glutamyl transpeptidase activity and presents later in childhood, more often displays portal fibrosis and ductular proliferation on liver biopsy, carries a higher risk of portal hypertension and gastrointestinal bleeding, and ends in liver failure at a later age than type I. An abnormal expression of the multidrug resistance 3 (*MDR3*) gene and a low biliary phospholipid concentration have been found in two such patients suggesting that, as in the *mdr-/-* mice, lack of micellar formation in bile, due to insufficient phospholipid secretion by the hepatocyte, could result in canalicular and ductular damage (Deleuze, Hepatol, 1996; 23:904). Ursodeoxycholic acid therapy is effective in about 40 per cent of these children but liver transplantation is necessary in the others. In a possible subgroup of children with type II progressive intrahepatic cholestasis, liver disease is associated with kidney disease of the nephronophthisis type (Witzleben, HumPath, 1982; 13: 728).

Benign neonatal cholestasis

In many cases, the cause of neonatal cholestasis cannot be identified, but the outcome is spontaneously good within a few months. These cases, formerly called 'neonatal hepatitis' of favourable outcome, are commonly but not exclusively seen in neonatal intensive-care units. Cholestasis is thought to result from the association of several factors, including prematurity resulting in increased immaturity of bile secretion, bacterial infection, ante- or perinatal trauma or shock (resulting in hepatic ischaemia because of the elective distribution of umbilical flow towards the brain through the ductus venosus under these circumstances), perinatal hepatic anoxia and/or ischaemia due to pulmonary disease and/or sepsis, and total parenteral nutrition, often required because of necrotizing enterocolitis, which further reduces the bile flow (Wolf, JPediatGastrNutr, 1989; 8:297; Jacquemin, EurJPaediatSurg, 1995; 5:259). In such cases there may be a low prothrombin time and defective coagulation factors during the first days of life, soon followed by cholestatic jaundice. Serum γ-glutamyl transpeptidase activity may initially be low for age but it usually increases during the second or third months. Liver histology displays non-specific signs such as giant-cell transformation, haemopoiesis, sometimes steatosis, and no or little fibrosis. Provided the associated conditions are cured, the outcome is good, but careful follow-up is needed to check for complete normalization of all clinical, biochemical, and ultrasonographic signs at age 1 year, as a few cases of familial progressive intrahepatic cholestasis may present initially in a very similar fashion.

Cholestasis may also be present in a few neonates with multinodular or solitary liver angiomas, or with adrenal or pituitary insufficiency, or after severe neonatal haemolytic disease. In such cases, cholestasis resolves spontaneously within a few months with no sequelae.

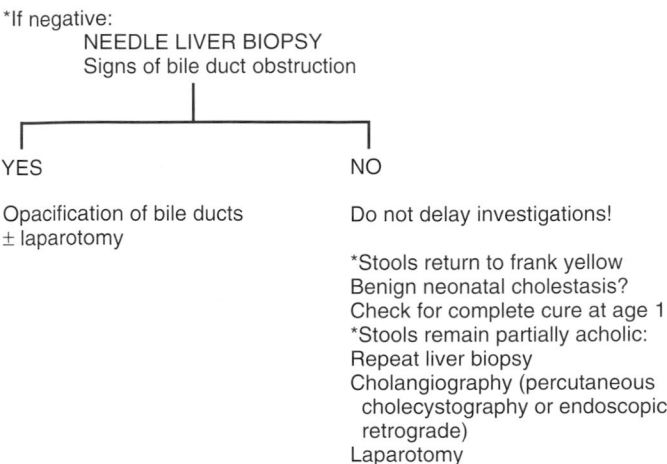

- Consider cholestasis in all jaundiced neonates after day 15
- Record clinical and biochemical signs of cholestasis
- Suspect biliary atresia from the outset

I. Permanently and completely acholic stools:
   BILIARY ATRESIA VERY LIKELY
(differential diagnosis: Alagille syndrome, α₁-antitrypsin deficiency cystic fibrosis, sclerosing cholangitis)
   LAPAROTOMY

II. Partially or temporarily acholic stools:
*Within 3 days   Ultrasound: dilation of bile ducts? Search for each intrahepatic cause by appropriate means

*If negative:
   NEEDLE LIVER BIOPSY
   Signs of bile duct obstruction

YES — Opacification of bile ducts ± laparotomy

NO — Do not delay investigations!

*Stools return to frank yellow
Benign neonatal cholestasis?
Check for complete cure at age 1
*Stools remain partially acholic:
Repeat liver biopsy
Cholangiography (percutaneous cholecystography or endoscopic retrograde)
Laparotomy

Fig. 1. A schematic approach to the aetiology of neonatal cholestasis.

Management
Primary objectives

The main objective of the management of a child with neonatal cholestasis is urgent identification of the cause (Fig. 1). This is of paramount importance because the prognosis of biliary atresia depends on the age at which corrective surgery is performed.[4]

The incidence of neonatal cholestasis is thought to be 1 in 2000 live births.[5] Presenting features are those of cholestatic jaundice in virtually all cases; in a few cases, haemorrhage due to vitamin K deficiency, acholic stools, sepsis, or the prenatal ultrasonographic finding of a cyst below the liver may be the initial features. The possibility of cholestasis must be considered in all jaundiced neonates after the age of 15 days. Diagnosis of cholestasis relies on the presence of pale or acholic stools, stained diapers (nappies), liver enlargement, presence of bilirubin or biliary salts (Matsui, JPediat, 1996; 129:306) in urine, and a raised serum conjugated bilirubin. All neonates with cholestasis must be investigated urgently, preferably in a hospital, and should immediately receive an injection of vitamin K to prevent the risk of haemorrhage. Within a few days, simple clinical findings and a few biochemical, ophthalmological, and radiological tests will allow identification of the cause in most cases. The main clinical points are a careful examination of the colour of each stool over a few days and an evaluation of the enlargement and consistency of the liver.[6] The significance of the stool discoloration is such that it should be examined under strict conditions: feeding the baby with mother's milk or normal formula, avoiding drugs that may alter the stool's colour, and, in case of doubt, studying the stool obtained by rectal examination to avoid contamination with stained urine.

Completely and permanently acholic stools lasting for more than 7 days strongly suggest biliary atresia; only the severe forms of Alagille syndrome, α_1-antitrypsin deficiency, cystic fibrosis, and sclerosing cholangitis may, in rare instances, result in prolonged acholic stools mimicking biliary atresia. Enlargement and firm consistency of the liver is also usually associated with biliary atresia. Thus the combination of permanently acholic stools with firm and hard hepatomegaly, and lack of signs in favour of one of the intrahepatic disorders just mentioned, should lead rapidly to laparotomy, best done before the age of 45 days by an experienced surgeon (McClement, BMJ, 1985; 290:345). If biliary atresia is confirmed, hepatic portoenterostomy or portocholecystostomy should be performed.

When the discoloration of the stools is not complete or permanent, a rapid search for the main extra- or intrahepatic causes of cholestasis should be made, with specific tests including abdominal ultrasonography. A few words of caution should be said about the interpretation of these tests. (1) Hepatobiliary scintigraphy is widely used (Spivak, JPediat, 1987; 110:855) but, in our experience, will not provide more accurate information than a careful examination of the colour of the stools. (2) Abdominal ultrasonography is more often misleading than useful: the number of cases with an obstruction restricted to the extrahepatic biliary tree and associated dilation of the bile ducts is very small at this age; the normal common bile duct is usually not visible ultrasonographically at this age, even less so when cholestasis limits the amount of bile in the bile ducts; a patent gallbladder may be present in biliary atresia when atresia is restricted to the hepatic ducts; conversely, a small gallbladder can be seen by ultrasonography when intrahepatic cholestasis is severe. Ultrasonography is therefore useful only in the rare cases of dilation of bile ducts, of liver angiomas, or when it shows cystic dilation or features of the polysplenia syndrome sometimes associated with biliary atresia. (3) The value of screening for cytomegalovirus infection is limited to cases when specific anticytomegalovirus IgM or viruria are found in the first week of life. In most cases when tests are positive for cytomegalovirus later on, they cannot be taken as proof of the role of the virus as the cause of cholestasis. Moreover, a true biliary atresia may be associated with antenatal infection with cytomegalovirus as well as other organisms.

If, after a few days of intensive investigation, the cause of cholestasis is not found, needle liver biopsy should be performed. If signs of bile-duct obstruction are present, such as bile-duct proliferation, portal fibrosis, and bile plugs in the bile ducts, cholangiography should be carried out, either operatively, or with percutaneous transhepatic cholecystography or endoscopic retrograde cholangiography. Biliary atresia or sclerosing cholangitis will be found in most of such cases.

If liver biopsy examination does not show signs of bile-duct obstruction and the cause is not found, investigation must go on and the child must be carefully followed, with two possible outcomes. (1) Complete normalization of stool colour within 1 or 2 weeks: a tentative diagnosis of benign neonatal cholestasis can then be made but the child must be followed until age 1 year to confirm that all indices of liver disease return to normal. (2) Persistence of partially acholic stools: in this case, biliary atresia cannot be excluded, so liver biopsy should be repeated and opacification of the bile ducts attempted, with eventual laparotomy in case of doubt.

Other aspects of management

The precise and early identification of the cause of neonatal cholestasis is essential for several reasons, as follows.

(1) In some cases there may be a specific treatment to be given—above all, early corrective surgery for biliary atresia—but also antibiotic therapy for a few ante- or postnatal infections, interventional radiology for lithiasis, surgery for choledochal cysts, steroid therapy for adrenal insufficiency, bile acids for deficiency of primary bile-acid synthesis, and ursodeoxycholic acid or biliary diversion for children with progressive familial intrahepatic cholestasis.

(2) Careful nutritional management is mandatory, especially when the disease is known to lead to long-lasting cholestasis. A hypercaloric diet is provided by supplementary feeding with dextrin–maltose and medium-chain triglycerides. In a few patients, mostly those with biliary atresia and Alagille syndrome with persisting jaundice, oral feeding is not sufficient and continuous enteral nocturnal feeding via a nasogastric tube may be necessary. In extreme cases, especially children with biliary atresia and early decompensation, parenteral nutrition is necessary to allow sufficient growth until the time of transplantation. In addition, as long as jaundice persists, supplementary lipid-soluble vitamins must be given with regular checking of their blood concentrations. One of the schedules that has been shown to prevent the consequences of lipid-soluble vitamin deficiency in these children (Alagille, SemLivDis, 1985; 5:254) consists of regular intramuscular injections as follows: cholecalciferol, 5 mg every 3 months, vitamin K_1, 10 mg/kg every 15 days, vitamin E, 10 mg/kg (never more than 200 mg) every 15 days, vitamin A, 50 000 IU every month. Alternative regimens use daily oral 25-hydroxycholecalciferol (Heubi, PediatRes, 1989; 27:26), oral vitamin K (Amédée-Manesme, JPediatGastrNutr, 1992; 14:160), and oral vitamin E (Sokol, JPediat, 1987, 111:830).

(3) Early identification and management of children who will eventually require liver transplantation is necessary. This is particularly important in children who may require liver transplantation before the age of 2 years, such as a few with biliary atresia, α_1-antitrypsin deficiency or progressive familial intrahepatic cholestasis. Conversely, it is essential to identify properly those diseases in which liver transplantation is contraindicated, such as Niemann–Pick disease type C or peroxisomal disorders, or those, such as cystic fibrosis or respiratory-chain disorders, for which transplantation should be undertaken only with caution.

(4) Finally, the parents should be provided with genetic information and the possibility of antenatal diagnosis should be offered when it is available.

Cholestasis in older children

Table 2 indicates the main causes of cholestasis in older children. Presenting symptoms are very variable and include, in isolation or associated, one or several of the following: jaundice, acholic stools, pruritus, abdominal pain, signs of malnutrition with deficiency of lipid-soluble vitamins, and the fortuitous finding of liver enlargement, of abnormal liver function tests or of abnormal ultrasonographic features. The approach to aetiological diagnosis,

Table 2 Aetiology of cholestasis after the neonatal period

Disorders of extrahepatic bile ducts
Congenital dilatation of the bile ducts (choledocal cyst)
Biliary stenosis
Cholelithiasis
Cancer (botryoid sarcoma, hepatoblastoma, neuroblastoma, lymphoma)
Blunt trauma
Pancreatitis
Retroperitoneal fibrosis

Disorders of intra- and extrahepatic bile ducts
Sclerosing cholangitis:
   Autoimmune
   Langerhans-cell histiocytosis
   Immune deficiencies (congenital or acquired)
   No identified cause

Disorders intrahepatic in origin
Syndromatic paucity of interlobular bile ducts (Alagille syndrome)
α_1-Antitrypsin deficiency
Cystic fibrosis
Autoimmune cholangitis of the small bile ducts
Kawasaki disease
Drug toxicity
Progressive familial intrahepatic cholestasis:
   with normal serum γGT activity
   with raised serum γGT activity
   with raised serum γGT activity and tubulointerstitial nephropathy/nephronophtisis
Prolonged hepatitis A
Benign recurrent intrahepatic cholestasis
3β-Hydroxy-C_{27}-steroid dehydrogenase/isomerase deficiency

γGT, γ-glutamyl transferase.

summarized in Fig. 2, relies initially on ultrasonography to look for dilated bile ducts and, if the bile ducts are not dilated, on serum γ-glutamyl transpeptidase activity. Indeed, in children, raised serum γ-glutamyl transpeptidase activity is a fairly reliable index of damage to bile-duct epithelium (Maggiore, JPediatGastrNutr, 1991; 12:21). Normal serum γ-glutamyl transpeptidase activity in a child with signs of cholestasis points to a hepatocytic disorder; absence of pruritus then suggests 3β-hydroxysteroid dehydrogenase/isomerase deficiency. Within the group of children with intrahepatic cholestasis and raised serum γ-glutamyl transpeptidase activity, a few causes will be found easily by non-invasive means (Alagille syndrome, α_1-antitrypsin deficiency, cystic fibrosis, drug toxicity, cholestasis associated with nephronophthisis or total parenteral nutrition). In the remaining cases, liver biopsy is necessary and will show, in most instances, portal fibrosis and ductular proliferation. Cholangiography (either percutaneous transhepatic cholecystography or endoscopic retrograde cholangiography) will identify sclerosing cholangitis, and if the bile ducts look normal, point to either autoimmune cholangitis with damage to the small bile ducts only, or to progressive familial intrahepatic cholestasis with raised serum γ-glutamyl transpeptidase activity, with a possible defect in *MDR3* gene expression. Further management will depend on the cause found.

Unconjugated hyperbilirubinaemia in infancy

Unconjugated hyperbilirubinaemia is rarely due to a disease involving the liver alone, except for the rare inherited disorders of bilirubin metabolism (see Chapter 20.6).[7,8]

The two main objectives of the management of an infant presenting with unconjugated hyperbilirubinaemia are to avoid the major complication of kernicterus, and to identify the cause. Physiological jaundice is a diagnosis of exclusion and jaundice is not 'physiological' if at the end of the first day the serum bilirubin is greater than 85 mmol/l, at the end of the second day greater than 170 mmol/l, or if it is more than 220 mmol/l at any time. An alternative cause should also be considered if the jaundice begins within 24 h of birth, if there is a conjugated bilirubin of more than 20 mmol/l, or if jaundice persists beyond 2 weeks.

The main causes are summarized in Table 3. The most frequent are related to increased bilirubin production and mainly to ABO incompatibility in view of the current prevention of Rh immunization. Erythrocyte enzyme defects and spherocytosis may present as neonatal jaundice; typical haematological findings may be absent in the neonatal period and must be sought later in life if the cause of the jaundice has not been identified. Prolonged elevation of indirect bilirubin was reported as the first clinical sign in some infants with hypothyroidism. Breast milk-related jaundice appears slowly, reaching a peak at about the second week. The interruption of breast-feeding for 24 to 72 h results in a fall in bilirubin, thus confirming the diagnosis. Kernicterus has never been observed. Resumption of breast-feeding may be allowed, and the bilirubin then usually rises only slightly and gradually falls to normal.

In the absence of the common causes of unconjugated hyperbilirubinaemia, the diagnosis of Crigler–Najjar syndrome must be considered. There is no widely available, simple clinical test to confirm the diagnosis, and during the period of testing the height and duration of serum bilirubin elevation may have led to the

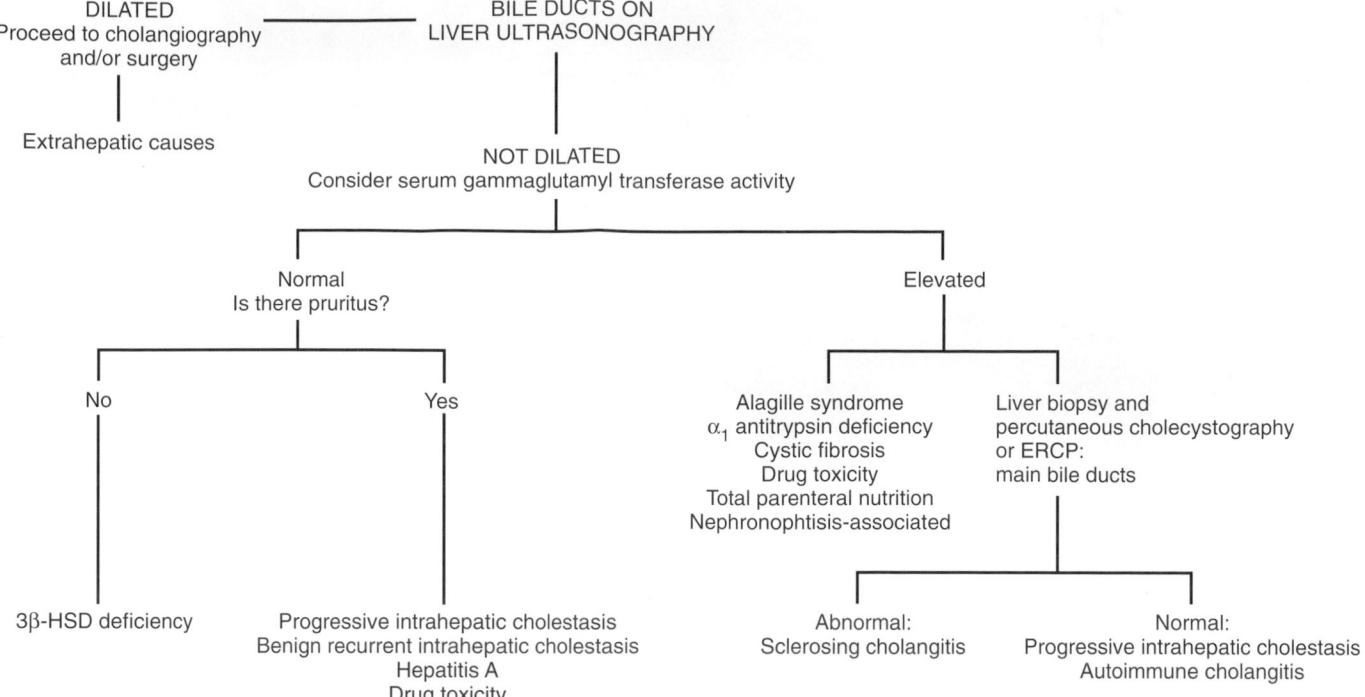

Fig. 2. A schematic approach to the aetiology of cholestasis in older children.

Table 3 Main causes of unconjugated hyperbilirubinaemia in infancy
Increased bilirubin production
Immune haemolytic disease:
Rh incompatibility
ABO incompatibility
Other (Lewis, Duffy, etc.)
Inherited haemolytic anaemia:
Spherocytosis
Elliptocytosis
Glucose 6-phosphate dehydrogenase deficiency
Pyruvate kinase deficiency
Infection
Enclosed haematoma
Diabetic mother
Fetal transfusion
Drugs
Decreased bilirubin uptake, storage or metabolism
Hypothyroidism or hypopituitarism
Congestive heart failure
Hypoxia
Infection
Drugs
Crigler–Najjar syndrome
Gilbert's syndrome
Enterohepatic recirculation
Breast-milk jaundice
Intestinal obstruction
Antibiotics

Adapted from ref. 8.

institution of phototherapy and/or exchange transfusion. A pheno-barbital test can differentiate Crigler–Najjar type 1 from type 2;

serum bilirubin decreases by at least 30 per cent after 5 days of treatment in type 2 and there is no response in type 1. Needle liver biopsy is required to measure bilirubin glycuronyltransferase activity since direct molecular diagnosis is hampered by the number of DNA mutations observed. The second goal is to prevent neuro-toxicity. Phototherapy and, when necessary, exchange transfusion remain the basis of therapy. Phototherapy must be pursued for a few years until liver transplantation is performed (Van der Veere, Hepatol, 1996; 24:311).

Liver-cell failure in infants

Acute liver-cell failure in neonates and infants is of special interest because of the variety of causes, many cases being due to genetic diseases, and because of the availability of specific treatment in some cases. Here, as in many areas of paediatric liver disease, the availability of liver transplantation has considerably altered the management.

Aetiology

The main causes of acute liver failure in neonates and infants are indicated in Table 4. Some of these diseases are described elsewhere in this book. Some others are briefly described here.

Neonatal haemochromatosis

So-called neonatal haemochromatosis is a severe liver disease of intrauterine onset characterized by parenchymal iron deposition in the liver, destruction of normal hepatic architecture, extrahepatic siderosis, and relative sparing of the reticuloendothelial system. This disorder is not a variant of HLA-linked haemochromatosis.

Table 4 Main causes of acute liver-cell failure in infancy

Metabolic disorders
Galactosaemia
Hereditary fructose intolerance
Hereditary tyrosinaemia
Ornithine carbamoyl transferase deficiency
Δ^4-3-Oxosteroid-reductase deficiency
Fatty acids oxidation disorders

Infections
Sepsis with shock
Extreme hyperthermia
Herpes simplex hepatitis
Hepatitis B
Hepatitis C*
Hepatitis A
Other viruses (adeno, echo, HHV6, EBV, coxsackie, etc.)

Drug toxicity
Na valproate**
Acetylsalicylic acid
Acetaminophen
Isoniazide

Vascular diseases
Left ventricular hypoplasia
Perinatal ischaemia/anoxia
Veno-occlusive disease
Budd–Chiari syndrome
Acute peliosis
Shock

Autoimmune hepatitis
Giant-cell hepatitis with autoimmune haemolytic anaemia
LKM$_1$ antibody-positive hepatitis

Malignancies
Familial lymphohistiocytosis
Acute leukaemia

Miscellaneous
Reye syndrome
Perinatal haemochromatosis

HHV, herpes hominis virus; EBV, Epstein–Barr virus; LKM, liver/kidney microsomal.
* Only one case reported so far; ** probably toxic in selected cases only.

The first cases were probably described in 1957 (Cottier, SchMedWoch, 1957; 37:39). In spite of several studies of iron metabolism in the infants and their mothers, there are no specific biochemical criteria and the diagnosis is one of exclusion. Studies of the few patients who have recovered do not show any evidence for abnormal iron metabolism later in life. Knisely, who has written extensively on this condition and has provided the definition and criteria for diagnosis, mentioned in his recent review that 'scepticism appears indicated when evaluating claims that iron storage peculiarly characterises specific kinds of neonatal liver disease'.[9]

The criteria for diagnosis of neonatal haemochromatosis are : (i) a rapidly progressive clinical course with death *in utero* or in the early neonatal period; (ii) increased tissue iron deposition in multiple sites especially the liver, pancreas, heart and endocrine glands, the reticuloendothelial system being relatively unaffected; (iii) no evidence of haemolytic disease, syndromes associated with haemosiderosis, or exogenous iron from transfusions (Knisely, AdvPediat, 1992; 39:383).

The presenting signs are those of liver failure, and most patients are either premature or small for gestational age. There is no specific biochemical finding and the diagnosis is most often made at autopsy. Indeed, concentrations of iron, transferrin saturation (78 per cent), ferritin in serum and stored iron in the liver are high enough even in the normal new-born infant to be misleading indicators, and the specific defect has not yet been identified (Knisely, AmJClinPath, 1989; 92:755). Liver biopsy is usually not performed because of severe coagulopathy, and it has been shown that iron deposition may be present in all infants with liver disease of prenatal onset (Silver, AmJPathol, 1993; 143:1312). Demonstration of iron deposits in salivary glands has been used as a diagnostic criterion (Knisely, JPediat, 1988; 113:871) and magnetic resonance imaging has been proposed as a non-invasive means of detecting iron *in utero* (Marti-Bonmati, AbdImag, 1994; 19:55). As mentioned above, neonatal haemochromatosis is a diagnosis of exclusion since iron overload has been described in inherited metabolic diseases such as Zellweger syndrome, tyrosinaemia, Δ^4–3-oxosteroid-5β-reductase deficiency, and in acquired infections such as cytomegalovirus (Kershisnik, HumPath, 1992; 23:1075), echovirus 9 (Bove, PediatPath, 1991; 11:389) or non-A, non-B hepatitis (Hoogstraten, Gastro, 1992; 98:1699). Considering that even if iron is not the primary cause of the disease it may be noxious for the liver, treatment with desferrioxamine associated with antioxidant therapy (vitamin E, selenium, *N*-acetyl-cysteine) may be beneficial (Shamieh, PediatRes, 1993; 33:109A; Jonas, JPediatGastrNutr, 1987; 6:984). Liver transplantation has been successful in a few cases (Rand, JPediatGastrNutr, 1992; 15:325; Lund, TransplProc, 1993; 25: 1068).

Genetic counselling remains very difficult, essentially because it cannot be stated whether neonatal haemochromatosis is one disease, several diseases or a spectrum (Witzleben, HumPath, 1989; 20:335; Collins, Hepatol, 1990; 12:176). Nevertheless, all children in a family may be affected. A recessive mode of inheritance has been suggested but seems unlikely because of the lack of parental consanguinity and also because two mothers are known who had infants with neonatal haemochromatosis by different men. So families may be informed that there is a risk for recurrence of the disease, that there is no relation to adult-onset haemochromatosis, that the genetic origin of the disease is not clear, and that we lack established methods for antenatal diagnosis (Ferrell, AmJMedGen, 1992; 44: 429).

Mitochondrial respiratory-chain disorders

Liver involvement in mitochondrial respiratory-chain disorders may present as mild liver disease manifested by raised serum aminotransferase activities and steatosis or neonatal cholestasis, but most often presents as liver-cell failure either in the neonatal period and/or later on during the first two years of life.[10] Often, but not always, signs of involvement of other organs, most notably the central nervous system, sensory organs or muscle, are associated and may be an early clue to the diagnosis. Further clues are provided by raised blood fasting and postprandial lactate:pyruvate ratios, presence of lactaturia and paradoxical hyperketonaemia after a glucose loading test (Munnich, EurJPed, 1996; 155:262). However, in about 20 per cent of cases of respiratory-chain disorders with liver involvement, these signs of abnormal redox status are absent. Definitive diagnosis is provided by the enzymatic study of the mitochondrial respiratory chain on liver homogenates; surgical liver biopsy is often necessary because of the low values of coagulation factors. Electron microscopy of the liver may show abnormal mitochondria, sometimes corresponding to the oncocytic appearance of hepatocytes by light microscopy; in other cases, liver histology shows non-specific changes such as steatosis and portal fibrosis. The spontaneous outcome is lethal within a few months in the cases reported so far. A remission may be observed after an initial phase of liver failure in the neonatal period, followed by a relapse after a few months. There is no satisfactory medical treatment. Dietary recommendations are a rather high-lipid and low-carbohydrate diet. Liver transplantation must be considered with the most extreme caution. It is not indicated when extrahepatic involvement is present. When the disease is apparently restricted to the liver an extensive check-up to look for possible involvement of other organs must be carried out, and should include: muscle histology, histochemistry and enzymatic study, assay for lactate:pyruvate ratio and protein in the cerebrospinal fluid, magnetic resonance imaging of the brain, bone marrow examination, sensory tests of ear and eye, echocardiography, and functional studies of the kidney tubule. When no apparent extrahepatic involvement is detected, liver transplantation may be performed successfully (Goncalves, JHepatol, 1995; 23:290), but careful follow-up is necessary because of the possible occurrence of signs of extrahepatic involvement late after transplantation. Because all modes of inheritance can be observed, genetic counselling is difficult; a secure prenatal diagnosis is currently only feasible by enzymatic study of cultured amniocytes when the enzyme deficiency is expressed in cultured skin fibroblasts from the patient (Munnich, EurJPed, 1996; 155:262).

Reye syndrome

More often seen in older children than in infants, Reye syndrome (Reye, Lancet 1963; ii: 749; Mowat, AdvDrugReactAcPoisRev, 1987; 4:211; Hardie, ArchDisChild, 1996; 74:400) is characterized clinically by a prodromic period suggesting mild viral infection, soon followed by vomiting and neurological involvement with coma with or without seizures, hepatomegaly, raised aminotransferase, prolonged prothrombin time, raised blood ammonia, and hypoglycaemia. Liver histology typically shows microvacuolar steatosis. The outcome of Reye syndrome is variable: it may proceed to brain death in a few hours or days and the mortality rate may be as high as 40 per cent; complete recovery is possible as well as neurological sequelae. Treatment in the acute phase is symptomatic and requires intensive care in specialized units, mostly directed at controlling intracranial pressure. There is no indication for liver transplantation. The precise mechanism is unknown; it may correspond to an acute and transient defect in mitochondrial function following viral (influenza, varicella) infection, drug intake (acetylsalicylic acid, sodium valproate) but clinical pictures resembling Reye syndrome have been described in inherited disorders such as deficiencies in fatty acid oxidation, carnitine deficiency, urea-cycle disorders, and organic acidurias. Thus, especially in infants, careful investigation to detect such disorders, both during the acute phase and after recovery, is necessary in all cases because they may relapse, may benefit from specific dietary treatment, and may require genetic counselling.

Investigation and management

Presenting features of acute liver-cell failure in infants are varied and include, singly or in association: jaundice, vomiting, sleepiness, changes in mood, convulsions, signs of hypoglycaemia, bleeding tendency, sepsis, ascites. Coagulation studies show a prolonged prothrombin time, low factors II and VII + X (below 30 per cent) and low factor V (below 50 per cent): the degree of diminution of factor V is of prognostic value, although it may be extremely low because of associated disseminated intravascular coagulation.

Investigations in search of the cause of liver failure are urgent and include the following. (1) Interview with the parents: looking for the country of origin, possible consanguinity, similar cases in sibship, distaste for sugar in parents or for protein in the mother, known viral hepatitis in the family, type of feeding, possible psychomotor retardation, and drug intake in the days before. (2) Clinical examination: jaundice is virtually always present in viral hepatitis but may be absent, even when signs of liver failure are apparently severe, in some metabolic diseases such as hereditary tyrosinaemia, or in Reye syndrome. Significant liver enlargement, early ascites and oedema suggest a metabolic or vascular cause. Signs of rickets are in favour of hereditary tyrosinaemia. Signs of extrahepatic involvement, neurological, sensory or muscular in particular, should point to a respiratory-chain disorder. (3) A few non-specific tests may be helpful. Serum aminotransferase activities are always high in viral hepatitis but may be only moderately raised or even normal in hereditary tyrosinaemia. Signs of renal tubular dysfunction suggest metabolic diseases. Very high blood ammonia concentrations should point to Reye syndrome or ornithine carbamoyl transferase deficiency. Very high serum α-fetoprotein suggests hereditary tyrosinaemia but is also seen in respiratory-chain disorders. Autoimmune haemolytic anaemia suggests autoimmune hepatitis with giant-cell transformation. Raised serum tyrosine, methionine and phenylalanine may be seen in all types of liver failure. (4) Specific tests (Table 5) allow identification of the cause and must be performed urgently; the choice of these tests should be dictated by the clinical findings and the results of non-specific biochemical tests.

An infant with acute liver failure must be admitted to hospital rapidly, having been started on a 10 per cent dextrose infusion to prevent hypoglycaemia, preferably to a specialized paediatric unit where there are hepatologists, intensive-care experts, and transplant surgeons. Regardless of the cause, a few therapeutic measures are necessary:

(1) intensive monitoring, vascular lines, prevention of hypoglycaemia, of gastrointestinal bleeding, of cerebral oedema;
(2) detection and treatment of bacterial infections;
(3) a normocaloric low-protein diet orally, or continuous enteral feeding with systematic exclusion of galactose and fructose until a precise diagnosis is made;
(4) specific treatment or diet is available for galactosaemia, hereditary fructose intolerance, ornithine carbamoyl transferase deficiency, a few metabolic Reye-like diseases, autoimmune hepatitis, herpes simplex hepatitis, paracetamol overdose, and hereditary tyrosinaemia; liver transplantation must be considered in viral or toxic hepatitis.

A careful aetiological check-up is necessary in all cases, not only for adequate treatment of the sick child, but also to decide upon the practical approach for other family members, present or future, such as vaccinations against hepatitis B or A, and antenatal diagnosis, which is available for most inborn metabolic diseases.

Table 5 Specific aetiological tests in infants with acute liver failure

Galactotransferase assay (heparinized whole blood or blood dried on filter paper; before any transfusion)
Mutations of the fructose 1-phosphate aldolase gene
Intravenous fructose-tolerance test (after a few weeks of diet; only if molecular screening is negative)
Urinary succinyl acetone
Urinary orotic acid
Chromatography of urinary organic acids
Fasting and postprandial blood lactate, pyruvate, β-hydroxybutyrate and acetoacetate
IgM antihepatitis A virus
HBs antigen, anti-HBs antibody, anti-HBc antibody (in child and mother)
Hepatitis C antibody, PCR for HCV RNA in blood (in child and mother)
Other virological studies
Non-organic-specific antibodies including LKM$_1$ antibody
Direct Coombs' test
Bone marrow examination
Search for toxins in urine and blood
Liver ultrasound
Echocardiography
Liver histology
Enzymatic studies on liver biopsy

HBs, hepatitis B surface antigen; HBc, hepatitis B core antigen; HCV, hepatitis C virus; LKM, liver/kidney microsomal; PCR, polymerase chain reaction.

When the child dies before a precise diagnosis is made, it is extremely important to store frozen urine, plasma and cerebrospinal fluid, to take a piece of liver in the immediate post mortem period for histopathological examination, transmission electron microscopy, enzymatic and genetic studies (on liver frozen in liquid nitrogen), and to take a skin biopsy for fibroblasts culture. Autopsy is necessary for the diagnosis of neonatal haemochromatosis.

Portal hypertension
Aetiology

The main causes of portal hypertension in children are indicated in Table 6. Portal vein obstruction, congenital hepatic fibrosis, and biliary cirrhoses are the most frequently encountered.

Portal vein obstruction

Obstruction of the portal vein (Alvarez, JPediat, 1983; 103:699) may be due to catheterization of the umbilical vein, omphalitis, intrahepatic or extrahepatic abdominal bacterial infections, or may be secondary to abdominal surgery. In most cases, however, the mechanism is unknown. Obstruction of the division of the portal trunk is present in virtually all cases, of the portal trunk itself in 90 per cent of cases, of the superior mesenteric vein in 13 per cent, and of the splenic vein in 7 per cent, resulting, in the last, in complete obstruction of the portal system. In 50 per cent of cases the obstruction extends into the intrahepatic branches of the portal vein. A 'cavernoma' is made up of the dilated pancreaticoduodenal and peribiliary veins by-passing the obstructed portal vein. The consequences of the obstruction are twofold. First and most importantly there is a high risk of gastrointestinal bleeding due to oesophageal or gastric varices. Secondly, the compression of the bile ducts by the cavernoma may result in chronic cholestasis.

Presenting symptoms, in almost all cases, are either the fortuitous finding of splenomegaly, or the onset of gastrointestinal bleeding; ascites may be present in infants or after a bleeding episode. Clinical examination shows splenomegaly; liver function tests are typically normal, except when post-transfusion hepatitis or cholestasis is present. A blood-cell count displays varying degrees of hypersplenism, often thrombocytopenia, rarely leucopenia. Co-agulation studies may show abnormal amounts of protein C, protein S, proaccelerin, and fibrinogen that are more consistent with activated coagulation than with liver failure (Alvarez, JPediat, 1983; 103:699; Dubuisson, JHepatol, 1997; 27:132).

Diagnosis relies on ultrasonography of the portal vein, and prognosis on the pattern of varices on upper gastrointestinal endoscopy. Gastrointestinal bleeding is frequent (80 per cent of children bleed before the age of 16), sometimes after acetylsalicylic acid intake or during a febrile episode; it occurs early (more than 50 per cent of children have bled once by the age of 4, but some will start bleeding at or after adolescence) and tends to recur (a mean number of five bleeding episodes) (Mitra, JPediatSurg, 1978; 13: 51); each bleeding episode may be life-threatening.

Cholestasis secondary to compression of the bile ducts may present with jaundice, but more commonly with raised serum aminotransferase and/or γ-glutamyl transpeptidase activities; colour duplex ultrasonography will show the dilated bile ducts; endoscopic retrograde cholangiography or percutaneous transhepatic cholangiography may confirm the abnormalities (Sultan Khuroo, Hepatol, 1993; 17:807).

Treatment is aimed at preventing relapses of gastrointestinal bleeding and is indicated after a first spontaneous episode of bleeding provided that no cause of bleeding other than the varices can be found. Two modes of treatment are available. (1) Surgical portosystemic shunts can be constructed safely, even in very young children, provided the surgeon has the necessary experience and that angiography of the portal system and inferior vena cava shows veins that can be used (Alvarez, JPediat, 1983; 103:703); jugular vein interpositions between the superior mesenteric vein or the splenic vein and the inferior vena cava or left renal vein, respectively, are commonly used. The advantage of the portosystemic shunt is that, once proved patent, it eliminates permanently the risk of bleeding and cures or prevents the cholestasis associated with

Table 6 Causes of portal hypertension in children

Arterioportal fistula
Splenic vein thrombosis
PORTAL VEIN OBSTRUCTION
Congenital hepatic fibrosis
Schistosomiasis
Idiopathic portal hypertension (a few familial cases)/hepatoportal sclerosis/nodular regenerative hyperplasia
CIRRHOSES
   BILIARY:
      Biliary atresia
      Cystic fibrosis
      α_1-*antitrypsin deficiency*
      Sclerosing cholangitis
      Progressive familial intrahepatic cholestasis with raised γGT
      Alagille syndrome
      Choledochal cysts
      Progressive familial intrahepatic cholestasis with normal γGT
      Deficiency in primary bile-acid synthesis
   Metabolic:
      Wilson disease
      Hereditary tyrosinaemia
      Respiratory-chain disorders
      Type IV glycogen-storage disease
      Cholesterol ester-storage disease
      Gaucher and Niemann–Pick diseases
      Type III glycogen-storage disease
   Chronic hepatitis:
      Autoimmune
      Viral hepatitis B, C, D
   Suprahepatic
      Veno-occlusive disease
      Budd–Chiari syndrome
      Cardiac abnormalities (mostly chronic pericarditis)
   Others:
      Indian childhood cirrhosis
      Perinatal haemochromatosis

γGT, γ-glutamyl transferase.
The most frequently encountered causes and those that present often with complications of portal hypertension are in italic or block capital letters. In other diseases, portal hypertension is rarely symptomatic.

compression of the bile ducts. Follow-up is necessary to detect the rare occurrence of benign hepatic tumours, or of cardiopulmonary complications. There is no risk of clinical portosystemic encephalopathy. A promising alternative to classical portosystemic shunts may be an interposition of the jugular vein between the superior mesenteric vein and the end of the left portal vein whenever ultrasonography shows it is still patent (De Ville de Goyet, Transpl, 1996; 62:71); this may obviate the risk of hepatic tumours and cardiopulmonary complications.

(2) Injection sclerotherapy is commonly used in the hope that, with increasing age, the risk of bleeding will diminish (Stamatakis, BrJSurg, 1982; 69:74; Stringer, Gut, 1994; 35:257). After a mean number of four to five sessions, eradication of varices is usually observed; strict endoscopic follow-up is necessary to detect a relapse of varices, which may require further sclerosis. Endoscopic sclerosis does not treat cholestasis due to bile-duct compression or allow regression of splenomegaly, and it does not prevent cardiopulmonary complications. Early results of variceal ligation in children seem promising in the short term (Price, JPediatSurg, 1996; 31: 1056). There are no published reports on the efficacy of treatment with β-blocking agents in children with portal vein obstruction.

Biliary cirrhoses

Among the numerous causes of cirrhosis in children, the biliary cirrhoses are the most prone to the complication of portal hypertension, for example biliary atresia, cystic fibrosis, α_1-antitrypsin deficiency, sclerosing cholangitis, and progressive familial intrahepatic cholestasis with raised γ-glutamyltransferase. All these diseases have in common significant damage to the bile ducts; indeed it has been suggested that abnormalities of the intrahepatic branches of the portal vein may be associated with bile-duct damage in such patients, as is the case in children with congenital hepatic fibrosis (Odievre, Radiol, 1977; 122:427). These portal vein lesions, consisting of interruption of branches and duplications, may correspond to localized thrombosis and increase the risk of portal hypertension and of gastrointestinal bleeding.[11]

Management of portal hypertension in children with cirrhosis uses mostly endoscopic sclerotherapy (Sokal, EurJPed, 1992; 151: 326) or variceal ligation for prevention of recurrence of bleeding. Portosystemic surgical shunts have been used in patients with good liver function, with satisfactory results.[11] Liver transplantation is indicated when gastrointestinal bleeding is not controlled by usual means, or when major varices with or without bleeding are associated with other significant signs of liver dysfunction. Transjugular intrahepatic portosystemic shunts have been used with short-term success in a few older children (Berger, Pediat, 1994; 153:721).

Indian childhood cirrhosis

This is a type of cirrhosis seen with a particularly high frequency in young children in India who present, from age 6 months to 3 to 4 years, with abdominal distension, liver and spleen enlargement, failure to thrive, sometimes jaundice, and a prolonged prothrombin time, resulting in endstage liver disease.[12] Liver histology is characterized by lesions of hepatocytes, intralobular and portal fibrosis, and the presence of numerous Mallory bodies. There is a striking increase in liver copper concentration and liver copper-associated protein. The mechanism of the disease is unknown; it has been suggested that excess dietary copper resulting from the use of copper-made utensils could be responsible for the increased copper content of the liver and thus the subsequent liver lesions, but this notion has been challenged (Sethi, AnnTropPaediat, 1993; 13:3). Early treatment with D-penicillamine may improve the prognosis of a condition that is otherwise spontaneously lethal (Bavdekar, ArchDisChild, 1996; 74:32). Diseases similar to Indian childhood cirrhosis have been described outside India (Maggiore, JPediat-GastrNutr, 1987; 6:980; Baker, JHepatol, 1995; 23:538; Muller, Lancet, 1996; 347:877), leading to the concept of idiopathic copper toxicosis with, in a few, but not all, cases, evidence that excess copper intake could result from contamination of water by copper. This proposition has been challenged as well and it has been suggested that some of these patients may in fact be affected by an inherited disorder (Scheinberg, Lancet, 1994; 344:1002). The reality of these entities must be viewed with caution since increased liver concentrations of copper are detectable in a number of patients with various kinds of liver disease (Reed, ArchPath, 1972; 93:249).

Cardiopulmonary complications

Regardless of its cause, all children presenting with portal hypertension are exposed to the occurrence of cardiopulmonary complications, as follows.

(1) Hypoxaemia due to pulmonary arteriovenous shunting may occur as early as 6 months of age[13] and is more frequent in children with biliary atresia and polysplenia syndrome (Fewtrell, ArchDisChild, 1994; 70:501). Children present with cyanosis and dyspnoea or both; in a few cases this complication may be detected by systematic examination. Pulmonary scintiscan with Tc-labelled macroaggregated albumin allows diagnosis when the brain:lung ratio of isotope fixation is above 2 (Grimon, JNuclMed, 1994; 35: 1328); the Pao_2 while breathing 100 per cent O_2 may have a prognostic value.[13] Liver transplantation allows complete regression of hypoxaemia and shunting, more easily when hypoxaemia is not too severe. However, extreme hypoxaemia may also regress after transplantation should the patient survive the first four postoperative weeks (Van Obbergh, AmRevRespDis, 1993; 148:1408). This pleads in favour of an early diagnosis by regular screening for this complication in children with portal hypertension. Interestingly, treatment with aspirin has been reported to result in the

disappearance of pulmonary arteriovenous shunting and hypoxaemia in two children with portal vein obstruction (Song, Pediat, 1996; 97:917).

(2) Pulmonary artery hypertension also occurs in children with portal hypertension, as early as 4 years of age.[14,15] Results of liver transplantation in adult patients suggest that pulmonary artery hypertension may be reversible in some instances. Pulmonary artery hypertension complicating liver disease in children may be fully reversible after liver transplantation provided the pulmonary lesions are not too advanced (Losay, JHepatol, in press). This again pleads for early detection by systematic echocardiography carried out at regular intervals in all children exposed to this complication.

Some inherited metabolic disorders
Hereditary tyrosinaemia

This disorder is due to an autosomal recessively inherited reduction in fumaryl acetoacetate hydrolase activity. The gene is located on chromosome 15. The condition is characterized by progressive hepatocellular damage, renal tubular dysfunction, hypophosphataemic rickets, and the excretion of succinylacetone to 100-fold excess. There is excess urinary excretion of metabolic products of tyrosine, such as p-hydroxyphenylacetic acid. Plasma tyrosine, phenylalanine, and methionine concentrations may be elevated, particularly in the acute case. It was first described in a 9-month-old in 1956 (Baber, ArchDisChild, 31:335), but was difficult to distinguish from other forms of severe liver injury in infancy until the specificity of the high urinary succinylacetone excretion was demonstrated in 1977 (Lindblad, PNAS, 74:4641) and the enzyme deficiency 2 years later (Falstrom, Pediat, 1979; 13:1). Tyrosinaemia, which has been reported in Europe, the Middle East and North America, appears to be rare except in north-east Quebec, where the estimated frequency is 15 cases per 10 000 population.

Pathogenesis and pathology

Liver injury is thought to be caused by succinylacetone and its immediate precursors interacting with sulphydryl groups in the liver and kidneys. The hepatocytes show intense fatty infiltration, necrosis, and cholestasis. There is gradually increasing fibrosis that progresses from a micro- to a macronodular cirrhosis. Hepatocellular carcinoma was found in 16 of 43 cases over the age of 2 years (Weinberg, JPediat, 1976; 88:434).

Clinical features

The acute form presents in the first weeks or months of life with failure to thrive, vomiting, diarrhoea, oedema, ascites, hepatosplenomegaly, and bleeding diathesis. Death from liver failure usually occurs by 8 months of age, with only 10 per cent of patients surviving beyond 12 months. The chronic form may evolve from the acute or present later with hypophosphataemic rickets, cirrhosis, and renal tubular dysfunction. Death usually occurs in the first decade but there can be survival to adulthood. The majority of, if not all, patients ultimately develop hepatocellular carcinoma. Evolution may be further aggravated by acute neurological crises resembling neuropathic porphyrias (Mitchell, NEJM, 1990; 322: 432).

Laboratory features

Hypoalbuminaemia, reduced cholesterol concentration, prolonged prothrombin time, markedly elevated α-fetoprotein (10–100-fold elevated), hypoglycaemia, as well as features of renal tubular and hepatic dysfunction are found, together with the diagnostic abnormalities noted above. The diagnosis is made by finding high amounts of succinylacetone in the urine.

Treatment

Management relies on 2-(2-nitro-4-trifluoromethylbenzoyl)-1,3-cyclohexanedione (**NTBC**) an inhibitor of 4-hydroxyphenyl-pyruvatedioxygenase, which prevents the accumulation of succinylacetone (Lindstedt, Lancet, 1992; 340:813). It is given at a starting dose of 1 mg/kg per day, together with a tyrosine-restricted diet. The efficacy of the drug has now been established in more than 100 children worldwide (Lindstedt, 1996, NTBC Study, interim report): liver function tests return to normal, serum α-fetoprotein decreases, kidney function improves, and neurological abnormalities regress. The long-term efficacy of the drug is not known yet, in particular whether NTBC will prevent hepatocellular carcinoma. Liver transplantation may remain necessary in case of strong suspicion of cancer or in case of persisting signs of liver failure in spite of NTBC treatment.

Prenatal diagnosis is available by assaying succinylacetone in amniotic fluid, assaying fumarylacetoacetate hydrolase in amniotic cells or chorionic villi, or looking for mutations in the fumaryl acetoacetate hydrolase gene.

Galactosaemia (galactose 1-phosphate uridyl transferase deficiency)

Since Mason and Turner first described galactosaemia in 1935 (AmJDisChild, 50:359) the clinical features have gradually been expanded. To the initial constellation of growth retardation, liver disease, cataracts, and mental retardation have been added extreme susceptibility to severe and frequently fatal septicaemia (Levy, NEJM, 1977; 297:823), renal tubular dysfunction, anorexia, vomiting, diarrhoea, and hypoglycaemia. More recently the high incidence of educational difficulties and of gonadal failure in females has been highlighted (Buist, SSIEM, 1989; 27:007). The reported incidence is from 1 in 10 000 to 1 in 60 000 births. The severity of enzyme deficiency varies from complete absence to 10 per cent of normal. The latter patients have less severe symptoms as they are able to metabolize some galactose. The gene is located on chromosome 9.

Pathogenesis and pathology

Patients are unable to metabolize galactose to carbon dioxide. Following galactose ingestion it accumulates as galactose 1-phosphate, some of which is metabolized to galactitol. The latter appears to cause cataract but does not contribute to the liver or renal injury. Galactose 1-phosphate accumulation causes a severe depletion of intracellular high-energy phosphate bonds. Exactly how this causes tissue damage is as yet unclear. There is impaired release of glucose from glycogen and reduced gluconeogenesis. The liver initially shows fatty change with periportal cholangiolar proliferation, followed within 2 weeks by pseudoglandular transformation of the hepatocyte plates, and, by 6 weeks, increased fibrosis, leading to cirrhosis by 3 to 6 months of age. Hepatocellular carcinoma is a long-term risk.

Clinical features

In its most severe forms, symptoms start soon after the first ingestion of milk, with a septicaemic state with inanition, reluctance to feed, vomiting, and diarrhoea. Death may occur within 48 h. More commonly there is a severe unconjugated hyperbilirubinaemia, with or without haemolysis, at 2 to 4 days of age, followed by clinical and biochemical evidence of hepatic dysfunction, hepatomegaly, a bleeding diathesis, and sometimes abdominal distension and ascites by 2 weeks of age. In milder cases, failure to thrive, vomiting, and less severe liver damage occur. The mildest present with developmental delay and cataracts, and are found to have firm hepatomegaly. Cataracts may be found by slit-lamp examination as early as 5 days of age.

Laboratory findings

As well as liver dysfunction there may be hyperchloraemic acidosis, albuminuria, and hyperaminoaciduria. Diagnosis is confirmed by demonstrating galactose 1-phosphate uridyl transferase deficiency in red blood cells. Note that the enzyme is stable for up to 3 months in transfused red cells. Galactosaemia or galactosuria in the face of a galactose load may occur in any severe liver disease.

Treatment

The essence of treatment is a galactose-free diet for life. Patients presenting with indirect bilirubin greater than 320 μmol/l or with prolonged prothrombin ratios unresponsive to parenteral vitamin K should be treated by exchange transfusion. Antibiotics should be given for suspected septicaemia. Within a few days of withdrawing galactose the clinical condition gradually improves and tissue damage stabilizes. Cataracts may regress slightly. Hepatocellular carcinoma can be a long-term sequel and may require treatment by liver transplantation (Otte, Transpl, 1989; 47:902). Brain damage may occur despite institution of a galactose-free diet from birth. Learning difficulties and an increased incidence of psychological problems occur in over 70 per cent of patients in whom a galactose-free regimen is recommended. Hypergonadotrophic hypogonadism occurs in 90 per cent of females. The age at which the diet is introduced does not influence the frequency of these complications.

Fructosaemia: hereditary fructose intolerance (fructose 1-phosphate aldolase deficiency)

This disorder was first described in 1956 (Chalmers, Lancet, ii: 340) and characterized one year later (Froesch, SchMedWoch, 1957; 87:1168). Hers and Joassin (EnzymolBiolClin, 1961; 1:4) showed that fructose 1-phosphate aldolase activity was reduced to between zero and 30 per cent (average 3 per cent) of normal. There is also a much smaller reduction in activity towards fructose 1,6-diphosphate. Immunologically reactive aldolase may be detected in tissues in concentrations that vary from 3 to 100 per cent of values from controls. Illness starts as soon as fructose is ingested. Vomiting, and hepatic, renal, and neuronal dysfunction are the features. If ingestion continues death from liver failure occurs. The incidence has been estimated as 1 in 20 000 births in Switzerland. The gene is located on chromosome 9.

Pathophysiology and pathology

All the manifestations are attributed to accumulation of fructose 1-phosphate and depletion of ATP, GTP, and inorganic phosphate. Many cellular functions are deprived of energy. Hypoglycaemia, hypophosphataemia, increased serum transaminase, lactic acidosis, and hyperuricacidaemia occur. Within 2 h of fructose ingestion, lysosomal hypertrophy is followed rapidly by lipid accumulation and hepatocellular necrosis with bile-duct proliferation. With chronic ingestion there is increased fibrosis that may proceed to cirrhosis and hepatocellular carcinoma (See, AnnPediat, 1984; 31:49)

Clinical features

The patient is well until fructose is ingested, usually on weaning. Drug 'sweeteners' or milks containing added fructose are other sources. Vomiting, failure to thrive, hepatomegaly, and disordered liver function are universal. Features of acute liver failure, particularly hypoglycaemia and a bleeding diathesis, are common with relatively acute exposure, while chronic exposure may give cirrhosis with ascites. Older children gradually develop aversion to fructose-containing food.

Laboratory findings

Biochemical evidence of liver and renal tubular dysfunction is frequently associated with hyperuricacidaemia and lactic acidosis. Anaemia, acanthocytosis, and thrombocytopenia may occur.

Diagnosis

When fructosaemia is suspected, diagnosis can be made rapidly in many instances by molecular genetics studies investigating one of the two most frequent mutations on the fructose-1-phosphate aldolase gene associated with the disease (Cox, 1994, FASEBJ; 8: 62). These two mutations account for over 80 per cent of European patients. When search for mutations is negative, an intravenous fructose tolerance test and assay for fructose-1-phosphate aldolase activity in liver biopsy are necessary.

Treatment and prognosis

A fructose-free diet must be maintained for life. It usually reverses the features of the disorder but hepatomegaly and steatosis usually persist and cirrhosis may continue to progress. Acute liver failure may require exchange transfusion.

References

1. Hadchouel M. Paucity of interlobular bile ducts. *Seminars in Diagnostic Pathology*, 1992; **9**: 24–30.
2. Jacquemin E, *et al.* A new cause of progressive intrahepatic cholestasis: 3β-hydroxy-C_{27} steroid dehydrogenase/isomerase deficiency. *Journal of Pediatrics*, 1994; **125**: 379–84.
3. Clayton RJ, Iber FL, Ruebner BH, and McKusick V. Byler's disease. Fatal familial intrahepatic cholestasis in an Amish kindred. *American Journal of Diseases of Children*, 1969; **117**: 112–24.
4. Mieli-Vergani G, Howard ER, Portmann B, and Mowat AP. Late referral for biliary atresia—missed opportunities for effective surgery. *Lancet*, 1989; i: 421–3.
5. Psacharopoulos HT and Mowat AP. Incidence and early history of obstructive jaundice in infancy in Southeast England. In Javitt NB, ed. *Neonatal hepatitis and biliary atresia*. Washington: US Department of Health, Education and Welfare Publications, 1978: 167–75.
6. Alagille D. Cholestasis in the first three months of life. *Progress in Liver Diseases*, 1979; **6**: 471–85.
7. Balistreri WF and Schubert WK. Liver disease in infancy and childhood. In Schiff L and Schiff ER, eds. *Diseases of the liver*. Philadelphia: Lippincott, 1993: 1099–203.
8. Jansen PL. Genetic diseases of bilirubin metabolism: the inherited unconjugated hyperbilirubinemias. *Journal of Hepatology*, 1996; **25**: 398–404.
9. Knisely AS. Iron and pediatric liver disease. *Seminars in Liver Diseases*, 1994; **14**: 229–35.
10. Cormier V, *et al.* Neonatal and delayed onset involvement in disorders of oxidative phosphorylation. *Journal of Pediatrics*, 1997; **130**: 817–22.
11. Bernard O, Alvarez F, Brunelle F, Hadchouel P, and Alagille D. Portal hypertension in children. *Clinics in Gastroenterology*, 1985; **14**: 33–55.
12. Tanner MS, Kantarjian AH, Bhave SA, and Pandit AN. Early introduction of copper-contaminated animal milk feeds as a possible cause of Indian childhood cirrhosis. *Lancet*, 1983; ii :992–5.
13. Barbe T, *et al.* Pulmonary arteriovenous shunting in children with liver disease. *Journal of Pediatrics*, 1995; **126**: 571–9.
14. Silver MM, Bohn D, Shawn H, Eich G, and Rabinovitch M. Association of pulmonary hypertension with congenital portal hypertension in a child. *Journal of Pediatrics*, 1992; **120**: 321–9.
15. Moscoso G, Mieli-Vergani G, Mowat AP, and Portmann B. Sudden death caused by unsuspected pulmonary arterial hypertension 10 years after surgery for extrahepatic biliary atresia. *Journal of Pediatric Gastroenterology and Nutrition*, 1991; **12**: 388–93.

27

Liver disease in the elderly

27 Liver disease in the elderly

O. F. W. James

Introduction

While there are no liver diseases specific to old age, the presentation, clinical course, and management of liver diseases in the elderly differ in important respects from that of younger individuals. Furthermore, age-related changes in morphology and function of the liver influence our understanding of the interaction between the liver and the organism in later life. Nowhere has this been more evident than in the advance of liver transplantation into patients in their eighth and, very exceptionally, ninth decade (Wall, Lancet, 1993; 341:121). It is only in the last 10 years that interest has grown in over 65-year-olds, despite the fact that this group now represents up to 18 per cent of the population in westernized countries and Japan. [1-4]

Morphology and function

Morphology

The liver attains maximum size in young adulthood and then steadily declines in weight, not only in absolute terms but in relation to body size. By the age of 90 one study of liver volume using ultrasound measurement showed a decline of estimated liver volume from 1475 ml at age 24 to approximately 930 ml at age 90—a fall of 37 per cent; this change is apparently more marked in women (44 per cent) than men (28 per cent) (Wynne, Hepatol, 1989; 9:297). Other non-invasive estimates have shown very similar findings (Swift, EurJClinPharm, 1978; 14:149; Marchesini, Hepatol, 1988; 8:1079). The largest postmortem study of liver weight found a fall of 46 per cent between the third and tenth decade (Galloway, JAmGeriatSoc, 1965; 13:20). In appearance the liver becomes a darker brown colour due to the accumulation of fluorescent brown-pigmented lipofuscin granules in lysosomes within the hepatocytes. Lipofuscin is largely composed of protein; Ivy and Kitani have recently suggested that its deposition in liver cells, as elsewhere in the body, is due to decreased intracellular proteolysis with age. Whether this is because of decreased protease activity or an age-related modification of proteins within the cell to make them more resistant to protease digestion is not clear (Ivy, Science, 1984; 226: 985).[5] In ageing many liver cells enlarge, and nuclei show more polyploidy with increased DNA per nucleus (Watanabe, VirchArchA, 1978; 27:307; Barz, ExpPath, 1977; 14:55). Cells contain more protein; as with the nuclei, mitochondria are also enlarged (Tauchi, JGeront, 1968; 23:454). It has been suggested that this increased protein is functionally inactive and represents the accumulation of 'junk' within the liver cells. It is important to emphasize, however, that observations of age-related morphometric and functional alterations in experimental animals must not be extrapolated to man.

Liver blood flow can only be estimated indirectly in man. Wynne et al. have recently used indocyanine green clearance to show that estimated liver blood flow falls by about 35 per cent between the third and tenth decades. In addition liver perfusion (liver blood flow per unit volume liver) also fell over this range by about 11 per cent (Wynne, Hepatol, 1989; 9:297). Such calculations depend upon the constancy of extraction of indocyanine green by the liver with advancing age (Vestal, Hepatol, 1989; 9:331). This has now been confirmed, thus validating the magnitude of estimated decline in liver blood flow.

Liver function tests and metabolism

Conventional liver blood tests do not change with age (Reed, ClinChem, 1972; 18:57). Thus, abnormalities of serum bilirubin, serum transaminases, hepatic alkaline phosphatase, and other liver blood tests should be regarded in the same way in an 80 year old as in a 20 year old. Nonetheless, a number of dynamic measurements of liver function probably do decline with age. Many pharmacokinetic studies in man suggest that the clearance of drugs predominantly metabolized by the cytochrome P-450 enzyme system is reduced by between 10 and 50 per cent with age (Greenblatt, NEJM, 1982; 306: 1081).[6] It seems probable that when other variables (diet, smoking, sex, nutrition) have been accounted for there is a decline in cytochrome P-450 related metabolism of between 5 and 30 per cent from early adulthood to senescence (Woodhouse, BrMedBull, 1990; 46:22). Studies in man and primates have hitherto shown few age-related decreases in the specific activities or affinities of individual cytochrome P-450s.[10] Nonetheless, it is very possible that there may be differential decline in some functions with age (Chandler, ClinPharmTher, 1988; 43:436). Galactose elimination has been shown to decline with normal ageing; it is suggested that this cytosolic function is reduced at the same rate as liver size (Marchesini, Hepatol, 1988; 8:1079).

Few studies of hepatic synthetic function have been carried out in man, but although basal urea nitrogen synthesis is unaltered, there is a significant negative correlation between peak urea synthesis and age (Marchesini, AgeAgeing, 1990; 19:4)—an example of the widespread phenomenon of the inability to respond to stress in old age. This group has now demonstrated that hepatic conversion of α-amino nitrogen into urea nitrogen—functional hepatic nitrogen clearance—was reduced by 50 per cent with advancing age and that this was considerably greater than the observed age-related decline in liver volume (Fabbri, Liver, 1994; 14:288). This confirms that some hepatic functions are independently impaired.

Response to stress

While it is well recognized that the liver has remarkable powers of regeneration. In old livers the rate of replacement of liver cells after injury may be reduced so that repair is probably slower.[11] One clue as to the possible mechanism of this impaired proliferative capacity of liver cells has been provided by the demonstration of an age-related decline in mitogen-activated protein kinase activity in epidermal growth factor stimulated rat hepatocytes (Liu, JBC, 1996; 271:3604).

Many studies in rodents have shown increased liver damage to a standard hepatic toxin with age, for example galactosamine,[11] increased production of an inactive form of protective enzymes in old age, for example superoxide dismutase (Gershon, PNAS, 1973; 70:909), and age-related inability of the Kupffer cells to inactivate endotoxin leading to increased mortality from hepatorenal failure (Brouwer, ArchGerontolGeriat, 1986; 5:317). These studies provide suggestive evidence of possible increased susceptibility to stress insult in old age, although there are no directly comparable human data.

In summary, reduction in liver size and blood flow probably accounts for much of the age-associated decline in hepatic metabolism of xenobiotics in healthy man and, hence, in most cases, for any reduction in dynamic liver tests. Furthermore, there is increasing understanding of age-related decline in the power of the liver to regenerate after cell damage or death. Far more important, however, may be the influence of coexistent disease, current nutritional status, genetic factors, and a lifetime variation in diet, smoking, and alcohol consumption. The sum of these parts leads to the far greater variance seen in many metabolic functions in elderly patient populations. These factors, combined with a poorly understood age-related failure of homeostatic response to stress, may well form the background for the age-related features of hepatobiliary disease described below.

Parenchymal liver disease

This chapter will seek to point out important areas in which there are special features or differences between old and young in respect of clinical liver disease and its management.

Viral hepatitis
Hepatitis A

The proportion of the older adult population without acquired immunity to hepatitis A virus, at least among affluent and western populations, is lower now than in previous decades (Vandervelde, BMJ, 1987; 294:1031). This is presumably, at least partly, a cohort effect due to improved sanitation. Now, in some groups only about 50 per cent of the over 50-year-old population possesses anti-HAV (Gust, JInfectDis, 1978; 138:425). We may, therefore, expect hepatitis A to become more frequent in the elderly. Mortality is age related. In Britain, while the ratio of deaths to notification of the disease was approximately 7 per 10 000 persons aged 15 to 24 it rose to more than 400 per 10 000 in those over age 65 (Forbes, JRoyCollPhys, 1988; 22:237). Forbes also reported that if fulminant hepatic failure developed then increased age was an adverse prognostic marker. Now that hepatitis A vaccination is widely available and with increased travel to areas of high endemicity of the disease, screening of elderly travellers for hepatitis A IgG antibodies and vaccination of those who are negative is strongly indicated although the effectiveness of the vaccine has not been tested in a specific elderly group.

Hepatitis B and D

The major risk groups for acute hepatitis B and D in Europe and the United States (homosexuals, IV drug abusers) are not highly represented in the elderly population but the disease may still occur. This disease is more cholestatic and the clearance of HBsAg is slower in the elderly but, although the short term prognosis is unaltered, one report of an outbreak of hepatitis B in a nursing home for old people reported a resultant carrier rate of 59 per cent (Condo, Hepatol, 1993; 18:768). In parallel with this finding hepatitis B vaccination appears progressively more unsatisfactory in older individuals with progressively lower antibody response. Both the possible increased carrier rate following acute infection and poor response to vaccination may be due to a lack of antibody-producing B cells—presumably a facet of the failure of the immune response in old age (Cook, CellImmunol, 1987; 109:86). In hepatitis D, progression to cirrhosis occurs in the majority of cases (Goodson, ArchIntMed, 1982; 142:1485; Chiaramonte, JMedVirol, 1982; 9: 247).

Hepatitis C

An Italian study has suggested that the prevalence of hepatitis C virus infection in the elderly is sixfold higher than in under 35-year-olds in the same region—unlike the findings for hepatitis B virus. Conceivably this is a cohort effect but the explanation is unknown (Osella, JHepatol, 1997; 27:30). The natural history of hepatitis C in older people is controversial. One epidemiologically-based study of community-acquired hepatitis C in the United States suggested that at least a proportion of mainly elderly patients have a rather benign course (Alter, NEJM, 1992; 327:1899). In contrast, in a hospital-based study of hepatitis C in Britain, of 25 patients presenting over age 65, 18 of the 20 patients who had liver biopsy showed cirrhosis (12 patients) or cirrhosis and hepatocellular cancer (six patients) at presentation, four further patients developed hepatocellular cancer, and two patients died of other diseases associated with hepatitis C virus infection—non-Hodgkin's lymphoma and fibrosing alveolitis (Brind, QJMed, 1996, 89:291). Putative factors for acquiring hepatitis C virus were identified in less than half.

Since elderly patients with hepatitis viruses frequently present with more cholestatic acute disease or chronic disease, which may be further advanced than in younger subjects, all older patients presenting with liver disease or abnormal liver function tests must be screened for possible hepatitis B or C and, where indicated, A, with appropriate serological tests before invasive investigations or procedures are carried out. The place of interferon treatment for elderly patients with hepatitis B virus or hepatitis C virus is still to be determined. At present the cost/benefit equation would not seem to favour treating elderly patients with established cirrhosis however.

Drug-induced liver disease

Drug-induced liver disease, or at least abnormality of liver function tests, may account for as much a third of the over 65-year-old patients presenting with an apparent acute hepatitis.[12] This is perhaps not as surprising as might have been thought since while over 65-year-olds account for 15 to 18 per cent of the population in most European countries, the United States, and Japan, they may consume over 30 per cent of prescribed medications and perhaps 40 per cent of non-prescription drugs. Furthermore, older people have more intercurrent illnesses, impaired cardiac or renal function for example, which may directly or indirectly potentiate the adverse effects of some drugs upon the liver. It is still unclear whether hepatic adverse drug reactions occur with a frequency out of proportion to the quantity of drugs prescribed to this group. Furthermore, the relevance of minor abnormalities of liver enzymes against the potential benefits of important medications must be considered. A major Swedish study of hepatic adverse drug reactions which did examine the effect of age, corrected for age-related prescribing variables, found no increased frequency of reported adverse drug reactions, nor any increased susceptibility to severe reactions. Unfortunately a number of important drugs—notably halothane—were excluded from this analysis. Two studies have found that hepatic failure and death are more common after halothane anaesthesia in older persons. Animal studies have indicated that this may not be due to age-related difference in metabolism of halothane but is conceivably due to other age-related, intrinsic factors such as decreased response to stress (Lind, Anesthesiol, 1989; 71:878). It is also suggested that a few other drugs, among them isoniazid, particularly in conjunction with rifampicin, may have increased severity of liver toxicity, should it occur in an elderly patient (Lewis, MedClinNAm, 1989; 73:775). Adverse effects of non-steroidal anti-inflammatory drugs—the model being benoxaprofen—do show a clear, age-related increased frequency as well as severity; while the mean age of individuals receiving benoxaprofen in the United Kingdom was 59, the mean age of those who sustained severe or fatal adverse drug reactions, usually hepatic, was 75.[13] Overall it is perhaps surprising that the age-related decline in clearance of many drugs, alluded to earlier, does not lead to more severe adverse consequences. This is presumably because, while mild dose-related abnormalities of liver enzymes may be frequent, severe adverse reactions are usually idiosyncratic, hence marginal age-related declining clearance is probably not relevant.

Autoimmune liver disease

Immune surveillance breaks down in advanced age—thus autoimmune markers, and some autoimmune diseases, hypothyroidism or rheumatoid arthritis for example, become more common. The effect of advancing age upon the presentation and prognosis of the autoimmune liver diseases has been unclear.

Primary biliary cirrhosis

All the major prognostic studies of the natural history of primary biliary cirrhosis have shown that increasing age is an independent prognostic indicator, even when liver deaths alone are considered (Roll, NEJM, 1983; 308:1; Christiansen, Gastro, 1985; 89:1084; Grambsch, Hepatol, 1989; 10:846). In a major recent epidemiological study of the incidence and prevalence of primary biliary cirrhosis in our region, we have shown that the average age of primary biliary cirrhosis at presentation is now about 60 although tertiary referral centres have a median referral age of around 55 (Metcalfe, IntJEpid, 1997; 26:830). Of 111 new incident cases of primary biliary cirrhosis diagnosed over age 65, at a mean follow-up of 5 years, 29 (26 per cent of the group) had died of liver-related causes. In this study, the point prevalence of primary biliary cirrhosis in over-65 year olds was 569 per million, or about 1 in 1000 women in 1994. Thus, in many populations up to a quarter of patients may present over age 65 and over one-third of prevalent cases at any one time may be above this age, including both those with severe disease, exceptionally requiring considering of transplantation, and those living into old age with prolonged mild disease.

Autoimmune hepatitis (AIH)

This has been thought to be uncommon (Selby, AgeAgeing, 1986; 5:350). Recently we have identified 12 individuals with a diagnosis of autoimmune hepatitis presenting over age 65; this was about 20 per cent of all patients in whom this diagnosis was made over a fixed period. The elderly group had more severe initial histological grade but their prognosis was no different from individuals presenting under age 65 (Newton, AgeAgeing, 1997; in press). Diagnostic scores (Johnson, Hepatol, 1993; 18:998) were slightly lower in the elderly group. It is the authors experience that there is a small group of autoimmune hepatitis elderly patients presenting with very aggressive disease, rapidly accompanied by the severe complications or portal hypertension and encephalopathy, with a larger group presenting with clinical autoimmune chronic hepatitis but without the full house of diagnostic criteria recently described by the International Association for the Study of the Liver (IASL). Conceivably, among these may be individuals with unrecognized, drug-related, chronic hepatitis.

Alcoholic liver disease

While there are no age-related changes in the specific activity of total hepatic alcohol dehydrogenase (Wynne, AgeAgeing, 1992; 21: 417), recent careful pharmacokinetic studies have shown that blood ethanol AUCs (areas under curve) among men are significantly greater in older subjects than younger in the oral fasted and intravenous fed states but not in the oral fed state. In women, there was a highly significant difference in the oral fasted state only. The authors suggest that the mechanism underlying the effect of age in reducing ethanol clearance is unlikely to be related to gastric metabolism or motility since average AUC was greater fasting than fed irrespective of intravenous or oral administration. The age-related difference, seen most clearly in the oral fasted state but not in the fed state, they suggest, implies decline in one or more mechanisms responsible for rapid ethanol metabolism within the first hour after ingestion.[14]

Although presentation of alcoholic liver disease is perceived as being most common in middle age, many patients present for the first time at an advanced age. Thus, in the United States one study from Baltimore showed that the peak decade for presentation with cirrhosis was the seventh (Garagliano, JChronDis 1979; 32:544). In a British series, 28 per cent of patients with alcoholic liver disease presented over age 60 and about 10 per cent over age 70 (Potter, Geront, 1987; 33:380). In France, a large retrospective study suggested that as many as 20 per cent of patients were over age 70 and there was no difference in their clinical features from patients with alcoholic liver disease as a whole (Aron, AnnGastroHep, 1979; 15: 558). In Italy, total mortality from alcoholic cirrhosis is highest around age 55 to 60, although it is not possible to say whether the reduced mortality thereafter merely reflects the fact that most alcoholic patients were dead before reaching an older age (Copocaccia, JClinEpidemiol, 1988; 41:347). In this study, age-specific mortality from cirrhosis of all causes in Italy rose strikingly. In our own series, older patients had a higher proportion of symptoms and signs suggestive of severe liver disease at presentation—ankle swelling, jaundice, and abdominal swelling—than young ones. All patients who presented over age 70 already had cirrhosis against about 50 per cent of younger patients. Prognosis was directly related to age. Mortality in those under 60 at presentation was 5 per cent at 1 year and 24 per cent at 3 years; in those over age 60 at presentation it was 34 per cent at 1 year and 54 per cent at 3 years; among those presenting over age 70 years, 75 per cent were dead at 1 year and 90 per cent at 3 years. Among the eldest patients, over half developed hepatocellular cancer. Among those without hepatocellular cancer the reasons for apparently increased severity of alcoholic liver disease is unclear. Patient selection for referral, greater length of history, or intrinsic age-related factors, could contribute to these results.

The only study to examine alcohol withdrawal in elderly versus young subjects suggested that older patients had more severe withdrawal and required higher doses of sedation (chlordiazepoxide) to control symptoms. The reasons for this increased severity are not clear (Liskow, JStudAlc, 1989; 50:414).

Other chronic liver disease

The proportion of patients with cryptogenic liver disease has decreased with improved diagnostic tools. Nevertheless, a recent major study of factors influencing survival in patients with cirrhosis has shown that the group with cryptogenic cirrhosis had the worst prognosis and that the most important single adverse factor in determining prognosis was increased age (Johnson, JHepatol, 1989; 9:549). One possible cause of cirrhosis in later life recognized recently is α-1 antitrypsin deficiency, usually in Z heterozygote (Roggli, AmJClinPath, 1981; 75:538; Battle, JClinGastro, 1982; 4: 269). While the diagnosis of haemochromotosis is usually made in middle-age men, occasionally old males and females can present with the complications of portal hypertension or liver failure superimposed upon evidence of cirrhosis, often associated with the development of hepatocellular cancer. In general, elderly patients presenting with cirrhosis usually present with, or rapidly develop, severe complications of portal hypertension and liver cell failure. Suspicion should be extremely high that these patients already have, or will shortly develop, hepatocellular cancers which have, in some instances, decompensated what has probably otherwise been long-term, well compensated cirrhosis regardless of cause. The concept of senile cryptogenic cirrhosis, favoured in years gone by, should now be discarded.

Liver transplantation in the elderly

Liver transplantation is increasingly an option for patients with chronic liver disease over age 60, even age 70 (Emry, TransplantProc, 1993; 25:1075). Several studies have now shown that in selected patients, over age 60, overall 1 year graft and patient survival rates equal those achieved in younger patients.[15] The important aspect is contained in the words 'carefully selected'. The experience of many transplant centres is now that much extra vigilance must be used in preoperative assessment of cardiac, respiratory, and renal function in patients over age 65 and that intercurrent illness or organ dysfunction aside from liver disease dramatically worsens prognosis. It has been suggested that a 'bonus' for elderly transplant recipients is that the impairment of immune function accompanying old age reduces the incidence of allograft rejection and may allow lower dosage of immunosuppressive drugs.[15] It has recently been implied that livers from older donors may impair short-term prognosis following transplantation. For this reason it may be considered appropriate in future to reserve livers from older donors for older recipients. This will be a matter for considerable discussion.

Primary hepatocellular cancer

It is increasingly clearly that primary hepatocellular cancer is a disease of ageing in western countries. In this respect it is of interest that, in experimental animals, there was an age-associated, marked (two fold) increase in DNA bases damaged by oxidative modification. This was similar to modification induced by carcinogens and seen in experimental hepatocellular cancers (Wang, ChemBiolInteract, 1995; 94:135). In Europe, hepatocellular cancer is largely associated with cirrhosis, regardless of cause, and probably also related to the length of time for which an individual has had cirrhosis (Melia, QJMed, 1984; 53:391). In a recent United Kingdom review of 110 cases of hepatocellular cancer, almost half presented age 65 or over; symptoms and signs at presentation were similar in the two age groups. At presentation only a quarter were previously known to have cirrhosis. This proportion rose to over 75 per cent after diagnosis. Survival from diagnosis was worse in the older age group (10.5 versus 18.5 weeks), the older patients having worse Okuda stage. Even in the United Kingdom, an area with a low prevalence of hepatitis B virus infection, 34 per cent of the younger patients showed hepatitis B virus markers versus only 23 per cent of the older group. Conversely, almost 40 per cent of the old patients had underlying cryptogenic disease (presumed hepatitis C, testing not being available) against 20 per cent in the younger patients (Collier, AgeAgeing, 1994; 23:22). In an eastern population a similar observation has been obtained. A Korean study of heptocellular cancer showed that the ratio of hepatitis B virus/hepatitis C virus among patients with hepatocellular cancer before age 50 was 29.7 whereas the ratio in patients presenting with hepatocellular cancer over 60 years was 0.9 (Lee, Cancer, 1993; 72:2564). This dramatically reflects the age of acquisition of hepatitis B virus (usually infancy) in this population whereas hepatitis C virus was presumably acquired in later life, as in Europe. Thus, among older individuals with hepatitis C virus cirrhosis the development of hepatocellular cancer should be anticipated and hence screened.

Liver abscess

Almost 50 per cent of patients from Europe and North America presenting with pyogenic liver abscess are age 70 or older (Smoger, AgeAgeing, 1997; in press). Several studies now show that older patients have less marked physical signs and present with more non-specific symptoms—epigastric pain, weight loss, shortness of breath, and malaise (Sridharan, AgeAgeing, 1990; 19:199). In a modern setting high quality ultrasound and/or computed tomography scan together with guided fine needle aspiration mean that the diagnosis can be made with increasing confidence. None the less, there is not infrequently a differential between possible liver abscess and malignancy or simple cyst within the liver. Such abscesses can appear as multiple, space-occupying lesions. Treatment with drainage and antibiotics is similar for elderly as for younger subjects; relatively few should need laparotomy and formal surgical drainage. Of the two major, recent series mentioned above one emphasized that in almost 50 per cent of these patients abscess was associated with gall stones, but this was the case in only 25 per cent of the second series, whereas the second series emphasized the relationship with diabetes in elderly patients (35 per cent). While some recent studies have suggested increased mortality in older patients with pyogenic liver abscess (Chou, JAmCollSurg, 1994; 179:727), this may be because of a slight increase in associated malignancy among older patients or because a proportion of liver abscess patients are only found at autopsy. Prognosis and hospital stay for elderly patients correctly diagnosed and managed and not associated with malignancy is now identical to that seen in younger patients.

Gallstones and their management

Studies from all over the world show that prevalence of gallstones increases with age. In Europe, the prevalence of gallstones/cholecystectomy in females over age 80 may be as much as 40 per cent. This can, therefore, be regarded as a truly age-related phenomenon (McDonald, Medicine, 1984; 64:291; Lindstrom, ScaJGastr, 1977; 12:341; Bateson, BMJ, 1975; 4:427; Thijs, NedTGeneesk, 1989; 133:110; Walker, AmJGastro, 1989; 84:1383). There are two apparent reasons. First, cholesterol saturation of bile rises with age; this is due to increasing hepatic secretion of cholesterol in both men and women and to decreased bile acid production (as measured by an isotope dilution technique) (Einarsson, NEJM, 1985; 313:277). Second, it is possible that the gallbladder is less sensitive to endogenous cholecystokinin with advancing age and, theoretically, this might lead to diminished gallbladder contraction following a meal (Poston, Gastro, 1990; 98:993). One study has, however, demonstrated that gallbladder contraction, as measured by ultrasound, is unimpaired in older subjects with fasting—maximally contracted gallbladder volumes being equal between young and old subjects. There was, however, a much higher fat-stimulated plasma concentration of cholecystokinin in the elderly group—the authors also suggested that this indicated diminished sensitivity of the gallbladder to cholecystokinin stimulation (Khalil, Surgery, 1985; 98:423). It has also been postulated that duodenal juxtapapillary diverticula, whose prevalence steeply increases with age, may be associated with biliary stasis, malfunction of the sphincter of Oddi,

and reflux of duodenal contents into the common bile duct (Grace, Gut, 1990; 31:571).

Not only do gallstones increase with age but, possibly due to decreased response to infection, the complications of biliary tract disease are age related and more severe in old age.

Age in relation to management of biliary disease

The management of biliary disease is fully dealt with elsewhere in this volume. However, a number of observations concerning the management of gallstone disease in old age are relevant. In general, mortality for the treatment of all forms of biliary disease rises with advancing age but this may be largely ascribed to other coincident conditions. For example in one series of over 80 year-olds treated surgically for acute cholecystitis, one-third had diabetes mellitus compared to only 5 per cent in a large younger group of patients from the same centre (Landau, DigSurg, 1994; 11:30). Furthermore, it is the impression from both the United States and Europe that acute biliary tract disease is becoming more common in elderly patients.[16] This may be because a higher proportion of the population is surviving to an advanced age to experience the complications of previously silent gallstones. In a retrospective study carried out in the 1960s, gallbladder disease appeared to have been an important contributor to death in 8.1 per cent of patients over age 70 in whom gallstones were discovered at autopsy (Amberg, Geriat, 1965; 20:539). Four main sets of circumstances may arise in an elderly patient with gallstones:

1. Acute or chronic cholecystitis—gallstones only in the gallbladder. Mortality or morbidity from early elective operative intervention is now said to be close to that in younger subjects. In experienced centres, after appropriate investigation (which may include endoscopic retrograde cholangiopancreatography) laparoscopic cholecystectomy may now be considered a treatment of choice in non-acute cases (NIH Consensus, JAMA, 1993; 269:1018). However, conventional cholecystectomy is certainly very safe and effective. In acute cholecystitis, early cholecystectomy with peroperative exploration of the bile duct is recommended (Piggott, AmJSurg, 1988; 155:408).
2. Cholangitis—stones in common bile duct. Endoscopic sphincterotomy is recommended and morbidity and· mortality in patients even over age 90 may be little higher than that in younger patients (Kasmin, GastrEnd, 1995; 41:A423).
3. Stones in the common bile duct and in the gallbladder. This is more controversial; it is suggested that, particularly in very frail old patients, endoscopic retrograde cholangiopancreatography with sphincterotomy alone may be sufficient (Siegal, DiagTherEndosc, 1994; 1:51).[15] If symptoms persist after clearance of the common bile duct then cholecystectomy or percutaneous cholecystostomy and gallstone removal may subsequently be carried out (Cuschieri, Gut, 1989; 30:1786).
4. Asymptomatic gallstones found by chance in an elderly person. The management of these patients is controversial. On the one hand, since such individuals have a relatively shorter life expectancy it might be argued that it is best to let sleeping dogs lie. On the other hand, complications of occult biliary disease are more severe in old age. The physician or surgeon should decide

each case on its merits (Donaldson, NEJM, 1982; 307:815). It should be remembered that biliary disease may present atypically in old people. The diagnosis should be considered in any elderly person with fever, fluctuating abnormal liver function tests, and confusion (Cobden, Lancet, 1984; 1:1062).

Acalculus cholecystitis represents an ischaemic inflammation of the gallbladder wall which can rapidly progress to necrosis and perforation if left untreated. It is increasing recognized as occurring particularly in elderly subjects and is often related to cardiovascular disease and atherosclerosis (Glenn, AnnSurg, 1982; 195:131).

References

1. Popper H. Aging and the liver. In: Popper H and Schaffner F, eds. *Progress in liver diseases*. Orlando: Grune and Stratton, 1986: 659–83.
2. Kitani K, ed. *Liver and aging—1982, liver and drugs*. Amsterdam: Elsevier/North Holland, 1982.
3. Kitani K, ed. *Liver and aging—1986, liver and brain*. Amsterdam: Elsevier Scientific Publishers, 1986.
4. Bianchi L, *et al.*, ed. *Aging in liver and gastrointestinal tract*. Lancaster: MTP Press, 1988.
5. Kitani K. Aging and the liver. In: Popper H and Schaffner F, eds. *Progress in liver diseases*. Philadelphia: W.B. Saunders, 1990: 603–23.
6. Arora S, *et al.* Effect of age on tests of intestinal and hepatic function in healthy humans. *Gastroenterology*, 1989; **96**: 1560–5.
7. James OFW, *et al.* The influence of frailty, liver blood flow and size upon hepatic oxidation and conjugation in aged man. In: Kitani K, ed. *Liver and aging—1990*. Amsterdam: Elsevier, 1990: 210–21.
8. Schnegg M and Lauterburg BH. Quantitative liver function in the elderly assessed by galactose elimination capacity, aminopyrine demethylation and caffeine clearance. *Journal of Hepatology*, 1986; **3**: 164–71.
9. Posner J, *et al.* The disposition of antipyrine and its metabolites in young and healthy elderly volunteers. *British Journal of Clinical Pharmacology*, 1987; **24**: 51–5.
10. Schmucker DL, Woodhouse KW, and Wang R. Effect of age and gender on invitro properties of liver microsomal mono-oxygenases. *Clinical Pharmacology and Therapeutics*, 1990; **48**: 365–74.
11. Platt D. Age dependent morphological and biochemical studies of the normal and injured rat liver. In: Platt D, ed. *Liver and ageing*. Stuttgart: F. K. Schattnauer, 1977: 75–83.
12. Benhamou JP. Drug induced hepatitis: clinical aspects. In: Fillastre JP, ed. *Hepatotoxicity of drugs*. Rouen: University of Rouen, 1986: 23–30.
13. James OFW. Parenchymal liver disease in the elderly. In Bianchi L, Holt P, James OFW, and Butler RN, eds. *Aging in liver and gastro-intestinal tract*. Lancaster: MTP Press, 1988: 359–69.
14. Beresford TP and Lucey MR. Ethanol metabolism and intoxication in the elderly. In: Beresford TP and Gomberg E, eds. *Alcohol and aging*. New York: OUP, 1995: 117–27.
15. Clain DJ. Liver disease in the elderly. In: Gelb AM, ed. *Clinical gastroentelogy in the elderly*. New York: Dekker, 1996: 167–83.
16. Kasmin FE and Siegal JH. Biliary disease in the elderly. In: Gelb AM, ed. *Clinical gastroenterology in the elderly*. New York: Dekker, 1996: 185–212.

28

Liver disease and pregnancy

28 Liver disease and pregnancy

A. K. Burroughs

The liver in normal pregnancy

During pregnancy the expanding uterus pushes the liver upwards so that mild enlargement of the liver may not be palpable. Spider naevi and palmar erythema are common. There is an increase in blood volume of approximately 45 per cent in the third trimester with a concomitant increase in central venous pressure and cardiac output (Walters, SGO, 1970; 131:765) which is most marked at 30 weeks gestation (Roy, AmJObsGyn, 1966:221). Hypertension is considered to be present if the diastolic pressure is more than 30 mmHg higher and systolic pressure more than 15 mmHg higher than the values in the first trimester. Blood pressure falls in the second trimester and returns to normal levels at term. Renal blood flow and glomerular filtration (measured by insulin clearance) also increase by 30 and 50 per cent, respectively (Sims, JCI, 1958; 37: 1764; Davidson, AmJKidneyDis, 1987; 9:248). Hepatic blood flow does not increase as measured by bromosulphthalein clearance (Munnell, JCI, 1947; 26:952) or indocyanine green clearance,[1] but the fractional blood flow to the liver decreases.[1] Due to compression of the inferior vena cava there is an increased flow in the azygous system which results in the development of small oesophageal varices in approximately 50 per cent of pregnant women. Gallbladder motility decreases with an increased residual volume. The lithogenic index of bile increases. There is an increase in hepatic cholesterol synthesis and cholesterol secretion in bile (Feingold, JLabClinMed, 1983; 101:256), and a decrease in cheno-deoxycholic acid synthesis in relation to cholic acid, with a reduction in the enterohepatic recirculation of bile acids. Fasting gallbladder volume is increased, even though there is a decrease in the proportion of biliary water.

Laboratory tests show a decrease in the haematocrit, and in serum urea, uric acid, albumin, and total protein values. Alkaline phosphatase is increased owing to a rise in placental and bone isoenzymes (Adeniyi, BrJObsGyn, 1984; 91:857); there is also an increase in the α_1-, α_2-, and β-globulins, fibrinogen, cholesterol, triglycerides (Svanborg, ActaMedScand, 1965; 178:615), and in the white cell count. There is no increase in total bilirubin, total bile acids, aminotransferases, gammaglobulin, and 5′-nucleotide concentrations. Compared with age-matched controls, total and free bilirubin concentrations are lower in all three trimesters, and conjugated bilirubin and γ-glutamyl transpeptidase levels are lower in the second and third trimesters, while 5′-nucleotidase is higher than normal (Bacq, Hepatol, 1996; 23:1030). Bromosulphthalein excretion decreases near term (Combes, JCI, 1963; 42:1431). Post-prandial cholylglycine concentrations increase during pregnancy from 0.3 mmol/1 at 15 weeks to 0.6 mmol/1 at 40 weeks, although the median peak value falls within the normal range (0 to 1.5 mmol/l); pruritus occurs in about half the women with elevated values but in only 20 per cent of those with normal values (Lunzer, Gastro, 1986; 91:825).

Liver histology is normal, with only non-specific reactive changes being seen, such as reactive Kupffer cells, variation in nuclear shape and size, and minimal bile ductular proliferation. Electron microscopy shows proliferation of the smooth endoscopic reticulum (Perez, AmJObsGyn, 1971; 110:428).

Liver disease in pregnancy

In a clinical setting it is useful to consider liver disease in pregnancy under three headings: those peculiar to pregnancy, liver diseases coincidental with pregnancy, and pregnancy in patients with already established liver disease. The incidence of jaundice (the most common clinical manifestation) is low, occurring in approximately 1 in 1500 pregnancies.[2]

Investigation of liver disease during pregnancy

Results of laboratory investigations should be interpreted in the light of the normal physiological changes described above. The risks of percutaneous liver biopsy are not increased and contraindications for a liver biopsy should be the same as for non-pregnant women. A CT scan (8-mm computed slice, 6 cm away from the liver) delivers less radiation than a single posteroanterior fetal radiograph (McKee, BMJ, 1986; 292:291). A single 10-mm section delivers an estimated skin dose of 80 mSv (Clements, BrJObsGyn, 1990; 97: 631). The fetus should be shielded. Ultrasound carries no risk.

Liver disease peculiar to pregnancy
Hyperemesis gravidarum

Nausea and vomiting frequently occur in normal pregnancy but are usually confined to the first trimester (Klebanoff, ObsGyn, 1985; 66:621) and are associated with faster gastric dysrhythmias than normal in terms of gastric myoelectric activity (Koch, DigDisSci, 1990; 35:961). When these symptoms are unusually prolonged and occur throughout the day, weight loss and dehydration may follow and jaundice (usually mild) may develop. Excessive salivation may be a feature and hyperthyroidism may be found (Bober, Ac-taEndoscop, 1986; 111:104). Hyperthyroidism has been suggested as a cause of jaundice (Colin, GastrClinBiol, 1994; 18:378). Amino-transferase values may be raised, usually no more than 250 u/l.[3] The syndrome is associated epidemiologically with young mothers (under 20 years), nulliparous women, obesity, and non-smokers. It is more frequent in patients with hydatidiform mole. The mean birth weight is reduced if the mother has severe hyperemesis gravidarum (Gross, AmJObsGyn; 1989; 160:906). As nausea and vomiting may be seen with acute viral hepatitis, the differential diagnosis for hyperemesis gravidarum is important. Repeated vom-iting is a presentation of hydatidiform mole. In rare cases recurrence occurs with subsequent pregnancies (Laurey, Gut, 1984; 25:1414).

Most of the epidemiological risk factors are associated with high oestrogen levels, suggesting a role for these in the pathogenesis. Gonadotrophins peak in the first trimester and may be another pathogenetic factor. Ketonuria is more severe (reflecting more severe starvation and dehydration) in those with abnormal liver enzymes. However, there is little correlation with the level of aminotransferases, suggesting that other mechanisms are responsible for this alteration (Morali, JClinGastro, 1990; 12:303).

Liver histology is usually normal or shows fatty change (Adams, ObsGyn, 1968; 31:659). Correction of the dehydration and mal-nutrition ensures a return to normal liver function. Ondansetron has been used with success (Guikontes, Lancet, 1993; 340:1223).

Intrahepatic cholestasis of pregnancy

This is the second most common cause of jaundice in pregnancy (the most common being acute viral hepatitis) and accounts for approximately 20 per cent of cases; it occurs in 0.5 to 1 per cent of pregnancies (Bacq, JHepatol 1996; 25(Suppl 1):209). It nearly al-ways occurs in the second or third trimester, although it can occur late in the first trimester (Svanborg, ActaGyn, 1954; 33:434; Jiang, ChinMedJ, 1986; 99:957). Pruritus appears first and, in very mild cases, jaundice is not seen (pruritus gravidarum). Other causes of itching, particularly if associated with skin lesions, need to be excluded (Dacus, SouthMedJ, 1987; 80:614). However, in many patients, clinically obvious jaundice follows the pruritus after about 2 weeks and is accompanied by the usual features of cholestasis, i.e. dark urine and pale stools with steatorrhoea (Reyes, Gastro, 1987; 93:584 and Hepatology, 1982; 2:87).[4] There may be right upper quadrant pain and tender hepatomegaly, but this is unusual and should lead to the consideration of alternative diagnoses. Itching can be severe and lead to lack of sleep, anorexia, and malnutrition. The syndrome lasts for the duration of pregnancy and resolves within 2 to 4 weeks of delivery with no sequelae. An increased incidence of postpartum haemorrhage has been reported, but it is not clear whether vitamin K was administered before delivery (Show, AmJObsGyn, 1982; 142:261; Jiang, ChinMedJ, 1986; 99: 957). Vitamin K should be administered parenterally.

The serum bilirubin increases and remains stable at a level that is usually less than 100 μmol/l, although concentrations as high as 600 μmol/l have been reported (Misra, AmJGastr, 1980; 73:54). Bile acids are raised. Aminotransferase values usually remain below 250 u/l but exceptions occur (Wilson, DigDisSci, 1987; 32:1665). γ-Glutamyl transpeptidase may be normal (Jacquemin, Gastr-ClinBiol, 1988; 12:768). Liver biopsy is not necessary to establish

the diagnosis; it shows centrilobular cholestasis, with no necrosis or inflammation. There is a twofold increase in the prevalence of gallstones (Furhoff, ActaMedScand, 1974; 196:181; Samsioe, Acta-ObGyn, 1975; 54:417). A low selenium and glutathione peroxidase activity are found, the significance of which is unclear (Kauppila, BMJ, 1987; 294:150). A higher postprandial glucose level has been found in intrahepatic cholestasis of pregnancy compared with controls matched for gestational age, demonstrating altered glucose metabolism (Wojcicka-Jacodzinska, AmJObsGyn, 1989; 161:959).

There is a higher incidence of miscarriage, premature labour, and perinatal mortality, perhaps related to illness in the mother. However, no direct relationship could be found between nutritional state and fetal prognosis (Reyes, Gastro, 1987; 93:584). Direct toxicity from bile salts crossing the placenta has been suggested by some authors (Laatikainen, AmJObsGyn, 1975; 122:852; Laa-tikainen, AmJObsGyn, 1983; 4:22), but has not been found by others (Sharr, AmJObsGyn, 1982; 142:621). An abnormal sensitivity of the myometrium has also been proposed (Israel, ActaObGyn, 1986; 65:581). There is an abnormal variability in fetal heart rate (Ammala, AmJObsGyn, 1981; 14:217). The placenta may be abnormal (Co-stoya, Placenta, 1980; 1:361) and intervillous flow has been shown to be decreased with cholestasis (Kaar, ActaObGyn, 1980; 59:7).

Itching has been treated by antihistamines or cholestyramine; however, these may not be tolerated by the patient, or they may be ineffective (Sharr, AmJObsGyn, 1982; 142:621, Laatikainen, AmJObsGyn, 1978; 132:501). Vitamin K should be administered and should also be given before delivery. Cholestyramine ex-acerbates vitamin K deficiency. Phenobarbitone has also been used (Laatikainen, AmJObsGyn, 1978; 132:501). Dexamethasone at 12 mg/day for 7 days, with tapering over 3 days, has been shown to improve pruritus, and also aids fetal lung maturation (Hirvioja, BrJObsGyn, 1992; 99:109), but one report suggested worsening of pruritus (Kretowicz, AustNZJObsGyn, 1996; 34:211). S-adenosyl-L-methionine (800 mg/day intravenously) has been shown to relieve the pruritus, lessen jaundice, and lower bile acids in controlled (Frezza, Hepatol, 1984; 4:274) and uncontrolled studies (Bon-fiarraro, DrugInvest, 1990; 2:125), without adverse effects on the fetus. Epomediol, a terpenoid, also reduced itching and in a pre-liminary study appeared to be safe (Gonzales, JHepatol, 1990; 11(Suppl 2):590). Ursodeoxycholic acid (1 mg/day) is safe and effective against pruritus and improves liver function (Palma, Hepa-tol, 1992; 15:1043; Davies, Gut, 1995; 37:580). A controlled trial found ursodeoxycholic acid to be more effective than S-adenosyl-L-methionine (Floreani, JHepatol, 1996; 25(Suppl. 1):136). Some authorities recommend delivery before 38 weeks gestation, while others only recommend induction if fetal distress occurs, or if jaundice is present at 36 weeks (Rioseco, AmJObsGyn, 1994; 170: 890).

The syndrome is caused by an increased sensitivity of the bile excretory system to oestrogen, whether of endogenous or exogenous origin. In a prospective study in France, orally administered pro-gesterone in early pregnancy was considered a possible trigger factor (Bacq, JHepatol, 1996; 25(Suppl. 1):138), and was also an independently predictive factor in another French study (Bronstein, JHepatol, 1996; 25(Suppl 1):209), together with twin pregnancy, in vitro fertilization, prematurity, and hypertension. It is more common in Scandinavia and in Araucanian Indians in Chile, and occurs in family clusters. In Chilean women there is a higher frequency of the HLA-DPB1 *0402 allele, but no association of the disease with DPB1 allele (Mella, JHepatol, 1996; 24:320). It is well documented in other ethnic groups such as the Chinese (Jiang, ChinMedJ, 1986; 99:957), but appears to be rare in black populations (Wilson, DigDisSci, 1987; 32:665). The exact mode of transmission is not known, but transmission through a male family member is described (Holzbach, Gastro, 1983; 85:175). It is more frequent in multiple gestations (Gonzalez, JHepatol, 1989; 9:84). Interestingly, among multiparous women who developed intrahepatic cholestasis of pregnancy with a twin pregnancy, it did not recur with single pregnancies but only with twin pregnancies, whereas the recurrence rate when the syndrome occurred with a singleton pregnancy was 70 per cent (Gonzalez, JHepatol, 1989; 9:84).

Pruritus usually reoccurs with subsequent pregnancies, or with menstrual disturbances associated with oestrogen excess or with ethinyloestradiol challenge (Kreek, AmJMed, 1967; 43:795), or with the oral contraceptive pill (Kreek, ScaJGastr, 1970; 7:123). A delay in the late clearance of bromosulphthalein occurs, is exaggerated following ethinyloestradiol in women with this condition, and is seen in male family members (Reyes, Gastro, 1981; 81:226). Thus Reyes et al. concluded that there is 'a constitutional abnormality in the metabolic interactions between estrogens and the liver, independent of pregnancy itself' (Vore, Gastro, 1987; 93:643). Impairment of sulphation could lead to retention of cholestatic compounds, as sulphation of oestrogens and monohydroxy bile acids attenuates their cholestatic potential. Pregnancy decreases sulphation capacity, thus possibly contributing to the cholestasis of pregnancy (Davies, JHepatol, 1994; 21:1127).

Ethinyloestradiol causes a decrease in the bile salt independent fraction of bile flow, which may be related to changes in membrane fluidity (Simon, Gastro, 1978; 75:512). S-adenosyl-L-methionine is thought to be effective in this condition by changing membrane fluidity through an increase in the methylation of the constituent phospholipids. It may also increase the O-methylation of catechol (2-hydroxylated) oestrogens, reducing the irreversible hepatic microsomal membrane binding of these oestrogens. This may increase the 2-hydroxylation, reducing the load of oestrogen metabolites (Schriber, Hepatol, 1983; 3:607). Dexamethasone may work by suppressing fetoplacental oestrogen synthesis. Ursodeoxycholic acid modifies the bile acid pool by increasing hydrophilic and less cytotoxic bile salts.

Intrahepatic cholestasis of pregnancy is associated with other forms of intrahepatic cholestasis. Women with cholestasis related to oral contraceptives have a history of cholestasis in pregnancy in 50 per cent of cases (Kreek, ScaJGastr, 1970; 7:123). Benign recurrent intrahepatic cholestasis can be associated with intrahepatic cholestasis of pregnancy in the same family (de Pagter, Gastro, 1976; 71:202). Lastly, in arteriohepatic dysplasia, in which cholestasis is associated with multiple organ defects, cholestasis worsens during pregnancy (Riely, AnnIntMed, 1979; 91:520; Romero, AmJObsGyn, 1983; 147:108).

Idiopathic acute fatty liver of pregnancy

The first case report was in 1934 (Stander, AmJObsGyn, 1934; 28:61), but it was described by Tarnier in 1857 (Tarnier, CRSocBio, 1857; 3:209). However, it was Sheehan who first described obstetric yellow atrophy as a specific cause of jaundice in pregnancy, distinguishing it from fulminant hepatitis (acute yellow atrophy) by

the absence of liver necrosis in the presence of microvesicular fat (within swollen hepatocytes with central nuclei), and by periportal sparing (Sheehan, JObstetGynaecolBrEmp, 1940; 47:49). This condition is now known as acute fatty liver of pregnancy. It occurs solely in the last trimester of pregnancy, usually presenting between the 34th and 36th weeks of gestation; earlier presentation is so exceptional (Buytaert, AmJGastr, 1996; 91:603) that other diagnoses must be entertained.

Tetracycline administration gives a similar clinical and histological picture in non-pregnant women (Peters, AmJSurg, 1967; 113:622) and in women at any stage of pregnancy (Schultz, NEJM, 1965; 63:851).

The incidence of acute fatty liver of pregnancy is approximately 1 in 14 000 pregnancies (Pockros, Medicine, 1984; 63:1), but milder cases are probably undiagnosed. The cause is unknown; defects in carnitine and fatty acid binding proteins have been invoked, but there is no good evidence for this. Recently, it was found that a defect in long-chain fatty oxidation (long-chain 3-hydroxyacyl coenzyme A dehydrogenase deficiency) in the fetus was associated with the picture of acute fatty liver of pregnancy and/or HELLP in the mother (Schoemann, Gastro, 1991; 100:544); when the fetus was not affected the mother was normal (Wilcken, Lancet, 1993; 341:407). Heterozygosity in the mother is probably necessary for the development of the syndrome (Treen, Hepatol, 1994; 19:399). The molecular basis has been identified as a single amino acid substitution, guanosine to cytosine, in the α-subunit that catalyses the last three steps of β-oxidation (Sims, PNAS, 1995; 92:841). Prenatal diagnosis by using amniocytes is now possible (Nada, PrenatalDiagn, 1996; 16:117). Pregnancy decreases in vivo mitochondrial oxidation of fatty acids in mice (Grimbert, Hepatol, 1993; 17:628), and this effect is mediated by oestrogens and progesterones (Gimbert, AmJPhysiol, 1995; 268:G107).

Burroughs et al., and later others, reported an increased frequency in this condition of signs of pre-eclampsia (approximately 50 per cent), and an increased incidence in primigravidae (50 per cent), and in twin pregnancies (10 to 15 per cent), features also found in toxaemia in pregnancy.[5] Earlier reports also confirmed the coexistence of pre-eclampsia and acute fatty liver of pregnancy (Nardone, AmJObsGyn, 1960; 80:258). There is a large degree of overlap and a spectrum of clinical disease which has been termed 'hepatic toxaemia' (Riely, AnnIntMed, 1987; 106:703). The **HELLP** syndrome (haemolysis, hepatic enzyme elevation, and low platelets) has been described in acute fatty liver of pregnancy (Riely, AnnIntMed, 1987; 106:203). One patient had pre-eclampsia with liver function test abnormalities in one pregnancy and acute fatty liver of pregnancy in her next one—each time only alkaline phosphatase was raised (Brown, AmJObsGyn, 1990; 183:1154). Male births are more common than female with this condition.[5,6]

In sheep, pregnancy toxaemia is also known as twin lamb disease and occurs in the last two-fifths of gestation, but it may also be associated with a single large lamb. The liver is yellow and friable, and fatty degeneration is seen in proximal renal tubules. A sudden change in food intake is sometimes observed (Ferris, JCI, 1969; 48:1643).[7]

The classic description of the clinical presentation is of a sudden onset of malaise progressing rapidly to persistent nausea, repeated vomiting, heartburn, and upper abdominal pain. This is followed by jaundice, usually within 2 weeks of onset of symptoms, and then coma, anorexia, and weight loss. Jaundice may be mild and thus overlooked, but hyperbilirubinaemia is absent in less than 10 per cent of cases. Persistent nausea and vomiting are the most frequent symptoms, occurring in approximately 90 per cent of cases. Haematemesis is not uncommon due to oesophagitis, gastric erosions, and/ or ulceration, or very occasionally, oesophageal varices (Duma, AnnIntMed, 1965; 63:851), and is part of a bleeding diathesis which is often fatal.

With the severity of illness described above there are usually stillbirths, and the mother often dies in hepatic and renal failure. However, it is now clear that the disease has a much wider spectrum with less severe cases occurring without symptom progression, so that maternal and fetal mortality now average 10 and 20 per cent, respectively. Other symptoms include headaches, ankle swelling, polyuria, and polydipsia (Bourliere, JGynObsBiolReprod, 1989; 18: 79; Reyes, Gut 1994;35:101). Transient diabetes insipidus has been described (Cammy, BrJObsGyn, 1987; 94:173; Mizuno, EndocrinolJpn, 1987; 34:449) and this diagnosis may be missed (Fukuda, JpnJAnesth, 1993; 42:1511). There may be a history of urinary tract or other infections. In more severe cases the patient may present in labour, or with antepartum haemorrhage or intrauterine death. The obstetric complications usually parallel the severity of liver disease.

Fever is unusual, and if present is mild. Abdominal tenderness is common and ascites may be present. Hepatosplenomegaly is not usually present but occasionally the liver is palpable. Unsuspected gastrointestinal bleeding must be looked for. Coma ranges in severity and may be absent; flap may be present. Peripheral oedema, hypertension, or proteinuria are found in approximately 50 per cent of cases and may lead to an initial diagnosis of pre-eclampsia.[5] Occasionally, acute fatty liver of pregnancy is diagnosed 'late' as a cause of postpartum jaundice (Douvres, AmJDigDis, 1965; 10:306; Breen, Gut, 1970; 11:822).

The complications of acute fatty liver of pregnancy are those of fulminant liver disease; they add to the clinical spectrum and are often the cause of death (Hatfield, DigDisSci, 1972; 17:167). They include disseminated intravascular coagulation, hypoglycaemia, bleeding (particularly postpartum), and acute pancreatitis. Severe oesophagitis with rupture of the oesophageal wall (Worms, SocMedHopPar, 1966; 17:999) and oesophageal stricture have been documented (O'Loughlin, JIrishMedAss, 1971; 64:45). Subcapsular haematoma (Roh, JForensicSci, 1986; 31:1509), rupture of the liver (Minuk, AmJGastro, 1987; 82:457), and fat emboli (Jones, AmJGastr, 1993; 88:791) have been described.

Laboratory investigations are variable and their alterations depend on the severity of the clinical presentation. Anaemia is not seen unless bleeding or disseminated intravascular coagulation is present. Neutrophilia, with or without toxic granulation, is almost universal (usually $15 \times 10^9/l$ or more) and is sustained postpartum, as is thrombocytopenia (usually less than $100 \times 10^9/l$). Normoblasts, giant platelets, and target cells are seen in the blood film and give a clue to the diagnosis, as this picture is not seen in viral hepatitis and is rare in pre-eclampsia.[5] Basophilic stippling has also been reported.[5] Bone marrow examination shows a hypercellular marrow.[5]

Liver function tests usually show modest elevations of aminotransferase values (rarely above 500 u/l). Occasionally, patients have higher values in the absence of shock, but usually there has been significant hypotension.[6] Aminotransferase values fall immediately following delivery. Bilirubin concentrations may be markedly raised and usually peak postpartum. Serum albumin values may be lower than that expected in the third trimester of pregnancy, and fall further postpartum. Gammaglobulin concentrations and quantitative immunoglobulin are not elevated or only minimally so[5]—this may be helpful in distinguishing acute fatty liver of pregnancy from acute viral hepatitis. Alkaline phosphatase concentrations are raised above the normal increase due to the elevation of placental phosphatase. However, the histological placental abnormalities seen in pre-eclampsia have not been described,[5] and alkaline phosphatase tends to be lower in pre-eclampsia (Adeniyi, BrJObsGyn, 1984; 91:857), so part of the abnormal alkaline phosphatase probably has a liver origin. There are no good data on abnormalities of 5′-nucleotidase or γ-glutamyl transpeptidase. Prothrombin and partial thromboplastin times may be increased, particularly if jaundice is present; skin bleeding time is increased.[5] Evidence for disseminated intravascular coagulation, decreased fibrinogen, fragmented red cells in a blood film, and fibrin degradation products may be found (Holzbach, ObsGyn, 1974; 43:740; Muldin, ActaObGyn, 1978; 57:178; Laursen, ActaObGyn, 1983; 62:403).

Antithrombin III concentrations are low at the time of delivery in normal pregnancy (Hyde, JObsGynBrCommonw, 1973; 80:1059) and have been found to be even lower in acute fatty liver of pregnancy (Mosvold, ScaJHaematol, 1982; 29:48; Liebman, Ann IntMed, 1983; 98:330). The antithrombin III concentrations correlate with maternal and fetal morbidity (Weenik, AmJObsGyn, 1984; 148:1092). Plasma urea, uric acid, and creatinine are usually elevated even in the absence of jaundice and rise until delivery. Urinary sodium excretion is low,[5] and hyponatraemia and hyperkalaemia may be present. Renal function improves postpartum with a return to a normal creatinine clearance about 2 weeks postpartum. Uric acid concentrations may increase days before symptoms of acute fatty liver of pregnancy (Quigley, SouthMedJ, 1974; 67:142) and may provide a pointer towards its early diagnosis (Hsiung, JGynObsBiolReprod, 1988; 17:901).[5] Serum ammonia concentrations are high,[5] and return to normal within 48 h of delivery. There is generalized hypoaminoacidaemia (Weber, JLabClinMed, 1978; 94:27),[5] which is not seen in acute or fulminant viral hepatitis (Morgan, Gut, 1982; 23:362). Serum cholesterol concentrations tend to be low or normal in contradistinction to the increased concentrations found in pregnancy.[5] Coeliac angiography on day 1 postpartum showed vascular narrowing and irregularity of the vessel wall which resolved by day 45 postpartum (Matsuda, ObsGyn, 1994; 84:678).

Pathology

As with the clinical characteristics there is a wide variation in histological findings, which are also dependent on the timing of the liver histology in relation to delivery; the fatty infiltration resolves rapidly following delivery.[5,6] Classically, there is microvesicular fatty infiltration, without displacement of the central hepatocyte nuclei, most prominently around the central veins. It may extend throughout the lobule. Macrovesicular fat may also be seen in more severe cases.[6]

The fat must be looked for using Oil Red O, or other appropriate fat stains, in unfixed sections (Brow, AmJGastr, 1987; 82:554).

Necrosis is often absent but can occur (Czernobilsky, ObsGyn, 1965; 26:792; Joske, Gut, 1968; 9:489)[5,6] and is usually seen as cell drop-out. Bridging necrosis is not seen. Lobular inflammation is usually mild but may be severe leading to a misdiagnosis of viral hepatitis.[5,6] Portal inflammation is mild. Cholestasis is frequent with canalicular bile plugs. In some patients, hepatocytes are ballooned without vesicular fat and this appears to be the initial stage of fatty degeneration.[6] Intrasinusoidal fibrin deposits and microhaemorrhages have been described (Hannah, AmJObsGyn, 1989; 161:322),[5] but this feature, which is characteristic of toxaemia, has not been found in an autopsy series, suggesting that the clinical overlap of toxaemia and acute fatty liver of pregnancy may not be mirrored by the histological findings.[6] However, microvesicular fat has been found in livers of women with toxaemia and earlier series suggest that fatty degeneration is not infrequent in toxaemia. Microvesicular fat is found in the HELLP syndrome (Minakami, AmJObsGyn, 1988; 159:1043). Extramedullary haemopoiesis is often found and may be responsible for the normoblasts commonly seen in the blood films.[5,6]

Misinterpretation of liver biopsies, for example diagnosis of viral hepatitis (Brown, AmJGastr, 1987; 82:554),[5] may result in failure to recognize acute fatty liver of pregnancy (Bernuau, Gut, 1983; 24:340; Hay, BrJObsGyn, 1973; 80:280). Electron microscopy confirms the fat as droplets that are not bound to the membrane. There is also dilated endoplasmic reticulum (Duma, AnnIntMed, 1965; 63:851) and mitochondrial pleomorphism with paracrystalline deposits (Bettram, Gastro, 1978; 74:1008; Weber, JClinLabMed, 1978; 94:27),[5] but these have been shown in normal pregnancy (Perez, AmJObsGyn, 1971; 110:428) and pre-eclampsia (Rolfes, AmJGastr, 1986; 81:1138). Cytoplasmic degeneration may be found (Lamontagne, UnionMedCan, 1970; 99:1083). In two reports the fat consisted of free fatty acids (Eisele, AmJPathol, 1975; 81:545; Weber, JLabClinMed, 1979; 94:27), but in a more recent case report only 10 per cent of the amount previously described was found (Ockner, Hepatol, 1990; 11:59).

Follow-up liver biopsies are normal (Whitacre, JAMA, 1942; 118:1358; Duma, AnnIntMed, 1965; 63:851; Breen, Gut, 1970; 11:822).[5] Livers at autopsy are macroscopically yellow and are usually shrunken, but normal liver weights may be found.[5] Kidneys can have fat in proximal convoluted tubules (Ober, AmJMed, 1955; 19:743; Slater, Histopath, 1984; 8:567).[5] Heart and pancreas may also show fatty infiltration. Fetal livers are normal.[5]

Diagnosis

The first step is to think about the possibility of acute fatty liver of pregnancy as it has such a wide clinical spectrum. Nausea and vomiting in the last trimester of pregnancy should always be fully investigated. As acute fatty liver of pregnancy occurs solely in the last trimester, the differential diagnosis lies between acute or fulminant viral hepatitis, drug hepatitis, or toxaemia of pregnancy as 'hepatic' diagnoses. Obstetric causes of renal failure should also be considered, i.e. the spectrum of haemolytic uraemic syndrome and thrombotic thrombocytopenic purpura. Haemolytic uraemic syndrome usually occurs postpartum and consists of renal failure and microangiopathic haemolytic anaemia (its principal features), as well as gastrointestinal bleeding, thrombocytopenia, and disseminated intravascular coagulation. Thrombotic thrombocytopenic purpura

results in thrombocytopenia and microangiopathic anaemia, but there are usually neurological abnormalities (including epileptic fits) without disseminated intravascular coagulation. These conditions may have similar haematological and renal indices to acute fatty liver of pregnancy and mildly abnormal liver function tests.

If the patient presents later on in the illness, then the syndrome of jaundice, renal failure, and a bleeding diathesis may be due to severe pre-eclampsia, acute fatty liver of pregnancy, fulminant hepatitis, haemolytic uraemic syndrome, or thrombotic thrombocytopenic purpura. The history may yield clues as to contact with hepatitis or inadvertent use of drugs (unlikely in pregnancy). Neutrophilia is a feature of acute fatty liver of pregnancy and pre-eclampsia but not of viral hepatitis. A blood film is diagnostic of microangiopathic haemolytic anaemia as seen in the haemolytic uraemic syndrome, and may show a typical picture in acute fatty liver of pregnancy, i.e. neutrophilia, normoblasts, giant platelets and thrombocytopenia.[5] Clearly, serological markers for the acute hepatitides must be looked for but, as yet, there is no test for the diagnosis of acute hepatitis C. Acute herpes hepatitis is not often considered: aminotransferase levels are usually very high, mucocutaneous herpetic lesions should be sought (Goyette, ObsGyn, 1974; 43:191; Wertheim, ObsGyn, 1983; 62:385); acyclovir can cure herpes hepatitis in pregnancy (Klein, Gastro, 1991; 100:239).

Ultrasound should exclude the presence of biliary obstruction or gallstones. A CT scan is mandatory. As first suggested by Burroughs et al.,[5] fatty infiltration can be diagnosed by CT scan, and several reports have confirmed this; others have found it to be of no use, particularly in less severe cases (Usta, AmJObsGyn, 1994; 171:1342).Ultrasound is often normal (Campillo, AnnIntMed, 1986; 105:383). The CT attenuation values are usually only half the lower limit of the normal range and less than those of the spleen, which is the converse of normal. Resolution can be followed with a return to normal values at 3 weeks postpartum (McKee, BMJ, 1986; 292:291; Goodacre, JClinGastro, 1988, 10:680; Mabie, AmJObsGyn, 1988; 158:142; Clements, BrJObsGyn, 1990; 97:631). However, normal CT and ultrasound scans do not exclude the diagnosis (Le Van, JReprodMed, 1990; 32:815).

A CT scan may also show intrahepatic or subscapular haemorrhage (Roh, JForensicSci, 1986; 31:1509) which may progress to rupture (Minuk, AmJGastr, 1987; 82:457). These are seen in pre-eclampsia (Manas, NEJM, 1985; 312:424) and eclampsia (Bis, ObsGynSurv, 1976; 31:763). Nuclear magnetic resonance imaging has also been used (Farine, AmJPerinat, 1990; 7:316), but appears less sensitive (Werth, Gastro, 1990; 99:552).

If clotting and bleeding times are normal, a liver biopsy should be performed to confirm the diagnosis. A portion should be processed for fat staining and not fixed. If haemostasis is so abnormal that a standard percutaneous liver biopsy is not possible, delivery should be induced in any case. If a caesarian section is indicated a biopsy can be taken or performed as soon as the clotting is sufficiently improved for biopsy. Alternatively, a transjugular route or plugged transhepatic route can be used after delivery. If the differential diagnosis only lies between toxaemia and acute fatty liver of pregnancy, then delivery should be undertaken as soon as possible as this is the primary treatment for both conditions. A liver biopsy can follow more safely after delivery.

Treatment of acute fatty liver of pregnancy

Immediate delivery is the key to managing acute fatty liver of pregnancy. Resolution of the syndrome can only begin once delivery occurs. There are no reports of recovery before delivery. The highest frequency of survival for both mother and baby is reported when delivery is made by caesarian section or induced (Ebert, DigDisSci, 1984; 29:453).[5] Because acute fatty liver of pregnancy usually occurs later in pregnancy, the fetus is mature and can be delivered. If symptoms of acute fatty liver of pregnancy are mild, careful fetal monitoring can be made to try and prolong gestation (Riely, AnnIntMed, 1987; 106:703). However, progression of illness in the mother may be unpredictable and rapid. Vaginal delivery should be attempted first. Caesarian section may be done under spinal anaesthesia if coagulation is close to normal, otherwise general anaesthesia is preferable to avoid bleeding due to spinal puncture. Uteroplacental insufficiency has been documented as a cause of fetal distress (Moise, ObsGyn, 1987; 69:482).

The management regimen for the mother is the same as for any cause of acute or fulminant liver failure. Hypoglycaemia may continue or it may present for the first time postpartum and requires constant monitoring. The most severe problem is postpartum haemorrhage, which may be severe, persist for a few days, and appears out of proportion to the abnormalities in coagulation (Torres, GastroHepato, 1981; 4:188), often occurring in the absence of disseminated intravascular coagulation. Deficiency in antithrombin III may be responsible (Liebmann, AnnIntMed, 1983; 98:330). Fresh frozen plasma (which has high concentrations of antithrombin III) and platelets are the mainstay of treatment, both therapeutically and prophylactically, although bleeding can be severe despite their use.[5]

Cryoprecipitate and antithrombin III have also been administered (Laursen, ActaObGyn, 1983; 62:403). Heparin should not be used. Tying-off the hypogastric arteries or a hysterectomy may be necessary (Pockros, Medicine, 1984; 63:1).[5]

Renal failure responds to haemodialysis or haemofiltration.[5,6] Liver transplantation has been successful in those very rare cases in which supportive therapy following delivery does not lead to recovery (Ockner, Hepatol, 1990; 11:59).

Further pregnancies

Three recent series report successful pregnancies without recurrence of acute fatty liver of pregnancy even when the pregnancy has lasted spontaneously to term (Pockros, Medicine, 1984; 63:1; Riley, AnnIntMed, 1987; 106:703).[5] There have only been a few case reports of recurrence in subsequent pregnancies (Barton, AmJObsGyn, 1990; 163:534; Shoeman, Gastro, 1991; 100:544; Reyes, Gut 1994; 35:101; Visconti, JClinGastro, 1995; 21:243), and these were probably related to an unsuspected urea cycle enzyme defect in the fetus.

Tetracycline-induced fatty liver of pregnancy

The first report of this condition was in 1956, although no connection was made between the chlortetracycline administration and fatty liver (Moore, JObstetGynaecolBrEmp, 1956; 63:189). The association was made in 1963 (Shultz, NEJM, 1963; 269:999; Clinico-pathologic Conference, AmJMed, 1963; 35:231). Fatty liver due to tetracycline administered intravenously has occurred in the second trimester (Kunelis, AmJMed, 1965; 38:359), in nonpregnant women (Peters, AmJSurg, 1967; 113:622), in men (Lepper, ArchIntMed, 1951; 88:271), and in children, including the fetus (Davis, AmJObsGyn, 1966; 95:523), whereas the liver of the fetus is not affected by idiopathic acute fatty liver of pregnancy.[5] Oral tetracyclines have also been implicated (Wenke, ReprodMed, 1981, 135:26).

Other microvesicular fat diseases of the liver and defects in urea cycle enzymes

Acute fatty liver of pregnancy shares the morphological feature of microvesicular fat infiltration as well as several clinical features, such as hypoglycaemia, hyperammoniaemia, and coma, with a number of other conditions. However, in Reye's syndrome, which is seen occasionally in adults (Ede, BMJ, 1988; 296:517), the mitochondrial changes at electron microscopy are not those of acute fatty liver of pregnancy. In Reye's syndrome there is a non-specific decrease in the activity of mitochondrial enzymes of the urea cycle, whereas different abnormalities have been found in acute fatty liver of pregnancy (Weber, JLabClinMed, 1979; 94:27). Hepatic fatty acid concentrations are increased in some cases of acute fatty liver of pregnancy (Eisele, AmJPathol, 1975; 81:545) as in Reye's syndrome, but minimal fatty acid changes have been found by others (Ockner, Hepatol, 1990; 11:59).

Hypoglycin A (in unripe ackee fruit) is a unique toxin that inhibits mitochondrial oxidation of long-chain fatty acids and causes Jamaican vomiting sickness. Valproic acid has a chemical structure similar to hypoglycin A and causes a similar clinical syndrome in susceptible patients. Defects in fatty acid oxidation also cause lipid accumulation in the liver (Stanley, AdvPediat, 1987; 34: 89). Medium–chain acyl-CoA dehydrogenase deficiency produces a secondary deficiency in carnitine, which is an essential cofactor in fatty acid transport into mitochondria for oxidation. There are other syndromes leading to carnitine deficiency (Rebouche, Mayo ClinProc, 1983; 58:533). Pregnancy leads to relative deficiency and may precipitate symptoms in those with a genetic deficiency of carnitine (Angelini, AnnNeurol, 1978; 4:558; Harpey, JPediat, 1983; 103:394). It is not surprising, therefore, that carnitine deficiency has been invoked as a pathogenic pathway in acute fatty liver of pregnancy (Feller, Gastro, 1983; 84:1150A). However, the small percentage of hepatic fatty acids described in a recent report (Ockner, Hepatol, 1990; 11:59) does not support this hypothesis.

Other genetic defects, such as mutations at the X-chromosome locus for ornithine carbamoyl transferase have been shown to cause hyperammoniac coma in the first 10 days postpartum (Arn, NEJM, 1990; 22:1652). It occurs in otherwise healthy women who deliver infants (usually female) who do not exhibit a homozygous deficiency in ornithine carbamoyl transferase. It is postulated that the healthy fetus *in utero* provides the enzymatic activity for the mother. Diagnosis is made by finding raised maternal plasma ammonia and glutamine concentrations. Early treatment with sodium benzoate, sodium phenylacetate, and arginine hydrochloride will reverse the syndrome by correcting ammonia concentrations (Brusilow, NEJM, 1984; 310:1630). The heterozygous state can be detected by an allopurinol stress test (Hauser, NEJM, 1990; 322:1641) or immunocytochemical staining of duodenal biopsy specimens (Hamano, NEJM, 1988; 318:1521).

Hypertension-associated liver dysfunction of pregnancy

Pre-eclampsia and eclampsia

In developed countries hypertension and pregnancy-induced hypertension are still the major cause of maternal death (Chesley, ClinObstetGynecol, 1984; 27:801). Pre-eclampsia is diagnosed when there is rapid weight gain indicative of oedema (often manifest by ankle oedema) together with proteinuria and hypertension, in the second or third trimester of pregnancy; a blood pressure above 140/90 mmHg in the absence of previous hypertension; or an increase in 30 mmHg systolic or 15 mmHg diastolic pressure when there is pre-existing hypertension. Eclampsia by definition requires the occurrence of fits. In between mild pre-eclampsia and eclampsia there is symptomatic end-organ disease (i.e. brain, kidney, and liver), with headache, visual disturbances, upper abdominal pain, and oliguria with renal failure. Cerebral haemorrhage is the major cause of death in eclampsia but hepatic complications may account for up to 16 per cent of deaths, usually due to hepatic rupture which was found in 18 per cent of cases.[8]

The hepatic abnormalities increase in severity with the severity of the pre-eclamptic process. The major symptom is epigastric or right upper quadrant pain with a tender but usually normal-sized liver. Surgical emergencies may be mimicked by the abdominal symptoms (Goodlin, AmJObsGyn, 1976; 125:747). With mild hypertension, 24 per cent of patients are said to have abnormal liver function tests[9] and this rises to over 80 per cent with severe hypertension. The principal hepatic abnormality is a rise in aminotransferase values. In most cases there is no bilirubin rise unless there is haemolysis or hepatic infarction associated with the severe pre-eclampsia or eclampsia. Antithrombin III concentrations are inversely correlated with outcome in severe pre-eclampsia (Weenink, AmJObsGyn, 1984; 148:1092). In mild pre-eclampsia there may be no hepatic histological abnormalities on light microscopy (Anita, Lancet, 1958; ii:776), but focal necrosis may be seen—17 per cent in one series (Maqueo, ObsGyn, 1964; 23:222). Immunofluorescence studies show fibrinogen deposition in sinusoids and the degree of staining is correlated with the increase in aspartate aminotransferase values (Arias, NEJM, 1976: 295:578). This lesion is found in asymptomatic patients. In severe cases the characteristic hepatic lesions are fibrin deposition in the space of Disse with associated haemorrhages—leading to hepatocyte necrosis. Periportal bleeding occurs with increased severity, probably due to the raised blood pressure which 'dissects' the portal connective tissue.

In the most severe cases large infarcts and haematomas may develop (Manas, NEJM, 1985; 312:424), and may rupture (Bis, ObsGyn, 1976; 31:763). Liver infarcts can also occur due to hepatic arterial thrombosis, which can resolve spontaneously, and this gives rise to very high aminotransferase values (Dammann, DigDisSci, 1982; 27:73).

The management for hepatic abnormalities is that of pre-eclampsia. Early delivery is the key to improvement for both the hypertensive and liver complications. The liver function tests show a typical pattern after delivery, with aminotransferase values falling after 24 h and bilirubin falling by 72 h, but alkaline phosphatase and γ-glutamyl transpeptidase rising on day 5 or 6, peaking on day 10, and returning to normal by 8 weeks (Rowan, Lancet, 1995; 345:1367). This cholestatic pattern is similar to the recovery following an ischaemic insult. A CT or ultrasound scan should be done to detect subclinical liver haematoma and infarcts (Kronthal, Radiol, 1990; 177:726). The pathogenesis of the liver lesions is still disputed. Fibrin deposition secondary to disseminated intravascular coagulation was thought to be the initiating event (McKay, AmJObsGyn, 1953; 66:507; Page, JObsGynBrCommonw, 1971; 79:883). However, only a few patients have evidence of disseminated intravascular coagulation. The other principal hypothesis is that of segmental vasospasm which progresses to a generalized vasculopathy due to endothelial cell injury.[8] If there is widespread damage the hepatic injury has been likened to the generalized Schwartzman reaction (Mori, VirchArchA, 1979; 382:179). There is a microangiopathy evidenced by an isolated thrombocytopenia (Bern, ObsGyn, 1981; 57:265). The latter is known to develop before hypertension (Romero, AmJPerinat, 1989; 6:32). The thrombocytopenia occurs without significant alteration of other coagulation factors (Gibson, SemThrombHaemost, 1982, 8:234). Abnormalities of coagulation factors have been documented in cord blood, suggesting that fetal hepatic synthesis is impaired (Lox, BiolNeon, 1990; 57:141).

Liver rupture

Liver infarcts, haematomas, and liver rupture in pregnancy are associated with severe pre-eclampsia and eclampsia in 80 per cent of cases (Neerhof, ObsGynSurv, 1989; 44:407), and have also been reported in acute fatty liver of pregnancy (Minuk, AmJGastr, 1987; 82:457) and with cocaine use (Moen, ObsGyn, 1993; 82:687). The first report occurred in 1844 (Abercrombie, LondMedGazz, 1844; 34:792). The management has changed in emphasis in recent years as the presence of haematomas without rupture has been recognized with ultrasound and CT scan (Herbert, NYStateJMed, 1986; 86:286). The haematoma is almost always confined to the right lobe, in the anterior or superior aspect, while ruptures occur from the interior margin. Penetration of the diaphragm with haemothorax has been reported (Castaneda, AmJObsGyn, 1970; 107:578), as well as concomitant rupture of a hepatic vein (Johanson, JObsGyn, 1990; 10:210).

Rupture occurs in the third trimester or postpartum. The risk of rupture is increased in older pregnant women and with late presentation of the underlying pre-eclampsia. It presents with sudden abdominal pain associated with nausea and vomiting, shock may develop very quickly (Editorial, BMJ, 1976; ii:1278) and the condition may mimic a perforated viscus. Mortality of hepatic rupture in early series was approximately 60 per cent for both mother and baby (Bis, ObsGynSurv, 1976; 31:763), with a lower mortality with surgical intervention (Stalter, Surgery, 1985; 98:112; Neerhof, ObsGynSurv, 1989; 44:407).[10] However, hepatic arterial embolization has also been successful (Loevinger, ObsGyn, 1985; 65:281; Terasaki, Radiol, 1990; 174:1039), as well as hepatic artery ligation (Naraynsingh, WIMedJ, 1984; 33:198; Stain, AnnSurg, 1996; 224:72). Conservative management of rupture has also been reported (Ekberg, AnnChirGyn, 1984; 73:350).

Conservative management of hepatic haematomas is now the initial therapy of choice, but very close monitoring is required

(Goodlin, JReprodMed, 1985; 30:368; Manas, NEJM, 1985; 312:424; Woodhouse, BrJObsGyn, 1986; 93:1097) and facilities for urgent laparotomy must be available. Liver transplantation may be necessary and has been successfully performed (Hunter, ObsGyn, 1995; 85:819). The baby should be delivered by caesarian section.[10] Infection may develop in the haematoma and associated infarcted area. Successful pregnancy has been reported after hepatic rupture (Salkala, ObsGyn, 1986; 68:124; Alleman, Eur-JObsGynReprodBiol, 1992; 47:76), but haemorrhage can recur with future pregnancies so these need to be monitored carefully (Greenstein, Gastro, 1994; 106:1668).

Other causes of hepatic rupture are adenoma (Hibbard, AmJObsGyn, 1976; 126:334), haemangioma (Bisk, ObsGynSurv, 1976; 31:763), hepatocellular carcinoma (Roddie, BMJ, 1957; i:31), choriocarcinoma (Barnard, GynOncol, 1986; 25:73), and amoebic abscesses (Yen, ObsGyn, 1964; 23:783). Spontaneous rupture of large spleens also occurs in pregnancy, mostly in the third trimester (Henderson, AustNZJObsGyn, 1979, 19:116).

HELLP syndrome

Pregnancy-associated hypertension has a wide spectrum of severity and so too has the presentation of liver abnormalities. A syndrome of haemolysis, abnormal liver function tests, and low platelet levels has been described (Fletcher, MedJAust, 1971; i:1065; Killam, AmJObsGyn, 1975; 123:823; Goodlin, AmJObsGyn, 1978; 132:595), which in 1982 was given the acronym HELLP syndrome—haemolysis, elevated liver enzymes, and low platelets (Weinstein, AmJObsGyn, 1982; 142:159). This presentation can be associated with hypertension (but has been recognized without it), may be found in the absence of proteinuria (Goodlin, ObsGyn, 1981; 58:743),[11] and may precede hypertension (Dantzer, RevFrGynObs, 1987; 82:243); it may also occur early in pregnancy as a complication of the antiphospholipid syndrome (Alsulyman, ObsGyn, 1996; 88:644). Liver haemorrhage can occur (Lee, ClinNuclMed, 1988; 9:635). The syndrome occurs more often in older Caucasian multiparous women who present late with their pre-eclamptic disease.[12]

There is a wide spectrum in the definition used to report the HELLP syndrome. A well-categorized series identified 112 cases out of 1153 (9.7 per cent) patients with pre-eclampsia over 8 years.[12] The evaluation was made only in patients with platelet counts below 100×10^9/l, a blood film which showed fragmented red cells, and elevated values of bilirubin, lactate dehydrogenase, and aspartate aminotransferase (4 standard deviations above normal). Amongst this group there were two maternal deaths, two ruptured livers, and a 37 per cent perinatal mortality, comprising a 19 per cent fetal mortality associated with a 20 per cent abruptio placentae; 38 per cent of mothers had intravascular coagulopathy. Only one recurrence was reported in a subsequent pregnancy. From this series a policy of early delivery was advocated. Another series, based simply on increase in aminotransferase values, a platelet count of less than 150×10^9/l, and serum haptoglobin of less than 0.7 g/l, gave a 19 per cent incidence (Abroug, IntensCareMed, 1992; 18:274).

In very severe cases liver transplantation has been performed (Erhard, ZblChir, 1994; 119:298). However, there are reports of spontaneous recovery (Clark, JReprodMed, 1986; 31:70). A good outcome has been reported with conservative management (Mackenna, ObsGyn, 1983; 62:751), use of plasma expansion (Goodlin, ObsGyn, 1981; 58:743) plasmapheresis (Martin, AmJObsGyn, 1990; 162:126), and steroids administered pre- (Magann, AmJObsGyn, 1994; 171:1148) and postpartum (Magann, AmJObsGyn, 1994; 171:1154). More recently, treatment with either 5-nitrosoglutathione (a nitric oxide donor with a potent inhibitory effect on platelet activation) used on the basis that pre-eclampsia may represent a systemic disorder of nitric oxide deficiency (de Belder, Lancet 1994; 345:124), and also prostacyclin and plasmapheresis (Huber, Lancet, 1994; 343:848) resulted in a good outcome. It is probable that mild cases can be monitored and delivery delayed for a day or two in order to try to mature the fetal lung. A recent report has shown that nifedipine (possibly by decreasing concentrations of thromboxane, and thus increasing the pro-stacyclin–thromboxane ratio which promotes prostaglandin I_2 synthesis) improves platelet counts, liver dysfunction, and high blood pressure in patients with HELLP syndrome (Lurie, JObsGyn, 1990; 10:492). The suggestion that the HELLP syndrome is part of the 'vasculopathy' of hypertensive disease of pregnancy is supported by a report of carotid artery thrombosis associated with the HELLP syndrome (Katz, AmJPerinat, 1989; 6:1360).

Overlap between acute fatty liver of pregnancy and hypertension-associated liver dysfunction of pregnancy

As discussed earlier, many patients with acute fatty liver of pregnancy have signs of pre-eclampsia. Acute fatty liver of pregnancy and the hepatic dysfunction associated with hypertension may be part of the same spectrum. Indeed both Sheehan and Lynch[13] and more recently Rolfes and Ishak[8] found fatty livers in a proportion of patients with eclampsia. A more interesting study showed that all of 41 patients with pre-eclampsia and liver dysfunction had microvesicular fat with Oil Red O staining; the density of fat staining correlated with serum urate concentration and was inversely correlated with platelet count; only 11 had fat visible by conventional stains (Minakami, AmJObsGyn, 1988; 159:1043). This was also shown in another series (Dani, AmJGastr, 1996; 91:292) in which laparoscopy did not show fatty infiltration. This may explain why a CT scan shows a normal density in HELLP syndrome (Mabie, AmJObsGyn, 1988; 158:142). A case report has shown HELLP syndrome in one pregnancy followed by acute fatty liver of pregnancy in a consecutive pregnancy, both manifested solely by a rise in serum alkaline phosphatase concentration (Brown, AmJObsGyn, 1990; 163:1154). Another case report has shown features of acute fatty liver of pregnancy and pre-eclampsia histologically, but without proteinuria or hypertension, the clinical syndrome resolving before delivery (Hannah, AmJObsGyn, 1989; 161:322).

Budd–Chiari syndrome

This syndrome has an increased incidence in pregnancy; most patients present during the immediate postpartum period but may present as late as 2 weeks postpartum (Ilan, AmJObsGyn, 1990; 162:1164). It is related to the increased hypercoagulable state which is probably due to lower antithrombin III concentrations at the time of delivery in normal pregnancy (Hyde, JObsGynBrCommonw, 1973; 80:1059). The fetus is unaffected but maternal mortality is high (Khuroo, AmJMed, 1980; 68:113; Oettinger, JObsGyn-BrCommw, 1970; 77:174; Tiliacos, PostgradMedJ, 1978; 54:686). Earlier recognition followed immediately by short-term anti-fibrinolytic therapy delivered through the hepatic artery, and then long-term anticoagulation, may improve maternal survival, but this has yet to be documented. Retrograde injection into the hepatic vein is technically difficult. A successful subsequent pregnancy has been reported in three patients, only one of whom had a shunt before conception (Powell-Jackson, QJMed, 1982; 201:79; Vons, Lancet, 1984; ii:975).

Gestational choriocarcinoma

Hepatic metastases may rupture (Barnard, GynOncol, 1986; 25:73; Alveyn, PostgradMedJ, 1988; 64:941; Wany, ChinMedJ, 1988; 101:637).

Pregnancy in pre-existing liver disease

As cirrhosis is associated with amenorrhoea and anovulation, pregnancy is rare in women with chronic progressive liver disease. The amenorrhoea is due to hypothalamic–pituitary dysfunction and is not directly related to the severity of the liver disease (Cundy, Gut, 1991; 32:2020). Pregnancy can be sustained without worsening of hepatic function, but there is a high fetal wastage due to stillbirths, low birth-weight babies, and prematurity (Cheng, AmJObsGyn, 1977; 128:812); however, there is no increase in fetal abnormalities (Whelton, ObsGyn, 1970; 36:31; Schieyer, ObsGynSurv, 1982; 37:304).

Unconjugated maternal bilirubin crosses the placenta and, in cases of severe maternal jaundice, neonatal kernicterus (Hsia, NEJM, 1952; 247:668) may develop requiring exchange transfusions (Cotton, ObsGyn, 1981; 57(Suppl):265; Waffarin, AmJDisChild, 1982; 136:416). However, no neurological deficit has been seen even when the bilirubin concentrations are very high (Waffarin, AmJDisChild, 1982; 136:416). There is no clear evidence for an increase in variceal bleeding, but if bleeding occurs the fetus may be lost. Pregnancies in patients with chronic liver disease should be closely monitored and followed in centres which have skills in critical neonatal care. The incidence of postpartum haemorrhage is increased in patients with cirrhosis, but not in those with extrahepatic portal venous obstruction (Cheng, AmJObsGyn, 1977; 128:812).

Chronic persistent and chronic active hepatitis

Chronic persistent hepatitis from any cause is a mild lesion and ovulation and fertility are not significantly altered. Normal pregnancy has been described in seven women during a 3- to 8-year follow-up (Infeld, Gastro, 1979; 77:524). Immunoprophylaxis at birth should be given to the fetus of a mother who has a viral aetiology.

Women with autoimmune or steroid-responsive chronic active hepatitis, who are properly treated, are fertile and have successful pregnancies, although there was a higher fetal wastage and up to 30 per cent prematurity in one series (Steven, QJMed, 1979; 48:519). The patients usually conceive in a period when the necroinflammatory activity is well controlled. There may be a higher

frequency of anovulatory cycles accounting for the infertility. Ovulation can be induced with clomiphene. There is no evidence that azathioprine is teratogenic (Steven, JMed, 1979; 48:519), but this drug is often discontinued during pregnancy. There is no evidence of an increased or decreased susceptibility to relapse of the hepatic inflammatory activity during pregnancy.

Primary biliary cirrhosis

Since the disease is usually diagnosed at the end of or after the reproductive age, there are no reports of pregnancy in patients with asymptomatic primary biliary cirrhosis, but, as many patients have had successful pregnancies before their diagnosis, this implies that some women with undiagnosed asymptomatic primary biliary cirrhosis have successful pregnancies. Indeed, the diagnosis may become apparent following pregnancy or during the last trimester (Ahrens, Medicine, 1950; 29:299; Rabinowitz, DigDisSci, 1995; 40:571).

Pregnancy has been reported with symptomatic primary biliary cirrhosis (Ahrens, Medicine, 1950; 29:299; Whelton, Lancet, 1968; ii:995; Nir, IntJGynObs, 1989; 28:279). Pruritus did not increase, but survival was short due to the severity of liver disease. If cholestyramine is used, vitamin K must be given before delivery. Ursodeoxycholic acid has been used without sequelae to control itching (Rudi, ZGastr, 1996; 34:188).

Primary sclerosing cholangitis

There are few reports of pregnancy in patients affected by primary sclerosing cholangitis. A similar picture to primary biliary cirrhosis exists, although in one case fetal compromise occurred with bile acid concentrations greater than 2000 mg/dl in the fetal circulation (Nolan, ObsGyn, 1994; 84:695).

Chronic viral hepatitis

For a discussion, see Section 12.

Alcoholic liver disease

The incidence of pregnancy in patients with alcoholic liver disease appears low, with very few reports of full-term pregnancies. The exact relationship of the fetal alcohol syndrome to liver disease is unknown.

Familial hyperbilirubinaemia

Gilbert's syndrome is unaffected by pregnancy (Friedlander, AmJObsGyn, 1967; 97:894). In the Dubin–Johnson syndrome the conjugated hyperbilirubinaemia increases during the third trimester, returning to prepregnancy levels after delivery (Cohen, Gastro, 1972; 62:1182). In Rotor syndrome there is no change in bilirubin concentration (Dizoglio, ObsGyn, 1973; 42:560).

Haemochromatosis and Wilson's disease

In women, haemochromatosis is usually diagnosed after the menopause. Many have had successful pregnancies before the diagnosis was made; they may have had a degree of iron overload, but probably no cirrhosis.

Pregnancy has been reported in treated Wilson's disease when necroinflammatory activity was controlled or absent, but rarely when the cirrhosis was decompensated (Nunns, Eur-JObsGynReprodBiol, 1995; 62:141). D-Penicillamine treatment must be continued during pregnancy. Cessation of the drug has resulted in haemolysis and worsening of liver function (Scheinbert, NEJM, 1975; 293:1300; Walshe, QJMed, 1977; 46:73). A reduction in dose to 250 mg/day in the last 6 weeks is advocated, but there is no clear rationale for this (Miehle, ZRheumatol, 1988; 47(Suppl. 1):20). Only one congenital malformation has been reported with D-penicillamine in a patient with cystinuria (Mjolnerod, Lancet, 1971; i:673). Trientine is also safe in pregnancy (Walshe, QJMed, 1986; 58:81; Devesa, JPediatGastrNutr, 1995; 20:102).

Liver tumours in pregnancy

Focal nodular hyperplasia (McMullan, AJR, 1973; 117:380; Whelan, AnnSurg, 1973; 177:150), adenomas (Kent, ObsGyn, 1978; 51:148; Rooks, JAMA, 1979; 242:644), hepatocellular carcinoma (Hayes, BMJ, 1977; ii:1394; Egwatu, TrRSocTropMedHyg, 1980; 74:793; Christensen, ActaObGyn, 1981; 60:519), and cholangiocarcinoma (Purtilo, AmJObsGyn, 1975; 121:41) have all been reported in pregnancy. Adenomas are the most common and are related to prior oral contraceptive use; they have a tendency to enlarge and to undergo haemorrhage and rupture during pregnancy, probably as a result of oestrogen stimulation. Pregnancy is thus contraindicated in the presence of an unresected adenoma, although there is a single case report of uneventful pregnancy (Kent, ObsGyn, 1978; 51:148). Successful pregnancy without recurrence of neoplasm has been reported (Check, ObsGyn, 1978; 52(Suppl):285). The median survival of pregnant women with hepatocellular carcinoma is shorter than for non-pregnant women (Lau, Cancer, 1995; 75:2669). Rupture may occur with hepatocellular carcinomas as well as adenomas (Roddie, BMJ, 1957; I:31; Hibbard, AmJObsGyn, 1964, 126:334), and with hepatic choriocarcinomas (Erb, AmJEmergMed, 1989; 7: 196), and testicular teratomas (Fidas-Kamini, AmJUrol, 1987; 60: 80).

Hepatic porphyrias

The effect of pregnancy on the course of acute intermittent porphyria is unpredictable (Hunter, JObsGynBrCommonw, 1871; 78: 746; Kanaan, ObsGynSurv, 1989; 44:244).[14] Hereditary coproporphyria may also worsen during pregnancy. However, serious or fatal complications are rare, as is also the case for variegate porphyria. Perinatal mortality is increased.

Schistosomiasis

Hepatic schistosomiasis is a common cause of portal hypertension worldwide. However, the reports of pregnancy in this disease are few (Fahmy, JKuwaitMedAssoc, 1971; 5:121; Britton, AmJSurg, 1982; 143:421; Soto-Albors, JReprodMed, 1984; 29:345).

Vascular abnormalities in the liver

Arteriovenous fistulas may lead to high-output cardiac failure when the already high cardiac output increases with pregnancy (Gong, ObsGyn, 1988; 72:440). Increased shunting, which reversed after

pregnancy, has been described in hereditary haemorrhagic telangiectasia (Livneh, SouthMedJ, 1988; 81:1047). Bleeding varices in pregnancy have been reported in a patient with portal cavernous haemangioma (Malaguarnera, Lancet, 1996; 347:727).

Variceal bleeding in pregnancy

Theoretically, the increase in circulating blood volume, cardiac output, central venous pressure, and azygous blood flow due to the pressure of the gravid uterus, should tend to increase portal pressure, and thus increase the probability of variceal bleeding in pregnant patients with varices, although the vasodilatation seen in pregnancy may tend to counteract this. Evidence for an increased risk of haemorrhage was not found in pregnant patients with varices in a large retrospective review (Cheng, AmJObsGyn, 1977; 128: 812; Britton, AmJSurg, 1982; 143:421), although some authors have reported more frequent variceal bleeding, particularly in non-cirrhotic portal hypertension (Varma, ObsGyn, 1977; 50:217).

Bleeding should be treated as in the non-pregnant patient except that vasoactive drugs should not be used because they may cause ischaemia of the placenta. Particular care should be taken to prevent hypotension. Sclerotherapy is as successful in stopping bleeding as in non-pregnant patients (Kochlar, AmJGastr, 1990; 85:1132), and does not interfere with subsequent conception (Salena, GastrEnd, 1988; 34:422; Kochlar, AmJGastr, 1990; 85:1132; Augustine, Gastr-End, 1989; 5:467).

Shunt surgery has been successfully performed during pregnancy without loss of the fetus (Chapis, AmJObsGyn, 1964; 90:272; Johnston, BrJObsGyn, 1965; 72:292; Brown, AmJSurg, 1971; 37: 441; Cheng, AmJObsGyn, 1977; 128:812; O'Leary, ObsGyn, 1982; 58:243; Chatoopadhyay, JpnJSurg, 1984; 14:405; Krol Van Stratten, NethJMed, 1984; 27:14). Pregnancy has been reported in patients after a portacaval shunt (Niven, AmJObsGyn, 1971; 110:1100); all cases had extrahepatic venous obstruction (Cheng, AmJObsGyn, 1977; 128:812). Prophylactic treatment with β-blockers may be indicated if the varices are large and have red signs, although propranolol may give rise to some intrauterine growth retardation (Rubin, NEJM, 1981; 305:1323). Rupture of splenic artery aneurysm may be more common in pregnancy (Barnett, ObsGyn, 1981; 157:255).

Contraception for women with chronic liver disease

Effective birth control should be used where clinically indicated. Although many recommend avoiding oral contraceptives, there is no evidence of increased susceptibility to side-effects in chronic liver disease and it remains the most effective female contraceptive method. The possible risks must be considered against the potential risk of pregnancy.

Liver disease not specific to pregnancy
Acute viral hepatitis

This is the most common cause of jaundice in pregnant women.[2] For all forms of viral hepatitis except epidemic non-A, non-B hepatitis, the clinical presentation, complications, course, and outcome are the same as in non-pregnant women. In this section the particular problems associated with pregnancy will be addressed.

The management should be conservative. Medication should be avoided. Serological diagnosis coupled with ultrasound is usually all that is necessary to establish a diagnosis. Amniocentesis is best avoided as it could be a source of infection for the fetus. Breast feeding is not contraindicated (Beasley, Lancet, 1975; i:740). Immunoprophylaxis of the fetus is the mainstay to prevent spread. There is a slight increase in prematurity (Hieber, JPediat, 1977; 91: 545), but no increased risk of malformation. Obstetric management should follow standard lines. Acute viral hepatitis may be misdiagnosed as acute fatty liver of pregnancy (Brown, AmJGastr, 1987; 82:554).[5]

Hepatitis A

There is no evidence that this is more common or more severe in pregnancy (Shalev, IntJGynObs, 1982; 20:73; Zhuang, ChungHua-FuChan, 1989; 24:136). The only risk to the fetus is if the mother is viraemic at the time of delivery, although anti-HAV appears early in the illness and does cross the placenta. Passive prophylaxis with 0.5 ml of immune serum globulin appears to protect the infant against infection, although there are no specific data to prove this. A single case report of fatal relapsing viral hepatitis A has been reported during pregnancy following the initial attack 5 months earlier (Lysy, IsrJMedSci, 1988; 24:681).

Hepatitis B

There is no evidence that the outcome of hepatitis B in the pregnant patient differs from that in non-pregnant women. Transmission to the fetus at birth occurs in 50 per cent of infants delivered to mothers with acute hepatitis (Gerety, JPediat, 1977; 90:368), and the risk is almost 70 per cent if the acute hepatitis started in the third trimester (Tong, Gastro, 1981; 80:999). Where the mother is a chronic hepatitis B carrier the risk of transmission is approximately 5 per cent. The risk of transmission is highest in Chinese due to the higher rate of HBeAg seropositivity;[15] indeed at least 90 per cent of infants born to HBeAg-positive mothers become infected and at least 80 per cent of these become chronic HBsAg carriers.[15] The child is usually asymptomatic until adult life. Spontaneous transient reactivation of chronic hepatitis B has been described in a mother positive for anti-HBe positive (Rawal, Lancet, 1991; 337:364).

All infants of HBsAg-positive mothers should receive immunoprophylaxis as the risk is not always correlated with the HBeAg status of the mother, and may be related to the presence of hepatitis B variants (with absent HBeAg expression). The regimen is hepatitis-B immunoglobulin at birth (0.5 ml intramuscularly), followed by HBV vaccine (10 mg) intramuscularly within 7 days of birth and 1 and 6 months later (Maupas, Lancet, 1981; i:289; Beasley, Lancet, 1983; ii:1099; Stevens, JAMA, 1985; 253:1750). A schedule of vaccination at birth, and at 1, 2, and 12 months results in higher anti-HBs titres (Anon, MMWR, 1990; 39:405). Effective prophylaxis depends on identification of HBsAg-positive mothers. A screening programme at 14 weeks gestation has been shown to be effective (Grosheide, BMJ, 1995; 311:1197). Postexposure prophylaxis of immunoglobulin and hepatitis B vaccine can be given

safely (Grosheide, EurJObsGynReprodBiol, 1993; 50:53). One report suggests that HBV replication in one mother decreased postpartum and then increased 1 to 2 months after delivery (Lin, JMedVirol, 1989; 29:1).

Hepatitis C

Studies in which acute non-A, non-B hepatitis was diagnosed by exclusion showed transmission to infants, evidenced by persistent aminotransferase elevations over a 10-month period (Tong, Gastro, 1981; 80:999); transmission was only shown with acute non-A, non-B hepatitis in the last trimester. Transmission with chronic non-A, non-B hepatitis has also been shown in a similar manner (Wejstal, ScaJInfectDis, 1989; 21:485). Seroconversion for anti-HCV antibodies (C-100 ELISA) has been shown in infants of 6 to 12 months of age born to mothers who had anti-HCV and anti-HIV antibodies (Giovanni, Lancet, 1990; 335:1166; Zanetti, Lancet, 1995; 345:289), but this is rare in mothers negative for anti-HIV and of the order of 0 to 2 per cent (Marcellin, DigDisSci, 1992; 38:2151; Meisel, Lancet, 1995; 345:1209), despite the presence of HCV-RNA in cord blood in many women (Silverman, AmJObstGyn, 1995; 173:1396). Chronic hepatitis C is not adversely affected by the pregnancy, and vice versa (Floreani, BrJObsGyn, 1996; 103:325).

Hepatitis D

Unlike hepatitis B this is rarely transmitted to the newborn (Zanetti, JMedVirol, 1982; 9:139), probably because the viral load of HBV is low. Anti-HDV antibodies are passively transmitted to the fetus and disappear within 3 months. Immunoprophylaxis for hepatitis B will prevent transmission of hepatitis D.

Hepatitis E

This epidemic, water-borne form of viral hepatitis has been recognized as having a worse prognosis and is more frequent in pregnancy. In India, mortality was 17.3 per cent in pregnant women, 2.1 per cent in non-pregnant women, and 2.8 per cent in men (Khuroo, AmJMed, 1981; 70:252). In Libya, non-B hepatitis has a very high mortality (Christie, Lancet, 1976; ii:827). In Algeria, the mortality was 100 per cent in those whose hepatitis was not serologically A or B (Belabbes, JMedVirol, 1985; 16:257). Infection with hepatitis E agent is the reason for the difference in mortality statistics for pregnant women with acute viral hepatitis in developed and developing countries (Khartoum, JGynObsBiolReprod, 1980; 9:887; Nouasria, AnnTropMed, 1986; 80:623). Nutritional factors are not important in this respect. Acute viral hepatitis is a leading cause of maternal mortality in developing countries (Kwast, Int JGynObs, 1987; 25:99). HEV has been detected in the liver of a patient with a fatal fulminant viral hepatitis in pregnancy who had anti-HEV in serum (Asher, JMedVirol, 1990; 31:229) and is the principal cause of the high mortality of viral hepatitis in the last trimester of pregnancy (Hamid, JHepatol, 1996; 25:20). Transmission to the fetus has not as yet been recognized. It is reasonable to give 0.5 ml of immune serum globulin intramuscularly at birth if hepatitis E is suspected or diagnosed in the mother.

Hepatitis G

Vertical transmission has been studied and seems higher than for HIV and HCV, but the clinical consequences are not known (Feucht, Lancet, 1996; 347:615).

Amoebiasis

Several cases of amoebic abscess have presented in pregnancy (Naidoo, SAMedJ, 1974; 48:1159; Wagner, ObsGyn, 1975; 45:562). Rupture of amoebic abscesses is well described (Yen, ObsGyn, 1964; 23:783; Cowan, SAMedJ, 1978; 53:460; Mitchell, BrJObsGyn, 1984; 91:393). Some consider that pregnancy confers an increased susceptibility to amoebiasis (Cowan, SAMedJ, 1978; 53:460) with an increased mortality (Abioye, TrRSocTropMedHyg, 1972; 66:754), but this is not generally accepted. Management and treatment with metronidazole is the same as for non-pregnant patients.

Herpes hepatitis and other infections

Herpes hepatitis is rare, but may be fulminant—mucocutaneous lesions must be looked for as acyclovir is an effective treatment (Flewett, JClinPath, 1969; 22:60; Goyette, ObsGyn, 1974; 43:191; Wertheim, ObsGyn, 1983; 62:385; Pauranik, JpnJMed 1987; 26:84; Klein, Gastro, 1991; 100:239; Jacques, HumPath, 1992; 23:183; Glorioso, DigDisSci, 1996; 41:1273). Leptospirosis has been described and has the same clinical features as in non-pregnant females.[16] Malaria may give rise to hepatitic liver dysfunction (Arya, JAssocPhysInd, 1988; 36:294). Pyogenic abscess (Kopernik, IsrJMedSci, 1988; 24:245) and hydatid cysts (Kain, AmJObsGyn, 1988; 159:1216) are treated with standard measures.

Drug toxicity

Drugs are normally avoided during pregnancy, and there is thus very little information as to whether drug hepatitis is more frequent or severe (Beeley, ClinObstetGynecol, 1981; 8:275). Theoretically this could be so as there is reduced hepatic clearance and inhibition of excretory function (Wood, ClinObstetGynecol, 1981; 8:255). Tetracycline can give rise to a syndrome similar to acute fatty liver of pregnancy (see above). Fulminant hepatitis due to drugs such as quinidine and phenylethylbarbiturate, used for obstetric indications, has been reported (Bourlier, JHepatol, 1988; 6:214), as well as more well-recognized drug reactions, such as methyldopa given for hypertension in pregnancy (Picaud, JGynObsBiolReprod, 1990; 19; 192), chlorpromazine (Read, AmJMed, 1961; 31:249), halothane (Holden, ObsGyn, 1972; 40:586), methoxyflurane (Ruginger, Anesthesiol, 1975; 43:593), hydralazine (Hod, IntJFert, 1986; 31:352), and isoniazid (Franks, PublHlthRep, 1989; 104:151). The use of β-sympathomimetics for premature labour has led to the use of relatively long- term drug therapy for pregnant women; there have been a few reports of drug-induced hepatitis due to terbutaline (Quinn, AmJGastr, 1994; 89:781) and ritodrine (Arcos, ActaObGyn, 1996; 75:340). Close monitoring of liver function is necessary to determine whether in the presence of mild abnormalities the drug could be continued to avoid the risk of premature labour.

Paracetamol overdose

Paracetamol is frequently recommended for analgesia if this is required in pregnancy. Overdoses have been described and N-acetylcysteine has been administered early in pregnancy without untoward effects. The fetal liver does not appear to be affected (Ludmin, ObsGyn, 1986; 67:750; Robertson, JFamPractice, 1986; 23:267; Kurzel, SouthMedJ, 1990; 83:983).

Biliary disease

A recent serial ultrasonographic study in 272 pregnant women updated a previous report showing that gallbladder sludge and gallbladder stones have a cumulative incidence of 31 and 9 per cent during pregnancy, but both spontaneously disappear in the first year after delivery in 87 and 30 per cent of cases, respectively ((Maringhini, JHepatol, 1987; 5:218; Maringhini, Hepatol, 1990; 12:900). The risk of developing gallstones in pregnancy is increased in those who previously took oral contraceptives (Evron, IntSurg, 1982; 67:448), but pregnancy itself leads to gallstone formation by stimulating cholesterol synthesis which increases delivery of cholesterol to the liver, and by impairing the ability to catabolize cholesterol to bile acid, increasing secretion of biliary cholesterol, reducing the cholesterol-carrying capacity of bile, and impairing contraction of the gallbladder with secondary stasis of bile (Everson, Hepatol, 1993; 17:159; Valdivieso, Hepatol, 1993; 17:1).

Biliary obstruction should be managed with standard protocols using endoscopic sphincterotomy and drainage, and/or stone removal, as the first therapeutic approach (Ballie, SGO, 1990; 171:1; Jamidar, AmJGastr, 1995; 90:1263). Cholecystectomy carries no extra risk in pregnancy, although in the first trimester there is increased fetal loss (Printen, AmJSurg, 1978; 20:432). Cholecystitis can be mimicked by severe pre-eclampsia (Friedenberg, WisMedJ, 1978; 77:117) and the HELLP syndrome. Choledochal cyst (Taylor, JRCollSurgEdinb, 1977; 22:424) and biliary carcinoma have been documented in pregnancy (Devoe, JReprodMed, 1983; 28:153).

Liver transplantation and pregnancy

Normal menstrual pattern returns quickly following successful transplantation (Laifer, MayoClinProc, 1995; 70:388). In one series comprising 44 women, all had a period within 10 months of transplant with a single exception—a patient who had polycystic ovaries (Cundy, Gut, 1990; 31:337). In another series, menstruation returned after a median of 8 weeks (range, 1 to 28 weeks) from transplant (de Koning, Digestion, 1990; 46:239). This emphasizes the need for contraceptive advice immediately after transplantation. Ideally pregnancy should be deferred for 1 year following liver transplantation as most complications and deaths occur in this period. An oral contraceptive may be prescribed; there are no data to suggest cholestatic reactions are more frequent in a transplanted liver. However, oral contraceptives can affect cyclosporin elimination (Scott, MedToxicol, 1988; 3:107) and potentiate cyclosporin hepatotoxicity (Deray, Lancet, 1987; i:58).

Oral contraceptives should not be used in patients transplanted for Budd–Chiari syndrome as these patients have an underlying thrombogenic tendency, although they routinely receive anticoagulants. Warfarin is teratogenic and therefore alternative contraceptive advice is even more important in this context (Hall, AmJMed, 1980; 68:122).

Successful pregnancies are increasingly reported in the literature, the first in 1978 (Walcott, AmJObsGyn, 1978; 132:340). Conception has occurred within 1 month, but the outcome was unsuccessful due to pre-eclampsia and premature delivery at 26 weeks (Laifer, ObsGyn, 1990; 76:1083), and as early as 4 months with a successful pregnancy (Haagsma, ObsGyn, 1989; 74:442; Hill, BrJObsGyn, 1991; 98:719).

Azathioprine is usually stopped in pregnant women; although there is no clear evidence for teratogenicity, it may cause pancytopenia in infants (Davidson, BrJObsGyn, 1985; 92:233). Prednisolone is safe and large doses of methylprednisolone given for acute cellular rejection are not thought to affect the fetus, although low birth-weight infants have been reported (Reinisch, Science, 1978; 202:436). Cyclosporin crosses the placenta and both the parent drug and metabolites have been found in the fetal circulation (Venkataramanan, Transpl, 1988; 46:468). Intrauterine growth retardation has been documented in renal transplant recipients given cyclosporin (Pickrell, BMJ, 1988; 296:825), and low birth-weight infants occur in liver transplant recipients (Hill, BrJObsGyn, 1991; 98:719); one intrauterine death has been attributed to cyclosporin (Cundy, Gut, 1990; 31:337). Clearly, fetal growth must be closely monitored.

No teratogenic effects with cyclosporin have been described. Children followed up to 12 years have had normal development (Scantlebury, Transpl, 1990; 49:317). No teratogenic effects have been described with tacrolimus, but the number of pregnancies on this drug is far smaller. Cyclosporin is nephrotoxic and almost 40 per cent of patients taking it will develop hypertension in pregnancy (Winter, JObsGyn, 1990; 10:396). Two overlapping series from the United States report a high incidence of hypertensive disease of pregnancy necessitating urgent delivery (Laifer, ObsGyn, 1990; 76:1083; Scantlebury, Transpl, 1990; 49:317); all patients were taking cyclosporin. However, this was not reported in a review of cases which excluded these two reports (Hill, BrJObsGyn, 1991; 98:719). It is possible that excess cyclosporin may be a contributing factor. Plasma concentrations of cyclosporin should be monitored very carefully. Divided doses may eliminate high maternal and fetal peaks (Varghese, BMJ, 1988; 296:1400).

Pregnancy does not increase the likelihood of graft rejection (Laifer, ObsGyn, 1990; 76:1083). There is a higher incidence of prematurity in the American reports, related to obstetric indications for early delivery, principally pregnancy-induced hypertension, which accounts for a caesarian section rate of over 50 per cent.

Liver transplantation has also been performed during pregnancy. Both cases reported have been in mothers with fulminant hepatitis B, transplanted at 21 weeks (Fair, Transpl, 1990; 50:534) and 26 weeks (Laifer, ObsGyn, 1990; 76:1083). Both required retransplantation within days of the first graft. In the first case, OKT3 monoclonal antibody was given and CMV hepatitis and pancreatitis occurred. Despite these insults a live baby was born by caesarian section, performed because of intrauterine growth retardation. Subsequent development was normal. In the second case, fetal distress on the seventh postoperative day required a caesarian section and the baby died.

References

1. Robson SC, Mutch, E, Boys RJ, and Woodhouse KW. Apparent liver blood flow during pregnancy: a serial study using indocyanine green clearance. *British Journal of Obstetrics and Gynaecology*, 1990; **97**: 720–4.

2. Hammerli UP. Jaundice during pregnancy with special reference on recurrent jaundice during pregnancy and its differential diagnosis. *Acta Medica Scandinavica*, 1966; **179** (Suppl. 444): 1.

3. Depue RH, Berstein L, Ross RK, Judd HL, and Henderson BE. Hyperemesis gravidarum in relation to estradiol levels, pregnancy outcome, and other maternal factors: a sero-epidemiologic study. *American Journal of Obstetrics and Gynecology*, 1987; **156**: 1137–41.

4. Reyes H. The enigma of intrahepatic cholestasis of pregnancy: lessons from Chile. *Hepatology*, 1982; **2**: 87–96.

5. Burroughs AK, Seong NH, Dojcinou D, Scheuer PJ, and Sherlock S. Idiopathic acute fatty liver of pregnancy in 12 patients. *Quarterly Journal of Medicine*, 1982; **204**: 481–97.

6. Rolfes DB and Ishak KG. Acute fatty liver of pregnancy: a clinico-pathologic study of 35 cases. *Hepatology*, 1985; **5**: 1149–58.

7. Parry HB. Toxaemias of pregnancy in domestic animals with particular reference to the sheep. In Sheehan HL, ed. *Toxaemias of pregnancy*. London: Ciba, 1950: 157.

8. Rolfes DB and Ishak KG. Liver disease in toxaemia of pregnancy. *American Journal of Gastroenterology*, 1986, **81**: 1138–44.

9. Chesley LC. *Hypertensive disorders in pregnancy*. New York: Appleton-Century Crofts, 1978: 268.

10. Henny Ch P, Lim AE, Brummelkamp WH, Buller HR, and Ten Cate JW. A review of the importance of the acute multidisciplinary treatment following spontaneous rupture of the liver in pregnancy. *Surgery, Gynecology, Obstetrics*, 1983; **158**: 593.

11. Aarnoudse JG, Hothoff HS, Weita S, Vellegnga E, and Hursies HJ. A syndrome of liver damage and intravascular coagulation in the last trimester of normotensive pregnancy. A clinical and histopathological study. *British Journal of Obstetrics and Gynaecology*, 1986; **932**, 145–55.

12. Sibai BM, Taslimi MM, El-Nazer A, Amon E, Mabie BC, and Ryan GM. Maternal–perinatal outcome associated with the syndrome of hemolysis, elevated liver enzymes, and low platelets in severe pre-eclampsia–eclampsia. *American Journal of Obstetrics and Gynecology*, 1986; **155**: 501–9

13. Sheehan HL and Lynch JB, eds. *Pathology of toxaemia of pregnancy*. Edinburgh: Churchill Livingstone, 1973.

14. Meyer UA and Schmid R. The porphyrias. In Stanbury JB, Wyngaarden JB, and Fredrickson DS, eds. *The metabolic basis of inherited disease*. New York: McGraw Hill, 1978: 1166.

15. Beasley RP, *et al*. The E antigen and vertical transmission of hepatitis B surface antigen. *American Journal of Epidemiology*, 1977; **105**, 94–8.

16. *Clinical Report for the National Maternity Hospital*. Dublin, 1979.

29

The management of liver disease

29.1 The general management of liver disease

Neil McIntyre

The general medical principles of management obviously apply to the management of patients with hepatobiliary problems. They include correct diagnosis of the underlying disease(s) and of its complications; proper monitoring; specific therapy (when available); relief of symptoms; prevention or management of complications; and sensible education of patients (and of their relatives and friends). It is also important to identify and treat other conditions which may be present, even if they are not causally related to the liver disease.

Diagnosis

The key to sound management is accurate diagnosis. This is particularly important when effective therapy is available, and when further hepatic damage can be prevented by stopping a hepatotoxic drug. Correct diagnosis also aids prognostication and the assessment of response to treatment. A general approach to diagnosis in liver disease is presented in Chapter 5.8, and specific aspects of the diagnosis of individual diseases are considered in the relevant chapters.

Unfortunately, the correct diagnosis is missed in many patients with liver disease. Often no action is taken when patients present with modest, often longstanding, abnormalities of liver function tests, even though serious liver disease may present with only minor abnormalities or even normal test results. Too often patients are told they drink too much, and are advised to reduce their alcohol intake. If they drink little or no alcohol this causes resentment. Even when chronic hepatitis or cirrhosis is found on biopsy there may be only a half-hearted attempt to find a cause; Wilson's disease, haemochromatosis, and autoimmune disease (particularly if associated with LKM-1 or LSA antibodies) are often missed, with delay in starting appropriate treatment and/or in the detection of the genetic disorder in close relatives.

There are two main reasons for an inadequate approach to diagnosis. One is ignorance of the many causes of liver disease; this restricts choice in differential diagnosis. The other is that hepatology is still a young speciality; the necessary diagnostic facilities and expertise are often unavailable even in large general gastroenterology units. Patients should be referred to a specialist liver unit if a firm diagnosis cannot be made.

We also need to look out for problems in other systems. They may be the cause or the consequence of liver disease (see Sections 24 and 25), or may be quite unrelated. They may cause symptoms which should be relieved, or which may adversely affect the overall prognosis. Their treatment may need modification because of the accompanying liver disease (see Chapter 29.3). Depression is common in patients with liver disease; it should be identified as it often responds to appropriate therapy.

Therapy, monitoring, and complications

The specific treatments for various diseases, monitoring of these conditions, relief of symptoms, and prevention and/or management of complications such as variceal bleeding, ascites, portalsystemic encephalopathy, hepatocellular carcinoma, and infections are discussed in the relevant chapters in this book.

Patients with chronic hepatobiliary disease require regular follow-up. They should be checked for deterioration in their general condition, for alteration of physical signs, and for unexpected changes in the results of laboratory tests. Their drug intake should be checked frequently, particularly if several doctors are involved in their care. Many of the causes of rapid deterioration in patients with chronic liver disease are correctable.

They should be advised to seek help quickly if they or their relatives become aware of deepening jaundice, fever and rigors, melaena, ankle or abdominal swelling, or signs of confusion, or if other symptoms and signs cause concern. We should try to avoid frightening patients when such advice is given, but they must appreciate the need to seek help early for complications such as bacteraemia, spontaneous bacterial peritonitis, and gastrointestinal bleeding. Cirrhotics should be checked regularly for the development of hepatocellular carcinoma, by ultrasound or computed tomography and by serial determination of serum α-fetoprotein levels.

When jaundice appears in patients with a primary or secondary hepatic malignancy it is often attributed to diffuse parenchymal involvement by the tumour and no further action may be taken. Occasionally jaundice is due to large bile duct obstruction; this can be relieved by biliary stenting, which may prolong life and lead to considerable improvement in the patient's general condition. Some hepatic secondaries respond well to appropriate antitumour therapy.

When managing patients with serious chronic liver disease, remember that liver transplantation may be considered at some stage. Procedures that might jeopardize transplantation should be done only if absolutely necessary, and after consideration of their likely consequences (see Chapter 30.5).

Patient education

Patients need a full explanation of their condition, even if they have only minor abnormalities of their liver function tests without clinical evidence suggesting significant liver damage, or if they have a relatively benign disorder such as non-alcoholic fatty liver or long-standing right upper quadrant discomfort without any detectable cause. Patients are often frightened by a diagnosis of chronic hepatitis C, even when it is in its early stages; their concern needs to be properly addressed and the reasons for follow-up made clear.

Patients with liver disease often ask what they should eat and drink (including alcohol), what drugs they should take, whether they can take exercise, travel abroad, drive a car, or whether they need to change their life style in other ways. They are often given erroneous advice; few publications cover these aspects of patient education.

We should aim for as little disruption as possible in the patients' daily lives; however, constraints are sometimes inevitable and advice must depend on individual circumstances.

The reasons for giving advice should be explained clearly; patients are more likely to follow it if they understand why it is being given. It helps to give patients informative handouts about their disease. Examples provided by the American Liver Foundation can be found in Appendix 6 to the first edition of this book; similar handouts are also available from other national associations, such as the British Liver Trust. They may need modification for patients in some countries, as there are often major cultural differences in the doctor–patient relationship.

Diet (Chapter 29.2)

Most patients with liver disease are given dietary advice of some kind; usually to avoid fatty foods and alcohol, to take a low or a high protein diet, a high carbohydrate diet, or a diet low in salt. There is rarely justification for such advice, particularly about fat intake. It has been known for 40 to 50 years or so that a high protein, high calorie intake is beneficial in acute viral hepatitis, and that fat restriction is unnecessary (Chalmers, JCI, 1955; 34:1163; Hoagland, AmJPublHlth, 1946; 36:1287).

Patients with liver disease should eat a normal mixed diet. The obese should lose weight; obesity is a common cause of abnormal liver function tests (Friedman, AnnIntMed, 1987; 107:137; Robinson, AnnClinBioch, 1989; 26:393), and may be associated with significant liver damage (Adler, AmJMed, 1979; 67:811); both may improve with weight loss.

Dietary fat reduction is necessary only for patients with trouble-some steatorrhoea (uncommon in acute or chronic liver disease) and those with cholecystitis (whose symptoms may be aggravated by fat intake). Low-fat diets are unpalatable and compound problems with anorexia. They may also be associated with a reduced intake of fat-soluble vitamins, whose absorption may be impaired with liver disease. Patients with cirrhosis tend to a deficiency of essential polyunsaturated fatty acids, which may impair renal function and platelet aggregation (see Chapters 2.12, 8.2, 25.3), and it has been suggested that arachidonic acid deficiency significantly increases the mortality risk in patients with advanced cirrhosis (Cabre, AmJ-Gastro, 1993; 88:718). Patients with liver disease should therefore be encouraged to take a normal fat intake, some of which should consist of plant fats, such as corn or safflower oil, which are rich in essential fatty acids. However, recent work suggests that the effects of lipid peroxidation (of polyunsaturated fatty acids) may contribute to hepatocellular damage; this issue needs to be resolved.

Patients with fluid retention (ascites and/or peripheral oedema) should not add salt to their diet; if they show avid sodium retention, they may benefit from a reduction in salt intake (see Chapter 8.1), but this must be done cautiously in patients from very hot countries. There may be advantages in treating patients with diuretics without salt restriction and without attempting complete removal of excess fluid; the diet can then be more palatable, and uraemia and hyper-uricaemia, which often complicate more vigorous regimens, are observed less frequently (Reynolds, Gut, 1978; 19:549) Patients with hepatic encephalopathy may need a low-protein diet but, if possible, chronic encephalopathy should be controlled with non-absorbable disaccharides (lactulose/lactitol) and avoidance of pre-cipitating factors, as cirrhotics tend to be protein depleted (see Chapter 29.2). It seems sensible to advise patients with oesophageal varices to avoid foods which might contain sharp-edged particles, for example bones or bone fragments, although there is nothing in the literature to support this suggestion.

Many patients with liver disease are advised to abstain from alcohol, even if they do not have alcoholic liver disease. Such advice is often given to patients with acute viral hepatitis; there is no good evidence that it affects outcome, but it is harmless advice which focuses patients' attention on the hepatotoxicity of alcohol at a time when they are likely to be receptive to the information. In those with chronic non-alcoholic liver disease, a little alcohol can be allowed but its consumption should not be encouraged. I advise complete abstention for patients with alcoholic hepatitis/cirrhosis, because there is a significant long-term reduction in mortality in those who give up drinking (Chapter 15.3), and because those who abuse alcohol often find it difficult or impossible to drink in moderation.

Rest and physical activity

Many patients with acute viral hepatitis are told to rest in bed, sometimes for long periods. Prolonged bed rest should be avoided; it has deleterious effects which delay convalescence and return to full activity. Bed rest may be sensible when patients feel ill; it is unnecessary when they start to improve, regardless of the degree of jaundice, although they should probably avoid undue exertion throughout the acute attack. In a classic study, freedom of move-ment, 'except for a one-hour rest period after each meal', caused no untoward effects either in the short (Chalmers, JCI, 1955; 34: 1163) or long term (Nefzger, AmJMed, 1963; 35:299). Mild, even relatively vigorous, exercise was well tolerated during the con-valescent phase, when the bilirubin was below 50 µmol/l or the aminotransferases below 300 µ/l (Chalmers, JCI, 1955; 34:1163; Edlund, ScaJInfectDis, 1971; 3:189), and no ill effects were observed when exercise was taken much earlier in the course of the disease (Repsher, NEJM, 1969; 281:1393), even from the day of hospital admission (Graubaum, DMedWoch, 1987; 112:47). This topic has been reviewed by Ritland (SportsMed, 1988; 6:121).

Patients usually recover fully from acute viral hepatitis and resume normal activities within a few months, regardless of the amount of rest they take initially. The question of physical activity is thus more important in patients with chronic liver disease. Many suffer asthenia and tend to tire easily; they often reduce physical activity and give up sports that they enjoy. Some doctors have recommended restriction of physical activity, believing exercise to be detrimental in chronic active hepatitis (Massarat, Gastroenterologia, 1962; 97: 231 (suppl.); Zwirner, ActaHepatoSplenol, 1970; 7:97; Anand, Gastro, 1971; 60:1739). There are few data about the consequences of reduced activity. However, it seems likely that a reduction of muscle mass due to inactivity might increase the sense of fatigue on mild effort, and that inactivity *per se* might result in thinning of bones.

Ritland *et al.* (ScaJGastr, 1983; 18:1083) studied nine patients with autoimmune chronic hepatitis in remission on steroid therapy (five with cirrhosis); they exercised 3 or 4 days each week for 12 weeks, each period lasting at least 30 min with 5 min of hard exercise. There were no significant changes in aminotransferases, alkaline phosphatase, or γ-glutamyltransferase; modest increases in lactate dehydrogenase and creatine kinase were thought to be of muscle origin. Before the study, most restricted their physical activity and had a reduced initial work capacity; this improved significantly with training, as did their oxygen consumption. Clinical deterioration was not observed in any of the patients. Six felt that their capacity for performing everyday duties had improved and wanted to continue exercise.

Muting *et al.* (MedKlin, 1987; 82:468; FortschrDMed, 1987; 105:65) exercised patients with liver diseases (including chronic active hepatitis and cirrhosis). Tolerance of fast walking and swimming was surprisingly good, as assessed by measurement of aminotransferases and other indices. Others have also found that appropriate training with aerobic exercise has beneficial effects on the patient with well-compensated cirrhosis (Ritland, SportsMed, 1988; 6:121; Kawase, ActaHepatolJpn, 1993; 34:950).

These studies suggest that patients with well-compensated chronic liver disease should be encouraged to engage in exercise, as it promotes general well-being. It seems likely that exercise would also minimize the development of osteoporosis, a common problem in patients with chronic liver disease, particularly those with cholestatic disorders such as primary biliary cirrhosis and those on long-term steroids. Studies are needed in this area.

It has been suggested that patients with oesophageal varices should avoid strenuous effort, for example lifting heavy weights, as this might increase intravariceal pressure and the risk of bleeding. However, there would also be an increase in intra-oesophageal pressure, and there is little to suggest that strenuous effort is an important precipitating factor for variceal bleeding.

As physical activity seems relatively harmless in patients with well-compensated liver disease, it seems sensible to encourage them to return quickly to work. Prolonged or repeated spells away from work may lead to loss of employment, creating financial and social problems. Particular problems arise with those suffering from encephalopathy (overt or latent); such patients should not return to work involving important decisions, or in which their encephalopathy may place them at risk of physical injury. Clearly, decisions must be based on individual circumstances.

Sexual activity

Impotence and loss of libido may occur with cirrhosis. In patients admitted for evaluation for liver transplant, impotence was more common in alcoholic than in non-alcoholic cirrhotics (Cornley, Hepatol, 1984; 4:1227). Their impotence was longer standing and more severe than that of non-alcoholic cirrhotics, even though their liver disease appeared to be less advanced on biochemical grounds. Sexual function improved spontaneously with abstinence in chronic alcoholics with normal sperm counts (about 25 per cent of those studied), and neither the presence of liver damage nor its severity (judged on biochemical and histological criteria) were predictive factors; fluoxymesterone (at high doses of 40–80 mg/day) led to return of potency in many subjects, but it was not clear how many had significant liver disease (Van Thiel, Gastro, 1982; 84:677). Gluud *et al.* (Gastro, 1988; 95:1582) also found spontaneous improvement of sexual function in alcoholic cirrhotic males who abstained from alcohol. Although reduced serum testosterone concentrations were significantly associated with sexual dysfunction at entry to the study, administration of testosterone appeared to be of no further benefit.

In women, liver disease *per se* seemed a relatively unimportant cause of sexual dysfunction (Bach, Hepatol, 1989; 9:698). Fatigue and depression were more important, and there was no statistical difference in sexual desire and function between women with and without liver disease (see Section 5). Women with liver disease should be reassured that they can, if they wish, maintain normal sexual relations. Mass *et al.* (Transpl, 1996; 62:476) studied gynaecological and reproductive function in 82 women before and after liver transplantation. There was little change in menstrual function after surgery. A total of 72 per cent of women were sexually active after transplantation, and six of 24 who had not been sterilized or had a hysterectomy conceived seven pregnancies. Regular cervical cytology is recommended after transplantation because of the recognized increase in cervical neoplasia in immunocompromised patients.

Younger women with liver disease often ask about pregnancy and its risks. Although there are many reports of successful pregnancy in women with chronic liver disease, there is a significant risk to the mother and the fetus. This topic is covered in Section 28.

Infectivity and sexual transmission of disease

Because the blood of carriers of hepatitis B, hepatitis C, and hepatitis D viruses is potentially infectious, they should not allow other persons to share a razor or any other instruments that may have been exposed to their blood (for example, toothbrushes, tweezers). If they cut themselves, they should clear up the blood carefully themselves, and exposed surfaces should be cleaned with a sodium hypochlorite bleach (which should be kept available). If uninfected persons have to clear up blood, they should wear rubber gloves. Sanitary towels or tampons contaminated with menstrual blood should be placed in a plastic bag prior to disposal. These precautions are most important in relation to infection with hepatitis B virus and hepatitis D virus.

Patients positive for HBsAg, HBeAg, and/or hepatitis B virus DNA are a particular risk to their sexual partners. Their partners should also be tested for markers of hepatitis B virus infection; if both antiHBs and antiHBc are positive, no further action is needed. If either or both are negative, then the partner may be at risk from unprotected vaginal intercourse, and from other forms of sexual contact (oral or anal), including 'deep kissing'; they should be vaccinated against hepatitis B virus and should use standard synthetic condoms until it can be shown that protective antibodies have appeared. If a patient develops acute hepatitis B, his/her sexual contact(s) should again be tested for hepatitis B virus markers and should receive an injection of hepatitis B (hyperimmune) gammaglobulin; those with negative markers should also receive hepatitis B vaccine. If the markers are positive, on blood taken before giving the immune-globulin, the contact may be the source of the hepatitis and should be investigated. Although it appears that hepatitis C may also be spread sexually (in heterosexuals and homosexuals), the risk is much lower than for hepatitis B. There seems little point in advising patients with chronic hepatitis C, who have usually carried the virus for many years, to abstain from unprotected intercourse with their wives or longstanding sexual partners. But condoms should clearly be used for casual sexual relationships in order to minimize the chance of the patient acquiring another contagious sexually transmitted disease.

Foreign travel and residence in underdeveloped areas

Patients with chronic liver disease often ask if it is safe for them to travel to, or live in, other countries; the risks have to be assessed in each case. They should appreciate the financial implications before visiting countries where medical care is expensive; they may not be able to get adequate insurance cover, and the cost of a prolonged hospital admission for complications of liver disease may be prohibitive.

Patients with portal hypertension and oesophageal varices are at risk of bleeding. I do not advise them to travel to or live in places lacking the facilities to deal with variceal haemorrhage, or places where the risks of contracting viral hepatitis (or AIDS) after blood transfusion are high. When patients come from such an area (and will return there) careful consideration should be given to some form of portal-systemic shunt surgery, as this will reduce the risk of subsequent variceal bleeding.

Patients with clear evidence of hepatic decompensation are also at risk of developing other serious complications while they are in another country, for example hepatic encephalopathy, ascites, or a severe infection such as bacteraemia or spontaneous bacterial peritonitis.

Those who travel far afield should carry with them a letter explaining the nature of their condition, and the telephone number of someone who can be contacted should they have any serious problems while they are away. Ideally they should be given the address of hepatologists practising in the areas that they will be visiting; these can be obtained from their local specialist liver units. It is sensible for some patients, particularly those who travel alone, to wear a MedicAlert bracelet indicating the nature of their disease. Those taking essential drugs (for example immunosuppressive therapy for autoimmune chronic hepatitis or following a liver transplant) should carry an adequate supply, or make sure that the drugs are available where they are to visit.

Patients with liver disease who travel to, or live in, areas in which malaria is endemic can take the standard antimalarial prophylaxis that is appropriate for the area to which they are travelling. There appears to be no danger, for patients with chronic liver disease, in active immunization against bacterial and viral diseases to which they may be exposed, but they may not have as good an immune response as normal persons.

Patients with chronic hepatitis and/or cirrhosis who are not immune to hepatitis A or hepatitis B should be vaccinated against these conditions if they are to visit high-risk areas (although, again, their antibody response may be suboptimal). If they have no immunity to hepatitis A, they should receive the first dose of the vaccine, ideally, a month or more before leaving, although protection is evident within 2 or 3 weeks; a booster dose should be given after 6 months (Lemon, NEJM, 1997; 336:196). The vaccine has little value after exposure, so immune globulin should be given (within 2 weeks) if there is close contact with someone suffering from hepatitis A. For travellers who are departing immediately, vaccine and immune globulin can be given together (at separate sites). Such protection is important because the clinical illness resulting from an attack of hepatitis A is likely to be more severe in those with underlying liver disease than in those who have a normal liver, and the mortality is higher (Keeffe, AmJGastr, 1995; 90:201); they also have an increased risk of fulminant hepatitis (Lemon, NEJM, 1997; 336:196).

Driving and liver disease

Patients with overt encephalopathy would clearly place themselves and others at risk if they were to drive a car or another large vehicle, and should be discouraged from doing so. If they have relatives who drive, there is rarely a problem, but if they do not, or if their work involves driving, then patients may refuse to accept advice not to drive. This creates a dilemma. To report them to the relevant licensing authorities would breach confidentiality, but this might be the only way of protecting the patient and others from serious injury. The survival of patients with cirrhosis who have suffered severe trauma is significantly reduced (Tinkoff, AnnSurg, 1990; 211:172).

Most patients with mild forms of chronic liver disease are capable of driving safely. However, Schomerus et al. (DigDisSci, 1981; 26: 622) studied 40 cirrhotics with portal hypertension but without clinical signs of portal-systemic encephalopathy (30 with a normal EEG—15 alcoholics, 15 non-alcoholic; 10 with minor EEG changes—seven alcoholics, three non-alcoholic), and 12 controls with chronic alcoholic pancreatitis; neuropsychologists with a particular interest in aptitude for driving used a variety of tests for assessment. Of the 15 non-alcoholics without EEG changes, only six were considered completely fit to drive; six were fit to drive with major restrictions (in terms of speed or range of driving) and three definitely unfit to drive. None of the 15 alcoholic patients with a normal EEG were considered completely fit to drive—three were thought fit to drive with restrictions and the others were definitely unfit to drive. Of the 10 patients with minor EEG abnormalities, nine were definitely unfit to drive, the other one was fit to drive with restrictions. By contrast, nine of the 12 alcoholics with pancreatitis were thought to be completely fit to drive, and only two unfit to drive.

More recently, Srivastava *et al.* (JHepatol, 1994; 21:1023) studied 15 cirrhotics using neuropsychological testing, driving tests in the laboratory, and driving on the road (assessed by a licensed Illinois state driving evaluator). As a group, patients with cirrhosis showed no significant differences in their performance on a simulator or during actual driving conditions when compared to matched controls. However 66 per cent of them had two or more abnormal neuropsychological tests, a criterion used to define the presence of subclinical encephalopathy; these patients showed no deficiencies in simulated or real driving performance when compared to cirrhotics with normal neuropsychological tests.

These papers have important implications for physicians caring for patients with cirrhosis; further studies are clearly needed.

Drugs and liver disease

Patients with liver disease often need to take drugs for unrelated conditions, and these should be prescribed with caution (Chapter 29.3). Drugs that commonly cause liver disease (Chapter 17) should, if possible, be avoided, as the diagnosis of drug-induced liver disease may be very difficult in the presence of pre-existing liver disease. Furthermore, even if the incidence of liver damage with a particular drug is no greater in patients with chronic liver disease than in healthy persons, one might expect a more severe reaction in such patients.

Simple analgesia is an exception to this principle. Paracetamol, despite its dose-dependent hepatotoxicity, is the drug of choice. It should not be used in a dose of more than 3 g/day (six tablets). As methionine, like *N*-acetylcysteine, protects against paracetamol hepatotoxicity, it is possible that the use of a combined preparation (500 mg paracetamol/250 mg methionine) may protect against liver damage even with larger doses; however, the administration of methionine may cause problems in patients with overt or latent encephalopathy.

Codeine may be useful in patients with liver disease. It has a much smaller first-pass uptake than most other opiates. Its analgesic effect may result from its demethylation to morphine; it may, therefore, have less analgesic effect in liver disease and does occasionally have a cerebral depressant effect in those who are particularly sensitive to opiates, and can cause coma.

Aspirin and other non-steroidal anti-inflammatory drugs (NSAIDs) should be avoided because of the risk of gastrointestinal bleeding, their antiplatelet effect, and their renal toxicity (particularly in patients with fluid retention). d-Propoxyphene is of doubtful efficacy and is hepatotoxic (Section 17).

Young women of childbearing age often ask whether they can take the contraceptive pill. Liver disease is widely considered a contraindication to such therapy, but there is little information on this topic. As long-term use of oral contraceptives may be associated with an increased (though small) risk of certain types of liver disease (hepatic vein thrombosis, gallstones, hepatic adenoma, and hepatocellular carcinoma), their use is probably best avoided in patients with chronic liver disease, as there may be diagnostic problems if one of these complications develops. Oestrogens also appear to have a dose-dependent effect on the hepatocyte surface membrane, including that lining the canaliculus. They reduce the excretory capacity for bilirubin, bile salts, and bromsulphthalein;

the liver has a large reserve capacity for excretion of these compounds and jaundice does not appear until the excretory capacity is below 10 per cent of normal.[1]

If a woman insists on using a contraceptive pill, because she finds other methods unacceptable, a low-dose oestrogen or a progestogen-only pill can be tried, although they are best avoided in jaundiced patients, or in those with clear evidence of biochemical abnormality. The risks should be explained, and liver function tests (bilirubin and aminotransferases) should be monitored regularly while the patient is taking the oral contraceptive; for example, weekly for the first month, monthly for the next 3 months, and every 3 months thereafter (Zimmerman, JAMA, 1983; 249:3241). Stop the drug if there is any deterioration of the test results.

A similar problem arises over hormone replacement therapy, particularly if menopausal symptoms are particularly severe or if the patient is osteoporotic. A therapeutic trial is justified, with careful monitoring of liver function tests; changes in test results are likely to be reversible on stopping the treatment. In one study ethinyl oestradiol appeared to reduce serum enzyme levels in patients with primary biliary cirrhosis, although the bilirubin rose in two who were already jaundiced (Guattery, Hepatol, 1987; 7: 737). In another case report transdermal oestrogen replacement therapy was given to a 41-year-old woman with autoimmune hepatitis who was being treated with corticosteroids; she had had an early and symptomatic menopause and a high rate of bone loss. The menopausal symptoms resolved completely, with no deterioration in her liver function tests, and no change in her corticosteroid requirement. Follow-up bone mineral measurements over 2 years showed improvement (Clements, Gut, 1993; 34:1639).

Subclinical vitamin deficiencies appear to be relatively common in patients with severe liver disease. While it is expensive to investigate for vitamin deficiencies, multivitamin therapy is cheap. The routine prescription of a water-soluble multivitamin preparation is probably sensible as these are harmless in the usual doses. This is not true for the fat-soluble vitamins; Vitamin A is potentially hepatotoxic (Minuk, Hepatol, 1988; 8:272; Kowalski, AmJMed, 1994; 97:523), and vitamins D and K can cause other clinical problems. Nor is it true for large doses of nicotinamide or nicotinic acid, which can cause hepatocellular necrosis[2] (Winter, NEJM, 1973; 289:1180).

Patients with liver disease are occasionally found to be taking herbal medicines on the advice of friends or homeopathic practitioners. They are rarely aware of the content of these medicines. Herbal remedies may cause liver disease in otherwise healthy individuals. Veno-occlusive disease has been attributed to the ingestion of comfrey (Kumana, Lancet, 1983; ii:1360; Weston, BMJ, 1987; 295:183) as well as plants of the genera *Heliotropium*, *Crotalaria*, and *Senecio*, and hepatitis to the ingestion of tablets containing mistletoe and skullcap (Harvey, BMJ, 1981; 282:186). More recently, hepatitis has been reported after ingestion of tablets containing skullcap alone, or skullcap and valerian (MacGregor, BMJ, 1989; 299:1156). Severe hepatitis has been described as a result of taking chapparal leaf (*Larrea tridentata*) which is sold in health-food shops (Katz, JClinGastro, 1990; 12:203; Alderman, JClinGastr, 1994;19:242; Gordon, JAMA, 1995; 273:489) and from Ma-Huang (Nadir, AmJGastr, 1996; 91:1436). Chronic hepatitis has been reported with the use of wild germander (Gastro, ClinBiol, 1993; 17:959). Acute hepatitis has also resulted in Japan from the use of *syo-saiko-to* (*xiao-chai-hu-tang* in China) (Itoh, DigDisSci, 1995; 40:1845).

Clearly, patients with existing liver disease should be strongly discouraged from taking herbal medicines.

Relatives and friends and serious illness

When managing patients with liver disease we must consider the possible impact on the family. When a genetic disorder is identified it may be important to check for its presence in relatives. This is true, for example, for Wilson's disease, hereditary fructose intolerance, and tyrosinaemia; early identification and appropriate therapy may prevent irreversible liver disease or other manifestations in younger siblings. Unfortunately, we often find that no firm diagnosis was made when children or young adults died of liver disease, and with no attempt to exclude a treatable genetic disorder in surviving siblings or other close relatives.

When a patient is found to carry hepatitis B or C viruses, one should check for evidence of infection in family members and sexual contacts; those without B markers should be vaccinated.

As a general rule, patients should be told the truth about their illness, even when suffering from a life-threatening condition. A decision to hide the truth from the patient is justifiable only under certain circumstances, for example if life expectancy is short, or if the patient has difficulty in understanding what he/she is told. Relatives often ask that the patient should be spared bad news; their wishes should clearly be taken into consideration, but usually both the patient and the family benefit when matters are brought out into the open. It is often important that the patient knows the truth in order that family and business affairs can be attended to properly. Furthermore, the management of serious illness is often made more difficult if the patient does not understand the nature of the underlying problem, particularly when the expected course is one of continuing deterioration. Clearly, discussion of the possibility of liver transplantation is impossible unless patients recognize the seriousness of their condition, and occasionally patients refuse transplantation because they have previously been given an overoptimistic view of their prognosis. Unfortunately, language problems may make it difficult to overcome cultural differences with relatives from some countries.

The good results that are now being achieved with liver transplantation have completely changed the approach to the management of endstage liver disease. If transplantation is feasible, then clearly every effort should be made to maintain the patient's condition in as good a state as possible until the operation can be performed. Every effort should also be made in treating complications in patients with liver disease, if there is a chance of their returning to an acceptable state of health. Sometimes, however, the successful management of complications may serve only to prolong an existence which is barely tolerable, and one in which further serious problems are inevitable. Under these circumstances there seems little point in prolonging life, particularly if methods employed are distressing to the patient, and if the costs of care are likely to ruin the family.

References

1. Anderson and Schrier. *Clinical use of drugs in patients with kidney and liver disease*. Saunders, 1981.
2. Stricker BHCh. *Drug induced hepatic injury*, 2nd edn. Amsterdam: Elsevier, 1992.

29.2 Nutritional aspects of liver and biliary disease

Marsha Y. Morgan

The liver plays a pivotal role in the metabolism of the nutrients essential for well being and for life. In individuals with hepatobiliary disease, nutrient metabolism may be disturbed, with detrimental consequences. Conversely, liver damage may result from dietary inadequacies, dietary excesses, and dietary contaminants or else as a result of various nutritional manoeuvres or therapies. The nutritional status of all patients with hepatobiliary disease should be assessed and monitored regularly. Dietary manipulation and specific nutrient therapy play an important role in the management of these individuals.

Nutrient metabolism and the effects of liver and biliary disease

Food may be broadly defined as any ingested substance which is capable of being assimilated and utilized for supporting growth, maintaining bodily function, repairing or maintaining cells and tissues, and satisfying energy requirements. The diet is the source of some 40 to 50 nutrients and these are classically divided into six categories—carbohydrate, fat, protein, vitamins, minerals, and water. The caloric requirements of the body can be met by the three bulk dietary components—carbohydrate, fat, and protein; of these only protein is indispensable. A number of other nutrients including certain amino acids, fatty acids, minerals, and the vitamins are termed essential because they cannot be synthesized *de novo*. Requirements differ from one individual to another and may change for a given individual with alterations in the composition and nature of the diet as a whole. For these reasons Reference Nutrient Intakes have been established which incorporate a margin of safety sufficient to meet the needs of approximately 97 per cent of the population and which take account of differences in requirements according to age, sex, levels of physical activity, pregnancy, and lactation.[1] Nutritional requirements and tolerances may change in patients with hepatobiliary disease.

Energy

Energy requirements depend on body size and composition, on sex, age, and on physical activity. The daily Estimated Average Requirement for energy is 1940 kcal (8.1 MJ) for women and 2550 kcal (10.6 MJ) for men;[1] dietary carbohydrate should ideally provide 50 to 55 per cent of total daily energy intake, fat 30 to 35 per cent, and protein 10 to 20 per cent.

The liver plays a central role in energy balance and fuel homeostasis, so that changes in the control of these variables might be expected in the presence of acute and chronic liver disease.

To date only one study has been undertaken in patients with acute hepatitis (Schneeweiss, Hepatol, 1990; 11:387), and this is open to criticism. Thus, although the authors reported that there was no appreciable change in energy expenditure or fuel utilization in these patients, except for a decrease in protein oxidation rates, few patient details were provided, and the dietary intakes of the patients and control subjects, in the period prior to the study, were likely to have differed significantly.

This same group of workers undertook metabolic studies in 12 patients with acute liver failure, predominantly of viral origin, and reported a 30 per cent increase in energy expenditure compared with healthy controls (Schneeweiss, Gastro, 1993; 105:1515). A number of factors could potentially have contributed to this increase including: pyrexia, which was present in an unspecified percentage of patients; glucose administration, which was used to counter hypoglycaemia in 58 per cent; renal failure, which was present in 25 per cent; and administration of dopamine by infusion to support renal function in 12 per cent. However, none of these factors, even in combination, would have been sufficient to account for the magnitude of the increase in energy expenditure observed. This hypermetabolic state most likely reflects the effects of sepsis, almost invariably present in these patients, and the acute-phase response to massive hepatic necrosis which may be mediated by the action of cytokines.

In the five patients who were studied in the fasting state, the glucose oxidation rates were reduced while the lipid oxidation rates were increased; the non-protein respiratory quotient was reduced reflecting utilization of a fat-enriched metabolic mixture. In the seven patients who were receiving intravenous glucose, no significant changes were observed in the glucose or lipid oxidation rates, nor in the non-protein respiratory quotient. Protein oxidation rates were unchanged in both groups of patients.

A large number of studies have been undertaken to assess energy expenditure and fuel utilization in patients with cirrhosis (Owen, JCI, 1983; 72:1821; Mullen, Hepatol, 1986; 6:662; Shanbhogue, JPEN, 1987; 11:305; Merli, Hepatol, 1990; 12:106; Schneeweiss, Hepatol, 1990; 11:387; Müller, AmJPhysiol, 1991; 260:E338;

Müller, Hepatol, 1992; 15:782; Campillo, Nutrition, 1997; 13:613). Many of these studies can be criticized for poor or inadequate patient characterization, lack of or inappropriate matching of control subjects, flawed methodology, and inadequate data collection (Heymsfield, Hepatol, 1990; 11:502). In the studies which were adequately controlled and performed, results were expressed variously in relation to either ideal, actual, or 'dry' body weight or else in relation to fat-free mass or body cell mass, making assessments and comparisons extremely difficult (Heymsfield, 1990).

In consequence, although most workers agree that the fasting, non-protein respiratory quotient is reduced in these patients indicating use, at least in the postabsorptive state, of a fat-enriched metabolic mixture, there is little consensus as to the effects of chronic liver disease on resting energy expenditure. Overall, it is likely that the majority of clinically stable patients with cirrhosis are normometabolic, 15 to 20 per cent may be hypermetabolic, while 15 to 20 per cent may be hypometabolic (Shanbhogue, JPEN, 1987; 11:305; Merli, Hepatol, 1990; 12:106; Müller, Hepatol, 1992; 15:782; Campillo, Nutrition, 1997; 13:613). Patients with high volume ascites (Dolz, Gastro, 1991; 100:738), and those with hepatocellular carcinoma (Merli, Nutrition, 1992; 8:321), are more likely to be hypermetabolic.

The hyper- and hypometabolic patients represent high-risk populations; those who are hypermetabolic are more likely to be severely malnourished, to have greater haemodynamic changes, and to have a poorer outcome following transplantation (Müller, ClinNutr, 1994; 13:131), while those who are hypometabolic have a generally poorer prognosis as they may show little or no improvement in either liver function or nutritional status even when adequately nutritionally supported (Campillo, Nutrition, 1997; 13:613).

Diet-induced thermogenesis is unchanged in patients with cirrhosis (Campillo, Metabolism, 1992; 41:476; Riggio, JPEN, 1992; 16:445), although the thermogenic response to food may be prolonged (Green, Hepatol, 1991; 14:464); the energy requirements for physical activity are also unchanged (Campillo, JHepatol, 1990; 10:163; De Lissio, JApplPhysiol, 1991; 70:210).

Total energy expenditure is normal in these patients when expressed in absolute terms but is reduced when expressed as a multiple of the sleeping metabolic rate (Verboeket-van de Venne, Gut, 1995; 36:110).

The changes observed in energy expenditure and fuel utilization in patients with acute and chronic liver failure can be attributed, at least in part, to changes occurring in carbohydrate and fat metabolism.

In healthy individuals, the net splanchnic glucose production rate, after an overnight fast, averages 8.6 mmol/min per 1.73 m^2 (Wahren, JCI, 1972; 51:1870). Approximately 80 per cent of glucose release is attributed to glycogenolysis while the remainder is attributed to gluconeogenesis from lactate, pyruvate, amino acids, and glycerol. The normal liver glycogen content, after an overnight fast, averages only 44 mg/g, so that the contribution of glycogenolysis to glucose production falls rapidly after 18 to 24 h without feeding.

The capacity to store hepatic glycogen is decreased in patients with cirrhosis because of spatial limitations secondary to fibrosis and/or because of parenchymal damage per se (Nilsson, ScaJCLI, 1973; 32:317; Owen, JCI, 1981; 68:240). Thus, in these patients, net splanchnic glucose production rates and the contribution of glycogenolysis to glucose production, after an overnight fast, might be expected to decrease. In addition, as circulating concentrations of gluconeogenic precursors (Dawson, Lancet, 1957; i:392), and of glucagon (Marco, NEJM, 1973; 289:1107), are increased in these patients, the contribution made by gluconeogenesis to glucose production might be expected to increase. Gluconeogenesis, unlike glycogenolysis, is an energy-requiring process (Flatt, Diabetes, 1972; 21:50); thus, if the contribution of gluconeogenesis to splanchnic glucose production, after an overnight fast, is increased, then hepatic oxygen consumption might increase, and this might be reflected by an increase in resting energy expenditure.

In an elegant catheterization study, Owen and colleagues (JCI, 1981; 68:240), showed that, after an overnight fast, the net splanchnic glucose production rate in patients with cirrhosis averaged 5.3 mmol/min per 1.73 m^2, which is only 62 per cent of the glucose release rate documented in healthy volunteers by Wahren and colleagues (JCI, 1972; 51:1870). The total net splanchnic extraction rate of gluconeogenic precursors in the patients with cirrhosis was about twofold greater than that reported in healthy volunteers. As glucagon levels were uniformly raised in the patients with cirrhosis, it is likely that the majority of gluconeogenic precursors were quantitatively converted to, and released as, glucose to account for, on average, 3.58 mmol/min per 1.73 m^2 of the splanchnic glucose production rate. Thus, after an overnight fast, gluconeogenesis accounted for 67 per cent of hepatic glucose release in these patients. Owen and colleagues (1981) also showed that the activities of key gluconeogenic enzymes in patients with cirrhosis, in vitro, were similar to those in healthy subjects and were more than sufficient to sustain the rates of hepatic gluconeogenesis observed in vivo.

If glucose production rates are reduced in patients with cirrhosis then fuel homeostasis can only be maintained if compensatory changes occur in the metabolism of other major fuels, and this has been shown to occur. Owen and colleagues (JCI, 1983; 72:1821) measured plasma free fatty acid concentrations and determined their oxidation and turnover rates using ^{14}C-palmitate, in eight patients with cirrhosis and ten healthy control subjects, after an overnight fast. Plasma free fatty acid concentrations were twofold greater in the patients with cirrhosis as a result of increased lipolysis, and an increase of similar magnitude was observed in the free fatty oxidation rate which, in the patients with cirrhosis, was equivalent to a mean (SEM) of 0.71 ± 0.07 kcal/min or to 67 ± 5 per cent of total energy requirements.

Thus, the primary mechanism for maintaining fuel homeostasis in patients with cirrhosis, in the fasting state, appears to be augmented lipolysis and free fatty acid oxidation which contribute about two-thirds of total energy requirements and almost 80 per cent of non-protein calorie requirements. Utilization of this fat-enriched 'metabolic mixture', in the fasting state, will be reflected in a reduction in the non-protein respiratory quotient.

These changes in energy expenditure and fuel utilization have obvious nutritional implications. In patients with clinically stable cirrhosis, the energy requirement for maintaining body composition is $1.3 \times$ resting energy expenditure, or 25 to 30 kcal/kg daily from non-protein sources. In patients who are malnourished, or who have decompensated disease, non-protein energy intake should amount to 35 to 40 kcal/kg daily. Protein intakes should be adjusted accordingly.

The inability of these patients to store glycogen in an effective manner results in utilization of a fat-enriched metabolic mixture, in the fasting state, and eventually to depletion of fat and protein stores. Provision of small frequent meals throughout the waking hours, together with a late-night snack, has been shown to improve fuel utilization and nitrogen economy in these patients (Swart, BMJ, 1989; 299:1202; Zillikens, JHepatol, 1993; 17:377; Verboeket-van de Venne, Gut, 1995; 36:110; Chang, JPEN, 1997; 21:96). Thus, patients with chronic liver disease should be encouraged to take between four and seven small meals throughout their waking hours together with a late-night snack of complex carbohydrates.

Carbohydrate

Glucose plays a central metabolic role as it is an optimal fuel for many tissues, and is an obligatory fuel for erythrocytes, fibroblasts, the renal medulla, and the brain, except during starvation. The phosphorylated forms of fructose are important intracellular intermediates in the metabolism of glucose.

The most important dietary sources of carbohydrate are bread, potatoes, pasta, rice, cereals, cakes, biscuits, milk, and the sugar added as a sweetener to foods and drinks. Sixty per cent of carbohydrate is ingested in the form of starch and 25 per cent as simple sugars. Carbohydrate should provide approximately half of total daily energy requirements with a high percentage from unrefined sources, thus ensuring an intake of dietary fibre of approximately 18 g (range 12 to 24 g); the intake of simple sugars should not exceed 60 g daily or 10 per cent of total dietary energy.[1]

Ingested carbohydrate is digested in the small intestine and the resulting monosaccharides are absorbed across the mucosa by simple diffusion, facilitated diffusion, or by an active transport system. The liver is of prime importance in the regulation of carbohydrate metabolism as it receives absorbed monosaccharides from the portal vein and provides an even and predictable supply of glucose to extrahepatic tissue, when required. The liver removes 25 to 50 per cent of ingested glucose, although probably less than 10 per cent is taken up on first passage (Radziuk, Metabolism, 1978; 27:657). Glucose diffuses rapidly into the liver, where it is used for energy, stored as glycogen, or converted to fat. The remaining 50 to 75 per cent enters peripheral tissues, where it is oxidized or stored as glycogen. As circulating concentrations of glucose fall, more is released from the liver. After an overnight fast, 75 per cent of released glucose is derived from glycogenolysis; the remainder is formed by gluconeogenesis using lactate, pyruvate, alanine, and glycerol as precursors. Glucose, glucose precursors, and hormones are all important in the regulation of glucogenesis, gluconeogenesis, and glycogenolysis. The major portion of fructose in the portal vein is removed by the liver on first pass. Approximately one-third is metabolized immediately to pyruvate and lactate; the remainder is rapidly phosphorylated.

Carbohydrate metabolism is disturbed in patients with liver disease, although the abnormalities are not as striking as might be anticipated. In fulminant hepatic failure, hypoglycaemia is common, presumably because of impairment of gluconeogenesis, glycogen synthesis, and breakdown; it should be managed by infusion of 10 per cent glucose intravenously at a rate of 1.5 to 2.0 litres daily or of 20 per cent glucose delivered centrally if fluid restriction is necessary; blood sugar levels should be monitored constantly as the hypoglycaemia may be asymptomatic. In chronic liver disease, hypoglycaemia is rare unless provoked by oral hypoglycaemic agents.

Glucose intolerance is commonly observed in patients with acute viral hepatitis, fatty liver, toxic liver damage, and autoimmune chronic active hepatitis. More patients show intolerance to oral than to intravenous glucose (Creutzfeldt, ProgLivDis, 1970; 3:371), which can be explained, but only in part, by portal–systemic shunting of blood (Holdsworth, Gut, 1972; 13:58; Radziuk, Metabolism, 1978; 27:657).

The majority of patients with cirrhosis show fasting hyperglycaemia and glucose intolerance; 15 to 37 per cent may have frank diabetes (Bianchi, Hepatol, 1994; 20:119; Müller, EurJClinChemClinBioch, 1994; 32:749); these patients have hyperinsulinaemia and exhibit insulin resistance (Müller, Gastro, 1992; 102:2033; Selberg, JCI, 1993; 91:1897).

Patients with mild glucose intolerance benefit from taking a diet in which 45 to 55 per cent of total daily energy requirements are provided by complex carbohydrates which have low glycaemic indices and are rich in soluble fibre (Jenkins, AmJGastr, 1989; 84:732; Barkoukis, Hepatol, 1997; 26 (Suppl.):380A abstr.).

Patients with cirrhosis may have high serum fructose concentrations after an oral load (Martin, ArchSurg, 1962; 85:783), most likely as a consequence of portal–systemic shunting of blood (Smith, JCI, 1953; 32:273); this is of no significant consequence.

Fat

Fat is a metabolic fuel and a major source of fat-soluble vitamins and essential fatty acids.

Dietary fat is mainly triglyceride and is available from such 'visible' sources as butter, margarine, cooking fat, vegetable oils, and meat fat, and from 'invisible' sources such as nuts, egg yolk, and lean meat. Cakes, biscuits, gravies, and sauces, because of their content of butter, cooking fat, milk, or eggs, are additional rich sources of dietary lipid. The main sources of dietary fat are fats and oils, meat and meat products, cereals, milk, and cheese.

Naturally occurring fat contains both saturated and unsaturated fatty acids. The most important are the long-chain fatty acids which have carbon chain lengths of 16 or more. They include: the common saturated fatty acids, palmitic (C16) and stearic (C18); the monounsaturated oleic (C18:1,n–9); and the polyunsaturated fatty acids, linoleic (C18:2,n–6) α-linolenic (C18:3,n–3), γ-linolenic (C18:3,n–6), and arachidonic (C20:4,n–6); of these linoleic and α-linolenic are essential. Medium-chain triglycerides contain fatty acids with chain lengths shorter than C16.

Total fatty acid intake should average 30 per cent of dietary energy including alcohol; of this, 10 per cent of total energy should be provided by saturated fatty acids, 12 per cent by monounsaturated fatty acids, and an average of 6 per cent by polyunsaturated fatty acids. When calculated as total fat, including glycerol, these figures amount to 33 per cent of total dietary energy including alcohol, or 35 per cent of energy from food.[1] Requirements for the fat-soluble vitamins are easily met with a palatable diet; the essential fatty acid requirement can be met by daily ingestion of 2 to 5 g of linoleic acid.[1]

Following ingestion, dietary fat is emulsified by bile salts. Pancreatic lipase splits the ester linkages of the long-chain triglycerides at positions 1 and 3 of the glycerol backbone to produce two fatty acids and a 2-monoglyceride. These associate with bile acids and phosphatidylcholine to form micelles which incorporate cholesterol and fat-soluble vitamins into their core. The micelles come into contact with small intestinal microvilli and their fatty acids, monoglyceride, cholesterol, and fat-soluble vitamins are taken up by the enterocytes. The monoglyceride and fatty acids are synthesized to triglyceride within the enterocyte, which is then, together with cholesterol, cholesterol esters, phospholipids, apoproteins, and fat-soluble vitamins, packaged into chylomicrons to leave the gut in intestinal lymph. Medium-chain triglycerides do not require bile salts or pancreatic lipase for their digestion; they pass directly through the mucosal cells into the portal blood and are bound to albumin for transport in unesterified form.

The major lipids of plasma are: cholesterol, which is an important constituent of all mammalian plasma membranes and a precursor of bile acids and steroid hormones; cholesterol esters, which store and transport cholesterol molecules; phospholipids, which are major constituents of membranes and take part in many important biochemical reactions, including intracellular signalling via breakdown of phosphoinositides; and triglyceride, which is the major form in which fat is transported in plasma and stored in adipose tissue.

Plasma lipids are associated with specific proteins. Unesterified fats and the phospholipid lysolecithin are bound to albumin or to specific proteins such as retinol-binding protein. However, the majority of plasma lipids are carried by lipoproteins; these are large macromolecular complexes which are manufactured in the liver or intestine and which contain cholesterol, phospholipid, one or more specific polypeptides, termed apoproteins, and small quantities of non-polar lipids. The lipoproteins are classified, on the basis of certain physicochemical properties, as chylomicrons, very low-density lipoproteins (**VLDL**), low-density lipoproteins (**LDL**) and high-density lipoproteins (**HDL**). Triglycerides are mainly transported in chylomicrons and in VLDL, while cholesterol is transported mainly in LDL.

The lipoproteins are subsequently broken down by peripheral and hepatic lipases and by lecithin cholesterol acyltransferase (**LCAT**). Once triglyceride has been released from chylomicrons and VLDL it is hydrolysed by lipoprotein lipase to free fatty acids which are available for uptake in the periphery. Fatty acids, particularly the polyunsaturated fatty acids, may be incorporated into cell structures and play an important role in membrane interchange, thus influencing the activity of certain key enzymes and receptors. In addition, polyunsaturated fatty acids with 20 carbon atoms are precursors of prostaglandins and related eicosanoids. The cholesterol released from LDL is not degraded in man; cholesterol losses from the body occur by shedding of cholesterol in skin cells and intestinal epithelia, and by faecal excretion of biliary and dietary cholesterol, bile salts, and metabolites of unabsorbed cholesterol.

In patients with parenchymal liver disease or chronic cholestasis the flow of bile salts is usually reduced and this interferes with fat emulsification and triglyceride hydrolysis by pancreatic lipase. However, some hydrolysis of triglyceride still occurs and free fatty acids and monoglyceride continue to be absorbed in relatively large amounts. Thus, steatorrhoea is usually modest; its severity is roughly proportional to the degree of hepatocellular damage or biliary obstruction. When luminal concentrations of bile salts are low, however, micelle formation is seriously disrupted and this will impair the absorption of fat-soluble vitamins, and occasionally essential fatty acids, as these depend on micellar solubility for their uptake.

A number of changes are observed in circulating lipid, lipoprotein, and fatty acid concentrations in individuals with both parenchymal liver disease and chronic cholestasis. Circulating cholesterol and triglyceride concentrations may increase due to the accumulation of biliary lecithin and a reduction in plasma LCAT activity secondary to impaired hepatic synthesis or defective enzyme release from the damaged liver (Agorastos, ClinSciMolMed, 1978; 54:369).

Changes may also occur in the structure, electrophoretic mobility, and composition of the lipoprotein fractions, predominantly in patients in whom plasma LCAT activity is reduced (Day, ClinSci, 1979; 56:575).

Total plasma fatty acid concentrations may be increased in patients with chronic liver disease (Owen, JCI, 1983; 72:1821; Merli, JHepatol, 1986; 3:348), and absolute and relative increases may be observed in the plasma concentrations of individual fatty acids (Szebeni, Alcoholism, 1986; 10:647). The constituent fatty acids of triglyceride, phospholipids, and cholesterol esters may show increased saturation and a concomitant decrease in polyunsaturated fatty acids, probably as a result of impaired hepatic essential fatty acid metabolism (Palombo, Gastro, 1987; 93:1170).

Cabré and colleagues (AmJGastr, 1988; 83:712; AmJGastr, 1990; 85:1597; JPEN, 1992; 16:359; Nutrition, 1996; 12:542) reported a reduction in total plasma concentrations of saturated fatty acids, linoleate, and polyunsaturated fatty acids in patients with alcoholic cirrhosis; the reduction in polyunsaturated fatty acids and linoleate was proportionally greater than the reduction in saturated and monoenoic fatty acids. The reductions observed in polyunsaturated fatty acids were greatest in those patients with the most severe liver disease, those most nutritionally compromised, and those actively abusing alcohol; creation of a portacaval shunt had no further effect on circulating polyunsaturated fatty acids levels but circulating concentrations of saturated and monounsaturated fatty acids increased (Cabré, JPEN, 1996; 20:168). Patients with cirrhosis who are deficient in arachidonic acid have a significantly higher mortality rate than those who are replete (Cabré, AmJGastr, 1993; 88:718); dietary supplementation with polyunsaturated fatty acids could be justified in decompensated patients with cirrhosis who are malnourished (Gonzalez, Metabolism, 1992; 41:954).

Xanthelasma may develop in patients with primary biliary cirrhosis and high circulating lipid levels; these typically appear around the eyes, on the palms and soles, and over bony prominences (Ahrens, JCI, 1949; 28:1565); rarely a xanthomatous peripheral neuropathy may develop (Thomas, Brain, 1965; 88:1079). Changes in the cholesterol and/or phospholipid content of erythrocyte membranes may occur in patients with liver disease, resulting in changes in red cell shape and possibly survival time. These patients may also show changes in membrane fluidity in many tissues in response to alterations in their lipoprotein profiles. Deficiency of polyunsaturated fatty acids may result in impaired synthesis of prostaglandins and related compounds.

Protein

Protein is an energy source and provides the body with amino acids for endogenous protein synthesis. The amino acids threonine, valine, methionine, leucine, isoleucine, phenylalanine, lysine, and tryptophan are 'essential' in both children and adults, while arginine and histidine are additionally essential during childhood.

Dietary protein is derived from animal sources such as meat, fish, eggs, milk, and cheese and from vegetable sources such as peas, beans, lentils, other pulses, cereals, and flour. In the United Kingdom approximately one-third of dietary protein is of animal origin. Daily protein requirements are influenced by the caloric intake and by the biological value of the proteins ingested. The biological value of a protein is defined as the proportion which is retained following absorption, and depends primarily on its content of essential amino acids. Animal proteins, in general, have higher biological values than vegetable proteins. If calories are deficient, then the daily protein requirement is inversely proportional to the energy intake. A diet which provides less than 10 per cent of total food energy as protein is likely to be unpalatable and may be deficient in other nutrients such as easily absorbable iron, vitamin B_{12}, riboflavin, nicotinic acid, and trace elements such as zinc and selenium. In adults, the Reference Nutrient Intakes for protein are 45 g/day for women and 55.5 g/day for men.[1]

During the process of digestion and intestinal absorption, dietary protein is completely hydrolysed to amino acids, which are released into the portal vein. There they mix with amino acids derived from the digestion and absorption of exfoliated intestinal cellular protein, secreted enzyme protein, and a small amount of exuded plasma protein.

Hepatocyte uptake of amino acids is governed by transport mechanisms which are stereospecific, saturable for certain amino acids, and which may exhibit cross-inhibition (Pardridge, AmJPhysiol, 1975; 228:1155). In consequence, there are selective differences in hepatic amino acid uptake and metabolism. Alanine uptake, for example, exceeds that of all other amino acids, while the branched-chain amino acids, leucine, isoleucine, and valine, are poorly extracted by the liver; their main site of metabolism is skeletal muscle.[2]

The liver plays a central role in protein and amino acid metabolism. It processes dietary amino acids and reprocesses amino acids released from muscle protein degradation. It regulates the supply of amino acids to peripheral tissues such as muscle, and converts excess amino acids into urea for excretion in urine. Ammonia derived from the intrahepatic deamination of amino acids and generated extrahepatically from the metabolism of nucleotides, from the metabolism of glutamine in the gut wall, and as a result of bacterial degradation of intestinal protein and urea, is efficiently eliminated, as urea, by the hepatic urea cycle enzymes. The liver utilizes amino acids, particularly alanine and glutamine, for gluconeogenesis and for protein synthesis. It is the exclusive or major site for synthesis of virtually all the plasma proteins and is an important site for the degradation of many proteins and hormones. The liver may modulate overall body protein metabolism because of its role in the metabolism of hormones which regulate peripheral amino-acid metabolism.

Changes occur in protein metabolism and requirements in patients with both acute and chronic liver disease. In severe viral hepatitis and fulminant hepatic failure, protein requirements are undoubtedly increased although this has not been formally documented; these patients are moderately to severely catabolic and should be provided with a protein intake of 1.2 to 1.5 g/kg daily. Patients with acute alcoholic hepatitis have increased protein requirements (Weber, DigDisSci, 1982; 27:103); they require daily protein intakes in excess of 1.2 g/kg to maintain nitrogen balance. Protein requirements are also increased in patients with cirrhosis (Gabuzda, AnnNYAcadSci, 1954; 57:776; Swart, ClinNutr, 1989; 8:329; Nielsen, BrJNutr, 1993; 69:665; Nielsen, BrJNutr, 1995; 74:557; Kondrup, BrJNutr, 1997; 77:197). The protein requirement for nitrogen balance is 0.83 g/kg daily; the recommended protein is, therefore, 1.0 to 1.5 g/kg daily depending on the degree of hepatic decompensation.

The increased protein requirements, in patients with chronic liver disease, may arise because these individuals cannot store hepatic glycogen (Nilsson, ScaJCLI, 1973; 32:317; Owen, JCI, 1981; 68:240), and in consequence show a reduction in the contribution of glycogenolysis to hepatic glucose release, at least in the fasting state, and a compensatory increase in gluconeogenesis (Owen, 1981). This results in additional loss of amino acids and depletion of tissue protein stores.

It has alternatively been hypothesized that the increase in protein requirements observed in these patients arises because of increased whole-body protein degradation, itself a reflection of a reduction in circulating concentrations of insulin-like growth factor (Kondrup, BrJNutr, 1997; 77:197). However, the studies on whole-body protein synthesis and breakdown in patients with cirrhosis have produced conflicting results mainly because of the effects of various confounding variables, such as the patients' nutritional status and dietary intakes in the weeks prior to study, and the fact that the tracers used may perform differently in patients with liver disease than in healthy volunteers. Thus, to date, whole-body protein synthesis and breakdown rates have been reported as increased (O'Keefe, Gastro, 1981; 81:1017; Swart, ClinSci, 1988; 75:101; McCullough, Gastro, 1992; 103:571; Kondrup, 1997), unchanged (Millikan, Surgery, 1985; 98:405; Mullen, Hepatol, 1986; 6:622; Petrides, Hepatol, 1991; 14:432; McCullough, Gastro, 1992; 102:1325), or reduced (Morrison, ClinSci, 1990; 78:613; Pacy, AlcAlc, 1991; 26:505). Protein turnover is increased in patients with alcoholic cirrhosis who are actively drinking (Hirsch, JAmCollNutr, 1995; 14:99).

Although protein requirements are increased in these patients, their diets are often suboptimal because of anorexia, nausea, abdominal distension, and/or ascites or else because of inappropriate dietary restrictions imposed for the management of the complications of their liver disease. In consequence, they may develop negative nitrogen balance (Swart, ClinNutr, 1989; 8:329; Fiaccadori, ItalJGastr, 1993; 25:336) and consequently a reduction in lean body mass and muscle wasting (McCullough, SemLivDis, 1991; 11:265; Müller, JHepatol, 1995; 23(Suppl.1):31; Kalman, NutrRev, 1996; 54:217). These patients can, however, tolerate protein intakes of 1.8 to 2.0 g/kg daily and retain 80 to 90 per cent of the excess ingested (Nielsen, BrJNutr, 1995; 74:557); every effort should therefore be made to furnish their requirements.

In patients with acute and chronic liver disease, synthesis of plasma proteins, for example albumin and prothrombin, may be reduced. Additionally, in patients with severe liver disease, qualitative changes may occur in certain proteins, for example fibrinogen, which alter or attenuate their function.

Blood urea concentrations may be low in patients with chronic liver disease reflecting a reduction in urea synthesis rates (Shambaugh, AmJClinNutr, 1978; 31:126). Conversely, blood ammonia concentrations may be elevated secondary to impaired hepatic function and portal–systemic shunting of blood. The increase in circulating ammonia concentrations has been implicated in the genesis of hepatic encephalopathy.

Significant changes occur in plasma amino-acid concentrations in patients with liver disease which appear to relate to the severity of the liver disease, its activity, and its aetiology. In patients with fulminant hepatic failure, plasma concentrations of all amino acids are high except those of the branched-chain amino acids, which are normal or low (Record, EurJClinInv, 1976; 6:387; Fiaccadori, DigDisSci, 1991; 36:801). These changes reflect release of amino acids into the plasma from peripheral tissues and from the necrosing liver, and failure of hepatic amino-acid uptake. The branched-chain amino acids are predominantly metabolized by muscle so that their plasma concentrations are largely unaffected. In patients with chronic liver disease, plasma concentrations of the branched-chain amino acids are reduced, while concentrations of one or both of the aromatic amino acids phenylalanine and tyrosine are increased, together with methionine (Morgan, Gut, 1982; 23:362; Montanari, Hepatol, 1988; 8:1034; Plauth, Hepatogast, 1990; 37:135; Petrides, Hepatol, 1991; 14:432). These changes result from a combination of impaired hepatic function, portal–systemic shunting of blood, hyperinsulinaemia, and hyperglucagonaemia.

In patients with minimal, potentially reversible liver damage, for example with alcoholic fatty liver or acute viral hepatitis, plasma concentrations of the branched-chain amino acids and proline are reduced (Morgan, Gut, 1982; 23:362). These changes are not readily explained, but indicate that amino-acid metabolism is disturbed even in the presence of minor liver injury.

Fat-soluble vitamins (Marcus, p.1573 in reference 4)[3]

Vitamin A (Marcus, p.1573 in reference 4; Blaner, p.529 in reference 5)[3,6]

Vitamin A originates in the diet in two forms: as preformed vitamin A or retinol, which is found in the tissues of animals and fish; and as plant carotenoids, mainly β–carotene, which are subsequently cleaved to retinol in the small intestinal epithelial cells. Fish liver oils are the richest source of vitamin A, but substantial amounts are present in mammalian liver, kidney, dairy produce, and eggs. β–Carotene is found in dark-green leafy vegetables such as parsley and spinach, and in carrots; approximately 25 to 30 per cent of dietary vitamin A is provided in this form. In adults, the Reference Nutrient Intakes for vitamin A are 600 μg/day for women and 700 μg/day for men. Regular intake should not exceed 7500 μg/day in women or 9000 μg/day in men.[1]

Retinol is present in the diet mainly in esterified form. Most of the retinyl esters are hydrolysed in the intestinal lumen by pancreatic enzymes and within the brush border before absorption. Although retinol is lipophilic and its absorption is linked to that of lipid and

is enhanced by bile, its uptake by intestinal cells is governed by a carrier-mediated process and is facilitated by the presence, in the cytosol, of cellular retinol-binding protein (**CRBPII**). The retinol is largely re-esterified in enterocytes before leaving the gut, incorporated in chylomicrons. Appreciable quantities of retinol are absorbed directly into the circulation. β–Carotene is less well absorbed, predominantly in the ileum; its uptake is, therefore, more affected by disorders of fat absorption and micelle formation. A proportion of β-carotene is converted to retinol in the intestinal wall; this is then esterified and transported via the lymphatic system to the liver. Some β–carotene is absorbed unchanged and circulates in association with lipoproteins.

Most of the absorbed retinyl esters are taken up by the liver through receptor-mediated internalization of chylomicron remnants. The concentration of retinyl esters in the liver is approximately 100 to 300 μg/g. Before release into the circulation, hepatic retinyl esters are hydrolysed and 90 to 95 per cent of the retinol formed is bound to an α_1-globulin, retinol-binding protein (**RBP**), which circulates in the blood complexed with transthyretin, a thyroxine-binding prealbumin. The formation of this complex prevents metabolism and excretion of the retinol-RBP moiety.

More than 95 per cent of plasma retinoids are bound to RBP; retinyl esters comprise less than 5 per cent of total retinoids in the blood; they are associated with lipoproteins. Plasma concentrations of retinol are maintained at the expense of hepatic reserves. Thus, plasma retinol concentrations do not provide an accurate assessment of overall vitamin A status, although low plasma retinol concentrations indicate a significant reduction in hepatic vitamin A reserves. The retinol–RBP complex reaches the cell membrane of various target organs where it binds to specific sites on the cell surface. The retinol is transferred to a membrane-bound protein which is closely related to soluble CRBP, and is converted to retinyl ester. Retinol is, in part, conjugated with β–glucuronide, which is excreted in bile and can be reabsorbed. It is also oxidized to retinal and retinoic acid, which together with other water-soluble metabolites are excreted in the urine and faeces.

Vitamin A plays an essential role in the function of the retina. It is necessary for the growth and differentiation of epithelial tissues and is required for bone remodelling, reproduction, and embryonic development. Vitamin A, together with certain carotenoids, appears to enhance the function of the immune system, to reduce the consequences of some infectious diseases, and to protect against the development of certain malignancies. Retinol also appears to have a specific biochemical function in the synthesis of mannose and galactose-containing glycoproteins and glycolipids.

In the retina, vitamin A forms a series of carotenoid proteins that provide the molecular basis for visual excitation. In order to be photochemically active, retinol must be converted to its aldehyde, retinal, which requires the zinc-dependent enzyme retinal dehydrogenase; vitamin E may be necessary to prevent peroxidation of vitamin A in the retina. Vitamin A, as retinal, also plays an important role in spermatogenesis; *in vitro* it acts synergistically with insulin, follicle-stimulating hormone, and testosterone to stimulate production of androgen-binding protein by Sertoli cells.

Symptoms and signs of vitamin A deficiency appear when the hepatic concentration of retinoid falls below 20 μg/g wet weight; plasma retinol concentrations are insensitive indicators of vitamin A status as homeostatic mechanisms maintain them at a reasonably constant level over a wide range of liver reserves. Plasma concentrations in individuals manifesting signs of vitamin A deficiency are usually less than 20 μg/100 ml (0.7 μmol/l.). Skin lesions such as follicular hyperkeratosis and infections are among the earliest signs of deficiency, but the most recognizable manifestation is impaired dark adaptation possibly leading to night blindness, even through it only develops when depletion is severe. Children in particular may develop xerophthalmia and keratomalacia. Deficiency in adults should be treated with oral retinol, 15 mg (50 000 IU) daily until stores are repleted; deficiency in children can be treated with a single intramuscular injection of 30 mg of the water-miscible palmitate followed by intermittent oral treatment with vitamin A in oil.

Vitamin A metabolism is disturbed in patients with chronic hepatobiliary disease. Absorption of the vitamin may be impaired whenever bile secretion is reduced. Hepatic synthesis and release of RBP may be impaired in patients with parenchymal liver damage, resulting in impaired release of vitamin A from hepatic stores (Kanai, JCI, 1968; 47:2025; Hirosowa, JElectronMicrosc, 1973; 22: 337; Smith, Lancet, 1975; i:1251; McClain, Alcoholism, 1979; 3: 135). In addition, synthesis of transthyretin may be significantly impaired resulting in urinary loss of the RBP–protein complex. In individuals chronically abusing alcohol, the microsomal cytochrome P450 enzyme system is induced, resulting in enhanced hepatic vitamin A metabolism and a reduction in retinoid stores (Leo, NEJM, 1982; 307:597). In addition, the dehydrogenase required to convert retinol to retinal has an affinity for ethanol which is 50 times that for retinol; therefore ethanol in the circulation could act as a competitive enzyme inhibitor.[7] Ethanol also increases urinary zinc excretion and this might further impair the function of vitamin A (Kalbfleisch, JCI, 1963; 42:1471).

Hepatic vitamin A and carotenoid stores are reduced in individuals with non-alcoholic liver disease (Schindler, IntJVitNutrRes, 1988; 58:146; Bell, JHepatol, 1989; 8:26; Leo, Hepatol, 1993; 17:977), and in individuals chronically abusing alcohol, whether or not they have significant liver injury (Leo, NEJM, 1982; 307:597; Johansson, BrJNutr, 1986; 55:227; Bell, 1989; Leo, 1993). Both groups of individuals may, therefore, develop vitamin A deficiency.

Circulating concentrations of retinol and the carotenoids are reduced in patients with cirrhosis irrespective of its aetiology; concentrations are lowest in patients with decompensated disease (Patek, JCI, 1939; 18:609; Leevy, AmJClinNutr, 1970; 23:493; Russell, AnnIntMed, 1978; 88:622; Herlong, Hepatol, 1981; 1:348; Schölmerich, Hepatogast, 1983; 30:119; Muñoz, Hepatol, 1989; 9: 525; Rocchi, JLabClinMed, 1991; 118:176; Leo, Hepatol, 1993; 17: 977; Goode, Hepatol, 1994; 19:354; Janczewska, ScaJGastr, 1995; 30:68; Madden, Hepatol, 1997; 26:40) (Fig. 1). Circulating concentrations of retinol, RBP, and carotenoids are also reduced in individuals chronically abusing alcohol; concentrations are lowest in those with significant liver injury (Horvath, ActaPhysiolHung, 1992; 80:381; Ward, AlcAlc, 1992; 27:359; Chapman, JAmCollNutr, 1993; 12:77; Leo, 1993; Ahmed, AmJClinNutr, 1994; 60:430).

Vitamin A deficiency is relatively common in patients with primary biliary cirrhosis; the lowest plasma concentrations are found in patients with the most severe cholestasis (Muñoz, Hepatol, 1989; 9:525). Deficiency is usually manifest as impaired dark adaptation; overt night blindness is unusual (Morrison, AmJClinNutr, 1978;

31:276; Herlong, Hepatol, 1981; 1:348). As individuals may be unaware of even severe impairment of dark adaptation, visual function should be checked routinely in all patients with chronic cholestasis. These patients should, if jaundiced, be given prophylactic intramuscular vitamin A in a dose of 30 mg (100 000 IU) every 3 months. However, as the disease progresses it would seem advisable to give oral supplements of 7.5 mg (25 000 IU) daily (Walt, BMJ, 1984; 288:1030). At present there is insufficient evidence to support the use of regular zinc supplementation.

Children with chronic cholestasis may show electrical abnormalities of the retina which could be attributed to lack of vitamin A, vitamin E, or both (Alvarez, Hepatol, 1983; 3:410). Studies in animals indicate that combined deficiency of these two vitamins accelerates the loss of photoreceptor cells (Robison, InvOphthalmolVisSci, 1980; 19:1030). Supplementation with both vitamins is, therefore, recommended.

Individuals chronically abusing alcohol may develop hypogonadism and impaired dark adaptation, possibly as a result of vitamin A deficiency (Patek, JCI, 1939; 18:609; McClain, Alcoholism, 1979; 3:135). Management involves abstinence from alcohol, the institution of a nutritionally sound diet, and oral vitamin A in a dose of 7.5 mg (25 000 IU) daily for a few days. There is no evidence that the hypogonadism responds to vitamin A supplementation alone. Severe, bilateral corneal manifestations of vitamin A deficiency have been reported in patients who chronically abuse alcohol and have significant liver disease (Sadowski, KlinMonatsblAugenheilkd, 1994; 205:76).

Vitamin A deficiency has been implicated in the abnormalities of taste perception observed in patients with cirrhosis; however, although improvement in gustatory activity has been reported in vitamin A-deficient individuals following supplementation (Garrett-Laster, HumNutrCN, 1984; 38C:203), the results of studies designed to examine the relationship between gustatory acuity and vitamin A status are conflicting (Smith, Gastro, 1976; 70:568; Garrett-Laster, 1984; Madden, Hepatol, 1997; 26:40).

Chronic ingestion of vitamin A can result in the development of liver injury (Russell, NEJM, 1974; 291:435; Hathcock, AmJClinNutr, 1990; 52:183; Geubel, Gastro, 1991; 100:1701; Kowalski, AmJMed, 1994; 97:523).

Vitamin D (Marcus, p. 1519 in reference 4; Holick, p.543 in reference 5)[3,8]

While many forms of vitamin D exist, only two are of nutritional or biological significance, vitamin D_2 (ergocalciferol), which is synthesized in the skin by ultraviolet irradiation of ergosterol derived from yeasts and fungi, and vitamin D_3 (cholecalciferol), which is synthesized in the skin by ultraviolet irradiation of 7-dehydrocholesterol derived from animal sources. The only structural difference between D_2 and D_3 is in the side chain; in the absence of a subscript the term vitamin D refers to either compound.

Vitamin D is unique among vitamins in that, with adequate sunlight, no dietary intake is needed, as the entire bodily requirements can be met by skin photolysis reactions. Only when skin irradiation is limited or insignificant is there a real need for dietary supplementation. The richest sources of dietary vitamin D are fish-liver oils, animal liver, and dairy produce; crystalline vitamin D is added to a variety of foods including milk, milk products, margarine,

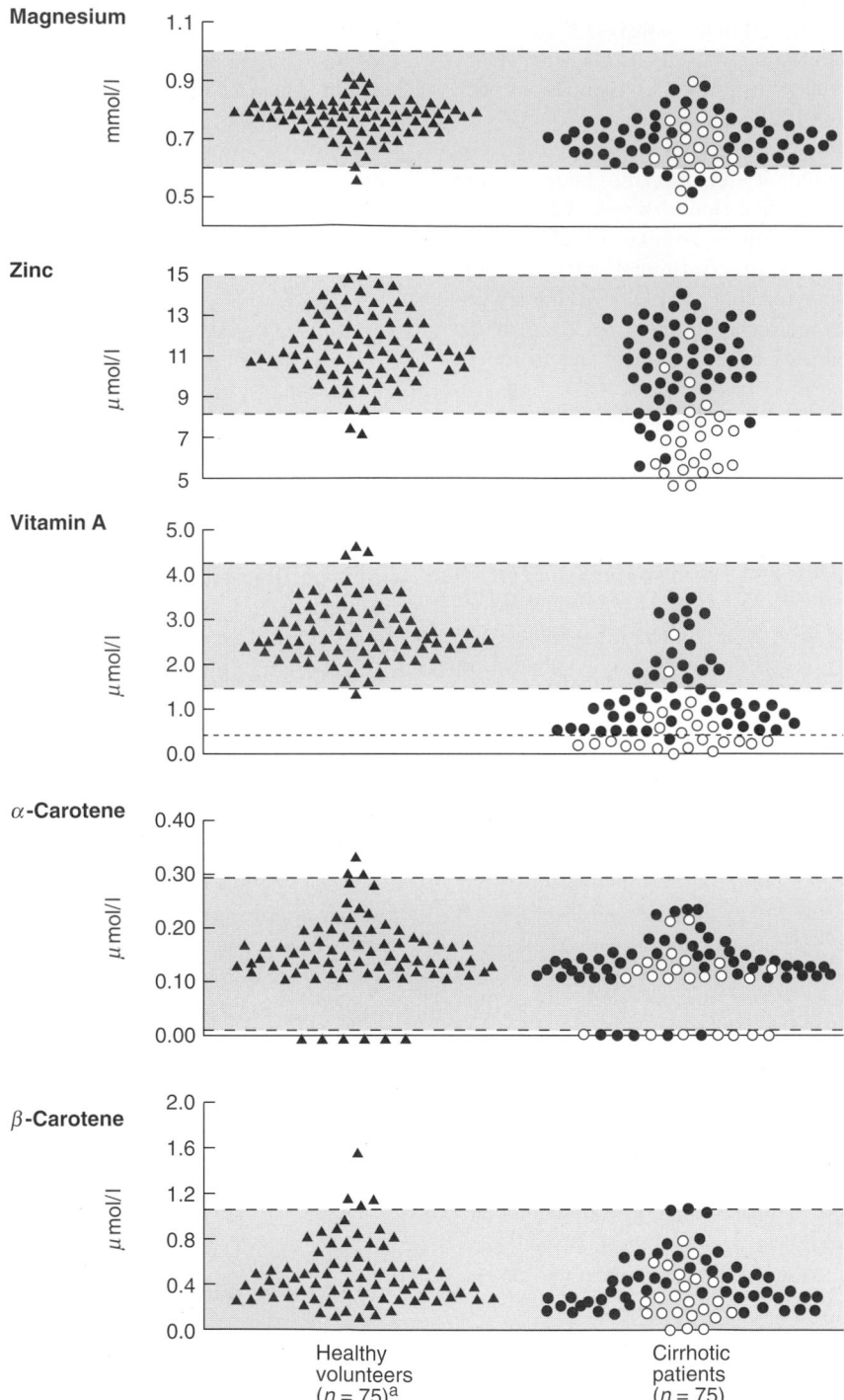

Fig. 1. Circulating concentrations of magnesium, zinc, vitamin A, and α- and β-carotene in healthy volunteers (▲; $n = 75$) and patients with cirrhosis with compensated (●; $n = 51$) and decompensated (○; $n = 24$) disease (Madden, Hepatol, 1997; 26:40). Shaded areas represent the reference ranges defined as mean ± 2SD of the values in the healthy volunteers. The single interrupted horizontal line represents the value that defines deficiency for vitamin A (Underwood, JNutr, 1990; 1205:1459). [a]Vitamin A and α- and β-carotene data from 74 healthy volunteers.

and cereals. No Reference Nutrient Intake has been set for healthy adults, although individuals over the age of 65 years or those permanently confined indoors may need to supplement their diet with 10 μg of cholecalciferol daily.[1]

Vitamin D is absorbed from the small intestine and requires micellar solubilization for its uptake. Newly absorbed vitamin D leaves the gut in the lymphatic system, primarily as a lipoprotein complex in the chylomicron fraction. Subsequently, the vitamin is either stored unchanged in the liver, skeletal muscle, or adipose tissue, or else converted to one of its biologically active, hydroxylated forms which circulate in plasma bound to a specific α–globulin designated vitamin D-binding protein (**DBP**). Vitamin D synthesized in the skin diffuses into the blood and is either deposited in fat or muscle or else transported to the liver bound to DBP.

Vitamin D is hydroxylated in the liver to 25-hydroxycholecalciferol (**25-OHD**) or calcifediol, which is the major circulating form of the vitamin. In healthy individuals there is marked seasonal variation in serum 25-OHD concentrations, which are maximal in autumn and minimal at the end of winter.

The calcifediol is transported to the kidney where it undergoes 1-α-hydroxylation to form 1,25-dihydroxycholecalciferol (1,25-[OH]₂D), or calcitriol, which is the active form of the vitamin. Calcitriol is hydroxylated to $1,24,25\text{-}(OH)_3D$ by a renal hydroxylase; this enzyme also hydroxylates 25-OHD to form $24,25\text{-}(OH)_2D$. These 24-hydroxylated compounds are less active than calcitriol and presumably represent metabolites destined for excretion. Vitamin D is inactivated by the hepatic microsomal enzyme oxidizing system or else is excreted unchanged in the bile to undergo enterohepatic recirculation.

The active forms of vitamin D, together with parathormone and calcitonin, play an important role in regulating calcium and phosphorus homeostasis, in particular the maintenance of plasma calcium and phosphorus concentrations. Vitamin D promotes calcium and phosphorus absorption from the small intestine, mobilizes calcium and phosphorus from bone, and increases calcium reabsorption by the kidney. Calcitriol also affects maturation and differentiation of mononuclear cells and influences cytokine production. It also inhibits proliferation and induces differentiation of malignant cells. Vitamin D may also have effects on skeletal muscle and brain function.

Vitamin D deficiency results in defective mineralization of bone with development of rickets in children and osteomalacia in adults. Oral cholecalciferol in a dose of 12.5 to 125 μg (500 to 5000 IU) daily is used to treat vitamin D deficiency; calcitriol should be used to treat vitamin D deficiency in patients with renal disease.

Patients with long-standing cholestasis or parenchymal liver disease may have low circulating serum 25-OHD concentrations (Herlong, Gastro, 1982; 83:103; Cuthbert, Hepatol, 1984; 4:1; Compston, Gut, 1986; 27:1073; Muñoz, Hepatol, 1989; 9:525; Guanabens, AmJGastr, 1990; 85:1356; Pietschmann, BoneMineral, 1990; 8:103; Floreani, JHepatol, 1991; 12:217; Sezai, ClinRadiol, 1991; 43:32; Chen, JGastHepatol, 1996; 11:417; Compston, JHepatol, 1996; 25:715; Riemens, OsteoporosisInt, 1996; 6:213; Monegal, CalcifTissInt, 1997; 60:148); the lowest concentrations are observed in the patients with the severest disease. Many of these patients have osteopenia; a small percentage will develop osteomalacia which is characterized by bone pain and fractures (Atkinson, QJMed, 1956; 25:299; Dibble, QJMed, 1982; 51:89; Sezai, 1991).

The aetiology of the vitamin D deficiency is multifactorial, but reduced exposure to sunlight, malabsorption, increased utilization, enhanced metabolic destruction, and increased urinary losses of water-soluble metabolites all play a role. In addition, malabsorption of calcium leads to increased production of $1,25\text{-}(OH)_2D$ and consequent depletion of vitamin D reserves by an action of $1,25\text{-}(OH)_2D$ in the liver which somehow enhances the metabolic destruction of 25-OHD (Clements, ClinEndoc, 1992; 37:17). It might be expected that, in the presence of severe liver disease, hydroxylation of vitamin D would be impaired, but there is little evidence that this occurs (Krawitt, Lancet, 1977; ii:1246; Posner, Gastro, 1978; 74:866).

Both vitamin D and its metabolites have been used to treat osteomalacia in patients with long-standing cholestasis and severe parenchymal liver disease (Long, BMJ, 1978; i:75; Compston, BMJ, 1979; ii:309; Compston, Gut, 1979; 20:133; Reed, Gastro, 1980; 78:512; Sezai, ClinRadiol, 1991; 43:32). Patients with primary biliary cirrhosis and those with long-standing biliary obstruction should receive prophylactic intramuscular vitamin D in a dose of 2.5 mg (100 000 IU) monthly; additional calcium supplements may be required.

Low serum 25-OHD concentrations are also found in individuals chronically abusing alcohol; the lowest levels are observed in the patients with significant liver disease (Posner, Gastro, 1978; 74: 866; Devgun, BrJNutr, 1981; 45:469; Mobarhan, Hepatol, 1984; 4:266; Diamond, AmJMed, 1989; 86:282; Hickish, ClinSci, 1989; 77:171; Peris, AlcAlc, 1992; 27:619); the aetiology is multifactorial and includes malabsorption, increased utilization, enhanced metabolic destruction, and increased urinary losses of water-soluble metabolites. Many such individuals have osteopenia but the percentage with osteomalacia is probably very small; once the individual has stopped drinking the osteomalacia will respond to vitamin D and its metabolites (Posner, 1978; Mobarhan, 1984).

Prolonged ingestion of vitamin D supplements is associated with the development of hypercalcaemia with metastatic tissue calcification.

Vitamin E (Marcus, p.1573 in reference 4)[3,9]

Vitamin E activity is manifest by two series of naturally occurring compounds, the more important being the tocopherols; the tocotrienols are less potent. The most active compound is α-tocepherol, which accounts for about 90 per cent of the vitamin E present in human tissues. The main sources of vitamin E in the diet are polyunsaturated vegetable oils, cereal products, and eggs. Daily α-tocopherol intakes of 3 mg/day for women and 4 mg/day for men are adequate.[1]

Ingested vitamin E requires intestinal solubilization by bile acids. Before absorption, most esterified tocopherols are hydrolysed in the intestinal lumen by pancreatic enzymes, or else within the brush border. Free tocopherol is transported from the intestine in chylomicrons and VLDL and is taken up by the liver in chylomicron remnants. It is then secreted in VLDL and perhaps HDL, and subsequently becomes associated with plasma β-lipoproteins. There does not appear to be a specific plasma transport protein. Circulating tocopherol is taken up slowly by tissues and stored in fat, skeletal muscle, and liver; tissue concentrations vary widely. Vitamin E is excreted by the liver; some metabolites appear in the urine.

Vitamin E is the most important antioxidant vitamin in the body, playing an essential protective role against free radical damage. It inhibits oxidation of unsaturated fatty acids, and other oxygen-sensitive compounds, by interacting with selenium and ascorbate. Its ability to prevent lipid peroxidation is of fundamental importance for all cells. It may have a cardioprotective effect by favouring redistribution of cholesterol in the HDL fraction and also influences cellular responses to oxidative stress.

Vitamin E deficiency is associated with the development of increased red cell fragility and haemolytic anaemia (Zipursky, Pediat, 1987; 79:61). While these changes may reflect alterations in lipid peroxidation, they may also indicate a role for the vitamin in normal haematopoiesis (Drake, AmJClinNutr, 1980; 33:2386). A neurological syndrome has been described in association with vitamin E deficiency; its features include muscle weakness, peripheral neuropathy, cerebellar degeneration, and abnormal eye movements (Muller, ArchDisChild, 1977; 52:209; Elias, Lancet, 1981; ii:1319; Rosenblum, NEJM, 1981; 304:503; Guggenheim, JPediat, 1982; 100:51; Harding, AnnNeurol, 1982; 12:419; Bieri, NEJM, 1983; 308:1063; Sokol, AnnRevNutr, 1988; 8:351). Vitamin E deficiency is treated with oral α-tocopherol preparations or else with tocopherol polyethylene glycol 1000 succinate (**TPGS**), which is water-soluble; the dose required relates to the aetiology of the deficiency.

Vitamin E deficiency may develop in patients with chronic hepatobiliary disease when the intraluminal bile salt concentrations falls below critical micellar concentration resulting in malabsorption (Muñoz, Hepatol, 1989; 9:525; Sokol, Gastro, 1989; 96:479). However, a number of other factors such as portal–systemic shunting of blood and impairment of the lymphatic circulation may also affect vitamin E metabolism in these patients (Rocchi, JLabClinMed, 1991; 118:176).

Hepatic vitamin E concentrations are reduced in patients with cirrhosis (Bell, AlcAlc, 1992; 27:39; Leo, Hepatol, 1993; 17:977), and in individuals chronically abusing alcohol with or without liver disease (Situnayake, Gut, 1990; 31:1311; Bell, 1992).

Serum vitamin E concentrations are reduced in patients with severe viral hepatitis (von Herbay, FreeRadRes, 1996; 25:461), and in patients with cirrhosis irrespective of its aetiology, although the lowest levels are often observed in those with alcohol-related disease (Jeffrey, JHepatol, 1987; 4:307; Muñoz, Hepatol, 1989; 9:525; Sokol, Gastro, 1989; 96:479; Arria, AmJClinNutr, 1990; 52:383; Bell, AlcAlc, 1992; 27:39; Ward, AlcAlc, 1992; 27:359; Clot, Gut, 1994; 35:1637; Goode, Hepatol, 1994; 19:354; von Herbay, JHepatol, 1994; 20:41; de la Maza, JAmCollNutr, 1995; 14:192).

Low serum vitamin E concentrations have also been observed in chronic alcohol abusers with or without liver disease (Bell, AlcAlc, 1992; 27:39; Horvath, ActaPhysiolHung, 1992; 80:381; Butcher, JHepatol, 1993; 19:105); the lowest levels are observed in the individuals with significant liver injury.

Children with chronic cholestasis develop a neurological syndrome which has been attributed to vitamin E deficiency (Elias, Lancet, 1981; ii:1319; Rosenblum, NEJM, 1981; 304:503; Sokol, AmJDisChild, 1985; 139:1211). These children also develop retinal degeneration which has been attributed to deficiency of vitamin E, vitamin A, or both (Alvarez, Hepatol, 1983; 3:410). Established deficiency can be treated with oral α-tocopherol acetate in a daily dose of 68 to 272 mg (50 to 200 IU)/kg; children who fail to respond may be given TPGS vitamin E in a dose of 25 IU/kg daily. If oral supplementation is unsuccessful, then DL-α-tocopherol may be given parenterally in a dose of 1 to 2 mg (1 to 2 IU)/kg daily, initially, and then at intervals determined by plasma concentrations.

In adults with chronic cholestatis or parenchymal liver disease, vitamin E deficiency, if present, tends to be mild or subclinical (Mills, AmJClinNutr, 1983; 38:849; Johansson, BrJNutr, 1986; 55:227; Mezes, IntJClinPharmRes, 1986; 6:333; Tanner, DigDisSci, 1986; 31:1307; Jeffrey, JHepatol, 1987; 4:307; Muñoz, Hepatol, 1989; 9:525; Arria, AmJClinNutr, 1990; 52:383).

Muñoz and co-workers (Hepatol, 1989; 9:525) found low vitamin E levels in 6 (13 per cent) of 45 patients with primary biliary cirrhosis, none of whom showed any neurological abnormalities.

Jeffrey and colleagues (JHepatol, 1987; 4:307) found biochemical evidence of vitamin E deficiency in 12 (15 per cent) or 80 patients with primary biliary cirrhosis; of these, six showed a mild sensorimotor peripheral neuropathy which did not, however, improve following restoration of circulating vitamin E concentrations.

Arria and associates (AmJClinNutr, 1990; 52:383) documented impaired psychomotor performance in 19 women with primary biliary cirrhosis who were vitamin E deficient; psychometric performance was also impaired, though to a lesser degree, in 15 similar patients who were vitamin E replete. Non-specific neurological abnormalities were observed in 47 per cent of the vitamin E-deficient patients and in 38 per cent of the vitamin E-replete patients.

An occasional patient with endstage primary biliary cirrhosis may exhibit severe vitamin E-associated neurological abnormalities (Knight, Gastro, 1986; 91:209).

Although red cell survival is shortened in these patients, its aetiology is multifactorial and lack of vitamin E is of only minor importance. The polyunsaturated fatty acid content of erythrocyte membranes is reduced in patients with jaundice and this may attenuate the effects of vitamin E deficiency.

Vitamin K (Marcus, p.1573 in reference 4; Furie, p.1217 in reference 5)[3,10]

Vitamin K activity is associated with at least two distinct natural substances: vitamin K_1 (phylloquinone), which is present in most edible vegetables, particularly spinach, broccoli, cabbage, Brussels sprouts, cauliflower, peas, and cereals; and vitamin K_2 (a series of menaquinones), which is produced in the mammalian intestine by Gram-positive bacteria. All other compounds which possess vitamin K-like activity are structurally related to the simpler compound, menadione. The richest source of vitamin K in the diet is green leafy vegetables although other vegetables, fruit, dairy produce, vegetable oils, cereals, and meats can provide significant amounts. Daily intakes of the order of 1 μg/kg body weight are adequate for adults.[1]

Vitamins K_1 and K_2 are dependent for their absorption on micellar solubilization, whereas menadione and its water-soluble derivatives are absorbed even in the absence of bile. Vitamin K_1 is absorbed by an active process in the proximal small intestine, while vitamin K_2 and the menadiones are absorbed by passive diffusion in the distal small intestine and colon. Following absorption, vitamins K_1 and K_2 leave the gut by way of the lymph, while menadione and its water-soluble derivatives enter the bloodstream directly. The plasma transport of vitamin K appears to be mediated entirely by lipoproteins. Vitamin K_1 is rapidly metabolized in the liver and its metabolites excreted in bile and urine. Body stores of vitamin K are small but take several weeks to deplete.

Vitamin K is responsible for the post-translational γ-carboxylation of glutamic acid residues on the vitamin K-dependent proteins (gla-proteins), so creating effective calcium-binding sites. It is, therefore, essential for the hepatic synthesis of the procoagulant factors II (prothrombin), VII, IX, and X, and for the production of protein C and protein S. Protein C, a serine protease, is synthesized in the liver and, in its activated form, functions as an anticoagulant by inactivating factors V and VII; it also facilitates clot lysis. Protein S, a glycoprotein, is synthesized in the liver and also in the bone, and in its free form acts as a cofactor in the inactivation of factors V and VII by protein C. Other vitamin K-dependent proteins are found in a number of tissues including cortical bone, renal tissue, lung, spleen, pancreas, and placenta; the function of the majority of these proteins is, as yet, unknown.

Deficiency of vitamin K is associated with a marked decrease in prothrombin and factor VII, IX, and X activities; this may be associated with a bleeding tendency. The prothrombin produced by the liver in the presence of vitamin K deficiency contains a considerably reduced number of γ-carboxyglutamic acid residues so that it is unable to bind calcium and to function normally (Perutz, Nature, 1976; 262:449). Similar abnormalities may occur in the other proteins which require vitamin K for post-translational modification. Vitamin K deficiency is treated with oral vitamin K supplements in a dose of 2.5 to 5.0 mg daily or, if the response is inadequate, with parenteral vitamin K_1 in a dose of 10 mg given daily for 3 days.

In patients with both acute and chronic liver disease, circulating concentrations of the blood-clotting proteins may be reduced and the prothrombin time prolonged. Several factors are responsible, including vitamin K deficiency due to malabsorption and cholestasis, diminished hepatic protein synthesis, and increased consumption of clotting factor following bleeding and fibrinolysis. Increased circulating concentrations of an abnormal protein, des-γ-carboxyprothrombin, are found in patients with hepatocellular carcinoma (Weitz, Hepatol, 1993; 18:990; Okuda, Hepatol, 1997; 26(Suppl.):171A abstr.).

Improvement may occur in the prothrombin time in patients with parenchymal liver disease following parenteral vitamin K_1, but in general, coagulation remains prolonged until liver function improves. Paradoxically, the administration of large doses of vitamin K_1 or its analogues to patients with severe parenchymal liver disease may result in further depression of the prothrombin concentration. The mechanism is unknown. Patients with obstructive jaundice absorb vitamin K poorly; defects in their clotting time can be corrected by parenteral administration of vitamin K_1. Patients with primary biliary cirrhosis, and those with long-standing biliary obstruction, should be given prophylactic intramuscular vitamin K_1 in a dose of 10 mg monthly; cutaneous hypersensitivity to injected vitamin K_1 may develop (Finkelstein, JAmAcadDermatol, 1987; 16:540; Lemlich, JAmAcadDermatol, 1993; 28:345; Bruynzeel, ContactDerm, 1995; 32:78).

Water-soluble vitamins (Marcus, p.1555 in reference 4; McCormick, p.563 in reference 5)

Thiamine

Thiamine is synthesized by a variety of plants and micro-organisms, but not by animal tissues. It is widely distributed in food; the richest dietary sources are whole-grain cereals, beans, seeds, and nuts; the main dietary sources are bread, flour, potatoes, and meat; eggs, fruit, vegetables, and fortified breakfast cereals provide useful contributions. A limited amount of thiamine may also be synthesized by intestinal bacteria. A large portion of the vitamin in vegetable products is in the form of thiamine itself, whereas in animal tissues

it is mainly present as phosphate esters. In adults, the Reference Nutrient Intake for thiamine is 0.4 mg/1000 kcal daily, or 0.8 mg/day for women and 1.0 mg/day for men.[1] Requirements increase in proportion to increases in metabolic rate and are greatest when carbohydrate is the main source of energy. Thiaminases present in raw fresh fish, shrimps, clams, mussels, and some raw animal tissues, and a thiamine antagonist present in tea, may reduce the amount of thiamine available for absorption.

At low or physiological concentrations, thiamine is absorbed from the small intestine by a sodium-dependent active transport process. At higher or pharmacological concentrations, transport across the intestine also occurs by passive diffusion. Absorption is usually limited to a maximum of 8 to 15 mg daily. Thiamine passes to the liver where it is phosphorylated to thiamine pyrophosphate. It is stored in the heart, liver, kidney, brain, and skeletal muscle, principally as the pyrophosphate. Thiamine is catabolized to a number of metabolites, some of which are excreted in urine, together with unchanged thiamine.

Thiamine pyrophosphate, the physiologically active form of thiamine, functions in carbohydrate metabolism as a coenzyme in the decarboxylation of α-keto acids, for example pyruvate and α-ketoglutarate, and as a cofactor for transketolase in the hexose–monophosphate shunt. It is also required to complete the metabolism of the branched-chain amino acids and for the interconversion of sugars of different chain lengths. Thiamine may have a specific role in neuromuscular transmission, independent of its function as a coenzyme in general metabolism (Cooper, NeurochemRes, 1979; 4:223; Schoffeniels, ArchIntPhysiolBioch, 1983; 91:233).

Thiamine deficiency leads to disorders of the cardiovascular system and both the central and peripheral nervous systems. Heart disease may develop acutely or chronically and usually results in high-output cardiac failure. Administration of thiamine rapidly restores peripheral vascular resistance, but as improvement of the myocardial abnormality is often delayed, treatment may be complicated by the development of low-output heart failure. The polyneuropathy associated with thiamine deficiency is of a peripheral sensorimotor type; it is non-specific and cannot be distinguished from other 'nutritional' neuropathies; it responds reasonably well to thiamine supplementation. The central nervous system manifestations of thiamine deficiency include: Wernicke's encephalopathy, which is characterized by a confusional state, variable degrees of ophthalmoplegia, and ataxia; and Korsakoff psychosis, which is characterized by a short-term memory deficit; confabulation may be present. Wernicke's encephalopathy and Korsakoff's psychosis are not separate clinical entities but represent successive stages of a single disease process. Treatment with oral or intramuscular thiamine hydrochloride, in doses of up to 600 mg daily, results in improvement in the features of the Wernicke's encephalopathy but the Korsakoff's psychosis improves in only 50 per cent of patients.

The factors which determine the manifestations of thiamine deficiency in individual patients are poorly understood. Several factors are, however, known to be important, including the duration and severity of the thiamine deficiency, the amount of physical activity undertaken, and the daily energy intake. Severe physical exertion coupled with a high carbohydrate intake and a moderate degree of chronic thiamine deficiency favours the development of cardiovascular disease. An equal deficiency coupled with caloric restriction and relative inactivity favours the development of peripheral neuropathy.

Biochemical evidence of thiamine deficiency is present in 9 to 80 per cent of individuals chronically abusing alcohol, irrespective of the presence of significant liver disease (Leevy, AmJClinNutr, 1965; 16:339; Fennelly, AmJClinNutr, 1967; 20:946; Leevy, AmJClinNutr, 1970; 23:493; Somogyi, BiblioNutrDiet, 1976; 23: 78; Rossouw, ScaJGastr, 1978; 13:133; Camilo, ScaJGastr, 1981; 16:273; Dancy, BMJ, 1984; 289:79; World, AlcAlc, 1985; 20:89; Graudal, Liver, 1987; 7:91; Baines, AlcAlc, 1988; 23:49; Tallaksen, AlcoholClinExpRes, 1992; 16:320). In the majority of patients, however, biochemical evidence of thiamine deficiency is unaccompanied by symptoms or signs of hypovitaminosis. The widely varying incidence of thiamine deficiency in the various reported series may be explained partly by the diversity of methods used to assess thiamine deficiency, and partly by differences in patient populations.

Several factors contribute to the development of thiamine deficiency in individuals chronically abusing alcohol, including reduced dietary intake, increased metabolic demands, and impaired intestinal absorption (Breen, AmJClinNutr, 1985; 42:121); additional factors play a role in patients with alcohol-related liver disease, including deficiency of the thiamine pyrophosphate apoenzyme (Fennelly, ClinRes, 1963; 11:182 abstr.), impaired conversion of the vitamin to its active form, and a reduction in hepatic storage capacity.

Camilo and coworkers (ScaJGastr, 1981; 16:273) found low erythrocyte transketolase activity in 19 (30 per cent) of 64 normally nourished alcohol abusers with well-compensated liver disease (Fig. 2). In six of the 19, addition of thiamine pyrophosphate *in vitro* (**TPP effect**) stimulated transketolase activity, indicating depleted thiamine stores. In the remaining 13 patients, the TPP effect was normal or low, suggesting a deficiency or an inability to use the transketolase apoenzyme, either as a result of long-standing thiamine deficiency or the presence of liver disease. A further eight patients (13 per cent) had normal transketolase activity but a low TPP effect, perhaps reflecting failure of the coenzyme TPP to recombine with the transketolase apoenzyme in the presence of normal thiamine stores.

Tallaksen and colleagues (AlcAlc, 1992; 27:523) measured plasma and whole blood concentrations of thiamine and its mono- and diphosphate esters, using high-performance liquid chromatography, in patients with alcoholic cirrhosis. The mean plasma thiamine concentration was elevated in the patients who were abstinent from alcohol; concentrations above the upper reference range were observed in 31 per cent of these individuals. However, the mean whole-blood concentrations of thiamine and its monophosphate ester were normal in this group while the whole-blood thiamine disphosphate concentration was significantly reduced. In the patients who were currently abusing alcohol, mean plasma and whole-blood concentrations of thiamine and its phosphorylated esters were significantly reduced.

The high plasma thiamine concentrations in a percentage of the patients who were abstinent from alcohol is not easily explained; these patients had decompensated disease, two dying shortly after completion of the study, and the authors postulate that alteration in protein-binding capacity might provide an explanation. The

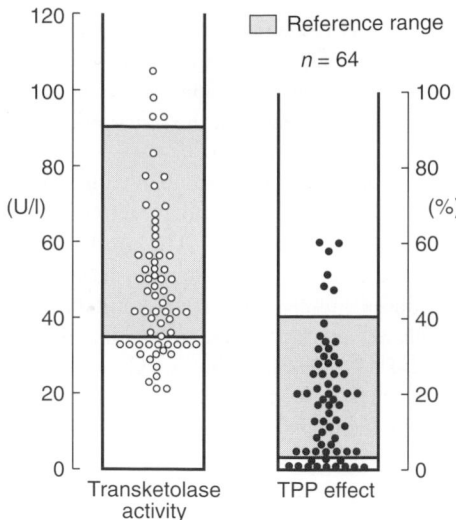

Fig. 2. Erythrocyte transketolase activity in 64 individuals with alcohol-related liver disease of varying severity both before and after stimulation *in vitro* with the coenzyme thiamine pyrophosphate (Camilo, ScaJGastr, 1981; 16:273).

reduction in circulating thiamine diphosphate concentrations, which were observed irrespective of drinking behaviour and which correlated significantly with plasma albumin concentrations, undoubtedly reflected the effect of liver disease on protein-binding capacity or on the phosphorylation process. The reduction in circulating concentrations of thiamine and its monophosphate undoubtedly reflected the effects of ethanol on intestinal absorption of the vitamin and its metabolism.

In the majority of alcohol abusers, subclinical thiamine deficiency can be corrected by use of oral thiamine hydrochloride, 30 to 100 mg daily in divided doses. In patients with overt deficiency, high-dose parenteral preparations should be used.

Subclinical thiamine deficiency has been described in patients with fulminant hepatic failure (Labadaros, IntJVitNutrRes, 1977; 47:17); biochemical abnormalities correct with thiamine supplements. The incidence of thiamine deficiency in patients with chronic non-alcoholic liver disease appears to vary. Morgan and co-workers (Gut, 1976; 17:113) found evidence of biochemical thiamine deficiency in only one (3 per cent) of 31 patients with cryptogenic cirrhosis or chronic active hepatitis, whereas Rossouw and colleagues (ScaJGastr, 1978; 13:133) found evidence of thiamine deficiency in six (43 per cent) of 14 patients with chronic non-alcoholic liver disease; the patients in the latter study were, however, severely ill and showed evidence of hepatic decompensation.

Riboflavin

Riboflavin is widely distributed in plants and animals but not in large amounts. The richest dietary sources are milk, milk products, and meat, especially liver, and eggs. The major dietary sources are milk, cheese, offal, whole-grain and enriched cereals and bread, and dark-green leafy vegetables. Requirements for riboflavin seem to relate to resting metabolic rate; in adults, the Reference Nutrient Intakes for riboflavin are 1.1 mg/day for women and 1.3 mg/day for men.[1]

Riboflavin is absorbed from the upper small intestine by a specific, active transport mechanism which involves phosphorylation of the vitamin to flavin mononucleotide (**FMN**). Both free and phosphorylated riboflavin enter the portal vein, where they bind to albumin and other plasma proteins. Within tissues, riboflavin is converted to FMN; riboflavin and FMN may undergo further phosphorylation, in the liver, to flavin–adenine dinucleotide (**FAD**). The main storage sites are the liver and kidney, but the stores are not extensive and are easily depleted. A small amount of riboflavin appears to be excreted in the bile and hence undergoes enterohepatic recirculation. However, the vitamin is mainly excreted in urine, predominantly in the free form.

FMN and FAD are the physiologically active forms of riboflavin. They serve a vital role in metabolism as coenzymes for a wide variety of respiratory flavoproteins; they are, for example, essential for oxidative phosphorylation, dehydrogenation of fatty acids, the conversion of folic acid to 5-*N*-methyltetrahydrofolic acid, the conversion of pyridoxine to its 5′-phosphate, and for the activity of the flavin-dependent purine enzyme, xanthine oxidase. In addition, covalently attached flavins are essential to the structure of enzymes such as succinate dehydrogenase and monoamine oxidase.

In man, riboflavin deficiency results in the development of cheilosis, angular stomatitis, glossitis, scrotal skin changes, seborrhoeic dermatitis of the face, a generalized dermatitis, a normochromic normocytic anaemia associated with pure red cell hypoplasia, and a neuropathy. In some individuals the cornea becomes vascularized and cataracts form. All of these features can be rapidly reversed with oral riboflavin in a dose of 5 to 10 mg daily. Deficiency of this vitamin rarely occurs in isolation and certain features of the riboflavin deficiency syndrome, such as cheilosis and glossitis, occur with deficiencies of the other B vitamins.

Biochemical evidence of riboflavin deficiency is present in 15 to 50 per cent of individuals abusing alcohol, with or without liver disease (Leevy, AmJClinNutr, 1965; 16:339; Rosenthal, AmJClinNutr, 1973; 26:858; Bayoumi, ClinChem, 1976; 22:327; Hell, DMedWoch, 1977; 102:962; Baines, AnnClinBioch, 1978; 15:307; Bonjour, IntJVitNutrRes, 1980; 50:425; Brown, AlcAlc, 1983; 18: 157). Several factors contribute to the deficiency, including poor dietary intake and reduced intestinal availability secondary to a direct effect of ethanol on the enzymes responsible for FMN and FAD hydrolysis (Pinto, AmJClinNutr, 1984; 39:685 abstr.). There is no evidence that riboflavin turnover is altered in patients with alcoholic cirrhosis (Zempleni, IntJVitNutrRes, 1996; 66:237). Despite the high incidence of biochemical riboflavin deficiency in alcohol abusers, clinical symptoms of hypovitaminosis are rare (Leevy, 1965; Rosenthal, 1973).

Very little information is available on riboflavin status in patients with non-alcoholic liver disease. The incidence of biochemical riboflavin deficiency reported in patients with non-alcoholic cirrhosis varies from 4 to 6 per cent (Chen, JVit, 1960; 6:171; Leevy, AmJClinNutr, 1970; 23:493; Morgan, Gut, 1976; 17:113). There is no evidence that riboflavin turnover is altered in patients with non-alcoholic cirrhosis (Zempleni, IntJVitNutrRes, 1996; 66:237).

Niacin

Niacin is the generic term for both nicotinic acid and nicotinamide. The richest dietary sources are liver, meat, fish, whole-grain and enriched breads and cereals, nuts, coffee, and tea; fruit, most vegetables, milk, and eggs are poor sources. Many foods, especially cereals, contain bound forms of niacin from which the vitamin is not available. The main dietary sources are meat, potatoes, and cereals. Niacin is not a vitamin, in the true sense, in that nicotinamide can be synthesized from the essential amino acid tryptophan. In adults, the Reference Nutrient Intake for niacin is 6.6 mg/ 1000 kcal daily, or 13 mg/day for women and 17 mg/day for men.[1]

Both nicotinic acid and nicotinamide are readily absorbed throughout the intestinal tract and the vitamin is distributed in all tissues. The principal route of metabolism is to N'-methylnicotinamide and its derivatives, which are, in turn, metabolized further. Otherwise little is known about the absorption, fate, and excretion of this compound.

Niacin is an essential component of nicotinamide–adenine dinucleotide (**NAD**) and nicotinamide– adenine dinucleotide phosphate (**NADP**), coenzymes for a multitude of important oxidation–reduction reactions essential for tissue respiration. NAD also participates, as a substrate, in the transfer of adenosine diphosphate (**ADP**)–ribosyl moieties to proteins (Gilman, AnnRevBioch, 1987; 56:615). Nicotinic acid will depress blood lipids and can prevent the rise in plasma triglycerides, phospholipids, and free fatty acids observed after acute alcohol ingestion (Kaffarnik, Atheroscl, 1978; 29:1). This latter effect has been attributed to inhibition of peripheral free fatty acid release and to inhibition of hepatic alcohol dehydrogenase, which prevents the shift in redox state associated with alcohol oxidation. However, if nicotinic acid is given to rats chronically fed with ethanol, then the development of hepatic steatosis is potentiated (Sorrell, BBActa, 1976; 450:231).

Niacin deficiency is one of the major factors in the development of pellagra. The clinical features of this condition include dermatitis, inflammation of mucous membranes, diarrhoea, and psychiatric disturbances. Skin changes, especially on the hands, may be useful in detecting early deficiency. The condition is treated with nicotinamide, 500 mg orally or 75 mg intravenously, daily, in divided doses.

Pellagra is rare in industrialized countries but when diagnosed is often associated with chronic alcohol abuse (Dogliotti, BrJDermatol, 1977; 97:25; Spivak, JohnsHopkMedJ, 1977; 140:295; Stratiagos, BrJDermatol, 1977; 96:99; Vannucchi, AmJClinNutr, 1989; 50:364).

Hepatic niacin concentrations are reduced in individuals abusing alcohol and the percentage reduction increases with increasing severity of liver injury (Baker, AmJClinNutr, 1964; 14:1; Leevy, AmJClinNutr, 1965; 16:339; Frank, ExpMolPath, 1971; 15:191). Biochemical evidence of niacin deficiency has been found in a percentage of individuals abusing alcohol in some series (Fennelly, BMJ, 1964; ii:1290; Dastur, BrJNutr, 1976; 36:143), but not in others (Kershaw, BrJPsychiat, 1967; 113:387; Nevill, AmJClinNutr, 1968; 21:1329; Rossouw, SAMedJ, 1978; 54:183).

Potential mechanisms for niacin deficiency in individuals chronically abusing alcohol include poor dietary intake, decreased conversion to active coenzyme forms, decreased hepatic storage, and increased requirements. In individuals chronically abusing alcohol, zinc deficiency may potentiate the development of pellagra, probably through an effect on pyridoxine metabolism (Vannucchi, IntJVitNutrRes, 1986; 56:355; Vannucchi, AmJClinNutr, 1989; 50: 364).

In patients with fulminant liver failure, blood levels of niacin vary (Rossouw, SAMedJ, 1978; 54:183). In patients with non-alcoholic chronic liver disease, biochemical niacin deficiency is rarely encountered (Morgan, Gut, 1976; 17:113).

Chronic ingestion of therapeutic doses of crystalline nicotinic acid can result in the development of hepatotoxicity; use of sustained-release preparations is associated with more severe hepatotoxicity which develops after ingestion of smaller doses over shorter time periods (McCreanor, BrJNutr, 1986; 56:577; Etchason, MayoClinProc, 1991; 66:23; Coppola, SouthMedJ, 1994; 87:30).[11]

Vitamin B_6

The biological activity of the vitamin B_6 group is displayed by pyridoxine, pyridoxal, and pyridoxamine and their 5'-phosphate esters, all of which are metabolically interconvertible. The vitamin is widely and uniformly distributed in all foods, but substantial losses occur during cooking; lean meat, liver, whole-grain breads and cereals, nuts, and bananas are among the richest sources. Intestinal bacteria synthesis large quantities of this vitamin, at least some of which is absorbed. In adults, the Reference Nutrient Intake for vitamin B_6 is 15 µg/g protein, or 1.2 mg/day for women and 1.4 mg/day for men.[1]

The vitamin B_6 ingested in food is released from its 5'-phosphate esters by intraluminal alkaline phosphatase. It is absorbed from the jejunum and ileum by passive diffusion and is then converted, predominantly in the liver, but also in skeletal muscle and kidney, to the active coenzyme form, pyridoxal-5'-phosphate. The coenzyme is transported in plasma bound to albumin. Release of free vitamin, mainly pyridoxal, occurs when the coenzymes are hydrolysed by non-specific alkaline phosphatases located on the plasma membranes of cells. The circulating pyridoxal can enter cells and is reutilized to synthesize pyridoxal-5'-phosphate. Ultimately, most pyridoxal-5'-phosphate is metabolized to 4-pyridoxic acid. The major circulating forms of the vitamin are pyridoxal-5'-phosphate, pyridoxal, and 4-pyridoxic acid.

Pyridoxal-5'-phosphate acts as a cofactor for a large number of enzymes involved in amino-acid metabolism including aminotransferases, decarboxylases, synthetases, and hydroxylases. It is of particular importance in humans in the metabolism of tryptophan, glycine, serine, glutamate, and the sulphur-containing amino acids. Pyridoxal-5'-phosphate is also required for the synthesis of the haem precursor 6-amino-laevulinic acid, for the breakdown of glycogen, for the conversion of linoleic acid to arachidonic acid, and for syringomyelin biosynthesis. A large percentage of the pyridoxine in the body is found in muscle phosphorylase, where it probably acts as an enzyme stabilizer. It also plays an important, although ill-understood role, in neuronal excitability, and modulates the actions of steroid hormones by interacting with steroid–receptor complexes.

Clinical symptoms of vitamin B_6 deficiency include neuromuscular irritability, peripheral neuropathy, dermatitis, cheilosis, stomatitis, anaemia, and impaired immunity. The vitamin is widely present in food; thus, dietary pyridoxine deficiency has never been recognized in human adults, although it can occur in infants fed highly-processed formula feeds. Pyridoxine deficiency can, however, arise in adults either during treatment with drugs such as isoniazid, cycloserine, hydralazine, and D-penicillamine, which act as pyridoxine antagonists, or as a result of genetically determined abnormalities in vitamin B_6 metabolism (Fowler, JInherMetDis, 1985; 8(Suppl. 1):76). Pyridoxine, in an oral dose of 30 mg daily, will correct the deficiency in patients taking isoniazid, while doses of up to 100 mg daily may be required in subjects taking D-penicillamine or in the presence of one of the genetically determined clinical states of 'pyridoxine dependency'. Vitamin B_6 should be given prophylactically to patients receiving pyridoxine antagonists in a dose of 25 mg daily.

Low circulating levels of pyridoxal-5'-phosphate have been eported in 30 to 50 per cent of alcohol abusers with minimal iver damage, but in 80 to 100 per cent of those with cirrhosis Leevy, AmJClinNutr, 1965; 16:339; Hines, NEJM, 1970; 283:441; Leevy, AmJClinNutr, 1970; 23:493; Lumeng, JCI, 1974; 53:693; Mitchell, Gastro, 1976; 70:988 abstr.; Labadarios, Gut, 1977; 18: 23; Bonjour, IntJVitNutrRes, 1980; 50:215; Diehl, Gastro, 1984; 86: 632; Henderson, Hepatol, 1986; 6:464; Ohgi, ClinBioch, 1988; 21:367).[12] This reduction in circulating pyridoxal-5'-phosphate concentrations occurs mainly because of increased degradation (Mitchell, 1976; Labadarios, 1977); the factors responsible are largely unknown, although acetaldehyde can produce this effect (Lumeng, JCI, 1974; 53:693). Ethanol per se interferes with the conversion of pyridoxine to pyridoxal-5'-phosphate (Hines, AnnNYAcadSci, 1975; 252:316), and this may contribute to the reduction in circulating pyridoxal-5'-phosphate concentrations.

In individuals with alcohol-related cirrhosis, circulating pyridoxal concentrations may be increased (Henderson, Hepatol, 1986; 6:464) or decreased (Ohgi, ClinBioch, 1988; 21:367). Similarly, 24-h urinary excretion of 4-pyridoxic acid may be increased (Ohgi, 1988) or unchanged (Henderson, 1986).

Deficiency, when present, may be corrected with oral pyridoxine hydrochloride, 50 to 150 mg daily, in divided doses. However, the plasma pyridoxal-5'-phosphate response to administered pyridoxine may be impaired in patients with cirrhosis (Henderson, Hepatol, 1986; 6:464).[12] Serum alkaline phosphatase activity is increased in these patients and this enzyme hydrolyses pyridoxal-5'-phosphate to pyridoxal (Anderson, Gut, 1980; 21:192; Whyte, JCI, 1985; 76: 752; Henderson, 1986; Merrill, AmJClinNutr, 1986; 44:461).

In patients with acute viral hepatitis, plasma pyridoxal-5'-phosphate concentrations are normal (Mitchell, Gastro, 1976; 70:988 abstr.), whereas in fulminant hepatic failure, plasma pyridoxal-5'-phosphate concentrations are more variable (Rossouw, SAMedJ, 1978; 54:183). Low plasma pyridoxal-5'-phosphate concentrations may also be found in patients with non-alcoholic chronic liver disease (Labadarios, Gut, 1977; 18:23; Zaman, BMJ, 1986; 293:175; Ohgi, ClinBioch, 1988; 21:367); increased pyridoxal-5'-phosphate degradation is the major aetiological factor, although reduced plasma albumin concentrations may be of additional importance. In these individuals, however, plasma pyridoxal concentrations and urinary excretion of 4-pyridoxic acid are normal, so that the plasma pyridoxal-5'-phosphate concentration may be an unreliable indicator of overall vitamin B_6 status (Ohgi, 1988). In these individuals the excess pyridoxal generated by dephosphorylation of pyridoxal-5'-phosphate, possibly under the influence of circulating alkaline phosphatase, may be taken up by tissues rather than being excreted. In consequence, although plasma pyridoxal-5'-phosphate concentrations are reduced in patients with non-alcoholic liver disease, tissue levels of pyridoxal-5'-phosphate are normal (Lumeng, JLab-ClinMed, 1984; 103:59; Henderson, Hepatol, 1986; 6:464; Ohgi, 1988).

Ingestion of high doses of pyridoxine of the order of 2 to 7 g/day for periods in excess of 6 months is associated with the development of a sensory peripheral neuropathy (Schaumburg, NEJM, 1983; 309:445; Dalton, ActaNeurolScand, 1987; 76:8).

Folate (Hillman, p.1311 in reference 4)

Folic acid (pteroylmonoglutamic acid) is the parent molecule for a large number of derivatives collectively known as folates. It is synthesized by many different plants and bacteria. Offal, yeast extract, green leafy vegetables, pulses, oranges, nuts, bananas, and bread are the richest sources. However, some forms of dietary folic acid are labile and may be destroyed by cooking. Thus, fruit and raw vegetables probably constitute the primary dietary sources of the vitamin. In adults, the Reference Nutrient Intake for folate is 200 µg/day.[1]

Food folates are present mainly as reduced polyglutamates and require deconjugation to mono- and diglutamates before absorption. Hydrolysis occurs in the gut lumen or else in the brush border of intestinal epithelial cells; the deconjugated folates are then actively transported across the intestinal epithelium by a carrier-mediated mechanism; passive transfer may also occur. The absorbed glutamates undergo reduction and methylation by the mucosal cell to the active form, 5-methyltetrahydrofolate, which then enters the portal circulation; some absorbed folate is transported unchanged. In plasma, folates circulate in the free form, or else are loosely bound to plasma proteins or firmly bound to high-affinity carriers. Folates appear to be taken up by tissues, including the liver, by a carrier-mediated transport mechanism; once internalized, the folates are retained partly through polyglutamylation but also through tight association with intracellular folate-binding proteins.

Folates are found in all body tissues; human liver contains 0.7 to 17 µg/g, mainly as the polyglutamate form of 5-methyl-tetrahydrofolate. 5-Methyltetrahydrofolate is excreted in the bile and undergoes enterohepatic circulation; intact folates and their cleavage products are excreted in the urine.

In the form of its tetrahydro derivatives, such as 5-form-iminotetrahydrofolate and 5,10-methylenetetrahydrofolate, folate functions as a participant in one-carbon transfer reactions; thus, it is involved in the synthesis of purine and pyrimidine nucleotides, in a number of amino-acid interconversions, and in the generation of formate for the 'formate' pool.

Folic acid deficiency results in reduced replication of rapidly dividing cells, especially those in the bone marrow and in the gastrointestinal tract. A macrocytic, megaloblastic anaemia may develop and is the major haematological manifestation of deficiency. The gastrointestinal manifestations include glossitis, cheilosis, and diarrhoea. Neurological abnormalities occur only rarely. Folic acid deficiency may arise during treatment with drugs which interfere with its absorption and conversion to 5-methyltetrahydrofolate such as phenytoin, phenobarbitone, and oral contraceptives, or with drugs which inhibit dihydrofolate reductase such as methotrexate, pyrimethamine, and triamterene. Deficiency is treated with oral folic acid, 10 to 20 mg daily, for 2 weeks; a maintenance dose of 5 to 10 mg daily may be required.

Folic acid deficiency is the most common vitamin deficiency observed in individuals abusing alcohol, although patients are rarely symptomatic. The incidence of low serum or red cell folate concentrations varies from 6 to 87 per cent in reported series (Jandl, AnnIntMed, 1956; 45:1027; Herbert, AnnIntMed, 1963; 58:977; Kimber, QJMed, 1965; 34:33; Klipstein, Blood, 1965; 25:443; Unger, AmJMedSci, 1974; 267:281; Wu, Lancet, 1974; i:829; Carney, BrJAddic, 1978; 73:3; Morgan, ClinLabHaemat, 1981; 3:35; World, AlcAlc, 1984; 19:281; Gimsing, JNutr, 1989; 119:416; Wickramasinghe, AlcAlc, 1994; 29:415);[13] the incidence of folic acid deficiency appears independent of the degree of liver injury. Factors important in the pathogenesis of folate deficiency in individuals abusing alcohol include dietary inadequacy, intestinal malabsorption, impaired delivery of circulating folate to tissues, decreased hepatic retention, increased urinary excretion, and, possibly, altered enterohepatic recycling (Halstead, AmJClinNutr, 1980; 33:2736; Russell, AmJClinNutr, 1983; 38:64; Weir, BiochemPharm, 1985; 34:1). Cessation of ethanol intake and oral folic acid supplements, in a daily dose of 5 to 15 mg, will correct the deficiency.

In acute viral hepatitis, the excretion of urinary folate is increased (Retief, BMJ, 1969; ii:150; Tamura, AmJClinNutr, 1977; 30:1378), presumably because of hepatic release of stored folate and exhausted plasma binding. Serum and red cell folate values are low in less than a quarter of patients with chronic non-alcoholic liver disease (Kimber, QJMed, 1965; 34:33; Klipstein, Blood, 1965; 25:443; Wu, BrJHaemat, 1975; 29:469; Morgan, Gut, 1976; 17:113; Morgan, ClinLabHaemat, 1981; 3:35); patients are rarely symptomatic.

Vitamin B$_{12}$ (Hillman, p.1311 in reference 4)

Vitamin B$_{12}$ is the name given to a group of compounds which consist of a corrinoid ring surrounding an atom of cobalt. These compounds are present in animal tissue but not in plant tissue; they can be synthesized by a number of micro-organisms, including a proportion of those normally present in the human intestine. Accordingly, the major dietary sources are liver, meat, fish, eggs, cheese, and milk. In adults, the Reference Nutrient Intake for vitamin B$_{12}$ is 1.5 µg/day.[1]

Vitamin B$_{12}$ is attached, in coenzyme form, to protein in food. During digestion, proteolysis occurs and the released vitamin B$_{12}$ forms a stable complex with R binder, which is one of a group of closely related glycoproteins found in intestinal secretions such as saliva, gastric juice, and bile acid, and also in granulocytes and plasma. The binding protein is removed in the presence of gastric acid and pancreatic proteases, releasing the vitamin, which then binds to intrinsic factor, a glycoprotein produced by the parietal cells of the stomach. The vitamin B$_{12}$–intrinsic factor complex is resistant to proteolytic digestion and travels to the distal ileum where it binds to specific receptors on the mucosal brush border. The vitamin B$_{12}$ is then transferred from the ileal receptor across the mucosa to the capillary circulation where it binds, initially, to a β-globulin, transcobalamin II.

The vitamin B$_{12}$–transcobalamin II complex is rapidly taken up by the liver, bone marrow, and other proliferating cells. Although transcobalamin II is the transport protein for newly absorbed vitamin B$_{12}$, most vitamin B$_{12}$ circulates bound to transcobalamin I, a glycoprotein closely resembling gastric R binder. This situation arises because the vitamin B$_{12}$ bound to transcobalamin II is rapidly cleared from the blood, while clearance of the vitamin B_{12} bound to transcobalamin I requires many days. The liver contains from 50 to 90 per cent of normal body stores of vitamin B_{12}, which range from 1 to 10 mg; the vitamin is stored as its coenzyme, 5-deoxy-adenosylcobalamin. Vitamin B_{12} is not catabolized; loss occurs by excretion, largely in the bile. Approximately 0.5 to 9.0 μg of vitamin B_{12} are excreted in bile daily, 65 to 75 per cent of which is reabsorbed.

Vitamin B_{12} is converted, in the liver, to its active coenzyme forms, methylcobalamine and 5-deoxyadenosylcobalamin. The co-enzymes are involved in many metabolic processes and, as they are necessary for nucleic acid synthesis, are important for maintaining growth, haematopoiesis, epithelial cell function, and possibly myelin integrity. Methylcobalamin is required for the transmethylation of homocysteine to methionine and its derivative, S-adenosyl-methionine. It acts as a cofactor for methyl transferase, which is essential for normal folate metabolism. 5-Deoxyadenosylcobalamin is also a cofactor for the enzyme methylmalonyl-CoA mutase in the oxidation of odd-numbered fatty acids.

Deficiency of vitamin B_{12} leads to haematological, gastro-intestinal, and neurological abnormalities. The main haematological manifestation is a macrocytic, megaloblastic anaemia; rarely thrombocytopenia may occur. The gastrointestinal manifestations are usually mild and include glossitis, cheilosis, and diarrhoea; malabsorption may lead to moderate weight loss. The neurological manifestations include a peripheral neuropathy, subacute combined degeneration of the spinal cord, a cerebellar syndrome, and dis-turbances of mentation which vary from mild irritability to severe dementia or frank psychosis. The haematological and gastro-intestinal manifestations respond well to parenteral vitamin B_{12}, but remission of the neurological features may be incomplete.

Plasma vitamin B_{12} concentrations are usually normal in in-dividuals abusing alcohol, irrespective of the presence of any as-sociated liver disease (Carney, BrJAddic, 1978; 73:3; Morgan, ClinLabHaemat, 1981; 3:35; Gimsing, JNutr, 1989; 119:416); hep-atic vitamin levels may, however, be reduced (Baker, AmJClinNutr, 1964; 14:1; Frank, ExpMolPath, 1971; 15:191). Ethanol has been shown to interfere with binding of the vitamin B_{12}–intrinsic factor complex, and may reduce *in vivo* uptake of vitamin B_{12}. However, neither of these factors appears to be of clinical significance.

Plasma vitamin B_{12} concentrations are low in only a very small percentage of patients with chronic, non-alcoholic liver disease (Leevy, AmJClinNutr, 1970; 23:493; Morgan, Gut, 1976; 17:113); the aetiology of the vitamin B_{12} deficiency in these patients is unclear as both absorption and transport of the vitamin are normal (Rosenthal, ProgLivDis, 1970; 3:118).

High circulating vitamin B_{12} concentrations have been reported in patients with viral hepatitis, fatty liver, alcoholic hepatitis, chol-angitis, liver abscess, metastatic carcinoma, and cirrhosis; this may reflect release of vitamin from injured hepatocytes or impaired clearance of the bound vitamin (Rachmilewitz, EurJClinInv, 1972; 2:239; Baker, AlcAlc, 1987; 22:1; Zhou, ChinJInternMed, 1992; 30: 625; Lambert, Digestion, 1997; 58:64).[14] Patients with pernicious anaemia may indeed undergo 'spontaneous remission' if they de-velop hepatitis, suggesting that under normal circumstances not all the hepatic stores of vitamin B_{12} are available for haematopoiesis.

Changes may also occur in the plasma binding of vitamin B_{12} in patients with liver disease. Patients with acute hepatitis, for example, have low plasma levels of vitamin B_{12}-binding capacity, possibly secondary to hyperbilirubinaemia, and, in consequence, have high levels of free plasma vitamin B_{12}; in patients with chronic liver disease, concentrations of the bound form increase (Jones, JLab-ClinMed, 1957; 49:910).

Increased circulating concentrations of the vitamin B_{12}-binding proteins, particularly transcobalamin I, have been reported in patients with hepatocellular carcinoma (Paradinas, BMJ, 1982; 285: 840; Fremont, TumBiol, 1991; 12:353).

Pantothenic acid

Pantothenic acid is a part of the coenzyme A molecule. It occurs widely in natural food and is probably an essential nutrient; offal, beef, and egg yolk are rich sources. Diets containing 3 to 7 mg of pantothenic acid daily are considered adequate.[1]

Pantothenic acid is readily absorbed from the small intestine by simple diffusion. It is present in tissues, probably in the bound form of coenzyme A, in concentrations ranging from 2 to 45 μg/g; the concentration in liver exceeds that in all other tissues. Pantothenic acid is not metabolized within the body to any extent and is largely excreted in the urine.

The vitamin is transformed within the body to 4′-phospho-pantetheine, which is then incorporated into the functional forms of the vitamin, coenzyme A and acyl carrier protein. Coenzyme A is a cofactor for a variety of enzyme-catalysed reactions involving transfer of two-carbon groups. Such reactions are important in the oxidative metabolism of carbohydrates, gluconeogenesis, de-gradation of fatty acids, and the synthesis of sterols, steroid hor-mones, and porphyrins. Pantothenate also participates in the post-translational modification of proteins, including N-terminal acet-ylation, acetylation of internal amino acids, and fatty acid acet-ylation. Such modifications influence the intracellular localization, stability, and activity of proteins.

Pantothenic acid deficiency has not been recognized in humans consuming a normal diet, presumably because of its ubiquitous presence in food. Experimental pantothenic acid deficiency results in the development of paraesthesias in the extremities, muscle cramps, impaired co-ordination, fatigue, headache, abdominal cramp, and vomiting (Fry, JNutrSciVitaminol, 1976; 22:339). The burning or electric foot syndrome which developed in prisoners in the Second World War responded to administration of pantothenic acid and probably, therefore, represents a specific feature of de-ficiency (Denny-Brown, Medicine, 1947; 26:41).

Hepatic pantothenic acid concentrations are reduced in in-dividuals with alcohol-related liver disease for reasons that are unclear (Baker, AmJClinNutr, 1964; 14:1). Plasma pantothenic acid concentrations vary in individuals chronically abusing alcohol (Leevy, JCI, 1960; 39:1005 abstr.; Baker, 1964; Leevy, AmJClin-Nutr, 1970; 23:493; Bonjour, IntJVitNutrRes, 1980; 50:425). The lowest values are observed in individuals with decompensated liver disease (Leevy, AmJClinNutr, 1965; 16:339; Leevy, 1970). No information is available on pantothenic acid status in patients with non-alcoholic liver disease.

Biotin

Biotin occurs widely in natural foods although in small amounts; offal, egg yolk, milk, fish, and nuts are the richest sources. Part of the biotin synthesized by intestinal bacteria is also available for absorption. The daily requirements of biotin are unknown but diets providing a daily intake of between 10 and 200 μg are considered adequate and safe.[1]

Ingested biotin is rapidly absorbed from the gastrointestinal tract and is readily excreted in the urine, predominantly in the form of intact biotin and to a lesser extent as its metabolites bis-norbiotin and biotin sulphoxide.

Biotin is a cofactor for the enzymatic carboxylation of pyruvate, acetyl coenzyme A, proprionyl coenzyme A, and β-methylcrotonyl coenzyme A; as such it plays an important role in carbon dioxide fixation in both carbohydrate and fat metabolism.

There is no evidence that spontaneous biotin deficiency can occur in man except in individuals who consume large quantities of raw egg white as this contains avidin, a glycoprotein which avidly binds biotin and prevents its absorption. The signs and symptoms of biotin deficiency, as observed in these individuals, include dermatitis, atrophic glossitis, hyperaesthesia, muscle pain, lassitude, anorexia, mild anaemia, and non-specific changes on the electrocardiogram. Symptomatic biotin deficiency has been reported in children and in adults receiving long-term total parenteral nutrition, manifest as severe exfoliative dermatitis and alopecia (Tanaka, NEJM, 1981; 304:839; Whitehead, ProcNutrSoc, 1981; 40:165; Gillis, JPEN, 1982; 6:308).

Low plasma and liver biotin concentrations have been found in individuals chronically abusing alcohol (Baker, AmJClinNutr, 1964; 14:1; Fennelly, BMJ, 1964; 2:1290; Leevy, AmJClinNutr, 1965; 16:339), but no clinical symptoms of deficiency have been recorded. The mechanism of the deficiency is unknown.

High serum biotin concentrations have been reported in patients with a variety of non-alcohol- related liver diseases, perhaps reflecting its release from damaged hepatocytes (Nagamine, JpnJGastro, 1990; 87:1168; Hashimoto, JpnJClinPath, 1996; 44:970). Low serum biotin concentrations have been reported in patients with fulminant hepatic failure, decompensated cirrhosis, and hepatocellular carcinoma (Nagamine, 1990; Nagamine, ScaJGastr, 1993; 28:899).

The serum activity of biotinidase, the enzyme which catalyses the hydrolysis of biotinides, is low in patients with decompensated cirrhosis and hepatocellular carcinoma (Nagamine, JpnJGastro, 1990; 87:1168; Nagamine, ScaJGastr, 1993; 28:899). Deficiency of this enzyme can result in organic acidaemia, and in some patients with severe decompensated liver disease, supplementation with biotin resulted in a reduction in the urinary excretion of propionate, lactate, and 3-hydroxybutyrate (Nagamine, 1993).

Vitamin C

Vitamin C is widely distributed in a variety of fruits and vegetables; orange and lemon juices are particularly rich sources. Storage of unprocessed fruits and vegetables for prolonged periods leads to loss of the vitamin; processed fruits and vegetables retain 50 per cent or more of their vitamin C content. In adults, the Reference Nutrient Intake for vitamin C is 40 mg/day.[1]

Vitamin C is readily absorbed from the intestinal tract via an energy-dependent process that is saturable and dose dependent. It is present in plasma and is ubiquitously distributed in all body tissues; the highest concentrations are found in glandular tissues, such as the pituitary and adrenal cortex; retinal concentrations are

20 to 30 times the plasma concentrations. The vitamin is partly metabolized and partly excreted unchanged in the urine. A major route of metabolism involves conversion to urinary oxalate.

Vitamin C functions as a cofactor in a number of hydroxylation and amidation reactions; for example, it is required for, or facilitates, the conversion of certain proline and lysine residues in procollagen to hydroxyproline and hydroxylysine in the course of collagen synthesis, the conversion of folic to folinic acid, microsomal drug metabolism, and the hydroxylation of dopamine to form noradrenaline. It also promotes the activity of an amidating enzyme thought to be involved in the processing of certain peptide hormones such as oxytocin, antidiuretic hormone, and cholecystokinin. In addition, it directly stimulates collagen peptide synthesis, promotes intestinal absorption of iron by reducing non-haem ferrous iron to its ferric state, and plays an ill-defined role in adrenal steroidogenesis.

Deficiency of vitamin C leads to scurvy. The main symptoms of this disorder arise from pathological lesions in the blood vessels and include: perifollicular hyperkeratosis and haemorrhage; purpura; haemorrhages into muscles and joints; swollen, friable, and bleeding gums in patients with teeth; poor wound healing; and anaemia. Haemorrhage may occur into the periosteum of long bones in infants and children, causing painful swelling and occasionally epiphysial separation. Treatment with oral vitamin C, 500 mg daily, in divided doses, will reverse these changes.

Individuals chronically abusing alcohol often have low leucocyte vitamin C concentrations (Leevy, AmJClinNutr, 1965; 16:339; Beattie, Gut, 1976; 17:571; Devgun, BrJNutr, 1981; 45:469; Mills, AmJClinNutr, 1983; 38:849; Dubey, IndJPhysiolPharmacol, 1987; 31:279), probably as a result of dietary deficiency.

Low leucocyte vitamin C levels have also been found in patients with viral hepatitis, cryptogenic cirrhosis, chronic aggressive hepatitis, Wilson's disease, primary biliary cirrhosis, and hepatocellular carcinoma (Beattie, Gut, 1976; 17:571; Morgan, Gut, 1976; 17:113; Dubey, IndJPhysiolPharmacol, 1987; 31:279; Ogihara, PediatRes, 1995; 37:219). Although poor dietary intake may play an important role in the development of deficiency, daily intakes of vitamin C were acceptable in the patients with primary biliary cirrhosis studied by Beattie and Sherlock (Gut, 1976; 17:571). These patients were, however, taking cholestyramine, which might interfere with vitamin C absorption. These authors also showed that vitamin C deficiency interfered with antipyrine metabolism and speculated that such deficiency might affect the microsomal oxidation of other drugs.

Minerals

Iron (Hillman, p.1311 in reference 4; Young, p.597 in reference 5)

Iron is present in many foods; the richest sources are offal, brewer's yeast, wheat germ, egg yolk, oysters, certain dried beans, and fruit; most lean meat, poultry, fish, green vegetables, and cereals contain moderate amounts. The main sources of dietary iron are meat, bread, flour, potatoes, and other vegetables. The average diet provides 10 to 20 mg (180 to 360 μmol) of iron daily; in healthy individuals only 10 per cent of ingested iron is absorbed. In adults, the Reference Nutrient Intake for iron is 14.8 mg (260 μmol)/day for women and 8.7 mg (160 μmol)/day for men.[1]

The rate of iron absorption is of prime importance in determining body iron status. However, the nature of the absorptive process is poorly understood (Charlton, AnnRevMed, 1983; 34:55); a carrier-mediated process is proposed (Simpson, BBActa, 1987; 898:181; Stremmel, EurJClinInv, 1987; 17:136). After acidification and partial digestion in the stomach, food iron is presented to the intestinal mucosa of the duodenum and proximal jejunum; it is then taken up by the absorptive cells and either transported directly into the plasma or stored as mucosal ferritin. Absorption is regulated by the relative activities of these two pathways which are in some way determined by the internal state of iron metabolism. Iron, derived from haemoglobin and other haem proteins of animal origin, is absorbed as the intact haem molecule. Most other forms of iron are more easily absorbed in the ferrous form. Phytates, polyphenols, phosphates, and oxalic acid in food form complexes with iron and reduce its absorption; achlorhydria and the administration of antacids and drugs which inhibit the gastric secretion of hydrochloric acid also decrease iron absorption. Reducing agents, such as ascorbic acid, facilitate iron absorption by converting ferric to ferrous iron; meat facilitates iron absorption by stimulating gastric acid production. Absorption is also increased when iron intake is deficient, when iron stores are depleted, or when erythropoiesis is enhanced; however, even under these circumstances, absorption is limited to between 3 and 4 mg (54 to 72 μmol) of dietary iron daily.

Absorbed iron is transported bound to transferrin, a β_1-glycoprotein synthesized in the liver. Iron is delivered from transferrin to intracellular sites by means of a specific transferrin receptor in the plasma membrane. A major proportion of the circulating iron is transported to the bone marrow for haemoglobin synthesis and to other sites for the manufacture of other essential iron-containing compounds, including myoglobin and a variety of iron-dependent enzymes. The remaining iron is stored either in the reticuloendothelial system or in liver and muscle. Approximately one-third of total storage iron is found in the liver as ferritin which exists as individual molecules or in an aggregated form, haemosiderin; over 95 per cent of hepatic iron is located in hepatocytes. The remaining two-thirds of storage iron is equally divided between reticuloendothelial cells in the spleen, bone marrow, and muscle. The body of a healthy man contains approximately 50 mg (900 μmol) iron/kg body weight; that of a healthy woman contains 37 mg (660 μmol) iron/kg. About two-thirds of body iron circulates in haemoglobin, while only 3 mg (54 μmol) circulates as transferrin. A small proportion of total body iron, perhaps 300 to 400 mg (5.4 to 7.2 mmol), is present in myoglobin and in the haem enzymes concerned with electron transfer. The remaining 1 g (16 mmol) in men and 100 to 400 mg (1.8 to 7.2 mmol) in women is stored in the liver, spleen, bone marrow, and muscle, complexed to protein, as ferritin and haemosiderin.

Daily iron losses average less than 1 mg (18 μmol) in men and 2 mg (36 μmol) in women who menstruate. The main loss occurs from desquamation of epithelial cells from the skin and gastrointestinal tract. In women, menstrual iron loss is highly variable but averages 17 mg (300 μmol) monthly. The net loss of iron during a normal pregnancy is about 700 mg (12.6 mmol).

Iron is essential for normal haematopoiesis and for the integrity of epithelial tissues. Most individuals with iron deficiency are asymptomatic; symptoms develop in proportion to the degree of anaemia and the constitution of the patient, and relate to the cause of the deficiency. In general, the clinical manifestations are those common to all chronic anaemias and include fatigue, headache, tachycardia, exertional dyspnoea, ankle oedema, and pallor. In occasional patients, abnormalities of epithelial tissues may occur, including glossitis, angular stomatitis, spooning of the nails, and dysphagia. Oral iron, for example ferrous sulphate, 600 mg daily, in divided doses, will correct the abnormalities, but the cause of the deficiency must be sought and ameliorated, if possible.

Abnormalities of iron metabolism are common in individuals abusing alcohol. Iron deficiency, with or without anaemia, is found in up to 25 per cent of such individuals (Kimber, QJMed, 1965; 34:33; Conrad, SemHemat, 1980; 17:149; Isa, ActaHaem, 1988; 80:85), and its presence is generally attributed to gastrointestinal bleeding and inadequate dietary intake.

Conversely, individuals abusing alcohol may have increased serum iron concentrations and increased saturation of their total iron-binding capacity (Sullivan, JCI, 1964; 43:2048; Lindenbaum, NEJM, 1969; 281:333; Chapman, DigDisSci, 1982; 27:909; Chapman, Gastro, 1983; 84:143). The mechanisms responsible for these findings are unclear, but as the abnormalities occur independently of the severity of any liver disease, they may represent a direct effect of alcohol on iron metabolism (Lindenbaum, 1969; Conrad, SemHemat, 1980; 17:149).

Liver iron concentrations are mildly to moderately increased in approximately one-third of alcohol abusers independently of the presence, or the degree, of alcohol-related liver injury (Barry, Gut, 1974; 15:324; Chapman, DigDisSci, 1982; 27:909). Several explanations have been suggested, but none is entirely satisfactory. The excess liver iron might reflect the iron content of the beverages consumed, but there is no relationship between the degree of hepatic siderosis and either the amount of alcohol or the amount of beverage iron ingested (Miralles Garcia, ActaHepatoGastroenterol, 1976; 23:10; Jacobovits, AmJDigDis, 1979; 24:305; Chapman, 1982). The high serum iron concentrations and increased transferrin saturations observed in these patients might enhance liver iron uptake (Wheby, NEJM, 1964; 271:1391), but although the uptake of transferrin-bound ^{52}Fe is increased in these individuals, independently of the degree of liver damage, it is also increased in patients with non-alcoholic liver disease (Chapman, Gastro, 1983; 84:143). Iron absorption might be increased in individuals chronically abusing alcohol, but studies have produced conflicting results (Chapman, DigDisSci, 1983; 28:321; Duane, AlcAlc, 1992; 27:539). The duodenal mucosa of alcohol abusers has an intrinsic ability to take up iron *in vitro*, but by a comparatively non-specific, low-affinity process (Duane, 1992). It is also possible that the hepatic siderosis might reflect defective release of transferrin-bound or non-transferrin-bound iron from tissue stores, perhaps as a direct effect of alcohol.

Serum iron (Rumball, Gastro, 1959; 36:219) and serum ferritin (Prieto, Gastro, 1975; 68:525) concentrations are often increased in patients with acute viral hepatitis. The mechanism is not clear, but release of transferrin from damaged cells, diminished haemoglobin synthesis, and impaired iron storage may all play a role.

Serum iron concentrations, transferrin saturation, and serum ferritin concentrations are also increased in 30 to 50 per cent of patients with chronic viral hepatitis, especially those infected with hepatitis C (Di Bisceglie, Gastro, 1992; 102:2108; Arber, DigDisSci, 1995; 40:2431; Haque, HumPath, 1996; 27:1277). The mechanism is unknown, but as serum ferritin concentrations correlate significantly with serum aspartate aminotransferase activities in these patients, iron release from necrotic hepatocytes might play a role (Di Bisceglie, 1992). Mild to moderate hepatic siderosis may be observed in these individuals (Di Bisceglie, 1992; Haque, 1996).

Evidence of iron deficiency, with or without anaemia, occurs in approximately 25 per cent of patients with cryptogenic cirrhosis and chronic active hepatitis (Morgan, Gut, 1976; 17:113). Its presence is attributed to either poor dietary intake or to occult gastrointestinal blood loss. Iron deficiency is uncommon in patients with non-alcoholic chronic liver disease in the absence of malabsorption, gastrointestinal haemorrhage, or a bleeding diathesis.

Hepatic siderosis, as observed in nutritional iron overload, idiopathic haemochromatosis, or as a complication of certain haematological disorders, can lead to the development of liver damage.[15–17]

Calcium (Marcus, p.1519 in reference 4)

Calcium is the most abundant mineral present in the body, accounting for about 40 per cent of the total mineral mass. The most important dietary sources of calcium are dairy produce, mainly milk and cheese, and bread. Varying quantities of calcium are present in domestic water supplies. In adults, the Reference Nutrient Intake for calcium is 700 mg (17.5 mmol)/day.[1]

Calcium from food and from intestinal secretions is absorbed by two different mechanisms. Active, vitamin D-dependent transport which occurs in the proximal duodenum, and facilitative diffusion which takes place throughout the small intestine. The efficacy of intestinal calcium absorption is inversely related to calcium intake; ingestion of a calcium-deficient diet results in an increase in fractional absorption; approximately 30 per cent of the calcium ingested is absorbed. Phosphates, phytates, and oxalates in food form complexes or insoluble salts with calcium and decrease its absorption; absorption may also decrease in the presence of steatorrhoea, while diarrhoea may be associated with increased faecal loss. Alcohol appears to depress duodenal calcium absorption, at least in experimental animals (Krawitt, JLabClinMed, 1975; 85:665).

Following absorption, calcium enters the plasma where it circulates either as free ions or bound to plasma proteins, primarily albumin, or, to a small extent, complexed with anionic buffers such as citrate and phosphate. The concentration of free calcium ions is of critical importance for a variety of functions and is subjected to precise hormonal control, largely via parathyroid hormone; circulating calcium concentrations are kept remarkably constant.

The body of a healthy adult contains 1.2 kg (300 mmol) of calcium, about 99 per cent of which is in the bones and teeth where its role is primarily structural; bone resorption and formation are usually tightly coupled, with approximately 500 mg (125 mmol) of calcium entering and leaving the skeleton daily. The remaining 1 per cent of body calcium is in the tissues and fluids where it is essential for cellular structure and inter- and intracellular metabolic function and signal transmission.

Calcium enters the gut in the bile, in pancreatic secretions, and in desquamated cells from the mucosal lining, and may be reabsorbed in the ileum and colon. Calcium is lost mainly through renal excretion; losses also occur via faeces, sweat, hair, and nails.

Calcium is essential for the functional integrity of the nervous and muscular systems; it has a major influence on excitability and release of neurotransmitters. Calcium is also necessary for normal cardiac function and is an important factor in maintenance of the integrity of membranes and blood coagulation. In addition it mediates the intracellular action of many hormones. Decrease in the concentration of free calcium ions secondary to, for example, reduced dietary intake of calcium and vitamin D, malabsorption of calcium and vitamin D, or hypoparathyroidism, is accompanied by increased neuromuscular irritability and the syndrome of tetany. Hypomagnesaemia and alkalosis lower the threshold for tetany, whereas hypokalaemia and acidosis raise the threshold. Hypercalcaemia secondary to, for example, hyperparathyroidism, vitamin D excess, sarcoidosis, or neoplasia is accompanied by anorexia, nausea, vomiting, constipation, polyuria and polydipsia, hypotonia, and depression and, when long-standing, by metastatic tissue calcification.

Bone density may be decreased in individuals chronically abusing alcohol as a result of a decrease in the mineral rather than the organic phase of bone (Saville, JBoneJtSurg, 1965; 47B:492; Nilsson, ClinOrthopRelRes, 1973; 90:229; Johnell, ClinOrthopRelRes, 1982; 165:253; Spencer, AmJMed, 1986; 80:393; Diamond, AmJMed, 1989; 86:282; Laitinen, CalcifTissInt, 1991; 49(Suppl.):70; Bilke, WRevNutrDiet, 1993; 73:53; Gonzalez-Calvin, AlcAlc, 1993; 28: 571; Holbrook, BMJ, 1993; 306:1506).[18] Several explanations have been suggested, including disturbances of calcium metabolism secondary to poor dietary intake, a direct effect of alcohol on absorption, fat malabsorption, and increased urinary losses of calcium and magnesium. There is, however, evidence that alcohol directly affects osteoblastic function, resulting in diminished bone formation and reduced bone mineralization (Johnell, 1982; Lalor, JMed, 1986; 59:497; Freitelberg, Metabolism, 1987; 36:322; Crilly, CalcifTissInt, 1988; 43:269; Diamond, 1989; Labib, AlcAlc, 1989; 24:141; Chappard, JStudAlc, 1991; 52:269; Lindholm, JClinEndoc, 1991; 73:118; Gonzalez-Calvin, 1993).

These changes in bone mass undoubtedly contribute to the increased prevalence of bone fractures in individuals abusing alcohol and their tendency to develop osteonecrosis of the femoral head. Although these individuals are more susceptible to bone fractures (Kristenson, ActaOrthScand, 1980; 51:205; Johnell, JSocMed, 1985; 13:95; Felson, AmJEpid, 1988; 128:1102; Hemenway, AmJPubHlth, 1988; 78:1554; Peris, CalcifTissInt, 1995; 57:111; Nordquist, ActaOrthScand, 1996; 67:364; Nyquist, AlcAlc, 1997; 32:91), healing times are generally not prolonged even when drinking continues (Nyquist, 1997). Similarly, although individuals chronically abusing alcohol are at increased risk of developing spontaneous osteonecrosis of the hip (Vignon, RevLyonMéd, 1980; 9:12; Jacobs, NYStateJMed, 1992; 92:334; Matsuo, ClinOrthopRelRes, 1992; 234:115), they show no increase in the risk of developing osteonecrosis after fracture of the femoral neck (Nyquist, AlcAlc, 1998; in press).

Up to 50 per cent of patients with either non-alcoholic chronic liver disease or chronic cholestasis develop osteoporosis as a result of an increase in bone reabsorption rates (Maddrey, ProgLivDis, 1990; 9:537; Crosbie, Hepatol, 1997; 26(Suppl.):347A abstr.).[18] Further significant bone loss may occur following orthotopic liver transplantation; losses of 20 to 30 per cent in the first 3 postoperative months have been reported (McDonald, Hepatol, 1991; 114:613), together with a high prevalence of vertebral fractures (Meys, AmJMed, 1994; 97:445). Several factors are of importance in the development of the bone disease, including calcium deficiency secondary to poor dietary intake and fat malabsorption, immobility, reduced muscle mass, and, in the transplant recipients, the use of immunosuppressive drugs, particularly corticosteroids.

Osteoporosis is not easily treated in this setting, but the provision of a high-protein diet together with calcium supplementation may lead to improvement; calcium provided in the form of hydroxy-apatite might be more beneficial than calcium provided as a simple salt (Epstein, AmJClinNutr, 1982; 36:426). Medium-chain triglycerides may be given to these patients not only as a fat source but also to promote calcium uptake. In postmenopausal women with primary biliary cirrhosis and osteoporosis, oestrogen replacement appears to improve lumbar spine bone mineral density (Lindor, SemLivDis, 1993; 13:367; Crippin, AmJGastr, 1994; 89:47). A gradual improvement is observed in bone mineral density in transplant recipients, but bone healing may take several years to complete (Crosbie, Hepatol, 1997; 26(Suppl.):347A abstr.; Feller, Hepatol, 1997; 26(Suppl.):347A abstr.).

A small number of patients with primary biliary cirrhosis experience severe bone pain despite provision of adequate amounts of vitamin D and calcium. The cause of the bone pain is uncertain, but it may respond to intravenous infusions of calcium (Ajdu-kiewicz, Gut, 1974; 15:788).

Zinc (Sternlieb, p.585 in reference 5)[19,20]

Zinc is widely distributed in food, particularly in meat, shellfish, liver, gelatin, bread, cereals, lentils, peas, beans, and rice. However, phytates in the diet will tightly bind zinc, thereby limiting its absorption; thus, the zinc from vegetable sources is generally un-available. Zinc uptake is also inhibited by polyphenols, oxalates, and folic acid. In adults, the Reference Nutrient Intake for zinc is 7.0 mg (110 µmol)/day for women and 9.5 mg (145 µmol)/day for men.[1]

Zinc is absorbed throughout the gut but since there is a large enteropancreatic circulation, net intestinal absorption occurs in the distal small intestine. Zinc is released from bound sources and attaches to amino acids which facilitates its absorption. Zinc com-petes for absorption with other divalent irons such as copper. Overall, only 30 per cent of ingested zinc is absorbed; the amount absorbed appears to be regulated by the zinc content of the intestinal mucosa and by metallothionein (Cousins, NutrRev, 1979; 37:97). Following absorption, zinc is transported from the intestine in the portal vein. After oral or parenteral administration, appreciable amounts of zinc accumulate in the liver bound to thioneines, which are proteins of low molecular weight synthesized in the presence of zinc.

The body of a healthy adult contains approximately 2 g (31 mmol) of zinc, 98 per cent of which is intracellular. Ap-proximately 60 per cent of body zinc is in skeletal muscle, 30 per cent in bone, and 4 to 6 per cent in the skin; the liver contains about 3 per cent of total body stores. In plasma, 60 per cent of circulating zinc is loosely bound to albumin, 30 to 40 per cent to a specific α_2-macroglobulin, and a small percentage to transferrin and γ-globulin; approximately 1 per cent is associated with amino acids such as histidine and cysteine (Boyett, Metabolism, 1970; 19:148). The major route of excretion is in faeces; faecal zinc is largely derived from pancreatic juice with a small contribution from bile (Lee, JLabClinMed, 1990; 166:283). In addition, approximately 0.66 mg (10 µmol) of zinc is excreted daily in urine and 10 mg/100 ml (1.5 mmol/l) in sweat.

Zinc is present in all tissues, and directly or indirectly par-ticipates in the major metabolic pathways involved in the meta-bolism of energy, proteins, carbohydrates, lipids, and nucleic acids. Zinc is a component of many metalloenzymes such as alkaline phosphatase, alcohol dehydrogenase, carbonic anhydrase, thym-idine kinase, deoxyribonucleic acid (**DNA**) and ribonucleic acid (**RNA**), polymerases, collagenase, carboxypeptidase, and superoxide dismutase. It is also a component of a number of metal–protein complexes, in particular metallothionein. It is important for micro-tubular and microfilament production, and for stabilization of microsomal and lysosomal membranes (Bettger, LifeSci, 1981; 28: 1425). It is also important for epithelial differentiation, immune responses, DNA and RNA synthesis and repair, prostaglandin metabolism, fatty acid metabolism, sensory functions, cerebral func-tion, and platelet aggregation. It plays a role in the storage and secretion of insulin. It is important for bone development, wound healing, growth and sexual maturation, for the conversion of retinol to retinal, and for hepatic secretion of retinol-binding protein.

Hypogonadal dwarfism, sometimes complicated by hepato-splenomegaly, has been described in rural Indian and Egyptian boys who subsist on diets of mainly bread and beans and very little animal protein. These youths have decreased zinc concentrations in plasma, erythrocytes, and hair, and decreased serum concentrations of the zinc-dependent enzyme, alkaline phosphatase. Growth and sexual maturation improve following a nutritionally adequate diet but the effect is enhanced by addition of zinc. Acrodermatitis enteropathica is an autosomal recessive disorder which manifests as severe chronic diarrhoea, wasting, alopecia, and roughened, thickened, and ulcerated skin around body orifices. Serum and hair zinc concentrations are extremely low and leucocyte chemotaxis is impaired. The condition responds promptly to administered zinc, although the exact mechanism of the zinc deficiency is unknown. Acrodermatitis enteropathica has also been observed in patients on long-term parenteral nutrition who are inadequately supplemented with zinc; the condition reverses quickly when zinc supplements are given. Wound healing is delayed in patients who are zinc deficient and is quickly restored following oral zinc sup-plementation. Zinc may also play a role in the maintenance of normal taste; patients with decreased taste acuity may improve following oral zinc sulphate, 660 mg daily, in divided doses.

The assessment of zinc status in man is difficult. Serum con-centrations can be affected by a variety of factors (Prasad, JAm-CollNutr, 1985; 4:591) and, even within individuals, tissue zinc concentrations may vary substantially (Schölmerich, LebMagDarm, 1984; 14:288). Thus, although marked changes occur in the zinc content of tissues, blood, and urine in many human diseases, the relationship of such alterations to the underlying condition is, for the most part, poorly understood.

Circulating concentrations of zinc are reduced and urinary zinc excretion increased in individuals chronically abusing alcohol, ir-respective of the presence or degree of any associated liver disease (Vallee, NEJM, 1956; 255:403; Kahn, AmJClinPath, 1965; 44:426; Halstead, Gastro, 1968; 54:1098; Keeling, ClinSci, 1982; 62:109; McClain, Alcoholism, 1983; 7:5; Ritland, JHepatol, 1987; 5:118; Bode, Hepatol, 1988; 8:1605; Goode, Gut, 1990; 31:694). In patients with alcoholic cirrhosis, circulating zinc concentrations are low (Sturniolo, JTraceElemElectrolHlthDis, 1992; 6:15; Rocchi, EurJClinInv, 1994; 24:149; Poo, DigDis, 1995; 13:136; Marchesini,

Hepatol, 1996; 23:1084; Perscovitz, ClinTranspl, 1996; 10:256; Madden, Hepatol, 1997; 26:40); the lowest circulating concentrations are observed in patients with the most severely decompensated disease (Fig. 1). However, although the fraction of circulating zinc bound to albumin is reduced in these patients; the amount bound to α_2-macroglobulin may be normal (Boyett, Metabolism, 1970; 19:148) or else increased (Schechter, EurJClin-Inv, 1976; 6:147). Leucocyte zinc concentrations may be reduced in these patients (Keeling, Gut, 1980; 21:561; Goode, 1990), but erythrocyte zinc concentrations are usually normal (Goode, 1990). Urinary zinc excretion is increased (Sturniolo, 1992; Rodriguez-Moreno, Liver, 1997; 14:39). Hepatic zinc concentrations are reduced in individuals with alcoholic liver disease irrespective of its severity (Vallee, 1956; Boyett, AmJDigDis, 1970; 15:797; Killerich, ScaJGastr, 1980; 15:363; Mills, ClinSci, 1983; 64:527; Milman, Liver, 1986; 6:111; Ritland, 1987; Bode, 1988; Adams, ClinInvestMed, 1991; 14:16; Rodriguez-Moreno, 1997).

Decreased circulating zinc concentrations have also been observed in patients with a variety of non-alcoholic liver diseases, including acute viral hepatitis (Kahn, AmJClinPath, 1965; 44:426), fulminant hepatic failure (Canalese, AustNZJMed, 1985; 15:7), chronic persistent and chronic active hepatitis (Keeling, ClinSci, 1982; 62:109; Bode, Hepatol, 1988; 8:1605; Goode, Gut, 1990; 31:694; Pramoolsinsip, JGastro, 1994; 29:610), primary biliary cirrhosis (Goode, 1990), cirrhosis (Solis-Herruzo, ZGastr, 1989; 27:335; Sturniolo, JTraceElemElectrolHlthDis, 1992; 6:15; Pramoolsinsip, 1994; Rocchi, EurJClinInv, 1994; 24:149; Poo, DigDis, 1995; 13:136; Marchesini, Hepatol, 1996; 23:1084; Perscovitz, ClinTranspl, 1996; 10:256), haemochromatosis (Brissot, Digestion, 1978; 17:469), Indian childhood cirrhosis (Misra, IndPaediat, 1989; 26:22), and schistosomiasis (Mikhail, HumNutrCN, 1982; 36:289). Reduced hepatic zinc concentrations have also been observed in patients with a variety of non-alcoholic liver diseases (Kiilerich, ScaJGastr, 1980; 15:363; Bhandari, JAssocPhysInd,1981; 29:641; Milman, Liver, 1986; 6:11; Bode, 1988; Kollmeier, PatholResPract, 1992; 188:942). Hepatic zinc concentrations are increased in patients with genetic haemochromatosis (Adams, ClinInvestMed, 1991; 14:16).

The mechanisms responsible for these changes in blood and tissue zinc concentrations in patients with liver disease are not entirely clear. Dietary zinc intake may be inadequate, particularly in the presence of anorexia. Alternatively, zinc absorption may be impaired (Dinsmore, Digestion, 1985; 32:238; Schölmerich, AmJClinNutr, 1987; 45:1487; Solis-Herruzo, ZGastr, 1989; 27:335), although there is evidence that absorption may be normal (Gohshi, Hepatogast, 1995; 42:487), or even increased (Mills, ClinSci, 1983; 64:527; Milman, ScaJGastr, 1983; 18:871). The low hepatic zinc concentrations observed in these individuals might reflect the presence of portal–systemic shunting and hepatocellular failure. However, hepatic zinc extraction has been reported to be normal or high in patients with liver disease (Keeling, ClinSci, 1981; 61:441), and the short-term kinetics of zinc turnover in patients with alcoholic cirrhosis are not significantly different from those in healthy volunteers (Lowe, ClinSci, 1993; 84:113). Finally, ethanol enhances urinary zinc excretion (Kalbfleisch, JCI, 1963; 42:1471) as will the use of thiazide diuretics.

A number of abnormalities have been reported in patients with liver disease which might reflect the presence of zinc deficiency.[19–21] Patients with long-standing cholestasis or with parenchymal liver disease may develop impaired dark adaptation as a result of vitamin A deficiency (Herlong, Hepatol, 1981; 1:348; Alvarez, Hepatol, 1983; 3:410). Zinc plays an important role in vitamin A metabolism as it is necessary for conversion of retinol to retinal and for hepatic secretion of retinol-binding protein. While most patients with liver disease and impaired dark adaptation respond to vitamin A alone, others require additional supplementation with zinc (Morrison, AmJClinNutr, 1978; 31:276; Herlong, 1981). Indeed, it has been suggested that patients with chronic liver disease and low leucocyte zinc concentrations may show photoreceptor dysfunction regardless of their vitamin A status (Keeling, ClinSci, 1982; 62:109).

Patients with liver disease may show abnormalities of taste and smell, which have been treated, with varying degrees of success, by zinc supplementation (Sullivan, AmJClinNutr, 1970; 23:170; Weismann, ActaMedScand, 1979; 205:361). However, no significant association between circulating zinc concentrations and gustatory or olfactory acuity has been demonstrated to date (Smith, Gastro, 1976; 70:568; Burch, ArchIntMed, 1978; 138:743; Sturniolo, JTraceElemElectrolHlthDis, 1992; 6:15; Madden, Hepatol, 1997; 26:40). Patients with cirrhosis and hypogonadism tend to have low serum zinc concentrations (Abdu-Gusau, EurJClinNutr, 1989; 43:53), but do not benefit in this regard from zinc supplementation (Goldiner, JAmCollNutr, 1983; 2:157).

Zinc deficiency may play a role in the pathogenesis of hepatic encephalopathy as serum zinc concentrations are reduced in patients with this syndrome and correlate inversely with blood ammonia concentrations (Reding, Lancet, 1984; ii:493; Grungrieff, ZGastr, 1988; 26:409); use of zinc supplements is associated with improvement in functional hepatic nitrogen clearance (Marchesini, Hepatol, 1996; 23:1084), but the effects on neuropsychiatric status are variable (Reding, 1984; Riggio, DigDisSci, 1991; 36:1204; van der Rijt, Gastro, 1991; 100:1114; Bresci, EurJMed, 1993; 2:414; Loomba, IndJGastro, 1995; 14:51; Marchesini, 1996). Patients with chronic liver disease may develop muscle cramps especially in their calves, mainly while sleeping. Zinc supplementation has been used with significant effect to treat these symptoms in patients with cirrhosis with low circulating zinc concentrations (Kugelmas, Hepatol, 1997; 26(Suppl.):386A abstr.).

Zinc deficiency has also been implicated in the pathogenesis of alcohol-related liver injury, particularly the development of fibrosis (Moussavian, Hepatol, 1981; 1:533; Panés, JHepatol, 1985; 1(Suppl. 2):300 abstr.; McClain, Alcoholism, 1986; 10:58S); no information is available currently on the potential benefits of zinc supplementation in individuals chronically abusing alcohol in relation to the development of liver injury. Finally, patients with cirrhosis show abnormal handling of sulphur-containing amino acids and decreased conversion of ornithine to citrulline; both abnormalities might reflect zinc deficiency.

Thus, while there is circumstantial evidence to suggest that zinc deficiency occurs in patients with liver disease, further study is needed to confirm its presence and its clinical significance.

Magnesium

Magnesium is the most abundant divalent intracellular ion in the body. It is widely distributed in ordinary foods; the richest sources are cocoa, nuts, barley, oats, oatmeal, wholemeal flour, soya flour, and lima beans; less than half of the magnesium ingested is absorbed. In adults, Reference Nutrient Intakes for magnesium are 270 mg (10.9 mmol)/day for women and 300 mg (12.3 mmol)/day for men.[1]

Magnesium is absorbed from the small intestine by an active transport system, which is vitamin D dependent, and by passive diffusion; it then enters the circulation. The body of a healthy 70-kg adult contains 2.5 g (1 mmol) of magnesium, of which approximately 60 per cent is found in bone, mainly in the mineral lattice. The remainder is located in skeletal and cardiac muscle, liver, kidney, brain, and interstitial fluid; the amount in extracellular fluid is extremely small. About two-thirds of plasma magnesium is present as the free ion while the rest is bound to proteins. Plasma magnesium concentrations are maintained within narrow limits but little information is available on the factors responsible for this. Plasma magnesium concentrations correlate best with those of the exchangeable magnesium of bone; a good correlation exists between plasma and intracellular magnesium concentrations. Magnesium is excreted mainly by the kidney, but over 90 per cent of the filtered cation is reabsorbed from the proximal renal tubule.

Magnesium acts as a cofactor for many enzymatic reactions, particularly those involved in high-energy phosphate metabolism. It is involved in the reversible association of intracellular particles and in binding of macromolecules to subcellular organelles. Body mechanisms for preserving magnesium are extremely efficient; thus, spontaneous magnesium deficiency is rarely encountered. Volunteers fed magnesium-deficient regimens develop hypomagnesaemia, inconsistently accompanied by hypokalaemia and hypocalcaemia. Clinically these subjects may develop neuromuscular disorders akin to those observed with hypocalcaemia, namely progressive muscle weakness, neuromuscular dysfunction, cardiac arrhythmias, and ultimately coma and death.

The incidence and implications of magnesium deficiency in patients with liver disease have received little attention, although magnesium has been incriminated in the fibrotic response of rat liver to carbon tetrachloride and alcohol (Rayssiguier, MedChirDig, 1981; 10:313), and in the neurological response to ammonia in patients with cirrhosis (Flink, JLabClinMed, 1955; 46:814). Magnesium deficiency has been documented in individuals chronically abusing alcohol, with or without liver disease, and may be accompanied by clinical signs of deficiency. Alcohol increases urinary magnesium excretion (Kalbfleisch, JCI, 1963; 42:1471), but other factors must also be important.

Hypomagnesaemia has also been reported in patients with cirrhosis, irrespective of its aetiology (Stutzman, JLabClinMed, 1953; 41:215; Wallach, JLabClinMed, 1962; 59:195; Rosner, JLabClinMed, 1968; 72:213; Cohen, JPediat, 1970; 76:453; Rocchi, EurJClinInv, 1994; 24:149; Skak, ClinTranspl, 1996; 10:157; Madden, Hepatol, 1997; 26:40), but clinical evidence of deficiency is said to be rare. However, Lim and Jacob (QJMed, 1972; 41:291) studied a group of patients with cirrhosis with anorexia, muscle weakness, and cramps and found that while plasma and bone magnesium concentrations were normal, muscle magnesium levels were low; magnesium supplementation over a period of 6 weeks resulted in resolution of the anorexia and muscle symptoms. Madden and colleagues (1997) reported a significant association between hypomagnesaemia and impaired gustatory function in patients with cirrhosis; the lowest serum magnesium concentrations and greatest impairment of gustatory acuity were observed in the most decompensated patients (Fig. 1); the effect of magnesium supplementation on gustatory acuity has not been studied in this population. The mechanism of magnesium deficiency in patients with liver disease, when it occurs, is unknown, although urinary magnesium concentrations may increase in patients with secondary hyperaldosteronism and in those taking loop diuretics.

Selenium

Selenium is present in a wide variety of foods. Cereal products, meat, poultry, and fish are the richest sources; milk, vegetables, and fruit contain only small amounts. Intakes may vary significantly between populations largely because of differences in the selenium content of soils and other soil–plant factors. Selenium in food is available in a number of forms mainly as the amino acids selenomethionine and selenocysteine and derivatives; not all forms of dietary selenium are equally available although information on bioavailability is incomplete. In adults, the Reference Nutrient Intake for selenium is 60 μg (0.8 μmol)/day for women and 75 μg (0.9 μmol)/day for men.[1]

Selenium is absorbed in the distal ileum. It is transported in plasma bound to a specific protein, probably produced in the liver (Motsenbocker, BBActa, 1982; 719:147). It is stored in the liver, spleen, heart, and nails. Newly absorbed selenium is rapidly excreted in the urine; it may also be excreted in sweat and bile.

Selenium is an essential component of a number of enzymes, most importantly glutathione peroxidase, which catalyses the breakdown of lipid peroxides and other organic peroxides generated during cellular metabolism. This enzyme, together with vitamin E, superoxide dismutase, and glutathione, is an antioxidant and serves to protect lipid membranes from oxidative stress and lipid peroxidation. Populations with low serum selenium concentrations may show reduced glutathione peroxide activity, but this has no obvious clinical consequences. However, in areas in China where the soil selenium is particularly low, two conditions develop which have been linked to low selenium status, namely Kershan disease, an endemic cardiomyopathy which affects mainly children and women of childbearing age, and Kashin-Bek disease, a degenerative disease of joints and cartilage also observed in children.

Serum, plasma, and erythrocyte selenium concentrations are reduced in individuals abusing alcohol, with or without liver disease (Aaseth, NEJM, 1980; 303:944 letter; Dutta, AmJClinNutr, 1983; 38:713; Valimäki, CCActa, 1983; 130:291; Dworkin, Alcoholism, 1984; 8:535; Dworkin, DigDisSci, 1985; 30:838; Korpela, AmJClinNutr, 1985; 42:147; Johansson, BrJNutr, 1986; 55:227; Tanner, DigDisSci, 1986; 31:1307; Casaril, CCActa, 1989; 182:221; Thuluvath, JHepatol, 1992; 14:176; Van Gossum, BiolTraceElemRes, 1995; 47:201; Buljevac, ActaMedCroatica, 1996; 50:11). Urinary selenium excretion is normal (Thuluvath, 1992). Hepatic selenium concentrations are reduced in patients with alcoholic cirrhosis (Milman, Liver, 1986; 6:111; Ritland, JHepatol, 1987; 5:118; Valimäki, CCActa, 1987; 166:171; Dworkin, DigDisSci, 1988; 33:1213; Thuluvath, 1992). Deficiency may arise because of a reduction in dietary intake or because of reduced hepatic production of the transport protein.

No changes have been observed in serum, plasma, or blood glutathione peroxide activity in individuals abusing alcohol, with or without liver disease (Johansson, BrJNutr, 1986; 55:227; Tanner, DigDisSci, 1986; 31:1307). However, platelet glutathione peroxide activity is reduced in patients with alcoholic cirrhosis (Johansson, 1986). Increased lipid peroxidation is thought to be a major pathogenic factor in the development of alcohol-related liver injury. Selenium deficiency is associated with reduced glutathione peroxidase activity and hence reduced antioxidant activity and enhanced lipid peroxidation. Selenium deficiency has, therefore, been implicated in the pathogenesis of alcohol-related liver injury (Dworkin, DigDisSci, 1988; 33:1213).

Much less information is available on selenium status in patients with non-alcoholic liver disease. Both reduced serum (Sullivan, JNutr, 1979; 109:1432; Aaseth, ClinBioch, 1983; 15:281; Valimäki, CCActa, 1983; 130:291; Aaseth, AnnClinRes, 1986; 18:43; Valimäki, CCActa, 1991; 196:7; Thuluvath, JHepatol, 1992; 14:176; Buljevac, ActaMedCroatica, 1996; 50:11) and hepatic (Milman, Liver, 1986; 6: 111; Thuluvath, 1992) selenium concentrations have been reported. Urinary selenium excretion is not increased (Valimäki, 1991; Thuluvath, 1992). Inadequate dietary intake is thought unlikely to be the sole cause of the selenium deficiency (Thuluvath, 1992).

Plasma selenium concentrations are reduced in children with biliary atresia (Thomas, JPediatGastrNutr, 1994; 19:213); deficient intake, malabsorption, and impaired hepatic synthesis of selenoprotein P, the major bioactive selenoprotein in plasma, have all been implicated. Plasma selenium concentrations correlate significantly with those of albumin and total bilirubin, and low circulating concentrations of selenoprotein P have been reported in these children (Schwarz, Hepatol, 1997; 26(Suppl.):387A abstr.). Selenium supplementation is associated with significant increases in plasma selenium concentrations but no significant change in circulating selenoprotein P levels (Schwarz, 1997). Supplements should, therefore, be used with caution.

'Nutritional' liver damage
Malnutrition and undernutrition[22]

Animals fed diets deficient in choline, protein, and/or vitamins develop fatty liver and cirrhosis (Hartcroft, ProgLivDis, 1962; 1: 68). As a result, the concept of nutritional liver injury arose and, for some considerable time, malnutrition was considered to be a factor in human cirrhosis, particularly in the tropics. In countries where malnutrition is endemic, however, environmental hygiene tends to be poor and large reservoirs of potentially hepatotoxic viruses, parasites, and food-borne contaminants are present. Thus, it is now considered unlikely that cirrhosis is related to malnutrition *per se* and 'nutritional' cirrhosis is a term of doubtful significance (Davidson, AmJClinNutr, 1970; 23:427; Thaler, ClinGastr, 1975; 4:273). Nevertheless, liver injury, short of cirrhosis, can accompany both malnutrition and undernutrition.

The term protein–calorie malnutrition is used to encompass the various clinical forms of malnutrition which result from an inadequate intake of calories, or protein, or both. These disorders are particularly common in the Third World where the food supply is often limited, but may also occur in the Western World, either as a consequence of disease or of unusual dietary habits or food fads (Chase, Pediat, 1980; 66:972; Sinatra, AmJDisChild, 1981; 135:21). In its most extreme forms, protein–calorie malnutrition manifests as one of two clinical syndromes, kwashiorkor and marasmus.

Kwashiorkor, first described in malnourished African children several decades ago, but still widely prevalent in tropical and subtropical regions, results from consumption of a diet severely restricted in protein but adequate in calories from carbohydrate and fat sources (Millward, ProcNutrSoc, 1979; 38:77). The syndrome classically develops when a child is weaned from breast milk, which provides a balanced intake of nutrients, to a diet composed mainly of starch. Kwashiorkor is characterized by growth failure, hair and skin changes, and peripheral oedema. Lean muscle mass and body fat stores are preserved, at least initially, but visceral protein production is seriously disturbed.

The liver is often grossly enlarged, containing 30 to 50 per cent fat by weight (Kirsch, SAMedJ, 1972; 46:2072), predominantly in the form of neutral fat or triglyceride (Chaudhuri, TrRSoc-TropMedHyg, 1972; 66:258). The intrahepatic accumulation of fat results from the combined effects of excess delivery of fatty acids to the liver and/or enhanced lipogenesis, combined with impaired lipid transport from the liver secondary to apoprotein deficiency. Although the liver may be markedly enlarged, serum enzyme abnormalities are usually mild, and often absent (Rao, TropGeogMed, 1985; 37:11), although coagulation defects have been described (Hassanein, TropGeogMed, 1973; 25:158).

All the features of kwashiorkor improve dramatically when protein is supplied; fat clears from the liver within a short period of time. If the disorder is severe and of long-standing, hepatic fibrosis may be observed, but it is never marked and cirrhosis does not develop (Ramalingaswami, Nature, 1964; 201:546; Cook, BMJ, 1967; iii:454).

Marasmus affects children in tropical and subtropical regions and arises when diets are deficient in both protein and calories. It is characterized by stunted growth, loss of fat stores, and generalized loss of lean body mass but maintenance of visceral protein production, at least initially. In contrast to kwashiorkor the liver in children with marasmus is not usually palpable and the changes that occur in liver histology are non-specific; neither fibrosis nor cirrhosis develop. Grossly undernourished adults show no signs of chronic liver disease and no important histological changes in the liver.[23] Institution of a normal diet results in reversal of any clinical or histological abnormalities.

Patients with anorexia nervosa may show abnormal biochemical test results but no histological evidence of liver disease; they may, however, develop significant alcohol-related liver damage with only modest intakes of alcohol because their body weight is so low (Catterson, IntJEatingDis, 1997; 21:303).

Most children and adults with protein–calorie malnutrition, both in the Third World and in the Western World, present with mixed features of kwashiorkor and marasmus, or more commonly still, with chronic mild to moderate malnutrition, which in children is manifest by retardation in height and weight and delayed psychomotor and mental development, but which in adults may be essentially asymptomatic.

Dietary excesses

Alcohol abuse is a well recognized cause of liver disease; excessive energy intake, resulting as it does in the development of obesity, may also result in liver injury. Liver damage may also develop in individuals consuming excessive amounts of vitamin A, niacin, and possibly dietary iron.

Alcohol[24–27]

Alcohol is not an essential nutrient but is a 'normal' constituent of the diet for many individuals. It is a metabolic fuel, which in Western diets supplies 6 to 10 per cent of total daily energy intake (Block, AmJEpid, 1985; 122:27; Cade, IntJEpid, 1988; 17:844).

Alcohol is the most important cause of liver disease in the Western World today. The majority of individuals abusing alcohol will develop fatty change in their liver at some stage of their drinking career. However, only 20 to 30 per cent will develop cirrhosis (Lelbach, ActaHepatoSplenol, 1966; 13:321; Leevy, MedClinNAm, 1968; 52:1445). An individual's susceptibility to develop significant alcohol-related liver injury is probably determined by a number of genetic, constitutional, and environmental factors.

In susceptible individuals, liver damage results from the prolonged daily intake of 60 g or more of alcohol, although daily intakes of 20 to 40 g may be sufficient in women (Coates, ClinInvestMed, 1986; 9:26; Norton, BMJ, 1987; 295:80; Batey, MedJAust, 1992; 156:413; Klatsky, AmJEpid, 1992; 136:1248; Carrao, JClinEpidemiol, 1993; 46:601; Becker, Hepatol, 1996; 23:1025). Alcoholic liver injury appears to progress from fatty liver through alcoholic hepatitis to cirrhosis (Lieber, AnnNYAcadSci, 1975; 252:63). Significant liver disease may not appear for 20 years but in some individuals may develop in as little as 5 years.

Fatty change is the most common liver lesion seen, but although fat accumulation represents a profound metabolic disturbance in the liver, it is not necessarily harmful. Certainly cirrhosis may develop in an alcohol abuser who has never had fatty change and isolated fatty change has not been shown to proceed directly to cirrhosis in man.

Alcoholic hepatitis develops in only a proportion of drinkers even after decades of abuse and is assumed to be a precirrhotic lesion, although its natural history is not well understood (Lelbach, AnnNYAcadMed, 1975; 252:85). Thus, in approximately 50 per cent of individuals, alcoholic hepatitis may persist for several years and in 10 per cent of individuals the lesion may heal despite continued alcohol abuse (Galambos, Gastro, 1972; 63:1026). It has, therefore, been suggested that although alcoholic hepatitis may contribute, when present, to the evolution to cirrhosis, it is not indispensable for such progression.

Cirrhosis is generally considered to be an irreversible lesion. Once established it may remain asymptomatic for many years but decompensation tends to develop at the rate of 10 per cent per annum (D'Amico, DigDisSci, 1986; 31:468); hepatocellular carcinoma develops in approximately 20 per cent of individuals with alcoholic cirrhosis (Lee, Gut, 1966; 7:77). Approximately 75 per cent of patients with alcoholic cirrhosis die as a result of their liver disease; the development of hepatocellular carcinoma accounts for one-third of the 'liver deaths' (Morgan, BMJ, 1977; i:939; Saunders, BMJ, 1981; 282:263; D'Amico, 1986).

The relative importance of alcohol toxicity and malnutrition in the pathogenesis of liver injury in alcohol abusers has been debated for years; both factors are probably important. Alcohol has been shown to be directly hepatotoxic, independently of dietary intake, in both individuals chronically abusing alcohol (Lieber, JCI, 1965; 44:1009), and in healthy volunteers (Rubin, NEJM, 1968; 278:869). In these early experiments, ethanol was substituted isocalorically for carbohydrate in diets that contained either normal or increased amounts of protein. Liver biopsies were obtained a maximum of 3 weeks later and the presence of fat taken to indicate hepatotoxicity. However, the fatty change observed might simply have reflected an adaptive response to obligatory ethanol metabolism. Also it might be argued that a diet which is adequate under normal circumstances might not be adequate when alcohol is substituted for carbohydrates to comprise 50 per cent of the total calorie intake. Such a sharp decrease in carbohydrate intake would limit glycogen reserves and gluconeogenesis,[28] and might lead to loss of the protein-sparing effect of carbohydrate. Additionally, the high fat to carbohydrate ratio of the diets might interfere with ethanol oxidation (Westerfeld, JAMA, 1959; 170:197), and fat metabolism (Jones, AmJClinNutr, 1966; 18:350; Lieber, AmJClinNutr, 1970; 23:474). Despite these reservations about the original studies, ample evidence has accrued to support the view that alcohol directly damages liver cells; the exact mechanism of damage remains in debate (Ishak, AlcoholClinExpRes, 1991; 15:45; Lieber, AnnMed, 1994; 26:325).

Although alcohol is believed to be directly hepatotoxic, it is of interest that in individuals with established alcoholic liver disease, alcohol in amounts up to 300 g daily does not impede recovery (Patek, JCI, 1941; 20:481; Volwiler, Gastro, 1948; 11:164; Summerskill, Lancet, 1957; i:335).[29] Indeed, provided that patients are adequately nourished, improvement occurs despite continued alcohol abuse. Patek and Post (JCI, 1941; 20:481) allowed a group of patients with decompensated alcoholic cirrhosis and severe malnutrition to stabilize in hospital on a nutritious, high-protein diet. Alcohol was then reintroduced, in quantities equivalent to one-third to one-half of a bottle of spirits daily, for up to 18 months. Improvement continued in both clinical signs and laboratory test results. Erenoglu and coworkers (AnnIntMed, 1964; 60:814) randomized patients recovering from liver failure to either high- or low-protein diets; all received approximately 160 g of alcohol daily. The majority of patients taking the high-protein diet showed clinical, biochemical, and histological improvements, while patients taking the low-protein diet showed either no change or a slight deterioration. These findings suggest that the patients' nutritional status might play an important role in limiting or repairing the liver damage caused by alcohol.

Alcohol provides 7.1 kcal (29 KJ)/g, so that a bottle of spirits provides 1500 kcal (6300 KJ) or more than one-half of the recommended daily energy requirement for a healthy individual. Alcohol does not, however, provide equivalent caloric value when compared, for example, to carbohydrate. In addition, alcoholic beverages contain only small amounts of nutrients which are inadequate to meet daily requirements (Table 1). Many individuals chronically abusing alcohol maintain food intake (Fig. 3), so that their total daily energy intakes equal or exceed those of healthy nondrinkers (Neville, AmJClinNutr, 1968; 21:1329; Morgan, ActaChirScandSuppl, 1981; 507:81; Mendenhall, AmJMed, 1984; 76:211). However, their body weights are invariably lower (Simko, AmJClinNutr, 1982; 35:197). This suggests that the calories derived from alcohol have little or no value in terms of maintaining body weight and hence nutritional reserves. Support for this suggestion is gained from a number of studies in which alcohol was fed to patients under carefully controlled conditions. Mezey and Faillace (JNervMentDis, 1971; 153:445) fed a diet which provided 2600 kcal daily to 56 alcohol abusers admitted to hospital, and noted that they all gained weight. Seventeen of these patients were provided with

Table 1 Alcohol, calorie, and nutrient content of various beverages

Constituent (per 100 ml)	Beer	Wine	Fortified wine (sherry, vermouth)	Spirits (70% proof)
Alcohol (g)	2.2–4.3	8.7–10.2	13.0–15.9	31.5
Energy (kcal)	25–39	66–94	116–157	222
Carbohydrate (g)	1.5–4.2	0.3–5.9	1.4–15.9	Trace
Protein (g)	0.2–0.3	0.1–0.3	Trace	Trace–0.3
Thiamine (mg)	Trace	Trace	Trace	—
Riboflavin (mg)	0.02–0.04	0.01	Trace–0.01	—
Nicotinic acid (mg)	0.30–0.51	0.06–0.09	0.04–0.10	—
Pyridoxine (mg)	0.012–0.023	0.012–0.023	0.004–0.010	—
Folic acid (µg)	4.0–8.8	0.1–0.2	Trace–0.1	—
Vitamin B_{12} (mg)	0.11–0.17	Trace	Trace	—
Iron (mg)	Trace–0.05	0.5–1.2	0.34–0.53	Trace
Calcium (mg)	4–11	3–14	4–9	Trace
Magnesium (mg)	6–10	6–11	4–13	Trace

Data from *McCance and Widdowson's The Composition of Foods.*[48]

an extra 1800 kcal daily in the form of spirits but gained no additional weight. Pirola and Lieber (Pharmacol, 1972; 7:185) showed that if alcohol were substituted isocalorically for up to 50 per cent of the carbohydrate in the diet then weight loss would occur. They also showed that addition of 2000 kcal daily, as alcohol, to the diet had no consistent effect on body weight, whereas addition of 2000 kcal daily, as chocolate, resulted in consistent weight gain (Fig. 4).

The calories provided by alcohol are, therefore, inefficiently utilized, probably because oxidation is not coupled by phosphorylation to produce adenosine triphosphate (ATP). Thus,

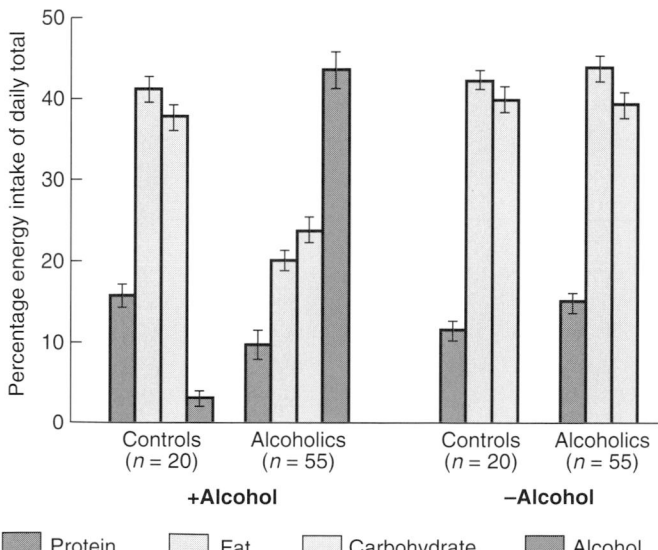

Fig. 3. Mean (± SEM) percentage contributions made by protein, fat, and carbohydrate to total daily energy intake in control subjects and alcohol abusers both with and without the energy contribution from alcohol. * Values significantly different from control values, $p < 0.01$ (Morgan, ActaChirScandSuppl, 1981; 507:81)

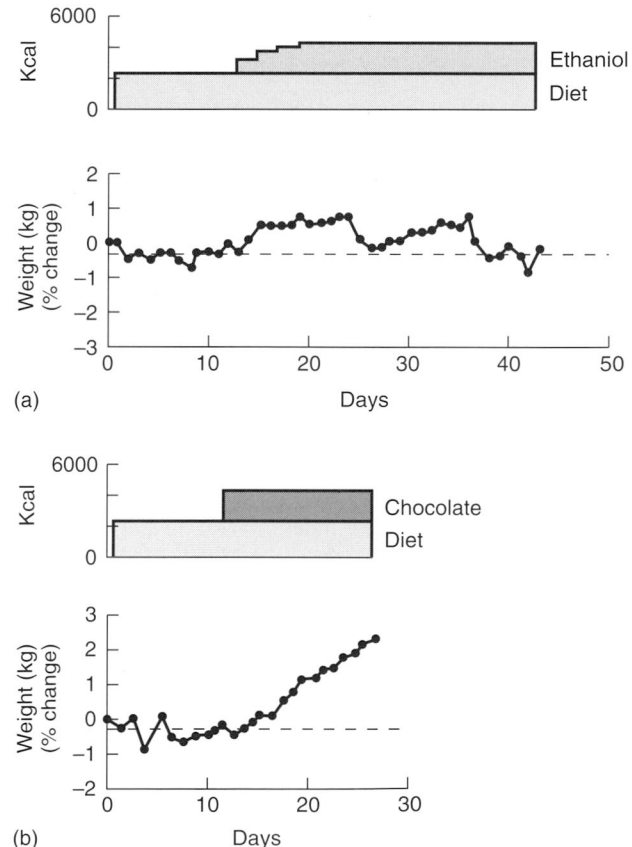

Fig. 4. (a) The effect on body weight of adding 2000 kcal/day as ethanol to the diet of one subject. (b) The effect on body weight of adding 2000 kcal/day as chocolate to the diet of the same subject. The dotted lines represent the mean weight change during the control period (Pirola, Pharmacol, 1972; 7:185).

although alcohol generates large amounts of reduced nicotinamide–adenine dinucleotide (**NADH**), much is wasted in shifting redox state. In addition, chronic alcohol intake causes mitochondrial dysfunction with the result that NADH reoxidation, electron transport, and phosphorylation processes may be impaired. Finally, chronic alcohol ingestion induces the activity of the microsomal ethanol oxidizing system, within the liver, thereby increasing its contribution to alcohol metabolism. Utilization of this process for metabolizing alcohol is energy wasting because it is not coupled with oxidative phosphorylation and so generates heat instead of conserving chemical energy (Pirola, AmJClinNutr, 1976; 29:90; Lands, AmJClinNutr, 1991; 54:47; Suter, NutrRev, 1997; 55:157). The induction of this energy-wasteful pathway for alcohol metabolism may explain, at least in part, the increase in resting energy expenditure observed in individuals chronically abusing alcohol (Levine, Hepatol, 1994; 20:318A abstr.). Alcohol is, therefore, at least in individuals who abuse it, an inefficient metabolic fuel (Suter, 1997).

Individuals chronically abusing alcohol may be malnourished not only because alcohol is a nutrient-poor, inefficient energy source but also because of its effects on nutrient absorption, metabolism, storage, and requirements. However, the relationship between malnutrition and the liver injury seen in individuals chronically abusing alcohol needs further clarification (French, AlcAlc, 1993; 28:97). While malnutrition may not initiate liver injury, it is undoubtedly important in limiting and repairing damage.

The mainstay of nutritional therapy in individuals with alcoholic liver disease is discontinuation of alcohol and provision of a well-balanced diet; specific deficiencies, for example of vitamins or trace metals, should be corrected.

Calories[30–36]

The basal energy expenditure of any given individual, in good health, is reasonably constant and can be met with a caloric intake of, on average, 1940 to 2550 kcal (8.1 to 10.6 MJ)/24 h. If body mass is to remain constant, then the caloric intake must match the energy expenditure. Calories ingested surplus to requirements are stored as triglyceride in adipose tissue. Body weight will increase if excess calories are consumed over time; the weight gain is proportional to the total excess energy consumed; approximately 30 per cent of the excess weight is lean body mass. Individuals are defined as overweight if their body mass index (weight/height^2) exceeds 24 if female, 25 if male; as obese if it exceeds 28.6 if female, 30 if male, and as morbidly obese if it exceeds 40. Obesity is associated with the development, in both adults and children, of parenchymal liver damage and the formation of gallstones.

The most common histological lesion observed in obese individuals is fatty change (Zelman, ArchIntMed, 1952; 90:141; Westwater, Gastro, 1958; 34:686; Rozental, AmJDigDis, 1967; 12:198; Drenick, NEJM, 1970; 282:829; Haines, Hepatol, 1981; 1:161; Andersen, IntJObes, 1984; 8:107; Klain, Hepatol, 1989; 10:873; Watanabe, JMed, 1989; 20:357; Silverman, AmJGastr, 1990; 85:1349; Andersen, JHepatol, 1991; 12:224); the fat comprises triglyceride, fatty acids, and mono- and diglycerides (Mavrelis, Hepatol, 1983; 3:226). While the most severe fatty change tends to be observed in morbidly obese patients, the amount of fat deposited in the liver does not invariably reflect the degree of obesity; 6 to 12 per cent of these individuals have normal liver histology (Andersen, 1984; Silverman, 1990). Mild to moderate degrees of hepatic inflammation and fibrosis are observed in 20 to 30 per cent of patients; the fibrosis is more severe and more extensive in individuals with morbid obesity of long standing who have severe fatty change (Watanabe, 1989; Silverman, 1990).

A small proportion of obese individuals develop steatohepatitis, which histologically mimics alcoholic hepatitis (Adler, AmJMed, 1979; 67:811; Ludwig, MayoClinProc, 1980; 55:434; Moran, AmJGastr, 1983; 78:374; Diehl, Gastro, 1988; 95:1056; Klain, Hepatol, 1989; 10:873; Lee, HumPath, 1989; 20:594; Powell, Hepatol, 1990; 11:74; Silverman, AmJGastr, 1990; 85:1349). There is no relationship between the development of non-alcoholic steatohepatitis and the degree of obesity. However, in individual patients the development of this liver lesion may be preceded by a period of rapid weight loss (Powell, 1990). Non-alcoholic steatonecrosis may progress to cirrhosis in a very small number of patients but generally it is a clinically mild, slowly progressive lesion (Lee, 1989; Powell, 1990; Silverman, 1990; Teli, Hepatol, 1995; 22:1714).

The abnormalities of liver function tests which arise in obese patients are non-specific; elevation of the serum alanine aminotransferase activity is the commonest abnormality observed (Palmer, Gastro, 1990; 99:1408). Liver function test results do not, however, correlate with the degree of liver damage, nor do 'functional' tests such as the bromsulphthalein retention. Overall, little correlation is observed between hepatic structural and functional abnormalities in obese individuals (Westwater, Gastro, 1958; 34:686; Drenick, NEJM, 1970; 282:829; Galambos, Gastro, 1978; 74:1191; Nakamura, TohokuJExpMed, 1980; 132:473; Haines, Hepatol, 1981; 1:161; Drenick, Gastro, 1982; 82:535).

The mechanism of the fatty change in obese individuals is not clear. These individuals tend to take diets low in protein but high in fat and carbohydrate, so that dietary imbalance may play a role (Drenick, NEJM, 1970; 282:829). Additionally, 50 per cent of obese subjects, or more, show carbohydrate intolerance which is a contributory factor (Zelman, ArchIntMed, 1952; 90:141; Westwater, Gastro, 1958; 34:686); indeed, the degree of fatty infiltration increases significantly with the degree of glucose intolerance (Silverman, AmJGastr, 1990; 85:1349).

Transient increases are observed in serum bilirubin and enzyme concentrations and bromsulphthalein retention in obese subjects who lose weight acutely through fasting or semistarvation; these abnormalities regress when dietary intake is resumed (Rozental, AmJDigDis, 1967; 12:198). Gradual weight loss, to within 15 per cent of ideal body weight, is associated with improvement in liver function test results (Westwater, Gastro, 1958; 34:686). For every 1 per cent reduction in body weight, the serum alanine aminotransferase activity decreases by 8 per cent; weight reduction of 10 per cent or more is associated with normalization of liver function test results (Palmer, Gastro, 1990; 99:1408).

Fatty infiltration of the liver decreases, to a degree, after moderate weight loss (Westwater, Gastro, 1958; 34:686), while after repeated short periods of fasting, fatty change diminishes, but fibrosis may become more prominent (Rozental, AmJDigDis, 1967; 12:198; Andersen, JHepatol, 1991; 12:224). More extensive and rapid weight loss results in a progressive reduction in the amount of fatty infiltration, and occasionally in a diminution of periportal fibrosis (Drenick, NEJM, 1970; 282:829). Near normal liver histology is observed in obese subjects who achieve and maintain substantial weight reduction (Drenick, 1970).

The presence of obesity increases the risk of gallstone formation, particularly stones of cholesterol or mixed type. In the general population the frequency of gallstones in individuals aged 18 years or older is approximately 11 per cent (Friedman, JChronDis, 1966; 19:273; Barbara, Hepatol, 1987; 7:913). In contrast, the frequency in obese subjects is 23 per cent and, in the morbidly obese, 30 to 35 per cent (Barbara, 1987).[33] Several factors are of importance in the genesis of gallstones in these individuals including increased bile saturation (Reuben, ClinSci, 1985; 69:71; Reuben, EurJClinInv, 1985; 16:133), impaired gallbladder motility (Fisher, DigDisSci, 1982; 27:1019; Marzio, DigDisSci, 1988; 33:4), and the ingestion of high-fat, high-carbohydrate diets (Scragg, BMJ, 1984; 288:1113).

Weight loss may be associated with an increased risk of gallstone formation if the saturation index of bile remains unchanged or else increases. This can be prevented by prophylactic use of ursodeoxycholic acid in a dose of 10 to 15 mg/kg daily (Broomfield, Gastro, 1987; 92:1721 abstr.). Both chenodeoxycholic acid and ursodeoxycholic acid, in daily doses of 15 mg/kg, have been used successfully to dissolve gallstones in obese adolescents (Podda, ArchDisChild, 1982; 57:956). The effectiveness of treatment may improve if weight is lost simultaneously (Wattchow, BMJ, 1983; 286:763; Reuben, EurJClinInv, 1985; 16:133).

Other nutrients

Excess intake or absorption of vitamin A (Marcus, p.1573 in[4]; Blaner, p.529 in[5]),[6] niacin,[11] and iron[15–17] may result in liver injury.

An intake of retinoids in excess of requirements results in the development of liver damage (Russell, NEJM, 1974; 291:435; Farrell, AmJDigDis, 1977; 22:724; Bendich, AmJClinNutr, 1989; 7:485; Hathcock, AmJClinNutr, 1990; 52:183; Geubel, Gastro, 1991; 100:1701; Kowalski, AmJMed, 1994; 97:523). Toxicity in children usually results from overenthusiastic 'vitamin' therapy and can arise with intakes as small as 7.5 to 15 mg (25 000 to 50 000 IU) daily, for 30 days. Toxicity in adults usually results from chronic ingestion of retinol or retinyl esters, not necessarily in very large quantities, but sufficient over time to increase hepatic reserves beyond the capacity of the liver to metabolize and/or store them. Regular intake should not exceed 7500 µg (25 000 IU) daily in women or 9000 µg (30 000 IU) daily in men.[1] Individuals chronically abusing alcohol are more susceptible to the hepatotoxic effects of vitamin A and may develop liver damage when taking only moderate amounts of supplements (Leo, Hepatol, 1983; 3:1).

The changes within the liver include hypertrophy of fat-storing cells, fibrosis, sclerosis of central veins, and cirrhosis. Geubal and colleagues (Gastro, 1991; 100:1701) examined 41 consecutive patients with vitamin A hepatotoxicity; 17 (41 per cent) had cirrhosis at the time of presentation, 10 (24 per cent) had mild chronic hepatitis, five (12 per cent) had non-cirrhotic portal hypertension, while the remaining nine (22 per cent) showed non-specific changes only; six (15 per cent) died as a result of their liver disease during a mean follow-up period of 4.6 years. The development of significant liver injury was associated with varying intakes and periods of exposure to vitamin A ranging from 7.5 mg (25 000 IU) daily for

6 years to 30 mg (100 000 IU) daily for 2.5 years. The diagnosis of vitamin A hepatotoxicity was suspected initially in only 13 (32 per cent) of the 41 patients; the typical histological feature on liver biopsy of fat-storing cell hyperplasia with fluorescent vacuoles was diagnostic in every case. The authors, therefore, speculated that, at least in some Western countries, vitamin A toxicity might be responsible for a significant proportion of occult or undiagnosed chronic liver disease.

In patients with hypervitaminosis A, increased concentrations of the vitamin are found in the serum mainly in the form of retinyl esters; concentrations of retinol in plasma in excess of 100 µg/100 ml (3.5 µM) are usually diagnostic. The concentration of retinol-binding protein is normal and the excess retinol circulates in association with lipoproteins. Serum alkaline phosphatase activity is high, reflecting increased osteoblastic activity; plasma triglyceride concentrations increase while the cholesterol of HDL decreases. Treatment consists of withdrawal of the retinoid.

Hypercarotenaemia is associated with biliary dyskinesia (Nishimura, JDermatol, 1993; 20:456).

Niacin (nicotinic acid) is widely used to treat hyperlipidaemias characterized by elevation of LDL and VLDL; it is available in both crystalline and sustained-release preparations. Hepatotoxicity is an infrequent but well-documented adverse effect of the crystalline preparation, usually only occurring when doses exceed 3 g daily (Patel, CleveClinJMed, 1994; 61:70). The biochemical picture is one of cholestasis and hepatocellular injury; the liver biopsy shows centrilobular cholestasis and parenchymal necrosis (Patterson, SouthMedJ, 1983; 76:239). Features are transient, and reverse when the preparation is withdrawn; the mechanism of the hepatic injury is unknown; current evidence implicates a dose-related phenomenon rather than a hypersensitivity reaction (Clements, JClinGastr, 1987; 9:582).

Sustained-release preparations of nicotinic acid were developed in order to minimize the skin-flushing reactions experienced with the crystalline preparations. However, their use has been associated with more frequent, more rapidly occurring, and more severe hepatotoxicity (Knopp, Metabolism, 1985; 34:642; Clements, JClinGastr, 1987; 9:582; Mullin, AnnIntMed, 1989; 111:253; Etchason, MayoClinProc, 1991; 66:23; Fischer, WestJMed, 1991; 155:410; Dalton, AmJMed, 1992; 93:107); toxicity occurring within days of changing from crystalline to sustained-release preparations and the development of fulminant hepatic failure have been described; focal defects on imaging studies thought to represent fatty infiltration of the liver have been reported (Lawrance, JClinGastr, 1993; 16:234; Coppola, SouthMedJ, 1994; 87:30).

Discontinuation of the slow-release preparation is associated with return of liver function to normal; challenge with the crystalline preparation is well-tolerated (Henkin, JAMA, 1990; 264:241; Etchason, MayoClinProc, 1991; 66:23). The mechanism of enhanced hepatotoxicity with the sustained-release preparation is unknown, but there is no doubt that in dosages that achieve the same reduction in serum lipids the likelihood of hepatic toxicity is greater with these preparations.

It has been suggested that the mandatory fortification of food with iron might lead to an increase in the incidence of iron-storage disease (Crosby, NEJM, 1977; 297:543). However, it is uncertain whether prolonged iron intake can result in excess iron accumulation, at least in healthy individuals. In Ethiopia, the daily ingestion of up to 200 mg (3.6 mmol) of iron, as dirt iron, causes only modest increases in reticuloendothelial iron stores (Hofvander, ActaMedScandSuppl, 1968; 494:11). Use of oral iron supplements is only rarely associated with the development of significant iron overload, although it has been reported in an individual who ingested a total of 1000 g of elemental iron, over a period of years, as a treatment for anaemia (Johnson, NEJM, 1968; 278:1100); significant iron overload is more likely to develop when iron is administered parenterally, for example when self-injected by disturbed individuals (al-Samman, SouthMedJ, 1995; 88:654).

Massive iron overload is nevertheless seen in the South African black population who use iron pots for cooking and for fermenting beer and, as a result, ingest up to 200 mg (3.6 mmol) of iron daily (Bothwell, AmJClinNutr, 1964; 14:47). Many of these individuals, however, show evidence of ascorbic acid deficiency (Seftel, BMJ, 1966; i:642), and this may have profound effects on iron metabolism (Bothwell, BrJHaemat, 1964; 10:50; Chapman, JClinPath, 1982; 35:487). Equally, non-HLA linked genetic factors may affect the degree of iron overload (Gordeuk, NEJM, 1992; 326:95). The hepatic iron overload observed in this so-called Bantu siderosis is a significant risk factor for death from hepatocellular carcinoma (Gordeuk, Blood, 1996; 87:3470). The excess iron can be removed by venesection but dietary iron intake must be reduced to prevent reaccumulation.

It is possible that as individuals in the Western World become more health conscious, other, as yet unrecognized, syndromes of 'dietary excess' or 'dietary imbalance' may arise as a result of self-administered dietary supplements.

Intestinal bypass[33,36]

Surgical bypass of the small intestine has been used in the treatment and control of severe obesity since the early 1960s. The procedure is undoubtedly efficacious, but is almost invariably complicated by increased fat deposition in the liver (Drenick, NEJM, 1970; 282:829; Snodgrass, NEJM, 1970; 282:870; Buckwald, AmJSurg, 1974; 127:48; Holzbach, NEJM, 1974; 290:296; Salmon, SGO, 1975; 141:75; Galambos, ArchPathLabMed, 1976; 100:299; Haines, Hepatol, 1981; 1:161; Drenick, Gastro, 1982; 82:535). Fatty change may regress within 1 to 2 years of surgery, but in many patients it persists for considerably longer (Galambos, 1976; Haines, 1981; Drenick, 1982). A minority of patients develop steatonecrosis, fibrosis, and frank cirrhosis (Galambos, 1976; Haines, 1981; Dean, AmJSurg, 1990; 159:118; Requarth, ArchSurg, 1995; 130:318); the morphology and the pathological sequence of these changes are indistinguishable from those observed in individuals chronically abusing alcohol (Peters, AmJClinPath, 1975; 63:318; Galambos, 1976; Diehl, Gastro, 1988; 95:1056). The development of cirrhosis is usually insidious and not heralded by any major changes in liver function test results (Drenick, 1970; Haines, 1981; Drenick, 1982); death may occur from hepatic failure (McGill, Gastro, 1972; 63:872; Brown, AmJSurg, 1974; 127:53; Mangla, AmJDigDis, 1974; 19:759; Spin, AmJSurg, 1975; 130:88; Braddeley, BrJSurg, 1976; 63:801; Iber, AmJClinNutr, 1977; 30:4; Maxwell, BMJ, 1977; ii:726; Requarth, 1995).

Haines and colleagues (Hepatol, 1981; 1:161) monitored hepatic function and morphology in 31 morbidly obese individuals undergoing intestinal bypass surgery. The initial liver biopsy showed varying degrees of fatty infiltration and portal fibrosis in the majority of individuals; mild pericentral fibrosis was noted in seven (26 per cent) and developing cirrhosis in one (4 per cent).

Following the surgical procedure, fatty infiltration increased in all patients, reaching maximum severity in 3 to 6 months and then gradually regressing; portal fibrosis increased in severity in 25 patients (93 per cent), while pericentral fibrosis persisted in the seven individuals in whom it was present preoperatively, and developed *de novo* in a further nine. More significant lesions such as steatonecrosis, central hyaline necrosis, and/or cirrhosis developed in seven patients (23 per cent) as early as 3 months and as late as 24 months after surgery. The patients who developed steatonecrosis and/or cirrhosis were older, had invariably shown pericentral fibrosis on the initial liver biopsy, and, 3 months after surgery, had lost significantly more weight and had significantly higher serum aspartate aminotransferase values and bromsulphthalein retention times than the individuals who had developed steatosis alone.

These authors suggest that the presence of pericentral fibrosis preoperatively identified patients at greater risk of developing significant liver disease following surgery. Similar conclusions were drawn by Clain and Lefkowich.[31] The incidence of significant liver injury in patients undergoing intestinal bypass surgery for the treatment of obesity is appreciable and about 7 per cent develop hepatic failure. Nevertheless, the associated mortality is only of the order of 1 to 2 per cent (Halverson, AmJMed, 1978; 64:461).

Gastric bypass procedures are better tolerated as a treatment for morbid obesity and their use is associated with fewer hepatic complications. Silverman and colleagues (AmJClinPath, 1995; 104:23) monitored a large group of morbidly obese individuals for between 2 and 61 months after gastric bypass surgery. The majority of individuals showed a reduction in hepatic steatosis and in perisinusoidal fibrosis. Similar findings have been reported by others (Ranloo, Digestion, 1990; 47:208).

Arrest, improvement, and at least partial recovery of the liver injury have been achieved by restoration of intestinal continuity, by enteral and parenteral hyperalimentation, and by use of metronidazole (Brown, AmJSurg, 1974; 127:53; Galambos, ArchPathLabMed, 1976; 100:229; Iber, AmJClinNutr, 1977; 30:4; Haines, Hepatol, 1981; 1:161; Drenick, Gastro, 1982; 82:535; Kirkpatrick, ArchSurg, 1987; 122:610; Dean, AmJSurg, 1990; 159:118).

The mechanism of the liver injury following bypass surgery remains speculative. Most observers believe that it results from complex nutritional deficiencies which arise during the period of rapid weight loss immediately following surgery (McClelland, SurgForum, 1970; 21:368; Moxley, NEJM, 1974; 290:921; Heimberger, AmJSurg, 1975; 129:229; Ames, JAMA, 1976; 235:1249; Galambos, ArchPathLabMed, 1976; 100:229; Lockwood, AmJClinNutr, 1977; 30:58). Others favour a hepatotoxic insult, directly or indirectly related to bacterial overgrowth of the bypassed intestinal segment (O'Leary, SurgForum, 1974; 25:356; Danö, ScaJGastr, 1975; 10:409; Drenick, Gastro, 1982; 82:535; Kirkpatrick, ArchSurg, 1987; 122:610).

The hepatic changes observed in these patients are similar to those of protein–calorie malnutrition and, indeed, following bypass surgery patients tend to favour low-protein diets high in carbohydrate and fat. The plasma amino-acid patterns observed following bypass surgery (Moxley, NEJM, 1974; 290:921) and in kwashiorkor (Saunders, Lancet, 1967; ii:795) are very similar and the hepatic lesions in both conditions have been shown to reverse with nutritional therapy (McClelland, SurgForum, 1970; 21:368; Ames, JAMA, 1976; 235:1249; Lockwood, AmJClinNutr, 1977; 30:58). In protein-deficient patients the liver is more susceptible to the toxic effects of various agents and impairment of the local immune response in the intestine facilitates its penetration by potentially hepatotoxic substances. Protein repletion may facilitate reversal of the liver lesion by improving host defence mechanisms. It could also be argued, however, that while the steatosis observed following bypass surgery is morphologically similar to that observed in protein–calorie malnutrition, it develops at a time when patients show no clinical or laboratory evidence of protein depletion and still have ample caloric reserves. Also, while nutritional therapy may have a favourable effect on the hepatic lesion, liver injury may progress despite provision of essential nutrients (Brown, AmJSurg, 1974; 127:53). Although the role of malnutrition in the genesis of hepatic steatosis, following intestinal bypass surgery, needs to be clarified, protein depletion is likely to be a permissive or potentiating factor.

The relationship between the development of liver injury and the presence of bacterial overgrowth in the bypassed segment is also debated. Colonic bacteria have been identified in the excluded small intestine (Corrodi, JInfDis, 1978; 137:1) and non-specific inflammatory changes develop in the mucosa of the bypassed segment (Drenick, AmJClinNutr, 1977; 30:76). Moreover, the hepatic steatosis has been shown to reverse with use of metronidazole (Drenick, Gastro, 1982; 82:535). However, significant bacterial overgrowth may not occur (Galambos, ArchPathLabMed, 1976; 100:229), and circulating bacterial endotoxin has not been found in these patients. Additionally, hepatic injury resembling alcoholic hepatitis may develop in obese subjects following gastroplasty in which the stomach is not bypassed but is merely partitioned (Hamilton, Gastro, 1983; 85:722; Cairns, JClinPath, 1986; 39:647).

Gallstones are prevalent in obese individuals and their incidence probably increases in those who undergo intestinal bypass procedures, irrespective of the surgical technique employed (Faloon, AmJClinNutr, 1977; 30:21; Wattchow, BMJ, 1983; 286:763; Thiet, SouthMedJ, 1984; 77:415; Deitel, SGO, 1987; 164:549).[32,36] Several pathogenic mechanisms have been proposed, including mobilization of cholesterol as a result of marked postoperative weight loss (Miettinen, CCActa, 1968; 19:341; Schaefer, AmJClinNutr, 1983; 37:749), increase in the saturation index of bile due to increased faecal bile acid loss and reduction in the bile acid pool (Barry, AmJClinNutr, 1977; 30:32; Faloon, 1977; Sørensen, ScaJGastr, 1977; 12:449), and reduction in biliary cholesterol solubilization secondary to changes in bile acid concentrations (Prakash, AmJClinNutr, 1987; 46:273). It is thought that the mechanism of gallstone formation after gastric operations for obesity might relate more directly to the weight loss.

Ursodeoxycholic acid may be absorbed in patients who have undergone ileal surgery (LaRusso, DigDisSci, 1981; 26:705) and appears to be well tolerated by patients with long-standing jejunoileostomies. It could be used prophylactically in patients undergoing jejunoileal bypass or gastric surgery for obesity to prevent gallstone formation. Some difficulty might be encountered in patients who have undergone gastric restrictive procedures, if the stomach outlet is small, because of the size of the capsules or tablets.

In view of the potentially serious hepatobiliary consequences associated with intestinal bypass surgery, great caution should be

exercised in using these techniques for treating and controlling obesity. The techniques of gastric restriction and gastric bypass surgery appear to be better tolerated and to have a lower associated morbidity, but long-term follow-up data are needed. It remains to be seen whether the newer techniques of pancreatobiliary diversion without intestinal exclusion will reduce hepatobiliary morbidity and mortality further (Brolin, AnnSurg, 1992; 215:387; Grimm, AmJGastr, 1992; 87:775).

Parenteral nutrition[37–43]

Total parenteral nutrition is an effective method of supplying energy and nutrients when oral or enteral feeding is impossible or contraindicated. Most total parenteral nutritional regimens supply energy in the form of carbohydrate, fat, and amino acids, with supplements of vitamins, minerals, and trace metals as required; glucose is the most commonly used carbohydrate and fat is usually supplied as the soybean emulsion, Intralipid.

Individuals receiving total parenteral nutrition may develop hepatobiliary abnormalities, for a number of reasons; they may, for example, have small bowel disease or have undergone small intestinal resection, or they may be septicaemic and/or suffer failure or dysfunction of multiple organ systems. However, there is clear evidence that the use of total parenteral nutrition, *per se*, may be associated with a number of abnormalities of hepatobiliary function which may result in significant morbidity and possibly even death; the spectrum of abnormalities includes asymptomatic biochemical abnormalities, hepatic steatosis with progression to steatohepatitis, fibrosis and cirrhosis, acalculous cholecystitis, cholelithiasis, and intrahepatic cholestasis.

Overall, the complications of total parenteral nutrition are more severe in infants than in adults. The most frequent and predictable hepatobiliary complication associated with use of total parenteral nutrition regimens is the development, in infants, especially those born prematurely, of cholestasis. The other common complications of this form of nutritional support, such as the development of fatty change or the accumulation of biliary sludge and stones, may occur in individuals of any age (Table 2).

Many individuals receiving total parenteral nutrition develop abnormal biochemical test results. However, it is often difficult to establish a cause and effect relationship because of the possible contribution of the patient's underlying disease process. Equally, it

Table 2 Hepatobiliary complications of total parenteral nutrition	
Infants	**Adults**
Cholestasis	Steatosis
Biliary sludge	Steatohepatitis
Cholelithiasis	Cholestasis
Fibrosis	Biliary sludge
Cirrhosis	Cholelithiasis
Hepatocellular carcinoma	Acalculous cholecystitis
	Fibrosis
	Cirrhosis

is difficult to assess the relevance of such changes in terms of hepatic morphology because liver biopsies are examined only infrequently.

Lindor and colleagues (JAMA, 1979; 241:2398) retrospectively reviewed the liver function test results of 48 patients who had received total parenteral nutrition for between 2 and 4 weeks, and found significant increases in serum concentrations of bilirubin in 10 (21 per cent), alkaline phosphatase in 26 (54 per cent), and aspartate aminotransferase in 32 (67 per cent); maximal values were observed between days 9 and 12. Liver biopsies were undertaken in four patients and showed periportal steatosis. Bengoa and coworkers (Hepatol, 1985; 5:79) examined liver function test results in 92 adults with inflammatory bowel disease during total parenteral nutrition. Twenty (22 per cent) had abnormal liver function test results from the outset. Within 2 weeks, serum alkaline phosphatase and aspartate aminotransferase activities had increased in the majority of patients, while hyperbilirubinaemia was observed in 23 (25 per cent). Liver biopsies were performed in the four patients with the highest serum aspartate aminotransferase activities and showed only minor, non-specific changes. Discontinuation of total parenteral nutrition was associated with a prompt return of biochemical abnormalities to baseline values. Finally, Robertson and colleagues (JPEN, 1986; 10:172) retrospectively assessed liver function test results in 127 general surgical patients who had received a course of intravenous nutrition. Test results were abnormal in 101 patients (80 per cent) at the outset. Serum concentrations of γ-glutamyl transferase increased in all patients by the fourth week of treatment but the changes were usually transient; the changes in serum alkaline phosphatase activity were more persistent. The incidence of biochemical abnormalities was significantly greater in individuals with major sepsis and in those who were malnourished; significant increases in serum bilirubin concentrations were only observed in individuals transfused more than 8 units of blood.

The alterations in liver function test results in patients receiving total parenteral nutrition may simply reflect 'infusate imbalance'. Certainly the use of high-calorie infusions in dextrose-based regimens is associated with a greater incidence of abnormalities than use of regimens in which 30 to 50 per cent of the calories are provided as lipid emulsion (Carpentier, ActaChirBelg, 1981; 80: 141; Meguid, ArchSurg, 1984; 119:1294; Buchmiller, JPEN, 1993; 17:301).

Fatty change is the most common liver lesion to develop in association with total parenteral nutrition; the accumulated lipid is almost entirely triglyceride (Kaminski, Surgery, 1980; 88:93). The clinical significance of the hepatic lipid accumulation is unknown. Thus, although it undoubtedly reflects abnormal liver cell metabolism, its presence does not predict progressive liver cell dysfunction or damage. Several mechanisms may be responsible for this change, reflecting metabolic alterations associated with the patients' nutritional status, their disease state, and the use of this form of nutritional support per se.

Calorie overload in excess of basal energy expenditure is thought to be a major factor in the development of hepatic steatosis in patients receiving total parenteral nutrition (Lindor, JAMA, 1979; 241:2398; Lowry, JSurgRes, 1979; 26:300; Wolfe, Metabolism, 1980; 29:892). Infusion of large amounts of glucose is thought to be the most likely contributor. At infusion rates as low as 4 mg/kg per min, less than half of the infused glucose is oxidized; higher rates of glucose infusion result in lipid and glycogen deposition in the

liver and may also affect fatty acid oxidation, thereby contributing to the steatosis (Wolfe, 1980; Stein, NutrRes, 1985; 5:1347; Sax, Surgery, 1986; 100:697). Provision of a proportion of non-protein calories, as fat, blunts the increase in hepatic lipids (Buzby, JSurgRes, 1981; 31:46), but administration of large amounts of lipid may also cause hepatic fat accumulation (Boelhouwer, JPEN, 1983; 7: 530; Martins, Lipids, 1984; 19:728). It has, therefore, been recommended that the non-protein calorie intake during total parenteral nutrition be reduced to provide a calorie to nitrogen ratio of 150 kcal to 1 g of nitrogen, and that 30 to 50 per cent of the non-protein calories be provided as lipid emulsion.

Carnitine is essential for long-chain fatty acid oxidation; carnitine deficiency is associated with the development of hepatic steatosis (Karpati, Neurology, 1975; 25:16). The fluids used for total parenteral nutrition do not contain carnitine but it can be synthesized from their contained methionine and lysine. Nevertheless, low circulating and hepatic carnitine concentrations have been documented in patients receiving total parenteral nutrition (Bowyer, AmJClinNutr, 1986; 43:85). Carnitine supplementation is associated with a restoration of carnitine concentrations in the blood and liver, but has little effect on liver structure or on hepatic lipid accumulation (Bowyer, Gastro, 1988; 94:434).

Choline is essential for the integrity of all membranes, the transport of lipids, and neural function; choline deficiency may be associated with the development of hepatic steatosis (Chawla, Gastro, 1989; 97:1514). The fluids used for parenteral nutrition do not contain choline although it can be synthesized de novo provided there is a supply of methionine. Plasma choline concentrations are low in individuals on long-term parenteral feeding regimens (Chawla, 1989; Buchman, Gastro, 1992; 102;1363; Buchman, Hepatol, 1995; 22:1399; Shronts, JAmDietAssoc, 1997; 97:639). Hepatic steatosis has been observed in 50 per cent of individuals receiving long-term parenteral nutritional support in whom plasma free choline levels are low (Buchman, 1992); treatment with orally administered lecithin increases plasma choline concentrations and is associated with a significant reduction in hepatic steatosis (Buchman, 1992); choline can be given intravenously with equal effect (Buchman, 1995). Choline must, therefore, be considered as a 'conditionally essential' nutrient in this situation.

Use of total parenteral nutrition may also be complicated by the development of intrahepatic cholestasis both in adults (Capron, Lancet, 1983; i:446; Pallares, Lancet, 1983; i:758) and in children, particularly preterm infants (Touloukian, ArchSurg, 1973; 106:58; Rager, JPediat, 1975; 86:264; Rodgers, AmJSurg, 1976; 131:149; Bernstein, JPediat, 1977; 90:361; Beale, Pediat, 1979; 64:342; Hughes, 1983). The histological changes in infants receiving total parenteral nutrition are non-specific and highly variable. The major component is intralobular cholestasis alone or in conjunction with bile-duct proliferation and occasionally periportal inflammation (Rager, 1975; Rodgers, 1976; Zarif, BiolNeon, 1976; 29:66; Cohen, ArchPathLabMed, 1981; 105:152; Hughes, Gut, 1983; 24:241). In adults, the histological picture is of a mixed portal and periportal inflammatory infiltrate, periportal canalicular bile plugs, and bile-duct proliferation (Sheldon, ArchSurg, 1978; 113:504; Salvian, JSurgRes, 1980; 28:547; Allardyce, SGO, 1982; 154:641).

The cholestasis which develops during total parenteral nutrition results from failure of bile secretion, or excretion, rather than from primary hepatocellular failure. Nevertheless, the mechanisms responsible for its development remain unclear (Roy, JAmCollNutr, 1985; 4:651; Whitington, Hepatol, 1985; 5:693; Merritt, JPediatGastrNutr, 1986; 5:9). In infants, the incidence of cholestasis during total parenteral nutrition correlates inversely with gestational age and body weight, suggesting that immaturity of hepatic excretory mechanisms must play a role. Equally, the requirements for certain essential nutrients such as taurine (Gaull, JAmCollNutr, 1986; 5: 121; Dahlstrom, JPediatGastrNutr, 1988; 7:748) and essential fatty acids (Richardson, AmJClinNutr, 1975; 28:258) may not be met, and immaturity of various biosynthetic enzyme systems might lead to deficiencies of nutrients such as carnitine and choline which are not usually considered essential; deficiencies of molybdenum, vitamin E, and selenium have also been proposed.

The basic components of the infusate have also been blamed for the development of cholestasis but the evidence is not entirely convincing (Postuma, Pediat, 1979; 63:110; Farrell, JPEN, 1982; 6: 30), although use of regimens in which lipid provides in excess of 60 per cent of non-protein calories is associated with the development of cholestasis (Allardyce, SGO, 1982; 154:641); the use of a mixture of medium- and long-chain triglycerides rather than long-chain triglycerides alone is associated with a lower incidence of hepatic complications (Baldermann, JPEN, 1991; 15:601). Other infusate components may cause liver injury; aluminium and iron, for example, can accumulate in the liver and are hepatotoxic (Klein, PediatRes, 1988; 23:275; Klein, JParentSciTech, 1989; 43:120; Ben Hariz, JPediat, 1993; 123:238).

Cholestasis has been observed in sick infants and adults after fasting and this led to the suggestion that lack of enteral nutrition with suppression or lack of hormone stimulation of the hepatobiliary system might be of aetiological importance in the development of cholestasis in relation to total parenteral nutrition (Rager, JPediat, 1975; 86:264; Hughes, Gut, 1983; 24:241). Finally, the possibility that the cholestasis might in some way relate to intestinal overgrowth with anaerobic bacteria must also be considered (Capron, Lancet, 1983; i:446; Pallares, Lancet, 1983; i:758); these individuals may be predisposed to intestinal bacterial overgrowth because of bowel inactivity.

The cholestasis observed in individuals receiving prolonged total parenteral nutrition regresses when treatment is discontinued. It can be ameliorated during treatment by stimulating bile flow with small lipid and protein meals or by use of cholecystokinin; a trial of metronidazole may be warranted (Capron, Lancet, 1983; i:446; Lambert, JPEN, 1985; 9:501; Kubota, JPediatSurg, 1990; 25:618; Teitelbaum, JPediatSurg, 1995; 30:1082).

The prolonged use of total parenteral nutrition is associated with the development of progressive liver injury including steatohepatitis, progressive cholestasis, fibrosis, and cirrhosis; children are more likely to be affected than adults; they may be asymptomatic or may develop symptoms and signs of progressive liver dysfunction and failure (Bowyer, JPEN, 1985; 9:11).

Benjamin (AmJClinPath, 1981; 76:276) observed hepatic periportal fibrosis and portal-to-portal bridging in eight (53 per cent) of 15 infants who had received parenteral nutritional support for more than 60 days; five (33 per cent) had established cirrhosis. In contrast, Bowyer and coworkers (JPEN, 1985; 9:11) found steatohepatitis on liver biopsy in eight (13 per cent) of 60 adults maintained on parenteral feeding regimens for, on average, 29 months; a further six (10 per cent) had central fibrosis/cholestasis, while one (2 per

cent) showed nodular regeneration; three of these individuals eventually developed significant symptomatic liver disease and one died in liver failure.

In infants, chronic liver disease appears to develop as a direct consequence of prolonged cholestasis and must be assumed to result from prolonged exposure to the factors proposed to be important in its genesis, but not necessarily to the parenteral nutritional support *per se*. The factors responsible for the development of chronic liver disease in adults are less well understood; deficiencies of carnitine, choline, and taurine, hypophosphataemia, and lithocholate toxicity have all been proposed.

Acalculous cholecystitis and cholelithiasis may develop in both adults (Anderson, MedAnnualDC, 1972; 41:438; Petersen, AmJSurg, 1979; 138:814; Messing, Gastro, 1983; 84:1012; Roslyn, Gastro, 1983; 84:148) and in children (Demarquez, Agressol, 1980; 21:137; Whitington, JPediat, 1980; 97:647; Benjamin, JPediatSurg, 1982; 17:386; King, JPediatSurg, 1987; 22:593). In a prospective evaluation of 21 children requiring total parenteral nutrition for a minimum of 3 months, nine (43 per cent) were found to have developed gallstones (Roslyn, Pediat, 1983; 71:789). In a prospective ultrasonographic study of the biliary tree of 41 neonates receiving total parenteral nutrition, gallbladder sludge was shown to develop in 18 (44 per cent), after a mean period of 10 days (Matos, JUSMed, 1987; 6:243). Evolution of sludge into 'sludge balls' was observed in five infants and two developed uncomplicated gallstones. Messing and co-workers (1983) also used ultrasonography to assess the prevalence of gallbladder sludge and lithiasis in 23 adults receiving total parenteral nutrition, who were free of hepatobiliary disease at the onset. The incidence of sludge formation during the first 3 weeks of treatment was 6 per cent, increasing to 50 per cent between weeks 4 and 6, and reaching 100 per cent with treatment periods in excess of 6 weeks. Gallstones were found, together with sludge, in six patients, three of whom required cholecystectomy after a mean of 43 days of treatment.

The biliary complications of total parenteral nutrition arise as a consequence of impaired biliary flow and gallbladder stasis. Such stasis can be prevented by administration of exogenous cholecystokinin (Doty, AnnSurg, 1985; 201:76; Sitzman, SGO, 1990; 170:25; Teitelbaum, JPediatSurg, 1995; 30:1082) or, if possible, by stimulating endogenous cholecystokinin release by intermittent oral or enteral feeding (Dunn, JPediat, 1988; 112:622; Slagle, JPediat, 1988; 113:526; Cohen, JPediatSurg, 1990; 25:163).

In general, total parenteral nutrition should be used for the shortest possible time; excess calories should be avoided and 30 to 50 per cent of non-protein calories should be provided as fat. Patients should be very carefully monitored throughout.

Inborn errors of metabolism
Tyrosinaemia, galactosaemia, and fructose intolerance

Children with hereditary tyrosinaemia (Mitchell, p.1077 in[44]), galactosaemia (Segal, p.967 in[44]), and hereditary fructose intolerance (Gitzelmann, p.905 in[44]) may develop liver damage in response to normal dietary constituents. They are autosomal recessive conditions which may present soon after birth. Successful management depends on early diagnosis and exclusion of the offending substance from the diet. The mechanism of the liver injury in these conditions is not understood but it is assumed to relate to the accumulation of toxic metabolites of tyrosine, galactose, or fructose.

Wilson's disease (Sternlieb, p.585 in reference 5; Danks, p.2211 in reference 44)[45]

Wilson's disease is a rare, autosomal, recessively inherited disorder of copper metabolism in which hepatic lysosomes fail to excrete copper into the bile. The gene for Wilson's disease is located on chromosome 13; it has been cloned and characterized; the gene product is a copper-transporting ATPase although its exact cellular location and function are still to be determined. The excess intracellular copper inhibits the formation of caeruloplasmin from apo-caeruloplasmin and copper; hence circulating concentrations of this glycoprotein are characteristically low. The capacity of hepatocytes to store copper is eventually exceeded; copper is released into the circulation and accumulates in the brain, kidney, and cornea. Toxicity occurs as a result of binding of the excess copper to various cellular proteins.

Fat and glycogen deposits are the earliest abnormalities observed in the liver biopsy on light microscopy. Mitochondrial abnormalities, said to be specific for this disorder, are seen on electron microscopy. At a later stage, necrosis, inflammation, fibrosis, bile-duct proliferation, and cirrhosis develop. The rate and mode of progression from steatosis, through fibrosis to cirrhosis, are variable.

Untreated, Wilson's disease is progressive and invariably fatal. Treatment consists of removing excess copper by use of a chelating agent. D-Penicillamine is the drug of choice and life-long therapy is required. Dietary copper intake should be kept as low as possible; patients should be advised to avoid shellfish, dried fruit, nuts, broccoli, chocolate, mushrooms, and liver and to restrict the amount of salt and pepper they use for flavouring. If local water supplies contain copper in excess of 0.1 mg/100 ml (1.6 μmol/l), demineralized water should be used. Domestic water softeners should not be used as they may substantially increase the copper content of the water.

Copper and zinc compete with one another for absorption in the small intestine (Festa, AmJClinNutr, 1985; 41:285); zinc supplementation could, therefore, be used to reduce copper absorption. Negative or neutral copper balance can be achieved in patients with Wilson's disease who received no treatment other than oral zinc, although not consistently (Brewer, AnnIntMed, 1983; 99:314; Brewer, Drugs, 1995; 50:240).

As D-penicillamine is a pyridoxine antagonist, patients receiving this drug should be given prophylactic pyridoxine in a dose of 25 mg daily.

Genetic haemochromatosis (Bothwell, p.2237 in reference 44)

Genetic haemochromatosis is a relatively common autosomal, recessively inherited, metabolic disorder of iron metabolism in which iron absorption is increased and excess iron gradually accumulates in various body tissues. The gene for haemochromatosis susceptibility, which has been designated HFE, is located on the short arm of chromosome 6 in proximity to the HLA A locus (Feder, NatureGen, 1996; 13:399). The most common HLA serotypes associated with this disorder are A3-B14, and A3-B7.

Although the control of iron absorption is known to be defective in this disease, the underlying metabolic defect has not been defined. After absorption, the excess iron is deposited in the parenchymal cells of the liver, pancreas, heart, and pituitary in the form of haemosiderin. The rate of accretion of absorbed iron is both slow and variable; an excess of 20 g of storage iron is needed to produce tissue damage. The precise cytopathological mechanisms by which excess iron causes cellular injury are unknown. However, several possible mechanisms have been proposed, including intracellular disruption of iron-laden lysosomes, increased lipid peroxidation, and stimulation of collagen biosynthesis.

Haemosiderin deposits in the liver appear first in the periportal parenchyma; over time, iron is deposited more extensively and a characteristic pattern of fibrosis emerges. Cirrhosis develops comparatively late in the disease. Hepatocellular carcinoma develops in about 35 per cent of patients; it is the most common cause of death in treated individuals.

Iron metabolism is disturbed in individuals chronically abusing alcohol; one-third of such individuals have increased hepatic iron concentrations (Chapman, DigDisSci, 1982; 27:909). Approximately 15 per cent of individuals with genetic haemochromatosis also abuse alcohol (Adams, Hepatol, 1996; 23:724); in these individuals, the accumulation of iron may be accelerated resulting in the development of more severe liver injury.

In individuals with genetic haemochromatosis, iron accumulates at the rate of 1.4 to 4.8 mg daily (Bomford, QJMed, 1976; 65:611); total body iron stores are of the order of 20 to 60 g. Iron can be removed by venesection; 1 unit of blood (500 ml) contains 250 mg (4.5 mmol) of iron. Based on weekly removal of this amount, it may take 2 to 3 years to remove the excess tissue iron stores; maintenance phlebotomy will be required, perhaps three to six times a year thereafter, to maintain the transferrin saturation at about 50 per cent. Iron depletion is accompanied by a reduction in the size of the liver and spleen, improvement in liver function test results and some regression of the hepatic damage observed histologically. Patients who have cirrhosis are at risk of developing hepatocellular carcinoma even when iron depleted.

While there is no need to restrict dietary iron intake, patients should be warned about the dangers of alcoholic excess, not only because alcohol may increase iron absorption (Charlton, BMJ, 1964; 2:1427; Chapman, DigDisSci, 1983; 28:321) but because it is hepatotoxic *per se*.

Hepatic siderosis arises in relation to a variety of dyserythropoietic anaemias (Schafer, NEJM, 1981; 304:319; Simon, BrJHaemat, 1985; 60:75; Massa, Haematologica, 1995; 80:398; Nielsen, BrJHaemat, 1995; 91:827); it is observed in both the sporadic and familial forms of porphyria cutanea tarda (Kushner, Gastro, 1985; 88:1232; Beaumont, Gastro, 1987; 92:1833; Rocchi, Dermatologica, 1991; 182:27), and in idiopathic neonatal iron storage disease (Silver, AmJPath, 1987; 128:538).

Toxic foods, dietary supplements, and contaminants[46]

Liver damage can be caused by the accidental ingestion of toxic agents. In addition, problems of toxicity have recently been observed with several commercially available herbal preparations (Table 3).[47]

Table 3 Medicinal plants associated with hepatotoxicity

Proven association
Plants containing pyrrolizidine alkaloids:
  Crotalaria
  Senecio
  Héliotropium
  Symphytum officinale
Atractylis gummifera L
Callilepsis laureola
Teucrium chamaedrys (germander)
Larrea tridentata (chaparral, creosote bush, grease wood)
Cassia angustifolia (senna)
Chinese herbs

Suspected association
Viscum album (mistletoe)
Scutellaria (skullcap)
Valeriana officinalis (valerian)
Teucrium polium
Mentha pulegium
Berberis vulgaris
Hedeoma pulegioides
Azadirachza indica
Sassafras albidum (sassafras)

The fungus *Amanita phalloides* contains a potent hepatotoxin; liver damage occurs in proportion to the amount ingested. After ingestion of small amounts of amitotoxin, the liver shows centrilobular necrosis with ceroid pigment in the surrounding Kupffer cells; if large amounts are ingested, severe steatosis and extensive or massive necrosis develop. No antitoxin is available and treatment is supportive.

Plants of the genera *Crotalaria*, *Senecio*, *Héliotropium*, and *Symphytum* contain pyrrolizidine alkaloids which have been linked to the development of veno-occlusive disease involving both small and medium-sized hepatic veins (Smith, JNatProd, 1981; 44:129; Valla, ClinGastroent, 1988; 2:481; Weston, BMJ, 1987; 295:183; Ridker, Lancet, 1989; i:657). Pyrrolizidine poisoning is endemic in areas such as Africa and Jamaica, where toxic alkaloids are ingested as infusions, herbal teas, decoctions, or used as enemas. Contamination of flour by plants containing pyrrolizidine alkaloids has also caused epidemic intoxication in India and Afghanistan. Recently, hepatotoxicity has been observed in individuals in Western countries following ingestion of toxic alkaloids in herbal teas, capsules, and dietary supplements (Ridker, Gastro, 1988; 88:1050; Larrey, Sem-LivDis, 1995; 15:183; Sperl, EurJPed, 1995; 1545:112).

Teucrium chamaedrys (germander) is a traditional herbal medicine used to facilitate weight loss. It is ingested in various forms including commercial herbal teas, capsules, and artisanal preparations. It has been implicated in more than 30 cases of liver injury in France, mainly in middle-aged women (Castot, GastrClinBiol, 1992; 16:916; Larrey, AnnIntMed, 1992; 117:129). Liver injury is characterized by the development of a mild to moderate hepatitis approximately 2 months after starting treatment. However, fatal fulminant hepatic failure (Mostefa-Kara, Lancet, 1992; 340:674), chronic hepatitis, and cirrhosis have also been observed (Ben Yahia, GastrClinBiol, 1993; 17:959; Dao, GastrClinBiol, 1993; 17:609). Germander has now been withdrawn from sale in France but cases of germander hepatitis continue to be reported from countries where it can still be obtained (Laliberte, CanMedAssJ, 1996; 154:1689).

Larrea tridentata (chaparral) is a dietary supplement made from desert shrubs which is used for its antioxidant properties. Several cases of chaparral-associated hepatotoxicity have been reported since the 1970s. The predominant pattern of liver injury is of a toxic or drug-induced cholestatic hepatitis; some exposed individuals have developed fulminant hepatic failure; cirrhosis has also been documented (Katz, JClinGastr, 1990; 12:203; Alderman, JClinGastr, 1994; 19:242; Batchelor, AmJGastr, 1995; 90:831; Gordon, JAMA, 1995; 273:489; Sheikh, ArchIntMed, 1997; 157:913).

Chinese herbal medicines have recently been shown to have beneficial effects on eczema and atopic dermatitis (Davies, Lancet, 1990; 336:177; Sheehan, Lancet, 1992; 340:13). However, their use in these conditions is associated with hepatotoxicity (Graham-Brown, Lancet, 1992; 340:673; Perharic-Walton, Lancet, 1992; 340:674).[47] Toxicity has also been reported with use of a number of other Chinese herbal preparations (Woolfe, AnnIntMed, 1994; 121:729; Itoh, DigDisSci, 1995; 40:1845; Kane, Gut, 1995; 36:146; But, VetHumTox, 1996; 38:280; Horowitz, ArchIntMed, 1996; 156:899; Nadir, AmJGastr, 1996; 91:1436).[47] The identification of the toxic substances is difficult; at least 7000 species of medicinal plants are used in China and preparations are often adulterated with substituted herbs, heavy metals, and Western medicines (Chan, Lancet, 1993; 342:1532).

Liver and biliary disease may also occur as a result of contamination of food or water supplies by viruses, parasites, and toxins. Hepatitis A and E are enterically transmitted. Epidemics of type A hepatitis have followed ingestion of infected clams, oysters, and other shellfish. Several outbreaks in the United Kingdom, in recent years, have been traced to soft fruits picked in open fields and frozen for storage without washing. The fruit was undoubtedly contaminated by excreta from fruit pickers or because human faeces had been used as fertilizer. Epidemics of type E hepatitis occur in developing countries almost invariably as a result of contamination of water supplies; infection resulting from contamination of Chinese herbal medicines has been reported (Isikawa, JGastr, 1995; 30:534).

A number of helminths enter the body via food and infest the liver and biliary tree. The roundworm *Ascariasis lumbricoides* is commonly found in Asia, especially in China. Infestation follows the ingestion of contaminated vegetables, usually in salads, but also in pickles. The adult ascaris may invade the entire biliary tree but is usually found in the common bile duct; cholangitis, lithiasis, and biliary obstruction may develop as a result. Eggs laid in the biliary tree may regurgitate into the portal tracts where they stimulate granuloma formation and eventual scarring. Pyogenic abscesses may develop within the liver and in some instances live ascaris migrate into the abscess cavities. Endoscopic worm extraction with or without sphincterotomy is the treatment of choice; antihelminthic chemotherapy will kill the ascaris but it will remain in the biliary tree.

The trematode *Clonorchis sinensis* is widely distributed in Eastern Asia. Infestation follows the ingestion of raw or inadequately cooked freshwater fish; a freshwater snail is the intermediate host. Larvae migrate from the duodenum into the peripheral bile ducts where they mature to adult worms; biliary obstruction, calculus formation, and cholangiocarcinoma may develop as a result. Antihelminthic drugs are generally ineffective although the response to drugs used in veterinary fascioliasis has been encouraging.

Infestation of the biliary tree by the trematode *Fascioliasis hepatica* occurs in mid- and Western Europe and the Caribbean. Cattle and sheep are the definitive hosts; a freshwater snail is the intermediate host. Humans become infested after ingestion of watercress (*Nasturtium officinale*) contaminated with the encysted metacercariae of the worm. If infestation is heavy, diarrhoea, prostration, fever, jaundice, tender hepatomegaly, and eosinophilia develop. Hepatic necrosis together with a marked cellular infiltration containing eosinophils, neutrophils, and lymphocytes may be seen; however, the liver lesion heals completely. The worms move to and fro in the intrahepatic ducts, damaging the biliary epithelium. Antihelminthic drugs may be used, but surgery may be necessary to relieve biliary obstruction.

Aflatoxins are derived from species of *Aspergillus* and are known to contaminate stored foods and groundnuts. A significant correlation has been found between aflatoxin ingestion and the incidence of hepatocellular carcinoma in several areas of Africa and Asia (van Rensburg, BrJCanc, 1985; 51:713; Wogan, CancerDetectPrev, 1989; 14:209). Danish workers exposed to aflatoxin via the respiratory route, while handling contaminated crops imported for animal feed production, show an increased risk of developing hepatocellular carcinoma, the magnitude of which increases in relation to the period of exposure (Olsen, BrJCanc, 1988; 58:392). In areas of the world such as Taiwan and the People's Republic of China, where hepatitis B virus infection is the major aetiological agent for hepatocellular carcinoma, there is no association between aflatoxin ingestion and development of this tumour (Campbell, CancerRes, 1990; 50:6882).

Nutritional management of hepatobiliary diseases

Nutritional deficiencies may arise in individuals with hepatobiliary disease and may adversely affect hepatic function, help perpetuate the liver injury, and detrimentally affect outcome (Calvey, JHepatol, 1985; 1:141; Mendenhall, AmJClinNutr, 1986; 43:213; Halliday, JPEN, 1988; 12:43; Lautz, ClinInvest, 1992; 70:479; Helton, SemLivDis, 1994; 14:140; Merli, Hepatol, 1996; 23:1041). Children with chronic liver disease may be particularly compromised because they develop resistance to the growth-promoting, diabetogenic, and lipolytic effects of growth hormone (Bucuvalas, JPediat, 1990; 117: 397). In consequence, they show growth failure, short stature, and if the onset of the disease is within the first few years of life, intellectual impairment (Stewart, Pediat, 1988; 82:167).

Individuals with hepatobiliary disease, therefore, require dietary advice and nutritional support. Specific dietary modifications may be necessary in patients with chronic parenchymal liver disease or chronic cholestasis, and specific dietary restrictions may be necessary in individuals with complications of chronic liver disease, such as fluid retention. Vigorous nutritional support may be necessary for patients with fulminant hepatic failure, severe alcoholic hepatitis, and endstage liver failure, particularly if they are candidates for liver transplantation (Goulet, TransplProc, 1987; 19:3249; Shronts, JAmDietAssoc, 1987; 87:441; DiCecco, MayoClinProc, 1989; 64: 95; Kaufman, SemLivDis, 1989; 9:176; Cabré, Gastro, 1990; 98: 715; Chin, JGastrHepatol, 1990; 5:566; Kearns, Gastro, 1992; 102: 200; Wicks, Lancet, 1994; 344:837; Hasse, JPEN, 1995; 19:437).

Aggressive nutritional support, beginning at the time of diagnosis, might help to offset the delays in growth and intellectual development in children with chronic liver disease (Stewart, Pediat, 1988; 82:167).

In order to provide a rational basis for dietary advice and therapy, nutritional status should be assessed initially and then again at suitable intervals. Careful and continual attention to diet is mandatory, as in many instances nutrient deficiencies arise as a result of inadequate or ill-conceived dietary advice.

Assessment of nutritional status

The methods used to determine nutritional status in patients with liver disease vary depending on whether the information is required in the clinical setting or for research purposes.

Clinical setting

Assessment of nutritional status is needed in the clinical setting: (i) to enable patients at risk to be identified, (ii) to document the nutritional consequences of disease progression, and (iii) to monitor the effects of treatment and nutritional intervention.

There are no 'gold standard' techniques for assessing nutritional status for clinical purposes. In practice, therefore, this assessment is made by combining the results of the clinical and dietary histories, physical examination, anthropometric measurements, and selected laboratory indices. However, problems arise in patients with liver disease, such as fluid retention and disturbances of protein and mineral metabolism, which may hinder the assessment process.

Information should be obtained from these patients on weight change, particularly in the preceding 6 months, and details of abdominal symptomatology such as anorexia, nausea, vomiting, discomfort or distension, and details of stool frequency, colour, and consistency should be sought. Case records should be scrutinized for information on the aetiology and severity of the liver disease, of any complications which may have arisen, such as gastrointestinal bleeding or fluid retention, and of other gastrointestinal diseases or surgery.

A diet history should be obtained by a trained observer using a dietary recall technique concentrating on the average nutrient intake in the week prior to review; this will provide information on food intake, eating habits, and meal consumption patterns. Patients abusing alcohol prior to admission and those who are moderately to severely encephalopathic may not be able to recall details accurately, but otherwise there is no reason why patients with liver disease should not be able to produce reasonably reliable information on their dietary habits.

As estimate of the number of grams of individual foods consumed daily can be made and the approximate intake of total energy, fat, carbohydrate, and protein assessed by reference to food composition tables;[48] this process is greatly facilitated by use of a computer program.

Calculated dietary intakes can then be compared with Reference Nutrient Intakes.[1] However, as these reference data are intended for use in healthy populations, their usefulness in individuals with liver disease and in individuals who take up to 50 per cent of their total daily calories as alcohol is limited.

Additional information on energy requirements can be obtained by reference to data on energy expenditure. However, accurate information on energy expenditure can only be obtained, in this patient population, by direct measurement, as the information obtained indirectly by use of prediction equations tends to be inaccurate. Thus, in patients with cirrhosis, values for energy expenditure predicted using the Harris–Benedict formulae[49] underestimate measured values by a mean of 13 per cent (Shanbhogue, JPEN, 1987; 11:305; Merli, Hepatol, 1990; 12:206; Müller, Hepatol, 1992; 15:782; Selberg, Hepatol, 1997; 25:652); in one study, measured values exceeded predicted values by more than 120 per cent in one-third of the patients (Selberg, 1997). However, even when facilities are available to measure energy expenditure directly, it is unclear whether actual, 'dry', or ideal body weight should be used in the calculations.

Nevertheless, even with these various provisos, the data obtained from the clinical and dietary history provide an invaluable baseline for therapy.

A detailed physical examination will provide an impression of overall nutritional status and furnish evidence of malnutrition such as muscle wasting, loss of subcutaneous fat, peripheral neuropathy, glossitis, cheilosis, and hair, skin, and nail changes.[50] If peripheral oedema and ascites are present they should be assessed semi-quantitatively.

An anthropometric assessment will provide information on body fat and muscle stores; the most frequently assessed variables are the body mass index, skinfold thicknesses, and mid-arm muscle circumference. This assessment should be undertaken by a skilled observer using standardized techniques;[51,52] repeat measurements should, whenever possible, be undertaken by the same individual.

In adequately nourished, non-obese individuals, the body mass index (weight/height^2) lies between 20 to 25; individuals with a body mass index of less than 20 may be at risk for malnutrition. Assessment of this variable may be of less value in patients with chronic liver disease as accurate estimates of weight are difficult to obtain in the presence of fluid retention. However, dry body weight can be estimated using previously documented weights and published guidelines,[53] and may facilitate a more accurate calculation of this variable.

Measurements of skinfold thicknesses are used to assess subcutaneous fat and hence, indirectly, body fat stores. The triceps skinfold (TSF) thickness is the one most frequently used. Measurement of the mid-arm circumference (MAC) allows calculation of the mid-arm muscle circumference (MAMC) using the formula:

$$MAMC = MAC - (TSF \times 0.3142)$$

Measurements of both TSF and MAMC are compared with published standards which are stratified for age and sex.[54,55] Values below the fifth percentile of the appropriate population bands are used to define malnutrition (Gray, JPEN, 1979; 3:366).

In patients with cirrhosis and fluid retention the presence of subcutaneous oedema may confound the measurement of skinfold thicknesses. In practice, this is difficult to evaluate both because of the errors inherent in remeasurement and because changes occurring in subcutaneous oedema over time may be accompanied by changes in fat stores. Skinfold thicknesses measured at the triceps and biceps sites are less likely to be affected by oedema than those made on the trunk or lower limbs, although even the triceps site, which is the most predictive of body fat stores, may be affected if the patient remains supine for long periods. The presence of skin oedema may result in an overestimation of fat stores and an underestimation of muscle stores.

Skinfold measurements can also be used to estimate total body fat using prediction formulae; the method of Durnin and Wormesley (BrJNutr, 1974; 32:77) is one of the more useful as it uses the logarithmic sum of skinfolds measured at triceps, biceps, subscapular, and suprailiac sites, thereby avoiding measurements in the lower limbs and waist circumference, which are included in other models, and which are more likely to be distorted by fluid retention. However, even use of this method for assessing total body fat may produce erroneous results in patients with gross ascites as the measurement of skinfolds at the suprailiac site may prove difficult or else may be precluded.

Great care must be taken when using anthropometric indices to assess nutritional status in children with chronic liver disease. Assessment of height and weight percentiles are often misleading; the weight of the enlarged liver and spleen, and of any fluid retained, may contribute substantially to total body weight, thereby producing erroneously high values, and hence underestimates of the degree of malnutrition; height is often reduced for age so weight/height comparisons may also produce underestimates of the degree of malnutrition. These measurements should, therefore, be converted to Z (standard deviation) scores using appropriate reference growth data.[56] The Z score is calculated from the formula:

$$Z = X - \bar{X}/SD^{\bar{X}}$$

where X is the patients' measured value, $\bar{X}$ is the mean standard deviation for age and sex, and $SD^{\bar{X}}$ is the standard deviation of the reference mean.

Measurements of TSF and MAC afford better estimates of nutritional status in children and should be used in preference to other indices (Sokol, AmJClinNutr, 1990; 52:203).

Provided that the difficulties which might arise in obtaining these measurements are appreciated, anthropometry may still play an important role in the assessment of nutritional status in this patient population.

The creatinine–height index is the ratio of measured 24-h urinary creatinine excretion to the expected excretion of a sex- and height-matched healthy adult, expressed as a percentage. It has been used to estimate muscle or body cell mass. Creatinine is the breakdown product of creatine, which is synthesized in the liver and stored in skeletal muscle. In patients with chronic liver disease, low urinary creatinine excretion may reflect depleted skeletal muscle but, equally, may reflect defective hepatic synthesis of creatine. As such, use of this index in the assessment of nutritional status in patients with chronic liver disease is not recommended.

Muscle protein stores can be evaluated by measurement of muscle strength using a number of techniques including hand-grip dynamometry. At present, no recommendation can be made about testing muscle function to evaluate nutritional status in patients with chronic liver disease as the available data are limited and conflicting (Lafleur, NutrRes, 1994; 16:545; Mendenhall, JPEN, 1995; 19:258; Tarter, AlcoholClinExpRes, 1997; 21:191).

Bioelectrical impedance analysis (BIA) has been used to estimate lean tissue mass and fat mass in patients with cirrhosis, but the

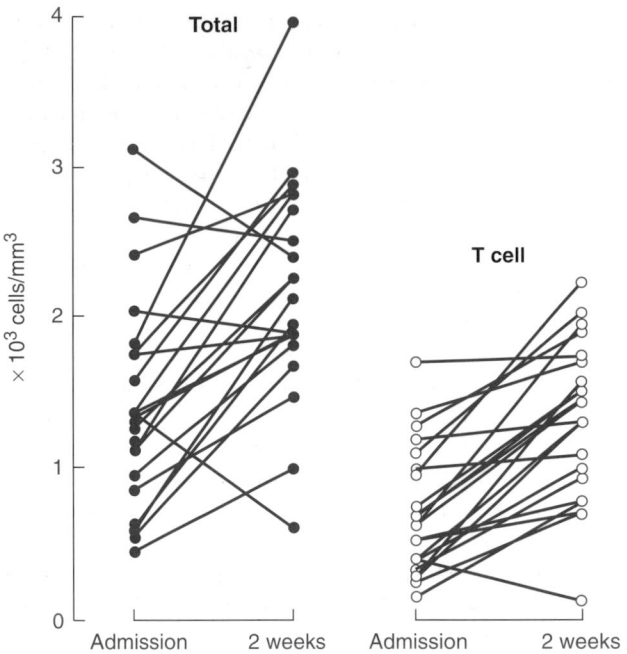

Fig. 5. Total peripheral blood lymphocyte and T-lymphocyte counts in individuals chronically abusing alcohol on admission to hospital and after 2 weeks in hospital (Mills, AmJClinNutr, 1983; 38:849).

validity of the measurements obtained has been questioned (Lautz, ClinInvest, 1992; 70:478; Bramley, BasicLifeSci, 1993; 60:211; Prijatmoto, Gastro, 1993; 105:1839; Holt, Nutrition, 1994; 10:211; Madden, JHepatol, 1994; 21:878; Schloerb, AmJClinNutr, 1996; 645:5105). Single-frequency techniques cannot be recommended for use in this population although multifrequency BIA might produce valid body composition data in patients not overtly retaining fluid (Borghi, BrJNutr, 1996; 76:325; Abergel, Hepatol, 1997; 26(Suppl):208A abstr.).

Circulating concentrations of albumin, transferrin, and RBP provide an estimate of visceral protein status, but these findings should be interpreted with caution in patients with liver disease, particularly if alcohol related. Plasma protein synthesis may be impaired in patients with liver disease *per se* irrespective of their nutritional status. In addition, alcohol directly inhibits protein synthesis (Rothschild, JCI, 1969; 48:344; Rothschild, Gastro, 1974; 67:1200); thus, in individuals actively abusing alcohol, circulating albumin and transferrin concentrations may be low but will return towards normal with abstinence from alcohol (Mills, AmJClinNutr, 1983; 38:849).

Total and T-lymphocyte counts and tests of delayed skin hypersensitivity are usually performed as part of the nutritional assessment, as an indirect measure of nutritional status. These data should also be interpreted with caution in individuals with liver disease, particularly if alcohol related. Lymphocyte counts are often significantly reduced in patients with cirrhosis with hypersplenism and are often low in individuals who are actively abusing alcohol although, in the latter, counts return quickly towards normal within days of alcohol withdrawal (Mills, AmJClinNutr, 1983; 38:849) (Fig. 5).

Deficiencies of specific nutrients such as vitamins and minerals may be detected using a variety of laboratory procedures. Again,

care must be taken in the interpretation of test results. Thus, many individuals who are abusing alcohol will show subnormal circulating concentrations of vitamins and minerals on admission to hospital, but levels may return towards normal following withdrawal from alcohol, without specific supplementation (Brown, AlcAlc, 1983; 18:157; Mills, AmJClinNutr, 1983; 38:849).

The technique of subjective global assessment in which data from the clinical history and physical examination are used to categorize patients' nutritional status, without recourse to a scoring system or any objective data, has been used with effect in general medical and surgical patients (Baker, NEJM, 1982; 306:969; Detskey, JPEN, 1987; 11:8).

Hasse and colleagues (Nutrition, 1993; 9:339) modified the subjective global assessment method for use in liver transplant candidates by highlighting clinical information of specific relevance in patients with chronic liver disease, such as variceal haemorrhage, fluid retention, and hepatic encephalopathy. Although this technique is reproducible, the assessments made are not valid when compared against anthropometric measures (Madden, JHepatol, 1997; 26(Suppl.1):267 abstr.).

Various modifications of the protein–calorie malnutrition score (Blackburn, JPEN, 1977; 1:11) have been used to assess nutritional status in patients with chronic liver disease (Mendenhall, AmJMed, 1984; 76:211; Abad, JClinNutrGastro, 1987; 2:63; Lautz, ClinInvest, 1992; 70:478). However, in this scoring system, anthropometric data are combined with variables such as the creatinine–height index, recall antigen testing, and circulating levels of visceral proteins which are of questionable value in the assessment of nutritional status in this patient population.

Similarly, the prognostic nutritional index which was devised to provide a global but objective assessment of nutritional status in surgical patients (Mullen, SurgForum,1979; 30:80; Buzby, AmJSurg, 1980; 139:160) is of no value for assessing nutritional status in patients with chronic liver disease (DiCecco, MayoClinProc, 1989; 64:95), as three of the four key index variables, namely serum albumin and transferrin concentrations and cutaneous hypersensitivity, are poor markers of nutritional status in this population.

A specific prognostic nutritional index has been devised for use in patients with chronic liver disease undergoing surgery in order to predict their risk of postoperative complications (Higashiguchi, JpnJSurg, 1995; 25:113). The key index variables are percentage ideal body weight, percentage weight change, percentage triceps skinfold thickness, and the International Normalized Ratio for prothrombin. Further evaluation of this potentially useful tool is warranted.

Thus, at present there is no general consensus on which technique(s) should be used to assess nutritional status in patients with chronic liver disease in the clinical setting. A reasonably reliable assessment can, however, be made by combining the data obtained from the clinical and diet histories, the physical examination, and the results of an anthropometric evaluation.

Research setting[57,58]

More accurate body composition data are required in a research setting: (i) to allow definition of the pattern of tissue loss in patients with chronic liver disease as this might provide insights into the disease process and might also affect the approach to nutritional therapy, its monitoring, and evaluation; (ii) metabolically active tissue compartments need to be accurately defined so that variables such as energy expenditure and protein synthesis can be correctly referenced; and (iii) 'bedside' techniques such as anthropometry need to be validated so that their use in the clinical setting can be optimized.

A number of so-called 'gold standard' techniques are available for measuring body compartments or subcompartments. These include: (i) densitometry, which provides a measure of body fat mass and is usually undertaken by underwater weighing; (ii) dual-energy X-ray absorptiometry (DEXA), which is used primarily to determine regional or whole-body mineral density and content, but which can also be used to determine regional or whole-body fat and fat-free soft tissue masses; (iii) total body potassium, measured by whole-body potassium-40 counting, which allows calculation of lean body mass; (iv) total body water, measured by isotope dilution, which also allows calculation of lean body mass; and (v) *in vivo* neutron activation analysis (IVNAA), which can be used to determine total body calcium, nitrogen, carbon, sodium, chloride, and phosphorus.

The majority of the body composition techniques currently employed, for example densitometry, water dilution, and total body potassium, are based on a two-component model (Keys, PhysiolRev, 1953; 33:245). In applying this model to body composition analysis a number of assumptions need to be made depending on the technique employed, *viz*: (i) the density of fat and fat-free mass, at 37°C, are 0.9 kg/l and 1.1 kg/l, respectively; (ii) the water content of fat-free mass remains constant at 72 to 74 per cent; (iii) the potassium content of lean tissue is constant at 60 mmol/l for women, and 66 mmol/kg for men; (iv) fat is anhydrous and potassium free; and (v) there is no variation in bone mineral density.

A number of theoretical difficulties arise when using the two-component model, which reflect uncertainties about the validity of these assumptions. Thus, it is possible that significant variation may occur in the hydration fraction and potassium content of fat-free mass, in both health and disease, which, if standard equations are employed in all instances, will result in under- or overestimates of body composition variables. In patients with fluid overload, for example, use of equations based on a two-component model would result in an overestimate of fat-free mass using water dilution, but an underestimate using densitometry or total body potassium.

In view of these difficulties, attempts have been made to combine the use of two or more techniques so that the components of the fat-free mass can be measured more directly and with greater certainty. These attempts resulted in the development of first three- and later four-component models of body composition (Heymsfield, AmJClinNutr,1990; 52:52).[59]

The three-component model of water, fat, and protein/mineral is based on measurements obtained from body densitometry and water dilution. This model overcomes some of the uncertainties over the hydration fraction of fat-free mass but it does assume a constant ratio of protein to mineral. The four-component model of water, fat, protein, and mineral incorporates direct measurement of total body mineral content using DEXA or total body calcium from IVNAA, as well as measurements of body density and water. This model removes the need for some of the assumptions inherent in two- and three-component models regarding the densities of the

different components of the fat-free mass and their relative proportions. However, the densities of fat and protein are assumed to be constant, as are both the density of total body mineral and the ratio of osseous to non-osseous mineral.

On theoretical grounds the use of three- and four-component models to assess body composition has clear advantages because the errors associated with variations in the proportions of water, protein, and mineral are less (Elia, ClinNutr, 1992; 11:114). In addition, analysis of the propagation of errors shows that the precision of the estimates is not compromised by the use of multiple techniques (Fuller, ClinSci, 1992; 82:687).

In practical terms the use of multicomponent models, and hence the use of several measurement techniques, increases the time and cost of assessments. Nevertheless, these models can be used as reference methods, particularly in disease states associated with altered hydration or bone density, and can be used to validate the individual component measurements and various of the 'bedside' techniques.

Very few specific attempts have been made to obtain information on body composition in patients with chronic liver disease using these 'gold standard' techniques, and where they have been used there are concerns that the methodological limitations have not been fully appreciated (McCullough, Hepatol, 1991; 14:1102; Bramley, BasicLifeSci, 1993; 60:211; Crawford, Gastro, 1994; 106:1611; Wicks, ClinNutr, 1995; 14:29).

Only two attempts have been made to assess body composition in patients with cirrhosis using modelling techniques. Oldroyd and colleagues (BasicLifeSci, 1993; 60:221) used DEXA to estimate total body lean tissue mass, total body fat mass, and total body bone mineral content, and potassium-40 to estimate body cell mass from total body potassium. A four-component model was then devised consisting of total body fat, extracellular water, extracellular solids, and body cell mass. This model was subsequently used to compare body composition variables in 54 healthy volunteers and 55 patients with cirrhosis, 23 (42 per cent) of whom had ascites. Mean body cell mass was reduced in the patients with cirrhosis independently of the presence of fluid retention. Extracellular water was significantly increased in patients with ascites while extracellular solids were increased selectively in male patients with cirrhosis and ascites.

These authors rightly caution against use of this model, however, because of doubts over the validity of measurements of total body potassium and, by extrapolation, the estimate of body cell mass.

Prijatmoko and colleagues (Gastro, 1993; 105:1839) used deuterium dilution to measure total body water (TBW), IVNAA to measure total body nitrogen (TBN), and DEXA to measure total body bone mineral (TBBM), body fat and fat-free mass. The data obtained were used to derive a multicomponent model which allowed calculation of fat-free mass (FFM) as the sum of the protein (TBP), intracellular and extracellular water (TBW), and mineral compartments (TBBM) from the equation:

$$\text{FFM} = (\text{TBN} \times 6.25) + (\text{TBW} - {}^2\text{H}) + (\text{TBBM} \times 1.235) + (\text{TBP} \times 0.044)$$

where TBP is TBN × 6.25.

This model was then used to assess body composition in 38 men with alcoholic cirrhosis, an unspecified proportion of whom had ascites, and in 16 age-matched male volunteers. The data obtained are confusingly reported and inadequately discussed. However, the

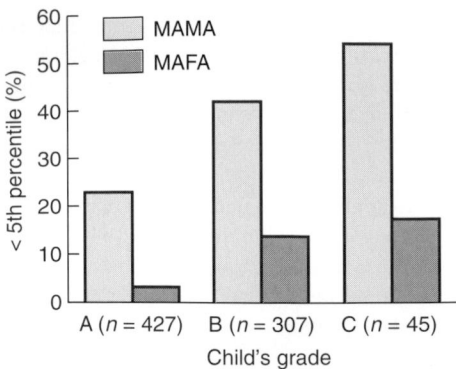

Fig. 6. Prevalence of depleted fat (MAFA) and muscle areas (MAMA) in male patients with cirrhosis by severity of liver disease (Italian Multicentre Co-operative Project, JHepatol, 1994; 21:317).

estimates of FFM derived using the multicomponent model were invariably higher than those obtained using anthropometry, BIA, and DEXA alone. Measurements of FFM made using anthropometry, BIA, and DEXA estimate both body water and body protein compartments and as total body water is increased in these patients, the body protein fraction of the FFM might be seriously underestimated. Thus, significant protein depletion may remain undetected if body composition is determined using these single techniques.

These findings serve to highlight the limitations of using 'bedside' or single techniques to assess body composition or nutritional status in this patient population and to reinforce the need to use multicomponent models.

Thus, in order to assess body composition accurately in patients with cirrhosis, a model is required which either takes into account, or else can be applied independently of changes in hydration and bone mineralization. A four-component model will enable measurements of fat, water, protein, and bone mineral to be made independently of these variables. The data are best compiled using DEXA to measure total body bone mineral, underwater weighing to determine body density, and deuterium dilution to determine total body water. Addition of a measure of extracellular water obtained, for example, by bromide dilution, would allow creation of a five-component model which would further refine the assessment process.

Prevalence of malnutrition

Despite the fact that it is now recognized that individuals with liver disease are at risk for developing malnutrition, surprisingly little information is available on the prevalence of nutritional deficiencies in this population. What data are available are of questionable value having been obtained either from very heterogeneous groups of patients or else by use of techniques inherently unsuitable for use in these individuals. The patient populations studied have, for example, varied from desocialized alcohol abusers (Leevy, AmJClinNutr, 1965; 16:339; Wood, JHumNutrDiet, 1992; 5:272) to liver transplant candidates (DiCecco, MayoClinProc, 1989; 64:95), while the assessment techniques used have been as diverse as measurement of circulating levels of individual vitamins (Leevy, 1965) to global methods using several objective variables (Higashiguchi, JpnJSurg,

1995; 25:113). It is not surprising, therefore, that the reported prevalence of malnutrition in patients with chronic liver disease varies from 10 to 100 per cent (McCullough, SemLivDis, 1991; 11: 265; Müller, JHepatol, 1995; 23(S1):31; Kalman, NutrRev, 1996; 54:217).

Some valuable information on the prevalence of malnutrition in patients with chronic liver disease can, however, be obtained from controlled studies where the assessment techniques used are considered to be reasonably valid in this patient population.

A number of studies in which nutritional status was assessed in patients with chronic liver disease using clinical criteria only meet these requirements (Patek, JAMA, 1948; 138:543; Morgan, Acta-ChirScandSuppl, 1981; 507:81; Abad, JClinNutrGastro, 1987; 2: 63; Hasse, TopClinNutr, 1992; 7:24; Nielsen, BrJNutr, 1993; 69: 665; Italian Multicentre Co-operative Project, JHepatol, 1994; 21: 317; Pikul, Transpl, 1994; 57:469; Ricci, Hepatol, 1997; 25:672), although in only one study was the methodology described in detail and its reproducibility examined (Hasse, 1992; Hasse, Nutrition, 1993; 9:339). Comparisons of studies are difficult, but overall between 21 and 88 per cent of patients assessed were categorized as adequately nourished and between 12 and 79 per cent as malnourished. Where categorization allowed, 19 to 59 per cent were classified as mildly malnourished, 21 to 43 per cent as moderately malnourished, and 10 to 26 per cent as severely malnourished.

Rather more studies have been undertaken in which nutritional status has been determined in patients with chronic liver disease using anthropometric variables (Morgan, ActaChirScandSuppl, 1981; 507:81; Simko, AmJClinNutr, 1982; 35:197; Mills, AmJClinNutr, 1983; 38:849; Mendenhall, AmJMed, 1984; 76:211; Jhangiani, AmJClinNutr, 1986; 44:323; Cabré, Gastro, 1990; 98:715; Dolz, Gastro, 1991; 100:738; Green, Hepatol, 1991; 14:464; Guglielmi, Hepatol, 1991; 13:892; Müller, AmJPhysiol, 1991; 260:E338; Wood, JHumNutrDiet, 1992; 5:275; Italian Multicentre Co-operative Project, JHepatol, 1994; 21:317; Madden, JHepatol, 1994; 21:878; Thuluvath, AmJClinNutr, 1994; 60:269; Wicks, ClinNutr, 1995; 14:29; Caregaro, AmJClinNutr, 1996; 63:602) (Table 4).

Comparisons of results between studies are extremely difficult, particularly as a number of different reference standards were used. However, overall, between 9 and 55 per cent of individuals showed significant reductions in TSF and between 9 and 50 per cent showed significant reductions in MAMC.

In general, the prevalence of malnutrition in patients with chronic liver disease, whether assessed clinically or anthropometrically, increases with increasing disease severity (Mendenhall, AmJMed, 1984; 76:211; Abad, JClinNutr, 1987; 2:63; Italian Multicentre Co-operative Project, JHepatol, 1994; 21:317; Wicks, ClinNutr, 1995; 14:29) (Fig. 6).

The changes in nutritional status in relation to disease aetiology are, however, less clear. Thus, while differences in the prevalence of malnutrition have been reported in some studies in relation to disease aetiology (Morgan, ActaChirScandSuppl, 1981; 507:8; Italian Multicentre Co-operative Project, JHepatol, 1994; 21:317; Thuluvath, AmJClinNutr, 1994; 60:269), no differences were reported in others (Caregaro, AmJClinNutr, 1996; 63:602). However, in only one of these studies (Italian Multicentre Co-operative Project, 1994) was account taken of the confounding effects of disease severity. Using stepwise regression analysis the Italian workers found no significant differences in the prevalence of malnutrition

Table 4 Anthropometric data from patients with liver disease included in the major studies available to date

First author	Date	Number (M:F)	Age (years)	Aetiology	Cirrhosis (%)	TSF (mm)	% Standard	MAMC (cm)	% Standard
Morgan	1981	43:12	48.8 ± 11.4	Alcohol	33	13.0 ± 5.0	—	23.0 ± 2.7	—
		1:19	57.7 ± 8.3	PBC	70	14.0 ± 5.0	—	20.4 ± 2.3	—
		4:13	45.5 ± 17.4	CAH	53	18.0 ± 7.0	—	22.5 ± 3.3	—
Simko	1982	57 M	49.9 ± 1.4	Alcohol	?	7.6 ± 0.6	10–25	24.0	5
Mills	1983	22:8	48.6	Alcohol	40	—	107	—	—
Mendenhall	1984	105	50.2 ± 0.5	Alcohol	41	8.1 ± 0.3	65	23.6 ± 0.3	93
Jhangiani	1986	8	47.5 ± 9.8	Alcohol	100	10.2 ± 6.7	—	24.8 ± 3.8	—
Cabré	1990	6:10	48.0 ± 3.0	Mixed	100	—	31	—	94
		9:10	53.0 ± 2.0		100	—	29	—	88
Dolz	1991	9 M	53.1 ± 9.9	Alcohol	100	8.4 ± 3.4	25–50	22.4 ± 2.5	<5
Green	1991	7 F	57.0 ± 12.0	PBC	?	9.9 ± 3.7	<5	21.8	25–50
Guglielmi	1991	36 M	55.0 ± 10.0	Mixed	100	11.0 ± 6.0	50	25.9 ± 3.4	10–25
Müller	1991	6 M	42.7 ± 4.5	Alcohol	100	8.1 ± 1.8	10–25	25.5 ± 2.8	10–25
		4 F	31.5 ± 5.1		100	6.0 ± 2.8	<5	18.9 ± 3.0	10
Wood	1992	34:5	39.0 ± 11.0	Alcohol	82	11.0	87	23.9	88
Italian MCP	1994	863 M	—	Mixed	100	11.6 ± 5.3	—	24.6 ± 3.1	—
		513 F	—		100	16.6 ± 7.1	—	23.3 ± 3.2	—
Madden	1994	40 M	51.7 ± 10.8	Mixed	100	11.2 ± 6.4	50–75	22.8 ± 2.9	<5
		20 F	47.8 ± 13.9		100	17.0 ± 9.2	10–25	21.0 ± 3.1	25–50
Thuluvath	1994	34 M	47.8 ± 10.8	Alcohol	?	16.7 ± 10.0	3%}	24.2 ± 3.3	44%}
		17 F	47.8 ± 10.8		?	16.9 ± 7.9	24%} <5th %ile	19.9 ± 1.5	18%} <5th %ile
		2:43	58.6 ± 9.5	Alcohol	?	17.1 ± 9.2	16%}	19.5 ± 2.4	18%}
Wicks	1995	3:5	49.6 ± 20.3	Cryptogenic	100	15.8 ± 5.7	25%}	20.7 ± 2.1	3%}
		34	55 (29–75)	PBC	100	11.9	47%} <5th %ile	24.6	38%} <5th %ile
Caregaro	1996	82 M	57.4 (29–75)	75% alcohol 26% viral	100	10.3 ± 6.5	94	24.1 ± 4.0	87
		38 F		42% alcohol 58% viral		16.9 ± 8.1	68	23.1 ± 3.2	103

Values expressed as mean (± 1SD, where available).
M:F, male:female; TSF, triceps skinfold; MAMC, mid-arm muscle circumference; PBC, primary biliary cirrhosis; CAH, chronic active hepatitis.

in relation to disease aetiology amongst men, but differences in prevalence were observed amongst women; thus, the greatest depletion of muscle stores was observed in women with hepatitis B-related liver injury, whilst the greatest depletion of fat stores was observed in those with alcohol-related disease.

Thus, the prevalence of malnutrition in patients with chronic liver disease varies from 10 to 80 per cent, depending on the severity and, to a degree, on the aetiology of the liver disease in the population under study.

Consequences of malnutrition

Patients with chronic liver disease who are moderately or severely malnourished tend to have higher serum bilirubin concentrations, lower serum albumin concentrations, and more prolonged prothrombin times than their adequately nourished counterparts. They are also more likely to have resistant ascites, to develop recurrent infections, and to have higher mortality rates (Mendenhall, AmJClinNutr, 1986; 43:213; Abad, JClinNutrGastro, 1987; 2:63; Lautz, ClinInvest, 1992; 70:478; Merli, Hepatol, 1996; 23:1041).

However, it is difficult to define the relationship between the presence of malnutrition and these outcome variables, and in particular to ascribe causality, because of the confounding effects of disease severity. Nevertheless, Merli and colleagues (Hepatol, 1996; 23:1041) attempted to do this in a multicentre study involving 1053 patients with cirrhosis followed for 5 years.

They found that the presence of moderate or severe malnutrition, assessed subjectively, and the presence of depleted fat and muscle stores, assessed anthropometry, were all associated with an increased risk of mortality. However, none of these nutritional variables was identified as an independent risk factor in multivariate analyses.

The Italian workers suggested that the presence of other factors, such as fluid retention and oesophageal varices, might obscure the importance of nutritional status as an outcome variable but they did not separately assess the relationship between the presence of malnutrition and the development of these features of hepatic decompensation.

There is very little information on the relationship between nutritional status and outcome following surgery in patients with chronic liver disease (Pitt, AmJSurg, 1981; 141:66; Garrison, AnnSurg, 1984; 199:648; Halliday, JPEN, 1988; 12:43),[60] although it would appear that malnourished patients are more likely to develop postoperative complications and are less likely to survive. However, the potential confounding effects of disease severity have not been examined.

Rather more information is available on the relationship between nutritional status and outcome following orthotopic liver transplantation in adults (Shaw, SemLivDis, 1985; 5:385; Pikul, Transpl, 1994; 57:469; Ricci, Hepatol, 1997; 25:672; Selberg, Hepatol, 1997; 25:652) and in children (Moukarzel, TransplProc, 1990; 22:1560; Shepherd, JPediatChildHlth, 1991; 27:295; Beath, Lancet, 1993; 307:825; Rodeck, Transpl, 1996; 62:1071). However, the methods used to assess nutritional status in two of the largest studies are somewhat questionable (Ricci, 1997; Selberg, 1997) and few if any controls have been exercised for confounding variables in the majority of the studies.

Nevertheless, it would appear that in both adults and in children, malnutrition is associated with prolonged ventilation, extended time in the intensive care unit and in hospital overall, a greater risk of postoperative complications, particularly infections, and a higher mortality rate.

Considerably more information is obviously needed on the relationship between nutritional status and outcome.

Nutritional therapy: general considerations[61–65]

Patients with liver disease are often given dietary advice of doubtful value, which may even prove harmful. High-calorie, low-protein diets are frequently prescribed for patients with uncomplicated hepatitis, but these diets may cause serious undernutrition with loss of lean body mass. Jaundiced patients are often advised to take low or fat-free diets even if they are fat tolerant; such diets are unpalatable, they often provide inadequate calories, and if continued for long periods, may lead to deficiencies of fat-soluble vitamins and essential fatty acids. Patients with liver disease are generally advised to abstain from alcohol irrespective of the aetiology of their liver damage; while this advice is essential for patients with alcohol-related liver injury, there is no contraindication to modest alcohol intake by others.

In general, patients with liver disease should take a diet which provides adequate intakes of calories, protein, vitamins, and minerals. However, it is likely that a diet which is adequate in healthy individuals may not be adequate in the presence of liver disease. For these reasons, dietary intake must be carefully monitored and adjusted to achieve positive nitrogen balance and correct deficiencies.

Many patients with chronic liver disease are anorexic or suffer from nausea or abdominal distension. Maintenance of an adequate oral intake may prove difficult under these circumstances. Patients should be encouraged to eat, and also to modify their eating pattern in order to take four to seven small meals throughout the day, including a late-night snack, as this regimen is better tolerated and improves nitrogen balance and substrate utilization (Swart, BMJ, 1989; 299:1202; Verboeket-van de Venne, Gut, 1995; 36:110). If a reasonable dietary intake can be achieved and body weight maintained, nothing further is required; periodic reassessment is recommended.

It is often difficult, however, to sustain an oral intake in patients with persistent anorexia and nausea, or to increase oral intake beyond a certain limit in malnourished patients. Under these circumstances, proprietary supplemental drinks can be used as a palatable adjunct to feeding, optimally taken between meals. Nutritionally complete, milk-based supplements include standard formulae providing 1 kcal/ml (e.g. Ensure [Abbott], Fresubin [Fresenius]) and more concentrated formulae providing 1.5 to 1.8 kcal/ml (e.g. Ensure Plus [Abbott], Entera [Fresenius], Fortisip [Nutricia Clinical], Resource [Sandoz]). Fruit juice-based supplements providing 1.25 kcal/ml are also available (e.g. Enlive [Abbott], Fortijuice [Nutricia Clinical]), which although nutritionally incomplete may prove more palatable and, hence, more acceptable to some patients. There is, at present, no compelling evidence that supplements enriched with branched-chain amino acids confer additional benefit.

Where individual requirements and tastes dictate, additional supplements may be prepared using separate proprietary modular components; carbohydrate can be supplied as glucose polymers (e.g. Maxijul [Scientific Hospital Supplies (SHS)], Polycal [Nutricia Clinical]), nitrogen as whey protein isolate (e.g. Maxipro Super Soluble [SHS]), and fat as emulsions of either long-chain fatty acids (e.g. Calogen [SHS]) or medium-chain fatty acids (e.g. Liquigen [SHS]). These supplements can be tailor-made to patients' requirements, particularly with regard to electrolyte and volume restraints; addition of vitamins, minerals, and trace elements will be necessary if these feeds are to provide the sole or major nutrient supply.

If oral intake remains inadequate despite supplementation, then enteral feeding via a fine-bore nasogastric tube should be instituted at the earliest opportunity; the presence of oesophageal varices is not a contraindication to the use of these tubes although they should be used with caution in the presence of oesophageal ulceration after injection sclerotherapy (Keohane, JPEN, 1983; 7:345). If the enteral feed is given at night, the patient can be encouraged to eat during the day.

If abdominal distension and vomiting continue, the nasogastric tube can be endoscopically repositioned in the jejunum. Standard, proprietary feeds providing 1 kcal/ml (e.g. Jevity [Abbott], Nutrison Standard [Nutricia Clinical]) are suitable for use in the majority of patients, but the volume of feed required to supply daily requirements may be excessive in those who are fluid overloaded. Under these circumstances a more concentrated feed providing 1.5 kcal/ml (e.g. Ensure Plus [Abbott], Nutrison Energy Plus [Nutricia Clinical]) or 2.0 kcal/ml (e.g. Nepro [Abbott], TwoCal HN [Abbott]) can be used, the choice being determined by the amount of protein required. The rate of feed administration and osmolarity can be manipulated to optimize tolerance.

Every attempt should be made to feed these patients either orally or enterally; the use of parenteral feeding should be avoided if at all possible. Dietary requirements for certain nutrients differ when given parenterally. More than 90 per cent of ingested carbohydrates, fats, sodium, potassium, and chloride are absorbed, so that recommended daily allowances apply whether nutrients are given enterally or parenterally. Other nutrients, in particular the essential minerals, are much less well absorbed, so that parenteral requirements are substantially less than enteral requirements. It is also likely that enteral and parenteral requirements for certain amino acids will differ. The timing of parenteral supply is also important. For example, if protein synthesis is to be supported, all the essential amino acids must be supplied simultaneously; if even one essential amino acid is administered at a different time to the others, protein assimilation is curtailed. Similarly, if amino acid, lipids, glucose, and minerals are infused at different times, assimilation of several nutrients may be impaired. For these reasons the parenteral requirements of many essential nutrients remain uncertain.

Several additional problems arise when providing parenteral nutrition in individuals with liver disease. They may be fluid intolerant so that the volume infused may need to be restricted to 1 litre or less. It may also be necessary to modify the amino-acid solutions used. Cysteine and tyrosine are synthesized in the liver from methionine and phenylalanine, and so under normal circumstances are non-essential. These amino acids are virtually insoluble in water and their concentrations in commercially available amino-acid mixtures are extremely low. In patients with cirrhosis, synthesis of cysteine and tyrosine may be impaired and deficiencies may arise during parenteral feeding (Rudman, Gastro, 1981; 81: 1025; Millikan, AnnSurg, 1983; 197:294; Chawla, Gastro, 1984; 87:770). Under these circumstances these amino acids become conditionally 'essential' and, without them, protein synthesis may become seriously impeded. Similar remarks can be made about choline (Chawla, Gastro, 1989; 97:1514; Buchman, Hepatol, 1995; 22:1399; Shronts, JAmDietAssoc, 1997; 97:639) and carnitine (Shapira, NutrInt, 1986; 2:334). In addition, many of the formulations used in patients with liver disease are nutritionally incomplete or else contain quantities of amino acids, such as glycine, proline, lysine, threonine, and arginine, which may not be adequately cleared when the liver's ureagenic capacity is limited (Vilstrup, EurJClinInv, 1982; 12:197).

For many years the presence of liver disease was considered as a contraindication to the use of intravenous lipid solutions, even by the manufacturers (Hallberg, PostgradMedJ, 1967; 43:307). Very little explanation was available other than that use of these preparations might lead to the accumulation of 'fat pigment' in liver cells, and early experiences with cotton-seed emulsions called for caution in their use in patients with hepatic dysfunction. Even so, several early reports showed that lipid solutions could be used safely in these patients (Kern, Metabolism, 1957; 6:743; Schuberth, BiblioNutrDiet, 1963; 5:387), and this has been confirmed more recently (Rössner, AmJClinNutr, 1979; 32:2022; Muscaritoli, JPEN, 1986; 10:599; Forbes, Gut, 1987; 28:A1347 abstr.; Nagayama, JSurgRes, 1989; 47:59; Fan, JPEN, 1992; 16:279; Druml, AmJClinNutr, 1995; 61:812); long-chain and medium-chain triglycerides are equally well tolerated (Druml, 1995). Thus, if patients with liver disease require parenteral nutrition, there is no contraindication to providing energy as glucose and fat, the latter constituting 35 to 50 per cent of the non-protein calories, and nitrogen as conventional amino acid solutions.

Several drugs prescribed for patients with liver disease cause malabsorption, impaired utilization, or urinary hyperexcretion of nutrients. Use of neomycin and cholestyramine may lead to malabsorption of several nutrients including fats, vitamins, and minerals. D-Penicillamine impairs the utilization of pyridoxine and increases the urinary excretion of zinc, pyridoxine, and copper. Diuretics increase the urinary excretion of several minerals. Careful note must, therefore, be made of all drugs prescribed for these patients.

Subclinical vitamin deficiencies may occur in patients with liver disease, more especially in individuals abusing alcohol. These are difficult to identify and their measurement often complex and expensive. Multivitamin therapy is cheap and is assumed to be harmless if recommended doses are not exceeded. Thus, the common practice of giving vitamin supplements to these patients has a reasonable therapeutic basis. If deficiencies are clinically overt, more specific therapy is required in higher dosage.

Nutritional management of individual disorders

Viral or drug-related hepatitis

Patients with few symptoms should be encouraged to eat normally. Even patients with anorexia, nausea, and vomiting can usually take some food by mouth and enough fluid to prevent dehydration. Patients tend to prefer small meals and these should be given frequently throughout the day. During the acute illness, requirements for protein and energy are similar to those of any moderately hypercatabolic illness; daily energy requirements increase to 2000 to 3000 kcal (8 to 12 MJ) and protein requirements to 100 to 120 g. Although early studies suggested that high-protein, high-calorie diets might benefit patients with hepatitis (Hoagland, AmJPublHlth, 1946; 36:1287; Chalmers, JCI, 1955; 34:1163), such diets should not be forced. Fat should not be restricted; low-fat diets are bulky, generally unappetizing, and may aggravate anorexia. If anorexia and vomiting persist, it may be necessary to institute enteral feeding. As patients with severe hepatitis may not be able to excrete a water load, very careful monitoring of fluid balance is necessary.

Patients with hepatitis are usually advised to abstain from alcohol during the acute illness and for 6 months afterwards. There is no good evidence, however, that alcohol in moderation has a deleterious effect on the liver either during the acute illness or during convalescence. Nevertheless, excessive amounts of alcohol are hepatotoxic in their own right and relapse of hepatitis following alcohol abuse has been reported (Damodaran, BMJ, 1944; ii:587).

Fulminant hepatic failure

Patients with fulminant hepatic failure may develop profound, recurrent hypoglycaemia because their glycogen stores are reduced and glycogenolysis and gluconeogenesis are impaired. They may also become rapidly malnourished because of the marked loss of nitrogen which occurs secondary to the endocrine response to massive hepatic necrosis. Additional nitrogen losses occur when artificial liver support systems, such as charcoal haemoperfusion or polyacrylonitrile membrane haemodialysis, are employed (Chase, Gastro, 1978; 75:1033).

These patients therefore need a constant supply of glucose that should be given intravenously as 10 to 20 per cent glucose solutions in a volume sufficient to provide 150 to 200 g over 24 h. They should, in addition, receive nutritional support designed to suppress protein catabolism, increase anabolism, and so optimize the conditions for hepatic regeneration. O'Keefe and colleagues (ActaChirScandSuppl, 1981; 507:91) showed that amino acid/glucose solutions infused intravenously to provide 3 g of amino acid and 5 g of glucose hourly were well-tolerated by these patients and their use was associated with decreased protein catabolism, improved plasma amino-acid profiles, and increased circulating insulin concentrations. Forbes and coworkers (Gut, 1987; 28:A1347 abstr.) have shown that lipid solutions can be safely incorporated into parenteral nutritional support regimens for these patients.

No formal trials of the use of parenteral nutrition in patients with fulminant hepatic failure have been published to date.

Acute alcoholic hepatitis[66]

Patients with acute alcoholic hepatitis have generally abused alcohol for many years and may have severely neglected their diet in the weeks or months before admission. Quite marked deterioration may occur in their clinical status after they have been admitted to hospital and this is generally attributed to loss of the calorie intake from alcohol (Hardison, NEJM, 1966; 275:61; Helman, AnnIntMed, 1971; 74:311; Lischner, AmJDigDis, 1971; 16:481; Sabesin, Gastro, 1978; 74:276; Marshall, Alcoholism, 1983; 7:312). These patients are frequently malnourished and this has a detrimental effect on outcome (Mendenhall, AlcoholClinExpRes, 1995; 19:635; Merli, Hepatol, 1996; 23:1041).

Very little information is available on the precise nutritional requirements of patients with alcoholic hepatitis. In one of the few studies available (Weber, DigDisSci, 1982; 27:103), seven patients with acute alcoholic hepatitis were investigated under metabolic ward conditions. Nitrogen balance became positive in three of five patients receiving 1 g of protein/kg per day and remained positive in the other two. The two remaining patients received 0.5 g of protein/kg per day and attained positive nitrogen balance within 2 weeks. The improvements in nitrogen balance reflected a reduction in urinary nitrogen excretion or more specifically in urinary urea nitrogen excretion. Thus, in patients with alcoholic hepatitis, daily protein intakes of 30 g are associated with negative nitrogen balance while intakes in the region of 70 to 100 g ensure positive nitrogen balance. It is also likely that daily energy requirements are increased in individuals chronically abusing alcohol (Levine, Hepatol, 1994; 20:318A abstr.).

There is, therefore, a clear rationale for the provision of nutritional support in this population. However, although a number of controlled trials of the efficacy and safety of nutritional supplementation have been undertaken in these patients, it is still unclear whether it influences the course of the disease.

A small number of studies have been undertaken in which nutritional supplements have been provided for patients with alcoholic hepatitis via oral or enteral routes (Calvey, Hepatol, 1985; 1:141; Mendenhall, JPEN, 1985; 9:950; Soberon, Hepatol, 1987; 7:1204; Keans, Gastro, 1992; 102:200).

Mendenhall and colleagues (JPEN, 1985; 9:590) assessed the effects of nutritional support on outcome in 57 patients with moderate to severe alcoholic hepatitis. Thirty-four patients received a routine hospital diet which provided 2500 kcal daily with the protein and sodium intakes adjusted to suit individual needs; the remaining 23 patients received a minimum of 1000 kcal daily as hospital food,

together with an enteral supplement, enriched with branched-chain amino acids, to provide an additional 2200 kcal daily; both groups were monitored for 30 days. Five (22 per cent) of the 23 patients given the nutritional supplement withdrew from treatment largely because of problems encountered with the enteral feed.

At the end of the trial period the patients who were enterally supplemented showed improvements in six of the nine variables used to assess nutritional status, whereas these variables remained unchanged or else deteriorated in the unsupplemented patients; mortality rates were, however, similar in both supplemented (17 per cent) and unsupplemented groups (21 per cent).

The two dietary regimens used in this study were neither isocaloric nor isonitrogenous. Thus, it is impossible to draw any conclusions from this study about the benefits of enteral supplementation over provision of a diet, adequate in calories and protein, consumed at will.

Calvey and co-workers (JHepatol, 1985; 1:141) undertook a detailed study of nutritional support in 64 patients with severe alcoholic hepatitis with or without cirrhosis. All patients were provided with a basic diet containing 40 to 80 g of protein, 1800 to 2400 kcal, and 20 mmol of sodium daily; 21 patients received an additional 10 g of nitrogen daily as 65 g of conventional protein, together with 2000 non-protein kcal; a further 21 patients received an additional 10 g of nitrogen daily as 45 g of protein and 25 g of branched-chain amino acids, together with 2000 non-protein kcal. The supplements were given orally, enterally, or, if necessary, parenterally, for approximately 3 weeks. Nitrogen balance studies were undertaken in the 49 patients with adequate renal function.

At the end of the trial period there was no significant difference in mortality rates between the control (32 per cent) and supplemented groups (38 per cent). Positive nitrogen balance was associated with daily nitrogen intakes of 10 g or more and was achieved by 53 per cent of control and 60 per cent of supplemented patients; overall, the mortality rate was 3.3 per cent in the patients who achieved positive nitrogen balance but 57.9 per cent in the patients who did not. No benefit was observed, in this respect, from supplementation, nor was there evidence of additional benefit in the subgroup receiving the supplements intravenously. These findings confirm those of Fiaccadori and colleagues (ItalJGastr, 1993; 25:336) that mortality rates are significantly increased in patients with chronic liver disease who are unable to maintain nitrogen equilibrium.

Soberon and associates (Hepatol, 1987; 7:1204) monitored metabolic balance over a 3-day period in 14 patients with moderately severe alcoholic hepatitis while they consumed a hospital tray diet designed to provide 35 kcal and 1.25 g of protein/kg ideal body weight, daily. The mean digestibilities (intake − faecal loss/intake) of energy and fat were subnormal in at least two-thirds of the group overall, whilst nitrogen balance was negative in at least half.

Six patients consumed 75 per cent or more of their calculated energy and protein requirements (group I); these individuals were continued on the hospital tray diet for a further 3 days and remained stable. Eight patients consumed less than 75 per cent of their calculated energy and protein requirements (group II); these individuals were fed enterally for 3 days with a formula feed which provided 35 kcal/kg ideal body weight daily, and as a result showed significant increases in the mean digestibilities of energy, protein, and fat and a fivefold increase in nitrogen balance. However, the improved digestibility and nitrogen balance figures observed in

Table 5 Randomized, controlled trials of parenteral nutrition in patients with alcoholic hepatitis

First author and date	Patients (n)	Trial period (days)	Control regimen (daily)	Test regimen (daily)	Short-term mortality	(%)	Other findings in trial group
Nasrallah 1980	35	25	Standard diet: 3000 kcal 100 g protein	Standard diet + IV 70–85 g a.a.	Control Trial *P<0.06	4/18 (22) 0/17 (0)*	Bilirubin ↓
Diehl 1985	15	30	Standard diet: 3000 kcal 98–139 g protein + IV 130 g glucose	Standard diet + IV 52 g a.a. and 130 g glucose	Control Trial	0/10 (0) 0/5 (0)	N$_2$ balance ↑
Naveau 1986	40	28	Standard diet: 2800 kcal 80 g protein	Standard diet + IV 90 g a.a and 2800 kcal as glucose/lipid	Control Trial	1/20 (5) 1/20 (5)	Bilirubin ↓
Achord 1987	28	21	Standard diet: 2800 kcal 100 g protein	Standard diet + IV 43 g a.a. and 200 g glucose	Control Trial	3/14 (21) 1/14 (7)	Bilirubin ↓ GEC ↑
Simon 1988	12 moderate 22 severe	28	Standard diet plus liquid feed: 3200 kcal 132 g protein	Standard diet plus liquid feed + IV 70 g a.a., 100 g glucose, 50 g lipid	Moderate Severe Control Trial	0 3/12 (25) 4/10 (40)	Albumin ↑ Transferrin ↑
Bonkovsky 1991	21	21	Standard diet: 2100 kcal 70 g protein	Standard diet + IV 70 g a.a. and 100 g glucose	Control Trial	0/12 (0) 0/9 (0)	—
Mezey 1991	54	30	Standard diet + IV 130 g glucose	Standard diet + IV 52 g a.a. and 130 g glucose	Control Trial 2-year mortality Control Trial	5/26 (19) 6/28 (21) (38) (42)	N$_2$ balance ↑ Aminopyrine clearance ↑ Bilirubin ↓ PT ↓

a.a., amino acids; GEC, galactose elimination capacity; IV, intravenous; N$_2$, nitrogen; PT, prothrombin time.

group II following enteral supplementation did not differ significantly from those observed in group I. Thus, while enteral feeding undoubtedly benefits patients with alcoholic hepatitis who are anorexic and in whom dietary intake is inadequate, it cannot be concluded, from this study, that enteral feeding would confer benefit in patients already consuming an adequate diet.

Finally, Keans and co-workers (Gastro, 1992; 102:200) randomized 31 patients with probable alcoholic hepatitis, with or without cirrhosis, to receive, over a 28-day period, either a standard hospital diet or else the same diet supplemented with a casein-based, enteral feed which provided an additional 40 kcal and 1.5 g of protein/kg ideal body weight daily; three patients in each group dropped out of the study.

During the trial period, patients in the supplemented group showed more rapid improvement in their encephalopathy, a significant fall in their mean serum bilirubin level, and a significant increase in their mean antipyrine clearance. The mortality rates in the supplemented (13 per cent) and unsupplemented (27 per cent) groups were not, however, significantly different.

This study has been criticized because the mean energy intake in the unsupplemented group met only 80 per cent of predicted requirements, whereas the mean energy intake in the supplemented group exceeded predicted requirements by 70 per cent; likewise, the mean daily protein intakes in the unsupplemented and supplemented groups were widely divergent, namely 50 and 103 g. Although the limitations of energy and protein intakes in the unsupplemented group were self-imposed, conclusions are, nevertheless, difficult to draw.

Several observations can be made based on the findings of these studies: (i) dietary intake is often suboptimal in patients with alcoholic hepatitis, even if they are provided with diets sufficient to meet their needs; (ii) enteral feeding can be used to improve nutrient intake in individuals who are consuming suboptimal diets and its use is associated with improvement in several nutritional variables; and (iii) outcome is determined by the patients ability, once adequately fed, to attain positive nitrogen balance.

A number of studies have also been undertaken in which nutritional supplementation has been provided for patients with alcoholic hepatitis via the parenteral route (Nasrallah, Lancet, 1980; ii:1276; Diehl, Hepatol, 1985; 5:57; Naveau, Hepatol, 1986; 6:270; Achord, AmJGastr, 1987; 82:871; Simon, JHepatol, 1988; 7:200; Bonkovsky, AmJGastr, 1991; 86:1200; Bonkovsky, AmJGastr, 1991; 86:1209; Mezey, Hepatol, 1991; 14:1090) (Table 5).

Overall, the number of treated patients is small. The majority of patients appear to have had mild to moderate alcoholic hepatitis as evidenced by the mortality rates in the control populations which ranged from 0 to 22 per cent. Histological confirmation of the diagnosis was obtained in 0 to 100 per cent of patients in the various studies; biopsies showed that between 0 and 100 per cent of the individuals had established cirrhosis. Inclusion and exclusion criteria varied between studies. All subjects were given a well-balanced hospital diet which provided at least 30 kcal and 1 g of protein/kg body weight daily, and received oral vitamin and mineral supplements. The experimental groups received, in addition, a parenteral infusion of a standard amino-acid solution with or without additional glucose and lipid. In two of the studies the control group received an intravenous infusion of glucose in addition to the standard diet (Diehl, Hepatol, 1985; 5:57; Mezey, Hepatol, 1991; 14:1090), while in a third study the control population received additional enteral supplements (Simon, JHepatol, 1988; 7:200). Nutritional support was provided for between 21 and 30 days. A wide range of variables was used to assess both liver function and nutritional status between studies; in all seven studies, however, the endpoint was death (Table 5).

The results of these studies are extremely difficult to interpret because it is often unclear what comparisons workers were trying to make. In several, the comparison made was ostensibly of the effects on outcome of a nutritionally adequate diet against a regimen providing excess protein and energy. However, in the majority of these studies, voluntary food intake was appreciably less than the amount offered and less than the amount required to satisfy nutritional requirements. In consequence, the comparisons made were effectively between regimens which were either nutritionally adequate or inadequate.

Because of the difficulties inherent in the interpretation of these data, conclusions cannot be drawn. However, a number of observations can be made: (i) voluntary food intake is likely to be poor in patients with moderate to severe alcoholic hepatitis, with the result that they may not be able to attain optimal nutrient intake unaided; (ii) provision of adequate energy and protein intakes will result in improvement in nutritional status and liver function even in patients who are severely ill, but has little effect on short-term mortality; and (iii) no appreciable adverse events are associated with the provision of high-energy, high-protein nutritional supplements—these regimens are well tolerated by even the most severely ill patients without exacerbation of fluid retention, azotaemia, or hepatic encephalopathy.

Thus, it would seem essential to ensure that all patients with alcoholic hepatitis are adequately nourished. They should receive a minimum of 1.2 to 1.5 g of protein/kg body weight daily and this should be given, whenever possible, by the oral or enteral route; if difficulties are encountered in meeting requirements, then a proportion of the required intake can be given parenterally, preferably via a peripheral vein.

Cholestasis

The severity of the nutritional disturbances associated with acute cholestasis depends on the degree of biliary obstruction and its reversibility. Steatorrhoea may occur but is rarely gross, as large amounts of fat can be absorbed from the intestine even when luminal concentrations of bile salts are low and the micellar phase reduced; severe reduction in micelle formation will, however, affect the absorption of fat-soluble vitamins. When the obstruction is easily remediable, there is little indication for specific dietary advice. Parenteral vitamin K_1 in a dose of 10 mg daily should be given for 3 days preoperatively, and dehydration and other obvious metabolic disturbances should be corrected as far as possible.

In patients with chronic cholestasis, as a result of primary or secondary biliary cirrhosis, sclerosing cholangitis, or biliary atresia, specific dietary advice is needed. If patients are fat intolerant, dietary fat should be reduced to tolerance levels and carbohydrate intake increased to balance the calorie loss. However, fat intake should not be restricted too rigorously as this will reduce the palatability of the diet. Medium-chain triglycerides may be given, preferably in the form of an emulsion (e.g. Liquigen [SHS]) which can be made into milk shakes. Circulating concentrations of vitamin A and D and the prothrombin time should be monitored in these patients and supplements provided as indicated. Replacement therapy may be given orally or intramuscularly depending on the degree of fat malabsorption, the severity of the depletion, and the response to treatment (Table 6). If vitamin status can not be assessed directly, then replacement should be provided on an empirical basis in jaundiced patients. Children with chronic cholestasis may develop vitamin E deficiency; this can be treated with oral α-tocopherol acetate in a daily dose of 68 to 272 mg (50 to 200 IU)/kg or TPGS vitamin E in a daily dose of 25 IU/kg; if oral supplementation is ineffective, DL-α-tocopherol may be given parenterally in a dose of 1 to 2 mg (1 to 2 IU)/kg daily, initially, and then at intervals determined by plasma concentrations.

Calcium supplements may be required by both children and adults. There is some evidence that calcium provided in the form of hydroxyapatite might be more beneficial than calcium provided as a simple salt (Epstein, AmJClinNutr, 1982; 36:426). Medium-chain triglycerides promote calcium uptake.

A sample high-protein, high-energy, low-fat diet to which medium-chain triglycerides can be added, and which would be suitable for patients with chronic cholestasis and steatorrhoea, is appended.

Chronic liver disease

Protein requirements are increased in patients with chronic liver disease; daily intakes of approximately 1.2 g/kg are required to maintain nitrogen equilibrium (Swart, ClinNutr, 1989; 8:329; Nielsen, BrJNutr, 1993; 69:665; Nielsen, BrJNutr, 1995; 74:557; Kondrup, BrJNutr, 1997; 77:197). Energy expenditure is also increased in a percentage of patients with decompensated disease (Shanbhogue, JPEN, 1987; 11:305; Schneeweiss, Hepatol, 1990; 11:387; Müller, Hepatol, 1992; 15:782). These patients are frequently malnourished (Mendenhall, AmJClinNutr, 1986; 43:213; Lautz, ClinInvest, 1992; 70:478; Italian Multicentre Co-operative Project, JHepatol, 1994; 21:317) and require nutritional support. However, the effects of nutritional support on outcome are not well documented.

To date, a total of 16 controlled studies have been undertaken which provide data on the efficacy and safety of oral or enteral nutritional supplementation in patients with cirrhosis (Table 7). Eight studies were specifically designed to address these questions (Bory, GastroHepato, 1982; 5:371; Watanabe, ActaMedOkayama, 1983; 37:321; Christie, JPEN, 1985; 9:671; Okita, JNutrSciVitaminol, 1985; 31:291; Rocchi, JPEN, 1985; 9:447; Bunout,

Table 6 Dose schedule for replacement of fat-soluble vitamins in patients with chronic cholestasis		
Vitamin	**Route of administration**	
	Oral	Intramuscular
A	7.5 mg (25 000 IU) daily	30 mg (100 000 IU) 3-monthly
D	10 to 100 μg (400 to 4000 IU) daily	2.5 mg (100 000 IU) monthly
K	10 mg daily	10 mg monthly

EurJClinNutr, 1989; 43:615; Cabré, Gastro, 1990; 98:715; Hirsch, JPEN, 1993; 17:119); the remaining eight trials were designed to assess the efficacy and safety of these supplements in patients with chronic hepatic encephalopathy, but also provide some nutritional data (Marchesini, Hepatol, 1982; 2:420; McGhee, AnnSurg, 1983; 197:288; Simko, NutrRepInt, 1983; 27:765; Egberts, Gastro, 1985; 88:887; Keans, Gastro, 1992; 102:200; Plauth, JHepatol, 1993; 17: 308; Guarnieri, p.193 in[68]).[67] All of the patients studied had cirrhosis, the majority having alcohol-related disease (Table 7). Many of the patients were protein depleted, but the exact numbers in any given study are poorly documented. In seven studies the patient numbers exceeded 30, but in the remainder the numbers were generally much smaller. In only five studies were patients treated beyond 30 days. In all studies patients received either a control or an experimental regimen in a randomized manner, except in the study undertaken by Okita and colleagues (1985) in which patients served as their own controls and received both the control and experimental regimens in set order. Seven studies included a cross-over phase in their design.

In six studies the control and experimental regimens were isonitrogenous, if not isocaloric, whereas in the remaining ten studies the experimental regimen invariably provided more energy and protein than the control regimen (Table 7). A proportion of the nitrogen in all but two of the experimental regimens was provided in the form of branched-chain amino acids.

The results of these studies are difficult to interpret because: (i) the variation in population size, trial duration, trial regimens, and control regimens make comparisons difficult, if not impossible; and (ii) outcome variables are poorly defined. In the majority of studies the main outcome variable is morbidity, usually in relation to some aspect of the nutritional assessment. However, in some studies the effects on morbidity are assessed in relation to dietary regimens which are clearly incomparable in their provision of energy and protein; in others, morbidity is assessed in relation to regimens which are comparable in their provision of energy and nitrogen, at least in theory, but in which the nitrogen sources differ. In a minority of studies, mortality is the main outcome variable. Finally, outcomes are not stratified by the nutritional status of the patient.

A number of conclusions can, however, be drawn: (i) patients with cirrhosis will tolerate high-protein, high-calorie diets without undue exacerbation of hepatic encephalopathy, azotaemia, or fluid retention; (ii) high-protein, high-calorie intakes are associated with improvements in nitrogen balance and 'nutritional indices' in the majority of patients with cirrhosis; (iii) improvements in nutritional status can be achieved in patients with stable cirrhosis, whatever the nitrogen source, provided that the amount given exceeds 10 g

daily ($\equiv$ 60 g of protein); and (iv) provision of adequate nutritional support *per se* does not significantly improve survival rates.

In 1997, the European Society for Parenteral and Enteral Nutrition (**ESPEN**) Consensus Group provided clear nutritional guidelines for the management of patients with chronic liver disease (Table 8).[65] In patients with clinically stable cirrhosis an intake of 1.3 times the resting energy expenditure or 25 to 30 kcal/kg of non-protein energy plus 1.0 to 1.2 g/kg of protein daily is recommended. Patients who are decompensated, malnourished, or otherwise compromised should take 35 to 40 kcal/kg of non-protein energy plus 1.5 g/kg of protein daily. It was further recommended that nutrients should be taken in small amounts frequently throughout the day, so that fasting periods should not exceed 6 h, and that whenever possible the oral or enteral route should be used.

Transplant candidates and recipients[69]

Malnutrition is uncommon in individuals transplanted for fulminant hepatic failure; these individuals must, however, be nutritionally supported prior to surgery to optimize outcome. A constant supply of glucose is needed to counter hypoglycaemia and this should be given intravenously as 10 to 20 per cent glucose solutions in a volume sufficient to provide 150 to 200 g over 24 h. A further 25 to 30 non-protein kcal/kg per day should be provided, preferably via the enteral route, together with approximately 1.2 g of protein/kg per day.

Malnutrition is frequently observed in transplant candidates with chronic liver disease (Hehir, JPEN, 1985; 9:695; DiCecco, MayoClinProc, 1989; 64:95; Chin, AmJClinNutr, 1992; 56:164; Hasse, TopClinNutr, 1992; 7:24; Lautz, ClinInvest, 1992; 70:478; Akerman, Nutrition, 1993; 9:350). Malnutrition is not a contraindication to transplantation *per se*, but it negatively affects outcome (Shaw, SemLivDis, 1985; 5:385; Moukarzel, TransplProc, 1990; 22:1560; Pikul, Transpl, 1994; 57:469; Rodeck, Transpl, 1996; 62:1071; Ricci, Hepatol, 1997; 25:672).

Very little information is available on the efficacy of nutritional support in patients with chronic liver disease awaiting transplantation; however, it is important that nutritional support is provided at this time as this may have an effect on outcome (DiCecco, Hepatol, 1997; 26(Suppl): 500A abstr.). Non-protein energy intakes of 35 to 40 kcal/kg per day and protein intakes of 1.2 to 1.5 g/kg per day would be appropriate. Nutrients should be provided by the oral or enteral route, preferably as four to seven small meals throughout the day; periods of 6 h or more without food should be avoided. Home enteral feeding is well tolerated if patients are encouraged and if they are made to understand the

Table 7 Controlled trials of 'nutritional therapy' in patients with chronic liver disease

First author and date	Patients (n)	Aetiology of cirrhosis	Trial duration (days)	Trial regimen (daily)	Alternative regimen (daily)	Outcome
Swart 1981	8	Chronic active hepatitis 50%	30; alternating 5-day regimens	Diet containing BCAA-rich protein (35% BCAA) 40, 60, 80 g at 10-day intervals	Diet containing mixed protein (20% BCAA) 40, 60, 80 g at 10-day intervals	Nitrogen balance positive on intakes of 60 and 80 g. Minimal protein requirements averaged 48 g/day on both regimens
Bory 1982	74	Alcoholic 63%	15	BCAA-enriched enteral feed	Standard hospital diet	24-h creatinine excretion, 'nutritional indices', serum albumin, and prothrombin time improved on enteral feed
McGhee 1983	4	Mixed	11 on each regimen	30 g Hepatic-Aid* 20 g casein + 260 g carbohydrate 80 g fat } 2000 kcal	50 g casein + 260 g carbohydrate 80 g fat } 2000 kcal	Nitrogen balance maintained on each regimen
Simko 1983	15	Alcoholic	90	Usual diet + 20–60 g Hepatic-Aid*	Usual diet + placebo powder	4 BCAA and 1 placebo patients dropped out. Calorie intake, fat stores, and serum transferrin concentrations increased significantly on BCAA
Watanabe 1983	2	Mixed	? 14 on each regimen	1600 kcal 40 g protein + 600 kcal 37 g protein } as BCAA supplement	2072 kcal 74 g protein	Nitrogen balance positive on BCAA
Guanieri 1984	8	Mixed	100–120	Calorie-reduced basal diet + 20 g Hepatic-Aid* Carbohydrate Fat } 1120 kcal	Calorie-reduced basal diet + Carbohydrate Fat } 1120 kcal	Fat stores, Plasma proteins, Cr/Ht index, Nitrogen balance, Muscle RNA/DNA } Increased with BCAA
Christie 1985	8	Alcoholic 75%	9 on each regimen	Diet containing 40 g protein + BCAA supplement 20 g increments × 3	Diet containing 40 g protein + casein supplement 20 g increments × 3	Significant increase in nitrogen balance on both regimens
Egberts 1985	22	Alcoholic 87%	7 on each regimen	Diet containing 1 g protein 35 kcal + BCAA 0.25 g/kg } /kg	Diet containing 1 g protein 35 kcal + casein 0.25 g/kg } /kg	Significant increase in nitrogen balance on both regimens
Okita 1985	10	Alcoholic 70%	14 control 14 trial 14 control } in order	Oral diet 40 g protein 1500 kcal + 40 g protein 630 kcal } Supplement rich in BCAA	Oral diet 80 g protein 2100 kcal	Improved nitrogen balance and serum prealbumin concentrations on supplemented regimen

Table 7 *Continued*

First author and date	Patients (n)	Aetiology of cirrhosis	Trial duration (days)	Trial regimen (daily)	Alternative regimen (daily)	Outcome
Rocchi 1985	36	Alcoholic 50%	5	A Oral diet + IV BCAA 0.5 g/kg; B Oral diet + IV BCAA 1.0 g/kg	C Oral diet + IV BCAA enriched 0.8 g/kg; D Oral diet + IV balanced AA 0.5 g/kg	Improved nitrogen balance in groups B, C, and D
Bunout 1989	36	Alcoholic	15–30	Diet containing BCAA-rich protein 1.5 g/kg energy 50 kcal/kg	Standard diet protein 0.8 g/kg energy 35 kcal/kg	No difference in nutritional status between groups
Cabré 1990	35	Alcoholic 66%	18–30	BCAA-enriched, energy-dense enteral feed 2115 kcal/day 40 mmol sodium/day	Standard low-sodium hospital diet 2200 kcal/day	Actual intake in control group 1370 kcal/day; Enteral feed withdrawn in two patients; Significant increase in serum albumin in enteral group
Marchesini 1990	64	Alcoholic 56%	90 on each regimen	Usual diet + 2.4 g BCAA/10 kg	Usual diet + 1.8 g casein/10 kg	Significant increase in nitrogen balance on both regimens after 6 months
Keans 1992	31	Alcoholic 100%	28	Standard hospital diet + casein-based enteral feed 40 kcal and 1.5 g protein/kg	Standard hospital diet	Significanly lower energy and protein intakes in control group; Serum albumin improved in both groups; Nitrogen balance more positive in trial group
Hirsch 1993	51	Alcoholic 100%	365	Usual diet + casein-based enteral feed ≡1000 kcal and 34 g protein	Usual diet + placebo tablet	Nutritional intake higher, MAC, serum albumin, and hand-grip strength improved earlier and hospital stay less in trial group; No significant difference in mortality
Plauth 1993	17	Alcoholic 88%	56 on each regimen	Unrestricted diet + BCAA 0.25 g/kg	Unrestricted diet + placebo	No difference in nutritional status between groups

* Hepatic-Aid: commercial BCAA-enriched supplement.
BCAA, branched-chain amino acid; Cr/Ht, creatinine–height; IV, intravenous; MAC, mid-arm circumference.

Table 8 The European Society for Parenteral and Enteral Nutrition Consensus Group recommendations 1997 for nutritional requirements in chronic liver disease[65]

Clinical condition	Non-protein energy (kcal/kg/day)	Protein or amino acids (g/kg/day)
Compensated cirrhosis	25–35	1.0–1.2
Decompensated cirrhosis	35–40	1.5
Malnourished } Anorexic	35–40	1.5
Oral or enteral routes		

importance of improving their nutritional status prior to surgery. Hyperglycaemia should be carefully controlled if present; vitamin and mineral deficiencies should be corrected.

Nitrogen requirements increase in transplanted patients in the early postoperative period as in all patients undergoing major abdominal surgery (Plevak, MayoClinProc, 1994; 69:225; Italian Society for Parenteral and Enteral Nutrition, 1996; 15:155). Glucose metabolism may also be disturbed. Blood glucose, lactate, and triglycerides should be monitored to ensure adequate substrate utilization.

Patients who are adequately nutritionally supported in the early postoperative period do better than those who are essentially unsupported (Reilley, JPEN, 1990; 14:386). Both enteral and parenteral regimens are efficacious and safe (Reilley, 1990; Wicks, Lancet, 1994; 344:837; Hasse, JPEN, 1995; 19:437; Mehta, ClinTranspl, 1995; 9:364; Pescovitz, Surgery, 1995; 117:642). However, use of the enteral route is associated with earlier institution of oral feeding, earlier attainment of optimal oral intake, and a lower incidence of postoperative ileus (Mehta, 1995). Nasojejunal tubes can be placed at the time of surgery and feeding can be instituted within 12 h.

The majority of the metabolic and nutritional abnormalities observed in these patients in the preoperative and early postoperative period will correct within weeks or months. However, some abnormalities take considerably longer to resolve; protein turnover, for example, may not return to normal for upwards of a year (Wicks, Lancet, 1994; 344:837), while bone healing may take several years to complete (Crosbie, Hepatol, 1997; 26(Suppl): 347A abstr.; Feller, Hepatol, 1997; 26(Suppl): 347A abstr.). Institution of a high-protein diet, calcium supplementation, use of oestrogen replacement in postmenopausal women, exercise, and early withdrawal of steroids may aid bone healing (Lindor, SemLivDis, 1993; 13:367; Crippin, AmJGastr, 1994; 89:47).

Excessive weight gain and hyperlipidaemia may develop, particularly during the first two postoperative years (Munoz, TransplProc, 1991; 23:1480; Palmer, Transpl, 1991; 51:797). Pretransplantation body mass index is the major determinant of subsequent obesity; the higher the initial body mass index, the greater the likelihood of significant weight gain (Everhart, Hepatol, 1997; 26(Suppl): 162A abstr.). Cyclosporin disturbs cholesterol metabolism and its use is associated with a higher incidence of obesity post-transplantation than use of tacrolimus (Everhart, 1997). Use of both cyclosporin and tacrolimus is associated with the development of hypomagnesaemia (McDiarmid, Transpl, 1993; 56:

847). These individuals therefore require long-term metabolic and dietary monitoring.

Dietary management of the complications of liver disease

Fluid retention[70]

Patients with both subacute and chronic liver disease may develop significant fluid retention which manifests as ascites and peripheral oedema. In general the development of ascites is associated with a poor prognosis (Arroyo, SemLivDis, 1986; 6:353). Fluid retention may develop gradually and spontaneously or its appearance may be precipitated by events, such as gastrointestinal bleeding, which further impair hepatic function. Spontaneous bacterial peritonitis may develop in patients with ascites; it is often subclinical and its development carries a high mortality.

The pathogenesis of the fluid retention observed in patients with chronic liver disease is multifactorial, but changes in renal function, in the systemic circulation, and in the vasoconstrictor and antinaturetic systems, all play key roles (Ginès, SemLivDis, 1997; 17: 175).

Sodium retention is the most frequent abnormality of renal function observed in these patients; it develops as a result of an increase in proximal and distal tubular reabsorption and leads to an increase in total body exchangeable sodium. Renal water excretion is also impaired, most probably due to an increase in circulating antidiuretic hormone (Ginès, Nephrol, 1994; 14:387); this leads to fluid retention, to an increase in total body water, and ultimately to dilutional hyponatraemia. These patients therefore present the paradox of hyponatraemia associated with a marked increase in total body exchangeable sodium. Manipulations of both dietary sodium and water intakes have therefore been used in the management of these patients, but dietary sodium restriction is the key element.[70]

The total amount of sodium retained reflects the balance between dietary sodium intake and urinary and non-urinary sodium losses. If dietary sodium is restricted to below total sodium losses, then fluid loss will ensue. Rigid restriction to a daily intake of 10 to 20 mEq (mmol) sodium will control ascites even in patients with little or no urinary sodium excretion (Eisenmenger, JLabClinMed, 1949; 34:1029). In practice, however, dietary sodium intake need only be restricted to between 60 and 80 mEq (mmol) daily if diuretics are used to increase urinary sodium excretion. Estimation of 24-h urinary sodium excretion will allow the dietary regimen to be adjusted in parallel with changes in diuretic requirements.

Further restriction of dietary sodium intake to 40 mEq (mmol) daily may be required as a temporary measure in patients with severe ascites; such regimens should not be used long-term; they are unpalatable and their use is associated with significant reductions in dietary energy and protein intakes and loss of lean body mass (Soulsby, Hepatol, 1997; 26(Suppl):203A abstr.).

Failure of seemingly adequate dietary and diuretic regimens to control fluid retention would suggest non-compliance, but care should be taken to eliminate the possibility that sodium is being ingested from non-food sources such as medication and herbal supplements.

Although fluid restriction has been used traditionally to treat fluid overload in patients with cirrhosis, no formal assessment of its efficacy has been undertaken. It is probably unnecessary to impose fluid restriction in the majority of patients with cirrhosis with ascites, but it should be considered, at least as a short-term measure, in patients with severe hyponatraemia.

Sample low-sodium diets are appended.

Hepatic encephalopathy

The treatment of hepatic encephalopathy is empirical and based on preventing the formation and absorption of gut-derived toxins, principally ammonia.

In the 1930s and 1940s patients with cirrhosis were encouraged to take high-protein, high-energy diets to counter the malnutrition they so often exhibited. The beneficial effects of this management approach were clearly appreciated at that time, and were carefully documented. Patek and colleagues (JAMA, 1948; 138:543), for example, recorded significant clinical improvement in 61 (50 per cent) of 124 patients with severely decompensated liver disease, 40 per cent of whom displayed 'mental change', following institution of a diet which provided 140 g of protein and 3500 kcal daily.

In the 1950s 'nitrogenous substances', including dietary protein, were implicated in the pathogenesis of the neuropsychiatric abnormalities associated with advanced chronic liver disease (Phillips, NEJM, 1952; 247:239; Schwartz, NEJM, 1954; 251:685; Sherlock, Lancet, 1954; ii:453). However, considerable variation was observed in the degree of tolerance to dietary protein in these early reports with the result that authors were very circumspect in their comments regarding the implications of their findings for the dietary management of these patients.

In the mid-1950s use of non-absorbable antibiotics was introduced as a treatment for hepatic encephalopathy, and it is noticeable that in the majority of reports authors stipulated that use of these agents would allow dietary protein to be continued or else to be reintroduced quickly if initially withdrawn (Dawson, Lancet, 1957; ii:1263; Summerskill, BMJ, 1958; ii:1322; Faloon, ArchIntMed, 1959; 103:43; Stormont, NEJM, 1959; 259:1145).

With this as background it is extremely difficult to understand why by the late 1950s and early 1960s the practice of withdrawing dietary protein in patients with cirrhosis, often for prolonged periods, was so widely advocated (Manning, NEJM, 1958; 258:55; Sherlock, AnnRevMed, 1960; 11:47). It may have resulted, however, from erroneous extrapolation of the results of two, well-publicized studies involving patients with the now rarely seen persistent form of hepatic encephalopathy (Sherlock, Lancet, 1956; ii:689; Summerskill, QJMed, 1956; 25:245). Such patients show little or

minimal disturbance of liver function but extensive portal–systemic shunting of blood; they may be truly protein-intolerant although daily intakes of 50 to 60 g of protein can usually be achieved.

It would appear, although it cannot be proved, that these studies, despite being confined to this specific subpopulation of patients with chronic liver disease, dictated the dietary management of all patients with cirrhosis with neuropsychiatric abnormalities, even if only transient, and later still of patients with cirrhosis who were neuropsychiatrically unimpaired but who might be at risk of developing this complication at some later stage.

In the mid-1960s the non-absorbable disaccharide lactulose was first used in the management of patients with hepatic encephalopathy (Bircher, Lancet, 1966; i:890), and by the 1980s it had become the agent of first choice for use in this syndrome. Throughout this time, however, patients continued to be protein restricted despite the obvious efficacy of this new agent.

In the late 1980s and early 1990s concern began to be expressed about the widespread practice of restricting dietary protein in patients with cirrhosis, first, because approximately 30 to 70 per cent of these patients are malnourished (Mendenhall, AmJClinNutr, 1986; 43: 213; Lautz, ClinInvest, 1992; 70:478; Italian Multicentre Co-operative Project, JHepatol, 1994; 21:317), and second, because their protein requirements were shown to be increased to 1.2 to 1.5 g/kg body weight daily (Swart, ClinNutr, 1989; 8:329; Nielsen, BrJNutr, 1993; 69:665; Nielsen, BrJNutr, 1995; 74:557; Kondrup, BrJNutr, 1997; 77:197). In addition, evidence began to accrue that patients with hepatic encephalopathy tolerate high-protein diets and can benefit from them (Kearns, Gastro, 1992; 102: 200; Morgan, JAmCollNutr, 1995; 14:152).

Keans and colleagues (Gastro, 1992; 102:200), for example, randomly assigned 31 patients with decompensated alcoholic liver disease, 55 per cent of whom had hepatic encephalopathy, to either a ward diet alone or to a ward diet plus a daily enteral supplement, and monitored their mental status over a period of 28 days. The mean protein intake was significantly higher in the enterally supplemented group, 103 g/day compared with 50 g/day, yet their mean mental state score significantly improved during the first 2 weeks of observation, while the mean mental score in the control group deteriorated; similar proportions of patients in each group were taking lactulose. These authors emphasized the beneficial effects of high- protein diets, commentating that lactulose could be used to offset any adverse effects on mental status which might develop.

Morgan and co-workers (JAmCollNutr, 1995; 14:152) examined the relationship between protein intake and hepatic encephalopathy in 136 patients with alcoholic hepatitis and/or cirrhosis followed as inpatients for 28 days. Low protein intake was shown to be independently associated with worsening hepatic encephalopathy, whereas high protein intake was associated with improving hepatic encephalopathy, but not as an independent variable.

In response to this evidence, the ESPEN Consensus Group have recommended not only that daily protein intakes in patients with cirrhosis should be of the order of 1.0 to 1.5 g/kg depending on their degree of decompensation (Table 8),[65] but that protein restriction should be avoided even in patients with established hepatic encephalopathy, although recognizing that in some patients a transient restriction of daily protein intake to 0.5 g/kg might be necessary. In the rarely encountered, truly protein-intolerant patient, some reduction of daily protein might be necessary although additional nitrogen should be provided in the form of an amino-acid supplement.[65]

Fuel utilization and nitrogen economy are optimized in these patients by provision of four to seven small meals throughout their waking hours together with a late-night snack of complex carbohydrate (Swart, BMJ, 1989; 299:1202; Zillikens, JHepatol, 1993; 17;377; Verboeket-van de Venne, Gut, 1995; 36:110; Chang, JPEN, 1997; 21:96). This feeding pattern should ensure even distribution of protein throughout the day, thereby avoiding protein loading.

Tolerance to dietary protein varies depending on its source. Thus, dairy protein is tolerated better than protein from mixed sources (Fenton, Lancet, 1966; i:164), while vegetable protein is tolerated better than meat protein (Greenberger, AmJDigDis, 1977; 22:845; Uribe, DigDisSci, 1982; 27:1109; De Bruijn, Gut, 1983; 24:53; Keshavarzian, AmJGastr, 1984; 79:945; Bianchi, JIntMed, 1993; 233:385).

The increased tolerance to vegetable protein diets reflects their high dietary fibre content and its effects on colonic function, namely decreased transit time, increased intraluminal pH, stimulation of microbial growth, and increased faecal ammonia excretion (Stephen, Nature, 1980; 284:283; Weber, Gastro, 1985; 89:538; García-Compean, Hepatol, 1987; 7:1034 abstr.; Herman, Gastro, 1987; 92:1795 abstr.). In addition, plasma arginine and citrulline concentrations tend to be higher in patients on vegetable protein diets (De Bruijn, Gut, 1983; 24:53), and this may facilitate ammonia removal via the Krebs–Henseleit cycle.

The acceptability of vegetable protein diets varies widely from population to population. In developed countries, where the fibre content of the staple diet is low, diets containing more than 50 g of vegetable protein are considered bulky and often produce early satiety, abdominal distension, flatulence, and diarrhoea. In under-developed countries, where the staple diet contains significant amounts of fibre, these diets tends to be better accepted. In general, patients should be encouraged to take as high a percentage of vegetable protein as they can, and provided that they are not also salt restricted, which makes the diet unpalatable, daily intakes of 30 to 40 g of vegetable protein can usually be achieved.

The use of oral, enteral, or intravenous supplements enriched with branched–chain amino acids for the treatment of hepatic encephalopathy remains controversial.[71] In patients with chronic liver disease, the plasma concentrations of the aromatic amino acids tend to be high, while those of the branched–chain amino acids are reduced (Morgan, Gut, 1982; 23:362; Petrides, Hepatol, 1991; 14:432). The aromatic amino acids serve as precursors for the physiological neurotransmitters and compete for passage across the blood–brain barrier with the other neutral amino acids, including the branched–chain amino acids. An increase in the free brain concentrations of the aromatic amino acids may result in neuro-transmitter imbalance. It therefore follows that correcting the plasma amino acid profile by use of oral or intravenous supplements enriched with branched-chain amino acids and low in aromatic amino acids might restore neurotransmitter balance and so benefit patients with this condition.

Several early studies using intravenous branched-chain amino acid-enriched solutions to treat episodes of hepatic encephalopathy in patients with cirrhosis were encouraging, but as they were generally uncontrolled, no firm conclusions could be made about the efficacy and safety of this form of treatment. Subsequently, a number of randomized, controlled clinical trials have been published (Rossi-Fanelli, DigDisSci, 1982; 27:929; Wahren, Hepatol, 1983; 3:475; Cerra, JPEN, 1985; 9:288; Fiaccadori, ItalJGastr, 1985; 17: 5; Michel, Liver, 1985; 5:282; Vilstrup, JHepatol, 1985; 1(Suppl.2): S347 abstr.; Strauss, NutrSupplSves, 1986; 6:18; Caballería Rovira, RevEspEnfermAparDig, 1987; 72:116; Hwang, ChinJGastro, 1988; 5:185), but they are not easily compared as the trial designs were not standardized to any great degree (Table 9). For example, there is wide variation in the aetiology and severity of the liver injury, in the cause and severity of the precoma/coma, and its duration before the trial. Equally, although in all nine studies the treatment groups received an infusion of a branched- chain amino-acid mixture and hypertonic glucose, the nature of the amino-acid solution varied from trial to trial. There is, in addition, little consensus on the nature of the control regimen or on the need for adjuvant therapy with lactulose and/or neomycin. The duration of treatment varies from trial to trial, although in most it was continued for 48 h after 'wake-up'. Endpoints for determining treatment outcome are not clearly defined, but in most the time to 'wake-up', generally to grade 0 or 1, is noted, and the percentage survival is recorded.

It is extremely difficult to interpret the results of these studies in view of the non-standardized way in which they were conducted. However, in six of the nine studies, infusion of branched-chain amino-acid mixtures had no significant effect on recovery or survival in comparison with the chosen control regimen. In one study the use of branched-chain amino acids had a significant effect on recovery from precoma but not on mortality (Cerra, JPEN, 1985; 9:288), while in another study, treatment with branched-chain amino acids was associated with an accelerated recovery from precoma (Strauss, NutrSupplSves, 1986; 6:18). In the final study (Fiaccadori, ItalJGastr, 1985; 17:5), treatment with branched-chain amino acids and/or lactulose was found to be more effective than treatment with lactulose alone.

These trials have been subjected to extensive review and re-analysis by two groups of workers, who unfortunately came to different conclusions. Eriksson and Conn (Hepatol, 1989; 10:228) reviewed seven of the nine studies and undertook an extensive reanalysis of one. They concluded that 'BCAA therapy, whether pure or combined with other amino acids, irrespective of the amount administered does not affect significantly the outcome of patients with acute hepatic encephalopathy'. Naylor and coworkers (Gastro, 1989; 97:1033) applied meta-analytical methods to review the results of seven of the nine studies, though unfortunately they seem to have used preliminary data, published earlier than the definitive studies, in three instances. They concluded that pooled analysis of five of the studies showed that treatment with branched-chain amino acids was associated with a highly significant improvement in mental recovery from severe encephalopathy over follow-up times varying from 5 to 14 days. The case–fatality data could not be pooled, although the most conservative interpretation of the data from three of the studies showed that treatment with branched-chain amino acids was associated with a significant reduction in mortality. However, the authors caution that although the study results to date are promising, they 'do not permit an unqualified conclusion in favour of the use of BCAA solutions and

Table 9 Randomized, controlled trials of intravenous branched-chain amino acids (BCAA) in the treatment of acute hepatic encephalopathy in patients with cirrhosis

First author and date	Patients (n)	Episodes treated (n)	Aetiology of cirrhosis (% alcoholic)	Coma grade (% III/IV)	Trial duration (days)	Treatment regimen (daily)	Control regimen (daily)
Rossi-Fanelli 1982	34	34	32	100	2–4	BCAA-rich (BS692) + 20% glucose	Lactulose + 20% glucose
Wahren 1983	50	50	76	96	<5	BCAA (KabiVitrum) + 50% glucose 20% lipid	5% glucose + 50% glucose 50% lipid
Cerra 1985	75	75	92	?	14	BCAA-rich (F080) + 25% glucose	Neomycin + 25% glucose
Fiaccadori 1985	48	48	52	50	7	BCAA-rich (BS666) + 30% glucose ± lactulose	Lactulose + 30% glucose
Michel 1985	70	70	81	64	5	BCAA-rich + 30% glucose 20% lipid	Conventional AA mixture + 30% glucose 20% lipid
Vilstrup 1985	65	65	91	69	<16	BCAA-rich (Pf 8) + Lactulose + 50% glucose	Lactulose + 50% glucose
Strauss 1986	29	32	75	34	?5	BCAA-rich (F080) + Hypertonic glucose	Neomycin
Caballería Rovira 1981	20	20	?	35	<5	BCAA-rich (F080)	Neomycin + Lactulose
Hwang 1988	55*	60*	15 (8/52)	89*	<5	BCAA-rich (Aminoleban) + Neomycin + Lactulose + 10% dextrose	Neomycin + Lactulose + 10% dextrose

Table 9 *Continued*

Oral intake (daily)	Response to treatment			Study mortality			Comments	Conclusion
	BCAA (n (%) improved)	Control	Combined	BCAA (n (%) deaths)	Control	Combined		
Nil	12/17 (71)	8/17 (47)	3/7 (43)	3/17 (18)	4/17 (24)	4/7 (57)	Patients failing to respond after 4 days given BCAA and lactulose	No significant effect of BCAA on recovery or mortality
Nil	14/25 (56)	12/25 (48)	—	10/25 (40)	5/25 (20)	—	Eight patients also received lactulose ± neomycin	No significant effect of BCAA on recovery or mortality
Nil until symptom-free	16/30 (53)	5/29 (17)	—	12/40 (30)	13/35 (37)	—	20% dropped out; 15% crossed to other regimen on Day 4. Results selectively analysed	Significant effect of BCAA on recovery but not on mortality
?	15/16 (94)	10/16 (63)	16/16 (100)	0	0	0	—	Treatment with BCAA ± lactulose significantly better than treatment with lactulose alone
Nil	12/36 (33)	10/34 (29)	—	7/36 (19)	7/34 (21)	—	—	No significant effect of BCAA on recovery or mortality
?	17/32 (53)	17/33 (52)	—	11/32 (30)	10/33 (34)	—	—	No significant effect of BCAA on recovery or mortality
Low protein when grade I/II	14/16 (88)	14/16 (88)	—	2/16 (13)	2/16 (13)	—	—	No significant effect of BCAA on recovery or mortality. Speed of recovery faster with BCAA
Protein-free diet?	6/10 (60)	6/10 (60)	—	2/10 (20)	2/10 (20)	—	—	No significant effect of BCAA on recovery or mortality
Nil days 0–3 <20 g protein days 3–5	19/27* (70)	15/28* (54)	—	10/27* (37)	14/28* (50)	—	—	No significant effect of BCAA on recovery or mortality

* Included three patients with fulminant hepatic failure.

hypertonic glucose as a nutritional support regimen for patients with cirrhosis with high-grade HE'. They stipulate that confirmatory randomized, controlled trials with longer follow-up periods are warranted.

Early studies showed that the use of oral amino-acid supplements enriched with branched-chain amino acids might be efficacious in treating persistent hepatic encephalopathy or in preventing recurrence of episodic encephalopathy in patients with chronic liver disease. However, the number of patients treated was small and the observations were uncontrolled. In recent years, a number of randomized, controlled clinical trials of this form of treatment have been undertaken (Schäfer, ZGastr, 1981; 19:356; Eriksson, Gut, 1982; 23:801; McGhee, AnnSurg, 1983; 197:288; Sieg, ZGastr, 1983; 21:644; Simko, NutrRepInt, 1983; 27:765; Horst, Hepatol, 1984; 4:279; Egberts, Gastro, 1985; 88:887; Marchesini, JHepatol, 1990; 11:92; Plauth, JHepatol, 1993; 17:308; Guarnieri, p.193 in[68]; Riggio, p.183 in[68])[67] (Table 10).

Many of the criticisms of the intravenous studies in acute hepatic encephalopathy can also be made of these studies. Thus, with few exceptions, the numbers of patients treated in the various studies is small and the treatment periods are short (Table 10). Wide variation is observed in the degree of encephalopathy on entry into the study, and in the trial and control regimens employed. In only one study was a branched-chain amino-acid mixture used as an alternative to treatment with lactulose (Riggio, p.183 in[68]), while in the others it was used either as an adjunct or as an alternative in individual patients depending on whether lactulose was given simultaneously. In several studies, the 'comagenic' potential of branched-chain amino acids mixtures was compared with that of isonitrogenous amounts of dietary protein or casein, although in only one study was lactulose discontinued (Riggio, p.183 in[68]). In seven of the 12 studies, a cross-over design was employed but, in general, wash-out periods between treatments were not allowed and the correct statistical analyses to allow separation of the effects of the two regimens were not employed. Overall, the endpoints of treatment were not clearly defined, although in most trials patients were monitored throughout by clinical examination, psychometric assessment, and measurements of blood ammonia concentrations and electroencephalogram mean cycle frequencies.

In eight of the 12 studies, no improvement was noted in mental status, psychometric test performance, or in electroencephalogram mean cycle frequencies in patients given branched-chain amino-acid mixtures. However, Horst and colleagues (Hepatol, 1984; 4:279) found that patients with cirrhosis with a history of chronic recurrent hepatic encephalopathy developed significantly less neuropsychiatric impairment when given an amino-acid supplement than when receiving isonitrogenous amounts of dietary protein. Likewise, Marchesini and coworkers (JHepatol, 1990; 11:92) reported significant improvements in mental status, psychometric test performance, and/or electroencephalogram mean cycle frequencies in patients with recurrent hepatic encephalopathy given oral branched-chain amino acids, but not in patients given oral casein. Egberts and associates (Gastro, 1985; 88:887) reported significant improvements in psychometric performance in patients with cirrhosis with subclinical hepatic encephalopathy when given branch-chain amino acids but not when given casein, while Plauth and coworkers (JHepatol, 1993; 17:308) reported improvements in the performance of three of 11 psychometric tests and in driving

capacity in patients with subclinical hepatic encephalopathy when receiving a branched-chain amino-acid supplement but not when taking a placebo preparation. Firm conclusions regarding the efficacy of oral branched-chain amino acids as a 'treatment' for hepatic encephalopathy cannot be made on the basis of the studies undertaken to date. An attempt at a meta-analysis of the trials undertaken in patients with cirrhosis with recurrent or persistent hepatic encephalopathy was made (Fabbri, JPEN, 1996; 20:159), but was unsuccessful because insufficient data were available from the published reports and the original trial data could not be obtained from the majority of the authors of the published studies.

It is clear that further, randomized, controlled studies are needed, preferably undertaken as large multicentre trials. In the meantime, branched-chain amino acids, if they are to be used at all, are best reserved for malnourished decompensated patients with cirrhosis with hepatic encephalopathy who are intolerant of dietary protein.

Sample vegetable protein diets are appended.

Carbohydrate intolerance

Glucose intolerance is commonly observed in patients with a variety of liver diseases. Individuals with chronic liver disease and mild glucose intolerance may benefit from dietary manipulation. They should be encouraged to take 45 to 55 per cent of their total energy intake as carbohydrate, predominantly unrefined, and approximately one-third as fat. Complex carbohydrates which have low glycaemic indices and which are rich in soluble fibre, such as pulses, pasta, and cereals, are recommended (Jenkins, AmJGastr, 1989; 84:732; Barkoukis, Hepatol, 1997; 26(Suppl):380A abstr.); sucrose intake should be limited to 30 g daily and its use as a sweetener in drinks should be avoided. The majority of dietary fat should be unsaturated. Provided that the postprandial blood glucose levels are not persistently elevated and that the immediate pre-prandial blood sugar concentrations do not exceed 6.0 mmol/l, no further measures are needed.

Patients with severe parenchymal liver disease complicated by hepatic encephalopathy and glucose intolerance have been shown to benefit from institution of a vegetable protein diet supplemented with dietary fibre (Uribe, Gastro, 1985; 88:901; Morán, Hepatol, 1997; 26(Suppl):282A abstr.).

A sample diet suitable for a patient with chronic parenchymal liver disease and mild to moderate glucose intolerance is appended.

Appendix*
High-protein, high-energy, low-fat diet

Approximately 80 g protein, 35 g fat, and 2400 kcal (10.8 MJ).

Daily	Skimmed milk (570 ml [1 pint]) (extra skimmed milk powder may be added to increase protein content)
Breakfast	Fruit or fruit juice
	Cereal or porridge with sugar and skimmed milk
	One egg, lean grilled bacon, lean ham, or fish
	Bread and scrape of very low fat spread such as Gold, Delight, or Outline
	Marmalade, honey, or jam

Table 10 Randomized, controlled trials of oral branched-chain amino acids (BCAA) in patients with chronic hepatic encephalopathy

First author, and date	Patients (n)	Mental state (grade)	Pretrial regimen	Trial period (days)	Trial regimen (daily)	Alternative/control regimen (daily)	Comments	Findings
Schäfer 1981	8	I–II	Protein restriction 8/8 Lactulose 5/8	30–60 on each regimen	Usual diet + 45 g protein (34% BCAA)	(a) Usual diet + 45 g milk protein (20% BCAA) (b) Usual diet + 125 g carbohydrate	Lactulose 5/8 BCAA-enriched protein well tolerated; milk protein poorly tolerated	No significant effect of BCAA on NCT results, or EEG mcf
Swart 1981	8	0	Protein restriction 8/8 Lactulose 8/8	30 alternating 5-day regimens	Diet containing BCAA-rich protein (35% BCAA) 40, 60, 80 g at 10-day intervals	Diet containing mixed protein (20% BCAA) 40, 60, 80 g at 10-day intervals	Lactulose 8/8	No significant effect of BCAA on mental state, NCT results, or EEG mcf
Eriksson 1982	7	I–II	Protein restriction 4/7 Lactulose 4/7	14 on each regimen	Usual diet + 30 g BCAA 15 g sucrose	Usual diet + 34 g maltodextrine 11 g sucrose	Lactulose 4/7 BCAA well-tolerated	No significant effect of BCAA on mental state, psychometric test results, or EEG mcf
McGhee 1984	4	0	Protein restriction 4/4	11 on each regimen	30 g Hepatic-Aid* 20 g casein + 260 g carbohydrate } 2000 kcal	50 g casein + 260 g carbohydrate } 2000 kcal	Both regimens well tolerated	No significant effect of BCAA on psychometric test results, or EEG mcf
Sieg 1983	14	0–I	Protein restriction 14/14 Lactulose 14/14	90 on each regimen	Usual diet + 44 g protein (30% BCAA) 80 g carbohydrate	Usual diet + 125 g carbohydrate	Lactulose 14/14 BCAA well tolerated	No significant effect of BCAA on NCT results, or EEG mcf
Simko 1983	15	0–I	Lactulose/neomycin ?/15	90	Usual diet + 20–60 g Hepatic-Aid*	Usual diet + placebo powder	Lactulose/neomycin ?/15 4 BCAA; 1 placebo dropped out	No adverse effect of BCAA on mental state or NCT results

Table 10 *Continued*

First author, and date	Patients (n)	Mental state (grade)	Pretrial regimen	Trial period (days)	Trial regimen (daily)	Alternative/control regimen (daily)	Comments	Findings
Guarnieri 1984	8	<II	Protein restriction 8/8 Lactulose/neomycin ?/8	100–120	Calorie-reduced basal diet + 29 g Hepatic-Aid* Carbohydrate }1120 kcal Fat	Calorie-reduced basal diet + Carbohydrate }1120 kcal Fat	Lactulose/neomycin ?/8 All patients malnourished; supplement well tolerated	No significant effect of BCAA on mental state or EEG mcf
Horst 1984	26	0–II	Protein restriction 26/26 Lactulose ± neomycin 25/26	30	Diet containing 20 g protein + Hepatic-Aid* 20 g BCAA added at weekly intervals	Diet containing 20 g protein + 20 g dietary protein added at weekly intervals	Lactulose 2/26 BCAA well tolerated	Incidence of encephalopathy significantly less with BCAA
Riggio 1984	28	0–II	Protein restriction 28/28 Lactulose 28/28	90	Diet containing 0.5 g/kg protein days 0–60 0.8 g/kg protein days 60–90 + 0.3 g/kg BCAA days 0–90	Diet containing 0.5 g/kg protein days 0–60 0.8 g/kg protein days 60–90 + Lactulose days 0–90	5/14 BCAA dropped out ? cause	One patient in each group developed grade II hepatic encephalopathy
Egberts 1985	22	0	Lactulose 14/22	7 on each regimen	Diet containing 1 g protein } /kg 35 kcal + BCAA 0.25 g/kg	Diet containing 1 g protein } /kg 35 kcal + casein 0.2 g/kg	Lactulose 14/22	Psychometric test results significant better on BCAA
Marchesini 1990	64	I–II	Protein restriction 64/64 Lactulose 64/64	90	Usual diet + 2.4 g BCAA/10 kg	Usual diet + 1.8 g casein/10 kg	Lactulose 64/64	Significant improvements in mental state, NCT results, and EEG mcf on BCAA
Plauth 1993	17	0	Unrestricted protein 17/17 Lactulose 14/17	56 on each regimen	Unrestricted diet + BCAA tablets 0.25 mg/kg	Unrestricted diet + placebo tablets	Lactulose 14/17	Psychometric tests and driving capacity significantly better on BCAA

* Hepatic-Aid: commercial BCAA-enriched supplement.
EEG, electroencephalogram; mcf, mean cycle frequency; NCT, number connection test.

	Tea or coffee with skimmed milk
Mid-morning	Skimmed milk-shake (skimmed milk, skimmed milk powder, and flavouring such as Nesquick or Crusha)
Lunch	Average portion lean meat, no visible fat, or large portion white fish or chicken
	Potatoes, rice, or spaghetti
	Vegetables or salad, no oil
	Skimmed milk pudding, fruit, jelly, or low-fat ice cream
	Stewed or tinned fruit
Tea	Tea with skimmed milk
	Plain biscuits
Supper	As lunch
Bedtime	Skimmed milk-shake

Energy intake may be increased by fruit drinks plus glucose, or a glucose polymer. The use of high-carbohydrate foods such as potatoes, rice, or spaghetti should be encouraged. Build-Up (Nestlé) is a useful protein supplement that is low in fat and palatable when made up with skimmed milk. Medium-chain triglycerides (**MCT**) can be added to a low-fat diet to increase the energy content. These should be introduced slowly into the diet over several days, as they may cause gastrointestinal disturbance in the early stages if administered rapidly. Medium-chain triglycerides are available as oil (MCT oil, [Bristol Myers, Cow & Gate]), an emulsion (Liquigen [SHS]), or powdered milk (Caprilon [Cow & Gate]). Adults will find the first two more useful, while infants and children will also require MCT milk. All products are available on prescription in the United Kingdom and patients will benefit most from individual practical advice from a dietitian on how to use them. The oil should not be taken undiluted but always mixed with at least an equal quantity of fluid or food.

Diets restricted in sodium

Intakes of 60 to 100 mEq (60 to 100 mmol) of sodium daily can be achieved by avoiding salt at table, minimizing the salt added to cooking, and avoiding the 'foods not allowed' listed below. All other foods may be taken freely.

The following regimen provides approximately 40 mEq (40 mmol) of sodium daily. Salt should not be used in cooking or added at table, and foods forbidden and allowed are given below.

Daily	Milk for tea, cereal, etc. (300 ml [approximately 0.5 pint])
Breakfast	Fruit or fruit juice, if desired
	Breakfast cereal (see under Foods allowed freely) or porridge made without salt
	One egg, tomatoes, mushrooms
	Two slices ordinary bread
	Salt-free butter
	Jam, marmalade, or honey
	Milk from allowance on cereal and in tea
Mid-morning	Tea or coffee, milk from allowance
Lunch	Meat or fish—home prepared without salt
	Potatoes, rice, or pasta
	Vegetables or salad
	Fruit, jelly, unsalted pastry

Tea	Tea with milk from allowance
	Salt-free cake or biscuit—home prepared using appropriate recipe
Supper	As lunch
Bedtime	Remainder of milk in tea or coffee
	Matzo bread, salt-free butter and ham, or salt-free cake or biscuit

Foods allowed freely

Fruit, fresh, canned, or frozen, dates
Fresh or frozen vegetables
Matzos, salt-free crispbread
Puffed Wheat, Shredded Wheat, Sugar Puffs, unsalted porridge
Plain rice, dried pasta, semolina, sago, tapioca
Sugar, glucose, honey, marmalade, jam
Boiled sweets, peppermints, chewing gum, dark chocolate
Pepper, herbs, spices, vinegar, powdered mustard
Meat, fish, eggs
Milk in limited quantities only
Tea, coffee, fresh fruit juice
Mineral waters, except Vichy water, Badoit, Ferrarelle
Salt substitutes (based on potassium chloride) may be used if serum potassium is normal or low, for example Ruthmol
Unsalted butter, all cooking oils, double cream

Foods not allowed

Ordinary biscuits, cakes
Ordinary bread above daily allowance
Self-raising flour, baking powder
Rice Krispies, Cornflakes, All-Bran, and all other cereals except those on the 'allowed freely' list
Cheese, ice-cream
Yoghurt—unless taken in place of milk
Evaporated or condensed milk
Sausages, beefburgers
Ham, bacon, tinned meats, meat paste
Tinned fish, smoked fish, fish paste, fish fingers, fish in sauce
All commercial ready-made meals
Meat extract, yeast extract
Tinned vegetables, including baked beans
Tinned or packet soups, instant mashed potato
Ketchup, pickles, ready-made mustard, soy sauce, all other bottled sauces
Milk chocolate, toffees, fudge, fruit gums, fruit pastilles
Lucozade, soda water, Vichy water, Badoit, Ferrarelle
Tomato juice
Sultanas, raisins
Potato crisps, salted nuts, and other savoury snacks
LoSalt, and other salt substitute containing sodium chloride

Vegetable protein diet

Approximately 80 g protein, 2600 kcal (11.7 MJ)

Daily	Milk for tea, cereal, etc. (300 ml [0.5 pint])
Breakfast	Orange juice (200 ml)
	Cereal or porridge and sugar

	Two slices wholemeal toast
	Butter, jam
Mid-morning	Peanuts (50 g)
	Orange juice (200 ml)
Lunch	Soya-protein meat substitute (100 g)
	Large serving of potatoes, rice, or pasta
	Vegetables or salad served with oil
	Wholemeal bread
	Butter
	Fruit, fresh, tinned, or cooked; or sponge pudding, or pastry with cream or custard (with additional milk)
Supper	Lentil soup (400 ml) or baked beans (300 g) on toast or with two slices of wholemeal bread and butter
	Side-salad or additional vegetables
	Fruit, fresh, tinned, or cooked
	Double cream

Low-sodium, vegetable protein diet

Approximately 80 g protein, 2600 kcal (11.7 MJ) and 40 mEq (mmol) sodium. No salt to be added in cooking or at table.

Daily	Milk for tea, cereal, etc. (300 ml [0.5 pint])
Breakfast	Orange juice (200 ml)
	Porridge or breakfast cereal (see foods freely allowed under diets restricted in sodium)
	Two slices wholemeal toast
	Salt-free butter
	Jam
Mid-morning	Unsalted nuts (50 g)
	Orange juice (200 ml)
Lunch	Pulses (400 g) cooked with oil and vegetables
	Large serving of potatoes, rice, or pasta (fried if desired)
	Vegetables or salad with oil or dressing without salt
	One slice of wholemeal bread
	Salt-free butter
	Tinned fruit in syrup
	Double cream
Supper	As lunch, or pulses (400 g) cooked and added to mixed salad
	Tinned, fresh or cooked fruit with sugar
	Double cream

Diet suitable for individuals with mild carbohydrate intolerance

Approximately 100 g protein, 73 g fat (two-thirds polyunsaturated fatty acids), 283 g carbohydrate, 46 g fibre, 2100 kcal (9.5 MJ). Approximately 52 per cent of total energy is supplied by carbohydrate and 30 per cent by fat.

Daily	Skimmed milk (570 ml [1 pint])
	Polyunsatured margarine (45 g)
Breakfast	Large bowl of high fibre cereal
	Two slices of wholemeal bread

	Margarine from allowance ± Marmite spread if desired
	Tea/coffee with skimmed milk
Mid-morning	Tea/coffee with skimmed milk or low calorie drink
	Piece of fresh fruit
Lunch	Average portion lean meat, chicken, or fish with no visible fat
	Large jacket potato
	Vegetables or salad, no oil
	Stewed or tinned fruit, unsweetened
	Low fat natural yoghurt or custard made from skimmed milk and artificial sweeteners
Tea	Tea with skimmed milk
Supper	Average portion lean meat, chicken, or fish with no visible fat
	Four slices of wholemeal bread
	Margarine from allowance
	Salad with up to 10 ml polyunsaturated oil as dressing
	Fresh fruit, or baked apple, no sugar added
Bedtime	Tea/coffee with skimmed milk
	One digestive or wholemeal biscuit

Saccharin or aspartame tablets, for example Sweetex, Hermesetas, or Canderel, may be used for sweetening.

References

1. Department of Health. *Dietary reference values for food energy and nutrients for the United Kingdom.* Report by the Committee on Medical Aspects of Food Policy. Report on Health and Social Subjects, No. 41. London: HMSO, 1991.
2. Miller LL. The role of the liver and the non-hepatic tissues in the regulation of free amino acid levels in the blood. In Holden JT, ed. *Amino acid pools.* New York: Dekker, 1961: 708–21.
3. Sokol RJ. Fat-soluble vitamins and their importance in patients with cholestatic liver diseases. *Gastroenterology Clinics of North America*, 1994; **23**: 673–705.
4. Hardman JG, Limbird LE, Molinoff PB, Ruddon RW, and Gilman AG, eds. *Goodman and Gilman's The pharmacological basis of therapeutics*, 9th edn. New York: McGraw-Hill, 1996.
5. Arias IM, Boyer JL, Fausto N, Jacoby WB, Schachter D, and Shafritz DA, eds. *The liver: biology and pathobiology*, 3rd edn. New York: Raven Press, 1994.
6. Bates CJ. Vitamin A. *Lancet*, 1995; **345**: 31–5.
7. Leathen JH. Nutrition. In Johnson AD, Gomes WR, and Vandemark NL, eds. *The testis*, Vol. 3. New York: Academic Press, 1970: 188–90.
8. Fraser DR. Vitamin D. *Lancet*, 1995; **345**: 104–7.
9. Meydani M. Vitamin E. *Lancet*, 1995; **345**: 170–5.
10. Shearer MJ. Vitamin K. *Lancet*, 1995; **345**: 229–34.
11. Rader JI, Calvert RJ, and Hathcock JN. Hepatic toxicity of unmodified and time-release preparations of niacin. *American Journal of Medicine*, 1992; **92**: 77–81.
12. Spannuth CL, Mitchell D, Stone WJ, Schenker S, and Wagner C. Vitamin B$_6$ nitriture in patients with uremia and liver disease. In National Research Council, ed. *Vitamin B$_6$ requirements.* Washington DC: National Academy of Science, 1978: 180–92.
13. Halstead CH and Tamura T. Folate deficiency in liver disease. In Davidson CS, ed. *Problems in liver disease.* New York: Grune & Stratton, 1979: 91–100.
14. Linnell J. The fate of cobalamins *in vivo*. In Babior BM, ed. *Cobalamin: biochemistry and pathophysiology.* New York: John Wiley, 1975: 287–333.

15. Gordenk VR, Becon BR, and Brittenham GM. Iron overload: causes and consequences. *Annual Review of Nutrition*, 1987; **7**: 485–508.

16. Stal P. Iron as a hepatotoxin. *Digestive Diseases*, 1995; **13**: 205–22.

17. Arthur MJ. Iron overload and fibrosis. *Journal of Gastroenterology and Hepatology*, 1996; **11**: 1124–9.

18. Honasoge M and Rao DS. Metabolic bone disease in gastrointestinal, hepatobiliary, and pancreatic disorders and total parenteral nutrition. *Current Opinions in Rheumatology*, 1995; **7**: 249–54.

19. Prasad AS. Clinical manifestations of zinc deficiency. *Annual Review of Nutrition*, 1985; **5**: 341–63.

20. Evans GW. Zinc and its deficiency diseases. *Clinical Physiology and Biochemistry*, 1986; **4**: 94–8.

21. Burch RF, Hahn HKJ, and Sullivan JF. Other metals and the liver with particular reference to zinc. In Powel L, ed. *Metals and the liver*. New York: Dekker, 1978: 333–61.

22. Quigley EMM and Zetterman RK. Hepatobiliary complications of malabsorption and malnutrition. *Seminars in Liver Disease*, 1988; **8**: 218–28.

23. Sherlock S and Walsh VM. Hepatic structure and function. In *Studies of undernutrition, Wuppertal 1946–1949*. Medical Research Council Special Report Series No. 275. London: Medical Research Council, 1951: 111–34.

24. Mitchell MC and Herlong HF. Alcohol and nutrition: caloric value, bioenergetics, and relationship to liver damage. *Annual Review of Nutrition*, 1986; **6**: 457–74.

25. Achord JL. 1987 Henry Baker lecture. Nutrition, alcohol and the liver. *American Journal of Gastroenterology*, 1988; **83**: 244–8.

26. Morgan MY and Levine JA. Alcohol and nutrition. *Proceedings of the Nutrition Society*, 1988; **47**: 85–98.

27. Marsano L and McClain CJ. Nutrition and alcoholic liver disease. *Journal of Parenteral and Enteral Nutrition*, 1991; **15**: 337–44.

28. Arky RA. The effect of alcohol on carbohydrate metabolism: carbohydrate metabolism in alcoholics. In Kissin B and Begleiter H, eds. *The biology of alcoholism*, Vol. I, *Biochemistry*. New York: Plenum Press, 1971: 197–227.

29. ReynoldsTB, Redeker AG, and Kuzma OT. Role of alcohol in pathogenesis of alcoholic cirrhosis. In McIntyre N and Sherlock S, eds. *Therapeutic agents and the liver*. Oxford: Blackwell, 1965: 131–42.

30. Kern, F. Epidemiology and natural history of gall-stones. *Seminars in Liver Disease*, 1983; **3**: 87–96.

31. Clain DJ and Lefkowitch JH. Fatty liver disease in morbid obesity. *Gastroenterology Clinics of North America*, 1987; **16**: 239–52.

32. Amaral JF and Thompson WR. Gallbladder disease in morbidly obese patients. *American Journal of Surgery*, 1988; **149**: 547–57.

33. Faloon WW. Hepatobiliary effects of obesity and weight-reducing surgery. *Seminars in Liver Disease*, 1988; **8**: 229–36.

34. Andersen T. Liver and gallbladder disease before and after very low-calorie diets. *American Journal of Clinical Nutrition*, 1992; **56**: 235S–9S.

35. Van Steenbergen W and Lanckmans S. Liver disturbances in obesity and diabetes mellitus. *International Journal of Obesity and Related Metabolic Disorders*, 1995; **19** (Suppl. 3): S27–36.

36. Ayub A and Faloon WW. Gallstones, obesity and jejunoileostomy. *Surgical Clinics of North America*, 1979; **59**: 1095–101.

37. Baker AL and Rosenberg IH. Hepatic complications of total parenteral nutrition. *American Journal of Medicine*, 1987; **82**: 489–97.

38. Klein S and Nealon WH. Hepatobiliary abnormalities associated with total parenteral nutrition. *Seminars in Liver Disease*, 1988; **8**: 237–46.

39. Fisher RL. Hepatobiliary abnormalities associated with total parenteral nutrition. *Gastroenterology Clinics of North America*, 1989; **18**: 645–66.

40. Balistreri WF and Bove KE. Hepatobiliary consequences of parenteral alimentation. *Progress in Liver Diseases*, 1990; **9**: 567–601.

41. Quigley EMM, Marsh MN, Shaffer JL, and Markin RS. Hepatobiliary complications of total parenteral nutrition. *Gastroenterology*, 1993; **104**: 286–301.

42. Fein BI and Holt PR. Hepatobiliary complications of total parenteral nutrition. *Journal of Clinical Gastroenterology*, 1994; **18**: 62–6.

43. Fleming CR. Hepatobiliary complications in adults receiving nutrition support. *Digestive Diseases*, 1994; **12**: 191–8.

44. Scriver CR, Beaudet AL, Sly WS, and Valle D, eds. *The metabolic and molecular bases of inherited disease*, 7th edn. New York: McGraw Hill, 1995.

45. Schilsky ML. Wilson's disease: genetic basis of copper toxicity and natural history. *Seminars in Liver Disease*, 1996; **16**: 83–95.

46. Rubin E and Farber JL. Environmental diseases of the digestive system. *Medical Clinics of North America*, 1990; **74**: 413–24.

47. Larrey D. Hepatotoxicity of herbal remedies. *Journal of Hepatology*, 1997; **26** (Suppl. 1): 47–51.

48. Holland B, Welch AA, Unwin ID, Buss DH, Paul AA, and Southgate DAT, eds. *McCance and Widdowson's The composition of foods*, 5th edn. London: The Royal Society of Chemistry, 1992.

49. Harris JA and Benedict TG. *Biometric studies of basal metabolism in man*. Washington, DC: Carnegie Institute of Washington, Publication No. 279, 1919.

50. Butterworth CE, Jr and Weinsier RL. Malnutrition in hospital patients: assessment and treatment. In Goodhart RS and Shils ME, eds. *Modern nutrition in health and disease*, 6th edn. Philadelphia: Lea & Febiger, 1978: 667–84.

51. Jelliffe DB. *The assessment of the nutritional status of the community*. WHO Monograph 53. Geneva: World Health Organization, 1966.

52. Blackburn GL, Bistrian BR, and Mainí BS. *Manual for nutrition/metabolic assessment of the hospitalized patient*. Chicago: American College of Surgeons, 1976.

53. Mendenhall CL. Protein-calorie malnutrition in alcoholic liver disease. In Watson RR and Watzi B, eds. *Nutrition and alcohol*. Boca Raton: CRC Press, 1992: 363–84.

54. Jelliffe DB and Jelliffe EFP. Age-dependent anthropometry. *American Journal of Clinical Nutrition*, 1971; **24**: 1377–9.

55. Frisancho AR. New norms of upper limb fat and muscle areas for assessment of nutritional status. *American Journal of Clinical Nutrition*, 1981; **34**: 2540–5.

56. United States Public Health Service Health Resources Administration. *NCHS growth charts*. Rockville, MD: HRA, 1976.

57. Morgan MY and Madden AM. The assessment of body composition in patients with cirrhosis. *European Journal of Nuclear Medicine*, 1996; **23**: 213–25.

58. Madden AM and Morgan MY. The potential role of dual-energy X-ray absorptiometry in the assessment of body composition in cirrhotic patients. *Nutrition*, 1997; **13**: 40–5.

59. Siri WR. The gross composition of the body. In Lawrence TH and Tobias CA, eds. *Advances in biological and medical physics*. New York: Academic Press, 1956:239–80.

60. Child CG, III and Turcotte JG. Surgery and portal hypertension. In Child CG, III, ed. *The liver and portal hypertension*. Philadelphia: WB Saunders & Co., 1964: 1–85.

61. Blendis LM. Nutritional management of patients with chronic liver disease. *Baillière's Clinical Gastroenterology*, 1989; **3**: 91–108.

62. McCullough AJ, Mullen KD, Smanik EJ, Tabbaa M, and Szanter K. Nutritional therapy and liver disease. *Gastroenterology Clinics of North America*, 1989; **18**: 619–43.

63. Schenker S and Halff GA. Nutritional therapy in alcoholic liver disease. *Seminars in Liver Disease*, 1993; **13**: 196–209.

64. Nompleggi DJ and Bonkovsky HL. Nutritional support in chronic liver disease: an analytical review. *Hepatology*, 1994; **19**: 518–33.

65. Plauth M, Merli M, Kondrup J, Weimann A, Ferenci P, and Müller MJ. ESPEN guidelines for nutrition in liver disease and transplantation. *Clinical Nutrition*, 1997; **16**: 43–55.

66. Morgan MY. The treatment of alcoholic hepatitis. *Alcohol and Alcoholism*, 1996; **31**: 117–34.

67. Swart GR, Frenkel M, and van den Berg JWO. Minimum portein requirements in advanced liver disease; a metabolic ward study of the effects of oral branched chain amino acids. In Walser M and Williamson JR, eds. *Metabolic and clinical implications of branched chain amino and ketoacids*. New York: Elsevier/North Holland, 1981: 427–32.

68. Capocaccia L, Fischer JE, and Rossi-Fanellis F, eds. *Hepatic encephalopathy in chronic liver failure*. New York: Plenum Press, 1984.

69. Driscoll DF, Palombo JD, and Bistrian BR. Nutritional and metabolic considerations of the adult liver transplant candidates and organ donor. *Nutrition*, 1995; 11: 255–63.

70. Runyon BA. Treatment of patients with cirrhosis and ascites. *Seminars in Liver Disease*, 1997; 17: 249–60.

71. Morgan MY. Branched chain amino acids in the management of chronic liver disease: facts and fantasies. *Journal of Hepatology*, 1990; 11: 133–41.

29.3 Drug treatment in patients with liver disease

Johannes Bircher and Waltraud Sommer

Introduction

Although relatively few drugs are currently available for the specific treatment of hepatic disorders, patients with liver disease often suffer from other conditions requiring drug treatment. In either case the liver plays a central role in drug disposition. Since most commonly used drugs are relatively lipophilic their elimination is dependent on biotransformation, a hepatic function which is often disturbed in liver disease (Bircher, SemLivDis, 1983; 3:275). Depending on the severity of the disease, physiological changes may also occur in other organ systems. As a result, the pharmacodynamic response to drugs may be increased, decreased, or changed in other ways. Consequently, the benefit–risk ratio of specific treatments may be markedly altered in such patients. In order to unravel such complex changes in individual cases, it is necessary to consider not only the specific physiological alterations induced by different liver diseases, but also the different mechanisms responsible for the specific pharmacological effects of each drug. Although incomplete, much work has been accomplished in this field in the past 20 years. It is therefore possible to combine clinical observations with modern pharmacological concepts in order to draw reasonable inferences about how to proceed in individual patients with liver disease. Several excellent reviews may be consulted.[1-4]

Relation between liver physiology and drug disposition (see also Chapters 2.4 and 2.5)

Relative hepatic and renal contribution to total drug clearance

Most drugs are cleared by both the liver and the kidneys but, depending on their lipophilicity, the relative contributions of the two organs to their removal varies enormously (Fig. 1). Water solubility (hydrophilicity) is a necessary condition for renal excretion. When urine is concentrated within the renal tubules lipophilic drugs diffuse back to the blood across the tubular epithelium.

The relative contribution of the renal clearance (Cl_{renal}) to the total clearance (Cl_{total}) may be estimated from the fraction of an intravenous dose which appears unchanged in the urine. The relative contribution of the extrarenal metabolic clearance, which is

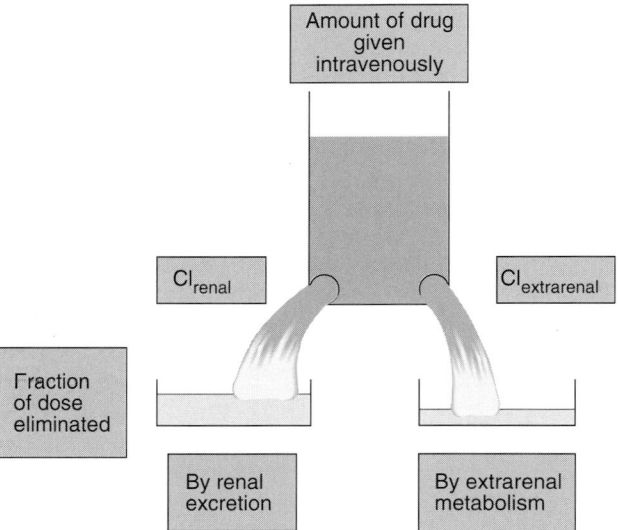

Fig. 1. The total clearance is the sum of the renal (Cl_{renal}) and the extrarenal clearance ($Cl_{extrarenal}$). The relative contribution of the renal clearance to the total clearance may be estimated from the fraction of an intravenous dose which is eliminated by renal excretion (f_{renal}), that appears as unchanged drug in the urine. The fraction eliminated by extrarenal metabolism corresponds to the difference between the dose and f_{renal} ($f_{extrarenal} = 1-f_{renal}$). If there is no extrahepatic metabolism, the extrarenal fraction represents hepatic metabolism. Under these circumstances the relative contribution of the liver ($Cl_{hepatic}$) to the total drug elimination (Cl_{total}) may be estimated as $Cl_{hepatic} = Cl_{total}-Cl_{renal}$. These relationships should be kept in mind when interpreting the data of Table 2.

mostly hepatic ($Cl_{hepatic}$), is then one minus this renal elimination fraction (see Table 2).

The simple relationship between extrarenal and renal clearance clearly shows that a reduction in hepatic clearance is only important for drug disposition if the hepatic clearance is a major fraction of total clearance. Thus, the disposition of drugs such as benzyl-penicillin or aminoglycosides, which are eliminated almost exclusively by the kidneys, is not affected if the metabolic capacity or the perfusion of the liver are disturbed. Similarly, alterations in liver physiology do not affect drugs which are metabolized extrahepatically. Such changes, however, determine the fate of compounds which are eliminated primarily by hepatic metabolism (see

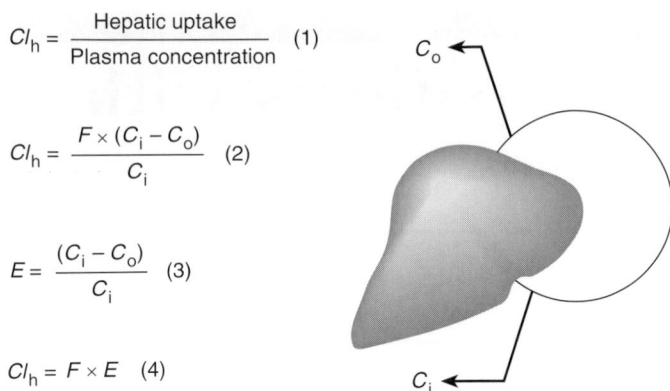

$$Cl_h = \frac{\text{Hepatic uptake}}{\text{Plasma concentration}} \quad (1)$$

$$Cl_h = \frac{F \times (C_i - C_o)}{C_i} \quad (2)$$

$$E = \frac{(C_i - C_o)}{C_i} \quad (3)$$

$$Cl_h = F \times E \quad (4)$$

Fig. 2. The relationship between hepatic blood flow and metabolic capacity becomes most apparent by considering the classical concept of hepatic clearance (Cl_h), which is the ratio of hepatic uptake (e.g. in μmol /min) to the inflowing plasma concentration (C_i in μmol/l, equation 1). Hepatic uptake is calculated as the product of plasma flow (F, in ml/min) and the difference in plasma concentration between the blood flowing into (C_i) and out (C_o) of the liver. In equation 2 the expression ($C_i - C_o$)/C_i corresponds to the definition of the hepatic extraction (E, equation 3). Consequently, the hepatic clearance may also be expressed as the product of flow and extraction (equation 4). From these relationships the following conclusions may be drawn: (1) If the metabolic capacity of the liver for a specific drug is very high, the hepatic extraction tends toward a value close to 1.0 (or 100 per cent), and the hepatic clearance is mainly determined by hepatic blood flow. (2) If the metabolic capacity is small, the hepatic extraction ratio tends toward a value close to zero (i.e. 0.1 to 30 per cent) and both flow and extraction may determine hepatic clearance.

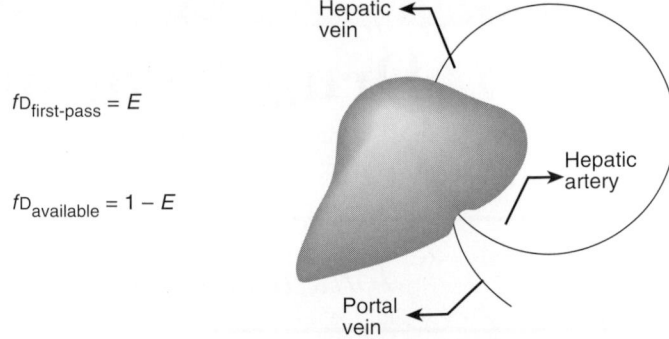

$$fD_{\text{first-pass}} = E$$

$$fD_{\text{available}} = 1 - E$$

Fig. 3. When drugs are given by mouth the whole dose reaches the liver through the portal vein and is subjected to 'first-pass' elimination. The fraction of the dose (fD) taken up by the liver during the first passage ($fD_{\text{first-pass}}$) corresponds for most of the drugs to the hepatic extraction (E, Fig. 2). Consequently, the fraction of the dose ($fD_{\text{available}}$) reaching the hepatic vein and corresponding to the systemic availability equals $1-E$. First-pass elimination may increase by enzyme induction and decrease by reduction of the metabolic capacity of the liver or by portal–systemic shunting. The systemic availability correspondingly changes in the opposite direction. In order to appreciate the potential role of altered first-pass elimination in liver disease, the hepatic extraction by the normal liver has been estimated from published data for many drugs and listed in Table 2.

Chapter 2.5). If functional renal failure accompanies hepatic failure, the renal clearance of a drug will also be correspondingly reduced.

These concepts are clinically important only for drugs which are pharmacologically active as such and which are transformed by the liver into inactive metabolites. Analogous considerations for drugs with pharmacologically active metabolites are currently too complex to be considered here (see Table 2).

Hepatic clearance of drugs

Hepatic handling of foreign compounds depends on hepatic blood flow, exchange between sinusoids and hepatocytes, hepatocellular uptake, cellular metabolism, and biliary excretion of the compounds. All of these factors may be abnormal to varying degrees in different liver diseases and may affect drug disposition in ways which depend on the type of physiological alteration and on the pharmacokinetic properties of the drugs. For clinical purposes, consideration of circulatory and metabolic changes are of prime importance (Fig. 2).

The clearance definition, as detailed in Fig. 2, shows that for drugs with a hepatic extraction close to 1.0 (or 100 per cent) hepatic clearance approaches blood flow. In real life there are no drugs with an extraction of 100 per cent, but only with a high extraction varying between 70 and 98 per cent. Nevertheless, for such compounds hepatic blood flow is the main determinant of hepatic clearance, and alterations of liver perfusion due to disease will change hepatic elimination of such compounds.

For drugs with low hepatic extraction, that is between 1 and 30 per cent, the above equations predict that both hepatic blood flow and extraction may be important. However, more detailed pharmacokinetic analyses (Wilkinson, ClinPharmTher, 1976; 18: 377; Winkler, ScaJGastr, 1979; 14:439) reveal that the metabolic capacity of the liver is the most relevant factor and that the contribution of hepatic blood flow may be neglected. Consequently, in patients with liver disease changes in metabolic capacity, rather than in liver blood flow, will be the major determinants of the rate of elimination of foreign compounds with a low hepatic extraction. The intact hepatocyte theory implies that a decrease in metabolic capacity in liver diseases does not result primarily from reduced function of each liver cell but from a reduced number of 'intact' hepatocytes (Branch, ClinPharmTher, 1976; 20:81). Whether or not this theory is valid probably depends on the type of liver disease.

The metabolism of drugs with an intermediate extraction, that is between 30 and 70 per cent, will be influenced by both blood flow and metabolic capacity.

First-pass elimination of drugs

When medicines are given by mouth, they reach the liver from the small bowel through the portal vein and are subjected to a 'first-pass effect' (Fig. 3). Ordinary dosage recommendations for drugs with a high extraction and a correspondingly substantial first-pass elimination take these losses into account. The proposed doses are usually much higher for the oral than for the parenteral route. In patients with liver disease such drugs carry a special risk. First-pass elimination may be reduced as a result of either decreased metabolic capacity of the liver or of portal–systemic shunting. In both cases, ordinary oral doses may result in serious toxicity, for example after ergotamine tartrate (Hanstein, EurJClinPharm, 1979; 16:425). These considerations apply to first-pass elimination only in regard to the liver. How liver disease affects first-pass metabolism by the intestinal mucosa is unknown.

Protein binding of drugs

In addition to blood flow and metabolic capacity, binding of drugs to plasma proteins may influence the rate of drug disposition by the liver. In principle, two situations may be distinguished. 'Restrictive' extraction of drugs by the liver implies that elimination from plasma is restricted to the free or unbound fraction of the drug. In contrast, 'non-restrictive' extraction implies that the liver clears plasma not only of the free but also of the protein-bound drug. The concept of restrictive and non-restrictive extraction is useful in practice but does not help us to understand the underlying physiological mechanisms. For practical purposes non-restrictive extraction is important only for drugs that have a high hepatic extraction and are therefore subject to a blood-flow-dependent clearance. This situation has already been described. In contrast, restrictive extraction is pertinent for drugs with a low extraction and points to an additional factor which may limit hepatic drug disposition. It is generally assumed that the sinusoidal cell membranes of hepatocytes are exposed only to the free concentration of a drug, which may be markedly influenced by protein binding. Reductions in protein binding due to liver disease becomes more important the higher the fraction bound, for example a change in binding from 98 to 96 per cent represents a doubling of the free concentration, whereas a change from 80 to 78 per cent represents only a 10 per cent increase in the free concentration of a drug.

Relation between liver physiology and pharmacodynamic drug actions

Pharmacological effects depend not only on the concentrations of free drugs in the relevant target tissues, but also on the physiological states of these tissues. These may be altered in liver disease and result either in hypo- or hyper-responsiveness. Some well described examples are as follows:

1. Disproportionate pharmacodynamic responses of the central nervous system have been observed in advanced cirrhosis with the benzodiazepine triazolam (Baktir, Hepatol, 1987; 7:629) and qualitatively abnormal results with diazepam (Branch, Gut, 1976; 17:975). Analogous abnormalities may also be inferred for other benzodiazepines, and for barbiturates and opiates.
2. Resistance to diuretics is a well-known complication of cirrhosis and the relative success of aldosterone antagonists depends on the degree of secondary hyperaldosteronism (Perèz-Ayuso, Gastro, 1983; 84:961).
3. Non-steroidal anti-inflammatory drugs (e.g. indomethacin) are more antidiuretic in cirrhotics with water retention than in subjects with normal renal physiology because they interfere with an important compensatory diuretic mechanism, that is the synthesis of prostaglandin E_2 (Laffi, Gastro, 1986; 90:182).
4. Angiotensin converting enzyme inhibitors have been used in cirrhotics in an attempt to prevent secondary hyperaldosteronism and to improve water retention. However, captopril dramatically lowered the blood pressure and had to be withdrawn (Daskalopoulos, JHepatol, 1987; 4:330).
5. Gentamicin nephrotoxicity is increased in patients with hepatic cirrhosis (Cabrera, Gastro, 1982; 82:97; Moore, AnnIntMed, 1984; 100:352) and in rats with extrahepatic cholestasis (Vakil,

Hepatol, 1989; 9:519). In this animal model, pretreatment with calcium, but not concurrent calcium administration, prevented this increase in nephrotoxicity.

Clinical conditions with altered physiological states relevant to drug disposition (Table 1)

Alterations of the metabolic capacity

Reductions in the metabolic capacity of the liver are not related to the aetiology of liver disease but to its severity. Consequently, the most severe reduction in metabolic capacity is found in fulminant hepatic failure (Saunders, BMJ, 1981; 282:263). Very dramatic reductions also occur in alcoholic hepatitis (Schneider, Gastro, 1980; 79:1145). In cirrhosis the Pugh score may be taken as a rough index of liver function, an increasing score indicating decreases in metabolic capacity. In general, a value of 8 or more suggests a severe reduction, to 30 per cent or less, of the normal metabolic capacity of the liver (Villeneuve, Hepatol, 1987; 7:660). In individual cases, however, the predictive value of the Pugh score may be limited.

A milder reduction in the metabolic capacity, of varying degree, may occur in patients with compensated cirrhosis. Furthermore, the metabolic capacity of the liver has been reported to be diminished in cholestasis and in hypothyroidism.

Slow metabolizers of debrisoquine and sparteine lack cytochrome P-450 2D6, an enzyme which is responsible for biotransformation of a whole group of drugs. Accordingly, the metabolism of most anti-arrhythmic drugs, several β-blockers, and tricyclic antidepressants may be very slow in such individuals (Secor, AdvIntMed, 1987; 32:379; Brosen, EurJClinPharm, 1989; 36:537). Interestingly, quinidine strongly inhibits the function of cytochrome P-450 2D6 and thereby transiently transforms phenotypically extensive metabolizers into slow metabolizers; the effect lasts for several days.

Inhibition of drug-metabolizing enzymes may occur in otherwise normal livers; this will reduce their metabolic capacity for foreign compounds. The inhibition may be relatively non-specific and result from concomitant administration of cimetidine, disulfiram, ethanol, ketoconazole, oral contraceptive steroids, or verapamil. In contrast, erythromycin and some other macrolide antibiotica specifically inhibit metabolism by cytochrome P-450 3A4 including, for example, the disposition of theophylline. Similarly, elimination of caffeine and theophylline metabolized by cytochrome P-450 1A2 may be affected by certain quinolone antibiotics, particularly enoxacin but also to some extent ciprofloxacine.

The metabolic capacity of the liver may also be increased, for example in mild hyperthyroidism and in acromegaly. More frequently enzyme induction increases only the drug-metabolizing enzymes. The most important enzyme inducers are phenobarbital, phenytoin, carbamazepine, and rifampicin. Chronic ingestion of ethanol also induces cytochrome P-450 2E1. Due to the inhibitory effects of ethanol itself, this enzyme induction becomes clinically most relevant during the first few days after alcohol withdrawal. These mechanisms increase the clearance of drugs which are primarily eliminated by this cytochrome. The effect of smoking on drug metabolism involves primarily the *CYP1* gene family and

Table 1 Clinical conditions with altered physiological states of the liver

Alterations of the metabolic capacity

Severe reductions
  Fulminant hepatic failure
  Decompensated cirrhosis of any aetiology
  Severe acute or chronic hepatitis of any aetiology
  Severe congestive heart failure (NYHA III/IV)
  Slow metabolism of sparteine, debrisoquine, and related drugs, either genetically or by inhibition after administration of quinidine

Mild reductions
  Old age
  Acute phase reactions
  Compensated cirrhosis
  Cholestasis of any cause
  Hypothyroidism
  Relatively non-specific enzyme inhibition by compounds such as cimetidine, disulfiram, ethanol, ketoconazole, oral contraceptives, verapamil
  Inhibition of specific enzymes, e.g. erythromycin and quinolone antibiotics for theophylline metabolism

Mild increases
  Hyperthyroidism, acromegaly
  Relatively non-specific enzyme induction by high protein diet, broiled meat, and brussel sprouts
  Relatively non-specific enzyme induction by phenobarbital, phenytoin, carbamazepine, rifampicin, chronic alcohol ingestion
  Relatively specific enzyme induction by smoking which accelerates theophylline metabolism for example

Changes in liver blood flow

Reductions
  Decompensated cirrhosis
  Portal or hepatic vein thrombosis
  Congenital hepatic fibrosis
  Congestive heart failure
  Treatment with β-adrenoceptor antagonists
  Hypothyroidism
  Postoperative state
  Firm liver of any cause (e.g. polycystic disease)

Increases
  After each meal
  Hyperthyroidism
  Arterioportal fistula

Portal–systemic shunting
  Portal hypertension of any cause

increases the elimination of caffeine and theophylline. In patients with early cirrhosis, enzyme induction may return an otherwise reduced metabolic capacity of the liver to normal, whereas in end-stage disease the effects of enzyme inducers are minimal.

Slowly-progressive, space-occupying lesions do not, *per se*, affect the metabolic capacity of the liver. Polycystic and hydatid disease of the liver are associated with a normal liver cell mass, even when the changes are massive. Similarly, hepatocellular carcinomas arising in otherwise normal livers do not impair liver function. In contrast, rapidly progressive lesions, such as hepatic metastases, are usually associated with reductions in the functioning liver cell mass.

Alterations in liver blood flow

There are two ways in which the effective blood flow may be reduced. They may occur independently or in combination. The first is a reduction of total flow to the liver; the second occurs when part of the blood flowing through the liver bypasses hepatic parenchyma via intrahepatic portal–systemic shunts. In the latter case, measurements of total blood flow are not helpful for understanding the mechanisms of hepatic clearance. In addition, hepatic extraction may not represent the functional capacity of the perfused liver parenchyma. To date, no non-invasive methods are available for measuring portal–systemic shunts and there is still controversy as to whether total or parenchymal flow should be assessed. For drug disposition, parenchymal flow is probably more pertinent. It can be measured non-invasively, for example by the sorbitol clearance technique (Zeeh, Gastro, 1988; 95:749), and is likely to be representative also of the disposition of other endo- and xenobiotics with high hepatic extraction.

Severe reductions in total liver blood flow occur primarily in congestive heart failure (NYHA III/IV), and in the Budd–Chiari syndrome. Lesser abnormalities may be seen postoperatively, in hypothyroidism and after portal vein thrombosis. Liver blood flow is also reduced in patients who are treated by β-adrenoceptor antagonists. Whenever, by palpation, a firm liver is found, irrespective of its cause, a reduction in portal flow and consequently in total perfusion of the liver, may be inferred. Since the portal bed is a low-pressure system, normal portal flow is dependent on normal compliance of the liver. Consequently, a clinically firm liver implies increased resistance to portal flow.

In alcoholic cirrhosis, intrahepatic portal–systemic shunts may lead to major discrepancies between measurements of total and

Table 2 Pharmacokinetic data, which may be used for dosage adjustment in patients with liver disease

Drug[1]	Estimated hepatic[2] extraction (%)[2]	Terminal half-lives (h)[3]		Fraction eliminated by extrarenal clearance[4] (%)
		Health	Liver disease	
Acebutolol	20	2.7	–	60
Acetylsalicylate*	50	0.3	–	99
Acyclovir	4	2.4		25
Alfentanil	20	4	5	100
Allopurinol*	55	0.8	–	92
Alprazolam*	5	11	20	85
Alprenolol	79	2.5	–	100
Amiloride	9	21	33	20
Amitriptyline*	65	16	38	98
Amoxicillin	5	1.0	–	25
Amphotericin B	2	360	–	97
Ampicillin	3	1.3	1.9	10
Amylobarbitone	7	21	39	100[a]
Antipyrine*	3	10	27	95[a]
Atenolol	1	5.0	6.0	10
Atropine	40	2.2	–	45
Azapropazone	1	12	62	38
Aztreonan	2	1.9	3.2	38
Betaxolol	25	12	–	99
Bromazepam	4	12	–	100
Bromocriptine	95	35	–	100
Bumetanide	4	1.1	2.3	36
Bunazosin	50	5.3	7.9	96
Buspirone*	90	2	6	100
Caffeine	4	5.2	6.1	80[a]
Captopril	33	1.9	–	50
Carbamazepine[b]*	7	15	–	99
Carvcdilol	80	5	9	99
Cefotaxim	15	0.8	2.4	40
Cefotaxime*	9	1.2	2.3	46
Cefprozil	12	1.3	2.2	35
Ceftazidime	0	1.6	–	16
Ceftriaxon	2	7	–	50
Cefuroxime	0	1.8	1.1	9
Cephalothin	2	0.8	0.9	60
Cephazolin	5	2.6	1.8	20
Cephoperazone	4	1.5	4.5	79
Cetirizin	2	9	14	30
Chloramphenicol	11	4.6	11	90
Chlordiazepoxide*	1	24	63	100[a]
Chlormethiazole	76	6.6	8.7	95[a]
Chloroquine	25	214	–	45
Chlorthalidone	3	44	–	35
Cimetidine	16	1.9	2.2	43
Ciprofloxacin	15	4.0	–	50
Clarithromycin*	40	3.5	5	75
Clindamycin	15	3.4	4.5	90[a]
Clofibrate	1	18	19	90
Clonazepam	8	23	–	99
Clonidine	1	8.5	–	38
Clotiazepam	17	10	10	100[a]
Cyclobarbital	3	13	35	100[a]
Cyclosporin	20	6.2	20	99
Desipramin	60	22	–	100
Desmethyldiazepam	1	51	108	100[a]
Dexamethasone	20	2.5	4	95
Diazepam*	2	47	105	100[a]
Dicloxacillin	5	0.9	–	44
Digitoxin	1	187	168	78
Digoxin	3	39	–	40
Dihydroergotamine	95	15	–	97
Diltiazem	58	3.2	–	96
Diphenhydramine	50	9.3	15	98
Dirithromycin	25	42**	74.7**	95
Disopyramide*	3	6.0	–	45
Doxepin*	74	17	–	100
Doxycycline	2	16	–	59

Table 2 continued

Drug[1]	Estimated hepatic[2] extraction (%)	Terminal half-lives (h)[3]		Fraction eliminated by extrarenal clearance[4] (%)
		Health	Liver disease	
Enalaprilat	1	35	–	60
Ergotamine	95	20	–	95
Erythromycin	37	1.4	2.2	87
Ethambutol	10	3.1	–	21
Ethosuximide	1	45	–	75
Famciclovir*[f]	10	2.3	2.5	<35
Famotidine	8	2.9	3.4	28
Fazadinium	6	1.4	2.6	50
Fentanyl	53	4.4	5.1	94
Flosequinan*	40	1.7	21	98
Flucytosine	1	4.2	–	3
Flumazenil	68	1.0	–	100
Flunarizine	33	96	–	100
Flunitrazepam*	10	29	–	100
Fluorouracil	82	0.2	–	97
Frusemide	2	1.2	2.2	24
Gemfibrozil	5	1.5	2.1	100
Gentamicin	0	53	–	10
Haloperidol	55	20	–	100
Hexobarbital	17	5.7	17	97
Hydrochlorothiazide	2	10	–	5
Ibuprofen	2	2.2	2.6	40
Imipramine*	77	18	–	98
Indomethacin	9	2.4	–	85
Isoniazid	14	1.1	–	71
Isosorbide dinitrate	90	0.8	–	99
Isosorbide 5-mononitrate	7	4.9	5.4	80[a]
Isradipin	80	5.1	11.9	100
Labetalol	80	5.2	–	95
Lidocaine*	72	1.5	1.6	96
Lincomycin*	4	4.9	8.9	60[a]
Lorazepam	4	22	32	100[a]
Lorcainide*	75	7.7	13	100[a]
Maprotilin*	75	40	–	100
Mercaptopurine	45	0.9	–	78
Methadone	14	19	36	60[a]
Methicillin	16	0.4	–	38
Methohexital	63	1.4	3.7	100[a]
Methotrexate	1	10	–	6
Methyldopa	20	1.8	–	72
Metoclopramide	20	4.5	–	40
Metoprolol	60	4.2	7.2	86
Metronidazole	3	7.9	19.9	77
Mexiletine	35	9.9	29	80[a]
Mezlocillin	12	0.9	2.6	65
Midazolam	24	2.3	–	24
Morphine	77	2.5	2.2	90[a]
Nadolol	4	16	–	27
Nafcillin	24	1.0	1.2	60[a]
Naftopidil*	85	5.4	17	95
Naproxen	1	14	–	99
Nefazodone*	40	2.7**	11.5**	100
Netilmicin	1	2.3	–	15
Nifedipine	50	1.9	7.0	100[a]
Nitrazepam	5	26	–	99
Nitrendipine	90	6.3	–	100
Norpropoxyphene	–	17	–	80
Nortriptyline	37	31	–	98
Ofloxacin	5	5	8	75
Ondansetron	60	3	21	90
Oxacillin	21	0.7	–	57
Oxazepam	9	5.6	5.8	100
Pancuronium	5	1.9	3.5	54
Paracetamol	31	2.0	3.1	96
Pefloxacin	9	11	35	91
Pefloxacin	15	11	46	90
Penicillin G	9	0.7	–	21

Table 2 continued

Drug[1]	Estimated hepatic extraction (%)[2]	Terminal half-lives (h)[3]		Fraction eliminated by extrarenal clearance[4] (%)
		Health	Liver disease	
Pentazocin	89	3.8	6.6	96
Pethidine*	55	5.2	11	98
Phenobarbital	1	99	–	76
Phenprocoumone	1	106	74	99
Phenylbutazone*	1	88	97	100[a]
Phenytoin[c]	1–3	14–50	13	95
Pindolol	20	3.6	–	46
Piperacillin	4	0.9	–	29
Pirenzepine	9	11	14	60
Piroxicam	1	38	–	90
Prednisolone	9	3.4	3.3	100[a]
Primidone*	2	17	18	75
Propafenone*	60	5	–	100
Propoxyphene	80	3	–	98
Propranolol	80	2.9	7.7	100[a]
Quinidine*	21	6.0	9.0	80[a]
Ranitidine	2	2.7	2.8	30[a]
Rifampicin[b]	17	2.8	5.4	93
Salicylate[c]	5	2.5	–	80
Spirapril*	35	1.5	1.5	95
Streptomycin	1	5.3	–	61
Sulphamethoxazole	1	10	–	77
Temazepam	1	16	13	20
Theophylline*	1	7.7	65	23
Thiopental	21	8.8	12	100[a]
Tocainide	8	14	27	60[a]
Tolbutamide	2	5.9	4.0	100[a]
Toremifene*	7	6 Tage	11 Tage	100
Trapidil	30	1.5	2.5	100
Triamteren	80	4.0	–	95
Triazolam	20	3.9	9.7	100
Trimethoprim	2	11	–	45
Valporic acid	1	12	19	95[a]
Vancomycin	1	2.6	37	3[a]
Verapamil*	85[d]	3.7	14	100[a]
Warfarin*	1	25	23	100[a]
Ximoprofen	12	1.6	2.2	75
Zidovudine	85	0.5	1.8	90

Limitations of data:
[1] Drugs transformed into pharmacologically active metabolites are indicated by an asterisk, when clinically important (*). The fate of metabolites must also be considered, but often is poorly known.
[2] Most hepatic extractions are only indirect estimates and may therefore be inaccurate. They were obtained as ratios of the non-renal clearances to an assumed hepatic blood flow of 19 ml/min/kg body weight and validated with the bioavailability, where available.
[3] Half-lives in patients with liver disease are mean values. In individual cases, they may be much longer.
[4] The fraction of the dose eliminated by extrarenal clearance is due to hepatic clearance in a majority, but not in all cases.
[a] Data taken from Dettli L. *Pharmakokinetische Daten für die Dosisanpassung. Arzneimittel-Kompendium der Schweiz.* Basel: Documed, 1989; 12: 3389–97.
[b] Induces microsomal enzymes, values are given for the induced state.
[c] Non-linear kinetics: half-lives prolonged at higher plasma concentrations.
[d] Lower upon repeated dosing.
[f] Famciclovir is a prodrug for penciclovir. The data refer to penciclovir.

parenchymal liver blood flow, the latter being normal, increased, or more often decreased. In other forms of cirrhosis, intrahepatic portal–systemic shunting may be less important. Recent studies indicate that, whatever the origin of cirrhosis, parenchymal flow decreases later and to a lesser extent than the metabolic capacity of the liver. Consequently, there are no simple clinical criteria to predict liver blood flow. If, however, a patient has a small cirrhotic liver and the disease is decompensated, it is reasonable to assume that liver blood flow is severely reduced.

It has been well documented that patients with hyperthyroidism have an increased liver blood flow which returns to normal after treatment. Increased hepatic perfusion has also been seen in patients with arterioportal fistulas.

Portal–systemic shunting

After oral administration, the fate of drugs with a high hepatic extraction is markedly affected by portal–systemic shunting. The resulting pharmacokinetic alterations are independent of the ana-tomical site of the shunts, for example intrahepatic (portal–hepatic venous) or extrahepatic, for example oesophageal varices or spleno-renal. Unfortunately, there is not, as yet, a satisfactory clinical method available for the measurement of portal–systemic shunting. Consequently, the clinical significance of this abnormality is in-sufficiently known. It is generally accepted, however, that the presence of portal–systemic encephalopathy implies a very im-portant degree of shunting.

The main consequence of shunting is an increase in systemic availability of drugs, the extent varying markedly from patient to patient. Nevertheless, in general, the increase will be more im-portant the higher the extraction of the drug by the normal liver; for example a change in first-pass elimination from 66 to 33 per cent implies only a doubling of the bioavailability, whereas a reduction from 92 to 33 per cent represents an eight fold increase in systemic availability with a correspondingly larger potential for toxicity. Unfortunately, the hepatic extraction of most drugs has not been measured in man and must be inferred indirectly from other pharmacokinetic properties, particularly from non–renal clearance and systemic availability. Unfortunately, the latter is often not reported explicitly, particularly if it is low. Furthermore, the relative importance of the factors affecting bioavailability, such as inadequate absorption, intestinal, and hepatic first-pass effects, cannot readily be separated. For this reason the data in Table 1 must be regarded as approximations. They indicate, however, for which drugs there may be risks due to shunting.

Hepatorenal syndrome

Functional renal failure—a well known complication of advanced chronic liver disease—further affects drug disposition by reducing renal elimination mechanisms. As shown above, this is important only for the fraction of the dose cleared by renal excretion. It will, therefore, particularly affect the fate of compounds which leave the organism, to a large extent, by unchanged renal elimination (Table 2). For such drugs the principles of dosage adjustments for patients with renal failure must then be followed.

Dosage recommendations based on a pharmacokinetic risk classification of drugs

Since in most patients with liver disease the severity of physiological abnormalities cannot be measured, it is impossible to formulate quantitative dosage recommendations. Consequently, an optimal dosage regimen cannot be more than a rough guess followed by a process of trial and error. Initial doses must be estimated clinically and their inaccuracy accepted. Thereafter, it is necessary to assess pharmacological responses by all available means and to adjust subsequent doses in order to obtain optimal pharmacological effects.

Risk 1: overdosage by single oral doses (Fig. 4)

This risk concerns the group of 'high extraction' drugs, since serious toxicity may result from the first dose if it is given by mouth. The potential for toxicity is related to the fact that conventional dosage

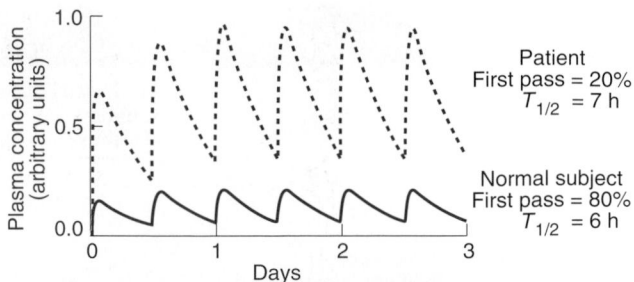

Fig. 4. Illustration of the pharmacokinetic risk which may occur with high extraction drugs (as detailed in Table 2 and Fig. 3). The assumptions are that in a normal subject the drug has a half-life of 6 h and an extraction of 80 per cent leading to a corresponding first-pass elimination. If such a patient has portal–systemic shunting such that the first-pass effect is reduced to 20 per cent and a hepatic blood flow which is not much reduced, leading to a half life of 7 h, the plasma concentrations after oral drug administration correspond to the interrupted line. It can be seen that already the first dose leads to a fourfold increase in plasma concentration and that subsequent doses further accentuate the potentially dangerous overdosage. Accordingly, when giving drugs with a high hepatic extraction, initial and repeated doses must be reduced.

recommendations take first-pass elimination by the normal liver into account. If, as a result of liver disease, first-pass elimination is reduced, an abnormally large fraction of the dose may become systemically available and lead to overdosage (the greater the hepatic extraction of a drug by the normal liver, the greater the fraction becoming systemically available in the presence of liver disease). A high extraction of a drug should be suspected when there is a large difference between the recommended oral and intravenous dose. Estimates of the hepatic extraction of various drugs are given in Table 2. Extractions above 50 per cent, and particularly above 70 per cent, are clinically pertinent. Consequently, dosage reductions should be planned accordingly.

Problems of systemic availability of this kind are not relevant for intravenous and intramuscular routes of drug administration.

Drugs with a low hepatic extraction are not subject to an important hepatic first-pass elimination. Consequently, portal–systemic shunting does not appreciably affect their fate and single doses need not be reduced. Generally, the purpose of single ('initial') doses is to 'fill up' the volume of distribution, which may be slightly enlarged in patients with liver disease because of ascites, but otherwise is affected to a lesser extent than the elimination processes.

Risk 2: overdosage after repeated administration (Fig. 5)

Obviously, dosage adjustments for increased bioavailability (as ex-plained above) are indispensable when a drug with a high extraction is administered repeatedly. In addition, however, attention must be paid to drug accumulation. The degree of accumulation is de-termined by the relationship between dosage interval and half-life of the drug. For instance, if both are equal, repeated administration will lead to a 'steady state' concentration which is approximately twice that following a single dose. More important drug ac-cumulation will occur if the half-life of a drug is much longer than

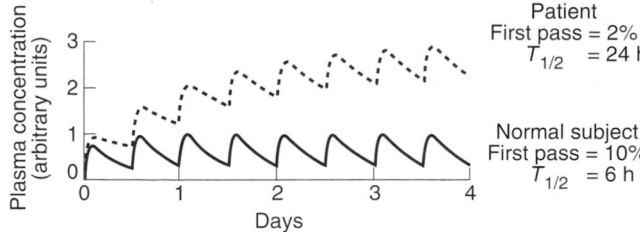

Fig. 5. Drugs with a low extraction show a different risk pattern. If a drug which normally has a half-life of 6 h is given twice a day, there is minimal accumulation (continuous line). When the metabolic capacity of the liver is reduced to 25 per cent because of the development of, for example, a cirrhosis, the half-life is presumably four times longer, that is 24 h. Yet, the bioavailability is not significantly increased. Single doses therefore are not followed by a clinically important increase in plasma concentration. Repeated dosing, however, leads to a significant degree of drug accumulation. Consequently, single doses of such drugs are not dangerous but repeated dosing renders dosage adjustments mandatory. For half-lives in cirrhosis see Table 2.

the dosage interval chosen by the physician. For a patient with liver disease, the risk of drug accumulation is therefore related to the degree of prolongation of the half-life which occurs in this case. Half-lives of drugs which have been studied in patients with liver disease are presented in Table 2. It should be noted, however, that the half-lives for patients with liver disease are mean values and that in many studies the severity of the liver disease was ill defined. Consequently in many patients with advanced disease, much more severe prolongations of terminal half-lives should be expected.

Risk 3: disproportionate pharmacological response

In general, the risks of toxicity due to disproportionate drug responses, as summarized in Table 3, depend on the extent of physiological abnormalities which prevail before the drugs are given. For instance, a patient with subclinical hepatic encephalopathy is more likely to respond excessively to sedatives than a patient with normal psychometric findings, and a patient with signs of water retention may become anuric, rather than oliguric after a dose of a non-steroidal anti-inflammatory drug. Unfortunately, the warning signs are often unapparent on routine clinical examination and can be detected only by special tests. In these instances disproportionate pharmacological responses may occur unexpectedly.

Drugs with low risks of overdosage

Drugs of this group are neither subject to significant pharmacokinetic abnormalities nor are they likely to produce a disproportionate pharmacological response in patients with liver disease. For these reasons they are obviously drugs of choice for hepatologists. Although they may be prescribed in normal doses, pharmacokinetic and pharmacodynamic variations still tend to be greater in patients with liver disease than in normal subjects. Consequently, even with this group of drugs, therapeutic effects must be monitored carefully and doses titrated individually.

The reasons why administration of drugs to patients with liver diseases may not be followed by excessive plasma concentrations are varied. Examples are as follows:

1. The fate of drugs which are mainly excreted by the kidneys without biotransformation is not altered as long as renal function remains normal. In Table 2 such drugs can be recognized from the small fraction of the dose eliminated by extrarenal clearance (20 per cent or less, e.g. atenolol, flucytosine, vancomycin).
2. Some drugs which are mainly glucuronidated are eliminated almost normally, even in severe liver disease, since glucuronidation may also take place extrahepatically and generally remains relatively well preserved in liver disease. Examples are morphine (Raschmi, Gastro, 1981; 81:1006), oxazepam (Shull, AnnIntMed, 1976; 84:420), and lorazepam (Kraus, ClinPharmTher, 1978; 24:411). Excessive pharmacological effects may, however, still occur due to hypersensitivity of the central nervous system to these drugs (Table 3).
3. An increased free fraction of the drug in plasma may facilitate hepatic clearance and thereby compensate for the decrease in metabolic capacity of the liver. This may be important, for example for phenprocoumon, temazepam, tolbutamide, or valproic acid.
4. The administered prodrug itself is pharmacologically inactive and the plasma concentrations of the pharmacologically active metabolite achieves 'normal' levels. In patients with liver disease, not only may the elimination of the pharmacologically active metabolite be slowed, but also its formation. A well documented example is encainide (Bergstrand, ClinPharmTher, 1986; 40: 148).
5. Other instances, such as clofibrate and methadone, remain unexplained.

Table 3 Altered pharmacological response in patients with liver disease	
Increased responsiveness ('hypersensitivity')	
Sedation:	Triazolam, probably all benzodiazepines, morphine, probably m-agonists, barbiturates
Antidiuresis:	Indomethacin and probably most non-steroidal anti-inflammatory drugs
Kaliuresis:	Loop diuretics
Hypotension:	Angiotensin-converting enzyme inhibitors
Decreased responsiveness ('hyposensitivity')	
Diuresis:	Benzothiadiazide and loop diuretics
Cardiovascular:	β-blockers
Increased toxicity	
Renal toxicity:	Aminoglycoside antibiotics

Table 4 Protein binding of drugs in healthy subjects and in liver disease		
Drug	**Fraction bound (%)**	
	Health	**Liver disease**
Alprazolam	71.0	76.8
Amylobarbitone	61.0	31.0
Azapropazone	99.6	93.9
Caffeine	31.3	25.2
Cephalothin	75.9	73.5
Cephazolin	88.6	72.3
Chlordiazepoxide	96.5	94.6
Chlormethiazole	64.4	55.8
Clindamycin	79.2	79.0
Clofibrate	97.2	92.8
Cyclophosphamide	12.5	12.5
Diazepam	97.8	95.3
Digitoxin	95.6	95.1
Diphenhydramine	78.1	66.7
Encainide	70.0	76.0
Erythromycin	69.5	42.7
Furosemide	96.0	89.8
Furosemide	95.6	93.5
Lorazepam	93.2	88.6
Lorcainide	83.3	80.5
Meperidine	58.3	56.0
Meperidine	64.3	64.9
Mexiletine	51.0	45.0
Morphine	19.8	16.0
Nifedipine	95.6	91.5
Nitrendipine	97.9	97.0
Oxazepam	89.3	87.6
Phenprocoumone	99.2	98.9
Phentytoin	90.3	87.4
Prednisone	77.0	69.0
Propoxyphene	76.0	69.0
Quinidine	77.0	64.0
Salicylate	91.5	81.4
Temazepam	96.1	93.4
Theophylline	65.0	29.0
Thiopental	85.5	74.8
Valporic acid	88.7	70.7
Warfarin	98.8	98.8

Therapeutic blood level monitoring

For a number of drugs with a small therapeutic index, it has become common practice to measure blood levels. In general, they will indicate if, for any reason, there is too much or too little drug in the blood. Since the concentration of free (i.e. not protein bound) drug is assumed to be in equilibrium with the tissue, it would be best to measure the concentration of free drug. However, for technical reasons the total concentration, that is the free plus the bound fraction, is measured. In patients with liver disease, protein binding of many drugs is often decreased (Table 4). This leads to a poorly predictable downward shift of the therapeutic range of blood levels, thereby complicating interpretation of the results. Lowered protein binding of drugs results either from a decrease in plasma albumin or an increase in competing ligands such as bilirubin and bile acids, for example in cholestasis or in advanced liver disease.

Changes in the therapeutic range in liver disease must be considered for drugs with relatively high protein binding, such as digitoxin, phenytoin, quinidine, tricyclic antidepressants, and valproic acid. There is no change in the therapeutic range in liver disease for aminoglycoside antibiotics, digoxin, or theophylline.

Cyclosporin

Cyclosporin is an example of a drug which exhibits many pharmacokinetic abnormalities in patients with liver disease. For example, the absorption of cyclosporin is heavily dependent on the presence of bile acids in the duodenum. Consequently, postoperative drainage of bile by an open T-tube dramatically impairs oral bioavailability of cyclosporin (Burckart, TransplProc, 1986; 18:129; Mehta, BrJClinPharm, 1988; 25:579). In such cases, the drug should be given intravenously.

In the plasma, cyclosporin is transported mainly by lipoproteins, and only 22 per cent remains in lipoprotein-deficient plasma obtained after ultracentrifugation (Gurecki, TransplProc, 1985; 17:1997). Consequently, changes in lipoprotein composition may affect the relation between the cyclosporin content and its pharmacologically active fraction. Cyclosporin is transformed to a large number of metabolites, which may accumulate in plasma (Sewing, BiblCardiol, 1988; 43:63; Christians, ClinChem, 1988; 34:34). A polyclonal radioimmunoassay cross reacts with some of these metabolites and therefore gives much higher values than measurements of cyclosporin by high pressure liquid chromatography (**HPLC**) (Keown, TransplProc, 1986; 18:160; Sewing, DMedWoch, 1988; 113:311). Although the pharmacological activity of the metabolites is not known in sufficient detail, it is generally assumed that they contribute relatively little to the immunosuppression (Wang, TransplProc, 1988; 20:591). Consequently, either a specific radioimmunoassay or HPLC should be used to monitor cyclosporin itself. This is particularly relevant after liver transplantation, when metabolism of cyclosporin may be disturbed and the relation between total immunoreactivity and cyclosporin measured by HPLC may be changed (Keown, TransplProc, 1986; 18:160; Sewing, DMedWoch, 1988; 113:311). Total body clearance may be markedly reduced in patients with liver failure and the half-life is correspondingly prolonged (Burckart, TransplProc, 1986; 18:129) (Table 2).

Unresolved problems

For drugs which are transformed into pharmacologically active metabolites, the fate of these metabolites must be taken into consideration. This has been well documented, for example in the case of diazepam and desmethyldiazepam. The latter has a much longer half-life than the former and tends to accumulate much more, particularly in cirrhotics with decreased metabolic capacity (Ochs, EurJClinPharm, 1986; 30:89).

For many years, it was hoped that drug clearance by the liver could become quantitatively predictable on the basis of some simple tests. Unfortunately, this goal has not, as yet, been achieved. The heterogeneity of drug-metabolizing enzymes with partly overlapping substrate specificities and their complex genetic and environmental regulation have remained almost insurmountable obstacles. Even in normal subjects these factors contribute to important interindividual variations in drug response and have rendered careful individualization of drug dosing necessary (see

Chapter 2.5). In view of these limitations every effort should be made to match each patient's therapy to his individual needs.

Some of the factors affecting the fate of drugs interact in a complex manner rendering any prediction impossible. Cholestasis is a good example. In general, cholestasis leads to a mild reduction in metabolic capacity. It may also be associated with a decrease in protein binding. For a highly protein-bound drug the final result may be a decrease, no change, or even an increase in overall drug clearance.

Treatment of specific medical conditions

Pain

Paracetamol in doses of 1 g twice to four times daily is the drug of choice for ordinary pain in adult patients with normal body weight. Even in patients with advanced cirrhosis the half-life of paracetamol is short enough to prevent significant accumulation, if a twice daily dosage is not exceeded. The risk of paracetamol hepatotoxicity appears not to be increased in patients with liver disease, except in alcoholics and those with other toxic damage to the liver. Aminotransferase levels should be followed regularly, although it may be difficult to relate changes in aminotransferase levels to paracetamol administration if they are elevated due to the liver disease itself.

Codeine in doses of 30 mg three times daily is an alternative to paracetamol, or it may be combined with 0.5 g doses of paracetamol. Its analgesic properties result from its metabolism to morphine, a metabolic pathway which is lacking in approximately 10 per cent of Caucasians who are slow metabolizers of the debrisoquine/sparteine type. When given codeine, patients with cirrhosis must be evaluated regularly for possible oversedation.

Although morphine may be eliminated normally, even in patients with advanced cirrhosis, excessive sedation after morphine administration is well documented and should be avoided by appropriate dose reduction. Presumably the central nervous system of patients with advanced cirrhosis may be hypersensitive to μ-agonists (Table 3).

Administration of aspirin to patients with cirrhosis carries an important risk of gastric haemorrhage and it should therefore be avoided. Non-steroidal anti-inflammatory drugs which inhibit cyclo-oxygenase activity not only increase the risk of gastric complications, but may also cause deterioration of renal function, particularly in patients with fluid retention. If they cannot be avoided, a non-steroidal anti-inflammatory drug with a short half-life (such as diclofenac or ibuprofen) should be tried and fluid balance should be supervised closely.

Cirrhotics with migraine headaches are at risk of severe ergotism if they ingest ergotamine tartrate (Hansteen, EurJClinPharm, 1970; 6:426) or dihydroergotamine, because both drugs are normally subjected to a high degree of first-pass elimination by the liver (Table 2). Consequently, in the case of portal–systemic shunting bioavailability may be increased up to 10 or 20 fold. If one of these drugs is indicated, it should be started at perhaps one-tenth of the normal dose and then adjusted subsequently in accordance with the response of the patient.

Sedation

Although 'hypersensitivity' of the brain to benzodiazepines has been well documented in patients with advanced cirrhosis (Branch, Gut, 1976; 17:975; Baktir, Hepatol, 1987; 7:629), benzodiazepines are probably to be preferred to the older drugs, because they have been studied more extensively. To be on the safe side, small initial doses of a benzodiazepine with a short half-life should be chosen. Oxazepam, lorazepam, and lormetazepam are eliminated by glucuronidation, which remains relatively normal in liver disease (Table 2). Consequently, when one of these three drugs is used the risk of prolonged sedation is decreased and adjustments of maintenance doses will become effective eventually. Other benzodiazepines are probably best avoided. In practice, 10 mg of oxazepam appears to be a reasonable first choice for oral dosing, and 0.2 mg of lormetazepam for intravenous administration. Further doses may then be adjusted according to the response of the patient. If oversedation becomes a clinical problem, it can be reversed by intravenous flumazenil (Klotz, ClinPharmacokin, 1988; 14:1).

Administration of neuroleptic and antidepressant drugs

Neuroleptic drugs exhibit a wide spectrum of pharmacological effects including sedation and antimuscarinic and antiadrenergic actions. With long-term administration different degrees of tolerance develop. In general, doses are titrated according to observed pharmacological effects. Since all neuroleptic drugs are eliminated mainly by hepatic metabolism, it is to be expected that their half-lives will be prolonged in patients with a reduced metabolic capacity of the liver, for example in cirrhosis. As a result, smaller maintenance doses are to be anticipated and the result of dosage adjustments will take longer than expected to become clinically apparent. These possible pharmacological changes in patients with liver disease call for caution. However, they influence neither the choice of neuroleptics nor the principle of dose titration.

Tri- and tetracyclic antidepressant drugs are also eliminated essentially by hepatic metabolism. For many of them their demethylated metabolites are equally effective as antidepressants but may be less sedative than the parent compound. In fact, excessive sedation has been noted in a patient with a portacaval shunt receiving amitriptyline (Hrdina, CanJPsychiat, 1985; 30:111). If antidepressants have to be given to patients with significant liver disease, it may be better to choose a demethylated compound such as nortriptyline or desipramine. In addition, in patients with established cirrhosis, it may be appropriate to initiate therapy with half of the usual dose, although firm quantitative recommendations cannot be given.

Tranylcypromine is a racemic mixture, the enantiomers of which are metabolized differently by the liver and also may contribute differently to pharmacological effects. In view of these complex conditions and of the lack of published experience, no recommendations for liver patients are possible.

Lithium administration to patients with cirrhosis of the liver may be uncomplicated, as long as the patient has normal renal function, no water retention, and is not in need of diuretics. Otherwise, the precautions established for such conditions are to be observed. Lithium therapy, however, may be associated with many adverse effects, which may be difficult to distinguish from consequences of the liver disease itself, for example reduced sexual potency, development of antinuclear antibodies, muscle weakness, tremor, and confusion.

Hypertension

Treatment of hypertension is usually started with a single drug. If necessary, combination therapy and increasing doses are prescribed. These principles apply also in patients with chronic liver disease, although with decompensated cirrhosis antihypertensive treatment is rarely needed. Most drugs may be prescribed with usual doses. Important exceptions, however, concern the calcium antagonists diltiazem, nifedipine, nitrendipine, and verapamil. These drugs have a first-pass elimination of 50 to 90 per cent and also exhibit prolonged half-lives in patients with cirrhosis of the liver (Table 2). Consequently, risks 1 and 2 apply and initial doses, as well as maintenance doses, should be started at one-half to one-quarter of the doses given to patients with normal livers.

The angiotensin-converting enzyme inhibitor enalapril is a model of a prodrug ester of the pharmacologically active agent. Its activation occurs in the liver and may be impaired in liver disease. Several newer drugs of this family are similar in this respect. Since angiotensin-converting enzyme inhibitors may interrupt regulatory mechanisms which tend to maintain blood pressure in cirrhosis, the administration of enalapril or captopril may result in excessive hypotension and should therefore be administered with the greatest caution (Table 3).

Antituberculous chemotherapy

In patients with cirrhosis, tuberculosis may be a relevant concomitant disease. Several important antituberculous drugs are metabolized by the liver and may also be hepatotoxic. Exceptions are streptomycin and ethambutol which are eliminated mainly by renal excretion and may be given in normal doses to patients with liver disease as long as renal function is adequate. Since the half-life of isoniazid is relatively short (1 and 3 h in rapid and slow acetylator phenotypes, respectively) compared to the conventional dosing interval of 24 h, drug accumulation will be minimal even if the metabolic capacity of the liver is reduced, and dosage adjustments for isoniazid are probably not essential. Nevertheless, it presumably is wise to choose relatively lower doses of 2 to 3, rather than 5 mg/kg per day. Generally, it is preferable to give divided smaller doses more frequently, that is two or three times daily, rather than a single large dose per day. Prophylactic administration of isoniazid is to be avoided. Maintenance doses of rifampicin, which is eliminated mainly by biliary excretion, must be reduced whenever serum bilirubin exceeds the upper limit of normal. In patients with severe liver impairments, doses of 6 to 8 mg/kg biweekly should not be exceeded (Curci, Chemother, 1973; 19:197). Pyrazinamide is usually given in single oral doses of 20 to 35 mg/kg per day, a dosage which is close to the limit of toxicity (increased aminotransferases or frank liver damage). In view of its relatively small margin of safety, pyrazinamide is to be avoided in patients with liver disease.

Treatment of common infections in outpatient departments

The most frequently used antibiotics in these situations are amino-penicillins (such as amoxicillin), the combination of sulpha-methoxazole and trimethoprim, doxycycline, and gyrase inhibitors such as ofloxacin or ciprofloxacin. Among these, amoxicillin is probably the safest choice for patients with advanced liver disease because it has a high therapeutic ratio and is excreted mainly by the kidneys (Table 2). Consequently, as long as renal function is maintained, ordinary doses of amoxicillin may be given. About 80 per cent of an oral dose of ofloxacin is eliminated by urinary excretion, and plasma protein binding is minimal. Advanced liver damage, therefore, will not substantially affect ofloxacin kinetics. This drug should therefore be given in ordinary doses, but patients should be supervised for possible central nervous system toxicity. Ciprofloxacin, sulphamethoxazole, and trimethoprim have renal elimination fractions of only 50, 25, and 50 per cent, respectively. If the renal function is normal and the metabolic capacity of the liver is moderately preserved, short-term administration of these drugs is unlikely to induce important toxicity, but in advanced cirrhosis some degree of accumulation appears unavoidable and should lead to a conservative dosing schedule. Tetracyclines have antianabolic properties and may therefore increase fatty changes in hepatocytes; in addition nitrogen balance may become negative and blood urea may increase (Gabuzda, ArchIntMed, 1958; 101:476; Shils, AnnIntMed, 1963; 58:389). These pharmacological effects are not desirable for patients with cirrhosis of the liver. Consequently, tetracyclines are to be avoided. To what extent similar considerations apply to moderate doses of the more modern tetracyclines such as doxycycline is not clear.

Oral contraceptives

Liver disease is generally considered to be a risk situation for the administration of oral contraceptive steroids. In particular, patients with recurrent cholestasis of pregnancy, Dubin-Johnson and Rotor syndrome may experience relapses or aggravations. Other drug-related effects are summarized in Section 17. In addition, some oestrogens and progestins used for oral contraception are subject to a significant first-pass metabolism in the liver and are eliminated from the systemic circulation mainly by hepatic metabolism. When there is portal–systemic shunting or a reduction of the metabolic capacity of the liver, plasma levels of the administered hormones are probably substantially higher than in persons with a normal liver. Excessive hormonal effects must therefore be feared. Since clinical evaluation of the metabolic capacity of the liver and of portal–systemic shunting is notoriously unreliable, it is difficult to assess the benefit/risk ratio of oral contraception in all patients with evidence for advanced cirrhosis or portal hypertension. In milder forms of liver disease this ratio probably is more favourable, and modern, low dose contraceptives are unlikely to create undue problems.

References

1. Bass NM and Williams RL. Guide to drug dosage in hepatic disease. *Clinical Pharmacokinetics*, 1988; **15**: 396–420.
2. Bircher J. Altered drug metabolism in liver disease—therapeutic implications. In McSween RNM and Thomas HC, eds. *Recent advances in hepatology*. London: Churchill Livingstone, 1983: 101–3.
3. Secor JW and Schenker S. Drug metabolism in patients with liver disease. *Advances in Internal Medicine*, 1987; **32**: 379–406.
4. Williams RL. Drug administration in hepatic disease. *New England Journal of Medicine*, 1983; **309**: 1616–22.

30

Surgery, anaesthesia, and the liver

30.1 General surgical aspects and the risks of liver surgery in patients with hepatic disease

Pietro E. Majno, Daniel Azoulay, and Henri Bismuth

Introduction

Although the first left lobectomy was performed by Caprio in 1932 and the first right hepatectomy by Lortat-Jacob and Robert in 1952, it is only since the publication of the remarkable anatomical works of Couinaud in 1957 that modern, anatomical liver surgery has evolved. The application of the segmental anatomy of the liver to surgery, made possible through the development of operative ultrasound, led to a new way of conceptualizing and performing liver resections.[1] During the past decade the principles of the segmental anatomy have been more widely applied. This, coupled with remarkable advances in techniques and tools, has allowed surgeons to perform resections with increasing safety and efficacy and to diminish the incidence of local complications such as per-operative bleeding, postoperative necrosis, and biliary fistula. Improved techniques of vascular control, in some cases derived directly from liver transplantation, have given access to the most awkwardly placed lesions.

The main challenge of contemporary liver surgery is the prediction, prevention, and treatment of postoperative liver insufficiency in patients in whom only massive resections can remove the tumuoral disease, and in patients with cirrhosis where the capacity for liver regeneration is greatly reduced. Techniques have been described for estimating preoperatively the risk of liver failure, allowing anatomical resections to be planed which preserve the maximum of functioning hepatic tissue. Experience has been gained in portal vein embolization, a technique to induce hypertrophy liver before the operation. Alternative methods of tumour destruction for deeply seated lesions, such as surgical cryotherapy, have been devised. The use of the bioartificial liver to provide temporary support to patients having undergone extensive liver resections appears as a concrete possibility.

The classification of liver resections

Hepatic resections can be divided into two broad categories:

1. *Anatomical resections* are performed following the segmental anatomy which identifies, according to the distribution of the

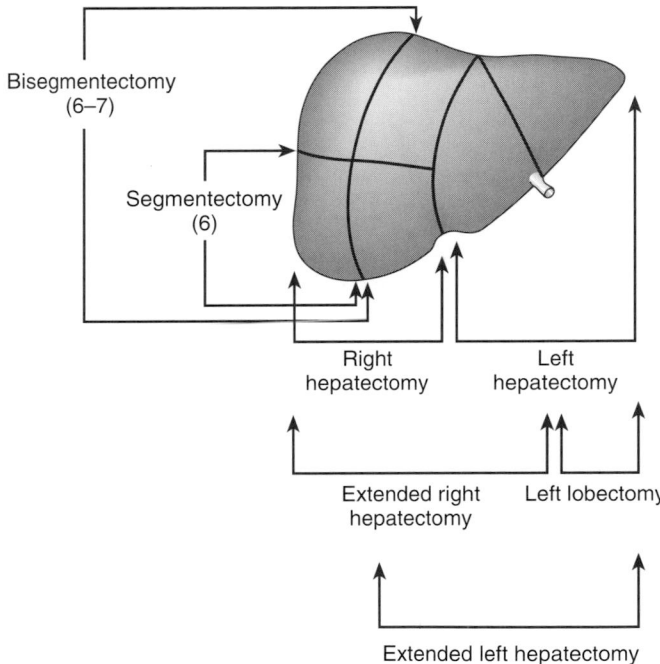

Fig. 1. Names of the anatomical hepatectomies according to the segmental anatomy. (By courtesy of Professor D. Castaing, Hepatobiliary Foundation, Hôpital Paul Brousse, Villejuif, Paris.)

branches of the portal vein and of the hepatic veins, eight segments, four sectors, and two livers (see Chapter 1.1). The names of the different types of resections according to the segmental anatomy are given in Fig. 1.

2. *Atypical resections* are not guided by the intrahepatic vascular anatomy.

The anatomical (or typical) hepatectomies can be divided according to the number of segments resected into minor or limited hepatectomies involving less than one, one, or two segments (Fig. 2) and major hepatectomies, involving three or more segments. Limited hepatectomies are particularly useful in patients with cirrhosis—they combine the advantages of being more economical in

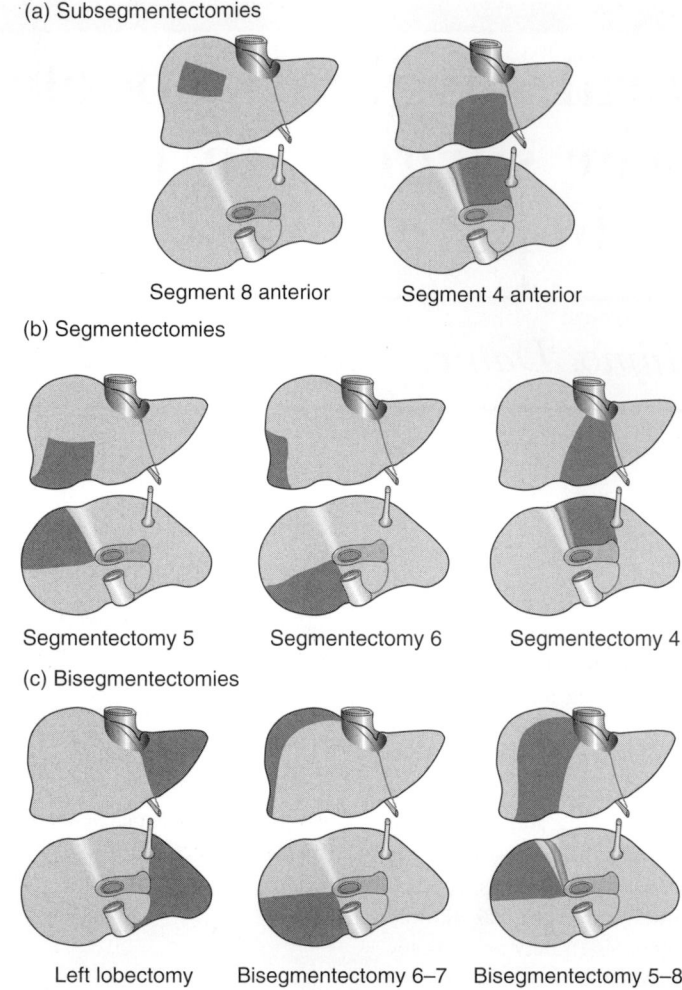

(a) Subsegmentectomies

Segment 8 anterior   Segment 4 anterior

(b) Segmentectomies

Segmentectomy 5   Segmentectomy 6   Segmentectomy 4

(c) Bisegmentectomies

Left lobectomy   Bisegmentectomy 6–7   Bisegmentectomy 5–8

Fig. 2. Limited hepatectomies, defined as resections involving less than three segments. They can be further divided into: subsegmentectomies (a), segmentectomies (b), and bisegmentectomies (c). The most common bisegmentectomy, left lobectomy, involves segments 2 and 3, on the left of the umbilical fissure. (By courtesy of Prof. D. Castaing, Hepatobiliary Foundation, Hôpital Paul Brousse, Villejuif, Paris).

the resection of functional liver tissue and of reducing the operative blood loss as they are in general performed under vascular control. Theoretically, each of the eight segments described by Couinaud can be resected separately—unisegmentectomy (Fig. 2)—although the elective resection of segment 2 or segment 3 has no practical value and a left lobectomy, involving segments 2 and 3 in which the line of transection is the umbilical fissure, is performed in preference (Bismuth, WorldJSurg, 1982; 6:10).

In right and left hepatectomies, the most common major hepatectomies (Fig. 3(a and b)), the line of transection is the plane of the middle hepatic vein (main portal scissura, as defined by the bifurcation of the portal vein) which separates the right and left liver. In the group of major hepatectomies it is now common to identify extended hepatectomies, involving five segments, and superextended hepatectomies, involving six segments (Fig. 4). The right lobectomy according to the macroscopical anatomy of the liver corresponds in the classification of Couinaud to a right hepatectomy extended to segment 4 and, to avoid confusion, we suggest that the term 'right lobectomy' should no longer be employed.

General and operative aspects of liver surgery

It is the meticulous attention to detail in the preoperative assessment of the patient, surgical technique, and postoperative care that have allowed the decrease the mortality and morbidity of liver surgery.

Preoperative care

Liver resections are major operations and every effort should be made in detecting and correcting any abnormalities in respiratory and cardiovascular function. Respiratory physiotherapy should be started before surgery. A programme of preoperative enteral or parenteral nutrition probably decreases the incidence of complications after liver surgery in patients with cirrhosis (Tat Fan, NEJM, 1994; 332:1547). Clotting function must be assessed and patients with obstructive jaundice should be treated with vitamin K until the prothrombin time returns to normal (about 2–3 days). The management of coagulation abnormalities in patients with cirrhosis

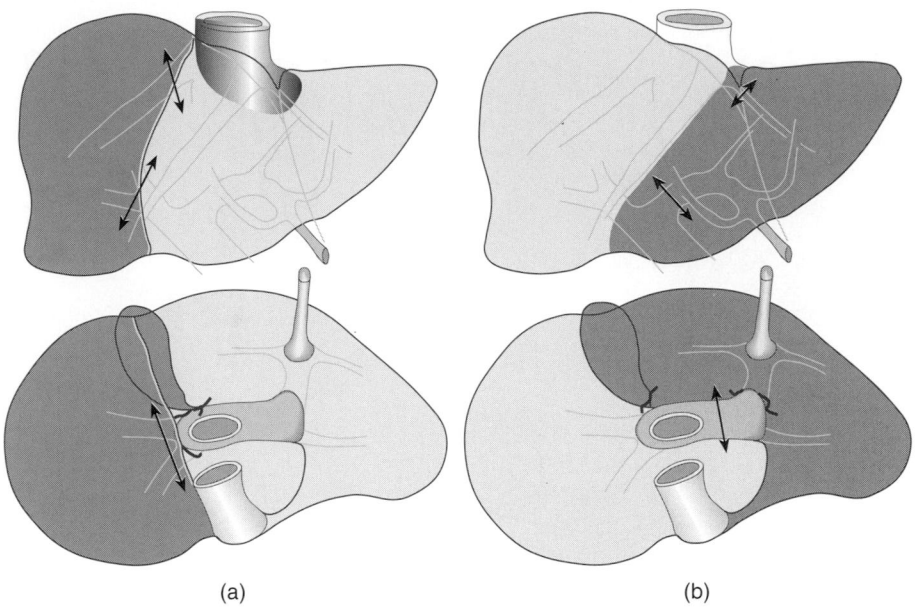

Fig. 3. The two most common major hepatectomies—right (a) and left (b) hepatectomy, as defined by the plane of the middle hepatic vein. Double headed arrows mark the site of transection of the portal and hepatic veins. (By courtesy of Professor D. Castaing, Hepatobiliary Foundation, Hôpital Paul Brousse, Villejuif, Paris.)

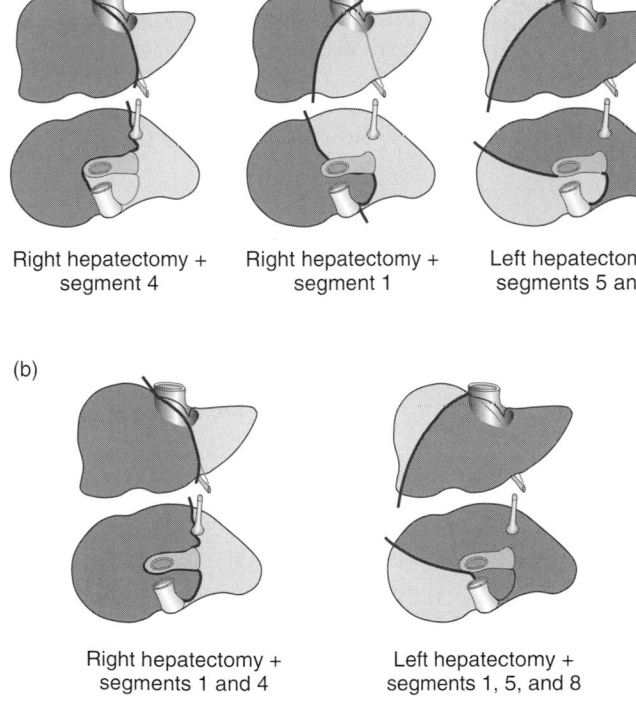

Fig. 4. Extended hepatectomies, involving five segments (a), and super-extended hepatectomies, involving six segments (b). (By courtesy of Professor D. Castaing, Hepatobiliary Foundation, Hôpital Paul Brousse, Villejuif, Paris.)

is more complex: platelets are low because of hypersplenism, and clotting factors are low because of diminished production and because of consumption in the ascitic fluid and in the spleen. There is no advantage in replacing clotting factors and platelets preoperatively as fresh frozen plasma and platelet concentrates can be used with success during and after the operation.

Surgical technique

Intraoperative ultrasound

Operative ultrasonography, first introduced into liver surgery by Japanese authors (Makuuchi, JpnJClinOncol, 1981; 11:367) is the indispensable tool allowing the surgeon to apply the principles of the segmental anatomy, which would otherwise be inaccessible because of the absence of surface markings corresponding to the intrahepatic vascular structures. A complete ultrasound examination consists of identifying the vascular landmarks, delineating the segments, and assessing the hepatic parenchyma within each segment.[2] The intraoperative use of ultrasonography provides the surgeon with an accurate three-dimensional picture of the intrahepatic vessels, thus preventing their inadvertent injury. Branches of the portal vein can be selectively cannulated and occluded to reduce bleeding or the risk of tumour spread. The surgical approach may be changed if major vessels run close to a tumour, are actually invaded by the neoplasm, or contain a tumoural thrombus. The anatomical boundaries of lesions can be identified and plotted on the liver surface, and the direction and depth of the excision can be monitored as the resection proceeds.

Techniques of resection

Operative blood loss has been recognized as the main factor associated with morbidity and mortality in liver resections.[3]

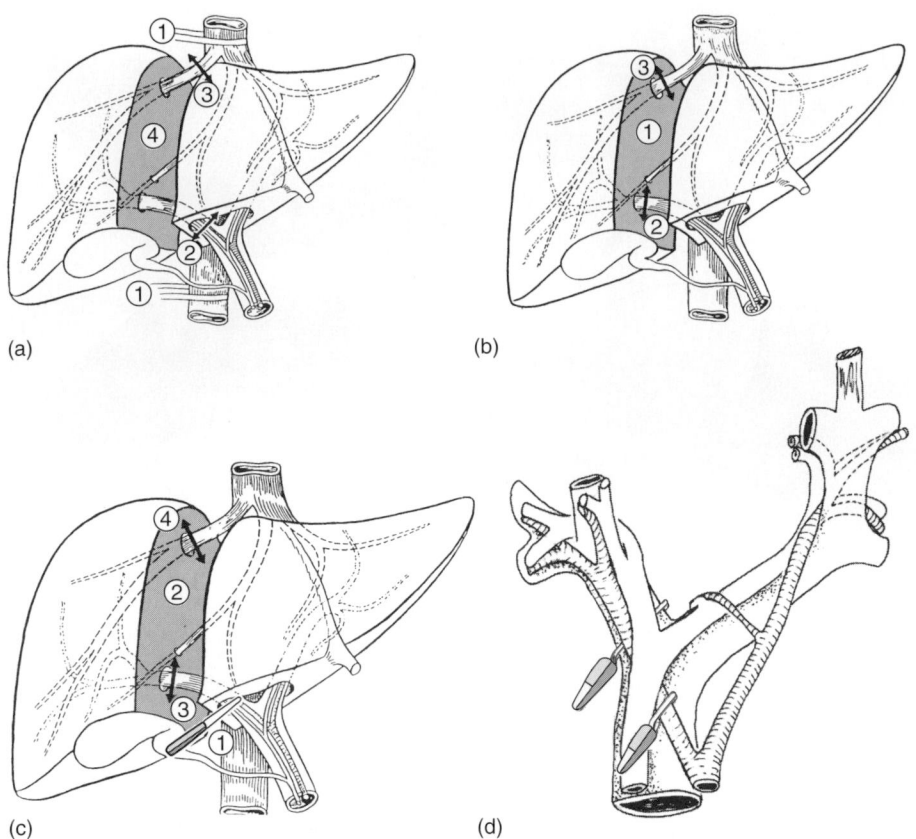

Fig. 5. The three basic techniques of right hepatectomy. (a) Primary division of the vessels (Lortat–Jacob's technique): (1) preliminary control of the suprahepatic and infrahepatic vena cava, (2) ligature and transection of the portal elements, (3) ligature and transection of the right hepatic vein, (4) parenchymatous transection. (b) Primary parenchymatous transection (Ton That Tung's technique): (1) transection of the hepatic tissue, followed by (2) intraparenchymal control of the portal pedicles and (3) of the hepatic veins. (c) Extrahepatic vascular control and intrahepatic ligation. The procedure combines the two techniques with temporary clamping of the right portal pedicle at the bifurcation (1), followed by parenchymatous transection (2), with intrahepatic ligation of the sectorial or segmental portal pedicles (3), and of the hepatic veins (4). (d) Schematic representation of the selective vascular control at the level of the hepatic hilum: bulldog forceps are applied to the right branch of the hepatic artery and portal vein. (By courtesy of Professor D. Castaing, Hepatobiliary Foundation, Hôpital Paul Brousse, Villejuif, Paris).

Techniques of parenchymal dissection and of vascular control have evolved so as to permit minimal blood loss associated with maximal security in dealing with the main blood vessels (Fig. 5).

Hepatectomy with preliminary vascular ligation

This technique was described by Lortat–Jacob at the time of the first typical right hepatectomy in 1952. With this technique, a right hepatectomy starts with the ligation and division of the right portal pedicle at the hilum, continues with the ligation and division of the right hepatic vein, and ends with division of the liver tissue (Fig. 5(a)). The dissection of the right hepatic vein is hazardous with a risk of entering either the vein itself or the inferior vena cava resulting in haemorrhage, which is difficult to control, or an air embolism. For this reason, in the initial technique of Lortat–Jacob, it was suggested that dissection of the right hepatic vein should be preceded by control of the inferior vena cava above and below the liver.

The technique of preliminary vascular control has two advantages: first, it reduces intraoperative blood loss and secondly, it shows clearly the line of separation between the ischaemic right liver and the normally-vascularized left liver. The disadvantage of the technique, beside the risk of injury to the right hepatic vein, is the danger of erroneous ligation of an element of the porta hepatis going to a part of the liver which has to be preserved (a risk increased by the frequency of anatomical variations in this area).

Hepatectomy by primary parenchymatous transection

In this technique, described by the Hanoi surgeon Ton That Tung, the hepatic tissue is divided along the line of the middle hepatic vein and the hilar vascular elements are then approached and ligated within the liver without prior vascular control (Fig. 5(b)). Section of the right hepatic vein is performed in the same fashion within the liver towards the end of the procedure. The technique has two advantages: firstly, liver tissue is excised 'as required' according to the nature and location of the lesion and secondly, there is less risk from anatomical variants as the portal elements are approached above the hilum and within the liver to be resected. The disadvantage of this technique is that bleeding can be considerable if the resection is not performed quickly, and clamping of the hepatic pedicle may be necessary.

Hepatectomy with extrahepatic vascular control and intrahepatic ligation

These two basic techniques of hepatectomy have been incorporated in the technique used at the author's institution,[1] aiming to profit from the advantages of both while seeking to avoid their disadvantages (Fig. 5(c)). The principle is to begin with the dissection of the hilar region to gain control of the arterial and portal elements of the right pedicle and to clamp but not ligate them (Fig. 5(d)). The right side of the retrohepatic vena cava is freed without dissecting the right hepatic vein. The liver is then opened along the main scissural line and, as in the technique of Ton That Tung, the portal elements are located as the parenchyma is transected. Ligation of these vessels, therefore, is performed distal to the clamps. At the end of the liver transection, the hepatic vein is ligated within the liver and the clamps are removed. This technique has the advantages of minimizing the blood loss by prior control of the vessels, as in Lortat–Jacob's technique, and of safe, accurate division and ligation of the vessels and biliary branches within the liver, as in the technique of Ton That Tung.

Techniques of vascular control

Liver resections are performed on richly-irrigated tissue and blood loss can be reduced by temporary interruption of the vascular supply to the liver. The interruption can be performed at various levels, from the hepatic pedicle in the hepatoduodenal ligament to the segmental portal branches. The definition of the indications for each particular type of vascular control and the tolerance of the liver to each has been one of the most important acquisitions in liver surgery during the past decade.

Clamping of the hepatic pedicle

Occlusion of the hepatic inflow by clamping the hepatic pedicle is the oldest method used to reduce bleeding from cut or torn liver tissue. Pringle used it first in three patients with liver trauma and reported it with the results of his experimental observations in a remarkable publication in 1908 (Pringle, AnnSurg, 1908; 48:541) (Fig. 6). Although not affecting bleeding from the hepatic veins, clamping of the hepatic pedicle alone is simple, quick, and usually not accompanied by haemodynamic instability despite some degree of congestion in the territory drained by the portal vein. The normal liver can tolerate continuous clamping of the hepatic pedicle for up to 70 min (Hannoun, BrJSurg, 1993; 80:1161) and periods exceeding 1 h have been reported in patients with cirrhosis (Kim, Hepatogast, 1994; 41:335). Although the experimental evidence in favour of intermittent clamping is not univocal (Isozaki, BrJSurg, 1992; 79: 310; Hardy, BrJSurg, 1995; 82:833) in most cases intermittent clamping is preferred, with 15-min periods of occlusion alternating with 5 to 10 min periods during which the pedicle is unclamped. In patients with cirrhosis or with abnormal liver function from previous chemotherapy the period of ischaemia is reduced to 10 min and although we prefer not to exceed a total clamping time of 30 min, intermittent occlusion has been repeated up to 10 times in some cases without harm.

Selective portal clamping

This method of hemihepatic vascular control as applied to right hepatectomy is illustrated in Fig. 5(d). The principle can be extended to a left hepatic resection, and has been applied to segmental liver resections in the region of the vascular control (Makuuchi, SGO, 1987; 164:155). It has the double advantage of allowing a virtually bloodless operative field and of diminishing the splanchnic congestion associated with the Pringle's manoeuvre.

Suprahilar vascular control and balloon occlusion of segmental portal branches

The perfusion of different sectors or segments can be interrupted at the suprahilar level by ligation or temporary occlusion of the portal pedicles by approaching the glissionian sheath surrounding them inside the liver. The manoeuvre requires incising the liver tissue above and below the location of the portal pedicles at the level of the hepatic fissuras (Takasaki, IntSurg, 1990; 75:73). The line of demarcation between the liver tissue deprived of blood flow and the normally perfused liver can be followed as the limit of the anatomical resection.

Balloon occlusion of segmental portal branches is the most refined application of the concept of intraparenchymal vascular control. Using intraoperative ultrasound the portal branch supplying the segment to be resected is punctured and through an introducer a balloon catheter is inserted over the needle into the portal vein and inflated (Fig. 7). This has the effect of stopping portal venous inflow into the segment; by clamping the appropriate branch of the hepatic artery at the hilum, total vascular exclusion of the segment is obtained. Methylene blue can be injected in the introducer, staining the portion of tissue supplied by the occluded portal branch, thus defining the boundaries of the segment.[4] The segmentectomy is then performed under relatively avascular conditions. This technique has the advantage of reducing the intraoperative haemorrhage while conserving the portal venous flow to the remaining liver. This is of particular importance in patients with cirrhosis in whom the maximum amount of functioning liver tissue must be preserved. A further advantage of segmental portal occlusion in the case of hepatocellular carcinoma which spreads primarily by the portal route, is that the risk of tumour dissemination at the time of the liver resection is minimized by the resection of the whole portal territory.

Total vascular exclusion

In the case of very large tumours when an extended hepatectomy is indicated and in the case of tumours in close relation to the retrohepatic vena cava or to the confluent of the hepatic veins, haemorrhage can be reduced by complete vascular exclusion of the liver. This procedure was first described by Heaney and Jacobson in 1975 (Heaney, Surgery, 1975; 78:138) and is achieved by simultaneous clamping of the hepatic pedicle and of the vena cava above and below the liver (Fig. 8). Heaney and colleagues (Heaney, AnnSurg, 1966; 163:237) showed in earlier experimental studies that normothermic ischaemia could be tolerated for at least 30 min and Huguet and co-workers[5] showed that the human liver will, in fact, withstand up to 65 min of ischaemia. This technique has been proven to be both efficient and safe during major hepatic resection in a series of 51 patients in whom the mean duration of vascular exclusion was 46.5 ± 5.0 min, with a mean transfusion requirement 1.4 ± 0.4 blood units and a mortality 2 per cent.[6] The main limitation to its use is the danger of haemodynamic instability associated

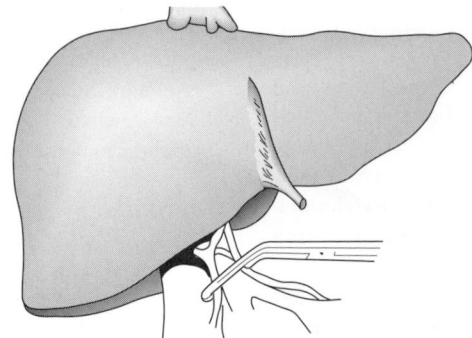

Fig. 6. Schematic representation of the occlusion of the hepatic artery and of the portal vein at the level of the hepatic pedicle (Pringle's manoeuvre). Note that the clamp is applied from the left side of the hepatoduodenal ligament so as to minimize the pressure on the bile duct.

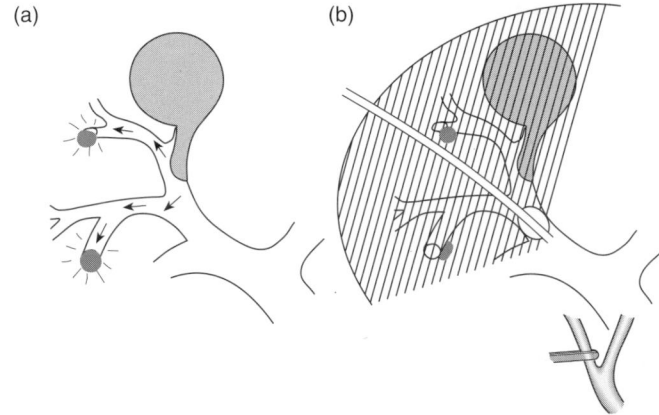

Fig. 7. (a) Mode of spread of hepatocellular carcinoma along the portal vein resulting in the formation of daughter nodules. (b) Selective occlusion of the anterior trunk of the right branch of the portal vein by a balloon catheter at the same time as selective occlusion of the right hepatic artery. Reproduced from Traynor O, Castaing D, and Bismuth H. Peroperative ultrasonography in the surgery of hepatic tumours. *British Journal of Surgery*, 1988; **75**:197–202, with permission of the publishers, Butterworth and Co.

with the diminished venous return to the heart from clamping both the portal vein and the inferior vena cava. The solution is an external venovenous bypass, indicated in particular for patients with altered cardiac and renal function. This in our experience has been necessary in 10 per cent cases of total vascular exclusion. Modifications of the technique by clamping of the hepatic veins and of the hepatic pedicle only, without interrupting the caval flow, has been recently described (Elias, BrJSurg, 1995; 82:1535). Although total vascular exclusion has been used with success in a small number of patients with cirrhosis (Yamaoka, ArchSurg, 1992; 127:276), the technique exposes the liver to an increased risk of portal thrombosis.

Ex situ surgery

Surgery on a liver totally removed from the patient and cooled with preservation solution (*ex situ ex vivo*), with the use of an external venovenous bypass, is the logical application of the techniques of liver transplantation to liver resection.[7] A simpler approach is the disconnection of the suprahepatic inferior vena cava only with perfusion cannulas inserted into the non-severed hepatic vessels (*ex situ in vivo*) (Delriviere, JAmCollSurg, 1995; 181:272). Although very useful in selected cases (tumours in which the dissection would be very haemorrhagic, or in close contact with the hepatic veins or the retrohepatic vena cava) the indications for these techniques

are in fact limited—only two of more than 1000 hepatectomies performed in the authors' institution.

Techniques of dissection and haemostasis
Dissection through the liver

The liver tissue may be divided by a number of methods including the finger-fracture technique (digitoclasy), the Kelly clamp ('Kellyclasy') or the use of the Cavitron ultrasonic dissector (Cavitron Surgical Systems, Stanford, Connecticut). The aim of all three methods is to divide only the parenchymal tissue, exposing the vessels and biliary structures. The ultrasonic dissector consists of a vibrating device which oscillates with a frequency of 23 kHz. It fragments tissue within a radius of 1 to 2 mm, preferentially destroying water-filled parenchymal cells that are removed by a coaxial irrigation–suction apparatus. The collagen and elastic tissue of the vessels is preserved so that they can be dissected clean before accurate coagulation or ligation.

Haemostasis and bilistasis of the cut surface

In the majority of cases nothing more is needed than meticulous suture or ligation of the larger vessels and coagulation of the finer vessels as the resection proceeds. After this has been done, spray

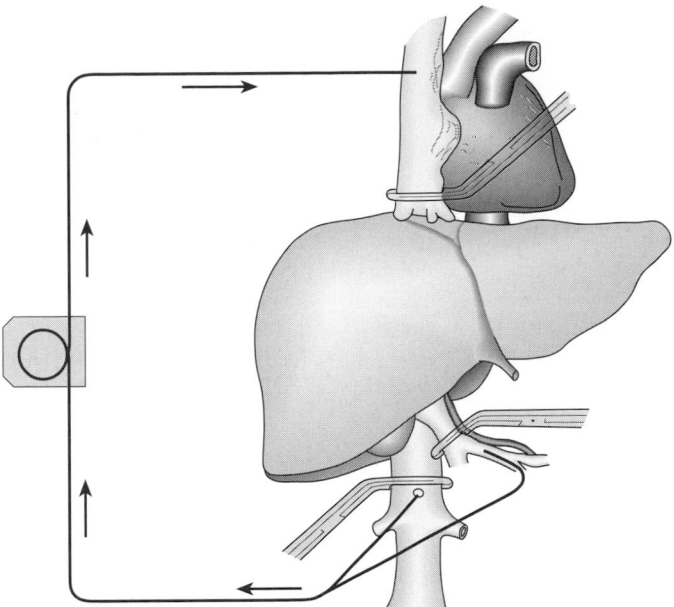

Fig. 8. Schematic representation of total vascular exclusion of the liver, in this case associated with venovenous extracorporeal bypass.

coagulation with the argon gas diathermy point can be most helpful (Postema, BrJSurg, 1993:1563). This is a modified monopolar coagulation device that transmits the cautery current through an electric arch in a plasma of ionized argon gas without direct contact with the tissue surface. Diffuse oozing from very small vessels, particularly in patients with altered clotting, can be more easily controlled with this device than with the use of contact coagulation. In some cases fibrin tissue adhesive (Tissucol, Biocol) can be applied with a syringe or sprayed on the raw liver surface. This is a concentrate of freeze-dried haemostatic factors prepared from human plasma and coagulated using thrombin. The adhesive reproduces the last phase of coagulation by the transformation of fibrinogen into soluble fibrin and its stabilization into an insoluble fibrin network under the influence of factor XIII. In practice its use is reserved for very large raw areas and in no way it should be considered a replacement for coagulation and ligation of vessels.

Bile channels run with the portal pedicles and are simultaneously dealt with by suture ligation during the resection. Small bile leaks on the raw surface should be actively looked for and under-run with fine sutures. Diluted methylene blue can be injected under slight pressure in the biliary system (through the gall bladder or the cystic duct, for instance) to reveal leaks which may otherwise escape detection.

Alternatives to surgical excision

In some patients with diminished hepatic reserve from cirrhosis or previous liver resection, especially in cases of lesions seated deeply inside the liver, conventional surgical resection may represent too big a sacrifice of functional hepatic tissue or an excessive operative risk. In some of these cases alcohol injection or surgical cryotherapy can be used. Surgical cryotherapy is performed by introducing into the tumour a probe which is cooled with liquid nitrogen to –196°C. The extent of the destruction can be monitored accurately by the progression of the area of frozen tissue which appears intensely

hypoechogenic on the ultrasound. This procedure has proven particularly useful as an adjunct to surgical excision in cases of multiple metastases and to increase the safety of the margins of resection for tumours in awkward intrahepatic locations (Adam, AnnSurg, 1997; 225:39).

Laparoscopic hepatic resections

Laparoscopic hepatic resection have been performed in anecdotal cases or small series. Although most of the technical problems can be solved, especially with the use of gasless laparoscopy which diminishes the risks of gas embolism, and with customized surgical tools such as the ultrasonic dissector and vascular staplers (Kaneko, Surgery 1996; 120:468) the indications for such an approach remain rare and the benefits unproven. Only lesions in the anterior segments of the liver or in the left lobe can be approached safely. Malignant tumours are generally too large to be confidently dealt with this technique and there is serious concern about the possibility of intra-abdominal or port-site implantation of neoplastic cells. Benign tumours, with the exception of adenomas, do not generally need surgery.

Postoperative care, complications, and mortality

The postoperative care after hepatic resections does not generally differ from the care of patients after other kinds of major abdominal surgery.[8] A characteristic profile of alteration of liver function tests has been described and involves transient elevation of transaminases, correlated with tissue damage from ischaemia, and a more persistent elevation of alkaline phosphatase and γ-glutamyl transferase, lasting for 2 to 3 months, correlated with liver regeneration.[9] Jaundice, prolonged clotting time, and ascites are generally short lived if enough functional liver tissue has been spared. Operative mortality, in centres with sufficient experience, is rare. In patients with normal preoperative liver function, figures as low as 2 per cent or less are possible[10–12] and to some extent depend on the aggressiveness with which tumour eradication is pursued. Mortality and morbidity are higher in patients with hepatocellular carcinoma, due to the high incidence of chronic hepatitis and cirrhosis, and operative mortality figures of 7 to10 per cent are reported in these patients (Ozawa, AmJSurg, 1991; 161:677; Bismuth, AnnSurg, 1993; 218:145).

The most common general complications concern the respiratory system, with right sided pleural effusion, atelectasis, respiratory infections, and pulmonary embolism from lower limb thrombophlebitis collectively reaching an incidence of 25 per cent in a recent series of 113 consecutive major hepatectomies without mortality at the university hospital of Geneva, Switzerland (G. Mentha, unpublished observation, 1995). Antithrombotic prophylaxis with elastic stockings is routinely applied and low molecular weight heparin is used after the operation unless clotting disfunction is anticipated.

The most common local complications are haemorrhage, biliary fistula, necrosis of devascularized tissue, and sepsis. These are directly related to the technique of liver resection and in general can be prevented by carefully following the recommendations described above. An average estimation of their incidence is difficult as it depends on the experience of the institution and the patient population undergoing surgery. The large series reported in the literature span a considerable period of time[11–13] which causes difficulties in interpreting the figures.

Haemorrhage

Postoperative bleeding requiring reoperation is fortunately rare if haemostasis is performed carefully at the time of surgery. Oversewing of all vascular pedicles is safer than simple ligatures or forceps coagulation and is particularly important in patients with cirrhosis because of impaired clotting and portal hypertension.

Biliary fistula

A persistent biliary leak or biliary fistula occurs if the surgeon fails to identify the orifice of a small bile duct at the resection margin. Bile leaks usually close spontaneously without the need for reoperation (as long as there is no distal obstruction) and therefore the presence of bile in an abdominal drain is generally not a cause for alarm. An inadequately drained biliary collection, however, is a potential source of sepsis. Abdominal ultrasonography is advisable before removal of abdominal drains to identify collections of blood or bile that should be evacuated by mobilization of the drains or percutaneously under ultrasound or computed tomography control.

Necrosis

If the principles of segmental liver surgery are followed, no devascularized tissue is left behind and this complication should be exceptional. After the vessels of the portal pedicle are occluded to give a line of demarcation between the ischaemic and viable liver, some surgeons advocate dividing the hepatic tissue 1 or 2 cm within the ischaemic zone. This may leave an area of devascularized tissue at the resection margin and we advise dividing the liver in close contact to the well-vascularized zone. Ischaemia and subsequent necrosis can also be caused by performing the haemostasis of the resection margin with tight sutures taking large bites. We consider

it unnecessary to close the resection margin and prefer to achieve haemostasis by under-running the individual bleeding points using fine sutures and occasionally with fibrin tissue adhesive (see above).

Sepsis

Sepsis is often the end result of insufficient treatment of the other complications, namely haemorrhage (failure to evacuate postoperative haematomata which then become secondarily infected) and the inadequate drainage of bile collections.

Postoperative hepatic insufficiency

This syndrome manifests as altered clotting, hyperbilirubinaemia, encephalopathy, ascites, and, in the most severe cases, with multiple organ failure and sepsis. The condition is fortunately self limited and uncommon, except in patients after very extensive liver resections or in patients with cirrhosis and limited capacities for liver regeneration. The consequences of this, usually predictable, complication can be limited by appropriate measures of prevention and postoperative management.

Postoperative hepatic insufficiency in non-cirrhotic patients

The main reason for postoperative liver insufficiency following surgery on a non-cirrhotic liver is a massive resection. The maximum volume of liver which can be safely resected in humans is unknown. In 1964, Monaco and coworkers (Monaco, AnnSurg, 1964; 139:513) reported the case of a 90 per cent hepatectomy in a patient who went on to have minimal postoperative liver dysfunction. However, the patient actually had an enormous benign adenoma of the right liver and the resection consisted almost totally of tumour with removal of a only a small amount of normal tissue. In addition, the patient had marked compensatory hypertrophy of the left liver. This case serves to make two important points. First, in liver tumours, there is destruction of liver parenchyma and the amount of functional tissue removed at hepatectomy does not always correlate with the anatomical extent of the liver resection. Secondly, there may be compensatory hypertrophy of the unaffected liver and this must be taken into account in the evaluation of the functional impairment following hepatectomy. The size of the resection is less important than the quantity and quality of the remaining functional hepatic tissue. The combination of experimental work and clinical experience indicates that there is a risk of severe postoperative hepatic insufficiency when resection exceeds 80 per cent of the functional (non-tumoural) liver tissue.

The second major cause of postoperative hepatic insufficiency is the interruption of blood perfusion such as may occur during total vascular exclusion. The liver is somewhat resistant to warm ischaemia, however, and under normothermic conditions total vascular exclusion can be safely extended to 65 min (see above). Hepatic regeneration and tolerance to vascular exclusion may be negatively affected by anticancer chemotherapy.

Postoperative hepatic insufficiency in cirrhotic patients

Patients with cirrhosis are particularly prone to postoperative hepatic insufficiency, especially if preoperatively they already have

Table 1 The Child–Paul Brousse classification

	One point	Two points
Bilirubin (mmol/l)	>30	
Albumin (g/l)	<30	
(PT + Factor II)/2	40–60	<40
Encephalopathy	Present	

Patients with no points are considered class A, patients with 1–2 points class B, and patients with ≥3 points class C.
PT = prothrombin time.
After Bismuth, AmJSurg, 1990; 160: 105.

appreciable manifestations of liver dysfunction. This complication can occur after any kind of surgery but the risk is increased in gastrointestinal surgery and especially so in procedures involving the biliary tree and the portal circulation. A mortality rate of 93 per cent has been reported following simple cholecystectomy if the prothrombin time is less than 60 per cent of normal (Schwartz, Surgery, 1981; 90:577).

There is also a risk of postoperative hepatic insufficiency in cirrhotic patients undergoing portal diversion to treat the complications of portal hypertension. The Child classification was initially developed to select patients suitable for portocaval shunts and has been extended to other forms of hepatobiliary surgery.[14] A modified form giving more weight to clotting function is used at the Paul Brousse Hospital (Table 1) (Bismuth, AmJSurg, 1990; 160: 105). Traditionally, the three groups (A, B, and C) have been considered to correspond to a reduction in hepatic function of 30, 50, and 90 per cent.

Prediction of hepatic insufficiency after liver resections in patients with cirrhosis

Patients with cirrhosis are at increased risk of developing hepatocellular carcinoma, and in patients in good clinical conditions (Child class A and occasionally class B) resection represents the mainstay of treatment. The prediction, prevention, and treatment of postoperative hepatic insufficiency in these patients is one of the main challenges of contemporary liver surgery and comprises:

(1) evaluation of preoperative hepatic function;
(2) estimation of the proportion of functional liver tissue which will remain after resection;
(3) prediction of the regeneration potential of the liver.

No single test can provide an unequivocal estimation of preoperative hepatic function and of the risk of postoperative insufficiency, which are best appreciated by a combination of factors.

Liver function tests

Serum levels of bilirubin, alkaline phosphatase, and transaminases have traditionally been thought to lack sensitivity in the estimation of hepatic function. In the cirrhotic liver, however, experience from Japan suggests that elevated serum bilirubin is an accurate predictor of liver dysfunction. Miyagawa and colleagues, in their experience of 172 hepatic resections in cirrhotic patients, used the preoperative level of serum bilirubin as an indicator of the possible extent of hepatic resection.[15] A serum bilirubin level greater than 2 mg/dl (35 μmol/l) was considered an absolute contraindication to surgery with levels between 1.6 and 2 mg/dl (27–34 μmol/l) allowing simple tumour enucleation (without resection of any functioning parenchyma), and levels between 1.1 and 1.5 mg/dl (18–25 μmol/l) allowing limited parenchymal resection (Fig. 9).

High transaminase levels in patients with cirrhosis, possibly as a correlation with chronic hepatitis status (Higashi, BrJSurg, 1994; 81:1342) have been associated with increased hospital mortality and complications in patients with Child's grade A cirrhosis (Farges, Gut, 1996; 39 (suppl 3):26)

Clotting factors and serum albumin

The synthetic function of the liver can be evaluated by measuring serum albumin and the hepatic-dependent clotting factors. Measurement of prothrombin time and the levels of factors II, V, VII, and X (as included in the commonly used modifications of the original Child's score) provide one of the most useful estimates of preoperative and postoperative hepatic function available to the surgeon.

Indocyanine green clearance

The measurement of the bloodstream clearance of the dye indocyanine green (ICG) is a very accurate means of predicting the risk of postoperative liver insufficiency, especially in patients belonging to class A of the Child classification (Hasegawa, JChir, 1987; 124:425; Noguchi, Hepatogast, 1990; 37:165; Hemming, AmJSurg, 1992; 163:515). The dye is non-toxic and after intravenous injection is cleared from the bloodstream exclusively by the liver without undergoing either intrahepatic conjugation or enterohepatic circulation. In these respects it has advantages over both bilirubin and bromosulphthalein as an indicator of hepatocyte function. Its clearance is, however, dependent upon liver blood flow.

The standard ICG test involves the intravenous injection of 0.5 mg/kg, with blood samples taken before injection and at 5 and 15 min after injection. From each sample, 1.0 ml of plasma is diluted with 3.0 ml of saline and the specimens analysed for ICG concentration in a spectrophotometer at 805 nm. In a patient with a normal liver, the amount of ICG remaining in the bloodstream 15 min after its injection (ICG R_{15}) will be less than 10 per cent. Miyagawa and colleagues consider that ICG R_{15} is an accurate marker of functional impairment in the cirrhotic liver and have used this parameter, together with serum bilirubin, to decide the volume of liver which can be safely resected (Fig. 9).[15] They consider that patients with an ICG R_{15} value of less than 10 per cent can safely undergo resection of two sectors of the liver (right hepatectomy for example) while a value between 11 and 20 per cent allows resection of only one sector and a value between 21 and 30 per cent resection of only one segment. For ICG R_{15} values greater than 30 per cent, enucleation of hepatic tumours or subsegmentectomy is all that can be safely performed.

The glucose tolerance test and the arterial ketone body ratio are an additional tests which have been validated as prognostic predictors in liver resection in patients with cirrhosis (Ozawa, JGastHepatol, 1990; 5:296; Mori, AnnSurg, 1990; 211:438).

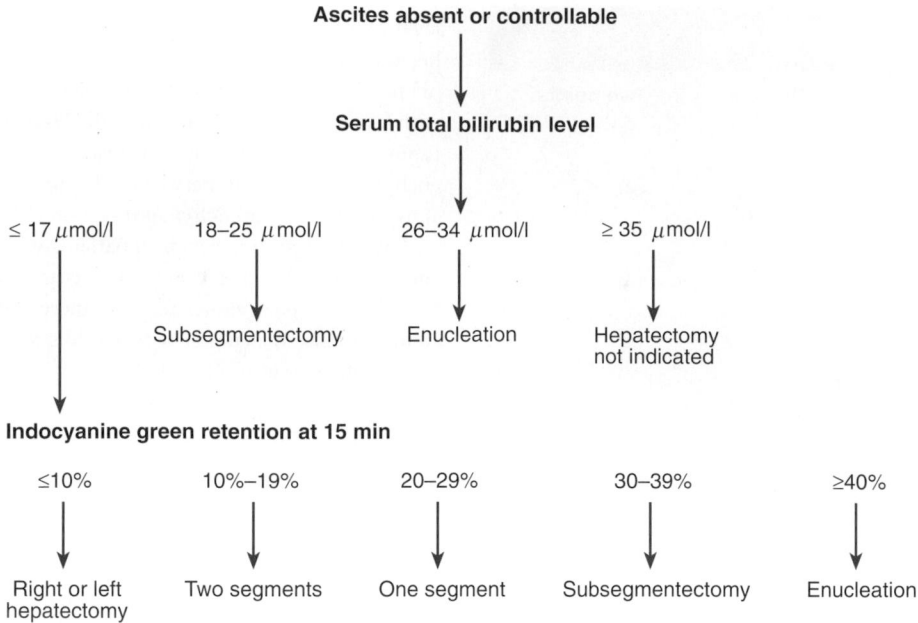

Fig. 9. Use of indocyanine green clearance as an indicator for the maximum extent of hepatic resection (after ref. 15 and modified to take into account the segmental classification of Couinaud).

Aminopyrine breath test

Measurement of the cleavage of the methyl groups of ^{14}C-labelled dimethyl aminopirine (amidopyrine), estimated from the recovery of radioactive CO_2 in the breath, provides a quantitative appreciation of hepatocyte cytochrome P-450 function and has been used as a predictor of outcome in patients with cirrhosis undergoing surgical operations (Gill, AnnSurg, 1983; 198:701). It has the advantage that it is not affected by portacaval shunts but it is considerably more expensive to use and does not appear as useful as indocyanine green clearance, which is the standard test in the authors' institution (Lau, BrJSurg, 1997; 84:1255).

Estimation of liver volume in the planning of hepatic resections

As has been discussed earlier, the determination of the volume and the function of the hepatic tissue likely to remain after hepatectomy is critical in the assessment of the risk of postoperative liver insufficiency and the planning of 'safe' liver surgery.

Over 20 years ago, Stone and colleagues (Stone, AmJSurg, 1969; 6:78) estimated the volumes of the various liver sectors and segments and expressed them as percentages of the whole organ. These figures have remained in general use ever since. The liver was divided thus:

posterolateral sector (segments VI and VII): 35 per cent
paramedian sector (segments V and VIII): 30 per cent
segments I and IV: 20 per cent
left lobe (segments II and III): 15 per cent

The surgeon can thus estimate the extent of a proposed hepatectomy simply by adding together the percentages of the resected segments (e.g. right hepatectomy = 65 per cent; right hepatectomy extended to segment IV = 85 per cent). These proportions, however, are based upon a normal liver and are inaccurate in the presence of a liver tumour (where the neoplastic tissue is not functional and there may be compensatory hypertrophy of the uninvolved liver).

Computed axial tomography (**CT**) can now measure the volume of the different liver sectors and the volume of a tumour as they are in a given patient at a given moment with outstanding accuracy. The tumoural tissue replacing a part of liver tissue should not be calculated in the estimation of the function of that part. Okamoto and colleagues (Okamoto, Surgery, 1984; 95:586) have devised a 'parenchymal hepatic resection rate' which is essentially an expression of the percentage of non-tumoural liver to be resected:

Parenchymal hepatic resection rate = 100 × [(volume of liver to be resected – volume of tumour) /

(total volume of liver – volume of tumour)]

This, combined with an estimation of the liver function and with the Child score in patients with cirrhosis, can provide an estimate of the amount of liver tissue that can be removed safely. At the authors' institution, for instance, a rule of thumb is that patients belonging to the Child's A class can be considered for resections of up to 50 per cent, patients classed Child B up to 25 per cent, and patient classed Child C, in the rare instances where surgery is indicated, for enucleation of the tumour only. A finer appreciation of the amount of liver tissue that can be resected can be obtained by including the indocyanine clearance (see above) and more complicated formulas have been developed (Yamanaka, AnnSurg, 1984; 200:658).

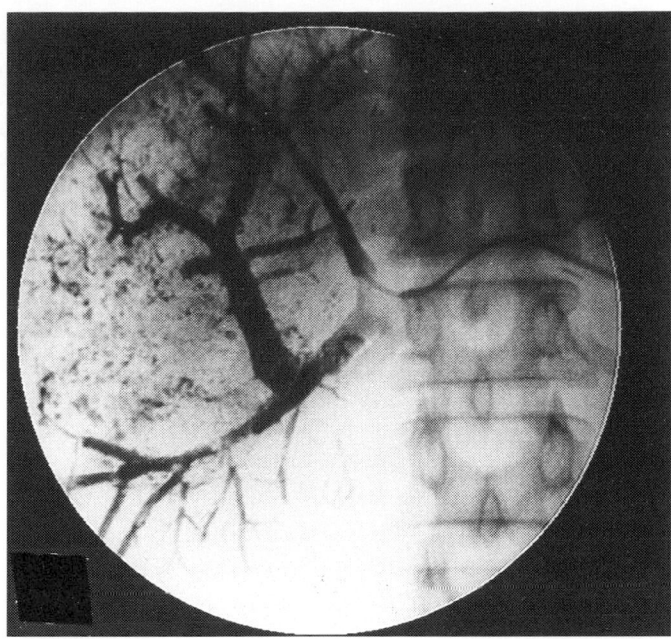

Fig. 10. Portal vein embolization of a patient with a large hepatocellular carcinoma involving the right anterior sector of the liver: a radio-opaque mixture of lipiodol and acrylic glue has been injected into the right sectorial branches of the portal vein. (The tumour had been treated previously by intra-arterial chemoembolization.)

New strategies in the prevention and management of postoperative hepatic insufficiency

A new and more specific method of prevention of postoperative liver insufficiency is the preoperative induction of contralateral liver hypertrophy by portal vein embolization. Unilateral portal vein thrombosis leads to unilateral atrophy of the liver and contralateral hypertrophy. In practice, to increase the volume of the left lobe before a right hepatectomy the right branch of the portal vein can be embolized percutaneously.[16] This technique was first employed by Kinoshita and coworkers (Kinoshita, WorldJSurg, 1986; 10:803) as a counter measure to the spread of tumour thrombi in the portal venous system in patients undergoing surgery for hepatocellular carcinoma. Liver hypertrophy was noted as a secondary effect.

Embolization is performed under ultrasound control by the percutaneous introduction of a catheter into either the right or left portal branch, as appropriate (Fig. 10). Portography is next performed and a mixture of lipiodol and biocompatible, non-absorbable glue is injected. Surgery should be performed approximately 6 to 8 weeks after portal embolization to allow sufficient time for the response to occur (Fig. 11). CT scanning and volumetric assessment can then be used to quantify the increase in volume of the contralateral liver. Six weeks after embolization, Kinoshita and colleagues reported an increase of 40 per cent in the volume of the contralateral lobe in one patient. This technique has now an established place in allowing liver resections for patients who were

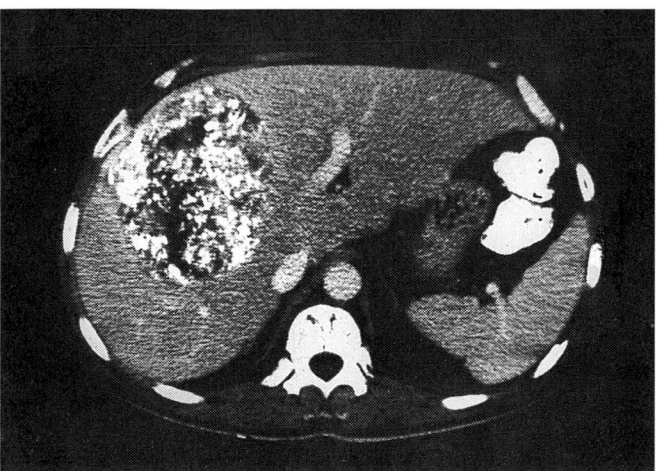
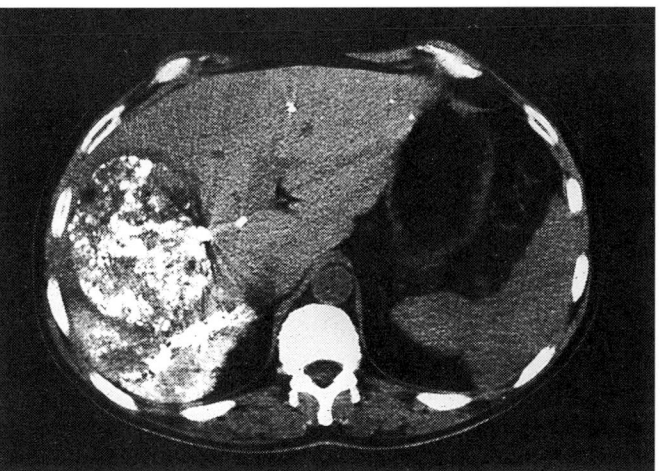

Fig. 11. CT scan of the patient (a) before portal vein embolization and (b) 6 weeks after the procedure. Note the hypertrophy of the left lobe, allowing an uncomplicated resection. (From Azoulay et al.[14] by permission of the *Journal of the American College of Surgeons*.)

previously considered inoperable because the volume of the remaining liver would have been too small to prevent postoperative liver insufficiency. A detailed review of the different hormonal mediators (Kogure, Gastro, 1995; 108:1136) and growth factors involved in liver regeneration is beyond the scope of this chapter and the reader will find the relevant information in specialized articles.[17,18]

When postoperative hepatic insufficiency is detected biologically or is foreseen from the magnitude of the liver resection or the poor state of preoperative liver function, supportive measures are aimed at preventing the complications which derive from the diminished liver function and at providing the best conditions for hepatic regeneration to occur. Infections have to be avoided or controlled. As glycogen storage is deficient, glucose is given to maintain adequate blood levels and to minimize protein breakdown. Fat emulsions, as part of parenteral nutrition, should be used sparingly in an effort to limit fatty infiltration of the liver.

Prevention of hepatic encephalopathy is particularly important after portal diversion or liver resection in patients with cirrhosis. Dietary protein restriction is an efficient short-term measure but has deleterious long-term nutritional consequences. Reduction of blood ammonia levels by lactulose, neomycin, or enemas continues to be of practical value.

A reduction in levels of the liver-dependent blood clotting factors occurs rapidly following hepatectomy and is proportional to the amount of functioning liver removed. Correction using fresh frozen plasma is often undertaken but is rarely necessary except in the event of postoperative haemorrhage.

The bioartificial liver has been used as a bridge to recovery of the hepatic function, brought about by liver regeneration, in a small number of patients with encouraging results (Rozga, AnnSurg, 1994; 219:538). It may prove to be an exciting new tool in the treatment of patients needing massive hepatic resection.

Conclusion

Sound knowledge of the functional liver anatomy (complemented by intraoperative ultrasound), experience with total and segmental vascular exclusion, new tools for parenchymal dissection, and haemostasis now allow modern liver surgery to be performed with very low mortality. Local complications such as haemorrhage, necrosis, biliary fistula, and sepsis have decreased in incidence and can be prevented, to a large degree, by the precise application of the modern techniques of liver surgery.

Postoperative hepatic insufficiency should no longer occur as an unexpected complication of liver resection. The accurate prediction of the risk of this complication is now possible by the combined use of indocyanine green clearance and volumetric (CT) measurement of liver sectors and segments. These techniques are particularly useful in planning (or avoiding) resections in patients cirrhosis who are most at risk from this complication. Preoperative portal vein embolization and postoperative assistance of liver function with the bioartificial liver open new exciting horizons in the surgical management of patients with hepatic disease.

References

1. Bismuth H. Surgical anatomy and anatomical surgery of the liver. *World Journal of Surgery*, 1982; **6**: 3–9.
2. Castaing D, Emond J, Kunstlinger F, and Bismuth H. Utility of operative ultrasound in the surgical management of liver tumors. *Annals of Surgery*, 1986; **204**: 600–5.
3. Ekberg H, Tranberg KG, Andersson R, Jeppsson B, and Bengmark S. Major liver resection: perioperative course and management. *Surgery*, 1986; **100**: 1–7.
4. Shimamura Y, Gunvén P, Takenaka Y, Shimizu H, Akimoto H, Shima Y, Arima K, Takahashi A, Kitaya T, Matsuyama T, and Hasegawa H. Selective portal occlusion by balloon catheter during liver resection. *Surgery*, 1985; **100**: 938–41.
5. Huguet C, Gavelli A, Chieco A, Bona S, Harb J, Joseph JM, *et al.* Liver ischemia for hepatic resection: where is the limit? *Surgery*, 1992; **11**: 251–9.
6. Bismuth H, Castaing D, and Garden OJ. Major hepatic resection under total vascular exclusion. *Annals of Surgery*, 1989; **210**: 13–19.
7. Pichlmayr R, Grosse H, Hauss J, Gubernatis G, Lamesh P, and Bretschneider HJ. Technique and preliminary results of extracorporeal liver surgery (bench procedure) and of surgery on the *in situ* perfused liver. *British Journal of Surgery*, 1990; **77**: 21–6.
8. Stone MD and Benoti PN. Liver resection: Preoperative and postoperative care. *Surgical Clinics of North America*, 1989; **69**: 383–92.
9. Suc B, Panis Y, Belghiti J, and Fékété F. 'Natural history' of hepatectomy. *British Journal of Surgery*, 1992; **79**: 39–42.
10. Bismuth H, Adam R, Lévi F, Farabos C, Waechter F, Castaing D, Majno P, and Engerran L. Resection of non resectable liver metastases from colorectal cancer following neoadjuvant chemotherapy. *Annals of Surgery*, 1996; **224**: 509–22.
11. Thompson HH, Tompkins RK, and Longmire WP. Major hepatic resections a 25 year experience. *Annals of Surgery*, 1983; **197**: 375–88.
12. Iwatsuki S and Starzl TE. Personal experience with 450 hepatic resections. *Annals of Surgery*, 1988; **208**: 421–34.
13. Scheele J, Stangl R, Altendorf-Hoffmann A, and Gall FP. Indication of prognosis after hepatic resection for colorectal secondaries. *Surgery*, 1991; **110**: 13–29.
14. Child CG and Turcotte JG. Surgery in portal hypertension. In Child CG, ed. *Major problems in clinical surgery. The liver and portal hypertension.* Philadelphia; WB Saunders, 1964: 1–85.
15. Miyagawa S, Makuuchi M, Kawasaki S, and Kakazu T. Criteria for safe hepatic resection. *American Journal of Surgery*, 1995; **169**: 589–94.
16. Azoulay D, Raccuia JS, Castaing D, and Bismuth H. Right portal vein embolization in preparation for major hepatic resection. *Journal of American College of Surgeons*, 1995; **181**: 267–9.
17. Francavilla A, Hagiya M, and Porter KA. Augmenter of liver regeneration: its place in the universe of hepatic growth factors. *Hepatology*, 1994; **20**: 747–57.
18. Boros P and Miller CM. Hepatocyte growth factor: a multifunctional cytokine. *Lancet*, 1995; **345**: 293–5.

S. V. Mallett

Surgery in the patient with liver disease can be associated with a high price in terms of perioperative morbidity and mortality (Doberneck, AmJSurg, 1983; 146:306). Careful preoperative preparation reduces mortality (Sirinek, ArchSurg, 1987; 122:271), but patients with advanced liver disease are still a major challenge to the skills and ability of the anaesthetist. One of the many benefits of the exponential increase in liver transplantation over the last 10 years has been the expertise gained as a result of managing these complex cases. Significant improvements and developments in perioperative monitoring, physiological manipulation, coagulation assessment, and transfusion technology have led to improved survival and reduced morbidity in patients undergoing major hepatic surgery.

The objective of this chapter is to review the specific problems posed by liver disease, to define the pathophysiological consequences of hepatic damage, and to identify potential risk factors. General guidelines for drug usage and the anaesthetic management of these patients will be presented, together with recommendations for the management of specific liver surgery including hepatic resection and liver transplantation.

Risk assessment

Child's classification,[1] although originally designed for patients undergoing portocaval shunt surgery, remains the standard by which patients with cirrhosis are assigned a risk assessment score preoperatively. The addition of the prothrombin time by Pugh[2] further increases the predictive accuracy of this scoring system (Table 1).

Anaesthesia and surgery in patients with advanced liver disease is associated with an extremely high morbidity and mortality. A mortality rate of 80 per cent occurred in patients with advanced cirrhosis undergoing cholecystectomy (Table 2), the major cause of death being uncontrolled haemorrhage (coagulopathy intraoperatively or postoperatively from variceal bleeding), sepsis, and multiorgan failure (Aranha, AmJSurg, 1982; 143:55).

An elegant study (Garrison, AnnSurg, 1984; 199:648) designed to clarify risk factors for abdominal surgery in patients with hepatic cirrhosis showed that (excluding Child's classification) the most important preoperative factors determining increased risk were the prothrombin time, serum albumin, and the presence of infection defined as a white blood-cell count in excess of 10 000. These three predicted survival with a 90 per cent accuracy and non-survival with a 70 per cent accuracy. Of 100 patients with biopsy-proven cirrhosis, 30 patients died and 30 developed major postoperative complications, sepsis with multisystem organ failure being the major cause of death. Operative factors associated with an increased risk included transfusion requirements, exploration of the common bile duct, and emergency surgery.

Major surgery in patients with even well-compensated liver disease (Child's A) can lead to clinically significant liver dysfunction postoperatively and in some cases marked decompensation. The perioperative death rate in patients with advanced cirrhosis is still excessive (up to 25 per cent), with the major causes being uncontrolled bleeding, sepsis, and liver failure.[3]

Improving the patients preoperative status can have a significant impact on outcome and reduce perioperative morbidity and mortality (Sirinek, ArchSurg, 1987; 122:271). This requires a multidisciplinary approach and liaison between hepatologists, anaesthetists, and the surgical team. Aspects of importance are, where time permits, improvement of nutritional status and careful control of ascites. In patients with uncontrolled ascites, there is

Table 1 Child–Pugh's risk grading

	Group A	Group B	Group C
Serum bilirubin	<40	40–50	>50
Serum albumin	>35	28–35	<28
Ascites	None	Mild	Moderate–severe
Encephalopathy	Absent	Grade I + II	Grade III + IV
PT (s) prolonged from control	1–4	4–6	>6
Surgical risk	Good	Moderate	Poor
Mortality	3–10%	10–30%	50–80%

PT, prothrombin time.

Table 2 Mortality following cholecystectomy

	PT (s)	Mortality (%)	Mean intraoperative transfusion	
			blood (ml)	FFP (ml)
Normal liver	Normal	1 (374/4)	35	10
Moderate cirrhosis	<2.5	9 (43/4)	450	975
Severe cirrhosis	>2.5	83 (12/10)	4500	4000

After Aranha, AmJSurg, 1982; 143:55.
PT, prothrombin time; FFP, fresh-frozen plasma.

some evidence that transjugular intrahepatic portosystemic shunt can lead to an improvement in the overall Child–Pugh score (Rossle, NEJM, 1994; 330:165).

Over the last decade, the experience and knowledge gained by anaesthetists in overcoming the numerous problems posed by liver transplantation have led to enormous improvements in the management of these high-risk cases and have made substantial inroads into reducing the excessive mortality associated with surgery in patients with advanced liver disease. The routine use of invasive cardiovascular monitoring allows much more precise assessment of physiological changes and enables a rapid response to adverse trends. Rapid infusion systems, serial assessment of coagulation and metabolic and electrolyte status, and avoidance of hypothermia have all had a part to play in limiting the development of serious physiological derangement and the potential for escalation to an irretrievable situation.

Pathophysiological consequences of liver disease
The relevance to intraoperative management
Cardiovascular system

The major consequences of liver disease are a hyperdynamic circulation with a high intravascular volume, a low systemic vascular resistance and an increased cardiac output.[4] These patients also exhibit a relative insensitivity to catecholamines (Fernandez-Seara, Gastro, 1989; 97:1304).

The increased intravascular volume is a result of sodium retention, while the low vascular resistance is due to vasodilatation, which may be caused by increased levels of vasodilator substances either produced or not detoxified by the liver. Many vasodilatory substances are possible mediators,[5] including vasoactive polypeptides, nitric oxide (Vallance, Lancet, 1991; 337:776), atrial natrietic peptide, bradykinin, and endotoxin.

Arteriovenous shunting may be extensive. Pulmonary shunts in patients with cirrhosis accounted for up to 70 per cent of the cardiac output (George, Lancet, 1960; i:852). In addition, the mediastinal and para-oesophageal pulmonary circulation may result in significantly increased cardiac work. Portal–systemic shunts may be both intra- and extrahepatic.[6] All shunts, whether arteriovenous or portosystemic, will decrease systemic vascular resistance and lead to an increase in cardiac output. The magnitude of the haemodynamic changes is related to the severity of the liver disease and becomes more marked as the disease progresses.[7] These changes

appear to reverse after successful liver transplantation (Glauser, Chest, 1990; 98:1210).

The increased cardiac output is often associated with normal filling pressures, but cirrhotic patients may have decreased myocardial contractility, which may only become apparent when afterload is increased and the myocardium is stressed. Alcoholic patients with alcoholic cardiomyopathy may demonstrate low-output cardiac failure.

Most cirrhotic patients have low/normal pulmonary artery pressures and pulmonary vascular resistance (Martini, ProgLivDis, 1972; 4:231). However, up to 2 per cent of patients presenting for assessment for liver transplantation have pulmonary hypertension, usually occurring in association with portal hypertension [portal hypertensive-associated pulmonary arterial hypertension (**PHPAH**)] (Lebrec, AmRevRespDis, 1979; 120:849). Evidence of pulmonary hypertension should always be sought during the preoperative assessment of potential liver transplant recipients as up to 60 per cent of patients with PHPAH are completely asymptomatic (Hadengue, Gastro, 1991;100:520). The electro- and echocardiograms may give some indication of right-ventricular pressure overload or hypertrophy. If there is evidence for PHPAH the patient requires right-heart catheterization to estimate the severity of the disease. The reactivity of the pulmonary vasculature to short-acting vasodilators such as prostacyclin and nitric oxide should also be assessed at this time, but many of these patients demonstrate little if any response (Mandell, Anesthesiol, 1994; 81:1538). Evidence of right ventricular hypertrophy is generally considered a contraindication to transplantation. Combined liver–lung or liver–heart–lung transplants may be considered in this group of patients (Wallwork, Lancet, 1987; ii:182). Mild to moderate degrees of pulmonary hypertension do not preclude transplantation but they are invariably associated with a stormy and difficult perioperative course. Evidence to date suggests that these changes are not reversible following liver transplantation (Prager, Anethesiol, 1992; 77:375).

All patients with liver disease who are to be anaesthetized should as a minimum have a chest radiograph and an electrocardiogram. Serum electrolytes, including magnesium (Ranasinghe, Anaesth, 1994; 49:394), must be measured.

If major surgery is contemplated in a patient with chronic liver disease it is wise to assess the cardiac function with echocardiography. Some degree of mitral regurgitation may be evident in individuals with a hyperdynamic circulation. Radionuclide studies (MUGA scans) at rest and during exercise may be helpful to detect wall-motion abnormalities and assess ejection fraction. Abnormal results are associated with a high risk of intraoperative cardiovascular instability (Berridge, EurJAnaesth, 1989; 1:25). Stress electrocardiograms are performed as part of the

Table 3 Pulmonary abnormalities associated with selected chronic liver disease

Liver disorder	Pathological or pathophysiological pulmonary findings
Cirrhosis	Intrapulmonary shunting
	Portopulmonary shunting
	Pleural shunting
	Pulmonary hypertension
	Pleural effusions
	Impaired hypoxic vasoconstriction
	Ventilation–perfusion mismatch
Primary biliary cirrhosis	Thoracic deformities
	Intrapulmonary granulomas
	Lymphocytic interstitial pneumonitis
	Obstructive airways disease
Chronic active hepatitis	Interstitial pneumonitis
	Pleuritis and pleural effusions
α_1-antitrypsin deficiency	Obstructive airways disease
	Intrapulmonary shunting
Primary sclerosing cholangitis	Suppurative bronchitis
	Bronchiectasis

From Cortese, MayoClinProc,1985; 60:407.

evaluation preceding transplantation. Where there is evidence of coronary vascular disease, coronary angiography is helpful and some patients may be considered for bypass grafting either before transplantation or as a combined procedure, depending on the severity of the underlying liver disease. Single-vessel disease (other than left main stem) does not appear to increase perioperative mortality.

In patients with liver disease, direct measurement of arterial pressure and central venous pressure is essential for all but the most minor of procedures.

A pulmonary artery flotation catheter is indicated if there is any evidence of abnormal cardiac function, and should be considered for major surgery. In hepatic transplantation and major liver surgery the measurement of cardiac output, left- and right-heart pressures, continuous mixed venous oxygen saturation, and systemic vascular resistance is a useful aid to the objective use and assessment of inotropic support and/or vasoconstrictors.

In individuals with serum bilirubin in excess of 2.7 mg/dl, measurement of oxygen saturation may be inaccurate (Chandhary, AmRevRespDis, 1978, 117:173).

Respiratory system

The pulmonary vascular and parenchymal disturbances associated with chronic liver disease may result in decreased arterial oxygen tension and saturation of haemoglobin (Chiesa, ClinSci, 1969; 37: 803). The various pulmonary abnormalities associated with liver disease are well described[8] and are listed in Table 3.

Intrapulmonary shunting in patients with liver disease, first reported in 1956 (Rydell, AmJMed, 1956; 21:450), may amount to 70 per cent of the cardiac output, and, combined with a shift in the oxyhaemoglobin dissociation curve,[9] results in the arterial desaturation so often seen in patients with chronic liver disease. The mechanism of the shunting might be due to an imbalance between vasoconstrictor and vasodilator substances that are abnormally metabolized by the impaired liver, and an unusual regulation of certain pulmonary vessels, which results in vasodilatation

during hypoxia and thus impaired hypoxic vasoconstriction (Daoud, JCI, 1972; 1:1076). In addition, a number of patients with intrapulmonary shunts may become more hypoxaemic in the upright position, presumably because most of the shunting occurs in the lung bases, to which the blood flow is increased in the upright position. Many of these patients become dyspnoeic in the upright position (orthodeoxia), while on assuming the supine position the dyspnoea lessens.

Hepatopulmonary syndrome describes the functional changes that occur in the pulmonary vasculature in association with cirrhosis.[10] There is a spectrum of abnormality from mild hypoxaemia associated with impaired hypoxic vasoconstriction and low pulmonary vascular tone to severe hypoxaemia from shunts and diffusion–perfusion defects (diffusion limitation due to massive dilatation of precapillary and capillary vessels, and rapid perfusion of venous blood through these abnormal vessels). Hypoxaemia due to diffusion limitation improves with an increased fraction of inspired oxygen and can be quantified by the DLCO lung function test (Hourani, AmJMed, 1991; 90:693). A number of reports describe reversal of hepatopulmonary syndrome after successful liver transplantation.[11]

The portal venous system may communicate with the pulmonary veins (para-oesophageal, azygous, and mediastinal veins). This postpulmonary anatomical shunt may become more significant in the presence of portal hypertension. Pulmonary parenchymal/pleural 'spiders' are sometimes found in chronic cirrhosis and must be considered as an anatomical shunt. However, it is generally agreed that these anatomical shunts are a cause of hypoxaemia in only a small percentage of cirrhotics.[12]

Pleural effusions are found in up to 10 per cent of patients with cirrhosis. They can be unilateral or bilateral. The pleural fluid may accumulate rapidly. This effusion is referred to as hepatic hydrothorax and biochemically it resembles ascitic fluid. The mechanisms involved in the formation of pleural effusions are discussed elsewhere (Morrow, ArchIntMed, 1958; 49:193), but it is now thought likely that small defects in the diaphragm act as conduits, with ascitic fluid under pressure passing into the pleural space, which is at a negative pressure (Vargas-Tank, ScaJGastr, 1984; 19: 294).

Before anaesthesia and surgery are contemplated a complete assessment of the respiratory system must be made. In addition to the alteration of blood flow within the lungs and its consequences, the movement of the diaphragm may be restricted by the ascites and pleural effusion.[8] Many alcoholic cirrhotics are heavy cigarette smokers and develop bronchitis and emphysema. Tidal volume, vital capacity and functional residual capacity are decreased, and a compensatory tachypnoea may result in a respiratory alkalosis (Heinemann, AmJMed, 1960; 28:234).

If necessary, attempts should be made to improve respiratory function with physiotherapy, antibiotics, and drainage of ascites and/or hydrothorax. Many cirrhotics are malnourished and have marked muscle wasting; therefore, particular attention should be paid to examination of the intercostal muscles. If marked muscle wasting is apparent, it is an indication that the patient may require ventilatory support postoperatively.

Renal system

Individuals with significant liver disease retain sodium, associated with the accumulation of water, resulting in the increased circulating intravascular volume, ascites, oedema, and pleural effusions. The mechanism of the sodium retention is not clear but several factors may interplay. There is enhanced tubular reabsorption of sodium, increased renin–angiotensin activity, decreased glomerular filtration rate, and decreased renal cortical perfusion. Urinary water excretion is impaired mainly because of increased antidiuretic hormone activity and excess water absorption at the proximal tubule. This combination of sodium retention and water retention may result in a low serum sodium because the water retention may be greater than the sodium retention even though the total body sodium stores are increased. In addition, prerenal insufficiency is not uncommon, owing to the use of diuretics and the presence of tense ascites.

The hepatorenal syndrome is a form of functional renal failure that is characterized by a progressive increase in the plasma creatinine, oliguria, and a low urinary sodium, in the presence of histologically normal kidneys. The disturbed haemodynamics associated with progressive liver disease play an important part in the pathogenesis of hepatorenal syndrome and there have been reports of complete reversal of hepatorenal syndrome following successful liver transplantation. Patients with hepatorenal syndrome are excessively sensitive to insults such as volume depletion or sepsis, and overt renal failure can rapidly ensue.

Jaundiced patients are also at increased risk of developing postoperative oliguric renal failure (Dawson, BrJSurg, 1965; 52:663; Dawson, BMJ, 1965; 1:82), which may be resistant to diuretics. Contributory factors are surgery, a high bilirubin (>120 μmol/l), endotoxaemia (especially Gram-negative bacteria), the use of some aminoglycoside antibiotics, aggressive diuretic therapy, and hypotension. The degree of impairment of liver function may not correlate.[13]

Acute tubular necrosis is more common than hepatorenal syndrome in cirrhotic patients (Shear, AmJMed, 1974; 56:695), and is associated with many of the factors that are associated with hepatorenal syndrome. Differential diagnosis to establish if the renal failure is prerenal or due to hepatorenal syndrome or acute tubular necrosis is important because the treatment for the three is so different. Impairment of renal function is a strong predictor of postoperative sepsis and mortality.

Careful preoperative assessment is essential. It should be remembered that the both the blood urea concentration and serum creatinine may be unreliable indicators of the extent of renal dysfunction in patients with liver disease, with misleadingly low values because of impaired hepatic urea synthesis and reduced muscle mass due to malnutrition. A creatinine clearance measured before major surgery gives helpful information on renal function.

The preoperative correction of hyponatraemia is complicated and requires close monitoring of biochemical and haemodynamic variables. Water restriction, albumin infusions, and reduced diuretic dosage are usually sufficient measures, but in cases of refractory hyponatraemia slow correction by haemofiltration has been advocated (Larner, BMJ, 1988; 297:1514). Rapid reversal of hyponatraemia can result in central pontine myelinolysis, which has been described following liver transplantation (Wzsolek, Transpl, 1989; 48:108).

Hypokalaemia is common, and can be associated with cardiac arrhythmias and muscle weakness. Causes include diuretic therapy, decreased intake, metabolic alkalosis, diarrhoea and vomiting, secondary hyperaldosteronism, and renal tubular defects. Attempts should be made to raise the serum and intracellular potassium before surgery if the hypokalaemia is symptomatic, e.g. cardiac arrhythmias. However, it should be remembered that during major liver surgery massive transfusion of banked blood, and in liver transplantation revascularization, are often associated with a rise in potassium.

Hypomagnesaemia is common in cirrhotics and alcoholic patients; contributory factors include poor diet, secondary hyperaldosteronism, direct effects of alcohol on magnesium excretion, and loop diuretics. Magnesium replacement is indicated to prevent the neuromuscular irritability, hyper-reflexia, and cardiac dysrhythmias that are associated with hypomagnesaemia (Ranasinghe, Anaesth, 1994; 49:394). Additionally, recent work in the animal model suggests that magnesium deficiency is associated with increased mortality in endotoxaemia and that supplementation with magnesium has a protective effect (Salem, CritCareMed, 1995; 23: 108).

Fluid administration in cirrhotic patients can be complicated because sodium-containing intravenous preparations may cause problems in a patient already retaining sodium, but against this must be balanced the fact that salt-free solutions given in excess can result in water intoxication. Because of this, judicious use of dextrose saline (0.18 per cent salt, 4.0 per cent glucose) or 5 per cent dextrose in water is recommended.

In patients with pre-existing renal disease, or those considered at increased risk of developing postoperative renal failure, biochemical and haemodynamic monitoring is essential. Maintenance of normovolaemia is critical and intravascular volume should be assessed by monitoring central venous pressure. An infusion of dopamine (Barnardo, Gastro, 1970; 58:524; Polsen, Anaesth, 1987; 42:15) is commenced and mannitol is given intravenously. As well as its osmotic diuretic effect, mannitol may be protective, as it has been shown in the animal model to restore normal pressure–flow relations at low arterial pressures and to increase glomerular filtration rate in both the intact and ischaemic kidney (Behnia, AnesthAnalg, 1996; 82:902).

Metabolic function

Three areas will be considered:

- glucose homeostasis
- acid–base balance
- nutrition.

Glucose homeostasis

The liver plays an essential part in glucose homeostasis. Hyperglycaemia is countered by glycogenesis (converting glucose to glycogen) and hypoglycaemia causes glycogenolysis (glycogen to glucose). When glycogen stores are depleted, gluconeogenesis (amino acids to glucose) takes place.

Hypoglycaemia, although common in fulminant liver failure, is rarely seen in patients with chronic liver disease, and mild hyperglycaemia and glucose intolerance are usual. Many cirrhotic patients tend to be insulin-resistant. Circulatory concentrations of insulin are elevated and there is an exaggerated increase in insulin in response to a glucose load. Despite this phenomenon, fasting glucose in cirrhotics is often normal and only becomes raised after a glucose load. The hyperglycaemia may be compounded by the frequent use of glucose-containing intravenous fluids in these patients. Diabetes mellitus can result from chronic liver disease, especially with autoimmune chronic active hepatitis and haemochromatosis.[14]

Hypoglycaemia can occur with acute viral hepatitis (Flag, NEJM, 1970; 283:1436), and is both common and frequently severe in preterminal liver failure and in patients with fulminant hepatic failure. These patients require prophylactic dextrose infusions; hypertonic (20–50 per cent) glucose solutions are often used to reduce the water load. Hyperglycaemia is seen more commonly than hypoglycaemia in hepatic transplantation, and this is discussed later.

Because of the liver's key role in glucose homeostasis, it is important to measure blood glucose before surgery and regularly during the operative procedure.

Acid–base balance

Acid–base disturbances are common, the most frequent finding being combined respiratory and metabolic alkalosis (Heinemann, AmJMed, 1960; 28:234). The respiratory component is due to tachypnoea and the metabolic component results from hypokalaemia, vomiting, and potassium-losing diuretics. Severe alkalosis causes hypokalaemia by increasing renal excretion of potassium in exchange for hydrogen ions, and may precipitate encephalopathy by facilitating the passage of ammonia into the brain.[15]

Hypochloraemic acidosis can be caused by potassium-sparing diuretics such as spironolactone, but in general a metabolic acidosis is a grave prognostic sign associated with renal failure, sepsis, or circulatory failure.

Lactate metabolism

Hepatic metabolism of lactate plays an important part in normal acid–base homeostasis, with over 70 per cent of lactate being removed by the liver, mainly by gluconeogenesis. With severe shock even the normal liver has an impaired capacity to dispose of lactate, owing to reduced liver blood flow, saturation of the transporter, and decreased gluconeogenesis due to intracellular acidosis.[16] Marked hyperlactaemia (>10 mmol/l) is a feature of fulminant liver failure or massive ischaemic injury (e.g. primary graft non-function or hepatic arterial thrombosis) and is usually preterminal unless the patient is urgently transplanted. In these circumstances not only is hepatic metabolism of lactate impaired, but also the liver actively produces lactate due to anaerobic glycolysis instead of directing the lactate into gluconeogenesis.

Lactate clearance in significantly impaired in severe liver failure and care should be exercised in the administration of intravenous solutions containing lactate as the liver will only slowly metabolize them to bicarbonate. Acidosis in patients with acute liver failure can be difficult to treat and large amounts of sodium bicarbonate may be required in association with haemofiltration, using lactate-free dialysis fluid.

Nutrition

Patients with endstage liver disease are frequently malnourished, with decreased muscle mass and low fat stores. This is due to reduced intake, malabsorption, impaired hepatic synthesis and degradation of protein and energy substrates, and a catabolic state. Nutrition is difficult because of the need to restrict dietary protein, and excessive glucose or fat can lead to fatty changes and cholestasis.

Severe malnutrition impairs respiratory muscle function and wound healing, and reduces resistance to infection. Dietary supplementation is important before surgery. Portal hypertension can be associated with significant malabsorption and parenteral nutrition may be required in these patients. Branched-chain amino acids may enable protein intake to be increased to adequate levels without precipitating encephalopathy.

Impaired albumin synthesis results in a decreased plasma albumin but with considerable quantities of albumin held in the ascites. The resultant oedema and decreased availability of albumin to carry drugs should be borne in mind. There is considerable debate as to the wisdom of albumin infusion in an attempt to raise the plasma albumin. The antagonists argue that the effect is short-lived, may damp down any albumin synthesis, and only fuels the oedema when much of the transfused albumin ends up in the intracellular pool. Recent studies show that giving albumin can maintain oncotic pressure, but does not decrease morbidity or mortality in critically ill patients. This may be due to continued extravascular leak of albumin (Golub, CritCareMed, 1994; 22:613).

Hepatic encephalopathy

Hepatic encephalopathy is a neuropsychiatric disorder associated with the accumulation of toxic substances that are not cleared by the failing liver. There are also changes in the blood–brain barrier, changes in neurotransmitter concentrations, and altered cerebral metabolism.

Hepatic encephalopathy leading to coma is a significant indicator of high mortality, although the overall survival from hepatic coma is better than any other form of non-traumatic coma (Levy, AnnIntMed, 1981; 94:293).

Hepatic encephalopathy is associated with an elevated plasma ammonia. The ammonia comes from the gastrointestinal tract and is not converted into urea in the liver. Alkalosis can worsen encephalopathy by increasing the conversion of ammonium ions (NH_4^+) into ammonia (NH_3), which is able to cross the blood–brain barrier (Morrow, ArchIntMed, 1958; 49:193).

The accumulation of other substances such as octopamine and mercaptans may be the result of decreased cellular oxidative metabolism. There is subsequent accumulation of amino acids, which are not incorporated into structural and secretory proteins necessary for defence and survival, or removed by gluconeogenesis and oxidation by the liver.[17] Hepatic coma in patients with cirrhosis is possibly a symptom of hyperaminoacidaemia but death is the result of impaired oxidative energy production and a deficiency of amino acid clearance for synthesis of protein required for survival.[17]

Although the mediators involved in the development of encephalopathy in acute and chronic liver disease may be similar, there are some important differences. In chronic liver disease, encephalopathy is usually associated with portosystemic shunting and there is generally an obvious precipitating cause such as gastrointestinal haemorrhage, protein loading, hypokalaemic alkalosis, or sepsis. Cerebral oedema is relatively unusual in chronic liver disease but occurs in up to 80 per cent of patients with acute liver failure. Both vasogenic and cytotoxic mechanisms are involved. Brainstem herniation caused by high intracranial pressure is a frequent cause of death in patients with acute liver failure, and monitoring of intracranial pressure is recommended if the patient is in grade IV coma or ventilated and awaiting transplantation (Cordoba, LiverTranspISurg, 1995; 3:187).

Several treatments will have been instituted before the anaesthetist is asked to see the patient before anaesthesia/surgery. Lactulose is used to acidify the gut, encouraging ammonia to convert to ammonium and remain in the gut. Neomycin is used to destroy bacteria in the gut that produce ammonia. However, it should be remembered that neomycin may be nephrotoxic as well as ototoxic, and may prolong the effect of neuromuscular blockers. Mannitol may be used to encourage and maintain urine output and reduce cerebral oedema. In some cases, tracheal intubation and ventilatory support may be indicated. Acidosis, hypoglycaemia, and hyperglycaemia are treated as required.

When anaesthetizing these individuals it is appropriate to use a minimum of drugs. More importantly, the patient will require continuous monitoring of haemodynamic and biochemical status, and support or treatment as indicated.

Coagulation

The liver is central to haemostasis: it is the primary site of synthesis of most of the coagulation factors and inhibitors of the coagulation cascade and also clears activated factors from the circulation. Liver disease can result in complex and variable coagulation disturbances, and also imbalances between the coagulation and fibrinolytic systems resulting in a bleeding diathesis. Impaired haemostatic function in patients with liver disease results from a number of factors, some or all of which may be present, depending on the nature and severity of the underlying disease process. These include vitamin K deficiency (factors II, VII, IX, and X), reduced hepatic synthesis of coagulation factors and inhibitors, a low-grade disseminated intravascular coagulation, enhanced fibrinolytic activity, and quantitative as well as qualitative platelet defects.

Patients with hepatocellular disease (cirrhosis, chronic active hepatitis) have much greater derangement of coagulation than those with cholestatic disease (Ritter, MayoClinProc, 1989; 64:216). Cirrhotic patients may have elevated concentrations of tissue plasminogen activator and reduced antiplasmin activity, resulting in accelerated fibrinolysis; in addition, the increased concentrations of thrombin–antithrombin and fibrin degradation products found in cirrhotics are evidence of coagulation activation in these patients (Paramo, BloodCoagFibrinol, 1991; 2:227).

In addition, many cirrhotic patients have a hypochromic microcytic (or macrocytic) anaemia caused by malabsorption of iron and folic acid, frequent variceal bleeding, and hypersplenism (Sheehy, JLabClinMed, 1960; 56:72). Thrombocytopenia is common and often there are qualitative abnormalities of platelet function. The total platelet count in a cirrhotic may be normal, but between 60 to 90 per cent of platelets can be sequestered in an enlarged spleen (Aster, JCI, 1966; 45:645).

Patients with endstage liver disease have an increased tendency to develop fibrinolysis and approx. 15 per cent of cirrhotic patients demonstrate a fibrinolytic state before surgery (Fletcher, JCI, 1964, 43:681). In some patients undergoing orthotopic liver transplantation the fibrinolytic activity may be increased to such an extent that it leads to clinically significant fibrinolysis and microvascular bleeding. Fibrinolysis is more frequent in patients with cirrhosis as opposed to cholestatic disease, and is maximal at the end of the anhepatic period and immediately following reperfusion of the grafted liver. Antifibrinolytic drugs such as ε-aminocaproic acid have been used both prophylactically and also to treat active fibrinolysis (Kang, Anesthesiol, 1987; 66:766). Aprotinin (Trasylol) is a naturally occurring inhibitor of human plasmin and kallikrein. It has been used with great success in cardiac surgery, where blood transfusions are markedly reduced (Royston, Lancet, 1987; 1289). A number of studies show that the use of aprotinin in liver transplantation results in a reduction in blood loss and transfusion of both red cells and blood products. The effects appear most marked on stage III (postreperfusion) blood loss, which is usually associated with severe coagulopathy (Mallett, TransplProc, 1991; 23:1931; Scudamore, AmJSurg, 1995; 169:546). The optimal dose regimen—that is, 'low dose', which will provide effective antiplasmin concentrations, or 'high dose', which is necessary for an antikallikrein effect—is still a subject of some debate (Marcel, AnesthAnalg, 1996; 82:1122).

Major abdominal surgery in patients with unsuspected liver disease

By way of a cautionary note it must be stressed that patients incubating viral hepatitis can have astronomically high morbidity and mortality when subjected to the stress of anaesthesia and surgery (Wataneeyawech, NYStateJMed, 1976; 7:1278). The mortality following surgery associated with hepatitis A infection approaches 35 per cent (compared to 0.1 per cent without surgery). The cause of death is generally either fulminant hepatic failure or sepsis. Consequently it is mandatory that patients with elevated transaminases and a history of prodromal infection should have serological testing done and elective procedures cancelled until the enzymes are back in the normal range (Kools, PostgradMed, 1987; 81:45).

One-quarter of jaundiced patients who are suspected on clinical grounds of having biliary obstruction are eventually diagnosed as having hepatocellular disease (O'Connor, Gastro, 1983; 84:1498). These patients should not be subjected to unnecessary anaesthesia and surgery. The Kings College Group (Powell-Jackson, BrJSurg, 1982; 69:499) reviewed the records of 36 patients referred to the liver unit after parenchymal liver disease had been found unexpectedly during laparotomy. The mortality was 30 per cent and morbidity 60 per cent. Complications included sepsis, renal failure, hepatic failure, and gastrointestinal bleeding. They concluded that careful history-taking, evaluation of liver function tests, and use of endoscopic retrograde cholangiopancreatography and percutaneous transhepatic cholangiography, in addition to ultrasound scanning, would provide the correct diagnosis in the majority of cases and avoid the need for exploratory laparotomy and its attendant risks.

Anaesthetic drugs and liver disease

Although the liver is a major site of drug biotransformation, the effect of hepatic dysfunction on drug elimination and disposition is inconsistent. Severe liver disease alters the pharmacokinetics and pharmacodynamics of many of the drugs used in anaesthesia, in some cases in a relatively unpredictable fashion. The overall effect depends on the nature of the drug, the enzymes involved in the reaction, the type and severity of hepatic disease, and any alterations in liver blood flow due to portosystemic and intrahepatic shunting. All drugs, therefore, should be used with thought and a degree of caution in patients with hepatic dysfunction.[20]

General factors that can cause substantial alterations in pharmacokinetics include: an increased distribution volume, lowered serum albumin that decreases some drug-binding sites, and reduced drug metabolism and excretion. Hepatic extraction of a drug is influenced by three independent factors: liver blood flow, drug protein binding, and the maximal intrinsic capability of metabolizing enzymes to clear a drug. Clearance of highly extracted drugs is dependent primarily on liver blood flow (e.g. lignocaine, propranolol). Clearance of poorly extracted drugs is limited by metabolizing activity and is independent of liver blood flow (e.g. phenytoin, warfarin). Obviously there are many drugs that fall somewhere in between these extremes. In general, drugs that undergo oxidative metabolism (phase I biotransformation) have their clearance reduced in proportion to the other indices of quantitative liver function. These reactions are mediated by cytochrome-P450 enzymes located mainly in hepatocytes around the central vein. Drugs that are conjugated (phase II biotransformation) usually have normal pharmacokinetics, even in the presence of severe liver disease.[21] Concomitant renal dysfunction in patients with advanced liver disease can further interfere with metabolism and elimination of drugs (Branch, Hepatol, 1987; 4:773).

Benzodiazepines

Liver disease is known to enhance cerebral sensitivity to psychotropic drugs. In the case of the benzodiazepines this is due to a potentiation of an underlying encephalopathic state and a direct enhancement of the response mediated at the benzodiazepine receptor (Branch, Hepatol, 1987; 4:773). There are increased circulating concentrations of γ-aminobutyric acid (**GABA**) in patients with hepatic encephalopathy (Hoyumpa, Hepatol, 1986; 6:1042) and a β_2-ligand is present in the cerebrospinal fluid of these patients, which enhances the susceptibility of the GABA receptor to respond to GABA (Mullen, Lancet, 1988; i:457). There have also been a number of case reports where encephalopathy has been effectively reversed with the benzodiazepine antagonist flumazenil (Burke, Lancet, 1988; 505).

Although the central nervous depressant effect of the benzodiazepines is increased and their metabolism may be altered (Macgilchrist, Gastro, 1981; 81:1006), it should be remembered that the benzodiazepines as a group have a wide therapeutic index, and they should not be arbitrarily avoided if they can contribute to the therapeutic management of the patient. Lorazepam and temazepam can be useful for preoperative anxiolysis, and midazolam can be very helpful in postoperative sedation if used with caution.

Narcotics

Many studies have been done on the pharmacokinetics of narcotic drugs in the presence of liver disease: however, there have been large variations in the reported effects. Much of this inconsistency may be a function of the heterogeneous pathophysiology of liver disease with respect to hepatocellular function, protein binding, and hepatic blood flow. Morphine and fentanyl have the most predictable effects and can be used safely in mild to moderate liver disease.[22] Pethidine should be used with care and reduced dosage (Klotz, ClinPharmTher, 1974; 16:667). Even moderate cirrhosis significantly reduces the clearance of alfentanil, which must also be used with care (Ferrier, Anesthesiol, 1985; 62:480).

The analgesic requirements of liver transplant patients immediately postoperatively are very much less than those of patients who have equivalent major surgery such as liver resection (Robertson, AnesthAnalg, 1996; 82: S381). The mechanisms involved are incompletely understood but include the effects of endorphins in cerebrospinal fluid, high-dose steroids, liver denervation, and the altered pharmacokinetics and dynamics of endstage liver disease.

Non-steroidal anti-inflammatory drugs

Although this group of drugs has many useful properties, the risk of causing gastrointestinal bleeding and renal dysfunction in patients with liver disease absolutely contraindicates their prescription.

Neuromuscular blockers
Depolarizing drugs (suxamethonium)

The reduction in plasma pseudocholinesterases that occurs with liver disease will result in some increased duration of action, but this is generally of little clinical significance.

Non-depolarizing drugs

Atracurium is the relaxant of choice in liver disease as its metabolism is independent of hepatic metabolism, occurring by Hoffman elimination and ester hydrolysis (Ward, BrJAnaesth, 1983; 55:1169). Clearance of its metabolite laudanosine is partially dependent on liver function, but even with prolonged infusions, concentrations do not reach those where neurological stimulation is of concern. Vecuronium is well tolerated in cirrhotics in small doses, but, with doses of 0.2 mg/kg, recovery of the twitch height is markedly prolonged (Bell, BrJAnaesth, 1985; 57:160). Increased volume of distribution will cause a relative resistance to the initial dose of all relaxants (i.e., higher dosage required). This may cause problems with reversal, especially with pancuronium and tubocurarine, where there is reduced elimination. Doxacurium, a newer muscle relaxant, appears to be a useful drug without prolonged effects in liver disease (Freeman, AnesthAnalg 1989; 68:590). Hepatobiliary clearance of rocuronium is high and prolonged duration of blockade can be anticipated. Whatever drug is used, it is advisable to monitor neuromuscular function in these patients with a peripheral nerve stimulator.

Inhalational agents

Of the available inhalational agents, isoflurane has many advantages in that it undergoes minimal biotransformation (<0.2 per cent) (Holaday, Anesthesiol, 1975; 43:323), and is potentially the least hepatotoxic. In addition, isoflurane maintained the relation between hepatic oxygen supply and uptake better than either halothane or enflurane (Matsumoto, Anesthesiol, 1987; 66:337). Sevoflurane has similar haemodynamic effects to those of isoflurane and may be a suitable alternative (Frink, Anesthesiol, 1992; 76:85). Although early studies on desflurane indicate it is a very useful agent in many circumstance (Merin, Anesthesiol, 1991; 74:568), the fact that it decreases both portal venous and hepatic arterial flow suggests that until further data are available it should perhaps be better avoided in patients with known hepatic dysfunction (Jones, BrJAnaesth, 1990; 64:482).

Halothane is best avoided because of its known hepatotoxicity (Brown, Anesthesiol, 1981; 55:93), which although very rare, occurs unpredictably and is dependent on a number of interrelated factors including age, genetics, hepatic oxygenation, degree of hepatic biotransformation, and previous exposure (Neuberger, BMJ, 1984; 289:1136).

Liver blood flow

Generally, the liver can tolerate cardiovascular insults to a greater degree than other critical organs, because of its dual blood supply and resultant increased oxygen delivery, its autoregulatory mechanisms, and the rapid readjustments in hepatic arterial flow to changes in portal flow. However, blood flow and oxygen supply may become critical in the presence of liver disease. It is well established that the inhalational agents and spinal anaesthetics will cause a reduction in hepatic flow.[23] However, the major changes in hepatic blood flow are apparently related more to the operation performed rather than to the anaesthetic agent used (Gelman, ArchSurg, 1976; II:881). Manipulating the intra-abdominal viscera can cause a 50 to 60 per cent fall in hepatic blood flow. It is well recognized that liver enzymes are significantly increased after major surgery but not after minor surgery (Harper, AnesthAnalg, 1982; 61:79). Thus, provided an adequate perfusion pressure and oxygen delivery are maintained, the effects of the inhalational agents are only of minor significance compared to the surgery itself.

Anaesthetic management of major liver surgery

The main anaesthetic problems related to liver surgery include deranged physiology as a result of hepatic disease, altered drug handling, electrolyte and metabolic changes, haemodynamic disturbances as a result of surgical manipulations, and the ever-present risk of sudden and massive blood loss. In addition, there are often major haemostatic defects resulting from impaired liver function, compounded by the effects of dilutional coagulopathy. In order to illustrate some of these problems and their management, the anaesthetic care of patients undergoing liver resection and orthotopic liver transplantation will be discussed in detail.

Liver resection

Elective resection is generally performed for either primary hepatomas or more commonly for solitary secondary deposits, usually from a carcinoma of the colon or rectum (Stimpson, AmJSurg, 1987; 153:189). A high proportion (60–85 per cent) of patients with primary liver tumours will have underlying cirrhosis. In many cases this will preclude resection because of the limited capacity of cirrhotic livers to regenerate and concern over the impaired functional status of the remaining liver postoperatively. Liver transplantation has been offered to some of these patients but metastatic recurrence of tumour is high.

In contrast, those with solitary metastatic lesions generally have normal liver function. Up to 80 per cent of the liver can be removed because of the superb regenerative capabilities of this organ, the liver regaining its original weight within 4 to 5 weeks. Surgical resection of metastatic tumour confined to the liver can be very successful, with survival rates of 70 per cent or more.

The major aspects to be considered with liver resection include:

(1) preoperative functional status of the liver;
(2) haemodynamic changes and monitoring;
(3) the possibility of massive and rapid blood loss;
(4) coagulation disturbances;
(5) fluid, electrolyte, and metabolic derangements.

Preoperative hepatic function

The majority of patients will have normal hepatic function, and intraoperative management is directed primarily at preserving haemodynamic stability and maintaining optimal hepatic blood supply and oxygen delivery to avoid compromising the liver and to minimize any postoperative dysfunction of the liver remnant. A few carefully selected patients with early cirrhosis may be considered for resection. They undoubtedly present an increased risk, especially of bleeding and developing coagulopathies intraoperatively, and inevitably exhibit a degree of deterioration of liver function postoperatively, sometimes aggressive and irreversible. There is some evidence that prostaglandin E_1 can protect against hepatic injury and consideration should be given to its use in cirrhotic patients (Peltekian, LiverTransplSurg, 1996; 2:171).

Thorough preoperative evaluation is essential to evaluate the risk to each patient, with particular attention to renal, cardiac, respiratory, and nutritional status, and derangements of coagulation. Patients who have received preoperative chemotherapy with Adriamycin should have a cardiac echography to assess ventricular function.

Haemodynamic changes and monitoring

Direct monitoring of arterial and central venous pressures is mandatory. A pulmonary artery flotation catheter for measurement of wedge pressure, cardiac output, and calculation of systemic vascular resistance is also necessary if the patient has a limited cardiovascular reserve or if the surgical technique will involve cross-clamping of the inferior vena cava or the use of a venovenous bypass. The risks of sudden massive haemorrhage and also the potential for air embolism during resection of the liver require that relatively high filling pressures (central venous pressure 12–14 mmHg) are maintained in order to attenuate the effects of either of these events.

Total vascular exclusion

This technique is being used with good results in some centres to minimize bleeding and facilitate resection of the liver. Most patients tolerate this procedure well and maintain an acceptable blood pressure, despite the reduction in venous return caused by caval clamping, by increasing their systemic vascular resistance and mounting a compensatory tachycardia. Cardiac output typically falls by less than 15 per cent[24] if the patient has been adequately volume-loaded before cross-clamping. Caution is required in patients with known cardiovascular disease because of the increased myocardial oxygen demand associated with these haemodynamic changes. Following release of the clamps, cardiac output increases and systemic vascular resistance falls, with the development of a hyperdynamic state that may necessitate diuretic therapy.

Blood loss

Because of the risk of massive blood loss, it is essential that adequate venous access is secured to facilitate transfusion. Using a Seldinger technique, wide-bore cannulas (8–10 FG) are inserted in a jugular vein and/or the antecubital fossa. Blood loss can be totally unpredictable and can vary from a few hundred millitres to 10 l or more. As in liver transplantation, postoperative morbidity and mortality correlate significantly with this variable (Sitzmann, AnnSurg, 1994; 219:13). Bleeding can be rapid and massive: with caval tears it can exceed 1000 ml/min; thus it is vital to have facilities to enable transfusion at very high flow rates. The rapid infusion system developed in Pittsburgh by Sassano (marketed by Haemonetics, Massachusetts, USA) enables controlled delivery of prewarmed and filtered blood at flow rates up to 1.5 l/min.[25]

Another aspect of concern is the association between recurrence of tumour and perioperative transfusion of banked blood (Yamoamoto, Surgery, 1994; 115:303). Autotransfusion (Cell Saver) systems salvage up to 30 to 40 per cent of red-cell loss and can significantly reduce banked blood requirements.[26] The current view is that their use is contraindicated in patients with malignant disease because of the risk of reinfusing tumour cells, but some interesting work is appearing to suggest that the use of leucocyte depletion filters may significantly reduce this risk. If the patient has a good preoperative haemoglobin (12 g or more), isovolaemic haemodilution is a useful technique for providing autologous blood and reducing red-cell loss.

Over the last decade, newer surgical techniques and equipment such as ultrasonic dissectors and argon-beam coagulators have done much to reduce the average blood loss during liver resection. There is increasing interest in vascular exclusion to minimize blood loss, both hepatic inflow occlusion and total vascular exclusion (porta hepatis and supra- and infrahepatic cava). On using total vascular

exclusion, 45 per cent of patients in a series required no red-cell transfusion at all.[24]

With massive, rapid transfusion, hypocalcaemia from citrate intoxication can become a problem even with normal hepatic function, resulting in myocardial depression. Ideally, ionized serum calcium measurements should be available; however, if haemodynamic depression becomes apparent in the face of normal filling pressures, then calcium chloride (0.06–0.1 mmol/kg) should be given.

Coagulation

The majority of patients presenting for liver resection will have normal liver synthetic function and normal coagulation preoperatively. There is a known association between malignant disease and hypercoagulability, and this has been demonstrated using thromboelastography in some patients undergoing liver resection (Howland, ArchSurg, 1974; 108:605). In cirrhotic patients, coagulation may be abnormal, with prolongation of the prothrombin time and a low platelet count, and fresh-frozen plasma and platelets should be available for them. In addition to the haemostatic defects associated with underlying cirrhosis, dilutional coagulopathy can develop as a result of massive transfusion and further blood-product support may be required. Therapy should be guided by regular clotting screens (prothombin time, partial thromboplastin time, fibrinogen, and platelet count), and also by thromboelastography where available (Mallett, BrJAnaesth, 1992; 69:307).

Fluid and electrolyte balance

Fluid management can be difficult in these cases. Third-space translocation of electrolyte-rich interstitial and extracellular fluid can be extensive in operations of this nature, because of surgical trauma and inflammation, particularly in the retroperitoneal space, and also because of the loss and reaccumulation of ascitic fluid in some cirrhotics. Fluid replacement must be guided by intravascular filling pressure and regular haematocrits. In cirrhotic patients, secondary hyperaldosteronism causes problems with salt and water retention, and salt-containing crystalloid solutions should be avoided or used sparingly. Dextrose–saline or 5 per cent dextrose should be used for background maintenance fluids. Hypoglycaemia can occur perioperatively and blood glucose must be checked regularly.

As mentioned earlier, jaundiced patients are at increased risk of developing postoperative oliguric renal failure (Dawson, BrJSurg, 1965; 52:663; Dawson, BMJ, 1965; 1:82). Maintenance of normovolaemia is essential and perioperative diuresis has been stressed as an important prophylactic measure. Renal-dose dopamine was effective in improving renal function in cirrhotics (Barnardo, Gastro, 1970; 58:524).

Orthotopic liver transplantation

There has been an exponential increase in both the number of centres performing liver transplantation and in the total number of patients receiving transplants. The transplant recipient will generally have been admitted to hospital some time before the operation for a full medical work-up, at which point an anaesthetic assessment is made, with particular emphasis on the cardiac, respiratory, renal, and coagulation systems, and on nutritional status. Many patients will be admitted from home when an organ becomes available; preoperative assessment at that time is necessarily brief, including a review of any recent changes and immediate preoperative chest radiograph, electrocardiograph, full blood count, clotting screen, and urea and electrolytes.

The introduction of University of Wisconsin preservation solution has extended the cold ischaemia time of liver grafts up to 18 to 20 h and has enabled liver transplants to be performed as semielective procedures in daylight hours, although the cold ischaemia time is limited to under 14 h where possible. In the case of fulminant liver failure or primary non-functional graft, transplantation is done as soon as a donor liver becomes available.

Surgical stages

The operation is divided into three stages as follows.

Dissection: stage I. From skin incision (bilateral subcostal extended to xiphisternum) to skeletonization of the hepatic vasculature. Previous upper abdominal surgery or portal hypertension can significantly increase blood loss in this stage.

Anhepatic: stage II. During this stage the major vessels are clamped and the native liver is removed. Clamping of the vena cava can have serious haemodynamic consequences and venovenous bypass may be used to alleviate this. The donor organ is placed in the recipient's hepatic fossa (beginning of warm ischaemia time) and anastomosed in place. The sequence of anastomoses is usually suprahepatic vena cava, portal vein, and then infrahepatic cava. Before reperfusion the liver is flushed through a cannula placed in the portal vein with 500 to 1000 ml of albumin to remove the perfusate solution and any air in the hepatic vasculature, and the effluent drained through the incomplete infrahepatic caval anastomosis. The anhepatic phase is also marked by significant metabolic changes and, in some patients, progressive deterioration in coagulation.

Postreperfusion: stage III. This begins with reperfusion of the grafted liver by release of the clamps on the infra- and suprahepatic inferior vena cava to restore normal caval flow, then the portal vein clamps are released. The early reperfusion stage is not infrequently characterized by both haemodynamic instability and also a sudden worsening of coagulation, which can be associated with microvascular ooze. Once the initial reperfusion stage is over, the hepatic artery is anastomosed and then the biliary tract reconstructed (duct-to-duct or roux-en-Y choledochojejunostomy). Early signs of graft functioning include spontaneous correction of coagulopathy and reversal of lactic acidosis. The latter part of surgery is usually a time of minimal blood loss and haemodynamic stability.

Anaesthesia for liver transplantation

Maintenance of physiological homeostasis and stability is the primary objective of the anaesthetist and techniques for the provision of anaesthesia, analgesia, and muscle relaxation should ideally be chosen for minimum intervention, for example by continuous intravenous infusions, so as not to detract from the overall task. This is essential in the face of the numerous physiological and metabolic insults that can occur both predictably and otherwise during the procedure.

Premedication

In the absence of encephalopathy, oral temazepam can be given approx. 2 h preoperatively. Ranitidine or omeprazole are usefully included in the premedication.

Induction and maintenance of anaesthesia

Preoxygenation and a rapid-sequence intravenous induction are required if the patient is in any way neurologically obtunded or has tense ascites. Both thiopentone and propofol are suitable induction agents, and suxamethonium may be used for intubation as prolongation of its action due to low plasma pseudocholinesterase is not a practical problem.

Maintenance is with an air/oxygen mixture together with isoflurane. Large tidal volumes (10–12 ml/kg) and 5 cm of positive end-expiratory pressure are used to minimize basal atelectasis. Nitrous oxide is avoided because of problems with bowel distension interfering with abdominal closure, the potential for air emboli (Mazzoni, TransplProc, 1979; 11:267; Prager, Anesthesiol, 1990; 72:198), depression of bone-marrow metabolism of vitamin B_{12} and folate with prolonged exposure, and possible detrimental effects on liver blood flow (Seyde, BrJAnaesth, 1986; 58:63).

Fentanyl is used for analgesia and atracurium for muscle relaxation, usually by infusion following an initial bolus. The potential for drug wash-out due to massive blood or fluid replacement should be borne in mind when giving any drug by infusion.

Vascular access

During liver transplantation there is always a possibility of massive blood loss and a requirement to be able to transfuse large volumes of fluid rapidly. Dedicated wide-bore (8 or 10 FG) transfusion cannulas, inserted in the jugular vein or antecubital fossa, are therefore essential. A triple-lumen central venous catheter is used for drug infusions and maintenance fluids. Two arterial lines are inserted, one for monitoring and one (non-heparinized) for blood sampling. An introducer sheath is also placed for the pulmonary artery flotation catheter. As an alternative to axillary vein cut-down, many centres now use large-bore cannulas inserted percutaneously into the left internal jugular vein for the return limb of the venovenous bypass circuit.

Monitoring

Basic monitoring includes electrocardiogram, capnography and agent analysis, airway pressure and volume, core temperature, hourly urinary output, central venous pressure, and direct arterial pressure. In adults an oximetric pulmonary artery flotation catheter is used to determine wedge pressures, cardiac output and mixed venous oxygen saturation, and to calculate systemic vascular resistance and oxygen delivery and consumption.

Some centres routinely use a right-ventricular ejection fraction catheter whilst others use rapid-response catheters that give a 'continuous' read-out of cardiac output. Inferior vena caval pressure is also often measured via a femoral vein cannula. The efficacy of venovenous bypass can be assessed by measuring the pressure gradient between the inferior vena cava and the right atrium (Peachey, TransplProc, 1989; 21:3526).

Specific anaesthetic problems related to liver transplantation

The major anaesthetic problems associated with orthotopic liver transplantation include massive blood loss, cardiovascular instability, coagulopathy, and electrolyte and metabolic disturbance.

Cardiovascular

The cardiovascular changes can be conveniently divided into the three stages of the operation as follows.

Dissection

The major changes associated with this stage are related to intravascular volume depletion as a result of blood loss and the drainage of large amounts of ascitic fluid. Blood loss depends to a large extent on the degree of coagulopathy, portal hypertension, and hepatic hilar scarring. Previous surgery involving the liver or biliary system, or shunt procedures, will significantly increase the likelihood of major blood loss.

Other causes of hypotension in this stage include surgical manipulations interfering with preload and, rarely pericardial effusion, which should be suspected in the presence of high filling pressures and low cardiac output.

Anhepatic stage

The major feature of this stage relates to the haemodynamic effects caused by cross-clamping of the inferior vena cava. On clamping, venous return drops by 50 per cent or more, particularly if there is not an extensive collateral network. Mean arterial pressure may not fall significantly, but is maintained at the expense of a two- to threefold increase in systemic vascular resistance, while cardiac output falls by 40 to 50 per cent (Pappas, Surgery, 1971; 70: 872). Most patients tolerate cross-clamping well, provided they are normovolaemic or slightly hypervolaemic before clamping and have a well-developed collateral circulation. It is essential to be cautious with transfusion during this stage as when the caval clamps are released and normal venous return restored the sudden volume loading may precipitate right heart failure. Patients with a limited cardiac reserve do not tolerate the increased afterload that results from clamping and caval bypass or preservation is necessary.

Venovenous bypass (femoral and portal veins to axillary vein) minimizes the haemodynamic changes that occur with occlusion of the major vessels, and, in addition, reduces the portal and systemic (renal and intestinal) congestion that results. In critical cases, venovenous bypass may provide improved haemodynamic control and decrease renal impairment postoperatively (Griffith, SGO, 1985; 160:271), but there is little objective evidence that the routine use of bypass improves results. The controversy over the benefits of venovenous bypass remains; some centres use it routinely and others not at all (Wall, Transpl, 1987; 43:56). Many centres use it only in selected patients for either medical indications, such as cardiac or renal dysfunction or pulmonary hypertension, or for surgical reasons. In patients with fulminant hepatic failure and raised intracranial pressure, the use of venovenous bypass is essential to limit the haemodynamic fluctuations and minimize fluid transfusion.

A significant fall in oxygen uptake (Vo_2) occurs on clamping (Svenson, TransplProc, 1987; 19(Suppl. 3):56). This is due to absent hepatic metabolic function and also to a reduction in oxygen supply to peripheral tissues, which is partly corrected by using venovenous bypass. Vo_2 increases in both groups after unclamping; this settles but remains at higher levels than during stage I, indicating a degree of oxygen debt incurred during stage II.

Ionized hypocalcaemia

Serum ionized calcium decreases progressively throughout the procedure, reaching the lowest concentrations in the anhepatic period and for a short while after reperfusion (Marquez, Anaesthesiol, 1986; 65:457). Citrate toxicity develops because of the combination of rapid blood transfusion in the presence of impaired or absent hepatic function, accentuated by hypothermia and acidosis. Ionized calcium below 0.56 mmol/l is associated with a decrease in left-ventricular stroke work index, despite adequate filling pressures and unchanged systemic vascular resistance.[27] Ionized Ca^{2+} must be measured regularly (half-hourly in the anhepatic period), and concentrations below 0.9 mmol/l treated with calcium chloride (0.06–0.1 mmol/kg). Hypercalcaemia has occurred following overcorrection of hypocalcaemia, but no ill effects were observed.[27]

Post-reperfusion

In order to reduce some of the effects of reperfusion it is essential to check blood gases, acid–base status, potassium and calcium, and to correct any abnormalities before the vascular clamps are released.

Profound haemodynamic changes can accompany reperfusion of the donor liver (Aggarwal, TransplProc, 1987; 19 (Suppl. 3):54). Typically there is a variable degree of hypotension associated with a profound fall in systemic vascular resistance and an increased cardiac index. Central venous and pulmonary arterial pressures also increase. There may also be myocardial depression, which can contribute further to hypotension. Dysrhythmias or bradyarrhythmias can also occur. In general these changes are short-lived, but may require treatment with sodium bicarbonate, calcium chloride, and small (5–10 µg) boluses of adrenaline or noradrenaline. The preload can be increased to treat hypotension, but aggressive transfusion will aggravate the already elevated filling pressures and also increase impedance to hepatic venous outflow, thus compromising hepatic perfusion and oxygen supply.

Although the haemodynamic effects generally subside within 10 to 15 min, pulmonary hypertension, high central venous pressure, and moderate hypotension may persist for some time and occasionally require continued support with adrenaline or noradrenaline. The profound haemodynamic changes at reperfusion are probably caused by the release of inflammatory mediators and cytokines from the ischaemic liver, and also by the release of vasoactive substances following decompression of the congested portal circulation. The cause of the acute increase in filling pressures is not entirely clear, but myocardial depression, right-ventricular strain from increased pre- and afterload, and air emboli may all play a part (Ellis, Anaesthesiol, 1987; 67S:A82; Lichtor, AnaesthAnalg, 1987; 66S:104).

Respiratory

These patients require ventilation with FIo_2 of 0.4–0.7, because there is frequently a degree of existing hypoxaemia. We use large tidal volumes (>10 ml/kg) and 5 cm positive end-expiratory pressure to reduce atelectasis. Pulmonary oedema may develop as a result of overzealous transfusion, especially following unclamping when normal venous return is restored, and is extremely difficult to treat.[26] Pleural effusions and pneumothorax may exist preoperatively or develop during the operation.

Renal

Renal impairment postoperatively is not uncommon and is associated with increased mortality.[30] Pre-existing renal dysfunction, hypotension, massive blood loss, graft dysfunction, and sepsis all increase the risk. A progressive decrease in glomerular filtration rate in the first few weeks post-transplant is common and related to the use of the immunosuppressant agents cyclosporin or FK506 (Tacrolimus).

Intraoperatively, the use of mannitol or low-dose dopamine as renal protection is often recommended, although their efficacy is unproven (Swygert, Anesthesiol, 1991; 75:571). There is some evidence that low-dose or continuous infusion of frusemide may also be effective in limiting renal dysfunction (Driscoll, CritCareMed, 1989; 17:1341). Although there are theoretical reasons for advocating the use of venovenous bypass (more stable haemodynamics and improved renal perfusion pressure) in patients with compromised renal function, a recent study failed to demonstrate any significant difference in postoperative renal function in patients who did or did not receive venovenous bypass (Veroli, AnesthAnalg, 1992; 75:489).

Electrolyte and acid–base balance

Repeated analysis of blood gases and determination of ionized calcium, magnesium, potassium, sodium, and glucose are essential during liver transplantation.

Potassium

Although many patients present with low potassium (<3.5 mmol/l), this should not be treated unless there is evidence of ventricular irritability, because of the sudden increase in potassium that can accompany reperfusion. A progressive increase in potassium can occur with the transfusion of large amounts of banked blood and products, acidosis, or renal impairment. If this becomes a problem, red cells should be washed using a cell saver (Ellis, TransplProc, 1987; 19 (Suppl. 3):73). Hyperkalaemia is treated in the usual way with sodium bicarbonate, calcium chloride, and insulin and glucose. Following reperfusion, when the graft liver starts to function, hypokalaemia may develop as the hepatocytes take up large quantities of potassium lost during ischaemic preservation (Abouna, Surgery, 1971; 69:419). It is essential to continue monitoring serum potassium regularly to detect severe hypokalaemia and treat it promptly.

Magnesium

Hypomagnesaemia is common in these patients and may increase the risk of intraoperative dysrhythmias. Ionized magnesium below 0.4 mmol/l should be corrected with magnesium sulphate, 20–40 mmol.

Calcium

Hypocalcaemia due to citrate toxicity is discussed above.

Sodium

Frequently these patients are found to be hyponatraemic preoperatively, the severity often reflecting the degree to which splanchnic and renal haemodynamics have been altered by progressive liver disease. Rapid increases in serum sodium and plasma osmolality due to transfusions, administration of sodium bicarbonate, and hyperglycaemia can be associated with adverse neurological outcomes (Holt, TransplProc, 1991; 23:1986).

Acid–base balance

Progressive metabolic acidosis and an increase in lactate occur during the anhepatic stage and early in stage III (Tulloch, Anaesthesiol, 1984; 61: A271). Because of the adverse effects of acidosis on myocardial function it is advisable to correct acidosis with bicarbonate to maintain a base deficit less than –8 before reperfusion. If graft function is good, the lactate acidosis will correct without treatment within a few hours. Persistence of acidosis is a grave prognostic sign suggestive of poor hepatic function and/or impaired tissue perfusion (Fortunato, TransplProc, 1987; 19(Suppl. 3):59).

Glucose metabolism

Hypoglycaemia is rarely a problem and glucose-containing solutions are generally unnecessary, except in the occasional case with extensive hepatic necrosis or fulminating hepatitis. Following reperfusion there is a often a sudden increase in blood sugar: this is due to administration of methylprednisolone, and also to the release of glucose from the donor liver (DeWolf, AnaesthAnalg, 1987; 66: 76; Mallett, AnesthAnalg, 1989; 68:182), and hormonal changes which occur at that time (Mallett, TransplProc, 1989; 21 (Suppl. 3):3529). This will generally resolve spontaneously, but occasionally insulin infusions may be required.

Thermal balance

Aggressive prevention of hypothermia is extremely important during liver transplantation. Potential causes of hypothermia include heat loss during presurgical preparation, evaporative loss from the exposed peritoneum and intestines, use of venovenous bypass, massive fluid replacement, and reperfusion of the cold donor graft in the recipient.

Hypothermia (<35°C) has a number of potentially serious adverse consequences, including potentiation of coagulopathy, impaired oxygen delivery, reduced renal concentrating ability, and reduced splanchnic blood flow. Myocardial contractility is reduced and there is an increased susceptibility to dysrhythmias. Recently, it has also been demonstrated that white-cell function is adversely effected by hypothermia.

Methods of minimizing heat loss include the use of humidified anaesthetic gases, warming all intravenous fluids, and heated underblankets. Warm-air convective warming blankets placed over the patient are particularly effective at maintaining core temperature.

Blood loss and red-cell transfusion

Early transplants were frequently complicated by massive blood loss and figures of 40 units or more were not unusual. Improved surgical experience and better management of coagulation have substantially reduced these figures and the average transfusion is now in the range of 4 to 6 units; some transplants are completed with no red-cell transfusion at all. However, the potential for major haemorrhage always exists and 20 to 30 units are routinely crossmatched for the procedure. Blood loss is not always predictable and depends on a number of factors including the severity and nature of the liver disease, the presence of portal hypertension, previous upper abdominal surgery, surgical technique and experience, and early graft function.

Blood loss is replaced using the rapid infusion system (see above) to maintain a haematocrit in the range 25 to 30 per cent. The transfusion mixture varies with the circumstances, but is usually a mixture of albumin (or fresh frozen plasma if there is a need for coagulation factors) and packed red cells. Blood loss estimates are totally inadequate for orthotopic liver transplantation, and transfusion requirements must be guided by intravascular filling pressures and serial haematocrit estimations.

Autotransfusion systems are useful in reducing banked blood requirements when blood loss is heavy. As blood loss can be rapid the blood salvage system should be capable of rapid processing of the red cells. In liver transplantation it is recommended that sodium citrate rather than heparin is used in the wash solution (Kang, AnesthAnalg, 1991; 72:94).

Coagulation

Major derangements in the coagulation system are a common feature of hepatic transplantation, due to the following factors.

Pre-existing coagulopathy

Typically there are decreased levels of all factors, except I and VIII, thrombocytopenia, and a 15 per cent incidence of primary fibrinolysis in cirrhotics (Bontempo, Transpl, 1985; 39:532). Patients with cholestatic disease such as sclerosing cholangitis or primary biliary cirrhosis often have relatively normal coagulation and may even develop evidence of hypercoagulability during the anhepatic stage. In the anhepatic stage and early in the neohepatic phase, no coagulation factors are produced and reduced clearance/production of inhibitors and activators increase the susceptibility to a fibrinolytic state.

Dilutional coagulopathy

Massive transfusion (in excess of one to two times the circulating blood volume) will significantly reduce the levels of coagulation factors, especially factors V and VII, and result in clinically significant thrombocytopenia.

Reperfusion coagulopathy

At the time of reperfusion there is often a marked deterioration in coagulation, including a 'heparin effect' and occasional 'explosive fibrinolysis', due in part to the massive increase in tissue plasminogen activator. Pathological fibrinolysis developing towards the end of the anhepatic period or after reperfusion can result in significant microvascular ooze and blood loss. This is more common in patients with advanced cirrhosis, and the prophylactic administration of antifibrinolytics such as tranexamic acid or aprotinin is useful in this group of patients (Mallett, TransplProc, 1991; 23:1931; Kang, AnaesthAnalg, 1985; 64:888). Protamine sulphate (50–100 mg) is given if a marked 'heparin effect' is demonstrated on the thromboelastograph (Bailey, BrJAnaesth, 1994; 73:840).

Once the liver graft starts to function these pathological coagulopathies start to correct spontaneously, and persistence of microvascular ooze from raw surfaces is often an early sign of poor graft function.

Coagulation monitoring

Because of the complexity of coagulation disorders and the rapidity at which changes can occur it is essential to monitor coagulation serially throughout the procedure. Conventional clotting screens (prothombin time, partial thromboplastin time, and platelet count) are totally inadequate for this purpose as they give little information on the quality or the stability of the blood clot, neither do they give a clear basis on which to direct replacement therapy or pharmacological intervention.

Whole-blood clot analysis by thromboelastography is used by many centres as the primary method of coagulation assessment (McNichol, AnaesthIntCare, 1994; 22:659). The technique enables assessment of the whole coagulation process from a single blood sample. Information about clotting factor activity, platelet function and number, and any fibrinolytic activity is obtained within 20 to 30 min (Kang, AnaesthAnalg, 1985; 64:888). Blood component therapy is guided by the various thromboelastographic variables, and the effects of antifibrinolytic agents and protamine can be tested *in vitro* before use in the patient (Fletcher, JCI, 1964, 43:681).

Conclusion

Much valuable knowledge and expertise in the field of hepatic anaesthesia has been gained in recent years as a result of meeting the challenges posed by liver transplantation. The competent management of anaesthesia in patients with liver disease demands a thorough appreciation of the pathophysiological consequences of hepatic disease, the variable effects on drug handling, and the implications of the surgical procedure to be undertaken.

References

1. Child CG. The liver and portal hypertension. In: Child CG ed. *Major problems in clinical surgery.* Vol. 1. Philadelphia: Saunders, 1965.
2. Pugh RNH, *et al.* Transection of the oesophagus for bleeding varices. *British Journal of Surgery*, 1973; 60: 646.
3. DeWolf AM and Kang Y. Major hepatic procedures. In: Park GR and Kang Y, eds. *Anesthesia and intensive care for patients with liver disease.* Oxford: Butterworth-Heinemann, 1995: 99–109.
4. Bayley TJ, Segel N, and Bishop JM. Circulatory changes in patients with cirrhosis of the liver at rest and during exercise. *Clinical Science*, 1964; 26: 227.
5. Kang Y. Anaesthesia for liver transplantation. *Anaesthesiology Clinics of North America*, 1989; 7: 551–80.
6. Huet PM, *et al.* Intrahepatic circulation in liver disease. *Seminars in Liver Disease*, 1986; 6: 277–86.
7. Biarhi DJ, Gimson AES, and Williams R. Disturbances in cardiovascular and renal function in fulminant hepatic failure. In: Williams R, ed. *Liver failure.* Edinburgh: Churchill Livingstone, 1986: 47–71.
8. Krowka MJ and Cortese DA. Pulmonary aspects of chronic liver disease and liver transplantation. *Mayo Clinic Proceedings*, 1985; 60: 407–18.
9. Caldwell PRB, Fritts HW Jr, and Cournand A. Oxyhaemoglobin dissociation curve in liver disease. *Journal of Applied Physiology*, 1965; 20: 316–20.
10. Eriksson, LS *et al.* Normalisation of ventilation/perfusion relationships after liver transplantation in patients with decompensated cirrhosis: evidence for a hepatopulmonary syndrome. *Hepatology*, 1990; 12: 1350–7.
11. Lange PM and Stoller JK. Hepatopulmonary syndrome: effect of liver transplantation. *Clinics in Chest Medicine*, 1996; 17: 115–23.

12. Brown BR Jr. *Anaesthesia in hepatic and biliary tract disease*. Philadelphia: Davis, 1988: 152–3.

13. Baldus WP and Summerskill WHJ. Liver–kidney interrelationships. In: Schiff L, ed. *Diseases of the liver*, 4th edn. Philadelphia: Lipincott, 1975.

14. Van Theil DH. The liver and its effects on endocrine function in health and diseases. In: Schiff L and Schiff ER, eds. *Diseases of the liver*. Philadelphia: JB Lippincott, 1987: 129–62.

15. Brown BR Jr. The patient with liver disease. *Clinics in Anaesthesiology*, 1986; **4**: 747–60.

16. Cohen RD. Roles of the liver and kidney in acid base regulation and its disorders. *British Journal of Anaesthesia*, 1991; **67**: 154–64.

17. Loda M, Clowes GHA Jr, Nespoli A, Bigatello L, Birkett DH, and Menzoian JO. Encephalopathy, oxygen consumption, visceral amino acid clearance and mortality in cirrhotic surgical patients. *American Journal of Surgery*, 1984; **146**: 542–50.

18. Fiore L, Levine J, and Deykin D. Alterations of haemostasis in patients with liver disease. In: Zakim D and Boyer TD, eds. *Hepatology: a textbook of liver disease*. Philadelphia: Saunders, 1990: 546–71.

19. Paramo JA and Rocha E. Haemostasis in advanced liver disease. *Seminars in Thrombosis and Hemostasis*, 1993; **19**: 184–90 .

20. Williams R. Drug administration in hepatic disease. *New England Journal of Medicine*, 1984; **309**: 1616–22.

21. Maze M. In Miller RD, ed. *Hepatic physiology in anaesthesia*. Edinburgh: Churchill Livingstone, 1986: 1199–221.

22. Shelley MP, Elston AC, and Park GR. Sedative and analgesic drugs. In: Park GR and Kang Y, eds. *Anaesthesia and intensive care for patients with liver disease*. Oxford: Butterworth-Heinemann, 1995: 57–77.

23. Lavson CP, *et al.* Effects of anaesthetics on cerebral, renal and splanchnic circulations: recent developments. *Anaesthesiology*, 1974; **41**: 169–78.

24. Edmond JC, Kelley SD, and Heffron TG. Surgical and anaesthetic management of patients undergoing major hepatectomy using total vascular exclusion. *Liver Transplantation and Surgery*, 1996; **2**: 91–8.

25. Sassano JJ. The rapid infusion system. In: Winter PM and Kang YG, eds. *Hepatic transplantation: anaesthetic and perioperative management*. New York: Praeger, 1986: 120–34.

26. Kang Y. Anaesthesia for liver transplantation. In: Scott Wheeler A, ed. *Anaesthesia and new surgical procedures (Anaesthesiology Clinics of North America)*. Philadelphia: Saunders, 1989: 551–80.

27. Kang YG and Gelman S. Liver transplantation. In: Gelman S, ed. *Anaesthesia and organ transplantation*. Philadelphia: Saunders, 1987: 139–85.

28. Carmichael FJ, Lindop MJ, and Farman JV. Anaesthesia for hepatic transplantation: Cardiovascular and metabolic alternations and their management. *Anesthesia and Analgesia*, 1985; **64**: 108–16.

29. Rettke SR, *et al.* Haemodynamic and metabolic changes in hepatic transplantation. *Mayo Clinic Proceedings*, 1989; **64**: 232–40.

30. Distant DA and Gonwa TA. The kidney in liver transplantation. *Journal of the American Society of Nephrology*, 1993; **4**: 129–36.

31. Lewis JH, Bontempo FA, and Kang YG. Intraoperative coagulation changes in liver transplantation. In: Winter PM and Kang YG, eds. *Hepatic transplantation: anaesthetic and perioperative management*. New York: Praeger, 1986: 142–50.

32. Porte RJ. Coagulation and fibrinolysis in orthotopic liver transplantation: current views and insights. *Seminars in Thrombosis and Hemostasis*, 1993; **19**: 191–6.

30.3 Postoperative jaundice

Juan M. Salmerón and Juan Rodés

Introduction

Postoperative jaundice is a common problem in daily clinical practice. Interest in this syndrome, first recognized in the nineteenth century with the initial use of chloroform (Guthrie, Lancet 1903; ii: 10), increased in the 1950s after the introduction of halothane in anaesthetic procedures. It has since become clear that hepatocellular dysfunction, both necrotic and cholestatic, can appear in association with most anaesthetic agents and major surgery. Different factors, such as drugs, underlying diseases, and acute complications related to surgery, can contribute to the development of this picture.[1] In addition, it is not uncommon for several situations, known to be potential causes of hepatocellular dysfunction, to coincide in the same patient at the time of evaluating postoperative jaundice.[2,3] In this context, it is not surprising that the exact aetiology of the process remains uncertain in a relatively high proportion of cases.

The real incidence of postoperative jaundice (bilirubin greater than 2 mg/dl (35 µmol/l)) is not known. It may vary according to the method used to determine bilirubin and the surgical population studied,[4] being more frequent after major surgery (especially cardiac surgery (Chu, Thorax, 1987; 39:52)), multiple traumas, prolonged interventions, and readministration of halothane. The expected incidence after elective abdominal surgery is less than 1 per cent.[4]

Increased production of bilirubin, hepatocellular damage, and extrahepatic biliary tract obstruction are the three main pathophysiological mechanisms leading to postoperative jaundice. Despite its difficult differential diagnosis, it is important to distinguish between obstructive and hepatocellular causes because of their different prognostic and therapeutic implications. Since most cases of postoperative jaundice usually resolve spontaneously, a conservative diagnostic approach is often appropriate.

Pathophysiology

Bilirubin overload

In normal conditions, the excretion of bilirubin by the liver is around 250 mg/day. This capability can be greatly increased in overload conditions. For this reason, only acute or massive haemolysis results in clinical jaundice, and it is often mild and transient. However, concurrence of diverse factors, such as multiple transfusions (haemolysis because of old erythrocytes) (Zuck, Transfusion, 1972; 17:374), resorption of haematomas,[5] underlying liver and haemolytic disease (liver cirrhosis, deficiency of glucose 6-phosphate dehydrogenase, sickle cell disease), and hepatocellular

Table 1 Causes of postoperative jaundice according to aetiopathogenesis

Bilirubin overload
  congenital
  secondary to drug administration
  prosthetic valves and extracorporeal circulation
  sepsis
Haemolysis of transfused blood
Resorption of haematomas
Hepatocellular dysfunction
Hepatitis-like pattern
  anaesthesia-induced hepatitis
  secondary to drug administration
  ischaemic-induced hepatitis
  pre-existing chronic liver disease
  viral hepatitis
Cholestatic pattern
  benign postoperative intrahepatic cholestasis
  secondary to drug administration
  sepsis
  ischaemic-induced cholestasis
Isolated unconjugated hyperbilirubinaemia
  Gilbert's syndrome
Extrahepatic biliary obstruction
Residual choledocholithiasis
Postoperative cholecystitis or pancreatitis

dysfunction related to surgical conditions, open heart surgery (Pirofsky, NEJM, 1965; 272:235) or prosthetic valves (Koff, MedClinNAm, 1975; 59:823), hypotension, and sepsis, and drug administration, may lead to overt jaundice. Impairment of renal function may contribute to the picture.

Haemolytic processes should be considered as a cause of postoperative jaundice when hyperbilirubinaemia, predominantly unconjugated, coexists with anaemia, reticulocytosis, and decreased levels of haptoglobin. The potential precipitating factors must be eliminated in order to facilitate its self-resolution and corticosteroid therapy may be useful when indicated.

Derangement of hepatocellular function

Impairment of hepatocellular function is the most frequent explanation for postoperative jaundice. Laboratory and histological features usually show hepatitis-like or cholestatic signs, with a mixture of both being more usual. Hepatobiliary disorders presenting as postoperative jaundice are listed in Table 1. Since most of them, including surgical problems in cirrhotic patients and in liver transplantation (see Chapter 30.5), are discussed in their specific chapters, the following exposition will be focused on the most frequent and relevant pictures.

Postoperative intrahepatic cholestasis

The most important operative risk factor for developing postoperative jaundice is bleeding which produces hypotension and requires blood transfusion. It now seems clear that the combination of both hypotension and multiple blood transfusions may be associated with a characteristic cholestatic postoperative syndrome, known as benign postoperative intrahepatic cholestasis. This picture was first described in patients who had undergone abdominal surgery and required blood transfusion (Caroli, ArchMalApp-DigNutr, 1950; 39:1057) and was later recognized in open heart surgery (Sanderson, AnnSurg, 1967; 165:217). Intrahepatic cholestasis has also been described in patients with severe trauma (Hartley, NZMedJ, 1977; 86:174) or burns (Sevitt, BrJSurg, 1958; 46:68), and after extensive haematoma formation. Jaundice, basically from conjugated bilirubin, typically occurs within 2 to 4 days after surgery, but may be delayed for up to 10 days. It reaches a peak that may be as high as 40 mg/dl (684 µmol/l), within a week, and then falls rapidly, disappearing in the first month (Kantrowitz, NEJM, 1967; 276:591).[2,6] Pruritus, fever and signs of hepatocellular failure are absent. Physical examination fails to find enlarged liver and spleen, or stigmata of liver disease. A mixed hyperbilirubinaemia with variable elevations of serum levels of alkaline phosphatase and almost normal serum aminotransferases without changes in serum albumin and prothrombin time are the characteristic findings in liver function tests. Morphological signs of cholestasis (canalicular bile plugs and staining of bile pigment in centrilobular liver cells) with preservation of the hepatic architecture without evidence of hepatocellular necrosis are the main histological features in this disorder (Kantrowitz, NEJM, 1967; 276:591).[2,6] Erythrophagocytosis by Kupffer cells has been seen in patients who have received multiple transfusions or have large haematomas (Kantrowitz, NEJM, 1967: 276:591). In some severe cases steatosis and swelling of centrilobular hepatocytes may be present. Although not completely clear, the pathophysiology is thought to be an acquired disorder of hepatic bilirubin transport. Subclinical degrees of impairment in excretory function evaluated by sulphobromophthalein excretion have been reported in up to 50 per cent of patients following general anaesthesia and surgery (Tagnon, NEJM, 1958; 238:556). The prognosis of this process depends on the severity of the associated illness, and the mortality, which correlates with the number of failing organs in the multiple organ failure syndrome, has been reported to be as high as 50 per cent.[3,6] Jaundice itself is a postoperative complication of little consequence, and does not influence the outcome.

Ischaemic liver damage

Arterial hypotension and hypoxaemia often coexist in surgical patients, whose hepatic blood flow may be reduced by anaesthetic agents,[7] leading to postoperative hepatic dysfunction due to ischaemia. The typical histological finding is centrilobular hepatic necrosis, the severity of which is related to the duration of hypoperfusion and to the degree of hypoxaemia. The incidence of hepatic dysfunction is particularly high after traumatic shock and open

heart surgery (Chu, Thorax, 1987; 39:52). Although cholestasis resembling benign postoperative jaundice is the most common pattern of injury following hypotension, a more serious event is ischaemic hepatitis, especially seen after open heart surgery and prolonged hypotension.[5] In this case, initial striking elevations of serum transaminases and marked decreases in prothrombin time are followed by a typically delayed hyperbilirubinaemia (Cohen, Gastro, 1978; 74:583). This biochemical picture appears within hours of surgery (Editorial, Lancet, 1985; i:1019) and returns rapidly to normal with restoration of oxygenation and perfusion of the liver when there has been no severe damage, or progresses to fulminant hepatic failure when there is massive centrilobular hepatic necrosis.

Sepsis

Sepsis may produce jaundice by a number of different mechanisms, including bacteriaemia-related haemolysis, septic shock with reduction in hepatic blood flow, endotoxaemia, and invasion of the liver by the infecting organisms. The typical biochemical pattern is cholestatic with minor changes in transaminase levels (Zimmerman, Gastro, 1979; 77:362). However, clinical jaundice occurs in less than 1 per cent of episodes of bacteraemia.[8] Jaundice usually appears within days after the onset of the infection. Hepatomegaly is detected in around 50 per cent of cases. Although hepatic dysfunction does not have clinical relevance, the bilirubin level 48 h after the onset of septic shock is the best predictor of outcome (Banks, JClinPath, 1982; 35:1249). In addition, the duration of the shock is an important factor determining the severity of the hepatic disturbance (Banks, JClinPath, 1982; 35:1249). The pathogenesis of this cholestatic process is unclear, but two aethiopathogenic mechanisms leading to an impairment in intrahepatic biliary excretory function have been proposed. Endotoxin, which is often present in portal blood, may inhibit sodium, potassium–ATPase (Utili, JInfDis, 1977; 136:523), and ischaemia could interfere with peribiliary vascular circulation (Rooney, AmJDisChild, 1971; 122: 39). Finally, pneumococcal pneumonia is a well-recognized cause of jaundice, and may be present in the postoperative period (Zimmerman, Gastro, 1979; 77:362).

Drug-induced postoperative jaundice

Although several drugs usually used in the perioperative period have been reported to be potentially hepatotoxic (see Section 17), drug-induced postoperative jaundice seems to be a rare condition.[3] However, it is important to note that diverse pharmacological combinations increase the individual risk of hepatotoxicity because of their interactions. In addition, clinical hepatotoxicity may appear when the toxic drug has already been withdrawn. Drug-induced hepatic injury is manifested clinically by either a hepatitis-like pattern or, less commonly, a cholestatic pattern. The drugs most frequently involved in liver dysfunction are listed in Table 2. The most frequent biochemical profile consists of striking elevations in serum transaminases and derangement of hepatic synthetic functions when there is severe liver damage. The cholestatic pattern is characterized by elevations in serum bilirubin and alkaline phosphatase, mimicking extrahepatic biliary obstruction. A detailed revision of the patient's history and medical record are the most

Table 2 Main drugs involved in postoperative jaundice

Predominantly cholestatic pattern
    Azathioprine
    Captopril
    Chlorpromazine
    Erythromycin
    Parenteral nutrition
    Nitrofurantoin
    Sulphonamide-related oral hypoglycaemic agents
Predominantly hepatitic pattern
    Acetylsalicylate
    Allopurinol
    Amiodarone
    Amoxycillin
    Halothane and related anaesthetic agents
    Ketoconazole
    Methyldopa
    Paracetamol
    Quinidine
    Sodium valproate
Mixed pattern
    Barbiturates
    Vitamin K
    Oleandomycin
    Non-steroidal anti-inflammatories
    Sulphonamides

valuable keys in making the diagnosis. Characteristic clinical symptoms, such as fever, chills, cutaneous rash, and arthralgias are often seen when autoimmune mechanisms are involved. In these cases, these symptoms are useful diagnostic clues. In other cases, when idiosyncratic reactions or direct toxic effects are responsible for the picture, only a rechallenge to the drugs, which cannot be recommended, may ensure that the aetiopathology of the process is understood. Since histological findings are usually non-specific, liver biopsy may not be useful in diagnosis.

Halothane-induced hepatitis (see Chapter 30.2) is the most controversial cause of postoperative drug-related hepatic injury, but it is very relevant because of the wide use of halothane and its potentially lethal effects as a cause of fulminant hepatic failure. The real incidence of halothane hepatitis remains uncertain, but it has been considered to be between 1 : 7000 and 1 : 30 000[9,10] (Fee, BrJAnaesth, 1979; 51:1133). In the past decade most centres haved replaced halothane by other anaesthesic agents, leading to a marked decrease in the incidence of this complication. The exact pathophysiological mechanisms have not been completely clarified. There is evidence that strongly supports participation of immunological mechanisms (increased risk and shortened asymptomatic period after repeated exposures, hepatic damage in rechallenge, cross-sensitization to anaesthetic agents, peripheral eosinophilia, and the presence of non-organ-specific antibodies) (Neuberger, BMJ, 1984; 289:1136). Alterations in halothane metabolism have been thought to play a role in its hepatotoxic effects (Nimmo, BrJClinPharm, 1981; 12:433). Halothane undergoes biotransformation by cytochrome P450 in the liver. Acetyl halide, an intermediate metabolite, may bind to liver cell surface proteins, turning them into antigenic proteins, and activating the immune response (Duvaldestin, ClinPharmTher, 1981; 29:61). It has also been suggested that a direct toxic effect of halothane metabolites in the hepatocytes is responsible. This hypothesis is supported by the histopathological

finding of centrilobular necrosis. Lipid membranes may be damaged by highly reactive free radicals from halothane metabolism under conditions of low oxygen tension (Dykes, BrJAnaesth, 1972; 44: 925)

Halothane-induced hepatitis mimics acute viral hepatitis but has a higher mortality rate. It preferentially affects patients aged from 40 to 70 years, and the risk seems to be higher in obese patients. The risk of developing halothane hepatitis is related to multiple exposures, and is more frequent when the exposures have been close in time. Patients first exposed to halothane develop fever between 1 and 2 weeks after its administration, presenting evident jaundice within 3 to 10 days later. When previously administered, fever may appear within the first week and jaundice as soon as a week after surgery. The physical examination may reveal mild hepatomegaly, but a decrease in liver volume is occasionally seen in fulminant hepatic failure. A cutaneous rash is noticed in some cases. Liver function tests show conjugated hyperbilirubinaemia, considerable elevations in serum transaminases, and a slight increase in alkaline phosphatase. Peripheral eosinophilia has been reported in one-third of the patients (Bottiger, ActaAnaesthScand, 1976; 20: 40), and the occurrence of autoantibodies is variable. The histological findings are similar to those in acute viral hepatitis. Centrilobular necrosis with a mononuclear infiltrate restricted to the damaged areas is characteristic (Peters, AmJMed, 1969; 47:748), with vacuolar changes in hepatocytes, acidophilic nuclei, and granular cytoplasm being additional changes. Occasionally, fatty and eosinophilic infiltration (Klion, AnnIntMed, 1969; 71:467), cholestasis, and bile duct proliferation may been seen. Regenerative features may be observed within 2 weeks. Prognosis depends on the signs of hepatocellular failure, with a prolonged prothrombin time, the appearance of hepatic encephalopathy, and a bilirubin greater than 10 mg/dl (171 μmol/l) being associated with poor survival. Treatment is only supportive, and liver transplantation may be indicated when fulminant hepatic failure is present.

Other halogenated anaesthetic agents, such as methoxyflurane and enflurane (Duvaldestin, ClinPharmTher, 1981; 29:61), have been implicated in liver damage similar to that caused by halothane. Since there is a cross-sensitization between these agents, patients who have developed hepatitis by exposure to any halogenated anaesthetic should be warned against future exposures to both.

Extrahepatic biliary tract obstruction

Although uncommon, postoperative jaundice may be due to extrahepatic biliary tract obstruction (see Chapter 23.4). It may be possible to find retained choledochal stones after cholecystectomy and exploration of the common bile duct. Biliary tract damage may occur in the same cases and in surgical manoeuvres to adjacent structures when there is an inadvertent ligation or transection of the common bile duct. Finally, postoperative pancreatitis (Saini, AmJSurg, 1963; 105:87) and cholecystitis (Johnson, ObsGyn, 1987; 164:197) may evolve with clinically evident jaundice in a variable number of cases. Abdominal ultrasonography and cholangiography, via a T-tube when it is placed, will provide the diagnosis and exact site of obstruction. Relief of obstructive matter and repair of damaged structures should solve the problem and avoid permanent liver damage.

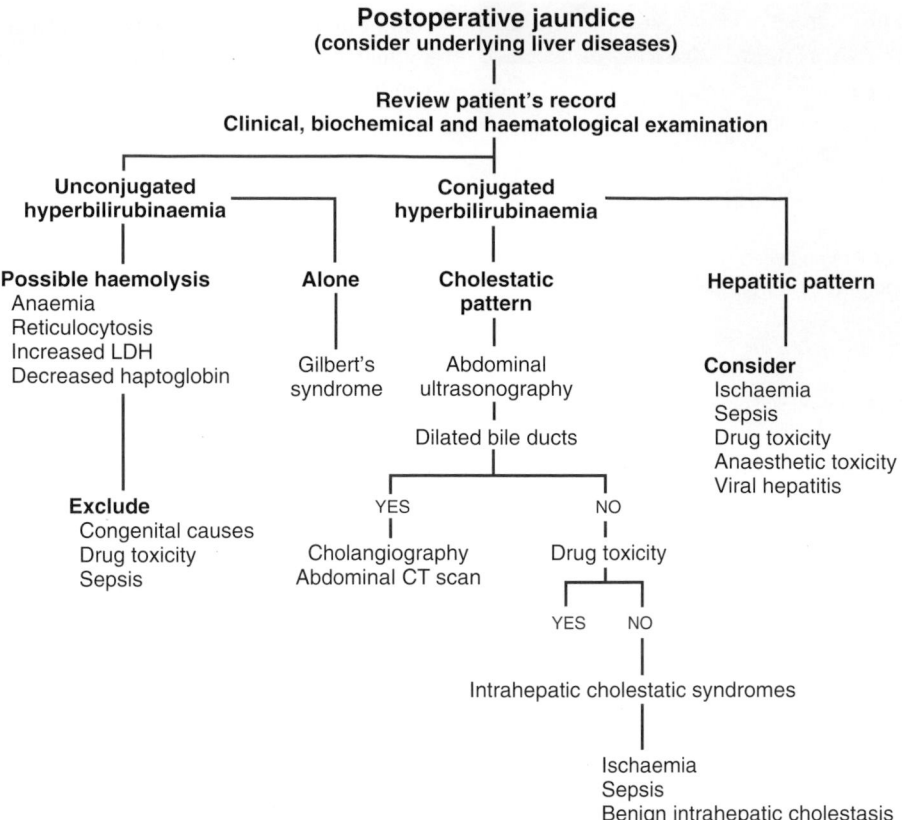

Fig. 1. Diagnostic approach to postoperative jaundice.

Investigation of postoperative jaundice

It should be possible to identify the cause of postoperative jaundice in most patients without excessive difficulty. Review of the patients' record and clinical examination give the most useful data. The pattern of liver injury assessed by liver function tests, the type of surgical intervention and its related conditions, the time of onset of jaundice,[11] and the knowledge of drugs used usually provide a correct approach. Abdominal ultrasonography is the most helpful procedure to ensure the patency of the extrahepatic biliary tree. More specific explorations are indicated only on the basis of clinical findings. Figure 1 provides a logical guide to the diagnostic process of postoperative jaundice.

When a hepatic profile is present in liver function tests, hypotensive liver injury, sepsis, drug toxicity, or viral hepatitis should be suspected as the cause. The timing of jaundice may help to distinguish between these factors. Drug toxicity and sepsis can develop at any time. Halothane-induced hepatitis and ischaemic hepatitis usually occur after the first week of exposure, but it should be kept in mind that previous exposures to halothane may shorten this period of time. Viral hepatitis takes some weeks for its clinical manifestations to develop when acquired from blood products.

A cholestatic pattern suggests biliary obstruction or functional cholestasis. Abdominal ultrasonography should always be performed in order to exclude structural abnormalities. When present, cholangiography, preferably endoscopic, may provide definitive diagnosis and may be therapeutic in some cases: When there is no biliary dilatation, drugs and benign postoperative intrahepatic cholestasis are the most probable aetiologies.

Finally, isolated unconjugated hyperbilirubinaemia may be present in patients with Gilbert's syndrome who have undergone surgical stress and prolonged fasting. A careful review of the history will probably allow recognition of previous episodes in the same patients or their relatives. Gilbert's syndrome is readily differentiated from haemolysis by its different biochemical and haematological pattern. When evidence of haemolysis is present, drug toxicity should once again be suspected.

Treatment

Depending on the aetiology, adequate treatment for postoperative jaundice ranges from an expectant attitude with supportive measures to invasive management, including liver transplantation for fulminant hepatic failure. It is important to note that in most cases the main cause of hepatic dysfunction may be remote from the liver (infection, cardiac and renal failure, drug reactions, haemolysis) and thus treatment may be quite different to that for liver diseases.

Specific treatment must be started as soon as the causes of postoperative jaundice are identified. Antibiotics are the treatment of choice for infectious postoperative complications, although surgical drainage of collected material should not be delayed because of impaired hepatic function.[12] Residual gallstones must be removed by endoscopic, solvent, or surgical procedures (see Chapter 23.4). Corticosteroids may be useful for the treatment of haemolytic processes and cholecystectomy for acalculous cholecystitis (see

Chapter 23.5). Withdrawal of potential hepatotoxic drugs is mandatory if they are thought to play a role.

General supportive measures should be applied to all patients, including maintenance of cardiocirculatory, respiratory, and renal functions, avoidance of the use of potentially hepatotoxic drugs, supply of adequate nutrition, prevention of severe complications, and correction of abnormalities from hepatic failure (coagulopathy, encephalopathy, hypoglycaemia, and cerebral oedema) when present. Finally, liver transplantation may be indicated when no response to conservative management of fulminant hepatic failure is achieved.

Prophylaxis or minimization of postoperative jaundice may be achieved through a meticulous analysis of the history and the patient's record for previous unexplained episodes of jaundice and data suggesting chronic liver disease, and treating all possible disturbances that may make the operative procedure difficult. Previous exposures to halothane should be investigated in order to rule out a possible hypersensitive. Screening of blood product donors decreases the risk of postransfusional hepatitis.

References

1. Evans C, Evans M, and Pollock AV. The incidence and causes of postoperative jaundice. *British Journal of Anaesthesiology*, 1974; **46**: 520–5.

2. La Mont JT and Isselbacher KJ. Postoperative jaundice. *New England Journal of Medicine*, 1973; **288**: 305–7.

3. Boekhorst Th, *et al.* Etiologic factors of jaundice in severely ill patients. A retrospective study in patients admitted to an intensive care unit with severe trauma or with septic intra-abdominal complications following surgery and without evidence of bile duct obstruction. *Journal of Hepatology*, 1988; **7**: 111–17.

4. Clarke RJS, Doggart JR, and Lavery T. Changes in liver function after different types of surgery. *British Journal of Anaesthesiology*, 1976; **48**: 119–28.

5. Nunes G, Blaisdell FW, and Margaretten W. Mechanism of hepatic dysfunction following shock and trauma. *Archives of Surgery*, 1970; **100**: 546–56.

6. Schmid M, *et al.* Benign postoperative intrahepatic cholestasis. *New England Journal of Medicine*, 1965; **272**: 546–50.

7. Cooperman LH, Wallman II, and Marsh ML. Anesthesia and the liver. *Surgical Clinics of North America*, 1977; **57**: 421–8.

8. Vermillion SE, *et al.* Jaundice associated with bacteremia. *Archives of Internal Medicine*, 1969; **124**: 611–18.

9. Bunker JP. Final report of the national halothane study. *Anesthesiology*, 1968; **29**: 231–2.

10. Toulokian J and Kaplowitz N. Halothane-induced hepatic disease. *Seminars in Liver Disease*, 1981; **1**: 134–42

11. Hayes PC and Bouchier AD. Postoperative jaundice. *Ballière's Clinical Gastroenterology*, 1989; **3**: 485–505.

12. Moody FG, and Potts JR. Postoperative jaundice. In Schiff L and Schiff ER, eds. *Diseases of the liver*, (7th edn). Philadelphia: Lippincott, 1993: 370–6.

30.4 Hepatobilary trauma

John Terblanche and J. E. J. Krige*

Definition

Liver trauma occurs as a result of open or closed injuries. Open injuries are caused by stab wounds, usually with a knife, or by missile wounds, usually with a bullet or shrapnel. Closed injuries are caused by blunt abdominal trauma, particularly due to high-speed motor vehicle accidents. Liver injuries can be classified as simple or complex. The majority are simple and easy to manage, whereas complex injuries often produce major challenges for the surgeon.

Biliary tract injuries due to external trauma are uncommon. The bile duct may also be injured due to surgical misadventure. These iatrogenic injuries occur during operative procedures on, or adjacent to, the biliary tract.

Introduction

Liver trauma

Major liver trauma has been recognized as a potentially fatal injury since ancient times. As the largest abdominal organ, it is not surprising that the liver is the most frequently injured organ in abdominal trauma. Even though it is protected by the rib cage, compression injury, particularly by the steering wheel in motor vehicle accidents, frequently causes rupture of liver and its capsule. Intrahepatically, the portal triad structures are protected by an investing layer of the glissonian sheath which tends to protect the major hepatic artery and portal vein branches within the liver. The unprotected major hepatic veins are more liable to damage and can result in life-threatening major haemorrhage. Changing concepts and improved management strategies have been outlined in major reviews.[1-7]

Many of the so-called modern concepts were proposed in Pringle's classic paper published in 1908.[8] He reported eight patients with major liver injuries and an experimental study in four rabbits. The four patients submitted to operation all died. After the first patient, he conceived the principle of inflow occlusion (today called the Pringle manoeuvre). This was used in the second patient and shown to control bleeding. After confirming its value in his experimental study in rabbits, he used inflow occlusion on the next two patients. Although his patients died, he was able to define the modern concepts of inflow occlusion, liver packing, and mobilization of the liver to deal with traumatic wounds.[8] One of his rabbits

* Financial assistance was received from the South African Medical Research Council and the Staff Research Fund, University of Cape Town.

had inflow occlusion for 1 h. All four animals survived. Nowhere did he refer to a limiting time factor for inflow occlusion. Subsequent publications suggesting that inflow occlusion should not be continued for longer than 15 min gave rise to the Pringle 'myth', which was a misinterpretation of his paper and an incorrect extrapolation to humans of later experimental work, mainly performed in dogs.

Considerable controversy still surrounds the management of major liver trauma. The controversies are outlined based on the literature and the authors' experience in Cape Town.

Biliary trauma

Isolated extrahepatic bile-duct or porta hepatis injuries due to external trauma are rare.[9] Injuries to other structures in the porta hepatis occur more often than isolated bile-duct injuries.[9] Tragic iatrogenic injuries of the bile duct are fortunately also uncommon but continue to occur.[10,11]

Incidence and prevalence

The incidence of liver trauma varies in different parts of the world. It is on the increase due to civilian violence and terrorist attacks and also due to misuse of the growing number of modern high-speed motor vehicles on our roads. Drug or alcohol abuse are frequent and important associated factors.

Biliary tract injuries due to external trauma are rare and are usually caused by penetrating injuries.[9] Some of the aetiological associations of iatrogenic biliary injuries have been defined in a major study from Sweden.[10] Although the incidence of iatrogenic injuries should lessen if only trained surgeons undertake biliary surgery, such injuries will still occur, albeit rarely, in skilled hands. There has been an increased incidence with the advent of laparoscopic cholecystectomy.[11]

Pathophysiology

Liver trauma

Types of injury

In the authors' opinion liver injuries are best classified as either simple or complex, depending on how difficult they are to manage. Patients with simple injuries are relatively easy to manage and have a low morbidity and mortality, whereas those with complex injuries are challenging and have a high morbidity and mortality. In an analysis of 1000 consecutive cases of liver trauma, the group from

Houston, Texas, noted that 88 per cent of patients fell into the simple category.[4] The Cape Town experience has been similar, with 80 per cent of patients presenting with simple injuries.[3] More comprehensive classifications, such as the American Association for the Surgery of Trauma (AAST) liver injury scale, which recognizes six grades, have been proposed.[12] In our view they do not help in the practical management of individual cases. We believe that retrohepatic vena caval and major hepatic vein injuries should be considered as a separate subcategory of complex injuries because of the controversies surrounding management and the previously reported prohibitively high mortality associated with these injuries.

Open injuries are caused by either stab or missile wounds. Stab wounds are usually simple unless a major blood vessel is damaged. Ninety-eight per cent of the stab wounds in Cape Town were classified as simple. Missile wounds may be more serious. Low-velocity bullet wounds frequently result in simple hepatic injuries (70 per cent in Cape Town). This applies to many civilian injuries. High-velocity missiles are seen in war injuries, but shrapnel wounds, which are becoming more common in civilian practice due to terrorist activity around the world, frequently result in high-velocity-type injuries which are very damaging, and may cause complex liver injuries.

Closed injuries due to blunt abdominal trauma are frequently caused by the rim of a motor vehicle steering wheel. These may be more serious, although 60 per cent of blunt injuries are simple to manage. Other causes of blunt injury include child abuse in paediatric practice and falls from a height on to the abdomen.

Pathological types

Small defects, which have frequently stopped bleeding at the time of laparotomy, are usually caused by stab wounds or low-velocity missiles. Such wounds only give rise to problems when a major blood vessel or bile duct is injured.

A subcapsular haematoma may be small or large and arises when the liver is disrupted under an intact Glisson's capsule. Delayed rupture, even of large subcapsular haematomas, is uncommon but fear of rupture has made management controversial.

The typical injury occurring in blunt trauma is a tear or split into the liver substance through the capsule. It occurs more commonly in the right lobe. It is frequently localized and minor. When extensive, the injury is often complex and difficult to manage. Occasionally, multiple complex tears occur in both lobes of the liver. The major intrahepatic branches of the portal triad structures are often spared because of the protecting covering of the glissonian capsule that ensheathes them in their intrahepatic course.

Deep-seated damage in a liver lobe may be due to a haematoma caused by a stab wound or even to an iatrogenic injury after a liver biopsy. It is usually of little consequence in management. On the other hand, severe trauma can disrupt the liver with disruption and pulping of a whole liver lobe. These injuries are difficult to treat.

Inferior vena cava and hepatic vein injuries are uncommon but pose problems in management and previously had a high associated mortality. They may be caused by stab or missile injuries or be due to major blunt trauma. They are often associated with severe liver tears and disruption of either the hepatic vein or vena cava, with attendant high mortality.

All of the above types of injuries occur in adults. In children most injuries are due to blunt trauma caused by motor vehicle accidents, falls, or occasionally child abuse.

Biliary injuries

The gallbladder may be injured by stab or missile injuries. It is usually associated with liver injuries and is treated together with these injuries. Isolated porta hepatis and extrahepatic biliary tract injuries are unusual and almost exclusively confined to stab and missile injuries. The vascular structures in the porta hepatis are more frequently damaged than the bile duct.[9]

The true incidence of iatrogenic injuries of the bile duct is not known because not all patients are reported. A comprehensive 8-year review from Sweden, made possible because of the insurance policy of that country, has highlighted some aetiological factors in the pre-laparoscopic cholecystectomy days. In this study bile-duct injury occurred more commonly in women, and the patients were younger when compared with a control group. Common bile-duct stones were usually not suspected and the patients were fit and not obese. Most surgeons were in training and 80 per cent had performed between 25 and 100 cholecystectomies before injuring a bile duct. These surgeons in training were seldom assisted by a more experienced surgeon. The commonly quoted problems of either severe inflammation or bleeding at the time of surgery did not occur. In almost all cases the duct was damaged either before the operative cholangiogram had been performed or while waiting to review the films. The authors of the paper consider most of these injuries to have been avoidable.[10]

The advent of laparoscopic cholecystectomy, particularly during the learning-curve phase, led to a significant increase in bile-duct injuries, which is beginning to level off now due to increasing experience.[11]

The definitive anatomical study of the blood supply of the bile duct, using a corrosion cast technique (Nonhover, BrJSurg, 1979; 66:379), has helped in understanding the cause and extent of iatrogenic bile-duct strictures. The intrahepatic bile ducts and the retropancreatic portion of the bile duct have a profuse blood supply, entering laterally from surrounding blood vessels. On the other hand, the supraduodenal bile duct between the duodenum and the porta hepatis has a tenuous blood supply, mostly coming up from below in longitudinal tiny medial and lateral vessels (the 3 o'clock and 9 o'clock arteries). In one-third of patients the blood supply from the 3 o'clock and 9 o'clock arteries is supplemented by a larger posterior retroportal artery. Damage to these main blood-supply vessels, with or without transection of the duct, can induce ischaemia and result in extensive stricturing of the extrahepatic biliary system. Dissection near the bile duct, with or without the use of diathermy, during laparoscopic cholecystectomy, may also damage these critical blood vessels. As a result of this study it is recommended that damaged bile ducts be repaired by an expert using bowel and performing a high anastomosis to well-vascularized bile duct at the porta hepatis (Fig. 1).[13]

Clinical features
Liver trauma

Liver injuries should be suspected in patients with penetrating wounds of the upper abdomen or lower chest and in patients with

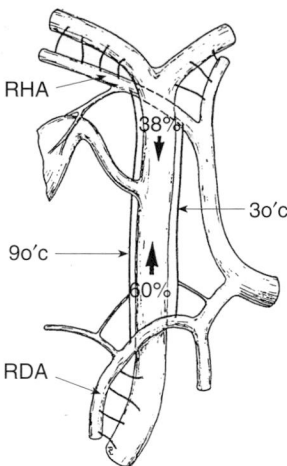

Fig. 1. Anterior view of the blood supply of the human bile duct. The blood supply to the bile ducts in the hilum of the liver (above) and the retropancreatic bile duct (below) from adjacent arteries is profuse. The supraduodenal bile-duct blood supply is axial and tenuous, with 60 per cent from below and 38 per cent from above. The small main axial vessels (3 o'clock and 9 o'clock arteries) are vulnerable and easily damaged. RHA, Right hepatic artery; RDA, retroduodenal artery. (Reproduced with permission from Terblanche J, Allison HF, and Nonhover JMA. An ischemic basis for biliary strictures. *Surgery*, July 1983; **94**:52–7.)

blunt abdominal trauma. A liver injury should also be suspected in patients with extensive blunt trauma who have a head injury or a spinal cord injury which might mask the relevant abdominal signs.

The main aim of the clinical examination is to diagnose those patients who require laparotomy as a life-saving measure or to prevent complications. The major cause of death in hepatic injuries is haemorrhage. Patients die either because of massive bleeding due to major blood-vessel injuries in or around the liver, or because of the development of a coagulopathy due to major haemorrhage having occurred during attempted surgical control. Occasionally patients die later due to septic complications. The other main cause of mortality is associated major non-hepatic injuries. With major blunt trauma this is frequently a severe head injury. Associated local abdominal injuries also increase the mortality. Mortality is increased by 50 per cent when four or more abdominal organs are involved (Walt, AmJSurg, 1978; 135:12). Associated colon injuries also play a major role in the development of subsequent intra-abdominal septic complications.

Most patients with an injured liver have a parenchymal injury which is usually simple and easy to manage. Extensive parenchymal injuries, or the rare injuries to the hepatic vein, vena cava, or portal triad, will be associated with major early haemorrhage and a potentially high mortality. These patients present with signs of hypovolaemic shock.

Major non-hepatic injuries need to be defined carefully and treated on their merits. The occurrence of signs of peritonitis in patients with either penetrating or blunt abdominal trauma suggests penetration of the bowel and the need for laparotomy. Patients presenting with shock and evidence of intra-abdominal bleeding require urgent laparotomy to confirm the cause of bleeding and to control haemorrhage.

The main clinical features which need to be looked for and which influence management in patients with suspected liver injuries are evidence of haemorrhage due to liver or other injuries, or peritoneal irritation due to associated bowel or other visceral injury. The decision to operate must be made on clinical grounds. Investigations merely assist in the assessment and decision making but should not be used in isolation to decide that an operation is required. Evidence of hepatic injury using modern imaging techniques is not an indication in its own right for operation.

Bile-duct injury

There are no specific clinical features of extrahepatic bile-duct injury. In the majority the injury to the biliary tree is due to penetrating trauma, but this is rare when compared with liver injuries.[9] Although bile-duct injuries are not frequently associated with vascular injuries to the porta hepatis, when this does occur the biliary injury would usually be diagnosed at the time of surgical management of the major vascular injury.[9]

Patients with iatrogenic injuries of the bile duct present in three main ways. First, the injury may be noted at the time it occurs during cholecystectomy or other surgery. Here the bile duct may have been divided or partially transected or clipped or clamped in error. Alternatively, if the lesion is missed initially, the patient usually becomes ill in the early postoperative period, with bile leakage either to the exterior or into the peritoneal cavity. Some patients present later with slowly increasing obstructive jaundice due to progressive bile-duct stricturing. Jaundice may be intermittent when there is an associated internal fistula into the bowel. There is continued controversy whether operative cholangiography helps to avoid bile-duct injury. The controversy has been revived in the laparoscopic era.[11]

Investigations and diagnosis
Liver trauma

A patient with a suspected localized hepatic injury who is not shocked can be investigated thoroughly. Ultimately, the decision about abdominal exploration should be made on clinical grounds, with additional help from the results of the investigations. On the other hand, a patient with severe shock and evidence of ongoing intraperitoneal haemorrhage should not undergo lengthy investigations. Here the most important diagnostic measure is immediate laparotomy, where the diagnosis of the source of bleeding should be made and the cause treated. In the majority of severe liver injuries presenting with massive haemorrhage, initial control of bleeding at laparotomy can be achieved by perihepatic packing, which allows time for resuscitation and for other injuries to be sought and treated.

Newer imaging techniques are very helpful in suspected liver trauma. Computed tomography (**CT**) scanning has been evaluated extensively.[1] The CT scan demonstrates parenchymal lacerations, intrahepatic haematomata, and free intraperitoneal blood[1] (Moon, Radiol, 1983; 141:309). A CT scan can also measure the size of the intrahepatic lesion and the amount of intraperitoneal bleeding. Intravenous contrast enhancement has improved the diagnostic capability of the CT scan.[1,2] The finding of a lesion on CT scan indicates that there is liver damage, but by itself is not an indication for operative intervention unless required on clinical grounds. Imaging merely provides additional information to assist in decision making.

Modern ultrasonography is an alternative which may be more readily available in trauma units outside major centres but it does not produce as clear a picture of the injury. Isotope scanning has been largely superseded by CT scanning. Hepatic angiography has a limited role in some patients to diagnose the cause of ongoing haemorrhage; it occasionally has a therapeutic role in treating arterial bleeding from a segmental or subsegmental intrahepatic artery by embolization. The major role of angiography is in managing patients with continued bleeding after therapeutic perihepatic packing,[3] and for recurrent bleeding after laparotomy. A chest radiograph is essential if there is any possibility of a pneumothorax or haemothorax. Patients with suspected renal injury or haematuria require a rapid intravenous pyelogram before laparotomy if the kidneys have not been adequately visualized on a contrast-enhanced CT scan.

The most important diagnostic test, after the initial evaluation of a patient, is repeated physical examination. This is particularly important in those patients in whom conservative management has been initiated. Evidence of continued intraperitoneal bleeding or of peritonitis due to suspected hollow muscular viscus injury necessitates a change in policy and is an indication for laparotomy.

The role of peritoneal lavage remains controversial. Many feel it to be helpful.[1,7] In the authors' view the finding of intraperitoneal blood in a patient who is otherwise stable is not an indication for laparotomy. An unstable patient requires laparotomy irrespective of the findings on peritoneal lavage. The authors advocate peritoneal lavage in patients with major head injuries or spinal cord injuries where the intra-abdominal injury may be masked. Here the finding of bowel content clearly necessitates laparotomy, as does the finding of gross intraperitoneal blood in a shocked patient where it had been suspected that other injuries might account for the shock.

The final arbitrator in the decision-making algorithm leading to conservative therapy or laparotomy is the overall clinical picture supplemented by the special investigations. Non-invasive imaging may well detect a liver injury in an otherwise asymptomatic patient. This has led to unnecessary laparotomies in the past. Liver injury *per se* does not make operative therapy obligatory unless there is major bleeding or other intra-abdominal injuries requiring surgical treatment. Surgery must not be undertaken on the basis of imaging data alone.

Biliary injuries

Diagnostic tests including imaging are not usually performed in patients with biliary tract injuries due to external trauma. These injuries are usually diagnosed during operative procedures for control of haemorrhage. The occasional patient may present late and an endoscopic retrograde cholangiogram (**ERCP**) may be helpful in diagnosis.

Patients with iatrogenic biliary strictures that are not diagnosed initially and who present with obstructive jaundice should have the diagnosis confirmed by ERCP or, more usually, by a combination of ERCP and percutaneous transhepatic cholangiography in cases presenting with a complete stricture of the bile duct. No patient with a suspected iatrogenic bile-duct injury should be operated upon until full imaging has been performed.[11]

Table 1 Principles of management of liver injuries
Do not overtreat minor injuries
Stop haemorrhage by:
Perihepatic packing
resuscitative packing
therapeutic packing
Temporary porta hepatis occlusion
Oversewing or repairing bleeding vessels
Oversew or repair damaged bile ducts
Resectional debridement rather than formal right or left hepatectomy

Management

Liver injuries

Principles of management

The principles of management are summarized in Table 1. They are as follows:

1. No treatment is required for minor or moderate parenchymal injuries that are not bleeding. There has been a tendency to overtreat in the past.
2. In major injuries with associated haemorrhage, bleeding must be stopped. Initial control is with resuscitative perihepatic packing and/or porta hepatis occlusion while the patient is resuscitated. Inflow occlusion should be avoided or used for the minimum time in liver trauma as it may be required later during definitive surgery. Inexperienced surgeons should rely on perihepatic packing until expert help arrives, or to allow for transfer of the patient to a specialist centre.[3] Subsequent definitive control of haemorrhage necessitates oversewing or repairing damaged blood vessels. Bleeding due to coagulopathy should also be controlled with perihepatic packing. Major hepatic vein and vena caval injuries or portal vein injuries require initial control with perihepatic packing during resuscitation and subsequent definitive repair using either inflow control or total hepatic vascular isolation. Even these major injuries may be controlled permanently with no further bleeding after therapeutic perihepatic packing.
3. Damaged or divided bile ducts in the liver parenchyma must be closed, either by oversewing or by repair of the bile ducts to prevent bile leaks.
4. Resectional debridement of all dead or devitalized liver tissue is required, leaving behind undamaged liver parenchyma.
5. Formal anatomical hepatic resection is very rarely required.

Advised management policy

The first step is thorough evaluation of associated injuries, particularly in multiply injured patients, in order to decide management strategy. Shocked patients require urgent resuscitation. If there is evidence of ongoing major intraperitoneal haemorrhage, immediate laparotomy is required for its control. Other injuries are assessed and treated on merit. Associated head injuries should be evaluated carefully and treated surgically if necessary.

The majority of patients with suspected liver injury have only a minor injury. If the injury is isolated, such patients should be treated conservatively. Laparotomy is only required to deal with

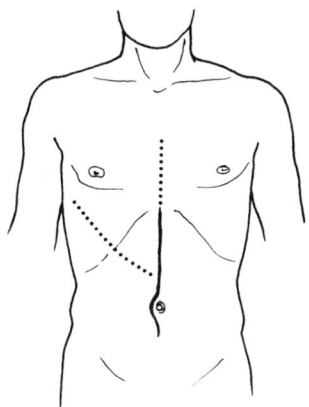

Fig. 2. Surgical exposure for patients with liver injury. The abdomen and lower chest are prepared and draped to allow extension of the incision. The primary exposure is by a long midline incision extended up to the xiphisternum. Upward extension into the lower mediastinum may rarely be required. Lateral extension into the chest is no longer used.

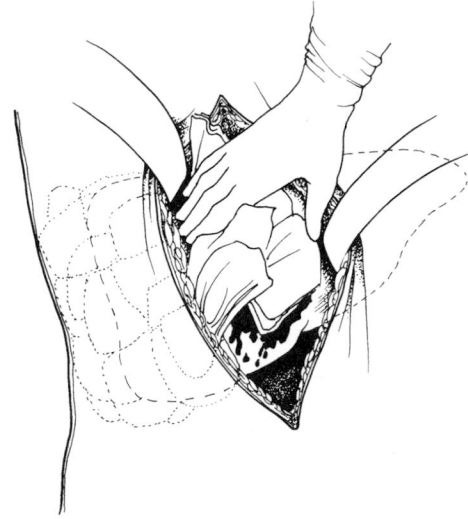

Fig. 3. Perihepatic packing: the 'six-pack' technique. Six or more large abdominal gauze swabs are packed between the liver and the chest wall and diaphragm to control bleeding by compression. The technique of resuscitative perihepatic packing is shown.

immediate or delayed haemorrhage or with other intra-abdominal organ injuries. Laparotomy or laparoscopy may also be indicated for suspected associated diaphragmatic injury.

Laparotomy for abdominal trauma, including suspected liver trauma, is best performed through a long midline abdominal incision extending up to the xiphisternum (Fig. 2). A fixed sternal retractor, as used for highly selective vagotomy, should be available. The patient is draped, with the abdomen widely exposed to allow for extension of the incision. Extension into the mediastinum via a lower median sternotomy may rarely be required to gain access to the inferior vena cava within the pericardium, although this is usually performed transabdominally via the diaphragm. Thoraco-abdominal incisions are virtually never used.

If the liver is bleeding either moderately or massively at the time of opening the abdomen, initial haemostasis should be secured by resuscitative perihepatic packing (Fig. 3).[3] Occasionally porta hepatis occlusion may also be required initially, but is usually only utilized later during the definitive operation on the liver. No procedure is required in the majority of patients in whom the liver injury is minor and not bleeding.

The next step is a full laparotomy to establish whether other injuries require treatment. These should be dealt with in order of priority to control haemorrhage and to deal with hollow viscus injuries.

The surgeon should then return his attention to the liver. Where major haemorrhage necessitated perihepatic packing, sternal retraction and mobilization of the liver may be required to assess fully the extent of injury. Full mobilization of the liver by dividing the falciform and right triangular ligament may even be necessary. This is usually delayed until a later definitive operation after initial therapeutic perihepatic packing.[3]

Bleeding usually stops spontaneously in liver lacerations from knife wounds and minor blunt trauma. No treatment is required. Non-bleeding wounds should not be explored with a finger or an instrument as this could initiate haemorrhage. The patient's abdomen should be closed without drainage. The controversies surrounding drainage are presented later. A contained subcapsular haematoma can be left alone as it will probably not extend or result in delayed rupture. Although this is current standard policy, the authors prefer to open subcapsular haematomas by incising Glisson's capsule. Haemostasis is then achieved by diathermy of the exposed liver surface, as described later. Deep stab wounds or bullet wounds with continued bleeding should be controlled initially by packing; if bleeding continues after resuscitative packing has been removed, direct suture ligation or repair of bleeding vessels should be performed under inflow occlusion using porta hepatis clamping (Pringle manoeuvre). The alternative is the use of therapeutic perihepatic packing, closure of the abdomen, and transfer of the patient to an intensive care unit.

Dead or devitalized liver tissue should be removed, either at the first operation, or at a later stage after therapeutic perihepatic packing. This is done by resectional debridement. Inflow occlusion with porta hepatis clamping is of great help in what would otherwise be a difficult and haemorrhagic surgical procedure. Formal hepatic resection is rarely indicated. Undamaged and non-devitalized tissue should be retained.

Major liver injuries, and particularly hepatic vein and vena caval injuries, should be identified early. After initial packing and resuscitation, haemorrhage will usually recur when the packs are removed. Porta hepatis compression will control inflow vessel haemorrhage but not vena caval or hepatic vein tears, which tend to bleed massively. This blood loss is aggravated on mobilizing the right liver despite the inflow occlusion. Such patients should be repacked, the inflow occlusion clamp removed, and further resuscitation initiated. At this point expert help should be sought or, alternatively, after other injuries have been dealt with, the patient can be left with packs *in situ*, the abdomen closed, and a transfer effected to an expert centre (Calne, BrJSurg, 1979; 66:338). Increasingly we have used therapeutic perihepatic packing as the definitive procedure. Frequently, no further procedure is required when the packs are removed at a later operation.[3]

Specific management options: indications and controversies

Conservative management

Conservative, non-operative management for patients with liver trauma was advocated initially in children and is being utilized increasingly in adults. Even in those patients where operative management is required, there has been a shift towards more conservative surgical procedures rather than radical surgical management of liver injuries.[1,2,14]

The introduction of conservative, non-operative management for children with blunt liver injury has brought therapy in line with the conservative management of blunt paediatric kidney and splenic injuries. A conservative policy for children with blunt liver injuries was initiated by the Cape Town group (Cywes, JPediatSurg, 1985; 20:14) and subsequently confirmed by others (Grisoni, JPediatSurg, 1984; 19:515; Oldham, Surgery, 1986; 100:542). The Cape Town study included 36 of 216 children with abdominal trauma who had liver trauma managed during an 11-year period. In the initial phase of the study all patients were subjected to laparotomy, which was the accepted management at that time internationally. On evaluation, all but two required no more than simple drainage, or suture and drainage. Because of this, in the second half of the study conservative management was practised in 23 consecutive children with blunt liver trauma seen after 1978. Only four ultimately required laparotomy. Complications were minimal and there was no mortality (Cywes, JPediatSurg, 1985; 20:14). Currently, worldwide, most blunt liver injuries in children are treated conservatively. Laparotomy is restricted to those children with concomitant injuries to abdominal organs requiring surgical management, or to those with continued haemorrhage.

The move to conservative management of liver trauma in adults followed approximately a decade later. We reviewed our adult liver injury experience in Cape Town during the period 1978 to 1985 and as a result of this analysis have adopted a more conservative approach.[14] During this period 345 adult patients with liver injury were evaluated and it was noted that all had been treated operatively, as was current policy. However, most patients had simple injuries that were treated by drainage alone and could therefore have been treated conservatively. Since that time we have adopted a more conservative approach to both stab wounds and blunt liver trauma, when this is not associated with clinical indications for laparotomy, such as injury to other abdominal organs requiring surgery or continued haemorrhage. Conservative management had been our previous standard approach to other abdominal injuries, although up until that time we had believed that liver injuries required laparotomy.

Even in those patients who require a laparotomy there has been a shift towards conservative surgical procedures.[1,2,14] Some of these conservative techniques are described below. The previous enthusiasm for formal right or left hepatectomy in liver trauma has been replaced largely by conservative techniques, some of which are described below.

Perihepatic gauze swab packing

Control of liver haemorrhage by perihepatic gauze packing is demonstrated in Fig. 3. Liver packing was proposed at the turn of the century,[8] but fell into disrepute because of problems with intracavity packing (in contra-distinction to perihepatic packing) which was used during the Second World War (Madding, ArchSurg, 1955; 70:748). At that time the pack, or packs, were placed into the cavity of the liver tear, which gave rise to problems. Intracavity packing can promote continued bleeding from hepatic or portal vein branches and is contra-indicated.

Liver packing has been reintroduced during the past two decades and is currently an accepted form of management. The packing must be perihepatic and not intracavity[1-3] (Feliciano, JTrauma, 1986; 26:738; Ivatury, JTrauma, 1986; 26:744). Perihepatic packing is achieved by placing six or more large abdominal gauze swabs (the 'six-pack' technique) between the liver and the diaphragm. Haemostasis is thus secured by compression (Fig. 3).

Our group recognizes two different forms of liver packing for trauma. The one is resuscitative perihepatic packing where packing is performed temporarily with the abdomen open to permit resuscitation or to enable expert help to be called (this is demonstrated in Fig. 3). The other is therapeutic liver packing where the packs are left in situ and the abdomen closed. This can either be used to allow the patient to be transferred to a major centre or as definitive therapy within a major centre, as described below. Our technique and early results with therapeutic perihepatic liver packing have been published.[3]

Resuscitative perihepatic packing with manual compression is utilized when massive bleeding occurs from a damaged liver at the time of opening the abdomen, and can be used later during the procedure to control bleeding while full resuscitation is instituted. This also allows time to obtain blood products, including fresh frozen plasma and/or platelets, if required. When severe bleeding occurs from the liver at the time of opening the abdomen, six to eight packs should be inserted over the liver and pressure applied (Fig. 3). No further procedures should be performed in the liver area until the patient has been fully resuscitated and additional blood products are available. A rapid laparotomy is undertaken to exclude other major bleeding lesions, which are immediately controlled. Defects in traumatized bowel should be closed temporarily, usually with a stapling device, and dealt with later. Once the patient has been fully resuscitated, the operation is recommenced and other injuries are dealt with definitively and finally the liver injury is reinvestigated. If bleeding from the liver has stopped, no further treatment is required. Continued bleeding should be treated by therapeutic perihepatic packing and the abdomen closed.

Temporary resuscitative packing is a life-saving measure and has, in our view, revolutionized the management of severe liver injuries. Not only is bleeding from the damaged liver controlled but all bleeding sites, including major hepatic vein and vena caval tears, can usually be controlled. Only a major arterial bleed (which is rare) will not be controlled by adequate packing. When this arises, inflow occlusion using the Pringle manoeuvre will confirm that there is a major arterial bleed that needs to be controlled surgically.

Therapeutic perihepatic packing is used either to permit transfer of the patient to a major centre, or within an expert centre when major bleeding recurs on removal of either resuscitative or therapeutic liver packs. It has been the general experience that this not only allows time for the patient's condition to be improved and for subsequent planned liver surgery to be undertaken, but also frequently no further bleeding occurs when the patient is returned to the operating room and the packs removed. Unlike the situation in the past, few patients require major surgical procedures, other than the removal of previously devitalized liver tissue.

Once the patient's abdomen has been closed after therapeutic perihepatic packing, the patient must be ventilated and should be cared for in an intensive care unit. In the intensive care unit the patient is fully resuscitated and coagulation defects corrected. Thereafter relevant investigations, including contrast-enhanced CT scanning, can be performed if required. The patient will require continued mechanical ventilation while the packs are *in situ*, because, if sufficient packs are inserted to achieve adequate compression and haemostasis, this will interfere with breathing.

The technique of therapeutic perihepatic packing is to place six or more large abdominal gauze swabs (the six-pack technique) between the liver and either the diaphragm and/or the abdominal wall.[3] The abdomen is closed and the patient is nursed in the intensive care unit on a ventilator. The timing of the reoperation to remove the packs has been controversial, but there is convincing data supporting early removal of the packs. We attempt to re-explore the patient's abdomen under general anaesthesia between 24 and 48 h after inserting the packs. If this is delayed beyond 72 h, infection becomes a major problem.[3] At the second laparotomy, additional resectional debridement of dead liver tissue may be necessary and rebleeding may have to be dealt with. Surprisingly, however, in most patients bleeding will have stopped and no further procedure will be required even when there is damage to major hepatic veins.

When a patient who has had therapeutic perihepatic liver packing is transferred to a major centre, he or she will also require ventilation and intensive care unit management. The timing of the removal of packs is the same. We usually obtain a contrast-enhanced CT scan to assess the extent of liver and major venous damage and to identify devitalized liver. As indicated above, bleeding will usually not recur when the packs are removed, but if it does, this will occur during a procedure undertaken semi-electively in daylight hours with senior staff and an experienced liver surgeon present to deal with whatever problems arise.

Liver suturing versus diathermy

Closure of liver tears by approximation with large mattress sutures has been largely abandoned. Occasionally large mattress sutures are used to deal with oozing from the raw liver surface after suture legation of vessels or resection of devitalized liver tissue. Large mass sutures are rarely necessary and may cause problems, including infection and later haematobilia. Occasionally, small lacerations with troublesome bleeding can be controlled by compressive mattress sutures.

Minor oozing from the raw liver surface or from underneath an opened subcapsular tear can usually be controlled by high-frequency diathermy. This is preferable to large mattress sutures. We use a metal sucker with the diathermy applied to the sucker as demonstrated in Fig. 4. Major vessels that have previously been ligated

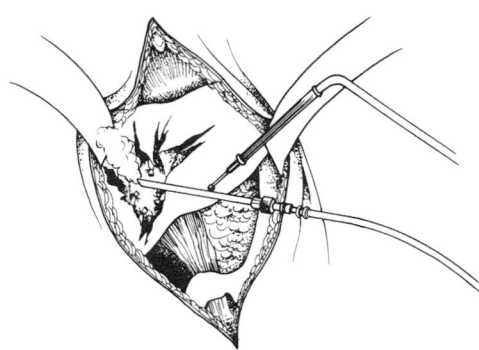

Fig. 4. Diathermy suction–coagulation. A metal sucker is used. High-frequency diathermy is applied to the sucker which coagulates the liver surface while removing both blood and smoke from the field. Previously suture-ligated vessels are avoided.

are avoided carefully. The sucker removes both blood and smoke while coagulating the raw liver surface.

Inflow occlusion with hepatotomy or resectional debridement

Inflow occlusion was advocated by Pringle at the turn of the century but was seldom used until recently, because of the fear of normothermic liver ischaemia.[8] The safety of inflow occlusion (the Pringle manoeuvre) in elective liver surgery, was demonstrated by Huguet (Huguet, ArchSurg, 1978; 113:1448) and has been confirmed by our group in an experimental study and in a patient who had 90 minutes of normothermic hepatic ischaemia (Kahn, EurSurgRes, 1986; 18:277). It has been applied increasingly in hepatic trauma management in major centres.[1,4,6] We occlude the porta hepatis with an aortic vascular clamp (Fig. 5).

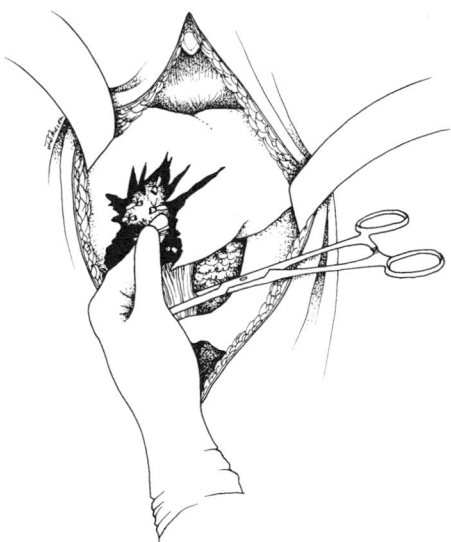

Fig. 5. Porta hepatis clamping (Pringle manoeuvre) and finger fracture technique. The porta hepatis is encircled with a tape and clamped with an aortic vascular clamp to achieve inflow vascular occlusion. Normal liver tissue is divided with a Kelly clamp or between finger and thumb, exposing major vessels and ducts which are suture ligated and divided. This exposes deep-seated bleeding vessels and traumatized bile ducts.

After commencing inflow occlusion by clamping the porta hepatis (Pringle manoeuvre), access to deep-seated bleeding vessels can be achieved relatively simply by performing a hepatotomy.[1,5,6] This means extending the liver injury by dividing normal liver tissue using the Kelly clamp or finger fracture technique (Fig. 5) until individual damaged vessels and bile ducts can be adequately visualized and suture ligated or repaired.[1,5,6] Transthoracic aortic clamping or temporary occlusion of the main mesenteric arteries are contra-indicated as they are unnecessary and associated with a prohibitive mortality.[4].

Hepatic inflow occlusion can be used continuously until haemostasis has been secured. Inflow occlusion appears to be safe for up to 60 min or longer (Kahn, EurSurgRes, 1986; 18:277), but occlusion should be used for the shortest possible time in each individual patient. Remember that the patient may have had pre-existing liver damage due to oligaemic shock before laparotomy. Most workers today use intermittent hepatic inflow occlusion. The occlusion periods are 15 to 20 minutes with breaks of between 10 and 15 minutes. While the occlusion is released, bleeding is controlled by temporary resuscitative perihepatic packing. This allows blood flow through the liver and, at the same time, further resuscitation of the patient can be continued if necessary.

After controlling the bleeding, the liver wounds should be left open. Postoperative drainage is controversial and is dealt with later. The insertion of an omental pack, which is sutured into the wound, has advocates (Stone, Ann Surg, 1975; 141:92) although it is no longer used by most groups. If major bleeding continues, because of a coagulopathy, the patient should be treated by therapeutic perihepatic packing and returned to an intensive care unit temporarily, as described above. Where inflow occlusion does not stop bleeding, major hepatic vein or vena caval injuries should be suspected and treated as described below.

Dead or devitalized liver tissue should be removed by resectional debridement while maintaining inflow occlusion. Only damaged liver tissue is removed. Vascularized liver is retained. Pre-existing tears are enlarged using the Kelly clamp or finger fracture technique to divide the remaining undamaged liver tissue and thereby to complete the resection (Fig. 5). Inflow occlusion is subsequently released to reveal additional bleeding vessels and open bile ducts which are oversewn. Diathermy may be used to achieve further haemostasis. Finally, our group usually spray tissue adhesive on to the cut liver surface while inflow occlusion is temporarily reapplied.

Formal right or left hepatectomy is very rarely indicated and should only be performed when the whole right or left liver has been devitalized. This is virtually never necessary in the authors' experience and then only in massive trauma, usually associated with major hepatic vein injuries.

Major vessel injuries: hepatic vein, vena caval, and porta hepatis injuries

Injuries to the porta hepatis blood vessels or bile duct are rare. Their management is presented below in the section on external trauma to bile ducts.

With hepatic vein or inferior vena caval injuries, inexperienced surgeons should utilize perihepatic packing and either await the arrival of an expert or transfer the patient. Definitive surgery should never be commenced until packs have been placed and the patient

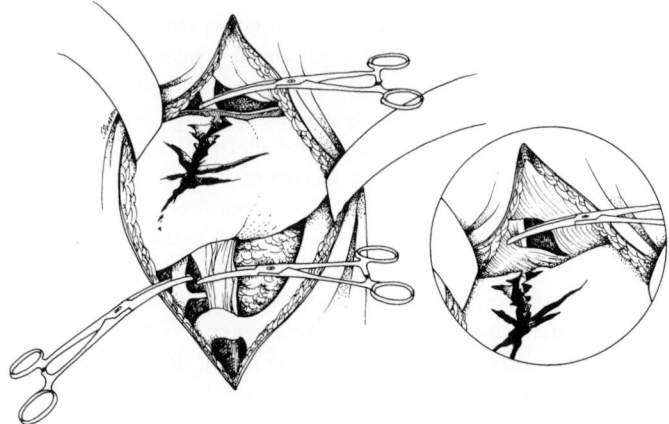

Fig. 6. Total hepatic vascular isolation. The vena cava above the liver is exposed within the pericardium, encircled, taped, and later clamped. The vena cava below the liver is similarly exposed and taped above the renal veins and then subsequently clamped. Hepatic vascular isolation is completed by porta hepatis occlusion. This clamp is applied first. Inset: the vena cava above the liver can be simply exposed inside the pericardium via a hockey-stick incision in the tendinous part of the diaphragm. This modification results in a purely abdominal approach.

fully resuscitated. Thereafter additional blood products should be available in the operating theatre before removing the packs. Additional exposure may be required and this is best achieved by dividing the tendinous portion of the diaphragm as depicted in Fig. 6 (insert) or by performing a lower sternal split (Miller, AnnSurg, 1972; 175:193) (Fig. 6).

Hepatic vein and vena caval injuries should be diagnosed when continued major bleeding occurs from the back of the right lobe of the liver despite clamping the porta hepatis (Pringle manoeuvre). When a major venous injury is confirmed the liver should be repacked. This should usually be therapeutic perihepatic packing, with the abdomen being closed and the patient returned to the intensive care unit. In an otherwise fit patient, and when an expert hepatic surgeon is available, definitive hepatic surgery can be undertaken.

Then the vena cava is exposed above and below the liver. Splitting the diaphragm gives direct access to the suprahepatic vena cava within the pericardium. The vena cava above the liver can either be encircled with a tape after dividing the posterior pericardial attachment or directly clamped without encircling (Fig. 6 insert) (Heaney, Surgery, 1975; 78:138). The vena cava below the liver is similarly exposed above the renal veins, encircled with a tape, and clamped. Total hepatic vascular isolation is completed by clamping the porta hepatis (Fig. 6).

Once the clamps have been applied, near total hepatic vascular isolation is achieved (Fig. 6) and this provides an almost bloodless field. The right liver is fully mobilized by dividing the falciform and right triangular ligaments. Then vena caval defects can be repaired directly and any hepatic vein defects can either be repaired or oversewn, depending on the extent of the injury and whether the right or left liver requires resection as well. The use of total vascular isolation has enabled the authors to salvage patients who would previously have had lethal liver injuries. The safe time-limit for total hepatic vascular isolation is unknown. The authors have used

60 min or longer (Krige, HPBSurgery, 1990; 3:39) but, as with porta hepatis occlusion, the least possible time should be used.

Total hepatic vascular isolation is preferable to the use of intracaval shunts as described in the past (Schrock, ArchSurg, 1968; 96: 698). Several years ago it was pointed out that there were more authors on the subject of hepatic vein and vena caval injuries than there were survivors of the various procedures described (Walt, AmJSurg, 1978; 135:12). We believe that intracaval shunts should be relegated to history as the mortality when they were used was prohibitive[1,4,5] (Burch, AnnSurg, 1988; 207:555).

The alternative to total hepatic vascular isolation for the control and repair of hepatic vein and vena caval injuries is the technique of hepatotomy with direct exposure, described by Pachter et al.[5, 6] Note that temporary occlusion of the aorta or mesenteric vessels is contra-indicated in association with either inflow occlusion or total hepatic vascular isolation.[4]

Drainage

A controlled trial has confirmed that the previously advocated T-tube drainage of a normal common bile duct to provide 'decompression' below a liver injury should not be used (Lucas, JTrauma, 1972; 12:925).

Abdominal cavity drains have been widely used in liver trauma patients because of the presumed likelihood of bile leakage from small divided bile ducts. This has been questioned, and most major groups seldom use abdominal drains[1] (Mullins, SouthMedJ, 1985; 78:259; Feliciano, CurrProbSurg, 1989; 26:459). Patients with liver trauma and no overt bleeding from the damaged liver should not be drained. If a drain is inserted, a closed suction drain system should be used and not open drainage as the latter will introduce infection into the abdominal cavity.

Other therapeutic options

Surgical hepatic artery ligation is virtually never required. It was popularized by Mays (Mays, JTrauma, 1972; 12:397) but has been abandoned since its limitations were recorded (Flint, JTrauma, 1979; 19:319).

Selective hepatic arterial embolization is the best method of treating continued bleeding from a segmental hepatic artery. The diagnosis is usually suspected when the patient continues to bleed after adequately placed therapeutic perihepatic packs and is confirmed angiographically. Selective hepatic arterial embolization is also the treatment of choice in patients who present later with post-traumatic haematobilia.

The role of mesh hepatorrhaphy using a synthetic absorbable mesh has yet to be defined, despite several enthusiastic reports[1] (Jacobson, Surgery, 1992; 111:455). In the authors' opinion, placing the mesh requires significant liver mobilization, therefore therapeutic perihepatic liver packing is simpler and likely to be more effective.

Liver transplantation has been advocated and utilized in patients with irreparable hepatic injuries (Ringe, BrJSurg, 1995; 82:837). It has been suggested that successful liver transplantation for trauma would first require liver resection to control haemorrhage and subsequently a transplant.[1] The authors believe that this will be a very unusual form of treatment for liver trauma.

High-velocity missile injuries

These produce extensive damage well beyond the missile tract due to the production of shock waves. Liver injuries in this setting are frequently either fatal in their own right or the patient dies because of other mortal injuries. In this exceptional case, formal hepatic resection is frequently required if the patient is to be salvaged. Major liver resection has been used successfully by the authors in this setting.

Mortality associated with management

Death in a patient with a liver injury is usually either due to bleeding, particularly from major hepatic vein, vena caval, or porta hepatis injuries, or due to lethal associated non-hepatic injuries. Late deaths are usually sepsis related and are no longer common. Surprisingly, mortality statistics in a unit which develops an interest and expertise in liver injuries may not improve. This has occurred in our own institution. The reason is that the ambulance services and the in-hospital resuscitation facilities are likely to be improved, and thus more mortally injured patients will arrive in the hospital or be referred to the surgical team before their inevitable death, and therefore be included in the mortality statistics (Walt, AmJSurg, 1978; 135:12).

Bile-duct injury

External trauma to the extrahepatic biliary tree is rare. Stab wounds of the gallbladder are usually associated with liver parenchymal injuries. A simple incision wound in the gallbladder should be repaired directly. More extensive lesions require cholecystectomy. In porta hepatis trauma bile-duct injuries are less common than portal vein injuries, but when they occur together the major vascular injury takes precedence in management.[9] Bleeding control is the priority. Penetrating injuries of the biliary tract are usually diagnosed at operation for intraperitoneal bleeding. A literature review[9] (Zollinger, JTrauma, 1972; 12:563; Busuttil, AnnSurg, 1980; 191:641; Parks, BrJSurg, 1995; 82:1303) has led us to recommend the following management policy in patients with porta hepatis injuries. A damaged hepatic artery should probably be ligated. Portal vein injuries should be repaired directly using finger and thumb control or using vascular clamps placed on either side of the injury. Bile-duct injuries should be repaired primarily by an expert hepatobiliary surgeon, using a hepaticojejunostomy (as for iatrogenic injuries) in haemodynamically stable patients in whom other organ injuries have been controlled. If expertise is not available, or when the patient has other severe injuries, the duct should be drained and delayed repair undertaken. Small defects in the bile duct can be treated by direct repair. Partially disrupted bile ducts can also be treated with an endoprosthesis inserted via the ERCP route.

A detailed analysis of the management of iatrogenic extrahepatic bile-duct injuries is beyond the scope of this presentation. Late recurrent strictures should be repaired by high hepaticojejunal anastomosis[11] (Andren-Sandberg, AnnSurg, 1985; 201:452). When the damage is noted at the time of the initial surgery we also advocate high hepaticojejunostomy by an expert, bearing in mind the tenuous blood supply of the supraduodenal bile duct.[13]

Stenting after high hepaticojejunostomy is controversial. Most authors only use stents in difficult high strictures where an adequate mucosa-to-mucosa anastomosis has not been achieved. In these circumstances the authors currently prefer an access loop (Krige, BrJSurg, 1987; 74:612) to allow later imaging and dilatation, if necessary. Although early data on the use of balloon dilatation of strictured bile ducts by either the percutaneous transhepatic route or the ERCP route have been encouraging (Huibregtse, Endoscopy, 1986; 18:133; Mueller, Radiol, 1986; 160:17), longer follow-up is required before balloon dilation can be advised routinely. Recent data reveal this to be largely unsuccessful.[11]

Subsequent monitoring

After treating a major hepatic injury, the patient needs to be followed carefully in the early postoperative period, watching for the development of a bile collection or of an intraperitoneal or subphrenic abscess. The best means of evaluation in patients suspected clinically of having an intra-abdominal collection is ultrasound or CT scanning. Abscesses or bile collections should be drained percutaneously under ultrasound or CT control. A second laparotomy is only required in the unusual event of unsuccessful percutaneous drainage.

Patients with major hepatic vein repairs should be reimaged at between 6 weeks and 3 months and again after a year, to ensure that they do not develop hepatic vein stenosis which may lead to the silent development of the Budd–Chiari syndrome. If hepatic vein narrowing is noted, the narrowing should be dilated using percutaneous balloon dilatation via the vena cava.

Patients who have had bile-duct injuries and who develop a raised alkaline phosphatase should have the biliary tract re-evaluated radiologically. If a direct bile duct to bile duct anastomosis has been performed, ERCP should be performed routinely at 6 months and at 1 year to ensure that no stenosis develops. Where a bowel to bile duct anastomosis has been performed and an access bowel loop is available, the anastomosis can be evaluated percutaneously (Krige, BrJSurg, 1987; 74:612). Where an access bowel loop has not been fashioned, imaging is difficult and should probably only be undertaken if the patient develops cholangitis or develops a raised alkaline phosphatase, when a percutaneous transhepatic radiological approach to the hepaticojejunostomy should be used.

References

1. Reed RL, Merrell RC, Meyers WC, and Fischer RP. Continuing evolution in the approach to severe liver trauma. *Annals of Surgery*, 1992; **216**: 524–38.
2. Croce MA, *et al*. Nonoperative management of blunt hepatic trauma is the treatment of choice for hemodynamically stable patients. Results of a prospective trial. *Annals of Surgery*, 1995; **221**: 744–55.
3. Krige JEJ, Bornman PC, and Terblanche J. Therapeutic perihepatic packing in complex liver trauma. *British Journal of Surgery*, 1992; **79**: 43–6.
4. Feliciano DV, Jordan GL, Bitondo CG, Mattox KL, Burch JM, and Cruse PA. Management of 1000 consecutive cases of hepatic trauma (1979–1984). *Annals of Surgery*, 1986; **204**: 438–45.
5. Pachter HL, Spencer FC, Hofstetter SR, Laing HC, and Coppa GR. The management of juxtahepatic venous injuries without an atriocaval shunt: preliminary clinical observations. *Surgery*, 1986; **99**: 569–75.
6. Pachter HL, Spencer FC, Hofstetter SR, and Coppa GF. Experience with the finger fracture technique to achieve intra-hepatic hemostasis in 75 patients with severe injuries of the liver. *Annals of Surgery*, 1983; **197**: 771–88.
7. Moore FA, Moore EE, and Seagraves A. Nonresectional management of major hepatic trauma: an evolving concept. *American Journal of Surgery*, 1985; **150**: 725–9.
8. Pringle JH. Notes on the arrest of hepatic hemorrhage due to trauma. *Annals of Surgery*, 1908; **48**: 541–9.
9. Sheldon GF, Lim RC, Yee ES, and Petersen SR. Management of injuries to the porta hepatis. *Annals of Surgery*, 1985; **202**: 539–45.
10. Andren-Sandberg A, Alinder G, and Bengmark S. Accidental lesions of the common bile duct at cholecystectomy. Pre- and perioperative factors of importance. *Annals of Surgery*, 1985; **201**: 328–32.
11. Stewart L and Way LW. Bile duct injuries during laparoscopic cholecystectomy. Factors that influence the results of treatment. *Archives of Surgery*, 1995; **130**: 1123–9.
12. Moore EE, *et al*. Organ injury scaling: spleen, liver, and kidney. *Journal of Trauma*, 1989; **29**: 1664–6.
13. Terblanche J, Allison HF, and Northover JMA. An ischemic basis for biliary strictures. *Surgery*, 1983; **94**: 52–7.
14. Terblanche J and Krige JEJ. Injuries to the liver and bile ducts. In Williamson RCN and Cooper MJ, eds. *Emergency abdominal surgery*, Vol. 17. London: Churchill Livingstone, 1990.

30.5 Liver transplantation*

Vijayan Balan, J. Wallis Marsh, and Jorge Rakela

Introduction

Liver transplantation is now an established treatment for endstage liver disease and fulminant hepatic failure. This accomplishment is due to the development of animal models for laboratory investigation of liver disease and liver transplantation, greater understanding of the pathophysiology and natural history of liver disease, and the establishment of multiorgan procurement and preservation techniques. Furthermore, the standardization of surgical techniques, advances in anaesthetic management and critical care medicine have contributed to this effort. Most importantly, the development of safer and more potent immunosuppressive agents has contributed to the long-term survival of liver transplant recipients.

The first report of experimental orthotopic liver transplantation was made by J. A. Cannon (TransplBull, 1956; 3:7) and C. S. Welch. C. S. Welch reported on attempts to transplant an auxillary liver heterotopically in the pelvis or the right paravertebral gutter in dogs. Subsequently, J. A. Cannon reported the first orthotopic liver transplant. The upshot of subsequent experimental efforts in the laboratory, mainly the development of the techniques of total hepatectomy and the orthotopic replacement of the liver, allowed for the initiation of human orthotopic liver transplantation in 1963. Seven such transplants were performed without success until 1967 when the first long-term survival was achieved in Denver, Colorado (Starzl, SGO, 1963; 117:659; Starzl, AnnSurg, 1968; 168:392). In the early years, a number of auxiliary liver transplantations were also attempted, and almost all failed. Despite these failures, auxiliary liver transplantation contributed to our knowledge of hepatic physiology, principally the importance of splanchnic venous flow in the maintenance of the grafted liver (Starzl, SGO, 1973; 137:179; Marchioro, SGO, 1985; 121:17). Thus, auxiliary liver transplantation was abandoned in favour of orthotopic liver transplantation.

The next stage of growth in liver transplantation was the development of safe and effective immunosuppressive regimens. The lack of safe and potent immunosuppressive agents was an important factor in the poor outcome of liver transplantation prior to 1979. The standard antirejection therapy prior to 1979 included azathioprine, steroids, and antilymphocyte globulin (Table 1). Unfortunately, the rates of rejection and infection were high with these agents.

* This chapter is an updated version of Chapter 31.4 published in the first edition of this textbook. The present authors wish to acknowledge the original authors and their contribution: Linda S. Sher, Todd K. Howard, Luis G. Podesta, Philip Rosenthal, John M. Vierling, Federico Villamil, Andreas Tzakis, Thomas E. Starzl, and Leonard Makowka.

Table 1 History of immunosuppression

Agent	Year reported
Azathioprine	1962
Combined azathioprine–steroids	1963
Polyclonal antibodies, antilymphocyte globulin	1966
Cyclophosphamide	1970
Cyclosporin used in humans	1978
Combined cyclosporin–steroids	1980
Monoclonal antibodies developed FK506	1981

In 1979, Calne demonstrated the efficacy of cyclosporin as the only immunosuppressant, in 34 patients receiving 36 cadaveric organ allografts (Lancet, 1979; ii:1033). He found it to be a more potent immunosuppressive agent than any previously used but also toxic, making it difficult to use. The true potential of cyclosporin was recognized when it was combined with prednisone by Starzl and colleagues. Regimens employing cyclosporin allowed a better balance between prevention of rejection and minimizing the liability of infection in the immunosuppressed patient. Better control of rejection and a more manageable postoperative course facilitated rapid progress in the field of liver transplantation. The number of liver transplantations performed each year since 1981 increased tremendously, as did the number of new transplantation centres throughout the United States and the world.

Immunosuppression entered a new level of sophistication with the introduction of monoclonal antibodies specific for T lymphocytes for the treatment of severe rejection. One such agent, OKT3, has successfully reversed unremitting rejection in many patients concurrently treated with steroids and cyclosporin, thereby averting retransplantation and even death.

Technical advances have also contributed to the success of liver transplantation. One of the most important advances was the introduction, in 1983, of heparin-free venovenous bypass (Griffith, SGO, 1985; 160:270). The use of venovenous bypass during the anhepatic phase has facilitated the maintenance of a stable haemodynamic state during completion of the recipient hepatectomy and implantation of the new allograft. It has allowed the most critical part of the transplantation procedure to be performed in a calm and safe atmosphere, thereby allowing the training of new transplantation surgeons, so important in the worldwide dissemination of this procedure. Other technical advances have included standardization of the biliary tract reconstruction, segmental liver transplantation, new applications of auxiliary liver transplantation, liver transplantation in continuity with other abdominal organs, and advances of the procedure in the very small paediatric patient. In addition, employment of vascular allografts has allowed transplantation to be performed in patients with portal vein thrombosis as well as inadequate hepatic arterial flow.

Liver transplantation is a multidisciplinary effort which has required advances in all fields of medicine. The technical growth has been made in parallel with advances in anaesthesiology, critical care, hepatology, radiology, and blood banking, as well as in most other medical specialties.

The standardization of the techniques of organ retrieval and the ability to procure multiple organs from a single donor have also been essential for the growth of liver transplantation. Furthermore, recent introduction of the new preservation solution, the University of Wisconsin Solution, has extended liver allograft preservation to 24 h (Todo, JAMA, 1989; 261:711). This has allowed more organs to be retrieved from greater distances and has contributed to an increased donor pool.

Liver transplantation has contributed to the understanding of normal hepatic physiology as well as to the pathophysiology of liver disease. Through the correction of specific inborn errors of metabolism, the genetics and molecular biology of many of these diseases have been defined. Through the study of the effects of the disease process on the new allograft, hepatology has been advanced. However, the most important contribution of liver transplantation is its ability to cure many hepatic diseases for which there had been no alternative treatment. Patients with liver failure have been restored to health and returned to a normal, active, and good quality of life.

Indications

Initially, liver transplantation was offered predominantly to patients for whom no other therapy was available and was the only alternative to imminent death. Theses candidates were patients with:

(1) unresectable hepatic malignancies;
(2) patients in fulminant hepatic failure;
(3) patients critically ill and debilitated from their endstage liver disease with its complications of encephalopathy, variceal bleeding, and coagulopathy;
(4) children with biliary atresia and failed Kasai procedures.

Not surprisingly the outcome and survival rates were poor in such patients, but better than if they were untreated. However, with the introduction of cyclosporin and the improved outcome after liver transplantation, the indications for it dramatically expanded to include many other liver diseases (Table 2).

Transplantation in adults

Common indications in adults for liver transplantation include advanced chronic liver disease, cholestatic liver disease such as primary biliary cirrhosis, and sclerosing cholangitis. The decision regarding the timing of transplantation for patients with these indications can often be difficult. Ideally, the patient should undergo

Table 2 Indications for orthotopic liver transplantation

Chronic active hepatitis
  Viral
  Drug-induced
  Autoimmune
  Cryptogenic
Alcoholic liver disease
Primary biliary cirrhosis
Sclerosing cholangitis
Biliary atresia
Cholestatic syndrome
Budd–Chiari syndrome
Unresectable hepatic malignancies
Fulminant hepatic failure
  Viral
  Drug-induced
  Metabolic liver disease
Inborn errors of metabolism
  Wilson's disease
  α_1-Antitrypsin deficiency
  Tyrosinaemia
  Glycogen storage disease type I
  Glycogen storage disease type IV
  Haemochromatosis
  Homozygous hyperlipoproteinaemia type II
  Crigler–Najjar syndrome I
  Neville's syndrome
  Protein C deficiency
  Haemophilia
  Urea cycle deficiency
  Cystic fibrosis
  Protoporphyria

transplantation at the time when morbidity and mortality would be minimized yet it is apparent that the patient's long-term survival is jeopardized by the liver disease. Although much is known about the natural history of these diseases, there is no substitute for early referral and close monitoring for subtle signs of deterioration.

Hepatic malignancy has become a much less common indication for transplantation, the major reason being the poor long-term survival. In most cases, there is an early recurrence of the malignancy with rapid progression to death. This has led to a closer look at the various types of malignancies for which transplantation has been performed. For certain pathological types there is a better prognosis than for others. Those malignancies with a better outcome include the fibrolamellar variant of hepatocellular carcinoma, epithelioid haemangioendothelioma, and the coincidental tumour found at the time of transplantation for chronic liver failure. Occasional long-term survivors with other types of malignancies, including hepatocellular carcinoma, have also been found (Koneru, GastrClinNAm, 1988; 17:177).

The reduced survival after transplantation for most hepatic malignancies compared to non-malignant diseases has led to variations in policy among different centres. Very careful evaluation is required preoperatively to determine the exact extent of the disease. In some centres this includes an exploratory laparotomy and lymph-node sampling prior to consideration of transplantation. Various auxiliary treatment modalities are being explored and it would appear that the future of transplantation for malignancies must include combinations of perioperative and adjuvant chemotherapy.

Cholangiocarcinoma has been found to recur rapidly following orthotopic liver transplantation (Koneru, GastrClinNAm, 1988; 17:

177). New and much more aggressive methods of surgical treatment for this disease are being explored. Recently, a new approach employing an upper abdominal exenteration, the so-called 'cluster procedure', with replacement of a liver or liver and pancreatic graft, has been employed (Starzl, AnnSurg, 1989; 210:374). The results for this procedure are preliminary and long-term follow up will be required to determine the efficacy of this approach.

Another important indication for which institutional policies have varied is for the patient with cirrhosis secondary to infection with hepatitis B virus. The 1- and 5-year survival rates for patients who are infected with hepatitis B virus have been uniformly inferior to those found with other liver diseases (Iwatsuki, TransplProc, 1988; 20:498). Recurrence is the rule. However, the natural history following transplantation spans a spectrum from fulminant hepatitis to recurrent bouts of hepatitis with spontaneous resolution, to recurrent cirrhosis requiring retransplantation; but there are many long-term survivors and, accordingly, attention is being focused on the perioperative management of these patients. Various protocols have been employed to prevent recurrence, including the use of α-interferon, hyperimmune hepatitis B immunoglobulin, and monoclonal antibodies against hepatitis B surface antigen. Prevention of allograft infection and management of patients with recurrence will remain important topics of future research.

Another controversial indication is alcoholic cirrhosis. The determination of candidacy relies heavily on the psychosocial evaluation. Cardiovascular evaluation to assess cardiomyopathy is also an important focus of the evaluation procedure. Although the accompanying physical and psychiatric stigmata of patients with alcoholic cirrhosis were once believed to result in poor outcome, it has been shown that success is common with proper patient selection. Indeed, recent results for transplantation of alcoholic cirrhosis have been as good as for other adult disease indications (Starzl, JAMA, 1988; 260:2542).

Transplantation is the therapy of choice for acute and subacute fulminant hepatic failure due to a variety of aetiologies. This is the most dramatic of all indications for transplantation. The decision to undertake transplantation must be made rapidly as these patients can progress rapidly to grade 4 coma, at which point transplantation may have a poor outcome (Stieber, GastrClinNAm, 1988; 17: 157). The decision is facilitated when there is evidence of rapid progression of encephalopathy and/or coagulopathy, as well as haemodynamic instability. Once it becomes clear that spontaneous recovery is unlikely, transplantation should be undertaken rapidly to prevent a poor neurological outcome or death.

Through modification of genetic disease processes, transplantation has provided benefits to patients and increased understanding of hepatic physiology. Transplantation has been performed for the purpose of treating liver failure, as well as for the correction of a single metabolic error in selected diseases. Metabolic diseases which have been cured by liver transplantation include Wilson's disease, tyrosinaemia, $α_1$-antitrypsin deficiency, galactosaemia, Crigler–Najjar type I disease, hyperlipoproteinaemia types II and IV, protoporphyria, sea-blue histiocyte syndrome, and several glycogen storage diseases. Equally striking is the correction of a number of coagulation defects following liver transplantation.

Hepatitis C infection accounts for approximately 50 to 60 per cent of adult chronic hepatitis. Hepatitis C may become the leading indication for liver transplant in the future. Prior to the availability of anti-hepatitis C virus testing, hepatitis C recurrence did not appear to be a frequent or severe complication after transplantation. Recurrent hepatitis C is a major complication post-transplant and is discussed in detail below.

Transplantation in children

The medical indications for adult and paediatric liver transplantation are comparable. Any child with endstage liver disease should be considered as a potential candidate for liver transplantation. Transplantation is indicated for life-threatening variceal bleeding, recurrent episodes of encephalopathy, coagulopathy, malnutrition, severe jaundice, profound growth retardation, or metabolic bone disease. When it is clear that survival for more than 1 year is unlikely, considerations for evaluation and candidacy for transplantation should be initiated. This is particularly important for small children for whom donor organ availability may be limited. Accurate assessment of the individual child's probability of survival may be difficult or impossible. If liver function is stable, specific therapy (such as sclerosis of oesophageal varices, diuretics, fluid restriction, or salt restriction) may be more appropriate. However, if liver function is progressively deteriorating, then transplantation therapy is indicated. The possibility of future transplantation must be considered whenever interventions are discussed. Any intervention which may jeopardize suitability for transplantation should be contemplated carefully. For example, a failed portacaval shunt with thrombosis of the portal system may make liver transplantation technically impossible.

Numerous hepatic diseases in children have been treated successfully with liver transplantation. In all series, extrahepatic biliary atresia remains the most frequent paediatric diagnosis requiring transplantation. Controversy surrounds the utility and the role of the Kasai portoenterostomy in the treatment of this disorder. In a significant percentage of individuals (25–30 per cent), if surgery is performed within the first 2 months of life, biliary drainage and successful outcome may be achieved. However, multiple attempts at revisions to establish bile flow, peritonitis, and intra-abdominal haemorrhage all contribute to technically more difficult subsequent surgery and a reduced likelihood of success if transplantation becomes necessary. Therefore an attempt to establish bile flow before 2 months of age in children with extrahepatic biliary atresia should be made by surgeons experienced in the Kasai procedure. If bile drainage is not established, evaluation for liver transplantation should quickly ensue. Even if bile drainage is incomplete, the Kasai procedure may facilitate improved survival by allowing the child to grow, thus increasing the availability of suitable donor organs.

Disorders in the formation and development of the biliary ductal system comprise the majority of the paediatric patients who undergo orthotopic liver transplantation. While extrahepatic biliary atresia represents the most common indication, Alagille's syndrome (arteriohepatic dysplasia), Byler's disease, and non-syndromatic intrahepatic biliary hypoplasia entities are included in this category (D'Alagille, TransplProc, 1987; 19:3242).

The next largest category requiring liver transplantation in paediatric patients consists of genetic disorders of metabolism (Putnam, Surgery, 1977; 81:258; Zitelli, TransplProc. 1983; 15:1284; Starzl, JPediat, 1985; 106:604). The more common inborn errors of metabolism requiring liver transplantation include $α_1$-antitrypsin deficiency, Wilson's disease, tyrosinaemia, glycogen storage disease, and galactosaemia. Rarer metabolic disorders for which hepatic transplantation has been utilized include Crigler–Najjar syndrome type I, hyperlipoproteinaemia types II and IV, protoporphyria, and the sea-blue histiocyte syndrome (Kaufman, Hepatol, 1986; 6:1259; Mowat, TransplProc, 1987; 19:3236).

α_1-Antitrypsin deficiency is inherited as an autosomal recessive disorder with a frequency of 1 in 2000 individuals. While not all homozygous individuals develop liver disease, of those who do, the majority will demonstrate cholestasis during infancy. Most of these infants will subsequently become anicteric, but the stigmata of significant liver disease will eventually ensue, usually during adolescence or early adulthood.

Liver transplantation corrects the enzyme deficiency, with the recipient acquiring the protease inhibitor type of the donor. Serum α_1-antitrypsin levels quickly return to the normal range after transplantation (Putnam, Surgery, 1977; 81:258). Long-term follow-up of children transplanted for α_1-antitrypsin deficiency has failed to disclose any evidence for pulmonary or other organ disease.

Evaluation for liver transplantation should proceed in any individual with the diagnosis of α_1-antitrypsin deficiency who manifests any signs of significant liver disease or demonstrates decompensation. While infusion of α_1-antitrypsin to adults with pulmonary complications of the disorder has been useful, this approach is not beneficial for hepatic complications. Since patients with mild liver disease at presentation may decompensate rapidly, careful observation and prompt referral for transplantation should be considered if jaundice or mild coagulopathy develops.

Wilson's disease remains one of the few hepatic disorders in which early diagnosis can lead to effective medical therapy, employing D-penicillamine or trientine therapy in conjunction with dietary copper restriction. Transplantation should be reserved for those patients with Wilson's disease who present with fulminant hepatic failure or failure of medical therapy. Transplantation cures the abnormal copper metabolism. It should be undertaken prior to the development of significant neurological deterioration, although reversal of severe neurological deficits has been observed following transplantation in patients with Wilson's disease.

Hereditary tyrosinaemia is an autosomal recessive disorder with a frequency of 1 in 100 000 births. The disease may present either acutely in the first weeks of life with fulminant hepatic failure, or after 6 months of life with cirrhosis, renal tubular defects, rickets, and failure to thrive. Onset of disease after 6 months of life has been associated with the development of hepatoma. Serum tyrosine and methionine levels are markedly elevated and succinylacetone is present in the urine. Transplantation results in the return of serum tyrosine levels to normal and prevention of hepatoma development; however, the effect on the status of metabolic derangements in other organs is not well characterized.

Glycogen storage diseases have been treated successfully by orthotopic liver transplantation (Mowat, TransplProc, 1987; 19: 3236). Long-term follow-up has demonstrated a return of glucose homeostasis to normal.

Unlike adults, in whom chronic liver disease secondary to viral aetiologies is a common indication for liver transplantation, in the paediatric group this is a much less common indication. Infants in this group may include those with the diagnosis of neonatal hepatitis, hepatitis B, and non-A, non-B hepatitis.

Fulminant hepatic failure signifies another group of paediatric patients who may undergo hepatic transplantation (Iwatsuki, SemLivDis, 1985; 5:325). This may be the result of a toxin-induced hepatic failure, a viral hepatitis, or a metabolic disorder (Wilson's disease, tyrosinaemia). Frequently, the aetiological agent remains unidentified. Development of hepatic encephalopathy in conjunction with coagulopathy is an immediate indication for referral to a transplant centre. Previous reports of poor results in patients with fulminant hepatic failure may be the consequence of waiting too long and attempting transplantation in individuals in deep coma.

Hepatic transplantation has also been utilized in the therapy of unresectable hepatic malignancies in children (Iwatsuki, AnnSurg, 1985; 202:401). The primary tumour type has been hepatoblastoma. As in adults, survival rates have not been encouraging and future approaches will include the use of peri-, intra-, and postoperative chemotherapy.

Many other disorders associated with liver failure in children have been treated with hepatic transplantation. For example, haemochromatosis, cystic fibrosis, sclerosing cholangitis, drug-induced cirrhosis, autoimmune hepatitis, and Budd-Chiari syndrome may all occur in paediatric patients and necessitate a transplant evaluation and procedure.[1–5] The indications and contra-indications for these patients are similar to those already discussed. Of course, each patient requires an individual assessment as circumstances will vary for each.

Evaluation for transplantation

The evaluation process is directed towards the determination of the need and urgency for the performance of an orthotopic liver transplant, as well as the feasibility of performing this procedure. The need and urgency are determined by obtaining a careful history, performing a physical examination, and obtaining various laboratory data, as well as reviewing any biopsies which may have been obtained in the past. The feasibility of transplantation requires evaluation of the entire medical status of the patient, including cardiovascular, pulmonary, and renal systems. Furthermore, the use of various radiological techniques permits definition of the vascular anatomy and size of the liver that is required for liver transplantation.

History

As with the approach to any medical disease, a careful history must first be obtained. Specific areas to be defined include possible aetiologies of the liver disease, prior complications secondary to liver disease, previous surgical procedures, and the current disability of the patient. Liver disease resulting from prior alcohol or illicit intravenous drug abuse will require further evaluation. A psychiatric and sociological evaluation should be performed to ascertain the patient's determination to abstain from further substance abuse, as well as his/her ability to comply with the postoperative medication regimen and medical follow-up.

The specific areas of concern regarding complications of the liver disease include episodes of encephalopathy, ascites, oedema, gastrointestinal bleeding, infections (particularly spontaneous bacterial peritonitis), and inability to perform daily chores. Prior complications in conjunction with ongoing hepatic disease, demonstrated by decreased synthetic function, are clearly indications for liver transplantation. The urgency must be determined based on the severity of the complications as well as the presence of current disabilities.

Laboratory data

Necessary laboratory data include a complete blood count, with special attention to signs of hypersplenism, and tests to define the electrolyte status and liver function. Elevated bilirubin levels indicate impaired hepatic excretory function, while an elevated prothrombin time and decreased serum albumin demonstrate impaired hepatic synthetic function. Hepatitis serological tests are obtained to identify those patients who are hepatitis B surface antigen positive, as these patients will require concurrent medical treatment in addition to liver transplantation. Levels of carcinoembryonic antigen, α-fetoprotein, and CA19–9 (in patients with primary sclerosing cholangitis) should be obtained and, if elevated, a search for occult malignancy or hepatocellular carcinoma must be undertaken. The combination of elevated carcinoembryonic antigen and CA19–9 is highly suggestive of the presence of cholangiocarcinoma in patients with primary sclerosing cholangitis (Ramage, Gastro, 1995; 108:865). A 24-hour urine collection for creatinine clearance is obtained to define the presence and degree of renal dysfunction, which may require adjustments in the dosage of postoperative immunosuppressive medications.

Various bacterial, viral, and fungal cultures and titres are obtained to establish a baseline for each patient as well as to identify those infectious disease processes which may require treatment prior to transplantation. A tuberculin skin test is performed with an appropriate control panel. In addition, an HIV antibody test is obtained.

Additional laboratory examinations, aimed at the determination of the aetiology of the liver disease, are tailored for each individual patient. These include antimitochondrial antibody, antinuclear antibody, antismooth muscle antibody, ceruloplasmin, urinary copper, iron, iron-binding capacity, iron saturation, ferritin, α1-antitrypsin level and phenotype, and drug screen.

Cardiac evaluation

Cardiopulmonary evaluation is tailored to each patient. An arterial blood gas and chest radiograph are obtained routinely. Should there be any indication, such as hypoxaemia, history of extensive smoking and/or prior pulmonary disease, pulmonary function tests are also performed. An ECG is obtained routinely and, once again, should there be an indication, a cardiac stress test, two-dimensional echocardiogram, and/or coronary angiogram may be required. Patients who are over 50 years of age with a history of coronary artery disease need a comprehensive cardiac evaluation to determine their eligibility for transplantation.

Radiological evaluation

The radiological imaging procedures are primarily directed towards the elucidation of the technical feasibility of transplantation as well as the collection of data which will be required for suitable donor-recipient matching. Doppler ultrasonography is performed to determine the patency of the hepatic veins, hepatic artery, and particularly the portal vein, as well as the presence of biliary tract

disease. Should portal vein patency be in question, an angiogram must be performed to define the portal system anatomy. Although previously thought to be a contra-indication to orthotopic liver transplantation, portal vein thrombosis is now no longer an absolute contra-indication. However, the presence of an adequate superior mesenteric vein is required for performance of the procedure.

A CT scan of the head and abdomen is performed. The presence of intracranial lesions must be determined prior to undertaking the transplantation procedure, as the presence of any vascular anomaly may lead to catastrophic events intraoperatively. Furthermore, the presence of encephalopathy requires the exclusion of other causes of altered mental status. The CT scan of the abdomen will demonstrate any intra- or extrahepatic malignancies and provide the measurement of liver volume which is important in the donor-recipient matching (Van Thiel, Gastro, 1985; 88:1812).

We are finding increasing value in the use of magnetic resonance imaging (**MRI**) in the evaluation process. This procedure provides us with similar data as the CT scan of the abdomen and demonstrates the presence of flow in the portal vein. With further studies confirming the reliability of this modality, MRI may become the primary radiological test in the evaluation of these patients.

Patients with primary sclerosing cholangitis are scheduled for endoscopic retrograde or percutaneous transhepatic cholangiography and brush biopsies when indicated. As previously stated, there is a 10 per cent coincidence of cholangiocarcinoma. Due to the dismal results of orthotopic liver transplantation for patients with a biliary tract malignancy, it is important to determine its presence prior to transplantation. In the presence of cholangiocarcinoma new alternative treatment methods, such as the cluster procedure, may prove to be of value.

Endoscopic evaluation

Endoscopic evaluation of the upper gastrointestinal tract is performed to determine the presence of, and potentially treat, oesophageal varices. Colonoscopy is performed in patients over 40 years of age or with a strong family history of colon cancer or polyposis.

Once the evaluation process is completed, the final determination for the need and urgency for transplantation is usually made by a multidisciplinary selection committee. Transplantation is indicated in the presence of endstage liver disease manifested by encephalopathy, ascites, impaired renal function, gastrointestinal bleeding, inability to perform daily chores, and decreased hepatic synthetic function. In the presence of these factors, a determination of feasibility is rendered.

Contra-indications for transplantation

Currently, the contra-indications for orthotopic liver transplantation are:

(1) presence of active infection outside the hepatobiliary system;
(2) acquired immune deficiency syndrome;
(3) technical impossibility;
(4) multiorgan system failure which is irreversible by orthotopic liver transplantation;
(5) irreversible brain damage; and
(6) inability to comply with the postoperative medication and medical follow-up regimen.

Table 3 Pretransplantation management problems

Hepatic encephalopathy
Infection
Refractory ascites
Renal failure
Variceal haemorrhage
Malnutrition

The evaluation and selection process for orthotopic liver transplantation has undergone major extensions to include aged patients, small infants, critically ill patients, and patients with portal vein thrombosis.

There are currently no age limits set for patients to be considered for transplantation. The oldest patient to have received an orthotopic liver transplant was a 76-year-old woman with primary biliary cirrhosis. Well-selected patients over 60 years of age have been shown to have a survival rate similar to that of younger patients (Starzl, NEJM, 1987; 316:484).

Improvements in the technical aspects of the transplant procedure have made it feasible to transplant very small infants. The youngest patient to have received a liver was a 3-week-old infant. Children under the age of 1 year can now be successfully transplanted with a good survival rate (Esquivel, JPediat, 1987; 110:545). Advances in critical care medicine and anaesthesiology, as well as in other medical specialties, have made it possible to maintain and transplant critically ill patients. Although patients who are ventilator dependent, require pressors or dialysis, or are in coma preoperatively constitute a high-risk population, many of these patients can be salvaged through transplantation and can go on to enjoy long-term survival with an excellent quality of life.

Preoperative management

The increased success of orthotopic liver transplantation has led to expansion of its indications and efforts to optimize timing for transplantation. The concept that an optimal time exists for transplantation, after which patients suffer increased morbidity or mortality, has now been validated (Shaw, ArchSurg, 1989; 124:895). Clinical and laboratory factors correlated with the success of transplantation have been codified into a risk stratification scoring system. Risk factors include degree of encephalopathy, presence of ascites, degree of malnutrition, serum bilirubin, age, requirement for transfusion during transplantation, and degree of coagulopathy. A prospective analysis from the University of Nebraska showed that patients with a low-risk score had an actuarial survival of 90.5 per cent for 1 year. Patients with intermediate- and high-risk scores had significantly diminished actuarial survivals of 85.2 and 44.5 per cent, respectively.

Although these results indicate that patients should be transplanted prior to the development of a high-risk profile, many patients continue to be referred late in the course of their illness and require meticulous management in the preoperative phase to countermand the adverse impact of the complications of terminal liver disease prior to transplantation. Table 3 lists the most significant management problems encountered in this preoperative population.

Hepatic encephalopathy

The degree of portal systemic encephalopathy at the time of transplantation is inversely related to survival. Stratification of 115 adult patients with chronic liver disease transplanted between 1985 and 1988 at the University of Nebraska showed actuarial survival rates of 89.6 per cent in the absence of preoperative encephalopathy. The actuarial survival rate diminished to 78.6 per cent in patients with mild encephalopathy (stages 1–2), and 33.6 per cent in patients with severe encephalopathy (stages 3–4).

The initial approach to management requires evaluation of reversible factors that may have precipitated or intensified encephalopathy. These factors include infection and fever, hypokalaemia, metabolic alkalosis, gastrointestinal bleeding, sedatives or narcotic analgesics, and constipation. Once precipitating factors are identified, specific measures should be taken to alleviate them. After treatment of precipitating factors, patients with stage 1 and 2 encephalopathy should receive lactulose orally in a dose sufficient to produce two to three soft bowel movements per day (Elkington, NEJM, 1969; 281:408). For patients with stage 3 or 4 encephalopathy, lactulose should be administered if intestinal peristalsis is present. Endotracheal intubation is required to protect the airway from possible reflux and aspiration pneumonia in patients with stage 3 or 4 encephalopathy. Oral or nasogastric administration of neomycin may also be utilized. However, the long-term use of neomycin should be avoided because of the chronic sequellae of midrange hearing loss and occasionally nephrotoxicity.

Although reports indicate that the administration of branched-chain amino acids may be of benefit in the treatment of chronic portal systemic encephalopathy (Fischer, Surgery, 1975; 78:276), studies evaluating this modality in patients awaiting transplant have not been reported. Similarly, studies using flumazenil to antagonize the GABA–benzodiazepine receptor complex have been reported in only a few patients with fulminant hepatic failure prior to transplant (Grimm, Lancet, 1988; ii:1392). Since these therapies do not improve hepatic function, they should have minimal impact on prognosis following transplantation.

Infections

Localized and systemic bacterial infections are common complications of endstage liver diseases in adults. Such patients are immunocompromised, both by their liver disease and the commonly accompanying state of malnutrition. Typical signs and symptoms, as well as laboratory tests indicative of infection, may be subtle or absent. Thus the clinician must be alert to the possibility of infection and prepared to treat it promptly.

Bacterial peritonitis

Spontaneous bacterial peritonitis may develop either insidiously or with evidence of fever, sudden hepatic decompensation, or onset or worsening of hepatic encephalopathy (Hoefs, DisMon, 1985; 31:1; Llach, Hepatol, 1992; 16:724). Abdominal findings of tenderness and rebound are infrequently present. Peripheral leucocytosis may also be absent, especially if a patient is leucopenic on the basis of hypersplenism. The clinical diagnosis is made by a diagnostic paracentesis in which 250 or more polymorphonuclear cells/mm^3 are present (Akriviadis, Gastro, 1990; 98:127). Although a variety of antimicrobial regimens have been advocated, a recent randomized controlled trial indicated the superiority of treatment with a third-generation cephalosporin (Felisart, Hepatol, 1985; 3:457). Subsequent adjustments in coverage can be made on the basis of culture and sensitivity results. In addition, single antibiotic coverage prevents potential nephrotoxicity associated with aminoglycosides.

Response to therapy can be monitored by subsequent paracenteses showing a substantially diminished total white count and a decreasing proportion of polymorphonuclear leucocytes. Since untreated bacterial peritonitis is an absolute contra-indication to transplantation, 4 to 5 days of antibiotic therapy with evidence of a clinical and ascitic fluid response are required prior to urgent transplantation. Patients transplanted after this abbreviated course should receive antibiotics postoperatively.

Spontaneous bacterial peritonitis must be distinguished from peritonitis secondary to intestinal perforation. Since patients with cirrhosis have a higher prevalence of peptic ulcer disease and may suffer complications associated with stress ulceration, this consideration is mandatory. Diagnostic evaluation, therefore, should include an upright posture chest film or decubitus abdominal film to identify free intra-abdominal air. Features suggestive of secondary bacterial peritonitis (Akriviadis, Gastro, 1990; 98:127) include:

(1) a rising ascites neutrophil count 48 h after the initiation of antibiotic treatment, and positive bacterial cultures from the ascitic fluid;
(2) multiple bacterial organisms; and
(3) continued culture positivity despite antibiotic therapy.

Further radiological investigations may be required to identify a perforation of the intestinal or biliary tract.

Ascending cholangitis

Ascending cholangitis is an infrequent complication in adult chronic liver disease, except in patients with sclerosing cholangitis, prior biliary tract surgery associated with the development of secondary biliary cirrhosis, and internal or external biliary prostheses. Clinical signs of cholangitis may be readily apparent with fever, leucocytosis, abdominal pain, and worsening liver tests. However, the presentation may be more insidious. Delay in the treatment of cholangitis predisposes to septicaemia and hepatic abscesses, which may preclude transplantation. Thus, aggressive empiric antibiotic therapy is warranted for suspected cholangitis following appropriate cultures of ascitic fluid and blood. In patients with a prior history of cholangitis and several course of antibiotics, the infecting organisms may include Gram-positive cocci, Gram-negative enteric bacilli, enterococci, and anaerobic species. Hence, initial antibiotic coverage should be broad spectrum. Prophylactic regimens of antibiotics for high-risk patients following the resolution of ascending cholangitis may be useful for a limited period of time before a donor organ becomes available.

Other infections

The immunosuppressed nature of endstage liver disease patients renders them susceptible to a variety of other bacterial, viral, and fungal infections (Dindzans, GastrClinNAm, 1988; 17:19). It may also be associated with the reactivation of previously quiescent infections, such as *Mycobacterium tuberculosis* or coccidiomycosis.

Changes in mental status or stages of encephalopathy may also indicate meningitis, which must be considered. Bacterial infections of the lung, abdominal abscesses, and pyelonephritis require a minimum of 7 to 10 days of therapy before transplantation. Viral infections, such as herpes simplex types 1 and 2 and cytomegalovirus, require antiviral therapy before and after transplantation. Active mycobacterial infections require prolonged therapy, while a history of untreated infection requires prophylactic treatment.

Ascites

Ascites, refractory to medical management, often necessitates recurrent admission to hospital prior to liver transplantation. Massive ascites may be associated with respiratory distress and compromise of the cardiovascular haemodynamics. If unrelieved, these situations may predispose to atelectasis, pneumonia, and azotaemia. Patients with tense ascites may be safely managed with a moderate volume paracentesis of 1 to 3l. The role for large-volume paracentesis (Gines, Gastro, 1987; 93:234) has not been evaluated in patients awaiting transplantation. However, the potential risks of hypotension and azotaemia appear unjustified.

Medical management includes sodium restriction, fluid restriction for hyponatraemia, and diuretics if renal function is normal. Diuretic regimens often include spironolactone or amiloride augmented with frusemide or bumetanide. The goal of diuretic therapy should be the maximum loss of 0.5 kg in weight per day. More aggressive diuresis may cause azotaemia or precipitate hepatorenal syndrome. For patients who cannot be managed with diuretics, periodic mild to moderate paracentesis and/or infusion of salt-poor albumin (75–150 g/day) may be used. If repeated paracenteses are performed, appropriate chemical studies and leucocyte counts should be ordered with each paracentesis to exclude iatrogenic contamination.

Hyponatraemia is the principal electrolyte disturbance accompanying refractory ascites and chronic endstage liver disease (Gines, Gastro, 1987; 93:234). Restriction of free water intake is often necessary to maintain a serum sodium of greater than 130 mmol/l. Intravenous electrolyte replacement may also be required. Severe hyponatraemia is to be avoided because of its effects on the mental status of the patient and its association with central pontine myelinolysis (Donovan, SemLivDis, 1989; 9:168).

Renal failure

Attention to fluid and electrolyte management, gentle diuresis, and avoidance of large-volume paracenteses help prevent prerenal azotaemia. However, if rising creatinine does occur in the face of ongoing diuresis or blood loss, intravascular volume should be replaced aggressively and diuretics discontinued. To evaluate suspected prerenal azotaemia, patients should receive a fluid challenge of normal saline or salt-poor albumin intravenously. The concentration of urinary sodium should also be measured, the expected concentration being 5 mmol/l or less. Failure to reverse the creatinine elevation or rapidly increasing creatinine are indicative of hepatorenal syndrome. Since this syndrome is refractory to medical management in the face of deteriorating liver function, patients awaiting transplantation with this complication should be maintained on haemodialysis. Typically, patients with hepatorenal syndrome recover normal renal function within days or weeks following successful liver transplantation (Wood, AnnSurg, 1987; 205:415). However, some patients have prolonged postoperative renal insufficiency that can often be attributed to prior nephrotoxic antibiotics, episodes of hypotension, or infusion of radiocontrast dyes. A peritoneovenous shunt should not be performed for hepatorenal syndrome prior to transplant because of unacceptable morbidity.

Chronic renal failure may also be evident in patients awaiting transplantation. Chronic renal failure poses an increased risk for early major bacterial infection, and is associated with increased mortality in liver transplantation (Rimola, Gastro, 1987; 93:148). Patients with chronic renal failure should undergo appropriate haemodialysis while awaiting transplantation. Selected patients should be evaluated as candidates for a combined kidney and liver transplantation procedure.

Variceal bleeding

Recurrent variceal haemorrhage is common in patients awaiting liver transplantation. The frequency of haemorrhage and risks of morbidity and mortality increase substantially with worsening coagulopathy and thrombocytopenia. The immediate goals of therapy are maintenance of intravascular volume with fluids and blood transfusion to maintain cardiac output and renal perfusion. Further attempts to stabilize or prevent recurrent bleeding may employ intravenous vasopressin, direct tamponade with a Sengstaken-Blakemore tube, sclerotherapy, or rubber-band ligation. Uncontrolled bleeding or bleeding from gastric, small bowel, or colonic varices requires urgent transplantation since medical therapy is ineffective. The role for sclerotherapy or rubber-band ligation as prophylaxis for recurrent variceal bleeding for inpatients awaiting liver transplantation remains controversial (Piai, Hepatol, 1988; 8:1495). Studies of β-blocker therapy in patients with endstage liver disease awaiting liver transplantation have not been reported (Conn, Hepatol, 1988; 8:167).

Nutrition

Malnutrition in adults undergoing orthotopic liver transplantation is an adverse prognostic indicator of survival (Shaw, ArchSurg, 1989; 124:895). Malnourished patients are particularly prone to infection and poor wound healing. Malnutrition is to be anticipated in 40 to 60 per cent of liver patients admitted to hospital (O'Keefe, Lancet, 1980; 2:615). Often, the malnutrition adds to the immunocompromised state of the patients, as evidenced by the high frequency of anergy in malnourished patients with endstage liver disease. Malnutrition in endstage liver disease may have many causes. Many patients are anorexic or unable to prepare adequate meals. Depending upon the type of liver disease, its complications, or necessity for hospitalization, excessive caloric expenditures may also be present. In patients with chronic cholestatic liver disease, fat malabsorption is common and may limit enteral nutritional capacity. Reduction in dietary fat to 40 g/day or use of medium-chain triglycerides may be of benefit. Such patients should be supplemented with parenteral or water-soluble forms of the fat-soluble vitamins A, D, K, and E.

The goal of nutritional therapy is to provide adequate calories while maintaining appropriate restrictions of total protein (for patients with chronic encephalopathy) and sodium (for patients with refractory ascites). A full nutritional analysis should be made by a dietitian. Enteral nutrition is preferable; however, peripheral venous or central venous parenteral nutrition may be required.

Surgery
Donor selection
General aspects

The transplantation process begins with the finding of a suitable donor. The criteria for donor selection are variable amongst different institutions and are changing rapidly. As liver transplantation becomes more universal and new programmes become established, each programme will determine its specific criteria for donor acceptance. It is not uncommon for a new programme to use more stringent criteria for blood pressure, arterial oxygenation, use of pressors, liver function tests, cause of death, and age, as well as other factors. However, the donor shortage has led to more liberal interpretation of these criteria. In more established programmes where the recipient waiting list may be long, it has been shown that with more liberal criteria the long-term outcome can be equally successful (Makowka, TransplProc, 1987; 19:2378).

The two major features that are required for appropriate donor-recipient matching are size and blood type; however, even these criteria are not absolute. The two major features that are required for appropriate donor–recipient matching are size and blood type; however, these criteria are not absolute. Appropriate size match requires the following information:

(1) recipient height and weight;
(2) donor height and weight;
(3) recipient chest circumference;
(4) donor chest circumference;
(5) recipient liver volume, calculated by radiological techniques; and
(6) estimated liver volume of the donor.

By using these figures, an appropriate size match can usually be made. One must keep in mind that, depending upon the liver disease, the recipient's liver volume may often be much smaller than the volume that can be placed in the hepatic fossa. A recipient with a small, shrunken liver who has a long history of ascites, can certainly take a larger liver than that calculated by his own volume. In these instances, it is important that the height, weight, and chest circumference of the recipient more closely match those of the donor.

In the case of the stable candidate, one can usually wait for a donor organ of the appropriate size. This becomes more difficult when faced with a critically ill patient or a small child. In these cases, it may be impossible to find an appropriately sized organ prior to further deterioration of the recipient. It is for this reason that size criteria have become more liberal to include the use of segmental livers.

Although transplantation of ABO-incompatible kidneys has been shown in many cases to result in hyperacute rejection, this has not been the case in liver transplantation. Despite the absence of hyperacute rejection, the survival for ABO-matched grafts still remains significantly higher than for ABO-incompatible or ABO-mismatched but compatible grafts (Gordon, GastrClinNAm, 1988; 17:53). In addition, in the presence of an ABO mismatch, a graft-versus-host reaction may develop between 2 and 3 weeks after transplantation. This is manifested by a haemolytic anaemia which is usually mild and resolves spontaneously. However, in some cases this reaction may be severe enough to warrant retransplantation.

Due to the decreased survival rates and the potential for graft-versus-host reactions, blood type remains an important criterion in donor–recipient matching. Once again, this is not an absolute criterion and ABO matching may be waived in the face of a severely ill patient.

Historically, due to the urgency imposed by a short cold-storage time, donor–recipient crossmatching has not been possible in liver transplantation. Retrospective review of donor-specific crossmatch has, however, revealed no significant effect on graft survival. The presence of a positive crossmatch or a high panel reactive antibody has not been shown to correlate with an increased graft loss due to rejection (Gordon, GastrClinNAm, 1988; 17:53).

HLA matching has also been studied retrospectively and histocompatibility has not been shown to increase graft survival (Markus, Transpl, 1988; 46:372). Clearly, as we become more able to preserve grafts for longer periods, it will become increasingly important to re-examine the effects of crossmatching and HLA matching on graft survival.

In the most perfect of circumstances, it would be preferable to use organs from only young haemodynamically stable donors with normal liver function tests. The shortage of donor organs, as well as the urgency of transplantation in critically ill patients, has made this situation impossible. Fortunately, however, through the use of imperfect donor organs, it has been shown that standard criteria for donor selection are not absolute and with some flexibility in the criteria, a good long-term outcome can still be obtained.

Upper age limits are increasing as we find satisfactory function obtained from donors older than 50 years of age with otherwise satisfactory criteria (Teperman, JAMA, 1989; 262:2837). Acceptable arterial blood gases, as well as haemodynamic status, vary from institution to institution. In the face of a questionable donor, it is always preferable to assess the liver intraoperatively. Much can be learned by direct examination of its consistency and colour. Furthermore, the bile can be inspected at the time of bile-duct transection. With the availability of the University of Wisconsin Solution, livers can be preserved for up to 24 h. This allows the procurement team to harvest a questionable liver and perform and evaluate a liver biopsy prior to undertaking the recipient operation. Through this method, many otherwise wasted organs can be salvaged and demonstrate good function.

Despite more liberal selection criteria, there do remain absolute contraindications to the use of an organ. These include:

(1) absence of heartbeat;
(2) presence of extracerebral malignancy;
(3) positive HIV antibody;
(4) positive hepatitis antigen status;
(5) systemic sepsis;
(6) presence of known liver disease; and
(7) presence of specific toxins.

Several other variables, including liver function tests, fluid and electrolyte status, use of pressors, and past medical history, must all be considered in donor selection. In the final analysis donor selection will vary from institution to institution and will depend heavily upon the judgement of the transplantation team. Clearly, a search for objective criteria will certainly be continued in the future of liver transplantation.

Surgical aspects

Donor hepatectomy

The first step in the performance of a liver transplantation is the procurement of the hepatic allograft. Co-ordination and co-operation are required among the various surgical teams to ensure the successful procurement of multiple organs from a single donor. Due to significant variations in technique for organ procurement among different transplant centres, the teams should discuss the methods and time requirements of the individual procedures prior to undertaking the operation, in order to assure optimal procurement of each organ with minimal ischaemia and injury. According to the preservation times which each organ can sustain, a priority order has been established for removal of organs once the circulation has been arrested. The heart and lungs are removed first, followed by the liver, and finally the kidneys.

A midline incision extending from the suprasternal notch to the pubic symphysis with good retraction provides sufficient exposure and access to the thoracic and abdominal organs. Upon entering the abdominal cavity, the different organs are carefully inspected to assess suitability for transplantation. This comprises evaluation of colour, consistency, and size of the various organs. The liver is mobilized by dividing the falciform ligament, left triangular ligament, and gastrohepatic ligament. When dividing the gastrohepatic ligament, it is important to check for the presence of a left hepatic artery arising from the left gastric artery. A left branch is present in approximately 15 per cent of donors and if found, must be preserved. The posterior aspect of the porta hepatis should also be inspected for the presence of a right hepatic artery originating from the superior mesenteric artery. Present in approximately 10 per cent of the donors, this branch can usually but not always be palpated and, if present, must be preserved to assure the viability of the liver.

Several techniques have been developed for liver procurement and the choice of technique depends upon the preference and experience of the recovery team as well as the haemodynamic stability of the donor (Starzl, SGO, 1984; 158:223; Starzl, SGO, 1987; 165:343). The three techniques currently employed are:

(1) the classic technique;
(2) the standard technique;
(3) the rapid-flush technique.

The techniques differ in the amount of dissection, especially of the hepatic hilum, prior to circulatory interruption. A long preliminary dissection may be time consuming and may require blood transfusions. It will, however, require a much less difficult and time-consuming extraction once the liver is perfused and cooled after circulatory arrest. Therefore, this is only suitable for a very stable donor. On the other hand, when there is less preliminary preparation, more dissection is needed after the liver has cooled and this requires a greater degree of skill and expertise for safe removal of the liver.

The three procedures have two common principles: the rapid and adequate core cooling of the liver following circulatory interruption, and preservation of all hepatic structures, including anomalous blood vessels.

Classic technique

This original technique is characterized by a thorough dissection of all the hepatic vessels. All the hilar structures, including the bile duct, hepatic artery, portal vein, and branches of the coeliac trunk, are dissected. The left gastric and splenic arteries are ligated and divided. The coeliac trunk and abdominal aorta are dissected. The superior mesenteric artery is identified and encircled at its origin. The liver is precooled with cold solution through a cannula inserted in the splenic vein. The supracoeliac aorta is encircled in preparation for cross-clamping. The infrahepatic vena cava, as well as the renal veins, are isolated. The distal aorta and inferior vena cava are both cannulated after full systemic heparinization. Following circulatory interruption, the liver is cooled rapidly through the cannulas placed in the aorta and the splenic vein. Following cooling, the liver can be removed with a minimum of further dissection.

Standard technique

The standard technique (Fig. 1) requires far less dissection than the classic technique. The hilum is freed by dividing the bile duct, and right gastric and gastroduodenal arteries. The left gastric and splenic arteries are ligated and divided distally. The portal vein is identified at its confluence and the splenic vein prepared for cannulation. The supracoeliac aorta is identified and prepared for cross-clamping. The distal aorta is dissected and cannulated after systemic heparinization. Following circulatory interruption, the supracoeliac aorta is cross-clamped and the intrathoracic vena cava divided. The liver is then cooled rapidly and the hepatectomy is performed. The superior mesenteric artery is approached by retracting the distal pancreas and, once identified, it is dissected down to the aorta. It is inspected carefully for the presence of a right branch and, depending on the anatomy, is either included or excluded in the aortic patch encompassing the coeliac trunk. The infrahepatic vena cava is then divided, allowing the liver to be removed.

Rapid flush technique

This technique requires the least time for preliminary dissection and is therefore suitable for unstable donors. The inferior mesenteric vein is dissected and cannulated. The distal aorta is then dissected and cannulated after heparinization. The supracoeliac aorta is prepared for cross-clamping prior to cannulation of the distal aorta. The remainder of the dissection is performed after circulatory interruption and cooling. The preparatory steps may take from 5 to 15 min. However, due to the minimal amount of previous dissection, this technique demands more skill and experience in the performance of the hepatectomy. Following division of the intrathoracic cava and cross-clamping of the supracoeliac aorta, the liver is cooled rapidly and hepatectomy undertaken. The right gastric and gastroduodenal arteries are divided to free the hepatic artery, and the bile duct is divided. The portal vein is identified at its confluence, and the splenic vein and superior mesenteric vein are then divided to free the portal vein. The left gastric and splenic arteries are divided. The superior mesenteric artery is approached in the same way as in the standard technique and an appropriate patch of aorta encompassing the coeliac axis is removed. Once again, the infrahepatic vena cava is divided and the liver removed with a cuff of diaphragm.

The iliac arteries and veins are routinely recovered after nephrectomy in the event that venous or arterial grafts will be required during the recipient liver procedure. Portions of spleen and mesenteric lymph nodes are removed for the purpose of donor–recipient crossmatching.

The remaining preparations of the donor liver prior to implantation are performed on the back-table at the recipient hospital. The liver is carefully prepared by completing the full dissection of the hepatic vasculature and performing any hepatic arterial reconstruction for anomalies. For livers with anomalous left gastric or superior mesenteric arteries, a single common arterial channel is created using various techniques in order to facilitate anastomosis to the recipient artery (Gordon, SGO, 1985; 160:474; Todo, TransplProc, 1987; 19:2406).

Recipient operation
Hepatectomy

The completed procedure (Fig. 2) consists of four vascular anastomoses and one biliary anastomosis. The vast majority of liver transplants have been performed in an orthotopic position; thus the first step is the recipient hepatectomy. The recipient surgeon must plan the hepatectomy based on individual considerations. These considerations include previous upper abdominal surgery, previous episodes of spontaneous bacterial peritonitis with resulting adhesions, the nature of the liver disease, patency of the portal vein, and the presence of portal-systemic shunts.

In order to devascularize the liver, the initial dissection is carried out in the hilum. With the exception of malignancies, the bile duct and the hepatic artery should be transected as proximal to the liver as possible to facilitate their reconstruction. The portal vein is skeletalized and prepared for venovenous bypass. The remaining liver attachments can be divided, before or during venovenous bypass, depending on the presence of coagulopathy and/or diffuse collaterals. A difficult hepatectomy can result in significant blood loss; therefore achieving haemostasis during the hepatectomy is essential in maintaining the stability of the recipient.

Liver implantation
Venovenous bypass

During the final stages of the recipient hepatectomy and ensuing liver implantation, the recipient portal vein and inferior vena cava are cross-clamped, diminishing blood return to the heart. Portal vein occlusion results in splanchnic hypertension, congestion of the bowel, increased lactate concentrations, and bleeding in the areas of dissection. Caval occlusion leads to renal hypertension, venous stasis, and decreased blood return to the heart. Since 1982, the use of heparin-free venovenous bypass has significantly improved these problems (Griffith, SGO, 1985; 160:270). Cannulas are inserted into the portal vein and inferior vena cava via the femoral vein. An atraumatic centrifugal pump channels blood through these cannulas

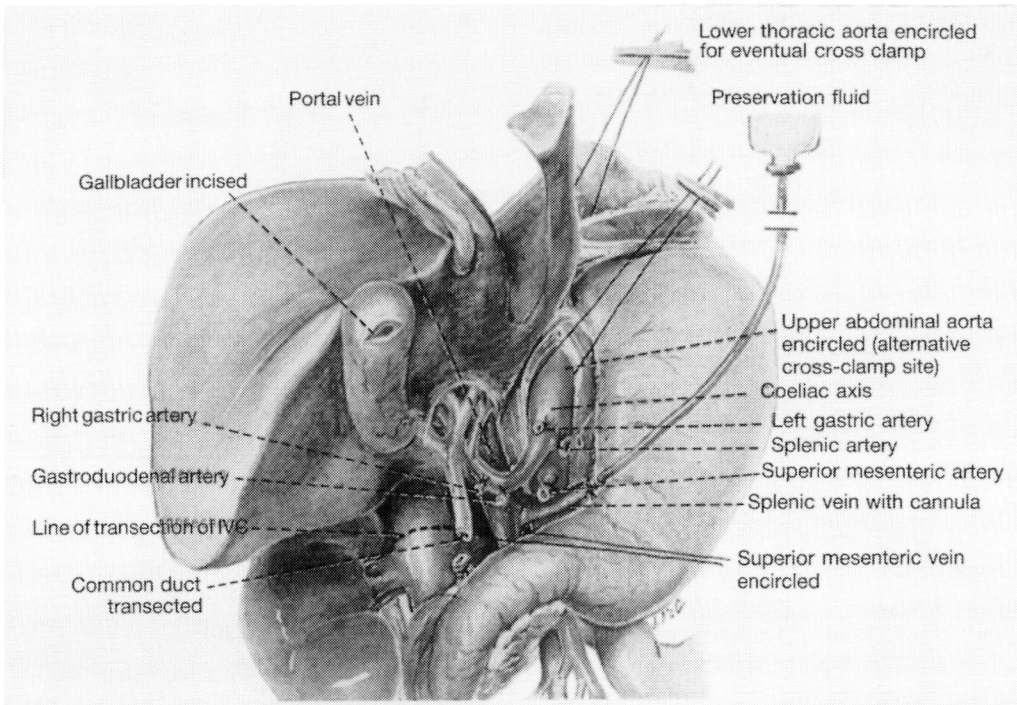

Fig. 1. Procurement of the hepatic allograft—standard technique. Common bile duct transected, splenic and left gastric arteries ligated, cannula in splenic vein for cold perfusion. (Reproduced by permission of *Surgery, Gynecology and Obstetrics*, 1984; 158:227.)

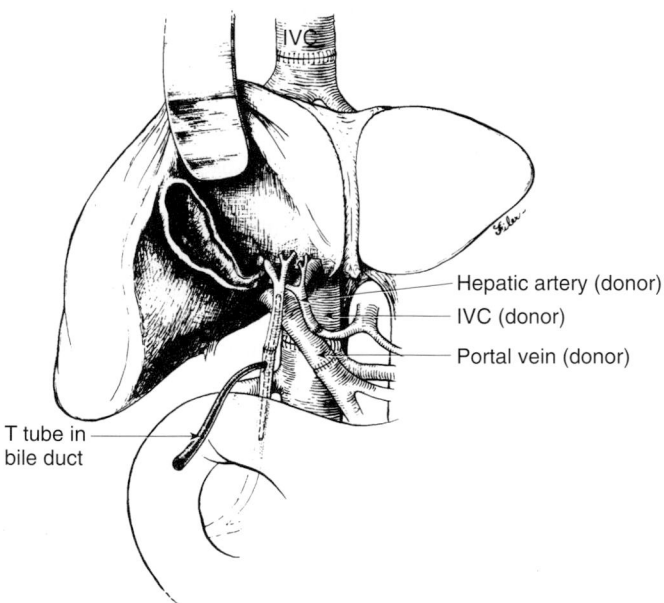

Fig. 2. Completed liver transplant including four vascular anastomoses and one biliary anastomosis. (Copyright 1989 by Matthew Bender and Co. Inc., and reprinted with permission from *New Developments in Medicine*.)

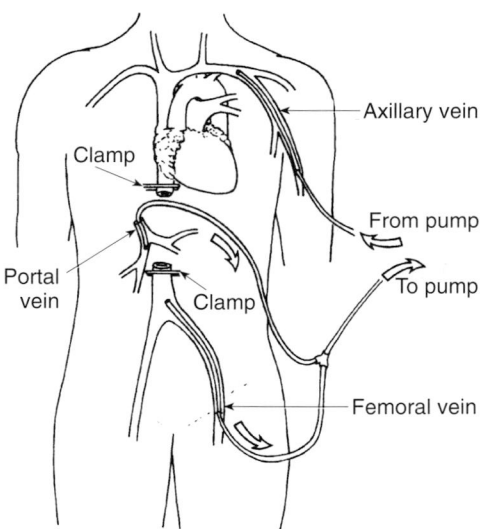

Fig. 3. Heparin-free venovenous bypass. (From Makowka L, Sher L, and Starzl TE. Liver transplantation: surgical considerations. In Bayless TM, ed. *Current Therapy in Gastroenterology and Liver Disease*, Vol. 3. Philadelphia: B. C. Decker, 1990.)

back to the heart via a cannula inserted in the axillary vein (Fig. 3). Venovenous bypass has facilitated the maintenance of recipient stability during this very critical time period. Good haemostasis is more readily achieved during the anhepatic phase because venovenous bypass allows the surgeon time to oversew any raw surfaces created during the hepatectomy. Use of venovenous bypass reduces

postoperative complications, including renal failure and sepsis, and allows a more rapid return of bowel function. Venovenous bypass is now used routinely in most adult and paediatric patients weighing over 30 kg.

In some instances, the retrohepatic vena cava can be completely preserved. This offers a further advantage in the maintenance of blood return to the heart and can be particularly useful for small paediatric recipients whose size makes the use of bypass practically impossible. Some adult recipients can also benefit from preservation of caval flow, i.e. those with portal systemic shunts who do not require portal bypass, or in cases of significant mismatch in the size of the donor and recipient organs. In the presence of severe portal hypertension in the retroperitoneum, this technique allows this area to remain intact. This is important for older patients and those with cardiac instability. In such cases, only suprahepatic vena cava anastomosis is performed and the donor infrahepatic cava is ligated. This technique has been termed the 'piggyback' technique (Tzakis, AnnSurg, 1989; 210:649).

Graft revascularization

Anastomosis of the vena cava above and below the liver is performed first. While the lower caval anastomosis is being sewn, the liver is flushed with cold saline solution to remove the highly concentrated potassium contained in the preservation fluid, and air from the major veins. Portal bypass is then interrupted and the portal vein anastomosis is performed. It is extremely important to match the lengths of donor and recipient portal veins accurately. This will prevent kinking and possible thrombosis. At this point, the liver is usually revascularized on portal flow only, major bleeding sources are controlled, and the venovenous bypass is terminated. The hepatic arterial anastomosis is then performed, preferably by anastomosing the recipient common hepatic artery to the donor's coeliac trunk, although there are many variations. An accurate match between donor and recipient hepatic arteries is essential. To prevent twisting, and to assure an adequate arterial blood flow to the liver, the lengths and positions of these arteries must be carefully examined before anastomosis.

When the recipient artery is severely diseased, injured, or exhibits poor inflow, an alternative source of inflow must be used. In most cases an aortohepatic graft is employed. A donor iliac graft is anastomosed to the intrarenal aorta, tunnelled either posteriorly or anteriorly to the pancreas, and anastomosed to the donor artery in the hilum. Other infrequent alternatives in cases where access to the intrarenal aorta is extremely difficult, include placement of the graft proximal to the coeliac trunk on the abdominal aorta, or anastomosis of the donor artery to a common orifice fashioned on the main coeliac trunk at the take-off of the splenic artery. Various techniques and reconstructions have been developed to handle the various hepatic arterial anomalies found in the donor liver. Usually performed on the back-table prior to implantation, these reconstructions are meant to produce a single orifice for anastomosis (Gordon, SGO, 1985; 160:474; Todo, TransplProc, 1987; 19:2406).

In the past, portal vein thrombosis has been a major contraindication to liver transplantation. Depending on the extent of thrombosis, different methods of venous grafting have been developed and employed with excellent results (Sheil, ClinTranspl, 1987; 1:18; Tzakis, Transpl, 1989; 48:530). If the clot obstructs only the main portal vein, the donor iliac vein graft is anastomosed to the confluence of the splenic and superior mesenteric veins. If the extension of the thrombosis includes the confluence, a jump graft is placed on the anterior surface of the superior mesenteric vein below the transverse mesocolon. This vein graft is brought anteriorly to the pancreas through the transverse mesocolon and into the hilum.

Careful collaboration between the surgeon and anaesthetist is then required to achieve appropriate haemostasis. This includes

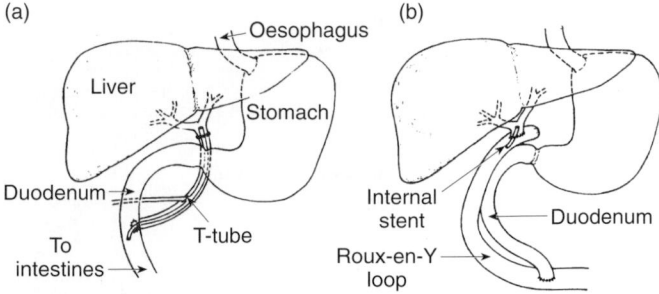

Fig. 4. Biliary tract anastomoses: (a) choledochocholedochostomy over a T-tube stent; (b) choledochojejunostomy over an internal stent. (From Makowka L, Sher L, and Starzl TE. Liver transplantation: surgical considerations. In Bayless TM, ed. *Current therapy in Gastroenterology and Liver Disease*, Vol. 3. Philadelphia: B. C. Decker, 1990.)

correction of coagulopathy and careful inspection of all surgical sites.

Bile-duct reconstuction

Standardization of bile-duct reconstruction has markedly reduced the incidence of postoperative complications, i.e. biliary tract leaks and strictures. There are two predominant methods of bile-duct reconstruction (Makowka, GastrClinNAm, 1988; 17:33):

(1) choledochocholedochostomy over a T-tube stent; and
(2) hepaticojejunostomy over an internal stent.

The preferred method is a choledochocholedochostomy over a T-tube stent (Fig. 4). The simplest of the two techniques, it provides an access for easy inspection of the bile and radiological evaluation of the biliary tree. It can only be used in the absence of malignancies, bile-duct diseases (e.g. sclerosing cholangitis), or significant discrepancies in the size of donor and recipient ducts. The T-tube is left in for approximately 3 months after the procedure.

The alternative procedure is a hepaticojejunostomy over an internal stent (Fig. 4(b)). A Roux-en-Y loop of jejunum is fashioned and brought up into the hepatic hilum either anti- or retrocolically. This is the anastomosis of choice in paediatric cases because of its reliability and extremely low complication rate. A third alternative, the so-called 'Waddell–Calne' technique, uses the gallbladder as an interpositional conduit between donor and recipient bile ducts (Waddell, Surgery, 1973; 74:524). This technique is rarely used, but can be employed when technical difficulties make it impossible to fashion a Roux-en-Y loop of jejunum.

Size-mismatched donor

In order to overcome the shortage of small donors in the paediatric liver transplant population, surgeons are currently exploring technical variations that would allow transplantation of grafts procured from size-mismatched donors. Such techniques may be needed when fulminant hepatitis or graft failure necessitates urgent transplantation and no appropriate donor can be found.

Reduced–size liver

The first such method to be used on a large scale is the reduced-size liver technique (Bismuth, Surgery, 1984; 95:367; Broelsch,

AnnSurg, 1988; 208:410; Otte, AnnSurg, 1990; 211:146). Reduced-size liver transplantation allows a weight ratio of 1 : 6, making possible a weight differentiation of 300 to 500 per cent between donor and recipient. The transplantation of a liver harvested from a large donor into a smaller recipient is accomplished by back-table resection of the right lobe, either by a bisegmentectomy using the left lobe or, more commonly, a trisegmentectomy using the left lateral segment. Both procedures require careful back-table dissection of the hilar structures and ligation of all of the structures transected in the liver parenchyma. Usually the left (and occasionally the middle) hepatic vein is preserved in continuity with the entire retrohepatic vena cava. The implantation is similar to that of an entire hepatic allograft, with exact positioning crucial to prevention of vessel torsion. In some cases, the recipient's retrohepatic vena cava can be preserved and the hepatic segment implanted in 'piggyback' fashion (see above). This avoids the need for cross-clamping of the vena cava in recipients who are typically too small for venovenous bypass.

Alternative liver transplantations
Split liver

The so-called split liver technique involves the division of the liver parenchyma and the partition of vascular and biliary structures. This technique addresses the shortage of suitable donor livers by allowing two viable grafts to be obtained from a single donor for implantation in different recipients. The split-liver technique continues to evolve with time and with the expanding, accumulative experience of transplant teams (Bismuth, BrJSurg, 1989; 76:722; Edmond, AnnSurg, 1990; 212:14; Otte, Surgery, 1990; 107:605).

Living related donor

Without considering, in this chapter, the ethical implications that have arisen, it is technically feasible to obtain a liver segment from a living relative for implantation into a paediatric recipient. The living related transplant procedure has been performed successfully in numerous cases (Strong, NEJM, 1990; 322:1505). The technique for donor segmentectomy includes hilar dissection, parenchymal transection, and isolation of the hepatic vein included with those segments. Once the vessels to this segment have been clamped, the hepatectomy is performed, and the organ is flushed and cooled on the back-table.

Auxiliary liver

Until recently, the technique of auxiliary liver transplantation was abandoned in favour of orthotopic transplantation. However, a few high-risk patients have recently undergone auxiliary transplantation with reports of some success (Terpstra, Transpl, 1988; 45:1003). In auxiliary liver transplantation, a segment of donor liver is implanted beneath the recipient's liver, which remains in place (Fig. 5). The usefulness of the procedure requires further evaluation and, in the future, may be considered under very special circumstances. An interesting approach reported in a few patients with acute hepatic failure is auxiliary liver transplantation in a heterotopic position with left segmentectomy or left lobectomy of the recipient liver. This approach may allow the permanent liver to regenerate and later the transplanted liver can be left to involute. This seems to

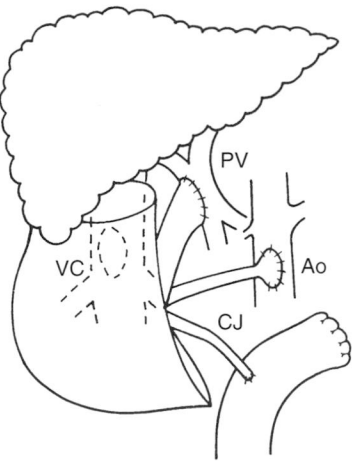

Fig. 5. Auxiliary liver transplant. VC, inferior vena cava; PV, portal vein; Ao, aorta; and CJ, choledochojejunostomy. (Reprinted by permission of *The New England Journal of Medicine*, 1988; 319:1508.)

be a suitable technique, with the additional potential of being reversible.

Postoperative care
Graft function

For purposes of postoperative evaluation, hepatic function can be divided conveniently into three general categories: synthetic, excretory, and metabolic. Synthetic function includes the production of coagulation factors, albumin, and other proteins such as transferrin and haptoglobin. Excretory function includes the excretion of bilirubin as well as the detoxification and excretion of drugs. Metabolic function includes glucose and lactate metabolism (including glycogenolysis and gluconeogenesis) and the intermediary metabolism of fat and protein. When evaluating the postoperative function of a hepatic allograft it is important to note that specific functions of the liver recover from cold preservation at different rates.

Synthetic function

Immediate hepatic synthesis of coagulation factors is necessary for haemostasis and successful completion of the transplant operation. With the addition of coagulation factors, in addition to the factors produced by the newly implanted liver, haemostasis can be attained. In the operating room, thromboelastography is used to assess the status of the interaction of platelets and coagulation factors.[6] In the postoperative period, platelet count, prothrombin time, and partial thromboplastin time are usually sufficient to monitor the coagulation status. The prothrombin time, which reflects ongoing synthesis of specific factors by hepatocytes, is an early indicator of graft function. Although return to normal is an encouraging sign, occasional prolongation occurs despite good graft function as a result of vitamin K deficiency. With the exception of vitamin K administration, aggressive correction of coagulation abnormalities with exogenous factors in the early postoperative period should be avoided so that graft function can be monitored by changes in the prothrombin time. Prothrombin times of even 20 to 25 s may not require treatment with fresh, frozen plasma as long as there is no evidence of bleeding or serious hypertension. If graft dysfunction requires factor supplementation, substantial improvement in prothrombin time with infusion of 7 to 10 ml/kg of fresh, frozen plasma indicates the likely recovery of synthetic function with time. If no improvement in the prothrombin time occurs, a severe preservation injury or technical complication should be suspected and investigated. Once the prothrombin time has corrected to within 2 s of normal, it is no longer a useful guide to graft function. An aggressive correction of a prolonged prothrombin time can be associated with development of thrombosis of hepatic artery and should be avoided. Thus, it is unnecessary to measure this parameter daily after the first week unless other signs of graft dysfunction are present. Activated partial thromboplastin time is rarely abnormal, and marked prolongation suggests the contamination of the specimen with heparin.

Excretory function

The production of bile in the operating room is the first indication of resumed excretory function. Because of the load of haemoglobin that accompanies transfusion during the procedure, increases in bilirubin in the first few days after the transplant are common, regardless of the function of the graft. Thus increases are not indicative of graft dysfunction. Paradoxical falls in bilirubin immediately after transplantation can result from dilution resulting from blood loss and fluid and blood replacement. However, such changes are limited to the first 24 to 48 h and subsequent changes in serum bilirubin are indicative of graft function.

If an end-to-end reconstruction of the biliary system has been performed, the bile excreted through the T-tube is an excellent gauge of liver function. The experienced clinician can derive a considerable amount of useful information about the graft from examination of recently produced bile. Both quality and quantity of bile produced are of considerable clinical value. Typically, bile is dark golden brown and very viscous, and up to 300 ml may be produced per day. As the quantity of bile produced increases, the colour may become lighter due to the increased content of water. Because the amount of bile passing into the gut rather than through the T-tube is unknown, a low quantity of bile output may not be a serious finding if the bile is of appropriate colour and viscosity. Light-coloured or water-clear bile indicates severe graft injury, most commonly due to preservation injury, primary non-function, or rejection.

Another important hepatic excretory function is the detoxification and clearance of anaesthetic agents as well as removal of the toxins of hepatic encephalopathy. Awakening from anaesthesia is an encouraging sign. To minimize confusion regarding the sensorium immediately after transplantation, analgesics are administered sparingly, if at all. Fortunately, the discomfort experienced by most patients during this stage is tolerable without a significant analgesic requirement. Once the patient is fully recovered from anaesthesia and encephalopathy has cleared, narcotics can be given with caution.

Metabolic function

Metabolic function of the liver is evident immediately after implantation. Two parameters which can be followed clinically both in the operating room and in the intensive care unit are serum lactate concentration and temperature. Liver metabolism produces significant heat, and rewarming frequently begins shortly after unclamping. Inability to rewarm or slow rewarming after closure of the wound raises concern about poor graft function. Similarly, the metabolism of lactic acid is an early sign of graft function (Fath, Surgery, 1984; 96:664). Generally, serum lactate concentration is normal within 6 to 12 h post-transplant. Increasing or persistent elevation of lactate indicates graft dysfunction. Glucose metabolism is an insensitive index of graft function; glucose levels generally remain high regardless of graft function. Hypoglycaemia occurs only in circumstances of severe graft injury.

Preservation injury

Some degree of injury occurs in the preservation of all hepatic allografts. Serum aminotransferase levels during the first 48 h are generally thought to reflect the degree of preservation injury. Interpretation of aminotransferase levels is not absolute and requires consideration of all clinical information. Aspartate aminotransferase (AST) levels less than 2000 and alanine aminotransferase levels less than 1500 suggest moderate preservation injury, while levels less than 600 indicate minimal preservation injury. With severe preservation injury, additional clinical indices of graft dysfunction can be expected. These include decreased clearance of bilirubin, delayed return to normal of prothrombin time, slowed awakening, and persistent encephalopathy. In severe cases, lactic acidosis and persistent hypothermia are observed. If the AST is over 4000, the survival of the graft is questionable. After careful serial evaluation and observation, retransplantation may be required.

Immunosuppression

Immunosuppression after liver transplantation requires continuous monitoring and adjustment. Although most centres follow a standardized immunosuppression protocol, great variation in treatment is required to respond to the needs of individual patients. Thus, immunosuppression protocols serve primarily as guidelines for the prescription of immunosuppression tailored to the individual. The need for immunosuppression is greatest during the first weeks after transplantation when the probability of rejection is the greatest.[7] After 2 to 3 months, the immunosuppressive regimen can be moderated as the host immune system accommodates to the graft. Although cyclosporin and steroids have been the mainstays of maintenance immunosuppression so far, tacrolimus is emerging as the preferred immunosuppressive agent in many large centres.

The need to provide adequate immunosuppression to prevent rejection must be weighed against the increased risk of subsequent infections (Wajszczuk, Transpl, 1985; 40:347; Oh, Transpl, 1988; 45:68). Unfortunately, the adverse effect of immunosuppression on host resistance is cumulative, and the onset of infections resulting from overimmunosuppression may occasionally be delayed by many months. Alternatively, insufficient immunosuppression resulting in rejection may require so much additional immunosuppression that the risk of unneccessary infectious complications is increased.

Tacrolimus (FK506)

Tacrolimus (FK506), is a macrolide antibiotic produced by the fungus, *Streptomyces tsukubaensis*. The molecular structure of

FK506 is unrelated to cyclosporin, and the two drugs have different cytosolic binding sites. However, both drugs inhibit T-lymphocyte activation, in part by suppressing the synthesis and expression of multiple cytokines, including interleukin-2 and γ-interferon. The availability of tacrolimus and its acceptance as the mainstay of immunosuppression allow many patients the initial use of tacrolimus and corticosteroids. After 1 year following transplantation many patients can be only on monotherapy with tacrolimus. Tacrolimus has three broad areas of liability which could limit its use or dictate its dosage: nephrotoxicity, neurotoxicity, and alterations in carbohydrate metabolism (Starzl, Lancet, 1989; ii:1000).

Cyclosporin

The introduction of cyclosporin in 1980 coincided with spectacular improvement in the results of liver transplantation. The acceptance of liver transplantation as standard therapy for endstage liver disease has accompanied the clinical introduction of cyclosporin (NIH, Hepatol, 1983; 4:107S; Starzl, TransplProc, 1985; 17:107). The dominant mechanism of action of cyclosporin is the inhibition of mitogen-induced production of interleukin-2. Additional effects may include reduced production of interleukin-1, γ-interferon, and interleukin-2 receptor.

Adverse effects of cyclosporin include renal impairment, hepatic dysfunction, hypertension, hyperkalaemia, CNS dysfunction, hirsutism, and gingival hypertrophy (Starzl, TransplProc, 1983; 15: 3103). The dosage of cyclosporin is determined ordinarily by measurement of levels in blood or serum. Many assays are available, and the desired target levels vary between centres. Furthermore, dosage may be limited by toxic effects. Unfortunately, manifestations of cyclosporin toxicity do not necessarily indicate achievement of an adequate therapeutic effect. Indeed, rejection and cyclosporin toxicity may coexist.

Steroids

Corticosteroids are the second major component of standard immunosuppression in liver transplantation. The action is primarily anti-inflammatory, although other specific activities have been proposed. Generally, high-dose steroids are the initial treatment and are tapered rapidly during the first 7 to 14 days, followed by maintenance doses which are slowly tapered during the ensuing 3 to 6 months. The usual side-effects of steroid therapy are reduced by this initial early pulse and subsequent tapering. Specifically, glucose intolerance, catabolism, susceptibility to infection, and fat accumulation are minimized, although they still remain substantial problems when the steroid requirements of individual patients remain high.

Azathioprine

Azathioprine is frequently used as an additional immunosuppressive agent in liver transplantation. It plays an important role in patients who are unable to tolerate adequate doses of cyclosporin due to side-effects, primarily renal failure or disturbances of CNS. At subtherapeutic doses it facilitates reduction of cyclosporin dosage while minimizing the adverse effects associated with full therapeutic doses of azathioprine. The mechanism of azathioprine is primarily cytotoxic, particularly on rapidly dividing cells. Thus, proliferating,

activated immune cells are susceptible to its action. Granulocytopenia, and occasionally thrombocytopenia, manifestations of toxicity, may require reduction of the dose. The dose may be reduced further when hypersplenism results in leucopenia or thrombocytopenia. Because of its relatively non-specific mode of action, the dose of azathioprine is generally reduced or the drug discontinued when infection is present. There is also concern regarding long-term hepatotoxic effects and predisposition to lymphoproliferative disorders.

Rejection

While the aim of maintenance immunosuppression is to prevent rejection, this is achieved in only about 30 per cent of liver transplant recipients.[7,8] Once rejection has developed, intensification of maintenance immunosuppression is insufficient to reverse the process and specific regimens of antirejection therapy are required. Generally, these regimens consist of high-dose steroids or specific T-cell cytotoxic therapy.

Virtually all rejection seen early after liver transplantation is acute cellular rejection mediated by the T cells. Acute cellular rejection is rarely seen in the first few days after transplantation. Most commonly, the onset of rejection occurs between the fourth and fourteenth postoperative day. There are few typical symptoms of hepatic rejection, although fever is not uncommon, and patients may report malaise on the first day of rejection. These non-specific signs and symptoms often have alternative explanations. Because the organ is free within the abdominal cavity, swelling does not usually cause pain, as seen with renal transplant rejection.

Antibody-mediated hyperacute rejection, more commonly seen in kidney transplantation, is extremely uncommon in liver transplantation. This is corroborated by the finding that cytotoxic crossmatching does not predict outcome in liver transplantation (Gordon, Surgery, 1986; 100:705). Although there are a few reports of hyperacute liver rejection (Hanto, ClinTranspl, 1987; 1:304; Olson, TransplProc, 1988; 20:667), it has been suggested that some cases of primary graft non-function may also represent hyperacute rejection.

Vanishing bile-duct syndrome may develop at virtually any time after transplantation, although it is rare during the first 1 or 2 months. Characteristically, there is a paucity or disappearance of bile ducts associated with non-suppurative destructive cholangitis and degenerative changes of bile-duct epithelial cells attributed to cytokine-mediated injury or ischaemia. There are several effective therapeutic options for acute cellular rejection, but standard regimens are ineffective for hyperacute or vanishing bile-duct syndrome.

The first signs of rejection are elevations of liver function tests.[8] Bilirubin usually increases, and aminotransferases and biliary enzymes may also increase. Fever and malaise as well as leucocytosis may also occur. The graft may become enlarged and firm on physical examination. Perhaps most important, the bile, if available for inspection, will be lighter and less viscous. Many centres perform routine biopsy on about the seventh postoperative day because of the frequency of rejection at this time; however, this is not our policy at the University of Pittsburgh.

The typical biopsy findings of rejection are expansion of the portal tracts by mononuclear cells, activated lymphocytes, and frequently eosinophils.[9] Polymorphonuclear leucocytes may also be present. The critical finding is invasion and damage of the bile ducts by the lymphocytes (Demetris, AmJPathol, 1985; 118:151). These findings can be spotty throughout the liver and should be noted in multiple portal tracts if the diagnosis of rejection is to be confirmed. Similar findings may be seen with cholangitis, but the predominance of polymorphonuclear leucocytes often provides the correct diagnosis.

Many laboratory tests have been proposed as aids to the diagnosis of rejection, but none has gained widespread acceptance or validation. Clinical judgment, standard laboratory tests of liver function, and liver biopsy remain the standard modalities for the diagnosis of rejection.

Steroid therapy of rejection generally consists of a brief course of very high doses of intravenous corticosteroids for 1 to 3 days or a bolus followed by tapering doses of corticosteroids.[5,7,8] A response is often seen within several hours of bolus injection. If there is no response to the steroid therapy, or if rebound rejection should occur after the steroid therapy, OKT3, a murine monoclonal antibody against T cells may be given daily for 7 to 14 days. This drug binds to the CD3 component of the CD3–T-cell receptor complex present on all mature T cells and causes T-cell inactivation, which interrupts the rejection process (Goldstein, Nephron, 1987; 46:5). Other antibody preparations that act similarly by binding to T cells include antilymphocyte, antilymphoblast, and antithymocyte antibodies.

Once rejection is controlled, maintenance immunosuppression is often intensified for several weeks or months to prevent recurrence. This may take the form of additional steroids or the conversion from dual drug (cyclosporin and steroids) to triple drug (addition of azathioprine) therapy or switch to tacrolimus-based immunosuppression. In some cases, rejection cannot be controlled by maximum therapy and retransplantation is required. Although the result of retransplantation for rejection is not as good as with the initial transplant, rejection does not necessarily recur (Shaw, TransplProc, 1985; 17:264).

Renal function

There is a close relationship between liver and kidney function, and many patients with endstage liver disease have significant renal impairment. In the setting of impaired renal function, the insult of operation, substantial blood loss, temporary occlusion of the vena cava, and large doses of intravenous cyclosporin results in some renal injury in the majority of liver transplant recipients. Fortunately, this injury is usually transient and dialysis is rarely needed. Oliguria is a common finding in the first two postoperative days and requires aggressive fluid administration guided by pulmonary artery pressure monitoring and haemodynamic evaluation. Once adequate volume expansion is achieved, as indicated by a pulmonary capillary wedge pressure of 14 to 17 mmHg, large doses of loop diuretics are indicated if urinary output does not improve. Typically, the blood urea nitrogen (**BUN**) and creatinine will rise for 48 to 72 h regardless of urinary output. The first sign of recovery from the perioperative renal injury is a decline in creatinine. The BUN usually rises for another 24 to 48 h before declining. Severe cyclosporin toxicity may sustain the elevated BUN despite improvement of creatinine and urine flow. As discussed below, postoperative bleeding may further impair urine output and cause oliguric acute renal failure in extreme instances.

Preoperative hepatorenal syndrome has prompted some centres to advocate simultaneous liver and kidney transplantation. Others have expected the prompt return of renal function with restoration of hepatic function and have deferred kidney transplantation for those who fail to respond to liver replacement alone (Gonwa, Transpl, 1989; 47:395). In those patients with pre-existing renal failure, hepatorenal syndrome, or perioperative renal failure, the timing of dialysis after liver transplantation is critical. It is wise to delay haemodialysis for as long as possible in order to avoid anticoagulation, platelet destruction, and subsequent bleeding. Continuous arteriovenous haemofiltration or venovenous haemofiltration can provide alternatives to haemodialysis for fluid removal as well as a very mild dialysis with minimal anticoagulation in the perioperative period. This is particularly useful in cases of severe volume overload or haemodynamic instability and can achieve significant volume losses over a period of several days.

Positive intraoperative fluid balance is expected during liver transplantation, and a gain of 10 per cent or more of the preoperative weight is not unusual even after significant losses of ascitic fluid. If substantial blood loss is encountered, weight gain of up to 20 per cent may be anticipated. Most or all of this volume is sequestered in the interstitial space and in the 'third space'. Much of this fluid can be mobilized and excreted in the third to fifth postoperative days if renal function is adequate. Removal of this fluid usually requires the use of diuretics even in the absence of renal injury. The addition of albumin to the diuretic regimen may increase the response if the serum albumin is low. As mentioned above, ultrafiltration is an option for fluid removal if the renal function is poor, but haemodialysis is otherwise not needed. If interstitial fluid is not removed as it is mobilized into the vascular space, pulmonary oedema may ensue. Careful management of volume status with central pressure monitoring may be necessary to manage difficult cases.

The common use of diuretic therapy in the first week after transplant often causes electrolyte imbalance with hypokalaemia, hypomagnesaemia, and alkalosis. Metabolic alkalosis may result from many causes (Driscoll, CritCareMed, 1987; 15:905; Fortunato, TransplProc, 1987; 19:59). The transfusion of large volumes of blood products supplies substantial amounts of citrate which are converted by the liver to bicarbonate for several days after transplantation. Acidosis during the hepatectomy and the anhepatic phase may occur because of accumulation of lactate, and requires infusion of sodium bicarbonate. Once the liver is reperfused and lactate metabolism is restored, the residual bicarbonate may also contribute to postoperative alkalosis. Nasogastric suction further aggravates alkalosis because of the loss of chloride, as does diuretic therapy which results in losses of potassium and chloride. The ensuing alkalosis may be quite severe and stimulate compensatory respiratory acidosis. This may result in small tidal volumes and, theoretically, may contribute to atelectasis. Systemic alkalosis also alters oxyhaemoglobin dissociation and impairs oxygen availability to the tissue, a potentially serious problem if arterial oxygenation is poor or tissue perfusion is impaired. In theory, this could contribute to further damage of grafts compromised by severe preservation injury.

Treatment of alkalosis usually begins with aggressive replacement of potassium deficits with potassium chloride. At the same time, ventilation is adjusted to return pH to normal and optimize oxygen delivery. Severe alkalosis constitutes a relative contraindication to extubation because of the risk of compensatory respiratory acidosis, hypoventilation, and atelectasis. Some patients maintain normal $Paco_2$ despite severe alkalosis rather than compensating with hypoventilation. In this case there is no contraindication to extubation in the face of metabolic alkalosis. If hypoventilation delays extubation, results in atelectasis or impaired tissue oxygenation, or if alkalosis results in pH above 7.5, treatment with intravenous hydrochloric acid is appropriate. Risks associated with infusion of concentrated hydrochloric acid include haemolysis and tissue injury resulting from extravasation. Carbonic anhydrase inhibitors are generally inadequate and may alkalinize the urine and enhance reabsorption of ammonia from the urine, potentially aggravating encephalopathy. Ammonium chloride is contraindicated to minimize the ammonia load requiring conversion to urea by the newly implanted liver.

Potassium deficits are common with the aggressive use of loop diuretics to maintain urine flow and achieve negative fluid balance. Because of the risk of oliguria or anuria during the early postoperative period, replacement has usually been given by intermittent infusions of potassium chloride. Addition of potassium to the maintenance fluid has traditionally been avoided because of potentially severe hyperkalaemia which might result from sudden graft failure and concomitant renal failure. This complication is now rarely seen, and addition of potassium to the maintenance fluid is probably safe if urine flow is adequate.

Maintenance of magnesium concentrations is particularly important because of the correlation between seizures during the early postoperative period of cyclosporin infusion and low or low-to-nominal magnesium levels. Prior to aggressive replacement of magnesium deficits, postoperative seizures were common while patients were receiving intravenous cyclosporin. Once the magnesium levels are regularly maintained at 1 mEq/l (>70.5 SI units) or more, seizures are rare.

Cardiovascular function

Cardiovascular complications of liver transplantation are fortunately quite rare. Significant cardiovascular disease has been considered a compelling contra-indication to liver transplantation. With improvement in anaesthesia, postoperative management, and relaxation of formerly rigid age limits, patients with pre-existing cardiovascular disease have more commonly become liver transplant candidates. Relatively mild degrees of cardiac impairment are acceptable among candidates, and satisfactory results have been obtained.

Pulmonary artery catheterization, thermodilution cardiac output, and intra-arterial monitoring have become standard practice in liver transplantation. Cardiac function is easily evaluated in the intensive care unit using standard techniques in those patients with pre-existing cardiac dysfunction or complications resulting from perioperative events. The effect of liver failure on altered haemodynamics must be appreciated. One should be aware of the reduction in afterload. Typically, cardiac output is high, resistance is low, ejection fraction is supranormal and mixed venous saturation is high. These changes are the result of marked peripheral shunting. After liver transplantation, the shunts persist for a considerable period of time before resolving. The rapidity of this change is uncertain since haemodynamic monitoring is ordinarily withdrawn within the first few days after transplantation and the hyperdynamic state persists beyond this time.

Pulmonary function

Pulmonary function is of paramount importance in the first few postoperative days. Pulmonary complications are frequent, but with careful management they are infrequently serious (Jensen, Transpl, 1986; 42:484). In contrast, minor respiratory complications, if not managed aggressively, can result in death. The typical postoperative patient returns to the intensive care unit intubated and requires several hours to several days of mechanical ventilation. The awakening process is delayed compared to other major surgical procedures, probably because of slow hepatic metabolism of anaesthetic agents and muscle relaxants and residual hepatic encephalopathy. Accordingly, prolonged awakening results in a substantial period during which the patient would be at risk for aspiration unless intubated.

All patients have impaired pulmonary mechanics resulting from the extensive upper abdominal incision which transects abdominal oblique muscles on the right as well as both rectus muscles. Many will have concomitant muscle atrophy resulting from malnutrition and prolonged hepatic failure. Finally, right, left, or bilateral phrenic nerve injury occasionally results from clamp placement or haemostatic sutures in the diaphragm.

Renal dysfunction, common in the first week after transplantation, often requires aggressive volume expansion which may contribute to pulmonary compromise because of volume overload with decreased pulmonary compliance, alveolar collapse, and increased respiratory effort.

Premature extubation of debilitated or encephalopathic patients may result in respiratory failure due to atelectasis or aspiration pneumonia. Careful evaluation of mental status, chest radiograph, and pulmonary mechanics prior to withdrawal of mechanical ventilatory support and airway protection can minimize these complications. Once pulmonary mechanics are adequate, the patient is evaluated for the ability to cough voluntarily and breathe deeply. A simple standardized test of cognitive function is performed to assess residual encephalopathy or persistent effects of anaesthesia. If all criteria are satisfied, the patient can be confidently weaned and extubated. This practice rarely prolongs by more than a few hours the period of intubation and permits detection of those patients at highest risk for aspiration, atelectasis, and pneumonia following premature extubation.

Right pleural effusion is a routine finding after liver transplantation (Olutola, Radiol, 1985; 157:594). Left-sided effusions are less common but not unusual. Effusions are transudative and may attain considerable volumes. If the volume of effusion impairs pulmonary mechanics or contributes to atelectasis, therapy is indicated. Although diuresis may reduce the volume of the effusion, thoracentesis provides a more rapid effect. Such drainage often allows earlier weaning and extubation, thus reducing the risk of nosocomial pneumonia.

Atelectasis is also a common postoperative pulmonary complication. The incidence of basilar atelectasis is probably no more common after liver transplantation than after other major upper abdominal procedures and resolves with mobilization of the patient and close attention to pulmonary toilet. Lobar or whole lung collapse is infrequent but requires aggressive management. Turning, bagging, and suctioning are important in prevention and treatment of atelectasis and may be sufficient treatment for minor collapse. More extensive collapse may result from major airway complications including malposition of the endotracheal tube, large mucous plugs, and blood clots. Such problems may be evaluated at the bedside and by portable chest radiograph and can frequently be treated appropriately without delay. Positive pressure manoeuvres can rapidly reinflate collapsed lung once obstruction is relieved. If pulmonary lavage, suctioning, and bagging with positive pressure do not quickly inflate the lung, prompt bronchoscopy is necessary.

Pneumonia is currently an infrequent complication of liver transplantation if the above precautions are observed. Pneumonia is most frequently bacterial in origin during the first 2 weeks. Subsequently, protozoal, fungal, and viral pneumonias are more common, with cytomegalovirus and *Pneumocystis* seen most frequently.

With improvement in anaesthetic management and a more stable intraoperative course, adult respiratory distress syndrome has also become an infrequent complication of liver transplantation. Treatment of adult respiratory distress syndrome resulting from liver transplantation is no different from its treatment when it results from other causes. However, the adverse effects of positive end-expiratory pressure on hepatic blood flow must be appreciated when treating adult respiratory distress syndrome. This may be particularly important when preservation injury or rejection produces oedema of the graft, and further reduction in blood flow resulting from positive end-expiratory pressure may exacerbate graft ischaemia (Matuschak, JApplPhysiol, 1987; 62:1377).

Late pulmonary complications are most commonly infectious and, as mentioned, cytomegalovirus and *Pneumocystis* are most frequently seen (Kusne, Medicine, 1988; 67:132). Adequate prophylaxis with sulphamethoxazole–trimethoprim or pentamidine has virtually eliminated *Pneumocystis* pneumonia. Cytomegalovirus remains a substantial problem but progress in the prevention and treatment of cytomegalovirus has reduced the clinical impact of this organism substantially. Both cytomegalovirus and *Pneumocystis* can present with a frank pneumonia, but more commonly the initial signs are subtle and may consist of isolated fever, mild dyspnoea, or tachypnoea. Hypoxaemia on room air has been a useful early sign of opportunistic infection and should prompt thorough evaluation of possible pulmonary infection. Bronchoalveolar lavage provides the diagnosis most consistently with minimal morbidity, and open lung biopsy is now rarely necessary. Other possible aetiologies for pneumonia should also be considered, including tuberculosis, legionella, and fungi. With aggressive and appropriate early detection and management, severe pulmonary compromise and intubation and mechanical ventilation are usually unnecessary.

Infections

Broad-spectrum antibacterial prophylaxis is given intravenously prior to operation and for 2 to 5 days afterwards. There has been a trend to shorten the duration of perioperative antibacterial therapy in an effort to minimize the selection of resistant organisms. The addition of oral antibacterial and antifungal therapy may decrease the colonization of the gut by yeast and opportunistic Gram-negative organisms (Wiesner, Transpl, 1988; 45:570). Patients receiving lactulose preoperatively, those undergoing prolonged operations (longer than 12 h), those undergoing second operations, and those cared for in the intensive care unit for more than 24 to 48 h prior to transplant have also received short courses of low-dose amphotericin B in an effort to reduce colonization and minimize fungal infections.

Pneumocystis carinii pneumonia has virtually disappeared with the introduction of low-dose trimethoprim–sulphamethoxazole therapy for 3 to 6 months after transplantation (Simmons, Transpl-Proc, 1988; 20:7). For those allergic to sulpha drugs, inhaled pentamidine is advocated (Montgomery, Lancet, 1987; ii:480). The prevention of cytomegalovirus infections has been less successful, although acylovir has proven to be an effective prophylactic agent (Balfour, NEJM, 1989; 320:1381). Intravenous human IgG has also shown promise in the prevention of cytomegalovirus infections (Snydman, NEJM, 1987; 317:1049). Finally, ganciclovir, a potent treatment for established cytomegalovirus infections has markedly reduced morbidity and mortality (Erice, JAMA, 1987; 257:3082).

Surgical complications
Bleeding

As noted earlier, initial graft function must be adequate for completion of the procedure with satisfactory haemostasis. The abdomen is not usually closed until the surgical team is satisfied that the entire surgical site is dry. Postoperative bleeding is most often the result of poor surgical haemostasis unless the graft is severely injured. Some blood loss from the surgical site is acceptable, but ordinarily drainage from the abdomen consists primarily of ascites and the haematocrit of such drainage is usually less than 5 per cent. Intra-abdominal drains are not infallible indicators of bleeding and a significant haematoma may develop without excessive drainage. Computed tomography may identify a large haemotoma when clinical findings are equivocal.

Significant bleeding is frequently associated with oliguria and, if the urine output is poor, the need for more than one or two units of transfusion in the first 12 h is cause for concern. If significant bleeding occurs, reoperation is often required to evacuate the blood clot even though active bleeding is infrequently observed at operation.

Hepatic artery thrombosis

The parenchymal tissue of the liver is capable of surviving on portal blood flow alone, making the early clinical detection of thrombosis of the hepatic artery difficult. In addition, the infrequent nature of hepatic artery thrombosis makes detection all the more challenging. Routine Doppler ultrasound can be used as a screening test for hepatic arterial flow (Segal, Transpl, 1986; 41:539). The test is very sensitive for detection of reduced or absent flow, but is relatively non-specific. Thus, if the sonographer is unable to demonstrate arterial flow, a confirmatory angiogram is necessary before corrective therapy is undertaken. If detected early, reoperation may restore flow and prevent the need for retransplantation. Alternatively, if flow is demonstrated, one can be confident of hepatic artery patency.

Several syndromes have been associated with untreated thrombosis of the hepatic artery (Tzakis, Transpl, 1985; 40:667). The earliest, and least common, occurs in those rare grafts which depend on arterial flow for survival. In such grafts, hepatic artery thrombosis produces a sudden graft failure with severe coagulopathy, renal failure, hyperkalaemia, encephalopathy, and hypoglycaemia. Urgent replacement of the graft is necessary if the patient is to survive. The other three syndromes result from dependency of the bile duct on hepatic artery blood flow. If the arterial thrombosis occurs early, the bile-duct anastomosis fails to heal and leakage develops. Should the artery thrombose later, multiple ischaemic intrahepatic bile-duct strictures may develop. Finally, intrahepatic bile ducts may undergo ischaemic necrosis with formation of multiple bile lakes or abcesses. Most of these complications are irreversible and require retransplantation. While waiting for a donor organ, abscesses or cholangitis should be treated by appropriate drainage and antibiotics.

Bile-duct complications

The blood supply of the common bile duct is quite tenuous and may explain the tendency of bilary anastomoses to scar and stricture when immunosuppression is withheld (Northover, BrJSurg, 1979; 66:379). Steroids and other immunosuppressive drugs prevent biliary sclerosis which may explain the relatively low incidence of biliary strictures in the transplant population. Biliary tract leaks usually result in signs and symptoms of an abdominal infection.[10] Diagnosis is usually made by cholangiogram. A cholangiogram is simple to perform via a T-tube or a transjejunal stent; a percutaneous transhepatic cholangiogram carries more risk. Leaks of the bile-duct anastomosis usually require surgery when detected as they rarely heal without reconstruction. If such a leak remains undetected until an abscess develops, immediate reconstruction is quite perilous. Cholangiography is also useful for detection of obstruction of the biliary system. Early on, ductal dilation is not always present, and a normal sonogram does not exclude biliary obstruction.

Simple strictures may be percutaneously dilated with a balloon catheter, although the beneficial effect can be transient (Molnar, Radiol, 1978; 129:59). Conversion of an end-to-end anastomosis to a Roux-en-Y or reconstruction of a Roux-en-Y provides a more durable result. It is important to note that bile-duct strictures can be misinterpreted as rejection on percutaneous liver biopsy. The presence of increased numbers of polymorphonuclear leucocytes around the bile ducts may be the only indication of biliary obstruction. When rejection is unresponsive to standard therapy, a bile-duct complication should be suspected and evaluated. Since bile leak or stricture may also result from hepatic artery thrombosis, discovery of a bile-duct complication warrants an investigation of the hepatic artery.

It is possible for the T-tube or internal stent to occlude the bile duct, thus producing chemical abnormalities. This is detected by cholangiogram. Removal of the T-tube or percutaneous removal of a retained stent can resolve this problem.

Intra-abdominal infections

Prolonged operation, perforation of the intestine, and immunosuppression all increase the risk for intra-abdominal infection in the liver transplant recipient. Poor nutritional status of the candidate preoperatively also increases the risk for infection. Bacterial infections are the most common and are most frequently associated with biliary complications. These infections usually occur during the first few weeks after transplantation, with fever, leucocytosis, or failure to thrive. Because of immunosuppression, patients may have minimal signs of infection despite large infected abdominal collections. For this reason, CT scanning and diagnostic aspiration of intra-abdominal fluid collections are important in those patients who appear to be failing without obvious cause.

Late intra-abdominal infections such as cholangitis and intrahepatic abscess are likely to be the result of occult occlusion of the hepatic artery or stricture of the bile duct. Diagnosis is based on appropriate imaging procedures and cultures obtained at the time of drainage. The surgical principle of adequate drainage coupled with appropriate antibiotics may be accomplished by percutaneous techniques, but open drainage may be necessary if a safe percutaneous route is unavailable or the response to percutaneous drainage is not prompt or complete. Caution should be exercised before routinely draining perihepatic fluid collections, since loculated perihepatic ascites is quite frequent and most often benign. Only if infection is clinically suspected and other sources of infection have been eliminated, should perihepatic fluid collections be aspirated.

Ascites

Ascites is almost universal after liver transplantation, even if none was present before the operation. This ascites has been attributed to open lymphatic vessels in the porta hepatis and the surface of the diaphragm. The ascites is usually worse in those patients with severe ascites prior to surgery. During the first few days after transplantation, the ascites is ordinarily drained by closed suction drainage systems. The amount of fluid which can be removed by these systems can be substantial and result in significant volume depletion.

Formation of ascites can increase dramatically when the graft is injured by rejection or portal vein thrombosis. A substantial increase in ascites should prompt an investigation of possible causes of graft dysfunction. Losses of ascites may require replacement with an appropriate solution, since fluid removed from the abdominal cavity is quite promptly replaced by the formation of new ascites at the expense of extracellular fluid and ultimately plasma volume. The protein losses associated with ascitic drainage can be formidable and some form of replacement, either by colloid infusions or parenteral nutrition, is necessary.

Occasionally, ascites will persist for more than 4 weeks and constitute a demanding patient management challenge with related problems of intravascular dehydration and renal failure.

Portal vein thrombosis

Portal vein thrombosis is a rare technical complication of liver transplantation (Lerut, AnnSurg, 1987; 205:404). If the anastomosis is technically adequate, and thrombosis occurs, intrahepatic obstruction of portal flow may sometimes be responsible. This may be due to oedema resulting from severe preservation injury or, less commonly, early severe cellular rejection. It has been suggested that portal vein thrombosis arising in the first few hours after implantation may be a manifestation of hyperacute rejection.

Another possible cause of portal vein thrombosis is clot forming within the donor portal system. Such thrombus may form within the portal system after a thrombectomy performed upon a clotted portal vein during the preparation for hepatic implantation. Alternatively, unsuspected pre-existing clot within the portal system may be a nidus for thrombus propagation within the portal system and subsequent portal vein thrombosis.

Finally, thrombosis due to poor flow in the portal system may be the result of high flow portal-systemic shunts arising spontaneously or surgically created prior to transplantation. Such a situation may be detected if portal vein flow is measured intra-operatively, and corrective action taken prior to closure.

The clinical findings associated with portal vein thrombosis are quite characteristic and should lead rapidly to the correct diagnosis after urgent study by Doppler ultrasound and confirmatory angiography, if necessary. The patient with complete thrombosis of the portal vein will suddenly become desperately ill, with hypotension, sudden and massive ascites, shock, and sepsis. Severe coagulopathy, marked elevation of aminotransferases, lactic acidosis, and hypoglycaemia are associated laboratory findings. Urgent re-transplantation is the only opportunity to salvage the patient with portal vein thrombosis, and survival for more than 24 h is unusual after the diagnosis is made.

Results

Liver transplantation has proved to be a successful treatment for endstage liver disease since the introduction of cyclosporin in the early 1980s. Introduction of this immunosuppressive agent was coincidental with other improvements in surgical techniques, anaesthesiology, critical care medicine, and hepatology. Currently, the 1-year survival rate for all indications is approximately 70 to 85 per cent (Krom, MayoClinProc, 1989; 64:84; Shaw, ArchSurg, 1989; 124:895; Starzl, TransplProc, 1989; 21:2197). The 5-year survival rate, similarly for all indications, is 60 to 70 per cent (Starzl, TransplProc, 1989; 21:2197). Survival rates for paediatric and adult recipients have been similar. It is very likely that the variations noted between centres are attributable to differences in patient selection. Those centres which have been more aggressive in transplanting patients with difficult anatomical situations and with more problematic indications (e.g. malignancy, hepatitis B), have lower survival rates than those centres transplanting carefully selected, good-risk patients.

The best survival is achieved for those adult patients transplanted for cryptogenic cirrhosis, primary biliary cirrhosis, sclerosing cholangitis without concomitant tumour, and inborn errors of metabolism. In the paediatric group of patients, the best results have been achieved for children transplanted for biliary atresia, cryptogenic cirrhosis, and inborn errors of metabolism. The indications for which survival is decreased are those diseases which can recur after transplantation. These include patients with hepatitis B surface antigen positivity and hepatic malignancies. Furthermore, patients with fulminant hepatic failure have shown a decreased survival following liver transplantation, most likely due to the advanced state of disease and coma with which these patients are often transferred to transplant centres (Stieber, GastrClinNAm, 1988; 17:157).

Clearly, early referral for patients with fulminant hepatic failure would improve the outcome and long-term survival.

Those patients transplanted for chronic hepatitis B who are hepatitis B surface antigen positive preoperatively, have, for the most part, developed recurrence of their disease following transplantation. The 1-year survival rate has been reported to be approximately 60 per cent, and the 5-year survival rate, approximately 50 per cent.[11] In comparison, patients transplanted for fulminant hepatic failure who are hepatitis B surface antigen positive have had 75 to 80 per cent 1- and 5-year survival rates.[11] Currently, clinical trials are under way in various centres exploring adjuvant therapy to prevent recurrent disease. These trials have included the use of large doses of hepatitis B hyperimmune globulin during the anhepatic phase and postoperatively, the use of hepatitis B vaccine in the perioperative period, and the use of nucleoside analogues such as lamivudine or famciclovir. Long-term follow-up of these patients is required before recommendations can be made as to the best perioperative treatment.

Transplantation for malignant disease has been, for the main part, disappointing. In the presence of hepatocellular carcinoma, survival has been poor with only occasional long-term survivors (Koneru, GastrClinNAm, 1988; 17:177). For the fibrolamellar variant of hepatoma, survival has been better, with many patients surviving for prolonged periods despite recurrence of the disease. Transplantation, in the face of cholangiocarcinoma, has been uniformly disappointing. The cluster operation, also termed the upper abdominal exenteration (Starzl, AnnSurg, 1989; 210:374), is currently being evaluated for this very difficult and frustrating indication. Epithelioid haemangioendothelioma has a 90 per cent 1-year and 50 per cent 5-year survival rate.

Although many centres have abandoned transplantation for hepatic malignancies, others continue to offer transplantation to these patients who have no other option for cure. However, most centres that continue to transplant patients for primary hepatic malignancies have instituted protocols employing perioperative chemotherapy to reduce the incidence of recurrence. The best survival can be obtained in those patients who undergo very careful preoperative assessment to exclude extrahepatic disease. This includes extensive radiological evaluation, radionuclear scans, pretransplantation laparotomy, and lymph-node sampling.

Patients transplanted for other indications and found to have small incidental tumours can attain similar survival rates as patients without tumours (Koneru, GastrClinNAm, 1988; 17:177).[11] With improvements in radiological techniques, small intrahepatic tumours can be diagnosed more readily than in the past, and what were previously considered incidental tumours may be diagnosed preoperatively. Clearly, it can be expected that results for liver transplantation for patients diagnosed with a tumour will improve in such situations.

Following liver transplantation, over 80 per cent of patients return to their normal life styles. Patients return to school, to their family responsibilities, to their employment, and to their normal social activities. Despite the use of long-term immunosuppressive therapy, many male patients have successfully fathered children, and many females have become pregnant and given birth to healthy children. In one report, 20 children were born to 17 female patients who had received a wide variety of immunosuppressive agents, including cyclosporin, Imuran®, steroids, polyclonal antibodies, and monoclonal antibodies (Scantlebury, Transpl, 1990; 49:317). Despite the increased incidence of Caesarean section and premature births, most of the children have done well.

Recurrence of disease after liver transplantation

As our experience with liver transplantation increases and with long-term follow-up of these patients, recurrence of disease in the grafted liver is increasingly being recognized. Recurrence of viral diseases is a major concern. Furthermore, chronic cholestatic diseases such as primary biliary cirrhosis and primary sclerosing cholangitis have also been reported to recur.

Recurrent primary biliary cirrhosis

The diagnosis of primary biliary cirrhosis in the pretransplant setting is based on clinical presentation, hepatic chemistries, and liver histology. In the initial stages, symptoms are non-specific, and with disease progression symptoms of chronic cholestasis, complications of portal hypertension, and decompensated liver disease develop. The hepatic chemistries reveal a cholestatic pattern with elevations in serum alkaline phosphatase and bilirubin. Hypergammaglobulinaemia (IgM) and presence of antimitochondrial antibodies are characteristic of primary biliary cirrhosis. On liver histology, the diagnostic finding is the 'florid duct lesion' or granulomatous bile-duct destruction.

After liver transplantation the diagnosis of recurrent primary biliary cirrhosis in the liver allograft is difficult as many of the clinical features may be due to other aetiologies. For instance, pruritus due to cholestasis may be secondary to medical or mechanical biliary complications. Cholestatic hepatic chemistries are often present after liver transplantation and may be related to bile-duct abnormalities, medications including cyclosporin and tacrolimus (FK506), sepsis, or rejection. Immunosuppressive agents may modify patterns of possible disease recurrence. Furthermore, immunosuppressive medications currently used following liver transplantation (azathioprine, corticosteroids, cyclosporin, and tacrolimus) have all been used in prospective trials in primary biliary cirrhosis patients and have been shown to have an effect on primary biliary cirrhosis.

Persistence of the immunological abnormalities, such as elevated IgM, positive antimitochondrial antibodies, and continuance or development of extrahepatic manifestations of primary biliary cirrhosis, do not prove disease recurrence. Therefore the diagnosis of recurrent disease depends mainly on histology. Histological interpretation in the allograft can be difficult as immune processes in the graft can target bile ducts. For example, rejection, cytomegalovirus infection and hepatitis C are associated with bile-duct damage. However, the use of strict histological criteria, such as the demonstration of the florid duct lesions with bile-duct damage and the presence of portal granulomas in the transplanted liver, is helpful in the diagnosis of recurrent primary biliary cirrhosis.

Neuberger et al., from King's College first reported (Neuberger, NEJM, 1982; 306:1) the development of a syndrome suggestive of recurrent primary biliary cirrhosis after liver transplantation in three patients. Their experience was later updated by Polson et al. (Polson, Gastro, 1989; 97:715) who reported the features compatible

with disease recurrence to be present in 9/10 patients with biopsies taken more than 1 year after liver transplantation. The diagnosis of recurrence was based on clinical and immunological changes with histological features suggestive of disease recurrence. Histological evidence of recurrent primary biliary cirrhosis included bile-duct damage with lymphocytic infiltrate arround irregular, enlarged portal tracts; development of septum formation; ductular proliferation; and the deposition of copper-associated protein in a periseptal distribution. However, these histological findings are not diagnostic of primary biliary cirrhosis.

In a study from the Mayo Clinic (Balan, Hepatol, 1993; 18: 1392), 60 consecutive patients with primary biliary cirrhosis with at least 1 year of follow-up after liver transplantation were studied. The immunosuppression regimen was either cyclosporin, prednisolone, and azathioprine, or FK506 and prednisolone. Hepatic biochemical parameters and protocol liver biopsy specimens were evaluated 1 week, 3 weeks, 4 months, and yearly after liver transplantation, and with hepatic dysfunction. Antimitochondrial antibodies and IgM levels were determined before liver transplantation, at 4 months, and yearly. Of the 72 patients grafted for primary biliary cirrhosis, 60 had survived for more than 1 year. The mean follow-up was 3.3 years.

At the time of the study, 55/60 (91 per cent) patients had normal hepatic chemistries, including serum levels of alkaline phosphatase, bilirubin, alanine aminotransferase, and IgM. In addition, all patients had significant decreases in antimitochondrial antibody titres and IgM levels at the time of last follow-up. On histological examination, 41/60 patients had a near normal liver histology. Of those with abnormal histology, five patients, 2 to 6 years after liver transplantation, had histological features typical of a 'florid duct lesion', suggesting recurrent primary biliary cirrhosis. All five with the presence of portal granulomas were asymptomatic with normal hepatic chemistries. Two of the five patients had persistent antimitochondrial antibodies. The HLA status of the five patients with recurrent primary biliary cirrhosis showed that all five had at least a single match, three at class I loci (A1 A2 Bw38), 1 at class II (DR4) and 1 in both class I and class II loci (B51 DQW1).

Subsequently, several other studies have also reported on recurrent primary biliary cirrhosis (Dietze, TransplProc,1990; 22: 1501; Nsien, SemLivDis, 1992; 12:93; Hubscher, JHepatol, 1993; 18:173; Wong, JHepatol, 1993 17:284). Hubscher et al. (Hubscher, JHepatol, 1993; 18:173) reported histological features suggestive of recurrent disease in 13 transplanted primary biliary cirrhosis patients between 12 and 100 months after liver transplantation. The main diagnostic features were mononuclear cell portal inflammatory infiltrate, portal lymphoid aggregates, portal epithelioid granulomas and bile-duct damage, ductopenia, ductular proliferation, portal fibrosis, and copper-associated protein deposition. Dietze et al. (Dietze, TransplProc, 1990; 22:1501) also reported primary biliary cirrhosis recurrence in two of eight patients. The diagnosis of recurrence was based on histological features of primary biliary cirrhosis in the allograft.

Several other studies have failed to find evidence for recurrent primary biliary cirrhosis. Many of these studies failing to identify recurrence have relatively few primary biliary cirrhosis patients with long-term histological follow-up.

At present recurrent primary biliary cirrhosis is not associated with significant clinical symptoms, and these patients, at least in the short to medium term seem to have a good quality of life. Longer-term studies will help in defining the clinical relevance of primary biliary cirrhosis recurrence in the allograft.

Recurrent primary sclerosing cholangitis

The issue of recurrent primary sclerosing cholangitis after liver transplantation is more complex than that of recurrent primary biliary cirrhosis as there is no diagnostic gold standard in primary sclerosing cholangitis. The diagnosis of primary sclerosing cholangitis in the native liver is made by a combination of: imaging the biliary tree, clinical presentation, hepatic chemistries, and hepatic histology. As with primary biliary cirrhosis, the clinical presentation initially includes non-specific symptoms and later signs of hepatic decompensation. Primary sclerosing cholangitis can occur alone; however, 70 per cent of cases are associated with inflammatory bowel disease. A cholestatic pattern is typical of the hepatic chemistries. Autoantibodies in primary sclerosing cholangitis are non-specific and infrequent. Anticolon, antineutrophil nuclear, and antineutrophil cytoplasmic antibodies have been described in primary sclerosing cholangitis. However, their association is variable and not specific for primary sclerosing cholangitis. The radiological features are characteristic and exhibit diffuse strictures, beading, and dilatation of the intra- and/or extrahepatic bile ducts. Similar radiological findings can also be seen in secondary sclerosing cholangitis due to sepsis, stones, rejection, and during the course of AIDS.

The diagnostic histological abnormality of primary sclerosing cholangitis is the fibrous obliterative cholangitis that results in the replacement of bile ducts by fibrous scars with the appearance of concentric rings of fibrosis around bile ducts. There have been some reports suggesting similar features in secondary sclerosing cholangitis as well.

After liver transplantation, imaging of the extrahepatic biliary tree is difficult as transplanted primary sclerosing cholangitis patients have a Roux loop with removal of the recipient bile duct. These patients have increased incidence of biliary problems such as anastomotic and non-anastomotic strictures which can radiologically and histologically be consistent with primary sclerosing cholangitis in the intrahepatic biliary tree. There are several reports of more frequent biliary complications in transplanted primary sclerosing cholangitis patients than in patients transplanted for other indications (Leturneau, Radio, 1988; 167:349; McEntee, TransplProc, 1991; 23:1563). These findings may be related to complications of the Roux-en-Y loop and are difficult to attribute to recurrent primary sclerosing cholangitis.

Iwatsuki (Gastro, 1991; 90:1736) from our institution initially found only 1/40 patients transplanted for primary sclerosing cholangitis who had biochemical and radiological features of recurrent primary sclerosing cholangitis 1 year after liver transplantation. A more recent review of this subject from our institution (Sheng, AmJRoent, 1996; 166:1109) found that radiological findings resembling primary sclerosing cholangitis occur more frequently in transplanted primary sclerosing cholangitis patients than in transplants for other diseases. A study group of 32 primary sclerosing cholangitis grafts with binary strictures was compared to a control group of 32 non-primary sclerosing cholangitis grafts with strictures. Both groups were matched for the type of biliary anastomosis and for the time interval between transplantation and

stricture diagnosis. The location, number, length of strictures, and ductal dilations were similar in the primary sclerosing cholangitis and non-primary sclerosing cholangitis groups. However, mural irregularities of bile ducts were present in 15/32 (47 per cent) of transplanted primary sclerosing cholangitis patients versus 4/32 (13 per cent) in the controls. Diverticulum-like outpouchings were seen in 6/32 (19 per cent) of transplanted primary sclerosing cholangitis patients versus 1/32 (3 per cent) in the controls. An overall resemblance to primary sclerosing cholangitis was seen in 8/32 (25 per cent) of transplanted primary sclerosing cholangitis patients versus 2/32 (6 per cent) in the controls. These findings are highly suggestive of recurrent primary sclerosing cholangitis.

As far as the histological findings of recurrent primary sclerosing cholangitis are concerned, Harrison et al. (Harrison, Hepatol, 1994; 20:356) suggested that the fibro-obliterative lesions (the onion-skin fibrosis) and the periductal lesions do occur in greater frequency in patients grafted for primary sclerosing cholangitis than in those grafted for other conditions. In a review of histological material from a series of 22 transplanted primary sclerosing cholangitis patients, 32 per cent had biopsies showing features of biliary obstruction, 27 per cent periductal fibrosis, and 14 per cent had the classical fibro-obliterative lesions. Of a control group of 22 patients transplanted for other diseases besides primary sclerosing cholangitis but having a Roux loop, 10 per cent had features of biliary obstruction, 5 per cent periductal fibrosis, but no fibro-obliterative lesions were noted. Thus, the histological features of primary sclerosing cholangitis are more common in the post-transplant setting. However, these features do not differentiate between primary and secondary sclerosing cholangitis, creating a dilemma in making the diagnosis of recurrent primary sclerosing cholangitis. In any case if the primary sclerosing cholangitis does recur, it appears to stay in an early stage. As with primary biliary sclerosis, longer and careful follow-up is required to determine the issue of recurrent primary sclerosing cholangitis.

Recurrent autoimmune hepatitis

Autoimmune hepatitis is a diagnosis of exclusion and is made on the basis of hepatic chemistries, autoantibodies, and histology. Hepatic chemistries reveal elevations of serum aminotransferases. Several autoantibodies have been described in the various types of autoimmune hepatitis, including antinuclear antibody, antiliver/kidney microsomal antibody class I, and antiactin (smooth muscle). Liver histology shows features of a chronic hepatitis with a portal cell infiltrate consisting of plasma cells, piecemeal necrosis, and bridging. Autoimmune hepatitis promptly responds to corticosteroids.

After liver transplantation the diagnosis of recurrent autoimmune hepatitis from acute rejection can be made easily by detecting elevated IgG levels and autoantibodies, characteristic of recurrent autoimmune hepatitis. The first report of recurrence of autoimmune hepatitis was by Neuberger et al. (Neuberger, Transpl, 1984; 37:363) in a female patient who developed clinical, biochemical, immunological, and histological features of recurrent autoimmune chronic active hepatitis when corticosteroids were discontinued. Re-introduction of steroids resolved the abnormalities. Of interest, the recipient was HLA B8 DR3 whereas the donor was negative for both these HLA antigens. In subsequent studies from our institution (Wright, Transpl, 1992; 53:136), based on a retrospective analysis of 43 transplanted autoimmune hepatitis patients, 11 cases of recurrent autoimmune hepatitis were reported. The diagnosis was made on the basis of histology. The recurrence was reported at a median of 18 months following transplantation, and all but one of the patients were female. Nine of the 11 patients were DR3 positive and, as with the initial patient, the graft was DR3 negative. Recurrence was not observed in those who had DR3-positive grafts. Autoimmune hepatitis can recur after liver transplantation and is readily controlled by increasing the dose of steroids.

Viral hepatitis C after liver transplantation

Endstage liver disease due to hepatitis C virus is rapidly emerging as the most prevalent indication for liver transplantation. However, following improvements in the identification of hepatitis C virus with the reverse transcriptase–polymerase chain reaction (RT–PCR), a more accurate assessment of liver transplantation for hepatitis C infection revealed a significant incidence of recurrent disease in transplant recipients.[6,7] The prognosis and treatment of recurrent hepatitis C virus infection have only recently been under investigation.

Hepatitis C virus reinfection following liver transplantation was believed to be 3 per cent or less during the late 1980s when testing for this virus was limited to anti-hepatitis C virus detection. With the development of RT–PCR for hepatitis C virus and more sensitive antibody assays, several studies reported universal reinfection of the liver allograft in recipients who have a positive serum or liver RT–PCR prior to transplantation. More recent studies utilizing both the RT–PCR test and histological examination of the liver have estimated the incidence of recurrent hepatitis to be 50 to 80 per cent by 2 years. This recurrent infection generally occurs as a mild increase in the serum aminotransferases anywhere from 2 weeks to 2 years postoperatively. The associated histological findings commonly include portal/lobular mononuclear infiltrates and hepatocyte necrosis. However, we have encountered recurrences characterized by severe cholestasis and by moderate bile-duct damage. Hepatitis C virus genotype 1b and the use of OKT3 have been associated with an early, more aggressive disease; however, additional confirmation of these and other predictors of aggressive, recurrent disease is needed.

Quantitation of the hepatitis C virus with the branched DNA (bDNA) assay in liver transplant recipients has demonstrated a dramatic increase in the viral load following transplantation. Transient increases in bDNA titre have recently been shown to correlate with increases in serum aminotransaminases and histological findings of hepatitis. However, the viral titre does not seem to correlate with the severity of hepatitis as determined histologically. Additionally a 'carrier state' with significantly elevated viral titre without histological evidence of hepatitis can be seen. However, a long-term comparison of viral titre and histological scores is needed.

Several studies have reported that the early survival of patients transplanted for hepatitis C virus infection is not significantly different from that of patients transplanted for non-viral diseases. However, these same studies have also reported the development of cirrhosis in patients within 2 years of transplantation, due to recurrent hepatitis C infection. A recent 10-year study involving 71 patients with hepatitis C virus following liver transplantation reported no differences in survival when compared to patients transplanted for other non-malignant diseases. However, this study also included de novo infections with hepatitis C virus, making interpretation difficult. In our own study involving 237 patients, preoperative hepatitis C infection was associated with a significant reduction in patient survival at 3 years—66 per cent 3-year survival for patients transplanted for hepatitis C virus infection versus 78 per cent for patients transplanted for other disorders. A recent study from the University of California at Los Angeles also found the survival in patients transplanted for hepatitis C virus infection to be reduced. In conclusion, a subset of patients will develop an aggressive recurrent infection leading to cirrhosis within 4 years of liver transplantation. As a result, patients undergoing liver transplantation for hepatitis C virus may experience a significant reduction in survival; however, liver transplantation is certainly justified since the long-term prognosis remains acceptable. Hopefully, future studies will allow us to identify patients with a poor prognosis.

Treatment of the candidate awaiting liver transplantation to prevent subsequent allograft infection has not been adequately examined. Obviously, neutropenia, thrombocytopenia, and hepatic decompensation pose limitations to treatment with interferon alone; however, combination therapy with interferon and nucleoside analogues, such as ribavirin, in candidates awaiting transplant warrants investigation. Prophylaxis treatment with this combination has recently been reported following liver transplantation. Mazzaferro et al. (Mazzaferro, TransplProc, 1997; 29:519) recently reported viral eradication in 9/21 (43 per cent) patients after a 6-month course of ribavirin/interferon given within 6 months of liver transplantation prior to the occurrence of hepatitis. Although this approach appears beneficial, a long-term analysis of survival benefit is needed to verify this and other prophylactic regimens. Once we are able to identify patients with a poor prognosis due to aggressive, recurrent disease, prophylactic regimens can be applied liberally.

Treatment of recurrent hepatitis C virus infection involves the use of interferon therapy as in the pretransplant setting. In the studies by Wright and Feray (Wright, Hepatol, 1994; 20:773), liver function tests returned to normal in 5 of 18 (28 per cent) and 2 of 14 (14 per cent) while undergoing treatment, and remained normal in four (22 per cent) and one (7 per cent) after cessation of therapy. No firm conclusions can be made concerning the histological response, since in the study by Feray (Hepatol, 1995; 22:1084) 2 of 14 showed evidence of histological improvement and Wright reported no improvement in histological scores. Reductions in viral RNA levels were observed in the majority of patients in the study by Wright (Hepatol, 1994; 20:773); however, upon the completion of therapy, viral RNA levels returned to pretreatment values in all patients. In the study by Feray (Hepatol, 1995; 22:1084) reductions in hepatitis C virus RNA by more than 50 per cent were observed in 4 of 14 (28 per cent), and in three of these four the reduction persisted up to 6 months after therapy was terminated. The fourth patient had a complete response and had negative bDNA and RT–PCR assays at 15 months after completion of therapy. We currently have enrolled 30 patients in a 6- to 9-month treatment protocol and, similar to the above studies, liver function tests have decreased to normal in approximately 25 per cent of patients during therapy. Hepatitis C virus RNA levels have displayed a consistent downward trend in almost all patients during therapy, but only one patient had undetectable RNA by RT–PCR assay at the end of therapy, and this patient had a low pretreatment RNA (7.0×10^5 genome Eq/ml).

Significant rejection did occur in both studies. Interferon therapy was terminated due to rejection in 1/18 patients in the study by Wright. However, in the study by Feray rejection occurred in 5/14, resulting in retransplantation in three patients. The authors do suggest that the low maintenance doses of cyclosporin utilized may have contributed to this high incidence of rejection. Other cases of interferon-induced rejection of hepatic allografts have been reported and patients need to be monitored closely for this infrequent but grave complication.

In immunocompetent patients, viral inhibition has been reported with ribavirin as a single agent, and when used in conjunction with interferon viral eradication has improved to almost 60 per cent. Gane et al. (Gane, TransplInt, 1995; 8:61) reported seven patients treated with a 6-month course of ribavirin for recurrent hepatitis C following liver transplantation. Three patients required a dosage reduction due to haemolysis and only four patients tolerated the full dose of 1200 mg/day. Reduction in aspartate aminotransferase to normal and improvement in histological grade occurred only in the four patients who tolerated the full dose while on therapy. Hepatitis C virus RNA remained detectable during therapy in all seven cases. Although long-term analysis is not provided, this study suggests that an extended regimen with ribavirin alone may be beneficial in patients with progressive, recurrent disease.

Although management options of recurrent hepatitis C in liver transplant recipients are currently limited, future therapies appear hopeful. Advancements in the treatment of AIDS should provide other antiviral agents possibly with anti-hepatitis C activity. Additionally, since proteases associated with the hepatitis C virus have recently been identified, protease inhibitors may also be available for trials in the near future. With these ongoing developments, control of, and possibly cure of, recurrent disease in the transplant recipient may be realized by the turn of the century.

The outcome for retransplantation for recurrent hepatitis C virus infection in patients who progress to liver failure is poor. In a study by Feray (Hepatol, 1995; 22:1084), the 1-year graft survival in patients retransplanted for hepatitis C-associated cirrhosis was 40 per cent. However, also in the study by Feray, the 1-year graft survival was 63 per cent in patients retransplanted for rejection with a coexisting diagnosis of hepatitis C. These poor results with retransplantation for allograft failure secondary to hepatitis C can likely be attributed to the debilitated condition of the recipient since recurrent hepatitis is unlikely to result in mortality within 1 year.

The use of anti-hepatitis C virus positive donors has now become more common due to the scarcity of suitable organ donors. Organs from anti-hepatitis C virus positive donors are being used for recipients with detectable serum hepatitis C virus RNA. Utilizing stored donor sera, studies have confirmed that the transmission of hepatitis C virus infection is essentially universal from this pool of donors. However, the survival of recipients of livers from anti-hepatitis C virus positive donors has been investigated in two studies, both of which suggest similar graft and patient survival when transplanted into anti-hepatitis C virus positive recipients. Additionally, the risk of the hepatitis C virus infected recipient developing recurrent hepatitis C does not appear to be increased by the use of an hepatitis C virus infected hepatic allograft. Certainly, some of these recipients are subjected to infection from a different hepatitis C virus genotype. However, until long-term studies suggest a survival disadvantage from this practice, we will continue to utilize suitable organs from hepatitis C virus infected donors.

Viral hepatitis B after liver transplantation

Hepatitis B almost always recurs following liver transplantation for hepatitis B infection. Transplant recipients reinfected with hepatitis B have a lower survival compared with patients receiving transplants for other causes of chronic liver disease (50 per cent versus 70–80 per cent at 2 years). The early fears of universal reinfection after liver transplantation for hepatitis B were tempered by several isolated case reports of patients who did not develop hepatitis B virus recurrence following liver transplantation.

The principle risk factor associated with hepatitis B virus recurrent disease following liver transplantation is the status of serum hepatitis B virus DNA prior to transplant. Patients that are hepatitis B virus DNA positive have a higher incidence of recurrence (92 per cent) compared to those that were hepatitis B virus DNA negative (32 per cent). Patient and graft survival are also adversely impacted by the presence of HBeAg (and correspondingly hepatitis B virus DNA positive), and short-term or no hepatitis B immunoglobulin (**HBIG**) therapy.

A large series of patients was analysed in a retrospective multicentre trial from Europe. Three hundred and seventy-two HBsAg patients underwent liver transplantation at 17 centres. Patients were divided according to the serological markers for hepatitis B, acute fulminant versus chronic, coexistent hepatitis D virus infection, and the length of HBIG therapy. The overall 3-year hepatitis B virus recurrence rate was 50 per cent. Recurrence occurred in 83 per cent of hepatitis B virus DNA positive patients; 66 per cent of the HBeAg positive, DNA negative; and 58 per cent of hepatitis B virus DNA negative, HBeAg negative. Patients who had coexistent hepatitis D virus infection in the chronic phase, had a 32 per cent incidence of recurrence, those that had both hepatitis B and D chronic disease had a 40 per cent recurrence rate, and those with fulminant hepatic hepatitis B virus had a 17 per cent recurrence rate. Recurrence as related to HBIG therapy revealed that no therapy was associated with the 75 per cent rate of recurrence, while those with short-term therapy (less than 6 months of HBIG) had a 74 per cent recurrence rate. Those that had longer than 6 months of HBIG had a 36 per cent recurrence rate. In addition, it appeared that most of the recurrence had occurred within 24 months of therapy. While no definitive statement could be made regarding the length of therapy, it appeared that 2 years of therapy should be sufficient to prevent long-term recurrence. Therefore, patients with coexisting hepatitis D infection, fulminant hepatitis B, HBeAg negative, serum hepatitis B virus DNA negative, and those who receive long-term (>6 months) passive immunoprophylaxis, experienced lower reinfection rates after liver transplantation.

HBIG therapy should be given for a period of a least 2 years, since the majority of those patients that become reinfected, do so within 24 months after transplantation.

Results of the use of α-interferon for treatment of hepatitis B virus in patients undergoing liver transplantation have been overwhelmingly poor, with only partial improvement in serum aminotransferase levels and temporary return to previous levels of response. The rationale for use of the interferons (α, β, and γ) is to increase leucocyte activity via the 2,5-oligoadenylate synthetase pathway, and also to up-regulate major histocompatibility complex (**MHC**) antigens on the surface of infected cells. While the rationale appears sound, the impact in these patients following liver transplantation has not been defined.

An exciting area for potential anti-hepatitis B virus therapy is to target specific antiviral mechanisms which interfere with hepatitis B virus replication. The DNA polymerase and reverse transcriptase that are required for hepatitis B virus replication are potential targets for blockade. Transient decreases in hepatitis B virus DNA were seen in patients with treated with foscarnet, which is a novel antiviral agent that inhibits viral-specific DNA polymerase. Use of nucleoside analogues, which either bind to reverse transcriptase or prevent RNA and DNA elongation, has also been proposed. Ganciclovir, which is a nucleoside analogue of 2′-deoxyguanosine, has also been reported to decrease hepatitis B virus DNA proliferation. Other agents, such as lamivudine and famciclovir, have been associated with encouraging preliminary results in terms of seroconversion to hepatitis B virus DNA negativity. However, there have been reports of the development of hepatitis B virus mutants that are resistant to lamivudine in association with long-term therapy.

Hepatitis B is still the leading cause of chronic liver disease throughout the world. Strategies for prevention and treatment of hepatitis B virus appear to be promising. It seems that patients with low or no active hepatitis B virus replication can benefit from liver transplantation. Use of HBIG can effectively reduce the chance of reinfection of the allograft in well-defined subsets of patients. Conversion of the actively replicating (high-risk) group of patients to a low-risk group can be the major area of interest for further investigation. It seems that different regimes of immunosuppression (i.e. FK506 versus cyclosporin) have no effect on the rate of recurrence of the disease.

Future directions

Despite the excellent results which have been obtained with liver transplantation, the field continues to evolve. Although various diseases can be cured with liver transplantation and have an excellent survival rate, other diseases will require development of efficacious adjuvant therapies before achieving equal survival rates. Research is in progress for those diseases that demonstrate recurrence following transplantation, including hepatitis B surface antigen positive cirrhosis and primary liver malignancies. A close collaboration between transplantation surgeons, hepatologists, virologists, and immunologists is required to devise perioperative management protocols for patients with hepatitis B. A major effort must be directed towards the definition of adjuvant therapy to prevent, or at least significantly alter, recurrent disease.

The efforts directed towards the management of patients with primary hepatic malignancies have many foci. The available data suggest that better results can be achieved through better patient selection, recognition of favourable tumour types, modification of the postoperative immunosuppressive regimen, administration of adjuvant chemotherapy, and the development of new operative approaches to these diseases. In the presence of hepatic malignancies that cannot be resected by conventional techniques, liver transplantation continues as the only hope for cure. Despite the occasional long-term survivor, the results for most hepatic malignancies remain poor. Carefully conducted trials of perioperative chemotherapy will be one area of focus to improve this situation.

Future research must address the supply of suitable and adequate donor organs. Improved preservation techniques and the development of segmental liver transplantation have alleviated a small part of the problem. The feasibility of organ transplantation across species has been demonstrated (Starzl, Lancet, 1993; 341:65). The survival is short, because these allografts succumb to an accelerated rejection process. It is anticipated that with improved techniques of immunosuppression and further studies to achieve immune tolerance, xenograft transplantation can become a reality. Although fraught with ethical and emotional issues, the ability to transplant across species would resolve the issue of the organ shortage and would render liver transplantation an elective procedure.

Although cyclosporin and now tacrolimus have helped revolutionize organ transplantation, rejection and infection remain among the most common postoperative complications.

Over the past three decades, the field of liver transplantation has made great strides. It has progressed from an experimental procedure to an accepted therapeutic modality for many patients with endstage liver disease. Survival rates and the quality of life have made this the treatment of choice for most patients with endstage liver disease and it can be anticipated that with further developments survival rates as well as quality of life will improve even further.

References

1. Iwatsuki S, Shaw BW, Jr, and Starzl TE. Liver transplantation for biliary atresia. *World Journal of Surgery*, 1984; **8**: 51–6.
2. Hiatt JR, *et al.* Pediatric liver transplantation at UCLA. *Transplantation Proceedings*, 1987; **19**: 3282–8.
3. Shaw BW, Jr., *et al.* Liver transplantation therapy for children: Part 1. *Journal of Pediatric Gastroenterology and Nutrition*, 1988; **7**: 157–66.
4. Starzl TE, Esquivel C, Gordon R, and Todo S. Pediatric liver transplantation. *Transplantation Proceedings*, 1987; **19**: 3230–5.
5. Starzl TE, Demetris AJ, and Van Thiel DH. Medical progress: liver transplantation (Part 1). *New England Journal of Medicine*, 1989; **321**: 1014–22,
6. Kang YG. Monitoring and treatment of coagulation. In Winter PM and Young YG, eds. *Hepatic transplantation*. New York: Praeger, 1986: 151–73.
7. Klintmalm GBG, *et al.* Rejection in liver transplantation. *Hepatology*, 1989; **10**: 978–5.
8. Emond JC, *et al.* Rejection in liver allograft recipients: clinical characterization and management. *Clinical Transplantation*, 1987; **1**: 143–50.
9. Ludwig J. Histopathology of the liver following transplantation. In Maddrey WC, ed. *Transplantation of the liver*. New York: Elsevier Science, 1988: 191–218.
10. Vicente E, *et al.* Biliary tract complications following orthotopic liver transplantation. *Clinical Transplantation*, 1987; **1**: 138–42.
11. Starzl TE and Demetris AJ. *Liver transplantation: a 31-year perspective.* Chicago: Yearbook Medical Publisher, Inc., 1990.

31

History of hepatology

31 History of hepatology

F. H. Franken and H. Falk

Liver diseases

Antiquity

Egypt and Greece

One of the earliest representations of the anatomy and physiology of the liver is to be found in the Ebers Papyrus, an Egyptian medical text written about 1550 BC. This text also states that liver diseases may be recognized by inspection and palpation of the abdomen. In Homer's *Iliad* and *Odyssey* (eighth and seventh centuries BC) (Table 1) there is a more precise identification of the topography of the liver. It was regarded as a vital organ, so that wounds to it were fatal.

Although the pre-Socratic philosophers had applied a rational mode of enquiry to produce more concrete and useful ideas of the structure and function of the liver, it was left to the Hippocratic school in the fifth and fourth centuries BC to lay the scientific foundation for an understanding of liver diseases. For example the *Corpus hippocraticum* describes liver abscesses, which were to be opened with a cautery (a hot iron); echinococcal infection of the liver is also mentioned. Icterus (jaundice) and ascites were brought into a causal relationship with diseases of the liver. Treatment included choleretic substances (stimulating bile flow), based on the idea that an excess of bile could be regarded as a cause of disease. Another principle of treatment was eating raw liver.

Herophilus of Chalcedon (circa 300–250 BC) was the first writer to recognize the portal venous system. Erasistratus, a contemporary of Herophilus, was responsible for the description of the hepatic parenchyma (παρέγχυμα—that which is poured out beside). He was trying to express the fact that the liver tissue arises by co-agulation of blood emerging from the vessels. He attributed ascites to hardening of the liver (ζκίςςοζ) and drained it by puncturing the umbilicus.

Rome

The greatest Roman physician of the first century AD was Aulus Cornelius Celsus. He had a profound knowledge of the anatomy of the liver, which he put to practical use in surgery, particularly in the treatment of trauma to the liver.

Aretaeus of Cappadocia, in the second century AD, described the pathogenesis of obstructive jaundice and its clinical symptoms. The first great milestone in the history of hepatology was the figure of Galen of Pergamum (AD 130–200). His scientific knowledge served as the basis of hepatologic thinking for more than a millennium

Galen described the form and structure of the liver on the basis of his studies of animals, and developed a true system of liver physiology. He regarded the liver parenchyma as the seat of the specific functions of the liver. He paid particular attention to the problem of jaundice and distinguished a number of forms of it, including obstructive, symptomatic, and haemolytic jaundice. Another of Galen's achievements was the founding of experimental hepatology. He performed elegantly logical animal experiments, producing, for instance, mechanical trauma to the liver or ligating blood vessels and studying the effects.

With Galen, the scientific hepatology of antiquity came to a temporary end. In Christian teaching, which was now to dominate European thinking for more than a millenium, such studies no longer had any place. So Galen's teaching on human anatomy and pathology was uncritically passed on down to the very Renaissance itself.

Renaissance

It was left to Leonardo da Vinci (1452–1519), the greatest universal genius in the history of mankind, to give the decisive impetus to modern ideas in hepatology. He can be regarded as the father of modern hepatology. Leonardo studied the anatomy of the liver in man and recognized the course of the portal vein, the intrahepatic vessels, and the biliary system. One of the liver diseases he described was cirrhosis. However, his studies did not directly influence the course of hepatology, as they remained unpublished for 300 years: this was a reason why it was Andreas Vesalius (1514–1564) who set his stamp on Renaissance hepatology. He sketched out an anatomical picture of the liver that is still largely valid today. He was less concerned with liver diseases, but he did draw attention to the relationship between cirrhosis and alcohol.

Seventeenth century

Hepatology received a new impetus with the discovery of the circulation of the blood in 1628, by William Harvey (1578–1657). It took some time for this discovery to make its mark, however. At first it was thought that the discovery meant that the liver could have no function beyond that of bile secretion, since the idea of the liver as a blood-forming organ—an idea passed down from antiquity—had to be abandoned.

Thomas Bartholinus (1616–1680) produced a specially composed dirge to mock the liver as having no more than a bile-forming function; but after this, its structure and function were illuminated

Table 1 Milestones in hepatology

Antiquity
Homer (*Iliad*, *Odyssey*)—topography of the liver, 8th century BC
Corpus hippocraticum—description of liver diseases; surgical and conservative liver treatment, 5th to 4th centuries BC
Galen of Pergamum—anatomy and physiology of the animal liver, experimental hepatology, different forms of jaundice, 2nd century BC

Renaissance
Leonardo da Vinci—anatomy of the human liver, description of cirrhosis, 15th century
Andreas Vesalius—anatomy of the human liver, 16th century

17th century
Francis Glisson—description of the liver capsule, 1659
Johann Jacob Wepfer—discovery of the liver lobules in pigs, 1664
Thomas Sydenham—epidemiology; descriptions of epidemic jaundice by Rayger, Löw, Stegmann, 1674–1697
John Browne—first clinical description of decompensated cirrhosis, 1685

18th century
Giovanni Battista Morgagni—histopathological findings in the liver; acute yellow atrophy of the liver, echinococcus, cirrhosis, 1761
Albrecht von Haller—comprehensive treatise on the physiology of the liver, 1764
Matthew Baillie—clinical description of alcoholic cirrhosis, 1793

19th century
René Th.H. Laennec—coined the term atrophic cirrhosis, 1819
Francis Kiernan—description of liver lobules in man, 1833
Robert Carswell and Eduard Hallmann—histological description of cirrhosis, 1838–1839
C. B. Chardon—proposed an infectious agent as the cause of epidemics of jaundice, 1842
Thomas Williams—histological description of acute yellow atrophy of the liver, 1843
Karl Joseph Horaczek—clinical description of hepatic coma (biliary dyscrasia), 1844
Claude Bernard—discovery of glycogen, 1848
Rudolf Virchow—icterus catarrhalis, 1858
Friedrich Theodor Frerichs—Klinik der Leberkrankheiten (2 Bde) (clinical features of liver diseases), 1858–1861
Victor Hanot—description of primary biliary cirrhosis, 1875
Paul Ehrlich—first diagnostic liver biopsy, 1884
Lürmann and Jehn—discovery of serum hepatitis following vaccination, 1885
Stephan Kartulis—discovery of amoebae as cause of liver abscesses, 1887
Luigi Lucatello—clinical use of liver biopsy, 1895

20th century
Georg Kelling—first laparoscopy, 1901
Otto Neubauer—Ehrlich's urobilinogen test as a liver function test, 1903
Richard Bauer—galactose test as liver function test, 1906
Gustav Embden—glucose and acetone formation in the liver, 1902–1913
Hyjmans van den Bergh—measurement of serum bilirubin, 1913
Heinz Kalk—systematic use of laparoscopy, 1923
Stanford Rosenthal—bromsulphthalein test, 1924
Maki Takata—first protein lability test, 1925
H. A. Krebs and K. Henseleit—discovery of urea cycle, 1932
Hans Eppinger—*Die Leberkrankheiten* (Liver diseases), 1937
H. Voegt, F. O. McCollum, and W. H. Bradley—Icterus catarrhalis = infectious hepatitis, 1942 and 1944
Grassmann and Hannig—protein electrophoresis, 1952
F. Wroblewski, A. Karmen, and S. La Due—serum transaminase measurements, 1955
B. S. Blumberg—discovery of Australia antigen, 1965
M. Schmid—systematic classification of chronic hepatitis, 1966
D. S. Dane *et al.*—electron-microscopic identification of hepatitis B virus, 1970
S. M. Feinstone *et al.*—electron-microscopic identification of hepatitis A virus, 1973
R. H. Purcell, F. Deinhard, A. M. Prince, *et al.*—hepatitis B immunization, 1976
M. Rizetto—delta hepatitis, 1977
G. Kuo *et al.*—discovery of hepatitis C virus, 1989

by one discovery after another, and it regained its rightful place. In 1664, Johann Jacob Wepfer (1620–1695) described the liver lobules in the pig and, in 1667, Marcello Malpighi (1628–1694) gave them the name 'lobuli'. He also demonstrated that the bile was formed not in the gallbladder but in the liver parenchyma. In 1659, Francis

Glisson (1597–1677) in his comprehensive monograph *Anatomia hepatis* described the liver capsule.

All these discoveries were accompanied by a change in clinical thinking. Thomas Sydenham (1624–1689) inaugurated the science of epidemiology and drew attention to the occurrence of icterus, the different forms of which were now more accurately described. Between 1674 and 1697, Rayger, Löw, and Stegmann reported three epidemics of icterus or jaundice. The first clinical description of decompensated hepatic cirrhosis was given by John Browne in 1685. Franciscus Rubeus is believed to have observed a case of acute yellow atrophy of the liver in 1660, and Frederik Ruysch in 1691 reported on a number of cases of echinococcal infection of the liver.

Eighteenth century

In the first half of the eighteenth century, ideas on the structure of the liver were influenced by the French anatomist Antoine Ferrein (1693–1769). According to him, the liver lobules were composed of a pale cortical substance and a dark medullary substance. Giovanni Battista Bianchi (1681–1761), in his *Historia hepatica* (1725), brought together a wide variety of inflammations of the liver under the heading of 'hepatitis'. Further epidemics of jaundice were described, including one in Augsburg in 1701 which only affected children, and one each in Ferrara in 1717 and Belgrade in 1734, which occurred among soldiers in mass billets.

Two personalities set their stamp on hepatology in the second half of the eighteenth century—the Swiss physician and scientist Albrecht von Haller (1708–1777) and Giovanni Battista Morgagni (1682–1771), the founder of pathological anatomy, who taught mainly in Padua. Haller, in Part 6 of his *Elementa physiologicae corporis humani* (1764) summarized contemporary knowledge of the physiology of the liver and supplemented it with his own experimental results. His work laid the foundation of hepatological thinking in the second half of the eighteenth century.

The 79-year-old Morgagni, in his work *De sedibus et causis morborum per anatomen indagatis* (published in 1761), reported some significant observations of histopathological findings in the liver. This book is a milestone in the history of medicine. In it he draws a vivid picture of acute yellow atrophy of the liver, as the morphological substrate of hepatic coma; of *Echinococcus* with its daughter cysts in the liver, and the compression of intrahepatic blood vessels in cirrhosis.

In 1793, Matthew Baillie (1761–1823) again gave a succinct description of the clinical picture of cirrhosis, 'which is most commonly seen in heavy drinkers'.

Nineteenth century

First half

The nineteenth century was marked by an explosive expansion of hepatology. More refined methods of scientific investigation, including the practical use of the microscope, led to new and fundamental discoveries. In 1833, Francis Kiernan (1800–1874) recognized the liver lobules in man, and described their structure in words that still hold true today. The brilliant physiologist Claude Bernard (1813–1878) discovered glycogen in the liver in 1848. This was a decisive turning point in liver research, because it finally refuted the idea that the main product of the liver was bile—the liver also produced sugar.

In 1819, René Th.H. Laennec (1781–1826) gave liver cirrhosis its name. Even today it is not clear whether he was trying to derive it from κιρρός, yellow, or from σκίρρος, hardened. Definitions of cirrhosis according to histological criteria were then provided by Robert Carswell (1793–1857) in 1838, and Eduard Hallmann (1813–1855) in 1839. No less important was the first histological description of acute yellow atrophy of the liver by Thomas Williams (1819–1865) in 1843; he accompanied this with a detailed analysis of cell necrosis. The term 'acute yellow liver atrophy' was actually coined by Carl von Rokitansky (1804–1878), but he did not know of the histological picture of cell necrosis.

On the clinical front, there were two works on acute yellow liver atrophy that established the close relationship between the morphological findings in this condition and hepatic coma: Karl Joseph Horaczek (dates unknown) produced his monograph *Die gallige Dyskrasie* (biliary dyscrasia) in 1844, and Charles Ozanam (1824–1890) published his description of 'icterus gravis' in 1849. William Bowman (1816–1892) in 1842 laid down the earliest histological criteria of fatty liver.

Great attention was paid to 'liver congestion', a term meant to indicate hyperaemia of the organ. This was seen as a consequence of a variety of external insults. It was distinct from 'tropical liver', a form of congestion to which Europeans who had settled in the tropics were supposed to be particularly susceptible. The teaching of Alfred Becquerel (1814–1862), who claimed that frequent and recurrent congestion of the liver led to cirrhosis, dominated therapeutic thinking for decades. But congestion was also seen as a precursor of liver abscess, 'hepatitis suppurativa'.

Since epidemics of jaundice were observed with increasing frequency, violent arguments arose about their causation, which was attributed to climatic influences, spoiled food, and other causes. In 1842, the French physician C. B. Chardon postulated the existence of a 'miasma', a disease-provoking agent, as a cause of these epidemics; he thus recognized their infectious origin.

Second half

In 1858, Rudolf Virchow (1821–1902) formulated the doctrine of 'icterus catarrhalis'. In this concept, he believed he had found an anatomopathological explanation of the epidemics of jaundice. The plug of mucus he claimed to have observed in the papilla of Vater continued, until late in our own century, to be regarded as the anatomopathological substrate of epidemic jaundice, although Carl von Liebermeister (1833–1901) had already criticized this notion in 1864. He considered that 'icterus catarrhalis' was caused by inflammation of the liver parenchyma due to an infection.

New knowledge on epidemic jaundice was provided in 1885 by the observations of Lürmann and Jehn. Lürmann had observed an epidemic of jaundice in factory workers in Bremen after smallpox vaccination, and Jehn had made a similar observation in a lunatic asylum in Merzig in the Saarland. They very acutely observed that the epidemics of jaundice had been transferred in a bloodborne manner by the vaccination, and that the incubation period was between 2 and 6 months. This led to the identification of 'serum hepatitis', later known as hepatitis B.

Hepatologists devoted themselves intensively to attempts to differentiate between various forms of cirrhosis. Adolphe Gubler (1821–1879) distinguished between an atrophic and a hypertrophic form as early as 1853. In 1875, Victor Hanot (1844–1896) described 'une forme de cirrhose hypertrophique', and considered that changes in the biliary canaliculi were specific to this form. He considered that this was 'une cirrhose biliaire, si on pouvait dire ainsi'. Eighty years were to pass before it was recognized that Hanot had diagnosed primary biliary cirrhosis. Arguments about the different forms of cirrhosis continued to rage irrespective of all this. The clearest view was taken by Carl von Liebermeister in 1892; he recognized only two forms, portal and biliary cirrhosis.

Armand Trousseau (1801–1867) drew attention, in 1865, to the simultaneous occurrence of diabetes mellitus and cirrhosis. Heinrich Quincke (1842–1922) had been the first, in 1877, to discover iron deposits in the liver in such patients, and had coined the term 'siderosis' for them. Hanot and Schachmann named this condition 'Le diabète bronzé'. The name 'haemochromatosis' was given to the condition by Friedrich Daniel von Recklinghausen (1833–1910) in 1889, since he regarded it as being due to pathological destruction of blood.

Physicians were greatly exercised by the consequences of a certain fashionable deformity, the 'laced-corset liver'. The use of laced corsets and bodices produced the most extraordinary deformities in the liver. These were classified in a wide variety of ways, and were used to explain all kinds of abdominal complaints. Noted surgeons such as the famous Theodor Billroth (1829–1894), Victor von Hacker (1852–1933), and Carl Langenbuch (1846–1901) devised operative procedures (such as hepatorrhaphy or ventrofixation) that were intended to deal with the problem of the 'laced-corset liver'.

The 'wandering liver' described by Cantani in 1866 was probably an error based on the apparent findings at palpation and percussion. In some cases it appears to have been a form of laced-corset liver, where corsets and laced bodices had forced the liver deep into the abdominal cavity.

As late as the second half of the nineteenth century, there was a belief in a causal relationship between head injury and the occurrence of liver abscesses. Von Bärensprung, in 1875, provided a statistical proof that no such relationship existed. But the hypothesis was not exploded until 1887, when Stephan Kartulis discovered *Entamoeba histolytica* in the pus of liver abscesses. Langenbuch, in 1894, formulated the idea 'that true dysentery takes its origin from one or more kinds of amoebae. From the intestine they penetrate via the portal vein to the liver and there give rise . . . to liver abscess'.

The most prominent personality in hepatology during the second half of the nineteenth century was Friedrich Theodor Frerichs (1819–1885). In his two-volume work *Klinik der Leberkrankheiten*, published in 1858 and 1861, he made a comprehensive survey of the state of hepatology at the time, supplemented with his own clinical observations and the diagnostic methods he had developed, such as the testing of urine for leucine and tyrosine crystals in acute yellow atrophy. He produced a detailed discussion of the various types of fatty change in the liver, not all of which he regarded as necessarily pathological. Like Virchow, he distinguished between coarse- and fine-droplet fatty change.

Treatment for the liver in the nineteenth century

The therapeutic options in liver disease were limited, and opinions about them were fettered by old-fashioned ideas based on humoral pathology, which generally did more harm than good. For the treatment of 'hepatitis' and liver abscess, the main remedies were venesection, cupping, and the application of leeches to withdraw blood. Although Thierfelder in 1878 denied that such measures had any therapeutic effect, the Englishman Harley, in 1889, actually recommended direct withdrawal of blood from the liver through a trocar advanced several centimetres deep into it.

Other treatments included emetics, laxatives, calomel, and acid of saltpetre. If a liver abscess was localized, it was laid open by scalpel or punctured. The mortality of such procedures was 80 to 90 per cent. With the introduction of antiseptic and aseptic techniques, the mortality could, according to Langenbuch, be reduced to not more than 50 per cent.

Echinococcal infection of the liver was treated with iodine preparations and mercurials. The first wedge resection of liver for multilocular echinococcal cysts was performed in 1896 by Paul von Bruns.

The treatment of hepatic cirrhosis also consisted of blood letting, cupping, and leeches. Another favourite remedy was that of drinking mineral spa water from spas such as Karlsbad, Marienbad, or Mergentheim. Paracentesis of ascites by puncturing the umbilicus was another time-honoured remedy. The importance of abstention from alcohol as the foundation-stone in the treatment of cirrhosis was generally accepted. Therapeutic measures were supported by an astonishing variety of dietary regimens, with emphasis on the avoidance of coffee and spices. This line was based on Becquerel's idea that hepatic congestion provoked by rich food and drink eventually led to cirrhosis.

Twentieth century
Laboratory diagnosis

After the systematic classification of liver diseases in the nineteenth century, the first half of our own century was marked by improved laboratory diagnostic methods. This was made possible by radical new insights into hepatic metabolism. Gustav Embden (1874–1933) investigated the complex processes of glucose synthesis and acetone body formation between 1902 and 1913. Hyjmans van den Bergh, in 1913, developed a method for measuring bilirubin in the serum; Krebs and Henseleit, in 1932, discovered the urea cycle. Liver function tests were introduced into clinical medicine: Otto Neubauer, in 1903 introduced Ehrlich's urobilinogen test, Richard Bauer introduced the galactose test; Stanford Rosenthal's bromsulphthalein dye test was introduced in 1924 and Quick's hippuric acid test in 1938. The large battery of protein reactions began with Maki Takata's colloid reaction in 1925. This was followed by Weltmann's serum test, the thymol turbidity test, and many other variants of the so-called protein flocculation tests, until in 1952 a new step forward was taken in the form of protein electrophoresis invented by Grassmann and Hannig and Wuhrmann and Wunderly.

However, these laboratory tests all suffered from the fault of being non-specific and providing only a rough picture of pathological changes in the liver. It was only the appearance of enzyme diagnostic techniques (transaminases) in the mid-1950s that provided a decisive improvement here. The pioneering works in this field were published by Wroblewski's group in New York and de Ritis' in Italy in 1955 and 1956.

Liver biopsy, laparoscopy, and ultrasound

The uncertain and non-specific nature of the so-called liver function tests left physicians still searching for direct diagnostic approaches based on morphological findings.

It was long held to be a matter of certain knowledge that the Italian Luigi Lucatello performed the first diagnostic liver biopsies, which he reported in 1895. It was forgotten that the famous scientist Paul Ehrlich (1854–1915) had anticipated him in puncturing the liver for the same purpose. Only Frerichs in a footnote to his book *Ueber den Diabetes* (1884) had related this fact. While Ehrlich and Lucatello had used thin cannulas to puncture the liver, enabling them to obtain only small amounts of tissue on which only cytological investigation was possible, Feruccio Schupfer shortly afterwards used needles with a diameter of up to 2 mm. In 1907, he was in a position to report on a whole series of hepatic and splenic punctures. Liver biopsy, however, only found more widespread clinical application with the work of Bingel (1923), Iversen and Roholm (1939), and Silverman (1938); the last used a split needle rather than an aspiration needle. The complication rate with all these biopsy techniques was relatively high and it was only the introduction of the far safer technique of one-second biopsy by Menghini in 1958 that brought a breakthrough with the widespread introduction of liver biopsy into clinical medicine.

In Germany in particular, morphological diagnosis of liver disease was based primarily on macroscopic inspection of the organ. In 1901, Georg Kelling reported on the possibility of imaging the abdomen after the introduction of air into the abdominal cavity. The Swede Hans Christian Jacobaeus introduced abdominal imaging into clinical practice in 1912. In 1923, quite independently, Heinz Kalk introduced the technique of 'laparoscopy' and stressed above all the importance of inspecting the surface of the liver. He supplemented his macroscopic diagnoses by directed puncture of the liver followed by histological examination of the core of tissue he obtained. In an overview of macroscopic and microscopic findings, he developed his own nomenclature for liver diseases, which became standard terminology on the continent of Europe but achieved only limited acceptance in English-speaking countries. At the beginning of the 1970s, abdominal ultrasound became part of routine liver diagnosis. Today, combined with ultrasound-assisted liver biopsy, it has replaced laparoscopy to a large extent.

Viral hepatitis

Virchow's teaching on 'icterus catarrhalis' overshadowed far more progressive views on the aetiology and pathogenesis of viral hepatitis in our own century. Even Hans Eppinger (1879–1946) in his well-known work *Die Leberkrankheiten* ('Liver disorders'), in 1937, obstinately denied the epidemic nature of hepatitis and claimed that it was due to a faulty diet. Yet even in 1919 Lindstedt in Sweden had put forward the term 'hepatitis' for icterus catarrhalis, and had tried to distinguish the epidemic form from serum hepatitis. But it was only the worldwide epidemics of hepatitis during the Second World War that led to the general recognition of the infective nature of Virchow's 'icterus catarrhalis'. In Germany, Voegt proved the point in 1942 by transmission experiments in man; the same was done in the United States by McCollum and Bradley in 1944, and Findlay and Willcox in 1945. The viruses responsible for hepatitis A and B however remained unknown, until hepatitis research

entered a new phase with the discovery of the Australia antigen by Blumberg in 1965. The crucial paper on the subject, for which Blumberg later received the Nobel Prize, was initially turned down by the publishers of a reputable specialist journal.

In 1970, Dane and his group identified the virus of hepatitis B under the electron microscope. The virus of hepatitis A was identified by Feinstone and his group in 1973. A further form, the delta agent associated with hepatitis B, was identified in 1977 by Rizetto. In 1989, Kuo and his group succeeded in identifying the virus of what used to be termed non-A, non-B hepatitis, and which is now termed hepatitis C.

Chronic liver diseases

In the last century, there was vigorous argument over the possibility of other causes besides alcohol abuse for the development of hepatic cirrhosis. In addition to a variety of foods and beverages, for example coffee and spices, it was believed that malaria, syphilis, and tuberculosis could produce cirrhosis. In the twentieth century, the possible relationship between viral hepatitis and cirrhosis has come to prominence. It took decades before it was demonstrated that acute hepatitis B and hepatitis C could become chronic, and that this was not the case of hepatitis A and hepatitis E which are transmitted by the intestinal route. The hypothesis that fatty liver and liver of undernutrition lead to cirrhosis was not confirmed.

The possibility of follow-up histological observations based on repeated biopsy influenced our models of liver disease, and these have thus become predominantly morphological rather than functional. With the wide variety of microscopic pictures, systematic classification has been difficult. The concept of the progression of acute viral hepatitis to a chronic form has been accepted on the European continent since the investigations carried out by Heinz Kalk in 1947. However, this only became established in the English-speaking world in the 1950s. In 1966, the Swiss hepatologist, Schmid, suggested subdividing chronic hepatitis into chronic persistent and chronic aggressive forms on the basis of morphological and clinical criteria. This soon gained universal acceptance. However, as the viruses of five different hepatitis forms have now been identified and can be serologically determined, this subdivision is now regarded as outdated.

Among all the personalities who have given a crucial impetus to experimental and clinical hepatology during this century, let us name just three representative figures: Hans Eppinger (1879–1946), Hans Popper (1904–1988), and Dame Sheila Sherlock (born 1918).

Treatments

At the beginning of the twentieth century, the accepted treatments were the traditional ones inherited from the nineteenth century, such as blood letting and leeches, laxatives, mineral waters, and various diets. The discovery of lipotropic substances by Best and Huntsman (1932) led to an entirely new line of therapeutic thinking in the 1930s. The amazing effects of choline and methionine in toxic liver damage in experimental animals were taken over into human pathology. With superstitious reverence, these substances were injected, infused, or administered orally. Even in hepatic coma, patients were still subjected to infusions of choline and methionine. It was even thought that alcoholic cirrhosis could be benefited by a

Table 2 Gallstone disease
Gentile da Foligno—first description of gallstones in man, circa 1400
Thomas Bartholinus—liver colic caused by gallstones, 1661
Albrecht von Haller—classification of gallstones, 1764
A. F. Fourcroy—first chemical analysis of gallstones, 1789
Etienne Frédéric Bouisson—inflammation of the gallbladder identified as a consequence of gallstones, 1843
Meckel von Hemsbach—*Ueber die Concremente im thierischen Organismus*, 1856; inflammation of the gallbladder identified as the cause of gallstones
Bernhard Naunyn—*Klinik der Cholelithiasis* (Clinical features of cholelithiasis), 1892; lithogenic catarrh
Carl Langenbuch—first cholecystectomy, 1882
E. A. Graham and W. H. Cole—first cholecystography, 1924
McCune *et al.*—first endoscopic retrograde cholecystography, 1924
J. S. Thistle and L. J. Schoenfield—*in vivo* gallstone dissolution, 1971
T. Sauerbruch *et al.* H. L. Greiner *et al.*—shock-wave lithotripsy, 1985/1986
E. Mühe and Mourat—laparoscopic cholecystectomy, 1986/1987

protein-rich diet (as suggested by Patek and Post in 1938). Curd diets were so popular that they bred an army of curd fanatics.

Effective treatment was only available for decompensated cirrhosis with ascites; the backbone of the treatment was the low-sodium diet introduced in 1903 by Strauss and Widal. The first drugs used were mercurial preparations followed by saluretics, and, from the 1960s onwards, aldosterone antagonists. Surgical treatments such as the omentopexy introduced by Talma in 1898, did not find favour. An entirely new approach was created by liver transplantation, first carried out by Starzl and his group in 1963.

The most important therapeutic advance may have been that of prophylaxis against hepatitis B by active immunization. A logical process of scientific research (by Purcell, Deinhard, Prince, and others) made this treatment generally available from 1976 onward. The availability of α-interferon opened up new treatment options, especially in the case of hepatitis B.

Gallstone disease
Earliest descriptions

Strangely enough, gallstones were not described by the physicians of antiquity, although the popular and widespread practice of inspection of the liver included an inspection of the gallbladder. The first description of gallstones in animals was given by the Arabian physician Rhazes about AD 900, who observed gallstones in oxen. Five hundred more years passed before Gentile da Foligno (d. 1438), working in Perugia, first observed gallstones in a human cadaver (Table 2). Some hundred years later, in 1506, Antonio Benivieni again described gallstones in humans. Further reports followed at short intervals, and in the seventeenth century the distinctive clinical features of gallbladder and bile duct stones were known. Thus, Scultet in 1622 pointed out that bile duct stones produced jaundice, and noted as a peculiar fact that this did not occur in one case he had observed. Fernel identified gallstones in the stool and Thomas Bartholinus, in 1661, explained the pain of 'liver colic' by the passage of gallstones through the common bile duct. Sydenham, however, still regarded 'liver colic' as being hysterical.

Eighteenth and nineteenth centuries

Systematic investigation of gallstone disease was undertaken in the eighteenth century. The English physician Thomas Coe (1704–1761), in his work *Treatise on biliary concretions: or stones in the gallbladder and ducts*, published in 1757, gave an overview of gallstone disease and put forward theories about its origin. Albrecht von Haller, in 1764, undertook a classification of gallstones based on their shape and composition. Samuel Thomas Sömmerring (1755–1830) followed with a review of more than 200 literary citations on the state of gallstone research. Friedrich August Walter, in his *Anatomical Museum* (1796), depicted gallstones in all their multifarious variations in a series of coloured engravings. The first chemical analysis of gallstones was performed by Fourcroy in 1789. By then it was already believed that immoderate eating and lack of exercise promoted gallstone formation, but emotional factors were also held to be responsible.

In the first half of the nineteenth century, Etienne Frédéric Bouisson (1813–1884) made a vital contribution to gallstone research in his treatise *De la bile, de ses variétés physiologiques et de ses altérations morbides* (1843). He saw inflammation of the gallbladder as a consequence, not a cause, of gallstone formation. His views were opposed by Robilier (1843) and Heim (1846), who saw an opposite causal sequence.

The most fundamental work on gallstones was written by Meckel von Hemsbach (1822–1856), who died at the age of 34 before completing his manuscript *Ueber die Concremente intramuscular thierischen Organismus*. Theodor Billroth published it in 1856, the year of Meckel's death. Meckel was of the opinion that gallstones arose from a catarrh of the gallbladder wall. He distinguished eight varieties of gallstones, including solitary cholesterol stones.

Further attempts at classification were undertaken by Frerichs in 1861 and Thudichum in 1863. The question of whether gallstones were formed first, followed by inflammation of the gallbladder, or vice versa, continued to dominate the discussion. In 1892 Bernhard Naunyn (1839–1925) in his work *Klinik der Cholelithiasis* brought matters to a temporary conclusion with his doctrine of 'lithogenic catarrh' as the cause of gallstone formation. Various experiments appeared to support his view. Naunyn's doctrine was refuted in

1909, when Ludwig Aschoff and Bacmeister produced the thesis that it was not lithogenic catarrh but biliary stagnation that was responsible for gallstone formation. Great attention has been paid in the past century to the clinical features of gallstone disease, with particular attention to biliary colic and to the question of whether gallstones could pass through the bile duct into the intestine without attacks of pain. Friedrich Hoffmann and Johann Peter Frank, in the eighteenth century, were already convinced that smaller stones could pass through the papilla of Vater without causing colic or jaundice. It was only after the middle of the nineteenth century that it was generally accepted that 'biliary colic' was identical with the old 'liver colic' which Sydenham had believed to be hysterical in origin.

Treatments

In the presurgical era, it was the principal concern of physicians to promote the passage of gallstones via the intestine, with the use of laxatives, choleretics, and mineral waters. The success of treatment was monitored with the stool sieve. Sieved-out gallstones were then subjected to physical and chemical analysis, and could easily be distinguished from faecoliths. Spas such as Marienbad, Karlsbad, and Mergentheim were popular places to go for 'cures' for the passage of gallstones, and this brought these places to prominence.

Attempts at *in-vivo* dissolution of stones date back to the seventeenth and eighteenth centuries. A favourite treatment was the grass cure, consisting of no more than eating raw grass. This was recommended not only by Morgagni but also by Maria Theresa's personal physician Gerhard van Swieten (1700–1772). This remedy was based on observations believed to have been made in oxen, who were supposed to develop gallstones in winter after feeding on hay, while these stones disappeared again in summer when the animals lived on grass. The French botanist Durande, in 1770, expressed the opinion that ingestion of a mixture of sulphuric ether and turpentine oil could achieve the dissolution of gallstones. This was immediately disputed by the famous chemist Thenard (1777–1857). Nevertheless, both 'Durande's treatment' and a variety of 'oil treatments' have survived to our own day, although since 1971 we have possessed effective treatments for the *in-vivo* dissolution of cholesterol stones, in the form of chenodeoxycholic and ursodeoxycholic acids.

The introduction of cholecystectomy by Carl Langenbuch in 1882 represented a turning-point in therapy. Although initially almost overlooked, this operative procedure had conquered the whole world by the 1890s. As early as 1884, Langenbuch also performed the first choledochotomy.

For several decades, cholecystectomy was considered to be the best treatment for gallstone disease. Advances occurred only in preoperative diagnosis, for example by cholecystography, described by Graham and Cole in 1924, and cholangiography, first successfully performed by Reich in 1918. Almost 50 years were to pass before the diagnostic repertoire was broadened by the addition of endoscopic retrograde cholangiography and soon after by ultrasound. Mechanical lithotripsy and endoscopic papillotomy (L. Demling, K. Kawai in 1972) brought about a renaissance with modern methods of attempts by earlier physicians to expel gallstones through the papilla of Vater. This reached a climax with shock-wave lithotripsy, developed in 1985 by Sauerbruch and 1986 by Greiner. Since then, it has faded into the background due to laparoscopic cholecystectomy which was first performed successfully in 1986 and 1987 by Mühe and Mourat respectively.

Bibliography

1. Beal JM. Historical perspective of gallstone disease. *Surgery Gynecology and Obstetrics*, 1984; **158**: 181–9.
2. Drossart R. *Historische Studien zum Problem der Fettleber*. Inaugural Dissertation, Düsseldorf, 1976.
3. Franken FH. *Die Leber und ihre Krankheiten. 200 Jahre Hepatologie*. Stuttgart: Enke, 1968.
4. Franken FH and Falk H. The history of liver therapy. In: Schaffner F, Sherlock S, and Leevy CM, eds. *The liver and its diseases*. New York: Intercontinental Medical Book Corporation, 1974: 117–25.
5. Franken FH. History of hepatology. In: Csomós G and Thaler H, eds. *Clinical hepatology*. Berlin: Springer, 1983: 1–15.
6. Franken FH. Geschichte der Therapie des Gallensteinleidens. *Therapeutische Umschau*, 1993; 50: 532–4.
7. Hinssen M. *Ein Beitrag zur Geschichte der Hepatitis-infectiosa-Epidemien in Europa vom Ende des 17. bis zur Mitte des 19. Jahrhunderts*. Inaugural Dissertation, Düsseldorf, 1966.
8. Lehr CH. *Geschichte der Laparoskopie und Biopsie der Leber*. Inaugural Dissertation, Düsseldorf, 1967.
9. Mani N. *Die historischen Grundlagen der Leberforschung. I. Teil: Antike. II. Teil: Von Galen bis Claude Bernard*. Basel: Schwabe, I. Teil, 1959, II. Teil, 1967.
10. Trüb HD. *Ein Beitrag zur Geschichte der Hepatitis-infectiosa-Epidemien in Europa in der 2. Hälfte des 19 Jahrhunderts*. Düsseldorfer Arbeiten zur Geschichte der Medizin. Düsseldorf: Triltsch Verlag, 1979.

32

Appendices

32.1 Geographic distribution of infections causing liver disease

Tom Doherty and A. J. Hall

The following pages contain tabulated data on the frequency of the important hepatic infections in different parts of the world. Since disease surveillance does not exist for most of these infections nor for the diseases that they may cause, the information is largely based on serological or parasitological surveys. The data may hide marked variation between different geographical groups and between social groups within the country. Thus, although malaria occurs in both Kenya and Argentina, almost every child on the Kenyan coast will experience at least one attack of malaria during each rainy season, while in Argentina malaria transmission is confined to one small area in the north of the country. Equally, not everyone in a specific geographical location is at risk of contracting a particular disease: people on package tours to Kenya are at relatively low risk of contracting schistosomiasis when compared to fishermen earning their livelihood from Lake Malawi.

'Frequency' is used to indicate the risk of infection between different countries, i.e., between rows in the table. The scale used for different diseases varies, so comparisons cannot be made between diseases, i.e., across the columns. The information can be used in two ways. First, it gives some indication of which infectious liver diseases exist in each country. Second, it gives some idea of the potential risk associated with travel to the country, risk that is influenced by behaviour. Hepatitis A is an ubiquitous virus, but people are only affected in conditions where standards of sanitation are poor. In general, hepatitis B and C can only be contracted through sexual contact or transfusion of blood products, although in much of Africa and Asia hepatitis B is transmitted from child to child by an unknown route. Yellow fever is a sporadic infection in Latin America; in Africa it occurs in epidemics in urban areas.

The data were compiled from various sources: the Centre for Disease Control in Atlanta, Georgia, United States, publishes annual handbooks containing advice for international travellers: the World Health Organization and World Bank publish annual reports; one invaluable book is *A world guide to infections* by Mary E. Wilson (Oxford University Press, 1991).

In each table, + + implies the disease is common; + implies it is quite frequent; ± implies it occurs, but is rare; – implies that the infection is not recognized as an important hazard, and ? implies that the information is not available.

Abbreviations included in the tables

HAV	hepatitis A virus
HBV	hepatitis B virus
HCV	hepatitis C virus
HEV	hepatitis E virus
Mal	malaria
SM	*Schistosoma mansoni*
Schisto	schistosomiasis (*haematobium, japonicum* or *mansoni*)
Lep	leptospirosis
YF	yellow fever
CS	*Clonorchis sinensis*
VL	visceral leishmaniasis
Hyd	hydatid disease (*Echinococcus granulosus*)
EH	*Entamoeba histolytica*

Table 1 Frequency of infectious liver diseases in Africa

	EH	HAV	HBV	HCV	HEV	Hyd	Lep	VL	Mal	SM	YF
Algeria	+	+	+	?	?	+ +	+	+	+	±	−
Angola	+	+	+ +	?	?	+	+	±	+ +	+ +	+
Benin	+	+	+	?	?	+	+	−	+ +	+ +	+
Botswana	+	+	+ +	?	+	±	+	−	+	+	−
Burkina Faso	+	+	+ +	?	?	−	+	±	+ +	+ +	+
Burundi	+	+	+	?	?	+	+	−	+ +	+ +	+
Cameroon	+	+	+ +	+	?	−	+	±	+ +	+ +	+
Central African Republic	+	+	+	+	?	−	+	±	+ +	+ +	+
Chad	+	+	+ +	?	?	±	+	+	+ +	+ +	+
Congo	+	+	+	?	?	−	+	−	+ +	+ +	+
Côte d'Ivoire	+	+	+ +	?	+	−	+	−	+ +	+ +	+
Democratic Republic of the Congo (formerly Zaire)	+	+	+	?	?	±	+	±	+ +	+ +	+
Egypt	+	+	+	+ +	?	+	±	+	+	+ +	−
Equatorial Guinea	+	+	+	?	?	−	+ +	−	+ +	+	+
Ethiopa	+	+	+ +	?	+	+ +	+	+ +	+	+ +	+
Gabon	+	+	+	+	?	−	+	−	+ +	+ +	+
Gambia	+	+	+ +	+	+	±	+	−	+ +	+ +	+
Ghana	+	+	+ +	?	+	±	+ +	−	+ +	+ +	+
Guinea	+	+	+ +	?	?	−	+ +	−	+ +	+ +	+
Guinea Bissau	+	+	+ +	?	?	−	+	+	+ +	+ +	+
Kenya	+	+	+	?	?	+ +	+	+ +	+ +	+ +	+
Lesotho	+	+	+	?	+	±	±	−	−	+	−
Liberia	+	+	+ +	?	?	−	±	−	+	+	+
Libya	+	+	+	?	+ +	+	+ +	+	±	+	−
Madagascar	+	+	+	?	?	+	+	−	+	+	−
Malawi	+	+	+	?	?	±	+	±	+ +	+	−
Mali	+	+	+ +	?	?	±	+	−	+ +	+ +	+
Mauritania	+	+	+	?	?	−	+	−	+	+	−
Mauritius	+	+	+	?	?	−	+	−	+	+	+
Morocco	+	+	+	?	?	+ +	+	±	±	±	−
Mozambique	+	+	+	?	?	±	+	±	+ +	+ +	−
Namibia	+	+	+	?	+	±	±	−	+	+	−
Niger	+	+	+ +	+	?	±	+	+	+ +	+ +	+
Nigeria	+	+	+ +	?	+	±	+	±	+ +	+ +	+
Rwanda	+	+	+	?	?	+	±	±	+ +	+ +	+
Senegal	+	+	+	+	?	−	+ +	−	+ +	+ +	+
Seychelles	+	+	+	?	?	−	±	−	−	−	−
Sierra Leone	+	+	+ +	?	?	−	+	−	+ +	+ +	+
Somalia	+	+	+ +	?	+	+ +	+	+	+ +	+	+
South Africa	+	+	+	?	+	−	±	−	+	+ +	−
Sudan	+	+	+ +	?	+	+	+	+ +	+ +	+ +	+
Swaziland	+	+	+	?	?	±	±	−	+	+ +	−
Tanzania	+	+	+	?	?	+	+	−	+ +	+ +	+
Togo	+	+	+ +	?	?	−	+	−	+ +	+ +	+
Tunisia	+	+	+	?	?	+ +	±	+	−	±	−
Uganda	+	+	+	?	?	±	+	±	+ +	+ +	+
Western Sahara	+	+	+	?	?	?	?	?	±	+	−
Zambia	+	+	+	?	?	±	+	±	+ +	+ +	+
Zimbabwe	+	+	+	?	?	±	+	−	+ +	+ +	−

Table 2 Frequency of infectious liver diseases in the Americas

	EH	HAV	HBV	HCV	HEV	Hyd	Lep	VL	Mal	SM	YF
Anguilla	±	+	+	?	?	−	+	−	−	−	−
Antigua	±	+	+	?	?	−	+	−	−	+	−
Argentina	+	+	+	?	?	+ +	+	±	±	−	−
Aruba	+	+	+	?	?	−	+	−	−	−	−
Bahamas	+	+	+	?	?	−	+	−	−	−	−
Barbados	±	+	+	?	?	−	+	−	−	−	−
Belize	+	+	+	?	?	−	+ +	−	+	−	−
Bolivia	+	+	+	?	?	+	−	±	+	−	±
British Virgin Islands	±	+	+	?	?	−	+	−	−	−	−
Brazil	+	+	+	?	?	+	+ +	+	+	+	±
Canada	−	+	+	+	−	+	−	−	−	−	−
Cayman	±	+	+	?	?	−	±	−	−	−	−
Chile	+	+	+	?	+	+	+	−	−	−	−
Columbia	+	+	+	?	?	−	+	±	+	−	±
Costa Rica	+	+	+	?	?	±	+	−	+	−	−
Cuba	+	+	+	?	?	−	+	−	−	−	−
Dominica	+	+	+	?	?	−	+	−	−	−	−
Dominican Republic	+	+	+	?	?	−	+	−	+	+	−
Ecuador	+	+	+	?	?	+	±	±	+	−	±
El Salvador	+	+	+	?	?	+	+	+	+	−	−
Grenada	+	+	+	?	?	−	+ +	−	−	−	−
Guadeloupe	+	+	+	?	?	−	+	−	−	+	−
Guatemala	+	+	+	?	?	+	+	±	+	−	−
Haiti	+ +	+	+	?	?	±	+	−	+	−	−
Honduras	+	+	+	?	?	+	+	±	+	−	−
Jamaica	+	+	+	?	?	−	+ +	−	−	−	−
Martinique	±	+	+	?	?	−	+	−	−	+	−
Mexico	+ +	+	+	?	+	+	+	+	+	−	−
Montserrat	±	+	+	?	?	−	+	−	−	+	−
Netherlands Antilles	±	+	+	?	?	−	+	−	−	−	−
Nicaragua	+	+	+	?	?	−	+	+	+	−	−
Panama	+	+	+	?	?	−	+	−	+	−	±
Paraguay	+	+	+	?	?	−	−	−	+	−	±
Peru	+	+	+	?	?	+	±	±	+	−	±
Puerto Rico	±	+	+	?	−	−	±	−	−	−	±
St Kitts and Nevis	±	+	+	?	?	−	+	−	−	−	−
St Lucia	±	+	+	?	?	−	+	−	−	±	−
St Vincent and the Grenadines	±	+	+	?	?	−	+	−	−	−	−
Surinam	±	+	+	?	?	−	+	±	+	+	±
Trinidad and Tobago	+	+	+	?	?	−	+ +	−	−	−	±
Turks and Caicos	±	+	+	?	?	−	±	−	−	−	−
United States	±	+	+	+	−	+	±	−	−	−	−
Uruguay	+	+	+	?	?	+	+	−	−	−	−
Venezuela	+	+	+	?	?	+	+	±	+	±	±
Virgin Islands	±	+	+	?	?	−	±	−	−	−	−

Table 3 Frequency of infectious liver diseases in Asia and Australasia

	EH	HAV	HBV	HCV	HEV	Hyd	VL	Mal	Schisto	CS
Afghanistan	+	+	+	?	+	+	±	+	−	−
Australia	−	±	±	+	−	±	−	−	−	−
Bangladesh	+ +	+ +	+	?	+	+	+	+	−	−
Bhutan	+	+	+	?	?	+	±	+	−	−
Brunei	+	+	+	?	?	−	−	−	−	−
China	±	+	+ +	+	+	+	±	±	±	+
Fiji	+	+	+	?	?	−	−	−	−	−
Hong Kong	±	+	+ +	?	?	−	−	−	−	+
India	+ +	+ +	+	?	+	+	+	+	±	−
Indonesia	+ +	+ +	+ +	?	+	±	−	+	+	+
Japan	±	+	+	+ +	+	−	−	−	−	+
Kampuchea	+	+	+	?	?	±	±	+	+	+
Korea (North)	+	+	+ +	?	?	−	−	−	−	+
Korea (South)	+	+	+ +	?	?	−	−	−	−	+
Laos	+	+	+ +	?	?	±	−	+	+	+
Malaysia	+	+	+	?	?	−	−	+	+	+
Mongolia	±	+	+	?	?	+	±	−	−	−
Micronesia	+	+	+	?	?	−	−	+	−	−
Myanmar	+	+ +	+ +	?	+	±	±	+	−	+
Nepal	+ +	+ +	+	?	+	+	+	+	−	−
New Zealand	−	±	±	+	−	±	−	−	−	−
Pakistan	+ +	+ +	+	?	+	+	±	+	−	−
Papua New Guinea	+ +	+ +	+ +	?	?	−	−	+	−	−
Philippines	+	+ +	+	?	?	±	−	+	+	+
Singapore	+	+ +	+	?	?	−	−	−	−	+
Sri Lanka	+	+ +	+	?	?	+	−	+	−	−
Taiwan	±	+	+ +	?	?	+	−	−	−	+
Thailand	+	+ +	+ +	?	?	±	−	+	±	+
Vietnam	+	+	+ +	?	?	±	−	+	−	+

Table 4 Frequency of infectious liver diseases in the Middle East

	EH	HAV	HBV	HCV	HEV	Schisto	Mal	Hyd
Bahrain	+	+	+	?	+	−	−	±
Cyprus	+	+	+	?	+	−	−	+ +
Democratic Yemen	+	+	+	?	+	±	+	±
Iran	+	+	+	?	+	+	+	+
Iraq	+	+	+	?	+	+	+	+ +
Israel	+	+	+	?	+	−	−	+
Jordan	+	+	+	?	+	±	−	+
Kuwait	+	+	+	?	+	−	−	±
Lebanon	+	+	+	?	+	±	−	+
Oman	+	+	+	?	+	±	+	±
Qatar	+	+	+	?	+	−	−	±
Saudi Arabia	+	+	+	+	+	+	+	+
Syria	+	+	+	?	+	+	±	+ +
Turkey	+	+	+	?	+	±	+	+ +
United Arab Emirates	+	+	+	?	+	−	±	±
Yemen	+	+ +	+ +	?	+	+	+	±

Table 5 Prevalence of infectious liver diseases in Europe

	EH	HAV	HBV	HCV	HEV	Hyd	Lep	VL	Mal
Albania	−	+	?	?	?	+	?	±	−
Armenia	−	±	±	±	−	−	−	−	−
Austria	−	±	±	±	−	−	−	±	−
Azerbaijan	−	±	+ +	±	+	+	+	−	±
Belarus	−	±	±	±	−	−	−	−	−
Belgium	−	±	±	±	−	−	−	−	−
Bosnia-Hercegovina	−	±	±	?	−	+	+	±	−
Bulgaria	−	±	+ +	±	−	−	+	±	−
Croatia	−	±	±	±	−	+	+	±	−
Czech Republic	−	±	±	±	−	+	+	±	−
Denmark	−	±	±	±	−	−	−	−	−
Estonia	−	±	±	±	−	−	?	−	−
Finland	−	±	±	±	−	−	−	−	−
France	−	±	±	±	−	±	+	±	−
Georgia	−	±	±	±	−	−	−	−	−
Germany	−	±	±	±	−	−	−	−	−
Gibraltar	−	±	+	+	−	−	+	±	−
Greece	−	±	+	?	−	+	?	±	−
Hungary	−	±	±	?	−	±	+	±	−
Iceland	−	±	±	±	−	−	−	−	−
Ireland	−	±	±	±	−	−	−	−	−
Italy	−	+	±	±	−	+	+	±	−
Kazakhstan	−	+	+ +	±	+	+ +	+	−	−
Kyrgyzstan	−	+	+ +	±	+	+	+	−	−
Latvia	−	±	±	±	−	−	−	−	−
Lithuania	−	±	±	±	−	−	−	−	−
Luxembourg	−	±	±	±	−	−	−	−	−
Malta	−	±	±	±	−	−	+	±	−
Moldova	−	±	+ +	±	−	−	?	−	−
Netherlands	−	±	±	±	−	−	−	−	−
Norway	−	±	±	±	−	−	−	−	−
Poland	−	±	±	±	−	±	−	−	−
Portugal	−	+	±	±	−	+	+	±	−
Romania	−	+	+ +	±	−	+	+	−	−
Russia	−	±	±	±	−	−	−	−	−
Serbia	−	±	±	±	−	+	+	±	−
Slovakia	−	±	±	±	−	+	+	±	−
Slovenia	−	±	±	±	−	+	+	±	−
Spain	−	+	±	+	−	+	+	±	−
Sweden	−	±	±	±	−	−	−	−	−
Switzerland	−	±	±	±	−	−	−	−	−
Tajikistan	−	+	+ +	±	+	+	−	−	±
Turkmenistan	−	+	+ +	±	+	+	−	−	−
Ukraine	−	±	±	±	−	−	−	−	−
Uzbekistan	−	+	+ +	±	+	+	−	−	−
United Kingdom	−	±	±	±	−	−	±	−	−

32.2 Liver injury in man ascribed to non-drug chemicals and natural toxins

Regine Kahl

Explanation of abbreviations

Column B

I Cross-sectional study

    (a) With control group; verification of exposure by:
        Detection of the chemical at the workplace
        And/or detection of the chemical in body fluids/tissues
        And/or presence of specific signs of intoxication
    (b) With control group; verification of exposure by anamnesis
    (c) Without control group; verification of exposure as Ia
    (d) Without control group; verification of exposure as Ib

II Screening at the workplace

    (a) With control group
    (b) Without control group

III Case report

IV Retrospective study

    (a) Case–control study
    (b) Without control
    (c) Cohort mortality study

V Report on epidemic outbreak

VI Register of cases

VII Report on correlation between disease incidence and exposure in large populations

Persons

In general this indicates number of persons exposed. A figure followed by an asterisk indicates total number of persons in the study.

Column D

One or several of the liver function tests indicated were abnormal
Abbreviations are used as below:

ALP = alkaline phosphatase
bili = bilirubin
BSP = sulphobromophthalein excretion
GlDH = glutamate dehydrogenase
GOT = serum glutamate oxalacetate (aspartate amino-transferase)
GPT = serum glutamate pyruvate (alanine aminotransferase)
GGT = γ-glutamyl transpeptidase
ICG = indocyanine green clearance
LDH = lactate dehydrogenase
LFT = liver function tests
OCT = ornithine carbamoyl transferase
SDH = sorbitol dehydrogenase
thymol = thymol turbidity test positive
\# = Biopsy or autopsy (diagnosis mostly as stated by the authors).

Column E

(a) Suggested by study protocol.
(b) Observed during the course of an acute disease for which other major causes were not obvious.
(c) Exposure history positive; chemical detected in body fluids/tissues and/or other specific signs of intoxication present. Other cause not excluded.
(d) Exposure history positive. Other cause not excluded.
(e) Very rare event in general population.
(f) Relief upon cessation of exposure.
(g) Recurrence on re-exposure.
(h) No causal relationship obvious.

A Chemical	B Type of study (no. of persons)	C Exposure	D Diagnosis (no. of persons)	E Causal relationship	F Reference
Acetone[1]	III (1)	Chronic/occupational Acetone recycling	bili	b, f	Sack, ArchGewerbepathGewerbehyg, 1941; 10:80
Acrylonitrile	Ia (102)	Chronic/occupational Acrylic fibre factory	Palpable liver (20%, control 13%) LFTs normal	a	Sakurai, BrJIndMed, 1941; 35:219
Aflatoxin B₁,	V (26)	Acute/alimentary Ingestion of mouldy rice	Palpable liver	b	Ling, JFormosanMedAss, 1967; 66: 517
	(397)	Ingestion of mouldy corn	Jaundice Bile duct proliferation Periportal fibrosis #	b	Krishnamachari, Lancet, 1975; i:1061
	III (1)	Ingestion of mouldy cassava	Diffuse necrosis #	b	Serck-Hanssen, ArchEnvironHlth, 1970; 20:729
	(1)	Ingestion of mouldy rice	Reye's syndrome[2] Fatty liver#	d	Bourgois, JMedAssThai, 1969; 52:553
	IVb (23)	Ingestion of mouldy food	Reye's syndrome	d	Shank, FoodCosmTox, 1971; 9:501
	III (1)	Ingestion of contaminated oil	Hepatomegaly GOT, GPT Microvesicular steatosis#	d	Sinniah, AmJGastr, 1982; 77:158
	VII	Chronic/alimentary	Encephalopathy; Reye's syndrome Hepatocellular carcinoma	d	Alpert, Cancer, 1971; 28:253 Peers, IntJCanc, 1976; 17:167 Peers, BrJCanc, 1973; 27:473 Shank, FoodCosmTox, 1972; 10:61 Shank, FoodCosmTox, 1972; 10:71 van Rensburg, SAMedJ, 1974; 48: 2508 Keen, TropGeogMed, 1971; 23:35 Campbell, JNCI, 1974; 52:1647
Allyl chloride	IIb (60)	Chronic/occupational Allyl chloride production	bili, thymol, GOT, GPT, LDH, GDH, SDH	d, f	Häusler, ArchToxicol, 1968; 23:209
Amanita phalloides	III (5)	Acute/alimentary Ingestion	GOT, GPT, LDH, ALP, bili Massive necrosis#	b, f	Harrison, AmJMed, 1965; 38:787
	III (8)		GOT,GPT Centrilobular necrosis#	b, f	Wepler, HumPath, 1972; 3:249
	III (1)		GOT, GPT, LDH	b	Plotzker, AmJMedSci, 1982; 283:79
	IVb (205)		Maximal values measured on day 2 of intoxication (means of 205 patients) GOT 1634; GPT 1599; LDH 1649; bili 5.6	b	Floersheim, SchMedWoch, 1982; 112: 1164
Aniline	III (1)	Chronic/suicidal Ingestion	Acute degenerative changes#	b	Janik-Kuryłcio, PolTygLek, 1973; 28: 1241

Agent	Code (no.)	Exposure	Effect	Note	Reference
Arsenic[3]	III (1)	Chronic/medicinal Fowler's solution	Portal hypertension#	c	Knolle, DMedWoch, 1974; 99:903
	(2)				Morris, Gastro, 1974; 64:86
	(1)				Chainuvati, DigDisSci, 1979; 24:70
	(1)				Cowlishaw, AustNZJMed, 1979; 9:310
	IVb (220)	Chronic/occupational Vintners	Hepatomegaly (70%) Cirrhosis (20%?)	d	Harren, DeutschArchKlinMed, 1943; 190:31
	(15)		Cirrhosis#	c	Liebegott, DMedWoch, 1949; 74:855
	(82)		Cirrhosis (28)#	d	Roth, ZblAllgPath, 1960; 100:34
	IVb (220)		Primary liver cell carcinoma (3)#	c	Liebegott, DMedWoch, 1949; 74:855
	III (1)	Chronic/occupational Arsenic plant		c	Jhaveri, BrJIndMed, 1959; 16:248
	(1)	Chronic/medicinal Fowler's solution		c	Cowlishaw, AustNZJMed, 1979; 9:310
	IVb (82)	Chronic/occupational Vintners	Haemangioendothelioma#	c, d, e	Roth, ZblAllgPath, 1960; 100:34 Roth, ZKrebsf, 1957; 61:468
	III (1)	Chronic/medicinal Fowler's solution		c, d, e	Regelson, Cancer, 1968; 21:514
	IVb (20)	Chronic/occupational Vintners	Angiosarcoma (2)#	c, d, e	Falk, AmJIndMed, 1981; 2:43
	(16)	Chronic/environmental Polluted drinking water	Primary liver cell carcinoma (4)#	c, d, e	Zaldívar, ArchToxicol, 1981; 47:145
	(163)	Chronic/occupational Vintners	Liver tumours (5)	d, e	Lüchtrath, JCancResClinOnc, 1983; 105:173
	IVa	Chronic/environmental Polluted drinking water	Liver tumours	d, e	Chen, BrJCanc, 1986; 53:399
Arsine	III (1)	Acute/occupational	GOT, GPT, bili	b	Hesdorfer, BrJIndMed, 1986; 43:353
Benzidine/β-naphthylamine	IVc (3322)	Chronic/occupational Not specified	Excess risk for cancer of liver, gall bladder, bile duct (3 vs. 0.35)	a	Morinaga, AmJIndMed, 1982; 3:243
Benzene[1]	IVb (65)	Chronic/occupational Chemical industry Shoe fabrication	GGT, GOT, GPT, ALP Steatosis, cirrhosis#	h[4]	Bittersohl, ZGesHyg, 1985; 31:168
Beryllium	IVb (20)	Chronic/occupational BeO alloys Ore reduction	Granuloma (2) # Centrilobular necrosis (1) #	d	Dutra, AmJPath, 1948; 24:1137
	(60)	Chronic/occupational Fluorescent lamp manufacture; experimental work; X-ray tube manufacture; Be extraction; Be alloys; aircraft industry	Hepatomegaly, BSP (12) Granulomatous infiltration (2) #	c, d	Stoeckle, AmJMed, 1969; 46:545
	III (1)	Chronic/environmental Patient lived near Be plant	Focal necrosis	h	DeNardi, AmJMed, 1949; 7:345

A Chemical	B Type of study (no. of persons)	C Exposure	D Diagnosis (no. of persons)	E Causal relationship	F Reference
Biphenyl	III/Ic (31)	Acute + chronic/occupational; Fruit paper production	Acute dystrophy (1) #; Incipient cirrhosis (1) #; Fatty metamorphosis (2) #	d	Häkkinen, ArchEnvironHlth, 1973; 26: 70
Boron hydrides	IVb (137*)	Acute or chronic/occupational	BSP (28); thymol (21); ALP (11)	d	Lowe, ArchIndHlth, 1957; 16:524
p-tert-Butylphenol (PTBH)	III (3)	Chronic/occupational; PTBH production	Minor parenchymal changes (1) #; GOT, GPT slightly; Mild steatosis (2) #	d	Rodermund, Hautarzt, 1975; 26:312
	IIa (12)	Chronic/occupational; PTBH handling; experimental work; solvent use	BSP (10)	d	Goldmann, Hautarzt, 1976; 27:155
Cadmium	III (1)	Chronic/occupational; Gold melting	Steatosis, fibrosis, cirrhosis#	c	Kaufmann, Leb MagDarm, 1984; 14: 103
Carbamate insecticide (isolan)	III (8)	Chronic/occupational/suicidal; Pesticide use	bili, BSP; LFTs abnormal	b	Lutterotti, MedWelt, 1961; 12:2430
Carbon disulphide[5] (CS$_2$)	IVb	Chronic/occupational; Spinning shop; CS$_2$ plant	Hepatomegaly (21%); Takata–Ara positive (75%)	d	Lysina, in: Brieger, ed., *Toxicology of carbon disulphide*, Amsterdam: Excerpta Medica Foundation,1967: 179
Carbonyl nickel	IVb (5)	Acute/occupational; Decanting, distillation	Hepatomegaly (3)	b,f	Kötzing, ArchGewerbepathGewerbehyg, 1933; 4:500
Chlordecone (kepone)	III (1)	Chronic/occupational	Postnecrotic cirrhosis#	d	Castano, MedLav, 1973; 64:401
	Ic (133)	Chronic/occupational; Chlordecone production	Hepatomegaly (9 of 23 persons with signs of intoxication)	c	Taylor, Neurology, 1978; 28:626
	(32)		Hepatomegaly (20); Minimal fatty metamorphosis, mild portal inflammatory changes, proliferation of smooth endoplasmic reticulum (12) #; Glucaric acid excretion; Antipyrine clearance	c,f	Guzelian, Gastro 1980; 78:206
Chromium	III (5)	Chronic/occupational; Chromium-plating factory	Icterus index, flocculation test, thymol, BSP; Toxic hepatitis#; Mild to moderate abnormalities (3)#	c	Pascale, JAMA, 1952; 149:1385
Cooking oil[6]					

Substance	Group	Exposure	Findings	Note	Reference
Copper sulphate	IVb (53)	Acute/accidental + suicidal Ingestion	Jaundice (11)	b	Chuttani, AmJMed, 1965; 39:849
	(30)	Chronic/occupational Vineyard sprayers	Kupffer cell proliferation (30), granuloma (7), fibrosis (8), cirrhosis (3), portal hypertension (2) # Angiosarcoma (1) #	d	Pimentel, Gastro, 1977; 72:275
	Ib (161)	Chronic/occupational Grape-garden sprayers	Hepatomegaly (7) ALP (16)	d, e	Habibullah, JAssocPhysInd, 1981; 29:735
Cyanamide[7]	VIb (9)	Chronic/medicinal Therapy of alcohol abuse	Granuloma (1 of 7 biopsies) Alcohol intolerance PAS–positive ground-glass hepatocytes#	d	Bruguera, Liver, 1987; 7:216
Cytostatics	III (3)	Chronic/occupational Nurses	GPT, ALP Portal hepatitis (1)# Fibrosis, fat accumulation (2)#	d, f	Sotaniemi, ActaMedScand, 1983; 214:181
1,2-Dibromoethane	III (1)	Acute/suicidal Ingestion	Aminotransferase, ALP, bili Flocculation test + massive necrosis#	b	Olmstead, ArchIndHlth, 1960; 21:525
Dichlorodiphenyl-trichloroethane (DDT)[8]	III (1)	Acute/accidental Ingestion	Centrilobular necrosis#	b[9]	Smith, JAMA, 1948; 136:469
	(1)	Acute/occupational Disinfection	Hepatomegaly bili, thymol, flocculation test	b, f	Klingemann, ÄrztlWschr, 1949; 4:465
	III (5)	Chronic/occupational Wood protection Pesticide bagging and application	GPT,GOT Steatosis (1)# Cirrhosis (2)# Chronic hepatitis (1)#	d[10]	Schüttmann, IntArchGewerbepath Gewerbehyg, 1968; 24:193
1,2-Dichloroethane[1]	III (2)	Acute/accidental Ingestion	bili Steatosis (1)#	b, f	Bloch, SchMedWoch, 1946; 42:1078
	(2)	Acute/occupational Repair of dichloroethane pipeline	Jaundice Steatosis, necrosis#	b	Brass, DMedWoch, 1949; 74:553
	(1)	Acute/accidental Ingestion	Steatosis	b	Hubbs, JAMA, 1955; 159:673
	(4)	Acute/occupational Paint application	Hepatomegaly bili, coagulation band	b, f	Menschik, ArchGewerbepathGewerbehyg, 1957; 15:241
	(1)	Acute/suicidal Ingestion	Acute dystrophy	b	Martin, DMedWoch, 1968; 93:2002
	(1)	Acute/accidental Ingestion	bili, ALP, LDH, GOT Midzonal necrosis#	b	Yodaiken, ArchEnvironHlth, 1973; 26:281
	(1)	Acute/occupational Tank cleaning	GOT, GPT, OCT, LDH Centrilobular necrosis#	b	Nouchi, IntArchOccupEnvirHlth, 1984; 54:111
Dichlorohydrin	III (1)	Acute/occupational Tank cleaning	Fatal fulminant hepatitis	b	Shiozaki, HumExpToxicol, 1994; 13:267

A Chemical	B Type of study (no. of persons)	C Exposure	D Diagnosis (no. of persons)	E Causal relationship	F Reference
Dichloropropanol	III (2)	Acute/occupational Tank cleaning	Fatal hepatic failure	b	Haratake, Liver, 1993; 13:123
1,3-Dichloropropene	III (41)	Acute/accidental Leak from tank due to a traffic accident	Submassive hepatic necrosis# GOT, GPT (11)	b	Gosselin, *Clinical toxicology of commercial products.* Baltimore: The Williams and Wilkins Co, 1976: 119
Diethylene glycol	V (14)	Acute/medicinal Ingestion of contaminated glycerol	Centrilobular necrosis#	b	Pandya, BM, 1988; 297:117
Dimethylacetamide[1]	Id (41)	Chronic/occupational Acrylic fibre factory	BSP (63%)	d	Corsi, MedLav, 1971; 62:28
+ 1,2-ethanediamine		Acute/occupational Inhalation and dermal exposure	bili, GPT, GOT, LDH, prothrombin	b, f	Marino, JOccMed, 1994; 36:637
Dimethyl formamide[1,11]	III (1)	Acute/occupational Solvent use	bili, GPT, GOT, BSP	b, f	Weiss, ZblArbMed, 1971; 21:345
	(1)	Acute/occupational Urethane fabric coating	bili, GPT, GOT	b, f	Potter, ArchEnvironHlth, 1973; 27:340
	(1)	Acute/occupational Solvent use	bili, GPT, GOT, ALP	b, f	Paoletti, MinMed, 1982; 73:3407
	(12)	Acute/occupational Polyacrylonitrile production	Hepatomegaly (4) Jaundice (4) Alcohol intolerance (4) GPT, GOT (6)	b, f	Reinl, IntArchGewerbpathGewerbehyg, 1965; 21:333
	Id (58)	Chronic/occupational Solvent use in fabric coating	GPT, GOT (62%) Alcohol intolerance (12) Microvesicular/mixed steatosis (3 of 4 biopsies)	d, f	Redlich, AnnIntMed, 1988; 108:680
	Ia (100)	Chronic/occupational	GGT	a	Cirla, GItalMedLav, 1984; 6:149
	IIb (11)	Chronic/occupational Chemical laboratory storing and handling	Flocculation test +	d	Shook, IndMedSurg, 1957; 56:333
1,2-Dimethyl-hydrazine	(1193)	Chronic/occupational Liquid rocket propellant	SGPT (46) Fatty degeneration (6 of 26 biopsies)	d	Petersen, BrJIndMed, 1970; 27:141
m-Dinitrobenzene	III (1)	Chronic/occupational Dinitrobenzene handling	Hepatomegaly, icterus	b	Ishihara, IntArchOccupEnvirHlth, 1976; 36:161
	(2)	Acute/occupational Dinitrobenzene production	Hepatomegaly (1) bili (2), thymol, ALP (1)	b, f	Beritic, BrJIndMed, 1956; 13:114
Dinitro-o-cresol		Acute/occupational Not specified	Jaundice bili, ALP	b, f	Gaultier, JEurTox, 1974; 7:9

Agent	Type (n)	Exposure	Findings	Code	Reference
Dinitrotoluene	IIb (154)	Chronic/occupational, Not specified	Jaundice (2)	d	McGee, AmJDigDis, 1942; 9:329
Dioxane[1]	III (5)	Subacute/occupational, Solvent use	Centrilobular necrosis#	b	Barber, Guy'sHospRep, 1934; 84:267
	(1)		Centrilobular necrosis#	b	Johnston, ArchIndHlth, 1959; 20:445
Diphenyl	III (1)	Chronic/occupational, Impregnated paper	GPT, GOT, GGT, ALP Inflammatory infiltrate#	d, f	Carella, JOccMed, 1994; 36:575
Ethylene chlorohydrin	III (1)	Acute/occupational, Solvent use	Areas of necrotic liver cells#	b	Dierker, JIndHygTox, 1944; 26:277
	(1)	Acute/occupational, Solvent use	Severe fatty infiltration	b	Bush, JIndHygTox, 1949; 31:352
	(1)	Acute/occupational, Rupture of a storage tank	bili, ALP, BSP, thymol Sporadic liver cell necroses and microvesicular steatosis#	b, f	Bleckat, IntArchGewerbepath-Gewerbehyg, 1968; 25:45
	(1)	Acute/accidental, Ingestion	Liver cell necrosis#	b	Miller, ArchDisChild, 1970; 45:589
Ethylene glycol	III (2)	Acute/accidental, Ingestion	Hydropic degeneration#	b	Smith, AMAArchPath, 1951; 51:423
Ethylene glycol monomethyl ester	III (1)	Acute/accidental, Ingestion	Fatty degeneration†#	b	Young, JIndHygTox, 1946; 28:267
Germander (*Teucrium chamaedrys*)	III (7)	Subacute/medicinal, For weight loss	bili, GPT, GOT Hepatocyte necrosis (3)#	d, f, g	Larrey, AnnIntMed, 1992; 117:129
	(826)	Subacute/medicinal, For weight loss	bili, GPT, GOT	d, f, g	Castot, GastrClinBiol, 1992; 16??
Glue thistle (*Actractylis gummifera*)	III (10)	Acute/accidental, Ingestion	bili, GOT, GPT	b, f	Lemaigre, NouvPresseMed, 1975; 4:2865
Hexachlorobenzene	V (>600)	Chronic/accidental, Ingestion of contaminated wheat	Porphyria cutanea tarda	d	Schmid, NEJM, 1960; 263:397
γ-Hexachloro-cyclohexane (γ-HCH)	III (1)	Acute/experimental	bili	b, f	Schmiedeberg, AnzSchaed, 1953; 26:129
	IVb (3)	Chronic/occupational, Pesticide use, γ-HCH production	GPT, GOT Cirrhosis, mixed steatosis (2)# Chronic hepatitis, Fibrosis (1)#	d	Schüttmann, IntArchGewerbepath-Gewerbehyg, 1968; 24:193
Hexafluorodi-chlorobutene (HFCB)	IVb (3)	Acute/occupational, HFCB production	bili, BSP Centrilobular necrosis#	b	Bertrand, PoumonCoeur, 1970; 26:941
Hornet's venom	III (1)	Acute/occupational, Multiple hornet stings (child)	Hepatomegaly bili, ALP, GGT, GOT, GPT, NH₃, encephalopathy Microvesicular steatosis#	b, f	Weizman, Gastro, 1985; 89:1407
Hydrazines[12]	IVb (140)	Chronic/occupational, Missile propellant handling	thymol, GPT (22) Fatty metamorphosis (2 of 3 biopsies)#	d	King, AerospaceMed, 1969; 40:315

A Chemical	B Type of study (no. of persons)	C Exposure	D Diagnosis (no. of persons)	E Causal relationship	F Reference
Kerosene	IVb (3)	Chronic/occupational Fuel handling	Hepatomegaly GPT, GOT, bili, BSP	d, f	Veljkov, MedicinskiArhiv, 1982; 36:19
Lead	III (4)	Acute/accidental Injection	GOT, ALP Hepatitis#	b	Beattie, ScotMedJ, 1979; 24:318
	(1)	Chronic/occupational Battery work-up	Nuclear inclusions Microvesicular steatosis#	c, f	Klinge, ActaHepatosplenol, 1970; 17:151
	Ia (135)	Chronic/occupational Metallurgic plant Tile manufacture Battery production Wire production Paint application	thymol, GPT, ALP (15)	a	Kosmider, ZblArbMed, 1967; 17:170
	III (1)	Acute/accidental Ingestion of red lead	bili, ALP, GOT, GPT, LDH	b, f	Nortler, VetHumTox, 1980; 22:145
Manganese	III (1)	Subacute/occupational Loading manganese ore	Hepatomegaly Takata positive	b, f	Ceresa, MedLav, 1951; 42:26
	(1)	Acute/suicidal Ingestion of potassium permanganate	BSP, LDH, ALP, GOT Mild fibrosis#	b, f	Lustig, ArchIntMed, 1982; 142:405
Mercury vapour	Ia (20)	Chronic/occupational Chemical laboratories	bili, thymol, GPT, ALP (4)	a	Kosmider, ZblArbMed, 1967; 17:170
	III (1)	Chronic/occupational Mercury distillation	Cirrhosis#	d	Martini, Zacchia, 1972; 8:31
	Ia (83)	Chronic/occupational Chlorine and acetaldehyde production	SDH (48%), GPT (28%), GOT(10%), ALP(8%), bili (17%), Fatty degeneration, Kupffer cell proliferation, Inflammatory infiltration (15 of 17 biopsies)	a	Pach, MatMedPol, 1985; 53:23
2-Methyl-4-chlorophenoxyacetic acid (MCPA)	III (1)	Chronic/occupational Pesticide application	GPT, GOT Liver cell necrosis, steatosis#	d, f[3]	Lun, ZKlinMed, 1986; 41:859
Methylenedianiline (4,4'-diamino-diphenylmethane)	V (84)	Acute/alimentary Contaminated bread (Epping jaundice)	Jaundice bili, ALP, GOT Cellular infiltration, cholestasis, damage to liver parenchyma, cholangitis#	b, f	Kopelman, BMJ, 1966; i:514
	IIb (6)	Acute/occupational Epoxy resin application	GPT, GOT, bili Cholestasis (1)#	d	Williams, NEJM, 1974; 291:1256

Substance	Code	Exposure	Findings	Note	Reference
	IVb (13)	Acute/occupational Use of epoxy resin hardener	Jaundice bili, ALP, GOT	b, f	McGill, NEJM, 1974; 291:278
	III (1)	Acute/occupational Not specified	Jaundice ALP, GPT, GOT Cholestasis, toxic hepatitis#	b, f	Brooks, JAMA, 1979; 242:1527
	(1)	Acute/accidental Ingestion	Jaundice bili, GOT	b	Roy, HumTox, 1985; 4:61
	(4)	Acute/occupational Laying an epoxy resin–based floor	Jaundice bili, ALP, GOT	b, f, g	Bastian, MedJAust, 1984; 141:533
Monobromomethane (methyl bromide)	III (2)	Acute/accidental Leakage from a defective insecticide cannister	Hepatomegaly NH_3 (2), bili (1), GOT, GPT, LDH (1)	b	Shield, Neurology, 1977; 27:959
	Ic (33)	Chronic/occupational Soil disinfection in greenhouses	ALP (2), GPT, GOT (1) Correlation between GOT, GPT and bromine in blood (GOT,GPT not exceeding upper limit in 32)	a	Verberk, BrJIndMed, 1979; 36:59
Monochloromethane (methyl chloride)	IVb (29)	Acute/accidental/ occupational Refrigerators	Icterus index; beginning fatty degeneration (1)#	b	Kegel, JAMA, 1929; 93:353
	III (2)	Acute/occupational Repair of air-conditioning plant	Jaundice, icterus index (1)	b	Weinstein, JAMA, 1937; 108:1603
	(4)	Acute/accidental Refrigerator	bili	b	Spevak, BrJIndMed, 1976; 33:272
	(1)	Acute/occupational Refrigeration engineer	Coproporphyrinuria	b	Chalmers, Lancet, 1940; ii:806
	III (1)	Chronic/occupational Refrigeration	thymol, ALP Cirrhosis#	d	Wood, Lancet, 1951; 260:508
	(1)		Hepatomegaly bili, ALP, thymol	d,f	Mackie, MedJAust, 1961; 48:203
	(1)		Porphyria cutanea tarda Cirrhosis	h[14]	Leurini, MedLav, 1982; 73:571
Mucochloric acid (2,3–dichloro–4–oxo–2–butenoic acid)	IIb (3)	Chronic/occupational Pyramin (weedkiller) production	Hepatomegaly	d,f	Kolesár, BratislLekListy, 1975; 64:132
Nickel	IVc (28261)	Chronic/occupational Production of high nickel alloys	Excess risk of primary liver cancer (SMR for males 1.82, $p < 0.01$)	a	Redmond, IARCSciPubl, 1984; 53:73
	(814)		Excess risk of primary liver cancer (SMR 3.87)	a	Cragle, IARCSciPubl, 1984; 53:57

A Chemical	B Type of study (no. of persons)	C Exposure	D Diagnosis (no. of persons)	E Causal relationship	F Reference
2-Nitropropane[1,15]	III (1)	Acute/occupational Paint application	Jaundice GOT, GPT, ALP	b	Gaultier, ArchMalProf, 1964; 25:425
	IVb (4)		Centrilobular degenerative hepatitis# Hepatomegaly, jaundice Hepatic failure	b[16]	Hine, JOccMed, 1978; 20:333
			GPT, GOT, LDH, ALP Centrilobular necrosis, fatty degeneration		
	III (1)		GOT, GPT, LDH, GlDH Acute hepatitis#	b[17]	Rondia, VetHumTox, 1979; 21:183
	III (2)	Acute/occupational Resin application	Hepatomegaly, hepatic failure, massive necrosis (1) GOT (1)	b[18]	Harrison, AnnIntMed, 1987; 107:466
Paraquat	III (2)	Acute/accidental/suicidal Ingestion	Centroacinar necrosis#	b	Bullivant, BMJ, 1966; i:1272
	(1)			b	Campbell, Lancet 1968; i:144
	(1)			b	Bronkhorst, NedTGeneesk, 1968; 112:310
	(1)		Liver epithelium degeneration#	b	Duffy, JIrishMedAss, 1968; 61:97
	(1)		Fatty liver epithelium degeneration#	b	Oreopoulos, BMJ, 1968; i:749
	(1)			b	Fenelly, BMJ, 1968; iii:722
	(1)		Intrahepatic cholestasis#	b	Matthew, BMJ, 1968; iii:759
	(1)		Fatty epithelium degeneration, slight cholestasis#	b	Tilling, DMedWoch, 1968; 93:2439
	(1)		Liver cell necroses#	b	Lanzinger, MünchMedWoch, 1969; 111:944
	(1)		Cholestasis#	b	McDonagh, ArchDisChild, 1970; 45:425
	(1)		Centroacinar necrosis, microvesicular steatosis#	b	von der Hardt, KlinWschr, 1971; 49:544
	(1)		bili, ALP, GOT, GPT	b	Hargreave, PostgradMedJ, 1969; 45:633
	(1)	Acute/occupational Herbicide application	Hepatomegaly bili, GPT, GOT	h	Guardascione, FolMed, 1969; 52:728
	IVb (14)	Acute/accidental/suicidal Ingestion	Jaundice (5) Centrilobular steatosis, centrilobular necrosis (6)#	b	Parkinson, Histopath, 1980; 4:171
	(14)		Jaundice GOT, GPT, LDH, ALP, bili Fatty metamorphosis (6)# Focal (5) or central (3) necrosis# Bile duct injury (3)# Portal inflammation (6)# Portal fibrosis (3)#	b	Matsumoto, ActaPathJpn, 1980; 30:859

Substance	Type (n)	Circumstances/exposure	Findings	Note	Reference
Parathion	IVb (4)	Acute/occupational/accidental Pesticide application Ingestion	bili, BSP (1)	b	Lutterotti, MedWelt, 1961; 12:2430
Pennyroyal oil (pulegone)	III (1)	Acute/accidental Ingestion	bili, ALP, GOT, GPT, LDH Centrilobular necrosis#	b	Sullivan, JAMA, 1979; 242:2873
Pentachlorophenol (PCP)[19,20]	III (10)	Chronic/occupational PCP production	thymol, coagulation band	d	Baader, IndMedSurg, 1951; 20:286
	IVb (80)	Chronic/occupational Herbicide production	Porphyria cutanea tarda (11) δ-aminolaevulinic acid and uroporphyrin excretion bili, GPT, GOT (11)	c	Jirásek, Hautarzt, 1976; 27:328
	Ia (23)	Chronic/occupational PCP production	GlDH (10)	a	Zober, IntArchOccEnvirHlth, 1981; 48:347
	Id (1107)	Chronic/occupational Sawmill workers	Liver-related symptoms by questionnaire	d	Sterling, IntJHlthServ, 1982; 12:559
	III (1)	Chronic/environmental Wood preservative	GOT, GPT, GGT, LDH, GlDH	g	Brandt, VerDtschGesInnMed, 1977; 83:1609
'Pesticides'[21]	Id (200)	Chronic/occupational Pesticide factory	Hepatomegaly (30%) GOT, GPT, GGT, ALP (40%) Steatosis (2/4), fibrosis (1/4), cirrhosis (1/4)#	d	Dal Monte, GClinMed, 1979; 60:624
	IIb (27)	Chronic/occupational	Follow-up: histological signs of liver damage ameliorated by concomitant cessation of exposure reduction of alcohol intake weight reduction	f	Erhardt, DtschGesundhwesen, 1981; 36:265
Petroleum distillates	IVb (14)	Chronic/occupational	Angiosarcoma	h, e	El Zayadi, Hepatogast, 1986; 33:148
	III (1)	Acute/accidental Ingestion	GPT, ALP, GGT	b, f	Janssen, IntensCareMed, 1988; 14:238
Phenol	III (1)	Chronic/occupational Laboratory	Hepatomegaly GOT, GPT, LDH	d, f	Merliss, JOccMed, 1972; 14:55
1-Phenyl-4,5-chloropyridason-6	IIb (4)	Acute/occupational Pyramin (weedkiller) production	Hepatomegaly GPT, LDH	d, f	Kolesár, BratislLekListy, 1975; 64:132
Phosphorus	IVb (56)	Acute/suicidal Ingestion	Jaundice (20)	b	Díaz-Rivera, Medicine, 1950; 29:269
	(45)	Acute/accidental Firecrackers Rat poison	Fatty change, necrosis[22] Portal fibrosis#	b	Salfelder, BeitrPath, 1972; 147:321
	(49)	Firecrackers	Fatty change, hydropic degeneration#	b	Marin, NEJM, 1971; 284:125
Polybrominated biphenyls (PBB)	Id	Chronic/occupational Soil contamination	Coproporphyrinuria Chronic hepatic porphyria	d	Doss, AnnNYAcadSci, 1987; 514:204
Polychlorinated biphenyls (PCB)[23]	V	Subacute/alimentary Ingestion of contaminated rice oil[24] (Yusho, Japan 1968)	Jaundice LFTs abnormal	c	Reggiani, EnvirHlthPerspect, 1985; 60:225[25] Kimbrough, AnnRevPharmTox, 1987; 27:87[25]

A Chemical	B Type of study (no. of persons)	C Exposure	D Diagnosis (no. of persons)	E Causal relationship	F Reference
	V (829)	(Yu-cheng, Taiwan 1979)	GOT, GPT, ALP	c	Lü, AmJIndMed, 1985; 5:81
	Ib (69)	Yu-cheng	δ-aminolaevulinic acid and uroporphyrin excretion	d	Chang, ResCommChemPathPharm, 1980; 30:547
	Ic (80)	Chronic/occupational Electrical capacitor manufacture	Hepatomegaly, GOT, GPT, GGT, OCT (16)	c	Maroni, BrJIndMed, 1981; 38:55
	(458)	Chronic/alimentary Ingestion of contaminated fish	Correlation between serum PCB and GGT	a	Kreiss, JAMA, 1981; 245:2505
	Ia (228)	Chronic/occupational Electrical capacitor manufacture	Correlation between serum PCB and GOT GGT (values within normal range)	a	Smith, BrJIndMed, 1982; 39:361
	Ia (120*)		Correlation between serum PCB and GOT	a	Chase, JOccMed, 1982; 24:109
	(67)		Porphyrinuria	a	Colombi, JApplTox, 1982; 2:117
	Ic (97)		ALP (11%). No correlation with PCB concentration in blood	d	Hara, EnvirHlthPerspect, 1985; 59:85
	(326)		Correlation between log LDH and log PCB (female) log GGT and log HPCB (male) [26] (values mostly within normal range) Follow-up: increased prevalence of abnormal GGT after 2.5 years	d	Fischbein, EnvirHlthPerspect, 1985; 60:145
	(194)		Correlation between serum PCB and GGT	d	Lawton, EnvirHlthPerspect, 1985; 60:165
	IVc (2567)		Excess mortality for liver cancer (3 vs. 1.07, NS)	a	Brown, ArchEnvirHlth, 1981; 36:120
	(120)	Subacute/accidental (Yusho)	Excess mortality for liver cancer Males: 9 vs.1.61 Females: 2 vs. 0.66 (NS) Excess mortality for chronic liver disease and cirrhosis (NS)	a	Kuratsune, Chemosphere, 1987; 16:2085
Polychloroprene	III (1)	Chronic/occupational Neoprene application	Angiosarcoma	e	Infante, EnvirHlthPerspect, 1977; 21:251
Pyrrolizidine alkaloids	IVb (6)	Chronic/alimentary Ingestion of contaminated food	Centrilobular haemorrhagic necrosis, occlusion of hepatic veins#[27]	d	Selzer, BrJExpPath, 1951; 32:14
	(100*)	Ingestion of bush tea possibly contaminated with Senecio spp.	Occlusion of hepatic veins (5)[27] cirrhosis (4)#	h	Bras, ArchPathol, 1954; 57:285

Code	Substance	Type / source	Findings		Reference
III (2)		Chronic/medicinal; Ingestion of folk medicine	Hepatomegaly, ascites; Centrilobular blood lagoons, occlusion of hepatic veins, cell necroses#[27]	f	Gupta, BMJ, 1963; i:1184
V (67)		Chronic/alimentary; Ingestion of cereals contaminated with *Crotolaria* spp.	Hepatomegaly, ascites; GOT, GPT, ALP; Centrilobular haemorrhagic necrosis, occlusion of hepatic veins#[27]	d	Tandon, Lancet, 1976; ii:271
(21)		Ingestion of wheat bread contaminated with *Heliotropium* spp.	Hepatomegaly, ascites; GPT, ALP; Centrilobular haemorrhagic necrosis, occlusion of hepatic veins#[27]	d, f	Mohabbat, Lancet, 1976; ii:269
III (1)		Chronic/medicinal; Ingestion of contaminated tea	Hepatomegaly, ascites; ALP; Centrilobular necrosis, occlusion of hepatic veins#[27]	d	McGee, JClinPath, 1976; 29:788
(1)		Ingestion of tea contaminated with *Crotolaria* spp.	Ascites; ALP, GOT; Sublobular hepatic vein obstruction#[27]	d, f	Lyford, Gastro, 1976; 70:105
(1)		Ingestion of tea contaminated with *Senecio* spp.	Hepatomegaly, distended abdomen; GOT; Distended sinusoids; 2 months later extensive fibrosis#[27]	d	Stillman, Gastro, 1977; 73:349
(4)		Ingestion of contaminated tea	Hepatomegaly, ascites; GOT, ALT, bili; Centrilobular haemorrhagic necrosis#[27]	d, f	Kumana, Lancet, 1983; ii:1360
IVa (440)	Silicon dioxide	Chronic/occupational	Uroporphyrinogen excretion (12; unexposed controls: 4/1362)	d	Hykes, CasLekCesk, 1981; 120:1190
Ic (23)	Styrene[1]	Chronic/occupational; Processing of storage pipes	Serum bile acids (11)	d	Edling, BrJIndMed, 1984; 41:257
(493)		Chronic/occupational; Styrene polymerization	GGT	d	Lorimer, ScaJWorkEnvirHlth, 1978; 4(Suppl.2):220
IIa (35)		Chronic/occupational; Manufacture of glass fibre-reinforced plastic products	GOT, GPT (8; 2/12 in controls); ALP (5; 1/12 in controls)	d	Axelson, ScaJWorkEnvirHlth, 1978; 4(Suppl.2):215
Ic (226)	2,3,7,8-Tetrachlorodibenzo-*p*-dioxin (TCDD)[28]	Acute/accidental; Explosion in TCP plant (Nitro, W.Virginia 1949)	GGT in persons with chloracne (as compared with persons without chloracne)	c	Moses, AmJIndMed, 1984; 5:161
(14)		(Derbyshire 1973)	thymol, zinc turbidity, GPT (9)	c, f	May, BrJIndMed, 1973; 30:276
(42)		(Ludwigshafen 1953)	Takata positive, thymol (4); Subacute hepatitis, slight steatosis (1)	c	Goldmann, ArbmedSozmedArbhyg, 1972; 7:12
(1029)		(Seveso 1976)	GGT, GOT, GPT (10%)	c	Homberger, AnnOccupHyg, 1979; 22:327

A Chemical	B Type of study (no. of persons)	C Exposure	D Diagnosis (no. of persons)	E Causal relationship	F Reference
	(1654)		Hepatomegaly (8-10%) GOT, GPT, GGT	c	Pocchiari, AnnNYAcadSci, 1979; 311[29]
	(164)		GPT, GGT (in children with chloracne as compared with those without chloracne)	c	Caramaschi, IntJEpid, 1981; 10:135
	Ia/b (31)		D-glucaric acid excretion[30] (in children with chloracne as compared with those without chloracne; 1976)	c	Ideo, CCActa, 1982; 120:273
	(67)		D-glucaric acid excretion (vs. control; 1979)		
	III (2)	Chronic/occupational 2,4,5-T[31] production	Porphyria cutanea tarda	d	Doss, AnnNYAcadSci, 1987; 514:204
	IVb (55)		Porphyria cutanea tarda (11) bili, thymol, GPT, BSP (11) Steatosis, periportal fibrosis#	d	Pazderova, ArchEnvirHlth, 1981; 36:5
	Id (154)	Chronic/environmental Soil contamination in mobile home park	Subclinical differences in LFTs	a	Stehr-Green, ArchEnvirHlth, 1988; 43:174
1,1,2,2-Tetrachloroethane[1]	III (1)	Acute/occupational Solvent use	Jaundice Subacute necrosis#	b	Willcox, Lancet, 1931; ii:57
	(277)	Chronic/occupational Solvent use	Palpable liver (55)	d, f	Gurney, Gastro, 1943; i:1112
Tetrachloroethylene[1,32]	III (1)	Acute/occupational Dry cleaning	Acute hepatitis	b, f	Meckler, JAMA, 1966; 197:144
	(1)	Solvent use	Centrilobular liver-cell degeneration#	b, f	Stewart, JAMA, 1969; 208:1490
	(1)	Dry cleaning	Mild hepatitis GOT	b	Trense, ZblArbMed, 1969; 19:131
	(1)		bili, GOT, GPT Centrilobular necrosis#	d	Hughes, JAMA, 1954; 156:234
	(1)	Subacute/occupational Dry cleaning	Acute hepatitis	d, f	Bagnell, CanMedAssJ, 1977; 117:1047
	(1)	Breast feeding[33]	Jaundice bili, GOT, ALP	d	Coler, ArchIndHyg, 1953; 8:227
	Id (7)	Chronic/occupational Degreasing	bili, BSP, flocculation (3)	a	Franke, MedWelt, 1969; 20:453
	Ia (113)	Dry cleaning	bili, thymol increased vs. control (values mostly within normal range)		
Tetrachloromethane[1]	III (3)	Acute/occupational Cleaning of clothes	Centrilobular necrosis#	b	Taubmann, MünchMedWoch, 1958; 47:1829
(carbon tetrachloride)	(2)	Machine degreasing	GOT (1), thymol (1) Liver cell necrosis (1)	b	Lachnit, ArchGewerbepath-Gewerbehyg, 1960; 18:337

Agent	Type (n)	Exposure	Findings	Code	Reference
	(1)	Relay cleaning	Jaundice; GPT, bili	b, f	Nielsen, ActaMedScand, 1965; 178: 363
	(1)	Motor degreasing	GOT, GPT, bili	b, f	Asshauer, MedWelt, 1969; 20:102
	(1)	Acute/accidental; Ingestion	GPT, LDH, ALP, bili	b, f	Alston, JClinPath, 1970; 23:249
	(1)	Chronic/occupational; Cloth cleaning	Chronic hepatitis, cirrhosis#	d	Poindexter, JAMA, 1934; 102:2015
	Ia (135)	Chronic/occupational	GPT, GOT, GGT, ALP (subclinical)	a	Tomenson, OccupEnvirMed, 1995; 52: 508
Thallium	IVb (4)	Chronic/accidental	thymol	d	Fischl, AmJMedSci, 1966; 251:78
Toluene[1,34]	III (1)	Acute/accidental; Glue sniffing	Jaundice; bili, ALP, GPT	b, f	O'Brien, BMJ, 1971; ii:29
	IIb (10)	Chronic/occupational; Construction work in a former laboratory	GOT, GPT	d	Pey, ArchMalProf, 1972; 33:584
	Id (27)	Chronic/occupational; Plastic and rotogravure industry	Hepatomegaly; GOT, GPT, bili	d	DeRosa, LavUmano, 1974; 26:144
	IIb (170)	Chronic/occupational; Not specified	GOT; Mitochondrial abnormalities (22)#	d	Szilard, MorphollgazOrvSz, 1978; 18: 117
	IVb (6)	Chronic/occupational; Shoemaker	GOT, GPT, GGT, ALP (5); Steatosis# (3)	d[35]	Lun, ZKlinMed, 1987; 42:671
	Id (262)	Chronic/occupational	Correlation of exposure history with GPT	d	Morck, DanMedBull, 1988; 35:196
	III (1)	Chronic/occupational	bili, prothrombin	d	Shiomi, ClinNuclMed, 1993; 18:655
Toxic oil syndrome, (Spain 1981)[36]	V (842)	Subacute/alimentary; Ingestion of adulterated rapeseed oil	GGT, ALP, LDH, GPT, GOT (203); Cholestatic hepatitis, ultrastructural changes#	d	Solis-Herruzo, Hepatol, 1984; 4:131
			Follow-up# of 124 persons: Cholestatic hepatitis (14); Chronic active hepatitis (13); Cirrhosis (4); Biliary cirrhosis (1); Liver-cell adenoma (1); Regenerative hyperplasia (8)		Solis-Herruzo, Gastro, 1987; 93:558
	(242)		GOT, GPT (99), ALP (34), bili (16); Hepatitis (10/14)#, cholestasis (3/14)#	d, f	Velicia, JHepatol, 1986; 3:59
1,1,1-Trichloroethane[1]	III (1)	Acute/accidental; Ingestion	bili (slightly)	b	Stewart, JAMA, 1966; 195:120
	(1)	Chronic/occupational; Degreasing	Cirrhosis#	d[37]	Thiele, Gastro, 1982; 83:926
	III (1)	Acute/accidental; Sniffing	bili, GOT	b, f	Nathan, BrJClinPharm, 1979; 8:2
	(4)	Chronic/occupational	GPT, GOT; Macrovesicular steatosis#	d	Hodgson, ArchIntMed, 1989; 149: 1793

A Chemical	B Type of study (no. of persons)	C Exposure	D Diagnosis (no. of persons)	E Causal relationship	F Reference
Trichloroethylene[38]	III (1)	Acute/occupational Solvent use	Jaundice bili, flocculation test Massive necrosis#	b	Joron, CanMedAssJ, 1955; 73:890
	(1)	Subacute/occupational Degreasing	Acute hepatic failure necrosis#	b	Priest, ArchEnvirHlth, 1965; 11:361
	(3)	Acute/accidental Sniffing	GOT, GPT	b	Baerg, AnnIntMed, 1970; 73:713
	(2)		Centrilobular necrosis, fibrosis (2)# bili, GPT, GOT, ALP Centrilobular necrosis		Clearfield, DigDis, 1970; 15:851
	(1)	Chronic/occupational Dry cleaning	Degenerative fatty metamorphosis#	d	Schollmeyer, ArchToxicol, 1960; 18:229
	IVb (14)	Chronic/occupational Various sources	Fatty liver (11)# Fibrosis (1)#	d	Schüttmann, DeutschZVerdauStoff, 1970; 30:43
Trichloromethane[1,39]	III (3)	Acute/medicinal Anaesthesia	Icterus gravis; degeneration of liver cells (1)#	b	Willcox, Lancet, 1931; ii:57
(chloroform)		Chronic/accidental Inhalation, bath additive	Cirrhosis (1)#, jaundice (1)	d	
	Id (68)	Chronic/occupational Pharmaceutical industry	Hepatomegaly GOT, GPT	a	Bomski, IntArchGewerbepath–Gewerbehyg, 1967; 24:127
2,4,5–Trichlorophenol (TCP)[40]	Id (29)[41]	Chronic/occupational TCP manufacture	Uroporphyrin excretion Porphyria cutanea tarda (11)	d	Bleiberg, ArchDermatol, 1964; 89:793
Triorthocresyl phosphate	III (6)	Chronic/occupational Car equipment industry	Vacuolar swelling of the cytoplasm, abnormalities of nuclear membrane#	c	Caudarella, LavUmano, 1975; 27:161
Trinitrotoluene	IVb (22)	Chronic/occupational Munition disposal	Toxic hepatitis (8) Degenerative changes, necrosis or acute yellow atrophy (12)#	d	McConnell, JIndHygTox, 1946; 28:76
	IIb (18)		Jaundice, GOT, GPT, bili (3)	d	Hassmann, SbornikVedPraciLek–HradKrá, 1968; 11(Suppl):339
	III (1)		Hepatomegaly Steatosis#	d	Hassmann, SbornikVedPraciLek–HradKrá, 1969; 12:561
	IIb (43)		GOT, LDH	d	Morton, AmIndHygAssJ, 1976; 37:56
Uranyl acetate	III (1)	Acute/suicidal Ingestion	Jaundice bili	b	Csapo, WienKlinWoch, 1958; 70:788
Vinyl chloride	VI (118)[42]	Chronic/occupational PVC production (especially autoclave workers)	Angiosarcoma	d, e	Forman, BrJIndMed, 1985; 42:750

	Exposure	Findings		Reference
IVa (26*)	Chronic/environmental[43] 5 women living near PVC plant		h, e	Brady, JNCI, 1977; 59:1383
III (14)	Chronic/occupational[44] Not specified	Portal fibrosis# Portal hypertension#	d	Thomas, NEJM, 1975; 292:17
IVb (49)	Chronic/occupational PVC production and processing	Hepatomegaly (31) BSP(38), bili(12), ALP(10), GOT(15), GPT(17) Capsular fibrosis Collagenization of sinusoidal walls; septal fibrosis; fatty change#	d	Marsteller, AnnNYAcadSci, 1975; 246: 95
(7)	Chronic/occupational Polymer reaction cleaning	ALP(l), GOT, GPT(2), BSP(4) Portal hypertension Fibrosis (6)#	d	Smith, Lancet, 1976; ii:602
III (2)	Chronic/occupational PVC industry	Portal hypertension, progression to angiosarcoma 5 and 10 years later	d	Jones, BrJIndMed, 1982; 39:306
Ic (271)	Chronic/occupational PVC production	bili (3), GPT (10), GOT (6), GGT (8), ALP (3) Hepatomegaly (8)	d	Ho, JSocOccupMed, 1991; 41:10
IVa (78*)	Chronic/occupational Not specified	Focal hepatocytic hyperplasia (17 vs. 4) Focal mixed hyperplasia or more advanced lesions (6 vs. 1) ICG, GGT, ALP, GOT, GPT	a	Tamburro, Hepatol, 1984; 4:413
III (2)	Chronic/occupational Not specified	Hepatocellular carcinoma#	d	Evans, Histopath, 1983; 7:377
III (1)	Chronic/occupational PVC production		d	Gokel, VirchArchA, 1976; 372:195
(3)			d	Dietz, KlinWschr, 1985; 63:325
Id (36)	Chronic/occupational Not specified	Coproporphyrin excretion Subclinical chronic hepatic porphyria BSP	d	Doss, KlinWschr, 1984; 62:175
Xylene[1] III (3)	Acute/occupational Paint application	GOT (2)	b, f	Morley, BMJ, 1970; iii:442

[1] For a discussion of potential tumour induction by solvents, see text.
[2] For a discussion of the causal relationship between aflatoxin B$_1$ and Reye's syndrome, see text.
[3] For a report on negative findings (chronic/occupational) see Hine, JOccMed, 1977; 19.391.
[4] Exposure also to other solvents.
[5] For a report on negative finding (chronic/occupational) see Vanhoorne, IntArchOccupEnvirHlth, 1992; 63:517.

6 See toxic oil syndrome.

7 Workers in farming occupation may be exposed to cyanamide calcium in fertilizers.

8 For a report on negative findings (chronic/occupational) see Laws, ArchEnvirHlth, 1973; 27:318.

9 Exposure also to xylene, kerosene.

10 Exposure also to γ–hexachlorocyclohexane.

11 For reports on negative findings (chronic/occupational) see Spassowski, EnvirHlthPerspect, 1976; 17:199; Lauwerys, IntArchOccupEnvinHlth, 1980; 45:189; Yonemoto, IntArchOccupEnvinHlth, 1980; 46:159; Cai, IntArchOccupEnvinHlth, 1992; 63:461.

12 See 1,2–dimethylhydrazine.

13 Exposure also to 2–chloroethyl phosphonic acid.

14 History of excessive alcohol consumption and viral hepatitis.

15 For a report on negative findings (chronic/occupational near exposure limit of 25 p.p.m.) see Crawford, AmIndHygAssJ, 1985; 46:45.

16 Drinking problem in 2/4. Exposure also to methyl ethylketone, cellosolve acetate, and toluene (2) or acetone (1).

17 Exposure also to acetone and dimethylformamide.

18 Exposure also to cyclohexane, toluene, 2,4,6–tri(dimethylaminomethyl)phenol, coal-tar pitch, bisphenol A, and epichlorohydrin.

19 PCP products may be contaminated with 2,3,7,8–TCDD.

20 For reports on negative findings (chronic/occupational) see Arsenault, ProcAmWoodPreservAss, 1976; 20:148; Fiedler, ToxRev, 1982; 5; and chronic/environmental > 5 μg/m^3 air see Aurand, SchrVerWaBoLufthyg, 1981; 52:293.

21 For a discussion of tumour induction by pesticides, see text.

22 In contrast to previous reports, necrosis was not restricted to lobular periphery.

23 For reports on negative findings (chronic/occupational) see Ouw, ArchEnvirHlth, 1976; 31:189; Baker, AmJEpid, 1980; 112:553; Takamatsu, AmJIndMed, 1985; 5:59.

24 Contaminated with polychlorinated dibenzofurans (PCDF) and polychlorinated quaterphenyls; toxicity ascribed to PCDF by most authors.

25 Most of the pertinent original literature is published in Japanese. Two reviews are cited here in which the information is briefly given.

26 Higher chlorinated biphenyls.

27 Veno–occlusive disease.

28 For reports on negative findings (chronic exposure) see Lathrop, cited in Webb, AmJPrevMed, 1986; 2:107; Stehr–Green, ArchEnvirHlth, 1986; 41:16.

29 Review.

30 Indicating enzyme induction.

31 2,4,5–Trichlorophenoxy acetic acid.

32 For a report on negative finding (chronic/occupational) see Szadkowski, IntArchGewerbepathGewerbehyg, 1969; 25:323.

33 Six–week–old child; tetrachloroethylene detected in the mother's milk.

34 For reports on negative findings (chronic/occupational) see Szadkowski, MedMonatschr, 1976; 30:25; Tähti, IntArchOccupEnvirHlth, 1981; 48:61; Waldron, Lancet 1982; ii:1276; Boewer, IntArchOccupEnvirHlth, 1988; 60:181.

35 Exposure also to other solvents.

36 The agent(s) responsible for the toxic effects have not been identified with certainty.

37 Exposure also to trichloroethylene which may have been the major cause of injury.

38 For reports on negative findings (chronic/occupational) see Szadkowski, IntArchGewerbepathGewerbehyg, 1969; 25:323.

39 For reports on negative findings (chronic/occupational) see Challen, BrJIndMed, 1958; 15:243; Gambini, MedLav, 1973; 64:432.

40 Later shown to be contaminated with 2,3,7,8–TCDD.

41 In a follow–up to this study, only one worker with elevated uroporphyrin excretion was found among 72 workers examined (Poland, ArchEnvirHlth, 1971; 22:316).

42 For a review of 20 epidemiological studies see Purchase, FoodChemTox, 1987; 25:187.

43 For a report on negative findings for angiosarcoma (chronic/environmental) see Barr 1982, cited in Purchase, FoodChemTox, 1987; 25:187.

44 For a report on negative findings for portal fibrosis (chronic/occupational) see Jones, ScaJWorkEnvirHlth, 1988; 14:153.

32.3 Rare diseases with hepatic abnormalities

Michael Baraitser and R. M. Winter

Disease	Features	Hepatic abnormalities	Reference(s)
Aagenae's syndrome (recurrent cholestasis with lymphoedema)	Oedema (lymphoedema)	Recurrent cholestasis from infancy. Later liver fibrosis	Aagenaes O. Hereditary recurrent cholestasis with lymphoedema—two new families. *Acta Paediatrica Scandinavica*, 1974; **63**: 465–71.
Adrenoleukodystrophy (neonatal, autosomal recessive)	Adrenal hypoplasia/insufficiency Agenesis/hypoplasia of corpus callosum Cataract Cerebral atrophy/myelin abnormality Deafness, sensorineural Dementia/psychosis Diffuse increased pigmentation of skin Hypotonia Lissencephaly/pachygyria/ polymicrogyria Mental retardation Migration abnormality/ heterotopia Nystagmus Optic atrophy Peripheral neuropathy Prominent forehead/frontal bossing Retinitis pigmentosa/ pigmentary retinopathy/ chorioretinitis Seizures/abnormal EEG Stippled or fragmented epiphyses	Enlarged liver	Braverman N, Dodt G, Gould SJ, and Valle D. Disorders of peroxisome biogenesis. (Review.) *Human Molecular Genetics* 1995; **4**: 1791–8. Paul DA *et al*. Neonatal adrenoleukodystrophy presenting as infantile progressive spinal muscular atrophy. *Pediatric Neurology*, 1993; **9**: 496–7. Poll-The BT *et al*. Infantile Refsum disease: an inherited peroxisomal disorder. Comparison with Zellweger syndrome and neonatal adrenoleukodystrophy. *European Journal of Pediatrics*, 1987; **146**: 477–83.
Adrenoleukodystrophy (pseudoneonatal)	Adrenal hypoplasia/insufficiency Buphthalmos Cerebral atrophy/myelin abnormality Club foot, varus Deafness, sensorineural Depressed/flat nasal bridge	Enlarged liver	Barth PG *et al*. Peroxisomal beta-oxidation defect with detectable peroxisomes: a case with neonatal onset and progressive course. *European Journal of Pediatrics*, 1990; **149**: 722–6.

Disease	Features	Hepatic abnormalities	Reference(s)
	Dolichocephaly/scaphocephaly Extrapyramidal disorder Glaucoma Hyperkeratosis Hypertonia Hypotonia Late puberty in male Mental retardation Muscle weakness/myopathy Nystagmus Optic atrophy Organicaciduria Palpebral fissures slant up Prominent forehead/frontal bossing Retina, general abnormalities Retinitis pigmentosa/ pigmentary retinopathy/ chorioretinitis Seizures/abnormal EEG Short stature, proportionate Stippled or fragmented epiphyses Storage cells/vacuolated lymphocytes Stridor		Mandel H *et al.* Zellweger-like phenotype in two siblings: a defect in peroxisomal beta-oxidation with elevated very long-chain fatty acids but normal bile acids. *Journal of Inherited Metabolic Disease*, 1992; **15**: 381–4. Santer R *et al.* Isolated defect of peroxisomal beta-oxidation in a 16-year-old patient. *European Journal of Pediatrics*, 1993; **152**: 339–42.
Aldolase A deficiency	Abnormal secondary sexual hair Anaemia/red cell abnormalities Congenital cardiac anomaly, unspecified Depressed/flat nasal bridge Epicanthic folds Flat face Hyperelastic skin Hypohidrotic or dry skin Joint laxity Low posterior/trident hairline Mental retardation Microcephaly Primary amenorrhoea Prominent ears Prominent vessels of skin Ptosis of eyelids Short nails Short neck Short stature, proportionate Small penis (including micro) Small teeth Spasticity/increased tendon reflex Telangiectasia of eyelids	Enlarged liver	Beutler E *et al.* Red cell aldolase deficiency and hemolytic anemia: a new syndrome. *Transactions of the Association of American Physicians*, 1973; **76**: 154–66. Hurst JA, Baraitser M, and Winter RM. A syndrome of mental retardation, short stature, hemolytic anemia, delayed puberty, and abnormal facial appearance: similarities to a report of aldolase A deficiency. *American Journal of Medical Genetics*, 1987; **28**: 965–70.
Alpers' progressive infantile poliodystrophy	Ataxia Camptodactyly Cerebral atrophy/myelin abnormality	Liver function is abnormal. Subacute hepatitis, fat infiltration, cell loss	Narkewicz MR *et al.* Liver involvement in Alpers disease. *Journal of Pediatrics*, 1991; **119**: 260–7.

Disease	Features	Hepatic abnormalities	Reference(s)
	Club foot, valgus Cryptorchid testes Deafness, sensorineural Dysphagia Extrapyramidal disorder Feeding problems in infants Flexion deformity of hip Flexion deformity of knee Hypospadias Hypotonia Joint contractures (including arthrogryposis) Limited movement of hip Limited movement/flexion deformity of elbow Mental retardation Microcephaly Muscle atrophy Recurrent infections Seizures/abnormal EEG Short neck Short stature, prenatal onset Sloping forehead Small mandible/micrognathia Spasticity/increased tendon reflex		Wilson DC, McGibben D, Hicks EM, and Allen IV. Progressive neuronal degeneration of childhood (Alpers syndrome) with hepatic cirrhosis. *European Journal of Pediatrics*, 1993; **152**: 260–2.
Apple-peel congenital intestinal atresia	Absent or hypoplastic hallux Absent toes Anal atresia/stenosis Atrial septum defect Brachydactyly Common mesentery Dilated ureters/ureteral atresia Feeding problems in infants Hydrocephaly/large ventricles, non-specific Intestinal duplication Intestinal malrotation Microphthalmia Skin syndactyly of fingers Small bowel atresia/absence/obstruction/short Small/hypoplastic/deep set nails Spina bifida occulta Syndactyly 2–3 of toes	Biliary atresia with secondary effects on the liver	Farag TI *et al.* Second family with 'apple peel' syndrome affecting four siblings: autosomal recessive inheritance confirmed. (Letter.) *American Journal of Medical Genetics*, 1993; **47**: 119–21.
Argininosuccinic aciduria	Ataxia Brittle hair Coarse hair Feeding problems in infants Mental retardation Seizures/abnormal EEG Sparse hair/alopecia areata Speech delay Trichorrhexis nodosa	Abnormal liver function, enlarged liver, fibrosis	Gerrits GPJM *et al.* Argininosuccinic aciduria: clinical and biochemical findings in three children with the late onset form, with special emphasis on cerebrospinal fluid findings of amino acids and pyrimidines. *Neuropediatrics*, 1993; **24**: 15–18. Renner C *et al.* Sodium citrate

Disease	Features	Hepatic abnormalities	Reference(s)
			supplementation in inborn argininosuccinate lyase deficiency: a study in a 5-year-old patient under total parenteral nutrition. *European Journal of Pediatrics*, 1995; **154**: 909–14. Zimmermann A, Bachmann C, and Baumgartner R. Severe liver fibrosis in argininosuccinic aciduria. *Archives of Pathology and Laboratory Medicine*, 1986; **110**: 136–40.
Arteriohepatic dysplasia (Alagille)	Anal atresia/stenosis Anterior chamber abnormalities, unspecified Atrial septum defect Cloudy corneas/sclerocornea Deep-set eyes Delayed bone age Depressed/flat nasal bridge Ectopic pupils Fallot tetralogy Hemivertebras High-pitched voice Hoarse voice Hypertelorism Hypothyroidism/small/absent thyroid Keratoconus Large spleen Late puberty in females Late puberty in male Mental retardation Palpebral fissures slant up Pointed chin Prominent forehead/frontal bossing Pulmonary stenosis Renal dysplasia Retinitis pigmentosa/ pigmentary retinopathy/ chorioretinitis Segmentation defects of spine Short phalanges Short stature, proportionate Spina bifida occulta Urethral fistulas Ventricular septal defect Vertebral interpedicular distance, narrow Xanthomas	Paucity of intrahepatic bile ducts resulting in prolonged neonatal jaundice	Elmslie FV *et al*. Alagille syndrome: family studies. *Journal of Medical Genetics*, 1995; **32**: 264–8. Hoffenberg EJ *et al*. Outcome of syndromic paucity of interlobular bile ducts (Alagille syndrome) with onset of cholestasis in infancy. *Journal of Pediatrics*, 1995; **127**: 220–4. Rand EB *et al*. Molecular analysis of 24 Alagille syndrome families identifies a single submicroscopic deletion and further localizes the Alagille region within 20p12. *American Journal of Human Genetics*, 1995; **57**: 1068–73.
Ataxia–ichthyosis– hepatosplenomegaly	Ataxia Hyperkeratosis Ichthyosis	Enlarged liver, but thought to be secondary to chronic congestion	Dykes PJ, Marks R, and Harper PS. A syndrome of ichthyosis, hepatosplenomegaly

Disease	Features	Hepatic abnormalities	Reference(s)
	Large spleen		and cerebellar degeneration. *British Journal of Dermatology*, 1979; **100**: 585–90. Harper PS *et al.* Ichthyosis, hepatosplenomegaly, and cerebellar degeneration in a sibship. *Journal of Medical Genetics*, 1980; **17**: 212–15.
Bardet–Biedl (Laurence–Moon–Bardet–Biedl) syndrome	Brachydactyly Cardiomyopathy Congenital cardiac anomaly, unspecified Diabetes mellitus/ hyperglycaemia Generalized obesity Glaucoma Glycosuria Hydronephrosis Hypogonadism Late puberty in females Late puberty in male Malformed uterus Mental retardation Multiple renal cysts Nephritis or nephropathy Nystagmus Pigmentary abnormality of macula Postaxial polydactyly of fingers Postaxial polydactyly of toes Renal dysplasia Retinitis pigmentosa/ pigmentary retinopathy/ chorioretinitis Secondary amenorrhoea Short stature, proportionate Small penis (including micro) Small testes Urethra, general abnormalities Urethral fistulas Vaginal atresia Vaginal septum/duplication/ hydrometrocolpos Vision, non-specific impairment	Congenital hepatic fibrosis	Carmi R, Elbedour K, Stone EM, and Sheffield VC. Phenotypic differences among patients with Bardet–Biedl syndrome linked to three different chromosome loci. *American Journal of Medical Genetics*, 1995; **59**: 199–203. Leppert M *et al.* Bardet–Biedl syndrome is linked to DNA markers on chromosome 11q and is genetically heterogeneous. *Nature Genetics*, 1994; **7**: 108–12. Nakamura F, Sasaki H, Kajihara H, and Yamanoue M. Laurence–Moon–Biedl syndrome accompanied by congenital hepatic fibrosis. *Journal of Gastroenterology and Hepatology*, 1990; **5**: 206–10.
Berardinelli syndrome (lipodystrophy, Lawrence-Seip)	Acanthosis nigricans Advanced bone age/large epiphyses Cardiomyopathy Deficient adipose tissue or fat/ lipodystrophy Diabetes mellitus/ hyperglycaemia Diffuse increased pigmentation of skin	Cirrhosis	Flier JS. Lilly Lecture: syndromes of insulin resistance. From patient to gene and back again. *Diabetes*, 1992; **41**: 1207–19. van der Vorm ER *et al.* Patients with lipodystrophic diabetes mellitus of the Seip–Berardinelli type, express normal insulin receptors.

Disease	Features	Hepatic abnormalities	Reference(s)
	Facial hirsutism Generalized hirsutism Glycosuria Hypohidrotic or dry skin Large kidneys Large penis Large spleen Mental retardation Ovarian cysts/tumours Prominent clitoris Prominent ears Protuberant abdomen Secondary amenorrhoea Sunken cheeks Tall stature, proportionate Thin		*Diabetologia*, 1993; **36**: 172–4.
Cantu syndrome (1976) (short stature; skeletal dysplasia)	Brachydactyly Depressed/flat nasal bridge Kyphosis Large ears Large spleen Lordosis Mesomelia of upper limbs Metaphyseal dysplasia Pectus carinatum Platyspondyly Prominent forehead/frontal bossing Prominent heels Proportionate shortening of lower limb Protuberant abdomen Sella turcica, J-shaped Short neck Short stature, prenatal onset Short stature, short limbs Short/hypoplastic metacarpals Small hands Small mandible/micrognathia Small/short nose Wide phalanges	Enlarged liver	Cantu JM *et al.* A distinct skeletal dysplasia in an infant from consanguineous parents. *Revista de Investigacion Clinica*, 1976; **28**: 255–61. Cantu JM *et al.* A distinct skeletal dysplasia in an infant from consanguineous parents. *Birth Defects, Original Article Series*, 1977; **13(3B)**: 139–47.
Carbohydrate-deficient glycoprotein syndrome type I	Abnormal labia Agenesis/hypoplasia of corpus callosum Arachnodactyly Ascites Ataxia Bleeding diatheses Cardiomyopathy Cataract Cerebellar abnormalities Cerebellar abnormalities (structural)	Cirrhosis, remodelling of parenchyma and intracellular lipid vacuoles	Conradi N *et al.* Liver pathology in the carbohydrate-deficient glycoprotein syndrome. *Acta Paediatrica Scandinavica*, 1991; **375**(Suppl.): 50–4. Hagberg BA, Blennow G, Kristiansson B, and Stibler H. Carbohydrate-deficient glycoprotein syndromes: peculiar group of new disorders. *Pediatric Neurology*,

Disease	Features	Hepatic abnormalities	Reference(s)
	Cerebral atrophy/myelin abnormality Cholesterol/lipids, abnormal Cryptorchid testes Dandy–Walker malformation Deficient adipose tissue or fat/lipodystrophy Extrapyramidal disorder Hypoplastic/inverted/absent nipples Hypotonia Joint contractures (including arthrogryposis) Large spleen Long toes Mental retardation Microcephaly Multiple renal cysts Muscle atrophy Oedema (including hydrops) Oedema of feet Oedema of hands Oedema of lower limbs Optic atrophy Patchy depigmentation of skin Patchy pigment of skin/café-au-lait spots Pericarditis (non-constrictive) Platelet abnormalities Prominent forehead/frontal bossing Recurrent infections Retinitis pigmentosa/pigmentary retinopathy/chorioretinitis Scoliosis Seizures/abnormal EEG Short stature, proportionate Small mandible/micrognathia Spasticity/increased tendon reflex Strabismus/gaze palsy Thin Truncal obesity		1993; **9**: 255–62. Hutchesson ACJ *et al.* Carbohydrate deficient glycoprotein syndrome; multiple abnormalities and diagnostic delay. *Archives of Diseases of Childhood*, 1995; **72**: 445–6. Jaeken J and Carchon H. The carbohydrate-deficient glycoprotein syndromes: an overview. *Journal of Inherited Metabolic Diseases*, 1993; **16**: 813–20.
Cardio-facio-cutaneous (CFC) syndrome	Atrial septum defect Brittle hair Cavernous haemangioma Cerebral atrophy/myelin abnormality Coarse facial features Cryptorchid testes Delayed bone age Depressed/flat nasal bridge Dystrophic nails Eczema/atopic dermatitis	Enlarged liver	Bottani A, Hammerer I, and Schinzel A. The cardio-facio-cutaneous syndrome: report of a patient and review of the literature. *European Journal of Pediatrics*, 1991; **150**: 486–8. Somer M *et al.* Cardio-facio-cutaneous syndrome: three additional cases and review of the literature. *American Journal of Medical Genetics*, 1992; **44**:

Disease	Features	Hepatic abnormalities	Reference(s)
	Epicanthic folds		691–5.
	Fine hair		
	Heart, general abnormalities		
	High frontal hairline		
	Hydrocephaly/large ventricles, non-specific		
	Hyperkeratosis		
	Hypertelorism		
	Hypohidrotic or dry skin		
	Hypoplasia/dysplasia of optic nerve		
	Hypoplastic supraorbital ridges		
	Hypotonia		
	Ichthyosis		
	Large spleen		
	Loose skin in neck		
	Macrocephaly		
	Mental retardation		
	Narrow forehead/temporal narrowing		
	Oedema (including hydrops)		
	Palpebral fissures slant down		
	Pectus carinatum		
	Pectus excavatum		
	Posteriorly rotated ears		
	Prominent ear helix		
	Ptosis of eyelids		
	Pulmonary stenosis		
	Scoliosis		
	Seizures/abnormal EEG		
	Short stature, proportionate		
	Sparse hair/alopecia areata		
	Webbed neck		
Cerebro-oculo-hepato-renal syndrome	Anaemia/red cell abnormalities	Enlarged liver with abnormal function and hyperechogenic, compatible with fat infiltration	Matsuzaka T *et al.* Cerebro-oculo-hepato-renal syndrome (Arima's syndrome): a distinct clinicopathological entity. *Journal of Child Neurology*, 1986; **1**: 338–46.
	Aplasia or dysplasia of retina		
	Blindness		
	Cataract		
	Cerebellar abnormalities (structural)		
	Depressed/flat nasal bridge		
	Dystopia canthorum (telecanthus)		
	Flexion deformity of knee		
	Hypotonia		
	Limited movement of ankle		
	Macrostomia		
	Mental retardation		
	Multiple renal cysts		
	Nystagmus		
	Optic atrophy		
	Ptosis of eyelids		
	Renal dysplasia		
Cerebrotendinous xanthomatosis	Absent/abnormal gallbladder	Hepatocytes contain a light golden pigment and bile cholestanol is significantly	Kim K-S *et al.* Identification of new mutations in sterol 27-hydroxylase gene in Japanese
	Ataxia		
	Cataract		

Disease	Features	Hepatic abnormalities	Reference(s)
	Cerebellar abnormalities Cerebral atrophy/myelin abnormality Cholesterol/lipids, abnormal Club foot, varus Dementia/psychosis Dysphagia Enlarged joints High arches of feet (pes cavus) Hypothyroidism/small/absent thyroid Malabsorption Mental retardation Muscle atrophy Peripheral neuropathy Pons/medulla/basal ganglia, abnormal Premature atherosclerosis Seizures/abnormal EEG Sensory abnormalities Spasticity/increased tendon reflex Speech defect/dysarthria Tremors Xanthomas	increased	patients with cerebrotendinous xanthomatosis (CTX). *Journal of Lipid Research*, 1994; **35**: 1031–9. Kuriyama M *et al.* Cerebrotendinous xanthomatosis: clinical and biochemical evaluation of eight patients and review of the literature. *Journal of the Neurological Sciences*, 1991; **102**: 225–32. Leitersdorf E *et al.* Cerebrotendinous xanthomatosis in the Israeli Druze: molecular genetics and phenotypic characteristics. *American Journal of Human Genetics*, 1994; **55**: 907–15.
Cholesterol ester storage disease	Adrenal calcification Ascites Cholesterol/lipids, abnormal Hypogonadism Large spleen Late puberty in females Late puberty in male Naevi or lentigines Premature atherosclerosis Respiratory abnormality, unspecified Short stature, proportionate	Enlarged liver, cirrhosis, lipid filled hepatocytes	Edelstein RA *et al.* Cholesteryl ester storage disease: a patient with massive splenomegaly and splenic abscess. *American Journal of Gastroenterology*, 1988; **83**: 687–92. Muntoni S *et al.* Homozygosity for a splice junction mutation in exon 8 of the gene encoding lysosomal acid lipase in a Spanish kindred with cholesterol ester storage disease (CESD). *Human Genetics*, 1995; **95**: 491–4.
Cumming syndrome (1986) (campomelia; polycystic dysplasia; polysplenia)	Absent or hypoplastic femur Bowed femur Bowed humerus Bowed radius Bowed tibia Bowed ulna Bowing of bones Cleft palate Club foot, varus Colon/caecum atresia Cranial sutures, wide Holoprosencephaly/arhinencephaly Hypoplastic or absent fibula Hypoplastic or absent humerus Hypoplastic or absent radii	Polycystic dysplasia	Cumming WA, Ohlsson A, and Ali A. Campomelia, cervical lymphocele, polycystic dysplasia, short gut, polysplenia. *American Journal of Medical Genetics*, 1986; **25**: 783–90. Urioste M, Arroyo A, and Martinez-Frias M-L. Campomelia, polycystic dysplasia, and cervical lymphocele in two sibs. *American Journal of Medical Genetics*, 1991; **41**: 475–7.

Disease	Features	Hepatic abnormalities	Reference(s)
	Hypoplastic or absent tibia Hypoplastic or absent ulna Lung hypoplasia/agenesis Multiple renal cysts Nuchal bleb/cystic hygroma of neck Oedema (including hydrops) Pancreatic cysts/tumours Polysplenia Proportionate short arms Short stature, prenatal onset Small bowel atresia/absence/obstruction/short		
Disseminated haemangiomatosis	Anaemia/red cell abnormalities Arteriovenous malformations Capillary haemangioma Cavernous haemangioma Facial haemangiomas Glaucoma Heart, general abnormalities Hydrocephaly/large ventricles, non-specific Intracranial calcification Large spleen Papules Platelet abnormalities Spasticity/increased tendon reflex Vascular malformations of brain	Hepatic haemangiomas	Byard RW, Burrows PE, Izakawa T, and Silver MM. Diffuse infantile haemangiomatosis: clinicopathological features and management problems in five fatal cases. *European Journal of Pediatrics*, 1991; **150**: 224–7. Gozal D *et al.* Diffuse neonatal haemangiomatosis: successful management with high dose corticosteroids. *European Journal of Pediatrics*, 1990; **149**: 321–4.
Erythropoietic protoporphyria	Abnormal scar formation Absent/abnormal gallbladder Anaemia/red cell abnormalities Bullas or vesicles Erythema/erythroderma Generalized hirsutism Localized hirsutism Patchy pigment of skin/café-au-lait spots Skin photosensitivity	Enlarged liver with progressive failure	Todd DJ. Erythropoietic protoporphyria. *British Journal of Dermatology*, 1994; **131**: 751–66.
Fanconi syndrome (ichthyosis–jaundice–diarrhoea)	Aminoaciduria Club foot, varus Dislocation of hip Feeding problems in infants Flexion deformity at wrist Flexion deformity of hip Flexion deformity of knee Glycosuria Hypotonia Ichthyosis Malabsorption Platelet abnormalities Proteinuria Recurrent infections	Enlarged liver, jaundice	Deal JE, Barratt TM, and Dillon MJ. Fanconi syndrome, ichthyosis, dysmorphism, jaundice and diarrhoea—a new syndrome. *Pediatric Nephrology*, 1990; **4**: 308–13.
Fetal congenital cytomegalovirus	Absent finger tips	Enlarged liver	Darin N, Bergstrom T, Fast A,

Disease	Features	Hepatic abnormalities	Reference(s)
infection	Absent fingers or oligodactyly Absent toes Ascites Brachydactyly Congenital cardiac anomaly, unspecified Cryptorchid testes Deafness, conductive Deafness, congenital Deafness, sensorineural Deafness, unilateral Glaucoma Hemiplegia High palate Hypoplastic toes (including phalanges) Hypotonia Inguinal hernia Intracranial calcification Large spleen Low birthweight (< 3rd centile) Mental retardation Microcephaly Optic atrophy Platelet abnormalities Pulmonary stenosis Retinitis pigmentosa/ pigmentary retinopathy/ chorioretinitis Seizures/abnormal EEG Spasticity/increased tendon reflex Strabismus/gaze palsy Umbilical hernia Ventricular septal defect		and Kyllerman M. Clinical, serological and PCR evidence of cytomegalovirus infection in the central nervous system in infancy and childhood. *Neuropediatrics*, 1994; **25**: 316–22. Fowler KB *et al.* The outcome of congenital cytomegalovirus infection in relation to maternal antibody status. *New England Journal of Medicine*, 1992; **326**: 663–7. Yow MD and Demmler GJ. Congenital cytomegalovirus disease—20 years is long enough. (Editorial.) *New England Journal of Medicine*, 1992; **326**: 702–3.
Fetal rubella	Anaemia/red cell abnormalities Anterior encephalocele/ meningocele Atrial septum defect Cardiomyopathy Cataract Cloudy corneas/sclerocornea Cryptorchid testes Deafness, sensorineural Diabetes mellitus/ hyperglycaemia Fontanelles, delayed closure/ large Glaucoma Hypopituitarism Hypospadias Intracranial calcification Large spleen Lung, general abnormalities Mental retardation	Prolonged jaundice, enlarged liver	Kaplan KM *et al.* A profile of mothers giving birth to infants with congenital rubella syndrome. *American Journal of Diseases of Childhood*, 1990; **144**: 118–23. McIntosh EDG and Menser MA. A fifty-year follow-up of congenital rubella. *Lancet*, 1992; **ii**:414.

Disease	Features	Hepatic abnormalities	Reference(s)
	Metaphyseal dysplasia Microcephaly Microphthalmia Patent ductus arteriosus Platelet abnormalities Pulmonary stenosis Retinitis pigmentosa/ pigmentary retinopathy/ chorioretinitis Ventricular septal defect		
Fetal toxoplasmosis	Anaemia/red cell abnormalities Hydrocephaly/large ventricles, non-specific Intracranial calcification Large spleen Low birthweight (< 3rd centile) Macules Mental retardation Microcephaly Microphthalmia Platelet abnormalities Polymorph abnormalities Purpura Retinitis pigmentosa /pigmentary retinopathy/ chorioretinitis Seizures/abnormal EEG Spasticity/increased tendon reflex	Enlarged liver, jaundice	Hall SM. Congenital toxoplasmosis. (Review.) *British Medical Journal*, 1992; **305**: 291–7. Mombro M *et al*. Congenital taxoplasmosis: 10-year follow up. *European Journal of Pediatrics*, 1995; **154**: 635–9.
Focal nodular hyperplasia of the liver (vascular malformations)	Aneurysms Brain tumours/cysts Vascular malformations of brain	Focal nodular hyperplasia	Albrecht S, Wanless IR, Bilbao J, and Frei JV. Multiple focal nodular hyperplasia of the liver associated with vascular malformations and neoplasia of the brain and meninges: a new syndrome. *Laboratory Investigation*, 1989; **60**: 2A. Goldin RD and Rose DSC. Focal nodular hyperplasia of the liver associated with intracranial vascular malformations. *Gut*, 1990; **31**: 554–5.
Fucosidosis	Absent or hypoplastic clavicles Beaked/wedged vertebrae Cardiomyopathy Cerebral atrophy/myelin abnormality Cloudy corneas/sclerocornea Coarse facial features Deafness, sensorineural Diaphyseal dysplasia Fullness of periorbital region Hypohidrotic or dry skin Joint contractures (including	Enlarged liver with foamy cytoplasm in some hepatocytes	Seo H-C, Willems PJ, and O'Brien JS. Six additional mutations in fucosidosis: three nonsense mutations and three frameshift mutations. *Human Molecular Genetics*, 1993; **2**: 1205–8. Willems PJ *et al*. Fucosidosis revisited: a review of 77 patients. *American Journal of Medical Genetics*, 1991; **38**: 111–31.

Disease	Features	Hepatic abnormalities	Reference(s)
	arthrogryposis) Kyphosis Large spleen Large tongue Long philtrum Mental retardation Mucopolysacchariduria/ oligosacchariduria Papules Prominent forehead/frontal bossing Proximal tapering of metacarpals Retinitis pigmentosa/ pigmentary retinopathy/ chorioretinitis Scoliosis Seizures/abnormal EEG Short stature, proportionate Spasticity/increased tendon reflex Storage cells/vacuolated lymphocytes Telangiectasia/angiokeratomas of skin Thick/stiff skin Umbilical hernia Vascular abnormalities of retina		
Galactosialidosis (neuraminidase and β-galactosidase deficiency)	Adrenal hyperplasia Ascites Beaked/wedged vertebrae Bulbous nasal tip Camptodactyly Cardiac situs inversus/ dextrocardia Cardiomyopathy Coarse facial features Dementia/psychosis Dolichocephaly/scaphocephaly Gibbus Hyperplastic supraorbital ridges Large kidneys Large spleen Macular red spot/cherry red spot Mental retardation Mucopolysacchariduria/ oligosacchariduria Oedema (including hydrops) Pectus carinatum Platyspondyly Scoliosis Seizures/abnormal EEG Sella turcica, J-shaped Single ventricle Storage cells/vacuolated	Enlarged liver with membrane-bound vacuoles on histology	Oyanagi K *et al.* Galactosialidosis: neuropathological findings in a case of the late-infantile type. *Acta Neuropathologica*, 1991; **82**: 331–9. Ozand PT and Gascon GG. Heterogeneity of carboxypeptidase activity in infantile-onset galactosialidosis. *Journal of Child Neurology*, 1992; **7**(Suppl.): S31–40. Strisciuglio P *et al.* Combined deficiency of beta-galactosidase and neuraminidase: natural history of the disease in the first 18 years of an American patient with late infantile onset form. *American Journal of Medical Genetics*, 1990; **37**: 573–7.

Disease	Features	Hepatic abnormalities	Reference(s)
	lymphocytes Subperiosteal new bone formation Telangiectasia/angiokeratomas of skin Thick lower lip Thick upper lip Thickened/oedematous eyelids		
Gardner syndrome	Aplasia or dysplasia of retina Brain tumours/cysts Cartilaginous/bony exostoses Colonic tumours Delayed tooth eruption/development Diffuse increased pigmentation of skin Gastrointestinal tumour/polyp/haemangioma Other tumours of skin Pancreatic cysts/tumours Retinitis pigmentosa/pigmentary retinopathy/chorioretinitis Skeletal cysts or tumours Skin cysts Spinal tumours Subperiosteal new bone formation Supernumerary teeth Thyroid tumours Tumour or cyst of the mandible	Hepatoblastomas	Hughes LJ and Michels VV. Risk of hepatoblastoma in familial adenomatous polyposis. *American Journal of Medical Genetics*, 1992; **43**: 1023–5. Perniciaro C. Gardner's syndrome. *Dermatologic Clinics*, 1995; **131**: 51–6.
Garrett–Tripp syndrome (mental retardation; polydactyly; hair absence; dermatitis; Perthe's disease)	Absent eyebrows Absent fingers or oligodactyly Absent or sparse eyelashes Alopecia totalis Capillary haemangioma Convex/beaked profile of nose Cutaneous pustules/ulcers Ear helix, general abnormalities Large spleen Mental retardation Perthe's/dysplastic hip Postaxial polydactyly of fingers Postaxial polydactyly of toes Recurrent infections Scalp, general abnormalities Seborrhoea Small penis (including micro) Syndactyly 2–3 of toes	Enlarged liver	Garrett C and Tripp JH. Unknown syndrome: mental retardation with postaxial polydactyly, congenital absence of hair, severe seborrhoeic dermatitis and Perthe's disease of the hip. *Journal of Medical Genetics*, 1988; **25**: 270–2.
Gaucher disease (neonatal)	Anteverted nares Ectropion of eyelids Flexion deformity of hip Flexion deformity of knee Ichthyosis Joint contractures (including	Enlarged liver with Gaucher cells in sinusoids (rather than in hepatocytes)	Horowitz M. Mutations causing Gaucher disease. *Human Mutation* 1994; **3**: 1–11. Sidransky E, Tayebi N, and Ginns EI. Diagnosing Gaucher disease. *Clinical Pediatrics*,

Disease	Features	Hepatic abnormalities	Reference(s)
	arthrogryposis) Large spleen Limited movement/flexion deformity of elbow Lung hypoplasia/agenesis Open mouth appearance Small ears/microtia Storage cells/vacuolated lymphocytes Thick/stiff skin		1995; **34**: 365–71.
Gaucher disease type II (infantile or acute neuronopathic type)	Anaemia/red cell abnormalities Dementia/psychosis Fetal finger pads Hypertonia Hypotonia Ichthyosis Incoordination Large spleen Mental retardation Pigmentary abnormality of macula Seizures/abnormal EEG Spasticity/increased tendon reflex Storage cells/vacuolated lymphocytes Strabismus/gaze palsy	Enlarged liver with Gaucher cells in sinusoids	Sidransky E, Tayebi N, and Ginns EI. Diagnosing Gaucher Disease. *Clinical Pediatrics*, 1995; 365–71. Walley AJ *et al.* Gaucher's disease in the United Kingdom: screening non-Jewish patients for the two common mutations. *Journal of Medical Genetics*, 1993; **30**: 280–3.
Gaucher disease type I (adult type)	Anaemia/red cell abnormalities Aortic stenosis Aseptic necrosis of epiphysis Ataxia Calcification of arteries Cloudy corneas/sclerocornea Cortical hyperostosis/thickening Dementia/psychosis Erythema/erythroderma Indifference to pain Large spleen Multiple fractures Oedema (including hydrops) Osteoporosis Patchy pigment of skin/café-au-lait spots Retinitis pigmentosa/pigmentary retinopathy/chorioretinitis Seizures/abnormal EEG Sensory abnormalities Skeletal cysts or tumours Speech defect/dysarthria Storage cells/vacuolated lymphocytes Subperiosteal new bone formation Wide metaphysis	Enlarged liver with Gaucher cells in sinusoids	Amaral O *et al.* Molecular characterisation of type 1 Gaucher disease families and patients: intrafamilial heterogeneity at the clinical level. *Journal of Medical Genetics*, 1994; **31**: 401–4. Beutler E. Modern diagnosis and treatment of Gaucher's disease. *American Journal of Diseases of Childhood*, 1993; **147**: 1175–83. Grabowski GA. Gaucher disease. Enzymology, genetics, and treatment. *Advances in Human Genetics*, 1993; **21**: 377–441.

Disease	Features	Hepatic abnormalities	Reference(s)
Gaucher disease type III (juvenile or norbottnian type)	Aseptic necrosis of epiphysis Ataxia Cortical hyperostosis/thickening Dementia/psychosis Dysphagia Hypotonia Large spleen Multiple fractures Muscle atrophy Osteoporosis Ptosis of eyelids Seizures/abnormal EEG Skeletal cysts or tumours Spasticity/increased tendon reflex Storage cells/vacuolated lymphocytes Strabismus/gaze palsy Subperiosteal new bone formation Wide metaphysis	Enlarged liver with Gaucher cells in sinusoids	Brady RO, Barton NW, and Grabowski GA. The role of neurogenetics in Gaucher disease. *Archives of Neurology*, 1993; **50**: 1212–24. Sidransky E and Ginns EI. Clinical heterogeneity among patients with Gaucher's disease. (Clinical conference.) *Journal of the American Medical Association*, 1993; **269**: 1154–7.
Geleophysic dysplasia	Abnormal/absent metatarsals Anteverted nares Aortic stenosis Brachydactyly Camptodactyly Coarse facial features Congenital cardiac anomaly, unspecified Coxa valga Delayed bone age Hypoplastic or absent carpals Joint contractures (including arthrogryposis) Large spleen Limited movement of fingers Limited movement of knee Limited movement/flexion deformity of elbow Long philtrum Macrostomia Mitral stenosis Perthes'/dysplastic hip Proximal tapering of metacarpals Round face Short bones Short stature, proportionate Short/hypoplastic metacarpals Simple/absent philtrum Small hands Small/short nose Thick/stiff skin Thin lower lip Thin upper lip Trachea or laryngeal anomalies	Enlarged liver, hepatocytes contain periodic acid–Schiff positive, diastase-resistant, inclusions	Rosser EM *et al.* Geleophysic dysplasia: a report of three affected boys—prenatal ultrasound does not detect recurrence. *American Journal of Medical Genetics*, 1995; **58**: 217–21. Shohat M *et al.* Geleophysic dysplasia: a storage disorder affecting the skin, bone, liver, heart, and trachea. *Journal of Pediatrics*, 1990; **117**: 227–32.

Disease	Features	Hepatic abnormalities	Reference(s)
Generalized gangliosidosis type 1	Wide metacarpals/modelling defect Wide nasal bridge Acromelia of upper limbs Beaked/wedged vertebrae Broad base to nose Cardiomyopathy Coarse facial features Depressed/flat nasal bridge Enlarged liver Epiphyseal dysplasia Full cheeks Generalized hirsutism Gum hypertrophy Joint contractures (including arthrogryposis) Joint stiffness/arthritis Kyphosis Large tongue Long philtrum Macrocephaly Macular red spot/cherry red spot Mental retardation Metaphyseal dysplasia Mucopolysacchariduria/ oligosacchariduria Osteoporosis Prominent forehead/frontal bossing Prominent maxilla Prominent/deep philtrum Proximal tapering of metacarpals Scoliosis Short stature, prenatal onset Stippled or fragmented epiphyses Storage cells/vacuolated lymphocytes Subperiosteal new bone formation Thick/wide alveolar ridges Thick/wide ribs Thickened/oedematous eyelids Trachea or laryngeal anomalies	Enlarged with vacuoles and diffuse foamy histiocytes	Boustany R-M, Qian W-H, and Suzuki K. Mutations in acid β-galactosidase cause GM1-gangliosidosis in American patients. *American Journal of Human Genetics*, 1993; **53**: 881–8. Nardocci N *et al.* Chronic GM1 gangliosidosis presenting as dystonia: clinical and biochemical studies in a new case. *Neuropediatrics*, 1993; **24**: 164–6.
Glutaric aciduria type 2	Biliary atresia/stenosis Brain, general abnormalities Club foot, varus Cryptorchid testes Dolichocephaly/scaphocephaly Fontanelles, delayed closure/ large Hamartoma of brain Hypoglycaemia Hypospadias	Enlarged liver with fatty infiltration	Colombo I *et al.* Mutations and polymorphisms of the gene encoding the β-subunit of the electron transfer flavoprotein in three patients with glutaric acidemia type II. *Human Molecular Genetics*, 1994; **3**: 429–36. Stockler S *et al.* Symmetric hypoplasia of the temporal

Disease	Features	Hepatic abnormalities	Reference(s)
	Large kidneys Lissencephaly/pachygyria/ polymicrogyria Low-set ears Macrocephaly Mental retardation Multiple renal cysts Organicaciduria Pancreas (exocrine), general abnormalities Rocker-bottom feet (see also vertical talus) Seizures/abnormal EEG Undermineralization of skull		cerebral lobes in an infant with glutaric aciduria type II (multiple acyl-coenzyme A dehydrogenase deficiency). *Journal of Pediatrics*, 1994; **124**: 601–4.
Goldstein syndrome (1988) (Sotos-like syndrome)	Advanced tooth eruption/ development Dolichocephaly/scaphocephaly Dystopia canthorum (telecanthus) Epicanthic folds Fontanelles, delayed closure/ large High birthweight (> 90th centile) Hypoplastic maxilla (excluding malar region) Hypotonia Large spleen Macrocephaly Mental retardation Narrow thorax/funnel chest Pectus excavatum Prominent forehead/frontal bossing Scoliosis Small/short nose Tall stature, proportionate Thin/long face Upturned nose	Enlarged liver	Goldstein DJ *et al.* Overgrowth, congenital hypotonia, nystagmus, strabismus, and mental retardation: variant of dominantly inherited Sotos sequence? *American Journal of Medical Genetics*, 1988; **29**: 783–92.
Growth retardation–alopecia–pseudoanodontia–optic atrophy (GAPO)	Alopecia totalis Bowed radius Bowed tibia Bowed ulna Cerebral atrophy/myelin abnormality Delayed bone age Delayed tooth eruption/ development Depressed/flat nasal bridge Diaphyseal dysplasia Fontanelles, delayed closure/ large Glaucoma Hypertelorism Hypogonadism	Enlarged liver	Moriya N *et al.* GAPO syndrome: report on the first case in Japan. *American Journal of Medical Genetics*, 1995; **58**: 257–61. Sandgren G. GAPO syndrome: a new case. *American Journal of Medical Genetics*, 1995; **58**: 87–90. Sayli BS and Gul D. GAPO syndrome in three relatives in a Turkish kindred. *American Journal of Medical Genetics*, 1993; **47**: 342–5.

Disease	Features	Hepatic abnormalities	Reference(s)
	Keratoconus Macrocephaly Macrocornea/megalocornea Mental retardation Nystagmus Oligodontia Optic atrophy Osteoporosis Papilloedema/optic neuritis Prominent eyes/proptosis Prominent forehead/frontal bossing Prominent upper lip Prominent/everted lower lip Sclerosis of skull Short stature, proportionate Small mandible/micrognathia Sparse/decreased eyebrows Tremors		
Haemangioendotheliomas–hemihypertrophy	Asymmetric arms Asymmetric face Asymmetric lower limbs Gastrointestinal tumour/polyp/haemangioma Hemihypertrophy Hypertrophy of lower limb Hypertrophy of upper limb Platelet abnormalities	Epithelial hepatoblastoma	Dehner LP and Ishak KG. Vascular tumors of the liver in infants and children. *Archives of Pathology*, 1971; **92**: 101. Geiser CF *et al*. Epithelial hepatoblastoma associated with congenital hemihypertrophy and cystathioninuria: presentation of a case. *Pediatrics*, 1970; **46**: 66. Wood BP, Putnam TC, and Chacko AK. Infantile hepatic hemangioendotheliomas associated with hemihypertrophy. *Pediatric Radiology*, 1977; **5**: 242–5.
Haemochromatosis (neonatal with multiple malformations)	Anteverted nares Aortic incompetence Apnoea or tachypnoea Blepharophimosis/blepharospasm Bulbous nasal tip Cardiomyopathy Cutis marmorata Horseshoe kidneys Hypoglycaemia Hypotonia Large spleen Postaxial polydactyly of fingers Postaxial polydactyly of toes Pulmonary stenosis Small mandible/micrognathia Syndactyly of toes (not 2–3) Ventricular septal defect	Enlarged liver, greenish brown in colour with architecture distorted by fibrous bands, cholestasis	Taucher SC, Bentjerodt R, Hubner ME, and Nazer J. Multiple malformations in neonatal hemochromatosis. (Letter.) *American Journal of Medical Genetics*, 1994; **50**: 213–14.
Haemolytic anaemia–polyendocrinopathy	Anaemia/red cell abnormalities Biliary atresia/stenosis	Chronic hepatitis	Colletti RB *et al*. Autoimmune enteropathy and nephropathy

Disease	Features	Hepatic abnormalities	Reference(s)
	Colon, general abnormalities Diabetes mellitus/ hyperglycaemia Hypothyroidism/small/absent thyroid Malabsorption Nephritis or nephropathy Proteinuria Recurrent infections		with circulating anti-epithelial cell antibodies. *Journal of Pediatrics*, 1991; **118**: 858–64. Hill SM, Milla PJ, Bottazzo GF, and Mirakian R. Autoimmune enteropathy and colitis: is there a generalised autoimmune gut disorder? *Gut*, 1991; **32**: 36–42. Satake N *et al.* A Japanese family of X-linked autoimmune enteropathy with haemolytic anaemia and polyendocrinopathy. *European Journal of Pediatrics*, 1993; **152**: 313–15.
Homocystinuria	Advanced bone age/large epiphyses Aminoaciduria Arachnodactyly Blood vessels, general abnormalities Cataract Dislocation of lens Fine hair Generalized depigmentation of hair Long toes Mental retardation Myopia Osteoporosis Pectus carinatum Pectus excavatum Platyspondyly Seizures/abnormal EEG Sparse hair/alopecia areata Thin	Enlarged and fatty liver (rare)	Hu FL *et al.* Molecular basis of cystathionine β-synthase deficiency in pyridoxine responsive and nonresponsive homocystinuria. *Human Molecular Genetics*, 1993; **2**: 1857–60. Keskin S and Yalcin E. Case report of homocystinuria: clinical, electroencephalographic, and magnetic resonance imaging findings. *Journal of Child Neurology*, 1994; **9**: 210–12. Kraus JP. Molecular basis of phenotype expression in homocystinuria. *Journal of Inherited Metabolic Diseases*, 1994; **17**: 383–90.
Hunter syndrome (mucopolysaccharidosis type II)	Aortic stenosis Beaked/wedged vertebrae Coarse facial features Deafness, sensorineural Delayed tooth eruption/development Depressed/flat nasal bridge Epiphyseal dysplasia Inguinal hernia Joint stiffness/arthritis Kyphosis Large nose Macrocephaly Mental retardation Mitral stenosis Mucopolysacchariduria/oligosacchariduria Pectus carinatum	Enlarged liver	Adinolfi M. Hunter syndrome: cloning of the gene, mutations and carrier detection. *Developmental Medicine and Child Neurology*, 1993; **35**: 79–85. Ben Simon-Schiff E, Bach G, Hopwood JJ, and Abeliovich D. Mutation analysis of Jewish Hunter patients in Israel. *Human Mutation*, 1994; **4**: 263–70. Yamada Y *et al.* Mucopolysaccharidosis type II (Hunter disease): 13 gene mutations in 52 Japanese patients and carrier detection in four families. *Human Genetics*,

Disease	Features	Hepatic abnormalities	Reference(s)
	Platyspondyly Sella turcica, J-shaped Short stature, proportionate Thick/wide ribs Umbilical hernia		1993; **92**: 110–14.
Hurler syndrome (mucopolysaccharidosis type IH)	Agenesis/hypoplasia of corpus callosum Aortic stenosis Beaked/wedged vertebrae Cardiomyopathy Cloudy corneas/sclerocornea Coarse facial features Deafness, conductive Depressed/flat nasal bridge Dolichocephaly/scaphocephaly Flared nares Gibbus Hydrocephaly/large ventricles, non-specific Inguinal hernia Joint stiffness/arthritis Limited movement of fingers Macrocephaly Mental retardation Mitral stenosis Mucopolysacchariduria/ oligosacchariduria Prominent forehead/frontal bossing Prominent upper lip Prominent/everted lower lip Proximal tapering of metacarpals Recurrent infections Short stature, proportionate Thick/wide alveolar ridges Wide metacarpals/modelling defect	Enlarged liver, fibrosis, swollen, empty or vacuolated hepatocytes and Kupffer cells	Clarke LA *et al.* Mutation analysis of 19 North American mucopolysaccharidosis type I patients: identification of two additional frequent mutations. *Human Mutation*, 1994; **3**: 275–82. Cleary MA and Wraith JE. The presenting features of mucopolysaccharidosis type IH (Hurler syndrome). *Acta Paediatrica*, 1995; **84**: 337–9.
Ichthyosis–biliary atresia	Biliary atresia/stenosis Ichthyosis	Enlarged liver, portal duct proliferation, bile plugging within bile ducts, cholestasis	Cunningham ML and Sybert VP. Idiopathic extrahepatic biliary atresia: recurrence in sibs in two families. *American Journal of Medical Genetics*, 1988; **31**: 421–6. Gunasekaran TS, Hassall EG, Steinbrecher UP, and Yong S-L. Recurrence of extrahepatic biliary atresia in two half sibs. *American Journal of Medical Genetics*, 1992; **43**: 592–4.
Ichthyosis–neutral lipid storage disease	Abnormal-coloured nails Aplasia or dysplasia of retina Ataxia Cataract Deafness, sensorineural Ectropion of eyelids	Enlarged liver, architecture in disarray, vacuolar fatty change	Angelini C *et al.* Multisystem triglyceride storage disorder with impaired long-chain fatty acid oxidation. *Annals of Neurology*, 1980; **7**: 5–10. Judge MR *et al.* Neutral lipid

Disease	Features	Hepatic abnormalities	Reference(s)
	Erythema/erythroderma Facial weakness High palate Hyperkeratosis Hypotonia Ichthyosis Large spleen Mental retardation Microcephaly Muscle weakness/myopathy Spasticity/increased tendon reflex Storage cells/vacuolated lymphocytes Thick/stiff skin Thickened nails		storage disease. Case report and lipid studies. *British Journal of Dermatology*, 1994; **130**: 507–10. Wessalowski R *et al.* Multisystem triglyceride storage disorder without ichthyosis in two siblings. *Acta Paediatrica*, 1994; **83**: 93–8.
Infantile Refsum	Ataxia Cataract Cholesterol/lipids, abnormal Deafness, sensorineural ECG abnormality/conduction defects Hypotonia Ichthyosis Malabsorption Mental retardation Microcephaly Muscle weakness/myopathy Nystagmus Osteoporosis Peripheral neuropathy Retinitis pigmentosa/ pigmentary retinopathy/ chorioretinitis Seizures/abnormal EEG Short stature, proportionate Spontaneous pain sensation Vascular malformations of brain	Enlarged liver, micronodular cirrhosis	Brown FR III, Voigt R, Singh AK, and Singh I. Peroxisomal disorders. Neurodevelopmental and biochemical aspects. (Review.) *American Journal of Diseases of Childhood*, 1993; **147**: 617–26. Chow CW *et al.* Autopsy findings in two siblings with infantile Refsum disease. *Acta Neuropathologica*, 1992; **83**: 190–5. Mandel H *et al.* Infantile Refsum disease: gastrointestinal presentation of a peroxisomal disorder. *Journal of Pediatric Gastroenterology and Nutrition*, 1992; **14**: 83–5.
Ivemark syndrome (asplenia or polysplenia)	Absent or hypoplastic spleen Atrioventricular septal defect Cardiac situs inversus/ dextrocardia Congenital cardiac anomaly, unspecified Holoprosencephaly/ arhinencephaly Hydranencephaly/ porencephaly/arachnoid cyst Hydrocephaly/large ventricles, non-specific Hypoplastic left heart Intestinal malrotation Malformation of the pancreas Meningocele/meningomyelocele Multiple renal cysts	Biliary atresia with secondary changes in the liver	Carmi R, Magee CA, Neill CA, and Karrer FM. Extrahepatic biliary atresia and associated anomalies: etiologic heterogeneity suggested by distinctive patterns of associations. *American Journal of Medical Genetics*, 1993; **45**: 683–93. Karrer FM, Hall RJ, and Lilly JR. Biliary atresia and the polysplenia syndrome. *Journal of Pediatric Surgery*, 1991; **26**: 524–7. Wainwright H and Nelson M. Polysplenia syndrome and congenital short pancreas.

Disease	Features	Hepatic abnormalities	Reference(s)
	Polysplenia Posterior encephalocele/ meningocele Pulmonary segmentation defects Single ventricle Situs inversus, abdominal Transposition of the great vessels Truncus arteriosus		*American Journal of Medical Genetics*, 1993; **47**: 318–20.
Jeune syndrome (asphyxiating thoracic dystrophy)	Acetabular spurs Cone-shaped epiphyses of phalanges Epiphyseal dysplasia Hydrocephaly/large ventricles, non-specific Metaphyseal dysplasia Multiple renal cysts Narrow thorax/funnel chest Nephritis or nephropathy Pancreas (exocrine), general abnormalities Postaxial polydactyly of fingers Preaxial polydactyly of fingers Proportionate short arms Proportionate shortening of lower limb Retinitis pigmentosa/ pigmentary retinopathy/ chorioretinitis Rhizomelia of lower limbs Rhizomelia of upper limbs Short ribs Short stature, proportionate Short stature, short limbs Trachea or laryngeal anomalies	Cirrhosis	Hudgins L, Rosengren S, Treem W, and Hyams J. Early cirrhosis in survivors with Jeune thoracic dystrophy. *Journal of Pediatrics*, 1992; **120**: 754–6.
Kahn syndrome (1987) (berry aneurysms; cirrhosis; emphysema; cerebral calcifications)	Clubbing of fingers (drumstick) Incoordination Intracranial calcification Large spleen Lung cysts Lung, general abnormalities Mental retardation Seizures/abnormal EEG Short stature, proportionate Speech defect/dysarthria Vascular malformations of brain	Cirrhosis	Kahn E *et al.* Berry aneurysms, cirrhosis, pulmonary emphysema, and bilateral symmetrical cerebral calcifications: a new syndrome. *American Journal of Medical Genetics*, 1987; Suppl. **3**: 343–56.
Kartagener syndrome	Bronchiectasis Cardiac situs inversus/ dextrocardia Congenital cardiac anomaly, unspecified Hydrocephaly/large ventricles, non-specific Polysplenia Situs inversus, abdominal	Situs inversus	Inamitsu M, Arima T, Nakashima T, and Uemura T. Ciliary ultrastructure in a child with Kartagener's syndrome. A transmission electron microscopic study using tannic acid staining. *European Archives of Oto-rhino-laryngology*, 1990; **248**: 49–52. Losa M *et al.* Kartagener

Disease	Features	Hepatic abnormalities	Reference(s)
			syndrome: an uncommon cause of neonatal respiratory distress? *European Journal of Pediatrics*, 1995; **154**: 236–8. Narayan D *et al.* Unusual inheritance of primary ciliary dyskinesia (Kartagener's syndrome). *Journal of Medical Genetics*, 1994; **31**: 493–6.
Katz syndrome (1973) (short stature; hepatomegaly; abnormal glucose tolerance)	Acanthosis nigricans Advanced bone age/large epiphyses Brachydactyly Clinodactyly Convex/beaked profile of nose Diabetes mellitus/ hyperglycaemia Dolichocephaly/scaphocephaly Late puberty in females Macules Primary amenorrhoea Prominent forehead/frontal bossing Short stature, proportionate Short/hypoplastic metacarpals Small mandible/micrognathia Sparse hair/alopecia areata Thick calvarium	Enlarged liver with abnormal function	Katz M. Case report 7. *Syndrome Identification*, 1973; **1(2)**: 6–9.
Keating syndrome (1985) (X-linked glycogen storage disease)	Joint stiffness/arthritis Late puberty in male Muscle weakness/myopathy Short stature, proportionate	Enlarged liver with glycogen storage in cytoplasm	Keating JP, Brown BI, White NH, and Dimauro S. X-linked glycogen storage disease: a cause of hypotonia, hyperuricemia, and growth retardation. *American Journal of Diseases of Childhood*, 1985; **139**: 609–13.
Larsen syndrome (1978) (cone dystrophy; liver disease; deafness; endocrine)	Aplasia or dysplasia of retina Deafness, sensorineural Diabetes mellitus/ hyperglycaemia Hypertension Hypothyroidism/small/absent thyroid Liver/biliary system, general abnormalities Night blindness Optic atrophy Sella turcica, large	Unspecified liver degeneration with fatty infiltration	Berg K, Larsen IF, and Hansen E. Familial syndrome of progressive cone dystrophy, degenerative liver disease, and endocrine dysfunction: III. Genetic studies. *Clinical Genetics*, 1978; **13**:190–200. Larsen IF, Hansen E, and Berg K. Familial syndrome of progressive cone dystrophy, degenerative liver disease and endocrine dysfunction. II. Clinical and metabolic studies. *Clinical Genetics*, 1978; **13**: 176–89.
Long-chain acyl-CoA dehydrogenase deficiency	Cardiomyopathy Feeding problems in infants Hypoglycaemia Hypotonia	Enlarged liver, lipid deposits, centrilobular necrosis	Aoyama T *et al.* Cloning of human very-long-chain acyl-coenzyme A dehydrogenase and molecular characterization

Disease	Features	Hepatic abnormalities	Reference(s)
	Mental retardation Microcephaly Muscle weakness/myopathy Organicaciduria		of its deficiency in two patients. *American Journal of Human Genetics*, 1995; **57**: 273–83. Coates PM. Very-long-chain acyl-CoA dehydrogenase deficiency: molecular genetics of a mitochondrial membrane enzyme. (Editorial.) *American Journal of Human Genetics*, 1995; **57**: 233–4.
Lutz–Richner syndrome (1973) (renal tubular insufficiency; jaundice; multiple anomalies)	Abnormal placement of anus Aminoaciduria Biliary atresia/stenosis Blepharophimosis/ blepharospasm Broad/barrel thorax Congenital cardiac anomaly, unspecified Dislocation of hip High palate Hypotonia Nephritis or nephropathy Polymorph abnormalities Proteinuria Recurrent infections Rocker-bottom feet (see also vertical talus) Small mandible/micrognathia Thin Wide-spaced nipples	Jaundice, pigment granules in hepatocytes (lipofuscin), periportal inflammatory cells, paucity of bile ducts	Horslen SP, Quarrell OWJ, and Tanner MS. Liver histology in the arthrogryposis multiplex congenita, renal dysfunction, and cholestasis (ARC) syndrome: report of three new cases and review. *Journal of Medical Genetics*, 1994; **31**: 62–4. Mikati MA *et al*. Renal tubular insufficiency, cholestatic jaundice, and multiple congenital anomalies—a new multisystem syndrome. *Helvetica Paediatrica Acta*, 1984; **39**: 463–71.
Mainzer–Saldino syndrome (retinal dysplasia; renal defects; skeletal anomalies)	Arachnodactyly Ataxia Cerebellar abnormalities (structural) Cone-shaped epiphyses of phalanges Delayed bone age Fine hair Hypotonia Joint laxity Mental retardation Metaphyseal dysplasia Nephritis or nephropathy Optic atrophy Ptosis of eyelids Renal dysplasia Retinitis pigmentosa/ pigmentary retinopathy/ chorioretinitis Short stature, proportionate Small kidneys Small penis (including micro) Small testes	Enlarged liver with hepatic fibrosis, histologically	Ellis DS *et al*. Leber's congenital amaurosis associated with familial juvenile nephronophthisis and cone-shaped epiphyses of the hands (the Mainzer–Saldino syndrome). *American Journal of Ophthalmology*, 1984; **97**: 233–9. Robins DG, French TA, and Chakera TMH. Juvenile nephronophthisis associated with skeletal abnormalities and hepatic fibrosis. *Archives of Diseases of Childhood*, 1976; **51**: 799–801.
Mannosidosis	Ataxia Beaked/wedged vertebrae	Enlarged liver	Bennet JK, Dembure PP, and Elsas LJ. Clinical and

Disease	Features	Hepatic abnormalities	Reference(s)
	Broad base to nose Cataract Cloudy corneas/sclerocornea Coarse facial features Deafness, sensorineural Depressed/flat nasal bridge Gibbus Joint stiffness/arthritis Kyphosis Large spleen Large tongue Mental retardation Mucopolysacchariduria/ oligosacchariduria Osteoporosis Platyspondyly Protuberant abdomen Short neck Short stature, proportionate Storage cells/vacuolated lymphocytes Thick calvarium Umbilical hernia Wide metacarpals/modelling defect		biochemical analysis of two families with type I and type II mannosidosis. *American Journal of Medical Genetics*, 1995; **55**: 21–6.
Maroteaux–Lamy syndrome (mucopolysaccharidosis type VI)	Aortic stenosis Beaked/wedged vertebrae Cardiomyopathy Cloudy corneas/sclerocornea Coarse facial features Deafness, conductive Deafness, sensorineural Depressed/flat nasal bridge Epiphyseal dysplasia Genu valgum Glaucoma Kyphosis Large nose Large spleen Large tongue Mitral incompetence Mucopolysacchariduria/ oligosacchariduria Platyspondyly Prominent forehead/frontal bossing Sella turcica, J-shaped Short stature, proportionate Storage cells/vacuolated lymphocytes Thick lower lip Thick upper lip Thick/stiff skin Thick/wide ribs Umbilical hernia	Enlarged liver	Isbrandt D *et al.* Mucopolysaccharidosis VI (Maroteaux–Lamy syndrome): six unique arylsulfatase B gene alleles causing variable disease phenotypes. *American Journal of Human Genetics*, 1994; **54**: 454–63. Jin W-D, Jackson CE, Desnick RJ, and Schuchman EH. Mucopolysaccharidosis type VI: identification of three mutations in the arylsulfatase B gene of patients with the severe and mild phenotypes provides molecular evidence for genetic heterogeneity. *American Journal of Human Genetics*, 1992; **50**: 795–800.

Disease	Features	Hepatic abnormalities	Reference(s)
Mathias syndrome (1987) (X-linked laterality sequence)	Abnormal placement of anus Absent or hypoplastic spleen Absent sacrum Anal atresia/stenosis Anomalous venous return Atrial septum defect Atrioventricular septal defect Cardiac situs inversus/dextrocardia Cerebellar abnormalities (structural) Duodenal stenosis Fallot tetralogy Holoprosencephaly/arhinencephaly Hydrocephaly/large ventricles, non-specific Hypertelorism Malformed uterus Meningocele/meningomyelocele Mitral incompetence Patent ductus arteriosus Polysplenia Pulmonary stenosis Single ventricle Situs inversus, abdominal Splenic abnormalities, unspecified Transposition of the great vessels Ventricular septal defect	Biliary atresia, situs inversus	Casey B, Devoto M, Jones KL, and Ballabio A. Mapping a gene for familial situs abnormalities to human chromosome Xq24-q27.1. *Nature Genetics*, 1993; **5**: 403–7. Mathias RS, Lacro RV, and Jones KL. X-linked laterality sequence: situs inversus, complex cardiac defects, splenic defects. *American Journal of Medical Genetics*, 1987; **28**: 111–16. Mikkila SP *et al.* X-linked laterality sequence in a family with carrier manifestations. *American Journal of Medical Genetics*, 1994; **49**: 435–8.
Meckel–Gruber syndrome (dysencephalia splanchnocystica)	Anal atresia/stenosis Cerebellar abnormalities (structural) Cerebral atrophy/myelin abnormality Cleft palate Cleft upper lip (non-midline) Dandy–Walker malformation Holoprosencephaly/arhinencephaly Hypospadias Lung hypoplasia/agenesis Mental retardation Microcephaly Microphthalmia Multiple renal cysts Neonatal teeth Pancreas (exocrine), general abnormalities Polydactyly/bifid thumb Polysplenia Postaxial polydactyly of fingers Postaxial polydactyly of toes Posterior encephalocele/meningocele	Enlarged liver, grossly fibrotic, cystic	Blankenberg TA *et al.* Pathology of renal and hepatic anomalies in Meckel syndrome. *American Journal of Medical Genetics*, 1987; Suppl. **3**: 395–410. Paavola P, Salonen R, Weissenbach J, and Peltonen L. The locus for Meckel syndrome with multiple congenital anomalies maps to chromosome 17q21-q24. (Letter.) *Nature Genetics*, 1995; **11**: 213–15. Wright C, Healicon R, English C, and Burn J. Meckel syndrome: what are the minimum diagnostic criteria? *Journal of Medical Genetics*, 1994; **31**: 482–5.

Disease	Features	Hepatic abnormalities	Reference(s)
Medium-chain acyl-CoA dehydrogenase deficiency	Posteriorly rotated ears Preaxial polydactyly of fingers Pulmonary segmentation defects Apnoea or tachypnoea Cardiomyopathy Cerebral atrophy/myelin abnormality Deafness, sensorineural Dementia/psychosis Feeding problems in infants Hypoglycaemia Hypotonia Muscle weakness/myopathy Organicaciduria Retinitis pigmentosa/ pigmentary retinopathy/ chorioretinitis Seizures/abnormal EEG	Steatosis	Andresen BS *et al.* Medium-chain acyl-CoA dehydrogenase (MCAD) deficiency due to heterozygosity for the common mutation and an allele resulting in low levels of MCAD mRNA. *Journal of Inherited Metabolic Diseases*, 1994; **17**: 275–8. Iafolla AK, Thompson RJ Jr, and Roe CR. Medium-chain acyl-coenzyme A dehydrogenase deficiency: clinical course in 120 affected children. *Journal of Pediatrics*, 1994; **124**: 409–15. Losty HC *et al.* Fatty infiltration in the liver in medium chain acyl CoA dehydrogenase deficiency. *Archives of Diseases of Childhood*, 1991; **66**: 727.
Mevalonic aciduria	Anaemia/red cell abnormalities Ataxia Cardiomyopathy Cataract Cerebellar abnormalities (structural) Dolichocephaly/scaphocephaly Fontanelles, delayed closure/ large Hypotonia Joint stiffness/arthritis Large spleen Long/prominent eyelashes Malabsorption Mental retardation Microcephaly Muscle weakness/myopathy Oedema (including hydrops) Organicaciduria Palpebral fissures slant down Papules Posteriorly rotated ears Prominent forehead/frontal bossing Protuberant abdomen Retinitis pigmentosa/ pigmentary retinopathy/ chorioretinitis Seizures/abnormal EEG Short stature, proportionate	Enlarged liver	Hoffmann GF *et al.* Clinical and biochemical phenotype in 11 patients with mevalonic aciduria. *Pediatrics*, 1993; **91**: 915–21. Mancini J *et al.* Mevalonic aciduria in 3 siblings: a new recognizable metabolic encephalopathy. *Pediatric Neurology*, 1993; **9**: 243–6.

Disease	Features	Hepatic abnormalities	Reference(s)
	Spasticity/increased tendon reflex Syndactyly of toes (not 2–3) Triangular face		
Mitochondrial cytopathy–diabetes mellitus–ataxia–renal tubular abnormalities	Anaemia/red cell abnormalities Ataxia Cardiomyopathy Cataract Deafness, sensorineural Diabetes mellitus/hyperglycaemia Enlarged liver Generalized hirsutism Multiple renal cysts Muscle weakness/myopathy Nephritis or nephropathy Parathyroid, absent/hypoparathyroidism Patchy pigment of skin/café-au-lait spots Retinitis pigmentosa/pigmentary retinopathy/chorioretinitis Seizures/abnormal EEG Short stature, proportionate	Enlarged liver, steatosis, liver failure	Cormier-Daire V, et al. Mitochondrial DNA rearrangements with onset as chronic diarrhea with villous atrophy. *Journal of Pediatrics*, 1994; **124**: 63–70. Luder A and Barash V. Complex I deficiency with diabetes, Fanconi syndrome and mtDNA deletion. *Journal of Inherited Metabolic Diseases*, 1994; **17**: 298–300. Tulinius MH et al. Atypical presentation of multisystem disorders in two girls with mitochondrial DNA deletions. *European Journal of Pediatrics*, 1995; **154**: 35–42.
Moore–Federman syndrome	Brachydactyly Detached retina Glaucoma Hoarse voice Hypermetropia Joint stiffness/arthritis Limited movement of fingers Limited movement/flexion deformity of elbow Platyspondyly Respiratory abnormality, unspecified Short stature, proportionate Thick/stiff skin	Enlarged liver	Fell JME and Stanhope R. Reviving the Moore–Federman syndrome. *Journal of the Royal Society of Medicine*, 1993; **86**: 52–3. Winter RM et al. Moore–Federman syndrome and acromicric dysplasia: are they the same entity? *Journal of Medical Genetics*, 1989; **26**: 320–5.
Mucolipidosis type IV	Agenesis/hypoplasia of corpus callosum Bulbous nasal tip Cloudy corneas/sclerocornea Coarse facial features Extrapyramidal disorder Hypertonia Hypotonia Kyphosis Large spleen Mental retardation Optic atrophy Photophobia Retinitis pigmentosa/pigmentary retinopathy/chorioretinitis	Enlarged liver	Casteels I et al. Mucolipidosis type IV. Presentation of a mild variant. *Ophthalmic Paediatrics and Genetics*, 1992; **13**: 205–10. Reis S et al. Mucolipidosis type IV: a mild form with late onset. *American Journal of Medical Genetics*, 1993; **47**: 392–4. Riedel KG et al. Ocular abnormalities in mucolipidosis IV. *American Journal of Ophthalmology*, 1985; **99**: 125–36.

Disease	Features	Hepatic abnormalities	Reference(s)
Mucopolysaccharidosis type VII (β-glucuronidase deficiency)	Scoliosis Spasticity/increased tendon reflex Storage cells/vacuolated lymphocytes Strabismus/gaze palsy Thick lower lip Thick upper lip Thickened/oedematous eyelids Anteverted nares Beaked/wedged vertebrae Cloudy corneas/sclerocornea Coarse facial features Craniosynostosis Depressed/flat nasal bridge Gibbus Joint stiffness/arthritis Large spleen Limited movement of fingers Macrocephaly Mental retardation Mucopolysacchariduria/oligosacchariduria Pectus carinatum Pectus excavatum Prominent forehead/frontal bossing Proximal tapering of metacarpals Seizures/abnormal EEG Short stature, proportionate Storage cells/vacuolated lymphocytes Thick/wide alveolar ridges Umbilical hernia Wide metacarpals/modelling defect	Enlarged liver, prolonged jaundice, giant cell hepatitis	de Kremer RD *et al.* Mucopolysaccharidosis type VII (β-glucuronidase deficiency): a chronic variant with an oligosymptomatic severe skeletal dysplasia. *American Journal of Medical Genetics*, 1992; **44**: 145–52. Yamada S *et al.* Four novel mutations in mucopolysaccharidosis type VII including a unique base substitution in exon 10 of the β-glucuronidase gene that creates a novel 5′-splice site. *Human Molecular Genetics*, 1995; **4**: 651–5.
Mucopolysaccharidosis type VII (di Ferrante)	Beaked/wedged vertebrae Coarse hair Deafness, conductive Generalized depigmentation of hair Generalized hirsutism Large spleen Mental retardation Mucopolysacchariduria/oligosacchariduria Odontoid hypoplasia/dysplasia Perthes'/dysplastic hip Short stature, proportionate Thick/wide ribs	Enlarged liver	Ginsberg LC *et al.* N-Acetylglucosamine-6-sulfate sulfatase in man: deficiency of the enzyme in a new mucopolysaccharidosis. *Pediatric Research*, 1978; **12**: 805–9. Matalon R *et al.* Keratan and heparan sulfaturia—a new mucopolysaccharidosis with N-acetylglucosamine-6-sulfatase deficiency. (Abstract.) *Pediatric Research*, 1978; **12**:453.
Mulibrey nanism	Cardiomyopathy Constrictive pericarditis Depressed/flat nasal bridge Fibrous dysplasia of bones High frontal hairline	Enlarged and cirrhotic liver	Balg S, Stengel-Rutkowski S, Dohlemann C, and Boergen K. Mulibrey nanism. *Clinical Dysmorphology*, 1995; **4**: 63–9. Lapunzina P *et al.* Mulibrey

Disease	Features	Hepatic abnormalities	Reference(s)
	Hydrocephaly/large ventricles, non-specific Hypertelorism Isolated growth hormone deficiency Medullary space stenosis Mental retardation Muscle weakness/myopathy Oligodontia Pericarditis (non-constrictive) Prominent forehead/frontal bossing Retinitis pigmentosa/ pigmentary retinopathy/ chorioretinitis Sella turcica, J-shaped Short stature, prenatal onset Short stature, proportionate Slender/thin bones Triangular face Underdevelopment of cranial sinus Wide nasal bridge		nanism: three additional patients and a review of 39 patients. *American Journal of Medical Genetics*, 1995; **55**: 349–55.
Multiple sulphatase deficiency	Aplasia or dysplasia of retina Ataxia Beaked/wedged vertebrae Cardiomyopathy Cloudy corneas/sclerocornea Coarse facial features Coarse hair Deafness, sensorineural Epiphyseal dysplasia Gibbus Hypoplastic ilia Ichthyosis Large spleen Macrocephaly Mental retardation Mucopolysacchariduria/ oligosacchariduria Optic atrophy Pigmentary abnormality of macula Retinitis pigmentosa/ pigmentary retinopathy/ chorioretinitis Seizures/abnormal EEG Sella turcica, J-shaped Spasticity/increased tendon reflex Stippled or fragmented epiphyses Storage cells/vacuolated lymphocytes Thick/wide ribs	Enlarged liver	Al Aqeel A *et al.* Saudi variant of multiple sulfatase deficiency. *Journal of Child Neurology*, 1992; **7**(Suppl.): S12–21. Harbord M *et al.* Multiple sulfatase deficiency with early severe retinal degeneration. *Journal of Child Neurology*, 1991; **6**: 229–35. Schmidt B *et al.* A novel amino acid modification in sulfatases that is defective in multiple sulfatase deficiency. *Cell*, 1995; **82**: 271–8.

Disease	Features	Hepatic abnormalities	Reference(s)
Mulvihill syndrome (1975) (progeria-like syndrome)	Blepharophimosis/ blepharospasm Brachydactyly Clinodactyly Cloudy corneas/sclerocornea Cryptorchid testes Deafness, sensorineural Deficient adipose tissue or fat/ lipodystrophy Diabetes mellitus/ hyperglycaemia Dolichocephaly/scaphocephaly Fontanelles, delayed closure/ large Hypohidrotic or dry skin Hypoplastic phalanges Hypospadias Immunoglobulin abnormality Irregular or crowded teeth Late puberty in male Low birthweight (< 3rd centile) Malocclusion of teeth Mental retardation Microcephaly Microstomia Naevi or lentigines Oligodontia Palpebral fissures slant down Pinched nose Premature ageing Prominent ears Recurrent infections Short stature, prenatal onset Small mandible/micrognathia Small/hypoplastic/deep-set nails Sparse hair/alopecia areata T-cell deficiency Telangiectasia/angiokeratomas of skin Thin Thin ear helix Thin skin/generalized skin atrophy Triangular face	Enlarged liver	Baraitser M, Insley J, and Winter RM. A recognisable short stature syndrome with premature aging and pigmented naevi. *Journal of Medical Genetics*, 1988; **25**: 53–6. Bartsch O, Tympner K-D, Schwinger E, and Gorlin RJ. Mulvihill-Smith syndrome: case report and review. *Journal of Medical Genetics*, 1994; **31**: 707–11.
Nezelof syndrome (1979) (arthrogryposis; renal dysfunction; hepatic disease)	Cataract Club foot, varus Flexion deformity at wrist Hypercalciuria Joint contractures (including arthrogryposis) Muscle atrophy Nephritis or nephropathy Polyuria Proteinuria Proximal placement of thumb	Pigment storage in hepatocytes, giant cell transformation, bile duct proliferation	Di Rocco M *et al.* Arthrogryposis, renal dysfunction and cholestasis syndrome: report of five patients from three Italian families. *European Journal of Pediatrics*, 1995; **154**: 835–9. Horslen SP, Quarrell OWJ, and Tanner MS. Liver histology in the arthrogryposis multiplex congenita, renal dysfunction,

Disease	Features	Hepatic abnormalities	Reference(s)
	Renal dysplasia Ulnar deviation of hand		and cholestasis (ARC) syndrome: report of three new cases and review. *Journal of Medical Genetics*, 1994; **31**: 62–4.
Niemann–Pick disease	Ataxia Dementia/psychosis Diffuse increased pigmentation of skin Large spleen Macular red spot/cherry red spot Mental retardation Papules Patchy pigment of skin/café-au-lait spots Pigmentary abnormality of macula Respiratory abnormality, unspecified Seizures/abnormal EEG Storage cells/vacuolated lymphocytes Strabismus/gaze palsy Thick/stiff skin	Prolonged jaundice, fibrosis, storage material in Kupffer cells	Kelly DA *et al.* Niemann–Pick disease type C: diagnosis and outcome in children, with particular reference to liver disease. *Journal of Pediatrics*, 1993; **123**: 242–7. Kristjansson K, Finegold MJ, Pentchev PG, and Belmont JW. Niemann–Pick-like liver disease and reduced cholesterol esterification in fibroblasts of two male infants. *European Journal of Pediatrics*, 1994; **153**: 347–51.
Oculo-encephalo-hepato-renal syndrome	Anteverted nares Ataxia Blepharophimosis/blepharospasm Cerebellar abnormalities (structural) Coloboma of retina/choroid Down-turned corners of the mouth Extrapyramidal disorder Hydrocephaly/large ventricles, non-specific Hypertelorism Low-set ears Mental retardation Multiple renal cysts Notched/hypoplastic alae nasi Posterior encephalocele/meningocele Prominent ears Prominent/everted lower lip Seizures/abnormal EEG Small kidneys Spasticity/increased tendon reflex Ulnar deviation of hand	Hepatic fibrosis	Lewis SME *et al.* Joubert syndrome with congenital hepatic fibrosis: an entity in the spectrum of oculo-encephalo-hepato-renal disorders. *American Journal of Medical Genetics*, 1994; **52**: 419–26.
Omenn syndrome (1965) (reticuloendotheliosis; eosinophilia)	Absent/hypoplastic thymus Bowed femur Bullas or vesicles Erythema/erythroderma	Enlarged liver, mild fibrosis, cholestasis, bile duct proliferation	Glastre C and Rigal D. Omenn syndrome: a review. (In French—summary in English.) *Pediatrie*, 1990; **45**: 301–5.

Disease	Features	Hepatic abnormalities	Reference(s)
	Flared ribs/anterior splaying Ichthyosis Immunoglobulin abnormality Large spleen Lymphadenopathy Lymphomas/leukaemias Metaphyseal dysplasia Papules Polymorph abnormalities Short bones Sparse hair/alopecia areata T-cell deficiency Thymus, general abnormalities Wide metaphysis		Gomez L *et al.* Treatment of Omenn syndrome by bone marrow transplantation. *Journal of Pediatrics*, 1995; **127**: 76–81.
Pearson's syndrome	Absent or hypoplastic spleen Anaemia/red cell abnormalities Cardiomyopathy Cloudy corneas/sclerocornea Delayed bone age Diabetes mellitus/ hyperglycaemia Hypotonia Low birthweight (< 3rd centile) Malabsorption Organicaciduria Osteoporosis Pancreatic insufficiency Platelet abnormalities Polymorph abnormalities Short stature, proportionate Splenic abnormalities, unspecified Storage cells/vacuolated lymphocytes Thick/wide ribs	Progressive enlargement of liver	Bernes SM *et al.* Identical mitochondrial DNA deletion in mother with progressive external ophthalmoplegia and son with Pearson marrow-pancreas syndrome. *Journal of Pediatrics*, 1993; **123**: 598–602. Mazziotta MRM *et al.* Fatal infantile liver failure associated with mitochondrial DNA depletion. *Journal of Pediatrics*, 1992; **121**: 896–901. Rotig A *et al.* Spectrum of mitochondrial DNA rearrangements in the Pearson marrow-pancreas syndrome. *Human Molecular Genetics*, 1995; **4**: 1327–30.
Pipecolic acidaemia	Aminoaciduria Hypotonia Mental retardation Nystagmus Optic atrophy Organicaciduria Seizures/abnormal EEG	Neonatal jaundice, large liver, periportal fibrosis, fat in hepatocytes, no peroxisomes seen, trilamina structures	Moser HW. Peroxisomal disorders. *Journal of Pediatrics*, 1986; **108**: 89–91. Moser HW. Hyperpipecolic acidemia. *Advances in Pediatrics*, 1989; **36**:17.
Polyneuropathy–organomegaly–endocrinopathy–M protein–skin changes (POEMS)	Anaemia/red cell abnormalities Ascites Calcification of arteries Capillary haemangioma Cavernous haemangioma Clubbing of fingers (drumstick) Diffuse increased pigmentation of skin Generalized hirsutism Gynaecomastia Hyperhidrosis Large spleen Lymphadenopathy	Enlarged liver, occlusion of hepatic veins (Budd–Chiari syndrome)	Jackson A and Burton IE. A case of POEMS syndrome associated with essential thrombocythaemia and dermal mastocytosis. *Postgraduate Medical Journal*, 1990; **66**: 761–7. Miralles GD, O'Fallon JR, and Talley NJ. Plasma-cell dyscrasia with polyneuropathy—the spectrum of POEMS syndrome. *New England Journal of Medicine*,

Disease	Features	Hepatic abnormalities	Reference(s)
	Muscle weakness/myopathy Oedema of lower limbs Osteosclerosis or osteopetrosis Papilloedema/optic neuritis Peripheral neuropathy Platelet abnormalities Thick/stiff skin		1992; **327**: 1919–23. Steinberg D and Harris NL. A 49-year-old woman with peripheral neuropathy, hepatosplenomegaly, and intermittent abdominal pain. *New England Journal of Medicine*, 1992; **327**: 1014–21.
Pseudo-Zellweger syndrome	Adrenal hypoplasia/insufficiency Cat cry/weak, high-pitched cry Cerebral atrophy/myelin abnormality Delayed bone age Depressed/flat nasal bridge Epicanthic folds Expressionless/dull face Feeding problems in infants Fontanelles, delayed closure/large High palate Hypertelorism Hypotonia Large kidneys Lissencephaly/pachygyria/polymicrogyria Low-set ears Mental retardation Multiple renal cysts Osteoporosis Persistent hyaloid artery Postaxial polydactyly of fingers Prominent upper lip Recurrent infections Seizures/abnormal EEG Ventricular septal defect	Mild steatosis	Nakada Y *et al.* A case of pseudo-Zellweger syndrome with a possible bifunctional enzyme deficiency but detectable enzyme protein. Comparison of two cases of Zellweger syndrome. *Brain and Development*, 1993; **15**: 453–6. Pietrzyk JJ *et al.* Two siblings with phenotypes mimicking peroxisomal disorders but with discordant biochemical findings. *Clinical Pediatrics*, 1990; **29**: 479–84. Schutgens RBH *et al.* A new variant of Zellweger syndrome with normal peroxisomal functions in cultured fibroblasts. *Journal of Inherited Metabolic Diseases*, 1994; **17**: 319–22.
Renal–hepatic–pancreatic dysplasia	Absent or hypoplastic spleen Biliary atresia/stenosis Cardiac situs inversus/dextrocardia Congenital cardiac anomaly, unspecified Diabetes mellitus/hyperglycaemia Hypothyroidism/small/absent thyroid Multiple renal cysts Pancreas (exocrine), general abnormalities Polysplenia Renal dysplasia Renal tubular acidosis Situs inversus, abdominal Transposition of the great vessels	Cholestasis resulting in fibrosis	Carmi R, Magee CA, Neill CA, and Karrer FM. Extrahepatic biliary atresia and associated anomalies: etiologic heterogeneity suggested by distinctive patterns of associations. *American Journal of Medical Genetics*, 1993; **45**: 683–93. Lurie IW, Kirillova IA, Novikova IV, and Burakovski IV. Renal–hepatic–pancreatic dysplasia and its variants. *Genetic Counseling*, 1991; **2**: 17–20. Pinar H and Rogers BB. Renal dysplasia, situs inversus totalis, and multisystem fibrosis: a new syndrome. *Pediatric Pathology*, 1992; **12**: 215–21.

Disease	Features	Hepatic abnormalities	Reference(s)
Renal–hepatic–pancreatic dysplasia with Dandy–Walker cyst	Absent/abnormal gallbladder Anomalous venous return Anophthalmia Atrial septum defect Cerebellar abnormalities (structural) Dandy–Walker malformation Duplicated/right aortic arch Fontanelles, delayed closure/large Heart, general abnormalities Hydrocephaly/large ventricles, non-specific Hypertelorism Low-set ears Lung hypoplasia/agenesis Malformation of the pancreas Malformed uterus Microphthalmia Multiple renal cysts Polysplenia Posterior encephalocele/meningocele Protuberant abdomen Small mandible/micrognathia	Enlarged liver, fibrosis	Genuardi M *et al.* Cerebro-reno-digital (Meckel-like) syndrome with Dandy–Walker malformation, cystic kidneys, hepatic fibrosis, and polydactyly. *American Journal of Medical Genetics*, 1993; **47**: 50–3. Hunter AGW, Jimenez C, and Tawagi FGR. Familial renal-hepatic-pancreatic dysplasia and Dandy–Walker cyst: a distinct syndrome? *American Journal of Medical Genetics*, 1991; **41**: 201–7. Summers MC and Donnenfeld AE. Dandy–Walker malformation in the Meckel syndrome. *American Journal of Medical Genetics*, 1995; **55**: 57–61. Walpole, *et al.* Dandy-Walker malformation (variant), cystic dysplastic kidneys, and hepatic fibrosis: a distinct entity or Meckel's syndrome? *American Journal of Medical Genetics*, 1991; **39**: 294–8.
Salla disease (lysosomal storage disorder)	Agenesis/hypoplasia of corpus callosum Ascites Ataxia Cerebellar abnormalities (structural) Cerebral atrophy/myelin abnormality Cloudy corneas/sclerocornea Coarse facial features Dementia/psychosis Depressed/flat nasal bridge Hypertonia Hypoplastic ilia Irregular endplates to vertebrae Large spleen Macrostomia Mental retardation Mucopolysacchariduria/oligosacchariduria Optic atrophy Proximal tapering of metacarpals Ptosis of eyelids Seizures/abnormal EEG Spasticity/increased tendon reflex Speech delay	Enlarged liver with numerous vacuolated cells. Membrane-bound vesicles containing granuloreticular material	Haataja L *et al.* The genetic locus for free sialic acid storage disease maps to the long arm of chromosome 6. *American Journal of Human Genetics*, 1994; **54**: 1042–9. Haataja L *et al.* Phenotypic variation and magnetic resonance imaging (MRI) in Salla disease, a free sialic acid storage disorder. *Neuropediatrics*, 1994; **25**: 238–44.

Disease	Features	Hepatic abnormalities	Reference(s)
Sanfilippo syndrome (mucopolysaccharidosis type III)	Storage cells/vacuolated lymphocytes Thick eyebrows Thick lower lip Thick upper lip Thickened/oedematous eyelids Acetabulum, general abnormalities Advanced bone age/large epiphyses Aggressive behaviour Aortic stenosis Beaked/wedged vertebrae Coarse facial features Generalized hirsutism Irregular endplates to vertebrae Large spleen Limited movement/flexion deformity of elbow Macrocephaly Medial eyebrow flare Mental retardation Mitral incompetence Mitral stenosis Mucopolysacchariduria/oligosacchariduria Spasticity/increased tendon reflex Stippled or fragmented epiphyses Synophrys Thick eyebrows Thick lower lip Thick upper lip Thick/stiff skin Thick/wide alveolar ridges Umbilical hernia	Enlarged liver	Di Natale P. Sanfilippo B disease: a re-examination of a particular sibship after 12 years. *Journal of Inherited Metabolic Diseases*, 1991; **14**: 23–8. Ozand PT *et al.* Sanfilippo type D presenting with acquired language disorder but without features of mucopolysaccharidosis. *Journal of Child Neurology*, 1994; **9**: 408–11. Wraith JE. The mucopolysaccharidoses: a clinical review and guide to management. *Archives of Diseases of Childhood*, 1995; **72**: 263–7.
Scheie syndrome (mucopolysaccharidosis type IS)	Aortic incompetence Aortic stenosis Beaked/wedged vertebrae Brachydactyly Camptodactyly Cloudy corneas/sclerocornea Coarse facial features Epiphyseal dysplasia Glaucoma Limited movement of fingers Mitral stenosis Mucopolysacchariduria/oligosacchariduria Prominent mandible Prominent upper lip Prominent/everted lower lip Retinitis pigmentosa/pigmentary retinopathy/	Enlarged liver	Scott HS *et al.* Identification of mutations in the α-L-iduronidase gene (IDUA) that cause Hurler and Scheie syndromes. *American Journal of Human Genetics*, 1993; **53**: 973–86. Tieu PT *et al.* Four novel mutations underlying mild or intermediate forms of α-L-iduronidase deficiency (MPS IS and MPS IH/S). *Human Mutation*, 1995; **6**: 55–9. Wippermann C-F *et al.* Mitral and aortic regurgitation in 84 patients with mucopolysaccharidoses. *European Journal of Pediatrics,*

Disease	Features	Hepatic abnormalities	Reference(s)
	chorioretinitis		1995; **154**: 98–101.
	Short neck		
	Umbilical hernia		
Shwachman syndrome (pancreatic insufficiency; neutropenia; metaphyseal dysplasia)	Anaemia/red cell abnormalities	Enlarged liver, extramedullary haematopoiesis, fatty infiltration, fibrosis	Danks DM *et al.* Metaphyseal chondrodysplasia, neutropenia, and pancreatic insufficiency presenting with respiratory distress in the neonatal period. *Archives of Diseases of Childhood*, 1976; **51**: 697–701. Dhar S and Anderton JM. Orthopaedic features of Shwachman syndrome. A report of two cases. *Journal of Bone and Joint Surgery*, 1994; **A76**: 278–82. Mortureux P, *et al.* Shwachman syndrome: a case report. *Pediatric Dermatology*, 1992; **9**: 57–61.
	Erythema/erythroderma		
	Ichthyosis		
	Macules		
	Malabsorption		
	Mental retardation		
	Metaphyseal dysplasia		
	Narrow thorax/funnel chest		
	Pancreatic insufficiency		
	Papules		
	Patchy pigment of skin/café-au-lait spots		
	Platelet abnormalities		
	Polymorph abnormalities		
	Recurrent infections		
	Short ribs		
	Short stature, proportionate		
	Sparse hair/alopecia areata		
Sialic acid storage disease, severe infantile type	Anaemia/red cell abnormalities	Enlarged liver, Kupffer cells with microvacuolated foamy cytoplasm	Berra B *et al.* Infantile sialic acid storage disease: biochemical studies. *American Journal of Medical Genetics*, 1995; **58**: 24–31. Paschke E, Gruber W, Ring E, and Sperl W. Storage material from urine and tissues in the nephropathic phenotype of infantile sialic acid storage disease. *Journal of Inherited Metabolic Diseases*, 1992; **15**: 47–56. Schleutker J *et al.* Lysosomal free sialic acid storage disorders with different phenotypic presentations—infantile-form sialic acid storage disease and Salla disease—represent allelic disorders. *American Journal of Human Genetics*, 1995; **57**: 893–901.
	Anteverted nares		
	Ascites		
	Cerebral atrophy/myelin abnormality		
	Club foot, varus		
	Coarse facial features		
	Erythema/erythroderma		
	Generalized depigmentation of hair		
	Gum hypertrophy		
	Hydrocephaly/large ventricles, non-specific		
	Hypotonia		
	Ichthyosis		
	Inguinal hernia		
	Large spleen		
	Macules		
	Malabsorption		
	Mental retardation		
	Mucopolysacchariduria/oligosacchariduria		
	Nephritis or nephropathy		
	Oedema (including hydrops)		
	Proteinuria		
	Short stature, prenatal onset		
	Short stature, proportionate		
	Sparse hair/alopecia areata		
	Stippled or fragmented epiphyses		
	Storage cells/vacuolated lymphocytes		
Sialidosis type 2	Ascites	Enlarged liver with foamy cells	Kanaka C *et al.* Mucocutaneous bleeding, a rare but severe
	Ataxia		

Disease	Features	Hepatic abnormalities	Reference(s)
	Beaked/wedged vertebrae Bulbous nasal tip Coarse facial features Dementia/psychosis Gibbus Hyperplastic supraorbital ridges Large spleen Macular red spot/cherry red spot Mental retardation Mucopolysacchariduria/ oligosacchariduria Nephritis or nephropathy Pectus carinatum Platyspondyly Proteinuria Scoliosis Seizures/abnormal EEG Sella turcica, J-shaped Short stature, proportionate Spasticity/increased tendon reflex Thick lower lip Thick upper lip		complication in nephrosialidosis. (Letter.) *European Journal of Pediatrics*, 1994; **153**: 703–4. Sasagasako N *et al.* Prenatal diagnosis of congenital sialidosis. *Clinical Genetics*, 1993; **44**: 8–11.
Sialuria	Coarse facial features Hypotonia Large spleen Large tongue Macrocephaly Mental retardation Mucopolysacchariduria/ oligosacchariduria	Enlarged liver, abnormal mitochondria containing unusual circular cristae and intramitochondrial cristalline arrays between the cristae	Don NA and Wilcken B. Sialuria: a follow-up report. *Journal of Inherited Metabolic Diseases*, 1991; **14**:942.
Siegler syndrome (1992) (cataract; malabsorption; renal and hepatic disease)	Anaemia/red cell abnormalities Cataract Malabsorption Nephritis or nephropathy Polyuria Recurrent infections Renal tubular acidosis Short stature, proportionate Small kidneys Strabismus/gaze palsy	Abnormal liver function, enlarged, fibrotic, cholestasis, fatty metamorphosis	Siegler RL, Brewer ED, and Carey JC. New syndrome involving the visual, auditory, respiratory, gastrointestinal, and renal systems. *American Journal of Medical Genetics*, 1992; **44**: 461–4.
Simpson–Golabi–Behmel syndrome	Acro-osteolysis/acral defects Advanced bone age/large epiphyses Broad base to nose Broad hands Cataract Caudal appendage Cleft of the lower lip Cleft palate Clinodactyly Coarse facial features Coloboma involving optic nerve Congenital cardiac anomaly,	Enlarged liver	Garganta CL and Bodurtha JN. Report of another family with Simpson–Golabi–Behmel syndrome and a review of the literature. *American Journal of Medical Genetics*, 1992; **44**: 129–35. Orth U *et al.* Gene for Simpson–Golabi–Behmel syndrome is linked to HPRT in Xq26 in two European families. *American Journal of Medical Genetics*, 1994; **50**: 388–90.

Disease	Features	Hepatic abnormalities	Reference(s)
	unspecified		
	Congenital hernia of diaphragm		
	Crease of ear lobule		
	Cryptorchid testes		
	Detached retina		
	Diffuse increased pigmentation of skin		
	Dystrophic nails		
	ECG abnormality/conduction defects		
	Furrowed tongue/prominent groove		
	Fusion of vertebrae		
	High birthweight (> 90th centile)		
	High palate		
	Hoarse voice		
	Hydronephrosis		
	Hypertelorism		
	Intestinal malrotation		
	Large kidneys		
	Large spleen		
	Large tongue		
	Macrocephaly		
	Macrostomia		
	Mental retardation		
	Mid-face hypoplasia (excluding malar region)		
	Multiple renal cysts		
	Open mouth appearance		
	Palpebral fissures slant down		
	Pectus excavatum		
	Polysplenia		
	Postaxial polydactyly of fingers		
	Prominent mandible		
	Renal tumours (including Wilms')		
	Scoliosis		
	Skin syndactyly of fingers		
	Small/hypoplastic/deep-set nails		
	Small/short nose		
	Submucous cleft palate		
	Supernumerary nipples		
	Tall stature, proportionate		
	Thick lower lip		
	Thick upper lip		
	Umbilical hernia		
	Ventricular septal defect		
	Wide nasal bridge		
Tay syndrome (1974) (mental retardation; facial/pigment abnormalities; cirrhosis; aminoaciduria)	Abnormally shaped teeth Aminoaciduria Deafness, conductive Large spleen Large/prominent teeth Long hallux	Enlarged liver with cirrhosis	Tay CH *et al.* A recessive disorder with growth and mental retardation, peculiar facies, abnormal pigmentation, hepatic cirrhosis and aminoaciduria. *Acta Paediatrica*

Disease	Features	Hepatic abnormalities	Reference(s)
	Mental retardation Microcephaly Microstomia Naevi or lentigines Notched/hypoplastic alae nasi Patchy depigmentation of skin Patchy pigment of skin/café-au-lait spots Pinched nose Prominent eyes/proptosis Short stature, proportionate Short toes Triangular face		*Scandinavica*, 1974; **63**: 777–82.
Tyrosinaemia type I	Aggressive behaviour Aminoaciduria Ascites Ataxia Glycosuria Hypertension Hypertonia Mental retardation Metaphyseal dysplasia Muscle weakness/myopathy Oedema (including hydrops) Peripheral neuropathy Platelet abnormalities Renal tubular acidosis Seizures/abnormal EEG Small bowel atresia/absence/obstruction/short	Enlarged liver, liver failure, macronodular cirrhosis and hepatocellular carcinoma	Barness L and Gilbert-Barness E. Pathological case of the month—hereditary tyrosinemia type I. *American Journal of Diseases of Childhood*, 1992; **146**: 769–70. Noble-Jamieson G *et al.* Neurological crisis in hereditary tyrosinaemia and complete reversal after liver transplantation. *Archives of Diseases of Childhood*, 1994; **70**: 544–5. Ploos van Amstel JK *et al.* Hereditary tyrosinemia type 1: novel missense, nonsense and splice consensus mutations in the human fumarylacetoacetate hydrolase gene; variability of the genotype–phenotype relationship. *Human Genetics*, 1996; **97**: 51–9.
Werner syndrome	Abnormal liver (including function) Calcification of arteries Calcification, subcutaneous Cataract Chromosome instability/breakage Convex/beaked profile of nose Deficient adipose tissue or fat/lipodystrophy Dementia/psychosis Diabetes mellitus/hyperglycaemia Full cheeks Glaucoma Gynaecomastia Hyperthyroidism Hyperkeratosis Lymphomas/leukaemias Muscle atrophy	Abnormal liver function	Goto M, *et al.* Genetic linkage of Werner's syndrome to five markers on chromosome 8. *Nature*, 1992; **355**: 735–8. Kakigi R *et al.* Accelerated aging of the brain in Werner's syndrome. *Neurology*, 1992; **42**: 922–4. Oshima J, *et al.* Integrated mapping analysis of the Werner syndrome region of chromosome 8. *Genomics*, 1994; **23**: 100–13.

Disease	Features	Hepatic abnormalities	Reference(s)
	Osteoporosis		
	Patchy depigmentation of skin		
	Patchy pigment of skin/café-au-lait spots		
	Peripheral neuropathy		
	Pinched nose		
	Premature ageing		
	Premature atherosclerosis		
	Retinitis pigmentosa/pigmentary retinopathy/chorioretinitis		
	Short stature, proportionate		
	Small feet		
	Small hands		
	Small penis (including micro)		
	Sparse hair/alopecia areata		
	Spasticity/increased tendon reflex		
	Telangiectasia/angiokeratomata of skin		
	Thin		
	Thin skin/generalized skin atrophy		
Wolman disease (acid lipase deficiency)	Adrenal calcification	Swollen foamy Kupffer cells	Anderson RA *et al. In situ* localization of the genetic locus encoding the lysosomal acid lipase/cholesteryl esterase (LIPA) deficient in Wolman disease to chromosome 10q23.2-q23.3. *Genomics*, 1993; **15**: 245–7.
	Anaemia/red cell abnormalities		
	Deficient adipose tissue or fat/lipodystrophy		
	Dementia/psychosis		
	Feeding problems in infants		
	Large spleen		Wolman M. Wolman disease and its treatment. *Clinical Pediatrics*, 1995; **34**: 207–12.
	Lymphadenopathy		
	Malabsorption		
	Mental retardation		
	Protuberant abdomen		
	Short stature, proportionate		
	Spasticity/increased tendon reflex		
	Storage cells/vacuolated lymphocytes		
	Thin		
	Xanthomas		
Zellweger (cerebro-hepato-renal) syndrome	Absent/hypoplastic thymus	Enlarged liver, prolonged jaundice, liver fibrosis	Braverman N, Dodt G, Gould SJ, and Valle D. Disorders of peroxisome biogenesis. (Review.) *Human Molecular Genetics*, 1995; **4**: 1791–8.
	Agenesis/hypoplasia of corpus callosum		
	Aminoaciduria		
	Brushfield spots		Brown FR III, Voigt R, Singh AK, and Singh I. Peroxisomal disorders. Neurodevelopmental and biochemical aspects. (Review.) *American Journal of Diseases of Childhood*, 1993; **147**: 617–26.
	Camptodactyly		
	Cataract		
	Cerebral atrophy/myelin abnormality		
	Depressed/flat nasal bridge		
	Epicanthic folds		Erdem G *et al.* Intestinal lymphangiectasia in a patient
	Feeding problems in infants		
	Flat face		
	Flat occiput		

Disease	Features	Hepatic abnormalities	Reference(s)
	Fontanelles, delayed closure/large High frontal hairline Hypoplastic supraorbital ridges Hypotonia Macrocephaly Migration abnormality/heterotopia Multiple renal cysts Pancreas (endocrine), general abnormalities Proteinuria Retinitis pigmentosa/pigmenatry retinopathy/chorioretinitis Seizures/abnormal EEG Small mandible/micrognathia Stippled or fragmented epiphyses Wide nasal bridge		with Zellweger cerebrohepatorenal syndrome. *American Journal of Medical Genetics*, 1995; **58**: 152–4.
Zimmermann–Laband syndrome (gingival fibromatosis; nail defects)	Absent nails Absent phalanges Acro-osteolysis/acral defects Bulbous nasal tip Dystrophic nails Flexion deformity of hip Flexion deformity of knee Generalized hirsutism Gum hypertrophy Large nose Large spleen Large tongue Macrostomia Mental retardation Retinitis pigmentosa/pigmentary retinopathy/chorioretinitis Scoliosis Synophrys Thick lower lip Thick upper lip Thickened ears	Enlarged liver	Bakaeen G and Scully C. Hereditary gingival fibromatosis in a family with the Zimmermann–Laband syndrome. *Journal of Oral Pathology and Medicine*, 1991; **20**: 457–9. Lacombe D *et al.* Congenital marked hypertrichosis and Laband syndrome in a child: overlap between the gingival fibromatosis-hypertrichosis and Laband syndromes. *Genetic Counseling*, 1994; **5**: 251–6.

32.4 The Cochrane Hepato-Biliary Group

Christian Gluud, on behalf of The Cochrane Hepato-Biliary Group Editorial Team*

'It is surely a great criticism of our profession that we have not organised a critical summary, by specialty or subspecialty, adapted periodically, of all relevant randomised controlled trials' (A.L. Cochrane 1931–1971: a critical review, with particular reference to the medical profession. In: *Medicines for the year 2000*. London: Office of Health Economics, 1997: 1–11)

The Cochrane Collaboration's task is to facilitate the preparation, maintenance, and dissemination of systematic reviews of randomized controlled trials, and reviews of other evidence evaluating health care when appropriate (Chalmers, BMJ, 1992; 305:736). The Cochrane Collaboration is named after Archie Cochrane (1909–1988), the epidemiologist who first emphasized that reliable information from randomized controlled trials is vital for making sound decisions in health care and research.[1]

The Cochrane Collaboration[2] started in 1992 and has since grown rapidly. By the end of 1997, 14 Cochrane Centres and more than 40 collaborative review groups had registered or were on the way to registration as components of the Collaboration. It seems likely that the infrastructure for covering almost all areas of health care will be in place before 1999.

The Cochrane Hepato-Biliary Group is the 20th collaborative review group registered within the Collaboration in March 1996. The scope of the Group is to perform the tasks of the Cochrane Collaboration within hepatobiliary disorders.

Problems facing medicine

Most clinical scientists who have tried to review the evidence for a particular intervention have been frustrated by the difficulties of finding out what randomized controlled trials have been done, and of interpreting their results critically. Further, the number of such trials is becoming so large that clinicians must increasingly rely on reviews of the primary research. More than 119 randomized controlled trials on portal hypertension have been published, and it is estimated that a new randomized controlled trial on the treatment of portal hypertension will appear every month.[3] Therefore, the quality, accuracy, and accessibility of reviews have become

increasingly important. Review articles prepared by experts may not take all the available evidence into consideration and may reflect the biases of their authors.[4] Cumulative meta-analyses of interventions preventing oesophageal variceal bleeding and re-bleeding, and of other interventions, have convincingly demonstrated that therapeutic recommendations in textbooks lack far behind the available evidence.[4,5]

The important disparities demonstrated between the recommendations made by experts in review articles and textbooks and the recommendations that could have been made on the basis of systematic reviews (i.e., prospective cumulative meta-analyses) underlined the need for an international collaboration such as the Cochrane.[2] There are several reasons for these disparities, as follows.

Reliance on electronic searching on MEDLINE and similar bibliographic electronic databases will reveal as few as 50 per cent of relevant, published, randomized controlled trials.[2,6]

The findings of randomized controlled trials with 'negative' results frequently remain unpublished.[2]

Reviews are frequently prepared without a sufficiently comprehensive search strategy to discover all relevant randomized controlled trials.

Reviews are frequently prepared without a formal research plan.

The review articles and textbooks are often out of date the moment they are published.

Current clinical practice among hospital-based specialists in gastro-enterology/hepatology varies considerably and significantly.[7] Physicians' reliance on incomplete, outdated, and biased reviews may have serious effects on the care of their patients.[8] Clinicians should have instantaneous, up-to-date assistance from an affordable, universally available database of systematic reviews of the best evidence from randomized controlled trials. The Cochrane Database of Systematic Reviews intends to provide such a service.[9]

The Cochrane Collaboration

The Cochrane Collaboration represents an international effort to prepare, maintain, and disseminate reviews of the effects of health-care interventions in a much more systematic and rigorous

*Christian Gluud, Co-ordinating Editor (DK), Torben Jørgensen, Editor (DK), Ronald L. Koretz (USA), Alberto Morabito, Statistical Editor (I), Luigi Pagliaro, Editor (I), Thierry Poynard, Editor (F), Robert Sutton, Editor (UK), Anne Gethe Hee, Review Group Co-ordinator (DK), Dimitrinka Nikolova, Review Group Co-ordinator (DK), and Nader Salasshahri, Data Manager (DK).

fashion. Each review contains the information needed for an analysis of the thoroughness and minimization of bias that were achieved in its preparation. Reference to all relevant randomized controlled trials (or other evidence) and a statistical summary of the results of the studies (meta-analysis when feasible) are presented. Conclusions are drawn as to whether the intervention does more good than harm and whether it should be adopted, rejected, or subjected to further research. The date of the review and the most recent amendments are specified. In this way the review process is a dynamic one, i.e., the review is modified as new information becomes available.

The Cochrane Collaboration is essentially a volunteer organization of individuals dedicated to the process of preparing high-quality, systematic reviews of the effects of health-care interventions, now and for the foreseeable future. The tasks of the collaborative review groups are to:

full-text search the specialist literature for randomized controlled trials, controlled clinical trials, and meta-analyses;

establish centralized libraries/databases of these articles;

prepare protocols for the systematic reviews;

prepare the systematic reviews as well as continually updating them.

The protocols and the systematic reviews are peer-refereed by other experts before acceptance. Once accepted the systematic reviews are included in the Cochrane Database of Systematic Reviews. The systematic reviews are disseminated electronically on floppy disks, CD-ROMs, and the Internet (available on the World Wide Web through Health Communications Network (http://www.hcn.net.au) and Synapse Publishing (http://www.medlib.com)), and will form the basis of an evidence-based health care. At the end of 1997, 253 protocols and 228 complete Cochrane reviews were available. The relevance of the Collaboration's output will grow as the number of systematic reviews becomes counted in thousands. The Cochrane Database of Systematic Reviews is one of the databases of the Cochrane Library, which also offers the Cochrane Collaboration Handbook[2] (describing the actions to take and how to proceed in the Collaboration), and the following databases: the York Database of Abstracts of Reviews of Effectiveness, the Cochrane Controlled Trials Register (now containing more than 150 000 articles on trials, of which almost 3 per cent is hepatobiliary), and the Cochrane Review Methodology Database. The Cochrane Library is available through Update Software Ltd. (tel: +44 1865 513902. FAX: +44 1865 516918. E-mail: info@update.co.uk).

The Cochrane Hepato-Biliary Group

A series of exploratory meetings and extensive correspondence led to the registration, in March 1996, of the Cochrane Hepato-Biliary Group. By November 1997, the Group comprised more than 160 hepatologists, hepatobiliary surgeons, and biostatisticians from 27 countries. Its members have expertise in clinical trials and in clinical epidemiology related to hepatobiliary diseases.

The Cochrane Hepato-Biliary Group has the task of full-text searching the specialist journals for randomized controlled trials and controlled clinical trials.[2] Members of the Group are at present involved in searching 26 out of the 190 identified specialist journals.

The Group has performed a MEDLINE search for randomized controlled trials, controlled clinical trials, and meta-analyses published during the period 1966 to 1996 pertinent to patients with hepatobiliary disorders. A total of 10 001 articles has been identified, of which 60 to 70 per cent seemed relevant. This corresponds to about 6500 published articles identifiable through MEDLINE, which is based on about 4500 of the most prestigious medical journals. However, there are probably another 25 000 medical journals in the world and a number of trials remain unpublished. If only half of the existing journal articles can be identified through MEDLINE, it is expected that another 6500 articles on trials exist. The Cochrane Hepato-Biliary Group has the task of identifying, registering, and filing the approximately 13 000 pertinent articles and distributing them to the relevant systematic reviewers. It is hoped that the Group will be at the top of this mountain of scientific articles before the end of the twentieth century.

How can I participate as a full-text searcher?

By contacting the Editorial Team Office, interested persons and groups can obtain information as to which specialist journals need full-text searching, and thereafter decide to register their search. The results of this full-text search for randomized controlled trials, controlled clinical trials, and meta-analyses are forwarded to the Cochrane Collaboration and articles dealing with hepatobiliary topics are forwarded to the Group.

Full-text searching takes time, but is certainly also rewarding. In addition to getting a good insight into the epidemiology of clinical research in a specific journal, one may be able to publish the results. Further, the full-text search is the chief foundation of all valid systematic reviews.

How can I participate as a systematic reviewer?

One can register a provisional title for a systematic review at the Cochrane Hepato-Biliary Group Editorial Team Office. One can choose to do this alone or preferably as a member of a group of systematic reviewers. Such groups should be international and have representation of specialists with different backgrounds (e.g. biostatisticians and surgeons or physicians and biostatisticians). Once the title has been registered, the systematic reviewer(s) will be allowed 6 months to finalize a protocol stating the background, materials, and methods of the review. After the protocol has been submitted to the Editorial Team, it will be subjected to peer-refereeing, normally involving two or more specialists from the Cochrane Hepato-Biliary Group or externally. Once the protocol has been accepted, the systematic reviewer(s) will be allowed 18 months to produce the review. When the systematic review has been submitted to the Editorial Team, it will be subjected to peer-refereeing, normally involving two or more specialists. Again these can be from the Cochrane Hepato-Biliary Group internally or external specialists.

Once the systematic review has been accepted by the Editorial Team, the text written in RevMan (Review Manager) will be incorporated into ModMan (Module Manager). Updated editions of ModMan are sent to the United Kingdom Cochrane Centre in Oxford (at present every third month). This Centre assembles the ModMans of the 34 existing collaborative review groups (ranging from groups on schizophrenia through stroke to musculoskeletal injuries) into the Cochrane Database of Systematic Reviews. The protocols and systematic reviews should be written in English language comprehensible to physicians and other health-care providers, consumers (i.e., persons who are or are at risk of becoming patients), and health-care purchasers.

Writing a protocol will normally take about 1 week and finalizing a systematic review can easily take several months.

Once the systematic review has been published it should be maintained, i.e., any criticism raised should be responded to and the review should be updated as new evidence appears. By choosing the electronic media for dissemination, it is easy to append criticism, which can be rebutted, and change the review when pertinent objections are raised.

How can I participate as a referee of protocols and systematic reviews?

Researchers who are not willing themselves to be systematic reviewers may enlist as potential candidates for peer referees of protocols and systematic reviews by forwarding to the Editorial Team Office information about their subject of interest and examples of research.

What can I expect of the Group as a patient?

The Group intends to provide patients and relatives with readable systematic reviews from which they can obtain up-to-date information on prevention, diagnosis, treatment, and care for their specific disease. Medicine can never, and must never, be performed according to cook books! It is the patient's right, in communication with health-care providers, to obtain the best form of intervention at the lowest risk (and cost). However, obtaining up-to-date information produced by international experts in a given area will surely assist the patient in making sound decisions. Furthermore, as an added benefit, the work of the Cochrane Collaboration may assist the public in better understanding, and thereby accepting, the conditions of health research. This could lead to a wider acceptance of the necessity of performing large, scientifically and ethically valid, randomized controlled trials.

What can I expect of the Group as a clinician?

At the bedside or in the practice, clinicians should have instantaneous, up-to-date assistance from an affordable, universally available database of systematic reviews of the best evidence from clinical trials.[9] The Cochrane Database of Systematic Reviews aims to provide this type of information.

At present, 60 titles of systematic reviews have been registered with the Cochrane Hepato-Biliary Group, 14 protocols have been submitted, and two systematic reviews have been published. It is hoped that before the year 2000 some 50 to 70 systematic reviews or more will have been prepared and that 600 to 800 reviews which fall within the scope of the Hepato-Biliary Group should be available

within the next 10 years or so. The speed of progress depends only on the amount of time dedicated to the Group, the collaborative spirit invested, and the understanding of universities, hospitals, health-care purchasers, and fund holders.

What do I get out of the Group as a researcher?

Each systematic review includes more than information on the steps required in the health-care system, i.e., to use the intervention or not. Each review also contains a recommendation as to whether more research should be done in the specific area or not. Accordingly, the reviews fuel ideas on what clinical research needs to be done and whether sufficient information exists. Likewise, researchers should not embark on a new randomized controlled trial without having performed a systematic literature review with, if feasible, a meta-analysis of previous research.[4]

In addition, the Cochrane Collaboration offers unique possibilities for easy access to informed specialists within a vast number of fields, areas, and interventions. Both nationally and internationally, the Collaboration offers free and unhindered communication, whether you want to contact a new collaborating centre in a randomized controlled trial, methodological advice on a meta-analysis or other matters, or a knowledgeable chairman of a Data Monitoring Committee.

Observational evidence is clearly better than opinion, but it is thoroughly unsatisfactory[1]

Opinion and observational evidence have their shortcomings.[1] On the other hand, one must also realize that systematic reviews and meta-analyses of randomized controlled trials are not free from problems.[10–13] In spite of these shortcomings, it would, by rephrasing Archie Cochrane's words, surely be a great criticism of our profession if we did not try to get an optimal outcome from exploring the information that may be obtained by systematic reviews and meta-analyses.

How can I assist?

The Cochrane Hepato-Biliary Group invites researchers to assist the collaborative review group in the number of tasks that must be dealt with. One may also help by informing the Group of the existence of any randomized controlled trials that may not have been published or about trials in progress. Such trials will be included in the database and could significantly influence the outcome of the systematic reviews of hepatobiliary interventions.

For further information, please contact the Editorial Team Office of the Cochrane Hepato-Biliary Group: Copenhagen Trial Unit, Institute of Preventive Medicine, H:S Kommunehospitalet, DK-1399 Copenhagen K, Denmark. Tel +45 3338 3742, fax +45 3332 4410, e-mail: CHBG<ctucph@inet.uni-c.dk>

References

1. Cochrane AL. *Effectiveness and efficiency. Random reflections on health services.* Cambridge University Press, 1972.

2. Sackett D and Oxman A (eds). *The Cochrane Collaboration handbook*. Oslo: Department of Health Services Research, National Institute of Public Health, 1994. Available through the Cochrane Library and the Internet (http://hirn.mcmaster.ca/cochrane/handbook/default.htm).

3. Becker U, *et al.* Trials in portal hypertension: valid meta-analyses and valid randomized clinical trials. In Franchis R de (ed.). *Portal hypertension II. Proceedings of the second Baveno International Consensus Workshop on definitions, methodology and therapeutic strategies.* Oxford: Blackwell Science, 1996: 180–210.

4. Antman EM, Lau J, Kupelnick B, Mosteller F, and Chalmers TC. A comparison of results of meta-analyses of randomized controlled trials and recommendations of clinical experts. Treatments for myocardial infarction. *Journal of the American Medical Association*, 1991; **268**: 240–8.

5. Pagliaro L, *et al.* Efficacy and efficiency of treatments in portal hypertension. In Franchis R de (ed.). *Portal hypertension II. Proceedings of the second Baveno International Consensus Workshop on definitions, methodology and therapeutic strategies.* Oxford: Blackwell Science, 1996: 159–79.

6. Gluud C, *et al.* Diagnosis and treatment of alcoholic liver disease in Europe. First report. *Gastrology International*, 1993; **6**: 221–30.

7. Poynard T and Conn HO. The retrieval of randomized clinical trials in liver disease from the medical literature. A comparison of MEDLARS and manual methods. *Controlled Clinical Trials*, 1985; **6**: 271–9.

8. Liberati A, *et al.* The role of attitudes, beliefs, and personal characteristics of Italian physicians in the surgical treatment of early breast cancer. *American Journal of Public Health*, 1991; **81**: 38–42.

9. Bero L and Rennie D. The Cochrane Collaboration. Preparing, maintaining, and disseminating systematic reviews of the effects of health care. *Journal of the American Medical Association*, 1995; **24**: 1935–8.

10. Friedman HP and Goldberg JD. Meta-analysis: an introduction and point of view. *Hepatology*, 1996; **23**: 917–28.

11. Taubes G. Looking for the evidence in medicine. *Science*, 1996; **272**: 22–4.

12. Christensen E and Gluud C. Glucocorticoids are ineffective in alcoholic hepatitis: a meta-analysis adjusting for confounding variables. *Gut*, 1995; **37**: 113–18.

13. Sharp SJ, Thompson SG, and Altman DG. The relation between treatment benefit and underlying risk in meta-analysis. *British Medical Journal*, 1996; **313**: 735–8.

Abbreviated journal titles as used in the text

AbdImag .... *Abdominal Imaging*
ActaAnaesthScand............... *Acta Anaesthesologica Scandinavica*
ActaAnat .... *Acta Anatomica (Basel)*
ActaBiolMedGerm............. *Acta Biologica et Medica Germanica*
ActaChemScand.................. *Acta Chemica Scandinavica*
ActaChirBelg .... *Acta Chirirurgica Belgica*
ActaChirScand .... *Acta Chirurgica Scandinavica*
ActaChirScandSuppl........... *Acta Chirurgica Scandinavica Supplementum*
ActaClinBelg.................... *Acta Clinica Belgica*
ActaCytol.................... *Acta Cytologica*
ActaDermVen .... *Acta Dermato-Venereologica*
ActaDiabetol .... *Acta Diabetologica*
ActaEnd.................... *Acta Endocrinologica*
ActaEndoscop .... *Acta Endoscopica*
ActaGastroBelg .... *Acta Gastroenterologica Belgica*
ActaGyn .... *Acta Gynecologica*
ActaHaem .... *Acta Haematologica (Basel)*
ActaHepatogastrBelg.......... *Acta Hepatogastroenterolgica Belgica*
ActaHepatoGastroenterol .... *Acta Hepato-Gastroenterologica*
ActaHepatolJpn.................... *Acta Hepatologica Japonica*
ActaHepatoSplenol .... *Acta Hepato-Splenologica*
ActaHistochem.................... *Acta Histochemica*
ActaMedAustr .... *Acta Medica Austriaca*
ActaMedCroatica .... *Acta Medica Croatica*
ActaMedOkayama .... *Acta Medica Okayama*
ActaMedScand.................... *Acta Medica Scandinavica*
ActaMedScandSuppl .... *Acta Medica Scandinavica Supplementum*
ActaMedSocUpsal .... *Acta Societatis Medicorum Upsaliensis*
ActaMorphHung................ *Acta Morphologica Academiae Scientiarum Hungaricae*
ActaNeurolBelg.................... *Acta Neurologica Belgica*
ActaNeurolScand .... *Acta Neurologica Scandinavica*
ActaNeuropath.................... *Acta Neuropathologica*
ActaObGyn.................... *Acta Obstetrica et Gynaecologica Scandinavica*
ActaOncol .... *Acta Oncologica*
ActaOphthalm.................... *Acta Ophthalmologica*
ActaOrthScand .... *Acta Orthopaedica Scandinavica*
ActaOtolaryngol .... *Acta Otolaryngologica*
ActaPaedScand.................... *Acta Paediatrica Scandinavica*
ActaPaedScandSuppl .... *Acta Paediatrica Scandinavica Supplementum*
ActaPaedSin.................... *Acta Paediatrica Sinica*
ActaPathJpn.................... *Acta Pathologica Japonica*
ActaPharmTox.................... *Acta Pharmacologica et Toxicologica*

ActaPhysiolHung .... *Acta Physiologica Academiae Scientiarum Hungaricae*
ActaPhysiolScand............... *Acta Physiologica Scandinavica*
ActaPMIScand.................... *Acta Pathologica, Microbiologica, et Immunologica Scandinavica*
ActaPMScandA .... *Acta Pathologica et Microbiologica Scandinavica, Section A: Pathology*
ActaPsychNeurol .... *Acta Psychiatrica et Neurologica*
ActaPsychScand.................. *Acta Psychiatrica Scandinavica*
ActaRadiol .... *Acta Radiologica*
ActaSocMedUps .... *Acta Societatis Medicorum Upsaliensis*
ActaUnioIntContra .... *Acta Unio Internationalis Contra Cancrum*
ActaUnioIntContra Cancrum *Acta Unio Internationalis Contra Cancrum*
AcuteCare .... *Acute Care*
AddicBiol.................... *Addiction Biology*
Addiction .... *Addiction*
AdvAlcSubstAb .... *Advances in Alcohol and Substance Abuse*
AdvBiochem .... *Advances in Biochemistry and Psychopharmacol* *Psychopharmacology*
AdvCarbChemBiochem....... *Advances in Carbohydrate Chemistry and Biochemistry*
AdvClinChem .... *Advances in Clinical Chemistry*
AdvClinEnzym .... *Advances in Clinical Enzymology*
AdvEnz.................... *Advances in Enzymology*
AdvEnzymReg .... *Advances in Enzyme Regulation*
AdvExpMedBiol .... *Advances in Experimental Medicine and Biology*
AdvImmunol.................... *Advances in Immunology*
AdvIntMed .... *Advances in Internal Medicine*
AdvLipRes.................... *Advances in Lipid Research*
AdvMyocardiol .... *Advances in Myocardiology*
AdvNephrol.................... *Advances in Nephrology*
AdvParasit .... *Advances in Parasitology*
AdvPediat .... *Advances in Pediatrics*
AdvPharmacol.................... *Advances in Pharmacology*
AdvProteinChem .... *Advances in Protein Chemistry*
AdvSurg .... *Advances in Surgery*
AdvVirusRes .... *Advances in Virus Research*
AerospaceMed .... *Aerospace Medicine*
Age .... *Age*
AgeAgeing .... *Age and Ageing*
AgentsActions.................... *Agents and Actions*
Agressol .... *Agressologie*
AIDS .... *AIDS*
AIDSRes.................... *AIDS Research*

AIDSResHumRV	*AIDS Research and Human Retroviruses*
AJR	*American Journal of Roentgenology*
AlcAlc	*Alcohol and Alcoholism*
AlcHealthResW	*Alcohol Health and Research World*
Alcohol	*Alcohol*
AlcoholClinExpRes	*Alcoholism: Clinical and Experimental Research*
Alcoholism	*Alcoholism*
AlcoholTreatQ	*Alcoholism Treatment Quarterly*
Alcologia	*Alcologia*
AlimPharmTher	*Alimentary Pharmacology and Therapeutics*
Alkfrag	*Alkoholfraagen*
AMAArchPath	*AMA Archives of Pathology*
AmFamilyPhysician	*American Family Physician*
AmHeartJ	*American Heart Journal*
AmIndHygAssJ	*American Industrial Hygiene Association Journal*
AmJAnat	*American Journal of Anatomy*
AmJCard	*American Journal of Cardiology*
AmJClinNutr	*American Journal of Clinical Nutrition*
AmJClinOnc	*American Journal of Clinical Oncology*
AmJClinOncCanClin Trials	*American Journal of Clinical Oncology and Cancer Clinical Trials*
AmJClinPath	*American Journal of Clinical Pathology*
AmJCritCareMed	*American Journal of Critical Care Medicine*
AmJDisChild	*American Journal of Diseases of Childhood*
AmJDrugAlcAb	*American Journal of Drug and Alcohol Abuse*
AmJEmergMed	*American Journal of Emergency Medicine*
AmJEpid	*American Journal of Epidemiology*
AmJGastr	*American Journal of Gastroenterology*
AmJHemat	*American Journal of Hematology*
AmJHospPharm	*American Journal of Hospital Pharmacy*
AmJHumGen	*American Journal of Human Genetics*
AmJHumMet	*American Journal of Human Metabolism*
AmJHypertension	*American Journal of Hypertension*
AmJIndMed	*American Journal of Industrial Medicine*
AmJInfecControl	*American Journal of Infection Control*
AmJKidneyDis	*American Journal of Kidney Diseases*
AmJMed	*American Journal of Medicine*
AmJMedGen	*American Journal of Medical Genetics*
AmJMedSci	*American Journal of the Medical Sciences*
AmJNephrol	*American Journal of Nephrology*
AmJObsGyn	*American Journal of Obstetrics and Gynecology*
AmJPathol	*American Journal of Pathology*
AmJPedHemOnc	*American Journal of Pediatric Hematology and Oncology*
AmJPerinat	*American Journal of Perinatology*
AmJPhysAnthropol	*American Journal of Physical Anthropology*
AmJPhysiol	*American Journal of Physiology*
AmJPrevMed	*American Journal of Preventive Medicine*
AmJPsychiat	*American Journal of Psychiatry*
AmJPublHlth	*American Journal of Public Health*
AmJReprodImmunol	*American Journal of Reproductive Immunology*
AmJRespirCellMolBiol	*American Journal of Respiratory Cell and Molecular Biology*
AmJRoent	*American Journal of Roentgenology*
AmJRoentRadTher NuclMed	*American Journal of Roentgenology, Radiation Therapy and Nuclear Medicine*
AmJSportsMed	*American Journal of Sports Medicine*
AmJSurg	*American Journal of Surgery*
AmJSurgPath	*American Journal of Surgical Pathology*
AmJSyphGonVenDis	*American Journal of Syphilis, Gonorrhea, and Venereal Disease*
AmJTropMedHyg	*American Journal of Tropical Medicine and Hygiene*
AmLabClinSci	*American Laboratory and Clinical Science*
AmRevRespDis	*American Review of Respiratory Disease*
AmSci	*American Scientist*
AmSurg	*American Surgeon*
AmyloidIntJExp ClinInvest	*Amyloid: The International Journal of Experimental and Clinical Investigation*
Anaesth	*Anaesthesia*
AnalBioch	*Analytical Biochemistry*
AnalChem	*Analytical Chemistry*
AnalQuantCytolHistol	*Analytical and Quantitative Cytology and Histology*
AnalSci	*Analytical Sciences*
AnatEmbryol	*Anatomy and Embryology*
AnatRec	*Anatomical Record*
Andrologia	*Andrologia*
AnEspPediatr	*Anales Espanoles de Pediatrica*
AnesthAnalg	*Anesthesia and Analgesia*
AnesthClinNAm	*Anesthesia Clinics of North America*
Anesthesiol	*Anesthesiology*
AnaesthIntCare	*Anaesthesia and Intensive Care*
AngewChemIntEdEngl	*Angewandte Chemie International Edition in English*
Angiol	*Angiology*

AnnAllergy .... *Annals of Allergy*
AnnBiolClin....................... *Annales de Biologie Clinique (Paris)*
AnnChir............................ *Annales de Chirurgie (Paris)*
AnnChirGyn...................... *Annales de Chirurgie Gynecologique*
AnnChirThoracCardiovasc.. *Annales de Chirurgie Thoracique et Cardio-Vasculaire*
AnnClinBioch .... *Annals of Clinical Biochemistry*
AnnClinLabSci .... *Annals of Clinical and Laboratory Science*
AnnClinRes .... *Annals of Clinical Research*
AnnDermatolVenereol........ *Annales de Dermatologie et de Venereologie*
AnnEmergMed .... *Annals of Emergency Medicine*
AnnEndocr .... *Annales d'Endocrinologie (Paris)*
AnnGastroHep................... *Annales de Gastroenterologie et d'Hepatologie (Paris)*
AnnHemat .... *Annals of Hematology*
AnnHumGenet .... *Annals of Human Genetics*
AnnInstPasteurMicrobiol .... *Annales de l'Institut Pasteur Microbiologie*
AnnIntMed........................ *Annals of Internal Medicine*
AnnItalMedInt................... *Annali Italiani di Medicina Interna*
AnnMed .... *Annals of Medicine*
AnnMedIntern .... *Annales de Médecine Interne (Paris)*
AnnMedInterna(Fenn)........ *Annales Medicinae Internae Fenniae*
AnnMedSectPolAcadSci ..... *Annals of the Medical Section of the Polish Academy of Sciences*
AnnNeurol......................... *Annals of Neurology*
AnnNuclMed .... *Annals of Nuclear Medicine*
AnnNutrAliment................ *Annals of Nutrition and Alimentation*
AnnNutrMetab .... *Annals of Nutrition and Metabolism*
AnnNYAcadMed .... *Annals of the New York Academy of Medicine*
AnnNYAcadSci.................. *Annals of the New York Academy of Sciences*
AnnOccupHyg.................... *Annals of Occupational Hygiene*
AnnOncol .... *Annals of Oncology*
AnnPath............................ *Annales de Pathologie*
AnnPediat .... *Annales de Pediatrie*
AnnPharmacother .... *Annals of Pharmacotherapy*
AnnProgrRepSEATO.......... *Annual Progress Report of the SEATO Medical Research Laboratory*
MedResLab
AnnRadiol.......................... *Annales de Radiologie*
AnnRCSurg .... *Annals of the Royal College of Surgeons*
AnnRepMedChem .... *Annals of Reproductive Medicine and Chemistry*
AnnRevBiochem .... *Annual Review of Biochemistry*
AnnRevCellBiol .... *Annual Review of Cell Biology*
AnnRevGenet .... *Annual Review of Genetics*
AnnRevImmunol................ *Annual Review of Immunology*
AnnRevMed .... *Annual Review of Medicine*
AnnRevMicro .... *Annual Review of Microbiology*
AnnRevNutr .... *Annual Review of Nutrition*
AnnRevPharmTox .... *Annual Review of Pharmacology and Toxicology*

AnnRevPhysiol .... *Annual Review of Physiology*
AnnRevRespDis................. *Annual Review of Respiratory Disease*
AnnRheumDis .... *Annals of the Rheumatic Diseases*
AnnSaudiMed..................... *Annals of Saudi Medicine*
AnnSocBelgeMedTrop .... *Annales de la Societé Belge de Médecine Tropicale*
AnnSurg .... *Annals of Surgery*
AnnThorSurg .... *Annals of Thoracic Surgery*
AnnTropMed...................... *Annals of Tropical Medicine and Parasitology*
AnnTropMedHyg .... *Annals of Tropical Medicine and Hygience*
AnnTropPaediat................. *Annals of Tropical Paediatrics*
AntibiotChemo .... *Antibiotics and Chemotherapy*
AntiCancDrugs .... *Anti-Cancer Drugs*
AntiCancerRes................... *Anticancer Research*
AntimicrobAgents .... *Antimicrobial Agents and Chemother Chemotherapy*
Chemother
AntiviralNews.................... *Antiviral News*
AntiviralRes .... *Antiviral Research*
AntiviralChemother .... *Antiviral Chemotherapy*
AnzSchaed .... *Anzeiger für Schaedlingskunde*
ApheresisBull.................... *Apheresis Bulletin*
Appetite .... *Appetite*
ApplBiochemBiotechnol...... *Applied Biochemistry and Biotechnology*
ApplEnvironMicrobiol .... *Applied Environmental Microbiology*
ApplPathol........................ *Applied Pathology*
ArbmedSozmedArbhyg .... *Arbeitsmedizin, Sozialmedizin, Arbeitshygiene*
ArchAnatCytolPath............ *Archives d'Anatomie et de Cytologie Pathologiques*
ArchBiochemBiophys.......... *Archives of Biochemistry and Biophysics*
ArchDermatol .... *Archives of Dermatology*
ArchDermRes .... *Archives of Dermatological Research*
ArchDisChild..................... *Archives of Diseases of Childhood*
ArchEnvironHlth .... *Archives of Environmental Health*
ArchExpPatholPharmakol ... *Archiv für Experimentelle Pathologie und Pharmakologie*
ArchFamMed .... *Archives of Family Medicine*
ArchFrancPediat .... *Archives Françaises de Pediatrie*
ArchFrMalAppDigNutr...... *Archives Françaises des Maladies de l'Appareil Digestif*
ArchGenPsychiatr.............. *Archives of General Psychiatry*
ArchGerontolGeriat .... *Archives of Gerontology and Geriatrics*
ArchGewerbepath .... *Archiv für Gewerbepathologie und Gewerbehyg Gewerbehygiene*
Gewerbehyg
ArchHistCyt .... *Archives of Histology and Cytology*
ArchIndHlth .... *Archives of Industrial Health*
ArchIndHyg....................... *Archives of Industrial Hygiene*
ArchInternatPharmTher ..... *Archives Internationales de Pharmacodynamie et de Thérapie*
ArchIntMed....................... *Archives of Internal Medicine*
ArchIntPhysiolBioch .... *Archives Internationales de Physiologie et de Biochemie*

ArchJpnChir	*Archiv für Japanische Chirurgie*
ArchMalAppDigNutr	*Archives des Maladies de l'Appareil Digestif et des Maladies de la Nutrition*
ArchMalCoeur	*Archives des Maladies du Coeur et des Vaisseaux*
ArchMalProf	*Archives de Maladies Professionelles, Hygiene et Toxicologie Industrielles*
ArchNeurol	*Archives of Neurology*
ArchGynaecolObstet	*Archives of Gynaecology and Obstetrics*
ArchOphthalmol	*Archives of Ophthalmology*
ArchOralBiol	*Archives of Oral Biology*
ArchPathLabMed	*Archives of Pathology and Laboratory Medicine*
ArchPathol	*Archives of Pathology*
ArchPediat	*Archives de Pédiatrie*
ArchPediatrAdolescMed	*Archives of Pediatrics and Adolescent Medicine*
ArchPharmacol	*Archives of Pharmacology*
ArchPharm	*Archiv der Pharmazie*
ArchSexBehav	*Archives of Sexual Behaviour*
ArchSurg	*Archives of Surgery*
ArchToxicol	*Archives of Toxicology*
ArchVirol	*Archives of Virology*
ArchVirolSuppl	*Archives of Virology. Supplementum*
ArkivKemi	*Arkiv foer Kemi*
ArqGastroSaoPaulo	*Arquivos de Gastroenterologia*
ArthRheum	*Arthritis and Rheumatism*
ArtifOrg	*Artificial Organs*
Artscler	*Arteriosclerosis*
ArzForsch	*Arzneimittel-Forschung*
Atheroscl	*Atherosclerosis*
ASAIOTrans	*ASAIO Transactions*
ATLA	*ATLA - Alternatives to Laboratory Animals*
AustAnnMed	*Australasian Annals of Medicine*
AustClinRev	*Australian Clinical Review*
AustDrugAlcRev	*Australian Drug and Alcohol Review*
AustJDermatol	*Australian Journal of Dermatology*
AustJExpBiolMedSci	*Australian Journal of Experimental Biology and Medical Sciences*
AustNZJMed	*Australian and New Zealand Journal of Medicine*
AustNZJObsGyn	*Australian and New Zealand Journal of Obstetrics and Gynaecology*
AustNZJSurg	*Australian and New Zealand Journal of Surgery*
AustPaedJ	*Australian Paediatric Journal*
AustRadiol	*Australian Radiology*
AustVetJ	*Australian Veterinary Journal*
AutoImmun	*Autoimmunity*
AvianDis	*Avian Diseases*
BacteriolRev	*Bacteriological Reviews*
BailClinGastr	*Bailliere's Clinical Gastroenterology*
BasicLifeSci	*Basic Life Sciences*
BBActa	*Biochimica et Biophysica Acta*
BBResComm	*Biochemical and Biophysical Research Communications*
BDOAS	*Birth Defects, Original Article Series*
BehavBrainRes	*Behavioural Brain Research*
BehavGen	*Behavior Genetics*
BehavResTher	*Behavior Research and Therapy*
BeitrPath	*Beitrage zur Pathologie*
BeitrPatholAnat	*Beitrage zur Pathologischen Anatomie und Allgemeinen Pathologie*
BiblCardiol	*Bibliotheca Cardiologica*
BiblioNutrDiet	*Bibliotheca 'Nutritio et Dieta'*
Biochem	*Biochemistry*
BiochemCellBiol	*Biochemistry and Cell Biology*
BiochemGen	*Biochemical Genetics*
BiochemGen	*Biochemical Genetics*
BiochemInt	*Biochemistry International*
BiochemJ	*Biochemical Journal*
BiochemMed	*Biochemical Medicine*
BiochemMolBiolInt	*Biochemistry and Molecular Biology International*
BiochemMolMed	*Biochemical and Molecular Medicine*
BiochemPharm	*Biochemical Pharmacology*
BiochemSocSymp	*Biochemical Society Transactions*
BiochemZ	*Biochemische Zeitschrift*
Biochim	*Biochimie*
BioconjugChem	*Bioconjugate Chemistry*
BioEssays	*Biological Essays*
BiolCell	*Biology of the Cell*
BiolChemHS	*Biological Chemistry Hoppe-Seyler*
BiolNeon	*Biology of the Neonate*
BiolPharmBull	*Biological and Pharmaceutical Bulletin*
BiolRepro	*Biology of Reproduction*
BiolTraceElemRes	*Biological Trace Element Research*
Biomark	*Biomarkers*
BiomedChromatogr	*Biomedical Applications of Gas Chromatography*
Biomedicine	*Biomedicine*
BiomedPharmacoth	*Biomedicine and Pharmacotherapy*
BioMedRes	*Biomedical Research*
Biometrika	*Biometrika*
BiopharmDrugDispos	*Biopharmaceutics and Drug Disposition*
BiophysJ	*Biophysical Journal*
BiosciRep	*Bioscience Reports*
Blood	*Blood*
BloodCells	*Blood Cells*
BloodCellsMolDis	*Blood Cells, Molecules and Diseases*
BloodCoagFibrinol	*Blood Coagulation and Fibrinolysis*
BloodRev	*Blood Reviews*
Blut	*Blut*
BMJ	*British Medical Journal*
Bone	*Bone*
BoneMTrans	*Bone Marrow Transplantation*
BoneMineral	*Bone and Mineral*
Brain	*Brain*
BrainDev	*Brain and Development*

BrainRes .... *Brain Research*
BratislLekListy .... *Bratislavske Lekarske Listy*
BrazJMedBiolRes............... *Brazilian Journal of Medical and Biological Research*
BrHeartJ .... *British Heart Journal*
BrJAddic.......................... *British Journal of Addiction*
BrJAlcAlc......................... *British Journal of Alcohol and Alcoholism*
BrJAnaesth....................... *British Journal of Anaesthesiology*
BrJCanc .... *British Journal of Cancer*
BrJClinPharm .... *British Journal of Clinical Pharmacology*
BrJClinPract .... *British Journal of Clinical Practice*
BrJDermatol .... *British Journal of Dermatology*
BrJDisChest...................... *British Journal of Disease of the Chest*
BrJExpPath .... *British Journal of Experimental Pathology*
BrJHaemat .... *British Journal of Haematology*
BrJHospMed...................... *British Journal of Hospital Medicine*
BrJIndMed .... *British Journal of Industrial Medicine*
BrJIntensCare .... *British Journal of Intensive Care*
BrJNutr .... *British Journal of Nutrition*
BrJObsGyn .... *British Journal of Obstetrics and Gynaecology*
BrJPharmacool .... *British Journal of Pharmacology*
BrJPsychiat .... *British Journal of Psychiatry*
BrJPsychol .... *British Journal of Psychology*
BrJRadiol .... *British Journal of Radiology*
BrJRheum .... *British Journal of Rheumatology*
BrJSportsMed.................... *British Journal of Sports Medicine*
BrJSurg............................ *British Journal of Surgery*
BrJUrol............................ *British Journal of Urology*
BrJVenerDis...................... *British Journal of Venereal Diseases*
BrMedBull........................ *British Medical Bulletin*
BrMedJClinRes.................. *British Medical Journal of Clinical Research*
BrVetJ .... *British Veterinary Journal*
BullAcadNatMed .... *Bulletin de l'Academie Nationale de Medicine (Paris)*
BullAssAnat .... *Bulletin de l'Association des Anatomistes*
BullCanc .... *Bulletin du Cancer (Paris)*
BullExpBiolMed .... *Bulletin of Experimental Biology and Medicine*
BullJHopkHosp.................. *Bulletin of the Johns Hopkins Hospital*
BullMemSocChirParis .... *Bulletin et Mémoires de la Societé des Chirurgiens de Paris*
BullMemSocMedHôp .... *Bulletins et Mémoires de la Societé*
  Paris   *Medicale des Hôpitaux de Paris*
BullNYAcadMed................ *Bulletin of the New York Academy of Medicine*
BullSocIntChir.................. *Bulletin de la Societé International de Chirurgie*
BullSocMedChir .... *Bulletin de la Societé Médicale des*
  Indochine   *Chirurgiens de Indochine*

BullSocPath .... *Bulletin de la Societé de Pathologie Exotique*
BullWHO .... *Bulletin of the World Health Organization*

CalcifTissInt .... *Calcified Tissue International*
CalcifTissRes .... *Calcified Tissue Research*
CalifMed........................... *Californian Medicine*
CanAnaesthSocJ................. *Canadian Anaesthetists Society Journal*
CancChemoPharm .... *Cancer Chemotherapy and Pharmacology*
CancChemoRep .... *Cancer Chemotherapy Reports*
Cancer .... *Cancer*
CancerBiochBiophys .... *Cancer Biochemistry Biophysics*
CancerCauseContr .... *Cancer Causes and Control*
CancerDetectPrev .... *Cancer Detection and Prevention*
CancerDrugDeliv............... *CancerDrugDelivery*
CancerGenetCytogen .... *Cancer Genetics and Cytogenetics*
CancerImmunTher .... *Cancer Immunology and Immunotherapy*
CancerInvest .... *Cancer Investigation*
CancerLett........................ *Cancer Letters*
CancerMetRev .... *Cancer Metastasis Reviews*
CancerRes......................... *Cancer Research*
CancerSurv .... *Cancer Survey*
CancerTreatRep................. *Cancer Treatment Reports*
CanJBiochCellBiol .... *Canadian Journal of Biochemistry and Cell Biology*
CanJBiochem .... *Canadian Journal of Biochemistry*
CanJCard .... *Canadian Journal of Cardiology*
CanJGastr .... *Canadian Journal of Gastroenterology*
CanJMicrobiol................... *Canadian Journal of Microbiology*
CanJNeurSci...................... *Canadian Journal of Neurological Sciebces*
CanJPhysPharm .... *Canadian Journal of Physiology and Pharmacology*
CanJPsychiat..................... *Canadian Journal of Psychiatry*
CanJSurg .... *Canadian Journal of Surgery*
CanMedAssJ .... *Canadian Medical Association Journal*
CarbohydrRes .... *Carbohydrate Research*
Carcinogenesis .... *Carcinogenesis*
Cardiol............................. *Cardiology*
CardiolClin .... *Cardiology Clinics*
Cardiologia........................ *Cardiologia*
CardiovascDrugRes............ *Cardiovascular Drug Research*
CardiovascDrugTher .... *Cardiovascular Drugs and Therapy*
CardvascIntRadiol.............. *Cardiovascular and Interventional Radiology*
CasLekCesk .... *Casopis Lekaru Ceskych*
CCActa .... *Clinica Chimica Acta*
CDCSurvSumm .... *CDC Survey and Summary*
CDR .... *Communicable Disease Reports*
Cell................................... *Cell*
CellBiolIntRep .... *Cell Biology International Reports*
CellBiolRep....................... *Cell Biology Reports*

CellCalcium .... *Cell Calcium*
CellDeathDiffer .... *Cell Death and Differentiation*
CellGrowthDiff................... *Cell Growth and Differentiation*
CellHepSin .... *Cells of the Hepatic Sinusoid*
CellImmunol...................... *Cellular Immunology*
CellMolecBiol .... *Cellular and Molecular Biology*
CellStructFunc .... *Cell Structure and Function*
CellTissKinet.................... *Cell Tissue Kinetics*
CellTissRes...................... *Cell Tissue Research*
CentrAfrMedJ................... *Central African Medical Journal*
ChemBiolInteract............... *Chemico-Biological Interactions*
Chemosphere .... *Chemosphere*
Chemother .... *Chemotherapy*
ChemPharmBull .... *Chemical and Pharmaceutical Bulletin*
ChemPhysLip .... *Chemistry and Physics of Lipids*
ChemResTox .... *Chemical Research in Toxicology*
Chest .... *Chest*
ChinJGastro...................... *Chinese Journal of Gastroenterology*
ChinJIntMed .... *Chinese Journal of Internal Medicine*
ChinJPhysiol .... *Chinese Journal of Physiology*
ChinMedJ .... *Chinese Medical Journal*
Chirurgie .... *Chirurgie*
ChungHuaFuChan.............. *Chung-Hua Fu Ch'an K'o Tsa Chih*
CibaSymp .... *Ciba Foundation Symposium*
CircRes .... *Circulation Research*
Circul.............................. *Circulation*
CircShock .... *Circulation and Shock*
CleveClinJMed .... *Cleveland Clinic Journal of Medicine*
CleveClinQ....................... *Cleveland Clinic Quarterly*
ClinAutonomRes................. *Clinical Autonomic Research*
ClinBioch......................... *Clinical Biochemistry*
ClinCard .... *Clinical Cardiology*
ClinChem .... *Clinical Chemistry*
ClinDiagVirol.................... *Clinical and Diagnostic Virology*
ClinEndMetab .... *Clinics in Endocrinology and Metabolism*
ClinEndoc......................... *Clinical Endocrinology*
ClinExpDerm .... *Clinical and Experimental Dermatology*
ClinExpImmun .... *Clinical and Experimental Immunology*
ClinExpMet .... *Clinical and Experimental Metastasis*
ClinExpPharmPhys............. *Clinical and Experimental Pharmacology and Physiology*
ClinExpRheumatol............. *Clinical and Experimental Rheumatology*
ClinGastroent .... *Clinics in Gastroenterology*
ClinGenet .... *Clinical Genetics*
ClinHaem .... *Clinics in Haematology*
ClinicsAnesthesiol .... *Clinics in Anesthesiology*
ClinImmunAllergy .... *Clinics in Immunology and Allergy*
ClinImmunPath .... *Clinical Immunology and Immunopathology*
ClinInfDis......................... *Clinical Infectious Diseases*
ClinInvest .... *Clinical Investigator*

ClinInvestMed .... *Clinical and Investigative Medicine*
ClinLabHaemat.................. *Clinical and Laboratory Haematology*
ClinMicroRev .... *Clinical Microbiology Reviews*
ClinNephrol....................... *Clinical Nephrology*
ClinNeurolNeurosurg .... *Clinical Neurology and Neurosurgery*
ClinNeuropathol .... *Clinical Neuropathology*
ClinNeuropharmacol .... *Clinical Neuropharmacology*
ClinNuclMed..................... *Clinical Nuclear Medicine*
ClinNutr .... *Clinical Nutrition*
ClinObstetGynecol............. *Clinical Obstetrics and Gynecol*
ClinOncol .... *Clinical Oncology*
ClinOrthopRelRes.............. *Clinical Orthopedics and Related Research*
ClinPediat .... *Clinical Pediatrics*
ClinPharmacokin................ *Clinical Pharmacokinetics*
ClinPharmTher................... *Clinical Pharmacology and Therapeutics*
ClinPhysiol .... *Clinical Physiology*
ClinPhysPhysiolMeas .... *Clinical Physics and Physiological Measurement*
ClinRadiol......................... *Clinical Radiology*
ClinRes .... *Clinical Research*
ClinRheum .... *Clinical Rheumatology*
ClinSci............................. *Clinical Science*
ClinSciMolMed .... *Clinical Science and Molecular Medicine*
ClinTher........................... *Clinical Therapeutics*
ClinToxicol .... *Clinical Toxicology*
ClinTranspl....................... *Clinical Transplantation*
ClinTropMedCommDis...... *Clinics in Tropical Medicine and Communicable Diseases*
Coagulation .... *Coagulation*
CollRelRes .... *Collagen and Related Research*
CompBiochPhys.................. *Comparative Biochemistry and Physiology*
Complement .... *Complement*
ConnMed........................... *Connecticut Medicine*
ConnTissRes...................... *Connective Tissue Research*
ContactDerm .... *Contact Dermatitis*
ContempSurg...................... *Contemporary Surgery*
ContribNephrol .... *Contributions to Nephrology*
ControlledClinTrials .... *Controlled Clinical Trials*
CRAcadSci......................... *Comptes Rendus de l'Academie des Sciences (Paris)*
CritCareMed...................... *Critical Care Medicine*
CritRevBiochem................. *Critical Reviews in Biochemistry and Molecular Biology*
CritRevClinLabSci............. *Critical Reviews in Clinical Laboratory Sciences*
CritRevDiagImag............... *Critical Reviews in Diagnostic Imaging*
CritRevImmunol................. *Critical Reviews in Immunology*
CritRevOnc/Hemat .... *Critical Reviews in Oncology/ Hematology*
CritRevTherDrugCarrSys... *Critical Reviews in Therapeutic Drug Carrier Systems*
CritRevTox........................ *Critical Reviews in Toxicology*

CRSocBio	*Comptes Rendus des Séances de la Société de Biologie et des Filiales (Paris)*
Cryobiology	*Cryobiology*
CryoLett	*Cryo Letters*
CSHarbSymQBiol	*Cold Spring Harbor Symposia on Quantitative Biology*
CurrAlc	*Currents in Alcoholism*
CurrBiol	*Current Biology*
CurrMedResOpin	*Current Medical Research and Opinion*
CurrModBiol	*Currents in Modern Biology*
CurrOpinCellBiol	*Current Opinion in Cell Biology*
CurrOpinGenetDevelop	*Current Opinion in Genetics and Development*
CurrOpinGastro	*Current Opinion in Gastroenterology*
CurrOpinLipidol	*Current Opinion in Lipidology*
CurrOpinImmunol	*Current Opinion in Immunology*
CurrOpinInfDis	*Current Opinion in Infectious Disease*
CurrOpinNephrolHypert	*Current Opinion in Nephrology and Hypertension*
CurrOpinRheum	*Current Opinion in Rheumatology*
CurrProbCardiol	*Current Problem in Cardiology*
CurrProbPediat	*Current Problem in Pediatrics*
CurrProbSurg	*Current Problems in Surgery*
CurrTherRes	*Current Therapeutic Research: Clinical and Experimental*
CurrTopHaemat	*Current Topics in Haematology*
Cutis	*Cutis*
Cytobios	*Cytobios*
Cytochem	*Cytochemistry*
CytogenetCellGenet	*Cytogenetics and Cell Genetics*
Cytokine	*Cytokine*
Cytopath	*Cytopathology*
DanMedBull	*Danish Medical Bulletin*
Dermatologica	*Dermatologica*
Dermatology	*Dermatology*
DeutschApothekZeit	*Deutsch Apotheka Zeitung*
DeutschArchKlinMed	*Deutsches Archiv für Klinische Medizin*
DeutscheZVerdauStoff	*Deutsche Zeitschrift für Verdaungs und Stoffwechselkrankheiten*
DeutschMedWoch	*Deutsche Medizinische Wochenschrift*
DeutschZNervenh	*Deutsche Zeitschrift für Nervenheilkunde*
DevBiol	*Developmental Biology*
Development	*Development*
DevDyn	*Developmental Dynamics*
DevelopBiolStandard	*Developments in Biological Standardization*
DevPharmacolTher	*Developmental Pharmacology and Therapeutics*
DiabetAnn	*Diabetes Annual*
DiabetCare	*Diabetes Care*
Diabetolog	*Diabetologia*
DiabeteMetab	*Diabetes Metabolism*
Diabetes	*Diabetes*
DiabetMed	*Diabetes Medicine*
DiabetMetabRev	*Diabetes-Metabolism Reviews*
DiabetNutrMetab	*Diabetes Nutrition and Metabolism*
DiabetRes	*Diabetes Research*
DiabetResClinPract	*Diabetes Research and Clinical Practice*
DiabetStoffw	*Diabetes und Stoffwechsel*
DiagCytopathol	*Diagnostic Cytopathology*
DiagIntervRadiol	*Diagnostic and Interventional Radiology*
DiagMicrobInfDis	*Diagnostic Microbiology and Infectious Disease*
DiagTherEndosc	*Diagnostic and Therapeutic Endoscopy*
DiagnosHistopath	*Diagnostic Histopathology*
DiagnosImagingClinMed	*Diagnostic Imaging in Clinical Medicine*
Differentiation	*Differentiation*
DigDis	*Digestive Diseases*
DigDisSci	*Digestive Diseases and Sciences*
Digestion	*Digestion*
DigSurg	*Digestive Surgery*
DisChest	*Diseases of the Chest*
DisColRec	*Diseases of the Colon and Rectum*
DisHeartCircul	*Diseases of the Heart and Circulation*
DisMon	*Disease-a-Month*
DMedWoch	*Deutsche Medizinische Wochenschrift*
DNA	*DNA*
DrugAlcDep	*Drug and Alchohol Dependence*
DrugDel	*Drug Delivery*
DrugDevRes	*Drug Development Research*
DrugInvest	*Drug Investigations*
DrugMetDisp	*Drug Metabolism and Disposition*
DrugRes	*Drug Research*
Drugs	*Drugs*
DrugSafety	*Drug Safety*
DrugsExpClinRes	*Drugs under Clinical and Experimental Research*
DrugsMetabolRev	*Drug Metabolism Reviews*
DtschGesInnMed	*Deutsche Gesellschaft fur Innere Medizin*
DtshGesundhwesen	*Deutsche Gesundheitswesen*
DtschZVerdau Stoffwechselkr	*Deutsche Zeitschrift fur Verdaungs- und Stoffwechselkrankheiten*
EcotoxEnvirSafety	*Ecotoxicology and Environmental Safety*
EdinburghMedJ	*Edinburgh Medical Journal*
EJPTox	*European Journal of Pharmacology, Environmental Toxicology and Pharmacology Section*
ElectroencephalogrClin Neurophys	*Electroencephalography and Clinical Neurophysiology*
Electroencephalogr Neurophysiol	*Electroencephalography and Neurophysiology*
Electrophoresis	*Electrophoresis*
EMBOJ	*EMBO Journal*

EndMetClinMedNAm .... *Endocrinology and Metabolism Clinics of North America*
Endocrinol .... *Endocrinology*
EndocrinolJpn .... *Endocrinologia Japonica*
EndocrRev .... *Endocrine Reviews*
Endoscopy .... *Endoscopy*
Endothelium .... *Endothelium*
EnfermInfecMicroClin .... *Enfermedades Infecciosas y Microbiologia Clinica*
EnvironHlthPerspect .... *Environmental Health Perspectives*
EnvirRes .... *Environmental Research*
Enzyme................................ *Enzyme*
EnzymolBiolClin................. *Enzymologia Biologica et Clinica*
EpidInf .... *Epidemiology and Infection*
EpidRev .... *Epidemiologic Reviews*
EurArchPsychNeurSci .... *European Archives of Psychiatry and Neurological Sciences*
EurCytokineNet.................. *European Cytokine Network*
EurHeartJ .... *European Heart Journal*
EurJAnaesth........................ *European Journal of Anaesthiology*
EurJBioch .... *European Journal of Biochemistry*
EurJCan .... *European Journal of Cancer*
EurJCanClinOnc .... *European Journal of Cancer and Clinical Oncology*
EurJCellBiol....................... *European Journal of Cell Biology*
EurJClinChemClinBioch ..... *European Journal of Clinical Chemistry and Clinical Biochemistry*
EurJClinInv .... *European Journal of Clinical Investigation*
EurJClinMicrobInfDis .... *European Journal of Clinical Microbiology and Infectious Disease*
EurJClinNutr .... *European Journal of Clinical Nutrition*
EurJClinPharm .... *European Journal of Clinical Pharmacology*
EurJDMPharm .... *European Journal of Drug Metabolism and Pharmacokinetics*
EurJEndocr........................ *European Journal of Endocrinology*
EurJEpid............................ *European Journal of Epidemiology*
EurJGastroHepatol.............. *European Journal of Gastroenterology and Hepatology*
EurJHumGenet.................. *European Journal of Human Genetics*
EurJImmunogenet.............. *European Journal of Immunogenetics*
EurJImmun........................ *European Journal of Immunology*
EurJNucMed .... *European Journal of Nuclear Medicine*
EurJObsGynReprodBiol...... *European Journal of Obsetrics, Gynaecology, and Reproductive Biology*
EurJPed .... *European Journal of Pediatrics*
EurJPaediatSurg.................. *European Journal of Paediatric Surgery*
EurJPharm......................... *European Journal of Pharmacology*
EurJRadiol .... *European Journal of Radiology*
EurJRespDis .... *European Journal of Respiratory Diseases*

EurJRheumInflamm .... *European Journal of Rheumatic Inflammation*
EurJSurg............................. *European Journal of Surgery*
EurJSurgOnc .... *European Journal of Surgical Oncology*
EurNeurol .... *European Neurology*
EurRespJ .... *European Respiratory Journal*
EurSurgRes........................ *European Surgical Research*
ExpAgeRes........................ *Experimental Ageing Research*
ExpCellRes .... *Experimental Cell Research*
Experientia .... *Experientia*
ExpBiol .... *Experimental Biology*
ExpGerontol .... *Experimental Gerontology*
ExpMolPath .... *Experimental Molecular Pathology*
ExpParasit.......................... *Experimental Parasitology*
ExpPath .... *Experimental Pathology*
EXS.................................... *EXS*
ExpToxPath .... *Experimental and Toxicologic Pathology*

FASEBJ .... *Federation of American Societies for Experimental Biology (FASEB) Journal*
FEBSLett .... *FEBS Letters*
FedProc .... *Federation Proceedings of American Societies for Experimental Biology*
FertSter .... *Fertilization and Sterilization*
FetDiagTher....................... *Fetal Diagnosis and Therapy*
Fibrinolysis .... *Fibrinolysis*
FOBrMedBull..................... *Foreign Office British Medical Bulletin*
FolHistochemCytol .... *Folia Histochemica et Cytochemica*
FolMed.............................. *Folia Medica*
FolPsychNeurolJapon .... *Folia Psychiatrica et Neurologica Japonica*
FoodChemTox.................... *Food and Chemical Toxicology*
FoodCosmTox .... *Food and Cosmetics Toxicology*
FoodNut............................ *Food and Nutrition*
FortschrMed....................... *Fortschritte der Medizin*
FortschrNeurolPsychiatr ..... *Fortschritte der Neurologie-Psychiatrie*
FortschrRoentg .... *Fortschritte der Roentgenologie*
FrankZeitschriPathol .... *Frankfurter Zeitschrift fur Pathologie*
FreeRadicBiolMed .... *Free Radical Biology and Medicine*
FreeRadRes........................ *Free Radical Research*
FreeRadicResComm........... *Free Radical Research Communications*
FrontGastrRes .... *Frontiers in Gastroenterological Research*
FundApplTox .... *Fundamental and Applied Toxicology*

Gann................................. *Gann*
GastrClinBiol...................... *Gastroenterologie Clinique et Biologique*
GastrClinNAm .... *Gastroenterological Clinics of North America*
GastrEnd .... *Gastrointestinal Endoscopy*
GastrInternat .... *Gastroenterology International*

GastrJap	*Gastroenterologia Japonica*
Gastro	*Gastroenterology*
Gastroenterologia	*Gastroenterologia*
GastroHepato	*Gastroenterologia y Hepatologia*
GastrRad	*Gastrointestinal Radiology*
GazIntMedChir	*Gazzetta Internazionale di Medicina e Chirurgia*
GClinMed	*Giornale di Clinica Medica (Bologna)*
GegenbaursMorphJahrb	*Gegensbaurs Morphologisches Jahrbuch*
Gene	*Gene*
GenesDevelop	*Genes Developments*
GenetEpid	*Genetic Epidemiology*
Genetics	*Genetics*
GenetRes	*Genetical Research*
GenitourinMed	*Genitourinary Medicine*
Genomics	*Genomics*
GenPharmacol	*General Pharmacology*
GenPractitioner	*General Practitioner*
GeogMed	*Geographia Medica*
Geriat	*Geriatrics*
Geront	*Gerontology*
GItalDermVener	*Giornale Italiano di Dermatologia e Venereologia*
GItalMedLav	*Giornale Italiano di Medicina del Lavoro*
GlycoconjugJ	*Glycoconjugate Journal*
Gut	*Gut*
Guy'sHospRep	*Guy's Hospital Reports*
GynecolObsInvest	*Gynecologic and Obstetric Investigation*
GynOncol	*Gynecologic Oncology*
Haematol(Pavia)	*Haematologica (Pavia)*
Haemostasis	*Haemostasis*
Hautarzt	*Hautarzt*
HealthEducJ	*Health Education Journal*
Heart	*Heart*
HelvChirActa	*Helvetica Chirurgica Acta*
HelvMedActa	*Helvetica Medica Acta*
HelvPaedActa	*Helvetica Paediatrica Acta*
HelvPharmActa	*Helvetica Pharmacologica Acta*
Hemat/OncolClinNAm	*Hematology/Oncology Clinics of North America*
HemOnc	*Hematological Oncology*
Hepatogast	*Hepato-Gastroenterology*
Hepatol	*Hepatology*
HiroshimaJMedSci	*Hiroshima Journal of Medical Sciences*
Histochem	*Histochemistry*
HistochemCytochem	*Histochemisty and Cytochemistry*
HistochemJ	*Histochemical Journal*
HistocompTest	*Histocompatibility Testing*
Histopath	*Histopathology*
HoppeSeylerZBiolChem	*Hoppe-Seylers Zeitschrift für Biologische Chemie*
HoppeSeyler ZPhysiolChem	*Hoppe-Seylers Zeitschrift für Physiologische Chemie*
HormCellReg	*Hormones Cell Regulation*
HormMetRes	*Hormone and Metabolic Research*
HormRes	*Hormone Research*
HospPract	*Hospital Practice*
HPBSurgery	*Hepato Pancreatico Biliary Surgery*
HumExpToxicol	*Human and Experimental Toxicology*
HumGenet	*Human Genetics*
HumGeneTher	*Human Gene Therapy*
HumHere	*Human Heredity*
HumImmunol	*Human Immunology*
HumMolGenet	*Human Molecular Genetics*
HumNutrAN	*Human Nutrition. Clinical Nutrition*
HumPath	*Human Pathology*
HumRepro	*Human Reproduction*
Hypertension	*Hypertension*
Hypotheses	*Hypotheses*
IARCEvalCarcinogRisk ChemHumMonogr	*IARC Evaluation of Carcinogenic Risk of Chemicals for Humans Monographs*
IARCSciPubl	*IARC Scientific Publications*
Iatriki	*Iatriki*
IEEETrBiomedEng	*IEEE Transactions on Biomedical Engineering*
Immunity	*Immunity*
Immunobiology	*Immunobiology*
Immunogenet	*Immunogenetics*
Immunol	*Immunology*
ImmunolAllergPract	*Immunology and Allergy Practice*
ImmunolCommun	*Immunological Communications*
ImmunoLett	*Immunology Letters*
ImmunolRev	*Immunological Reviews*
ImmunolToday	*Immunology Today*
IndJGastro	*Indian Journal of Gastroenterology*
IndJMedRes	*Indian Journal of Medical Research*
IndJMedSci	*Indian Journal of Medical Sciences*
IndJPhysiolPharmacol	*Indian Journal of Physiology and Pharmacology*
IndMedGaz	*Indian Medical Gazette*
IndMedSurg	*Indian Medical Survey*
IndPaediat	*Indian Paediatrics*
Infec	*Infection*
InfectImmun	*Infection and Immunity*
InnMed	*Innere Medizin*
IntAbstrSurg	*International Abstracts of Surgery*
IntArchAllApplImmunol	*International Archives of Allergy and Applied Immunology*
IntArchOccupEnvirHlth	*International Archives of Occupational and Environmental Health*
IntensCareMed	*Intensive Care Medicine*
IntensCareWorld	*Intensive Care World*
Internist	*Internist*
Intervirology	*Intervirology*

IntHepatolComm .... *International Hepatology Communications*
IntJAddict .... *International Journal of Addiction*
IntJArtifOrg .... *International Journal of Artificial Organs*
IntJAndrol .... *International Journal of Andrology*
IntJBiochem .... *International Journal of Biochemistry*
IntJBiochemCellBiol .... *International Journal of Biochemistry and Cell Biology*
IntJCanc .... *International Journal of Cancer*
IntJCardiol .... *International Journal of Cardiology*
IntJClinLabRes .... *International Journal of Clinical and Laboratory Research*
IntJClinPharmacol.............. *International Journal of Clinical Pharmacology*
IntJClinPharmRes.............. *International Journal of Clinical Pharmacological Research*
IntJDermatol...................... *International Journal of Dermatology*
IntJEatingDis .... *International Journal of Eating Disorders*
IntJEpid .... *International Journal of Epidemiology*
IntJExpPathol .... *International Journal of Experimental Pathology*
IntJFert............................ *International Journal of Fertility*
IntJGynObs .... *International Journal of Gynecology and Obstetrics*
IntJHlthServ .... *International Journal of Health Services*
IntJObes........................... *International Journal of Obesity*
IntJParasitol .... *International Journal of Parasitology*
IntJPediatriNephrol .... *International Journal of Pediatric Nephrology*
IntJPeptProteinRes .... *International Journal of Peptide and Protein Research*
IntJPharmaceut .... *International Journal of Pharmaceutics*
IntJRadiatBiol .... *International Journal of Radiation Biology*
IntJRadiatOncolBiolPhys..... *International Journal of Radiation, Oncology, Biology, Physics*
IntJSportsMed .... *International Journal of Sports Medicine*
IntJSystBacteriol .... *International Journal of Systematic Bacteriology*
IntJVitNutrRes.................. *International Journal for Vitamin and Nutrition Research*
IntMed .... *Internal Medicine*
IntRevCytol .... *International Reviews of Cytology*
IntRevExpPath................... *International Reviews of Experimental Pathology*
IntSurg .... *International Surgery*
IntUrolNephrol.................. *International Urology and Nephrology*
IntVirol .... *International Virology*
InvasMetast....................... *Invasion and Metastasis*
InvestRadiol...................... *Investigative Radiology*
InvestUrol........................ *Investigative Urology*

Invitro.............................. In Vitro *Cell Development Biology*
InvOphthalmolVisSci .... *Investigative Ophthalmology and Visual Science*
IRCSJMedSci .... *IRCS Journal of Medical Science*
IrJMedSci .... *Irish Journal of Medical Science*
IrMedJ............................. *Irish Medical Journal*
ISIAtlasSci:Pharmacol .... *ISI Atlas of Science: Pharmacology*
IsrJMedSci........................ *Israeli Journal of Medical Sciences*
ItalJGastr .... *Italian Journal of Gastroenterology*
ItalJNeurolSci................... *Italian Journal of Neurological Sciences*
ItalJPediat .... *Italian Journal of Pediatrics*
ItalJSurgSci...................... *Italian Journal of Surgical Sciences*

JAIDS.............................. *Journal of Acquired Immune Deficiency Syndromes and Human Retrovirology*
JAllClinImmunol .... *Journal of Allergy and Clinical Immunology*
JAMA .... *Journal of the American Medical Association*
JAmAcadDermatol............. *Journal of the American Academy of Dermatology*
JAmCollCard .... *Journal of the American College of Cardiology*
JAmCollNutr .... *Journal of the American College of Nutrition*
JAmCollSurg .... *Journal of the American College of Surgeons*
JAmDietAssoc................... *Journal of the American Dietetics Association*
JAmGeriatSoc................... *Journal of the American Geriatrics Society*
JAmMedWomAssoc........... *Journal of the American Medical Women's Association*
JAmSocNephrol................. *Journal of the American Society of Nephrology*
JAnat .... *Journal of Anatomy*
JAntimicChemo .... *Journal of Antimicrobial Chemotherapy*
JApplPhysiol .... *Journal of Applied Physiology*
JApplTox .... *Journal of Applied Toxicology*
JAssocPhysInd .... *Journal of the Association of Physicians of India*
JAutonNervSyst................. *Journal of the Autonomic Nervous System*
JAutonPharmacol .... *Journal of Autonomic Pharmacology*
JBacteriol .... *Journal of Bacteriology*
JBC................................. *Journal of Biological Chemistry*
JBehavTherExpPsych .... *Journal of Behavior Therapy and Experimental Psychiatry*
JBioch .... *Journal of Biochemistry*
JBiochem(Tokyo) .... *Journal of Biochemistry (Tokyo)*
JBioenergBiomembr .... *Journal of Bioenergetics and Biomembranes*
JBiolStandard.................... *Journal of Biological Standardization*
JBoneJtSurg...................... *Journal of Bone and Joint Surgery*

JBoneMinRes...................... *Journal of Bone and Mineral Research*
JCanAssocRadiol................ *Journal of the Canadian Association of Radiologists*
JCanMedAssoc.................... *Journal of the Canadian Medical Association*
JCancResClinOnc............... *Journal of Cancer Research and Clinical Oncology*
JCardiolPharmacol .... *Journal of Cardiology and Pharmacology*
JCardiovascSurg................. *Journal of Cardiovascular Surgery*
JCellBiochem .... *Journal of Cellular Biochemistry*
JCellBiol .... *Journal of Cell Biology*
JCellPhysiol .... *Journal of Cellular Physiology*
JCellSci............................. *Journal of Cell Science*
JCerebBloodFlowMetab ...... *Journal of Cerebral Blood Flow and Metabolism*
JChildNeurol .... *Journal of Child Neurology*
JChir................................. *Journale de Chirurgie*
JChromatogr .... *Journal of Chromatography*
JChromatogrB .... *Journal of Chromatography, B. Biomedical Applications*
JChronDis......................... *Journal of Chronic Diseases*
JCI.................................... *Journal of Clinical Investigation*
JClinChemClinBioch.......... *Journal of Clinical Chemistry and Clinical Biochemistry*
JClinDysmorph.................. *Journal of Clinical Dysmorphism*
JClinElectronMicrosc......... *Journal of Clinical Electron Microscopy*
JClinEndoc .... *Journal of Clinical Endocrinology and Metabolism*
JClinEndocrinol .... *Journal of Clinical Endocrinology*
JClinGastro....................... *Journal of Clinical Gastroenterology*
JClinEpidemiol .... *Journal of Clinical Epidemiology*
JClinImmunol................... *Journal of Clinical Immunology*
JClinInvest....................... *Journal of Clinical Investigation*
JClinLabAnal .... *Journal of Clinical Laboratory Analysis*
JClinLabImmunol.............. *Journal of Clinical and Laboratory Immunology*
JClinMicrobiol .... *Journal of Clinical Microbiology*
JClinNeurophys .... *Journal of Clinical Neurophysiology*
JClinNutrGastro .... *Journal of Clinical Nutrition and Gastroenterology*
JClinOncol........................ *Journal of Clinical Oncology*
JClinPath .... *Journal of Clinical Pathology*
JClinPharm .... *Journal of Clinical Pharmacology*
JClinPsych .... *Journal of Clinical Psychology*
JClinPsychpharm .... *Journal of Clinical Psychopharmacology*
JClinSurg.......................... *Journal of Clinical Surgery*
JClinUltrasound................. *Journal of Clinical Ultrasound*
JCommDis.......................... *Journal of Communicable Diseases*
JComputAssistTomogr .... *Journal of Computer Assisted Tomography*
JCutPath .... *Journal of Cutaneous Pathology*
JDermatol .... *Journal of Dermatology*
JDrugDevel........................ *Journal of Drug Development*

JDrugTarget....................... *Journal of Drug Targeting*
JEgyptSocParasitol............. *Journal of the Egyptian Society of Parasitology*
JElectronMicrosc .... *Journal of Electron Microscopy*
JEMTech .... *Journal of Electron Microscopy Techniques*
JEmbrExpMorph .... *Journal of Embryology and Experimental Morphology*
JEndocr............................. *Journal of Endocrinology*
JEndocrMetab.................... *Journal of Endocrinology and Metabolism*
JEndocrInv .... *Journal of Endocrinological Investigation*
JEpidCommHlth................. *Journal of Epidemiology and Community Health*
JEukaryotMicrobiol............ *Journal of Eukaryotic Microbiology*
JEurTox............................. *Journal Européen de Toxicologie*
JExpBiol .... *Journal of Experimental Biology*
JExpImmunol .... *Journal of Experimental Immunology*
JExpMed .... *Journal of Experimental Medicine*
JExpPath........................... *Journal of Experimental Pathology*
JFamPractice..................... *Journal of Family Practice*
JForensicSci...................... *Journal of Forensic Science*
JFormosanMedAss............. *Journal of the Formosan Medical Association*
JGastHepatol .... *Journal of Gastroenterology and Hepatology*
JGastro .... *Journal of Gastroenterology*
JGenPhysiol .... *Journal of GeneralPhysiol*
JGenVirol.......................... *Journal of General Virology*
JGeront............................. *Journal of Gerontology*
JGynObsBiolReprod .... *Journal de Gynecologie Obstetrique et Biologie de la Reproduction*
JHeartLungTranspl............. *Journal of Heart and Lung Transplantation*
JHepatobilPancrSurg.......... *Journal of Hepatobiliary and Pancreatic Surgery*
JHepatol............................ *Journal of Hepatology*
JHered .... *Journal of Heredity*
JHistochemCytochem .... *Journal of Histochemistry and Cytochemistry*
JHospInf............................ *Journal of Hospital Infection*
JHumNutrDiet .... *Journal of Human Nutrition and Dietetics*
JHyg .... *Journal of Hygiene*
JHypert.............................. *Journal of Hypertension*
JikeikaiMedJ .... *Jikeikai Medical Journal*
JImmunol........................... *Journal of Immunology*
JImmunolMethods............. *Journal of Immunological Methods*
JImmunother .... *Journal of Immunotherapy with Emphasis on Tumor Immunology*
JIndHygTox....................... *Journal of Industrial Hygiene and Toxicology*
JInfDis.............................. *Journal of Infectious Diseases*
JInfect............................... *Journal of Infection*
JInherMetDis..................... *Journal of Inherited Metabolic Diseases*

JIntChir	*Journal International de Chirurgie*
JInterferonRes	*Journal of Interferon Research*
JIntMed	*Journal of Internal Medicine*
JIntMedRes	*Journal of International Medical Research*
JInvDermatol	*Journal of Investigative Dermatology*
JIrishMedAss	*Journal of the Irish Medical Association*
JJapSurgSoc	*Journal of the Japanese Surgical Society*
JKurumeMedAssoc	*Journal of the Kurume Medical Association*
JKuwaitMedAssoc	*Journal of the Kuwait Medical Association*
JLabClinMed	*Journal of Laboratory and Clinical Medicine*
JLeukBiol	*Journal of Leukocyte Biology*
JLipRes	*Journal of Lipid Research*
JMed	*Journal of Medicine*
JMedAssThai	*Journal of the Medical Association of Thailand*
JMedChem	*Journal of Medicinal Chemistry*
JMedEntomol	*Journal of Medical Entomology*
JMedGenet	*Journal of Medical Genetics*
JMedMicrobiol	*Journal of Medical Microbiology*
JMedPrimatol	*Journal of Medical Primatology*
JMedVirol	*Journal of Medical Virology*
JMembrBiol	*Journal of Membrane Biology*
JMentalDeficRes	*Journal of Mental Deficiency Research*
JMicrosc	*Journal of Microscopy*
JMolBiol	*Journal of Molecular Biology*
JMolEndocr	*Journal of Molecular Endocrinology*
JMolMed	*Journal of Molecular Medicine*
JMorph	*Journal of Morphology*
JMRI	*Journal of Magnetic Resonance Imaging*
JNatProd	*Journal of Natural Products*
JNCI	*Journal of the National Cancer Institute*
JNepalMedAss	*Journal of the Nepalese Medical Association*
JNervMentDis	*Journal of Nervous and Mental Disease*
JNeuroch	*Journal of Neurochemistry*
JNeurol	*Journal of Neurology*
JNeurolNeurosurgPsych	*Journal of Neurology, Neurosurgery, and Psychiatry*
JNeurolSci	*Journal of the Neurological Sciences*
JNeuropathExpNeurol	*Journal of Neuropathology and Experimental Neurology*
JNeurosci	*Journal of Neuroscience*
JNeurosurg	*Journal of Neurosurgery*
JNuclMed	*Journal of Nuclear Medicine*
JNutr	*Journal of Nutrition*
JNutrSciVitaminol	*Journal of Nutritional Science and Vitaminology*
JObsGynBrCommonw	*Journal of Obstetrics and Gynaecology of the British Commonwealth*
JObstetGynaecolBrEmp	*Journal of Obstetrics and Gynaecology of the British*
JOccMed	*Journal of Occupational Medicine*
JOklStatMedAssoc	*Journal of the Oklahoma State Medical Association*
JohnsHopkHospBull	*Johns Hopkins Hospital Bulletin*
JohnsHopkHospRep	*Johns Hopkins Hospital Reports*
JohnsHopkMedJ	*Johns Hopkins Medical Journal*
JObsGyn	*Journal of Obstetrics and Gynaecology*
JOralPathol	*Journal of Oral Pathology*
JParasitol	*Journal of Parasitology*
JParentSciTech	*Journal of Parenteral Science and Technology*
JPath	*Journal of Pathology*
JPatholBacteriol	*Journal of Pathology and Bacteriology*
JPediat	*Journal of Pediatrics*
JPediatChildHlth	*Journal of Pediatrics and Child Health*
JPediatGastrNutr	*Journal of Pediatric Gastroenterology and Nutrition*
JPediatSurg	*Journal of Pediatric Surgery*
JPEN	*Journal of Parenteral and Enteral Nutrition*
JPerinatMed	*Journal of Perinatal Medicine*
JPharmacbioDyn	*Journal of Pharmacobiodynamics*
JPharmaceutSci	*Journal of Pharmaceutical Sciences*
JPharmacokinBiopharm	*Journal of Pharmacokinetics and Biopharmaceutics*
JPharmExpTher	*Journal of Pharmacology and Experimental Therapeutics*
JPharmPharmacol	*Journal of Pharmacy and Pharmacology*
JPhysiol	*Journal of Physiology*
JPhysiolPharmacol	*Journal of Physiology and Pharmacology*
JpnJAllergy	*Japanese Journal of Allergology*
JpnJAnesth	*Japanese Journal of Anesthesiology*
JpnJCancerChemother	*Japanese Journal of Cancer and Chemotherapy*
JpnJCancerRes	*Japanese Journal of Cancer Research*
JpnJClinMed	*Japanese Journal of Clinical Medicine*
JpnJClinOncol	*Japanese Journal of Clinical Oncology*
JpnJClinPath	*Japanese Journal of Clinical Pathology*
JpnJClinRadiol	*Japanese Journal of Clinical Radiology*
JpnJExpMed	*Japanese Journal of Experimental Medicine*
JpnJGastro	*Japanese Journal of Gastroenterology*
JpnJMed	*Japanese Journal of Medicine*

JpnJNuclMed	*Japanese Journal of Nuclear Medicine*
JpnJPhysiol	*Japanese Journal of Physiology*
JpnJStudAlc	*Japanese Journal of Studies in Alcoholism*
JpnJSurg	*Japanese Journal of Surgery*
JPostgradMed	*Journal of Postgraduate Medicine*
JPsychiatRes	*Jouranl of Psychiatric Research*
JRadioanalChem	*Journal of Radioanalytical Chemistry*
JRadiol	*Journal de Radiologie*
JRArmyMedCorp	*Journal of the Royal Army Medical Corps (London)*
JRCollSurgEdinb	*Journal of the Royal College of Surgeons Edinburgh*
JReprodMed	*Journal of Reproductive Medicine*
JRheum	*Journal of Rheumatology*
JRoyCollPhys	*Journal of the Royal College of Physicians*
JRSM	*Journal of the Royal Society of Medicine*
JSocMed	*Journal of Social Medicine*
JSterBioch	*Journal of Steroid Biochemistry*
JStructBiol	*Journal of Structural Biology*
JStudAlc	*Journal of Studies on Alcohol*
JSubsAbus	*Journal of Substance Abuse*
JSubsAbuseTreat	*Journal of Substance Abuse Treatment*
JSupramolStruct	*Journal of Supramolecular Structure*
JSurgOncol	*Journal of Surgical Oncology*
JSurgRes	*Journal of Surgical Research*
JTheorBiol	*Journal of Theoretical Biology*
JThoracCardiovascSurg	*Journal of Thoracic and Cardiovascular Surgery*
JTraceElemMedBiol	*Journal of Trace Elements in Medicine and Biology*
JTrauma	*Journal of Trauma*
JTropMedHyg	*Journal of Tropical Medicine and Hygiene*
JTropPed	*Journal of Tropical Pediatrics*
JUltrastructRes	*Journal of Ultrastructural Research*
JUrol	*Journal of Urology*
JUrologie	*Journal d'Urologie*
JUSMed	*Journal of Ultrasound in Medicine*
JVascSurg	*Journal of Vascular Surgery*
JVirol	*Journal of Virology*
JViralHepat	*Journal of Viral Hepatitis*
JVirolMethods	*Journal of Virological Methods*
JVit	*Journal of Vitaminology*
KeioJMed	*Keio Journal of Medicine*
Khirurgia	*Khirurgia*
KidneyInt	*Kidney International*
KlinMonatsblAugenheilkd	*Klinische Monatsblatter für Augenheilkunde*
KlinPadiatr	*Klinische Pädiatrie*
KlinWschr	*Klinische Wochenschrift*
LabInvest	*Laboratory Investigation*
Lancet	*Lancet*
Lakartid	*Läkartidningen*
LangArchChir	*Langbecks Archiv für Chirurgie*
LavUmano	*Lavoro Umano*
LebMagDarm	*Leber, Magen, Darm*
LifeChem Rep	*Life Chemistry Reports*
LifeSci	*Life Sciences*
LilleMed	*Lille Medical*
Lipids	*Lipids*
Liver	*Liver*
LiverTransplSurg	*Liver Transplantation and Surgery*
LondMedGaz	*London Medical Gazette*
Lupus	*Lupus*
LymphokineRes	*Lymphokine Research*
Lymphology	*Lymphology*
LyonChirurg	*Lyon Chirurgical*
Maandschr Kindergeneeskd	*Maandschrift voor Kindergeneeskunde*
MagnesBull	*Magnesium Bulletin*
Magnesium	*Magnesium*
MagResImag	*Magnetic Resonance Imaging*
MammGenome	*Mammalian Genome*
MatMedPol	*Materia Medica Polona*
Matrix	*Matrix*
MatrixBiol	*Matrix Biology*
MayoClinMonogr	*Mayo Clinic Monographs*
MayoClinProc	*Mayo Clinic Proceedings*
MedAnnualDC	*Medical Annual DC*
MedBiol	*Medical Biology*
MedChirDig	*Médecine et Chirurgie Digestives*
MedClinNAm	*Medical Clinics of North America*
MedHypothes	*Medical Hypotheses*
MedicinaClin	*Medicina Clinica*
Medicine	*Medicine*
MedicinskiArhiv	*Medicinski Arhiv*
MedJAust	*Medical Journal of Australia*
MedJMalaysia	*Medical Journal of Malaysia*
MedJOsakaUniv	*Medical Journal of Osaka University*
MedKlin	*Medizinische Klinik*
MedLav	*Medicina del Lavero*
MedMicrobiolImmunol	*Medical Microbiology and Immunology*
MedMonatschr	*Medizinische Monatsschrift*
MedOncTumPharm	*Medical Oncology and Tumour Pharmacology*
MedPediatOncol	*Medical and Paediatric Oncology*
MedSentinel	*Medical Sentinel*
MedSciSportsExer	*Medicine and Science in Sports and Exercise*
MedTher	*Médecine Thérapeutique*
MedToxicol	*Medical Toxicology*
MedWelt	*Die Medizinische Welt*
MemInstOswaldoCruz	*Memorias do Instituto Oswaldo Cruz*
MetabolBrainDis	*Metabolic Brain Disease*
Metabolism	*Metabolism: Clinical and Experimental*
MethodsEnz	*Methods in Enzymology*

Microbiology	*Microbiology*	Nephrol	*Nephrology*
MicrobiolRev	*Microbiological Reviews*	NephrolDialTranspl	*Nephrology Dialysis Transplantation*
MicrovascRes	*Microvascular Research*	Nephron	*Nephron*
MilitMed	*Military Medicine*	Nervenarzt	*Nervenarzt*
MinDietGastro	*Minerva Dietologica e Gastroenterologica*	NethJMed	*Netherlands Journal of Medicine*
		NeurochemRes	*Neurochemistry Research*
MinElecMetab	*Mineral and Electrolyte Metabolism*	Neurology	*Neurology*
MinMed	*Minerva Medica*	Neuropediatrics	*Neuropediatrics*
MittGrenzgebMedChir	*Mitteilungen aus den Grenzgebieten der Medizin und Chirurgie*	Neuropharmacol	*Neuropharmacology*
		Neuroradiol	*Neuroradiology*
MittOstGestTrop MedParas	*Mitteilungen der Österreichischen Gesellschaft für Tropenmedizin und Parasitologie*	NeurosciLett	*Neuroscience Letters*
		NewCompBiochem	*New Compounds in Biochemistry*
		NIHBull	*National Institutes of Health Bulletin*
MMWR	*Morbidity and Mortality Weekly Report*	NipponGekaGakkaiZass	*Nippon Geka Gakkai Zasshi*
ModPathol	*Modern Pathology*	NipponKyobuShikkai GakkaiZass	*Nippon Kyobu Shikkai Gakkai Zasshi*
MolAspMed	*Molecular Aspects of Medicine*		
MolBiochemParasitol	*Molecular and Biochemical Parasitology*	NipponShokGakkaiZass	*Nippon Shokakibyo Gakkai Zasshi*
		NorthwestMed	*Northwest Medicine*
MolBiolEvol	*Molecular Biology and Evolution*	NoShinkeiGeka	*No Shinkei Geka*
MolBiolMed	*Molecular Biology and Medicine*	NouvPresseMed	*Nouvelle Presse Medicale*
MolBiolRep	*Molecular Biology Reports*	NouvRevFrHemat	*Nouvelle Revue Française d'Hématologie*
MolCarcinog	*Molecular Carcinogenesis*		
MolCellBiochem	*Molecular and Cellular Biochemistry*	NucAcidRes	*Nucleic Acids Research*
MolCellBiol	*Molecular and Cellular Biology*	Nucleonics	*Nucleonics*
MolCellEndocrinol	*Molecular and Cellular Endocrinology*	NuclMedComm	*Nuclear Medicine Communications*
		NutrBioch	*Nutrition and Biochemistry*
MolCellProbes	*Molecular and Cellular Probes*	Nutrition	*Nutrition*
MolEndocrin	*Molecular Endocrinology*	NutrCanc	*Nutrition and Cancer*
MolImmunol	*Molecular Immunology*	NutrMetab	*Nutrition and Metabolism*
MolMed	*Molecular Medicine*	NutrRepInt	*Nutrition Reports International*
MolMembBiol	*Molcular and Membrane Biology*	NutrRes	*Nutrition Research*
MolPharm	*Molecular Pharmacology*	NutrResRev	*Nutrition Research Reviews*
MonatsschrKinderheilkd	*Monatsschrift fur Kinderheilkunde*	NutrRev	*Nutrition Reviews*
MonogrCancerRes	*Monographs in Cancer Research*	NutrRevInt	*Nutrition Reviews International*
MonogrVirol	*Monographs in Virology*	NYStateJMed	*New York State Journal of Medicine*
MonthlyJMedSci	*Monthly Journal of Medical Science*	NZMedJ	*New Zealand Medical Journal*
MorpholIgazOrvSz	*Morphologiai es Igazsagugyi Orvosi Szemle*		
		ObsGyn	*Obstetrics and Gynaecology*
MovementDisorders	*Movement Disorders*	ObsGynSurv	*Obstetrics and Gynaecology Survey*
MtSinaiMedJ	*Mount Sinai Medical Journal*	OccupEnvironMed	*Occupational and Environmental Medicine*
MunchMedWoch	*Munchener Medizinische Wochenschrift*		
		OkajimasFAnatJap	*Okajimas Folia Anatomica Japonica*
Mutagenesis	*Mutagenesis*	Oncogene	*Oncogene*
Mycopathologia	*Mycopathologia*	OncogeneRes	*Oncogene Research*
		Oncol	*Oncology*
NatlCancerInstMonogr	*National Cancer Institute, Monograph*	Ophthalmologica	*Ophthalmologica*
		OralSurg	*Oral Surgery*
Nature	*Nature*	OsteoporosisInt	*Osteoporosis International*
NatureGen	*Nature Genetics*		
NatureMed	*Nature Medicine*	Pancreas	*Pancreas*
NatureNewBiol	*NatureNewBiol*	PapuaNGuineaMedJ	*Papua and New Guinea Medical Journal*
Naunyn-Schmiedb ArchPharm	*Naunyn-Schmiedberg's Archives of Pharmacology*		
		ParasiteImmunol	*Parasite Immunology*
NedTGeneesk	*Nederlands Tijdschrift voor Geneeskunde*	ParasiticProtozoa	*Parasitic Protozoa*
		Parasitol	*Parasitology*
NEJM	*New England Journal of Medicine*	ParasitolRes	*Parasitology Research*
Neoplasma	*Neoplasma*	ParasitolToday	*Parasitology Today*

Pathobio.......................... *Pathobiology*

Pathology .... *Pathology*

PatholAnn......................... *Pathology Annual*

PathInt............................ *Pathology International*

PatholResPract .... *Pathological Research Practice*

Pediat............................. *Pediatrics*

PediatAnn......................... *Pediatric Annals*

PediatClinNAm .... *Pediatric Clinics of North America*

PediatInfectDis .... *Pediatric Infectious Disease*

PediatPath........................ *Pediatric Pathology*

PediatrDermatol.................. *Pediatric Dermatology*

PediatRes .... *Pediatric Research*

Pediatria.......................... *Pediatria*

PediatrNeurol .... *Pediatric Neurology*

PediatrPulmonol .... *Pediatric Pulmonology*

PediatrRadiol .... *Pediatric Radiology*

Peptides .... *Peptides*

PerspectPedPathol.............. *Perspectives of Pediatric Pathology*

PfleugersArchPhysiol .... *Pfleugers Archiv für die Gesamte Physiologie des Menschen und der Tiere*

PharmaceuWeekbl .... *Pharmaceutisch Weekblad*

Pharmacogenet................... *Pharmacogenetics*

Pharmacol .... *Pharmacology*

PharmacolToxicol................ *Pharmacology and Toxicology*

PharmBiochBehav .... *Pharmacology, Biochemistry, and Behavior*

PharmRes......................... *Pharmaceutical Research*

PharmResComm .... *Pharmacological Research Communications*

PharmRev .... *Pharmacology Reviews*

PharmTher .... *Pharmacology and Therapeutics*

PhTrRoySoc .... *Philosophical Transactions of the Royal Society*

Physiologist....................... *Physiologist*

PhysiolRev .... *Physiological Reviews*

PhysMedBiol .... *Physics in Medicine and Biology*

PhysSportsMed................... *Physician and Sports Medicine*

Placenta........................... *Placenta*

Plasma............................ *Plasma*

PNAS .... *Proceedings of the National Academy of Sciences*

PolTygLek .... *Polski Tygodnik Lekarski*

PoliclinicoSezMed.............. *Policlinico- Rome-Sezione Medica*

PopTrends .... *Population Trends*

PostgradMed...................... *Postgraduate Medicine*

PostgradMedJ .... *Postgraduate Medical Journal*

PoumonCoeur .... *Poumon et le Coeur*

PracovLek......................... *Pracovni Lekarstvi*

Praxis.............................. *Praxis*

PrenatalDiagn .... *Prenatal Diagnosis*

PrescribersJ....................... *Prescribers' Journal*

PressMed .... *Presse Medicale*

PrevMed .... *Preventive Medicine*

ProbRéan .... *Problèmes de Réanimation*

ProcAmAssocCancerRes ..... *Proceeding of the American Association for Cancer Research*

ProcAmSocClinOncol .... *Proceedings of the American Society of Clinical Oncology*

ProcAmSocTransplSurg...... *Proceedings of the American Society of Transplant Surgery*

ProcAmWoodPreservAss..... *Proceedings of the American Wood Preservative Association*

ProcAnnMeetAmAssoc .... *Proceedings of the Annual Meeting of* CancerRes *the American Association for Cancer Research*

ProcAssResNervMentDis.... *Proceedings of the Association for Research into Nervous and Mental Disorders*

ProcBostonSocNatHist........ *Proceedings of the Boston Society of Natural History*

ProcEDTA......................... *Proceedings of the European Dialysis and Transplant Association*

ProcMayoClinic .... *Proceedings of the Mayo Clinic*

ProcNatlSciCounc.............. *Proceedings of the National Science* RepubChina *Council of the Republic of China*

ProcNutrSoc...................... *Proceedings of the Nutrition Society*

ProcRoySocB .... *Proceedings of the Royal Society. Series B: Biological Sciences*

ProcRoySocMed .... *Proceedings of the Royal Society of Medicine*

ProgBiochemPharm .... *Progress in Biochemical Pharmacology*

ProgChemFibrinThromb .... *Progress in Chemical Fibrinolysis and Thrombolysis*

ProgClinBiolRes................. *Progress in Clinical and Biological Research*

ProgCollPolymerSci .... *Progress in Colloid and Polymer Science*

ProgGrowthFactorRes .... *Progress in Growth Factor Research*

ProgLivDis .... *Progress in Liver Diseases*

ProgMedVirol .... *Progress in Medical Virology*

ProgNeurobiol .... *Progress in Neurobiology*

ProgNucAcidResMolBiol .... *Progress in Nucleic Acid Research and Molecular Biology*

ProgPediatSurg .... *Progress in Pediatric Surgery*

ProgrCardiovascDis .... *Progress in Cardiovascular Disease*

ProgrDerm........................ *Progress in Dermatology*

ProgrHepatol .... *Progress in Hepatology*

ProsLeukMed .... *Prostaglandins, Leukotrienes and Medicine*

Prostagl............................ *Prostaglandins*

ProteinSci .... *Protein Science*

PSEBM .... *Proceedings of the Society for Experimental Biology and Medicine*

Psychodynamics .... *Psychodynamics*

Psychopharm .... *Psychopharmacology*

PublHlthRec .... *Public Health Record*

PublHlthRep...................... *Public Health Reports*

PublHlthRepWash .... *Public Health Report Washington*

QJExpPhysiol...................... *Quarterly Journal of Experimental Physiology*

QJMed............................. *Quarterly Journal of Medicine*

QJStudAlc .... *Quarterly Journal of Studies on Alcohol*

Radiol .... *Radiology*
RadiolClinNA .... *Radiological Clinics of North America*
RadiothOnc....................... *Radiotherapy and Oncology*
RCollSurg(Edin) .... *Royal College of Surgeons of Edinburgh*
ReanimUrg .... *Reanimation Urgences*
ReaSoinsIntensMedUrg ...... *Réanimation, Soins Intensifs et Médecine d'Urgence*
RecDevAlc......................... *Recent Developments in Alcoholism*
Receptor .... *Receptor*
RecProgHormRes............... *Recent Progress in Hormone Research*
RecProgMed...................... *Recenti Progressi in Medicina (Roma)*
RecResCancRes.................. *Recent Results in Cancer Research*
RegulPeptides .... *Regulatory Peptides*
RenFail .... *Renal Failure*
ReprodMed....................... *Reproductive Medicine*
ResAging .... *Research on Aging*
ResCommChemPath Pharm .... *Research Communications in Chemical Pathology and Pharmacology*
ResCommMolPathPharm.... *Research Communications in Molecular Pathology and Pharmacology*
ResExpMed .... *Research in Experimental Medicine*
ResImmunol....................... *Research in Immunology*
RespEnfApDig.................... *Revista Espanola de las Enfermadades del Aparato Digestivo*
RespirCircul...................... *Respiration and Circulation*
RespirPhysiol .... *Respiratory Physiology*
ResPublResNervMentDis ... *Research Publications - Association for Research in Nervous and Mental Disease*
ResVetSci.......................... *Research in Veterinary Science*
ResVirol .... *Research in Virology*
Retina .... *Retina*
RevAssMedBras .... *Revista da Associacao Medica Brasileira*
RevBiochTox .... *Reviews in Biochemical Toxicology*
RevClinEsp........................ *Revista Clinica Espanola*
RevEspEnfermAparDig....... *Revista de las Enfermedades del Aparato Digestivo*
RevEspFisiol...................... *Revista Espanola de Fisiologia*
RevFrGynObs..................... *Revue Francaise de Gynecologie et d'Obstetrique*
RevFrMalResp.................... *Revue Francaise des Maladies Respiratoires*
RevGastrMex..................... *Revista de Gastroenterologia de Mexico*
RevInfDis .... *Reviews of Infectious Diseases*
RevInstAdolfoLutz.............. *Revista do Istituto Adolfo Lutz*
RevInstMedTropSP............ *Revista do Instituto de Medicina Tropical de Sao Paulo*

RevIntHep .... *Revue Internationale d'Hepatologie*
RevInvestClin(Mex)............ *Revista de Investigacion Clinica (Mexico City)*
RevLyonMed .... *Revue Lyonaise de Médecine*
RevMaladEnfance .... *Revue des Maladies de l'Enfance*
RevMedChile...................... *Revista Medica de Chile*
RevMedChirMalFoie .... *Revue Medico-Chirurgical des Maladies du Foie*
RevMedInt........................ *Revue de Médecine Interne*
RevMedMicrobiol.............. *Reviews in Medical Microbiology*
RevMedVirol..................... *Reviews in Medical Virology*
RevNeurol .... *Revue Neurologique*
RevPhysiolBiochem Pharmacol............. *Reviews of Physiology, Biochemistry, and Pharmacology*
RevSaúdePúbl .... *Revista de Saúde Pública*
RheumDisClinNAm .... *Rheumatic Disease Clinics of North America*
RheumInt.......................... *Rheumatology International*
Rhumatologie .... *Rhumatologie*
RicClinLab .... *Ricerca in Clinica e in Laboratorio*
RinshoByori .... *Rinsho Byori*
RinshoShin .... *Rinsho Shinkeigaku*
ROFO............................... *Fortschritte auf dem Gebiete der Rontgenstrahlen und der Nuklearmedizin*
RPARNMD .... *Research Publications – Association for Research in Nervous and Mental Disease*

SAJSurg............................ *South African Journal of Surgery*
SAMedJ............................ *South African Medical Journal*
Sante................................ *Sante*
Sarcoid............................. *Sarcoidosis*
SbornikVedPraciLek HradKra .... *Sbornik Vedeckych Praci, Lekarske Fakulty Karlovy University v Hradci Kralove*
ScaJCLI............................ *Scandinavian Journal of Clinical and Laboratory Investigation*
ScaJGastr .... *Scandinavian Journal of Gastroenterology*
ScaJHaematol.................... *Scandinavian Journal of Haematology*
ScaJImmunol .... *Scandinavian Journal of Immunology*
ScaJInfectDis .... *Scandinavian Journal of Infectious Diseases*
ScaJRheum .... *Scandinavian Journal of Rheumatology*
ScaJStatist......................... *Scandinavian Journal of Statistics*
ScaJThorCardiovascSurg .... *Scandinavian Journal of Thoracic and Cardiovascular Surgery*
ScaJUrolNephrol .... *Scandinavian Journal of Urology and Nephrology*
ScaJWorkEnvirHlth .... *Scandinavian Journal of Work Environment and Health*
ScandStudCriminol............ *Scandinavian Studies in Criminology*
ScanMicrosc .... *Scanning Microscopy*
SchMedWoch .... *Schweizerische Medizinische Wochenschrift*

SchRundMed	*Schweizerische Rundschau für Medizin*
SchrVerWaBoLufthyg	*Schriftenreihe des Vereins für Wasser-, Boden-, und Lufthygiene*
SciAm	*Scientific American*
Science	*Science*
SciTotalEnv	*Science of the Total Environment*
ScotMedJ	*Scottish Medical Journal*
SEAsianJTropMed PubHlth	*South East Asian Journal of Tropical Medicine and Public Health*
SemaineMed	*Semaine Medicale*
SemArthrRheum	*Seminars in Arthritis and Rheumatism*
SemCellBiol	*Seminars in Cell Biology*
SemDiagPath	*Seminars in Diagnostic Pathology*
SemGastroDis	*Seminars in Gastrointestinal Disease*
SemHemat	*Seminars in Hematology*
SemHepatol	*Seminars in Hepatology*
SemHopPar	*Semaine des Hôpitaux Paris*
SemImmunopathol	*Seminars in Immunopathology*
SemIntRadiol	*Seminars in Interventional Radiology*
SemLivDis	*Seminars in Liver Disease*
SemNuclMed	*Seminars in Nuclear Medicine*
SemOnc	*Seminars in Oncology*
SemPediatSurg	*Seminars in Pediatric Surgery*
SemRoent	*Seminars in Roentgenology*
SemSurgOncol	*Seminars in Surgery and Oncology*
SemThrombHaemost	*Seminars in Thrombosis and Haemostasis*
SeronoSymposiaRev	*Serono Symposia Review*
SGO	*Surgery, Gynecology and Obstetrics*
SkeletalRadiol	*Skeletal Radiology*
SocNeurosciAbstr	*Abstracts - Society for Neuroscience*
SomCellMolGen	*Somatic Cell and Molecular Genetics*
SouthMedJ	*Southern Medical Journal*
SouthMedSurg	*Southern Medicine and Surgery*
SovHlthcareKirgiz	*Soviet Healthcare Kirgizii*
SportsMed	*Sports Medicine*
SpringerSem Immunopathol	*Springer Seminars in Immunopathology*
SSIEM	*Society for the Study of Inborn Errors of Metabolism*
StatMed	*Statistics in Medicine*
Steroids	*Steroids*
Stroke	*Stroke*
SubcellBioch	*Sub-cellular Biochemistry*
SubsAlcActMis	*Substance and Alcohol Actions/ Misuse*
SurgAnnu	*Surgery Annual*
SurgClinNAm	*Surgical Clinics of North America*
SurgEndosc	*Surgical Endoscopy*
Surgery	*Surgery*
SurgForum	*Surgical Forum*
SurgGastr	*Surgical Gastroenterology*
SurgLapEndosc	*Surgical Laparoscopy and Endoscopy*
SurgToday	*Surgery Today*
SympSocExpBiol	*Symposia of the Society for Experimental Biology*
SyndIdent	*Syndrome Identification*
TexasMed	*Texas Medicine*
Therapie	*Therapie*
Therapiewoche	*Therapiewoche*
TherDrugMonit	*Therapeutic Drug Monitoring*
Thorax	*Thorax*
ThrombDiathHaemorrh	*Thrombosis et Diathesis Haemorrhagica*
ThrombHaem	*Thrombosis and Haemostasis*
ThrombRes	*Thrombosis Research*
Thymus	*Thymus*
TIBS	*Trends in Biological Sciences*
TissAnt	*Tissue Antigens*
TohokuJExpMed	*Tohoku Journal of Experimental Medicine*
TopClinNutr	*Topics in Clinical Nutrition*
ToxApplPharmacol	*Toxicology and Applied Pharmacology*
Toxicol*InVitro*	*Toxicology* in Vitro
Toxicology	*Toxicology*
ToxicolLett	*Toxicology Letters*
ToxicolPath	*Toxicologic Pathology*
ToxRev	*Toxicity Review*
TrAAP	*Transactions of the Association of American Physicians*
TraceElemElectrol	*Trace Elements and Electrolytes*
TraceElemMed	*Trace Element Medicine*
TraceSubEnvirHlth	*Trace Substances Environment and Health*
TrAmNeurolAss	*Transactions of the American Neurological Association*
TrAmSocArtOrg	*Transactions – American Society for Artificial Internal Organs*
TransConfChemother Tuberc	*Transactions – Conference on Chemotherapy of Tuberculosis*
TransfusMed	*Transfusion Medicine*
Transfusion	*Transfusion*
TransfusMedRev	*Transfusion Medicine Reviews*
TransJpnPathSoc	*Transactions of the Japanese Pathological Society*
Transpl	*Transplantation*
TransplBull	*Transplantation Bulletin*
TransplImmunol	*Transplantation Immunology*
TransplInt	*Transplantation International*
TransplMediz	*Transplantationsmedizin*
TransplSci	*Transplantation Science*
TransplProc	*Transplantation Proceedings*
TransplRev	*Transplantation Review*
TreatConnTissDis	*Treatment of Connective Tissue Diseases*
TrendsBiochemSci	*Trends in Biochemical Sciences*
TrendsCellBiol	*Trends in Cell Biology*
TrendsEndocrinMetab	*Trends in Endocrinology and Metabolism*
TrendsNeurosci	*Trends in Neurosciences*

TrendsPharmacolSci	*Trends in Pharmacological Sciences*
TrNYAcadSci	*Transactions of the New York Academy of Sciences*
TropGastr	*Tropical Gastroenterology*
TropGeogMed	*Tropical and Geographical Medicine*
TropMedParas	*Tropical Medicine and Parasitology*
TrRSocTropMedHyg	*Transactions of the Royal Society of Tropical Medicine and Hygiene*
Tubercle	*Tubercle*
TumBiol	*Tumour Biology*
TumTarg	*Tumor Targeting*
UltrastructPathol	*Ultrastructural Pathology*
UnionMedCan	*Union Médicale du Canada*
UpdateIntensCare EmergMed	*Update in Intensive Care and Emergency Medicine*
Urol	*Urology*
UrolClinNAm	*Urology Clinics of North America*
UrolRes	*Urological Research*
USImag	*Ultrasonic Imaging*
USMedBiol	*Ultrasound in Medicine and Biology*
Vaccine	*Vaccine*
VerDschGesInnMed	*Verhandlungen der Deutschen Gesellschaft für Innere Medizin*
VerDschGesPath	*Verhandlungen de Deutschen Gesellschaft für Pathologie*
VetHumTox	*Veterinary and Human Toxicology*
VetPathol	*Veterinary Pathology*
VetRec	*Veterinary Record*
ViralHepatRev	*Viral Hepatitis Reviews*
VirchArchA	*Virchows Archiv. A Pathological Anatomy and Histopathology*
VirchArchCP	*Virchows Archiv. B Cell Pathology*
VirolMon	*Virology Monographs*
Virology	*Virology*
VirRes	*Virus Research*
VitHorm	*Vitamins and Hormones*
VoprVirusol	*Voprosy Virusologii*
VoxSang	*Vox Sanguinis*
WestJMed	*West Indian Journal of Medicine*
WHOChron	*World Health Organization Chronicle*
WienKlinWoch	*Wiener Klinische Wochenschrift*
WienMedWoch	*Wiener Medizinische Wochenschrift*
WIMedJ	*West Indian Medical Journal*
WisMedJ	*Wisconsin Medical Journal*
WklyEpidemiolRec	*Weekly Epidemiological Record*
WorldMedJ	*World Medical Journal*
WorldJSurg	*World Journal of Surgery*
WRevNutrDiet	*World Review of Nutrition and Dietetics*
Xenobiot	*Xenobiotica*
YaleJBiolMed	*Yale Journal of Biology and Medicine*
Zacchia	*Zacchia*
ZblAllgPath	*Zentralblatt für Allgemeine Pathologie und Pathologische Anatomie*
ZblArbMed	*Zentralblatt für Arbeitsmedizin und Arbeitsschutz und Prophylaxe*
ZblBakteriol MikrobiolHyg	*Zentralblatt für Bakteriologie, Microbiologie, und Hygiene (Stuttgart)*
ZblBaktHyg	*Zentralblatt für Bakteriologie und Hygiene*
ZblChir	*Zentralblatt für Chirurgie*
ZGastr	*Zeitschrift für Gastroenterologie Verhandlungsband*
ZGesamExpMed	*Zeitschrift für die Gesamte Experimentalle Medizin*
ZGesHyg	*Zeitschrift für Gesundheitstechnik und Staedtehygiene*
ZImmunitat	*Zeitschrift für Immunitatsforschung*
ZKardiol	*Zeitschrift für Kardiologie*
ZKinderchir	*Zeitschrift für Kinderchirurgie*
ZKinderheilk	*Zeitschrift für Kinderheilkunde*
ZKlinChemKlinBiochem	*Zeitschrift für Klinische Chemie und Klinische Biochemie*
ZKlinMed	*Zeitschrift für Klinische Medizin*
ZKrebsf	*Zeitschrift für Krebsforschung*
ZMikroskAnatForsch	*Zeitschrift für Mikroskopisch-Anatomische Forschung*
ZPhysiolChem	*Zeitschrift für Physiologische Chemie*
ZRheumatol	*Zeitschrift für Rheumatologie*

Index

Page numbers in **bold** refer to major sections of the text.

Page numbers in *italics* refer to pages on which tables may be found.

Indexing style / conventions used

Alphabetical order. This index is in letter-by-letter order, whereby hyphens, en-rules and spaces within index headings are ignored in the alphabetization. Terms in brackets are excluded from initial alphabetization.

Cross-references. Cross-reference terms in *italics* are either general cross-references, or refer to subentry terms within the same main entry (the main entry term is not repeated, in order to save space) i.e. they are not main entry terms.

Abbreviations used without explanation

DNA	deoxyribonucleic acid	HDV	hepatitis D virus
EGF	epidermal growth factor	NADP	nicotine–adenine diphosphate
HBV	hepatitis B virus	RNA	ribonucleic acid
HCV	hepatitis c virus		